W9-BRS-014

List of Nursing Skills

FUNDAMENTALS OF NURSING

The Art and Science of Nursing Care

FUNDAMENTALS OF NURSING

The Art and Science of Nursing Care

Fifth Edition

Carol Taylor, CSFN, RN, MSN, PhD
Director, Center for Clinical Bioethics
Assistant Professor, Nursing
Georgetown University
Washington, DC

Carol Lillis, RN, MSN
Dean, Allied Health and Nursing
Delaware County Community College
Media, Pennsylvania

Priscilla LeMone, RN, DSN, FAAN
Associate Professor Emeritus
Sinclair School of Nursing
University of Missouri–Columbia
Columbia, Missouri

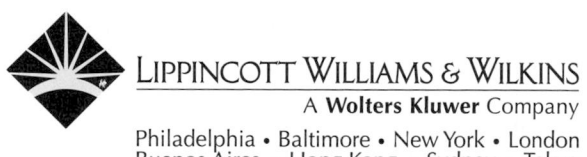

LIPPINCOTT WILLIAMS & WILKINS
A **Wolters Kluwer** Company
Philadelphia • Baltimore • New York • London
Buenos Aires • Hong Kong • Sydney • Tokyo

Senior Acquisitions Editor: Elizabeth Nieginski
Senior Developmental Editor: Danielle DiPalma
Editorial Assistant: Josh Levandowski
Senior Production Editor: Rosanne Hallowell
Copy-editors: Barbara Ryalls and Wendy Walker
Director of Nursing Production: Helen Ewan
Managing Editor / Production: Erika Kors

Art Director: Carolyn O'Brien
Illustration Coordinator: Brett MacNaughton
Cover Designer: Anthony Groves
Senior Manufacturing Manager: William Alberti
Indexer: Coughlin Indexing Services, Inc.
Compositor: Circle Graphics
Printer: R. R. Donnelley / Willard

Fifth Edition

9 8 7 6 5 4 3 2 1

Library of Congress Cataloging-in-Publication Data

Taylor, Carol, CSFN.
  Fundamentals of nursing : the art & science of nursing care / Carol Taylor, Carol Lillis, Priscilla LeMone.—5th ed.
    p. ; cm.
  Includes bibliographical references and index.
  ISBN 0-7817-4480-6 (hardback : alk. paper)
  1. Nursing. I. Lillis, Carol. II. LeMone, Priscilla. III. Title.
  [DNLM: 1. Nursing. 2. Ethics, Nursing. 3. Health Promotion. 4. Nurse-Patient Relations. 5. Nursing Process. WY 16 T239f 2005]
RT41.T396 2005
610.73—dc22

                    2004002964

Care has been taken to confirm the accuracy of the information presented and to describe generally accepted practices. However, the authors, editors, and publisher are not responsible for errors or omissions or for any consequences from application of the information in this book and make no warranty, express or implied, with respect to the content of the publication.

The authors, editors, and publisher have exerted every effort to ensure that drug selection and dosage set forth in this text are in accordance with the current recommendations and practice at the time of publication. However, in view of ongoing research, changes in government regulations, and the constant flow of information relating to drug therapy and drug reactions, the reader is urged to check the package insert for each drug for any change in indications and dosage and for added warnings and precautions This is particularly important when the recommended agent is a new or infrequently employed drug.

Some drugs and medical devices presented in this publication have Food and Drug Administration (FDA) clearance for limited use in restricted research settings. It is the responsibility of the health care provider to ascertain the FDA status of each drug or device planned for use in his or her clinical practice.

LWW.com

To my mother, Mildred Taylor, who continues to teach me the art of human caring.

—*Carol Taylor*

To my grandchildren who bring so much love, joy and laughter into my life.

—*Carol Lillis*

To all the students who will be the nurses of the future. May you always love this profession as much as I do.

—*Priscilla LeMone*

Contributors to Current and Previous Editions

Mary Brekke, PhD, RN, CHTP, HNC
Associate Professor
School of Nursing
Metropolitan State University
Minneapolis, Minnesota
Chapter 28: Complementary and Alternative Modalities

Annemarie Dowling-Castronovo, RN, MA, CS-GNP
Coordinator Nursing Science IV Medical-Surgical/Elder
New York University Division of Nursing
New York, New York
Gerontology Consultant

Pamela Evans-Smith, MSN, RN, CS, FNP
Instructor of Clinical Nursing
Sinclair School of Nursing
Columbia, Missouri
Chapter 27: Asepsis and Infection Control
Chapter 29: Medications
Unit 8: Promoting Healthy Physiologic Responses

Geralyn Frandsen, EdD, MSN, RN
School of Nursing
Maryville University
St. Louis, Missouri
Chapter 21: Communicator
Chapter 34: Sensory Stimulation

Mary Jane Mastorovich, MS, RN
Instructor in Nursing
School of Nursing and Health Studies
Georgetown University
Washington, DC
Chapter 23: Leader and Manager

Judith Ann Rogers, RNC, MSN, PhD(c)
Assistant Professor
Marymount University
Arlington, Virginia
Faculty Associate
Center for Clinical Bioethics
Georgetown University Hospital
Washington, DC
Chapter 22: Teacher and Counselor
Chapter 35: Sexuality

Jane Rothrock, RN, CNOR, DNSc, FAAN
Professor and Program Consultant
Perioperative Program
Delaware County Community College
Media, Pennsylvania
Chapter 30: Perioperative Nursing (4th edition)

Theodora Sirrota, PhD, APRN, BC
Adjunct Clinical Associate Professor
The Steinhardt School of Education
New York University
New York, New York
Chapter 31: Self-Concept

Teneer Veneema, PhD, MPH, MS, CPNP
Associate Professor
School of Nursing
University of Rochester
Rochester, New York
Chapter 26: Safety, Security, and Emergency Preparedness

Reviewers

Lynn Allchin, RN, PhD
Department of Nursing
University of Connecticut
Storrs, Connecticut

Celeste M. Baldwin, PhD, RN, CNS
Director of Nursing
The University of Toledo
Toledo, Ohio

Carole Bomba, RN, MSN
Assistant Professor of Nursing
William Rainey Harper College
Palatine, Illinois

Jeanie Burt, MA, RN, MSN
Assistant Professor of Nursing
School of Nursing
Harding University
Searcy, Arkansas

Danette Birkhimer, RN, MS, OCN
Clinical Instructor
Ohio State University College of Nursing/James Cancer
  Hospital
Dublin, Ohio

Jean Cox, RN, MSN
Nursing Lab Coordinator
Northwest State Community College
Archibald, Ohio

Marianne Craven, MN
Associate Professor
Utah Valley State College
Orem, Utah

Loretta Delargy, RN, MSN
Faculty
Department of Nursing
North Georgia College & State University
Dahlonega, Georgia

Emily Donato, RN, MEd
Assistant Professor
Laurentian University
Sudbury, Ontario
Canada

Cheryl Fenton, RN, BHSc
Professor
Mohawk College
Hamilton, Ontario
Canada

Donna Funk, RN, MN/E, ONC
Nursing Instructor
Brigham Young University
Department of Nursing
Rexburg, Idaho

Alfreda Harper-Harrison
Assistant Professor
Macon State University
Macon, Georgia

Karen A. Hecomovich, MS, RN, CS
Arapahoe Community College
Littleton, Colorado

Karen Hoffman, RN, BS, MS
Assistant Professor
Indiana Wesleyan University
Marion, Indiana

Ellen S. House, RNC, CLNC, DNSc
Nursing Professor
Truckee Meadows Community College
Reno, Nevada

Norlyn B. Hyde, RN, C, MSN, CNS
Associate Professor of Nursing
Louisiana Tech University
Ruston, Louisiana

Merilyn Hunter
Garland Community College
Hot Springs, Arizona

Joan Jinks, RN, MSN
Associate Professor
Eastern Kentucky University
Richmond, Kentucky

Carolyn S. Jones, RNC, MEd, MSN
Director of Health Care Programs
Craven Community College
New Bern, North Carolina

Linda Ann Kucher, MSN, RN
Assistant Professor of Nursing
Gordon College
Barnesville, Georgia

Susan J. Lamanna, RN, MA, MSN, ANP
Associate Professor
Onondaga Community College
Syracuse, New York

Gayle Lee, PhD, RNC, CCRN
Nursing Instructor
Brigham Young University
Department of Nursing
Rexburg, Idaho

Debbie McCoy, BSN, MSN, RN
Program Coordinator
Assistant Professor
Mercy College of Northwest Ohio
Toledo, Ohio

Susan O'Dell, MSN, APRN-BC, FNP
Faculty Nursing Instructor
Mercy College of Northwest Ohio
Toledo, Ohio

Lauren O'Hare, EdD, RN
Associate Professor
Department of Nursing
Wagner College
Staten Island, New York

Caroline A. Ostand, RNBC, MSN
Professor
University of Charleston
Charleston, West Virginia

Winnie Pickering, MS, RNCS
Associate Professor
Rhodes State College
Lima, Ohio

Diane Sheets, MS, RN
Professor
Ohio State University College of Nursing
Dublin, Ohio

Nancy York, RN, MSN
Ballantine University
Bloomington, Indiana

Preface

Today's competitive, market-driven healthcare environment is challenging the very nature of professional nursing practice. *Fundamentals of Nursing: The Art and Science of Nursing Care,* fifth edition, promotes nursing as an evolving art and science, directed to human health and well-being. It challenges students to focus on the blended skills they will need to serve patients and the public well. Our aim is to prepare nurses who combine the highest level of scientific knowledge and technologic skill with responsible, caring practice. We want to challenge students to identify and master the cognitive and technical skills as well as the interpersonal and ethical/legal skills they will need to effectively nurse the patients in their care. We refuse to allow accountability and caring relationships to become relics of a bygone era.

Those new to nursing can quickly become overwhelmed by the demands placed on the nurse's knowledge, technical competence, interpersonal skills, and commitment. Therefore, much care has once again gone into the selection of both the content in this edition and the manner of its presentation. We strive to capture the unique essence of both the art and science of nursing, distilling what the person beginning the study and practice of nursing needs to know. We invite students to identify with the profession, to share in its pride, and to respond to today's challenges competently, enthusiastically, and accountably.

Those familiar with earlier editions of this text will note that we have chosen to replace the term "client" with "patient." The term client was initially used to highlight the active role that most individuals prefer to play in directing their healthcare. From the very first edition of this text, students were encouraged to actively partner with patients and their family caregivers in designing and implementing care. Today we have witnessed the healthcare "industry" transform patients to "customers" who buy healthcare (if they are able) as a commodity in the marketplace. We do not believe that a "customer-orientation" serves patients or nurses well. One of our students shared her belief that she owes less to a "customer" and even to a "client" than she does to a "patient." We therefore have chosen to reclaim the term *patient*—in its most positive sense—to designate the recipient of nursing care.

Efforts have been made to highlight nursing strategies for actively engaging patients, family caregivers, and the public in the development of health goals and strategies to achieve these goals. Patients may be individuals, families, or communities. Care has been taken to communicate that both nurses and patients may be male or female and that they come from every racial and ethnic background and socioeconomic group. Whenever possible we have tried to avoid male/female distinctions in personal pronouns.

ORGANIZATION

Fundamentals of Nursing: The Art and Science of Nursing Care, fifth edition, is organized into eight units. Ideally, the text is followed sequentially, but every effort has been made to respect the differing needs of diverse curricula and students. Thus, each chapter stands on its own merit and may be read independently of others.

Unit I, Foundations of Nursing Practice

Unit I opens with a description of contemporary nursing. Successive chapters introduce content foundational to nursing practice: human needs (individual, family, and community), culture and ethnicity, health and illness, nursing theory, research and evidence-based practice, ethics, values, advocacy, and law.

Unit II, Community-Based Settings for Patient Care

Unit II introduces the multiple settings in which nursing is practiced and prepares students to ensure continuity of care in what could be a fragmented healthcare system. Chapters address the variety of community-based healthcare settings; continuity of care as the patient enters a healthcare facility, is transferred within the facility, and is discharged into another setting within the community; and care provided within the home.

Unit III, The Nursing Process

Presented earlier in the fifth edition, Unit III offers a detailed, step-by-step guide to each component of the nursing process. Practical guidelines and examples are included in each chapter. Separate chapters address the nursing process as a whole, nursing's blended skills, critical thinking, assessing, diagnosing, planning, implementing, and evaluating. A chapter on documentation, reporting, and conferring highlights these nursing responsibilities.

Unit IV, Promoting Health Across the Life Span

Unit IV provides the basis for understanding growth and development across the life span and acknowledges nursing's differing requirements arising from the various developmental stages and abilities to meet developmental tasks.

Unit V, Roles Basic to Nursing Care

Unit V describes major roles in which nurses function as they interact holistically with patients. Chapters focus on the communicator, teacher and counselor, and leader and manager roles of the nurse as caregiver.

Unit VI, Actions Basic to Nursing Care

Unit VI introduces the foundational skills used by nurses: measuring vital signs, assessing health, promoting safety, maintaining asepsis, incorporating complementary and alternative modalities, administering medication, and caring for surgical patients.

Unit VII, Promoting Healthy Psychosocial Responses

Unit VII explores the nurse's role in helping patients meet basic psychosocial needs: self-concept, stress and adaptation, loss, grief and dying, sensory stimulation, sexuality, and spirituality. In each chapter, guidelines are included for assessing and diagnosing unhealthy responses and for planning, implementing, and evaluating appropriate care strategies. Chapters conclude with a *Nursing Plan of Care* illustrating the use of the nursing process and nursing's blended skills to resolve selected nursing diagnoses.

Unit VIII, Promoting Healthy Physiologic Responses

Unit VIII uses the same format as Unit VII to focus on the physiologic needs of patients: hygiene, skin integrity and wound care, activity, rest and sleep, comfort, nutrition, urinary elimination, bowel elimination, oxygenation, and fluid, electrolyte, and acid–base balance.

THEMES

In this edition, we capitalize on the strengths of the first four editions and address new priorities. The following themes are interwoven throughout the text to provide a broad knowledge base of nursing essentials while emphasizing holistic care.

Integrated Nursing Process

After the nursing process is introduced in Unit III, it provides the organizational framework for successive chapters. Chapters in Units VII and VIII, which deal with psychosocial and physiologic responses, begin with a succinct background discussion of the concept, followed by an identification of factors

that influence how different individuals respond to these needs. Steps in the nursing process are used to describe related nursing responsibilities. Throughout these chapters, students will find numerous practical examples of how to conduct focused assessments, develop and write diagnostic statements, identify goals and outcomes, and select, implement, and evaluate appropriate nursing interventions. These examples will reinforce the student's mastery of nursing process skills. Each chapter in Units VII and VIII concludes with a *Nursing Plan of Care* that illustrates each step of the nursing process and a sample documentation of nursing assessment or intervention.

Assessing

Common elements of both a comprehensive and problem-focused nursing assessment are presented; sample interview questions are included within *Focused Assessment Guides* and specific physical assessment techniques are described. Students will learn the what, why, and how of assessment.

Diagnosing

North American Nursing Diagnosis Association (NANDA)-approved nursing diagnoses related to the human need being discussed are identified. *Examples of NANDA Diagnoses* boxes illustrate the relationship between related factors and the problem statement, and provide sample defining characteristics.

Outcome Identification and Planning

Sample expected outcomes are suggested based on patient health problems and strengths within Unit III: The Nursing Process and *Nursing Plans of Care*. Nursing Outcomes Classification (NOC) is also discussed within Unit III.

Implementing

Nursing interventions are clearly explained and are illustrated when this is deemed helpful. *Skills* have been streamlined to facilitate mastery. Age and home health considerations are included. A sufficient variety of nursing interventions is provided to foster the development of a repertoire of nursing actions that makes practicing the art of nursing possible. *Examples of Nursing Interventions Classification (NIC)* provide a sampling of potential nursing interventions for specific topics.

Evaluating

Criteria for evaluating the effectiveness of the plan of care are suggested.

Nursing as an Art and Science

Nursing, as a science, is characterized by a growing body of knowledge that links technical and interpersonal interventions to desired patient outcomes; as an art, nursing demands of its practitioners sufficient competency to creatively design individualized strategies to assist patients to reach personal health goals. A unique spirit of caring always must prevail.

Health Orientation

A health rather than an illness orientation provides a framework for presentation of content. *Promoting Health* boxes highlight assessment checkpoints for specific components of high-level health and include suggestions for designing a self-care prescription. These boxes serve a twofold purpose as a self-care model for the learner and an invaluable aid to the individual who is developing the role of patient healthcare educator. *Teaching to Promote Health at Home* boxes also focus on health and wellness by providing health topics and strategies for home care.

Aims of Nursing

Learners are gradually introduced to the theory and blended skills that will enable them to work successfully with patients to promote health, prevent illness, restore health, and facilitate coping with altered functioning. Early attention to these broad aims of nursing will prepare learners to meet the needs of patients in diverse healthcare settings.

Basic Human Needs

Common to all people and communities, and essential to health and survival, are basic human needs. The clinical chapters in Unit VII, Promoting Healthy Psychosocial Responses, and Unit VIII, Promoting Healthy Physiologic Responses, prepare the learner to assist patients and family members in meeting these needs. Learners are encouraged to explore human responses to health and illness as indicators of how well an individual is functioning to meet basic human needs.

Holistic Care Across the Life Span

A holistic orientation to basic human needs exists across the life span. This orientation is emphasized through information about growth and development in Unit IV, Promoting Health Across the Life Span; through developmental considerations and related tables and displays in Unit VII, Promoting Healthy Psychosocial Responses, and in Unit VIII, Promoting Healthy Physiologic Responses; through age consideration in many *Skills;* and through the diverse ages and needs of patients represented in numerous features. Wherever appropriate, cultural considerations are included.

Attention to Special Needs of the Older Person

Because the age of the population is increasing, nurses encounter growing numbers of older patients in all practice settings. The section on older adults in *Chapter 20, The Aging Adult,* the *Focus on the Older Adult* boxes, and general considerations for the older patient that appear within the text aim to sensitize students to the special nursing needs of this population. The textbook has been reviewed by a gerontology consultant to ensure the material complies with guidelines for addressing the needs of older adults.

Critical Thinking

The critical thinking content is expanded in *Chapter 11, Blended Skills and Critical Thinking Throughout the Nursing Process* and in the Nursing Process chapters that follow. There are more *Focused Critical Thinking Guides.* The new *Reflective Practice* boxes and *Developing Critical Thinking Skills* material in each chapter challenge students to use new knowledge and experience to "think through" learning exercises designed to demonstrate how critical thinking can change outcomes.

Personal Accounts

Delighted with the response to the personal accounts in previous editions, we invited students, patients, and family caregivers to share their experiences. Boxes entitled *Through the Eyes of a Student, Through the Eyes of a Patient,* and *Through the Eyes of a Family Caregiver* speak eloquently of nursing's power to "make a difference." The new *Reflective Practice* boxes are written by students and are designed to engage readers in real-life scenarios encountered by their peers. These personal accounts will evoke smiles, pride, and empathy, and they will unite nurse caregivers in their struggles to perfect their caregiving skills as they make a difference in the lives of others.

Nursing Skills

Skills are presented in a concise, straightforward, and simplified format that is intended to facilitate competent performance of nursing skills. A scientific rationale accompanies each nursing action, and many color photographs and illustrations further reinforce mastery. Special considerations, including modifications and age and home care considerations, are given where appropriate. *Guidelines for Nursing Care* provide a quick reference for additional nursing actions. A companion skills textbook, a skills video series, and an interactive CD-ROM are now part of the teacher–learner package. Available as separate purchases, these products expand upon the skills provided in this Fundamentals text and, additionally, address numerous basic, intermediate, and advanced skills.

Broad Scope of Nursing Practice

Fundamentals of Nursing: The Art and Science of Nursing Care, fifth edition, is written to encompass fundamental skills in a laboratory as well as in actual clinical settings where nurses care for both well and ill patients. To acquaint students of nursing with many exciting career options in nursing, numerous examples are given to illustrate nurses interacting with patients of all ages and backgrounds and in traditional and nontraditional settings.

Focus on Community and Expanded Nursing Roles

Patients today spend fewer days in the hospital, are frequently transferred both within the hospital and between healthcare institutions and home, and need to rely on rapidly proliferating community-based healthcare resources. Content, photos, and illustrations throughout the text highlight both traditional and innovative nursing roles in institutional and community-based practice settings. This text encourages students to dream about new ways nurses can serve the public by creatively responding to health needs and problems.

Research as a Strength to Practice

Content on research and evidenced based practice has been updated and moved to Unit I for increased emphasis early in the learning experience. Updated *Research in Nursing: Making a Difference* boxes, appearing throughout the book, promote the value of research and apply its relevance to nursing practice. Students are challenged to become informed participants in, or consumers of, clinical research.

Up-to-date Clinical Information

Revisions in each clinical chapter will help educators and students remain current. Sample new content includes:

- Increased emphasis on research, evidence-based practice, and nursing management
- New chapter on Complementary and Alternative Modalities
- New bioterrorism content
- JCAHO 2003 National Patient Safety Goals, with reference to accurate patient identification, safe medication and IV administration, and reducing risk of nosocomial infection
- CDC Hand Hygiene Guidelines
- Safe Patient Handling and Movement Practices, including discussion of current research related to identifying high-risk lifting and movement activities for caregivers and promotion of a safe working environment
- Updated ANA Standards of Practice, ICN Definition of Nursing, and Healthy People 2010
- Content on what to do for a mercury spill (*Teaching to Promote Health at Home* box)
- New health interview topics for each body system
- New first aid content
- New content on Concept Mapping

Emphasis on Partnering with Patients, Family, and Professional Caregivers

Careful attention is paid to directing students to identify, value, and develop the interpersonal skills that will allow them to effectively partner with patients, family, and professional caregivers. This will set a tone for successful practice.

Self-Assessment Guides

Fundamentals of Nursing has always encouraged students to be independent learners. Checklists throughout the text (eg,

blended skills assessment, use of nursing process, health assessments) allow students to evaluate their personal strengths and limitations and develop related learning goals.

RECURRING FEATURES

Chapter Opening Features

New! Patient Scenarios

Chapter openers present three medical "charts" with patient photos and a short description of their cases. The learner is then asked to anticipate how he/she will apply the four blended skills of nursing to each scenario. To reinforce learning and engage the reader, the three "patients" are mentioned throughout the chapter to support clinical examples from the text.

Focusing on Blended Skills

These chapter openers offer students everyday nursing challenges and invite them to identify the cognitive, technical, interpersonal, and ethical/legal skills they would need to meet the challenge. Sample responses highlight examples of these skills. Students will begin reading each chapter with an understanding of why the content is important and with their intellectual curiosity piqued! The emphasis on blended skills prepares nurses who combine the highest level of scientific knowledge and technologic skill with responsible, caring practice.

Learning Outcomes and Key Terms

By beginning each chapter with the chapter objectives, we are offering a valuable learning checklist to assess mastery of essential content. Students can use these outcomes as a basis for learning outlines or self-testing, or the instructor may use them for evaluating student knowledge and abilities. The key terms for each chapter also appear in the beginning of the chapter. When these terms are defined in the chapter, they are in bold type for clarity. A Glossary appears at the back of the book for easy studying of these terms.

In-Text Features

- **New! Reflective Practice Boxes.** These exercises are written by students to describe a challenge to their blended skills: cognitive, technical, interpersonal, or ethical/legal. Students identify possible courses of action and *the criteria they would use to identify a successful outcome,* and then described what they learned after reflecting on their response. The readers are asked if they think they would respond in the same way; what this tells them about themselves and the adequacy of their blended skills; and whether the criteria for a successful outcome were appropriate.
- **Nursing Process Demonstrations.** *Fundamentals of Nursing* continues to set the standard for practical demonstrations of each step of the nursing process. As they read through clinical chapters, students see multiple examples of assessment questions and skills, diagnostic statements,

plans of care, documented nursing interventions, evaluative statements, and discharge and teaching plans. For visual learners, these tools greatly facilitate mastery of the complex behaviors students must master quickly when beginning clinical experiences.

- **Case scenario extracts** provide real-world examples and lend significance to conceptual content. These extracts refer back to the chapter-opening patient scenarios for a cohesive learning experience.
- **Through the Eyes of a Student, Through the Eyes of a Patient,** and **Through the Eyes of a Family Caregiver** offer personal anecdotes from different perspectives in order to help students relate to their patients
- **Promoting Health** boxes highlight assessment checkpoints for various health and wellness issues and include suggestions for patient and self-care.
- Nursing **Skills** show both actions and rationales, and highlight special considerations.
- **Guidelines for Nursing Care** boxes outline important points to remember in practice.
- **Examples of NANDA Nursing Diagnoses** and **Examples of Nursing Interventions Classification (NIC)** boxes highlight nursing diagnoses and nursing interventions for quick and easy reference.
- **Focused Assessment Guides** provide sample interview questions to foster independent learning.
- **Focused Critical Thinking Guides** help students follow the step-by-step critical thinking process and develop critical thinking skills.
- **New! Teaching to Promote Health at Home** boxes provides patient teaching tips for nurse-patient communication.
- **Research in Nursing: Making a Difference** boxes highlight recent findings in nursing care.
- **Focusing on the Older Adult** boxes emphasize geriatric care.
- **Nursing Plans of Care with Patient Case Studies.** Each clinical chapter concludes with a Nursing Plan of Care that opens with a patient case study. Students will find concrete examples of each step of the nursing process (assessment, diagnosis, planning, implementation, and evaluation), as well as related examples of documentation. The diagnoses that are worked up in these studies illustrate common health problems and the wide variety of independent and collaborative interventions nurses manage in different practice settings.

Chapter Ending Features
Developing Critical Thinking Skills

These exercises challenge students to synthesize, rather than just reiterate, the information they have learned. By thinking through various scenarios to a final outcome, students will begin to see how their decisions influence end results.

Practicing for NCLEX

In response to requests for "more test questions," sample test questions now appear at the end of *every* chapter to facilitate mastery of chapter content. These exercises will assist students who are attempting to improve their objective test-taking skills. Students who want additional practice with NCLEX-type questions will find the student study guide useful.

Bibliography

Bibliographies at the end of each chapter help make students aware of the variety of resources for information on nursing and give additional reference materials for instructors or students.

Summary of New Features

These features have already been discussed, but we list them here so that you can see at a glance which recurring features are new to the book:

- An increased emphasis on the blended skills (cognitive, technical, interpersonal, and ethical/legal) nurses need to practice effectively into today's world
- An increased emphasis on application to practice through the use of opening chapter case scenarios, which are used as examples throughout the chapters to reinforce content
- New *Reflective Practice* boxes
- Revised *Nursing Process* content and presentation
- New *Teaching to Promote Health at Home* boxes showing an increased emphasis on patient teaching
- Additional *Practicing for NCLEX* review questions in each chapter

TEACHING/LEARNING PACKAGE

To facilitate mastery of this text's foundational content, a comprehensive teaching/learning package has been developed to assist faculty and students.

Instructor's Resource CD-ROM

This all-in-one resource features an Instructor's Manual, Brownstone Test Generator, WebCT/BlackBoard-ready material, and Image Bank

- The Instructor's Manual contains Lecture Outlines, Lesson Plans, PowerPoint Slides, Sample Quizzes, and assignments for every chapter.
- The Test Generator lets you create new, innovative exams based on your own curriculum to help you evaluate your students' progress. This test generator comes with a bank of over 900 questions.
- Web-CT/BlackBoard-ready material allows you to post the material on your learning management system.
- The Image Bank provides free access to the textbook's illustrations and photos for use in POWERPoint Slides, handouts, etc.

Contact your sales representative or check out LWW.com/ Nursing for more details and ordering information.

Student Resources

Students resources include a free back-of-book CD-ROM, Study Guide, Skills Checklist, and Interactive CD-ROM.

- FREE back-of-book CD-ROM features a link to NCLEX-type questions on the web, a Fluid and Electrolyles tutorial, and a tutorial on the NCLEX's new innovative items.
- *Study Guide to Accompany Fundamentals of Nursing: The Art and Science of Nursing Care,* 5th edition, by Carol Taylor, Carol Lillis, Priscilla LeMone, and Marilee LeBon. This guide reinforces the Taylor Fundamentals suite by offering exercises and study review tools to enhance the learning process. It also includes hundreds of NCLEX®-style questions in both multiple choice and the alternate format.
- *Skills Checklist to Accompany Fundamentals of Nursing: The Art and Science of Nursing Care,* 5th edition, by Carol Taylor, Carol Lillis, Priscilla LeMone, and Marilee LeBon. This checklist is designed to accompany the comprehensive fundamentals textbook and promote proper technique while increasing confidence.

Check out your college bookstore or LWW.com/Nursing for more details and ordering information.

TAYLOR SUITE OF PRODUCTS

From traditional texts to video and interactive products, the Taylor Fundamentals suite is tailored to fit every learning style. This integrated suite of products offers students a seamless learning experience you won't find anywhere else. The following products accompany *Fundamentals of Nursing: The Art and Science of Nursing Care,* fifth edition:

- *Taylor's Clinical Nursing Skills* by Pamela Evans-Smith, MSN, FNP. This text covers all of the *Skills* and *Guidelines for Nursing Care* identified in *Fundamentals of Nursing* as well as additional skills, at the basic, intermediate, and advanced levels. Each Skill follows the nursing process format and includes "unexpected situations" followed by an explanation of how best to react.
- *Taylor's Video Guide to Clinical Nursing Skills.* Hosted by a nurse mentor, this video series offers engaging reality-based footage, detailed step-by-step demonstration of skills, and unexpected situations with related interventions. Each module corresponds with a unit of the parent text so students can refer to the Fundamentals or Skills text as they follow along with the video.
- *Taylor's Interactive Nursing Skills (CD-ROM).* This high-quality interactive electronic product provides a consistent learning structure for both Skills and Fundamentals. *Taylor's Interactive Nursing Skills CD-ROM* is divided into two parts:
  - Interactive Skills: students develop skills by answering critical thinking questions, as well as NCLEX-type questions.
  - Interactive Tutorials: students engage in tutorials covering fundamentals concepts.

Contact your sales representative or check out LWW.com/ Nursing for more details and ordering information.

Carol Taylor, CSFN, RN, MSN, PhD
Carol Lillis, RN, MSN
Priscilla LeMone, RN, DSN, FAAN

Letter to the Student

Dear Student,

Congratulations on choosing an exciting and rewarding profession! All of us who have been part of the writing of this text welcome you warmly to our profession and prize our role as your guides to excellent practice! We have tried in this text to present in a readable and enjoyable format the scientific and technical knowledge you will need to design safe and effective nursing care. But we want to do more than prepare you intellectually and technically. You will also find narratives that will teach you valuable interpersonal skills, and content specifically designed to prepare you to meet the ethical and legal challenges in today's practice. So take a deep breath and dig in! Your patients are counting on you and so are we!

How to Use
Fundamentals of Nursing

LOOK AHEAD!

Before reading the chapter content, read the **Learning Outcomes**. These roadmaps help you understand what is important and why. Review the **Key Terms** lists to become familiar with new vocabulary presented throughout the narrative.

FOLLOW THE STORY LINES!

Get to know your patients by reading the chapter opening **Case Scenarios** (see below). Review **Focusing on Blended Skills** to relate the four blended skills of nursing to each scenario. This feature challenges you to consider cognitive, technical, interpersonal, and ethical/legal skills you will need to care for your patients. Specific examples related to the Case Scenarios are provided. Read **Reflective Practice** boxes and discover how other nursing students confront challenging situations related to the Case Scenarios. After reading these boxes, consider how you would respond to similar situations. Stop and think! **In-text references to Case Scenarios** (below right) allow you to consider how the chapter content applies to care of real patients.

Focusing on Blended Skills

The types of blended skills you'll need to respond to the case scenarios include:

Cognitive Skills
- Knowledge of the anatomy and physiology underlying vital signs and the significance of normal and abnormal findings
- Knowledge of nursing responsibilities in assessing temperature, pulse, respirations, and blood pressure
- Knowledge of how to tailor vital-signs technology to meet the individualized needs of patients (eg, best means to assess the temperature of a 2-year-old, the fact that a larger cuff is needed to accurately assess the blood pressure of the overweight man)
- Knowledge of how to teach patients and their family caregivers how to assess vital signs and how to respond to significant findings
- Ability to incorporate factors affecting vital signs into a patient's plan of care
- Ability to use critical-thinking skills to intervene appropriately in situations involving an upset toddler, an inquiring daughter, and a middle-aged man requiring infection-control precautions

Technical Skills
- Ability to ...
- Ability ...
- Ability ...
- Ability ...
- Ability ...

Interpersonal Skills
- Strong people skills to establish a trusting relationship with a toddler, a daughter seeking information, and a middle-aged man who is irritable and requires infection-control measures
- Ability to communicate and interact effectively with patients and their caregivers while assessing vital signs and teaching others how to assess vital signs accurately
- Confidence in own abilities and interpersonal competence to interact with other healthcare personnel, confronting the appropriate persons when help is needed
- Ability to demonstrate respect for the patient's human dignity throughout the patient's care

Ethical and Legal Skills
- Commitment to safety and quality nursing care
- Strong sense of responsibility and accountability
- Ability to put the need for accurate assessment over own

Reflective Practice
Challenge to Ethical and Legal Skills

At clinical 2 weeks ago, I had four patients for the first time and I was very busy. One of my patients, Tomas Esposito, required specialized infection-control precautions, so every time I entered his room, I had to put on a gown and gloves. It was getting to be late in the morning and I still had not completed this patient's full assessment, including his vital signs. Upon entering the patient's room, I discovered that the separate stethoscope usually found in isolation rooms was not there. As a result, I had to remove my gown and gloves and go find the nurse to help me locate the stethoscope. Ultimately, the nurse had to get me a new isolation stethoscope set and put it together for me. Unfortunately, these stethoscopes are poor in quality.

I went back to the patient's room and put on a new gown and gloves. By this time, Mr. Esposito was very irritable and just wanted me to do the assessment quickly and leave him alone. I attempted to listen to his heart sounds but I couldn't hear them. I played with the stethoscope for a few minutes and tried again, but I still couldn't hear his heart or lung sounds. My patient kept telling me to leave him alone. Being a 4th-year nursing student and self sufficient in doing the basic patient assessment, I felt stupid going to get the nurse or my instructor and telling her I couldn't hear anything. I was really pressed for time and now was faced with a critical decision.

Thinking Outside the Box: Possible Courses of Action
- Remove my gown and gloves, get my instructor and the nurse and tell them that I was unable to hear heart and lung sounds, and request their assistance.
- Leave the patient alone as he requested, saving precious time, pretending that I completed the assessment, and charting the same findings as the previous shift's assessment.
- Explain to the nurse that the patient wasn't cooperating and ask her to do the assessment without my instructor knowing about it.
- Try to complete the assessment using my own stethoscope and risk passing the patient's infections on to my other patients.

Evaluating a Good Outcome: How Do I Define Success?
- Patient receives the highest quality of care.
- Professional integrity of all healthcare team members involved is maintained.
- All information charted is accurate.
- Ethical and legal principles are maintained.

Personal Learning: Here's to the Future!
Luckily my conscience and my desire to always give the best care to my patients pushed me to the right decision. I took the time to remove my gown and gloves and went to find my instructor and the nurse. I told the nurse that I was having trouble hearing the patient's heart and lung sounds. She was very understanding and came to the room with me and tried herself. Upon further investigation, we found that the problem was a broken stethoscope, not my incompetence to complete an assessment. After assessing the patient with a properly functioning stethoscope, I found expiratory wheezing and documented it. This finding also provided a clue that I should probably keep a very close eye on this patient. Mr. Esposito ended up experiencing increasing difficulty breathing and his oxygen saturation levels began to drop into the 80% range. As a result, I realized just how important the initial assessment is when caring for a patient throughout the day. Hopefully, the lesson about how important it is to do the "right" thing for the patient will stick with me forever.

Reflection
How do you think you would respond in a similar situation? Why? What does this tell you about yourself and about the adequacy of your skills for professional practice? Can you think of other ways to respond? Regarding the nursing student have done to prevent the numerous trips in and out of the patient's room? To determine whether the stethoscope was functioning properly? How do you think the nursing student's time management and organizational skills affected the situation? What other skills (cognitive, interpersonal, technical, ethical/legal) would you need to respond well in this situation? What ethical principles did the nursing student incorporate into the response to the situation? What responses related to the patient's irritability would have been appropriate by the nursing student? Do you agree with the criteria to evaluate a successful outcome? Did the nursing student meet these criteria? Please explain.

Catherine Barrell, Georgetown University

Noah Shoolin is a 2-year-old who is brought to the emergency department by his mother. When the nurse attempts to obtain a tympanic temperature, the child begins to scream uncontrollably, crying and pushing the device away from his ear.

Doretha Renfrow brings her 65-year-old hypertensive husband to the clinic for evaluation. He is 5'10 and overweight. Mrs. Renfrow states "I really would like to learn how to take my husband's blood pressure so that I can keep track of his progress. Can you teach me how to do it?"

Tomas Esposito is a middle-aged man admitted to the hospital. He is placed in a private room with specialized infection-control precautions, requiring staff to don a gown and gloves when entering the room each time. A morning assessment, including vital signs, is needed.

Recall Tomas Esposito, the patient requiring initial assessment described in the Reflective Practice display? The nurse's inability to auscultate heart and lung sounds would be an important finding that requires additional assessment. The nurse would need to evaluate these findings in conjunction with the patient's vital signs.

DEVELOP CRITICAL THINKING SKILLS!

Learn how critical thinking can change patient outcomes. Like nursing care, critical thinking follows a process. Study the **Focused Critical Thinking Guides** to gain skill in working through the step-by-step critical thinking process. Challenge yourself! Use the new knowledge you've gained to "think through" learning exercises presented in **Developing Critical Thinking Skills.**

Developing Critical Thinking Skills

1. You are providing the immediate preoperative care for a woman scheduled for surgery to remove a brain tumor. She tells you she does not want the surgery because she knows she is dying and just wants to go home to be with her husband and children. She also knows that her husband cannot accept the fact that she is dying and wants her to have the surgery. What do you do?

2. You are assigned to discharge a woman from your same-day surgery unit to her home. You strongly believe that she is not ready to go home, and there is no caretaker in her home. When you voice your concern to the surgeon, you are told that this is not your problem and that there is nothing anyone can do about the situation because her insurer will not approve hospitalization. How do you respond?

Focused Critical Thinking Guide 38-1

Wound Care:
Promoting Acceptance of Changes in Body Image

During both clinical days in one week you (a female student) have been assigned to care for a middle-aged woman who has had a breast removed because of cancer. The patient, Mrs. Nola, is an attractive woman who is usually cheerful and eager to get better and return home. However, on both days she turned her head away and would not look at the incision when her dressing was changed. She tells you that she "just can't stand to look at herself." Her husband was in the room during the dressing changes after telling you that "it makes me sick to see what happened to my wife." Mrs. Nola is to be discharged to her home the next day and needs to learn how to provide self-care for her wound. What do you do?

1. **Identify Goal of Thinking**
   Determine the most effective way of ensuring wound care and at the same time assisting Mrs. Nola in accepting her altered self-image.

2. **Assess Adequacy of Knowledge**
   Pertinent circumstances: The diagnosis of cancer was made only one day before the surgical removal of the breast. The wound from her mastectomy has not completely healed and will require dressing changes for another 3 or 4 days. Mrs. Nola has had a disfiguring surgery and is coping with not only a change in body image but also the diagnosis of cancer. She has never before been seriously ill nor had surgery. She has a strong, loving relationship with her husband, but he is unable to deal with the physical disfigurement at this time.
   Prerequisite knowledge: Before you decide what to do in this situation, you need to know at what level Mrs. Nola is in coping with the diagnosis of cancer. If she is still in denial about the disease, it is likely that she is also denying the surgical procedure and the changes in her body. You will need to review responses to the diagnosis of cancer as well as the stages of grief and loss. You will have to learn what her sources of support are and how she can best access and use them. You will need to assess how best to help her achieve wound care in the face of her continued refusal even to look at the wound.
   Room for error: If she is forced to look at the wound or made to feel inadequate because of her inability to do so,

she will feel threatened and most likely will become angry in response to the perceived threat.
   Time constraints: Some decision about wound care must be made before her discharge the next day.

3. **Address Potential Problems**
   There are several potential obstacles to critical thinking in this situation. As a student, you want to exhibit safe, knowledgeable care, and the importance of teaching for home care has been an emphasis in this course. As a woman, you have a sense of what the loss of a breast must mean. Having had a family member die of cancer, you find yourself wanting to do everything for Mrs. Nola. As a novice in nursing, you find it difficult to handle these emotional components of patient care and find yourself wanting to scold both the patient and her husband for being so silly about something as simple as a dressing.

4. **Consult Helpful Resources**
   You must first understand the loss and grief Mrs. Nola is experiencing, and you must then relate that to her response to self-care of the wound. Your best source of information about her coping methods and sources of personal strength is Mrs. Nola herself. You also discuss the most effective way of providing wound care at home with your instructor and the case manager for Mrs. Nola.

5. **Critique Judgment/Decision**
   After talking with Mrs. Nola, your instructor, and the case manager, you mutually agree that Mrs. Nola cannot be hurried into acceptance of her medical diagnosis or her body changes. The case manager consults with Mrs. Nola's physician, who writes an order for a home health nurse to visit for the next 4 days and complete the dressing change. After talking with Mrs. Nola, you identify that she is still very much in denial. You discuss with her the possibility of having a visitor from "Reach to Recovery," a support group for women with breast cancer who have had a mastectomy. Mrs. Nola tells you that she thinks she would like to talk to someone with the same problem, and you call a referral for her. When you tell Mrs. Nola that a home health nurse will be visiting her for the first few days at home to change her dressing, tears come into her eyes. She says "I am so scared, I just don't know what to do." You realize that insisting that Mrs. Nola do her own dressing would have been extremely stressful for her, and that you would have considered the wound as more important than the patient. When you share the situation in postconference, your clinical group supports your decision.

MASTER NURSING PROCESS!

Throughout the clinical chapters, follow the step-by-step organization of the **Nursing Process** to understand nursing responsibilities. Review the sample interview questions within **Focused Assessment Guides** to strengthen your assessment skills.

THE NURSING PROCESS FOR OXYGENATION

Assessing

The patient's health history is an essential component for assessing respiratory functioning. Either the patient or a family member can provide this information. The nursing examination combined with laboratory findings can provide information to identify a patient's strengths, the nature of the problem, its course, related signs and symptoms, and its onset, frequency, and effects on activities of daily living. The nurse decides, based on these findings, what problems can be treated independently by nursing. Other problems are referred to a physician for decisions on treatment.

Nursing History

The nursing history, an important clinical tool in the early steps of the nursing process, always includes a respiratory component. The information gained provides data about why the patient needs nursing care and what kind of care is required to maintain a sufficient intake of air. Interview questions help identify current or potential health deviations, actions performed by the patient for meeting respiratory needs and the effects of such actions, contributing factors, the use of any aids to improve the intake of air, and effects on the patient's lifestyle and relationships with others.

Before starting the interview, ascertain that the patient is not in acute distress and that family members are comfortable. If the patient is experiencing any respiratory distress, initiate appropriate actions immediately to help relieve symptoms. Enlist the aid of family members or others to help answer questions. When the patient is able, interview the patient to expand this initial database. If no emergency interventions are necessary for the patient's clinical condition, obtain a comprehensive history at this time.

When a health deviation is noted during the data collection, collect as much descriptive information as possible, including whether the problem evolved suddenly or slowly. The accompanying Focused Assessment Guide 45-1 provides some appropriate questions for assessment.

Physical Assessment

The basic examination of the lungs and respiratory status is discussed in Chapter 25. Always proceed in a well-organized manner through a sequence of inspection, palpation, percussion, and auscultation.

Recall Mr. Kim, the 57-year-old man who is receiving oxygen therapy and mechanical ventilation via an endotracheal tube. A complete assessment is necessary to identify specific problems related to oxygenation as well as to determine the effectiveness of current treatments.

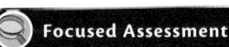
Focused Assessment Guide 45-1

Respiration and Oxygenation

Factors to Assess	Questions and Approaches
Usual patterns of respiration	How would you describe your breathing patterns?
	Do you have allergies?
	Do you smoke?
	Do you live with a smoker or are there smokers or other pollutants in your workplace?
Recent changes	Have you noticed any changes in your breathing pattern (out of breath, cough, pain)?
	Do you have chest pain?
Cough	How much and how often do you cough?
	Is the cough related to the time of day or any activity?
	What is it like (dry, bubbly, hoarse)?
	Do you have a history of allergies?
	Do you ever wheeze?
	Are you exposed to dust? Fumes?
	Where do you work? What kind of work?
	How are you treating the cough?
Sputum	Do you ever cough up and spit out mucus?
	How much do you spit out and do you associate it with anything (time of day, environment)?
	What color is it? Is it ever blood tinged?
	What is its odor?
Chest pain	On a scale of 0 to 5 (5 being very painful), how severe is the pain?
	Where is the pain?
	Is the pain worse with inspiration? Expiration? Cough?
	Does the pain radiate?
	What measures are you using to relieve the pain?
Dyspnea	Is it constant or remittent or related to any activity?
	How do different positions affect it?
	How does it affect your daily activities?
	Is any part of your body bluish during the breathing problem?
	What do you do during and after the breathing attack?
	Have you ever been told that you have asthma? Emphysema? Tuberculosis? Heart disease?
	Do you think the problem is getting worse or staying the same?
Fever	Have you had pneumonia recently?
	Do you have any contact with people who have tuberculosis?
	Do you have night sweats?
	Are others in your household well or ill?
	Have you traveled anywhere recently?
	What medications are you using?
	Have you been exposed to any pollutants?
Fatigue	Have you noticed you feel more tired lately?
	Are you getting your normal amount of sleep at night?
	Has your sleep at night been affected by any difficulty breathing?
	Do you become easily fatigued when you climb stairs?
	Has your pattern of daily activity changed lately?
	Can you sleep lying flat? How many pillows do you use?

Discover how to develop and write diagnostic statements in **Examples of NANDA Nursing Diagnoses.** Learn to select, implement, and evaluate appropriate nursing interventions in **Examples of Nursing Interventions Classification (NIC)** boxes. Carefully follow the concise, straightforward, and simplified format of the nursing **Skills** and **Guidelines for Nursing Care** to gain competence in performing nursing skills. Put it all together! Apply chapter content to clinical practice through studying **Nursing Plan of Care** boxes. These boxes represent a broad range of the health problems you might encounter in different settings. The patient case study introduces a specific case, and the related Care Plan follows through the interventions. Each step of the nursing process is covered, and related documentation is included.

Examples of NANDA Nursing Diagnoses — Oxygenation

Nursing Diagnoses	Related Factors	Sample Defining Characteristics
Ineffective Airway Clearance	Thick yellow secretions, fever, fatigue, dehydration, poor nutrition	"I never feel as though I am getting enough air." Seventy-year-old man with a 20-year history of COPD, recent development of pneumonia. He is pale with circumoral cyanosis. His respiratory rate is 40 breaths/min and shallow. Coarse crackles are auscultated bilaterally. He does not sit quietly in chair or on bed. He cannot walk length of room without coughing episode, which produces little sputum.
Impaired Gas Exchange	Smokes one pack per day; works with asbestos in auto factory; has had a cold for 7 days	Cyanotic 50-year-old man. Using pursed-lip breathing while sitting on emergency room stretcher. Sitting hunched forward with overbed table supporting arms. Altered blood gases show respiratory acidosis. Admits to shortness of breath, nausea, and ankle edema for 1 week.
Ineffective Breathing Pattern	Anxious about results of cardiac catheterization and possible cardiac surgery	Hyperventilating, tachypneic (40 minutes). "I have a tingling feeling in my fingers."

Examples of Nursing Interventions Classification (NIC) — Oxygenation Ventilation Assistance

- Maintain a patent airway
- Auscultate breath sounds, noting areas of decreased or absent ventilation, and presence of adventitious sounds
- Initiate and maintain supplemental oxygen, as prescribed
- Administer appropriate pain medication to prevent hypoventilation
- Ambulate three to four times per day, as appropriate
- Monitor respiratory and oxygenation status
- Administer medications (eg, bronchodilators and inhalers) that promote airway patency and gas exchange
- Teach pursed-lip breathing techniques, as appropriate
- Teach breathing techniques as appropriate
- Initiate a program of respiratory muscle strength and/or endurance training, as appropriate

(From McClosky, J., & Bulechek, G. [2000]. *Nursing interventions classification [NIC]* [3rd ed.]. [p. 697]. St. Louis: C. V. Mosby. A full listing of nursing activities for each nursing intervention can be found in this book.)

SKILL 45-2 Administering Oxygen by Nasal Cannula

EQUIPMENT
Flowmeter connected to oxygen supply | Humidifier with sterile distilled water (optional with low-flow system) | Nasal cannula and tubing | Gauze to pad tubing over ears (optional)

ACTION	RATIONALE
1. Explain procedure to patient and review safety precautions necessary when oxygen is in use. Place No Smoking signs in appropriate areas.	Oxygen supports combustion.
2. Perform hand hygiene.	Hand hygiene deters the spread of microorganisms.
3. Connect the nasal cannula to the oxygen setup with humidification, if one is in use. Adjust the flow rate as ordered by physician (see photo). Check that oxygen is flowing out of prongs.	Oxygen forced through a water reservoir is humidified before it is delivered to the patient, thus preventing dehydration of the mucous membranes. Low-flow oxygen does not require humidification.
4. Place the prongs in the patient's nostrils (see photo). Adjust according to type of equipment. a. Over and behind each ear with adjuster comfortably under chin; or b. Around the patient's head	Correct placement of the prongs and fastener facilitates oxygen administration and comfort for the patient.

Nasal cannula.   Action 3: Adjusting flow rate.
Action 4: Placing cannula prongs in nostrils.   Action 4: Adjusting for comfort.

(continued)

NURSING PLAN OF CARE 45-1 for Freddie Taft

Freddie Taft is a 1-year-old, alert, well-developed child who has been a patient on the pediatric unit for 3 days with status asthmaticus. He has had two other hospitalizations for acute asthma, during which he responded quickly to intravenous and inhalation bronchodilators. During this hospitalization, either his mother, a teacher, or his father, a psychologist, has stayed with him. Other relatives are caring for Freddie's 9-year-old sister and 5-year-old brother.

Freddie interacts happily with staff as long as a parent is within sight. Gross and fine motor coordination are appropriate for his age. His vocabulary consists of 25 words. The history is from his mother, who is a reliable source. He has had a clear nasal discharge with slight, intermittent, nonproductive cough for 3 days with no change in appetite or activity pattern.

On the day of admission, he attended the day-care center as usual. After being there for 3 hours, his cough became more frequent, and his respirations became more labored. The caregivers were not alarmed because he continued to eat, drink, nap, and play in his usual pattern. His mother states that when she arrived in the afternoon to pick up the boys, she discovered him to be using his intercostal and neck muscles excessively with every breath. His respirations were 50 breaths/min, labored, and accompanied by a grunt. By the time she arrived home, he was pale and fitful and was crying weakly. Respirations were 60 breaths/min, and peripheral cyanosis was noted. The pediatrician advised lung evaluation in the emergency department. While there, three subcutaneous injections of epinephrine were administered 5 minutes apart. The child did not

respond satisfactorily, so he was admitted for intravenous aminophylline and steroid administration.

In addition to a history of asthma, Freddie is allergic to eggs and peanuts and has eczema on his face, arms, legs, and upper back. His current medications include albuterol every 8 hours; a topical steroid (Lidex Cream); and a multivitamin and mineral supplement (Poly-Vi-Sol drops). No one in the family smokes. The caregivers at the day-care center smoke outside the building. The day-care center is clean and had the rugs shampooed the night before this child's illness. This child had no sputum production or fever. Immunizations are current. A comprehensive assessment revealed the following findings:
Respiratory rate, 44 breaths/min
Irregular rhythm
Excessive use of accessory muscles
Nonproductive, frequent cough
Gurgles and expiratory wheezes noted
Pale, no cyanosis
Blood pressure, 100/60 mm Hg; heart rate, 120 beats/min
Restless child who naps for only 20 to 30 minutes at intervals day and night
Arterial blood gases: normal values
Chest radiograph: normal
Poor appetite, vomiting one or two times
Up early in morning
Sweat test: negative for cystic fibrosis

(continued)

...ated to exposure to allergens, viral infection, broncho-... as manifested by: nonproductive frequent cough, pres-...chi) and sibilant wheezes on expiration, restlessness,

...g and no vomiting

Evaluative Statement
3/19/06 Outcome met. Freddie has not vomited in 2 days and has 2-hour intervals between coughing episodes.
M. Jones, RN

...ts will:
• Remove dust-collecting toys

Nursing Interventions	Rationale	Evaluative Statement
Give parents allergy pamphlets from American Lung Association.	Adequate information reinforces instruction given by healthcare providers.	3/17/06 Outcome met. Parents removed furry toys from hospital room. M. Jones, RN
Review with both parents methods to reduce exposure to possible allergens at home.	Constant exposure to allergens (dust, mold, mildew, and so forth) and irritants (perfume, smog, cleaners, and so forth) produces bronchospasm and stimulates copious mucus production. Medications are most effective when allergens are removed.	
Encourage parents to examine day-care environment. Explore options with them.	Environment in day-care may contain allergens. The least irritating setting is desirable.	

SAMPLE DOCUMENTATION   3/17/06 Nursing

Family and staff conference to discuss Freddie's respiratory disturbance initiated by primary nurse's concern. Present were Freddie's mother; MJ (primary nurse); TK (clinical coordinator); TR (head of respiratory department); and MM and LQ (staff nurses). Primary nurse presented findings from assessment and nursing examination. Discussion centered on strategies to control airway edema and reduce wheezes, reduce coughing episodes and control vomiting, and prevent further bronchospasms and edema resulting from exposure to allergens in environment. See plan of care. Patient progress will be evaluated in 4 days during nursing grand rounds, 3/21/06.
M. Jones, RN

Guidelines for Nursing Care 45-1 Monitoring a Patient With a Chest Tube

- Assess the patient's respiratory status, vital signs, and breath sounds. Monitor for any indication of change in respiratory status.
- Observe the dressing around the chest tube insertion site and ensure that it is occlusive. All connections should also be securely taped.
- Check that the drainage tube has no dependent loops or kinks. The drainage collection device must be positioned below the tube insertion site to facilitate drainage.
- Keep drainage collection device secure so that it does not tip over.
- Check that two padded Kelly clamps are available and secured at the bedside. If the drainage unit requires changing, one clamp is positioned 1½ to 2½ inches from the insertion site, and the second clamp is placed 1 inch down from the first one until the unit has been switched. The physician may order a chest tube clamped before its removal to observe the patient's tolerance when it is discontinued or the chest tube may be clamped to assess for an air leak.
- Keep bottle of sterile saline or water at bedside. If chest tube disconnects from drainage unit, submerge end in water. This is done instead of clamping to prevent another pneumothorax. Air is still allowed to escape.

- Never clamp the tube if the patient leaves the unit for a test or moves away from the bed. Disconnect the suction tubing from the drainage system, allowing the unit to continue to collect drainage by gravity. Take bottle of sterile normal saline or water with patient.
- Avoid milking or stripping the tube to promote drainage. This creates excessive negative pressure that can damage delicate lung tissue.
- Assess the suction control chamber if suction is in use. If water suction is used, ensure that water is at the appropriate level (fluid can evaporate); water must be added to ensure that suction is adequate. Gentle bubbling in the suction chamber indicates that suction is being applied to assist drainage.
- Assist the patient to remain in high Fowler's position (if hemothorax is present) or semi-Fowler's position (for pneumothorax) for improved drainage.
- Measure drainage output at the end of each shift by marking the level on the container or placing a small piece of tape at the drainage level to indicate date and time. Drainage is never emptied from the collection chamber. Document color and consistency of drainage. Drainage exceeding 100 mL/hr or a change in drainage to a bright red color that indicates fresh bleeding requires immediate notification of the physician.

PROMOTE HEALTH!

Learn not only to treat illness but also to promote the health and wellness of your patients. Check out the **Promoting Health** boxes, which include assessment checkpoints for specific health and wellness topics and suggestions for designing a self-care prescription. Use the Promoting Health boxes for yourself as well as your patients. After all, it is important to take care of yourself and serve as a role model for your patients. Review the teaching strategies presented in **Teaching to Promote Health at Home** boxes to develop your role as patient educator. Study the **Focus on the Older Adult** boxes, which provide general considerations for older patients and address their special nursing needs.

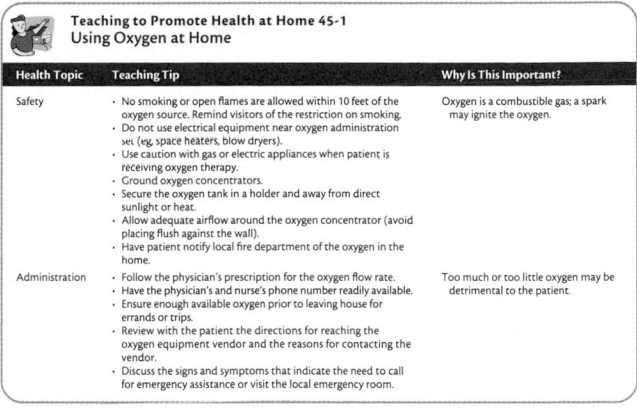

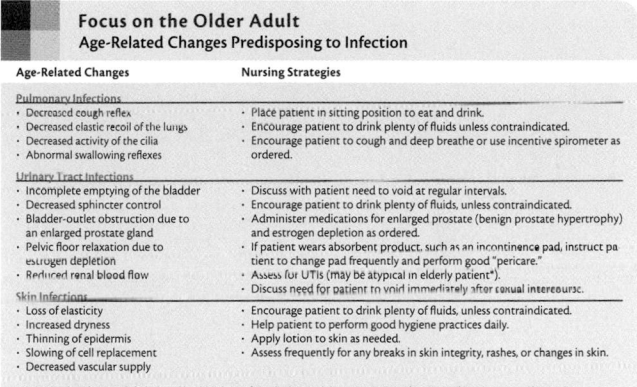

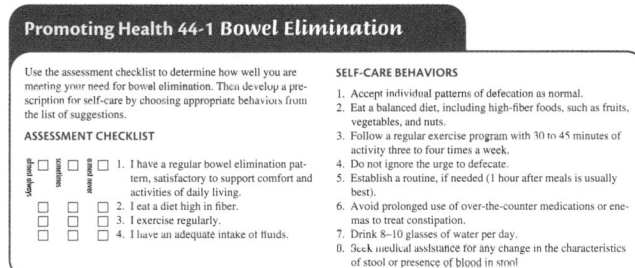

GAIN NEW INSIGHTS!

Read **Through the Eyes of a Patient/Family Caregiver/Student** to gain insight into nursing care from various perspectives. These real-life stories demonstrate how nursing can make a difference in the lives of patients and their families. Gain insight into the "why" behind nursing care. Consider **Research in Nursing: Making a Difference** boxes to discover recent findings in nursing care and relate their relevance to nursing practice.

Research in Nursing Making a Difference
Enhancing Medication Compliance in Elderly People Living in the Community

Noncompliance with a medical regimen places an individual at risk for complications from disease, leading to an increase in physician visits and hospitalizations. Many previous studies have documented that elderly individuals living at home who require medication for chronic diseases are particularly at risk for noncompliance with their medication schedules. Managed care and the accompanying cuts in home care reimbursement limit the nurse's ability to improve compliance, yet simple measures that serve as reminders for this population can have a positive effect on management of symptoms and overall well-being.

Related Research
Winland-Brown, J., & Valiante, J. (2000). Effectiveness of different medication management approaches on elders' medication adherence. *Outcomes Management for Nursing Practice, 4*(4), 172–176.

Participants, ranging in age from 70 to 100 years old, who lived in an independent living facility and had a chronic illness were recruited to participate in the study. All participants were cognitively intact and had a previous hospitalization due to a medication noncompliance issue or medication management concern. The participants were randomly placed in three groups. The con-

trol group performed self-administration of medications. The second group used the pillbox method as the approach to medication management. During the study, the number of doses of medications taken by the patient was recorded, as well as the effect of medication compliance on the medical diagnosis. The voice-activated medication dispenser showed the highest rate of medication compliance, with the pillbox method coming in second. The lowest rate of medication compliance was with the self-administration of medications. This study demonstrated the need for individualized medication administration methods for elderly persons living in the community.

Relevance to Nursing Practice
Interventions that enable the nurse to increase medication compliance in a group such as the elderly can lead to a direct decrease in the number of hospitalizations and physician visits as well as a higher quality of life for the patient. The interventions studied here not only increased compliance but also allowed the subjects to continue to feel independent. The nurse can play an essential role in helping elderly people to remain compliant with their medications while keeping their independence.

Through the Eyes of a
Student

The first time I took care of a patient with "multiple tubes," I was horrified at the thought of actually touching the patient. I hadn't really been exposed to that many critically ill patients until my last semester as a student nurse. I remember being assigned a patient in the cardiothoracic intensive care unit in the hospital where I trained. The patient was a "fresh heart"—a cardiopulmonary bypass graft patient who had just been operated on that morning.

I remember walking into the room and thinking, "What do I do with all of these tubes?" and then with horror thinking, "What if one of them falls out?" Needless to say, I was overwhelmed and frightened but at the same time excited at the challenge that faced me. I asked my preceptor what each tube was for and where it was hooked up and whether it would fall out if I touched it. She answered all my questions with patience and understanding and asked me if I wanted to handle the lines. I looked at her as if she were insane, but went ahead and did it. Would you believe that nothing fell out! I must admit that the experience taught me a lot, but it also got me over the fear of tubes.

I now chuckle every time I see a nursing student's face with that same look of horror as I had, and I try to answer every question with the same degree of patience and understanding that my preceptor had for me.

—Lynda L. Ullmer, RN
Gaithersburg, MD

PREPARE FOR NCLEX!

Start preparing for NCLEX right from the beginning of your nursing education. Familiarize yourself with the multiple-choice format of test taking. Multiple-choice questions presented in **Practicing for NCLEX** test your knowledge of basic through complex concepts.

▪ Practicing for NCLEX

1. The smallest infectious agents capable of causing an infection are:
   a. Bacteria
   b. Viruses
   c. Molds
   d. Yeasts
2. Your patient has developed a low-grade fever and states that she has felt very tired lately. This phase of an infection is known as the:
   a. Incubation period
   b. Prodromal stage
   c. Full stage of illness
   d. Convalescent period
3. The highest mortality rate is associated with nosocomial infections that involve the:
   a. Respiratory tract
   b. Integumentary system
   c. Urinary tract
   d. Intestines
4. A patient develops a urinary tract infection after an indwelling urinary catheter has been inserted. This would most accurately be termed:
   a. A viral infection
   b. A chronic infection
   c. An iatrogenic infection
   d. An opportunistic infection
5. The nurse has opened the sterile supplies and donned two sterile gloves to complete a sterile dressing change. Maintaining surgical asepsis requires the nurse to:
   a. Keep splashes on the sterile field to a minimum
   b. Cover the nose and mouth with gloved hands if a sneeze is imminent
   c. Use the dominant hand to cleanse the incision with a moist saline sponge and then apply the dry dressing
   d. Consider the outer 1 inch of the sterile field as contaminated
6. The CDC standard precaution recommendations apply to:
   a. Only patients with diagnosed infections
   b. Only blood and body fluids with visible blood
   c. All body fluids including sweat
   d. All patients receiving care in hospitals
7. In addition to standard precautions, the nurse caring for a patient with rubella would plan to implement:
   a. Droplet precautions
   b. Airborne precautions
   c. Contact precautions
   d. Universal precautions
8. When caring for a patient with latex allergy, the nurse creates a latex-safe environment by:
   a. Carefully cleaning the wall-mounted blood pressure device before using it
   b. Donning latex gloves outside the room to limit powder dispersal
   c. Using a latex-free pharmacy protocol
   d. Placing the patient in a semiprivate room
9. The guidelines for minimum protection standards for infection prevention and control were initially developed by:
   a. OSHA
   b. Individual healthcare facilities
   c. The state governing body
   d. The CDC
10. The recommended sequence for removing soiled personal protective equipment when the nurse prepares to leave the patient's room is to remove:
    a. Gown, goggles, mask, gloves, and exit the room
    b. Gloves, wash hands, remove gown, mask, and goggles
    c. Gloves, mask, gown, goggles, and wash hands
    d. Goggles, mask, gloves, gown, and wash hands

Acknowledgments

This revision is the work of many talented and committed people, and we wish to gratefully acknowledge the assistance of all who have contributed in any way to the completion of this project. Our first debt of gratitude is to all the nurse educators and students who have adopted the text and shared with us their experiences in using the teaching and learning package. We are deeply grateful for their revision suggestions and trust they will enhance the learning experiences of others.

The work of this revision was superbly facilitated by our new and seemingly tireless Developmental Editor, Danielle DiPalma, in the Nursing Editorial division of Lippincott Williams & Wilkins. A fierce advocate for this text and each element of the new state-of-the art teaching/learning package, Danielle somehow managed to become a respected friend while using her wiles to keep us "at the top of our game" and "on schedule"! Our very special thanks to her and to Elizabeth Nieginski, Editor, and Sarah Kyle and Maryann Foley, Development Editors, for their support and guidance throughout the project. To the members of the production department, who patiently pulled everything together to form a completed book: Helen Ewan, Director of Production, Rosanne Hallowell, Senior Production Editor, Carolyn O'Brien, Art Director, and Brett MacNaughton, Illustration Coordinator.

We thank all who generously gave their time, ideas, and resources, and we gratefully acknowledge the special contributions of the following:
- Rick Brady, Joe Mitchell, Ken Kasper, Barbara Proud, Gates Rhodes, and Kathy Sloane, photographers
- Marie Clark, who developed the math problems and solutions in the "Medications" chapter

We gratefully acknowledge the influence of our mentors and teachers who have influenced our thoughts and writing; each person we have been privileged to care for as nurses; our students, who continually challenge us to find more effective means to teach nursing; our professional colleagues; and perhaps most important, our families and friends, whose love sustained us through the long hours of research and writing.

Finally, we are grateful to the reviewers and contributors of this edition and of the previous four editions, whose expertise broadened both the scope and depth of the text. A special thank you to Pamela Evans-Smith for her extensive contributions to this edition.

Carol Taylor
Carol Lillis
Priscilla LeMone

Expanded Contents

Unit II Community-Based Settings for Patient Care, 141

Chapter 8 Healthcare Delivery Systems, 143

Chapter 9 Continuity of Care, 161

FUNDAMENTALS
OF NURSING
The Art and Science of Nursing Care

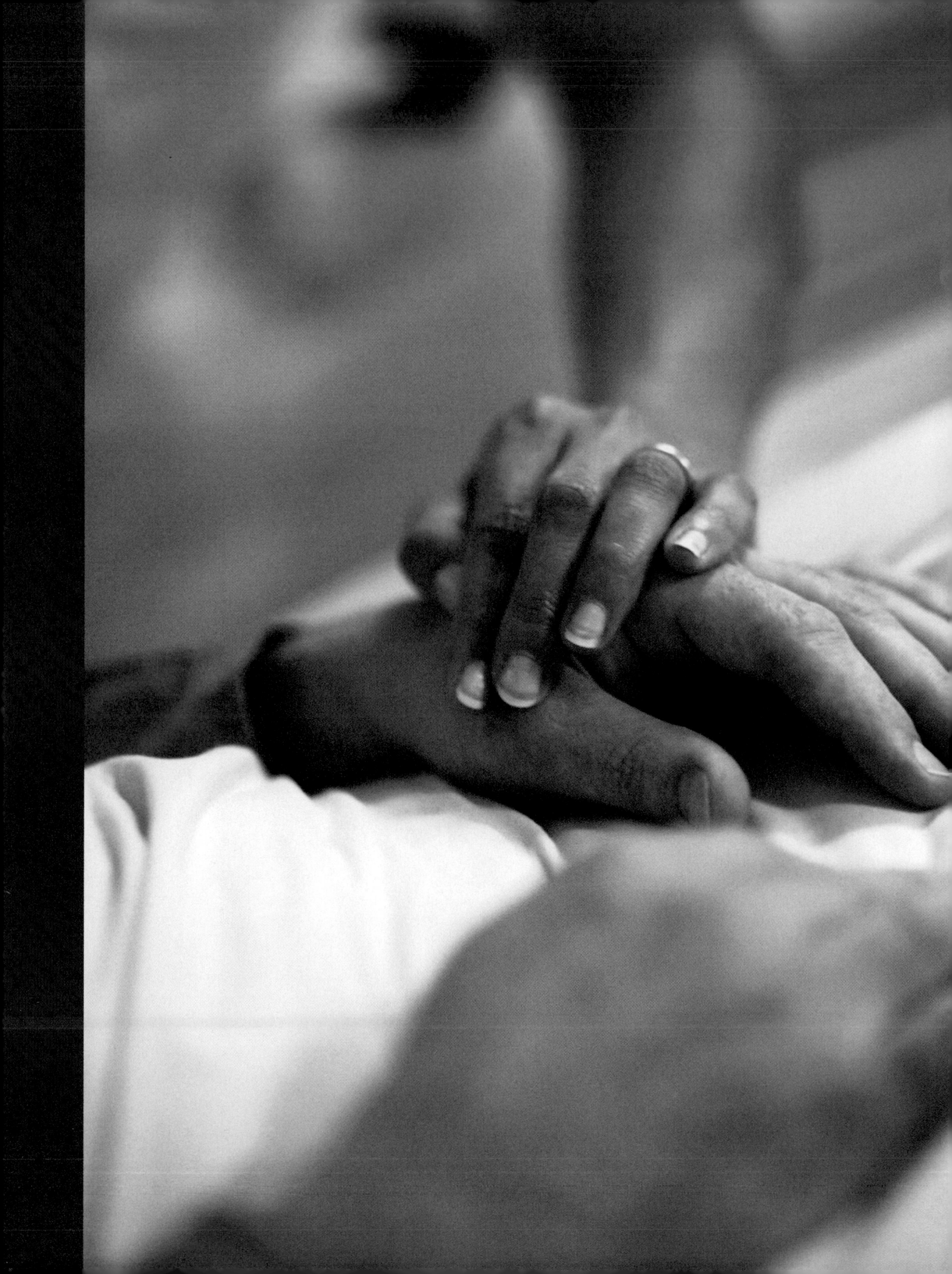

Foundations of Nursing Practice

"Basic to any philosophy of nursing seems to be these three concepts: (1) reverence for the gift of life; (2) respect for the dignity, worth, autonomy, and individuality of each human being; (3) resolution to act dynamically in relation to one's beliefs."

Ernestine Wiedenbach (1900–)
a faculty member at Yale University School of Nursing, where she developed her model of nursing from years of experience in various nursing positions

Nursing is both an art and a science. It is a profession that uses specialized knowledge and skills to care for people in both health and illness and in a variety of practice settings. Unit I introduces concepts that provide the foundation for nursing practice by defining nursing as a whole. Chapters in this unit introduce the profession of nursing; basic needs of individuals, their families, and the community; culture and ethnicity; promotion of wellness in both health and illness; the theoretical base for nursing; and ethical and legal implications for nursing practice.

Historical perspectives, educational preparation, professional organizations, and guidelines for professional nursing practice serve as a base for understanding what nursing is and how it is organized. An understanding of basic human needs and the individualized definitions of wellness and illness prepare the nurse to integrate the human dimensions—the physical, intellectual, emotional, sociocultural, spiritual, and environmental aspects of each person—into the care given to promote wellness, prevent illness, restore health, and facilitate coping with altered function or death. Knowledge of the varied methods of care delivery is necessary in today's complex healthcare system.

Nursing theories and nursing research provide a foundation for evidence-based nursing practice, defining the rationale for nursing actions and offering a focus for nursing care. An understanding of the influence of values on human behavior and of the ethical dimensions of nursing practice is essential to responsible and accountable patient care. Finally, sensitivity to the legal implications of professional nursing practice is imperative in today's culture.

Unit I explores the foundations for nursing practice from both the perspective of the nurse and a holistic understanding of the patient. Students of nursing are introduced to a challenging and rewarding profession, and are provided with a knowledge base to ground the development of caregiving skills and professional relationships and behaviors.

Introduction to Nursing

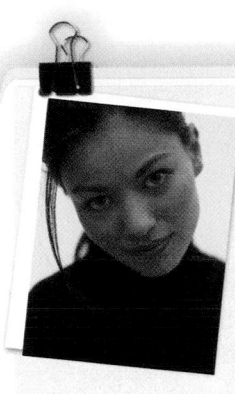

Michelle Fine, a 19-year-old first-time mother who was discharged with her healthy 7-lb 8-oz baby girl 2 days ago, calls the nursery. She reports, "My baby isn't taking to my breast and she hasn't had any real feeding for 24 hours."

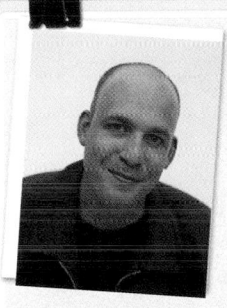

Roberto Pecorini is a 38-year-old man diagnosed with metastatic colon cancer. Having undergone radiation treatments and chemotherapy, he is extremely weak and malnourished, receiving numerous intravenous fluids via a central venous catheter. He has two pressure ulcers on his sacrum, each approximately 1½" in diameter, requiring wound care. He also has a colostomy that he cannot care for independently.

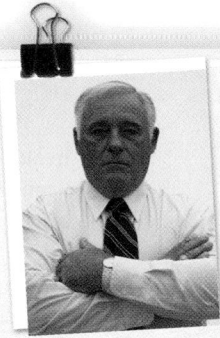

Albert Rowlings, a 62-year-old male who is at risk for heart disease, is being taught about lifestyle modifications, such as diet, exercise, and stress reduction. He states, "Just save your breath. Why should I bother about all that? I'd be better off dead than living like I am now, anyway!"

Focusing on Blended Skills

The types of blended skills you'll need to respond to the case scenarios include:

Cognitive Skills
- Knowledge of breastfeeding, and factors and variables that affect newborn nutrition
- Knowledge of risk factors for heart disease, and factors that can and cannot be modified
- Ability to incorporate knowledge of the influence of values on behavior, especially involving maternal–newborn attachment, and nutrition and lifestyle modifications
- Ability to identify the principles for and reasons underlying necessary interventions when caring for a patient with multiple needs associated with colon cancer
- Ability to incorporate knowledge of pertinent scope of practice guidelines, standards of care, and agency and institutional policies when providing care
- Ability to use critical-thinking skills to intervene appropriately to meet patients' needs
- Knowledge about designing an effective teaching program for patients

Technical Skills
- Strong assessment skills to identify difficulties with breastfeeding and the patient's beliefs about health and illness
- Ability to demonstrate competence in specific skills and tasks related to patient care within the scope of practice
- Ability to identify limitations in performance of skills, asking for assistance as necessary when performing skills and tasks
- Ability to use appropriate teaching strategies and adapt these strategies as needed

Interpersonal Skills
- Strong people skills, to establish trusting relationships with the new mother, patients with risk factors associated with disease, and patients with multiple needs related to cancer

- Special interpersonal competence to interact with other healthcare personnel, confronting appropriate persons when necessary
- Ability to communicate to the patient that your first concern is the patient's status, rather than rote implementation of the plan of care—for example, when instructing a new mother dealing with a newborn's feeding or when interacting with a patient who feels as if changes in lifestyle would be worthless
- Ability to demonstrate respect for the patient's human dignity throughout the patient's care

Ethical and Legal Skills
- Demonstration of a strong sense of accountability for the health and well-being of patients, which translates into a commitment to get them the help needed to achieve their health goals—within the scope of nursing responsibilities and available resources
- A willingness to hold one's self accountable for safe and high-quality practice
- Skill in working collaboratively with colleagues to ensure safe, effective care
- Knowledge of the ethical and legal principles related to situations such as telephone instructions for the new mother, a patient's reluctance or refusal to engage in lifestyle modifications, or the care of patients with multiple needs, in addition to other practice responsibilities

Learning Outcomes

After completing the chapter, the learner should be able to accomplish the following:

1. Describe the historic background of nursing, definitions of nursing, and the status of nursing as a profession and as a discipline.
2. Identify the aims of nursing as they interrelate to facilitate maximal health and quality of life for patients.
3. Describe the various levels of educational preparation in nursing.
4. Discuss the effects on nursing practice of nursing organizations, standards of nursing practice, nurse practice acts, and the nursing process.
5. Identify current trends in nursing.

Key Terms

health
licensure
nurse practice act
nursing
nursing process
profession
standards

What is nursing? Consider the following examples of who nurses are and what they do:

- Delton Nix, RN, graduated from an associate degree nursing program 3 years ago. He is now working full-time as a staff nurse in a hospital medical unit while attending school part-time toward a baccalaureate degree in nursing; his goal is to become a nurse anesthetist.
- Jeiping Wu, RN, MSN, FNP, specializes as an advanced practice family nurse practitioner. She has an independent practice in a rural primary health clinic.
- Samuel Cohen, LPN, decided to follow his life's dream to become a nurse after 20 years as a postal worker. After examining all his options and goals, he completed a practical nursing program and is now a member of an emergency ambulance crew in a large city.
- Amy Orlando, RN, BSN, graduated 2 years ago and recently began a new job in an urban community health service.
- Roxanne McDaniel, RN, PhD, with a doctorate in nursing, teaches and conducts research at a large university.

These examples show how difficult it is to describe nursing simply. If everyone in your class were asked to complete the sentence, "Nursing is . . . ," there would be many different responses because each person would answer based on his or her own personal experience and knowledge of nursing at that time. As you progress toward graduation and as you practice nursing after graduation, your own definition will reflect changes within you as you learn about and experience nursing.

Basically defined, **nursing** is the care of others. That care may involve any number of activities, from carrying out complicated technical procedures to something as seemingly simple as holding a hand. Nursing is focused on the person receiving care and is a blend of the science and the art of nursing. The science of nursing is the knowledge base for the care that is given, and the art of nursing is the skilled application of that knowledge to help others reach maximum health and quality of life.

This chapter introduces you to nursing, including a brief history of nursing from its beginnings to the present, and provides definitions of nursing. Educational preparation, professional organizations, and guidelines for professional nursing practice are discussed to help you better understand what nursing is and how it is organized. (For an example demonstrating nursing practice and responsibilities, see the accompanying Reflective Practice box.) Because nursing is a part of an ever-changing society, current trends in nursing also are discussed.

HISTORIC PERSPECTIVES ON NURSING

Development of Nursing in Early Civilizations

Most early civilizations believed that illness had supernatural causes. The theory of animism attempted to explain the cause of mysterious changes in bodily functions. This theory was based on the belief that everything in nature was alive with invisible forces and endowed with power. Good spirits brought health; evil spirits brought sickness and death. The roles of the physician and the nurse were separate and distinct. The physician was the medicine man who treated disease by chanting, inspiring fear, or opening the skull to release evil spirits (Dolan, Fitzpatrick, & Herrmann, 1983). The nurse usually was the mother who cared for her family during sickness by providing physical care and herbal remedies. This nurturing and caring role of the nurse has continued to the present.

As civilizations grew, temples became the centers of medical care because of the belief that illness was caused by sin and the gods' displeasure (ie, disease literally means "dis-ease"). Priests were highly regarded as physicians, but neither human life nor women were valued by society. In some societies, the nurse was viewed as a slave, carrying out menial tasks based on the orders of the priest-physician. During the same period, the ancient Hebrews developed rules through the Ten Commandments and the Mosaic Health Code for ethical human relationships, mental health, and disease control. Nurses cared for sick people in the home and the community and also practiced as nurse-midwives (Dolan et al., 1983).

In the early Christian period, nursing began to have a formal and more clearly defined role. Led by the belief that love and caring for others were important, women called deaconesses made the first organized visits to sick people, and members of male religious orders gave nursing care and buried the dead. Both male and female nursing orders were founded during the Crusades (11th to 13th centuries). Hospitals were built for the enormous number of pilgrims needing healthcare, and nursing became a respected vocation. Although the early Middle Ages ended in chaos, nursing had developed purpose, direction, and leadership.

Development of Nursing from the 16th to 19th Centuries

At the beginning of the 16th century, many Western societies changed from having a religious orientation to emphasizing warfare, exploration, and expansion of knowledge. Many monasteries and convents closed, leading to a tremendous shortage of people to care for the sick. To meet this need, women who had committed crimes were recruited into nursing in lieu of serving jail sentences. In addition to having a poor reputation, nurses received low pay and worked long hours in unfavorable conditions.

From the middle of the 18th century to the 19th century, social reforms changed the roles of nurses and of women in general. It was during this time that nursing as we now know it began, based on many of the beliefs of Florence Nightingale. Born in 1820 to a wealthy family, she grew up in England, was well educated, and traveled extensively. Despite strong opposition from her family, Florence Nightingale undertook nurse's training at the age of 31. The outbreak of the Crimean War and a request by the British to organize nursing care for a military hospital in Turkey gave Nightingale an opportunity for achievement (Kalish & Kalish, 1995). As she successfully

Reflective Practice
Challenge to Ethical and Legal Skills

A few years ago, I was working as a nurse's aide on a busy oncology unit. It was here that I met Roberto Pecorini, a 38-year-old man diagnosed with metastatic colon cancer. He had undergone radiation treatments and chemotherapy and was extremely weak and malnourished. He was receiving numerous intravenous fluids via a central venous catheter. In addition, he had developed two pressure ulcers on his sacrum, each approximately 1½" in diameter, that required wound care. He also had a colostomy that he could not care for independently.

Although the staff was very helpful, the orientation I received to the unit was brief because they were very short staffed. During one occasion, shortly after I had been oriented to the floor, I was working a night shift and was the only nurse's aide on the unit. The nurses I was working with asked me to care for Mr. Pecorini, including performing several tasks and skills with which I was unfamiliar. In addition to my lack of familiarity with skills such as changing central line dressings and performing blood draws and wound care, I was not licensed to perform these tasks. I felt uncomfortable performing these skills on my own. However, the nurses were extremely busy and I wanted to help them as much as possible. If I performed these skills on my own, I could be putting the patient at risk. Moreover, I could be threatening the license of the nurses.

Thinking Outside the Box: Possible Courses of Action

- Perform the tasks requested despite the fact that I had little experience with them.
- Inform the nurses that I did not feel comfortable completing these skills on my own and ask that they assign me other tasks within my scope of duty.
- Ask the nurses to be present when I performed these tasks so that they could observe my skills and intervene if necessary.
- Refrain from performing these tasks and alert the nurse manager the following day that I was assigned to tasks outside my scope of duty.

Evaluating a Good Outcome: How Do I Define Success?

- The patient received safe, comprehensive care without being placed at risk.
- I performed tasks and skills within my scope of practice.
- The nurses understood my job duties and properly delegated the necessary tasks.
- The nurses' licensure was not put in jeopardy.
- I felt comfortable and competent in my job performance.

Personal Learning: Here's to the Future!

Since I felt uncomfortable in performing the duties assigned to me by the nurses, I confronted them and told them that I had recently been oriented to the floor and did not have experience with these skills. Although somewhat surprised that I didn't have the experience, they understood, not wanting me to do anything I felt uncomfortable with. The nurses were used to having an LPN as a night aide, and the LPN's scope of practice was broader than mine. Throughout the night, I observed the nurses performing the skills and tasks, with the nurses walking me through several of the skills that I was allowed to perform but in which I did not feel proficient. In the morning, we spoke with the nurse manager, who realized the need for clarifying the job duties of the nurse's aides and the appropriate delegation of tasks. I feel that I made the right decision in speaking with the nurses because patient safety could have been compromised by my inexperience. The nurses' licensure also could have been put at risk. As a result of our conversation with the nurse manager, the orientation for new nurse's aides was reorganized, helping greatly to define the scope of duties for the aides.

Reflection

How do you think you would respond in a similar situation? Why? What does this tell you about yourself and about the adequacy of your skills for professional practice? Can you think of other ways to respond? How was the nursing student's action ethical? Legal? Please explain. What other skills (cognitive, interpersonal, technical, ethical/legal) would you need to respond well in this situation? Do you agree with the criteria to evaluate a successful outcome? Based on the nursing student's personal learning, were the criteria met? Please explain why or why not.

Colleen Kilcullen, Georgetown University

overcame enormous difficulties, Nightingale challenged prejudices against women and elevated the status of all nurses. After the war, she returned to England, where she established a training school for nurses and wrote books about healthcare and nursing education. Florence Nightingale's contributions include:

- Identifying the personal needs of the patient and the role of the nurse in meeting those needs
- Establishing standards for hospital management
- Establishing a respected occupation for women
- Establishing nursing education
- Recognizing the two components of nursing: health and illness
- Believing that nursing is separate and distinct from medicine
- Recognizing that nutrition is important to health
- Instituting occupational and recreational therapy for sick people
- Stressing the need for continuing education for nurses
- Maintaining accurate records, recognized as the beginnings of nursing research

Florence Nightingale elevated the status of nursing to a respected occupation, improved the quality of nursing care, and founded modern nursing education. Florence Nightingale, other historically important nurses, and images of nursing are shown in Figure 1-1; people important to the development of nursing are listed in Table 1-1.

Development of Nursing from the 19th to 21st Centuries

Both the work of Florence Nightingale and the care provided for battle casualties during the Civil War focused attention on the need for educated nurses in the United States. Schools of nursing, founded in connection with hospitals, were established on the beliefs of Nightingale, but the training they provided was based more on apprenticeship than on educational principles. Hospitals saw an economic advantage in having their own schools, and most hospital schools were organized to provide more easily controlled and less expensive staff for the hospital. This resulted in a lack of clear guidelines separating nursing service and nursing education. As students and as graduates, female nurses were under the control of male hospital administrators and physicians. The lack of educational standards, the male dominance in healthcare, and the pervading Victorian belief that women depended on men combined to contribute to several decades of slow progress toward professionalism in nursing (Kalish & Kalish, 1995).

World War II had an enormous effect on nursing. For the first time, large numbers of women worked outside the home. They became more independent and assertive. These changes in women and in society led to an increased emphasis on education. The war itself had created a need for more nurses and resulted in a knowledge explosion in medicine and technology, which broadened the role of nurses. After World War II, efforts were directed at upgrading nursing education. Schools of

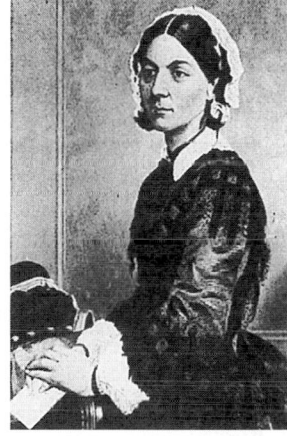

Florence Nightingale, initiator of major reforms in health care and nursing training in England

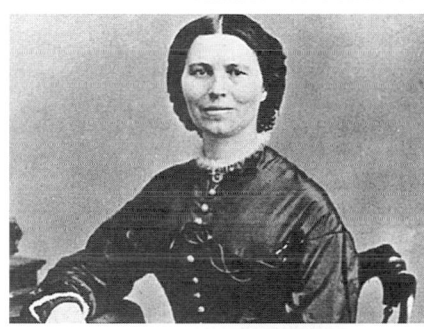

Clara Barton, founder of the American Red Cross in 1882

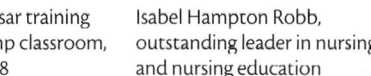
Vassar training camp classroom, 1918

Isabel Hampton Robb, outstanding leader in nursing and nursing education

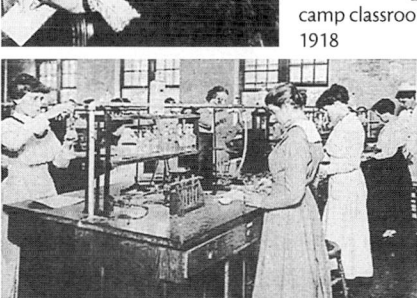
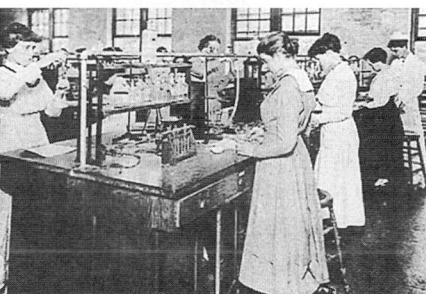

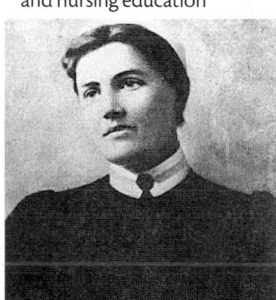

Post-WWII nursing school poster

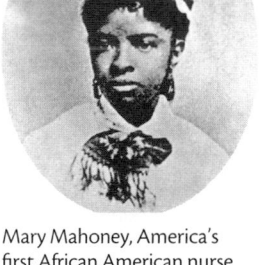

Mary Mahoney, America's first African American nurse to graduate from a school of nursing

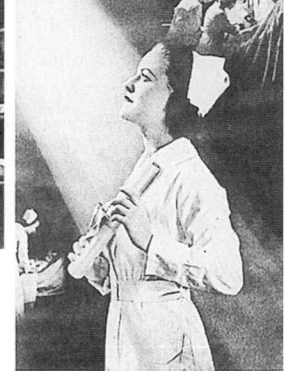

Philadelphia General Hospital nurse, late 1800s

FIGURE 1-1 Images of nurses spanning more than 100 years of service. (Courtesy of the Center for the Study of the History of Nursing, University of Pennsylvania.)

TABLE 1-1 People Important to the Development of Nursing in North America

Person	Contribution
19th Century	
Florence Nightingale	Defined nursing as both an art and a science, differentiated nursing from medicine, created freestanding nursing education; published books about nursing and healthcare; is regarded as the founder of modern nursing (see text for further information)
Clara Barton	Volunteered to care for wounds and feed Union soldiers during the Civil War; served as the supervisor of nurses for the Army of the James, organizing hospitals and nurses; established the Red Cross in the United States in 1882
Dorothea Dix	Superintendent of the Female Nurses of the Army during the Civil War; was given the authority and the responsibility for recruiting and equipping a corps of army nurses; was a pioneering crusader for the reform of the treatment of the mentally ill
Mary Ann Bickerdyke	Organized diet kitchens, laundries, and an ambulance service and supervised nursing staff during the Civil War
Louise Schuyler	A nurse during the Civil War, she returned to New York and organized the New York Charities Aid Association; this organization worked to improve care of the sick in Bellevue Hospital; one recommendation was to have standards for nursing education.
Linda Richards	The first trained nurse in the United States; a graduate of the New England Hospital for Women and Children in Boston, Massachusetts in 1873. She became the night superintendent of Bellevue Hospital in 1874 and began the practice of keeping records and writing orders.
Jane Addams	Provided social services within a neighborhood setting; a leader for women's rights; recipient of the 1931 Nobel Peace prize
Lillian Wald	Established a neighborhood nursing service for the sick poor of the Lower East Side in New York City; the founder of public health nursing
Mary Elizabeth Mahoney	Graduated from the New England Hospital for Women and Children in 1879 as America's first African American nurse
Harriet Tubman	A nurse and an abolitionist, she was active in the underground railroad movement before joining the Union Army during the Civil War.
Nora Gertrude Livingston	Established a training program for nurses at the Montreal General Hospital (the first 3-year program in North America)
Mary Agnes Snively	Director of the nursing school at Toronto General Hospital and one of the founders of the Canadian Nurses Association
Sojourner Truth	A nurse who not only provided care to soldiers during the Civil War but also worked for the women's movement
Isabel Hampton Robb	A leader in nursing and nursing education, she organized the nursing school at Johns Hopkins Hospital, where she initiated policies that included limiting the number of hours in a day's work and wrote a textbook to help student learning; was the first president of the Nurses Associated Alumnae of the United States and Canada (which later became the American Nurses Association).
20th Century	
Mary Adelaide Nutting	As a member of the faculty of Teachers' College, Columbia University, she became the first professor of nursing in the world and, with Lavinia Dock, published the four-volume *History of Nursing*.
Elizabeth Smellie	A member of the original Victorian Order of Nurses for Canada (a group who provided public health nursing); organized the Canadian Women's Army Corps during World War II
Lavinia Dock	A nursing leader and women's rights activist who was instrumental in the Constitutional amendment giving women the right to vote
Mary Breckenridge	Established the Frontier Nursing Service and one of the first midwifery schools in the United States

nursing were based on educational objectives and were increasingly developed in university and college settings, leading to degrees in nursing for both men and women.

Nursing has broadened in all areas, including practice in a wide variety of healthcare settings, the development of a specific body of knowledge, the conduct and publication of nursing research, and recognition of the role of nursing in promoting health. Increased emphasis on nursing knowledge as the base for nursing practice has led to the growth of nursing as a professional discipline. See the section entitled "Current Trends in Nursing" for a detailed discussion of how nursing is changing and developing in the 21st century.

DEFINITIONS OF NURSING

The word *nurse* originated from the Latin word *nutrix,* meaning "to nourish." Most definitions of nurse and nursing describe the nurse as a person who nourishes, fosters, and protects and who is prepared to take care of sick, injured, and aged people. With the expanding roles and functions of the nurse in today's society, however, any one definition is too limited.

The International Council of Nurses published a full definition of nursing in 1987, followed by this shorter, more succinct version in 2002:

> *Nursing encompasses autonomous and collaborative care of individuals of all ages, families, groups and communities, sick or well and in all settings. Nursing includes the promotion of health, prevention of illness, and the care of ill, disabled, and dying people. Advocacy, promotion of a safe environment, research, participation in shaping health policy and in patient and health systems management, and education are also key nursing roles.*
>
> (*International Council of Nurses, 2002*)

> *Recall Roberto Pecorini, the 38-year-old patient with metastatic cancer described in the Reflective Practice box. When providing care for Mr. Pecorini, the nurse assumes the role of caregiver, maintaining the patient's safety throughout, and explaining to the patient all interventions being performed, thereby educating the patient.*

The American Nurses Association's Nursing's Social Policy Statement (1995) describes the values and social responsibility of nursing, provides a definition and scope of practice for nursing, and discusses nursing's knowledge base and the methods by which nursing is regulated. Nurses focus on human experiences and responses to birth, health, illness, and death within the context of individuals, families, groups, and communities. The knowledge base for nursing practice includes diagnosis, interventions, and evaluation of outcomes from an established plan of care. In addition, the nurse integrates objective data with knowledge gained from an understanding of the patient's or group's subjective experience, applies scientific knowledge in the nursing process, and provides a caring relationship that facilitates health and healing.

> *Recall Michelle Fine, the young mother with a newborn who is having difficulty breastfeeding. The nurse, having a knowledge base about newborn care and nutrition, would integrate this information with subjective and objective data gained from Michelle to arrive at potential solutions to her current problems.*

The central focus in all definitions of nursing is the patient (the person receiving care) and includes the physical, emotional, social, and spiritual dimensions of that person. Nursing is no longer considered to be concerned primarily with illness care. Nursing's concepts and definitions have expanded to include the prevention of illness and the promotion and maintenance of health for individuals, families, and communities.

> *Think back to Albert Rowlings, the 62-year-old male at risk for heart disease who was described at the beginning of the chapter. The nurse participates in illness prevention, thus promoting healthier behavior by instructing the patient in lifestyle changes necessary to reduce his risk for developing heart disease.*

AIMS OF NURSING

Four broad aims of nursing practice can be identified in the definitions of nursing:
1. To promote health
2. To prevent illness
3. To restore health
4. To facilitate coping with disability or death

To meet these aims, the nurse uses knowledge, skills, and critical thinking to give care in a variety of traditional and expanding nursing roles (Box 1-1). To provide knowledgeable care, the nurse uses cognitive, technical, interpersonal, and ethical/legal competencies essential to nursing practice. The primary role of the nurse as caregiver is given shape and substance by the interrelated roles of communicator, teacher, counselor, leader, researcher, and advocate. These competencies and roles are described in Table 1-2 and are fully discussed in Unit V. The nurse carries out these roles in many different settings, with care increasingly provided in the home and in the community. Examples of settings for care are listed in Box 1-2 and are fully described in Chapters 8 and 10.

Promoting Health

Health is a state of optimal functioning or well-being. As defined by the World Health Organization, one's health includes physical, social, and mental components and is not merely the absence of disease or infirmity. Health is often a subjective state—a person may be medically diagnosed with an illness but still consider himself or herself healthy. Wellness is another term with essentially the same meaning as health, and both terms are used in this text. Models of health and wellness are described in Chapter 2.

Health promotion is motivated by the desire to increase a person's well-being and health potential (Pender, Murdaugh, & Parsons, 2002). A person's level of health is affected by many different interrelated factors that either promote health or increase the risk for illness. These factors include genetic inheritance, cognitive abilities, educational level, race and ethnicity, culture, age and gender, developmental level, lifestyle, environment, and socioeconomic status.

Health is an essential part of each of the other aims of nursing. Every patient, no matter how ill, has strengths. Nurses promote health by maximizing the patient's own individual strengths. Identifying and analyzing the patient's strengths are a component of preventing illness, restoring health, and facilitating coping with disability or death. The nurse identifies and uses these strengths to help the patient reach maximum function and quality of life or meet death with dignity.

BOX 1-1 **How Can You Be a Nurse?**

How can you be a nurse? How can you bear to watch children suffer?
Wait until you've rocked and soothed a suffering child into peaceful sleep, and you feel the child's relief washing over you like a blessing. Then you won't need to ask.

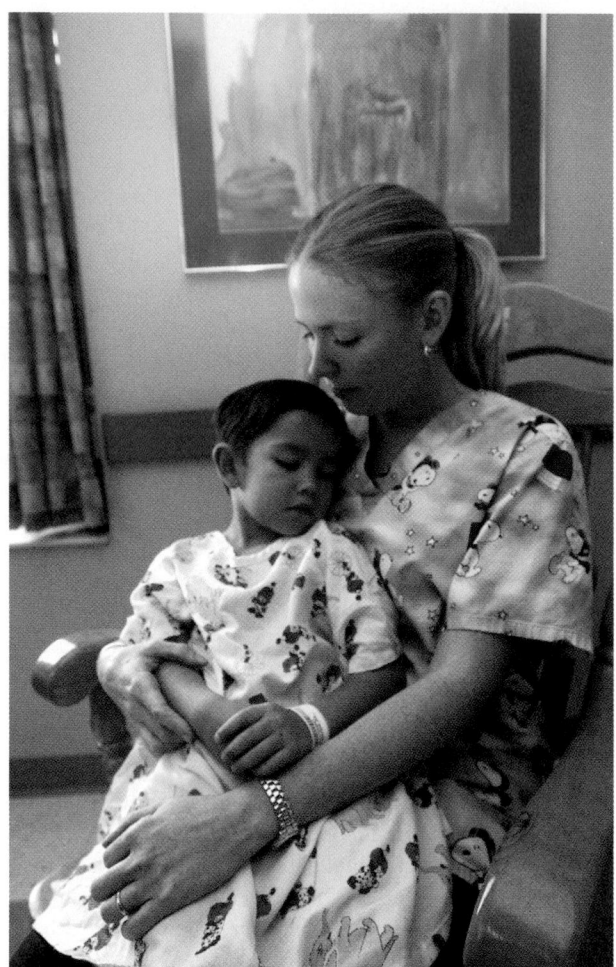

Photo by Joe Mitchell.

How can you be a nurse? So many of your patients are so old, so sick, these days. How can you bear the thought that, in the end, your care may make no difference?
Wait until you've used your hands and eyes and voice to dispel terror, to show a helpless person that his life is respected, that he has dignity. Your caring helps him care about himself . . .

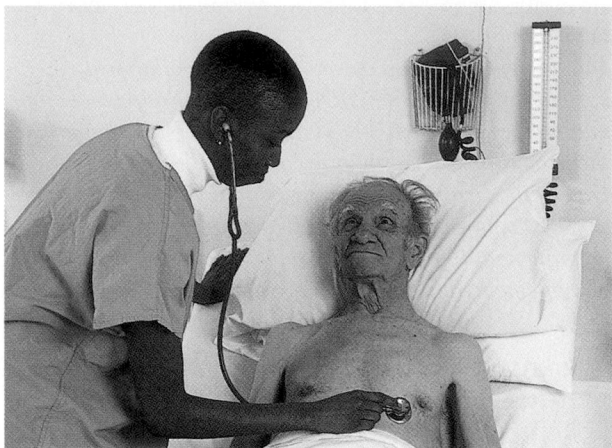

Photo © Barbara Proud.

How can you be a nurse? How can you bear to care for frustrating, confused Alzheimer's patients?
Wait until you've devised a combination of strategies that provide exercise and permit safe wandering, and you see a lift, almost a spring, in a patient's shuffling gait. You'll feel the lightness of Baryshnikov in your own step that day.

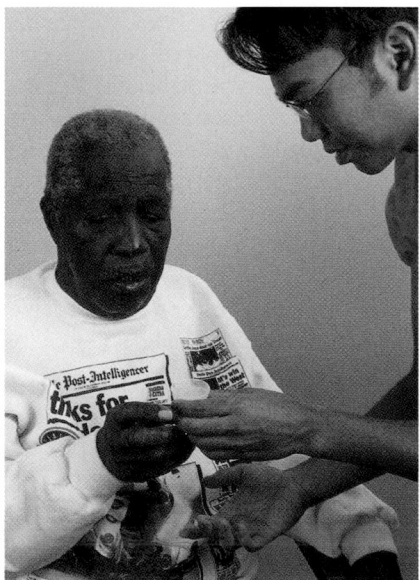

BOX 1-1 (Continued)

How can you be a nurse? How can you bear the sound of babies crying?
Wait until your combination of vigilance, bulldog advocacy, and gentle handling has given a preemie's lungs the time they needed to develop, and you hear his first lusty cry. You'll laugh out loud!

So you keep choosing to be a nurse. You have days of frustration, nights of despair, terrible angers. Your highs and lows are peaks and chasms, not hills and valleys. The defeats come more than often enough to keep you humble: the problems you can't untangle, the lives that seep away too fast, the meanings that elude your understanding. But you keep working at it, learning from it, knowing the next peak lies ahead.

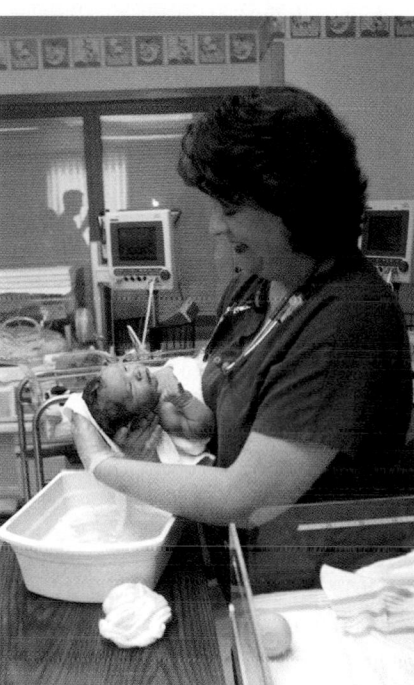
Photo by Joe Mitchell.

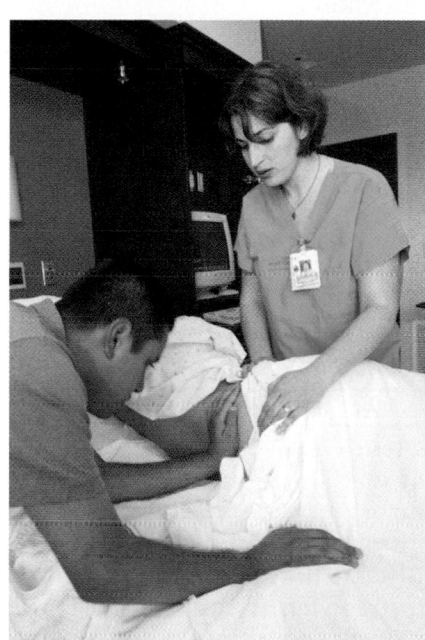
Photo by Joe Mitchell.

Mary Mallison
Editorial, April 1987
American Journal of Nursing

TABLE 1-2 Nursing Roles in All Settings

Role	Function
Caregiver	The provision of care to patients that combines both the art and the science of nursing in meeting physical, emotional, intellectual, sociocultural, and spiritual needs. As a caregiver, the nurse integrates the roles of communicator, teacher, counselor, leader, researcher, and advocate to promote wellness through activities that prevent illness, restore health, and facilitate coping with disability or death. The role of caregiver is the primary role of the nurse.
Communicator	The use of effective interpersonal and therapeutic communication skills to establish and maintain helping relationships with patients of all ages in a wide variety of healthcare settings
Teacher/Educator	The use of communication skills to assess, implement, and evaluate individualized teaching plans to meet learning needs of patients and their families
Counselor	The use of therapeutic interpersonal communication skills to provide information, make appropriate referrals, and facilitate the patient's problem-solving and decision-making skills
Leader	The assertive, self-confident practice of nursing when providing care, effecting change, and functioning with groups
Researcher	The participation in or conduct of research to increase knowledge in nursing and improve patient care
Advocate	The protection of human or legal rights and the securing of care for all patients based on the belief that patients have the right to make informed decisions about their own health and lives

---

BOX 1-2 Examples of Settings for Nursing Care

Hospitals
Ambulatory surgery centers
Emergency helicopter services
Clinics
Homes
Educational programs
Public health offices
Doctors' offices
Industry
Long-term care facilities
Mobile healthcare units
Schools
Offices
Hospice
Mental health facilities
State health programs
Skilled-care facilities
Churches
Prisons

When teaching Mr. Rowlings, the patient described at the beginning of the chapter with risk factors for heart disease, the nurse would focus the teaching plan to rely on the patient's strengths. Although his statements reflect a reluctance to learn and change, emphasizing the patient's strengths would help increase the patient's awareness of them and thus, hopefully, spur him to make the necessary changes.

The U.S. Department of Health and Human Services has established health promotion guidelines for the nation as a whole in *Healthy People 2010.* The guidelines are focused on meeting two overarching goals: (1) to increase quality and years of healthy life, and (2) to eliminate health disparities. The guidelines contain 10 Leading Health Indicators, which are being used to measure the health of the nation over 10 years. The Leading Health Indicators (Box 1-3) reflect the major health concerns in the United States at the beginning of the 21st century. They were selected on the basis of their ability to motivate action, availability to measure progress, and importance as public health issues.

Health promotion is the framework for nursing activities. The nurse considers the patient's self-awareness, health awareness, and use of resources while providing care. Through knowledge and skill, the nurse accomplishes the following:

- Facilitates decisions about lifestyle that enhance quality of life and encourage acceptance of responsibility for one's own health
- Increases health awareness by assisting in the understanding that health is more than just not being ill, and by teaching that certain behaviors and factors can contribute to or diminish health
- Teaches self-care activities to maximize achievement of goals that are realistic and attainable; serves as a role model

- Encourages health promotion by providing information and referrals.

Preventing Illness

The objectives of illness-prevention activities are to reduce the risk for illness, to promote good health habits, and to maintain optimal functioning. The motivation for illness prevention is to avoid or achieve early detection of illness or to maintain function within the constraints of an illness (Pender et al., 2002). Nurses prevent illness primarily by teaching and by personal example. Such activities include the following:

- Educational programs in areas such as prenatal care for pregnant women, smoking-cessation programs, and stress-reduction seminars
- Community programs and resources that encourage healthy lifestyles, such as aerobic exercise classes, "swimnastics," and physical fitness programs
- Literature, television, radio, or Internet information on diet, exercise, and the importance of good health habits
- Health assessments in institutions, clinics, and community settings that identify areas of strength and risks for illness

Restoring Health

Activities to restore health encompass those traditionally considered to be the nurse's responsibility. These focus on the individual with an illness and range from early detection of a disease to rehabilitation and teaching during recovery. Such activities include the following:

- Performing diagnostic measurements and assessments that detect an illness (eg, taking blood pressure, measuring blood sugars)
- Referring questions and abnormal findings to other healthcare providers as appropriate
- Providing direct care of the person who is ill by such measures as giving physical care, administering medications, and carrying out procedures and treatments

---

BOX 1-3 Healthy People 2010: Leading Health Indicators

- Physical Activity
- Overweight and Obesity
- Tobacco Use
- Substance Abuse
- Responsible Sexual Behavior
- Mental Health
- Injury and Violence
- Environmental Quality
- Immunization
- Access to Healthcare

U.S. Department of Health and Human Services. Office of Disease Prevention and Health Promotion. (2000). *Healthy people 2010.* Washington, DC: U.S. Department of Health and Human Services.

- Collaborating with other healthcare providers in providing care
- Planning, teaching, and carrying out rehabilitation for illnesses such as heart attacks, arthritis, and strokes
- Working in mental health and chemical-dependency programs

Facilitating Coping With Disability and Death

Although the major goals of healthcare are promoting, maintaining, and restoring health, these goals cannot always be met. Nurses also facilitate patient and family coping with altered function, life crisis, and death. Altered function decreases an individual's ability to carry out activities of daily living and expected roles. Nurses can facilitate an optimal level of function through maximizing the person's strengths and potentials, through teaching, and through referral to community support systems. Nurses provide care to both patients and families during end-of-life care, and they do so in hospitals, long-term-care facilities, and homes. Nurses are active in hospice programs, which assist patients and their families in preparing for death and in living as comfortably as possible until death occurs.

NURSING AS A PROFESSIONAL DISCIPLINE

As definitions of nursing have expanded to describe more clearly the roles and actions of nurses, increased attention has been given to nursing as a professional discipline. Nursing uses existing and new knowledge to solve problems creatively and meet human needs within ever-changing boundaries. Nursing is recognized increasingly as a **profession** based on the following criteria:
- Well-defined body of specific and unique knowledge
- Strong service orientation
- Recognized authority by a professional group
- Code of ethics
- Professional organization that sets standards
- Ongoing research
- Autonomy

Nursing involves specialized skills and application of knowledge based on an education that has both theoretical and clinical practice components. Nurses uphold standards set forth by professional organizations and follow an established code of ethics. Nursing focuses on human responses to actual or potential health problems and is increasingly focused on wellness, an area of caring that encompasses nursing's unique knowledge and abilities. Nursing is increasingly recognized as scholarly, with academic qualifications, research, and publications specific to nursing accepted and respected widely. In addition, nursing interventions are focused on evidence-based practice, which is practice based on research and not intuition.

Nursing has evolved through history from a technical service to a person-centered process that maximizes potential in all human dimensions. This has been an active process as nursing has developed, using lessons from the past to gain knowledge for practice in the present and in the future.

EDUCATIONAL PREPARATION FOR NURSING PRACTICE

Educational preparation for nursing practice involves several different types of programs. Students may choose to enter a practical nursing program and be licensed as a licensed practical nurse (LPN), or they may enter a diploma, an associate degree, or a baccalaureate program to be licensed as a registered nurse (RN). State laws in the United States recognize both the LPN and the RN as credentials to practice nursing. Increasingly, various levels of nursing education are providing programs for educational advancement. For example, the LPN can complete an associate degree and become an RN, and the RN prepared at the diploma or associate degree level can attain a bachelor of science in nursing (BSN) degree. There are also programs that provide RN to master's degrees as well as BSN and master's degree to PhD. Graduate programs in nursing provide masters and doctoral degrees.

Educational preparation for the nurse has become a major issue in nursing; the multiple methods of preparation are confusing to employers, consumers of healthcare services, and nurses themselves. Nursing organizations are working hard to answer questions such as "What is technical nursing?" and "What is professional nursing?" as well as "Should graduates of different programs take the same licensing examination and have the same title?" These questions are likely to be resolved during your nursing career. The following sections discuss education for LPNs and RNs, as well as graduate nursing education, continuing education for nurses, and in-service education.

Practical and Vocational Nursing Education

Practical (also labeled vocational) nursing programs were established to teach graduates to give bedside nursing care to patients. Schools for practical nursing programs are located in varied settings, such as high schools, technical or vocational schools, community colleges, and independent agencies. Most programs are 1-year programs divided into one-third classroom hours and two-thirds clinical laboratory hours. On completion of the program, graduates can take the National Council Licensure Examination (NCLEX-PN) for licensure as a licensed practical nurse (LPN). LPNs work under the direction of a physician or RN to give direct care to patients, focusing on meeting healthcare needs in hospitals, nursing homes, and home health agencies.

Registered Nursing Education

Three primary types of educational programs lead to licensure as an RN: (1) diploma, (2) associate degree, and (3) baccalaureate programs. Graduates of all three programs take the NCLEX-RN examination. Although it is a national examination, it is administered by, and the nurse is licensed in, each state. It is illegal to practice nursing unless one has a license verifying completion of an accredited (by state) program in nursing and has passed the licensing examination. Nurses gain legal rights to practice nursing in another state by applying to that state's board of nursing and receiving reciprocal **licensure.** Table 1-3 summarizes the types of education for RNs.

Diploma in Nursing

Many nurses practicing in the United States received their basic nursing education in a 3-year, hospital-based diploma school of nursing (Ellis & Hartley, 2003). The first schools of nursing established to educate nurses were diploma programs, and until the 1960s they were the major source of graduates. In recent years, the number of diploma programs has decreased greatly.

Graduates of diploma programs have a sound foundation of the biologic and social sciences, with a strong emphasis on clinical experience in direct patient care. Graduates work in acute, long-term, and ambulatory healthcare facilities (Ellis & Hartley, 2003).

Associate Degree in Nursing

Associate degree nursing (ADN) education is based on a research project that was carried out by Dr. Mildred Montag in the 1950s. At that time there was a shortage of nurses, and the project was created to meet the needs of society by preparing nurses in less time than was required in diploma programs. The emphasis of this type of program was education rather than service.

Currently, most associate degree programs are in community or junior colleges. These 2-year educational programs attract more men, more minorities, and more nontraditional students than do the other types of programs. Associate degree education prepares nurses to give care to patients in various settings, including hospitals, long-term care facilities, and home healthcare settings. Graduates of these programs are technically skilled and well prepared to carry out nursing roles and functions. Competencies of the ADN on entry into practice, as de-

TABLE 1-3 Summary of Types of Educational Programs for Registered Nurses (RNs)

	Diploma	Associate Degree	Baccalaureate
Location	Hospital	Community college	Senior college or university
Length	24–36 mo	2 academic or calendar years	4 academic years
Course work	Biologic science Physical science Nursing theory Nursing practice	Basic sciences Social sciences General education Nursing theory Nursing practice	Basic sciences General education Social sciences Nursing theory Nursing practice Nursing research Community health Management
Clinical component	Both hospital and community settings	Both hospital and community settings	A variety of settings in which healthcare and nursing care are provided
Further education opportunity	If affiliated with a college, may transfer some credit toward a BSN	Credits often apply toward a bachelor of science in nursing (BSN) degree	Base for advanced education at the master's and doctoral levels
Competencies on graduation	Plans and gives direct care to patients in structured settings Works with other members of the healthcare team to plan and provide care to ill patients	Plans and gives direct care to patients in structured settings Works with other members of the healthcare team to plan and provide care to ill patients	Plans and gives direct care to individual patients, groups, and communities Directs other members of the healthcare team in planning and providing care to ill and well patients in a variety of settings; assumes beginning leadership roles; provides comprehensive healthcare, including health promotion, illness prevention, and rehabilitative, educational, and health counseling

fined by the National League for Nursing (NLN), encompass the roles of provider of care, manager of care, and member of the discipline of nursing.

Baccalaureate in Nursing

The first baccalaureate nursing programs were established in the United States in the early 1900s. The number of programs and the number of enrolling students, however, did not increase markedly until the 1960s. Most graduates receive a bachelor of science in nursing (BSN).

Recommendations by national nursing organizations that the entry level for professional practice be at the baccalaureate level has resulted in increased numbers of these programs. Although BSN nurses practice in a wide variety of settings, the 4-year degree is required for many administrative, managerial, and community health positions.

In BSN programs, the major in nursing is built on a general education base, with concentration on nursing at the upper level. Students acquire knowledge of theory and practice related to nursing and other disciplines, provide nursing care to individuals and groups, work with members of the healthcare team, use research to improve practice, and have a foundation for graduate study. Nurses who graduate from a diploma or associate degree program and wish to complete requirements for a BSN may choose to enroll in an RN-to-BSN pro-

gram or may complete requirements through an external degree program.

Graduate Education in Nursing

The two levels of graduate education in nursing are the master's and doctoral degrees. A master's degree prepares advanced practice nurses to function in educational settings, in managerial roles, as clinical specialists, and in various advanced practice areas, such as nurse midwives and nurse practitioners (Table 1-4). Many master's graduates gain national certification in their specialty area, for example, as family nurse practitioners (FNPs). Nurses with doctoral degrees meet requirements for academic advancement and are prepared to carry out research necessary to advance nursing theory and practice.

Continuing Education

In its *Scope and Standards of Practice for Nursing: Professional Development* (2000), the ANA defines continuing education as those professional development experiences designed to enrich the nurse's contribution to health. Colleges, hospitals, voluntary agencies, and private groups offer formal continuing education through courses, seminars, and workshops. In some

TABLE 1-4 Expanded Educational and Career Roles of Nurses

Title	Description
Clinical nurse specialist (eg, enterostomal therapist, geriatrics, infection control, medical–surgical, maternal–child, oncology, quality assurance, nursing process)	A nurse with an advanced degree, education, or experience who is considered to be an expert in a specialized area of nursing; carries out direct patient care; consultation; teaching of patients, families, and staff; and research
Nurse practitioner	A nurse with an advanced degree, certified for a special area or age of patient care; works in a variety of healthcare settings or in independent practice to make health assessments and deliver primary care
Nurse anesthetist	A nurse who completes a course of study in an anesthesia school; carries out preoperative visits and assessments, administers and monitors anesthesia during surgery, and evaluates postoperative status of patients
Nurse midwife	A nurse who completes a program in midwifery; provides prenatal and postnatal care, and delivers babies for women with uncomplicated pregnancies
Nurse educator	A nurse, usually with an advanced degree, who teaches in educational or clinical settings; teaches theoretical knowledge and clinical skills; conducts research
Nurse administrator	A nurse who functions at various levels of management in healthcare settings; is responsible for the management and administration of resources and personnel involved in giving patient care
Nurse researcher	A nurse with an advanced degree who conducts research relevant to the definition and improvement of nursing practice and education
Nurse entrepreneur	A nurse, usually with an advanced degree, who may manage a clinic or health-related business, conduct research, provide education, or serve as an adviser or consultant to institutions, political agencies, or businesses

states, continuing education is required for an RN to maintain licensure.

In-Service Education

Many hospitals and healthcare agencies provide education and training for employees of their institution or organization, called in-service education. This is designed to increase the knowledge and skills of the nursing staff. Programs may involve learning, for example, a specific nursing skill or how to use new equipment.

PROFESSIONAL NURSING ORGANIZATIONS

One of the criteria of a profession is having a professional organization that sets standards for practice and education. Nursing's professional organizations are concerned with current issues in nursing and healthcare, and influence healthcare policy and legislation. The benefits of belonging to a professional nursing organization include networking with colleagues, having a voice in legislation affecting nursing, and keeping current with trends and issues in nursing.

International Nursing Organization

The International Council of Nurses (ICN), founded in 1899, was the first international organization of professional women. By sharing a commitment to maintaining high standards of nursing service and nursing education and by promoting ethics, the ICN provides a way for national nursing organizations to work together.

National Nursing Organizations

Professional nursing organizations in the United States include the American Nurses Association (ANA), the National League for Nursing (NLN), and the American Association of Colleges in Nursing (AACN). The National Student Nurses' Association (NSNA) prepares students to participate in professional nursing organizations.

ANA

The ANA is the professional organization for RNs in the United States. Founded in the late 1800s, its membership is comprised of the state nurses' associations to which individual nurses belong. The ANA establishes standards of practice, encourages research to advance nursing practice, and represents nursing for legislative actions.

NLN

The NLN is an organization open to all people interested in nursing, including nurses, nonnurses, and agencies. Established in 1952, its objective is to foster the development and improvement of all nursing services and nursing education.

The NLN conducts one of the largest professional testing services in the United States, including pre-entrance testing for potential students and achievement testing to measure student progress. It also serves as the primary source of research data about nursing education, conducting annual surveys of schools and new RNs. The organization also provides voluntary accreditation for educational programs in nursing.

AACN

The AACN is the national voice for baccalaureate and higher degree nursing education programs. The organization's goals focus on establishing quality educational standards; influencing the nursing profession to improve healthcare; and promoting public support of baccalaureate and graduate education, research, and nursing practice. National accreditation for collegiate nursing programs is provided (based on meeting standards) through AACN by the Commission on Collegiate Nursing Education (CCNE).

NSNA

The NSNA is the national organization for student nurses. Established in 1952 with the assistance of the ANA and NLN, its members are students enrolled in nursing education programs. Through voluntary participation, students practice self-governance, advocate for student and patient rights, and take collective, responsible action on social and political issues.

Specialty Practice and Special Interest Nursing Organizations

A wide variety of specialty practice and special interest nursing organizations are available to nurses. These organizations provide information on specific areas of nursing, often have publications in the specialty area, and may be involved in certification activities. Examples of these organizations are listed in Box 1-4.

BOX 1-4 Examples of US Specialty Practice and Special Interest Nursing Organizations

- American Academy of Nurse Practitioners
- American Assembly for Men in Nursing
- American Association for the History of Nursing
- American Association of Nurse Attorneys
- American Holistic Nurses' Association
- Association of Nurses in AIDS Care
- Dermatology Nurses Association
- Hospice Nurses Association
- Oncology Nurses Society
- Sigma Theta Tau International
- Transcultural Nursing Society

Note: Access to many nursing organizations is available through the World Wide Web at http://www.nsna.org/resources/weblinks/associate.html and http://www.nursingworld.org/affil/index.htm.

GUIDELINES FOR NURSING PRACTICE

As previously described, nursing continues to evolve and change to meet the needs of society. The ANA Congress for Nursing Practice (1973) stated that a profession must control its practice to guarantee the quality of its service to the public, and that "a profession that does not maintain the confidence of the public will soon cease to be a social force." Nursing controls and guarantees its practice through standards of practice, nurse practice acts and licensure, and the use of the nursing process. Each of these will guide your nursing education as a student and your nursing practice after graduation.

Standards of Nursing Practice

The ANA's 2003 *Nursing: Scope and Standards of Practice* define the activities of nurses that are specific and unique to nursing. **Standards** allow nurses to carry out professional roles, serving as protection for the nurse, the patient, and the institution where healthcare is given. Each nurse is accountable for his or her own quality of practice and is responsible for the use of these standards to ensure knowledgeable, safe, and comprehensive nursing care.

Remember Roberto Pecorini, the patient described in the Reflective Practice display. The nurse in the capacity of a nurse's aide realized the limitations of this role, and asked for assistance when delegated duties that were outside the scope of practice in this current role.

The 2003 ANA standards outlined in Box 1-5 apply to the practice of all RNs and lay the foundation for the practice of professional nursing in all settings.

Nurse Practice Acts and Licensure

Nurse practice acts are laws established in each state in the United States to regulate the practice of nursing. They are broadly worded and vary among states, but all of them have certain elements in common, such as the following:
- Protect the public by defining the legal scope of nursing practice, excluding untrained or unlicensed people from practicing nursing
- Create a state board of nursing or regulatory body having the authority to make and enforce rules and regulations concerning the nursing profession
- Define important terms and activities in nursing, including legal requirements and titles for RNs and LPNs
- Establish criteria for the education and licensure of nurses

The board of nursing for each state has the legal authority to allow graduates of approved schools of nursing to take the licensing examination. Those who successfully meet the requirements for licensure are then given a license to practice nursing in the state. The license, which must be renewed at specified intervals, is valid during the life of the holder and is registered in the state. The license and the right to practice

---

BOX 1-5 ANA Standards of Nursing Practice

Standards of Practice
- Assessment: The nurse collects comprehensive data pertinent to the patient's health or the situation.
- Diagnosis: The nurse analyzes the assessment data to determine the diagnoses or issues.
- Outcomes Identification: The nurse identifies expected outcomes for a plan individualized to the patient or the situation.
- Planning: The nurse develops a plan that prescribes strategies and alternatives to attain expected outcomes.
- Implementation: The nurse implements the identified plan, coordinates care delivery, employs strategies to promote health and a safe environment (the APRN* also provides consultation and uses prescriptive authority and treatment).
- Evaluation: The nurse evaluates progress towards attainment of outcomes.

Standards of Professional Performance
- Quality of Practice: The nurse systematically enhances the quality and effectiveness of nursing practice.
- Practice Evaluation: The nurse evaluates one's own practice in relation to professional practice standards and guidelines, relevant statues, rules, and regulations.
- Education: The nurse attains knowledge and competency that reflects current nursing practice.
- Collegiality: The nurse interacts with and contributes to the professional development of peers and colleagues.
- Collaboration: The nurse collaborates with patient, family, and others in the conduct of nursing practice.
- Ethics: The nurse integrates ethical provisions in all areas of practice.
- Research: The nurse integrates research findings into practice.
- Resource Utilization: The nurse considers factors related to safety, effectiveness, cost, and impact on practice in the planning and delivery of nursing services.
- Leadership: The nurse provides leadership in the profession and the professional practice setting.

*APRN=Advanced Practice Registered Nurse
American Nurses Association. (2003). *Nursing: Scope and Standards of Practice.* Washington, DC: Nursesbooks.org. Reproduced with permission of the American Nurses Association.

nursing can be denied, revoked, or suspended for professional misconduct (eg, incompetence, negligence, chemical impairment, or criminal actions).

As nursing roles continue to expand, and as issues in nursing are resolved, revised nurse practice acts will reflect those changes. Discussion is under way about the possibility of national licensure. All nurses must be knowledgeable about the specific nurse practice act under which they practice.

Nursing Process

The **nursing process** is one of the major guidelines for nursing practice. Nurses implement their roles through the nursing process, which integrates both the art and the science of nursing—that is, the nursing process is nursing made visible.

The nursing process is used by the nurse to identify the patient's healthcare needs and strengths, to establish and carry out a plan of care to meet those needs, and to evaluate the effectiveness of the plan to meet established outcomes. The nursing process allows nurses to use critical thinking when providing care that is individualized and holistic, and to define those areas of care that are within the domain of nursing. Critical thinking and the nursing process are fully described in Unit III.

CURRENT TRENDS IN NURSING

Nursing changes continually in response to the needs and resources of society as a whole. Nursing also changes in response to factors such as definitions of nursing, the aims of nursing, the educational preparation for nursing, and expanded practice roles. The trends discussed below are currently affecting nursing education and nursing practice. These trends and many others provide the background for nursing in the new century. As nurses continue to define their own practice, the special and distinctive role of nursing in caring for others will become increasingly recognized in society.

Nursing Shortage

Registered nurses are the largest group of healthcare providers in the United States, numbering nearly 2.7 million, with 2.2 million employed in nursing (U.S. Department of Health and Human Services, 2002). However, various forces may decrease that number. By 2010, an anticipated national shortage of nurses will put the nursing workforce in critical condition, with the Bureau of Labor Statistics projecting the need for new and replacement nurses by that time. This reduction in the workforce continues to occur at the same time as the population ages and develops chronic illnesses and disabilities that require skilled nursing care. The Nurse Reinvestment Act of 2002 contains many programs to improve the nursing shortage, increase career options for nurses, and improve governance of healthcare facilities in which nurses work (Washington Watch, 2003).

Evidence-Based Practice

Although nurses have conducted and published research since the 1950s, only recently has the importance of using scientific evidence to develop guidelines for nursing care been recognized. By identifying and analyzing the best available scientific evidence, nurses are steadily developing further guidelines for clinical practice that are useful nationally and internationally. Additional information about evidence-based practice provided in Chapter 5.

Community-Based Nursing

Healthcare is increasingly provided in community-based settings, such as clinics, outpatient settings, and homes (discussed in Unit II). The impetus for this change has largely been the implementation of a system of managed care to control and monitor healthcare services to minimize costs.

Decreased Length of Hospital Stay

Though patients who require in-hospital care are more acutely ill or injured than in the past, their length of stay in the hospital has decreased. This trend affects nursing in several ways. Nurses employed in hospital settings must have the knowledge and skills to provide often complex care to very ill patients. In the home, nurses may find themselves providing much the same type of care, as well as teaching patients and their families how to provide self-care.

> *Recall Michelle Fine, the young mother with a new baby who calls the nursery for help with breastfeeding. Making a referral for home care follow-up before Michelle's discharge from the hospital would have been appropriate to offer support, guidance, and additional teaching.*

Aging Population

The older adult population is expanding more rapidly than any other age group, with the greatest increase in those older than 75 years of age. This population trend means that patients in all healthcare settings increasingly are older and require teaching and nursing interventions designed to meet needs different from those of younger patients. Older healthcare consumers are also demanding more disease-prevention interventions, new building designs to meet their housing needs, and a focus on communities of care. Nursing will continually need to research health issues related to the oldest old, ethnically diverse populations, quality of life, and innovative systems of care.

Increase in Chronic Health Conditions

Chronic health conditions, such as heart disease, cancer, respiratory diseases, and acquired immunodeficiency syndrome (AIDS), are major health problems in our society. As the population ages, it has been projected that by the year 2030, nearly 150 million people will have a chronic health condition. Meet-

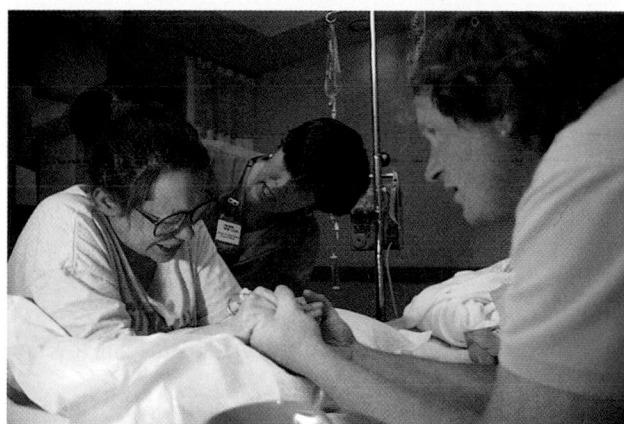
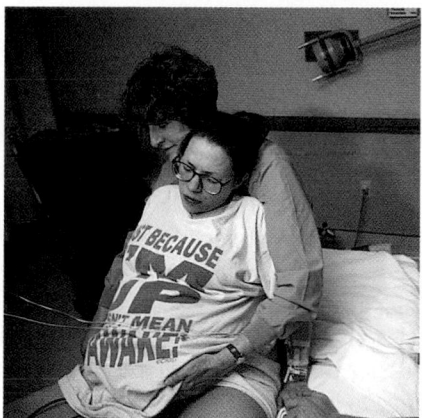

FIGURE 1-2 Growing numbers of women's health centers staffed with certified nurse practitioners and nurse midwives provide affordable health maintenance care.   (Photo by B. A. Rupert.)

ing the healthcare needs of so many people will be more difficult for society, particularly for those who live in poverty, are homeless, are mentally ill, or are of different cultures.

Independent Nursing Practice

Advanced practice nurses, such as nurse practitioners and nurse midwives, are increasingly establishing independent practices in which they diagnose and treat illnesses, promote health, provide well-women care, and deliver babies (Fig. 1-2). Depending on state certification requirements, they may practice in collaboration with a physician.

Culturally Competent Care

The importance of culturally competent care and the use of alternative or complementary therapies to treat illnesses are recognized as crucial to providing holistic, individualized care. Nurses must become more culturally diverse as our society becomes increasingly global.

■ Developing Critical Thinking Skills

1. Consider the roles and functions of professional nursing (see Table 1-2). Interview several nurses in different settings to see how much value they attach to these roles and how much time they are able to devote to them.
2. Describe how a nurse would meet the aims of nursing as described in this chapter (promoting health, preventing illness, restoring health, and facilitating coping) when caring for the following patients:
   • A single mother who has just delivered her first child and is scheduled to be discharged 12 hours after delivery
   • An 82-year-old woman who wants to begin an exercise program
   • A 32-year-old man dying of AIDS at home

As you consider these situations, try to identify factors that either promote or inhibit the fulfilling of these aims.

■ Practicing for NCLEX

1. Which term best describes the science of nursing?
   a. The skilled application of knowledge
   b. The knowledge base for care
   c. Hands-on care, such as giving a bath
   d. Respect for each individual patient
2. Which nurse in history is credited with establishing nursing education?
   a. Clara Barton
   b. Lillian Wald
   c. Lavinia Dock
   d. Florence Nightingale
3. What historic event in the 20th century led to an increased emphasis on nursing and broadened the role of nurses?
   a. Religious reform
   b. Crimean War
   c. World War II
   d. Vietnam War
4. Which of the following phrases describes one of the purposes of the ANA's Nursing Social Policy Statement?
   a. To describe the nurse as a dependent caregiver
   b. To provide standards for nursing educational programs
   c. To regulate nursing research
   d. To describe nursing's values and social responsibility
5. You are teaching a class of junior-high students about the effects of smoking. This educational program will meet which of the aims of nursing?
   a. Promoting health
   b. Preventing illness
   c. Restoring health
   d. Facilitating coping with disability or death
6. Which of the following nursing degrees prepares a nurse for advanced practice as a clinical specialist or nurse practitioner?
   a. LPN
   b. ADN

c. BSN

d. Master's degree

7. Which nursing organization was the first international organization of professional women?

a. ICN

b. ANA

c. NLN

d. NSNA

8. What is the purpose of the ANA's Standards of Clinical Nursing Practice?

a. To describe the ethical responsibility of nurses

b. To define the activities that are special and unique to nursing

c. To establish nursing as an independent and free-standing profession

d. To regulate the practice of nursing

9. What type of authority regulates the practice of nursing?

a. International standards and codes

b. Federal guidelines and regulations

c. State nurse practice acts

d. Institutional policies

10. Who are the largest group of healthcare providers in the United States?

a. Registered nurses

b. Physicians

c. Physical therapists

d. Social workers

■ Answers With Rationale

1. The correct response is *b*. The science of nursing is the knowledge base for care that is provided. In contrast, the skilled application of knowledge is the art of nursing.

2. The correct response is *d*. Florence Nightingale established nursing education.

3. The correct response is *c*. During World War II, large numbers of women worked outside the home. There was an increased emphasis on education and a knowledge explosion in medicine and technology, broadening the roles of nurses.

4. The correct response is *d*. The Nursing's Social Policy Statement describes the values and social responsibility of nursing.

5. The correct response is *b*. Educational programs, such as the risks of smoking, can reduce the risk of illness and promote good health habits.

6. The correct response is *d*. A master's degree prepares advanced practice nurses.

7. The correct response is *a*. The ICN, founded in 1899, was the first international organization of professional women.

8. The correct response is *b*. The ANA's Standards of Clinical Nursing Practice define the activities of nurses that are specific and unique to nursing.

9. The correct response is *c*. Nurse practice acts are established in each state to regulate the practice of nursing.

10. The correct response is *a*. Numbering nearly 2.7 million, registered nurses are the largest group of healthcare providers in the United States.

Bibliography

Alfaro, R. (2002). *Applying nursing process: Promoting collaborative care* (5th ed.). Philadelphia: Lippincott Williams & Wilkins.

American Nurses Association. (2003). *Nursing: Scope and standards of practice: Professional development.* Washington, DC: Author.

American Nurses Association, Committee on Education. (1965). *A position paper.* New York: ANA.

American Nurses Association. (1995). *Nursing's social policy statement.* Washington, DC: ANA.

Bulechek, G. M., & McCloskey, J. C. (2000). *Nursing interventions: Treatments for nursing diagnoses* (3rd ed.). Philadelphia: W. B. Saunders.

Carpenito, L. J. (2002). *Nursing diagnosis: Application to clinical practice* (9th ed.). Philadelphia: Lippincott Williams & Wilkins.

Chitty, K. (2001). *Professional nursing: Concepts & challenges* (3rd ed.). Philadelphia: W. B. Saunders.

Deloughery, G. (1998). *Issues and trends in nursing* (3rd ed.). St. Louis: C. V. Mosby.

Dolan, J. A., Fitzpatrick, M. L., & Herrmann, E. K. (1983). *Nursing in society: A historical perspective.* Philadelphia: W. B. Saunders.

Ellis, J., & Hartley, C. (2003). *Nursing in today's world: Challenges, issues, trends* (8th ed.). Philadelphia: Lippincott Williams & Wilkins.

International Council of Nurses. (2002). *The ICN definition of nursing.* Geneva: Imprimeries Populaires.

Kalish, P., & Kalish, B. (1995). *The advance of American nursing* (3rd ed.). Philadelphia: J. B. Lippincott.

Nightingale, F. (1992). *Notes on nursing: What it is and what it is not.* (Commemorative ed.). Philadelphia: J. B. Lippincott.

Pender, N. J., Murdaugh, C., & Parsons, M. A. (2002). *Health promotion in nursing practice* (4th ed.). Upper Saddle River, NJ: Prentice Hall.

U.S. Department of Health and Human Services. (2002). *Projected supply, demand, and shortages of registered nurses 2000–2020.* Available at http://bhpr.hrsa.gov/healthworkforce/rnproject/default.htm.

U.S. Department of Health and Human Services. Office of Disease Prevention and Health Promotion. (2000). *Healthy people 2010.* Washington, DC: U.S. Department of Health and Human Services.

Washington Watch. (2003). What can the nurse reinvestment act mean for you? *American Journal of Nursing, 102*(12), 14.

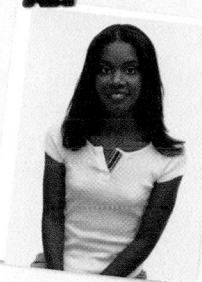

Rolanda Simpkins, a sexually active 16-year-old girl, comes to the clinic seeking information about contraception. She states, "My mother would 'kill me' if she knew I was asking about this."

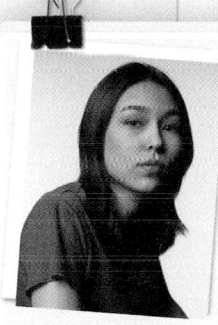

Carlotta Rios is a 17-year-old girl who was brought to the mental health–psychiatric unit because of attempted suicide. She does not speak English very well and lives with her sister because of the recent death of her mother. Further assessment reveals possible verbal abuse by her sister and a desire to "disappear" and not return to her sister's home.

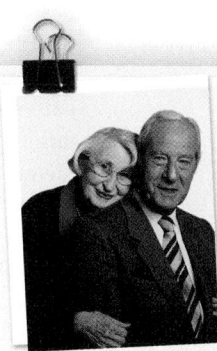

Samuel Kaplan is the 80-year-old husband of a 76-year-old woman diagnosed with Alzheimer's disease 1 year ago. Visibly tearful, he states, "I don't think that I can continue to care for my wife at home anymore. But how can I even consider putting her in a nursing home?"

Focusing on Blended Skills

The types of blended skills you'll need to respond to the case scenarios here include:

Cognitive Skills
- Knowledge of contraception and reproductive decision making; Alzheimer's disease, associated family burdens, and community resources; and adolescent suicide
- Ability to incorporate knowledge of Maslow's hierarchy of needs to determine patient priorities
- Knowledge of risk factors for the family and community
- Ability to incorporate knowledge of family-centered nursing care and associated rationales when providing care to an adolescent who has attempted suicide
- Ability to use critical-thinking skills to intervene appropriately to meet patients' needs at various developmental stages
- Ability to use knowledge about available community resources to assist patients in adapting to changes in health

Technical Skills
- Strong assessment skills related to sexual development and reproductive decision making, family caregiver needs, and adolescent suicide
- Ability to demonstrate competence in specific skills, such as teaching how to use contraceptive aids effectively
- Ability to adapt procedures and skills appropriately when dealing with different age groups

Interpersonal Skills
- Strong interpersonal skills to establish trusting relationships with an adolescent, an older adult, and an adolescent who has attempted suicide
- Special interpersonal competence to mobilize the suicidal adolescent to make effective, sound, safe decisions
- Ability to communicate to the patient a greater concern about the patient's status, for example, an older adult facing the possibility of no longer being able to care for his wife or a patient with threats to self-esteem who has attempted suicide
- Ability to demonstrate respect for the patient's human dignity and autonomy throughout the patient's care

Ethical and Legal Skills
- Demonstration of a strong sense of accountability for the health and well-being of individuals of differing age groups, with a commitment to getting patients the help needed—within the scope of nursing responsibilities and available resources
- Skill in working collaboratively with colleagues and others in the community to advocate for the health needs of specific populations, such as adolescents or older adults with health-care needs
- Incorporation of the ethical and legal principles that guide decision making related to adolescent contraception, adolescent suicide, and provision of safe care in the home
- Ability to practice nursing in an ethically and legally defensible manner, consistent with nursing code of ethics and within the scope of legal practice

Learning Outcomes

After completing the chapter, the learner should be able to accomplish the following:

1. Describe each level of Maslow's hierarchy of basic human needs.
2. Discuss nursing care necessary to meet needs for each level of Maslow's hierarchy.
3. Discuss family concepts, including family roles, structures, functions, developmental stages, tasks, and health risk factors.
4. Identify aspects of the community that affect individual and family health.
5. Describe nursing interventions to promote and maintain health of the individual as a member of a family and as a member of a community.

Key Terms

basic human needs
blended family
community
extended family
family
hierarchy of basic human needs
love and belonging needs
nuclear family
physiologic needs
safety and security needs
self-actualization needs
self-esteem needs

Humans are complex organisms, influenced by and responsive to both the internal and external environments. Our behaviors, our feelings about ourselves and others, our values, and the priorities we set for ourselves all relate to our physiologic and psychosocial needs. These needs are common to all people, and meeting these needs is essential to the health and survival of all people; hence, they are labeled **basic human needs.** Basic human needs can be met or unmet in a variety of ways. A person can meet some needs independently, but most needs require relationships and interactions with others for partial or complete fulfillment. Satisfying one's needs often depends on the social and physical environment, especially one's family and community.

Holistic nursing care, which is based on considering all the patient's dimensions that affect how basic human needs are met in health and in illness, allows the nurse to provide individualized and health-oriented care. This chapter discusses how basic human needs, the family, and the community environment affect the health of the individual. (For an example, see the accompanying Reflective Practice box.) Chapter 3 introduces the cultural dimension, and Chapter 4 discusses concepts of health and illness, models of health and illness, factors affecting health and illness, and nursing care to promote health and prevent illness.

THE INDIVIDUAL'S BASIC HUMAN NEEDS

In nursing, we consider both the physical and psychosocial needs of each individual patient. Abraham Maslow (1968) developed a **hierarchy of basic human needs** (Fig. 2-1) that can be used to consider which needs of a person are the most important at any given time. Certain needs are more basic or essential than others and must be at least minimally met before other needs can be considered.

Maslow's hierarchy is useful for understanding the relationships of basic human needs and for establishing priorities of care. The hierarchy is based on the theory that something is a basic need if it has the following characteristics:

- Its absence results in illness.
- Its presence helps prevent illness or signals health.
- Meeting it restores health.
- It is preferred over other satisfactions when unmet.
- One feels something is missing when the need is unmet.
- One feels satisfaction when the need is met.

Maslow arranged the hierarchy to show that certain needs are more basic than others. Although all people have all the needs all the time, people generally strive to meet certain of the needs (at least to a minimal level) before attending to other needs. The five levels of needs, with physiologic being the most basic, are as follows:

Level 1: Physiologic needs
Level 2: Safety and security needs
Level 3: Love and belonging needs
Level 4: Self-esteem needs
Level 5: Self-actualization needs

Nursing care is often directed toward meeting unmet or threatened needs. Maslow's hierarchy provides a framework for nursing assessment and for understanding the needs of patients at all levels, so that interventions to meet priority needs become a part of the plan of care. Many of the nursing interventions that you learn as you progress through your education are aimed at meeting patients' basic human needs. The following sections describe each level of need in more detail.

Physiologic Needs

Physiologic needs—oxygen, water, food, temperature, elimination, sexuality, physical activity, and rest—must be met at least minimally to maintain life. These needs are the most basic in the hierarchy of needs, are the most essential to life and therefore have the highest priority. Most healthy children and adults meet their physiologic needs through self-care, but physiologic needs are often a major part of the nursing care plan for young, old, disabled, and ill people who require assistance in meeting them.

Oxygen is the most essential of all needs because all body cells require oxygen for survival. Oxygenation of body cells is carried out primarily by the respiratory and cardiovascular systems, and any alteration in their structure or function can result in an increased need for oxygen. This need may be acute (such as when cardiopulmonary resuscitation is needed) or chronic (requiring special positioning, treatments, and teaching). Nurses evaluate patients' oxygen needs by assessing skin color, vital signs, anxiety levels, responses to activity, and mental responsiveness.

A balance between the intake and elimination of fluids is essential to life. Healthy people drink fluids to satisfy thirst, and maintain fluid balance through various physiologic processes. Either dehydration or edema (the collection of fluid in body tissues) evidences changes in the water balance of the body. Dehydration occurs from conditions such as severe diarrhea or vomiting, whereas causes of edema include diseases of the cardiovascular or renal system and trauma. Measuring intake and output, testing the resiliency of the skin, checking the condition of the skin and mucous membranes, and weighing the patient assesses water balance.

Food is a physiologic need, with balance maintained through digestive and metabolic processes. The need for food is manifested through hunger. Insufficient nutrient intake results in nutrient and electrolyte imbalances and weight loss. A component of the digestive processes that is also a physiologic need is elimination. Waste products are eliminated from the body through the skin, lungs, kidneys, and intestines. Nutritional status is assessed with a variety of indicators, including weight, muscle mass, strength, and laboratory values.

The human body functions best within a narrow range of temperatures, usually considered as plus or minus 98.6°F (37°C). Homeostatic mechanisms and adaptive responses, such as shivering, maintain this temperature. Nurses assess body temperature as a vital sign (discussed in Chap. 24).

Sexuality is an integral component of each individual and may be affected by physical and emotional illnesses. Sexual

Reflective Practice
Challenge to Ethical and Legal Skills

Junior year was full of excitement and new experiences. I was both nervous and excited about our mental health clinical rotation. Although the staff was very helpful and cooperative in providing as great an experience as they could, I found this clinical rotation to be difficult. I was going to be speaking with patients who had mental-health problems and developing nurse–patient relationships that were different from the ones that I had been exposed to in the past. To tell the truth, I was fearful. I was afraid I would say the wrong thing, causing the person to react, possibly injuring himself or others.

One patient really made an impression on me—Carlotta Rios, a 17-year-old girl who was brought to the unit because of attempted suicide. She did not speak English very well and lived with her sister because her mother had recently passed away. The nurses asked me to speak with her because I spoke Spanish.

When talking with her, I found out that Carlotta did not like living with her sister because the sister verbally abused her, always putting her down and constantly reminding Carlotta that the only reason she was here was because of her sister. Carlotta reported that her sister constantly told her about all of the sacrifices that she was making just so that Carlotta could be with her. According to Carlotta, her sister said that Carlotta did not appreciate everything that her sister was doing. The sister constantly reminded Carlotta of everything she bought for her, making sure to keep a record so that Carlotta would pay her back. Carlotta said that she was not happy and figured that the only way she would stop feeling bad and that her sister would be happy again would be if Carlotta disappeared. Carlotta no longer wanted to exist.

Talking with Carlotta further, I found out that she did not want to return home, which currently was her sister's home. Unfortunately, this was a problem because legally she was not considered an adult. Therefore, Carlotta's sister would have to be contacted. Yet, it seemed that Carlotta's current family and living situation was not the safest. At the same time, it also seemed to be the cause of Carlotta's desperate attempt to take her life. If she chose not to return to her sister's house, Carlotta would be taken to court in handcuffs and placed in a foster home. Although this placement would only be until she turned 18 years old, which was at the end of the month, it also meant that once she was 18 years old, she would be on her own. It was apparent that she was not ready for such a drastic change.

Thinking Outside the Box: Possible Courses of Action

- Call her sister and have her pick her up, because legally she was responsible for the patient.
- Gain the trust of the patient by speaking to her as an adult and informing her of all the options, ultimately assisting her with carrying them out.
- Call someone with whom she felt comfortable to provide support and also to hear the options available; in this way, the patient would have the opinion of someone she knew and trusted before she made a decision on which course of action to take.

Evaluating a Good Outcome: How Do I Define Success?

- Patient's safety is ensured.
- Patient benefits from the course of action decided upon.
- The patient's human dignity is respected.
- No violations of the American Nurses Association's Code of Ethics occur.
- Patient makes the most appropriate decision, resulting in the best outcome for her.
- The ethical and legal obligations for myself and those of the hospital are met.

Personal Learning: Here's to the Future!

I figured the best way to approach this situation was to develop a trusting relationship. So, after getting Carlotta up, we went to a brighter, better-lit room, where we had breakfast. I started by asking simple questions, eventually progressing to those that pertained to why she was in the hospital. Throughout our talks, I reinforced that her sister was considered the person legally responsible for Carlotta, explaining that if Carlotta decided not to call home, she would be taken in handcuffs to court, where she then would be placed in a foster home. I told her that this would only be until she turned 18 years' old; upon turning 18, she then

would be on her own. After listening to all of her options, she decided that she would call her sister to let her know where she was. She also told her sister that she would be staying with a best friend until she had figured things out. For Carlotta, this was the best decision to make because she felt safest. As a result of informing her sister, Carlotta would not have to go to court. Subsequently, any upset or disruption for her sister would be minimized, further adding to Carlotta's feelings of being safe. The priority for Carlotta was a safe environment. We were able to establish a trusting relationship and work together towards this end.

Reflection

How do you think you would respond in a similar situation? Why? What does this tell you about yourself and about the adequacy of your skills for professional practice? Can you think of other ways to respond? How might the death of Carlotta's mother have impacted her "desire to disappear"? What family risk factors were evident here? Were they addressed in this scenario? If so, how; if not, then how could they be? What community resources might have been helpful for Carlotta? How were the nursing student's actions legal? Ethical? Please explain. What other skills (cognitive, interpersonal, technical, ethical/legal) would you need to respond well in this situation? Do you agree with the criteria to evaluate a successful outcome? Were the stated criteria met? Why or why not?

Stephanie Cuellar, Georgetown University

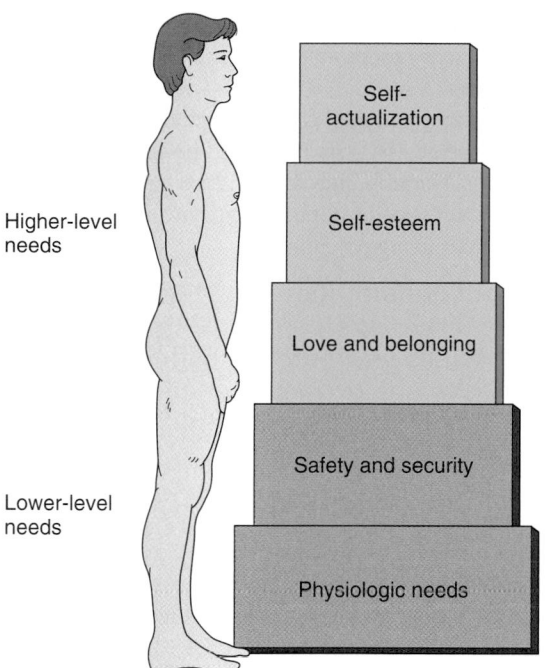

FIGURE 2-1 Maslow's hierarchy of basic human needs.

practices are dependent on a variety of factors, such as a person's age, sociocultural background, self-esteem, and level of health. There is increasing awareness in healthcare that the consideration of sexuality is a vital part of holistic care.

Recall Rolanda Simpkins, the 16-year-old girl described at the beginning of the chapter requesting information about contraception. The nurse would use knowledge about Rolanda's sexuality and sexual practices in helping to determine to the most appropriate method of contraception for her.

Physical activity and rest are also basic physiologic needs. Physical activity can be accomplished with intact and functioning neuromuscular and skeletal systems. Rest and sleep allow time for the body to rejuvenate and be free of stress. Individual requirements for rest and sleep vary widely, but the effects of deprivation have been well documented as significant. Factors that influence sleep are age, environment, exercise, stress, and drug use.

Think back to Samuel Kaplan, the older adult man caring for his wife with Alzheimer's disease at home. The nurse would assess the effect of providing this care on his activity, rest, and sleep patterns, thereby developing an appropriate plan of care for Mr. Kaplan to ensure that his needs are met.

Safety and Security Needs

Safety and security needs come next in priority and involve both physical and emotional components. Physical safety and security means being protected from potential or actual harm.

Nurses carry out a wide variety of activities to meet patients' physical safety needs, such as the following:

- Using proper handwashing and sterile techniques to prevent infection
- Using electrical equipment properly
- Administering medications knowledgeably
- Using skill when moving and ambulating patients
- Teaching parents about household chemicals that are dangerous to children

Emotional safety and security involves trusting others and being free of fear, anxiety, and apprehension. Patients entering the healthcare system often fear the unknown and may have significant emotional security needs. Nurses can help meet such needs by encouraging spiritual practices that are a source of strength and support, by allowing as much independent decision making and control as possible, and by carefully explaining new and unfamiliar procedures and treatments.

Remember Carlotta Rios, the adolescent described in the Reflective Practice display? The nurse fosters the development of a trusting relationship to promote emotional safety and security. Doing so would assist Carlotta in her decision-making process about going home.

Love and Belonging Needs

All humans have a basic need for love and belonging. After physiologic and safety and security needs, this is the next priority and is often called a higher-level need. **Love and belonging needs** include the understanding and acceptance of others in both giving and receiving love, and the feeling of belonging to families, peers, friends, a neighborhood, and a community.

People who believe that their love and belonging needs are unmet often feel lonely and isolated. They may withdraw physically and emotionally, or they may become overly demanding and critical. Often, these behaviors are a signal (or cue) that the person has unmet love and belonging needs. Nurses should always consider love and belonging needs when developing a plan of care. Some nursing interventions to help meet this need are as follows:

- Including family and friends in the care of the patient
- Establishing a nurse–patient relationship based on mutual understanding and trust (by demonstrating caring, encouraging communication, and respecting privacy) (Fig. 2-2)
- Referring patients to specific support groups (such as a cancer support group or Alcoholics Anonymous)

Think back to Samuel Kaplan, the 80-year-old man caring for his wife with Alzheimer's disease. The nurse could refer Mr. Kaplan to a support group for caregivers of patients with Alzheimer's disease to help in meeting Mr. Kaplan's needs for love and belonging.

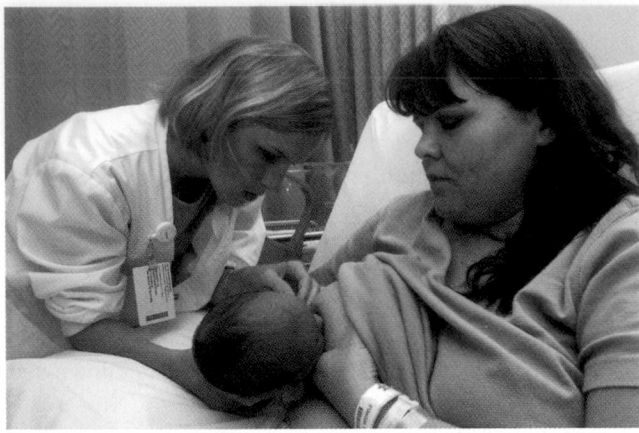

FIGURE 2-2 By teaching the mother to care for her infant, the nurse is helping to fulfill the need for love and belonging of both mother and child.   (Photo by Joe Mitchell.)

Self-Esteem Needs

The next highest priority on the hierarchy is **self-esteem needs,** which include the need for a person to feel good about himself or herself, to feel pride and a sense of accomplishment, and to believe that others also respect and appreciate those accomplishments. Positive self-esteem facilitates the individual's confidence and independence.

Many factors affect self-esteem. When a person's role changes (eg, through a job change or through the death of a spouse), self-esteem can be seriously altered because the person's responsibilities and relationships have also changed. Other changes that may affect self-esteem include a change in body image, such as the loss of a breast, an injury, or a growth spurt during puberty. Nurses must remember that the person's perception of the change—rather than the actual change itself—is what affects that individual's self-esteem.

Nurses can help meet patients' self-esteem needs by respecting their values and beliefs, encouraging patients to set attainable goals, and facilitating support from family or significant others. These actions promote a sense of worth and self-acceptance.

Self-Actualization Needs

The highest level on the hierarchy of needs is **self-actualization needs,** which include the need for individuals to reach their full potential through development of their unique capabilities. In general, each lower level of need must be met to some degree before this need can be satisfied. The process of self-actualization is one that continues throughout life. Maslow lists the following qualities that indicate achievement of one's potential:
- Acceptance of self and others as they are
- Focus of interest on problems outside oneself
- Ability to be objective
- Feelings of happiness and affection for others
- Respect for all people

- Ability to discriminate between good and evil
- Creativity as a guideline for solving problems and pursuing interests

To help meet patients' self-actualization needs, the nurse focuses on the person's strengths and possibilities rather than on problems. Nursing interventions are aimed at providing a sense of direction and hope and providing teaching that is aimed at maximizing potentials.

Recall Carlotta Rios, the 17-year-old who had attempted suicide. By focusing on her strengths as well as providing her with a sense of direction through decision making, the nurse helps to meet Carlotta's self-actualization needs.

Applying Maslow's Theory

Nurses can apply Maslow's hierarchy of basic needs in the assessment, planning, implementation, and evaluation of patient care. The hierarchy can be used with patients at any age, in all settings where care is provided, and in both health and illness. It helps the nurse identify unmet needs as they become healthcare needs. The hierarchy of basic needs allows the nurse to locate the patient on the health–illness continuum and to incorporate health models into meeting needs (these concepts are discussed in Chap. 4).

As the nurse identifies and carries out interventions to help meet patients' needs, it is important to remember that this is only a framework or guideline and that, in actuality, each individual sets priorities for meeting needs on levels most important to that person. Additionally, basic human needs are interrelated and may require nursing actions at more than one level at a given time. For example, in caring for a person coming into the emergency department with a heart attack, the nurse's immediate concern is the patient's physiologic needs (ie, oxygen and pain relief). At the same time, however, safety needs (eg, following proper precautions with oxygen use and ensuring the person does not fall off the examining table) and love and belonging needs (eg, letting a family member stay with the person, if possible) are still major considerations. You will learn about how nurses meet basic human needs throughout the rest of this book.

THE FAMILY

Almost every person is a member of a number of groups, such as groups of friends, colleagues at work, or members of a church or school class. Each of these groups involves a specific part of the person's life and is important to the person. Only one group, however, is concerned with all parts of a person's life and with meeting his or her basic human needs to promote health. That group is the family.

A **family** can be defined simply as any group of people who live together. Families exist in all sizes and configurations and are essential to the health and survival of the individual family members, as well as to society as a whole. The family is a buffer between the needs of the individual member and the demands and expectations of society. The role of the family is to help meet the basic human needs of its members while also meeting the needs of society (Friedman, Bowden, & Jones, 2003).

Duvall (1977) defined a family as two or more people who are related through blood, marriage, adoption, or birth. Friedman (1992) expanded that definition by including two or more people who are emotionally involved with each other and live together. The latter definition includes more of the different types of current family structures in which members may be unrelated either biologically or legally.

Family Structures

There is no single, commonly accepted form of family structure. Nurses must remember that there are no absolute "rights" or "wrongs" about what makes a family, and one person's values must not be imposed on another person. Your respect for of all kinds of family members and relationships is essential to holistic, individualized patient care. The following sections briefly introduce many different types of family structures.

Nuclear Family

The **nuclear family,** also called the traditional family, is composed of two parents and their children. The parents might be heterosexual or homosexual, are often married or in a committed relationship, and all members of the family live in the same house until the children leave home as young adults. The traditional family may be composed of biologic parents and children, adoptive parents and children, surrogate parents and children, and stepparents and children.

In the classic nuclear family, the father was the family member who went to work, providing economic security, whereas the mother stayed at home, providing physical and emotional safety and security. This family group usually lived in close geographic proximity to relatives, such as aunts, uncles, and grandparents, who are a part of the **extended family.** Although many people still consider the nuclear family the ideal, it is no longer the dominant structure in our society.

The contemporary nuclear family still has the same basic form, but the roles of the members have changed considerably. The two major causes of this change are increased education and career opportunities for women and changes in our economy resulting in a need for additional income to maintain a desired standard of living. As a result, two-career families, in which both parents work outside the home, have become the norm instead of the exception. When both parents work, there is usually a blending of tasks, with both parents taking a more active role in housework and childcare as well as economic support.

Couples without children and couples with grown children who no longer live at home are considered traditional families as well. The **blended family** is also a traditional family, formed when parents bring unrelated children from previous relationships together to form a new family.

With changes in family structure have come other influences on the basic human needs of family members. Consid-erations for the family, and for nursing care, include support systems (in our mobile society, family members may live hundreds or thousands of miles away), availability of childcare, time for leisure and recreation, and changing role models.

Single-Parent Family

Single parents may be separated, divorced, widowed, or never married. Increasing numbers of never-married men and women are choosing to become parents. It is estimated that more than one fourth of all children in North America live in single-parent families. Most single-parent families are African American and headed by women. Single parents have special problems and needs, including financial concerns and role shifts (ie, having the roles of both parents, often looking to re-marriage or new relationships). These problems are important considerations when planning and implementing nursing care.

Other Family Structures

In addition to traditional and single parent families, cohabiting adults and single adults are other family structures. Cohabiting families are individuals who choose to live together for a variety of reasons—relationships, financial need, or changing values. Cohabiting families include unmarried adults (of any age, including retired people who choose not to marry because it would impose financial hardship) living together, and communal or group marriages. Other family structures include binuclear (where divorced parents assume joint custody of children) and dyadic nuclear (in which the couple chooses not to have children).

Single adults may not be living with others, but they are part of a family of origin, usually have a social network with significant others, or may even regard a pet as family. Most single adults living alone are either young adults who achieve independence and enter the workforce or older adults who never married or are left alone after the death of a spouse.

Family Functions

Families have functions that are important in how individual family members meet their basic human needs and maintain their health. The family provides the individual with the necessary environment for development and social interactions. Families also are important to society as a whole because they provide new and socialized members for society. Five major functions of the family are as follows:

1. Physical
2. Economic
3. Reproductive
4. Affective and coping
5. Socialization

Physically, the family provides a safe, comfortable environment necessary for growth, development, and rest or recuperation. Economically, the family provides financial aid to family members and also helps meet monetary needs of society. The reproductive function of the family is raising children. The affective and coping function of the family involves providing emotional comfort to family members. It also helps members to establish an identity and to maintain that identity in times of stress. Finally, through socialization, the family teaches; transmits beliefs, values, attitudes, and coping mechanisms; provides feedback; and guides problem-solving society (Friedman et al., 2003).

Developmental Tasks of Families

Duvall (1977) identified critical family developmental tasks and stages in the family life cycle. Duvall's theory, based on Erikson's theory of psychosocial development (described in Chap. 18), states that all families have certain basic tasks for survival and continuity and specific tasks related to the sequential stages of development throughout the life of the family.

These stages and related developmental tasks are outlined in Table 2-1. If the family does meet certain developmental tasks, societal disapproval may be lead to intervention by children's services, social services, police departments, welfare agencies, or health departments (Edelman & Mandle, 2002). The successful mastery of each developmental stage is important to the family's adaptation and growth through successive stages.

The Family in Health and Illness

Individuals learn healthcare activities, health beliefs, and health values in the family. In health and illness, as well as in other areas of life, the individual reflects behaviors learned from the family. When patients enter the healthcare system, they bring their own personal behaviors and needs, but they also bring (in a sense) their family too.

Friedman and associates (2003) identified the importance of family-centered nursing care, based on four rationales. First, the family is composed of interdependent members who affect one another. If some form of illness occurs in one member, all other members become a part of the illness. Second, a strong relationship exists between the family and the health status of its members; therefore, the role of the family is essential in every level of nursing care. The third rationale is that the level of health of the family and, in turn, each member, can be significantly improved through health promotion activities. Finally, illness of one family member may suggest the possibility of the same problem in other members; through assessment and intervention, the nurse can assist in improving the health status of all family members.

Remember Carlotta Rios, the 17-year-old described in the Reflective Practice display? The nurse would incorporate knowledge of these rationales when providing care to Carlotta, such as when helping her determine viable options and when assisting her with decision making.

Illness may precipitate a health crisis in a family. Brief changes in family tasks may occur if an illness is relatively minor, such as a viral infection in a child. If an injury or illness to a family member is serious, roles and responsibilities, as well as functions, of individual family members change. This is especially true if the illness is chronic and long-term, or results in disability. Some families find it difficult to adapt to the stress of changes in financial, social, and caregiving resources, whereas other families experience renewed family closeness and stability. Regardless of how the family adapts, members of the family must constantly adjust roles and responsibilities to manage the needs of the ill family member and the family.

Remember Samuel Kaplan, the 80-year-old man caring for his wife with Alzheimer's disease? Now the primary caregiver, Mr. Kaplan's role has changed. Adapting to this role change in conjunction with adjusting to the long-term nature of his wife's illness can seriously impact the family's ability to function. The nurse would incorporate knowledge of this when developing the most appropriate plan for Mr. Kaplan and his wife.

Nursing interventions for the family in a health crisis include provision of information via teaching that is honest, open, and respectful; use of therapeutic communication skills; knowledge of family dynamics; and referral to community healthcare and financial resources to support realistic hope. In addition, it is important to involve family members in the plan of care and the implementation of care.

Family Risk Factors

Family patterns of behavior, the environment in which the family lives, and genetic factors can all place family members at risk for health problems. It is important for nurses to assess these factors before developing nursing care plans. Typical questions that should be part of a family assessment include the following:

- What is the family structure?
- What is the family's socioeconomic status?
- What are the ethnic backgrounds and religious affiliations of family members?
- Who cares for children if both parents work?
- What health practices are common (eg, types of foods eaten, meal times, immunizations, bedtime, exercise)?
- What habits are common (eg, do any family members smoke, drink to excess, or use drugs)?
- How does the family cope with stress?
- Do close friends or family members live nearby, and can they help if necessary?

These questions would be extremely important to ask when assessing Carlotta Rios, the adolescent described in the Reflective Practice display, and Samuel Kaplan, the older adult caring for his ill wife at home. Each patient's answers to these questions would provide the nurse with valuable information about determining the best way to meet each patient's needs. For Carlotta, this would include information about viable options for her living

TABLE 2-1 Family Stages, Tasks, Health Risk Factors, and Nursing Interventions to Promote Health

Family Stage*	Tasks	Risk Factors	Nursing Interventions/Referrals
Couple and family with children	Establish a mutually satisfying marriage Plan to have or not to have children Have and adjust to infant Support needs of all family members Adjust to cost of family life Adapt to needs and activity of children Cope with loss of energy and privacy Encourage and support growth and development, educational achievements	Inadequate knowledge of contraception and family Inadequate knowledge of sexual and marital roles Lack of knowledge about child safety and health Child abuse and neglect First pregnancy before age 16 Inadequate nutrition; obesity Drug and alcohol abuse Sexually transmitted diseases Rubella	Family planning clinics Prenatal classes Well-child clinics Immunization information Vision and hearing screenings Dental health information Parent support groups Communicable disease control Safety in the home, daycare, school, neighborhood, and community
Family with adolescents and young adults	Maintain open communications Support moral and ethical family values Balance teenagers' freedom with responsibility Maintain supportive home base Strengthen marital relationships	Family of origin Low socioeconomic status Family value of aggressiveness Dependence on welfare Inadequate problem-solving abilities Conflict between family members Physical or sexual abuse Use of drugs or alcohol Sexually transmitted diseases	Alcohol and drug information Accident prevention programs Sex education Nutrition support groups Mental health programs Screening for chronic illness
Family with middle-aged adults	Maintain ties with younger and older generations Prepare for retirement	Diet high in fat, sugar, salt Obesity Use of drugs or alcohol Physical inactivity Depression Exposure to environmental or work-related health risks, such as sunlight, asbestos, radiation, coal dust, air or water pollution	Blood pressure screenings Screening for chronic illness Nutrition information Support groups (eg, for loss, grief, smoking cessation, alcohol or drug abuse)
Family with older adults	Adjust to retirement Adjust to loss of spouse May move from family home	Increasing age with loss of physical function Chronic illness Poor nutrition Lack of exercise Depression Death of spouse Limited income Past lifestyle	Screening for chronic illness Nutrition information Exercise information Home safety information Retirement information Pharmacology information

Data from Duvall, E. (1977). *Marriage and family development* (5th ed.). Philadelphia: J. B. Lippincott; Aldous, J. (1975). *The developmental approach to family analysis*. Minneapolis: University of Minnesota Press.
* Family includes all forms: nuclear, extended, single-parent, etc.

arrangements that provide physical and emotional safety. For Mr. Kaplan, answers would provide information about available sources of help so that he can continue to care for his wife at home, or if necessary, ease the transition and adjustment to moving his wife to a long-term care facility.

When conducting a health assessment for a family, the nurse should consider the risk factors for altered health described in Box 2-1.

Nursing Interventions to Promote Health

The role of the nurse in reducing risk factors involves activities that promote health for all family members at any level

---

BOX 2-1 Risk Factors for Altered Family Health

Lifestyle Risk Factors
- Lack of knowledge about sexual and marital roles, leading to teenage marriage and pregnancy; divorce; sexually transmitted diseases; child, spouse, or elder abuse; and lack of prenatal or child care
- Alterations in nutrition—either more or less than body requirements at any age
- Chemical dependency, including the use of alcohol, drugs, and nicotine
- Inadequate dental care and hygiene
- Unsafe or unstimulating home environment

Psychosocial Risk Factors
- Inadequate childcare resources, when both parents work, for preschool and school-aged children
- Inadequate income to provide safe housing, food, clothing, and healthcare
- Conflict between family members

Environmental Risk Factors
- Lack of knowledge or finances to provide safe and clean living conditions
- Work or social pressures that cause stress
- Air, water, or food pollution

Developmental Risk Factors
- Families who have new babies, especially if support systems are unavailable
- Older people, especially those living alone or on a fixed income
- Unmarried adolescent mothers who lack personal, economic, and educational resources

Biologic Risks
- Birth defects
- Mental retardation
- Genetic predisposition to certain diseases, including cardiovascular diseases and cancer

---

of development. Each person has his or her own definition of health, based on family beliefs and values about health and illness. Through interventions that emphasize health, the nurse assists both the individual and the family to meet their basic human needs. See Examples of NANDA Nursing Diagnoses: Family and Community for examples of diagnoses that might be appropriate when planning care for the patient as a member of the family or community. Examples of nursing interventions to promote health in the family are shown in Table 2-1. Nurses may carry out such activities themselves or may refer the individual or family to other healthcare providers for additional education.

The family is the primary educational and support structure for the individual. The family, as a social unit, provides the environment and relationships necessary for members to meet their basic human needs. Health beliefs and practices are learned within the family context and are influenced by the family's developmental level. Health promotion activities and nursing actions can reduce the risk for illness and facilitate healthy behaviors at any age within the family life cycle.

Consider Rolanda Simpkins, the adolescent seeking contraceptive information. The nurse would need to evaluate further Rolanda's statement that her mother would "kill her," questioning Rolanda further to determine the family's health beliefs and practices. For example, is it that Rolanda is 16 and sexually active that would upset her mother, is it that contraception violates the family's beliefs, or is it something else?

THE COMMUNITY

A person, as an individual and as a member of a family, is also a member of a community. The community environment also affects the ability of the individual to meet basic human needs. This section discusses the relationship of the community to basic human needs, including influences on health and illness.

A **community** can be defined in a variety of ways, but the most basic definition is that a community is a specific population or group of people living in the same geographic area under similar regulations and having common values, interests, and needs. A community may be a small neighborhood in a major urban city or a large rural area encompassing a small town. Communities are formed by the characteristics of people, area, social interaction, and common familial, cultural, or ethnic heritage and ties. Within a community, people interact and share resources. See the accompanying Research in Nursing box.

Many community factors affect the health of residents. A healthy community provides elements that enable people to maintain a high quality of life and productivity. For example, as defined in *Healthy People in Healthy Communities* (2001), a healthy community:

Examples of NANDA Nursing Diagnoses

Family and Community

Nursing Diagnoses	Related Factors
Family	
Risk for Caregiver Role Strain	Long-term home care of spouse with Alzheimer's disease
Impaired Parenting	History of child abuse by primary caretaker
Dysfunctional Family Processes: Alcoholism	Maternal refusal to accept need for help for persistent and excessive alcohol intake
Readiness for Enhanced Family Coping	Request for information about cancer support groups
Health Seeking Behaviors	Visit to local wellness center
Community	
Ineffective Community Coping	Inadequate medical and social support systems
Readiness for Enhanced Community Coping	Active planning by community leaders to provide resources

- Offers access to healthcare services for all members of the community, which provide both treatment for illnesses and activities to promote health
- Has roads, schools, playgrounds and other services to meet needs of the people in the community
- Provides and maintains a safe and healthy environment

Health of the residents of a community is affected by the social support systems, the community health structure, environmental factors, and types of agencies providing assistance for those in need of shelter, housing, and food. Examples of community factors affecting health are listed in Box 2-2 and are discussed further in the following sections.

Social Support Systems

The social support systems of an individual are made up of all the people who help meet financial, personal, physical, and emotional needs. In most instances, family, friends, and neighbors provide the best social support within a community. To understand the social support systems of a community, it is

Research in Nursing Making a Difference

Older Adults Living With Chronic Illness in Rural Communities

Chronic illness is a major health problem in the United States. As people age, they are at a greater risk of developing one or more chronic illnesses that may make living independently more difficult. This is especially true for older adults who live in rural communities, where incomes are typically lower and access to healthcare services is more limited. Nurses participate in and plan nursing care for the chronically ill, and must be able to identify how the healthcare system and the community facilitate or inhibit the ability of rural older adults to manage their own care.

Related Research

Davis, R., & Magilvy, J. (2000). Quiet pride: The experience of chronic illness by rural older adults. *Journal of Nursing Scholarship*, 32(4), 385–390.

This study was conducted to describe the experience and management of chronic illness by rural older adults; the interactions of those people in the rural healthcare system and community; and problems with health services from the perspectives of the older adults, their families, healthcare providers, and community

members. Findings of the study were five interrelated themes that illustrated the values and beliefs of finding meaning in life. The themes were managing life daily, support from faith and family, balance through negotiation, self-care, and belonging to community. Study participants saw the formal healthcare system as complex, confusing, and constantly changing, even when care was satisfactory. All of the participants were sustained while managing their chronic illness through their traditions, families, faith, and sense of community.

Relevance to Nursing Practice

Nurses care for many patients who live in rural areas of the United States. Findings from this study provide information about problems in healthcare and changes that are needed to better provide care to rural people with chronic illness. Nursing care must include health-promoting interventions to enhance individual independence and self-care for older adults with chronic illness. When planning and providing care in community settings, nurses must also consider individual strengths and values, family dynamics, and sense of community.

BOX 2-2 Examples of Community Factors Affecting Health

- Number and availability of healthcare institutions and services
- Housing codes
- Police and fire departments
- Nutritional services for low-income infants, mothers, school-aged children (eg, lunch programs), and older people
- Zoning regulations separating residential and industrial areas
- Waste disposal services and locations
- Air and water pollution
- Food sanitation
- Health education services and dissemination
- Recreational opportunities
- Violent crimes or drug use

important to know who and what provides support (such as family, neighbors, friends, church, and organizations).

Community Healthcare Structure

The healthcare structure of a community has a direct effect on the health of the people living within it. The size and location of the community often determine the types of services available. For example, urban residents have various means of transportation to a variety of healthcare providers, whereas rural residents might need to travel long distances for care. In addition, the county and state funding for community healthcare services also determines the type and number of healthcare institutions and agencies that are available.

Economic Resources

Financial and insurance coverages affect an individual's access to healthcare services within a community. As private health insurance costs continue to escalate, fewer citizens have it. Many part-time and unskilled jobs provide no insurance benefits at all, resulting in a substantial number of citizens who do not have any financial assistance for healthcare screenings or care for illnesses.

Environmental Factors

The environment of the community in which an individual lives and works might have both helpful and harmful effects on health. The quality of air and water differ across communities. Large urban areas are often affected by air pollution, whereas smaller communities may be at risk for water pollution from run-off of chemical or livestock wastes. Environmental barriers to accessing healthcare within a community include lack of transportation, distance to services, and location of the services.

The community has a strong influence on health promotion and illness-prevention activities of individuals and families in the community (Fig. 2-3). Just as there are family risk factors for the health of individual members, so are there community risk factors involving resources, economics, and services. For nursing assessments and interventions to be comprehensive and individualized, the nurse must also consider the community's influence.

To illustrate how the community can affect the individual's and family's needs, consider the following examples. Maria, 20 years old, lives in an inner-city, two-room apartment with her 6-month-old baby girl. The apartment lacks adequate heat and plumbing. Maria has no family living nearby, and her husband has left her. Maria rarely leaves her apartment because she fears the street gangs and drug addicts. She has never taken her baby to a local clinic for checkups because she doesn't know how to get there.

Anne, 22 years old, lives in a small house in a rural area with her 2-year-old son. She is a single mother and works as a secretary at an insurance agency. Anne often sees her family members, who live nearby. Anne and her son have regular health assessments.

These two different examples illustrate that the community plays a major role in the health of people who live there. Maria and her baby are at much greater risk for illness than are Anne and her son. Even if the two women had identical healthcare needs, their care plans would have different interventions because of their different community environments.

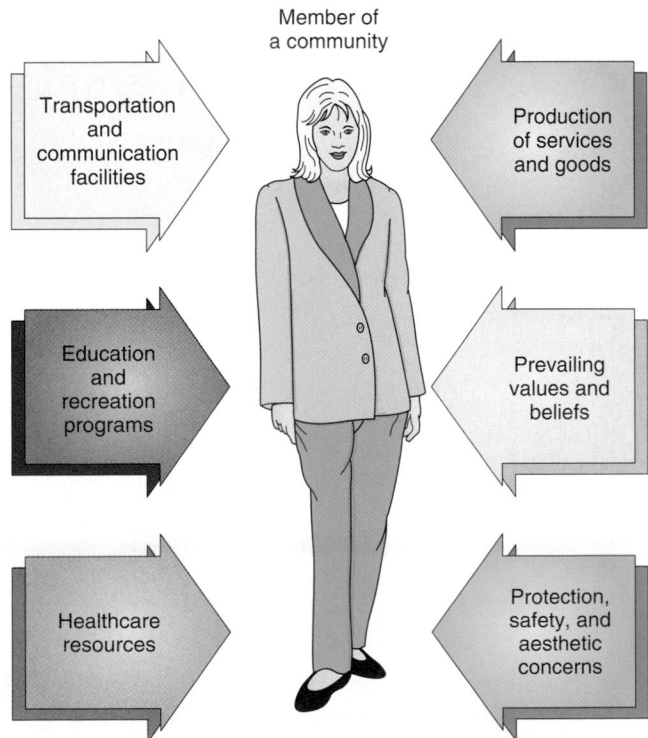

FIGURE 2-3 Many characteristics of a community influence the health of its members. This diagram shows six categories of characteristics that influence the health of a member of a community.

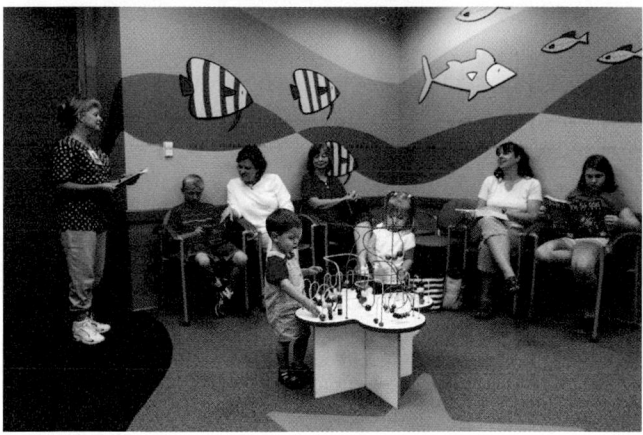

FIGURE 2-4 A nurse at work in an occupational (work-site) setting. (Photo by Joe Mitchell.)

Nursing in the Community

In contrast to community health nursing, which focuses on populations within a community, community-based nursing is centered on individual and family healthcare needs. The nurses practicing community based nursing provide interventions to manage acute or chronic health problems, promote health, and facilitate self-care. The nursing care provided within a community must be culturally competent and family-centered.

Nurses providing community-based care must know about the location and specialty of healthcare providers, the availability and accessibility of services and supplies, and public health services. Other factors to consider include facilities (such as day care or long-term care), housing, and the number and type of agencies providing services.

Nurses carry out a variety of activities that involve the community, designed to promote health and prevent illness. Nurses promote health as individuals, as caregivers within institutional settings, and as community-based healthcare providers. Nurses also provide community services as volunteers in health-related activities (eg, screenings, educational programs, and blood drives), and as role models for health practices and lifestyles. Nurses working in a variety of healthcare settings consider community influences when developing individualized nursing care plans and when making referrals to community agencies and support groups (see Examples of NANDA Diagnoses: Family and Community). Community-based nurses are employed in many different kinds of practice settings, including home healthcare, community health centers, school nursing, occupational nursing (Fig. 2-4), and independent nursing practice. Community-based care is discussed in more detail in Chapter 8.

■ Developing Critical Thinking Skills

1. What do you believe to be the most important basic human need that is actually or potentially unmet in the following situations?
   - A toddler falls into a swimming pool.
   - An elderly woman falls at home and is not found for 3 days.
   - A preschooler is admitted to the hospital with multiple bruises and burn marks.
   - A teenager is constantly told "you are no good" by his parents.
   - A nursing home resident says "I never did anything right in my life."
2. Our own family experiences often affect the way we relate to the families of our patients. Describe at least two possible responses to the families described below.
   - Suspecting child abuse, a nurse asks a mother about her child's bruises. The woman says "In our family, we believe in 'spare the rod and spoil the child'."
   - A single woman wants to have a child and comes to a fertility clinic for information on artificial insemination.
   - Several members of a patient's large, extended family are in the patient's long-term facility room and are trying to do everything for the patient.

■ Practicing for NCLEX

1. Maslow's hierarchy of basic human needs is useful when planning and implementing nursing care as it provides a structure for:
   a. Making accurate nursing diagnoses
   b. Establishing priorities of care
   c. Communicating concerns more concisely
   d. Integrating science into nursing care
2. Which of the following levels of basic human needs is most basic?
   a. Physiologic
   b. Safety and security
   c. Love and belonging
   d. Self-actualization
3. Of all the physiologic needs, which one is the most essential?
   a. Food
   b. Water
   c. Elimination
   d. Oxygen
4. Careful handwashing and using sterile techniques are ways in which nurses meet which basic human need?
   a. Physiologic
   b. Safety and security
   c. Self-esteem
   d. Love and belonging
5. Of the following statements, which one is true of self-actualization?
   a. Humans are born with fully developed self-actualization.
   b. Self-actualization needs are met by having confidence and independence.
   c. The self-actualization process continues throughout life.
   d. Loneliness and isolation occur when self-actualization needs are unmet.

6. What is the best broad definition of a family?
   a. A father, a mother, and children
   b. Members are biologically related
   c. Includes aunts, uncles, and cousins
   d. A group of people who live together
7. Where do individuals learn their health beliefs and values?
   a. In the family
   b. In school
   c. From school nurses
   d. From peers
8. John and Mary, each parents of one child, are both divorced. When they marry, the family structure that is formed will be:
   a. Nuclear family
   b. Extended family
   c. Blended family
   d. Cohabiting family
9. One of the developmental tasks of the older adult family is to:
   a. Maintain a supportive home base
   b. Prepare for retirement
   c. Cope with loss of energy and privacy
   d. Adjust to loss of spouse
10. One element of a healthy community is that it:
    a. Meets all the needs of its inhabitants
    b. Offers access to healthcare services
    c. Has mixed residential and industrial areas
    d. Is little concerned with air and water quality

Answers With Rationale

1. The correct response is *b*. Maslow's hierarchy of basic human needs is useful for establishing priorities of care.
2. The correct response is *a*. Physiologic needs are the most basic and must be met at least minimally to sustain life.
3. The correct response is *d*. Oxygen is the most essential of all needs because all body cells require oxygen for survival.
4. The correct response is *b*. By carrying out careful handwashing and using sterile technique, nurses provide safety from infection.
5. The correct response is *c*. Self-actualization, or reaching one's full potential, is a process that continues through life.
6. The correct response is *d*. Although all the responses may be true, the best definition is a group of people who live together.
7. The correct response is *a*. Healthcare activities, health beliefs, and health values are learned within one's family.
8. The correct response is *c*. A blended family is formed when parents bring unrelated children from previous relationships together to form a new family.

9. The correct response is *d*. A developmental task of the older adult family is adjusting to the loss of a spouse.
10. The correct response is *b*. A healthy community offers access to healthcare services to treat illness and to promote health.

Bibliography

Acton, G., & Malathum, P. (2000). Basic need status and health-promoting self-care behavior in adults. *Western Journal of Nursing Research, 22*(7), 796–811.

Aldous, J. (1975). *The developmental approach to family analysis.* Minneapolis: University of Minnesota Press.

Bell, J., Swan, N., Taillon, C., McGovern, G., & Dorn, J. (2001). Learning to nurse the family. *Journal of Family Nursing, 7*(2), 117–127.

Crawford, D. (2002). Reflection. Keep the focus on the family. *Journal of Child Health Care, 6*(2), 133–146.

Davis, R., & Magilvy, J. (2000). Quiet pride: The experience of chronic illness by rural older adults. *Journal of Nursing Scholarship, 32*(4), 385–390.

Duvall, E. (1977). *Marriage and family development* (5th ed.). Philadelphia: J.B. Lippincott.

Ebersole, P., Hess, P., & Luggen, P. (2004). *Toward healthy aging: Human needs and nursing response* (6th ed.). St. Louis: Mosby.

Edelman, C., & Mandle, C. (2002). *Health promotion throughout the lifespan* (5th ed.). St. Louis: Mosby.

Feeley, N., & Gottlieb, L. (2000). Nursing approaches for working with family strengths and resources. *Journal of Family Nursing, 6*(1), 9–24.

Friedman, M. (1992). *Family nursing: Theory and assessment* (3rd ed.). Norwalk, CT: Appleton & Lange.

Friedman, M., Bowden, V., & Jones, E. (2003). *Family nursing: Research, theory, and practice* (5th ed.). Upper Saddle River, NJ: Prentice Hall.

Healthy people in healthy communities: A community planning guide using Healthy People 2010. (2001). Available at http://healthypeople.gov/Publications/HealthyCommunities2001/Chapter_1.htm.

Hesketh, J. (2002). Community nursing—the last 25 years. *Nursing Times, 16*(7), 4–5.

Maslow, A. (1968). *Toward a psychology of being* (2nd ed.). New York: Van Nostrand–Reinhold.

Pender, N. J., Murdaugh, C., & Parsons, M. A. (2002). *Health promotion in nursing practice* (4th ed.). Upper Saddle River, NJ: Prentice Hall.

Stanhope, M., & Lancaster, J. (2002). *Foundations of community health nursing—community oriented practice.* St. Louis: Mosby.

U.S. Department of Health and Human Services. Office of Disease Prevention and Health Promotion. (2000). *Healthy people 2010.* Washington, DC: U.S. Department of Health and Human Services.

Cultural Diversity

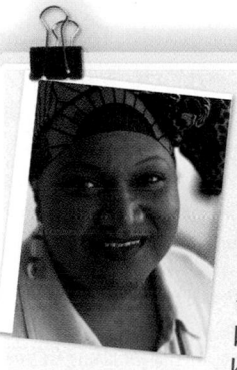

Danielle Dorvall is an immigrant from Haiti who has been in the United States for approximately 8 months. She recently had surgical repair of a fractured femur and is now confined to bed in skeletal traction. She asks that a Haitian folk healer from her neighborhood be allowed to come to the hospital to help heal her broken leg.

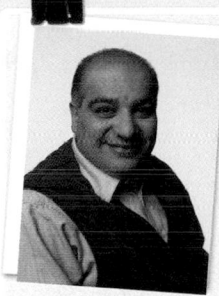

Khalifa Abdul Hakim, the husband of a Muslim patient, requests that only female healthcare practitioners care for his wife. In the Muslim culture, it is deemed immodest for the body of a married woman to be seen by any male other than her husband.

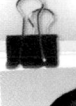
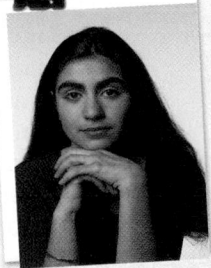

Janice Goldberg, a 23-year-old woman of Jewish ancestry, comes to the women's health clinic for a routine examination. During the visit, she asks "I've been dating this man who also is Jewish, and we're thinking about getting married and having children. But I've heard about this hereditary disorder called Tay-Sachs disease that occurs in Jews. Should I be concerned?"

Focusing on Blended Skills

The types of blended skills you'll need to respond to the case scenarios here include:

Cognitive Skills
- Knowledge of how culture and ethnicity influences a person's beliefs and values, daily living, health behaviors, decision making, and disease risk; for example, the Haitian patient's request for a faith healer and confidence in that healer's intervention, knowledge about Eastern European Jews and hereditary disease to facilitate decisions about marriage and childbearing, and the request by a patient's husband that his wife receive no care by male practitioners
- Knowledge that people from different cultures and ethnic groups can think differently about what is right in any given situation
- Knowledge of acculturation and ethnocentrism and effects on persons of various cultures
- Knowledge of physiologic and psychological characteristics of various cultures that may affect the client's health; for example, a person's increased risk for a hereditary disorder such as Tay-Sachs disease
- Ability to incorporate knowledge of specific cultural beliefs and values to plan appropriate care for the client; for example, allowing a folk healer to participate in the care of a patient with a fractured femur
- Ability to demonstrate knowledge of transcultural care when providing nursing care

Technical Skills
- Strong assessment skills related to culture and its influence on health
- Ability to demonstrate competence in cultural assessment skills

- Ability to adapt procedures and skills appropriately when dealing with different cultural groups, such as teaching a young adult about the risk of Tay-Sachs disease in her children

Interpersonal Skills
- Respect that individuals from different cultural and ethnic groups may believe, value, choose, and behave differently than you do
- Ability to establish trusting relationships with colleagues, patients, family members, and others who are different from you
- Ability to communicate to the patient a greater concern about the patient's status; for example, respecting the wishes of a patient's husband that no male healthcare providers be involved with his wife's care

Ethical and Legal Skills
- Commitment to securing the best possible care for patients from different cultures that is respectful of their beliefs and preferences but that does not violate your conscience or the practice of good nursing
- Ability to advocate for the Haitian patient, who has the right to be visited by a folk healer, and for the husband of a Muslim woman requesting care by female practitioners, as long as this does not harm other patients or result in harm while she is entrusted to the institution's care
- Ability to provide accurate information about the patient's risk for passing on a hereditary disease within the scope of nursing practice
- Ability to practice transcultural nursing care in an ethically and legally defensible manner, consistent with nursing code of ethics and within the scope of legal practice

Learning Outcomes

After completing the chapter, the learner should be able to accomplish the following:

1. Discuss concepts of cultural diversity.
2. Describe cultural influences that affect culturally competent healthcare.
3. Identify diversity in health and illness care, including culturally based traditional care.
4. Practice cultural competence when assessing and providing nursing care for patients from diverse cultural groups.
5. Discuss factors in the healthcare system and in nursing that facilitate or impede culturally competent nursing care.

Key Terms

cultural assimilation
cultural blindness
cultural diversity
cultural imposition
culture
culture conflict
culture shock
ethnicity
ethnocentrism
personal space
race
stereotyping

Our society is made up of people from many different culturally diverse backgrounds. Included in **cultural diversity** are people of varying racial classification and national origin, religious affiliation, language, physical size, gender, sexual orientation, age, disability, socioeconomic status, occupational status, and geographic location (Campinha-Bacote, 2003). Nurses provide care to culturally diverse people, and must develop the knowledge and practice the skills necessary for culturally competent care. (For an example, see the accompanying Reflective Practice display.) This chapter focuses on the concepts of culture and discusses the influence of cultural diversity on nursing care.

CONCEPTS OF CULTURAL DIVERSITY

Cultural diversity is an integral component of both health and illness because of genetic characteristics and the cultural values and beliefs we learn in our families and communities. To be able to provide culturally competent care to people from diverse backgrounds, nurses must be sensitive to culturally diverse needs, characteristics, and values of individuals, families, and groups. Definitions of concepts related to culture are summarized in Table 3-1.

Reflective Practice
Challenge to Intellectual Skills

I had thought that I'd pretty much gotten used to all sorts of questions from patients about why a guy like me would go into nursing. Today, however, I was surprised when Khalifa Abdul Hakim, the husband of a newly admitted patient, demanded that I leave his wife's room immediately. Stepping into the corridor with me, he explained that he and his family were Muslim, and that in their culture it was deemed immodest for the body of a married woman to be seen by any male other than her husband. He asked me to make sure that his wife's chart made it clear that there were to be no male nurses. He also asked about female physicians. Since we were short-staffed and all trying to cover for one another to get through the day, I wasn't sure that I could make that promise, especially since our unit has three or four male nurses. I wasn't clear if this was just a personal preference, a religious or cultural matter or both, or if this mattered at all. I have to admit that I had absolutely no clue as to how to respond. I remembered classes about the importance of culturally appropriate care, but didn't remember ever learning about how to respond to requests such as this one. I also wasn't sure if the hospital had a policy about these types of requests.

Thinking Outside the Box: Possible Courses of Action

- Find someone to swap patients with me and forget about having to deal with the situation (probably the simplest response).
- Use the opportunity to research the Muslim culture and talk with the patient's male family members about what is important to them. Since our Muslim patient population seems to be growing, suggest an in-service program on this topic for everyone.

- Explain to Mr. Hakim that his wife is in a U.S. hospital, and that while here they should observe U.S. customs, meaning she may have male nurses or other male healthcare practitioners.
- Check the hospital's policy on these sorts of requests and then follow it.

Evaluating a Good Outcome: How Do I Define Success?

- I need to know enough to do whatever is necessary to ensure the patient's health and well-being, as well as respect the integrity of all participants involved within the scope of my responsibilities.

- The patient and her family feel sufficiently comfortable in our environment (culturally appropriate care) for healing to be maximized.
- I know more at the end of the experience than when I started.

Personal Learning: Here's to the Future!

I was pretty surprised when two of the older, more experienced nurses said they had never encountered such a request, and that they didn't know if the hospital had a policy on these sorts of matters. Luckily, one of them referred me to our patient-relations person, and she came right up to the unit. I had never met her before, but I was impressed with her knowledge and her strong commitment to patient advocacy. She showed me the hospital policy that obligates all workers to respect the beliefs and values of patients unless this entails compromising their own integrity

or the safety of other persons. She said that we will be seeing more Muslim patients because of a new influx into our community and recommended a website to get more information. I have to admit that I haven't checked it out yet, but I did talk some with the patient's family and have a better understanding of why these things matter to them. I'm thinking of trying to cultivate the attitude that each patient and family could be an important learning opportunity for me if I'm open to what they have to teach!

Reflection

How do you think you would respond in a similar situation? Why? What does this tell you about yourself and about the adequacy of your skills for professional practice? Can you think of other ways to respond? What type of information would you need to respond in a different manner? Imagine if the nurse had been

female. Would this situation have arisen? Explain why or why not? What other skills (cognitive, interpersonal, technical, ethical/legal) would you need to respond well in this situation? Do you agree with the criteria to evaluate a successful outcome? Did the nursing student meet the criteria?

TABLE 3-1 Definitions of Concepts Related to Cultural Diversity

Concept	Definition
Cultural Diversity	Diverse groups in society, with varying racial classification and national origin, religious affiliation, language, physical size, gender, sexual orientation, age, disability, socioeconomic status, occupational status, and geographic location
Culture	A shared system of beliefs, values, and behavioral expectations that provide social structure for daily living. Includes beliefs, habits, likes and dislikes, and customs and rituals.
Subculture	A large group of people who are members of a larger cultural group but have certain ethnic, occupational, or physical characteristics not common to the larger culture
Dominant Group	The group within a country or society that has the most authority to control values and sanctions
Minority Group	Most often has some physical or cultural characteristic that identifies the people within it as different
Cultural Assimilation	When members of a minority group live within a dominant group and lose the cultural characteristics that made them different
Culture Shock	The feelings a person experiences when placed in a different culture
Ethnicity	The sense of identification with a collective cultural group, largely based on the group's common heritage. Includes language and dialect, religious practices, literature, music, folklore, political interests, food preferences, and employment patterns.
Race	Racial categories are based on specific physical characteristics
Stereotyping	Assuming that all members of a culture, subculture, or ethnic group act alike
Cultural Imposition	The belief that everyone should conform to the majority belief system
Cultural Blindness	The result of ignoring differences and proceeding as though they do not exist
Culture Conflict	The state that occurs when people become aware of cultural differences, feel threatened, and respond by ridiculing the beliefs and traditions of others to make themselves feel more secure
Personal Space	The area around a person regarded as part of the person; varying among people and cultural and ethnic groups
Ethnocentrism	The belief that one's ideas, beliefs, and practices are the best, are superior, or are most preferred to those of others

Culture

Culture may be defined as a shared system of beliefs, values, and behavioral expectations that provide social structure for daily living. Culture defines roles and interactions with others as well as within families and communities, and is apparent in the attitudes and institutions unique to particular groups. Culture includes the beliefs, habits, likes and dislikes, and customs and rituals learned from one's family (Andrews & Boyle, 2002b). The characteristics of culture include the following:

- Culture guides behavior into acceptable ways for people in a specific group. It is shared by, and provides an identity for, all members of the same cultural group.
- Culture is learned by each new generation through both formal and informal life experiences. Language is the primary means of transmitting culture.
- The practices of a particular culture often arise because of the group's social and physical environment.
- Cultural practices and beliefs may evolve over time, but they mainly remain constant as long as they satisfy a group's needs.
- Culture influences the way people of a group view themselves, have expectations, and behave in response to certain situations. Because a culture is made up of individuals, there are differences both within cultures and among cultures.

Recall Mr. Hakim, the Muslim man described in the Reflective Practice display? The nurse's knowledge of his culture and beliefs would be important in determining staffing needs, as well as ensuring culturally appropriate care. The nurse would need to understand how Mr. Hakim views himself and his wife, as well as understand actions and behaviors that would be acceptable to Mr. Hakim and his wife.

Within most cultures are subgroups, or subcultures. A subculture is a large group of people who are members of a larger cultural group, but have certain ethnic, occupational, or physical characteristics that are not common to the larger culture. For example, nursing is a subculture of the larger healthcare system culture, and teenagers and older adults are often regarded as subcultures of the general population in the United States.

Cultures include both dominant groups and minority groups. A dominant group is the group within a country or society that has the most authority to control values and sanctions of the society. The dominant group usually is (but does not have to be) the largest group in a society. The dominant group in the United States is currently composed of white middle-class people of European ancestry. The values of this cultural group have strongly influenced the value system of our society as a whole. Some of the dominant values include the following:

- Youth, thinness, and beauty
- Success and achievement
- Independence and self-reliance
- Technology
- Work
- Ownership
- Duty and conscience

A minority group usually has some physical or cultural characteristic (such as race, religious beliefs, or occupation) that identifies the people within it as different. When minority groups live within a dominant group, many of their members lose the cultural characteristics that once made them different. This process is called **cultural assimilation** or acculturation. Assimilation occurs when one's values are replaced by the values of the dominant culture. When people immigrate, their values are on one end of the spectrum and the values of the dominant culture are on the other end. As immigrants go to work, go to school, move out of the community, and learn the dominant language, they often move closer to the dominant culture. The process and the rate of assimilation are individualized.

Consider Danielle Dorvall, the immigrant from Haiti who has been in the United States for 8 months. Because she has been in the U.S. for a relatively short period of time, the nurse would need to determine the amount of acculturation she has experienced and plan Mrs. Dorvall's care accordingly, without discounting her desire for a folk healer.

Mutual cultural assimilation does occur, with some characteristics of both groups being traded. For example, Hispanic immigrants to the United States learn to speak English, and Americans learn and use traditional Hispanic foods. In this way, we gain from the many cultures with which we live. Although we seldom think about it, the clothes we wear, the foods we eat, the music we enjoy, many of the words we use, and the leisure activities we practice are all characteristics in which we have become acculturated.

Culture shock, or the feelings a person experiences when placed in a different culture that the person perceives as strange, may result in psychological discomfort or disturbances. The patterns of behavior a person found acceptable and effective in his or her own culture are often not adequate in the new one. The effect of colliding cultures often results in stress, as described in the accompanying Research in Nursing box. The person may then feel foolish, fearful, incompetent, inadequate, embarrassed, humiliated, or inferior. These feelings eventually can lead to frustration, anxiety, and loss of self-esteem.

Ethnicity

Ethnicity is the sense of identification with a collective cultural group, largely based on the group's common heritage. One belongs to a specific ethnic group either through birth or through adoption of characteristics of that group. People within

Research in Nursing Making a Difference
Stress in Immigrant Women

Changes in international political and economic patterns have, in turn, resulted in changes in global migration patterns. Large numbers of immigrants from the former Soviet Union have entered and now live in the United States. These immigrants tend to be older, with more than one fourth of them women over the age of 50 years. For many of these women, the ongoing stress of acculturating into a new culture and the effects of a lifetime of inadequate healthcare contribute to high levels of psychological distress.

Related Research
Miller, A., & Chandler, P. (2002). Acculturation, resilience, and depression in midlife women from the former Soviet Union. *Nursing Research, 51*(1), 26–32.

> The purpose of this study was to explore the effect of immigration on Soviet midlife women, as measured by acculturation, demands of immigration, resilience, and psychological distress. The researchers found that these women experienced frequent symptoms of depression during their first few years in the United States. However, working and living near those who speak En-

glish, as well as exposure to media and cultural events, improved English proficiency and enhanced psychological well-being. Although these results corroborate findings of previous studies, additional validation is suggested to differentiate depressed mood from clinical depression.

Relevance to Nursing Practice
Acquisition of language skills when one migrates to a new country and culture has proven to be a critical prerequisite for securing employment and for communicating with healthcare and social service providers. Nurses who work in communities with new residents who have recently immigrated should explore referral options for new language development, and recommend those that are appropriate. Nurses also should understand that cultural differences in willingness to report symptoms exist and may hinder assessments. Further research is necessary to begin to understand which strengths and resources protect immigrants from the stress of acculturation and enhance transition to a new country.

an ethnic group generally share unique cultural and social beliefs and behavior patterns, including language and dialect, religious practices, literature, folklore, music, political interests, food preferences, and employment patterns. Ethnicity largely develops through day-to-day life with family and friends within the community.

Race

Although the term ethnicity often is used interchangeably with **race,** these terms are not the same. Racial categories are typically based on specific physical characteristics, such as skin pigmentation, body stature, facial features, and hair texture. Although there has been a blending of physical characteristics through the centuries, the three major race classifications are Caucasian, Negroid, and Mongoloid.

Factors Affecting Cultural Sensitivity

A variety of factors may affect sensitivity to other cultures. When one assumes that all members of a culture or ethnic group act alike, **stereotyping** is at work. Common stereotypic beliefs are that all Italians are emotional, that all Germans are stoic, that men never cry, and that the elderly are senile. Stereotyping may be positive or negative. Negative stereotyping includes racism, ageism, and sexism. These are beliefs that certain races, an age group, or one gender is inherently superior to others, leading to discrimination against those considered inferior. Stereotyping is often done by members of the dominant group about the minority group in a culture (Fig. 3-1).

Cultural imposition is the belief that everyone should conform to the majority belief system. **Cultural blindness** occurs when one ignores differences and proceeds as though they do not exist. This has been true of the healthcare system, especially in regard to what are considered nontraditional methods of care. **Culture conflict** occurs when people become aware of cultural differences, feel threatened, and respond by ridiculing the beliefs and traditions of others to make themselves feel more secure about their own values (Andrews & Boyle, 2002b).

CULTURAL INFLUENCES ON HEALTHCARE

The US is multicultural, multiethnic, and multiracial. Therefore, it is important for nurses to be aware of, and sensitive to, the needs of a culturally diverse patient population. Table 3-2 describes selected cultural variations in the concepts of health and health promotion. The following sections describe general considerations in culturally competent care.

Physiologic Characteristics

Researchers theorize that in the past, cultural groups adapted slowly to their environment. For example, dark-skinned people developed lighter skin as early populations moved to colder northern climates, where there is less sunlight throughout the year compared with equatorial climates. Lighter skin is better able to use vitamin D from sunlight than darker skin. It also is theorized that a group's nose shape and size evolved according to the climate in which they lived (Henderson & Primeaux, 1981). From a scientific and anthropologic point of view, these adaptations were natural changes that helped improve the lives and well-being of human beings. Some of these biologic variations were effective adaptations for a particular period or for living in a certain environment.

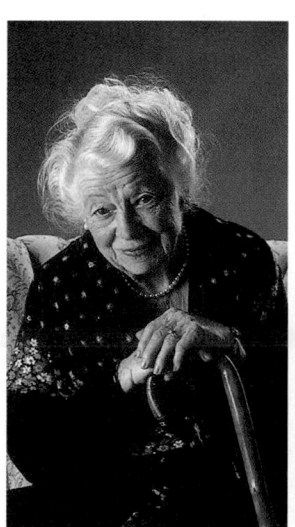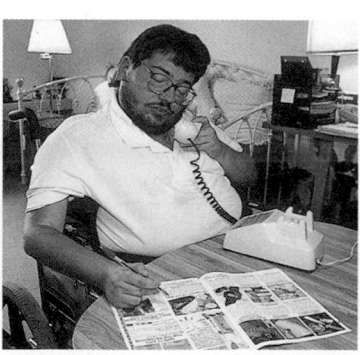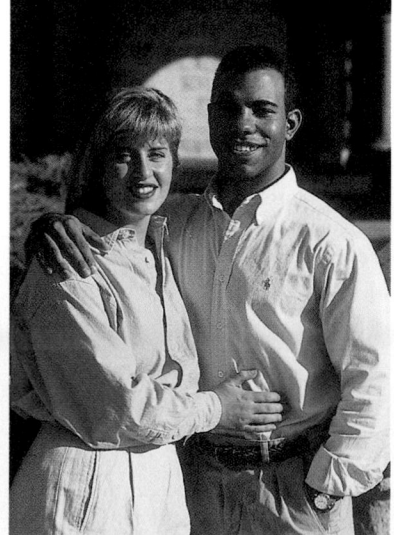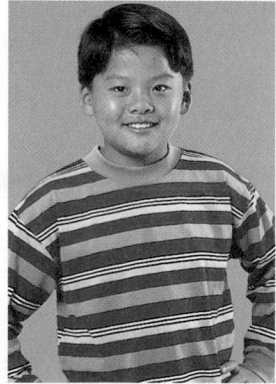

FIGURE 3-1 Identifying one's own prejudices is the first step toward eliminating them. Think about the assumptions you make about the people in these images.   (*Left to right,* Photo © Christopher Briscoe, Science Source/Photo Researchers; Photo © Jeff Isaac Greenberg, Science Source/Photo Researchers; Photo © Renee Lynn, Science Source/Photo Researchers; Photo © Ken Cavanagh, Science Source/Photo Researcher)

TABLE 3-2 Cultural Variations in Health Concept and Promotion

Cultural Group	Concept of Health	Health Promotion
Native American	Traditional health beliefs are holistic and health oriented	Traditional health practices include physical stamina (running), relaxation (meditation), cleansing (sweats), self-sufficiency, and harmonious living. Participation in religious ceremonies and prayer promotes health of self and family.
African American	Maintaining feelings of well-being, ability to fulfill role expectations, freedom from pain and excessive stress	Proper diet, proper behavior, and exercise in fresh air are prescription for maintaining health; protect against excessive cold
Cambodian	Being healthy is seen as being in equilibrium. Health needs to be individually maintained but is influenced by family and community.	Illness is seen as preventable. Nutrition is important, but not physical activity.
Chinese American	Maintaining balance between *yin* and *yang* influences in the body and in the environment. Harmony is important to maintain body, mind, and spirit.	One should eat a diet balanced with *yin* and *yang* foods and maintain harmony with friends and family.
Gypsies (Roma)	Maintaining moral purity, keeping upper and lower body separate, and practicing good behavior. Good health, prosperity, large families, and good appearance are intertwined.	Staying clean (*wuzho*) and avoiding unclean (*mahrime*)
Hmong	Being able to perform expected routines and duties.	Not a priority if considered from Western perspective
Hispanic	Feeling well and being able to maintain role function	Orientation to the present and belief that the future is in God's hands mean that health screenings and routine checkup may not be scheduled by traditional Hispanics.
Puerto Rican	Absence of mental, spiritual, or physical discomforts as well as *lenities y limpios* (not being too thin and being clean) are perceived as healthy	Eating well and drinking fruit beverages Multivitamins are commonly used
Samoan	Holistic approach, including aspects of body, mind, and spirit. Includes relationships with family, environment, and spiritual world.	Concept of preventive health not well established in Samoa
Vietnamese	Principles of harmony and balance within self. Overweight a positive sign of good economic status and contentment.	Encompasses physical, spiritual, emotional, and social factors. Consuming lots of fresh vegetables, fruit, fish, and meat. Keeping clean and warm.

Data from Lipson, J., Dibble, S., & Minarik P. (Eds.). (1996). *Culture & nursing care: A pocket guide.* San Francisco: UCSF Nursing Press, pp. 21, 42, 62–63, 80–81, 136–137, 168, 219–220, 236–237, 262–263, 289.

When a person no longer is in the environment that encouraged the biologic variation, the variation might then have a detrimental effect on the person's health and well-being. Various studies have shown that certain racial groups have particular characteristics that make them more prone to developing specific diseases and conditions. For example, a hereditary disorder, Tay-Sachs disease, is associated with individuals of Eastern European Jewish descent. Although the incidence of this disorder has declined over the years due to improved and earlier testing, it is still a concern.

Recall Janice Goldberg, the young adult woman described at the beginning of the chapter? Knowledge of the disorder and screening and early detection methods would be im-portant for the nurse to use as a foundation when counseling and teaching Janice.

Three examples of these conditions, which may result from environmental factors or through inheritance, include:
1. Keloids
2. Lactase deficiency and lactose intolerance
3. Sickle cell anemia

Keloids result from an overgrowth of connective tissue during the healing process that forms a scar after an injury, surgery, or burn. People with dark skin are much more likely to develop keloids. Rather than healing level with the surrounding skin tissue, the wound of a person with a tendency toward keloid formation heals with a rough, lumpy, or elevated scar.

Milk and many milk products contain lactose, a sugar. The enzyme lactase must be present in the body to break down lactose during digestion. Without lactase, the lactose ferments in the intestines, resulting in gas (flatus), diarrhea, and abdominal bloating and cramping. Lactase deficiency and lactose intolerance are more common in Hispanic women and in both men and women of African, Chinese, and Thai ancestry (Andrews & Boyle, 2002b).

People with sickle cell anemia have sickle-shaped red blood cells (RBCs) that break down more rapidly than normal-shaped RBCs. The sickle shape also prevents the RBCs from moving easily through the smaller blood vessels in the body. This factor can lead to these blood vessels being clogged by RBCs, which can cause many potentially serious problems. Sickle cell anemia is most common in people of African or Mediterranean origin.

Psychological Characteristics

In most situations, a person interprets the behaviors of another person in terms of her or his own familiar culture. This process usually is multidirectional; for example, in a healthcare setting, the patient evaluates the attitudes and actions of the healthcare provider at the same time the healthcare provider interprets the behavior of the patient. Remember that what may seem reasonable and important to a patient may seem ridiculous and irrelevant to a nurse. The reverse is also true; practices a nurse perceives as logical and effective may seem senseless, incompetent, or even dangerous to a patient.

Consider Danielle Dorvall, described at the beginning of the chapter. She might view skeletal traction as senseless, while the nurse may view her request for a folk healer in the same way. The nurse needs to be aware of these possible attitudes and beliefs to ensure maximum effective care while still meeting the patient's cultural needs.

Reactions to Pain

Healthcare researchers have discovered that many of the expressions and behaviors exhibited by people in pain are culturally prescribed. Some cultures allow and even encourage the open expression of emotions experienced by a person in pain, whereas other cultures frown on the open and free expression of emotions.

The main issue for nurses in this area of cultural expression is their attitude toward the "ideal patient." Nurses often assume that a patient who does not complain of pain is not having pain. A patient who deals with pain quietly and stoically may have pain-reduction needs ignored by nurses. Nurses should be sensitive to other signals of discomfort, such as holding or applying pressure to the painful area, self-restriction of activities that intensify the pain, and uncontrollable, spontaneous expressions of discomfort, such as facial grimacing and moaning. Nurses should not consider patients who freely express their discomfort as constant complainers whose requests for pain relief seem excessive. Pain is a warning from the body that something is wrong. Pain is what the patient says it is, and every complaint of pain should be assessed carefully.

Nursing care for the patient in pain is always individualized (see Chap. 41), but important culture-sensitive considerations include the following:
- Recognize that culture is an important component of individuality and that each person holds (and has the right to hold) various beliefs about pain.
- Respect the patient's right to respond to pain in whatever manner is culturally and individually appropriate.
- Never stereotype a patient's perceptions or responses to pain based on the person's culture.

Mental Health

Most mental health norms are based on research and observations made of white, middle-class people. Many ethnic groups have their own norms or acceptable patterns of behavior for psychological well-being and normal psychological reactions to certain situations. For example, many Hispanic people deal with problems within the family and would view it as inappropriate to tell problems to a stranger. Traditional Chinese people often consider mental illness a stigma; therefore, seeking psychiatric help would be a disgrace to the family. Chinese people traditionally have been taught that the expression of strong emotions results in disharmony and imbalance between the body's energy forces (yin and yang) and is considered a sign of weakness. In times of high stress or anxiety, some Puerto Ricans may demonstrate a hyperkinetic seizure activity known as *ataques*. This behavior is a culturally accepted reaction.

Gender Roles

In many cultures, the man is the dominant figure and generally makes decisions for all family members. For example, if approval for medical care is needed, the man gives it regardless of which family member is involved. In male-dominant cultures, women are usually passive. On the other hand, in many African American and Caucasian families, the woman is often dominant.

Knowing who is the dominant member of the family is an important consideration when planning nursing care. If the dominant member is ill and can no longer make decisions, for example, the whole family may be anxious and confused. If a nondominant family member is ill, he or she may require help in verbalizing needs, particularly if they differ from those the dominant member perceives as being important.

Think back to Mr. Hakim, the Muslim man concerned about his wife's care providers being male. Since Mr. Hakim, and not his wife, was the person who made the request about no male care providers, the nurse would interpret this as indicating that Mr. Hakim is the dominant family member.

Language and Communication

When people from another part of the world move to the United States, they may speak their own language fluently but have difficulty speaking English. This is especially true for the women or older adults in the family if they do not work outside the home, or for people who live in proximity to others who speak the same language. Thus, assimilation is slower for people who stay at home, especially if they live in communities of their ethnic culture. Children usually assimilate more rapidly and learn the language of the dominant culture quickly because they leave home each day to go to school, making new friends in the dominant culture. Wage earners also tend to learn a new language more quickly through the work setting. Language acquisition is thus tied to necessity and assimilation rather than to degree of difficulty.

Most Americans do not know a language other than English. As a result, communication problems can arise during healthcare activities. This problem is not unique to non–English-speaking patients; even in different regions of the US, certain dialects or word meanings can cause differences in understanding. Consider how difficult it must be to describe symptoms or give a personal health history when you do not understand the questions being asked. Something as simple as showing the nurse where you hurt is impossible if you do not know what you are being asked. In addition, patients may forget English words or revert to their more familiar language when experiencing the stress of an injury, illness, or pain.

Nurses who work in a geographic area with a high population of residents who speak a language other than English should learn pertinent words and phrases in that language. See the accompanying box Through the Eyes of a Student. Many agencies have a qualified interpreter, or one can be found in the community. To avoid misinterpretation of questions and answers, it is important to use an interpreter who understands the healthcare system. Sometimes a family member or friend can translate for the nurse, but such a person may be protective and not the most reliable means of transferring information. Nurses may find themselves talking in a louder tone of voice to a patient who does not understand what they are saying; remember that this is a communication problem, not a hearing problem.

Eye contact, as a nonverbal communication behavior, is one of the most culturally variable forms of communication. The American dominant culture emphasizes eye contact while speaking, but other cultures regard this behavior in different ways. For example, direct eye contact may be considered impolite or aggressive by Asians, Native Americans, Indochinese, Arabs, and Appalachians; these groups of people tend to avoid direct eye contact and avert their eyes while speaking with another. Native Americans often stare at the floor during conversations, a behavior that indicates they are carefully listening. Hispanics look downward in deference to age, gender, social position, economic status, and authority. Muslim–Arab women indicate modesty by avoiding eye contact with men, and Hasidic Jewish men tend to avoid direct eye contact with women (Andrews & Boyle, 2002b).

Through the Eyes of a Student

I was doing my maternity rotation and was assigned to labor and delivery. I was assigned a woman who spoke no English—she and her husband were from Central America and had been in the United States for only 2 months.

When I arrived at 7 am, the night nurse was giving a report about my patient to the day nurse. The night nurse was frantic—no one understood the couple, all efforts to locate a translator had come up empty, and, quite frankly, she had no idea exactly what condition this woman was in.

I quickly began to think back on my 2 years of Spanish. Could I be of any help to this couple? I wondered. Would I remember enough to communicate with them about giving birth? Then I decided that any little bit of communication at this point was better than none, so I spoke up. I told both nurses that I spoke some Spanish and asked if I could be of any help. The night nurse literally hugged me!

I began by telling the expectant couple that I was a nursing student and that I spoke some Spanish. We exchanged introductions and then I asked the woman some assessment questions. Nothing I said was complicated—all of my sentences were short and simple, but who needed more than that?

Then the couple asked me some questions. They had heard about "cutting open the stomach" to deliver a baby. I naturally assumed that they meant a cesarean delivery. They looked so afraid but I had to be honest. They wanted to know how it was done and why. The words I could not remember or did not know I acted out. They looked so relieved when I was finished.

The man said that they thought *all* babies were born this way in our country. He said that they had never heard of this procedure until coming to the United States. No wonder they were so frightened!

The doctor came in, examined the woman, and said she was fully dilated. The doctor asked if I could teach a crash course in Lamaze breathing to the woman. She also asked me if I would stay throughout the delivery because she would need assistance in translating directions to the woman. Of course I said yes.

The woman was terrified. I told her that it was normal to be afraid and that I would be with her during the delivery. She took my hand and whispered, "Muchas gracias." I never felt more useful than I did at that moment.

—A. Kelly Gaylor,
Holy Family College, Philadelphia

When caring for culturally and ethnically diverse patients, it is it important to perform a transcultural assessment of communication (adapted from Andrews and Boyle, 2002b):

- What language does the patient speak during usual activities of daily living?
- How well does the patient speak and write in English?
- Does the patient need an interpreter? Are family members or friends available? Are there people the patient would not want to serve as an interpreter?

- How does the patient prefer to be addressed?
- What cultural values and beliefs of the patient may change your techniques of communication and care (such as eye contact, space, or social taboos)?
- How does the patient's nonverbal behavior affect the responses of members of the healthcare team?
- How does the patient feel about healthcare providers from other cultures; would the patient prefer a healthcare provider of the same culture, gender, or age?
- What are the cultural characteristics of the patient's communications with others?

> *Think back to Mr. Hakim, the man described in the Reflective Practice display. Answers to these questions would be important to provide a baseline from which to develop the plan of care for Mr. Hakim and his wife, thus providing culturally effective care.*

Chapter 21 provides additional information on communicating with non–English-speaking patients.

Orientation to Space and Time

Personal space is the area around a person regarded as part of the person. This area, individualized to each person and to different cultures and ethnic groups, is the area into which others should not intrude during personal interactions. If others do not consider a person's personal space, that person may become uncomfortable or even angry. When providing nursing care that involves physical contact, you should know the patient's cultural personal space preferences. For example, people of Arabic and African origin commonly sit and stand close to one another when talking, whereas people of Asian and European descent are more comfortable with some distance between themselves and others.

Many people and almost all institutions in the US value promptness and punctuality. When arriving for an appointment, doing a job, or carrying out an activity, being on time and getting the job done promptly are viewed as important. This is not true in some other cultures. For example, in some South Asian cultures, being late is considered a sign of respect. In addition, although most of the US middle-class is future oriented (including activities that promote health not only in the present but also in the future), other cultures are more concerned with the present or the past.

Food and Nutrition

Food preferences and how foods are prepared often are related culturally. Certain food groups serve as staples of the diet based on culture and remain so even when members of that culture are living in a different country. For example, rice and vegetables are the staples of Asians and Chinese, and pasta is a staple of Italians. Hispanics favor beans and tortillas, whereas Puerto Ricans try to eat a balance of hot, cold, and cool foods (the classification is based on type of foods, not cooking temperatures). These are only examples and should not be used to

select patient foods; the nurse should always ask the patient about individual food preferences.

Patients in a hospital or long-term care setting often do not have much of a choice of foods. This means that people with cultural food preferences may not be able to select appealing foods and thus may be at risk for inadequate nutrition. When assessing the cause of decreased appetite in patients, the nurse should determine whether the problem may be related to culture. It may be possible for family or friends to bring in foods that satisfy the patient's nutritional needs while still meeting dietary restrictions. Dietary teaching must be individualized according to cultural values about the social significance and sharing of food. A culturally sensitive assessment of nutrition is provided in Box 3-1.

Family Support

In many cultural and ethnic groups, people have large, extended families and consider the needs of any family member to be equal to or greater than their own. They may be unwilling to share private information about family members with those outside the family (including healthcare providers). Other cultural groups have great respect for the elders in the family and would never consider institutional care for them. Including the family in planning care for any patient is a major component in nursing care to meet individualized needs, especially if those needs can be met only through consideration of all members of the family.

BOX 3-1 Culturally Sensitive Nutrition Assessment

1. Which foods are considered edible and which are not?
   - In France, corn is considered an animal feed, whereas corn is a commonly eaten vegetable in the United States.
   - Religious beliefs prohibit some Jewish, Muslim, and Seventh-Day Adventist patients from eating pork.
   - Patients who follow a vegetarian diet do not eat pork, beef, or chicken.
2. What times and types of food are considered meals?
   - Anglo-Americans typically eat three meals a day, with foods such as bacon and eggs or cereal for breakfast, sandwiches and soup for lunch, and meat with potatoes and vegetables for dinner.
   - Vietnamese may eat soup for every meal.
   - Beans are a staple for meals among Mexican people.
   - People from Middle Eastern countries often eat cheese and olives for breakfast.
   - Native American and Latin American people usually eat two meals a day.
   - Rural southern African Americans may eat large amounts of food on weekends and less food at meals during the week.
   - Holy days or religious holidays influence food choices for almost all cultures.

Socioeconomic Factors

Low income is a major problem in the United States, and is often described as having created a culture of poverty. Recent statistics noted that the number of poor—32.9 million—increased by 1.3 million from 2000 to 2001 (Poverty in the United States, 2002). There has been much debate about how to define poverty. In terms of economics, a person or family whose income falls below the poverty line is considered poor. The US Bureau of the Census defines poverty by using a set of money/income guidelines that vary by family size and composition. If the family's total income is less than that family's threshold, the family, as well as each member of that family, is considered poor. Others have stated that poverty is a relative term that reflects a judgment on the basis of community standards. Such standards vary at different times and in different places; what is judged poverty in one community might be regarded as wealth in another (Spector, 2000). No matter how poverty is defined, it is an increasingly devastating epidemic that has evolved into a culture of its own. At highest risk are children, older people, families headed by single mothers, and future generations of those now living in poverty. The amount of money a person or family has affects how they meet their basic needs and maintain their health. Poverty leads to other problems, such as lack of health insurance, care of infants and children, and homelessness. All these areas are of concern to nursing.

The feminization of poverty threatens to increase the number of people who are living at poverty level. The number of female-headed households is increasing as a result of divorce, abandonment, unmarried motherhood, and changes in abortion laws. Because it is now common in many households that two incomes are required for economic survival, a single woman supporting a household is at a financial disadvantage. The number of single-parent families headed by women is associated closely with the increasing number of children living in poverty and the number of homeless families with children.

The expanding population of older people has also raised problems associated with poverty. Many older people live on fixed incomes that often do not keep up with inflation, and many (particularly widows) are on the borderline of poverty or have already slipped below the poverty level. Socioeconomic status often differs by the cultural group of the older adult. For example, Pacific/Asian, African American, Native American, and Hispanic elders generally have lower incomes than do elders in the Anglo-American majority population. The work history of the cultural group, especially those who have worked all their lives as agricultural workers, often means an individual has no Social Security or Medicare benefits.

In some cases, the culture of poverty is passed from generation to generation. This appears to be especially true in such groups as migrant farm workers, families living on welfare, and people who live in isolated areas of Appalachia. Poverty cultures have the following characteristics:

- Feelings of despair, resignation, and fatalism
- Day-to-day attitude toward life, with no hope for the future
- Unemployment and need for financial or government aid
- Unstable family structure, possibly characterized by abusiveness and abandonment
- Decline in self-respect and retreat from community involvement

Poverty has long been a barrier to adequate healthcare. It prevents many people from consistently meeting their basic human needs. The lack of affordable or adequate housing is a problem experienced frequently by poor people. When low-income housing is available, it sometimes lacks such necessities as running water, heat, and electricity. To stretch their available money and to pool resources, many poor people live in crowded conditions, with several families living together in one household.

Research has demonstrated that crowded living conditions foster depersonalization, correlate with higher crime rates, and lead to psychological problems, such as schizophrenia, alienation, and feelings of worthlessness (Spector, 2000). Such conditions also contribute to an increased incidence of disease and illness because of the proximity of people, the sharing of utensils and belongings, poor sanitation, and poor health habits. The health effects of such conditions include a higher incidence and severity of illness in poor people than in people of higher income groups.

Accessing healthcare facilities frequently requires transportation, which many times is neither affordable nor available to poor people. Their access to health insurance also is frequently limited, and commonly they must choose between purchasing food and purchasing healthcare. Those in upper-income groups tend to live longer and to experience less disability than those in lower-income groups. Other barriers to healthcare include isolation, language or communication difficulties, seasonal occupations, migration patterns, depersonalization, and institutional prejudice (Spector, 2000).

CULTURAL INFLUENCES IN ILLNESS CARE

People's values and beliefs about health, illness, and care for an illness develop as a direct result of cultural and ethnic influences. For example, in some groups, illnesses are classified as natural or unnatural. Dangerous agents, such as cold air or impurities in the air, water, or food, cause natural illnesses. Unnatural illnesses are punishments for failing to follow God's rules, resulting in evil forces or witchcraft causing physical or mental health problems.

In some cultures, the power to heal is thought to be a gift from God bestowed on certain people. People in these cultures believe that these folk or traditional healers know what is wrong with them through divine intervention and experience. A patient used to traditional healers may think of healthcare providers as incompetent because they have to ask many questions before they can treat an illness. A healer may prescribe boiled herbal tea as a treatment, and someone who is accustomed to this type of treatment may find it difficult to take pills that are not even steeped in hot water. Traditional healers speak the patient's language, often are more accessible, and are usually more understanding of the patient's cultural and personal needs.

> *Think back to Danielle Dorvall, the immigrant from Haiti asking for a folk healer. Allowing the use of a folk healer as appropriate demonstrates respect for and an understanding of the patient's cultural beliefs.*

Herbs are a common method of treatment in many cultures. In fact, many medications used today have a basis in herbs or other plant sources that have been used for centuries to cure illnesses. If a patient traditionally drinks an herbal tea to alleviate symptoms of an illness, there is no reason why both the herbal tea and prescribed medications cannot be used, as long as the tea is safe to drink and the ingredients do not interfere with or exaggerate the action of the medication.

Other types of traditional therapies include the use of cutaneous stimulation, therapeutic touch, acupuncture, and acupressure. Cutaneous stimulation by massage, vibration, heat, cold, or nerve stimulation reduces the intensity of the sensation of pain. Therapeutic touch is an intentional act that involves an energy transfer from the healer to the patient to stimulate the patient's own healing potential. Acupuncture, long used in China, is a method of preventing, diagnosing, and treating pain and disease by inserting special needles into the body at specified locations. Acupressure involves a deep-pressure massage of appropriate points of the body.

CULTURALLY COMPETENT NURSING CARE

Providing culturally competent nursing care means that care is planned and implemented in a way that is sensitive to the needs of individuals, families, and groups from diverse cultural populations within society. The nurse who recognizes and respects cultural diversity has cultural sensitivity and provides nursing care that accepts the significance of cultural factors in health and illness. See Examples of NANDA Nursing Diagnoses. To provide culturally competent care, the nurse must be aware that the healthcare system itself is a culture and that cultural imposition and ethnocentrism must be avoided.

The healthcare system is a culture with customs, rules, values, and a language of its own. As you progress through your education, you will be acculturated into the culture of the healthcare system and will develop values related to health and healthcare. Many of the customs and rules are typical of the society in which we live; for example, cleanliness and punctuality are valued behaviors. Box 3-2 lists some common cultural norms of the healthcare system.

Nursing is the largest subculture of the healthcare system. Most nurses are members of, and have the same value systems as, the dominant middle class in the US. According to Andrews and Boyle (2002b), the typical American nurse is "white, middle-class, Anglo-Saxon, Protestant, female, and socialized into a subculture labeled 'healthcare professional, subdivision nurse' " (p. 37). When the nurse, with a particular set of cultural values about health, interacts with a patient who has his or her own particular set of cultural values about health, the following factors affect this interaction:

- The cultural background of each participant
- The expectations and beliefs of each about healthcare
- The cultural context of the encounter (eg, hospital, clinic, home)
- The degree of agreement between the two persons' sets of beliefs and values (Andrews & Boyle, 2002b)

Cultural imposition is the tendency for health personnel to impose their beliefs, practices, and values on people of other cultures because they believe that their ideas are superior to those of another person or group. When health professionals assume that they have the right to make choices and decisions for patients, patients respond in the same way that minority cultures often respond to an attitude by the dominant culture: by becoming passive, resistive, angry, or resistant to treatment.

Examples of NANDA Nursing Diagnoses | Cultural Diversity

The following nursing diagnoses are examples of those that might be appropriate for providing culturally competent care:

- Impaired Verbal Communication related to inability to speak English and interpreter unavailable
- Impaired Social Interaction related to recent move away from neighborhood and friends of same ethnic group
- Impaired Parenting related to use of culturally based discipline considered inappropriate or abusive by current country of residence

- Spiritual Distress related to inability to take part in significant culturally based rituals regularly
- Family Coping: Potential for Growth related to request for information about child care
- Ineffective Management of Therapeutic Regimen (Individual) related to mistrust of traditional healthcare personnel
- Low Self-Esteem related to language difficulties and inability to secure employment
- Powerlessness related to inability to make healthcare providers understand the importance of dietary and social values and beliefs

BOX 3-2 Cultural Norms of the Healthcare System

Beliefs
- Standardized definitions of health and illness
- Omnipotence of technology

Practices
- Maintenance of health and prevention of illness
- Annual physical examinations and diagnostic procedures

Habits
- Documentation
- Frequent use of jargon
- Use of a systematic approach and problem-solving methodology

Likes
- Promptness
- Neatness and organization
- Compliance

Dislikes
- Tardiness
- Disorderliness and disorganization

Customs
- Professional deference and adherence to the pecking order found in autocratic and bureaucratic systems
- Use of certain procedures attending birth and death

Closely related to cultural imposition is **ethnocentrism,** the belief that one's own ideas, beliefs, and practices are the best, are superior, or are most preferred to those of others (Leininger & McFarland, 2002). To avoid this practice, the nurse must carefully and critically examine his or her own values and beliefs and be willing to understand health and illness from the viewpoint of the patient receiving care.

Nursing care can become complicated when the patient and the nurse have distinctly different cultural norms. The nurse's role is to understand the patient's needs and to adapt care to meet those needs.

> *Think back to Mr. Hakim, the man described in the Reflective Practice display. With an understanding of Muslim culture, the nurse would ensure that adequate female staff is available to provide care for Mr. Hakim's wife.*

Unless the nurse is willing to examine carefully and clarify his or her own attitudes and values and to be sensitive to others who are "different," the use of cultural concepts to provide care will be unsuccessful.

Sometimes a nurse is placed in a cultural bind: the nurse's cultural upbringing influences values and beliefs, and the nurse is expected to adopt the customs of the nursing profession and at the same time accommodate the folkways and norms of individual patients. A careful merging of modern and traditional cultural beliefs is a necessary prerequisite for safe, considerate, and successful nursing care of all patients.

Cultural Assessment

When caring for patients who are from a different culture than the nurse, it is important to first ask the patients how they want to be treated based on their cultural values and beliefs. An effective way to identify specific factors that influence a patient's behavior is to perform a cultural assessment. The primary informant should be the patient, if possible. If the patient is not able to respond to the questions, a family member or a friend can be consulted.

The nurse can anticipate a patient's values, religion, dietary practices, family lines of authority, family life patterns, and beliefs and practices related to health and illness. The nurse can obtain this information through research before initiating contact with the patient, with the reminder that information about any culture is general, and that the nurse must individualize this information for the specific patient once interaction begins. One part of the Andrews and Boyle Transcultural Nursing Assessment Guide (2002B) is illustrated in Box 3-3.

Guidelines for Nursing Care

Cultural competence is a process in which "the nurse continuously strives to achieve the ability and availability to effectively work within the cultural context of an individual, family or community" (Campinha-Bacote, 1998, p. 6). Cultural competence takes time. It involves developing awareness, acquiring knowledge, and practicing skills. As defined by Campinha-Bacote (2003), the nurses should answer the following questions when caring for culturally diverse patients:

- Am I aware of my personal biases and prejudices towards cultural groups different from mine?
- Do I have the skill to conduct a cultural assessment in a sensitive manner?
- Do I have knowledge of the patient's worldview?
- How many encounters have I had with patients from diverse cultural backgrounds?
- What is my genuine desire to be culturally competent?

Box 3-4 lists health practices of selected diverse cultures to illustrate similarities and differences. It is important to remember that these are only general guidelines and that each patient must be considered a unique individual.

When providing care to different people from different cultures, it is important to use past experiences as a guide, but never as the answer to all cultural solutions. Learn from your mistakes and do not repeat them. All nurses make mistakes at some time when caring for culturally different patients. Inadvertent mistakes are just that, but repeated mistakes are careless and disrespectful; they will adversely affect your interaction with patients and coworkers.

Another important cultural guideline is to treat each person as an individual. What was true of one person will not be true of another, even if they are from the same cultural background. The following sections provide additional guidelines that are useful in providing appropriate nursing care.

(text continues on page 53)

BOX 3-3 Transcultural Assessment: Health-Related Beliefs and Practices

1. To what cause(s) does the patient attribute illness and disease (eg, divine wrath, imbalance in hot/cold or yin/yang, punishment for moral transgressions, hex, soul loss, pathogenic organism)?
2. What are the patient's cultural beliefs about the ideal body size and shape? What is the patient's self-image compared to the ideal?
3. What name does the patient give to his or her health-related condition?
4. What does the patient believe promotes health (eating certain foods; wearing amulets to bring good luck; sleep; rest; good nutrition; reducing stress; exercise; prayer; rituals to ancestors, saints, or intermediate deities)?
5. What is the patient's religious affiliation (eg, Judaism, Islam, Pentacostalism, West African voodooism, Seventh-Day Adventism, Catholicism, Mormonism)? How actively involved in the practice of this religion is the patient?
6. Does the patient rely on cultural healers (eg, curandero, shaman, spiritualist, priest, minister, monk)? Who determines when the patient is sick and when the patient is healthy? Who influences the choice/type of healer and treatment that should be sought?
7. In what types of cultural healing practices does the patient engage (use of herbal remedies, potions, massage; wearing of talismans, copper bracelets, or charms to discourage evil spirits; healing rituals, incantations, prayers)?
8. How are biomedical/scientific healthcare providers perceived? How does the patient and his or her family perceive nurses? What are the expectations of nurses and nursing care?
9. What comprises appropriate "sick role" behavior? Who determines what symptoms constitute disease/illness? Who decides when the patient is no longer sick? Who cares for the patient at home?
10. How does the patient's cultural group view mental disorders? Are there differences in acceptable behaviors for physical versus psychological illnesses?

From Andrews, M., & Boyle, J. (2002b). *Transcultural concepts in nursing care* (4th ed.). Philadelphia: Lippincott Williams & Wilkins.

BOX 3-4 Cultural Factors That Affect Nursing Care

White Middle Class

Family
- Nuclear family is highly valued.
- Elderly family members may live in a nursing home when they can no longer care for themselves.

Folk and Traditional Healthcare
- Self-diagnosis of illnesses
- Use of over-the-counter drugs (especially vitamins and analgesics)
- Dieting (especially fad diets)
- Extensive use of exercise and exercise facilities

Values and Beliefs
- Youth is valued over age
- Cleanliness
- Orderliness
- Attractiveness
- Individualism
- Achievement
- Punctuality

Common Health Problems
- Cardiovascular diseases
- Gastrointestinal diseases
- Some forms of cancer
- Motor vehicle accidents
- Suicides
- Mental illness
- Chemical abuses

Nursing Considerations
- Careful assessment of client's use of over-the-counter medications (observe for signs and symptoms of toxic medication levels, especially fat-soluble vitamins)
- Nutritional assessments of dietary habits

African American

Family
- Close and supportive extended-family relationships
- Strong kinship ties with nonblood relatives from church or organizational and social groups
- Family unity, loyalty, and cooperation are important.
- Usually matriarchal

Folk and Traditional Healthcare
- Varies extensively and may include spiritualists, herb doctors, root doctors, conjurers, skilled elder family members, voodoo, faith healing

Values and Beliefs
- Present oriented
- Members of the African American clergy are highly respected in the black community.
- Frequently highly religious

Common Health Problems
- Hypertension (precise cause unknown, may be related to diet)
- Sickle cell anemia

(continued)

BOX 3-4 (Continued)

- Skin disorders; inflammation of hair follicles, various types of dermatitis and excessive growth of scar tissue (keloids)
- Lactose enzyme deficiency, resulting in poor toleration of milk products
- Higher rate of tuberculosis
- Diabetes mellitus
- Higher infant mortality rate than in the white population

Nursing Considerations

- Many African American families may still use various folk healing practices and home remedies for treating particular illnesses.
- Special care may be necessary for the hair and skin.
- Special consideration should be given to the sometimes extensive and frequently informal support networks of patients (ie, religious and community group members who offer assistance in a time of need).

Asian

(Beliefs and practices vary, but most Asian cultures share some characteristics.)

Family

- Welfare of the family is valued above the person.
- Extended families are common.
- A person's lineage (ancestors) is respected.
- Sharing among family members is expected.

Folk and Traditional Healthcare

- Theoretical basis is in Taoism, which seeks a balance in all things.
- Good health is achieved through the proper balance of yin (feminine, negative, dark, cold) and yang (masculine, positive, light, warm).
- An imbalance in energy is caused by an improper diet or strong emotions.
- Diseases and foods are classified as hot or cold, and a proper balance between them will promote wellness (eg, treat a cold disease with hot foods).
- Many Asian healthcare systems use herbs, diet, and the application of hot or cold therapy. Also, many Asians believe that there are points on the body that are located on the meridians or energy pathways. If the energy flow is out of balance, treatment of the pathways may be necessary to restore the energy equilibrium.

  Acumassage—Technique of manipulating points along the energy pathways

  Acupressure—Technique for compressing the energy pathway points

  Acupuncture—Technique by which fine needles are inserted into the body at energy pathway points

Values and Beliefs

- Strong sense of self-respect and self-control
- High respect for age
- Respect for authority
- Respect for hard work
- Praise of self or others is considered poor manners
- Strong emphasis on harmony and the avoidance of conflict

Common Health Problems

- Tuberculosis
- Communicable diseases
- Malnutrition
- Suicide
- Various forms of mental illness
- Lactose enzyme deficiency

Nursing Considerations

- Some members of Asian cultures may be upset by the drawing of blood for laboratory tests. They consider blood to be the body's life force, and some do not believe that it can be regenerated.
- Some members believe that it is best to die with the body intact, so they may refuse surgery except in dire circumstances.
- Members of many Asian cultures seldom complain about what is bothering them. Therefore, the nurse must carefully assess the patient for pain or discomfort by observing for nonverbal signs of discomfort, such as facial grimacing or wincing and holding of the painful area.
- Some Asians consider it polite to give a person the responses the person is expecting. Therefore, misinformation may be transmitted to the questioner in an effort, on the client's part, to be respectful.
- Some members may move from physician to physician in an attempt to be cured of an illness, but to avoid insulting or embarrassing a physician, they will not inform him or her that they are going to another physician. This can result in confusion, inaccuracies, and overmedication.
- Some Asians may refuse to have diagnostic studies done because they believe that a skilled and competent physician can diagnose an illness solely through a physical examination.
- Some members may have a difficult time understanding the importance of taking a regimen of medications because many of their folk treatments involve the ingestion of one dose of herbal mixtures.
- Dietary counseling may be necessary if the patient is on a salt-restricted diet because many Asian foods have a high salt content related to the use of soy sauce.

Hispanic

Family

- Familial role is important.
- *Compadrazgo:* special bond between a child's parents and his or her grandparents
- Family is the primary unit of society.

Folk and Traditional Healthcare

- *Curanderas(os):* frequently folk healers who base treatments on humoral pathology—basic functions of the body are controlled by four body fluids or "humors":

  Blood—hot and wet

  Yellow bile—hot and dry

  Black bile—cold and dry

  Phlegm—cold and wet

- The secret of good health is to balance hot and cold within the body; therefore, most foods, beverages, herbs, and medications are classified as hot (*caliente*) or cold (*fresco, frío*) (a cold disease will be cured with a hot treatment).

Values and Beliefs

- Respect is given according to age (older) and sex (male).
- Roman Catholic Church may be very influential.

(continued)

BOX 3-4 (Continued)

- God gives health and allows illness for a reason; therefore, may perceive illness as a punishment from God. An illness of this type can be cured through atonement and forgiveness.

Common Health Problems
- Diabetes mellitus and its complications
- Poverty and resultant problems, such as poor nutrition, inadequate medical care, poor prenatal care
- Lactose enzyme deficiency

Nursing Considerations
- It may be difficult to convince an asymptomatic patient that he or she is ill.
- Special diet considerations are necessary if the patient believes in the hot/cold theory of treating illnesses.
- Diet counseling may be necessary at times because many members have a normal diet that is high in starch.

Puerto Rican
(Since the Jones Act of 1917, all Puerto Ricans are American citizens.)
Family
- *Compadrazgo*—same as in Hispanic culture

Folk and Traditional Healthcare
- Similar to that of other Spanish-speaking cultures

Common Health Problems
- Parasitic diseases, such as dysentery, malaria, filariasis, and hookworms
- Lactose enzyme deficiency

Values and Beliefs
- Place a high value on safeguarding against group pressure to violate a person's integrity (may be difficult for Puerto Ricans to accept teamwork)
- Close-mouthed about personal and family affairs (psychotherapy may be difficult to achieve at times because of this belief)
- Proper consideration should be given to cultural rituals such as shaking hands and standing up to greet and say goodbye to people.
- Time is a relative phenomenon; little attention is given to the exact time of day.
- *Ataques*—culturally acceptable reaction to situations of extreme stress, characterized by hyperkinetic seizure activity

Nursing Considerations
- It may be difficult to teach Puerto Rican patients to follow time-oriented actions (eg, taking medications, keeping appointments).

Native American
(Each tribe's beliefs and practices vary to some degree.)
Family
- Families are large and extended.
- Grandparents are official and symbolic leaders and decision makers.
- A child's namesake may become the same as another parent to the child.

Folk and Traditional Healthcare
- Medicine men (*shaman*) are heavily used.
- Heavy use of herbs and psychological treatments, ceremonies, fasting, meditation, heat, and massages

Common Health Problems
- Alcoholism
- Suicide
- Tuberculosis
- Malnutrition
- Communicable diseases
- Higher maternal and infant mortality rates than in most of the population
- Diabetes mellitus
- Hypertension
- Gallbladder disease

Values and Beliefs
- Present oriented. Taught to live in the present and not to be concerned about the future. This time consciousness emphasizes finishing current business before doing something else.
- High respect for age
- Great value is placed on working together and sharing resources.
- Failure to achieve a personal goal frequently is believed to be the result of competition.
- High respect is given to a person who gives to others. The accumulation of money and goods often is frowned on.
- Some Native Americans practice the Peyotist religion, in which the consumption of peyote, an intoxicating drug derived from mescal cacti, is part of the service. Peyote is legal if used for this purpose. It is classified as a hallucinogenic drug.

Nursing Considerations
- The family is expected to be part of the nursing care plan.
- Note-taking often is taboo. It is considered an insult to the speaker because the listener is not paying full attention to the conversation. Good memory skills often are required by the nurse.
- Indirect eye contact is acceptable and sometimes preferred.
- It often is considered rude or impolite to indicate that a conversation has not been heard.
- A low tone of voice often is considered respectful.
- A Native American patient may expect the caregiver to deduce the problem through instinct and not through asking many questions and history taking. If this is the case, it may help to use declarative sentences rather than direct questioning.

Hawaiian
Family
- Familial role is important.
- *Ohana*, or extended families, are jointly involved in childrearing.
- Hierarchy of family structure, each gender and age have specific duties
- Closely knit families in small, isolated communities

Folk and Traditional Healthcare
- *Kahuna La'au Lapa'nu* is the ancient Hawaiian medical practitioner.
- View patient's illness as part of the whole.
- Relationships between the physical, psychological, and spiritual
- Emphasis on preventive medicine

(continued)

BOX 3-4 (Continued)

- Treatment uses more than 300 medicinal plants and minerals

Values and Beliefs
- Aloha: a deep love, respect, and affection between people and the land
- Respect given to people and land
- Christian gods replaced the myriad of Hawaiian gods.
- Lifestyle more revered than compliance with healthcare issues
- Present oriented, less initiative and drive rather than direction and achievement
- Death seen as part of life and not feared

Common Health Problems
- Diabetes mellitus and its complications
- Hypertension (unknown cause; perhaps related to diet)
- Gout (perhaps related to diet)
- Respiratory disorders: asthma, allergies, tuberculosis
- Skin disorders: bacterial, fungal, cancer
- Obesity
- Smoking, alcoholism, drug abuse

Nursing Considerations
- Many Hawaiians may still use folk healing practices and home remedies.
- Special consideration given to the extensive family network during hospitalization
- Acceptance from healthcare practitioners of current health practices and lifestyle

Appalachian

Family
- Intense interpersonal relations
- Family is cohesive, and several generations often live close to each other.

- Elderly are respected as providers.
- Tend to live in rural, isolated areas

Folk and Traditional Healthcare
- "Granny" woman, or folk healer, provides care and may be consulted even if receiving traditional care.
- Various herbs, such as foxglove and yellow root, are used for common illnesses, such as malaise, chest discomfort, heart problems, and upper respiratory infections.
- Elderly may have had only limited contact with healthcare providers and be skeptical of modern healthcare.

Values and Beliefs
- Independence and self-determination
- Isolation is accepted as a way of life.
- Person-oriented
- May be fatalistic about losses and death
- Belief in a divine existence rather than attending a particular church

Common Health Problems
- Cardiovascular disorders
- Respiratory disorders
- Nutritional disorders
- Smoking, alcoholism

Nursing Considerations
- Treat each person with regard for personal dignity.
- Allow family members to remain with patient as support system
- Acceptance from healthcare providers of current health practices and lifestyle
- Allow patients to make decisions about care.

Develop Cultural Self-Awareness

Become aware of the role of cultural influences in your own life. Objectively examine your own beliefs, values, practices, and family experiences. As you become more sensitive to the importance of these factors, you will also become more sensitive to cultural influences in others' lives. Identify biases in your own life. How do they affect your feelings about others? How could they affect your nursing care of others?

Develop Cultural Knowledge

Learn as much as possible about the belief system and practices of people in your community and of patients in the area in which you work. Practice techniques of observation and listening to acquire knowledge of the beliefs and values of patients for whom you are caring. Some people, especially those of minority cultures, may have been belittled and subjected to ridicule and may be hesitant to discuss their beliefs and practices. Approach this topic with patients carefully. If you are motivated by sincerity, respect, and concern, your attitude will convey this, and most patients will respond positively. On the other hand, if you are motivated by curiosity and have a condescending attitude, most patients will respond negatively.

Accommodate Cultural Practices in Healthcare

Incorporate factors from the patient's cultural background into healthcare whenever possible and when the practices are not considered harmful to health. To ignore or contradict the patient's background may result in the patient refusing care or failing to follow prescribed therapy. Modify care to include traditional practices and practitioners as much as possible, and be an advocate for patients from diverse cultural groups.

Accommodate the cultural dietary practices of patients as much as possible. Dietary departments in many hospitals and long-term care facilities can supply patients with meals that are consistent with special dietary practices. Families may be encouraged to bring food from home for patients with particular preferences when this practice does not violate policy. Teaching patients and families about therapeutic diets can also be done within the framework of particular cultural practices.

Respect Culturally Based Family Roles

Take into consideration the cultural role of the family member who makes most of the important decisions. In some cultures, it is the husband or father, whereas in others, it is the grandmother or another respected elder. To disregard this fact or to proceed with nursing care that is not approved by this person can result in conflict or in disregard for what has been taught. Be careful to involve this person in the nursing care planning.

Avoid Mandating Change

Keep in mind that health practices are part of the overall culture and that changing them may have widespread implications for the person. You need to provide the necessary support and reinforcement for the patient if a change in a health practice with a cultural basis is considered necessary.

Do not force the patient to participate in care that conflicts with his or her values. If the patient is forced to accept it, the care may become harmful because resulting feelings of guilt and alienation from a religious or cultural group are likely to threaten the patient's well-being.

Seek Cultural Assistance

Seek assistance of a respected family member, member of the clergy, or traditional healer, as indicated, so that the patient is more likely to accept healthcare services. Acknowledging the role of the person's traditional healer can be an important way of building trust. If invited, folk medicine practitioners can work closely with professional health practitioners in the interest of the patient and family. Such efforts promote mutual understanding, respect, and cooperation.

■ Developing Critical Thinking Skills

1. Analyze the following situations, identifying potential sources of cultural imposition:
   - A young Ethiopian woman with terminal breast cancer requests that all treatment decisions be made by her uncle, who is the family elder. Her primary nurse is an active feminist.
   - A Native American woman refuses a life-saving amputation of her leg because she believes it is essential to enter the next world "whole."
2. Interview family members or friends who have recently received healthcare, such as for a health screening, diagnostic testing, emergency care, routine checkup, office/clinic visit, or hospitalization. What aspects of the healthcare culture were most distressing to them? What factors were most helpful? Do their answers vary according to the setting for care? If so, why do you think they felt as they did?

■ Practicing for NCLEX

1. Which of the following phrases best defines culture?
   a. A dominant group within a society
   b. A shared system of beliefs, values, and behaviors
   c. One's values are replaced by the values of the dominant culture.
   d. Categories are based on specific physical characteristics.

2. Minority groups living within a dominant culture may lose the cultural characteristics that made them different. This process is called:
   a. Cultural diversity
   b. Cultural imposition
   c. Cultural assimilation
   d. Ethnocentrism
3. The sense of identification with a collective cultural group is defined as:
   a. Ethnicity
   b. Race
   c. Cultural acquisition
   d. Culture shock
4. When one assumes that all older adults are too old to learn, what is being done?
   a. Cultural imposition
   b. Clustering
   c. Cultural competency
   d. Stereotyping
5. A young Hispanic mother comes to the local clinic because her baby is sick. She speaks only Spanish and you speak only English What would you do?
   a. Use short words and talk more loudly.
   b. Ask an interpreter to help you.
   c. Tell your instructor you can't care for her.
   d. Give her instructions in writing.
6. Which of the following questions would be considered culturally sensitive in regard to food preferences for a hospitalized patient?
   a. "Do you think you will be able to eat the food we have here?"
   b. "Do you understand that we can't prepare special meals?"
   c. "What types of food do you eat for meals?"
   d. "Why can't you just eat our food while you are here?"
7. What group is the largest subculture of the healthcare system?
   a. Nurses
   b. Physicians
   c. Social workers
   d. Physical therapists
8. Healthcare providers often believe their beliefs and practices are superior to those of the patient. What is this practice called?
   a. Cultural assimilation
   b. Racism
   c. Ethnocentrism
   d. Stereotyping
9. How can the nurse gain knowledge of a specific culture before actually assessing and caring for a patient of that culture?
   a. Talk to coworkers
   b. Review literature
   c. Talk to family members of the patient
   d. Ask others with more experience for help

10. Although all of the following are important to culturally competent nursing care, which one is most basic?
    a. Learning another language
    b. Having significant information
    c. Treating each person as an individual
    d. Recognizing the importance of family

■ Answers With Rationale

1. The correct response is *b*. Culture may be defined as a shared system of beliefs, values, and behavioral expectations that provide social structure for daily living.
2. The correct response is *c*. When minority groups live within a dominant group, many members lose the cultural characteristics that once made them different.
3. The correct response is *a*. Ethnicity is the sense of identification with a collective cultural group, largely based on the group's common heritage.
4. The correct response is *d*. Stereotyping is assuming that all members of a group are alike.
5. The correct response is *b*. Many agencies have a qualified interpreter who understands the healthcare system and can reliably provide assistance.
6. The correct response is *c*. Asking patients what types of foods they eat for meals is culturally sensitive.
7. The correct response is *a*. Nurses are the largest subculture of the healthcare system.
8. The correct response is *c*. Ethnocentrism occurs when one believes that one's own ideas and practices are superior to those of others.
9. The correct response is *b*. Reviewing the literature about a specific culture can provide the nurse with information about cultural values, dietary practices, family lines of authority, and health and illness beliefs and practices.
10. The correct response is *c*. In all aspects of nursing, it is important to treat each patient as an individual. This is also true in providing culturally competent care.

Bibliography

American Nurses Association. (1998). *Position statement on discrimination and racism in health care.* Available at http://nursingworld.org/readroom/position/ethics/etdisrac.htm.

American Nurses Association. (1998). *Position statement on cultural diversity in nursing practice.* Available at http://nursingworld.org/readroom/position/ethics/etcldv.htm.

Andrews, M. M., & Boyle, J. S. (2002a). Transcultural concepts in nursing care. *Journal of Transcultural Nursing, 13*(3), 178–180.

Andrews, M. M., & Boyle, J. S. (2002b). *Transcultural concepts in nursing care* (4th ed.). Philadelphia: Lippincott Williams & Wilkins.

Campinha-Bacote, J. (1998). *The process of cultural competence in the delivery of healthcare services: A culturally competent model of care* (3rd ed.). Cincinnati, OH: Transcultural C.A.R.E. Associates.

Campinha-Bacote, J. (2003). Many faces: Addressing diversity in health care. *Online Journal of Issues in Nursing, 8*(1), Manuscript 2. Available at http://nursingworld.org/ojin/topic20/tpc20_2.htm.

Clark, C., & Robinson, T. (2000). Multiculturalism as a concept in nursing. *Journal of the Black Nurses Association, 11*(2), 39–43.

D'Avanzo, C. E., & Geissler, E. M. (2003). *Cultural health assessment* (3rd ed.). St. Louis: Mosby.

Hagey, R., Choudry, U., Guruge, S., et al. (2001). Immigrant nurses' experience of racism. *Journal of Nursing Scholarship, 33*(4), 389–394.

Henderson, G., & Primeaux, M. (1981). *Transcultural health care.* Menlo Park, CA: Addison-Wesley.

Leininger, M., & McFarland, M. (2002). *Transcultural nursing: Concepts, theories, research and practice* (3rd ed.). New York: McGraw-Hill.

Leonard, B. J. (2001). Quality nursing care celebrates diversity. *Online Journal of Issues in Nursing, 6*(2). Manuscript 3. Available at http://www.nursingworld.org/ojin/topic15/tpc15_3.htm.

Lipson, J., Dibble, S., & Minarik, P. (Eds.). (1996). *Culture & nursing care: A pocket guide.* San Francisco: UCSF Press.

Lowe, J., & Struthers, R. (2001). A conceptual framework of nursing in Native American culture. *Journal of Nursing Scholarship, 33*(3), 279–283.

Miller, A., & Chandler, P. (2002). Acculturation, resilience, and depression in midlife women from the former Soviet Union. *Nursing Research, 51*(1), 26–32.

Spector, R. E. (2000). *Cultural diversity in health and illness* (5th ed.). Upper Saddle River, NJ: Prentice Hall.

Steefel, L. (2002). Treat pain in any culture. *Nursing Spectrum (New England Edition), 6*(5), 8–9.

U.S. Census Bureau. (2002). *Poverty in the United States: 2001.* Washington, DC: U.S. Department of Commerce.

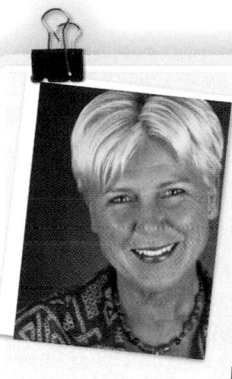

Ruth Jacobi is a 62-year-old woman who was hospitalized after a "mini-stroke." She has now returned to her pre-event level of functioning and is being prepared for discharge. She states "I know that I have an increased risk for a major stroke, so I want to do everything possible to stay as active and as healthy as I possibly can."

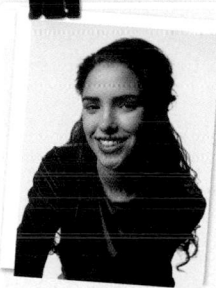

Sara Gelbart, a college freshman, is encouraged to visit the student health center by her roommate because she rarely visits the dining hall for meals, runs 5 to 8 miles a day, and has recently lost a significant amount of weight. Sara states "I'm plenty healthy, just a bit 'nuts' about being fit!"

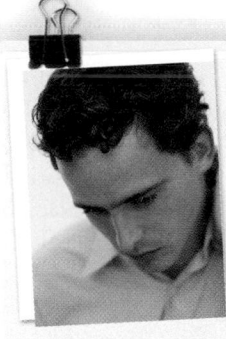

Daniel Sternman is a 27-year-old man with history of schizophrenia. He comes to the mental health clinic, loudly demanding relief from the voices who are telling him to hurt himself. Mr. Sternman is well known by the clinic staff. His medical record reveals that he has had numerous visits to the clinic, and also that he has difficulty interacting and dealing with various staff members.

Focusing on Blended Skills

The types of blended skills you'll need to respond to the case scenarios here include:

Cognitive Skills

- Knowledge of definitions of health, disease, and illness; models of health and illness; and factors influencing health and illness
- Knowledge of risk factors associated with health and illness
- Ability to identify ways to modify lifestyles to promote health and prevent disease
- Knowledge of how to implement competently a plan of nursing care for the woman with the mini-stroke, the man with schizophrenia, and a young adult with an eating disorder
- Ability to differentiate acute and chronic illness; knowledge of the stages of acute illness
- Ability to integrate knowledge of the effects of illness on the family when providing care to the individual

Technical Skills

- Strong assessment skills related to health, factors affecting health and illness, and alterations in health that can lead to illness
- Ability to provide the technical nursing assistance necessary to meet the needs of the woman with the mini-stroke, the man with schizophrenia, and the young adult with an eating disorder
- Ability to adapt measures to provide care to individuals experiencing acute and chronic illness
- Ability to perform nursing care safely based on sound scientific rationales
- Ability to demonstrate competent use of teaching skills to promote healthy lifestyles

Interpersonal Skills

- Ability to establish caring relationships with individuals experiencing various levels of health and illness, such as the woman with the mini-stroke, the man with schizophrenia, and the young adult woman with an eating disorder
- Ability to work collaboratively with the interdisciplinary team
- Ability to assess health-related beliefs, goals, and practices
- Ability to demonstrate respect for the patient's human dignity and autonomy
- Ability to communicate concern about a patient's status; for example, a patient with schizophrenia who is considered to be a difficult patient or a young adult woman who is unwilling to talk about her nutritional health and eating habits

Ethical and Legal Skills

- Strong commitment to self-care, demonstrating the ability to balance responsibilities to self with care demands of others
- Demonstration of a strong sense of accountability for the health and well-being of patients, which translates into a commitment to getting patients the help that they need to achieve their health goals; demonstration of accountability for all actions performed, including the ability to practice nursing in an ethically and legally defensible manner consistent with the nursing code of ethics and within the scope of legal practice
- Ability to participate as a trusted and effective patient advocate, including a commitment to securing the best possible care for the patients and families assigned to your care
- Ability to mobilize the appropriate mental health services for the man with schizophrenia or a young adult with an eating disorder
- Knowledge of the nurse's legal responsibilities when providing care, including caring for patients with physical and mental illnesses

Learning Outcomes

After completing the chapter, the learner should be able to accomplish the following:

1. Define health, illness, and wellness.
2. Compare and contrast acute illness and chronic illness.
3. Describe how the human dimensions, basic human needs, and self-concept influence health and illness.
4. Summarize the role of the nurse in promoting health and preventing illness.
5. Describe the levels of preventive care.

Key Terms

acute illness
chronic illness
disease
exacerbation
health
illness
remission
risk factor
wellness

The primary roles of the nurse as caregiver are to promote health, to prevent illness, to restore health, and to facilitate coping. These activities help maximize the health of patients of all ages, in all settings, and in both health and illness. Health is more than just the absence of illness; it is an active process in which an individual moves toward wellness by reaching his or her maximum potential. (See the accompanying Reflective Practice box for an example.) This chapter discusses how nursing care is influenced by the patient—the person receiving care. To give holistic care, the nurse must understand and respect each person's individual definition of health and responses to illness and should be familiar with models of health and illness. In addition, the nurse must be familiar with factors affecting health and illness. One's health is influenced by a variety of factors, including risk factors for illness, the human dimensions, how well one's basic human needs are met, and the person's self-concept. Finally, the nurse needs to understand how to provide nursing care to promote health

and prevent illness. The nurse's knowledge of health and illness, as well as a philosophy of health, is even more important because of the continuing trend toward care being provided in the home and community, the increasing numbers of older adults, and the growing incidence of chronic illnesses.

DEFINING HEALTH AND ILLNESS

Meguni Kuni, 4 years old, was born with cystic fibrosis. Although she requires ongoing treatment for this illness, she is now an active member of her preschool class, takes gymnastics lessons, and wants to be a doctor when she grows up. Shondra Cole, 34 years old, is married and has two school-aged children. She has chronic rheumatoid arthritis and is in a wheelchair. Shondra takes care of her house and family and uses a specially designed car to get to her part-time job. Samuel Cohen is

Reflective Practice
Challenge to Intellectual Skills

My first college roommate, Sara Gelbart, seemed the ideal roommate when I first met her. A good student, she was thoughtful, outgoing, and fun. By October, however, I was really worried about her. I noticed that she rarely wanted to come to the dining hall with our group of friends. When she did come, she just seemed to pick at her food. She also spent a lot of time at the athletic center, running 5 to 8 miles almost daily. I wasn't surprised when she started losing significant amounts of weight. What worried me was her lack of willingness to talk about her nutritional habits and health. She told me that she was plenty healthy, just a bit "nuts" about being fit! She also kidded that I'd be healthier if I worked out more often with her. While she was certainly right about that, I was worried that she had a serious eating disorder and wasn't sure what I could do to help. She politely told me to "mind my own business" when I asked her if she had ever spoken with anyone about her health and eating.

Thinking Outside the Box: Possible Courses of Action

- Respect Sara's wishes and simply try to be a good friend without continuing to confront her about her nutritional status.
- Tell Sara I am concerned that she has a serious eating disorder, and then plan the next steps with her, fully respecting her right to seek or refuse professional help.
- Tell Sara that if she fails to get professional help, I will contact her parents or a counselor at school.

Evaluating a Good Outcome: How Do I Define Success?

- Sara gets whatever help she needs to address her eating problems and regain health.
- Sara's right to make her own decisions is respected.
- My obligations as a friend are fulfilled.
- My beginning ability to identify and correctly respond to health problems affirms my choice for nursing.

Personal Learning: Here's to the Future!

Unfortunately, I did not intervene because (1) I failed to recognize how serious a problem this would become, and (2) I wasn't sure what I could do after Sara refused my initial offers of help. Sara dropped out of school at the end of our freshman year and she has not returned my calls, so I'm not sure how she is doing. I've read more about eating disorders, and I now know how important it is to get professional help early. I learned too late that Sara had been in treatment for anorexia during high school and that the pressures of college life had led to a relapse. I think I valued her friendship more than I valued getting her the help that she needed to address a serious health problem.

Reflection

How do you think you would respond in a similar situation? Why? What does this tell you about yourself and about the adequacy of your skills for professional practice? What pressures of college life might have impacted the nursing student's actions? Sara's actions? Please explain. How did the nursing student view health and illness? How did Sara view it? Can you think of other ways to respond? How might the student's and Sara's developmental level affected their responses? What other skills (cognitive, interpersonal, technical, ethical/legal) would you need to respond well in this situation? Do you agree with the criteria to evaluate a successful outcome? Are there any other criteria that could have been used? Please explain.

67 years old. He was diagnosed with type II diabetes and high blood pressure last year and takes medications for both health problems. Samuel is retired but volunteers 3 days a week in a local hospital as a transport technician. Would you define Meguni, Shondra, and Samuel as well? Although they each have a physical condition that might lead them to define themselves as being ill, they are all productive members of their society and would say they are healthy.

Health

Because **health** is individually defined by each person and is affected by so many factors, a standard definition is difficult. See the accompanying Through the Eyes of a Student. The most widely accepted definition of health is that health is a state of complete physical, mental, and social well-being, not merely the absence of disease or infirmity (World Health Organization, 1946). This definition was expanded as other models of health were developed. On a personal level, most individuals define health according to how they feel ("I feel really sick"); the absence or presence of symptoms of illness ("I have a terrible pain in my stomach"); or their ability to carry out activities of daily living ("I felt so much better that I got up and cooked supper").

Each person defines health in terms of his or her own values and beliefs. The family, community, and society in which one lives also influence one's personal perception of health.

Think back to Sara Gelbart, the college freshman who rarely eats and runs several miles almost daily. According to her statement, she considers herself to be healthy. However, her roommate is concerned because of what she views as excessive exercise and Sara's poor nutrition. The nurse needs to investigate each person's views a bit further to determine exactly what each believes to be healthy. Doing so provides a foundation on which to develop an appropriate plan of care.

Health, as defined by each person, integrates all the human dimensions—the physical, intellectual, emotional, sociocultural, spiritual, and environmental aspects of the whole person. The nurse giving holistic nursing care must equally consider all these interrelated and interdependent dimensions of the whole person (Fig. 4-1).

Illness

Illness is also defined individually by each person who experiences an alteration in health. It is also difficult to make a standard definition of illness because disease and illness are often used to mean the same process. **Disease** is a medical term, meaning that there is a pathologic change in the structure or function of the body or mind. Box 4-1 lists examples of causes of disease. An **illness** is the response of the person to a disease; it is an abnormal process in which the person's level of functioning is changed when compared with a previous level. This

Through the Eyes of a Student

Carrie was a 17-year-old brunette who attended my high school, dated my best friend Ricky, and participated in many of the same clubs and activities as me. By looking at her, I never would have guessed anything was wrong. However, once I got to know her, I learned that she was diagnosed with cancer and that the disease had spread through her heart and lungs. The situation, as doctors continually told her, did not look promising. Yet she never once let that slow her down, and she lived each day to the fullest. It was almost 1 year ago I watched this friend pass away from bone cancer. However, until the days before her last breath, in my eyes she was a happy and healthy girl. She never once let the disease get the best of her, and she fought for life every second of every day. Her constant optimism and determined smile touched and moved so many others. So you ask me, was Carrie healthy?

Health to me is a state of mind, not the physical condition of a person's body. Carrie, in my opinion, was the definition of healthy; she was happy, she lived her life to the fullest, and she continually inspired others to embrace life. The dictionary may state that health is the absence of a disease; however, for me it is the way a person thinks and reacts to life. A person's health consists of being able to work to the best of her capability, look out for herself, and her ability to respond to life enthusiastically. In my eyes, a person like Carrie can be physically unwell, but in terms of living, is healthy. Perhaps this is where heath and wellness differ in that, to me, health means the person's entire state of being and is decided by the individual, whereas wellness refers more to the physical condition of a person and is determined more readily by society. The words illness and disease also correspond with these words. I believe that illness, like health, is a matter of thinking, while disease is a medical term that relates to physical condition and wellness. All of these states are constantly changing, and I have probably experienced the best and worst of all of them. However, as I embark on this new and exciting journey of college, I consider myself extremely healthy. I am living each day to the fullest, trying to impact other people's lives, and am filled with optimism. This all may change shortly, but as I look back on Carrie's life and the effect she has had on me, I will always try to live my life in a healthy and grateful way.

—Molly Proskine, Georgetown University

response is unique for each person and is influenced by self-perceptions, others' perceptions, the effects of changes in body structure and function, the effects of those changes on roles and relationships, and cultural and spiritual values and beliefs. Always remember that a person may have a disease but still achieve maximum functioning and quality of life.

Consider Ruth Jacobi, the 62-year-old woman who is being prepared for discharge after a "mini-stroke." Although she most likely has cerebrovascular disease, she wants to stay as active and as healthy as she can. The nurse would

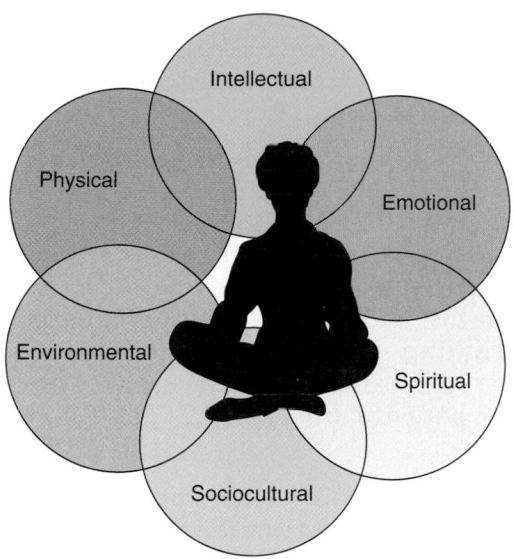

FIGURE 4-1 The human dimensions. All of these interdependent parts compose the whole person.

integrate knowledge of the disease process and work with the patient to achieve this goal.

Nurses often care for people entering the healthcare system because of an illness. Definitions of acute and chronic illness, illness behaviors, and the effects of illness on the family are discussed in this section. Physiologic and psychosocial homeostasis and adaptation to injury and illness are discussed in Chapter 32.

Illnesses are classified as either acute or chronic. A person may have an acute illness, a chronic illness, or both at the same time; for example, an adult with diabetes (a chronic illness) may also have appendicitis (an acute illness).

Acute Illness

An **acute illness** generally has a rapid onset of symptoms and lasts only a relatively short time.

Think back to Ruth Jacobi, the 62-year-old woman described at the beginning of the chapter. Her mini-stroke signaled an acute illness that required her to be hospitalized. However,

---

BOX 4-1 **Causes of Diseases**

- Inherited genetic defects
- Developmental defects resulting from exposure to such factors as virus or chemicals during pregnancy
- Biologic agents or toxins
- Physical agents such as temperature, chemicals, and radiation
- Generalized tissue responses to injury or irritation
- Physiologic and emotional reactions to stress
- Excessive or insufficient production of body secretions (hormones, enzymes, and so forth)

---

the patient has improved and is ready for discharge. The nurse would incorporate knowledge of the acuity of the situation to develop an appropriate discharge teaching plan for this patient.

Although some acute illnesses are life threatening, many do not require medical attention. If medical care is required, a specific treatment with medications (eg, antibiotics for pneumonia) or surgical procedures (eg, an appendectomy for appendicitis) usually return the person to normal functioning. With self-treatment and use of over-the-counter medications, simple acute illnesses, such as the common cold or diarrhea, do not usually require medical treatment.

When a person becomes acutely ill, certain illness behaviors may occur in identifiable stages (Suchman, 1965). These behaviors are the way people cope with alterations in function caused by the disease. Illness behaviors are unique to the individual and are influenced by age, gender, family values, economic status, culture, educational level, and mental status.

There is no specific timetable for the stages-of-illness behaviors. The stages may occur rapidly or slowly. Nursing roles throughout the stages remain constant. In all stages, the nurse accepts the patient as an individual, gives nursing care based on prioritized needs, and facilitates recovery through physical care, emotional support, and health education (Fig. 4-2).

Stage 1: Experiencing Symptoms

How do people define themselves as "sick"? The first indication of an illness usually is recognizing one or more symptoms that are incompatible with one's personal definition of health. Although pain is the most significant symptom indicating illness, other common symptoms include a rash, fever, bleeding,

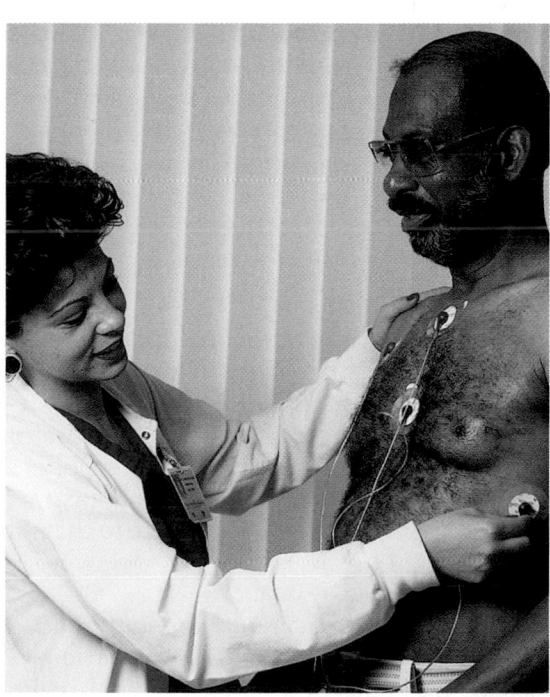

FIGURE 4-2 The nurse is assessing the patient as a basis for teaching healthy heart behaviors.

or a cough. If the symptoms last for a short time or are relieved by self-care, the person usually takes no further action. If the symptoms continue, however, the person enters the next stage.

Stage 2: Assuming the Sick Role

The person now defines himself or herself as being sick, seeks validation of this experience from others, gives up normal activities, and assumes a "sick role." At this stage, most people focus on their symptoms and bodily functions. Depending on individual health beliefs and practices, the person may choose to do nothing, may buy over-the-counter medications to relieve symptoms, or may seek out a healthcare provider for diagnosis and treatment. In our society, an illness becomes legitimate when a healthcare provider diagnoses it and prescribes treatment. When help from the healthcare provider is sought, the person becomes a patient and enters the next stage.

> *Recall Daniel Sternman, the young man with schizophrenia. His arrival at the mental health clinic indicates that he is seeking help from a healthcare provider. The nurse would interpret this behavior as signaling his assumption of the sick role.*

Stage 3: Assuming a Dependent Role

This stage is characterized by the patient's decision to accept the diagnosis and follow the prescribed treatment plan. The person conforms to the opinions of others, often requires assistance in carrying out activities of daily living, and needs emotional support through acceptance, approval, physical closeness, and protection.

If the disease is serious (such as a heart attack or stroke), the patient may enter the hospital for treatment. If the symptoms can be managed by the patient or family alone or with the assistance of home care providers, the patient is cared for at home. To facilitate adherence to the treatment plan, the patient needs effective relationships with caregivers, knowledge about the illness, and an individualized plan of care. The patient's responses to care depend on a variety of factors, including the seriousness of the illness, the patient's degree of fear about the disease, the loss of roles, the support of others, and previous experiences with illness care. The patient is expected by both caregivers and family to get well and resume normal roles.

> *Consider Daniel Sternman, the patient with schizophrenia described at the beginning of the chapter, who has had difficulty interacting and dealing with various staff members. The nurse needs to be aware of these past difficulties when planning his care to ensure that the staff and patient will adhere to the plan of care.*

Stage 4: Achieving Recovery and Rehabilitation

Recovery and rehabilitation might begin in the hospital and conclude at home, or may be totally concluded at a rehabilitation center or at home. Most patients complete this final stage of illness behavior at home. In this stage, the person gives up the dependent role and resumes normal activities and responsibilities. If the plan of care included health education, the individual may return to health at a higher level of functioning and health than before the illness.

> *Remember Ruth Jacobi, the woman being prepared for discharge after a mini-stroke. The patient's stated desire to be as active and as healthy as she possibly can reflects her desire to give up the dependent role. The nurse would use this knowledge as a basis for the patient's teaching plan, thereby fostering a return to health, possibly at a level higher than before the patient's mini-stroke.*

Chronic Illness

Chronic illness is a broad term that encompasses many different physical and mental alterations in health, with one or more of the following characteristics:

- It is a permanent change.
- It causes, or is caused by, irreversible alterations in normal anatomy and physiology.
- It requires special patient education for rehabilitation.
- It requires a long period of care or support.

Chronic illnesses usually have a slow onset and many have periods of **remission** (when the disease is present, but the person does not experience symptoms) and **exacerbation** (the symptoms of the disease reappear). Examples of common chronic illnesses are heart problems, diabetes mellitus, lung diseases, and arthritis.

> *Recall Daniel Sternman, the young man with schizophrenia? The nurse would integrate knowledge of this disorder, understanding that it is a chronic illness that can be controlled with treatment. The patient's arrival at the clinic with reports of hearing voices would indicate to the nurse that symptoms of the disorder have reappeared, necessitating treatment.*

Chronic illnesses are the leading health problem in the world. Current trends that result in an increase in chronic illnesses include growing numbers of older adults, lifestyle choices (such as smoking and drug use), environmental factors (increasing air and water pollution), and the AIDS epidemic. Nursing care of more patients with chronic illnesses will be required in the future. Although not all people with a chronic illness require care, all who are chronically ill must accept certain conditions of life to be able to live with the illness on a day-to-day basis for the rest of their lives. People with a chronic illness often grieve over losses or changes in physical structure and function, worry about finances, status, roles, and dignity, and must face the possibility of an earlier death.

To successfully adapt to the chronic illness, the individual must learn to live as normally as possible and maintain a positive self-concept and sense of hope, despite symptoms and treatments that may make an individual feel different from others. Activities of daily living, relationships, and self-care activities must often be modified, and it is important that the person maintain a feeling of being in control of his or her own life and the prescribed treatments.

As a nurse, you will care for individuals of all ages with chronic illnesses, and you will provide that care in all types of settings, including homes, hospitals, clinics, nursing homes, and institutions. Regardless of the age of the patient or the effects and demands of the illness or the setting, the nurse must make every effort to promote health for patients with chronic illness, with a focus of care that emphasizes what is possible rather than what can no longer be.

Effects of Illness on the Family

Most nursing care is given to patients with some form of support system, usually the family. When an illness occurs, roles change for both the patient and the family. For example, a chronic illness creates stress for the patient and family because it might require lifelong alterations in roles or lifestyle, frequent hospitalizations, economic problems, and decreased social interactions among family members. The responses of family members to an illness are also individualized. Some family members want to be with the patient all the time, while others might avoid visiting. Parents of a sick child often react with blame, overprotection, and severe anxiety, and family members of patients requiring intensive care often feel alone and frightened. In both cases, they might also feel guilty and imagine the worst possible outcome. See Chapter 2 for more information on the family in health and illness.

MODELS OF HEALTH AND ILLNESS

Because it is difficult to provide universal definitions of health and illness, models have been developed to help describe the concepts and relationships involved. The models described in this chapter are:

- Agent–host–environment model
- Health–illness continuum
- High-level wellness model
- Health belief model
- Health promotion model

The Agent–Host–Environment Model

The agent–host–environment model of health and illness for community health, developed by Leavell and Clark (1965), is useful for examining the causes of disease in an individual. The agent, host, and environment interact in ways that create risk factors, and understanding these is important for the promotion and maintenance of health. An agent is an environmental factor or stressor that must be present or absent for an illness to occur. For example, the factor may be bacteria or a virus, a chemical substance, or a form of radiation whose presence,

excessive presence, or absence (such as in a vitamin-deficiency disease) is necessary for an illness. A host is a living organism capable of being infected or affected by an agent. The host reaction is influenced by family history, age, and health habits. The environment includes all the factors external to the host that make illness more or less likely. The factors can include any that influence health, including physical, social, biologic, and cultural factors.

For example, a person who has poor nutritional habits and gets little sleep is at increased risk for infection during an outbreak of influenza. If that person also is immune deficient (as in AIDS), the risk is even greater. The triangle in Figure 4-3 shows that each of the agent–host–environment factors affects and is affected by the others. These factors are constantly interacting, and a combination of factors may increase the risk of illness. When the factors are balanced, health is maintained; when they are out of balance, disease occurs. Thus, health is an ever-changing state.

The Health–Illness Continuum

The health–illness continuum is one way to measure a person's level of health. This model views health as a constantly changing state, with high-level wellness and death being on opposite ends of a graduated scale, or continuum (Fig. 4-4). This continuum illustrates the dynamic (ever changing) state of health, as a person adapts to changes in the internal and external environments to maintain a state of well-being. A patient with a chronic illness may view himself or herself at different points on the continuum at any given time, depending on how well the patient believes he or she is functioning with the illness.

> *Think back to Sara Gelbart, the college freshman described in the Reflective Practice display. The nurse could apply the health–illness continuum model when assessing this patient, recognizing that the stressors of college life have resulted in a shift along the continuum for this patient away from high-level wellness.*

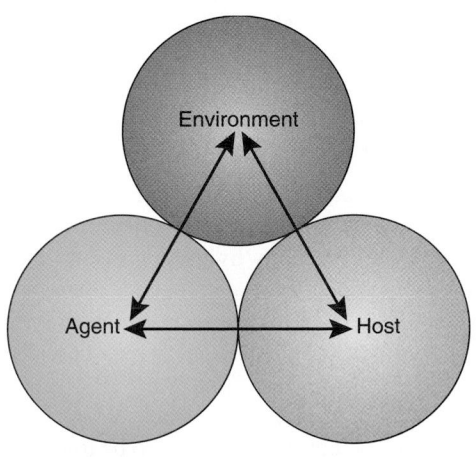

FIGURE 4-3 The agent–host–environment triangle.

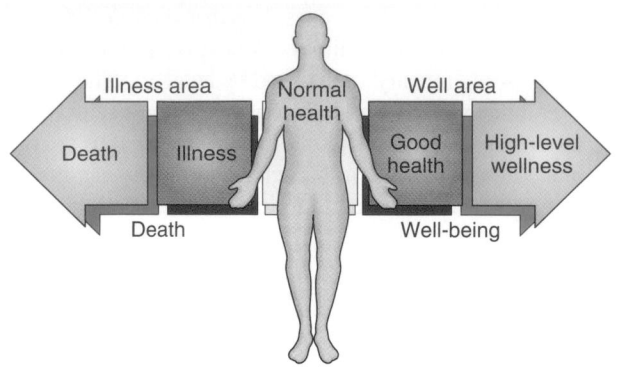

FIGURE 4-4 The health–illness continuum.

The High-Level Wellness Model

Halbert Dunn (1961) described his model of high-level wellness as functioning to one's maximum potential while maintaining balance and a purposeful direction in the environment. Dunn differentiated "wellness" from "good health," believing that good health is a passive state wherein the person is not ill. **Wellness** is a more active state, oriented toward maximizing the potential of the individual, regardless of his or her state of health. Dunn also defined processes that help a person know who and what he or she is. These processes, which are a part of each individual's perception of his or her own wellness state, are being (recognizing self as separate and individual); belonging (being part of a whole); becoming (growing and developing); and befitting (making personal choices to befit the self for the future).

Dunn's model encourages the nurse to care for the total person, with regard for all factors affecting the person's state of being while striving to reach maximum potential.

> *For example, when planning and giving care to Sara, the college freshman with a suspected eating disorder, the nurse would include nursing interventions to meet her educational needs (intellectual dimension); incorporate friends and family (sociocultural dimension); provide or refer for counseling (emotional dimension); and ask the institution's chaplain to visit (spiritual dimension).*

The Health Belief Model

Free or low-cost screens and health information are available in most areas to help in the early detection of disease and to educate people about healthy living to prevent illness. Why, then, don't more people take advantage of these services or change their lifestyles? This question can be answered with the widely used health belief model, which describes health behaviors.

The health belief model (Rosenstock, 1974) is concerned with what people perceive, or believe, to be true about themselves in relation to their health. This model is based on three components of individual perceptions of threat of a disease: (1) perceived susceptibility to a disease, (2) perceived seriousness of a disease, and (3) perceived benefits of action.

Perceived susceptibility to a disease is the belief that one either will or will not contract a disease. Perceived susceptibility ranges from being afraid of contracting a disease to completely denying that certain behaviors will result in illness. For example, one person who smokes cigarettes may believe he or she is at danger for lung cancer and may stop smoking, while another person may believe smoking poses no serious threat and continues to smoke.

Perceived seriousness of a disease concerns the perception of the seriousness of the disease and its effect on the person's lifestyle. This component is related to how much the person knows about the disease and can result in a change in health behavior. If a person who smokes believes that lung cancer can lead to physical disability or death and would therefore affect his or her ability to work and care for the family, the person is more likely to stop smoking.

Perceived benefits of action is concerned with how effective the individual believes preventive measures will be in preventing illness. This factor is influenced by the person's conviction that carrying out a recommended action will prevent or modify the disease and by the person's perception of the cost and unpleasant effects of performing the health behavior (compared with not taking any action). For example, the person may believe that stopping smoking will prevent future breathing problems and that the initial withdrawal symptoms can be overcome; therefore, the person may stop smoking.

Modifying factors for one's health beliefs include demographic variables (such as age or race), sociopsychological variables (such as personality and peer group pressure), and structural variables (such as knowledge and prior contact with the disease). These factors interact to influence the perceived benefits of preventive action minus the perceived barriers to preventive action. Cues to action are also modifying factors and are provided by activities such as others' advice, mass-media campaigns, literature, appointment-reminder telephone calls or postcards, and illness of a significant other. The likelihood of taking a recommended preventive health action is thus a composite of individual perceptions and modifying factors.

This model is useful when teaching individuals about health and illness. The nurse can assess the patient's health beliefs and mutually structure goals to help realistically meet health needs. Teaching and health promotion activities are ineffective, however, unless the patient believes they are important and necessary.

> *Consider Ruth Jacobi, the woman being discharged after a mini-stroke. The patient's statement indicates that she is positively motivated to achieve health, providing the nurse with valuable information about the patient's health beliefs. Together, the nurse and patient can determine realistic goals. The nurse, then, could use this model to develop the patient's teaching plan, including information about*

the underlying disease process, risk factors for stroke, and ways to reduce the patient's risk for a major stroke.

The Health Promotion Model

The health promotion model (Pender, 1996) was developed to illustrate the "multidimensional nature of persons interacting with their environment as they pursue health" (p. 53). The model incorporates individual characteristics and experiences and behavior-specific knowledge and beliefs, to motivate health-promoting behavior. The components of the model can be used to design and provide nursing interventions to promote health for individuals, families, and communities.

Individual characteristics and experiences can be useful in predicting if an individual will incorporate and use health-related behaviors. If a behavior has been used before and becomes a habit, it is more likely to be used again. Personal biologic, psychological, and sociocultural factors, including age, gender, strength, self-esteem, perceived health status, definition of health, race, acculturation, and socioeconomic status are all predictive of a given health-related habit. For example, the person who has high self-esteem, defines self as healthy, and has an adequate income might be less likely to use alcohol or tobacco and more likely to follow a healthy diet and take part in regular exercise. Conversely, a person with low self-esteem, a fatalistic attitude toward health, and a low socio-economic base might be more likely to have poor nutrition, never exercise, and use addictive substances.

Behavior-specific knowledge, beliefs, and relationships are considered to be major motivators for engaging in health-promoting behaviors. These include the belief that there will be a positive outcome from a specific health behavior, that one has the skill and competence to engage in health behaviors, and that one is affected by the interpersonal influences of others (especially family, peers, and healthcare providers). Situational influences, such as no-smoking policies, also influence health behaviors. Barriers to action, which include perceptions of un-availability, inconvenience, expense, difficulty, or time, usually result in avoidance of a behavior.

A health-related behavior is initiated by committing to a plan of action, accompanied by developing associated strategies to perform the valued behavior. Failure to sustain the behavior may result from competing demands. For example, a person may begin a low-fat diet but "give in" to the desire for fast foods. Health-related behavior is the outcome of the model and is directed toward attaining positive health outcomes and experiences throughout the life span.

FACTORS AFFECTING HEALTH AND ILLNESS

Many factors influence a person's health status, health beliefs, and health practices. These factors may be internal or external to the individual and may or may not be under the person's conscious control. To plan and provide holistic care, the nurse must understand how these factors influence behavior in both healthy and ill patients. This section describes those factors that affect health status, health beliefs, and health practices, including risk factors for illness; factors in the human dimensions that influence health–illness status, beliefs, and practices; basic human needs; and self-concept.

Risk Factors for Illness

A **risk factor** is something that increases a person's chance for illness or injury. The six general types of risk factors are described in Table 4-1. Risk factors for each developmental level across the life span are included in Unit II, and cultural influences on health are discussed in Chapter 3.

Like other components of health and illness, risk factors are often interrelated. As the number of risk factors increases, so does the possibility of illness. For example, an overweight executive, under pressure to increase sales, smokes and drinks alcohol in excess. These factors, combined with a family history of heart disease, place this person at higher risk for illness.

The Human Dimensions

The factors influencing a person's health illness status, health beliefs, and health practices relate to the person's human di-

TABLE 4-1 Major Areas of Risk Factors

Risk Factor	Examples
Age	School-aged children are at high risk for communicable diseases. After menopause, women are more likely to develop cardiovascular disease.
Genetic factors	A family history of cancer or diabetes predisposes a person to developing the disease.
Physiologic factors	Obesity increases the possibility of heart disease. Pregnancy places increased risk on both the mother and the developing fetus.
Health habits	Smoking increases the probability of lung cancer. Poor nutrition can lead to a variety of health problems.
Lifestyle	Multiple sexual relationships increase the risk for sexually transmitted diseases (eg, gonorrhea or acquired immunodeficiency syndrome). Events that increase stress (eg, divorce, retirement, work-related pressure) may precipitate accidents or illness.
Environment	Working and living environments (such as hazardous materials and poor sanitation) may contribute to disease.

mensions (see Fig. 4-1). Each dimension interrelates with each of the others, and influences the behaviors of the person in health and in illness. Nursing assessments of strengths and weaknesses in each dimension are used to develop a plan of care that is individualized and holistic. The nursing process, used to plan, implement, and evaluate plans of care, is discussed in Unit III.

Physical Dimension

The physical dimension includes genetic inheritance, age, developmental level, race, and gender. These components strongly influence the person's health status and health practices. Inherited genetic disorders include Down syndrome, hemophilia, cystic fibrosis, and color blindness. The toddlers at greater risk for drowning and the adolescent and young adult male are at greater risk for automobile crashes from excessive speed. There are specific racial traits for disease, including sickle cell anemia, hypertension, and stroke. A young woman who has a mother and grandmother with breast cancer is more likely to have an annual clinical breast examination and mammogram.

Emotional Dimension

How the mind affects body function and responds to body conditions also influences health. Long-term stress affects body systems, and anxiety affects health habits; conversely, calm acceptance and relaxation can actually change body responses to illness. As examples of the negative effects of emotions, a student always has diarrhea before examinations and an adolescent with poor self-esteem begins to experiment with drugs. The positive effects of emotions include reducing surgical pain with relaxation techniques and reducing blood pressure with biofeedback skills.

> *Knowledge of the emotional dimension would be important when planning care for Sara Gelbart, the college freshman described at the beginning of the chapter. The nurse would need to examine how she responds to stress and anxiety.*

Intellectual Dimension

The intellectual dimension encompasses cognitive abilities, educational background, and past experiences. These influence responses to teaching about health and reactions to nursing care during illness. They also play a major role in health behaviors. Examples of situations involving this dimension include a young college student with diabetes who follows a diabetic diet but continues to drink beer and eat pizza with friends several times a week, and a middle-aged man who quits taking his high-blood-pressure medication after developing unpleasant side effects.

Environmental Dimension

The environment has many influences on health and illness. Housing, sanitation, climate, and pollution of air, food, and water are elements in the environmental dimension. A few ex-

amples of environmental causes of illness are deaths in older adults from inadequate heating and cooling, increased incidence of asthma and respiratory problems in large cities with smog, and increased incidence of skin cancer in people who live in hot, sunny areas of the world.

Sociocultural Dimension

Health practices and beliefs are strongly influenced by a person's economic level, lifestyle, family, and culture. In general, low-income groups are less likely to seek medical care to prevent illness, and high-income groups are more prone to stress-related habits and illness. The family and the culture to which a person belongs influence the person's patterns of living and values about health and illness; such patterns are often unalterable. All of these factors are involved in personal care, patterns of eating, lifestyle habits, and emotional stability. Examples of other sociocultural situations that influence health and illness are an adolescent who sees nothing wrong with smoking or drinking because her parents smoke and drink, parents of a sick infant who do not seek medical care because they have no health insurance, a single parent (abused as a child) who in turn physically abuses her own small son, and a person of Asian descent who uses herbal remedies and acupuncture to treat an illness.

Spiritual Dimension

Spiritual beliefs and values are important components of a person's health and illness behaviors (see Chapter 36). It is important that the nurses respect these values and understand their importance for the individual patient. Examples of the influences of the spiritual dimension on healthcare include the Roman Catholic requirement of baptism for both live births and stillborn babies; Kosher dietary laws, prohibiting the intake of pork and shellfish, practiced by Orthodox and Conservative Jews; and opposition to blood transfusion common to Jehovah's Witnesses.

Basic Human Needs

A need is something that is essential to the emotional and physiologic health and survival of humans. Basic human needs, discussed in Chapter 2, are essential and are common to all people. A person whose needs are met may be considered to be healthy, and a person with one or more unmet need is at increased risk for illness. Needs are an integral part of each person's human dimensions, as illustrated in Table 4-2.

Self-Concept

Another variable influencing health and illness is a person's self-concept (see Chapter 31), which incorporates both how the person feels about self (self-esteem) and the way he or she perceives his or her physical self (body image). Self-concept has both physical and emotional aspects and is an important factor in the way the individual reacts to stress and illness, follows self-care health practices, and relates to others.

TABLE 4-2 The Human Dimensions and Basic Human Needs

	Basic Human Need	Examples
Physical dimension	Physiologic needs	Breathing Circulation Temperature Intake of food and fluids Elimination of wastes Movement
Environmental dimension	Safety and security needs	Housing Community/ neighborhood Climate
Sociocultural dimension	Love and belonging needs	Relationships with others Communications with others Support systems Being part of a community Feeling loved by others
Emotional dimension	Self-esteem needs	Fear Sadness Loneliness Happiness Accepting self
Intellectual and spiritual dimensions	Self-actualization needs	Thinking Learning Decision-making Values Beliefs Fulfillment Helping others

For example, consider Sara Gelbart, the college freshman with a suspected eating disorder. Although she has lost a significant amount of weight, she states that she is healthy, but just "nuts" about being fit. Her self-concept is most likely one of being overweight. Subsequently she rarely eats.

In contrast, a person who is overweight may feel that nothing will change the way he or she looks and refuse to follow a diet and exercise program.

A person's self-concept results from a variety of past experiences, interpersonal interactions, physical and cultural influences, and education. It includes a person's perceptions of his or her own strengths and weaknesses. Illness can alter a person's self-concept as it affects roles, independence, and relationships with important others.

NURSING CARE TO PROMOTE HEALTH AND PREVENT ILLNESS

The current focus of healthcare at local, state, national, and global levels is on preventing disease and illness. This focus is important to nursing. Chapter 1 provides information about *Healthy People 2010,* a national agenda to promote health. Nursing interventions to promote health in the community are discussed in Chapters 2 and 8. Chapters 19 and 20 discuss recommended screenings, immunizations, and safety practices across the lifespan. This section discusses levels of preventive care and how nurses are role models for health.

Levels of Preventive Care

The levels of preventive care, described by Leavell and Clark (1965) are summarized below. Examples of nursing activities for each level are discussed below and listed in Table 4-3.

Primary Preventive Care

Primary preventive care is directed toward promoting health and preventing the development of disease processes. Health-risk assessments are an important part of primary preventive

TABLE 4-3 Examples of Nursing Activities by Level of Preventive Care

Level	Topic
Primary Prevention	Diet Exercise Smoking cessation Alcohol consumption Drugs Farm safety Seat belts and child safety seats Immunizations Water treatment Safer sex practices Parenting
Secondary Prevention	Screenings: Blood pressure, cholesterol, glaucoma, HIV, skin cancer Pap smear Mammograms Testicular examinations Family counseling
Tertiary Prevention	Medications Medical therapy Surgical treatment Rehabilitation Physical therapy Occupational therapy Job training

care. A health-risk assessment is an assessment of the total person. The "picture" of the individual resulting from this assessment indicates areas of risk for disease or injury as well as areas that support health. A variety of formats are used to perform the assessment, but all of them take a broad approach to health, focusing on lifestyle and health behaviors. Promoting Health 4-1 contains an example of a health-risk assessment that is completed by the patient.

Nursing activities at the primary preventive level may focus on individuals or groups. Activities are focused on promoting health and preventing illness or injury. Examples of primary-level activities are immunizations, family planning services, teaching breast self-examination, poison-control information, and accident-prevention education. Examples of recommended lifestyle practices that support health are listed in Promoting Health 4-1.

Promoting Health 4-1 A *Health Style* Self-Test

All of us want good health, but many of us do not know how to be as healthy as possible. Health experts now describe *lifestyle* as one of the most important factors affecting health. In fact, it is estimated that as many as 7 of the 10 leading causes of death could be reduced through common-sense changes in lifestyle. That's what this brief test, developed by the Public Health Service, is all about. Its purpose is simply to tell you how well you are doing to stay healthy. The behaviors covered in the test are recommended for most Americans. Some of them may not apply to people with certain chronic diseases or disabilities, or to pregnant women. Such people may require special instructions from their physicians.

CIGARETTE SMOKING

If you never smoke, enter a score of 10 for this section and go the next section on Alcohol and Drugs.

2 1 0 1. I avoid smoking cigarettes.

2 1 0 2. I smoke only low-tar and nicotine cigarettes *or* I smoke a pipe or cigars.

Smoking score: _____

ALCOHOL AND DRUGS

4 1 0 1. I avoid drinking alcoholic beverages *or* I drink no more than one or two drinks a day.

2 1 0 2. I avoid using alcohol or other drugs (especially illegal drugs) as a way of handling stressful situations or the problems in my life.

2 1 0 3. I am careful not to drink alcohol when taking certain medicines (eg, medicine for sleeping, pain, colds, and allergies), or when pregnant.

2 1 0 4. I read and follow the label directions when using prescribed and over-the-counter drugs.

Alcohol and drugs score: _____

EATING HABITS

4 1 0 1. I eat a variety of foods each day, such as fruits and vegetables, whole-grain breads and cereals, lean meats, dairy products, dry peas and beans, and nuts and seeds.

2 1 0 2. I limit the amount of fat, saturated fat, and cholesterol I eat (including fat on meats, eggs, butter, cream, shortenings, and organ meats such as liver).

2 1 0 3. I limit the amount of salt I eat by cooking with only small amounts, not adding salt at the table, and avoiding salty snacks.

2 1 0 4. I avoid eating too much sugar (especially frequent snacks of sticky candy or soft drinks).

Eating habits score: _____

EXERCISE AND FITNESS

3 1 0 1. I maintain a desired weight, avoiding overweight and underweight.

3 1 0 2. I do vigorous exercises for 15 to 30 minutes at least three times a week (examples include running, swimming, brisk walking).

2 1 0 3. I do exercises that enhance my muscle tone for 15 to 30 minutes at least three times a week (examples include yoga and calisthenics).

2 1 0 4. I use part of my leisure time participating in individual, family, or team activities that increase my level of fitness (such as gardening, bowling, golf, and baseball).

Exercise/fitness score: _____

STRESS CONTROL

2 1 0 1. I have a job or do other work that I enjoy.

2 1 0 2. I find it easy to relax and express my feelings freely.

2 1 0 3. I recognize early, and prepare for, events or situations likely to be stressful for me.

2 1 0 4. I have close friends, relatives, or others whom I can talk to about personal matters and call on for help when needed.

2 1 0 5. I participate in group activities (such as church and community organizations) or hobbies that I enjoy.

Stress control score: _____

(continued)

Promoting Health 4-1 A Health Style Self-Test (Continued)

SAFETY

almost always 2   sometimes 1   almost never 0   1. I wear a seat belt while riding in a car.

2   1   0   2. I avoid driving while under the influence of alcohol and other drugs.

2   1   0   3. I obey traffic rules and the speed limit when driving.

2   1   0   4. I am careful when using potentially harmful products or substances (such as household cleaners, poisons, and electrical devices).

2   1   0   5. I avoid smoking in bed.

Safety score: _____

WHAT YOUR SCORES MEAN TO YOU

Scores of 9 and 10
Excellent! Your answers show that you are aware of the importance of this area to your health. More important, you are putting your knowledge to work for you by practicing good health habits. As long as you continue to do so, this area should not pose a serious health risk. It's likely that you are setting an example for your family and friends to follow. Because you got a very high test score on this part of the test, you may want to consider other areas where your scores indicate room for improvement.

Scores of 6 to 8
Your health practices in this area are good, but there is room for improvement. Look again at the items you answered with "Sometimes" or "Almost never." What changes can you make to improve your score? Even a small change can often help you achieve better health.

Scores of 3 to 5
Your health risks are showing! Would you like more information about the risks you are facing and about why it is important for you to change these behaviors? Perhaps you need help in deciding how to make the changes you desire. In either case, help is available.

Scores of 0 to 2
Obviously, you were concerned enough about your health to take the test, but your answers show that you may be taking serious and unnecessary risks with your health. Perhaps you are unaware of the risks and what to do about them. You can easily get the information and help you need to improve, if you wish. The next step is up to you.

(Adapted with permission of the National Health Information Clearinghouse.)

SUGGESTED SELF-CARE BEHAVIORS

Start by asking yourself a few frank questions: *Am I really doing all I can to be as healthy as possible? What steps can I take to feel better? Am I willing to begin now?* If you scored low in one or more sections of the test, decide what changes you want to make for improvement. You might pick that aspect of your lifestyle where you feel you have the best chance for success and tackle that one first. Once you have improved your score there, go on to other areas.

Lifestyle practices that promote health include:
- Sleeping regularly, 7 to 8 hours per night
- Eating regular meals, which include recommended food groups
- Maintaining ideal body weight
- Having a regular schedule of exercise
- Using alcohol in moderation, if at all
- Not smoking
- Maintaining positive mental health and self-concept
- Practicing safer sex
- Wearing seatbelts, using car seats for children, and wearing bicycle helmets
- Having recommended screenings and checkups by your medical and dental healthcare providers

If you already have tried to change your health habits (to stop smoking or exercise regularly, for example), don't be discouraged if you haven't yet succeeded. The difficulty you have encountered may be due to influences you've never really thought about—such as advertising—or to a lack of support and encouragement. Understanding these influences is an important step toward changing the way they affect you.

There's help available. In addition to personal actions you can take on your own, there are community programs and groups (such as the YMCA or the local chapter of the American Heart Association) that can assist you and your family to make the changes you want to make. If you want to know more about these groups or about health risks, contact your local health department or the National Health Information Clearinghouse. There's a lot you can do to stay healthy or to improve your health—and there are organizations that can help you. Start a new "health-style" today!

For assistance in locating specific information on these and other health topics, write to the National Health Information Clearinghouse:

National Health Information Clearinghouse
P.O. Box 1133
Washington, DC 20013

Secondary Preventive Care

Secondary preventive care focuses on early detection of disease, prompt intervention, and health maintenance for patients experiencing health problems. The goal of secondary preventive care is to reverse or reduce the severity of the disease or to provide a cure (Stanhope & Lancaster, 2004). Examples of activities at this level are carrying out direct nursing actions (eg, providing wound care, giving medications, or exercising arms and legs); assessing children for normal growth and development; and encouraging regular medical and dental screenings and care.

> *Consider Daniel Sternman, the young man with schizophrenia. Secondary preventive care would encompass medication administration to control the symptoms of schizophrenia and appropriate psychotherapeutic techniques.*

Tertiary Preventive Care

Tertiary preventive care begins after an illness is diagnosed and treated to reduce disability and to help rehabilitate patients to a maximum level of functioning. Nursing activities on a tertiary level include teaching a patient with diabetes how to recognize and prevent complications, using physical therapy to prevent contractures in a patient who has had a stroke or spinal cord injury, and referring a woman to a support group after removal of a breast because of cancer. Nurses are important in monitoring the responses of the patient to the prescribed therapy and in providing services to patients to facilitate recovery or improve quality of life while living with the effects of an illness or injury.

> *Think back to Sara Gelbart, the college freshman with a suspected eating disorder. The nurse would use tertiary preventive care by referring the patient to a eating disorders support group. For Ruth Jacobi, the woman being discharged after a mini-stroke, tertiary preventive care would include educating her about the warning signs and symptoms of a major stroke and about measures to reduce her risk for a major stroke.*

Nurses as Role Models for Health

Nurses must take care of their own health to be able to give effective nursing care to others. Good personal health not only enables nurses to practice more efficiently but also enables them to serve as role models for patients and families. Nurses can help patients acquire new health behaviors by modeling the very behaviors that are important to the patients' well-being.

It is difficult for nurses to be sincerely attentive to the needs of patients when their own needs are not being met. Because no one is perfectly healthy all of the time, it is important for nurses, as they prepare for professional practice, to spend time getting to know themselves. From this self-knowledge should come a commitment to pursue holistic health actively. To help you increase your self-knowledge, complete the health-style self-test in Promoting Health 4-1. As you work with patients to provide care, you can use this self-test to help your patients assess their state of health and health risks, and learn a new health style.

The health promotion guides highlighted throughout the text may be useful to you as well as to your patients. Use these guides to assess and identify both strengths and risks for alterations in health. The guides can also serve as a basis for teaching self-care to patients.

■ Developing Critical Thinking Skills

1. Identify a family in which someone has a chronic illness. Interview as many of the other family members as possible, and discuss the effect of the illness on them. What do you observe about the effects of the illness in relation to the patient's age, type of illness (eg, AIDS versus cancer), gender, and family role?
2. List the six human dimensions described in this chapter, and identify your personal strengths and weaknesses in each area. For example, you may have inherited a genetic tendency toward overweight (a weakness), but have controlled your weight through nutrition and exercise (a strength). After considering your strengths and weaknesses, develop a personal plan for health promotion.

■ Practicing for NCLEX

1. Of the following statements, which is most true of health and illness?
   a. Health and illness are the same for all people.
   b. Health and illness are individually defined by each person.
   c. People with acute illnesses are actually healthy.
   d. People with chronic illnesses have poor health beliefs.
2. Of the following terms, which would be defined as a disease?
   a. Excess fluid volume
   b. Risk for infection
   c. Rheumatoid arthritis
   d. Altered body image
3. Your neighbor, Alan, asks you to come over because he has a high temperature, feels "awful," and did not go to work. What stage of illness behavior is Alan exhibiting?
   a. Experiencing symptoms
   b. Assuming the sick role
   c. Assuming a dependent role
   d. Achieving recovery and rehabilitation
4. Of the following characteristics, which one is not a part of chronic illness?
   a. Permanent change in body structure or function
   b. Self-treatment that relieves symptoms
   c. Long period of treatment and care
   d. Often has remissions and exacerbations

5. The agent–host–environment model of health and illness is based on the concept of:
   a. Risk factors
   b. Infectious diseases
   c. Behaviors to promote health
   d. Stages of illness

6. What do both the health–illness continuum and the high-level wellness models demonstrate?
   a. Illness as a fixed point in time
   b. The importance of family
   c. Wellness as a passive state
   d. Health as a constantly changing state

7. Following the birth of his first child and after reading about the long-term effects of nicotine, John decides to stop smoking. This behavior change is most likely based on John's perceptions of all but one of the following. Which one is not true?
   a. His susceptibility to lung cancer
   b. How serious lung cancer would be
   c. What benefits his stopping smoking will have
   d. Personal choice and economic factors

8. Of the following clinic patients, which one is most likely to have annual breast examinations and mammograms based on the physical human dimension?
   a. Jane, because her best friend had a benign breast lump removed
   b. Sarah, who lives in a low-income neighborhood
   c. Tricia, who has a family history of breast cancer
   d. Nancy, because her family encourages regular physical examinations

9. You are asked to teach a group of preschool parents about poison control in the home. This activity is an example of what level of preventive care?
   a. Lowest
   b. Tertiary
   c. Primary
   d. Secondary

10. As a nurse, you follow the guidelines for a healthy lifestyle. How can this promote health in others?
   a. By being a role model for healthy behaviors
   b. By not requiring sick days from work
   c. By never exposing others to any type of illness
   d. By not being overweight

■ Answers With Rationale

1. The correct response is *b*. Each person defines health and illness individually, based on a number of factors.

2. The correct response is *c*. Rheumatoid arthritis is a disease; the other responses are nursing diagnoses labeling an actual or potential response to a disease.

3. The correct response is *b*. When people assume the sick role, they define themselves as ill, seek validation of this experience from others, and give up normal activities.

4. The correct response is *b*. Acute illnesses are often self-treated to relieve symptoms.

5. The correct response is *a*. The interaction of the agent–host–environment creates risk factors that increase the probability of disease.

6. The correct response is *d*. Both these models view health as a dynamic (constantly changing state).

7. The correct response is *d*. Responses *a*, *b* and *c* are components of the health belief model.

8. The correct response is *c*. A family history of breast cancer is a major risk factor.

9. The correct response is *c*. Teaching poison control in the home is an example of primary preventive care.

10. The correct response is *a*. Good personal health enables the nurse to serve as a role model for patients and families.

Bibliography

Allen, J. (2002). What will it take to promote healthy lifestyles among all Americans? *American Journal of Health Promotion, 17*(2), 4–5.

Austin, L., Ahmad, F., McNally, M., & Stewart, D. (2002). Breast and cervical cancer screening in Hispanic women: A literature review using the Health Belief Model. *Women's Health Issues, 12*(3), 122–127.

Clemen-Stone, S., McGuire, S., & Eigsti, D. (2002). *Comprehensive community health nursing* (6th ed.). St. Louis: Mosby.

Dunn, H. (1961). *High level wellness.* Arlington, VA: Beathy.

Edelman, C., & Mandle, C. (2002). *Health promotion throughout the life span* (5th ed.). St. Louis: Mosby.

Goodshall, M. (2003). Caring for families of chronically ill kids. *RN, 66*(2), 31–35.

Hawranik, P., & Pangman, V. (2002). Perceptions of a senior citizens' wellness center: The community's voice. *Journal of Gerontological Nursing, 28*(11), 38–44.

Kearney, M., & O'Sullivan, J. (2003). Identity shifts as turning points in health behavior change. *Western Journal of Nursing Research 25*(2), 134–152.

Leavell, H., & Clark, E. G. (1965). *Preventive medicine for the doctor in the community* (3rd ed.). New York: McGraw Hill.

Maslow, A. (1968). *Toward a psychology of being* (2nd ed.). New York: Van Nostrand Reinhold.

Miller, J. F. (2000). *Coping with chronic illness: Overcoming powerlessness* (3rd ed.). Philadelphia: F. A. Davis.

Murray, R. B., & Zentner, J. P. (2001). *Health promotion strategies through the lifespan* (7th ed.). Upper Saddle River, NJ: Prentice Hall.

Pender, N. (1966). *Health promotion in nursing practice* (3rd ed.). Stamford, CT: Appleton & Lange.

Pender, N. J., Murdaugh, C., & Parsons, M. (2002). *Health promotion in nursing practice.* (4th ed.). Upper Saddle River, NJ: Prentice Hall.

Pollock, S. E. (1986). Human responses to chronic illness: Physiologic and psychosocial adaptation. *Nursing Research, 35*(2), 90–95.

Raphael, D. (2002). Models of illness, models of health, models of society. *Health Promotion: Global Perspectives, 5*(1), 2p.

Rosenstock, I. (1974). Historical origin of the health belief model. *Health Education Monographs, 2,* 334.

Stanhope, M., & Lancaster, J. (2004). *Community & public health nursing* (6th ed.). St. Louis: Mosby.

Suchman, E. (1965). Stages of illness and medical care. *Journal of Health and Human Behavior, 6,* 114.

World Health Organization. (1946). Preamble to the Constitution of the World Health Organization as adopted by the International Health Conference, New York, 19–22 June, 1946; signed on 22 July by the representatives of 51 states (Official Records of the World Health Organization, no. 2, p. 100) and entered into force on 7 April, 1948.

Theory, Research, and Evidence-Based Practice

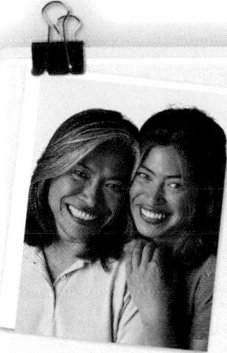

Charlotte Horn, the daughter of a 57-year-old patient being discharged with an order for intermittent nasogastric tube feedings, is being taught how to perform the procedure. During one of the teaching sessions, Charlotte asks "How will I know that the tube is in the right place?"

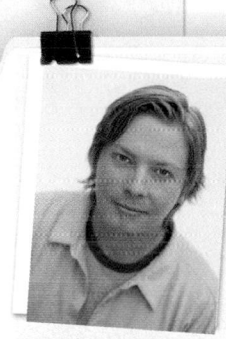

Joe Wimmer, a first-time father of a healthy 8-lb baby girl delivered several hours ago, is visiting with his wife and new daughter. He asks "Why is my daughter wearing that funny little cap on her head?"

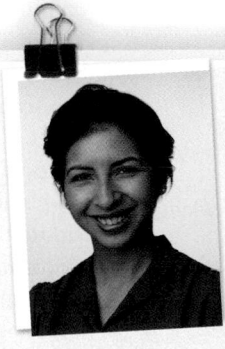

Maribella Santos, who had just arrived back on the unit after undergoing abdominal surgery, is complaining of nausea. A while later, she states "My nausea is gone. The nurse did something with her hands and the feeling just went away."

The types of blended skills that you'll need to respond to the case scenarios include:

Cognitive Skills

- Demonstration of understanding about the sources and types of knowledge, nursing theories, nursing research, and evidence-based practice
- Knowledge of nasogastric tube feedings and associated care, newborn heat-loss mechanisms, and therapeutic touch
- Knowledge of appropriate research sources, including ability to read published research
- Ability to incorporate knowledge of nursing models and theories when developing the plan of care for clients with different needs
- Ability to demonstrate knowledge of how nursing models and theories dictate assessment, planning, and research design

Technical Skills

- Ability to access computerized searches to facilitate selection of appropriate nursing literature to direct your work
- Ability to provide technical nursing assistance based on sound scientific rationales to meet the needs of a woman learning about tube feedings, a new father with questions, and a woman with postoperative nausea
- Ability to adapt measures to provide care to patients with different needs

Interpersonal Skills

- Ability to work collaboratively with nursing colleagues and the interdisciplinary team from the perspective of nursing's theoretical base, with the goal of helping others understand nursing's unique perspective and voice as healthcare is planned, implemented, and evaluated
- Ability to establish caring relationships with patients and their families with different needs at various stages in the life cycle
- Ability to demonstrate respect for the patient's human dignity and autonomy
- Demonstration of ability to translate theoretical information and scientific rationales for practice measures for patients and their families asking questions

Ethical and Legal Skills

- Ability to be trusted to bring the best that nursing has to offer to the research, design, implementation, and evaluation of healthcare for different population groups
- Knowledge of the nurse's legal responsibilities when researching, designing, implementing, and evaluating healthcare
- Ability to participate as a trusted and effective patient advocate, including a commitment to securing the best possible care for patients, such as the woman experiencing a relief of nausea from therapeutic touch intervention
- Demonstration of a strong sense of accountability for the health and well-being of patients and their families based on integration of knowledge, theory, research, and evidence-based practice
- Ability to practice in an ethically and legally defensible manner consistent with the nursing code of ethics and within the scope of legal practice

Learning Outcomes

After completing the chapter, the learner should be able to accomplish the following:

1. Explain the various types of knowledge.
2. Define concept, theory, philosophy, and process.
3. Explain how theories from other disciplines have influenced nursing theory.
4. Identify the four concepts common to all nursing theories.
5. Discuss historical and societal influences on the development of nursing knowledge.
6. Discuss the significance, importance, and evolution of nursing research.
7. Explain the differences between quantitative and qualitative research methods.
8. Outline the steps of the quantitative research process.
9. Define informed consent as it applies to research.
10. Describe evidence-based practice in nursing, integrating the relevance of nursing theory and nursing research.
11. Read and understand, on a beginning level, a published research article.

Key Terms

applied research
basic research
concept
conceptual framework or model
data
deductive reasoning
evidence-based practice
inductive reasoning
informed consent
nursing research
nursing theory
philosophy
process
qualitative research
quantitative research
research
science
theory

Nursing is a unique healthcare discipline in which nurses provide a service based on knowledge and skill. Nursing has two essential aspects: a body of knowledge and the application of that knowledge through clinical nursing practice. This body of knowledge, called a knowledge base or the science of nursing, provides the rationale for nursing interventions. As you learn and practice nursing, you will use rationales from many different disciplines, such as anatomy, physiology, chemistry, nutrition, psychology, and sociology. You will also use the knowledge base developed specifically for nursing through theory development and research. (See the accompanying Reflective Practice display for an example.) This chapter will discuss the concepts of nursing knowledge, nursing theory, nursing research, and evidence-based practice separately, despite the fact that in practice they are often intertwined.

NURSING KNOWLEDGE

Knowledge is an awareness of the reality one acquires through learning or investigation. Every individual collects, organizes, and arranges facts to build a knowledge base relevant to his or her personal reality.

Sources of Knowledge

Knowledge comes from a variety of sources, and may be traditional, authoritative, or scientific.

Traditional Knowledge

Traditional knowledge is that part of nursing practice passed down from generation to generation. When questioned about the origin of such nursing practices, nurses might reply "We've always done it this way." Changing bedclothes is an example of how traditional knowledge has affected nursing practice. It is customary in acute care settings to change a patient's bedclothes daily, whether soiled or not. There are no research data to support this, yet virtually millions of hospital beds are changed daily because this practice is accepted as a necessary component of quality patient care. Until this practice is challenged scientifically and its assumed value disproved, it will remain a traditional part of patient care.

Authoritative Knowledge

Authoritative knowledge comes from an expert and is accepted as truth based on the person's perceived expertise—for example, when a senior staff nurse teaches a new graduate nurse an easier way of doing a technical procedure such as inserting an

Reflective Practice
Challenge to Cognitive Skills

One of the nurses, Danielle, on a surgical floor where I was assigned, took a course in therapeutic touch. When she returned to work, she was eager to use her new "intervention." My patient, Maribella Santos, had come back to the unit after undergoing abdominal surgery. Upon her return, she complained of nausea. Danielle used her "unruffling" technique to calm the patient, whose nausea then "disappeared." Excited, I reported this in postconference, only to learn from my instructor that therapeutic touch was "a lot of bunk" without scientific support.

Thinking Outside the Box: Possible Courses of Action

- Accept my instructor's dismissal of therapeutic touch.
- Learn more about therapeutic touch from my colleague Danielle and professional literature.
- Become an advocate for therapeutic touch if it DOES work!

Evaluating a Good Outcome: How Do I Define Success?

- Patient is not harmed by anyone using an unproven therapy.
- Patient benefits from my openness to new (potentially beneficial) therapies.
- I rely on research, not hearsay, as a basis for my clinical judgments and actions.

Personal Learning: Here's to the Future!

I was surprised to find the literature so inconclusive about the benefits of therapeutic touch. Obviously its adherents claim that they can measure its efficacy. Others find these claims unsupported. Since this event happened at the beginning of my clinical rotation, I decided to observe Danielle throughout my rotation. What I saw made me a believer in this technique. Danielle was using therapeutic touch as an adjuvant to other therapies and it seemed to be working. I want to learn more about this technique. My goal is to attend a workshop on therapeutic touch to see if is something I can incorporate into my practice.

Reflection

How do you think you would respond in a similar situation? Why? What does this tell you about yourself and about the adequacy of your skills for professional practice? Can you think of other ways to respond? What sources of knowledge did the nursing student use? Did the nursing student use theory and research? If so, please explain how? Would you consider therapeutic touch to be evidence-based practice? Why or why not? How might the patient's culture have affected the response? What other skills (cognitive, interpersonal, technical, ethical/legal) would you need to respond well in this situation? Propose possible reasons for the instructor's response? Do you agree with the criteria to evaluate a successful outcome? Did the nursing student meet the criteria? Please explain your answer.

Katherine Figliala, Georgetown University

intravenous catheter. The senior nurse has gained knowledge through experience, and the new graduate nurse accepts it as truth based on the perceived authority of the experienced nurse. Authoritative knowledge generally remains unchallenged as long as the presumed authority maintains his or her perceived expertise.

> *Consider Charlotte Horn, the patient's daughter who is being taught how to give nasogastric tube feedings. In this situation, the nurse performing the teaching would be considered the expert. Here the nurse would provide the daughter with some helpful hints based on experience to make the tube feeding procedure less overwhelming. In doing so, the nurse is using authoritative knowledge.*

Scientific Knowledge

Scientific knowledge is that knowledge arrived at through the scientific method (implying through research). New ideas are tested and measured systematically using objective criteria.

> *Think back to Maribella Santos, the woman complaining of nausea after undergoing abdominal surgery. The nurse would integrate scientific knowledge about the effects of surgery on the body to develop the postoperative plan of care. Additionally, the nurse would use this scientific knowledge as a basis for determining the underlying cause of the patient's complaint of nausea.*

Is one source of knowledge better than another? All sources of knowledge are useful in the collective body of knowledge that constitutes the nursing profession. Although these three sources provide nursing with important contributions, each has inherent strengths and limitations. Both traditional and authoritative knowledge are practical to implement but are often based on subjective data, limiting their usefulness in a wide variety of practice settings. For this reason, nurses often focus on scientific knowledge, commonly called evidence-based practice or research-based practice.

Types of Knowledge

Some of the types of knowledge include science, philosophy, and process.

Science

Science implies a body of knowledge. Science is observing, identifying, describing, investigating, and explaining events and occurrences that are perceived in the world. The science of nursing is the knowledge in and of nursing.

Philosophy

Philosophy is the study of wisdom, fundamental knowledge, and the processes we use to develop and construct our perceptions of life. Philosophy provides a viewpoint and implies a system of values and beliefs. Each individual develops a per-

sonal philosophy to give meaning to experiences and to guide behavior and attitudes. We develop personal philosophies by learning from interpersonal relationships, through formal and informal educational experiences, through religion and culture, and from the environment.

Every nurse's philosophy, developed through education and practice, forms the basis for providing nursing care. Nurses demonstrate both a personal and a professional philosophy through their values and beliefs about concepts such as goodness, health, illness, accountability, and ethics. In the same way, nursing education and nursing practice settings provide education or patient care based on philosophic beliefs about humans, health, teaching and learning, and quality patient care.

Process

A **process** is a series of actions, changes, or functions intended to bring about a desired result. During a process, one takes systematic and continuous steps to meet a goal and uses both assessments and feedback to direct actions to meet the goal. A particular theory or conceptual framework directs how these actions are carried out. The delivery of nursing care within the nursing process (described in Unit III) is directed by the way specific conceptual frameworks and theories define the person (patient), the environment, health, and nursing.

Historical Influences on Nursing Knowledge

The development of nursing knowledge has been influenced by the work of Florence Nightingale and by societal changes.

Nightingale's Contributions

Nightingale influenced nursing knowledge and practice by demonstrating efficient and knowledgeable nursing care, defining nursing practice as separate and distinct from medical practice, and differentiating between health nursing and illness nursing.

Although both men and women have given comfort and assistance to sick people through history, nursing essentially was considered "women's work" until the 1970s. In the 18th and 19th centuries, women were viewed as subservient and inferior to men in many societies. After Nightingale established an acceptable occupation for educated women and improved society's attitudes toward nursing, the role of women as nurses became more favorably accepted.

Despite Nightingale's belief in the uniqueness of nursing, the training of nurses was initially carried out under the direction and control of the medical profession (Kalish & Kalish, 1995). Because the conceptual and theoretical basis for nursing practice came from outside the profession, nursing struggled for years to establish its own identity and to receive recognition for its significant contributions to healthcare.

Societal Influences on Nursing Knowledge

Most schools of nursing established in the United States were adapted from Nightingale's model. There was no planned educational curriculum; instead, knowledge was acquired from lectures by physicians and by practical experience through caring for sick people in hospitals. This service orientation for nursing education remained the strongest influence on nursing practice until the 1950s. Rather than developing a body of knowledge specific to nursing, nursing care was carried out under the control and direction of the hospital administration and physicians practicing in that hospital. Nursing care was based on traditional ideas about following orders, as well as on common wisdom about caring for others based on either "common sense" or widely accepted scientific principles (Chinn & Kramer, 2004). As a result, nursing knowledge remained undeveloped and fragmented.

During the first half of the 20th century, a change in the structure of society resulted in changed roles for women and, in turn, for nursing. As a result of World Wars I and II, women increasingly entered the workforce, became more independent, and sought higher education. At the same time, nursing education began to focus more on education than hands-on training, and nursing research was conducted and published. As women became more assertive, nursing's need for a clearly defined identity based on unique contributions to the healthcare system emerged. In the mid-20th century, the idea of nursing as a science became more generally accepted, and philosophic beliefs and a knowledge base for nursing practice began to evolve.

NURSING THEORY

A **theory** is composed of a group of concepts that describe a pattern of reality. A theory is a statement that explains or characterizes a process, an occurrence, or an event and is based on observed facts. However, a theory cannot be proved directly or absolutely as can a fact. Theories arrange a group of related statements or concepts so that they give meaning to a series of events. Theories can be tested, changed, or used to guide research or to provide a base for evaluation. They are derived through two principal methods: **deductive reasoning,** in which one examines a general idea and then considers specific actions or ideas, and **inductive reasoning,** in which the reverse process is used—one builds from specific ideas or actions to conclusions about general ideas.

Concepts, like ideas, are abstract impressions organized into symbols of reality. Concepts describe objects, properties, and events and relationships among them. A group of concepts that follows an understandable pattern makes up a **conceptual framework or model.** Concepts can be thought of as the individual bricks and boards used to build a house, with the conceptual framework being the blueprint that specifies where each brick and board should go.

Nursing theory, as defined by Barnum (1998), "attempts to describe or explain the phenomenon (process, occurrence, or event) called nursing." Nursing theory differentiates nursing from other disciplines and activities in that it serves the purposes of describing, explaining, predicting, and controlling desired outcomes of nursing care practices. Theories thus provide a means of testing knowledge through research and, for

nursing, expanding its knowledge base to meet the healthcare needs of patients in an ever-changing society.

Interdisciplinary Base for Nursing Theories

Nursing theories are often based on, and influenced by, other broadly applicable processes and theories. The ideas and principles of the theories described briefly in the following sections are basic to many nursing concepts and are a part of the nursing literature. Nurses need to understand these theories and terminologies as they develop their own knowledge base in nursing.

General Systems Theory

General systems theory has been used in a wide range of disciplines since it emerged in the 1920s. Its primary theorist, Ludwig von Bertalanffy, developed the theory for universal application. This theory describes how to break whole things into parts and then to learn how the parts work together in "systems." It emphasizes relationships between the whole and the parts and describes how parts function and behave. These concepts may be applied to different kinds of systems, for example, to molecules in chemistry, cultures in sociology, organs in anatomy, and health in nursing. Key points in general systems theory are outlined in Box 5-1.

Recall Maribella Santos, the woman described in the Reflective Practice display who received therapeutic touch? The nurse would need to integrate knowledge of systems theory, including system communication, open systems, and energy transfer to better understand the goal of this technique.

BOX 5-1 Key Points in General Systems Theory

- A system is a set of interacting elements, all contributing to the overall goal of the system. The whole system is always greater than the sum of its parts.
- Systems are hierarchical in nature and are composed of interrelated subsystems that work together in such a way that a change in one element could affect other subsystems as well as the whole.
- Boundaries separate systems both from each other and from their environments.
- A system communicates with and reacts to its environment through factors that enter the system (input) or are transferred to the environment (output).
- An open system allows energy, matter, and information to move freely between systems and boundaries, whereas a closed system does not allow input from or output to the environment (no totally closed systems are known to exist in reality).
- To survive, open systems maintain balance through feedback.

Adaptation Theory

Adaptation theory defines adaptation as the adjustment of living matter to other living things and to environmental conditions. Adaptation is a continuously occurring process that effects change and involves interaction and response. Human adaptation occurs on three levels: the internal (self), the social (others), and the physical (biochemical reactions). Chapter 32 describes adaptation in relation to stress.

Developmental Theory

Developmental theory outlines the process of growth and development of humans as orderly and predictable, beginning with conception and ending with death. Although the pattern has definite stages, the progress and behaviors of an individual within each stage are unique. Heredity, temperament, emotional and physical environment, life experiences, and health status influence the growth and development of an individual.

Several theorists have made important contributions to developmental theory, but only two are mentioned here because their work is often used to develop nursing theory and to organize nursing practice. Eric Erikson based his theory of psychosocial development on the process of socialization, emphasizing how individuals learn to interact with the world. Erikson recognized the role of social, biologic, and environmental factors in development, and defined specific tasks or conflicts that people accomplish or overcome during what he defined as the eight stages of life. Chapters 18, 19, and 20 present more information on developmental theory.

Abraham Maslow developed his theory of human needs in terms of physical and psychosocial needs considered essential to human life, rather than by chronologic age as Erikson did. As described in Chapter 2, Maslow defined five levels of need in a hierarchy, with different needs existing simultaneously.

> *Think back to Joe Wimmer, the new father of a baby girl. When explaining about the use of the cap on the baby's head, the nurse would incorporate knowledge of Maslow's hierarchy of needs, specifically physiologic needs, and the need to minimize heat loss as a priority.*

As you continue in your nursing education and practice, you will learn how systems, adaptation, and developmental theories are used in planning and giving holistic care to patients. The following sections on specific nursing theories will help you better understand the knowledge base used to develop the concepts unique to nursing.

Nursing Theories

Even though nurses have difficulty agreeing on precise definitions of nursing, theory-based nursing directs nurses toward a common goal, with the ultimate outcome being improved patient care. Nursing theory provides rational and knowledgeable reasons for nursing actions, based on organized, written descriptions of what nursing is and what nurses do. Additionally, nursing theory gives nurses the knowledge base necessary for acting and responding appropriately in nursing care situations, provides a base for discussion, and, ideally, helps resolve current nursing issues. Theory gives nurses who know and practice theory better problem-solving skills, so that nursing actions are better organized, considered, and purposeful. Nursing theory also prepares nurses to question assumptions and values in nursing, thus further defining nursing and increasing the knowledge base.

Nursing theories are valuable in research, education, and practice. Nursing theories identify and define interrelated concepts important in nursing and clearly state the relationships between and among these concepts. Nursing theories should be simple and general; simple terminology and broadly applicable concepts ensure their usefulness in a wide variety of nursing practice situations. Nursing theories should also increase the nursing profession's body of knowledge by generating research to guide and improve practice. Overall, nursing theory guides nurses by providing a knowledge base, organizing concepts, providing guidelines for practice, and identifying nursing care goals.

Nursing theories may be descriptive or prescriptive (Meleis, 1997). Descriptive theories describe a phenomenon, an event, a situation, or a relationship. They further identify the properties and components of each of these as well as the circumstances in which it occurs. Prescriptive theories address nursing interventions and the consequences of those interventions; they are designed to control, promote, and change clinical nursing practice.

The aims of nursing, described in Chapter 1, are the same for all nursing theorists, but the values, assumptions, and beliefs individualize each theory when it is applied to the giving of nursing care. Theoretical frameworks of nursing provide a focus for nursing care activities. The person receiving care is the central theme, but the way each theorist defines that person, the environment, health, and nursing gives a unique focus specific to a particular theory. The ultimate goal of each framework, however, is holistic patient care, individualized to meet needs, promote health, and prevent or treat illness.

Common Concepts in Nursing Theories

Four concepts common in nursing theory that influence and determine nursing practice are (1) the person (patient), (2) the environment, (3) health, and (4) nursing. Each of these concepts is usually defined and described by a nursing theorist, often uniquely; and although these concepts are common to all nursing theories, both the definitions and the relations among them may differ from one theory to another. Of the four concepts, the most important is that of the person. The focus of nursing, regardless of definition or theory, is the person (Fig. 5-1).

Historical Influences on Nursing Theory

Florence Nightingale developed and published a philosophy and a theory of health and nursing that has served as a solid foundation for the nursing profession (Fig. 5-2). Her contributions to nursing theory include identifying the role of the nurse in meeting the patient's personal needs, recognizing the impor-

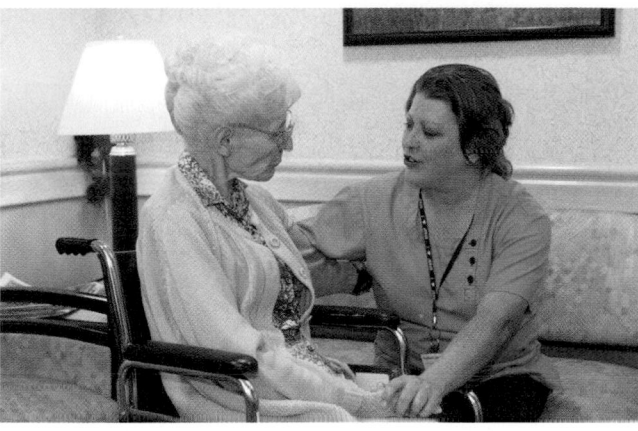

FIGURE 5-1 Four concepts common to all nursing theories are person, environment, health, and nursing. The most important concept, and the focus of nursing, is the person.   (Photo by Rick Brady.)

tance of environmental influences on the care of sick people, and elevating the standards and acceptance of nursing by developing sound principles of nursing education. Nightingale developed her theories of nursing in the late 1800s. Her foundational work is what nursing theorists expanded upon, starting in the 1950s until the present time (see Table 5-1).

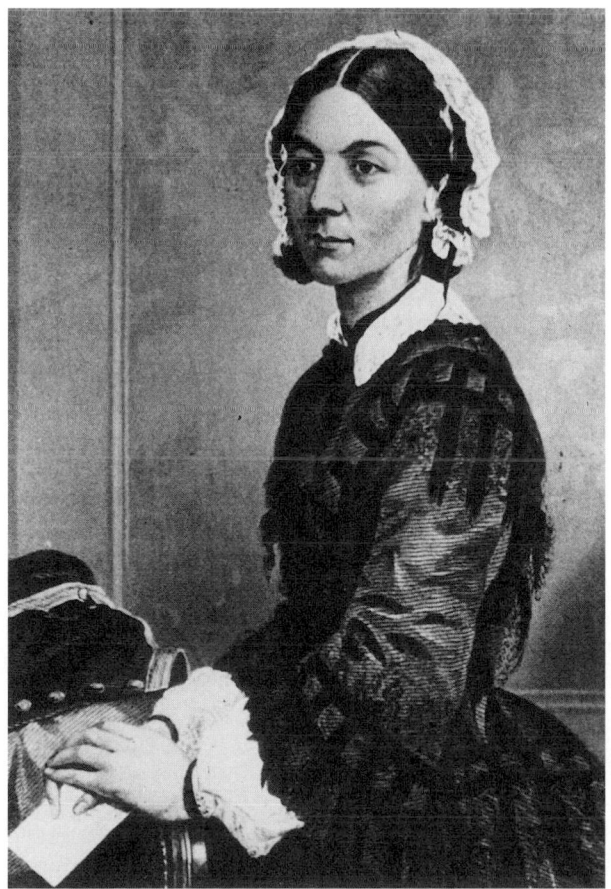

FIGURE 5-2 Florence Nightingale developed and published a philosophy and theory of health and nursing that has served as a solid foundation for the nursing profession.   (Photo courtesy of the Center for the Study of the History of Nursing, University of Pennsylvania.)

Applying Nursing Theory in Clinical Practice

As a discipline, nursing is increasingly defining its own independent functions and contributions to healthcare. The development and use of nursing theory provide autonomy (independence and self-governance) in the practice of nursing in many ways. As nurses demonstrate that nursing care does indeed make a difference and that nursing services are valuable, the discipline becomes more independent. Having a body of knowledge specific to the discipline allows members to be viewed by others as experts; this, in turn, gives nurses authority to carry out actions. In addition, interventions carried out and based on sound rationales are trusted and respected.

Today, it has become even more necessary and important for nurses to demonstrate efficient, cost-effective, high-quality care within organized healthcare delivery systems. By practicing theory-based nursing combined with critical thinking skills, nurses are able not only to deliver care that meets those criteria but also to describe and document what it is they do. Professional nurses use theories from nursing and from the behavioral sciences to collect, organize, and classify patient data and to understand, analyze, and interpret patients' health situations. Theoretical concepts and theories guide all phases of the nursing process, including planning, implementing, and evaluating nursing care, while also describing and explaining desired responses to and outcomes of care.

The major concepts of a chosen model or theory guide each step of the nursing process. The concepts serve as categories to guide the nurse in determining what information is relevant and should be collected to make assessments and to formulate nursing diagnoses. The concepts also suggest the appropriate types of nursing interventions and patient outcomes to be included in the care plan. Table 5-1 presents the purpose and clinical application of selected nursing theories. It is important to realize that as the focus of nursing changes, so does the applicability of the concepts within a specific theory.

NURSING RESEARCH

Research most simply defined means to examine carefully or to search again. Research as scientific inquiry is a process that uses observable and verifiable information (**data**), collected in a systematic manner, to describe, explain, or predict events. Research is conducted to validate and refine current knowledge or to develop new knowledge. The goals of research are to develop explanations (in theories) and to find solutions to problems.

Consider Charlotte Horn, the daughter who is being taught how to give tube feedings and is asking about ensuring proper tube placement. The nurse would incorporate information about various methods used to check for tube placement, emphasizing the rationale for doing so. In addition, the nurse would

TABLE 5-1 Selected Theorists and Theories of Nursing

Nursing Theorist and Date of Theory	Central Theme	Application to Clinical Practice
Florence Nightingale (1860)	Meeting the personal needs of the patient within the environment	Concern for the environment of the patient, including cleanliness, ventilation, temperature, light, diet, and noise
Hildegard Peplau (1952)	Nursing is a therapeutic, interpersonal, and goal-oriented process.	Nursing interventions are directed toward developing the patient's personality toward productive personal and community living.
Virginia Henderson (1955)	The patient is an individual who requires help to reach independence.	Nursing practice is independent; autonomous nursing functions are identified, and self-help concepts are described.
Faye Abdullah (1960)	Nursing is a problem-solving art and science used to identify the nursing problems of the patients as they move toward health and cope with illness-related health needs.	The 21 nursing-care problems identified were based on research and can be used to determine patient needs and formulate nursing-focused care.
Ida Jean Orlando (1961)	The nurse reacts to the patient's verbal and nonverbal expression of needs both to understand the meaning of the distress and to know what is needed to alleviate it.	Uses the nursing process to provide solutions to problems as well as to prevent problems
Ernestine Wiedenbach (1964)	Nursing as an art; nursing is providing nurturing care to patients.	Clinical nursing includes a philosophy, a purpose, the practice, and the art. Care is directed toward a specific purpose to meet the patient's perceived healthcare needs.
Lydia E. Hall (1966)	A focus on rehabilitation, encompassing nursing's autonomy, is therapeutic use of self, treatment within the healthcare team (cure), and nurturing (care).	The major outcome of nursing care is rehabilitation and feelings of self-actualization by the patient.
Myra E. Levine (1967)	Emphasis is on the ill person in the healthcare setting; describes detailed nursing skills and actions	The patient is the center of nursing activities, with nursing care provided based on four conservation principles to help patients adapt to their environment.
Martha Rogers (1970)	Emphasis on the science and art of nursing, with the unitary human being central to the discipline of nursing	Nursing interventions are directed toward repatterning human environment fields or assisting in mobilizing inner resources.
Dorothea Orem (1971)	Self-care is a human need, self-care deficits require nursing actions	Nursing is a human service, and nurses design interventions to provide or to manage self-care actions for sustaining health or recovering from illness or injury.
Imogene King (1971)	The patient is a personal system within a social system; the nurse and the patient experience each other and the situation, act and react, and transact.	Nursing is a process of human interactions as nurses and patients communicate to mutually set goals, and explore and agree on the means to reach those goals.
Sr. Callista Roy (1974)	Humans are biopsychosocial beings existing within an environment. Needs are created within interrelated adaptive modes: physiological self-concept, role function, and interdependence.	Nursing interventions are required when individuals demonstrate ineffective adaptive responses.
Madeline Leininger (1978)	Caring is the central theme of nursing care, nursing knowledge, and nursing practice.	Provides the foundation of transcultural nursing care. Caring improves human conditions and life processes.
Jean Watson (1979)	Nursing is concerned with promoting and restoring health, preventing illness, and caring for the sick.	Clinical nursing care is holistic to promote humanism, health, and quality of living. Caring is universal, and is practiced through interpersonal relationships.

(continued)

TABLE 5-1 (Continued)

Nursing Theorist and Date of Theory	Central Theme	Application to Clinical Practice
Margaret A. Newman (1979)	Nursing interventions are purposeful, using a total-person approach to patient care to help individuals, families, and groups attain and maintain wellness.	Nursing care is directed toward reducing stress factors and adverse conditions that increase the risk for or actually affect optimal patient functions.
Dorothy E. Johnson (1980)	Nursing problems arise when there are disturbances in the system or subsystem or the level of behavioral functioning is below an optimal level.	Nursing interventions are designed to support/maintain, educate, counsel, and modify behavior.
Rosemarie Parse (1981)	The individual continually interacts with the environment and participates in maintaining health.	Health is a continual, open process (rather than an absence of illness), with nursing care planned based on the patient's perspective of health and care.
Nola Pender (1982)	The goal of nursing is the optimal health of the individual, with a focus on how individuals make healthcare decisions.	Factors significant to health-promoting behaviors include an individual's beliefs about the importance of health, the perceived benefits of and perceived barriers to those behaviors. Participation in health-promoting behaviors is modified by one's demographic and biologic characteristics, interpersonal influences, and situational and behavioral factors.
Patricia Benner & Judith Wrubel (1989)	Nursing practice within a context of caring and skill development. Caring is a common bond of persons situated in a state of being that is essential to nursing.	A systematic description of stages of nursing practice: novice, advanced beginner, competent, proficient, and expert

recommend the best method to use based on scientific evidence from research.

Nursing research, broadly defined, encompasses both research to improve the care of people in the clinical setting and also the broader study of people and the nursing profession, including studies of education, policy development, ethics, and nursing history. Nurses should be concerned with the advancement of nursing as a profession. One of the many ways to promote nursing's development of greater autonomy and strength is nursing research. Nurses, depending on their level of education, conduct or participate in research to improve their efforts to deliver high-quality, cost-efficient care. Nurses also increasingly use the findings of research to provide evidence-based nursing practice (discussed in the next section).

Nursing research is fundamental to the recognition of nursing as a profession. As an occupation, nursing has existed since the beginning of human history. Many argue, however, that the profession of nursing is still in its infancy. One of the essential elements that differentiates a profession from an occupation is the existence of a unique and distinct knowledge base. The ultimate goal of expanding nursing's body of knowledge is to learn improved ways to promote and maintain health. As healthcare and illness patterns change, nursing interventions must change. Ongoing practice-based research reflects the nursing profession's commitment to meet the ever-changing demands of healthcare consumers.

Remember Joe Wimmer, the new father described at the beginning of the chapter? Before responding to Mr. Wimmer, the nurse would need knowledge of nursing research studies dealing with newborn heat loss and methods to minimize it. A review of the literature would provide theoretical information necessary to explain the scientific rationale for using caps on the heads of newborns to reduce heat loss.

The Evolution of Nursing Research

While caring for victims of the Crimean War, Florence Nightingale kept careful and objective records. These records provided baseline data that she later used to determine which nursing interventions were most effective in treating her patients. Since that time, nursing research has taken many different pathways, and all nurses are involved with research either as consumers (nurses who use and evaluate research findings) or as actual investigators who design and implement research studies.

Although nurses have always provided care through nursing interventions and have evaluated the response of the patient, for a long time those interventions were primarily intuitive or based on a philosophy of "It's always been done that way." Despite the initial work by Nightingale, this persisted until the mid-20th century. As advances were made in technology and medical research during the 20th century, nursing leaders realized that research about the practice of nursing was necessary to meet the health needs of modern society. Increasing numbers of nurses began to conduct research and write articles telling other nurses how to conduct nursing research.

During the 1950s and 1960s, research was increasingly recognized as important. Early studies provided the basis for the development of nursing practice standards and the most effective educational preparation for registered nurses. The American Nurses Association (ANA) sponsored a series of nursing research conferences. A focus on clinical studies to examine quality of care and the development of outcomes of care grew out of the newly developed intensive care units.

The 1970s and 1980s focused on clinical research, with published studies of such clinical interventions as vital signs and treatment procedures. Primary patient care was a popular method of nursing care, with research investigating outcomes and quality of care. The nursing process also was studied, with research into assessment and effective nursing diagnosis of patient responses to the effects of illness. Studies of nursing education were concerned with student learning experiences and clinical evaluation methods, as well as differentiation of practice by educational preparation. In addition, models, conceptual frameworks, and theories were developed to guide nursing practice. More nurses were prepared at the doctoral level, and federal funding for nursing research increased. Journals specific to nursing research and nursing research in specialty areas were published. Of major importance was the creation of the National Center for Nursing Research (NCNR) by the ANA in 1985.

From the 1990s to the present, nursing research has continued to expand. The NCNR was promoted to the National Institute of Nursing Research (NINR) in 1993, gaining equal status with all other National Institutes of Health. The research themes for the future developed by NINR are listed in Box 5-2. Research is included as an essential component of nursing by the ANA, by the International Council of Nurses, and by nursing specialty organizations. Further contributing to a focus on research in the clinical setting are the increased numbers of graduates from nursing masters' and doctoral programs.

Methods of Nursing Research

Two primary methods of conducting nursing research are quantitative and qualitative. Each method is summarized here to facilitate understanding published research so that findings may be used in clinical practice.

Recall Maribella Santos, the woman with postoperative nausea relieved by therapeutic touch? To gain insight into this technique and better patient teaching, the nurse would need to review the literature for related published research studies. Based on the information found, the nurse would then integrate it into the teaching plan for this patient.

BOX 5-2 National Institute of Nursing Research Themes for the Future

Panels of nursing research experts developed the following themes. They encompass cross-cutting issues, including ethnic and cultural sensitivities, family and community considerations, a multidisciplinary approach, biologic and behavioral mechanisms and their interrelationships, the clinical setting in which care is provided, and the cost-effectiveness of research interventions. The themes are:

- Changing Lifestyle Behaviors for Better Health
- Managing the Effects of Chronic Illness to Improve Quality of Life
- Identifying Effective Strategies to Reduce Health Disparities
- Harnessing Advanced Technologies to Serve Human Needs
- Enhancing End-of-Life Experience for Patients and Their Families

(National Institute of Nursing Research, National Institutes of Health. [2003]. *Mission statement and research themes for the future.* The full document may be found at http://www.nih.gov/ninr/.)

Quantitative Research Methods

Quantitative research involves the concepts of basic and applied research. **Basic research,** sometimes called pure research, is designed to generate and refine theory and the findings are often not directly useful in practice. **Applied research,** also called practical research, is designed to directly influence or improve clinical practice.

The types of quantitative research depend on the level of current knowledge about a research problem. The various types are described in Table 5-2. The steps of quantitative research are followed carefully, although they may be designed in different ways. The basic steps of the quantitative research process are outlined and described briefly in Table 5-3. Important terms in quantitative research are defined in Box 5-3.

Qualitative Research Methods

Qualitative research is a method of research conducted to gain insight by discovering meanings. It is based on the belief that reality is based on perceptions, which differ for each person and change over time. The research design follows many of the same steps as does quantitative research, but differs in that the researcher primarily analyzes words rather than numbers. The methods of qualitative research are outlined and briefly described in Table 5-4.

Protecting the Rights of Human Subjects

Many nurses work in healthcare institutions in which patients are invited to participate in clinical research. With their focus on the overall well-being of the patient, nurses play an impor-

TABLE 5-2 **Types of Quantitative Research**

Type	Purpose
Descriptive Research	To explore and describe events in real life situations, describing concepts and identifying relationships between and among events. Often used to generate new knowledge about topics with little or no prior research.
Correlational Research	To examine the type and degree of relationships between two or more variables. The strength of the relationship varies from a -1 (perfect negative correlation, in which one increases as the other decreases) to a $+1$ (perfect positive correlation, with both variables increasing or decreasing together).
Quasi-experimental Research	To examine cause-and-effect relationships between selected variables. Often conducted in nursing to examine the effects of nursing interventions on patient outcomes.
Experimental Research	To examine cause-and-effect relationships between variables under highly controlled conditions. These are often conducted in a laboratory setting.

tant role in ensuring that patient interests are not sacrificed to research interests. Nursing priorities on research units include determining that research studies have met appropriate scientific and ethical criteria before their implementation, and protecting patient rights. Specific patient rights include **informed consent,** the patient's right to consent knowledgeably to participate in a study without coercion (knowing that this consent may be withdrawn at any time) or to refuse to participate without jeopardizing the care that he or she will receive;

the right to confidentiality; and the right to be protected from harm.

Federal regulations require that institutions receiving federal funding or conducting studies of drugs or medical devices regulated by the Food and Drug Administration establish institutional review boards (IRBs). The IRBs review all studies conducted in the institution to determine the risk status of all studies and to ensure that ethical principles are followed (see Chapter 6 for full discussion of values and ethics in nursing).

TABLE 5-3 **Steps of the Quantitative Research Process**

Step	Description
1. State the research problem.	Often stated as a question, the problem should be focused narrowly on the problem being studied. For example: "What is the optimal time for taking a rectal temperature with a glass thermometer?"
2. Define the purpose of the study.	The purpose explains "why" the problem is important and what use the findings will be.
3. Review related literature.	The literature review provides information about what is already known, provides information about concepts and how the concepts have been measured. It also identifies gaps in knowledge that will be studied.
4. Formulate hypotheses and variables.	Hypotheses are statements about two or more concepts or variables. Variables are concepts of varying levels of abstraction that are measured, manipulated, or controlled in a study.
5. Select the research design.	The design is a carefully determined, systematic, and controlled plan for finding answers to the question of the study. This provides a "road map" for all aspects of the study, including how to collect and analyze the data.
6. Select the population and sample.	The population is the group to be studied. The sample refers to specific people or events in the population from which data will be collected.
7. Collect the data.	Sources of data may include people, literature, documents, and findings (for example, from sources such as laboratory data or measurements of vital signs). Data may be collected from interviews, questionnaires, direct measurement, or examinations (such as physical or psychological tests).
8. Analyze the data.	Statistical procedures are used to analyze the data and provide answers to the research question.
9. Communicate findings and conclusions.	Through publications and presentations, the researcher explains the results of the study and links them to the existing body of knowledge in the literature. The researcher also describes the implications of the study and suggests directions for further research.

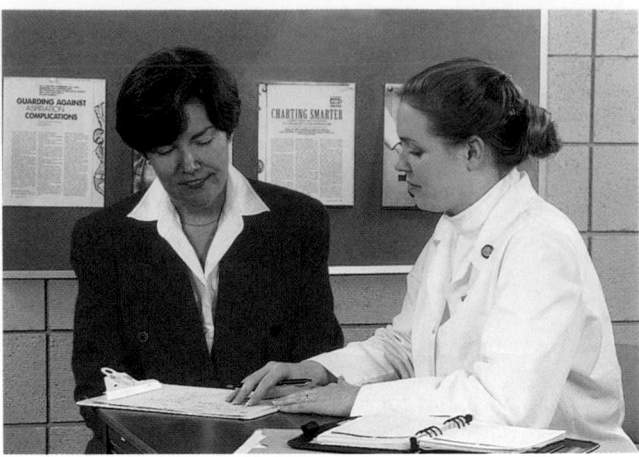

FIGURE 5-3 A student questions her instructor about the discrepancy between what she sees staff nurses doing to treat a wound and what her text and literature search recommend.

Relating Research to Practice

Research about nursing education, administration, and practice all affect patient care directly or indirectly. Too often, practicing nurses mistakenly think research is far removed from caring for patients at the bedside. This false impression has slowed the progress of practice-based nursing research. Yet much of what bedside nurses routinely do constitutes research. The nursing process (ie, assessing, diagnosing, planning, implementing, and evaluating) represents the basic framework of the research process. The most common impediments to nursing research include restricted access to resources, limited time to participate in research-related activities, and lack of educational preparation needed by nurses for research.

Unless the research findings of nurse researchers are used by practicing nurses to improve the quality of patient care, clinical nursing research is useless. Nursing students developing clinical skills must understand the scientific rationale that makes one course of action preferable to another (Fig. 5-3). Throughout this text, Research in Nursing boxes highlight current studies that have the potential to make a positive difference in nursing practice and patient outcomes.

EVIDENCE-BASED PRACTICE

Evidence-based practice (EBP) is nursing care provided that is supported by reliable research-based evidence. The nursing care may be of specific interventions (such as the most effective and safe method of inserting and caring for nasogastric tubes) or guidelines established for the care of patients with specific illnesses, treatments, or surgical procedures.

The foundation of the current emphasis on EBP is evidence-based medicine, a clinical learning strategy at a medical school in Canada. Evidence-based nursing practice originated outside

TABLE 5-4 Qualitative Research Methods

Method	Description
Phenomenology	The purpose of phenomenology (both a philosophy and a research method) is to describe experiences as they are lived by the subjects being studied. Analysis of data provides information about the meaning of the experience within each person's own reality (for example, the experience of health or of having a heart attack).
Grounded Theory	The basis of grounded theory methodology is the discovery of how people describe their own reality and how their beliefs are related to their actions in a social scene. The findings are grounded in the data from subjects and are used to formulate concepts and to generate a theory of the experience, supported by examples from the data (for example, coping with a seriously ill child).
Ethnography	Developed by the discipline of anthropology, ethnographic research is used to examine issues of a culture that are of interest to nursing.
Historical	Historical research examines events of the past to increase understanding of the nursing profession today. Many historical studies focus on nursing leaders, but there is increasing interest in the historical patterns of nursing practice.

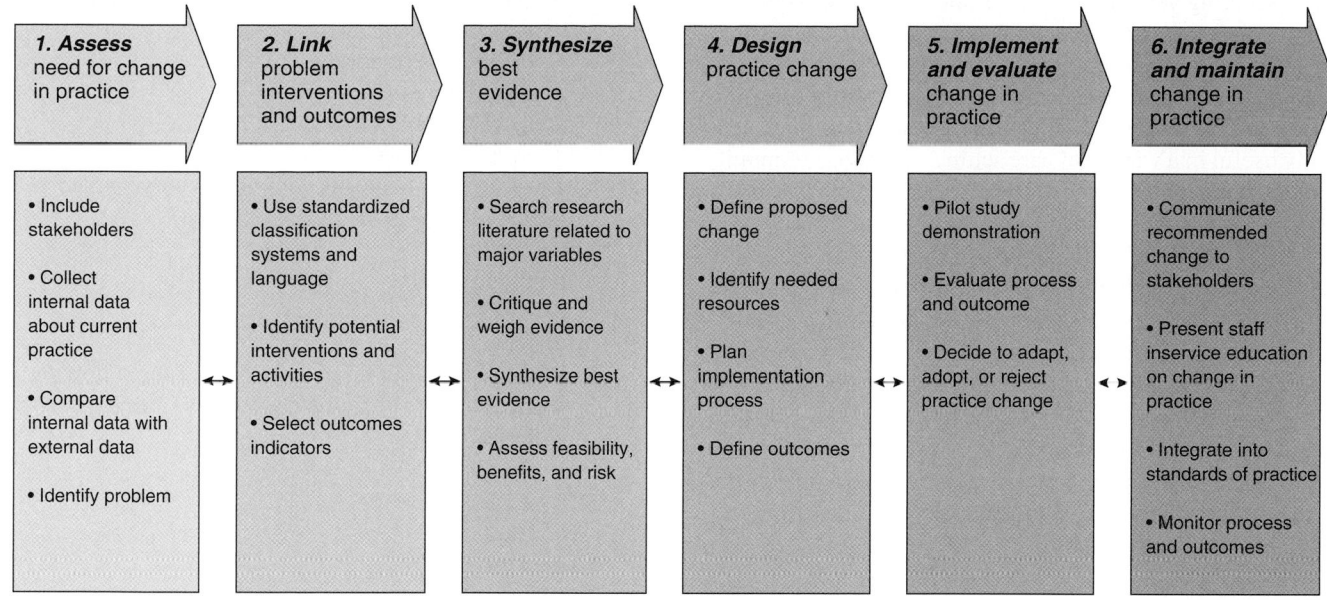

FIGURE 5-4 A model for evidence-based practice. (Used with permission from Rosswurm, M. A., & Larrabee, J. H. [1999]. A model for change to evidence-based practice. *Image: The Journal of Nursing Scholarship, 31*[4], 318.)

the United States, with evidence-based nursing organization now in Canada, the United Kingdom, Australia, and the United States. Definitions of EBP are variable. Two definitions follow.

- "Evidence-based nursing is practice that relies on information generated from results of scientific research (Stevens & Pugh, 1999, p. 155)."
- "Evidence-based nursing practice is the conscientious, explicit, and judicious use of theory-derived, research-based information in making decisions about care delivery to

individuals or groups of patients and in consideration of individuals' needs and preferences (Ingersoll, 2000, p. 152)."

Although this is a fairly new movement in nursing, and one that is not clearly understood, it is important that nurses understand that using research and practicing research-based practice are a part of EBP (Jennings & Loan, 2001).

Those interested in quality and cost control want evidence that the services and interventions being funded are effec-

TABLE 5-5 **Reading a Research Journal Article**

Sections (in usual order)	Description
Abstract	The abstract is at the beginning of the article. It summarizes the entire article and usually provides the purpose of the study, a description of the subjects, data collection and data analysis, and a summary of important findings.
Introduction · Review of the literature · Statement of the purpose	The literature review discusses relevant studies that have been conducted in the area of this study. A statement of the specific goals or purpose of the study often follows the review.
Method · Subjects · Design · Data collection · Data analysis	The methods section provides in detail how the study was conducted, including who and how many subjects, what research design was used, what data were collected and how, and types of analysis done. There should be enough information so that the study could be replicated (repeated).
Results	The results (findings) are often presented both in words and in charts, tables, or graphs. It is important to understand what the results were and if they are meaningful.
Discussion (Conclusions)	The discussion section reports what the results mean in regard to the purpose of the study and the literature review. It may also include suggestions for further research and application to nursing education or practice as appropriate.
References	The references are at the end of the article and include a list of articles and books used by the researcher.

tive in securing valued goals. Scientific research, designed to achieve high levels of objectivity, may be costly and time-consuming, and can be impractical given the complexities surrounding patient care. The control and objectivity of scientific knowledge, however, allow it to be generalized, making it highly useful in a variety of care settings. Nursing's commitment to acquiring new knowledge is one reason why nurses must become more aware of and involved in the research process. Rosswurm and Larrabee (1999) designed the model illustrated in Figure 5-4 to guide nurses and other healthcare professionals through a systemic process for change to EBP.

The use of EBP mandates critical analysis and extensive, systematic reviews of research articles and findings. As beginning students, you will not yet have acquired the knowledge to complete that task. The first step for you as a student is to be able to read and understand a research article. To help you, the typical format of a research journal article with a description of each part is outlined in Table 5-5.

Developing Critical Thinking Skills

1. Describe your own beliefs about the patient, the nurse, health, and what nursing is. Compare and contrast your answers with another student. How are they different, and how are they alike? How do you think such differences might influence nursing practice for each of you?
2. In preparation for your clinical assignment, you read three research articles about positioning and moving patients who are at risk for pressure ulcers (bed sores). The staff nurse responsible for the patient tells you "Oh, I don't pay any attention to that stuff." What would you do?

Practicing for NCLEX

1. When you ask an older student why it is necessary to change the patient's bed every day, he says "I guess we have always done it that way." This answer is an example of:
   a. Unsubstantiated knowledge
   b. Scientific knowledge
   c. Authoritative knowledge
   d. Traditional knowledge
2. One method of developing a theory is by first examining a general idea and then considering specific actions or ideas. What is this method called?
   a. Inductive reasoning
   b. Deductive reasoning
   c. Conceptual modeling
   d. Concept development
3. What word may be used to describe a concept?
   a. Fact
   b. Science
   c. Idea
   d. Truth

4. Which of the following types of nursing theory focuses on clinical nursing practice?
   a. Prescriptive theory
   b. Descriptive theory
   c. Developmental theory
   d. Systems theory
5. There are four concepts common to nursing theories. Which concept is the most important?
   a. Person
   b. Environment
   c. Health
   d. Nursing
6. When conducting research, which of the following terms is used to describe the information that is collected?
   a. Subject
   b. Analysis
   c. Data
   d. Abstract
7. What is the name of the type of quantitative research conducted to directly influence or improve clinical practice?
   a. Basic research
   b. Applied research
   c. Experimental research
   d. Descriptive research
8. A researcher is studying the effects of exercise and sleep on blood pressure. What type of variable is the blood pressure in this study?
   a. Exploratory
   b. Correlational
   c. Dependent
   d. Independent
9. Of the following types of qualitative research, which method developed in anthropology?
   a. Historical
   b. Ethnography
   c. Grounded theory
   d. Phenomenology
10. What type of clinical nursing practice is becoming increasingly important to healthcare and nursing today?
    a. Primary care nursing
    b. Community-based nursing
    c. Authoritative nursing
    d. Evidence-based nursing

Answers With Rationale

1. The correct response is *d*. Traditional knowledge is the part of nursing practice passed down from generation to generation, often without research data to support it.
2. The correct response is *b*. Moving from a general idea to specific ideas is deductive reasoning.
3. The correct response is *c*. A concept, like an idea, is an abstract impression of reality.

4. The correct response is *a.* Prescriptive theories address nursing interventions and are designed to control, promote, and change clinical nursing practice.

5. The correct response is *a.* Of the four concepts, the most important is the person.

6. The correct response is *c.* Data are observable and verifiable information collected to describe, explain, or predict events.

7. The correct response is *b.* Applied research, a type of quantitative research, is designed to directly influence or improve clinical practice.

8. The correct response is *c.* The dependent variable is the variable being studied and is determined by manipulating conditions (the independent variables).

9. The correct response is *b.* Ethnographic research was developed by the discipline of anthropology and is used to examine issues of culture of interest to nursing.

10. The correct response is *d.* An increasing trend in healthcare, including nursing, is the use of research-supported, evidence-based clinical nursing practice.

Bibliography

Alligood, M., & Marriner-Tomey, A. (1999). *Nursing theory: Utilization & application.* St. Louis: C. V. Mosby.

American Nurses Association. (1997). *Position statement: Education for participation in nursing research.* Available at http://nursingworld.org/rcadroom/position/research/rseducat.htm.

Barnum, B. (1998). *Nursing theory: Analysis, application, and evaluation* (5th ed.). Philadelphia: Lippincott Williams & Wilkins.

Burns, N., & Groves, S. (2003). *Understanding nursing research* (3rd ed.). Philadelphia: W. B. Saunders.

Chinn, P., & Kramer, M. (2004). *Integrated knowledge development in nursing* (6th ed.). St. Louis: C. V. Mosby.

Frisch, N., & Kelley, J. (2002). Nursing diagnosis and nursing theory: Exploration of factors inhibiting and supporting simultaneous use. *Nursing Diagnosis, 13*(2), 53–61.

Gortner, S. (2000). Knowledge development in nursing: Our historical roots and future opportunities. *Nursing Outlook, 48*(2), 60–67.

Ingersoll, G. (2000). Evidence-based nursing: What it is and what it isn't. *Nursing Outlook, 48*(4), 151–152.

Jennings, B., & Loan, L. (2001). Misconceptions among nurses about evidence-based practice. *Journal of Nursing Scholarship, 33*(2), 121–127.

Kalish, P., & Kalish, B. (1995). *The advance of American nursing* (3rd ed.). Philadelphia: J. B. Lippincott.

Krause-Bachand, J. (2002). Ethical considerations in nursing research. *SCI Nursing, 19*(3), 136–137.

Marriner-Tomey, A., & Alligood, M. (2001). *Nursing theorists and their work* (5th ed.). St. Louis: Mosby.

McElroy, D., & Walker, C. (2001). On theories and evidence-based practice. *Journal of Nursing Scholarship, 33*(4), 306–307.

Meleis, A. I. (1997). *Theoretical nursing: Development and progress* (3rd ed.). Philadelphia: Lippincott-Raven.

National Institute of Nursing Research, National Institutes of Health. (2003). *Research themes for the future.* Available at http://www.nih.gov/ninr/.

Polit, D., Beck, C., & Hungler, B. (2002). *Essentials of nursing research: Methods, appraisal, and utilization.* Philadelphia: Lippincott Williams & Wilkins.

Rosswurm, M., & Larrabee, J. (1999). A model for change to evidence-based practice. *Image: Journal of Nursing Scholarship, 31*(4), 317–322.

Stevens, K., & Pugh, J. (1999). Evidence-based practice and perioperative nursing. *Seminars in Perioperative Nursing, 8*(3), 155–159.

Values, Ethics, and Advocacy

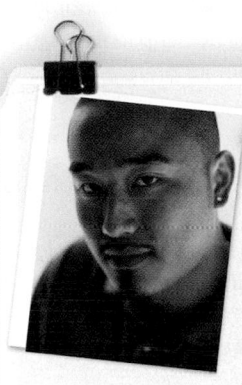

Chengyu Zhang is an alert 32-year-old man in the intensive care unit who is begging to be removed from the ventilator. He understands that it is highly unlikely that he will be able to breathe on his own without the ventilator. He writes on the communication board "If I die, I die. I can't keep living like this."

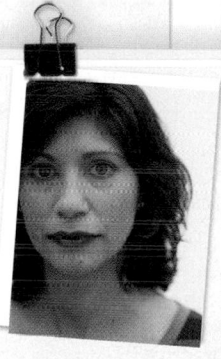

Marissa Sandoval, a 44-year-old woman who has just recently undergone extensive surgery to treat uterine cancer, is experiencing several serious postoperative complications. She states "I don't know why all of these things are happening. I ask the doctors. So does my family. But we get no answers. We just want to know what is happening." The nurse is surprised to observe that not only does the surgeon not answer Marissa's questions, but that he also dismisses her fears without any explanation.

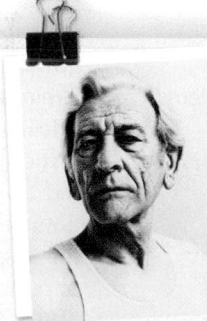

William Raines, a homeless, 68-year-old indigent man diagnosed with schizophrenia, developmental delays, and uncontrolled hypertension, was admitted for control of moderately severe elevated blood pressure. A review of his medical record reveals that Mr. Raines was getting samples of medications for blood pressure treatment from the pharmaceutical representatives at the clinic, but recent policy changes stopped this practice approximately 4 weeks ago. Mr. Raines is about to be discharged with several prescriptions for medications and no way to fill them.

Focusing on Blended Skills

The types of blended skills you'll need to respond to the case scenarios here include:

Cognitive Skills

- Basic knowledge of how values influence behavior
- Ability to identify the factors affecting the development of values, such as culture and environment
- Ability to incorporate knowledge of values transmission and clarification, theories of ethics, codes of professional ethics, and ethical standards for practice when developing a client's plan of care
- Knowledge of the patient's bill of rights and ethical principles of the nurse–patient relationship
- Ability to integrate ethical principles and use an ethical framework and decision-making process to resolve ethical problems

Technical Skills

- Ability to integrate ethical agency to provide the technical nursing assistance necessary to meet the needs of patients
- Ability to use correctly the equipment and protocols necessary to promote advocacy and address ethical problems

Interpersonal Skills

- Ability to establish trusting professional relationships with both patients and colleagues—relationships that are respectful of value differences and that enhance dignity and worth
- Ability to demonstrate respect for patient's autonomy and self-determination throughout the nurse–patient relationship
- Ability to advocate for patients whose preferences may be different from personal ones

Ethical and Legal Skills

- Ability to use values clarification techniques in professional practice
- Ability to prevent and resolve ethical conflict by employing ethical principles, and appropriately using ethics consultations and other resources
- Ability to practice nursing consistent with nursing's code of ethics
- Ability to recognize and respond appropriately to ethical issues in practice

Learning Outcomes

After completing the chapter, the learner should be able to accomplish the following:

1. List five common modes of value transmission.
2. Describe seven steps in the valuing process.
3. Use values clarification strategies in clinical practice.
4. Compare and contrast the principle-based and care-based approaches to bioethics.
5. Describe nursing practice that is consistent with the code of ethics for nursing.
6. Describe the purpose of the Bill of Rights for Registered Nurses.
7. Recognize ethical issues as they arise in nursing practice.
8. Use an ethical framework and decision-making process to resolve ethical problems.
9. Identify four functions of institutional ethics committees.
10. Describe three typical concerns of the nurse advocate.

Key Terms

advocacy
autonomy
beneficence
bioethics
care-based approach
clinical ethics
deontologic
ethical agency
ethical dilemma
ethical distress
ethics
feminist ethics
fidelity
justice
morals
nonmaleficence
nursing ethics
paternalism
principle-based approach
utilitarian
value
value system
values clarification

The unique nature of nursing places nurses both at the bedside and in groups of professionals where critical decisions are made about the best way to treat injury and illness and to solve healthcare problems. Often, the question confronting the nurse is not "How do I do this?" but, rather, "Should I do this?" The more that science and technology increase the options available to patients and healthcare professionals, the more frequently nurses will find themselves asking "We can do this, but should we, here and now, for this patient?" "Should the professionals in the intensive care unit keep Mr. Zhang on ventilatory support?"

Nurses also are increasingly distressed by the failure of society to provide adequate care for its most vulnerable members. Nothing is more disturbing for professional nurses than seeing firsthand the consequences of unmet healthcare needs. When nurses care for patients like Mr. Raines, who lack the financial resources to obtain the medications and treatment they need, they have special advocacy obligations. A shortage of nurses further complicates the nursing work environment, creating the necessity for nurses to be skilled advocates for safety, quality care, and their own needs. Never has it been more important for nurses to grasp the ethical dimensions of professional practice and to be confident in "doing the ethically right thing simply because it's the right thing to do!" With their moral integrity on the line every day, nurses understand the need to be as skilled ethically as they are intellectually, interpersonally, and technically.

Ethics, or morality, poses questions about how we ought to act and how we should live. It is an inquiry into the justification of particular actions (eg, Are these actions right or wrong?), as well as a search for traits of moral character that promote more human growth.

This chapter explores the influence of values on human behavior and the ethical dimensions of nursing practice. Chapter 11 describes specific ethical competencies, or skills, that are essential to nursing practice. Nurses who understand how patients' values and their own values shape nurse–patient interactions, and who continually develop sensitivity to the ethical dimensions of nursing practice, are best able to provide quality care and advocate for their patients. (For an example, see the accompanying display, Reflective Practice: Challenge to Ethical and Legal Skills.)

VALUES

A **value** is a belief about the worth of something, about what matters, that acts as a standard to guide one's behavior. If you think back to how you spent your last weekend, you may observe something about your values. The amount of time and money you devote to relationships, work, study, fitness activities, leisure, and other experiences reveals something about the importance (value) you attach to these endeavors.

A **value system** is an organization of values in which each is ranked along a continuum of importance, often leading to a personal code of conduct. A person's values influence beliefs about human needs, health, and illness; the practice of health behaviors; and human responses to illness. For example, individuals who place a high value on health and personal responsibility often work hard to reach their fitness goals. Individuals who value high-risk leisure activities may attach less value to life and health. Nurses who work effectively with patients are sensitive to how a patient's values and their own values influence their interactions.

Development of Values

An individual is not born with values; rather, values are formed during a lifetime from information from the environment, family, and culture.

> Recall Chengyu Zhang, the 32-year-old man in the intensive care unit asking to be removed from the ventilator, even if it means that he will die. The nurse can integrate knowledge of the patient's culture and family and their influence on the patient's value of independence as a key aspect in planning his care.

As children observe the actions of others, they quickly learn what has high and low value for family members. If the parents spend a good portion of each day cooking, and the family spends a long time eating and talking at the table, the children learn to value food and the good times it represents. Similarly, children learn that helpfulness is a good and respected quality if praised when helping parents, grandparents, and siblings. Common modes of value transmission include:

- Modeling
- Moralizing
- Laissez-faire
- Rewarding and punishing
- Responsible choice

Through modeling, children learn what is of high or low value by observing parents, peers, and significant others. Thus, modeling may lead to socially acceptable or unacceptable behaviors. Children whose caregivers use the moralizing mode of value transmission are taught a complete value system by parents or an institution (eg, church or school) that allows little opportunity for them to weigh different values.

Those who use the laissez-faire approach to value transmission leave children to explore values on their own (no one set of values is presented as best for all) and to develop a personal value system. This approach often involves little or no guidance and can lead to confusion and conflict.

Through rewarding and punishing, children are rewarded for demonstrating values held by parents and punished for demonstrating unacceptable values. Finally, caregivers who follow the responsible-choice mode of value transmission encourage children to explore competing values and to weigh their consequences. Support and guidance are offered as children develop a personal value system.

Reflective Practice
Challenge to Ethical and Legal Skills

A common ethical dilemma that I have faced both as a student in the clinical area and as a nurse extern during the summers involves my lack of confidence preventing me from being a patient advocate. My lack of status in the unit makes it very difficult for me to stand up to more senior, experienced staff to act as a patient advocate. However, patient advocacy is a crucial duty for any nurse. I feel that when I neglect this duty, I am being unethical because I am not fulfilling one of the most important nursing roles. An example of this dilemma occurred during one of my first weeks on the gynecologic surgical floor where I was an extern this summer.

Mrs. Marissa Sandoval was a 44-year-old woman who had just recently undergone extensive surgery for treatment of newly diagnosed uterine cancer. She also developed several postoperative complications. Mrs. Sandoval and her family were unhappy about the lack of answers they were getting from the attending surgeon and the residents about the complications she was experiencing from the surgery. After observing the surgeon interacting with the patient and her family in her room, I could easily understand the patient's distress. In addition to the surgeon not answering any of the family's questions, he dismissed all of her legitimate fears without an explanation. I felt this was a terrible way to treat a patient and that as patient advocate, I had an ethical and professional duty to make sure the patient and her family received adequate answers.

Thinking Outside the Box: Possible Courses of Action

- Confront the surgeon, explaining the patient's anxiety and asking him to return to her room to answer the questions.
- Try to answer the patient's questions to the best of my ability.
- Pretend that the doctor was acting appropriately. Tell the patient that the doctor will return tomorrow during rounds, and that she will have the opportunity to ask questions then.
- Ask another, more experienced nurse to answer my patient's questions.
- Tell the patient not to worry so much, because the doctors and nurses will take good care of her.

Evaluating a Good Outcome: How Do I Define Success?

- The patient receives satisfactory answers to her questions.
- The situation is handled in a respectful manner for all parties involved.
- The American Nurses Association's Bill of Rights is followed: "Nurses have the right to freely and openly advocate for themselves and their patients, without fear of retribution."
- No one involved in the situation suffers from a violation of integrity.
- The ANA Code of Ethics is followed: "The nurse promotes, advocates for, and strives to protect the health, safety, and rights of the patient."

Personal Learning: Here's to the Future!

In retrospect, when I examine the situation, I don't think that I handled the situation in the most ethical manner. Rather than dealing with the situation myself, I sought out the help of a more experienced nurse to answer the patient's questions to the best of her ability. Unfortunately, because of the complexity of the case, the more experienced nurse was not able to answer all of the questions adequately. I should have spoken with the surgeon and expressed my concern regarding the patient's questions going unanswered. However, I was greatly intimidated by this surgeon, and thus, I did not want to confront him. My actions demonstrate that I was compromising my role as a patient advocate. I compromised this role because of personal anxiety and lack of confidence associated with confronting the surgeon.

I do feel that I am trying to base my personal practice on a strong ethical foundation, with my personal actions reflective of this, as I hold my own actions to a high ethical standard. However, I am not a very confrontational person. This, coupled with my great insecurities about working in the hospital setting, make it difficult for me to confront other healthcare providers when I think they are acting in an unethical manner. Therefore, while I think my personal actions have a strong ethical foundation, I have a lot of room for growth when acting in an ethical manner when needing to confront coworkers. I hope that as I grow more comfortable in the hospital setting, I will not compromise my role as a patient advocate because of my personal fears.

Reflection

How do you think you would respond in a similar situation? Why? What does this tell you about yourself and about the adequacy of your skills for professional practice? How might the surgeon's values have influenced his actions? Please explain. Did the student adhere to the ANA's Bill of Rights? ANA Code for Nurses? Canadian Nurses Association Code of Ethics? Explain your answer. Evaluate whether the patient's rights as stated in the American Hospital Association's Bill of Rights were respected. How did the student use or not use ethical agency? What ethical principles were involved in this situation? How did the student attempt to use these principles? Can you think of other ways to use these principles or respond? What other skills (cognitive, interpersonal, technical, ethical/legal) would you need to respond well in this situation? Do you agree with the criteria to evaluate a successful outcome? Was anyone's integrity violated? Please explain.

Elizabeth Nalli, Georgetown University

Values Essential to the Professional Nurse

Professional values provide the foundation for nursing practice and guide the nurse's interactions with patients, colleagues, and the public. In 1998, the American Association of Colleges of Nursing identified five values that epitomize the caring, professional nurse. Box 6-1 lists these values and sample behaviors illustrating each of these values. Every nurse should critically examine his or her personal values to see if they match these essential professional values. For example, if I value self-promotion to the extent that I won't make the sacrifices demanded by a genuine commitment to the welfare of the patients entrusted to my care, I will never be successful as a nurse. Similarly, if I attach low value to respecting people who are different from me, I may interact with patients and colleagues in a way that is demeaning and unprofessional. It is helpful to identify nurses in your practice setting who epitomize nursing's essential values and to learn from observing their behavior.

To encourage healthcare professionals to respect and accept the individuality of patients, some educators have advised that professionals be "value neutral" and "nonjudgmental" in their professional roles. Thus, the nurse has a "commitment to patients whether or not the nurse and the patients hold the same values. The nurse does not assume that her personal values are right and should not judge the patient's values as right or wrong depending on their congruence with the nurse's personal value system" (Steele & Harmon, 1983, p. 27). This kind of thinking encourages effective care for patients with values different from the nurse's. For example, a nurse who strongly believes that any premarital or extramarital sex is wrong can still offer competent and compassionate nursing care to a young woman prostitute with active herpes lesions. On the other hand, if the same patient, after receiving education, indicates that she is unconcerned about whom she might infect in future sexual encounters, the nurse has an ethical obligation to protect the patient and others from the harm the patient's values may cause.

Values Clarification

Values clarification is a process by which people come to understand their own values and value system. "It is a process of discovery and allows the person to discover through feelings and analysis of behavior what choices to make when alternatives are presented, and to identify whether or not these choices are rationally made or are the result of previous conditioning" (Steele & Harmon, 1983, p. 13). Values clarifica-

---

BOX 6-1 Professional Values

Altruism is a concern for the welfare and well-being of others. In professional practice, altruism is reflected by the nurse's concern for the welfare of patients, other nurses, and other healthcare providers. Sample professional behaviors include the following:

- Demonstrates understanding of cultures, beliefs, and perspectives of others
- Advocates for patients, particularly the most vulnerable
- Takes risks on behalf of patients and colleagues
- Mentors other professionals

Autonomy is the right to self-determination. Professional practice reflects autonomy when the nurse respects patients' rights to make decisions about their healthcare. Sample professional behaviors include the following:

- Plans care in partnership with patients
- Honors the right of patients and families to make decisions about healthcare
- Provides information so that patients can make informed choices

Human dignity is respect for the inherent worth and uniqueness of individuals and populations. In professional practice, human dignity is reflected when the nurse values and respects all patients and colleagues. Sample professional behaviors include the following:

- Provides culturally competent and sensitive care
- Protects the patient's privacy
- Preserves the confidentiality of patients and healthcare providers
- Designs care with sensitivity to individual patient needs

Integrity is acting in accordance with an appropriate code of ethics and accepted standards of practice. Integrity is reflected in professional practice when the nurse is honest and provides care based on an ethical framework that is accepted within the profession. Sample professional behaviors include the following:

- Provides honest information to patients and the public
- Documents care accurately and honestly
- Seeks to remedy errors made by self or others
- Demonstrates accountability for own actions

Social justice is upholding moral, legal, and humanistic principles. This value is reflected in professional practice when the nurse works to assure equal treatment under the law and equal access to quality healthcare. Sample professional behaviors include the following:

- Supports fairness and nondiscrimination in the delivery of care
- Promotes universal access to healthcare
- Encourages legislation and policy consistent with the advancement of nursing care and healthcare

From American Association of Colleges of Nursing. (1998). *The essentials of baccalaureate education for professional nursing practice.* Washington, DC: American Association of Colleges of Nursing.

tion has a beneficial application to nursing. When nurses understand the values that motivate the decisions and behaviors of patients, they can tap these values when teaching and counseling patients. For example, a man who does not value his own health and well-being may be motivated by the value he attaches to being a good father for his children to make needed lifestyle changes.

Values theorists most often describe the process of valuing as having seven steps focusing on three main activities (Raths, Simon, & Harmin, 1978; Simon, 1972):

1. Choosing
2. Prizing (treasuring)
3. Acting

When one values something, one chooses freely from alternatives after careful consideration of the consequences of each alternative. Prizing something one values involves pride, happiness, and public affirmation. Finally, the person who values something acts by combining choice into one's behavior with consistency and regularity on the value.

> *Remember Chengyu Zhang described at the beginning of the chapter? Understanding the patient's values would aid the nurse in developing an appropriate plan of care for the client based on his request to be removed from the ventilator.*

Example of Values Clarification by the Nurse

If respect for human dignity is a value that characterizes your nursing practice, you choose freely to believe in the worth and uniqueness of each individual; to realize that you have other options (eg, you could treat with dignity only those people who are most like you); and to believe that respecting each person's human dignity yields the best consequences for you and for all of society.

You also will prize your choice. For example, you especially enjoy when patients let you know they appreciate your care and when nursing colleagues and supervisors compliment you on interpersonal skills. You also prize your ability to defend this value when someone's human dignity is being ignored.

Clarifying this value of respect for human dignity will motivate you to incorporate this value into your practice. You strive to respect human dignity consistently in your personal as well as professional life.

As you become more conscious of this value, you will be sensitive to your actions that are inconsistent with it. For example, you may feel uncomfortable gossiping with other nurses during break about a patient no one likes, realizing that this behavior contradicts your basic respect for human dignity.

Clinical Applications

Box 6-2 illustrates how the steps in the valuing process can be used to help a patient with high blood pressure take charge of his health and manage his medications. Other clinical examples follow here.

Patient Places Low Value on Health and Health Behaviors

You become frustrated when repeated attempts to teach or counsel a 26-year-old pharmaceutical salesperson meet with failure. Although hospitalized with a serious duodenal ulcer, all he can talk about is his job and meeting his sales quota.

Values Clarification. First help this patient identify his basic life values. Ask him "What three things are most important to you in life?" or have him rank the following behaviors in terms of how he would most likely spend an unexpected free day:

_____ Enjoy some quiet time alone (eg, thinking, reading, listening to music)
_____ Spend time with family, friends
_____ Do something active (eg, hiking, playing ball, swimming)
_____ Watch television
_____ Volunteer time and energy to help someone else
_____ Use time for my job
_____ Other

Discuss with the patient what these rankings suggest about his values. Determine whether his rankings would be different if he were asked how he *wished* he could spend the free day versus how he would *most likely* spend it.

Values of Patient and Family Members Conflict

You sense a growing tension while counseling the young parents of a child with asthma. Questioning them ("You seem uncomfortable with what I'm saying now. Is there something wrong?") reveals that the wife is a smoker and cat lover who has told her husband that even if these behaviors are hurting their child, she is unwilling to give them up.

Values Clarification. Suggest that both parents complete the following exercise, and then talk with them about their different responses:

Where do you stand on the following issues? (Indicate your responses in the following manner: SA, strongly agree; A, agree; D, disagree; SD, strongly disagree; U, undecided.)

_____ A parent's primary obligation is to meet the needs of his or her child.
_____ Each member of a family is entitled to pursue personal pleasures, even if these are not in the best interest of all.
_____ Pleasure is more important than health.
_____ The choices one family member makes can dramatically affect other family members (positively or negatively).

This exercise will help the parents to evaluate their basic values, explore areas of conflict, and, perhaps, move toward joint choosing, prizing, and acting on several health-promoting values.

ETHICS

Ethics is systematic inquiry into principles of right and wrong conduct, of virtue and vice, and of good and evil as they relate to conduct. The ability to be ethical, to make de-

BOX 6-2 **Steps in the Valuing Process**

Situation: Mr. Jefferson is a 49-year-old man with uncontrolled high blood pressure

Choosing

1. *Freely.* Rehospitalized for high blood pressure after abruptly stopping his antihypertensive medication, Mr. Jefferson decides from now on to take his medication as prescribed.
2. *From Alternatives.* After a teaching–learning session with a nurse, Mr. Jefferson understands he has basically three options:
   - Comply with prescribed treatment regimen
   - Refuse to take the medication but try harder to control his blood pressure through diet, exercise, and stress management
   - Refuse to take the medication and assume a "we'll see" attitude
3. *After Consideration of the Consequences.* Mr. Jefferson understands the *probable* consequences of these options:
   - Compliance with the treatment regimen will yield the best control of high blood pressure (but may cause some annoying side effects).
   - Diet, exercise, and stress management may reduce his blood pressure somewhat but did not yield sufficient control in the past.

- High blood pressure may result in serious complications such as stroke, kidney disease, or impaired vision.

Prizing

4. *With Pride and Happiness.* Mr. Jefferson states, "Now that I understand high blood pressure better and know what I can do to control it, I feel more in charge of my life—and I like that!"
5. *With Public Affirmation.* Mr. Jefferson states to his wife, "I guess I was wrong to stop taking that medicine when I blamed it for how lousy I was feeling. You can bet that won't happen again. If you ever hear me complaining about my pills, remind me to see my doctor right away."

Acting

6. *With Incorporation of the Choice Into One's Behavior.* After discharge from the hospital, Mr. Jefferson takes the medication as prescribed.
7. *With Consistency and Regularity on the Value.* Mr. Jefferson seeks to understand any new medication he is prescribed (ie, reason for the medication, possible side effects, consequences of the noncompliance) and successfully manages the treatment regimen; he feels proud of his new knowledge and self-care abilities.

cisions, and to act in an ethically justified manner, begins in childhood and develops gradually. See Chapter 18 for a description of two popular accounts of moral development, Kohlberg's justice-based account and Gilligan's care-based account.

Many people use the term ethics when describing the systematic ethics incorporated into a code of professional conduct, such as nursing codes of ethics. The term **morals,** although similar in meaning to ethics, usually refers to personal or communal standards of right and wrong. It is important to distinguish ethics from religion, law, custom, and institutional practices. For example, the fact that an action is legal or customary does not in itself make the action ethically or morally right.

Since values are beliefs about what is important, they are intimately related to and direct ethical conduct. If I place a high value on patient safety and well-being, I am more likely to inconvenience myself to secure the patient's safety and well-being—even when this entails sacrifice—than a nurse who places less value on securing the patient's interests.

Types of Ethics

There are many types of ethics. Those of particular concern to the nurse are bioethics, clinical ethics, and nursing ethics. The *Encyclopedia of Bioethics* describes the scope of **bioethics** as encompassing a number of fields and disciplines grouped broadly under the rubric "the life sciences":

They encompass all those perspectives that seek to understand human nature and behavior, characteristically the domain of the social sciences, and the natural world that provides the habitat of human and animal life, primarily the population and environmental sciences. Yet it is the medical and biological sciences in which bioethics found its initial impetus and in which it has seen the most intense activity.

(Callahan, 1995, p. 255)

Issues in bioethics include responsible research conduct, genetic enhancement, environmental ethics, and sustainable healthcare.

Clinical ethics is that branch of bioethics literally concerned with ethical problems "at the bedside," that is, ethical concerns that arise within the context of caring for actual patients, wherever they are found. Clinical ethics developed in response to three criticisms of bioethics.

1. The need for a contextual approach to ethical inquiry that takes more careful account of the variety of contexts in clinical care and the special needs of ill and suffering patients
2. The need to emphasize the relevance of clinical experience that draws on the knowledge available only through the intimacy of the clinician–patient relationship when doing clinical ethics
3. The need for an orientation toward service in clinical ethics that addresses ethics education, policy-making to address ethical issues in patient care, ethics consultation, and clinical ethics research (Fletcher, Miller, & Spencer, 1997, p. 4)

Examples of issues in clinical ethics include informed consent, and how one ought to respond to requests for medically futile treatment or assisted suicide.

Nursing ethics, which is a subset of bioethics, is the formal study of ethical issues that arise in the practice of nursing and of the analysis used by nurses to make ethical judgments.

As nurses assume increasing responsibility for managing care, it is critical that we are prepared to recognize the ethical dimensions of our practice and to participate competently in ethical decision making. Common ethical issues encountered by nurses in daily practice include cost-containment issues that jeopardize patient welfare, end-of-life decisions, breaches of patient confidentiality, and incompetent, unethical, or illegal practices of colleagues.

Recall Mr. Raines, the 68-year-old indigent, homeless man who is being discharged with several medication prescriptions. Due to policy changes, this patient is no longer able to receive his medications at the clinic free of charge. Whether healthcare is a commodity that can be bought and sold in the marketplace ("too bad Mr. Raines if you don't have insurance to cover your meds or money in your pocket . . .") or a social good owed everyone is a basic question in bioethics. Clinical ethics might evaluate whether or not the institution should have a policy to cover patients like Mr. Raines who are too poor to buy the treatment they need. Nursing ethics will ask about the moral obligations of the nurse case manager caring for Mr. Raines.

Theories of Ethics

Ethical theories are systems of thought that attempt to explain how we ought to live and why. These theories may be broadly categorized as action-guiding theories that answer the question "What ought I to do?" or character-guiding theories that answer the question "What kind of person ought I to be?" Action-guiding theories fall into two main categories:

• **Utilitarian.** The rightness or wrongness of an action depends on the consequences of the action.
• **Deontologic.** An action is right or wrong independent of its consequences.

These distinctions are important because they form the basis of many ethical conflicts we experience in practice. For example, one nurse may believe that abortion is ethically justified in situations that result in the best consequences for the woman, child, and society (utilitarian argument). Another nurse may agree that certain abortions yield better consequences than allowing an unplanned and unwanted pregnancy to continue, but believe that the act of abortion is nonetheless ethically wrong because no consequences justify the taking of innocent life (deontologic argument).

Nurse ethicists frequently use two popular theoretical and practical approaches to "doing ethics"—the principle-based approach and the care-based approach.

Principle-Based Approach

The **principle-based approach** to doing ethics combines elements of both utilitarian and deontologic theories and offers specific action guides for practice. The Beauchamp/Childress principle-based approach to bioethics (2001) identifies four key principles: **autonomy, nonmaleficence, beneficence,** and **justice** (Table 6-1). Many nurses add **fidelity,** veracity, accountability, privacy and confidentiality to this list, because they play a central role in the tradition of nursing (and medical) ethics and guide the behavior of healthcare professionals toward patients and their families.

Recall Marissa Sandoval, the 44-year-old woman who developed complications following extensive surgery for uterine cancer? The nurse would likely feel that the surgeon and residents are not being faithful (principle of fidelity) to their responsibility to address the patient's questions and fears. Unless the nurse can effectively advocate for Marissa with the medical team, her own ability to be faithful to Marissa and accountable for her well-being will be compromised.

The principles offer general guides to action. All things being equal, we ought to act at all times in a manner that respects the autonomy of others, does not harm, does benefit others, treats others fairly, and is faithful to the promises we make to others. Rarely is this as simple as it sounds. Be sensitive to the fact that individuals (patients, family members, and professional caregivers) may identify benefits and harms differently. A benefit to one may be a burden to another.

Review the request by Mr. Zhang, the 32-year-old man described at the beginning of the chapter. Although the nurse may view the request for removal from the ventilator as harmful, most likely leading to the patient's death, the patient's view differs, that is, he does not want to be dependent on a ventilator to live. When conflict about how to apply these principles cannot be resolved, the nurse can request an ethics consult, which is described at the end of this chapter.

Ethical dilemmas arise when attempted adherence to basic ethical principles results in two conflicting courses of action. There is no foolproof method for identifying which principle is most important when there is conflict between competing principles. Popularized versions of the principle-based approach to bioethics have too frequently resulted in a type of "quandary ethics" that diminishes in importance the everyday ethical concerns of nurses (Taylor, 1997), and misleadingly suggests that how ethical dilemmas are resolved is unimpor-

TABLE 6-1 Principles of Bioethics

Principle	Moral Rule	Implications for Nursing Practice
Autonomy (self-determination)	Respect the rights of patients or their surrogates to make healthcare decisions.	Provide the information and support patients and families need to make the decision that is right for them; at times, this may mean collaborating with other members of the healthcare team to advocate for the patient.
Nonmaleficence	Avoid causing harm.	Seek not to inflict harm; seek to prevent harm or risk of harm whenever possible.
Beneficence	Benefit the patient, and balance benefits against risks and harms.	Commit yourself to actively promote the patient's benefit (health and well-being). Be sensitive to the fact that individuals (patients, family members, and professional caregivers) may identify benefits and harms differently. A benefit to one may be a burden to another.
Justice	Give each his or her due; act fairly.	Always seek to distribute the benefits, risks, and costs of nursing care justly. This may involve recognizing subtle instances of bias and discrimination.
Fidelity	Keep promises.	Be faithful to the promise you made to the public to be competent and to be willing to use your competence to benefit the patients entrusted to your care. Never abandon a patient entrusted to your care without first providing for their needs.

tant, as long as one can justify one's recommendation with recourse to a principle. Thus, many healthcare professionals equate ethics with decisions about whether to "pull the plug," ignoring the ethical challenges involved in daily decisions about what constitutes an honest day's work, how respectful we are to others, how truthful, and how compassionate.

Care-Based Approach

Dissatisfaction with the principle-based approach to bioethics led many nurses to look to care as the foundation for nursing's ethical obligations. The nurse–patient relationship is central to the **care-based approach,** which directs attention to the specific situations of individual patients viewed within the context of their life narrative. The care perspective directs that how you choose to "be" and act each time you encounter a patient or colleague is a matter of ethical significance. Ethics is not reduced to a decision to withhold or withdraw life-sustaining treatment. Characteristics of the care perspective include the following:

- Centrality of the caring relationship
- Promotion of the dignity and respect of patients as people
- Attention to the particulars of individual patients
- Cultivation of responsiveness to others and professional responsibility
- A redefinition of fundamental moral skills to include virtues like kindness, attentiveness, empathy, compassion, reliability (Taylor, 1993)

Feminist Ethics

Feminist ethics is a particular type of ethical approach popular among nurses. It aims to critique existing patterns of op-

pression and domination in society, especially as these affect women and the poor. There are many forms of feminist ethics and their subjects range from gender-related inequities to concern for the least well-off. Nurses working within a feminist framework promote social policy that reflects a fundamental trust in the moral agency of women and those on the margins. This is a recognition that all persons deserve the opportunity to make legitimate choices about conditions that affect their lives, and are deserving of respect whenever they exercise such agency. This approach reflects a full commitment to full personhood for marginalized persons and provides for basic human needs that are consistent with one's capacity to flourish; and that honors human dignity and relationality (Holland, 2001, pp. 74–75).

An excellent example of feminist ethics is Holland's critique of human embryonic stem cell research:

It is true that women, the poor, persons of color and marginals could benefit from the regenerative medical therapies and drug therapies heralded by hES (human embryonic stem) cell and EG (embryonic germ) cell research, but it is not at all likely that they will be the ones who do benefit. Such therapies, when they are perfected, are likely to be cost-prohibitive for all but the wealthy and the well-insured, assuming that insurance companies agree to such coverage, a big assumption in any case. The poor, who are primarily women and most persons of color, will simply be marginalized from these therapies, even as it is possible that their eggs are commercialized downstream for profit.

(Holland, 2001, p. 83)

ETHICAL CONDUCT

Nurses committed to high-quality care base their practice on professional standards of ethical conduct. The study of professional ethical behavior begins in nursing school, continues in formal and informal discussions with colleagues and peers, and culminates when nurses "try on" and adopt the behaviors of role models who practice professional nursing consistent with high ethical standards. How do nurses learn the standards for professional ethical behavior? At the very least, nurses should identify and develop the essential elements of ethical agency, cultivate the virtues of nursing, understand ethical theories that dictate and justify professional conduct, and be familiar with bioethical standards for professional nursing conduct.

Ethical Agency

It is unrealistic to assume that the simple desire to be a nurse is accompanied by the natural ability to behave in an ethical way and to do the ethically right thing because it is the right thing to do. This ability, **ethical agency,** must be cultivated in the same way that nurses cultivate the ability to do the scientifically right thing in response to a physiologic alteration. Nurses who appreciate the ethical challenges in professional practice value their ethical development sufficiently to work hard to develop these skills. Essential elements of ethical agency include:

- *Ethical sensibility:* Ability to recognize the "ethical moment" when an ethical challenge presents itself
- *Ethical responsiveness:* Ability and willingness to respond to the ethical challenge
- *Ethical reasoning and discernment:* Knowledge of and ability to use sound theoretical and practical approaches to "thinking through" ethical challenges, to ultimately decide how to respond to this particular situation after identifying and critiquing alternative courses of action; these approaches are used to inform as well as to justify moral behavior
- *Ethical accountability:* Ability and willingness to accept responsibility for one's ethical behavior and to learn from the experience of exercising ethical agency
- *Ethical character:* Cultivated dispositions that allow one to act as one believes one ought to act
- *Ethical valuing:* Valuing in a conscious and critical way that which squares with good ethical character and ethical integrity
- *Transformative ethical leadership:* Commitment and proven ability to create a culture that facilitates the exercise of ethical agency, a culture in which people do the right thing because it is the right thing to do
    Box 6-3 illustrates these elements of ethical agency in action.

The Virtues of Nurses

Virtues are human excellencies, cultivated dispositions of character and conduct that motivate and enable us to be good human beings. Clinical virtues enable nurses to provide good care to patients. While there is no official list of essential virtues of nurses, the following virtues are frequently named:

- Competence
- Compassionate caring
- Subordination of self-interest to patient care
- Self-effacement
- Trustworthiness
- Conscientiousness
- Intelligence
- Practical wisdom
- Humility
- Courage
- Integrity

Since these human qualities cannot be "put on" the way one puts on a uniform or identity badge, it is important that they are part of the nurse's character, part of who the nurse is. They form an important basis of what allows patients to trust us!

Nursing Codes of Ethics

A professional code of ethics provides a framework for making ethical decisions and sets forth professional expectations. Nursing codes of ethics inform both nurses and society of the primary goals and values of the profession. These should be compatible with the nurse's personal value system and moral code. Other functions of professional nursing codes (American Nurses Association, 1985, pp. i–iv) include the following:

- Indicating nursing's acceptance of the responsibility and trust with which it has been invested by society
- Providing guidance for conduct and relationships in carrying out nursing responsibilities consistent with the ethical obligations of the profession and with high-quality nursing care
- Providing a means for the exercise of professional self-regulation

    Codes are effective in accomplishing their goals only to the extent that members of the profession uphold them. Code requirements may exceed legal requirements. Violations of the law subject a nurse to civil or criminal liability (see Chap. 7), and violations of the code of ethics may result in reprimands, censure, suspension, and expulsion.

    Codes of ethics for nursing include the International Council of Nurses (ICN) *ICN Code for Nurses* (adopted in 1953 and revised in 1965 and 1973) (Box 6-4); the *ANA Code for Nurses With Interpretive Statements* (adopted in 1950 and revised in 1968, 1976, 1985, and 2001) (Box 6-5); and the Canadian Nurses Association (CNA) *Code of Ethics for Registered Nurses* (adopted in 1980 and revised in 2002) (Box 6-6).

Nursing Standards of Practice

When the American Nurses Association revised its Standards of Clinical Nursing Practice in 1991, it developed standards of professional performance as well as standards of care. Standard V of professional performance, Ethics, describes the nurse's ethical obligations; the nurse's decisions and actions on behalf of patients are determined in an ethical manner. Measurement Criteria for Standard V (American Nurses Association, 1998, pp. 13–14) are:

BOX 6-3 Ethical Agency

Situation: A 75-year-old patient with end-stage lung cancer suffers a respiratory arrest and is coded, ventilated, and admitted to the intensive care unit (ICU). When the receiving nurse reviews his chart, she discovers that upon admission, his nurse documented that he "did not want to be resuscitated" and that he wanted to prepare an advance directive specifying "no heroics." There is no do-not-resuscitate order on the chart, and the nurse can find no advance directive.

Ethical Sensibility
The ICU nurse notes the discrepancy between the patient's documented preferences and the care that he has received. She senses personal discomfort about this disregard for his wishes.

Ethical Responsiveness
The nurse can decide to ignore her discomfort and simply provide excellent technologic care or acknowledge her discomfort and respond. She decides to talk with the attending physician about his knowledge concerning the patient's preferences and learns that the attending was unaware of the patient's documented preferences and has no personal knowledge of these. She contacts the nurse who originally admitted the patient and learns that although the patient was quite clear about his preference, no one followed up and translated this conversation into orders on his chart. She calls an ethics consult when the attending says that there is "nothing to be done now that treatment is initiated."

Ethical Reasoning and Discernment
During the ethics consult, family members agree that the patient would not be happy to find himself on a ventilator and request that he be weaned—even if this results in his death. The ethicist explains that weaning him from an ineffective treatment (the ventilator will not cure his lung cancer) that is disproportionately burdensome is an ethically justified action.

Ethical Accountability
The nurse initiated the ethics consult because she believed that she could not be an advocate for this patient and merely provide good physical care. Once she knew (or suspected) that his preferences had been ignored, she felt accountable for determining how the system had failed this patient and for remedying the problem. The nurse prides herself on being responsible and accountable and therefore could not "stick her head in the sand" and pretend that this was not her problem! After the ethics consult, she participates in plans to find an optimal time and conditions to wean the patient from the ventilator and makes sure that his family is present. The patient does not survive the weaning, and although they are grieving, his family members are grateful to the nurse for her care for the patient and for them.

Ethical Character
Because she had cultivated the virtues of responsibility and fidelity, the nurse's course of action was natural.

Ethical Valuing
Because she places a high value on being an effective patient advocate, the nurse was willing to confront the attending physician and initiate an ethics consult, even though these actions caused her some discomfort and the expense of time and inconvenience.

Transformative Ethical Leadership
When her colleagues asked her where she got the "guts" to follow through with this course of action, the nurse knew that the culture within the hospital had to change so that more nurses would choose to do the same thing she did without fearing negative consequences. She asks the nurse educator on her unit to explore the possibility of pursuing this theme in a future Nursing Grand Rounds and is willing to work to make this happen.

---

1. The nurse's practice is guided by the Code for Nurses.
2. The nurse maintains patient confidentiality within legal and regulatory parameters.
3. The nurse acts as a patient advocate and assists patients in developing skills so they can advocate for themselves.
4. The nurse delivers care in a nonjudgmental and non-discriminatory manner that is sensitive to patient diversity.
5. The nurse delivers care in a manner that preserves or protects patient autonomy, dignity, and rights.
6. The nurse seeks available resources to help formulate ethical decisions

Remember Marissa Sandoval, the 44-year-old woman who wants answers but is not getting them? Integration of these standards would be essential for the nurse to act professionally and ethically when obtaining the needed answers.

A Patient's Bill of Rights

The American Hospital Association developed *A Patient's Bill of Rights* in 1972 (revised in 2003 as *The Patient Care Partnership;* see Chap. 7, Box 7-5). The bill of rights includes the rights and responsibilities of the patient while receiving care in the hospital, and range from "the right to considerate and respectful care" to "the right to be informed of hospital policies and practices that relate to patient care, treatment and responsibilities." With care moving increasingly from the hospital to the community, nurses must be familiar with how different institutions and professional groups define patient rights and responsibilities. Other bills of rights include Pregnant Patient's Bill of Rights, Indian Patient's Bill of Rights, Nursing Home Bill of Rights, and Veterans Administration Code of Patient Concern. Each emphasizes a specific aspect of patient rights within a particular health agency and implies a code of ethics the nurse observes professionally.

BOX 6-4 International Council of Nurses Code for Nurses

- The fundamental responsibility of the nurse is fourfold—to promote health, to prevent illness, to restore health, and to alleviate suffering.
- The need for nursing is universal. Inherent in nursing is respect for life, dignity, and rights of humans. It is unrestricted by considerations of nationality, race, creed, age, sex, politics, or social status.
- Nurses render health services to the individual, the family, and the community and coordinate their services with those of related groups.

Nurses and People

- The nurse's primary responsibility is to those people who require nursing care.
- The nurse, in providing care, promotes an environment in which the values, customs, and spiritual beliefs of the individual are respected.
- The nurse holds in confidence personal information and uses judgment in sharing this information.

Nurses and Practice

- The nurse carries personal responsibility for nursing practice and for maintaining competence by continual learning. The nurse maintains the highest standards of nursing care possible within the reality of a specific situation.

- The nurse uses judgment in relation to individual competence when accepting and delegating responsibilities.
- The nurse, when acting in a professional capacity, should at all times maintain standards of personal conduct that reflect credit on the profession.

Nurses and Society

- The nurse shares with other citizens the responsibility for initiating and supporting action to meet the health and social needs of the public.

Nurses and Coworkers

- The nurse sustains a cooperative relationship with coworkers in nursing and other fields. The nurse takes appropriate action to safeguard the individual when his or her care is endangered by a coworker or any other person.

Nurses and the Profession

- The nurse plays the major role in determining and implementing desirable standards of nursing practice and nursing education.
- The nurse is active in developing a core of professional knowledge.
- The nurse, acting through the professional organization, participates in establishing and maintaining equitable social and economic working conditions in nursing.

Adapted with permission from International Council of Nurses. (1973). *ICN Code for nurses: Ethical concepts applied to nursing.* Geneva: Imprimeries Populaires.

BOX 6-5 American Nurses Association Code for Nurses

1. The nurse, in all professional relationships, practices with compassion and respect for the inherent dignity, worth, and uniqueness of every individual, unrestricted by considerations of social or economic status, personal attributes, or the nature of health problems.
2. The nurse's primary commitment is to the patient, whether an individual, family, group, or community.
3. The nurse promotes, advocates for, and strives to protect the health, safety, and rights of the patient.
4. The nurse is responsible and accountable for individual nursing practice and determines the appropriate delegation of tasks consistent with the nurse's obligation to provide optimum patient care.
5. The nurse owes the same duties to self as to others, including the responsibility to preserve integrity, to maintain competence, and to continue personal and professional growth.

6. The nurse participates in establishing, maintaining, and improving healthcare environments and conditions of employment conducive to the provision of quality healthcare and consistent with the values of the profession through individual and collective action.
7. The nurse participates in the advancement of the profession through contributions to practice, education, administration, and knowledge development.
8. The nurse collaborates with other health professionals and with the public in promoting community, national, and international efforts to meet health needs.
9. The profession of nursing, as represented by associations and their members, is responsible for the articulating of nursing values, for maintaining the integrity of the profession and its practice, and for shaping social policy.

Reprinted with permission from American Nurses Association. (2001). *Code for nurses.* Washington, DC: Author.

Safe, Competent and Ethical Care—Nurses value the ability to provide safe, competent and ethical care that allows them to fulfill their ethical and professional obligations to the people they serve.

Health and Well-Being—Nurses value health promotion and well-being and assisting persons to achieve their optimum level of health in situations of normal health, illness, injury, disability or at the end of life.

Choice—Nurses respect and promote the autonomy of persons and help them to express their health needs and values and also to obtain desired information and services so they can make informed decisions.

Dignity—Nurses recognize and respect the inherent worth of each person and advocate for respectful treatment of all persons.

Confidentiality—Nurses safeguard information learned in the context of a professional relationship, and ensure it is shared outside the health care team only with the person's informed consent, or as may be legally required, or where the failure to disclose would cause significant harm.

Justice—Nurses uphold principles of equity and fairness to assist persons in receiving a share of health services and resources proportionate to their needs and in promoting social justice.

Accountability—Nurses are answerable for their practice, and they act in a manner consistent with their professional responsibilities and standards of practice.

Quality Practice Environments—Nurses value and advocate practice environments that have the organizational structures and resources necessary to ensure safety, support and respect for all persons in the work setting.

*This represents only one element of the code—values. Obligations, which provide more specific direction for conduct than do values by spelling out what a value requires under particular circumstances, and limitations, which describe exceptional circumstances in which a value or obligation cannot be applied, are provided with each value in the publication.
Reprinted with permission from Canadian Nurses Association. (2002). *Code of ethics for registered nurses*. Ottawa, Ontario: Author.

The nurse could use knowledge of the Patient's Bill of Rights to ensure that the questions from Marissa Sandoval, the woman described at the beginning of the chapter, and those of her family, are answered.

Bill of Rights for Registered Nurses

Two of the chief reasons nurses cite for the declining quality of nursing care at their facilities are inadequate staffing and decreased nurse satisfaction. Advocacy on behalf of nurses and the profession has resulted in a tangible tool, the Bill of Rights for Registered Nurses, to aid in improving workplaces and ensuring nurses' ability to provide safe, quality patient care. The Bill of Rights is intended to empower nurses by making it

clear what is absolutely nonnegotiable in the workplace. "The ANA and its constituent member organizations will continue their longstanding work, through political and legislative activism, collective bargaining, workplace advocacy, and public education, to ensure that the basic tenets of this Bill of Rights are a reality for nurses across the country" (Wiseman, 2001).

The seven basic tenets of the Bill of Rights for Registered Nurses are:
1. Nurses have the right to practice in a manner that fulfills their obligations to society and to those who receive nursing care.
2. Nurses have the right to practice in environments that allow them to act in accordance with professional standards and legally authorized scopes of practice.
3. Nurses have the right to a work environment that supports and facilitates ethical practice, in accordance with the Code of Ethics for Nurses and its interpretive statements.
4. Nurses have the right to freely and openly advocate for themselves and their patients, without fear of retribution.
5. Nurses have the right to fair compensation for their work, consistent with their knowledge, experience, and professional responsibilities.
6. Nurses have the right to a work environment that is safe for themselves and their patients.
7. Nurses have the right to negotiate the conditions of their employment, either as individuals or collectively, in all practice settings.

(ANA, 2001; used with permission)

ETHICAL DECISION MAKING

Two types of ethical problems commonly faced by nurses are ethical dilemmas and ethical distress. In an ethical dilemma, two (or more) clear moral principles apply but support mutually inconsistent courses of action. **Ethical distress** occurs when the nurse knows the right thing to do but either personal or institutional factors make it difficult to follow the correct course of action. Nurses need sound analytic skills and the ability to engage in ethical reasoning to resolve ethical dilemmas and ethical distress. Resources for ethical decision making are highlighted in Box 6-7.

Using the Nursing Process to Make Ethical Decisions

Every nurse needs to be confident in using a process of ethical decision making. One process with which nurses are familiar and thus can use to make ethical decisions is the nursing process. Using the nursing process to make ethical decisions involves following the steps discussed below. The accompanying patient care study illustrates this five-step model of ethical decision making that is based on the nursing process (Box 6-8).

Assess the Situation (Gather Data)
Recognize and then describe the situation and contextual factors that give rise to the ethical problem. This involves the main people involved (their views and interests); the patient's

BOX 6-7 Ethics Resources

The following are ethics resources for healthcare professionals:

American Nurses Association Center for Ethics and Human Rights
http://www.nursingworld.org/ethics/index.htm
     In September 1990, the Center for Ethics and Human Rights was established, with the following guiding objectives:

- *Promulgate* in collaboration with ANA constituents a body of knowledge, both theoretical and practical, designed to address issues in ethics and human rights at the state, national and international level.
- *Develop and disseminate* information about and advocate for public policy to assure that ethics and human rights are addressed in healthcare.
- *Assure* that short- and long-range objectives regarding ethics and human rights will be addressed within the Association, and expressed to appropriate bodies external to the Association.

The American Society for Bioethics and Humanities
http://www.asbh.org/
     This is a professional society of more than 1500 individuals, organizations, and institutions interested in bioethics and humanities. Their website serves as a source of information for members, prospective members, and anyone interested in bioethics and humanities. There is a special interest group for nurses.

The American Society for Law, Medicine and Ethics
http://www.aslme.org/
     Within this site you will find information about two nationally acclaimed peer-reviewed journals, *The Journal of Law, Medicine & Ethics* and *The American Journal of Law & Medicine*. You will be able to search for information from hundreds of articles that have been published. You will also be able to register for ASLME educational conferences and connect to relevant web links from the ASLME site.

The Medical College of Wisconsin's Center for the Study of Bioethics
http://www.mcw.edu/bioethics/

The Medical College of Wisconsin's Center for the Study of Bioethics is dedicated to nationally and internationally recognized innovation and excellence in:

- *Bioethics Education:* Educating healthcare professionals, researchers, policy makers, and students in bioethics
- *Bioethics Research and Scholarship:* Advancing current knowledge through research in bioethics and health policy
- *Bioethics Consultation:* Assisting ethics committees and healthcare providers in shared bioethical decision making with patients and their representatives
- *Bioethics Community Service:* Fostering greater understanding of bioethics issues locally, regionally, nationally, and internationally, through conferences, programs, and the development and dissemination of resource materials

National Reference Center for Bioethics Literature
http://www.georgetown.edu/research/kie/
     A specialized collection of library resources concerned with contemporary biomedical issues in the fields of ethics, philosophy, medicine, nursing, science, law, religion, and the social sciences. Call for bioethics information, BIOETHICS-LINE searches (computerized database), search strategies, reference help, and publication orders.

The Hastings Center
http://www.thehastingscenter.org/
     The Hastings Center is an independent, nonpartisan, and nonprofit bioethics research institute, founded in 1969 to explore fundamental and emerging questions in healthcare, biotechnology, and the environment. Publishes *The Hastings Center Report.*

Centre for Applied Ethics
http://www.ethics.ubc.ca/resources/
     Provides links to many ethics resources in healthcare and other disciplines

---

overall nursing, medical, and social situation; and relevant legal, administrative, and staff considerations.

Diagnose (Identify) the Ethical Problem

State the problem clearly. Identify your relationship to the decision. Identify time parameters. Make sure that the problem is an ethical problem as opposed to a communication or legal problem. Some suggest that whenever human dignity is being threatened, you have an ethical problem.

Plan

Identify options and explore the probable short-term and long-term consequences of each for each stakeholder. Use ethical reasoning to decide on a course of action that you can justify ethically. Decide on the course of action you are best able to support. Consultation with a respected and wise colleague or an institutional ethics committee may be helpful at this point.

Implement Your Decision

Implement your decision and compare the outcome of your action with what you considered and hoped for in advance.

Evaluate Your Decision

What have you learned from this process that will help you in the future? How can you improve your reasoning and decision making in the future?

Ethically Relevant Considerations

Fletcher, Miller, and Spencer recommend attention to eight ethical considerations that have the greatest weight and relevance in the care of patients, which bridge between ethical principles, an ethics of caring, and the clinical situation (1997, pp. 13–15).

BOX 6-8 Patient Care Study Using a Five-Step Process for Resolving Ethical Conflict

Jean Watts is a labor and delivery room nurse in a small community hospital that serves both private and clinic patients. Jean has always felt that certain members of the obstetrics–gynecology medical staff have treated these two groups of clients differently. On this particular morning, Jean is caring for a woman who is scheduled for an elective cesarean delivery. The woman (who is a clinic patient) has made it very clear that she wants to be awake for the delivery and has requested epidural or spinal anesthesia. Jean is dismayed when the anesthesiologist enters the delivery room because the anesthesiologist's success rate with epidural anesthesia is poor. The anesthesiologist unsuccessfully attempts to perform an epidural block. After waiting 20 minutes for results, the obstetrician is growing impatient and instructs the anesthesiologist to put the patient to sleep. Jean feels the rights of this patient are being violated but is unsure of what her response should be.

Step 1: Assess the Situation (Gather Data)
The patient is in stable medical condition (elective cesarean delivery, not an emergency) and has made it very clear that she wishes to be awake for the delivery. The patient is not a private paying patient of the obstetrician. The nurse believes her role is to promote and protect the patient's interests; she knows of no reason in this case why the patient's preferences should be disregarded.

The anesthesiologist has a poor success record with epidural anesthesia.

The obstetrician seems to want to complete delivery quickly. In the past, he has seemed to give more weight to following wishes of private patients as opposed to clinic patients. He is the head of the obstetrics–gynecology department; he believes nurses should obey physicians unquestioningly.

Nurses have in the past expressed dissatisfaction with the different levels of care being provided to private and clinic patients, but no one to date has formally addressed the concern.

Step 2: Diagnose (Identify) the Ethical Problem
Jean objects to the obstetrician's intent to disregard the patient's wish to be awake for her delivery; she is aware of no good reasons justifying this course of action.

The nurse will be a participant in carrying out the decision.

The decision for this case must be made immediately; it would be helpful to plan to avoid situations like this in the future.

Step 3: Plan
a. Identify Options
The nurse can say nothing to the obstetrician and help with the delivery. If asked by the patient later why she needed to be put to sleep, the nurse can (1) tell the truth, (2) refer her to the obstetrician, (3) express sympathy that she could not be awake, or (4) say nothing. *Outcome:* The patient's wishes are disregarded; delivery occurs in record time, and the obstetrician is happy; the nurse fulfills obligation to physician and hospital but feels she has betrayed the patient's trust. *Long-term outcome:* There is a good probability the same problem will happen again.

Or

The nurse can remind the obstetrician that the patient was adamant about wanting to be awake and suggest that a different anesthesiologist be called in. If the obstetrician agrees, the patient may get her wish and everyone is satisfied with the outcome (the nurse must still decide how to prevent recurrence of this dilemma). If the obstetrician refuses and insists that the patient be put to sleep, the nurse can (1) refuse to participate (if another nurse is unavailable or unwilling to replace her, the nurse has abandoned the patient and harm may ensue); or (2) participate and proceed as above or resolve to speak to the obstetrician in a "cool moment" after the delivery to see how to avoid this problem in the future. If the nurse does not get satisfaction with the obstetrician, then she must decide whether to move through the proper administrative channels. Depending on the institution and people involved, the nurse may be affirmed or censored for this move. *Long-term outcome:* Future patients may be helped by the nurse following through with her concerns.

Or

The nurse can say nothing and assist with this delivery, believing it to be the wisest course of action for the time being, but resolve to take the steps above to correct the perceived injustice. *Outcome:* There is no benefit for the present patient but potential benefit to future patients.

b. Think the Ethical Problem Through
Basic moral principles: The good of patients (beneficence) should be the nurse's primary concern; this strongly suggests that the nurse should act, but it does not address the nurse's obligation to do so if she feels it would jeopardize her own good (job security).

Respect for persons would suggest that the patient's autonomy (right to self-determination) should be respected unless there is strong justification for not doing so.

Justice would suggest that whether a patient pays the obstetrician privately should have no bearing on the quality of care received.

Care-based ethics would obligate Jean to serve as an effective advocate for her patient, respecting the nurse's commitment to be faithful to the nurse–patient relationship.

c. Make a Decision
Jean feels from past interactions with this obstetrician that her speaking up will not influence his decision to have the patient put to sleep. She decides to speak with the obstetrician after the delivery and follow up with whatever approach is necessary to avoid recurrence.

Steps 4–5: Implement and Evaluate Your Decision
Jean will never know if speaking up would have resulted in the patient's wishes being respected. Although she is dissatisfied with the outcome of this case, she hopes to prevent this from happening to other clinic patients in the future. In this instance, a hospital committee was formed to study the problem and make recommendations. If Jean had been told to "mind her own business" unless she wanted trouble, she would have to make a decision weighing patient benefit on one hand with potential personal risk or harm on the other.

The Balance Between Benefits and Harms in the Care of Patients

Nurses are superbly positioned to contribute to reasoning about what counts as the benefits or burdens of treatment and what are the related harms, since their relationships with patients enable them to see more than physiologic effects.

Disclosure, Informed Consent, and Shared Decision Making

There are three basic models of healthcare decision making. In the paternalistic model, clinicians acting to benefit the patient decide what ought to be done and inform the patient, and the patient's role is to comply. In the patient sovereignty model, patients or their surrogates, expressing their right to be autonomous, tell the clinician what they want, and the clinician's role is to comply. Most ethicists reject these models in their extremes and recommend a model of shared decision making, which respects and uses the preferences of the patient and the expertise and judgment of the clinician. *The object of all clinical decision making is decisions that secure the health and well-being of the patient and that honor and respect the integrity of all participants in the decision-making process.* Nurses can play an important role in ensuring that patients and their surrogates receive the information and support they need to make healthcare decisions that secure their interests.

Norms of Family Life

Most patients do not present as isolated individuals. Nurses who are sensitive to how a patient's injury or illness influences family members and significant others will be better able to appreciate how this influences decisions about care, and can bring this information to the interdisciplinary team.

The Relationship Between Clinicians and Patients

The healing encounter is central to nursing ethics. As nurses reason ethically about what ought to be done, it is always in the context of the relationships, which hold us accountable to patients and their families, and the professional caregivers with whom we work. Much ethical distress for nurses results from the strong conviction that we owe individual patients more than present work environments allow us to deliver.

The Professional Integrity of Clinicians

While the 2001 ANA Code of Ethics for Nurses clearly states that the primary commitment of the nurse is the patient, it also states that the nurse owes the same duties to self as to others—including the responsibility to preserve integrity, to maintain competence, and to continue personal and professional growth. Nurses should think long and hard when they find themselves asked to sacrifice personal integrity to meet the needs of another.

Cost-Effectiveness and Allocation

The increasing awareness of how difficult it is to make valued and scarce health resources available to all in need has resulted in new appreciation for the moral relevance of cost-effectiveness. Nurses who are committed to patient advocacy bridge the sometimes overwhelming needs of patients and their families and the limited resources available to professional caregivers. Justice is the principle of bioethics that speaks to distributing the benefits and burdens or healthcare delivery fairly. Nurses are uniquely positioned within the interdisciplinary team to speak to what it means to give patients or patient cohorts "their due."

Issues of Cultural and/or Religious Variation

Since many conflicts about what ought to be done are rooted in different cultural or religious beliefs and values, nurses who are sensitive to the cultural and/or religious identity of patients and caregivers can help mediate these conflicts.

Considerations of Power

Differences in power underlie many of the ethical challenges encountered in clinical practice. Injury and illness create vulnerabilities in the most sophisticated consumer of healthcare and mandate vigilance on the part of the nurse and other caregivers to challenge any abuses of power by clinicians. Clinicians who believe they lack power to influence care settings and delivery may also experience ethical conflict and distress.

A Final Note About Trustworthiness

Common to all of the standards discussed above is the obligation for nurses to be competent and willing to use their competence to secure the health and well-being or good dying of the patient. Whom nurses choose to be on any day they arrive for practice literally has the power to influence how people are born, live, and die. When nurses become aware that something is interfering with patients getting the care they need, they are responsible for responding within the scope of their power and responsibility. If they cannot independently resolve the problem, they are responsible for alerting the appropriate party, who may be the attending physician, a nursing supervisor, or a medical director. While some nurses believe "the problem is out of their hands" once they notify the next person in the chain of command, the problem remains theirs until appropriate action is taken. Thus, you should know and use the chain of command, and continue to refer a problem upwards until it is resolved and the patient's needs are met.

Examples of Ethical Problems

Ethical problems commonly arise between nurses and patients, nurses and physicians, nurses and other nurses, and nurses and their employing institutions. Moreover, nurses are often most conflicted when good practice seems to require acting against their personal moral convictions. As you read through the following mini-cases, try to determine how you would respond. The process of ethical decision making described above should prove helpful.

Nurses and Patients

Troublesome nurse–patient situations that can result in ethical problems for nurses include **paternalism** (acting for patients without their consent to secure good or prevent harm), deception, confidentiality, allocation of scarce nursing resources, informed consent, and conflicts between the patient's and nurse's values and interests.

Paternalism

An alert older resident who lives in a nursing home and who is now at high risk for falls refuses to call the nurse for assistance when getting out of bed. The nurse must decide whether to obtain an order to restrain the patient. Does preventing potential harm justify violating the patient's right to autonomy and make it acceptable for the nurse to act as a "parent" and choose an action the patient does not want because the nurse believes it to be in the patient's best interest?

Deception

A postoperative patient asks the student nurse, who is about to administer an intramuscular injection for pain, "Is this your first shot?" It does happen to be the student's first injection and the student is anxious. Would the student's intent to decrease the patient's anxiety justify telling the patient "No, I've given several before"?

Confidentiality

A nurse asks a middle-aged woman who is crying quietly "Would you like to share what's troubling you?" The woman tells the nurse she has no idea how she will pay for this clinic visit because she entered the country illegally 2 months ago and is trying to earn enough money to help her family back home. She begs the nurse not to tell anyone. If the nurse believes this anxiety is interfering with the patient's ability to obtain needed healthcare, would it be ethical to break the woman's confidence to obtain help for her?

Allocation of Scarce Nursing Resources

A nurse has just been pulled from your unit, leaving it understaffed. Among your patients is a 33-year-old man recovering from a heart attack who is being discharged in the morning (he tells you he still has many questions); an older patient who is close to death; and a woman with cancer who has been vomiting all day and who is in severe pain. You know you cannot meet everyone's needs well. How do you "distribute" your nursing care? (You really like the patient who is going home in the morning.)

Advocacy in Market-Driven Environment

A hospitalized 57-year-old woman who underwent two lengthy bowel resections has just been informed by her health plan that she has exceeded her allowable length of stay and needs to be discharged immediately. She lives alone and has no family members or friends who are able to assist with her care. You believe that she would benefit immensely from extra hospital days so that she could regain her strength and learn how to provide necessary self-care. She does not have the money to pay for more days. What do you do?

A resident is attempting to perform a spinal tap on an adolescent who you know dislikes the resident. After one failed attempt, the adolescent tells the resident to stop. The resident asks you to administer an antianxiety medication to the patient so the resident can get the spinal tap done quickly. Should you administer the medication knowing the patient no longer consents to the procedure?

Conflicts Between the Patient's and Nurse's Interests

Home health nurses are taking turns being assigned to care for new patients who test positive for the human immunodeficiency virus (HIV). One nurse, who is nursing her 8-month-old infant, refuses to take her turn, fearing she will transmit the disease to her baby. The other nurses tell her she must accept the assignment of this HIV-positive patient because none of them is willing to take her turn. Is a nurse ever justified in refusing to nurse a patient assigned to his or her care?

Conflicts Concerning the Appropriate Use of Technology

An infertile woman asks you what you think about in vitro fertilization. She tells you that she is "desperate to produce a child for her husband and in-laws" but also has grave reservations about the whole process. "I've read about couples who end up with seven frozen embryos, and I think that would kill me, thinking I've got seven potential kids 'on ice.'"

Nurses and Physicians

Nurse–physician situations can also result in ethical distress for nurses. Common problems include disagreements about a proposed medical regimen, conflicts regarding the scope of the nurse's role, and physician incompetence.

Disagreements About the Proposed Medical Regimen

In the nursing home where you work, any patient who loses a significant amount of weight (more than 10% of usual body weight) is automatically subjected to an exhaustive battery of tests (including a complete gastrointestinal [GI] series) to determine whether there are any physical causes for the weight loss (eg, a tumor). You strongly object to one patient being put through these tests because she has made it clear that she wants to die and will starve herself to death if that is the only way she can do it. The medical director insists that the patient undergo the diagnostic studies because there is a long history of patient family dissatisfaction with the facility's medical care. The director wants to avoid causing further dissatisfaction. Are you responsible for preparing the patient for these diagnostic studies and scheduling them? Are there grounds for refusing to participate?

Conflicts Regarding the Scope of the Nurse's Role

A young woman needing surgery that will result in a permanent colostomy tells the nurse how afraid she is and how much she dreads depending on "the thing." The nurse is certain this patient would benefit greatly from the help of the young staff enterostomal therapist (ET), who also has a colostomy. When this suggestion is mentioned to the surgeon, however, the surgeon tells the nurse that he does his own teaching and counseling for all his patients and does not "believe" in ETs. He points out that the nurse's duty here is to carry out his orders. Does it fall within the scope of nursing to recommend the ET to the woman? Is the nurse obligated to make this recommendation to the patient?

Unprofessional, Incompetent, Unethical, or Illegal Physician Practice

A nurse who works in the operating room notices that a pediatric surgeon who has been on the staff for several years and done excellent work suddenly seems not to be concentrating during surgery and to be making more mistakes than usual. Rumors have been circulating about the surgeon having a problem with cocaine abuse after his recent divorce. The parents of one pediatric patient are dissatisfied with the progress the patient is making and ask the nurse for an opinion about the surgeon. Should the nurse voice personal concerns? Is the nurse obligated to report the physician to the proper hospital authority for investigation?

Nurses and Other Nurses

Some of the most difficult ethical problems nurses encounter result from nurse–nurse interactions, which may be complicated by obligations of friendship. Problems include claims of loyalty and nurse incompetence.

Claims of Loyalty

A nurse working the 11 p.m. to 7 a.m. shift tells the other nurse on the unit "I just made rounds and everyone is OK. Please cover for me while I catch an hour of sleep. I had an awful day." She neglects to tell the other nurse that a report mentioned that one patient needed special monitoring. This patient dies unexpectedly while the nurse sleeps. When she wakes up and discovers what happened, she begs the other nurse, her friend, never to tell anyone she was sleeping. "That patient could have died anyway between my rounds" she says.

Unprofessional, Incompetent, Unethical, or Illegal Nurse Practice

When you make your morning rounds, a patient tells you that one of the nurses fondled her body and made suggestive remarks during the previous night shift. You suspect that the patient may simply be trying to cause trouble, and because you like the nurse in question, you find it hard to believe the patient. What should you do?

Nurses and Institutional and Public Policy

As nurses assume increased responsibility for decision making at all levels of care, the institutional and public policy arenas offer unique dilemmas. Three current examples are short staffing, whistle-blowing, and healthcare rationing.

Short Staffing and Whistle-Blowing

Restructuring has resulted in chronic understaffing on the unit where you work. You believe that patients are now at risk be-

cause there simply are not enough nurses to provide quality care. Some nurses are talking about forming a union and going on strike. Because yours is the only major hospital in a rural area, you are unsure whether striking is a morally legitimate option. Because efforts to get management involved in addressing the issues have repeatedly failed, you are also contemplating "going public" with your concerns. Your brother works for the local newspaper, and you are pretty sure he would be willing to do a story about the situation at the hospital. What do you do?

Healthcare Rationing

In the United States, as many as 43 million people are uninsured or underinsured and have limited access to healthcare. Whether each person has a "right" (is entitled to) basic healthcare continues to be the subject of debate. There are plans for rationing healthcare that could limit the options available to the elderly, the poor, the terminally ill, and those in society whom many view as having limited "social value." What moral obligation do you have to contribute to this debate? How might you ensure that your voice and the nursing viewpoint are heard?

Nurses' Personal Moral Convictions and Institutional or Professional Ethics

Nurses sometimes experience a challenge to their personal ethical integrity because what they believe ought to be done in a particular situation is forbidden by the ethics of their place of employment or profession.

Beginning-of-Life Issues

You are a psychiatric mental health nurse working in a Catholic hospital whose ethical and religious directives forbid abortion and abortion counseling. You are talking with a single woman recently hospitalized with bipolar disorder who is in the first trimester of an unplanned pregnancy and who is expressing great ambivalence about continuing the pregnancy. You personally believe that your ethical obligation is to explore abortion as an option with this woman and to refer her to outside resources if she elects to abort. The charge nurse tells you that these are not appropriate options within this hospital.

End-of-Life Issues

You are the nurse case manager for a woman with a history of breast cancer whose cancer recurred (metastasis to the spine) after she had been cancer free for 7 years. She frequently tells you when you come to visit her at home that she is unwilling to fight anymore and wants to die with some dignity while she is still in control. She begs you to get her something that will "put me gently to sleep once and for all before my pain gets worse." You believe that this is her sincere wish, not just depression speaking, and you honestly believe that she would be better off spared the last stage of her illness. Your religious beliefs, however, tell you that assisted suicide is wrong under any circumstances. Moreover, the American Nurses Association has a position statement that claims that nurse-assisted suicide is incompatible with the ethics of nursing. How do you reconcile your desire to help this woman with your profession's ethical code and your religious conviction that what she is asking for is intrinsically wrong? For a fuller discussion of ethical issues at the end of life, see Chapter 33.

Nurses and Ethics Committees

An increasing number of healthcare institutions have developed ethics committees whose chief functions include education, policy making, case review, consultation, and, in some cases, research. Some committees focus on clinical ethics and some on organizational ethics. These committees are uniquely equipped to deal with the complexities of modern healthcare because they are multidisciplinary and provide a forum in which radically divergent views can be aired without fear of repercussion. Nurses bring an important voice to the ethics committee. When clinical issues are being reviewed, nurses can help to ensure that the technical facts are understood, that the appropriate decision makers have been identified, that the patient's medical and overall best interests have been identified, and that the course of action selected from the alternatives is justified by sound ethical principles. Nurses' strong backgrounds in interpersonal communications allow us to contribute unique knowledge about the patient and family to the discussion and to facilitate the ethics committee's group dynamics.

Nurses also play an important role in policy making. They are frequently able to identify what policies are needed to address recurring ethical concerns and to suggest needed modifications of existing policies.

ADVOCACY IN NURSING PRACTICE

Bridging vulnerable patients and the resources they need to secure health outcomes, nurses have always been strong patient advocates. **Advocacy** is the protection and support of another's rights. This role is increasingly important because of patients' changing expectations and demands, and because the public has learned that in our increasingly market-driven healthcare economy there are no guarantees that the healthcare system will work to secure their safety and health.

Nurses who value patient advocacy:
- Make sure that their loyalty to an employing institution or colleague does not compromise their primary commitment to the patient
- Give priority to the good of the individual patient rather than to the good of society in general
- Carefully evaluate the competing claims of the patient's autonomy (self-determination) and patient well-being

When respecting autonomy, the nurse respects and supports the patient's right to make decisions. Informed consent is described in Chapter 7. When promoting patient well-being, the nurse acts in the best interests of the patient. Ideally, both autonomy and patient well-being are promoted in every nurse–patient interaction; however, conflicts sometimes arise.

For example, when Mr. Zhang, the 32-year-old man described at the beginning of the chapter, requests to be removed from the ventilator, the principle of autonomy demands respect for his treatment preferences at the same time that the principle of nonmaleficence obligates us to prevent the harm of his likely death. Nurses sensitive to the need to promote both patient autonomy and well-being may often experience conflict, but they are more likely than other nurses to succeed in securing the patient's genuine best interests.

Representing Patients

Most nurses would agree that a great deal of nursing time is spent representing patients' interests or guiding patients in protecting their own rights. The nurse is often involved as an intermediary between the patient and the family, especially when the patient and family have conflicting ideas about the management of healthcare situations (Fig. 6-1). For example, a patient with terminal cancer may want to go home to die. He tells this to his nurse. The patient's family, however, tells the nurse that they cannot care for him at home. As an advocate, the nurse recognizes the rights of both the patient and his family. The nurse then works to assist them in finding a solution that benefits both the patient and them. By informing the family of the availability of home care and hospice care, the nurse gives them knowledge that may help satisfy the patient's right to a dignified death. Working alone, most people would be unable to get the financial help needed for such care. Nurses have the resources available to help them and can arrange referrals from other healthcare workers, such as social workers, to achieve the desired outcomes.

Nurses may also serve as intermediaries between patients and the medical profession. Nurse ethicist Patricia Murphy

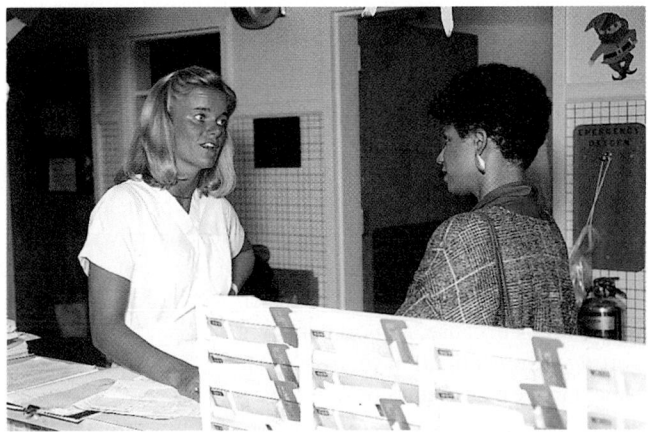

FIGURE 6-1 The nurse acts as a patient advocate in discussing all aspects of the patient's healthcare with family members.

(1990) documented a moving account of how nurses interceded for a 43-year-old woman with amyotrophic lateral sclerosis who was on a ventilator but wished to die. The patient's primary physicians refused to help remove her from the ventilator, and more than 20 other physicians declined to accept her as a patient when they learned what she wanted to do. After unsuccessful appeals for help to the county medical society and her own attorney, the patient's visiting nurse, working with a supportive social worker, contacted her state nurses association and finally secured the assistance she needed to help the patient achieve her goal of a dignified death.

Patients with special advocacy needs include those who are uninformed concerning their rights and opportunities, those with sensory impairment, those who do not speak English well or at all, the very young and the elderly, those who are seriously ill, those who are mentally or emotionally impaired, those with physical disabilities, and those who lack adequate financial or human resources.

Consider Mr. Raines, the 68-year-old man described at the beginning of the chapter. Awareness of his special needs would be critical in developing his discharge plan of care.

Promoting Self-Determination

Advocacy is linked to the belief that making choices about health is a fundamental human right that promotes the individual's dignity and well-being. Ethical dilemmas may arise when people are unable or unwilling to make choices or when they are not given the opportunity to do so. Faulty communication among patients, family members, and caregivers frequently contributes to these dilemmas. Nurses have an important advocacy role in educating the public about the value of written advance directives (described in Chapter 33).

Nurses as advocates must realize that they do not make ethical decisions for their patients. Instead, they facilitate patients' decision making. Nurses interpret findings for their patients; inform them of various aspects to be considered; help them verbalize and organize their feelings; call in those people who should be involved in the decision making (eg, family, primary nurse, physician, or clergy); and help patients assess all of their options in relation to their beliefs. In this way, nurses advocate for the right of patients to make their own decisions concerning their health. Not all individuals want to make their own treatment decisions, however, and you should not violate the spirit of autonomy (self-determination) by forcing it on anyone. Nurses sometimes advocate for patients by helping them to delegate decisions to a preferred decision maker whom they trust. In addition, when claiming to be a patient advocate, nurses must be careful to clarify exactly what it is they mean by advocacy because, in most instances, this is not simply supporting patients in all of their preferences. For example, if a patient in the early stages of Alzheimer's disease, with the support of her husband, asks a nurse for help in terminating her life, the nurse would have strong ethical grounds for refusing to advocate for this particular request.

Being Politically Active

No discussion of nursing advocacy would be complete without noting nursing's continuing voice in the political arena on behalf of those least well served by the existing healthcare system, including homeless people, minorities, women, and children. As the government becomes more involved in the delivery and funding of healthcare services, and as those designing rationing plans speak seriously of age and other variables as criteria for limiting care, nurses must continue to advocate for the healthcare needs of those least empowered to do so for themselves. Nurses are a powerful block of voters whose potential for influencing healthcare legislation is just beginning to be tapped.

■ Developing Critical Thinking Skills

1. Students choose nursing as a career because of different values. A desire to help others, a love of money, wanting a career that allows you to work anywhere at any time, a commitment to provide for your children's well-being, a love of science and technology, and respect for your parents' wishes are all values that may lead to choosing nursing as a career.
   - Interview your classmates and identify the values that brought everyone to nursing. When a classmate lists more than one value, ask him or her to rank these in order of their importance. Compare your lists.
   - Discuss which values, if any, provide the best motivation for professional nursing. Are there certain values that are incompatible with professional nursing and that ought to be grounds for rejecting candidates for professional nursing?
   - Make a judgment about how well your personal values equip you for professional nursing. Are any modifications needed?
2. Make a list of all the values that might positively or negatively influence someone's ability to lose weight. Think about how you could use this knowledge when counseling obese patients.
3. Another student tells you "Who I am outside of school is no one's business and has no effect on my nursing." Do you agree? Why or why not?
4. Take any current ethical issue (assisted suicide, human cloning, how to allocate scarce organs for transplantation, everyone's right to healthcare) and poll your class to see the range of opinions among your classmates. Reflect on what it is that causes people to reach different conclusions about what is the ethically right thing to do. How might you use this knowledge as you experience ethical conflict in your professional practice?

■ Practicing for NCLEX

1. Five-year-old Bobby has dietary modifications related to his diabetes. His parents want him to value

good nutritional habits and they decide to deprive him of a favorite TV program when he becomes angry after they deny him foods not on his diet. This is an example of what mode of value transmission?
   a. Modeling
   b. Moralizing
   c. Laissez-faire
   d. Rewarding and punishing
   e. Responsible choice

2. Which of the following is the best professional response to a patient who tells you that she believes that "white nurses are smarter than nurses of color" and then asks if you agree?
   a. "You are right!" (The patient/customer is always right!)
   b. "What I think doesn't matter. What's important is whatever you believe." (Value neutrality)
   c. "I don't believe being smart is related to race or ethnicity." (Commitment to human dignity)

3. The American Association of Colleges of Nursing identified five values that epitomize the caring professional nurse. Which of these is best described as acting in accordance with an appropriate code of ethics and accepted standards of practice?
   a. Altruism
   b. Autonomy
   c. Human dignity
   d. Integrity
   e. Social justice

4. A professional nurse with a commitment to social justice is most apt to:
   a. Provide honest information to patients and the public
   b. Promote universal access to healthcare
   c. Plan care in partnership with patients
   d. Document care accurately and honestly

5. When an older nurse complains that nurses just aren't ethical anymore, the reply that reflects the best understanding of moral development is:
   a. "The ability to behave ethically must be carefully cultivated; maybe we don't value this sufficiently to pay it the attention it deserves."
   b. "I don't agree that nurses were more ethical in the past. It's a new age and the ethics are new!"
   c. "Ethics is genetically determined . . . it's like having blue or brown eyes. Maybe we're evolving out of the ethical sense you and your generation had."
   d. "No kidding! Who could be ethical in a practice setting like this!"

6. A home health nurse who performs a careful safety assessment of the home of a frail elderly patient to prevent harm to the patient is acting in accord with which of the principles of bioethics?
   a. Autonomy
   b. Beneficence
   c. Justice
   d. Fidelity
   e. Nonmaleficence

7. A professional nurse committed to the principle of autonomy would be careful to:
   a. Provide the information and support a patient needed to make decisions to advance her own interests
   b. Treat each patient fairly, trying to give everyone his or her due
   c. Keep any promises made to a patient or another professional caregiver
   d. Avoid causing harm to a patient

8. A friend asks you about the new Bill of Rights for nurses. What can you tell her that accurately reflects the concerns of the drafters of these rights?
   a. The Bill of Rights was drafted by nurses who care more about themselves than they do about patients.
   b. The Bill of Rights was drafted by union nurses who are always looking for a reason to strike.
   c. The Bill of Rights was drafted to empower nurses and to improve conditions in the workplace.

9. Janie wants to call an ethics consult to clarify treatment goals for a patient no longer able to speak for himself. She believes his dying is being prolonged painfully. She is troubled when the patient's doctor tells her that she'll be fired if she raises questions about his care or calls the consult. This is a good example of:
   a. Ethical uncertainty
   b. Ethical distress
   c. Ethical dilemma

10. Nurse advocates often are conflicted about respecting a patient's right to be self-determining, while at the same time wanting to do everything in their power to promote the patient's best interests. Which is the best general guideline for situations like these?
   a. Patient rules! "It's my life!"
   b. Nurse rules! "It may be your life but in this instance you don't know enough to make the right choice!"
   c. When in conflict, weigh the benefits and risks of following each option and then choose wisely.

■ Answers With Rationale

1. The correct response is *d.* When rewarding and punishing are used to transmit values, children are rewarded for demonstrating values held by parents and punished for demonstrating unacceptable values.

2. The correct response is *c.* While it is true that value neutrality commits nurses to care for patients whether or not the nurse and patient hold the same value, it is not true that nurses should sacrifice their moral integrity and compromise their beliefs or values to please a patient.

3. The correct response is *d*. The American Association of Colleges of Nursing defines integrity as acting in accordance with an appropriate code of ethics and accepted standards of practice.

4. The correct response is *b*. The American Association of Colleges of Nursing lists promoting universal access to healthcare as an example of social justice. Providing honest information and documenting care accurately and honestly are examples of integrity, and planning care in partnership with patients is an example of autonomy.

5. The correct response is *a*. The ability to be ethical, to make decisions, and to act in an ethically justified manner, begins in childhood and develops gradually.

6. The correct response is *e*. Nonmaleficence is defined as the obligation to prevent harm. Autonomy is respect for another's right to make decisions, beneficence obligates us to benefit the patient, justice obligates us to act fairly, and fidelity obligates us to keep our promises.

7. The correct response is *a*. The principle of autonomy obligates us to provide the information and support patients and their surrogates need to make decisions that advance their interests.

8. The correct response is *c*. The drafters of the American Nurses Association's Bill of Rights for Registered Nurses was a result of advocacy on behalf of nurses, to aid in improving workplaces and to ensure that nurses would have what they needed to provide safe, quality patient care. It is not true that these nurses cared more for themselves than patients (*a*) nor that these were nurses looking for reasons to strike (*b*).

9. The correct response is *b*. Ethical distress results from knowing the right thing to do but finding it almost impossible to execute because of institutional or other constraints (in this case, fear of losing her job). Ethical uncertainty (*a*) results from feeling troubled by a situation but not knowing if it is an ethical problem. Ethical dilemmas occur when the principles of bioethics justify two or more conflicting courses of action (*c*).

10. The correct response is *c*. Neither respecting and supporting patient preferences (*a*) nor ignoring patient preferences to achieve a medical benefit (*b*) routinely trump all other considerations. When a nurse cannot do both simultaneously, she must carefully weigh the benefits and risks of each option and then choose wisely.

Bibliography

American Association of Colleges of Nursing. (1998). *The essentials of baccalaureate education for professional nursing practice.* Washington, DC: Author.

American Nurses Association. (1985, 2001). *Code for nurses with interpretive statements.* Washington, DC: Author.

American Nurses Association. (1988). *Ethics in nursing: Position statements and guidelines.* Kansas City, MO: Author.

American Nurses Association. (1991, 1998). *Standards of clinical nursing practice.* Washington, DC: Author.

American Nurses Association's Code of Ethics Task Force. (July 2000). A new code of ethics for nurses. *AJN, 100*(7), 69, 71–72.

Beauchamp, T. L., & Childress, J. F. (2001). *Principles of biomedical ethics* (5th ed.). New York: Oxford University Press.

Bishop, A. H., & Scudder, J. R. (1990). *The practical, moral, and personal sense of nursing.* Albany: State University of New York Press.

Callahan, D. (1995). Bioethics. In W. T. Reich (Ed.), *Encyclopedia of bioethics* (rev. ed., pp. 247–256). New York: Macmillan.

Canadian Nurses Association. (2002). Code of ethics for registered nurses. Ottawa, Ontario: Author.

Corley, M. C., Elswick, R. K., Gorman, M., & Clor, T. (2001). Development and evaluation of a moral distress scale. *Journal of Advanced Nursing, 33*(2), 250–256.

Daly, B. J. (1999). Why a new code? *American Journal of Nursing, 99*(6), 64, 66.

Edwards, B. S. (1993). When the physician won't give up. *American Journal of Nursing, 93*(9), 34–37.

Edwards, B. S. (1994). When the family can't let go. *American Journal of Nursing, 94*(1), 52–56.

Fletcher, J. C., Miller, F. G., & Spencer, E. M. (1997). Clinical ethics: History, content, and resources. In J. C. Fletcher, et al., (Eds.), *Introduction to clinical ethics* (2nd ed., pp. 3–20). Hagerstown, MD: University Publishing Group.

Fowler, M. (1999). Relic or resource? The Code for Nurses. *American Journal of Nursing, 99*(3), 56, 58.

Holland, S. (2001). Beyond the embryo: A feminist appraisal of the embryonic stem cell debate. In S. Holland, K. Lebacqz, & L. Zoloth (Eds.), *The human embryonic stem cell debate* (pp. 73–86). Cambridge, MA: A Bradford Book.

International Council of Nurses. (1973). *ICN code for nurses: Ethical concepts applied to nursing.* Geneva: Imprimeries Populaires.

Jameton, A. (1993). Dilemmas of moral distress: Moral responsibility and nursing practice. *AWHONN's Clinical Issues in Perinatal and Women's Health Nursing, 4*(4), 542–551.

Kirschbaum, H. (1977). *Advanced values clarification.* La Jolla, CA: University Associates.

Murphy, D. (1990). A profile in courage. *Nursing 90, 20*(11).

Penticuff, J. H., & Waldron, M. (2000). Influence of practice environment and nurse characteristics on perinatal nurses' responses to ethical dilemmas. *Nursing Research, 49*(2), 64–72.

Raths, L. E., Simon, S. B., & Harmin, M. (1978). *Values and teaching* (2nd ed.). Columbus, OH: Charles E. Merrill.

Redman, B., & Fry, S. T. (2000). Nurses' ethical conflicts: What is really known about them? *Nursing Ethics, 7*(4), 360–366.

Simon, S. B. (1972). *Values clarification.* New York: Hart.

Steele, S. M., & Harmon, V. M. (1983). *Values clarification in nursing* (2nd ed.). Norwalk, CT: Appleton-Century-Crofts.

Taylor, C. (1993). Nursing ethics: The role of caring. *AWHONN's Clinical Issues in Perinatal and Women's Health Nursing, 4*(4), 552–560.

Taylor, C. (1997). Everyday nursing concerns: Unique? Trivial? Or essential to healthcare ethics? *HEC Forum, 9*(1), 68–84.

U.S. General Accounting Office. (July 2001). *Nursing workforce: Emerging nurse shortages due to multiple factors. Report to Chairman, Subcommittee on Health, Committee on Ways and Means, House of Representatives.* (Publication No. GAO-01-944). Washington, DC: Author.

Uustal, D. B. (1978). Values clarification in nursing: Application to practice. *American Journal of Nursing, 78*(12), 2058–2063.

White, G. (October 2001). The code of ethics for nurses. *AJN, 101*(10), 73, 75.

Wiseman, R. (November 2001). The ANA develops Bill of Rights for Registered Nurses. *AJN, 101*(11), 55, 57.

Legal Implications of Nursing

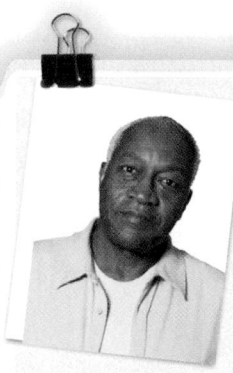

Ramone Scott, a 66-year-old man, had surgery to repair a fractured hip earlier in the day. He just received a dose of an intravenous antibiotic that was prescribed for another patient.

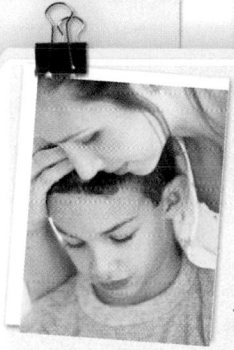

Meredith Bedford is the mother of a terminally ill child with a brain tumor who is admitted to the pediatric oncology unit for a pain management program. One morning she comes out to the nurses' station and firmly states, "I'm very unhappy with the care my son is receiving. I'm going to talk with my attorney as soon as possible to press charges against the hospital."

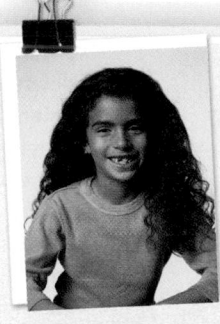

Ella Rodriguez, an 8-year-old girl, comes to the emergency department with a right forearm fracture. She requires diazepam (Valium) sedation for a closed reduction procedure. The protocol for administration to a child states that a physician must be present throughout the entire sedation procedure. One of the physicians has been working his 14th hour, and the ED is overflowing. He orders the nurse to begin the sedation protocol, stating that he will be back in the room in 10 minutes.

Focusing on Blended Skills

The types of blended skills you'll need to respond to the case scenarios include:

Cognitive Skills

- Knowledge of law and the sources of laws
- Ability to incorporate knowledge of standards and credentialing into nursing practice activities
- Knowledge of how to practice nursing in a legally defensible manner
- Ability to identify potential areas of liability in nursing
- Knowledge of how to write an incident (or variance) report
- Knowledge of the elements of liability and how malpractice litigation works
- Knowledge of legal safeguards for nurses

Technical Skills

- Ability to provide the technical nursing assistance necessary to meet the needs of the patients entrusted to your care
- Ability to use appropriate documentation systems and tools to record practice
- Ability to adapt technical nursing assistance for patients at different developmental stages such as an older adult, a woman with a terminally ill child, and a young child
- Ability to use equipment correctly, competently, and safely when implementing a patient's plan of care
- Ability to ask for assistance as necessary when performing new or complex procedures or faced with new situations

Interpersonal Skills

- Ability to establish trusting and respectful professional relationships with patients and colleagues
- Demonstration of integrity and honesty in all actions, including interactions with patients, patients' families, and other healthcare team members
- Ability to demonstrate respect for the patient's and family's human dignity when implementing the plan of care, such as with the mother of a terminally ill child
- Ability to work collaboratively with other members of the healthcare team, using clear, accurate, and professional communication skills

Ethical and Legal Skills

- Ability to evaluate personal areas of liability and to use appropriate legal safeguards
- Ability to identify errors in personal action
- Knowledge of how to challenge unsafe patient situations, such as not adhering to agency protocols for drug administration, with competence in using this knowledge to effect change
- Consistent use of appropriate legal safeguards when implementing a patient's plan of care
- Commitment to implementing nursing care within the standards of care and scope of nursing practice

Learning Outcomes

After completing the chapter, the learner should be able to accomplish the following:

1. Define law and describe its four sources.
2. Describe the professional and legal regulation of nursing practice.
3. Identify the purpose of credentialing, using as examples accreditation, licensure or registration, and certification.
4. Identify grounds for suspending or revoking a license or registration.
5. Differentiate intentional torts (assault and battery, defamation, invasion of privacy, false imprisonment, fraud) and unintentional torts (negligence).
6. Evaluate personal areas of potential liability in nursing.
7. Describe the legal procedure once a plaintiff files a complaint against a nurse for negligence.
8. Describe the roles of the nurse as defendant, fact witness, and expert witness.
9. Use appropriate legal safeguards in nursing practice.
10. Explain the purpose of incident reports.
11. Describe laws affecting nursing practice.

Key Terms

accreditation
assault
battery
certification
common law
credentialing
crime
defamation of character
defendant
expert witness
fact witness
felony
fraud
liability
licensure
litigation
malpractice
misdemeanor
negligence
plaintiff
sentinel event
statutory law
tort

As the roles and duties of nurses expand, so also does their legal accountability. In the past, many nurses worked under the supervision of a physician, few carried liability insurance, and even if a nurse's actions were the direct cause of harm to a patient, the primary liability for the nursing action fell on the employing agency or physician. In modern practice, nurses assess and diagnose patients and plan, implement, and evaluate nursing care independently. Full legal responsibility and accountability for these nursing actions rest with the nurse. (See the accompanying Reflective Practice box for an example.) Nurses are increasingly the subjects of both civil and criminal negligence cases and are being brought to court to defend their practice.

Although many nurses continue to work in traditional settings like hospitals and nursing homes, more nurses are working in nontraditional community settings, such as home care agencies, clinics, day care centers, and nurse-managed health centers. Advanced practice nurses may have independent practices. It has never been more important for nurses to document their actions carefully and act in ways to prevent malpractice accusations. Nurses who wish to avoid legal conflicts need to develop trusting nurse–patient relationships (satisfied patients rarely sue), practice within the scope of their competence, and identify potential liabilities in their practice and work to prevent them.

LEGAL CONCEPTS

As you begin professional practice, it is essential to understand how the law defines the nurse's legal responsibilities and duties.

Definition of Law

A law is a standard or rule of conduct established and enforced by the government. Laws are intended chiefly to protect the rights of the public. Public law is law in which the government is involved directly. It regulates relationships between individuals and the government. Public law, for example, describes the powers of the government. Private law, also called civil law, regulates relationships among people. Civil law includes laws relating to contracts, ownership of property, and the practice of nursing, medicine, pharmacy, and dentistry. Criminal law concerns state and federal criminal statutes, which define criminal actions such as murder, manslaughter, criminal negligence, theft, and illegal possession of drugs.

Sources of Laws

Four sources of laws exist at both the federal and state level: constitutions, statutes, administrative law, and common law.

Constitutions

Federal and state constitutions indicate how the federal and state governments are created and are given authority and state the principles and provisions for establishing specific laws.

Although they contain relatively few laws (called constitutional laws), constitutions serve as guides to legislative bodies.

Statutes

A legislative body enacts **statutory law.** Statutory laws must be in keeping with both the federal constitution and the state constitution. Nurse Practice Acts are an example of statutory laws. (Nurse Practice Acts are discussed fully in the section "Professional and Legal Regulation of Nursing Practice.")

Administrative Law

Executive officers (eg, the president of the United States, state governors, or city mayors) administer agencies that, among other functions, are responsible for law enforcement. These agencies have the power to make administrative rules and regulations, in conformity with enacted law, that act as laws and are enforceable. Boards of nursing are administrative agencies at the state level. The rules and regulations they adopt are administrative laws. An example of a municipal administrative agency is the city board of health.

Common Law

The government provides for a judiciary system, which is responsible for reconciling controversies. It interprets legislation at the local, state, and national levels as it has been applied in specific instances and makes decisions concerning law enforcement. A body of law known as **common law** has evolved from these accumulated judiciary decisions. Common law is thus court-made law. Most law involving malpractice is court-made law.

Common law is based on the principle of *stare decisis,* or "let the decision stand." After a decision has been made in a court of law, the principle in that decision becomes the rule to follow in similar other cases. The case that first sets down the rule by decision is called a precedent. Court decisions can be changed, but only with strong justification. Common law helps prevent one set of rules from being used to judge one person and another set to judge another person in similar circumstances.

Litigation

A lawsuit is a legal action in a court. **Litigation** is the process of bringing and trying a lawsuit. The person or government bringing suit against another is called the **plaintiff.** The one being accused of a crime or tort (defined later) is called the **defendant.** The defendant is presumed innocent until proved guilty of a crime or tort.

> *Recall Meredith Bedford, the mother of the terminally ill child threatening to bring charges against the hospital. The mother would be considered the plaintiff, while those named in the lawsuit would be considered the defendants.*

The two levels of courts in the United States are trial courts and appellate courts. The trial court, the first-level court, hears all the evidence in a case and makes decisions based on facts,

Reflective Practice
Challenge to Ethical and Legal Skills

This past summer I worked in the emergency department of a very reputable hospital. Overall I felt that the department was a desirable working environment and that the relationships between physicians and nurses were very open. However, one incident occurred that I felt put the patient's safety at risk.

Ella Rodriguez, an 8-year-old girl, had come to the emergency department with a right forearm fracture. She required diazepam (Valium) sedation for a closed reduction procedure. The protocol for administration for a child states that a physician must be present throughout the entire sedation procedure. One of the physicians had been working his 14th hour, and the ED was overflowing. He ordered the nurse to begin the sedation protocol, stating that he would be back in the room in 10 minutes. The nurse taking care of the patient was a new graduate and did not feel comfortable giving the drug alone, but also did not feel comfortable speaking up to the doctor. She proceeded to go into the room and inject the first dose of diazepam (Valium), against protocol.

This nursing action completely undermined the patient's safety because she not only stated previously that she did not feel comfortable with the sedation procedure but she also went against protocol. Although the physician was also responsible for giving the nurse orders against protocol, her obligation to herself and the patient should have been the priority, and thus she should have refused to give the drug until the physician was in the room.

Thinking Outside The Box: Possible Courses of Action

- Hope and pray that nothing happens to the patient until the physician comes back into the room.
- Get the physician back into the room; if he refuses an invitation to be present, report this to someone in a leadership position.
- Ask the nurse why she is violating protocol.
- Seek the help of my preceptor immediately.

Evaluating a Good Outcome: How Do I Define Success?

- Patient is benefited or at the very least not harmed.
- The physician, nurse, and unit leaders accept responsibility for safely implementing protocols.
- All healthcare team members demonstrate accountability for failures to adhere to protocols.
- Patient safety is put first, even when this means challenging other members of the team.

Personal Learning: Here's to the Future!

My preceptor, the charge nurse, realized that the nurse was in the room administering the medication. Once he realized this, he immediately got the physician to go into the patient's room. After the procedure was completed successfully, he discussed the implications of both the nurse's and the doctor's actions with each of them together and separately. I did not have time to respond to this incident because the charge nurse had acted so quickly and appropriately.

Obviously, I think that the nurse should have spoken to the physician and refused to give the medication, but I can understand her feelings, especially being a new graduate. The entire situation can be very intimidating, but as nurses our responsibility is to the patient. By not standing up for the patient and herself, the nurse put the patient in danger and herself in danger, and did nothing to change the climate of the ED. The experienced and exceptionally capable charge nurse was not afraid to stand up to the doctor. Not only did his actions put the patient's safety first, but he also demonstrated to the nurse, myself, and other nurses that it is imperative that nurses stand up for themselves and patients.

I believe that no matter what the circumstance is, nurses need to stand up for themselves and their patients, especially now, when our healthcare climate yields to nurses' voices being heard. The only way that nurses' roles and reputations will change is if we, the nurses, speak up, and speak loudly. Right now we have a unique opportunity to change the way medicine is practiced to benefit both patients and nurses. If all nurses grab this opportunity and make something of it, we can really make a difference, but it needs to be a collective effort to be successful. Regardless of how small the problem is, it must be addressed.

Reflection

How do you think you would respond in a similar situation? Why? What does this tell you about yourself and about the adequacy of your skills for professional practice? Can you think of other ways to respond? Do you think that the nurse would be able to admit that she made a mistake by not following the protocol? How was the nurse's integrity compromised? The nursing student's integrity? What legal principles were violated by not following the sedation protocol? What influence, if any, might the patient's age have had on the nurse's action? What types of leadership skills did the charge nurse demonstrate? What other skills (cognitive, interpersonal, technical, ethical/legal) would you need to respond well in this situation? Suppose the charge nurse had not intervened. What might have occurred? Do you agree with the criteria to evaluate a successful outcome? Did the nursing student meet the criteria?

Julia Strobel, Georgetown University

usually through a jury. The appellate court hears only cases questioning a point of law decided by the trial court. No witnesses testify at the appellate court level. The opinions of appellate judges are published and become common law.

PROFESSIONAL AND LEGAL REGULATION OF NURSING PRACTICE

Nurses who practice safely respect both the voluntary and legal controls that map the boundaries of nursing practice. Both of these controls are designed to ensure quality healthcare and to protect society from unsafe actions.

Nurse Practice Acts

Your state's Nurse Practice Act is the most important law affecting your nursing practice. Each state has a Nurse Practice Act that protects the public by broadly defining the legal scope of nursing practice. You should obtain a copy of this act from your state Board of Nursing and study it carefully. Each nurse is expected to care for patients within defined practice limits. Practicing beyond those limits (eg, performing an appendectomy) makes you vulnerable to charges of violating the state Nurse Practice Act.

> Consider Ella Rodriguez, the 8-year-old with the fractured arm requiring administration of sedation based on a protocol. The nurse would need to integrate knowledge of the state's Nurse Practice Act when administering the medication, understanding the need to adhere to the protocol that requires a physician to be present throughout the administration.

Nurse Practice Acts list the violations that can result in disciplinary actions against a nurse and also serve to exclude untrained or unlicensed people from practicing nursing. Table 7-1 illustrates different sources of rules affecting nursing practice, examples of issues covered, where these rules are documented, and suggestions for initiating change. Sharp (2003, p. 12) claims that gaining power and influence for nurses is easier than we think: "Simple as it seems, the written word can get us exactly what we want and what our patients need—more nurses and improved working conditions. . . . To get what we want, we have to make sure our legislators hear us loud and clear. What easier way to do this than with a letter or e-mail?" Examples of a letter and an e-mail to members of Congress to support funding for the Nurse Reinvestment Act (NRA) are provided in Box 7-1.

Standards

Voluntary standards, developed and implemented by the nursing profession itself, are not mandatory but are used as guidelines for peer review. Professional nursing organizations continually reassess the functions, standards, and qualifications of their members. These organizations are guided by their own assessment of society's need for nursing and by the public's expectations of nursing. Examples of voluntary standards include the American Nurses Association (ANA) standards of practice (see Chap. 1), professional standards for the accreditation of education programs and service organizations, and standards for the certification of individual nurses in general and specialty areas of practice.

Legal standards, on the other hand, are developed by a legislature and are implemented by authority granted by the state to determine minimum standards for the education of nurses, to set requirements for licensure or registration, and to decide when a nurse's license may be suspended or revoked. Examples of legal standards include state Nurse Practice Acts and rules and regulations of nursing.

Credentialing

Nursing has taken several steps to ensure the competence of its practitioners, including the credentialing process. **Credentialing** refers to ways in which professional competence is ensured and maintained.

Three processes are used for credentialing in nursing. The first is **accreditation,** which is the process by which an educational program is evaluated and recognized as having met certain standards. The second is **licensure,** which is the process by which a state determines that a candidate meets certain minimum requirements to practice in the profession and grants a license to do so. The third is **certification,** which is the process by which a person who has met certain criteria established by a nongovernmental association is granted recognition in a specified practice area.

Accreditation

State constitutions give states a responsibility for the public welfare. State legislative bodies have used this principle to enact laws controlling occupational and professional groups. One function of these laws is to see that schools preparing practitioners maintain minimum standards of education. Nursing is one of the groups operating under state laws that promote the general welfare by determining minimum standards of education through accreditation of schools of nursing. State-approved, or accredited, educational programs in nursing include practical or vocational, associate degree, diploma, baccalaureate, and graduate programs in nursing.

Legal accreditation of a school preparing nursing personnel by the state Board of Nursing should not be confused with voluntary accreditation. The National League for Nursing Accrediting Commission (NLNAC) and the American Association of Colleges of Nursing (AACN) are voluntary agencies that accredit schools when they meet certain criteria. Most schools choose to seek this voluntary accreditation, and many prospective students prefer selecting accredited schools. Accreditation by NLNAC or AACN is not a legal requirement for a school to exist; state accreditation is a legal requirement.

TABLE 7-1 Who Makes Nursing Practice Rules?

Source of Practice Rules	Examples of Issues Covered	Where Rules Are Documented	How to Initiate Change
Federal legislation	• Medicare and Medicaid provisions related to reimbursement for nursing services	• Federal statutes	• Review documents. • Draft desired legislative changes. • Obtain support of colleagues, nursing organizations, other healthcare providers, and the public, if appropriate. • Obtain support and sponsorship from a US congressperson or senator, who will introduce the bill. • Lobby for the bill's passage.
State legislation	• Scope of practice for RNs, LPNs, advanced practice nurses • Nursing educational requirements • Composition and disciplinary authority of board of nursing	• Nurse practice act • Medical practice act • Other statutes	• Review documents. • Draft desired legislative changes. • Obtain support of colleagues, nursing organizations, other healthcare providers, and the public, if appropriate. • Obtain support and sponsorship from a state legislator, who will introduce the bill. • Lobby for the bill's passage.
Board of nursing	• Delegation • Medication administration • Unprofessional conduct • Licensing	• Rules and regulations • Position statements • Declaratory rulings (as found in meeting minutes or newsletters), which may be specific to a particular setting or institution	• Review documents. • Initiate a formal query to the licensing board. • Obtain board support for change. • The board may issue a position statement or declaratory ruling or hold a formal public hearing before voting to promulgate new rules or change existing ones.
Healthcare institution	• Clinical procedures, such as wound dressing changes • Policies specific to the institution, specialty, or practice setting • Personnel and employment policies	• Unit-based policies • Institutional policies • Institutional credentialing policies	• Review institutional policies. • Follow institutional policies or the chain of command to make inquiries or propose change.

From Laskowshi-Jones L. (1998). Reaching beyond the rules: Understanding—and influencing—your scope of practice. *Nursing, 28*(9), 45.

Licensure

Licensure is a specialized form of credentialing based on laws passed by a state legislature. A license is a legal document that permits a person to offer to the public skills and knowledge in a particular jurisdiction, where such practice would otherwise be unlawful without a license. Licensure is discussed in Chapter 1.

The State Board of Nurse Examiners in the United States may revoke or suspend a nurse's license or registration for drug or alcohol abuse, which is currently the most frequent reason. Other reasons for revocation or suspension of a license

or registration include fraud, deceptive practices, criminal acts, previous disciplinary action by other state boards, gross or ordinary negligence, and physical or mental impairments, including those resulting from aging.

Once earned, a license to practice is a property right and may not be revoked without due process. This includes notice of the investigation, a fair and impartial hearing, and a proper decision based on substantial evidence. Crucial to a nurse's successful defense are early legal counsel, character and expert witnesses, and thorough preparation for all proceedings.

BOX 7-1 Examples of a Letter and an E-Mail to Congress to Support Funding for the Nurse Reinvestment Act (NRA)

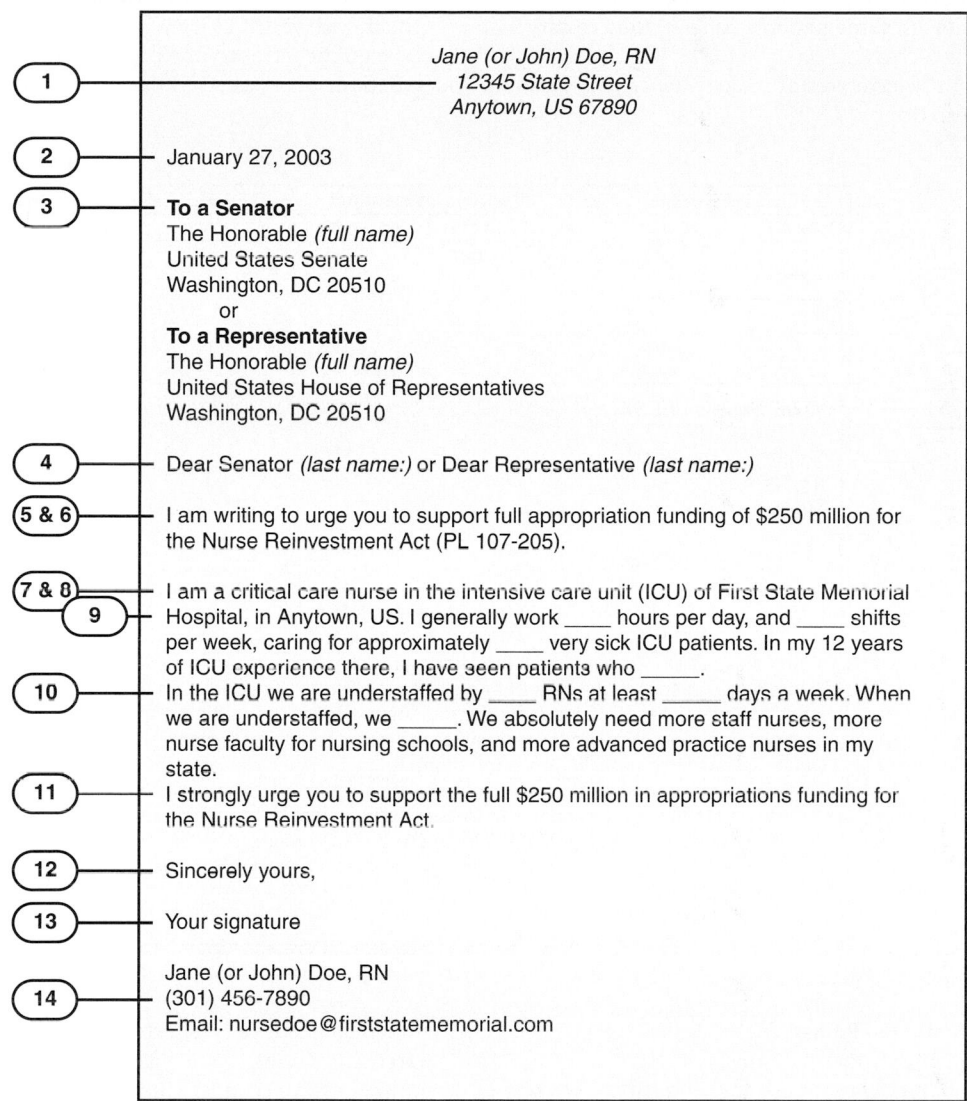

1 — Jane (or John) Doe, RN
12345 State Street
Anytown, US 67890

2 — January 27, 2003

3 — **To a Senator**
The Honorable *(full name)*
United States Senate
Washington, DC 20510
          or
To a Representative
The Honorable *(full name)*
United States House of Representatives
Washington, DC 20510

4 — Dear Senator *(last name:)* or Dear Representative *(last name:)*

5 & 6 — I am writing to urge you to support full appropriation funding of $250 million for the Nurse Reinvestment Act (PL 107-205).

7 & 8
9 — I am a critical care nurse in the intensive care unit (ICU) of First State Memorial Hospital, in Anytown, US. I generally work ____ hours per day, and ____ shifts per week, caring for approximately ____ very sick ICU patients. In my 12 years of ICU experience there, I have seen patients who ____.

10 — In the ICU we are understaffed by ____ RNs at least ____ days a week. When we are understaffed, we ____. We absolutely need more staff nurses, more nurse faculty for nursing schools, and more advanced practice nurses in my state.

11 — I strongly urge you to support the full $250 million in appropriations funding for the Nurse Reinvestment Act.

12 — Sincerely yours,

13 — Your signature

14 — Jane (or John) Doe, RN
(301) 456-7890
Email: nursedoe@firststatememorial.com

Letter to Congress.

Explanation of Numbered Points

1. Use either letterhead stationery of your own, or just type your name and address (centered) at the top of the sheet.
2. Write the month, day, and year you are writing the letter.
3. Find the names of your members of Congress (two senators and one representative) at http://www.house.gov or http://www.senate.gov. Just type in your state and ZIP code, and the names will come up. Write to each member of Congress separately.
4. Use the appropriate title—either "Senator" or "Representative"—along with the member of Congress' last name in your salutation.
5. State your purpose for writing briefly and clearly in the first paragraph. If you know the specific piece of legislation, identify it accordingly as shown (PL 107-205) or make your subject clear (for example, "Nurse Reinvestment Act").
6. Talk about only one legislative issue in each letter.
7. State clearly that you are a nurse.
8. Name the city and state where you live to identify that you are a voter, live in the legislator's district, and are therefore eligible to vote (this may not be where you practice). Be sure that you are contacting the legislator in the place you are eligible to vote. If you decide also to contact a legislator in the place where you work—for instance, if you live in one state or district and work in another—write the letter to show the impact the legislation will have on the legislator's constituents, who are your patients.
9. Be courteous and to the point, and include key information.

(continued)

BOX 7-1 (Continued)

10. Talk about what you know and what you do in your own words. Use specific examples from your workplace to support your position. For example, "As a result of having too few nurses, some patients suffered unnecessary complications such as . . ."

11. At the end of the letter, restate exactly what you want the legislator to do.

12. Closing

13. Sign you name in blue or black ink.

14. Be sure to list all your contact information, including your e-mail address, in case the legislator wants to get in touch with you.

Try to keep the letter to one page. Check your spelling and punctuation.

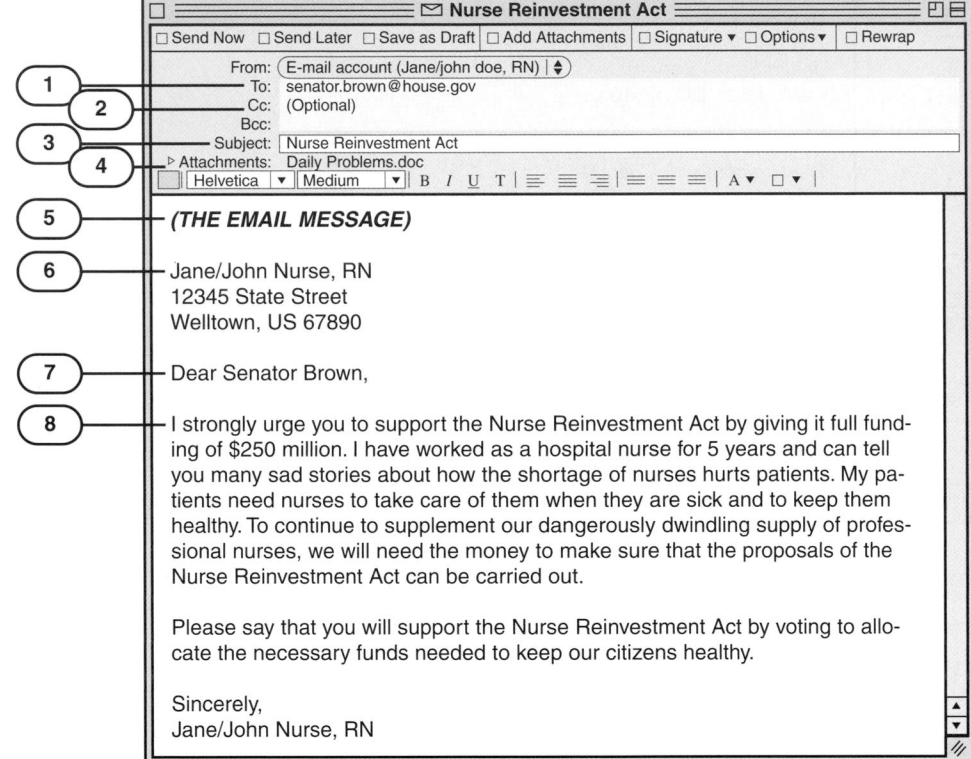

E-mail to Congress.

Explanation of Numbered Points

1. Use your member of Congress' e-mail address, which can be found at http://www.house.gov and http://www.senate.gov. Send an individual e-mail to each member of Congress separately, with only one e-mail address in the "To:" line. You may want to send an e-mail to the member who represents voters from the place where you work, if you live in a different state or district from where you work. If you do this, be sure to write the e-mail to describe the impact the legislation will have on your patients, who are the legislator's constituents.

2. You can copy this e-mail to a professional nursing organization or leave this blank. Do not copy it to another member of Congress.

3. State as clearly as possible the legislation you are addressing (eg, nursing shortage). Although not necessary, you can use the bill number, if known.

4. If you want to attach a letter you have written that is longer and more fully explains your position, you may do so here.

5. An e-mail needs to be shorter and more succinct than a letter. The person reading it should be able to view your entire message on one screen without scrolling down. If you want to write more, attach a letter (see above).

6. Put your name and address at the top to show the legislator that you are a voter in his or her district or state.

7. The legislator's title—either "Representative" or "Senator"—and last name make up the salutation.

8. Body of the e-mail:
   - State what you want the legislator to do in the first sentence.
   - Identify yourself as a concerned nurse.
   - Tell why the legislator should do what you are asking.
   - Ask the legislator to vote for/support what you are asking.

Finally, use spell-check and reread the e-mail to make sure the message you want to get across is clear and concise.

Used with permission. Sharp, N. (Jan. 27, 2003). The "write stuff." *Nursing Spectrum, 13*(2), 12–13.

Certification

Whereas licensure measures entry-level competence, certification validates specialty knowledge, experience, and clinical judgment. Nursing certification is offered by many U.S. professional organizations, including two primary organizations: the American Association of Critical-Care Nurses, which represents the specialty with the largest number of certified nurses, and the ANA, which began certifying nurses in 1974. According to Cary (2001), there are now 410,000 nursing certifications in 134 specialties from 67 certifying organizations with at least 95 different credentials. Although certification, which involves special testing, is voluntary, nurse specialists are increasingly becoming certified.

Certification is one means to demonstrate advanced proficiency and a commitment to ensuring competence in the context of the current U.S. healthcare crisis, with daily reports of unsafe care, rising litigation, escalating costs, and a worsening nursing shortage. A call to action was issued in 2002 in a white paper drafted by the American Association of Critical-Care Nurses and AACN Certification Corporation: "Today's critically ill patients require heightened vigilance and extraordinarily intricate care. As skilled and responsible health professionals, the 403,000 critical care nurses in the United States must acquire the specialized knowledge and skills needed to provide this care and demonstrate their competence to the public, their employers and profession. Recognizing that nurses can validate specialty competence through certification, this white paper . . . puts forth a call to action for all who can influence and will benefit from nurses' contributions to patient care."

CRIMES AND TORTS

Crime

A **crime** is a wrong against a person or his or her property, but the act is considered to be against the public as well. In a criminal case, the government, called "the people," prosecutes the offender. When a crime is committed, the factor of intent to commit wrong is present in most cases. Nonetheless, people who break certain laws are guilty of a crime regardless of whether they intended it. For example, failure to observe the Federal Food, Drug, and Cosmetic Act may constitute a crime.

Criminal law is in most cases statutory law (eg, federal Controlled Substance Acts and kidnapping laws or state criminal codes that define murder, manslaughter, criminal negligence, rape, fraud, illegal possession of drugs, theft, assault and battery); only infrequently is it common law. Examples of common law are informed consent and the right to refuse treatment. Crimes are classified as felonies (rape, murder) or misdemeanors. A **misdemeanor** is a less serious crime than a felony. Misdemeanors are commonly punishable with fines, imprisonment for less than 1 year, or both, or with parole. A **felony** is punishable by imprisonment in a state or federal penitentiary for more than 1 year.

Torts

A **tort** is also a wrong committed by a person against another person or his or her property. A tort is subject to action in a civil court; a crime is a violation punishable by the state. In most instances, the court in a civil case settles the damages with money; rarely is imprisonment involved. Torts may be intentional or unintentional acts of wrongdoing. Some of the intentional torts for which nurses may be held liable include assault and battery, defamation of character, invasion of privacy, false imprisonment, and fraud. A person committing an intentional tort is considered to have knowledge of the permitted legal limits of his or her words or acts. Violating these limits is grounds for prosecution. For example, although there are policies that specify when a nurse may use restraints to protect an incompetent patient, restraining a competent patient to enable you to administer medications forcefully while the patient is refusing is assault and battery. Unintentional torts are referred to as negligence. A nurse who fails to initiate proper precautions to prevent patient harm (falls, skin breakdown) is subject to the charge of negligence.

An act that is a tort may also be a crime. For example, gross negligence that demonstrates the offender is guilty of complete disregard for another's life may be tried as both a civil and a criminal action. It is then prosecuted under both criminal and civil law. By its very nature, a wrong tried as a crime is considered a more serious offense, with more legal implications, than a tort.

Intentional Torts
Assault and Battery

Assault is a threat or an attempt to make bodily contact with another person without that person's consent. **Battery** is an assault that is carried out and includes every willful, angry, and violent or negligent touching of another person's body or clothes or anything attached to or held by that other person. Forcibly removing a patient's clothing, administering an injection after the patient has refused it, and pushing a patient into a chair are all examples of battery. Threatening to do any of these actions if the patient does not cooperate would be assault. When a nurse needs to defend himself or herself or others from an aggressive patient, only actions necessary for self-protection or the aid of another are permitted.

Every individual has the right to be free from invasion of his or her person, and adult patients who are alert and oriented have the right to refuse any treatment. The fact that treatment is desirable does not allow the nurse or physician to proceed without the consent of the patient or to go beyond the limits to which the patient has consented (see "Informed Consent" within "Legal Safeguards for the Nurse").

Defamation

Defamation of character is an intentional tort in which one party makes derogatory remarks about another that diminish the other party's reputation. Slander is oral defamation of character; libel is written defamation. Defamation of character is grounds for an award of civil damages. Damages are awarded to the plaintiff based on the amount of harm done to the plaintiff. Nurses who make false or exaggerated statements about their patients or coworkers run the risk of being sued for slander or libel. A person charged with slander or libel may be found not liable if it can be proved that the statement was made not to injure another but for a nonmalicious, justifiable purpose (eg, proof of consent, truth, privilege, or fair comment).

Invasion of Privacy

The U.S. Supreme Court has interpreted the right against invasion of privacy as inherent in the U.S. Constitution. The Fourth Amendment gives citizens the right of privacy and the right to be left alone. State courts have also been strong in protecting a patient's right to have information kept confidential. What is confidential? All information about patients is considered private or confidential, whether written on paper, saved on a computer, or spoken aloud. This includes their name and all identifiers such as address, telephone and fax number, Social Security number, and any other personal information. It also includes the reason the patient is sick or in the hospital, office, or clinic, the treatments he or she receives, and information about past health conditions. Protected health information may be found in the patient medical record, computer systems, telephone calls and voice mails, fax transmissions, e-mails that contain patient information, and conversations about patients between clinical staff.

Congress passed the Health Insurance Portability and Accountability Act (HIPAA) in 1996; the final regulations were published in December 2000, modified by the Bush administration, and released in August 2002. Most agencies now require workers to undergo HIPAA training and to review and sign a confidentiality agreement when hired and at each performance review. As a student in a healthcare setting, it is important for you to discuss privacy guidelines with your instructor and nurse mentors. According to HIPAA, patients have a right:

- To see and copy their health record
- To update their health record
- To get a list of the disclosures a healthcare institution has made independent of disclosures made for the purposes of treatment, payment, and healthcare operations
- To request a restriction on certain uses or disclosures
- To choose how to receive health information

If a health institution wants to release a patient's health information for purposes other than treatment, payment, and routine healthcare operations, the patient must be asked to sign an authorization. Box 17-2 in Chapter 17 gives a list of permitted disclosures of patient health information and incidental disclosures.

The doctrine of privileged communication specifies that individuals in a protected relationship, such as a doctor and patient, cannot be forced, even during legal proceedings, to reveal communication between them unless the person who benefits from the protection agrees to it. State laws determine which relationships are protected by the privilege doctrine, and not all states privilege nurse–patient communication. Disclosure of confidential information, such as inappropriately

discussing a patient's problem with a third party, may be construed as invasion of privacy and may subject the nurse to liability. The nurse's intimate knowledge of the patient increases legal risk in this regard.

HIPAA includes punishments for anyone caught violating patient privacy: those who do so for financial gain can be fined as much as $250,000 or go to jail for up to 10 years. Even accidentally breaking the rules can result in penalties—and embarrassment—for you and your organization.

Certain acts by nurses could constitute invasion of privacy, as the following examples illustrate:

- Unnecessary exposure of patients while moving them through a corridor or while caring for them in rooms they share with others
- Talking with patients in rooms that are not soundproof
- Discussing patient information with people not entitled to the information (eg, with the patient's employer or the press)
- Pressing the patient for information not necessary for care planning
- Interacting with the patient's family in ways not authorized by the patient
- Using tape recorders, dictating machines, computers, and the like without taking precautions to ensure the patient's confidentiality (see Chap. 17 and Box 7-2)
- Preparing written or oral class assignments about patients without concealing their identity
- Carrying out research without taking proper precautions to ensure the anonymity of patients

At times, an individual's right to privacy may conflict with other rights, such as the public's right to information. When in doubt about disclosing confidential information, consult the nursing supervisor, ethics committee, or public relations department of the institution.

False Imprisonment

Unjustified retention or prevention of the movement of another person without proper consent can constitute false imprisonment. For example, only a reasonable amount of restraint should be used in circumstances that warrant it. The indiscriminate and thoughtless use of restraints on a patient can constitute false imprisonment.

A person cannot be legally forced to remain in a health agency, such as a hospital, if he or she is of sound mind, even when health practitioners believe the person should remain for additional care. Health agencies have special forms to use when a patient insists on being discharged against medical orders. The patient signs to indicate that he or she does not hold the agency responsible for any harm that may result from leaving. People who are mentally ill may be committed to a psychiatric institution for treatment without their consent (involuntary commitment) only when it can be proved that they may be harmful to themselves or others.

Fraud

Fraud is willful and purposeful misrepresentation that could cause, or has caused, loss or harm to a person or property.

BOX 7-2 Privacy and Confidentiality of Healthcare Records

Security measures that a nurse can be aware of, particularly when using computerized healthcare records, include the following:

- Authorized users of an automated information system should have individual passwords and identification codes that are changed frequently.
- Terminals, including those at the point of care, should have key locks as an additional measure to prevent unauthorized access to data.
- The computer system should "time out" when not in use for a specific period of time. The authorized user would need to reenter the password and identification code to regain access.
- Temporary employees, such as traveling nurses, should have temporary passwords assigned.
- Employees who leave the organization should have their passwords and IDs terminated.

- The system should be able to track which users viewed, deleted, or updated patient information.
- Some information, such as results of acquired immunodeficiency syndrome testing, should not be stored on a computer.
- Computer printouts must be discarded appropriately because they may contain sensitive data about a patient.
- Your organization should have a policy regarding the use of patient data in research. Patient identifiers should be removed before the data are analyzed.
- Every nurse must be aware of the laws and statutes that protect the confidentiality of medical records. Most states have guidelines on the sharing of medical information. Your State Board of Nursing may revoke your license for serious breaches of patient confidentiality.

Protecting the privacy and confidentiality of healthcare records is the duty of every nurse (McMullen & Philipsen, 1996).

Misrepresentation of a product is a common fraudulent act. A person fraudulently misrepresenting himself or herself to obtain a license to practice nursing may be prosecuted under the state's Nurse Practice Act. Also, misrepresenting the outcome of a procedure or treatment may constitute fraud.

Unintentional Torts

Negligence and Malpractice

Negligence is defined as performing an act that a reasonably prudent person under similar circumstances would not do or, conversely, failing to perform an act that a reasonably prudent person under similar circumstances would do. As the definition implies, an act of negligence may be an act of omission or commission. **Malpractice** is the term generally used to describe negligence by professional personnel.

Elements of Liability

Liability involves four elements that must be established to prove that malpractice or negligence has occurred: duty, breach of duty, causation, and damages. Duty refers to an obligation to use due care (what a reasonably prudent nurse would do) and is defined by the standard of care appropriate for the nurse–patient relationship. Breach of duty is the failure to meet the standard of care. Causation, the most difficult element of liability to prove, shows the failure to meet the standard of care (breach) actually caused the injury. Damages are the actual harm or injury resulting to the patient. Examples of these four elements are presented in Table 7-2.

Standards of Care

Whether negligence has occurred depends on a standard of care—what a reasonably prudent person would or would not have done under similar circumstances. All nurses are responsible for following the standards of care for their particular areas of practice. For example, labor and delivery nurses must understand how standards for nursing practice differ from

those for medical obstetric practice (according to the state's Nurse Practice Act), must be familiar with specific standards for obstetric nursing (eg, standards of the Nurses' Association of the American College of Obstetricians and Gynecologists), and must carry out the nursing responsibilities detailed in the

TABLE 7-2 Proof of Malpractice

An example of how a plaintiff (person bringing the lawsuit) proves that the nurse defendants are guilty of malpractice.

Element	Example
Duty	Hospital staff nurses are responsible for • Accurate assessment of patients assigned to their care • Alerting responsible healthcare professionals to changes in a patient's condition • Competent execution of safety measures for patients
Breach of duty	• Failure to note and report that an elderly patient assessed as alert on admission is exhibiting periods of confusion • Failure to execute and document use of appropriate safety measures (eg, upper and lower bedside rails, use of restraints if necessary, assisted ambulation)
Causation	• Failure to use appropriate safety measures; this failure causes the patient to fall while attempting to get out of bed, resulting in a fractured left hip
Damages	• Fractured left hip, pain and suffering, lengthened hospital stay, and need for rehabilitation

hospital's policies and procedures and in their job description. If hospital policy dictates an assessment of each woman in the early stages of labor every 30 minutes, nurses must adhere to this standard unless they document a reason for doing otherwise.

> *Consider Ramone Scott, the man who received the wrong medication. Should a lawsuit be filed related to this incident, proof that the nurse failed to adhere to the standards of care for administering intravenous medications would be necessary.*

Table 7-3 lists areas of potential liability associated with each of the ANA standards of clinical nursing practice. Nursing errors can result in serious outcomes for the patient, as these examples show. To read more about standards, see Chapter 14, Outcome Identification and Planning, and Chapter 16, Evaluating.

Malpractice Litigation

When a patient believes that he or she has been injured because of the negligence of a nurse or other healthcare professional and pursues legal action, one of three outcomes usually occurs:

- All parties work toward a fair settlement.
- The case is presented to a malpractice arbitration panel (in the United States).
- The case is brought to trial court.

The steps involved in malpractice litigation are as follows:

1. The basis for the claim is appropriate and timely; all elements of liability are present (duty, breach of duty, causation, and serious damages).
2. All parties named as defendants (nurses, physicians, healthcare agency), as well as insurance companies and attorneys, work toward a fair settlement.
3. The case is presented to a malpractice arbitration panel. The panel's decision is either accepted or rejected, in which case a complaint is filed in trial court
4. The defendants contest allegations (believe there is no basis for alleging deviation from the appropriate standard of care or for proving causation and damages).
5. Pretrial discovery activities: review of medical records and depositions of plaintiff, defendants, and witnesses
6. Trial
7. Decision or verdict reached
8. If the verdict is not accepted by both sides, it may be appealed to an appellate court.

The nurse may be involved in legal proceedings as a defendant, a fact witness, or an expert witness.

Nurse as Defendant

A nurse who is named a defendant should work closely with an attorney while preparing the defense. The attorney representing the nurse's interests is secured by either the nurse (if carrying personal liability insurance) or the employing agency. Recommendations for the nurse defendant include the following:

- Do not discuss the case with anyone at your agency (with the exception of the risk manager), with the plaintiff, with the plaintiff's lawyer, with anyone testifying for the plaintiff, or with reporters.
- Do not alter the patient's records. Tampering with a chart is the worst mistake you can make—you may well ruin your defense.
- Cooperate fully with your attorney. Do not hide any information from him or her. Make sure you are fully prepared before you go on the witness stand.
- Be courteous on the witness stand. Do not volunteer any information.

Nurse as Fact Witness

Either the defense or the prosecuting attorney may call a nurse who has knowledge of the actual incident prompting the legal case to testify as a **fact witness.** Fact witnesses, who are placed under oath, must base their testimony on only firsthand knowledge of the incident and not on assumptions. The nurse will be asked if the testimony is based on independent recollection of the incident or on documentation in the patient record. The nurse may testify, "I do not remember Ms. Jones, but I see from review of her record that I cared for her on the evenings of June 10, 13, 14, and 17." When in doubt about facts, the nurse should simply testify, "I do not remember that." New research into memory is showing that people often remember things differently from the way they were; this challenges the value of eyewitness memory. Thus, accurate documentation remains the nurse's best defense.

Nurse as Expert Witness

A nurse may be called by either attorney to testify as an **expert witness:** to explain to the judge and jury what happened based on the patient's record and to offer an opinion about whether the nursing care met acceptable standards. Nurse expert witnesses need a solid educational background and strong clinical experience comparable with those of the nurse defendant. The expert witness also needs an understanding of the legal aspects of nursing and malpractice liability and knowledge of the state Nurse Practice Act and the standard of nursing care where the incident occurred.

LEGAL SAFEGUARDS FOR THE NURSE

Informed Consent

Every person is granted freedom from bodily contact by another person unless consent is granted. In all healthcare agencies, informed and voluntary consent is needed for admission (for routine treatment), for each specialized diagnostic procedure or medical or surgical treatment, and for any experimental treatments or procedures. The consent must be written, designated for the procedure to be performed, and signed by the patient or person legally responsible for the patient. A signed consent is not needed in an emergency if

TABLE 7-3 Areas of Potential Liability for Nurses

Areas of Potential Liability	Examples
Standard I: Assessment The nurse collects patient health data. • Incomplete database obtained (occurs frequently when patient is too ill at admission to respond to questions) • Significant omissions or errors in recording database • Failure to note in the patient's plan of care (and to execute) need for more frequent nursing assessments • Failure to recognize and to report significant changes in the patient's condition	• Child too weak to be weighed on admission; chart contains no record of patient's weight; dosage of postoperative antibiotic therapy (which should be calculated on child's weight) too small to prevent infection; abscess develops • Nurse fails to detect and report observable signs that an older patient is at risk for abuse in her home from her granddaughter • Previously alert patient was exhibiting periods of confusion; found beating roommate with a hairbrush • Mother's labor is failing to progress, nurses unaware of signs of fetal distress; obstetrician not informed; irreversible cerebral damage to fetus • Healthy patient making slower than usual postanesthesia recovery; signs of developing cerebrovascular accident (slurred speech, difficulty moving extremities, falling to one side) present and unnoted
Standard II: Diagnosis The nurse analyzes the assessment data in determining diagnoses. • Failure to identify priority nursing diagnosis critical to the patient's care • Nursing diagnosis incorrectly developed and "labels" the patient negatively	• Nowhere in the resident's plan of care was it noted that the patient had a history of choking on food ("impaired swallowing") and that close supervision was indicated during meals; patient aspirated Brussels sprout and died. • Homosexual male patient without acquired immunodeficiency syndrome (AIDS) admitted for gallbladder surgery questions the few interactions he has with staff, nursing diagnosis on Kardex reads "High Risk for Violence: Directed at Others (AIDS), related to homosexuality"
Standards III and IV: Outcome Identification and Planning The nurse identifies expected outcomes individualized to the patient. • No indication in nursing care plan that nurses were aware of and sensitive to the patient's healthcare priorities	• The nurse develops a plan of care that prescribes interventions to attain expected outcomes. • Obese patient with a history of impaired circulation continually refuses to ambulate after major abdominal surgery; patient dies after a massive pulmonary embolism; plan of care showed no concern or attempt to compensate for patient's lack of mobility; family states no nurse consulted them to encourage mobility
Standard V: Implementation The nurse implements the interventions identified in the plan of care. • Patient's record contains no documentation of attempts to teach appropriate self-care measures to patient and family • Nursing interventions deviate from usual standard of care (understaffing, indifference on part of nurse, inexperience of nurse, faulty or scarce equipment or resources)	• Male patient discharged from short-procedure unit on crutches; falls first day home, refracturing leg; alleges his not receiving instructions for crutch-walking caused fall; patient record contains no documentation of client education • Skin breakdown on frail, older homebound patient worsens with eventual muscle deterioration; sepsis; nurses seem confused about treatment regimen for pressure ulcers; treatment is inconsistent
Standard VI: Evaluation The nurse evaluates the patient's progress toward attainment of outcomes. • No evidence in plan of care and nursing notes that nurses evaluated whether the patient achieved target goals • Patient discharged before key goals are met and without follow-up instruction	• Male patient, newly started on insulin therapy, discharged after giving himself the insulin only once, and without understanding the relationship among food, exercise, and insulin. No referral made to visiting nurse; patient readmitted after 2 weeks with dangerously low blood sugar after overdose with insulin

American Nurses Association (2003). *Nursing scope and standards of practice.* Kansas City, MO: Author.

there is an immediate threat to life or health, if experts would agree that it is an emergency, and if the patient is unable to consent and a legally authorized person cannot be reached. Although some value informed consent mostly as a protection against lawsuits, the central values underlying informed consent include promoting the patient's well-being and respecting the patient's self-determination (President's Commission for the Study of Ethical Problems in Medicine and Biomedical and Behavioral Research, 1982). Elements of informed consent include disclosure, comprehension, competence, and voluntariness (Box 7-3).

Obtaining informed consent is the responsibility of the person who will perform the diagnostic or treatment procedure or the research study. The nurse's roles are to confirm that a signed consent form is present in the patient's chart and to answer any patient questions about the consent. In some instances, a nurse may be responsible for having a patient sign the consent form after a physician has explained to the patient the procedure, its risks and benefits, and alternative treatments.

The documentation of the consent process through the use of a printed consent form should not be confused with the actual explanation given to the patient and the informed consent itself. When documenting consent, the nurse should assess whether the patient understands what he or she is signing and report to the physician any problems. Having patients describe in their own words what they understand they are consenting to is the best way to make sure they understand. Nurses often find themselves in a position in which they question the patient's understanding of the proposed procedure and its risks or the patient's ability to consent voluntarily to the procedure.

Impediments include the effects of anxiety, pain, medication, depression, and temporary or permanent states of disorientation and confusion. Unless a nurse is actually obtaining consent for a nurse-prescribed and -initiated intervention, the nurse signs the consent form as a witness to having seen the patient sign the form, not as having obtained the consent (Fig. 7-1).

Consequences of not obtaining a valid consent include the possibility of charges of battery against the nurse, the doctor, and the healthcare agency, which has a duty to protect patients and is responsible for its employees' actions. A patient's refusal to sign a consent should be documented, and the patient should be informed of the possible consequences of the refusal. The patient should sign a release form indicating his or her refusal to consent and releasing the nurse, physician, and agency from responsibility for outcomes of this act. This statement should be witnessed.

Contracts

A contract may be defined as the exchange of promises between two parties. The agreement may be in writing or oral, although oral contracts may be more difficult to prove. The law of contracts provides a remedy for a breach of contract so that the person who suffers from a broken contract may be compensated for any resulting loss. For a contract to be legally enforceable, it must involve real consent of the parties, a valid consideration, a lawful purpose, competent parties, and the format required by law.

Practicing nurses enter into legally valid and binding contracts with both their employers and their patients. It is thus important that they understand and are able to fulfill the terms of their agreement before giving consent. Your employment contract should specify what it is reasonable for you to expect of your employer and what the employer can expect of you. An employer that repeatedly expects you to assume supervisory responsibilities without benefit or who fires you without just cause is most likely guilty of contract violations. Simi-

---

BOX 7-3 Checklist to Ensure Informed Consent

Disclosure
Patient/surrogate has been informed of the (1) nature of the procedure, (2) risks (nature of the risk, magnitude, probability that the risk will materialize) and benefits, (3) alternatives (including the option of nontreatment), (4) fact that no outcomes can be guaranteed.

Comprehension
Patient/surrogate can correctly repeat in his or her own words that for which they are giving consent.

Competence
The patient understands the information needed to make *this* decision, is able to reason in accord with a relatively consistent set of values, and can communicate a preference.

The surrogate (if needed) meets the above criteria, knows the patient's wishes to the extent that this is possible, and is free from undue emotional stress and conflict of interests.

Voluntariness
The patient is voluntarily consenting or refusing. Care has been taken to avoid manipulative and coercive influences.

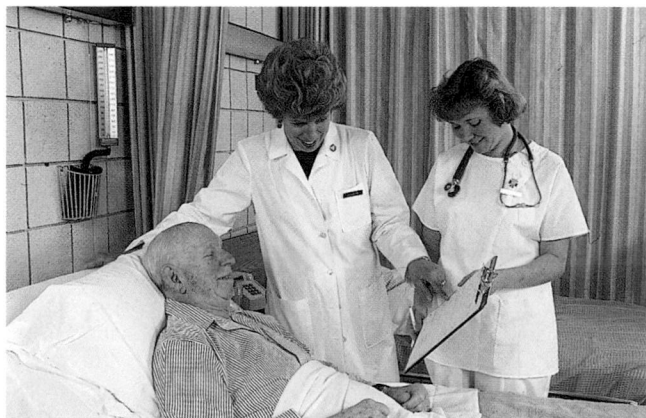

FIGURE 7-1 Elements of informed consent include disclosure, comprehension, competence, and voluntariness. The documentation of the consent process through the use of a printed consent form does not substitute for the actual explanation given to the patient and the informed consent itself.   (Photo © B. Proud.)

larly, you may be guilty of contract violations if you refuse to accept reasonable assignments, repeatedly fail to arrive on time for work, or are habitually unable to complete reasonable work assignments. Any action by your employer that violates a federal or state law would be the basis of a grievance, even if the employment contract permits the action. Examples include a female nurse receiving less pay for performing the same work as a male nurse or a supervisor's failure to promote on the basis of race. When discrimination is suspected, complaints should be filed with the Equal Employment Opportunity Commission (EEOC).

Contracts with patients are often implied. There may not be a written contract specifying what is reasonable for patients to expect of nurses, but courts will uphold that an implied contract exists obligating the nurse to be competent and to provide responsible care.

Remember Meredith Bedford, the mother of the terminally ill child threatening to sue the hospital. The nurse would need to understand about the implied contract between the patient (and his family) and the healthcare team.

Collective Bargaining

The 2001 revision of the American Nurses Association's Code of Ethics for Nurses states that the nurse "participates in establishing, maintaining and improving health care environments and conditions of employment conducive to the provision of quality health care and consistent with the values of the profession through individual and collective action."

Although individual contracts serve many nurses adequately, an increasing number of nurses have joined other groups of workers in finding their interests better protected when contracts are negotiated for them as a group. Collective bargaining is a legal process in which representatives of organized employees negotiate with employers about such matters as wages, hours, and conditions. Arbitration, strikes, and threats of strikes may be used to enhance the terms of employment and to enforce contracts. Many nurses choose their state nurses' association, versus a trade organization, as their collective bargaining representative. Other nurses question whether collective bargaining is an appropriate role for a professional organization to play. The *Nurse's Legal Handbook* (Shaw, 1996, p. 261) recommends asking the following questions before deciding whether to participate in collective bargaining:

- Will collective bargaining help my professional and economic status?
- Can I address my professional concerns through collective bargaining?
- Can I devote the time and effort that such organized activity demands?
- Can I change my working conditions as an individual, or do I need to organize with other nurses?

Competent Practice

Competent practice remains the nurse's most important and best legal safeguard (Fig. 7-2). Each nurse is responsible for making sure that his or her educational background and clinical experience are adequate to fulfill the nursing responsibilities described in the job description. Legal safeguards include the following:

- Respecting legal boundaries of practice
- Following institutional procedures and policies
- "Owning" personal strengths and weaknesses; seeking means of growth, education, and supervised experience to ensure continued competence for new and evolving responsibilities
- Evaluating proposed assignments; refusing to accept responsibilities for which the nurse is unprepared
- Keeping current
- Respecting patient rights and developing rapport with patients
- Keeping careful documentation
- Working within the agency to develop and support management policies

Think back to Ella Rodriguez, the girl with a fractured arm requiring the administration of sedation according to the agency's protocol. The nurse would need to incorporate knowledge of the legal safeguards for competent practice when preparing to administer the medication and knowledge of the unit's protocol. In addition, the nurse would need to identify personal limitations and confront the physician, stressing the need for his presence to ensure the patient's safety.

Competent practice includes developing sensitivity to common sources of patient injury, such as falls, restraints, and malfunctioning equipment, and then taking specific measures to prevent patient injury. Box 7-4 lists the most frequent allegations against nurses and related prevention tips.

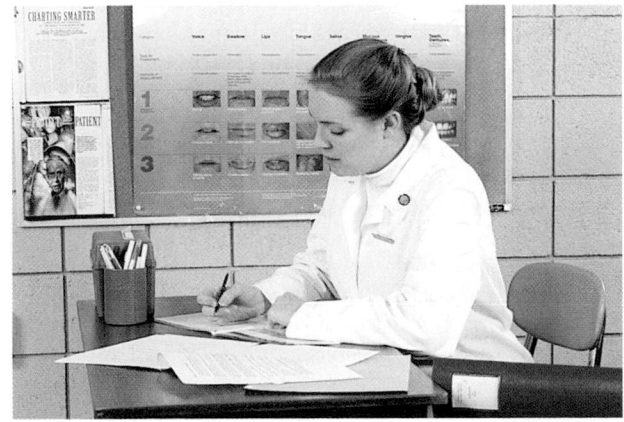

FIGURE 7-2 Competent practice is the nurse's most important legal safeguard. Careful documentation is the key to competent practice. (Photo © B. Proud.)

BOX 7-4 Nursing Malpractice Prevention

Most Frequent Allegations Against Nurses and Related Prevention Tips

1. Failure to ensure patient safety
- Monitor patients in a timely manner. Assess and document potential for injury. Incorporate safety needs into plan of care.
- Clearly define criteria for use of restrictive devices. Ensure that the use of restrictive devices is consistent with agency policy. Use the least restrictive devices that will be effective in preventing injury.
- Update knowledge on patient safety and new interventions to prevent and reduce injury.
- Evaluate whether patients at high risk for injury are routinely being identified before injury results.

2. Improper treatment or performance of treatment
- Question treatments you believe are improper. Know your agency's policy for questioning a problematic order.
- Use proper techniques when performing procedures, and follow agency procedures.
- Seek assistance when unsure of a new procedure. Never perform an intervention until you know what you are doing, why you are doing it, and your ongoing assessment and teaching responsibilities.
- Update your clinical skills through continuing education classes, conferences, and workshops.

3. Failure to monitor and report
- Follow physician orders regarding monitoring of patients unless changes in the patient's condition necessitate a change in the frequency of monitoring; report need for change to the physician.
- Report any requested information or significant changes in a patient's condition. If unsure of the significance of an observed change, consult with an experienced colleague.
- Perform appropriate and timely nursing assessments.
- Ensure that the nurse–patient ratio is adequate.

4. Medication errors and reactions
- Verify any questionable medical orders.
- Verify patient's name before administering medication.
- Listen to patients objections regarding medication and investigate patient's concerns *before* administering the medication.
- Refer to a drug reference for any questions about appropriate dosages, side effects, and reactions.
- Know your agency's policies on verbal and written medication orders and on medication administration.
- Update your knowledge of medications and new medication administration protocols.

5. Failure to follow agency procedure
- Know your agency's procedures. Ensure that your orientation to new responsibilities familiarizes you with pertinent policies and procedures.
- If you must deviate from a procedure, discuss the incident with your supervisor and decide on appropriate action.

- Advise the appropriate person of procedures that need to be revised.

6. Documentation
- Document significant information about your patients objectively and factually.
- Know and follow the agency's documentation policies.
- Be time-specific about the information, such as when you performed actions, made observations, or performed patient assessments.
- Document legibly when writing, spell correctly, and use only agency-approved abbreviations.
- Be sensitive to privacy considerations when documenting on a computer.
- Routinely evaluate the quality of documentation and update your knowledge of new documentation methodologies.

7. Equipment use
- Learn how to operate equipment in a safe and appropriate manner. Never operate equipment with which you are unfamiliar.
- Use predetermined procedures when teaching patients how to use equipment and ensure that all the nurses involved in client education are teaching the same procedures.
- Provide home care patients with the telephone number of a 24-hour backup hospital or home care service available in case of emergency.
- Have patients demonstrate their competence with equipment before allowing them to use it.
- Attend orientations and in-services on the use of new or modified equipment.

8. Adverse incidents
- When adverse incidents occur, complete the appropriate documentation and report the incident to the designated individual after agency policy.
- Do not assume, voice, or record any blame for the incident.
- Know the institutional chain of command for reporting instances when patient care is at issue.
- Support agency loss prevention programs that identify potential liabilities, guard against patient injuries, and maximize the defense of the agency and its employee nurses.

9. Clients with human immunodeficiency virus (HIV)
- Be conscious of actions that could result in a lawsuit:
  - Discrimination in treatment
  - Nosocomial (in-hospital) transmission of virus
  - Breach of confidentiality
  - Participation in testing a patient for HIV without first obtaining informed consent.
- Know and follow agency policies and procedures for the care of patients with infectious diseases.
- Update your knowledge of HIV infection; be familiar with national standards (such as those established by the Centers for Disease Control) and pertinent state/province laws.

Adapted in part from *American Nurse*, June 1989, p. 28.

Patient Education

U.S. courts affirm the patient's right to know and view patient education as the legal duty of the nurse. Standards for patient education are derived from national professional standards and from state Nurse Practice Acts as well as the local standards described in agency policies, procedure manuals, and job descriptions. Special forms for documenting the nurse's assessment of the patient's learning needs and for subsequent teaching are available in some agencies. Failure to conduct or document the assessment of learning needs and teaching may later be construed as negligence.

Determine in your practice setting what specific aspects of patient education are the responsibility of nursing. Consult your job description, and be familiar with agency policies regarding patient education and its documentation. Remember that an important aim of nursing is to assist patients in managing their own care. Discuss the nursing plan of care with patients and family members, and identify their learning needs and learning readiness. Document the teaching plan as part of the nursing plan of care. Document all nursing efforts to educate the patient and family about healthcare management, and also document the patient's response. If a patient refuses health education or refers the nurse to a family member (eg, "Talk to my wife about my pills; she'll be giving them to me at home"), document this in the patient's record. If patient education greatly increases the patient's anxiety and the patient requests not to be given any more information, document the patient's initial response to teaching, the patient's request that it be stopped, and, if the nurse complied, the reason for doing so.

Because a lack of time is a frequently offered reason for failing to document patient education, assess what type of patient documentation is performed routinely. If possible, develop forms or checklists that will facilitate rapid documentation. For example, preoperative checklists have greatly facilitated the recording of preoperative teaching and are often introduced as evidence in court that preoperative teaching was done. Other successful models include forms for documenting diabetic patient teaching, teaching after a myocardial infarction, and teaching postpartum and baby care to mothers. The teaching role of the nurse is discussed in Chapter 22, Teacher and Counselor.

Executing Physician Orders

Nurses are legally responsible for carrying out the orders of the physician in charge of a patient unless an order would lead a reasonable person to anticipate injury if it were carried out. Guidelines when executing orders follow:

1. Be familiar with the parties designated in your state's Nurse Practice Act who can legally write orders for the nurse to execute (in many states, a physician's assistant cannot legally write orders for the nurse).
2. Be familiar with your institution's or agency's policy regarding physician orders.
3. Attempt to get all physicians' orders in writing. Verbal and telephone orders should be countersigned within 24 hours. See Chapter 17, Documenting, Reporting, and Conferring, for additional guidelines on executing verbal, telephone and fax orders. Take the following steps to eliminate errors caused by telephone orders:
   a. Limit telephone orders to true emergency situations in which there is no alternative.
   b. Designate which nurses may take telephone orders (eg, those who have more education and experience, such as primary nurses).
   c. Repeat a telephone order back to the physician for confirmation.
   d. Document the order, its time and date, the situation necessitating the order, the physician prescribing and reconfirming the order as it is read back, and your name; indicate if the order is a VO (verbal order) or TO (telephone order).
   e. When telephone extensions make this possible, have two nurses listen to a questionable telephone order, with both nurses countersigning the order.
4. Question any physician order that is:
   a. Ambiguous
   b. Contraindicated by normal practice (eg, dose of medication that is abnormally high)
   c. Contraindicated by the patient's present condition (eg, as a patient's present condition improves, he or she may no longer need aggressive forms of treatment)

Remember Ella Rodriguez, the young girl requiring a sedation protocol for closed reduction of her fracture. The nurse would understand that the child is at risk for complications if the physician was not present during the drug administration. Therefore, the nurse would need to question the physician's order to ensure the patient's safety.

It is good practice for the nurse to double-check any order that a patient questions. See Chapter 17 for another discussion of orders.

Documentation

Documentation is discussed in Chapter 17; this chapter addresses only the legal implications of documentation.

Although most nurses prefer to spend their time interacting with patients rather than writing in a patient's record, careful documentation is a crucial legal safeguard for the nurse. Documentation must be factual, accurate, complete, and entered in a timely fashion. The presumption of the law is that if something was not documented, it was not done. This includes even routine acts, such as taking vital signs, repositioning patients, and ensuring the patient's safety.

Nurses should be sure that the nursing plan of care is part of the patient's permanent record. Agencies should have flow sheets or some type of documentation form that enables nurses to check off routine aspects of care rapidly and completely. The nurse should write a comprehensive nursing note for each patient problem the nurse addressed during his or her time of duty. The note should include the current nature of the problem, how the nurse intervened, the patient's response, and, when appropriate, future priorities for care. After a problem is noted, nursing documentation should demonstrate continuity of care until the problem is resolved.

A common problem reported by nurses is not knowing how to document an incident—for example, when the nurse believes the patient needs medical attention and intervention but the responsible physicians are not responding to calls for assistance. In this case, the best legal safeguard for the nurse is to document the facts of the incident, being careful not to make incriminatory statements, such as, "Anyone could see we were losing this patient rapidly" or "Once again, Dr. Jones was unavailable when her patient needed her." The note should document the time the physician was called, the time of response or lack of response, and the subsequent nursing response (eg, nursing supervisor notified). Such a note documents that the nurse is carefully assessing the patient, recognizing significant cues, and reporting them appropriately. The nursing supervisor should write the next note after reviewing the case and choosing a course of action. Patient noncompliance with a treatment also should be documented, along with the nurse's attempts to increase compliance.

Adequate Staffing

Understaffing is a problem that results in reduced quality of nursing care and may jeopardize patient safety. Temporary management solutions to understaffing, such as floating nurses from one unit to another or asking (or mandating) nurses to work overtime or double (back-to-back) shifts, are ineffective because they can further jeopardize patient safety. A nurse in an understaffed agency will be held to a professional standard of judgment with respect to accepting responsibility for work and for delegating nursing responsibilities to others. Thus, if a patient claims negligent care, a nurse who claims that she was overworked that evening because of an unrealistic assignment does not have adequate grounds for a legal defense. If patient injury results, the agency and nurse employee will most likely be named as codefendants. Some state nursing associations are using "protest of assignment forms" to track employer practices of routine understaffing.

Professional Liability Insurance

Although a nurse's best legal safeguard is always competent practice, the increasing number of malpractice claims naming nurses as defendants makes it wise for nurses to carry their own liability insurance. Nurses may obtain this insurance through ANA and other nursing associations and other sources.

Reasons the ANA (1993) lists for purchasing a personal professional liability insurance policy are as follows:

- Protection of the nurse's best interests. If the nurse is named as a defendant in a malpractice action along with the agency, a conflict of interest could arise between the nurse and the agency. Nurses have no assurance that their best interest will be represented unless they have their own coverage, which provides their own attorney.
- Limitations of employer's coverage. Most healthcare facilities carry "claims made" insurance, which means that if the nurse is no longer working there or the facility closes, the nurse is not covered when a claim is filed.
- Care or advice given outside of work. An employer's policy covers the nurse only within the confines of the work setting.

Risk Management Programs

Hoping to reduce malpractice claims, many healthcare agencies have initiated risk management programs designed to identify, analyze, and treat risks. Elements of a comprehensive risk management program include the following:

- Safety program. The aim is to provide a safe environment in which the basic safety needs of patients, employees, and visitors are met.
- Product safety program. The aim is to ensure safe and adequate equipment; this involves ongoing equipment evaluation and maintenance.
- Quality assurance program. The aim is to provide quality healthcare to patients; this involves ongoing evaluation of all systems used in the care of the patient.

Nurses with legal questions often find risk managers a helpful resource.

Incident, Variance, or Occurrence Reports

An incident report, also called a variance or occurrence report, is used by healthcare agencies to document the occurrence of anything out of the ordinary that results in, or has the potential to result in, harm to a patient, employee, or visitor (Fig. 7-3). These reports are used for quality improvement and should not be used for disciplinary action against staff members. They are a means of identifying risks. More harm than good results from ignoring mistakes. Incident reports improve the management and treatment of patients by identifying high-risk patterns and initiating in-service programs to prevent future problems. These forms also make all the facts about an incident available to the agency in case of litigation.

The nurse responsible for a potentially or actually harmful incident or who witnesses an injury is the one who fills out the incident form. This form should contain the complete name of the person or people involved and the names of all witnesses; a complete factual account of the incident; the date, time, and place of the incident; pertinent characteristics of the person or people involved (eg, alert, ambulatory, asleep) and of any equipment or resources being used; and any other variables believed to be important to the incident.

Think back to Ramone Scott, the patient who received the wrong medication. The nurse would document the incident, including the actions taken upon finding the error, such as

Medication Occurrence Information Report/PI
Send completed form to Risk Management
This document is part of a quality improvement process
CONFIDENTIAL: Do Not PHOTOCOPY
Do Not File in Patient Record
All Sections Must Be Completed

ADDRESSOGRAPH

Patient age:_____

Definition of occurrence: Any preventable event that may cause or lead to inappropriate medication use or patient harm while the medication is in the control of the healthcare professional, patient, or consumer. Such events may be related to professional practice, healthcare products, procedures and systems, including prescribing, order communication, product labeling, packaging and nomenclature; compounding; dispensing; distribution; administration; education; monitoring; and use.

Section A: Report filed by (please print): _____ Title: _____ Date/Time: _____
Location of event
Floor/Unit: _____ Date of event: _____ Time of event (24 hour): _____ ☐ Inpatient   ☐ Outpatient

Error discovered: ☐ Within same shift   ☐ Within 24 hours   ☐ Greater than 24 hours

Staff involved in initial error: ☐ Staff RN ☐ Agency RN ☐ Pharmacist ☐ NP ☐ House staff ☐ Attending MD   Name: _____
Other staff also involved (ie perpetuated the error): ☐ Staff RN ☐ Agency RN ☐ Pharmacist ☐ Physician

Staff that discovered error: ☐ Staff RN ☐ Agency RN ☐ Pharmacist ☐ Physician

Physician notified? ☐ No ☐ Yes Date: _____ Time: _____ Attending: _____

Section B: Medication type: Medication(s) involved: Incident documented in medical record? ☐ Yes   ☐ No
        ☐ IV   A. _____   Patient/family aware of incident? ☐ Yes   ☐ No
        ☐ Non-IV   B. _____   *(If yes, please comment below)*

TYPE OF ERROR *(See reverse for definitions)*	BREAKDOWN POINT *(Where in process did the <u>initial</u> error occur?)*	BREAKDOWN POINT *(Where in process did the <u>initial</u> error occur?)* *(continued from the previous column)*

☐ Prescribing
☐ Omission—Total #
_____ Schedule: _____
☐ Monitoring error
☐ Wrong patient
☐ Wrong time
☐ Wrong route
☐ Wrong dose/quantity/extra dose
• dose ordered _____
• dose given _____
☐ Medication D/C'd, given
• extra doses:
_____
☐ Wrong drug
• med ordered _____
• med given _____
☐ Medication not ordered
• med given _____
• dose _____
☐ Wrong drug preparation
☐ Wrong rate of administration
☐ Given to patient with known allergy
☐ Investigational protocol not followed
☐ Other _____
	☐ Prescribing
	circle:
	• illegible handwriting
	• wrong chart/order sheet
	• incorrect order
	• incomplete order
	• other, please describe below
	☐ Order processing
	circle:
	• carbon not pulled/pulled late
	• order not transcribed
	• transcribed incorrectly
	• other, please describe below
	☐ Dispensing
	circle:
	• incorrectly entered into computer by pharmacist/not entered at all
	• wrong strength sent
	• wrong med sent
	• label incorrect/unclear
	• delay in delivery of medication
	• other, please describe below
	
	(continued next column)
		☐ Administration
		circle:
		• med given, but not charted
		• med charted, but not given
		• held med given
		• incorrect medication taken from floorstock/Pyxis and given
		• incorrect dose/rate calculation
		• pump error
		  –tubing clamped
		  –incorrect rate setting
		  –pump malfunction
		  –pump turned off
		☐ Other, please describe below

ERROR SEVERITY/OUTCOME

☐ **Category A:** Circumstances or events that have the capacity to cause error
☐ **Category B:** Error occurred; medication not given
☐ **Category C:** Medication given but did not cause patient harm
☐ **Category D:** Resulted in the need for increased patient monitoring but no harm
☐ **Category E:** Resulted in the need for treatment or intervention and caused temporary patient harm
☐ **Category F:** Resulted in initial or prolonged hospitalization and caused temporary patient harm
☐ **Category G:** Resulted in permanent patient harm
☐ **Category H:** Resulted in a near-death event (eg anaphylaxis, cardiac arrest)
☐ **Category I:** Resulted in patient death

COMMENTS/DESCRIBE EVENT (include any intervention/treatment given and outcome):
_____
_____
_____

FIGURE 7-3 Medication occurrence information report. (From Georgetown University Medical Center. Used with permission.) *(continued)*

Section C: ANALYSIS/RECOMMENDATIONS/ACTION PLAN *(Manager to complete):*
Possible causes: ☐ abbreviation ☐ calculation error ☐ communication confusing/intimidating/lacking
☐ computer order entry ☐ decimal point/leading zero missing/trailing zero ☐ equipment design ☐ facsimile order ☐ handwriting
illegible ☐ inexperienced staff ☐ staffing level ☐ labeling (GUMC) confusing/incomplete/inaccurate ☐ labeling (manufacturer)
confusing/incomplete/inaccurate ☐ similar name ☐ patient identification ☐ shift change ☐ floating staff ☐ poor lighting
☐ performance deficit ☐ preparation error ☐ procedure/protocol not followed ☐ reference manual confusing/inaccurate/unclear/outdated
☐ verbal order confusing/incomplete/misunderstood ☐ written order confusing/incomplete/misunderstood ☐ other _____

_____

_____

_____

Signature of Manager: _____   Date: _____

FIGURE 7-3 *Continued*

immediately stopping the medication, assessing the patient, and notifying the physician. In addition, the nurse would need to document continued follow-up assessments and interventions taken to ensure the patient's safety.

A physician completes the incident form with documentation of the medical examination of a patient, employee, or visitor with an actual or potential injury.

In some states, incident reports may be used in court as evidence. The nurse documenting a patient incident should include a complete account of what happened in the patient's record and should also prepare the incident report. Documentation in the patient record, however, should not include the fact that an incident report was filed.

Sentinel Events

The Joint Commission on Accreditation of Healthcare Organizations (JCAHO) implemented its Sentinel Event Policy in 1996 and has made revisions since that time. The JCAHO defines a **sentinel event** as an unexpected occurrence involving death or serious physical or psychological injury, or the risk thereof. Serious injury specifically includes loss of limb or function. The phrase "or the risk thereof" includes any process variation for which a recurrence would carry a significant chance of a serious adverse outcome. Such events are called "sentinel" because they signal the need for immediate investigation and response. Accredited organizations are expected to identify and respond appropriately to all sentinel events occurring in the organization or associated with services that the organization provides, or provides for. Appropriate response includes a thorough and credible root cause analysis, implementation of improvements to reduce risk, and monitoring of the effectiveness of those improvements. Nurses play a critical role in responding to sentinel events. Doni Haas, RN, director of risk management, described in 1998 her hospital's response to a medication error that caused the death of a 7-year-old boy: "Every step in any process needs to be viewed as an opportunity for error. Opportunities for error are opportunities for improvement that must not be ignored. It does not matter how long a process has been 'the standard.' Challenge it."

Patient's Bill of Rights

The American Hospital Association developed "A Patient's Bill of Rights" in 1972 (revised in 1992 and 2003) (Box 7-5). The bill of rights addresses the expectations, rights, and responsibilities of the patient while receiving care in the hospital and ranges from "high-quality hospital care" to "helping prepare you and your family for when you leave the hospital." With care moving increasingly from the hospital to the community, nurses must be familiar with how different institutions and professional groups define patient rights and responsibilities. Other bills of rights include the Pregnant Patient's Bill of Rights, the Indian Patient's Bill of Rights, a Nursing Home Bill of Rights, and the Veterans Administration Code of Patient Concern. Each emphasizes a specific aspect of patient rights within a particular health agency and implies a code of ethics the nurse observes professionally.

Good Samaritan Laws

Good Samaritan laws are designed to protect health practitioners when they give aid to people in emergency situations. For example, a physician at the scene of an automobile accident may give emergency care without fear of legal suit if such care appears necessary, unless care is given in a grossly negligent manner.

Forty-eight states and the District of Columbia have Good Samaritan laws, although the laws vary considerably. Nurses are covered in some states but not in others. Except in employment situations, no person has a legal obligation to help another, and a health practitioner, like any other person, may choose to help or to leave the scene of an emergency. In many situations, however, there would appear to be an ethical responsibility to assist. When health practitioners assist a person in an emergency situation and obtaining consent for the care is impossible, they are expected to use good judgment in determining whether an emergency exists and to give care that a rea-

BOX 7-5 The Patient Care Partnership: Understanding Expectations, Rights, and Responsibilities

When you need hospital care, your doctor and the nurses and other professionals at our hospital are committed to working with you and your family to meet your health care needs. Our dedicated doctors and staff serve the community in all its ethnic, religious, and economic diversity. Our goal is for you and your family to have the same care and attention we would want for our families and ourselves.

The sections below explain some of the basics about how you can expect to be treated during your hospital stay. They also cover what we will need from you to care for you better. If you have questions at any time, please ask them. Unasked or unanswered questions can add to the stress of being in the hospital. Your comfort and confidence in your care are very important to us.

What to Expect During Your Hospital Stay

- **High-quality hospital care.** Our first priority is to provide you the care you need, when you need it, with skill, compassion, and respect. Tell your caregivers if you have concerns about your care or if you have pain. You have the right to know the identity of doctors, nurses, and others involved in your care, as well as when they are students, residents, or other trainees.
- **A clean and safe environment.** Our hospital works hard to keep you safe. We use special policies and procedures to avoid mistakes in your care and keep you free from abuse or neglect. If anything unexpected and significant happens during your hospital stay, you will be told what happened and any resulting changes in your care will be discussed with you.
- **Involvement in your care.** You and your doctor often make decisions about your care before you go to the hospital. Other times, especially in emergencies, those decisions are made during your hospital stay. When they take place, making decisions should include:
  - *Discussing your medical condition and information about medically appropriate treatment choices.* To make informed decisions with your doctor, you need to understand several things.
    - The benefits and risks of each treatment
    - Whether it is experimental or part of a research study
    - What you can reasonably expect from your treatment and any long-term effects it might have on your quality of life
    - What you and your family will need to do after you leave the hospital
    - The financial consequences of using uncovered services or out-of-network providers

    Please tell your caregivers if you need more information about treatment choices.
  - *Discussing your treatment plan.* When you enter the hospital, you sign a general consent to treatment. In some cases, such as surgery or experimental treatment, you may be asked to confirm in writing that you understand what is planned and agree to it. This process protects your right to consent to or refuse a treatment. Your doctor will explain the medical consequences of refusing recommended treatment. It also protects your right to decide if you want to participate in a research study.
  - *Getting information from you.* Your caregivers need complete and correct information about your health and coverage so that they can make good decisions about your care. That includes:
    - Past illnesses, surgeries, or hospital stays
    - Past allergic reactions
    - Any medicines or diet supplements (such as vitamins and herbs) that you are taking
    - Any network or admission requirements under your health plan
  - *Understanding your health care goals and values.* You may have health care goals and values or spiritual beliefs that are important to your well-being. They will be taken into account as much as possible throughout your hospital stay. Make sure your doctor, your family, and your care team know your wishes.
  - *Understanding who should make decisions when you cannot.* If you have signed a health care power of attorney stating who should speak for you if you become unable to make health care decisions for yourself, or a "living will" or "advance directive" that states your wishes about end-of-life care, give copies to your doctor, your family, and your care team. If you or your family need help making difficult decisions, counselors, chaplains, and others are available to help.
- **Protection of your privacy.** We respect the confidentiality of your relationship with your doctor and other caregivers, and the sensitive information about your health and health care that are part of that relationship. State and federal laws and hospital operative policies protect the privacy of your medical information. You will receive a Notice of Privacy Practices that describes the ways that we use, disclose, and safeguard patient information and that explains how you can obtain a copy of information for our records about your care.
- **Help preparing you and your family for when you leave the hospital.** Your doctor works with hospital staff and professionals in your community. You and your family also play an important role. The success of your treatment often depends on your efforts to follow medication, diet, and therapy plans. Your family may need to help care for you at home.

  You can expect us to help you identify sources of follow-up care and to let you know if our hospital has a financial interest in any referrals. As long as you agree we can share information about your care with them, we will coordinate our activities with your caregivers outside the hospital. You can also expect to receive information and, where possible, training about the self-care you will need when you go home.
- **Help with your bill and filing insurance claims.** Our staff will file claims for you with health care insurers or other pro-

(continued)

sonably prudent person with a similar background and in similar circumstances would give.

STUDENT LIABILITY

Student nurses are responsible for their own acts of negligence if these result in patient injury. Moreover, they are held to the same standard of care that would be used to evaluate the actions of a registered nurse. The legal responsibilities of student nurses include careful preparation for each new clinical experience and a duty to notify their clinical instructor if they feel in any way unprepared to carry out a nursing procedure. For no reason should a student attempt a clinical procedure if he or she is unsure of the correct steps involved. Student nurses are responsible for being familiar with agency policies and procedures.

A hospital may also be held liable for the negligence of a student nurse enrolled in a hospital-controlled program because the student is considered an employee of the hospital. The status of students enrolled in college and university programs is less clear, as is the liability of the educational institution in which they are enrolled and the healthcare agency offering a site for clinical practice.

Nursing instructors may share a student's responsibility for damages in the event of patient injury if the student's assignment called for clinical skills beyond the student's competency or the instructor failed to provide reasonable and prudent clinical supervision. Because the status of patients can change rapidly, especially in an acute care setting, students should notify their instructor or a staff member of any significant changes in the patient's condition, even if they are unsure of the meaning of these changes.

Most nursing programs require students to carry personal professional liability insurance. *School policies provide coverage only for clinical nursing done for educational purposes at the direction of the school.* Moreover, student nurses who work as nursing assistants or in some other healthcare role are legally permitted to offer only the services contained in their job description. Even if they feel confident with medication administration, catheter insertion, and other professional nursing acts, they risk disciplinary action when they perform these procedures outside the supervised clinical practice setting.

LAWS AFFECTING NURSING PRACTICE

Occupational Safety and Health

The Occupational Safety and Health Act of 1970 set legal standards in the United States in an effort to ensure safe and healthful working conditions for men and women. The act, intended to reduce work-related injuries and illnesses, has affected healthcare agencies and has increased certain responsibilities for many nurses. In December 1991, the Occupational Safety and Health Administration (OSHA) published a rule establishing safety standards for workers who may be exposed to bloodborne pathogens in the course of their employment. The following examples illustrate situations that could violate standards, if care is not taken, because of the potential threat to worker safety:

- Use of electrical equipment
- Use of isolation techniques for patients with infectious diseases and the management of contaminated equipment and supplies
- Use of radiation, such as infrared or ultraviolet radiation, sound or radio waves, and laser beams
- Use of chemicals, such as those that are toxic or flammable

The law, which continues to be updated, is specific in its applications, and fines can be severe when infractions are noted. Nurses can assist in implementing this law by promoting health and safety precautions wherever they work. Nurses employed in industrial settings have a particularly important role in conforming to the law's requirements. The U.S. Labor Department created a new Office of Occupational Health Nursing at OSHA to underscore the major role such nurses play in striving for safe and healthful workplaces.

National Practitioner Data Bank

The Health Care Quality Improvement Act of 1986 was enacted to encourage healthcare practitioners to identify and discipline practitioners who engage in unprofessional conduct and to restrict the ability of incompetent practitioners to move from state to state without disclosure of the practitioner's previous performance. When a state licenses, certifies, or registers practitioners, they become subject to the National Practitioner Data Bank requirements. The Act contains two major provisions: (1) immunity from civil damages for peer review and (2) establishment of the National Practitioner Data Bank as an information clearinghouse. Nurses may be reported to the National Practitioner Data Bank for medical malpractice payments, adverse licensure actions, or adverse professional actions.

Reporting Obligations

The unique nature of nurse–patient interactions frequently results in the nurse's having knowledge that a state requires to be reported, such as child abuse, rape, or a communicable disease. Legislation varies in this regard, and the nurse is responsible for knowing what needs to be reported in the local area and to what authority.

Nurses are frequently the first members of the public to detect abuse. Abuse includes physical, verbal, sexual, and emotional attack; neglect; and abandonment. Targets of abuse include infants, children, and adult men and women of all ages. Abusers are men and women of all ages, races, socioeconomic groups, and religious backgrounds. Nurses are obligated both ethically and legally to report abuse. In many states, the failure to report actual or suspected abuse is a crime in itself. Nurses are protected by law against suits from alleged abusers if they erroneously but in good faith filed a report of suspected abuse.

Controlled Substances

The United States has special laws governing the distribution and use of controlled substances (drugs with abuse potential), such as narcotics, depressants, stimulants, and hallucinogens. Drug abuse laws are specific, and violations are considered criminal acts. Nursing responsibilities for controlled substances include storing them in special locked compartments and adhering to specific documentation responsibilities.

Impaired Nurses

The stresses involved in nursing and healthcare and the availability of controlled substances combine to make nurses prime candidates for alcohol and drug addiction problems. In earlier days, nurses with substance abuse problems were promptly punished by firing and license suspension. Today, substance abuse is recognized as a treatable disorder, and the objective is to detect problems early and get nurses into treatment. Students should recognize their level of risk and know to seek help promptly if they suspect a personal problem or a problem on the part of a classmate or colleague. The public's trust and well-being and the well-being of the nurse are both at stake.

Discrimination and Sexual Harassment

Title VII of the Civil Rights Act of 1964 protects employees from discrimination based on race, color, religion, sex, or national origin and provides that pregnant women receive the same protection as other employees and applicants. The EEOC, which enforces Title VII, defines sexual harassment as "unwelcome sexual advances, requests for sexual favors, and other verbal or physical conduct of a sexual nature" occurring in the following circumstances:

- Submission to sexual advances is implicitly or explicitly considered a condition of employment.
- Submission to sexual advances is used as a basis for employment decisions.
- Sexual harassment interferes with job performance even if it only creates an intimidating, offensive, or hostile atmosphere. (EEOC, 1980, sections 3950.10 to 3950.11).

People With Disabilities

Noting that there are at least 43 million Americans with physical or mental disabilities and that discrimination against such individuals persists in such crucial areas as employment, housing, public accommodations, education, transportation, communication, and health services, in 1990 Congress passed the Americans With Disabilities Act (ADA). The ADA provides a broad definition of "disability"; it covers any individual who has a physical or mental impairment that substantially limits one or more major life activities or who has a record of such impairment. In addition to covering people who have impairments that have traditionally been perceived as disabilities, the ADA also specifically protects people who have communicable diseases, such as AIDS or HIV infection; people who are recovering from drug or alcohol addiction; and people who are regarded as being disabled, whether or not they are in fact disabled. The ADA imposes two requirements on businesses covered by the Act. First, it prohibits such entities from discriminating against disabled people. Second, it requires covered entities to "reasonably accommodate" individuals who are protected by the Act.

Wills

State and provincial laws regulate requirements for wills. The person who makes a will is called the testator. A will describes the intentions of a testator to be carried out upon his or her death. A person who receives money or property from a will is called a beneficiary. Nurses are occasionally asked to witness a testator's signing of his or her will and should be familiar with the following guidelines:

- The witness should feel sure that the testator is of sound mind—that is, that the testator knows what he or she is doing and is free of the influence of drugs that could distort his or her thinking.
- The witness should feel sure that the testator is acting voluntarily and is not being coerced in any way concerning the terms of his or her will.
- Witnesses should watch the testator sign the will, and they should sign in the presence of each other. State law indicates how many witnesses must acknowledge the testator's signature on a will; two or three witnesses are most commonly required.

- Witnesses to the signature on a will do not need to read it, but they should be sure that the document being signed is a will and not some other type of document.
- In most states, a person who is a beneficiary in a will is disqualified from acting as a witness to the testator's signature.

Legal Issues Related to Dying and Death

Legal responsibilities for the dying or deceased patient are discussed in Chapter 33, Loss, Grief, and Dying. Legal issues include advance directives, do-not-resuscitate orders, assisted suicide, direct voluntary euthanasia, organ donation, autopsy, and inquest.

■ Developing Critical Thinking Skills

1. Part of nursing's collaborative responsibilities are to help other practitioners obtain informed and voluntary consent for treatment in difficult situations. How might a nurse facilitate the process of obtaining informed consent in the following situations?
   - A 15-year-old boy with cancer who is tired of therapy needs a new course of chemotherapy.
   - Vietnamese parents who speak little English are being asked to consent to surgery for their newborn.
   - An older adult who has had pain with eating for 6 months is being offered an exploratory laparotomy. She tells the surgeon, "I don't care what you do, just get rid of this pain."
   - Rehabilitation options are being considered for an elderly man who is intermittently confused.
2. You are caring for a recently hospitalized patient who had been living in a retirement community. When his daughters, who tend to be critical, come to visit, they tell you that they hope their father's care here will be better than it is in the retirement community, which they are in the process of suing. How would you respond to the daughters, and what, if anything, would you share with other nurses about this incident?
3. Recent layoffs have reduced the number of professional nurses on your unit, and you are growing increasingly concerned about safety as well as quality issues. What would you do about your concern for your personal liability for inadequate care?
4. When you bring an antipsychotic medication to your alert nursing home resident, she refuses to take it, saying, "I don't like the way it makes me feel." When you report this to one of the nurses, she tells you that they always crush the medication and administer it in food so that the resident doesn't know what she is getting. How do you respond?

■ Practicing for NCLEX

1. When a state attorney decides to charge a nurse with manslaughter for allegedly administering a lethal medication order, this is an example of:
   a. Public law
   b. Private law
   c. Civil law
   d. Criminal law
2. If you wanted to find a list of the violations that can result in disciplinary actions against a nurse, you should read:
   a. Nurse Practice Act
   b. Code of Ethics for Nurses
   c. Nurses' Bill of Rights
   d. *American Journal of Nursing*

Questions 3 through 7 refer to the following scenario:
"Jean," a veteran nurse, pleaded guilty to a misdemeanor negligence charge in the case of a 75-year-old woman who died after slipping into a coma during routine outpatient eye surgery at an eye surgery center. Jean admitted she failed to monitor the woman's vital signs during the procedure. The surgeon who performed the procedure called the nurse's action pure negligence, saying the patient could have been saved. The patient was a vibrant grandmother of 10 who had walked three quarters of a mile the morning of her surgery and had sung in her church choir the day before. As part of her plea arrangement, the nurse agreed to serve 6 months of probation—the first 2 months on house arrest—and surrender her nursing license.

3. Those bringing the charges against Jean are called:
   a. Appellates
   b. Defendants
   c. Plaintiffs
   d. Attorneys
4. Jean's attorney was careful to explain in her defense that Jean had specialty knowledge, experience, and clinical judgment and had met certain criteria established by a nongovernmental association, as a result of which she was granted recognition in a specified practice area. This sort of credential is called:
   a. Accreditation
   b. Licensure
   c. Certification
   d. Board approval
5. If review of this patient's record revealed that she had never consented to the eye surgery, of which intentional tort might the surgeon have been guilty?
   a. Assault
   b. Battery
   c. Invasion of privacy
   d. False imprisonment
6. What must be established to prove that malpractice or negligence has occurred in this case?
   a. The surgeon who performed the procedure called the nurse's action pure negligence, saying the patient could have been saved.

b. The fact that this patient should not have died—she was a vibrant grandmother of 10 who had walked three quarters of a mile the morning of her surgery and had sung in her church choir the day before.

c. The nurse intended to harm the patient and was willfully negligent.

d. The nurse had a duty to monitor the patient's vital signs, failed to do so, the patient died, and it was Jean's failure to do her duty that caused the patient's death.

7. When the attorney representing the patient's family calls Jean and asks to talk with her about the case so that he can better understand her actions, how should Jean respond?

a. "I'm sorry, but I can't talk with you. You'll have to contact my attorney."

b. Answer the attorney's questions honestly and make sure that he understands her side of the story.

c. Appeal to the attorney's sense of compassion and try to enlist his sympathy by telling him how busy it was that morning.

d. "Why are you doing this to me? This could ruin me!"

8. If you harm a patient by administering a medication (wrong drug, wrong dose, etc.) ordered by a physician, which of the following is true?

a. You are not responsible, since you were merely following the doctor's orders.

b. Only you are responsible, since you actually administered the medication.

c. Only the physician is responsible, since he or she actually ordered the drug.

d. Both you and the physician are responsible for your respective actions.

9. A friend tells you not to even think about carrying your own insurance because "you'll be a magnet for attorneys trying to make a buck." When you seek the advice of the American Nurses Association, you are likely to read which of the following reasons for purchasing a personal professional liability insurance policy?

(1) Protection of the nurse's best interests
(2) Limitations of employer's coverage
(3) Care or advice given outside of work
(4) Protection of the institution's best interests
  a. (1)
  b. (1) and (2)
  c. (1), (2), (3)
  d. All of the above

10. A fellow student asks you about your legal liability when you do your clinical practice. Which of the following are true?

(1) Student nurses are responsible for their own acts of negligence if these result in patient injury.

(2) Students nurses are held to the same standard of care that would be used to evaluate the actions of a registered nurse

(3) A hospital may also be held liable for the negligence of a student nurse enrolled in a hospital-controlled program because the student is considered an employee of the hospital.

(4) Nursing instructors may share a student's responsibility for damages in the event of patient injury if the instructor failed to provide reasonable and prudent clinical supervision.

  a. (1) and (3)
  b. (2) and (4)
  c. (1), (2), (3)
  d. All of the above

Answers With Rationale

1. The correct answer is *d*. Criminal law concerns state and federal criminal statutes, which define criminal actions such as murder, manslaughter, criminal negligence, theft, and illegal possession of drugs. Public law (*a*) is law in which the government is directly involved. It regulates relationships between individuals and the government. Private law (*b*), also called civil law (*c*), regulates relationships among people. Civil law includes laws relating to contracts, ownership of property, and the practice of nursing, medicine, pharmacy, and dentistry.

2. The correct answer is *a*. Each state has a Nurse Practice Act that protects the public by broadly defining the legal scope of nursing practice. Practicing beyond those limits makes you vulnerable to charges of violating the state Nurse Practice Act. Nurse Practice Acts list the violations that can result in disciplinary actions against a nurse and also serve to exclude untrained or unlicensed people from practicing nursing.

3. The correct answer is *c*. The person or government bringing suit against another is called the plaintiff. The one being accused of a crime or tort is called the defendant (*b*).

4. The correct answer is *c*, certification. Three processes are used for credentialing in nursing. The first is accreditation (*a*), which is the process by which an educational program is evaluated and recognized as having met certain standards. The second is licensure (*b*), which is the process by which a state determines that a candidate meets certain minimum requirements to practice in the profession and grants a license to do so. The third is certification (*c*), which is the process by which a person who has met certain criteria established by a nongovernmental association is granted recognition in a specified practice area.

5. The correct answer is *b*. Assault (*a*) is a threat or an attempt to make bodily contact with another person without that person's consent. Battery (*b*) is an assault that is carried out. Every person is granted freedom from bodily contact by another person unless consent is granted.

6. The correct answer is *d*. Liability involves four elements that must be established to prove that malpractice or negligence has occurred: duty, breach of duty, causation, and damages. Duty refers to an obligation to use due care (what a reasonably prudent nurse would do) and is defined by the standard of care appropriate for the nurse–patient relationship. Breach of duty is the failure to meet the standard of care. Causation, the most difficult element of liability to prove, shows that the failure to meet the standard of care (breach) actually caused the injury. Damages are the actual harm or injury resulting to the patient.

7. The correct answer is *a*. One of the cardinal rules for nurse defendants is: Do not discuss the case with anyone at your agency (with the exception of the risk manager), with the plaintiff, with the plaintiff's lawyer, with anyone testifying for the plaintiff, or with reporters.

8. The correct answer is *d*. Nurses are legally responsible for carrying out the orders of the physician in charge of a patient unless an order would lead a reasonable person to anticipate injury if it were carried out. If the nurse should have anticipated injury and did not, both the prescribing physician and the administering nurse are responsible for the harms to which they contributed.

9. The correct answer is *c*. The ANA (1990) lists reasons (1), (2), and (3) for purchasing a personal professional liability insurance policy.

10. The correct answer is *d*. All of the answers are true.

Bibliography

Aiken, T. D., & Catalano, J. T. (1994). *Legal, ethical and political issues in nursing.* Philadelphia: F. A. Davis.

American Association of Critical Care Nurses and AACN Certification Corporation. (2002). *Safeguarding the Patient and the Profession: Executive Summary.* Aliso Viejo, CA: Author.

American Nurses Association. (1990). *Liability prevention and you: What nurses and employers need to know.* Washington, DC: ANA.

American Nurses Association. (1994). *Guidelines on reporting incompetent, unethical or illegal practices.* Washington, DC: ANA.

American Nurses Association. (2003). *Nursing scope and standards of practice.* Kansas City, MO: Author.

Brent, N. J. (1997). *Nurses and the law: A guide to principles and application.* Philadelphia: W. B. Saunders.

Brown, S. M. (1999). Good Samaritan laws: Protections and limits. *RN, 62*(11), 65–68.

Calfee, B. E. (1995). Going before the board: How to prepare yourself. *Nursing, 25*(3), 56–58.

Calfee, B. E. (1995). Was it really wrongful termination? *Nursing, 25*(4), 65.

Calfee, B. E. (1996). Labor laws: Working to protect you. *Nursing, 26*(2); 34–40.

Cary, A. (2001). Certified registered nurses: Results of the study of the certified workforce. *American Journal of Nursing, 1*(1), 44–52.

Creighton, H. (1986). *Law every nurse should know* (5th ed.). Philadelphia: W. B. Saunders.

Editors of Nursing '94. (1994). Confronting sexual harassment. *Nursing, 24*(10), 48–50.

Equal Employment Opportunity Commission. (1980). Sex discrimination guidelines. In: *EEOC rules and regulations.* Chicago: Commerce Clearing House.

Eskreis, T. R. (1998). Seven common legal pitfalls in nursing. *American Journal of Nursing, 98*(4), 34–41.

Fickeissen, J. L. (1990). 56 ways to get certified. *American Journal of Nursing, 90*(3), 50–57.

Fiesta, J. (1988). *Law and liability for nurses* (2nd ed.). Albany: Delmar Publishers.

Gallagher, R. M., Kany, K. A., Rowell, P. A., & Peterson, C. (1999). ANA's nurse staffing principles. *American Journal of Nursing, 99*(4), 50–53.

Grant, A. (1994). Instructor, students and the law. *Canadian Nurse, 90*(10), 53.

Haas, D. (February 27, 1998). *In memory of Ben: a case study.* Sentinel Events Alert. Joint Commission on Accreditation of Healthcare Organizations. Retrieved from the Internet July 16, 2003. Available at: http://www.jcaho.org/about+us/news+letters/sentinel+event+alert/sentinel+event+alert+index.htm

Helm, A. (1998). Liability, UAPs, and you. *Nursing, 28*(11), 52–53.

Hutcherson, C., Sheets, V. R., & Williamson, S. H. (1998). What five regulatory trends mean to you. *Nursing, 28*(5), 54–57.

LaDuke, S., & Spital, J. K. (1999). What you should expect from your attorney . . . and what your attorney expects from you. *Nursing, 29*(6), 62–64.

Lammer, M. (1994). Nurses alert! Nurses and the Good Samaritan act. *Concern, 23*(2), 8–9.

Laskowshi-Jones, L. (1998). Reaching beyond the rules: Understanding—and influencing—your scope of practice. *Nursing, 28*(9), 42–48.

Mandell, M. (1986). Ten legal commandments for nurses who get sued. *Nursing Life, 6*(3), 18–21.

Martin, K., & Cepero, K. (1999). You're being deposed? Remain calm. *Nursing, 29*(3), 60–61.

McMullen, P. C., & Philipsen, N. C. (1996). Confidentiality: Computer security and data protection. In B. R. Heller, M. E. Mills, & C. A. Romano (Eds.). *Information management in nursing and health care.* Springhouse, PA: Springhouse.

Moore, G. M. (1993). Surviving a malpractice lawsuit. *Nursing, 23*(10), 55–57.

Polston, M. D. (1999). Whistleblowing: Does the law protect you? *American Journal of Nursing, 99*(1), 26–32.

President's Commission for the Study of Ethical Problems in Medicine and Biomedical and Behavioral Research. (1982). *Making healthcare decisions: A report (Vol. 1).* Washington, DC: US Government Printing Office.

Sharp, N. (January 27, 2003). The "write stuff." *Nursing Spectrum, 13*(2), 12–13.

Shaw, M. (ed.). (1996). *Nurse's legal handbook* (3rd ed.). Springhouse, PA: Springhouse Corporation.

Smetzer, J. L. (1998). Lesson from Colorado: Beyond blaming individuals. *Nursing, 28*(5), 48–51.

Sorich, M. P. (1994). Nursing malpractice litigation: A personal journey. *MCN, 19*(5), 249–254.

Wilkinson, A. D. (1998). Nursing malpractice. *Nursing, 28*(6), 34–39.

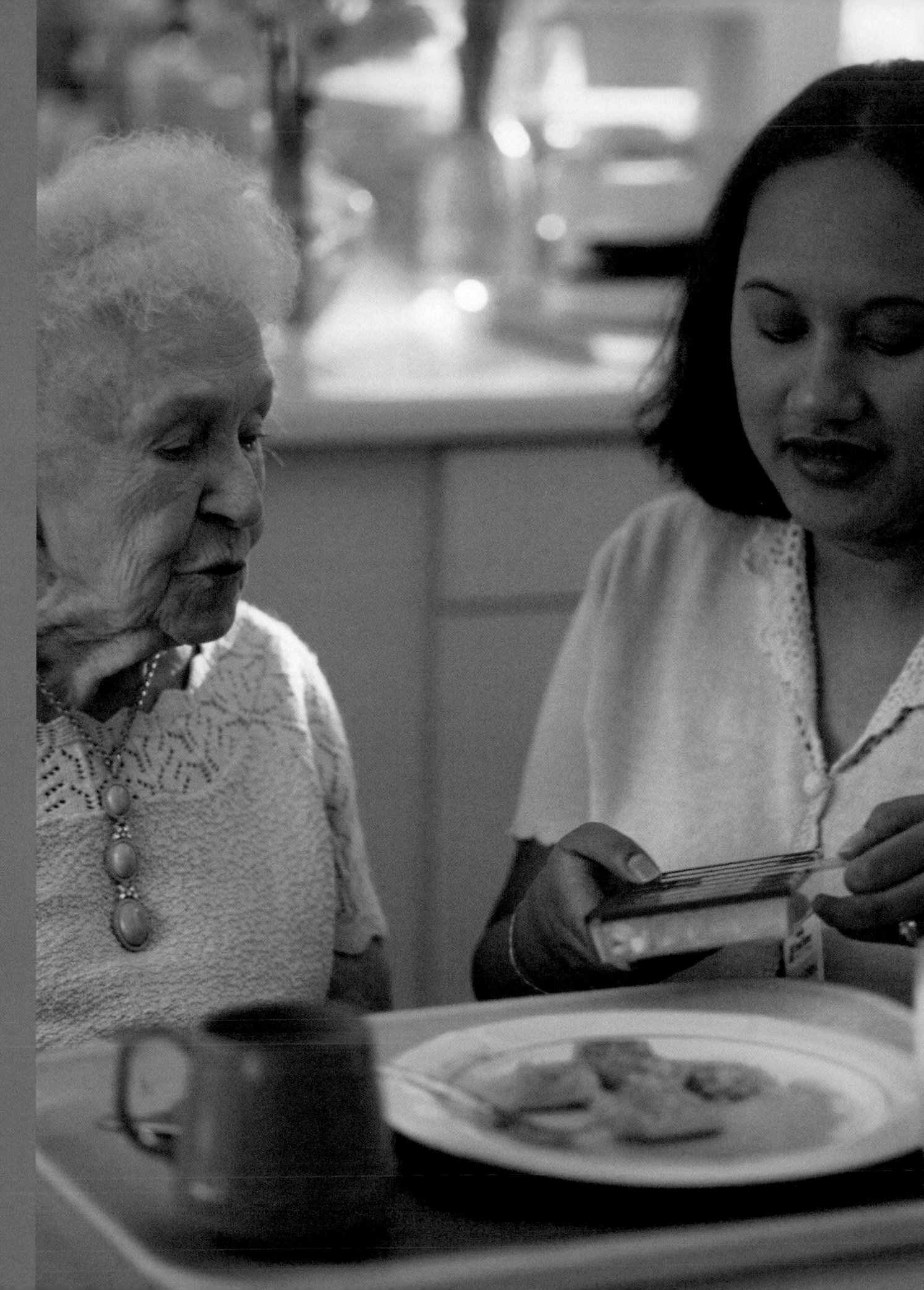

Community-Based Settings for Patient Care

Unit II

"... a realization that the call to the nurse is not only for the bedside care of the sick, but to help in seeking out the deep-lying basic causes of illness and misery, that in the future there may be less sickness to nurse and to cure."

Lillian Wald (1867–1940)
a visionary humanitarian who initiated child-labor law revision, improved housing conditions in tenements, supported education for the mentally handicapped, originated public health nursing, and founded the Visiting Nurse Service at the Henry Street Settlement House, in New York City

Nurses care for patients in a wide variety of settings. As the healthcare environment changes, nurses increasingly provide care to promote wellness and restore health outside the traditional hospital setting. Patients may receive healthcare services as inpatients or ambulatory outpatients in a hospital, through voluntary or public health agencies, in day-care centers and schools, in offices and clinics, in their home, or through crisis intervention centers. A healthcare team often provides care to meet physical, psychological, sociocultural, economic, and spiritual needs. Healthcare services may be financed through federal funding, health maintenance organizations, or private insurance. These factors, combined with increasing concern about healthcare provision, have raised questions about cost containment, consumer rights, fragmentation of care, and changing patient populations and needs.

As patients move among healthcare settings, the nurse is most often the member of the healthcare team responsible for coordinating care and teaching so that continuity of care is maintained. Unit II provides information about the various settings in which nursing care is provided and the resources for that care. Chapter 8 discusses the healthcare system as a whole, including settings and services, services for caregivers and end-of-life care, healthcare agencies, members of the collaborative healthcare team, methods of healthcare delivery, financial aspects of healthcare, and selected trends and issues. Chapter 9 provides information for the nurse in providing continuity of care as patients are admitted, transferred, and discharged from healthcare settings. Because more and more healthcare is provided to patients in their own homes, Chapter 10 describes the characteristics and roles of the home healthcare nurse as well as the components of a home visit. The information in this unit enables the nurse to work within the healthcare system to meet individualized patient needs and provide holistic, patient-centered care.

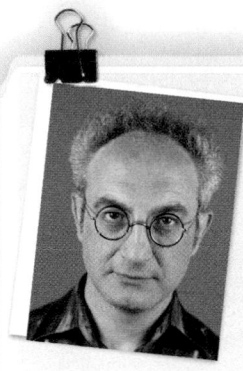

Paul Cochran, a 38-year-old man with a history of mental illness and numerous visits to mental health inpatient and outpatient facilities, comes to the mental health clinic for follow-up. He says "I ran out of my medications last week, but I feel fine. Do I still need to take them?"

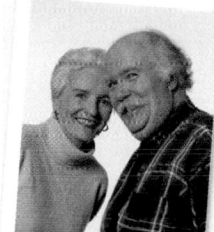

Margaret Ritchie, a 63-year-old woman, is caring at home for her 67-year-old husband who has been diagnosed with amyotrophic lateral sclerosis (ALS, or Lou Gehrig's disease). She states "All of the help from the home care agency has been a blessing. But I need more help and some other equipment now that our insurance won't cover. Plus, now the doctor says that his condition has really worsened, and he probably has 6 months or less to live."

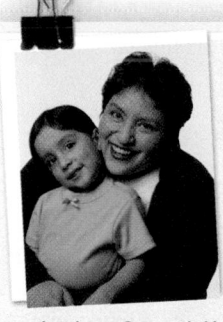

Maritza Cortes, a 37-year-old Hispanic woman, brings her daughter to the emergency department. The child is diagnosed with a strep throat and is given a starting dose of penicillin. After receiving discharge instructions, including information about possible complications, and a prescription for additional doses of penicillin, she says "I can't afford to get the prescription filled. Exactly what are these problems and what are my son's chances for also having these same problems?"

Focusing on Blended Skills

The types of blended skills you'll need to respond to the case scenarios include:

Cognitive Skills

- Knowledge of the various types of healthcare services and settings available to meet the needs of a patient with a mental illness, an elderly woman caring for a terminally ill husband at home, and a mother with financial difficulties needing medication for her daughter
- Knowledge of psychiatric–mental health disorders, including medications, amyotrophic lateral sclerosis, and strep throat and its possible complications
- Ability to incorporate knowledge of available resources to assist patients in meeting their needs
- Ability to integrate understanding of cultural and societal factors affecting health and healthcare services when developing a plan of care for a mother of a child with a streptococcal infection
- Knowledge of how finances and health policy affect the types of healthcare available to people in your community
- Knowledge of how to intervene politically to secure needed healthcare reform
- Knowledge of how to develop community resources responsive to unmet healthcare needs
- Ability to use critical thinking skills to intervene appropriately when meeting patient needs at various stages of illness

Technical Skills

- Strong assessment skills related to mental illness and effectiveness of medications, needs of patients with terminal illness, and patient knowledge deficits of possible complications associated with a streptococcal infection
- Ability to provide the technical assistance necessary to meet the needs of patients and families in various settings
- Ability to demonstrate competence in specific skills, such as teaching about medications and disorders
- Ability to ask for assistance as necessary when faced with new or unfamiliar situations
- Ability to adapt interventions to meet the needs of patients from different cultures or at different life stages

Interpersonal Skills

- Ability to establish trusting professional relationships with patients and colleagues in various healthcare settings
- Ability to work with different available resources to ensure everyone's access to safe, quality healthcare
- Demonstrate respect for a patient's human dignity and autonomy throughout the patient's care
- Ability to communicate to the patient a greater concern about the patient's status; for example, assisting the wife of a terminally ill patient or the mother of a patient needing medication but having limited financial resources
- Special interpersonal competence to interact with other healthcare personnel, confronting appropriate persons when help is needed
- Ability to communicate effectively with healthcare team members to ensure safe, effective patient care

Ethical and Legal Skills

- Strong sense of accountability for the health and well-being of patients, which translates into a commitment to getting patients the help that they need within the scope of nursing responsibilities and available resources
- A willingness to hold one's self accountable for safe, high-quality care in any practice setting
- Commitment to healthcare reform to ensure that everyone gets, at the very least, a "basic decent minimum" of healthcare
- Ability to practice in an ethically and legally defensible manner, regardless of the practice setting
- Knowledge of ethical and legal principles related to mental healthcare, terminal illness, and medication teaching and follow-up
- Skill in working collaboratively with other members of the healthcare team in different settings
- Ability to mobilize the appropriate services and resources needed for a patient with mental illness, a woman caring for a terminally ill husband, and a mother with limited finances who cannot afford the cost of antibiotic therapy

Learning Outcomes

After completing the chapter, the learner should be able to accomplish the following:

1. Compare and contrast agencies and settings in which healthcare are provided.
2. Describe the members of the collaborative healthcare team.
3. Explain managed care, case management, and primary healthcare.
4. Discuss various methods of financing healthcare.
5. Discuss selected trends and issues affecting healthcare delivery.
6. Describe the role of nursing in meeting the challenges of healthcare reform.

Key Terms

ambulatory care	long-term care
bereavement care	managed care
case management	Medicaid
consumer	Medicare
diagnosis-related group (DRG)	outpatient
	palliative care
hospice	primary healthcare
inpatient	respite care

The healthcare system is comprised of institutions, agencies, policies, payment plans, providers, patients, families, and caregivers. This chapter introduces healthcare delivery systems, facilities and frameworks for care, members of the healthcare team, financial aspects, selected trends and issues affecting the healthcare system, and nursing's role in healthcare reform. See the accompanying Reflective Practice display for an example of care in one type of healthcare system setting.

HEALTHCARE SETTINGS AND SERVICES

Healthcare is provided within many different types of facilities to meet the needs of people. There are 5,800 hospitals, 17,000 long-term care facilities, and more than 20,000 home care providers in the United States. Figure 8-1 illustrates examples of the various settings for healthcare. When one considers that only patients who require complex surgery, who are acutely ill or seriously injured, or who are having babies are hospitalized—and then only for a minimum period of time—it is apparent that most healthcare services are provided in settings outside the hospital. Some examples of these settings are clinics, homes, schools, prisons, and day-care centers for children and older adults. Other healthcare settings include crisis-intervention centers, mental health centers, drug and alcohol rehabilitation programs, storefront clinics, and churches.

Some healthcare agencies provide immunizations for infants and children, screenings for sexually transmitted diseases (STDs) or tuberculosis, and verification of need and voucher distribution for milk and food for women and children with low incomes through the Women, Infants, and Children (WIC) program. Healthcare facilities may also focus on patients with special needs, such as older adults or terminally ill patients. Nurses are involved in caring for patients and families in all of these agencies and in many other settings. Box 8-1 lists examples of nursing activities in different types of healthcare agencies.

Hospitals

Hospitals have become the acute care provider for people who are too ill to care for themselves at home, who are severely injured, who require surgery or complicated treatments, or who are having babies. Traditionally, individuals were admitted to the hospital and were not discharged until they fully recovered or until they had used all of the services available within the hospital. As a result of federal regulations and other healthcare reimbursement policies, this is no longer true. As patients are discharged earlier, most hospitals focus on the acute care needs of the patient.

Inpatient and Outpatient Care

People requiring care may be classified as inpatients or outpatients. An **inpatient** is a person who enters a healthcare facility, such as a hospital, and remains for more than 24 hours. In addition to providing acute care, hospitals have many services for **outpatients**—those who require healthcare but do not need to stay in the facility. Individuals who do not require inpatient care can receive treatment, care, and education on an outpatient basis. Examples of outpatient services include surgical procedures, diagnostic tests, medications, physical therapy, counseling, and health education. A form of outpatient care provided by hospitals occurs in short-stay units, where patients having diagnostic tests or surgery enter the hospital, have the procedure, and then return to the hospital room for a brief (1–6 hours) recovery period before going home. Patients may also be categorized as outpatients when they are admitted, treated, and discharged within a 23-hour period of time.

Size and Services

Hospital size ranges from as few as 20 beds to large medical centers with hundreds of beds. Various services are provided, depending on the size and location of the hospital. Most hospitals provide emergency care, inpatient care, surgery, diagnostic tests, and patient education. Other hospital services might include urgent care, intensive care, obstetrical care, social services, outpatient clinics and surgery, educational programs, and long-term skilled nursing care facilities. Hospitals may provide care for all types of illnesses and trauma or may specialize in the treatment of certain types of illness. Specialty hospitals, or special units in general hospitals, meet the varied needs of certain patient groups, including children, patients needing rehabilitation, patients requiring psychiatric or drug-dependency care, and patients with severe burns.

Classification

Hospitals are classified as public or private, and as for-profit or nonprofit. Public hospitals, which are nonprofit institutions, are financed and operated by local, state, or national agencies. Patients admitted to a public hospital may not have health insurance, and services are provided at no cost or little cost to the patient. Tax revenue or public funds cover the cost. Private hospitals may be for-profit or nonprofit and are operated by communities, churches, corporations, and charitable organizations. Many patients cared for in private hospitals have some type of personal health insurance or healthcare plan.

Nurses' Role in Hospitals

Although the trend is changing, hospitals still employ more nurses than any other type of facility. The percentage of RNs working in hospitals is declining, but more than half (59.1%) of all RNs are employed in hospitals (ANA, 2003a). Nurses employed in hospitals have many roles. Although many nurses are direct care providers, other roles include manager of other members of the healthcare team providing patient care, administrator, nurse practitioner, clinical nurse specialist, patient educator, in-service educator, and researcher.

Reflective Practice
Challenge to Cognitive Skills

Maritza Cortes, a 37-year-old Hispanic woman came into the emergency department (ED) this summer with her daughter, who was diagnosed with strep throat, using a rapid strep test. The child was given an initial dose of penicillin and was getting ready for discharge. When I entered the patient's room to give her mother the discharge instructions and the prescription for 10 more doses of penicillin, Ms. Cortes said that she could not afford the medication and probably would not be able to have the prescription filled. I told her that it is essential to fill the medication because strep throat can lead to rheumatic fever and glomerulonephritis. She then asked me to elaborate, requesting exact information about the chances of her son also developing these complications. She wanted exact numbers and did not settle for my answer of "No matter what the percentage is, the medication is still necessary." She also wanted me to elaborate on the disease processes of rheumatic fever and glomerulonephritis. Although I do know basic information about these conditions, I did not feel comfortable being the primary and sole informer.

Thinking Outside the Box: Possible Courses of Action

- Make up a percentage to tell the mother and give a partial explanation of the diseases so that she would sign the discharge papers.
- Look up the answer in books available in the ED or on the Internet.
- Try to persuade her that numbers don't matter and that the possible diseases are very severe.
- Ask the nurse to inform me or explain the information to me while we were with the patient.
- Ask the physician to inform me or provide the information to me while we were with the patient.

Evaluating a Good Outcome: How Do I Define Success?

- Ms. Cortes receives adequate information regarding the medication and the conditions that may follow strep throat.
- Ms. Cortes obtains medication and gives it to her daughter as prescribed.
- The standards of nursing care and protocols of the hospital are maintained.
- I am able to acknowledge that I need the help of others, seeking out their help; in return, those individuals help me.

Personal Learning: Here's to the Future!

Because I was working under my preceptor's license and he had to cosign my signature, I decided that he would be the best person to go to first. My preceptor said that this situation is a common occurrence in this ED because many people come in to get checked, even though they know that they cannot afford the medication if necessary. As a justification to themselves, patients often want to know what are the exact chances for developing complications, which will likely influence whether or not they go ahead and fill the prescription.

My preceptor and I returned to the room, where he was able to explain rheumatic fever and glomerulonephritis in detail in Spanish. Because he was able to do this at the education level of the patient's mother and be very direct and persuasive, she was no longer concerned about exact numbers. She stated that she would try to get the medication filled, and then she signed the discharge document. Unfortunately, there is no way to follow-up in these situations. I still wonder if the patient was able to get her medications.

Medical information is always changing, and what people held as standards of practice years ago differ from what we practice today. Similarly, what we hold today may be obsolete and even wrong in the years ahead. As a student, I find overwhelming the vast information that is necessary to be a competent nurse, especially in pharmacology. In this example, I should have probably been able to give the patient a comprehensive explanation of rheumatic fever and glomerulonephritis. However, I didn't feel comfortable. I do feel that I have learned a lot in the past years as a student, but I know that the knowledge I need to act as a professional nurse is much greater! While it is overwhelming and very challenging at times, I think continued learning is one reason why nursing is such a wonderful profession. I think it will never get boring.

Reflection

How do you think you would respond in a similar situation? Why? What does this tell you about yourself and about the adequacy of your skills for professional practice? Can you think of other ways to respond? What, if any, effect do you think the preceptor's culture had on the situation? His gender? His position or title in the ED? Please explain your answers. Reread the preceptor's statement about this type of situation being common in the ED. Do the statements reflect culturally competent nursing? Or are the statements judgmental? Support your response. Did the nursing student seek out the most appropriate resource for information? Why or why not? What other resources could have been helpful? What other skills (cognitive, interpersonal, technical, ethical/legal) would you need to respond well in this situation? Do you agree with the criteria to evaluate a successful outcome? Did the nursing student meet the criteria? Explain your answer.

Julia Strobel, Georgetown University

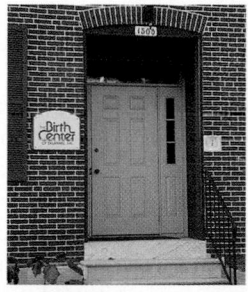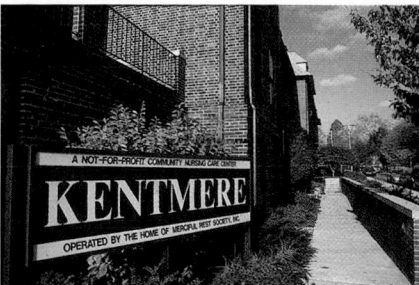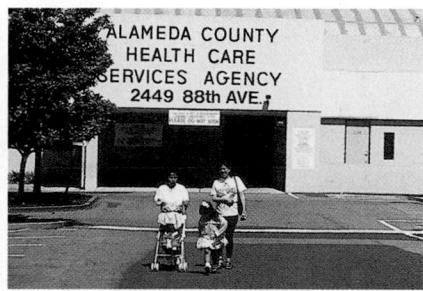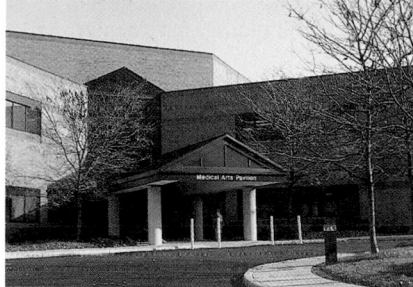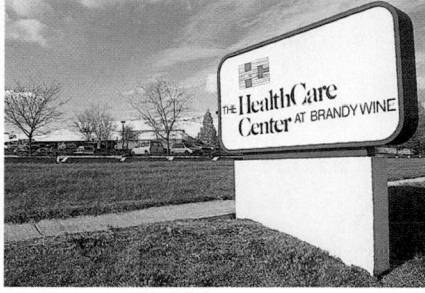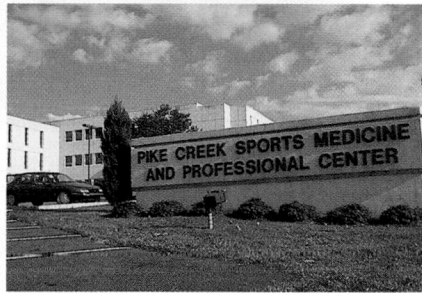

FIGURE 8-1 In recent years, the number and variety of healthcare settings have increased dramatically. (Photos © B. Proud.)

Think back to Maritza Cortes, the mother who brings her daughter to the emergency department for care. The nurse, in this situation, acts primarily in the caregiver role. However, the nurse also plays a major role in education, using knowledge about the infection for teaching the mother about possible complications and the need for continued antibiotic treatment.

The current emphasis on cost containment and restructuring has made and will continue to make changes in where and how nurses work.

Primary Care Centers

Physicians and advanced practice nurses provide primary healthcare services in offices and clinics. Services include the diagnosis and treatment of minor illnesses; performing minor surgical procedures; and providing obstetrical care, well-child care, counseling, and referrals (Fig. 8-2). Many offices have laboratory and radiographic facilities. Although some physicians are general practitioners who treat all types of illness, many physicians specialize in one type of illness or surgery.

A nurse in a physician's office makes health assessments, performs technical procedures, assists the physician, and provides health education. Nurse practitioners or clinical nurse

---

BOX 8-1 **Examples of Nursing Activities in Various Healthcare Settings**

Home
- Assesses the home environment and the patient
- Develops the relationship based on mutual trust
- Plans, implements, and evaluates the plan of care
- Provides direct care
- Coordinates care of others
- Teaches patient and family
- Provides support for family members
- Makes referrals

Hospitals
- Serves as administrator or manager
- Assesses and monitors patient's health status
- Provides direct care
- Coordinates the care provided by others
- Teaches patients and families
- Plans, implements, and evaluates the plan of care
- Provides staff information
- Coordinates discharge planning to ensure continuity of care

- Provides specialized care
- Makes referrals

Ambulatory Care
- Makes assessments of health status of patients
- Assists (or is) the primary care provider
- Provides direct patient care
- Coordinates care provided by others
- Teaches patients and family
- Plans, implements, and evaluates the plan of care
- Serves as patient advocate

Long-Term Care
- Serves as administrator
- Coordinates the care provided by others
- Provides direct care
- Teaches patients and families
- Plans, implements, and evaluates the plan of care
- Makes referrals

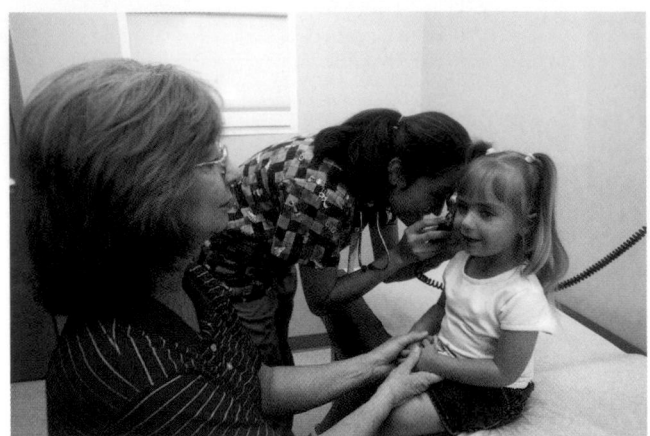

FIGURE 8-2 A nurse assesses a patient during a well-child visit at a primary care center.   (Photo by Joe Mitchell.)

specialists work collaboratively with physicians to make assessments and care for patients who require health maintenance or health promotion activities. Nurse practitioners also have their own offices and clinics to provide primary care and treatment to patients and only refer complex health problems to a physician.

> *Recall Maritza Cortes, the mother of the child with a strep throat? When thinking about healthcare for usual childhood illnesses, one might commonly think of primary healthcare services. However, in this case, Ms. Cortes uses the emergency department. The nurse would need to determine the rationale for this decision. Possibly the mother thought that the child was too ill and needed to be seen immediately. In this case, the nurse would develop a teaching plan for Ms. Cortes about typical childhood illnesses. Maybe she did not know of anywhere else to obtain services. Here, the nurse could contact social services to obtain information about community clinics for Ms. Cortes. Finances on the mother's part may have led to her decision to use the emergency department. In this case, the nurse also could contact social services to assist in this area and arrange for financial assistance. However, regardless of the reason for Ms. Cortes choosing the emergency department, the nurse provides safe, quality care.*

Ambulatory Care Centers and Clinics

Ambulatory care centers and clinics may be located in hospitals, may be a free-standing service provided by a group of healthcare providers who work together, or may be managed by a nurse practitioner. Ambulatory care centers and clinics are often located in convenient areas such as shopping malls or other community agencies. Many ambulatory care centers and clinics offer walk-in services so that appointments are unnecessary, and they are also open at times other than traditional office hours.

Nurses in ambulatory care centers and clinics provide technical services (eg, administering medications), determine the priority of care needs, and provide teaching about all aspects of care. A special type of ambulatory care center is an urgent-care center, which provides walk-in emergency care services. Nine and one half percent of RNs work in ambulatory care centers (ANA, 2003a). Ambulatory surgical centers, discussed in Chapter 30, are another form of ambulatory care center.

Home Healthcare

Home healthcare is one of the most rapidly growing areas of the healthcare system. (See Chap. 10 for a full discussion of this type of community-based nursing care.) Home healthcare may be provided through community health departments, visiting nurses' associations, hospital-based case managers, and home health agencies. These agencies provide many different health-related services, including skilled nursing assessment, teaching and support of patients and family members, and direct care for patients.

The importance of home healthcare is evidenced by many factors. The prospective payment system of reimbursement (diagnosis-related groups, or DRGs, discussed later), encourages early discharge from the hospital, and has created a new, acutely ill population that needs skilled care at home. Increasing numbers of older people are living longer and have multiple chronic illnesses, and with sophisticated technology, people can be kept alive and relatively comfortable in their own homes. Healthcare consumers demand that services be humane and that provisions be made for a dignified death at home.

Nurses who provide care in the home make assessments and provide physical care, administer medications, teach, and support family members. They also collaborate with other healthcare providers, such as physicians, physical therapists, occupational therapists, respiratory therapists, and social workers to plan and provide patient care.

> *Consider Margaret Ritchie, the older adult woman caring for her husband at home. She is receiving home care services to help provide for her husband at home. In addition to nursing, physical therapy, respiratory therapy, and social services may be provided, based on an assessment of the patient's needs.*

Long-Term Care Facilities

Long-term care facilities provide healthcare and help with the activities of daily living for people of any age who are physically or mentally unable to care for themselves independently. Long-term care may extend for periods ranging from days to years. Agencies that provide long-term care are often independent but may be associated with a hospital. Long-term care facilities include transitional subacute care, intermediate and long-term care, nursing homes, retirement centers, and residential institutions for mentally and developmentally or physically disabled patients of all ages. One of the newest concepts in long-term care is called "aging in place." In this type of care, patients move to a living space, such as an apartment, while they are still physically able to care for themselves, and then have access to more healthcare services as needed as long as they live.

Long-term care facilities have proliferated in recent years for two reasons. First, as many patients are discharged from the hospital earlier in their recovery period, they require care that is beyond the scope of home care. These patients receive transitional, subacute care in a long-term facility. Second, many older adults do not have caregivers available and are no longer be able to carry out activities of daily living independently. As the services available through home healthcare increase, however, more people are able to remain in their own homes; thus the number of older adults in nursing homes has declined in the past decade.

Although long-term facilities, especially nursing homes, have had a negative image in the past, much has changed. Most nursing homes focus on maintaining residents' quality of life and function and independence, with concern for the living environment as well as the healthcare provided. A focus on maximizing quality of life for residents has led to surroundings that include plants and animals as part of the home. Many of the overall improvements in long-term care resulted from the 1987 Omnibus Budget Reconciliation Act (OBRA), which included legislation to maintain standards of quality assurance in the nursing home industry.

Because patients entering long-term care facilities require so many different levels of care, it is difficult to generalize about the services provided (see Chap. 20 for a listing of different types of housing choices for older adults). Those entering convalescent centers remain only until they have recovered. In some instances, an older adult may choose to move into a retirement or assisted-living center that provides healthcare services only when needed. Other people who enter a nursing home may require complete care as long as they live. The nurse's roles in long-term care facilities may include being a provider of direct care, supervisor, administrator, or teacher (Fig. 8-3). Because most patients are older, increasing numbers of gerontology nurse specialists are contributing their knowledge and expertise to the care of these patients. Almost all long-term care facilities require that skilled nursing care be available at all times. The care given to patients can be performed only by or under the direct supervision of a licensed nurse.

Specialized Care Centers and Settings

Specialized care centers and settings provide services for a specific population or group. They are usually located in easily accessible locations within a community.

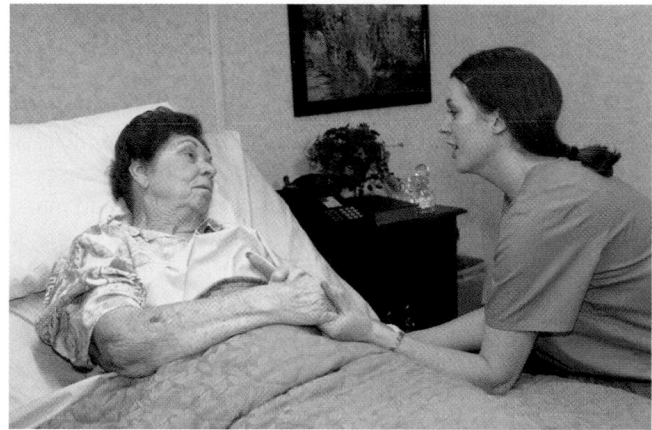

FIGURE 8-3 A nurse provides care and counseling at a long-term care facility.

Day-Care Centers

Day-care centers have a variety of purposes. Some centers care for healthy infants and children whose parents work; some also care for children with minor illnesses. Eldercare centers and senior citizen centers provide a place for older adults to socialize and to receive care while family members work. Some day-care centers provide health-related services and care to people who do not need to be in a healthcare institution but cannot be at home alone. Such centers provide services to older people for physical rehabilitation and special needs (eg, cerebral palsy), and for chemical dependency and mental health.

Nurses who work in day-care centers administer medications and treatments, conduct health screenings, teach, and counsel.

Mental Health Centers

Mental health centers may be associated with a hospital or may provide services as an independent agency. The services provided may be crisis centered or may involve long-term counseling. Patients receive outpatient care through a variety of interventions, including individual and group counseling, medications, and assistance with independent living. Crisis intervention centers are also mental health centers. They typically provide 24-hour services and hotlines for people who are suicidal, abusing drugs or alcohol, or in abusive situations. These centers also provide information and services for victims of rape and abuse.

Nurses who work in mental health centers must have strong communication and counseling skills and must be thoroughly familiar with community resources specific to the needs of patients being served in order to make appropriate referrals.

Remember Paul Cochran, the patient with a mental illness who ran out of his medications? The nurse needs knowledge of local mental health centers to ensure continuity of care, including follow-up with medication regimen.

Rural Health Centers

Rural health centers are often located in geographically remote areas that have few healthcare providers. Many rural health centers are run by nurse practitioners, who serve as the patient's primary health provider for the care of minor acute illnesses as well as chronic illnesses. Patients who are seriously ill or injured are given emergency care and then transported to the nearest large hospital. Nurses who practice independently usually do so in collaboration with a physician who approves protocols for care. Many rural hospitals, physicians, and nurse practitioners now have immediate access to information about diagnosis and treatment of illness through telecommunication and computers.

Schools

School nurses are often the major source of health assessment, health education, and emergency care for the nation's children. The role of the school nurse reflects changes in society itself: children in schools today are from many different racial and ethnic groups, have varying socioeconomic backgrounds, and have more complex disabilities that require expert knowledge and skills for management during school hours. School nurses provide many different services, including maintaining immunization records, providing emergency care for physical and mental illnesses, administering prescribed medications, conducting routine health screenings (eg, vision, hearing, and scoliosis), and providing health information and education.

Industry

Many large industries have their own ambulatory care clinic, staffed primarily by nurses. Occupational health nurses in industrial clinics focus on preventing work-related injury and illness by conducting health assessments, teaching for health promotion (eg, stopping smoking, eating sensibly, using safety equipment, and exercising regularly), caring for minor accidents and illnesses, and making referrals for more serious health problems.

Homeless Shelters

Homeless shelters are usually living units, such as an apartment building or home, that provide housing for people who do not have regular shelter. The homeless are at increased risk for illness or injury because of factors such as exposure to the elements, exposure to violence, drug and alcohol addiction, poor nutrition, poor hygiene, and overcrowding. Services provided by nurses in homeless shelters include immunizing children, teaching pregnant women, treating infections and illnesses, referring for diagnosis and treatment of STDs, and providing information about maintaining health.

Rehabilitation Centers

Rehabilitation centers specialize in services for patients requiring physical or emotional rehabilitation and for treatment of chemical dependency. These centers may be either freestanding or associated with a hospital. The goal is to return patients to optimal health and to return them to the community as independent members of society. Rehabilitation centers often use a multidisciplinary team composed of physicians, nurses, physical therapists, occupational therapists, and counselors. The role of the nurse includes direct care, teaching, and counseling. The practice of rehabilitation nursing is based on a philosophy of encouraging independent self-care within the patient's capabilities.

Healthcare Services for Caregivers and End-of-Life Care

Healthcare services are provided for the caregivers of those that are chronically ill and for patients and caregivers as a part of end-of-life care. These services include respite care and hospice services.

Respite Care

Respite care is a type of care provided for caregivers of homebound ill, disabled, or elderly patients. The main purpose is to give the primary caregiver some time away from the responsibilities of day-to-day care. Professionals or volunteers may provide care in an adult day-care center or in the patient's home.

> Recall Margaret Ritchie, the woman caring for her ill husband at home? The nurse visiting Mrs. Ritchie in her home might determine that she needs some relief from caring for her husband. This relief could be something as short as an afternoon out with friends or possibly a weekend away with friends or family.

In most instances, the care is provided by trained nursing assistants or volunteers. Professional nurses provide information about how to access respite care and may make referrals. Medicaid and most insurance providers do not cover the costs of respite care.

Hospice Services

Hospice is a program of palliative and supportive care services providing physical, psychological, social, and spiritual care for dying persons, their families, and other loved ones (National Center for Health Statistics, 2002). This care is most often provided in the home, but hospital-based hospice services are also available. The hospice agency may be public or private.

Hospice care usually begins when the patient has 6 months or less to live and ends with the family 1 year after the death. This continuation of care for the family after the death is bereavement care. Nurses providing hospice care work with an interdisciplinary team of other health professionals, such as social workers, pastoral counselors, home health aides, and volunteers to provide comprehensive palliative care (care that is provided to relieve or reduce the intensity of uncomfortable symptoms).

> Again, think back to Margaret Ritchie, who is caring for her husband at home. The physician recently informed her of her husband's prognosis. The nurse might anticipate that hospice care would be appropriate for Mrs. Ritchie and her husband.

The hospice nurse combines the skills of the home care nurse with the ability to provide daily emotional support to dying patients and their families. Hospice nurses are especially skilled in pain and symptom management. Their focus is on improving quality of life, as opposed to prolonging the length of it, and on preserving dignity for the patient in death. After the death, the nurse continues to care for the patient's family during the bereavement period for up to 1 year. Nurses use this time to help families work through the grief process after their loss.

The American hospice movement was originally led by volunteers (many of whom were nurses) who wanted to make life better for those who were dying. These devoted volunteers promoted the dignity of dying patients and decreased their institutionalization. Dr. Elizabeth Kubler-Ross published *On Death and Dying* in 1969, which describes the five stages that many terminally ill patients experience (see Chap. 33). She promoted the use of home care as a more effective means of providing support and care to dying patients and their families. In 1986, Congress passed the Medicare Hospice Benefit and also gave states the option of including hospice services in their Medicaid programs. Since then, patients who are dying of cancer or any other terminal illness may receive hospice care in the comfort of their homes with the family nearby.

Healthcare Agencies

Many different types of agencies provide healthcare services. This section includes discussion on voluntary agencies, religious agencies, and government agencies.

Voluntary Agencies

Community agencies are often nonprofit voluntary agencies. These agencies are financed by private donations, grants, or fundraisers (although some may charge minimal fees). Examples of volunteer agencies are Meals on Wheels, which supplies meals to older and homebound people; transportation services for older and physically disabled people; and shopping or house-cleaning services. Other nonprofit voluntary community agencies include the American Heart Association and the American Lung Association. Physicians and nurses are often active members of these organizations and provide health screenings and educational programs.

Voluntary agencies may also provide a setting for support groups. These groups provide an education and support system for patients who are adjusting to their health problems. Members of these support groups have experienced the same type of problem. By sharing experiences, members learn to solve problems when dealing with a stressful or crisis situation. Professional nurses most often provide information about and make referrals to these agencies to patients and family members. The following are some examples of support groups:

- Alcoholics Anonymous—an international organization for recovering alcoholics. The purpose of this support group is to help individuals stop drinking and remain sober. Meetings are held in accessible community locations such as churches and hospitals.
- Cancer support groups—focus on support and solving problems experienced by people diagnosed with cancer. Most cancer support group meetings are held at hospitals.

- Reach to Recovery—for women who have had a breast removed for cancer or have had breast reconstruction surgery. Among other activities, members visit women before surgery, teach exercises to prevent muscle atrophy, and provide information about prostheses and clothing.

Parish Nursing

Parish nursing is an expanding area of nursing practice that emphasizes holistic healthcare, health promotion, and disease-prevention activities. Activities are often volunteer services and are based within a church. Parish nurses function as health educators, resource and referral aids, and facilitators of lay volunteer and support groups. Parish nurses reach out to those most vulnerable, such as the elderly, those who have suffered a loss or change, single parents, and children.

Government Agencies

National, state, or local taxes finance government agencies. City and county taxes help support hospitals and public health clinics, state taxes help support state mental health hospitals, and national taxes help finance national health and welfare programs.

Veterans Administration and Military Agencies

Veterans Administration (VA) hospitals and military hospitals all come under the umbrella of government-supported and government-operated healthcare. VA hospitals provide healthcare services to veterans, and military hospitals provide care to active members of the armed forces and their immediate families. Nursing services provided in military hospitals are the same as those in other types of hospital settings.

Public Health Service

The Public Health Service (PHS) is a federal health agency under the direction of the U.S. Department of Health and Human Services. The PHS is a multifaceted program with a wide range of services. It is the medical branch of the U.S. Coast Guard and the principal source of Native American healthcare through the Indian Health Services. The PHS supplies funds to health centers that provide care to migrant workers and to community agencies that supply healthcare to the poor and uninsured. The principal budget of the PHS goes to grant programs for poor and uninsured people.

The Centers for Disease Control and Prevention (CDC) in Atlanta and the National Institutes of Health (NIH) are both part of PHS. The CDC focuses on the epidemiology, prevention, control, and treatment of communicable diseases, such as STDs. The NIH is engaged in both funding and conducting various health research activities.

The PHS also supplies healthcare professionals (eg, nurses, physicians, dentists, and pharmacists) to the U.S. Department of Justice to provide care in federal prisons. The service is also involved to some extent in drug and alcohol abuse and mental health programs within the state. PHS activities focus on community needs whenever possible. Nurses practicing in these settings provide direct care, provide information, and serve as patient advocates within the community.

Public Health Agencies

Public health agencies are local, state, and federal agencies that provide public health services at the local, county, state, or federal level. They are usually funded by taxes and run by elected or appointed administrators. Local agencies provide services and programs to promote health and prevent illness, such as screening for tuberculosis and STDs, and immunizations. Public health agencies work collaboratively with state and local departments to ensure public health through activities such as inspections of restaurants and water supplies. They also provide educational programs and may provide direct care services for low-income people or people living in rural, isolated areas. Nurses who practice in public health agencies focus on prenatal care, well-child care, screening programs, education, and outreach into the community (Fig. 8-4).

COLLABORATIVE CARE: THE HEALTHCARE TEAM

In any type of agency, setting, or framework, nurses collaborate with other members of the healthcare team to plan, provide, and evaluate patient care. For example, a nurse may request a consult with a dietitian for a patient who is not eating well or for a patient who needs to lose weight. After the dietitian talks with the patient and mutually determines a plan of care, the nurse can reinforce the plan and evaluate its effectiveness. The primary goal of each member of the healthcare team is to promote and restore health. The following sections describe members of the healthcare team with whom nurses work most often.

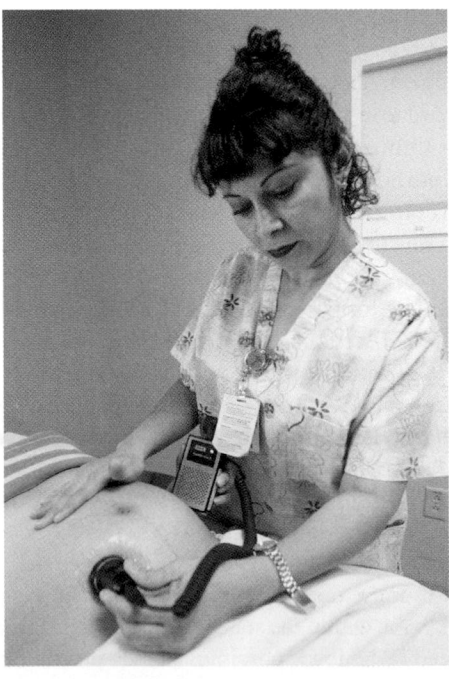

FIGURE 8-4 A nurse provides prenatal care at a public health clinic. (Photo by Joe Mitchell.)

Physician

The physician is primarily responsible for the diagnosis of illness and the medical or surgical treatment of that illness. Physicians are granted the authority to admit patients to a healthcare agency by the healthcare agency or institution itself and to practice care within that setting through such actions as prescribing medications, interpreting the results of laboratory and diagnostic tests, and performing procedures and surgery. Individuals become physicians after extensive education and clinical practice and a licensing examination. Depending on the curriculum completed, a physician may graduate from a medical school and become a Doctor of Medicine (MD) or from a college of osteopathy and become a Doctor of Osteopathy (DO). MDs and DOs have similar educations and areas of practice, but osteopathic medicine emphasizes the study of mechanical changes in tissues as a cause of illness and treatment that involves manipulation of body structures. Physicians may choose to be general practitioners or to specialize in the treatment of one type of illness or body system (such as a cardiologist) or a specific type of surgery (such as an orthopedic surgeon).

Physician's Assistant

A physician's assistant (PA) has completed a specific course of study and a licensing examination in preparation for providing support to the physician. The PA's responsibilities usually depend on the supervising physician and might include conducting physical examinations and suturing lacerations. In most states, nurses are not legally bound to follow a PA's orders unless the orders are cosigned by a physician. This is an important aspect to investigate if PAs are employed by hospitals in your area.

Physical Therapist

A physical therapist (PT) seeks to restore function or to prevent further disability in a patient after an injury or illness. PTs use various techniques to treat patients, including massage, heat, cold, water, sonar waves, exercises, and electrical stimulation. Most PTs are also educated in the use of psychological strategies to motivate patients.

Respiratory Therapist

A respiratory therapist (RT) is trained in techniques that improve pulmonary (lung) function and oxygenation. RTs may also be responsible for administering a variety of tests that measure lung function and for educating the patient about the use of various devices and machines prescribed by the physician.

Occupational Therapist

An occupational therapist (OT) assists physically challenged patients to adapt to limitations. OTs use a variety of adaptive devices and strategies to aid patients in carrying out the activities of daily living.

Speech Therapist

A speech therapist is trained to help hearing-impaired patients speak more clearly, to assist patients who have had a stroke to relearn how to speak, and to correct or modify a variety of speech disturbances in children and adults. Speech therapists also diagnose and treat swallowing problems in patients who have had a head injury or a stroke.

Dietitian

A registered dietitian (RD) manages and plans for the dietary needs of patients, based on knowledge about all aspects of nutrition. RDs can adapt specialized diets for the individual needs of patients, counsel and educate individual patients, and supervise the dietary services of an entire facility.

Pharmacist

A pharmacist is licensed to formulate and dispense medications. The pharmacist is also responsible for keeping a file of all patient medications and for informing the physician when a potential or actual medication error in prescribing has occurred or when prescribed drugs may interact adversely. The pharmacist is an excellent resource for information related to medications for both patients and nurses.

Social Worker

A social worker counsels patients and family members and also informs them of and refers them to various community resources. Social workers are involved in many activities, such as counseling, reporting suspected drug addiction or abuse, assisting with decisions about life-sustaining treatments, placing patients in long-term care facilities, and providing support to dying patients and their family members.

> *Think about Maritza Cortes, the woman who brought her daughter to the emergency department. The statement by Ms. Cortes about not having the money needed to have the prescription filled would alert the nurse to the need for consulting social service. The social worker could provide Ms. Cortes with information about financial assistance for her and her family, and community resources available to her.*

Unlicensed Assistive Personnel

Unlicensed assistive personnel (UAPs) help nurses provide direct care to patients. As defined by individual state boards of nursing, UAPs may have the title of certified nursing assistants, orderlies, attendants, or technicians.

FRAMEWORKS FOR HEALTHCARE DELIVERY

Different methods are used to ensure continuity of care and cost-effective care as a patient moves through the healthcare system. These methods include managed care systems, case management, and primary healthcare.

Managed Care Systems

Managed care systems are a way of providing care that is designed to control the cost while still maintaining the quality of that care. The care of the individual is carefully planned and monitored by the primary care provider, sometimes referred to as the case manager or "gatekeeper," from the initial contact to discharge from a healthcare episode. A managed care system limits the choice of care provider and requires approval for specialty care.

Planning and monitoring activities are conducted to ensure that standards are followed and costs minimized. Health maintenance organizations and insurance companies are increasingly changing to managed care systems. A form of managed care has been proposed as a national healthcare plan; in general, large "umbrella" organizations would provide all aspects of care and compete for the consumer's business. Consumers would be able to choose only among managed care organizations, not among individual healthcare providers.

Case Management

Case management is a method used by some managed care systems to coordinate a patient's healthcare to maximize positive outcomes and contain costs (Rossi, 1999). Case managers are often nurses who maintain continuity of care across settings for patients who are seriously ill or have chronic illnesses. In this role, the nurse monitors the care provided and ensures that appropriate referrals are made and that the plan of care follows established standards.

Although there are different forms of case management, all focus on enhancing continuity of care and effectively using healthcare resources. The primary objective in many case management systems is to identify specific protocols and timetables for care and treatment in a format called a critical pathway. These written critical paths (also called clinical pathways, care maps, or anticipated recovery paths) incorporate independent and collaborative nursing interventions to reach desired patient outcomes within a specific time frame.

Nursing case management is an important method of coordinating care, controlling costs, and improving access to healthcare. The nurse case manager is responsible for these goals and may follow the patient from diagnosis of an illness to hospitalization and then back to home care. During the healthcare episode, the nurse case manager is responsible for managing the patient's interactions with the entire healthcare system. Nurses who are case managers do not give direct care; rather, they coordinate the care provided by others. In this role, nurse case managers have increased autonomy and power within the healthcare system in a variety of settings, including hospitals, long-term care facilities, and clinics.

Primary Healthcare

Primary healthcare was originally conceptualized in 1978 by the World Health Organization (WHO) and the United Nations International Children's Emergency Fund (UNICEF). The concept was developed based on decreases in illness and death in member countries that were achieved by simple, local, inexpensive solutions to health problems, especially when combined with economic and social development. Further discussion led to a focus on a global health strategy called primary healthcare. **Primary healthcare** is defined as essential healthcare based on practical, scientifically sound, and socially acceptable methods and technology, made universally accessible to individuals and families in the community through their full participation and at a cost the community can afford. It brings healthcare as close as possible to where people live and work.

Primary *healthcare* should not be confused with primary *care*. Primary care is the delivery of healthcare services, including the initial contact and ongoing care. Included in primary care is the responsibility for referral to other providers based on patient needs. Both physicians and nurse practitioners provide primary care, which focuses on the individual patient and is directed by the provider. In contrast, primary healthcare has a community-based philosophic base that emphasizes universal access and affordability of healthcare, health of the whole population, and consumer involvement. However, primary care and case management can both be practiced within a primary healthcare philosophy.

FINANCIAL ASPECTS OF HEALTHCARE

Many questions have been raised about the present healthcare system. Most questions involve access to, cost of, and quality of care. These questions are debated at the local, state, and federal level, as well as by healthcare providers and consumers of healthcare services. Healthcare reform plans have been proposed at both the federal and state levels, but as yet, no one plan has been accepted. Federal legislation up through the 1996 Health Insurance Portability and Accountability Act has improved access to insurance for employed persons and prohibits denial of coverage for an existing illness. Increased options for health insurance for children who do not live in poverty are available. Despite these measures, the number of people without access to private insurance continues to increase.

Healthcare is very expensive, and costs continue to increase. Few citizens can afford to pay for healthcare from their own resources. The costs of most people's healthcare are covered by federally funded programs, prepaid plans, and/or private insurance.

Federally Funded Healthcare Programs

The primary federally funded healthcare programs are Medicare and Medicaid.

Medicare

The 1965 **Medicare** amendments to the Social Security Act established national and state health insurance programs for the elderly under Title 18. Within a decade, almost all citizens older than 65 years of age held Medicare insurance for hospital care, extended care, and home healthcare. Medicare coverage was increased in 1972 to include permanently disabled workers and their dependents, if they also qualified for Social Security benefits.

In 1983, Medicare converted to a prospective payment plan based on **diagnosis-related groups** (DRGs). This plan pays the hospital a fixed amount that is predetermined by the medical diagnosis or specific procedure rather than by the actual cost of hospitalization and care. The federal government implemented DRGs in an effort to control rising healthcare costs. The plan pays only the amount of money preassigned to a treatment for the diagnosis (eg, an appendectomy); if the cost for hospitalization is greater than that assigned, the hospital must absorb the additional cost. If the cost is less than that assigned, the hospital makes a profit.

Medicare was again expanded in 1988 to include catastrophic care costs and expensive medications. People who receive Medicare pay both a deductible cost and a monthly premium for full insurance coverage. Part A of Medicare, which pays most inpatient hospital costs, is paid by the federal government. Part B of Medicare, which is voluntary, is paid by monthly premium; it covers most outpatient costs for physician visits, medications, and home health services. Because the full cost of some services is not covered by Medicare, a supplemental insurance policy offered by a private insurance company is recommended. Also, because Medicare is federally funded, benefits may change annually according to decisions related to the federal budget.

Remember Margaret Ritchie, the older adult woman caring for her husband at home? Most likely, she and her husband have Medicare. Medicare does pay for home healthcare services if the patient meets specific criteria. However, Medicare does not cover all equipment that may be necessary. For example, Mrs. Ritchie may need a wheelchair to help get her husband around the house. Often, Medicare does not routinely cover the cost of this device. As a result, the family may rent or purchase it, ultimately leading to an additional outlay of money by the family.

Medicaid

Medicaid was also established in 1965 under Title 19 of the Social Security Act. Medicaid is a federally funded public assistance program for people of any age who have low incomes; for the blind, elderly, and disabled covered by supplemental security benefits; and for beneficiaries of Aid to Families With Dependent Children. The coverage depends on individual state regulations.

Current budgetary considerations are forcing state and federal agencies to trim Medicaid expenditures. The rapid growth of an aging population and an increase in the number of poor people, many of whom are women and children, are draining the Medicaid budget. In an attempt to survive, Medicaid programs are implementing changes such as reduced benefits or placing patients into managed care programs.

> *Remember Maritza Cortes, the woman who brought her daughter to the emergency department for treatment? The nurse would investigate Ms. Cortes situation, possibly consulting social services for assistance in obtaining Medicaid for Ms. Cortes and her daughter.*

Group Plans

The major group plans for financing healthcare are managed care plans, such as health maintenance organizations (HMOs), preferred provider organizations (PPOs), and private insurance. Enrollment in these plans is voluntary. An individual pays a fixed rate on a monthly or annual plan and, in turn, receives coverage for most healthcare services to maintain health and treat illness.

Because group plans such as HMOs and PPOs pay the direct costs of the healthcare services used by their subscribers, they encourage preventive healthcare to avoid the higher costs of illness and hospitalization. For the same reason, they carefully monitor the quality and quantity of the healthcare delivered to their subscribers. They also place limitations on the use of high-cost procedures and require certain guidelines to be followed when a costly procedure is recommended by a physician. Some people do not like these plans because they use a selective contracting approach that mandates subscribers use specific institutions and healthcare providers. Some consumers dislike not being able to control decisions about their own or their family's health.

Health Maintenance Organizations

Health maintenance organizations (HMOs) are prepaid, group-managed care plans that allow subscribers to receive all the medical services they require through a group of affiliated providers. There may be no additional out-of-pocket costs, or subscribers may pay only a small fee, called a copayment. An HMO may employ all its providers (including physicians) or may be a group of physicians in alliance who provide care as independent practitioners. In most HMOs, the patient does not have a choice about healthcare providers but receives all services from physicians who are associated with or are part of the HMO. HMOs are becoming popular with large employers who support the concept of managed care.

Preferred Provider Organizations

Preferred provider organizations (PPOs) allow a third-party payer (agencies that pay healthcare providers for services provided to individuals, such as a health insurance company) to contract with a group of healthcare providers to provide services at a lower fee in return for prompt payment and a guaranteed volume of patients and services. Although patients are encouraged to use specific providers, they may also seek care outside the panel without referral by paying additional out-of-pocket expenses. One type of PPO is called a preferred provider arrangement, in which a contract is made with an individual healthcare provider rather than with a group of providers. Similarly, a point-of-service plan encourages the use of specified physicians and services but pays a portion of expenses if referrals are made to physicians outside the organization by the patient's primary care physician.

Private Insurance

Personal healthcare can be financed by private insurance through large, nonprofit, tax-exempt organizations or through smaller, private, for-profit insurance companies. To be insured, members pay monthly premiums either by themselves or in combination with employer payments. These plans are called third-party payers because the insurance company pays all or most of the cost of care. The premiums on private insurance plans tend to be higher than those for managed care plans, but members can choose their own physician and services desired.

Long-Term Care Insurance

Increasing numbers of people are enrolling in long-term care (LTC) insurance. Most LTC insurance (about 90%) is paid for by Medicaid and out-of-pocket spending. Medicare and private insurance pays for only a minimal amount of LTC insurance. Some commercial insurance companies offer LTC benefits. Promoters of LTC insurance have developed plans that cover a variety of services, such as nursing home care and home care, as well as other services that help prevent the institutionalization of older, debilitated, and chronically ill people. Adult daycare centers and respite care are also LTC services and would be covered by such benefits.

TRENDS AND ISSUES IN HEALTHCARE DELIVERY

This section discusses some current issues and trends in healthcare. In your career as a nurse, you may find that some issues are resolved, whereas other new challenges arise. It is important for you both personally and professionally to be knowledgeable about all healthcare trends affecting the healthcare delivery system (Box 8-2).

BOX 8-2 **Trends to Watch in Healthcare Delivery**

· Changing demographics
· Increasing diversity
· Technology explosion
· Globalization of economy and society
· Educated consumers
· Increasing complexity of patient care
· Costs of healthcare
· Effect of health policy and regulation
· Current nursing shortage

Focus on Self-Care and Health

Health awareness and the desire to be involved in one's own healthcare have strongly influenced the delivery of healthcare services in our society. Stress management programs, nutritional awareness, exercise and fitness programs, and antismoking and antidrug campaigns are all examples of this trend. Equally important to health are measures such as legislating the use of seat belts, promoting automobile and airplane safety, controlling smog, controlling handguns, and eliminating hazardous wastes.

Knowledgeable Consumers

A **consumer** is someone who uses a commodity or service. Healthcare consumers are increasingly knowledgeable about health, prefer to control and make decisions about their own health, and want to be active participants in planning and implementing their healthcare. Consumers of healthcare services are better educated about the services they require and the services that are available, largely because so much health information is available on the Internet. They also are concerned about access to services, the cost of those services, and the quality of the care received for services. Consumers have questioned escalating costs and the proliferation and duplication of services. Consumers have become actively involved in the administration of healthcare agencies and have helped develop standards for care, patient rights, and cost-containment measures as protection for patients when they enter a healthcare setting.

Cost Containment

The U.S. healthcare system has been experiencing a financial crisis. Costs have increased dramatically, and some analysts believe that cost-containment measures were implemented too late to reverse the rise in health costs. The actual short-term and long-term results of cost-containment measures remain to be seen.

Historically, the ways healthcare was paid for encouraged the use of expensive and sometimes inappropriate or ineffective services. In the past, healthcare also focused primarily on the treatment of illnesses rather than prevention because preventive strategies were not covered by health insurance. The system of third-party reimbursement effectively insulated patients, who seldom saw the bills, from knowing the actual cost of their healthcare.

Competition among hospitals has further fueled the increase in health costs. To attract patients, hospitals have invested huge sums of money in technologically advanced equipment. As new machines and more advanced procedures have been developed and used, patients' expectations of the availability and use of those resources have also tended to increase. Supporters of cost-containment measures are encouraging hospitals to cooperate and share resources rather than compete. Other efforts at cost containment include hospital restructuring and multiple hospitals joining together as one system.

Fragmentation of Care

Expanded healthcare research has led to an upward spiral of new technology and knowledge. Because many healthcare providers can no longer keep up with all of the advances being made in all areas, specialization in smaller areas has become almost the rule rather than the exception. What does this mean for patients?

A general practitioner physician diagnoses and treats a variety of common health problems; however, a patient who requires diagnosis and treatment for a more complex problem is usually referred to a specialist physician. For example, a patient with diabetes and a heart condition may be cared for by the family physician, a cardiologist, and an endocrinologist. Hospitalized patients not only come in contact with many different healthcare providers (eg, RNs, LPNs, nursing assistants, nurse specialists, PTs, RDs, and students) but also are frequently seen by other physician specialists who are called in on consultation or to do surgery. This can cause patients to become confused about care and treatments. This fragmentation of care can lead to a loss of continuity of care, resulting in conflicting plans of care, too much or too little medication, and higher healthcare costs.

Remember Paul Cochran, the patient with a history of mental illness and numerous visits to inpatient and outpatient facilities? The nurse would be alert for possible fragmentation of care with this patient based on this history. As a result, the nurse would need to obtain a thorough assessment of the patient's medications to ensure the most accurate information from which to develop a plan of care.

Healthcare: A Right or a Privilege?

Two major factors influencing the provision of healthcare in the United States are the ability to pay and the location of facilities. Poor or uninsured people, minorities, residents of rural areas, and older people often have inadequate access to healthcare services. In the United States, millions of people have in adequate insurance or none at all. Although many people assume that everyone has a right to healthcare, consider these questions that pose ethical dilemmas for nurses who provide care, as well as for consumers of healthcare services:

- Do uninsured people who do not take care of themselves deserve the same healthcare as employed people with insurance, even if they cannot pay for it?
- Who provides funds for the healthcare needs of the homeless?
- Is someone who pays for national television coverage to ask for an organ donation for his or her child any more deserving than someone who has been waiting months for just such a transplant?
- Are you willing to pay higher insurance premiums or taxes so that drug addicts who overdose can have intensive care?
- If 20 people need a heart transplant and only one heart is available, who decides who gets another chance at life?

These are only a few of the questions being raised, and there are no easy answers.

NURSES' ROLE IN HEALTHCARE REFORM

Changes taking place in healthcare give nurses the opportunity to help shape healthcare for the future. Although it is impossible to predict exactly the roles of future practitioners, projections have outlined expected competencies (listed in Box 8-3) for the 21st century (Pew Health Professions Commission, 1991, 1998). These projections, coupled with the national health promotion and disease prevention objectives outlined in the *Healthy People 2010* project (American Public Health Association, 2000), emphasize the importance of nursing's role in improving access to care, quality of care, and cost of care.

The goals of healthcare reform focus on cost containment, improved access, and increased quality of services for all citizens. Where do nurses fit into the reform movement? First, nurses are becoming a stronger voice in protesting health-related problems in our nation. Second, nurses in greater numbers are increasing their education and becoming advanced practice nurses (APNs). As such, more nurses now provide primary healthcare services in areas and to people long neglected: the elderly, women, infants, the poor, and those living in rural areas. In addition, the focus of nursing care provided by all nurses is holistic care essential to promoting health and preventing illness.

"Nursing's Agenda for the Future" (American Nurses Association, 2003b) is a strategic plan focused on the means to ensure safe, quality patient care and address the causes of the acute shortage of RNs, predicted to worsen in the next decade. "Decades of research have consistently shown that high quality nursing care reduces the rate of complications and length of hospital stays" (p. 8). As discussion continues about the goals of this important document, the common themes for all nurses emerged: collaborating with other nurses (as individuals and as groups), developing leaderships and public communication skills, increasing collaboration with policy-makers and business leaders, and communicating successes to the public. There are many ways nurses can become involved in shaping healthcare reform and healthcare policy. Selected examples are listed in Box 8-4.

The issues of who gets healthcare and who pays the bills continue to have major importance for society in the 21st century. These issues will present both challenges and opportunities for nurses of the future.

BOX 8-3 Competencies for Healthcare Practitioners of the Future

Practitioners for the future should undertake the following:

- Care for the community's health
- Expand access to effective care
- Provide contemporary clinical practice
- Emphasize primary care
- Participate in coordinated care
- Ensure cost-effective and appropriate care
- Practice prevention
- Involve patients and families in the decision-making process
- Promote healthy lifestyles
- Access and use technology appropriately
- Improve the healthcare system
- Manage information
- Understand the role of the physical environment
- Provide counseling on ethical issues
- Accommodate expanded accountability
- Participate in a racially and culturally diverse society
- Continue to learn

(From Pew Health Professions Commission. [1991]. *Healthy America: Practitioners for 2005.* Durham, NC: Author; and Pew Health Professions Commission. [1998]. *Twenty-one competencies for the twenty-first century.* Durham, NC: Author.)

BOX 8-4 Nurses Can Make a Difference in Healthcare Policy and Reform

- Stay informed about current issues and pending legislation.
- Make your voice heard by writing or e-mailing members of Congress to support legislation to improve nursing and patient care.
- Belong to and participate in key nursing organizations.
- Document the outcomes of nursing care and develop a database to influence healthcare costs and quality of care.
- Be a leader in local, state, and national nursing and consumer groups.
- Advocate for the rights of all individuals for equal, affordable, accessible, and knowledgeable healthcare.

(From The Fourth Report of the Pew Health Professions Commission, Chapter IV: Recreating Health Professional Practice for a New Century, December, 1998. San Francisco: University of California.)

Developing Critical Thinking Skills

1. Make a list of the different types of healthcare settings where you have received care. How many different healthcare providers did you come in contact with? How did the structure and organization of the settings differ, and how were they alike?
2. How might prenatal and well-child care differ for two women—one without health insurance and the other with a good health insurance plan? Why do you think this happens? What can nurses do?

Practicing for NCLEX

1. Of the following descriptors, which one does not accurately pertain to care in a hospital?
   a. Acute care provider
   b. Inpatient
   c. Outpatient
   d. Parish nursing
2. Which type of healthcare facility employs the largest percentage of RNs?
   a. Ambulatory care centers
   b. Long-term care
   c. Hospitals
   d. Clinics
3. What is the most rapidly growing area of healthcare services?
   a. Hospitals
   b. Home care
   c. Nursing homes
   d. Parish nursing
4. Which healthcare provider is a major source of health assessment and health education for children?
   a. Hospital emergency department
   b. Community center
   c. Nurse practitioner
   d. School nurse
5. How is respite care best defined?
   a. A service that allows time away for caregivers
   b. A special service for the terminally ill and their family
   c. Direct care provided to individuals in nursing homes
   d. Living units for people without regular shelter
6. Of the following healthcare agencies and services, which one is a government agency?
   a. Alcoholics Anonymous
   b. Public Health Service
   c. Rural health center
   d. Ambulatory care center
7. Which purpose best describes managed care as a framework for healthcare?
   a. Designed to control the cost of care while maintaining the quality of care
   b. Coordinates care to maximize positive outcomes and contain costs

   c. The delivery of services from initial contact through ongoing care
   d. Based on a philosophy of ensuring death in comfort and dignity
8. Your newly employed friend is a part of the company's HMO. This means he:
   a. Can have healthcare services from a provider of his choice
   b. Will be unable to have emergency care
   c. Receives all healthcare from providers within the HMO
   d. Must pay an additional monthly premium
9. Private insurance most often is called a third-party payer. What does this mean?
   a. You pay no monthly premium and pay all healthcare costs yourself.
   b. You belong to a preferred provider organization.
   c. You are at risk if your healthcare provider is not a part of the plan.
   d. You pay a monthly premium, and the insurance company pays the bills.
10. What type of technology has increased the number of knowledgeable healthcare consumers?
    a. Television
    b. Computers
    c. Cell phones
    d. Informatics

Answers With Rationale

1. The correct response is *d.* Hospitals are acute care providers, providing services to both inpatients and outpatients.
2. The correct response is *c.* Despite a downward trend, the largest percent of RNs are employed by hospitals.
3. The correct response is *b.* Home care services are the most rapidly growing area of healthcare.
4. The correct response is *d.* School nurses do provide much of the health assessment and health information for the nation's children.
5. The correct response is *a.* Respite care is provided to enable a primary caregiver time away from the day-to-day responsibilities of homebound patients.
6. The correct response is *b.* The Public Health Service is a government agency.
7. The correct response is *a.* Managed care is a way of providing care, designed to control costs while maintaining the quality of care.
8. The correct response is *c.* In most HMOs, the patient does not have a choice of healthcare providers and receives all services from providers within the HMO.
9. The correct response is *d.* You (and your employer, if appropriate) pay monthly premiums, and the insurance company pays all or most of the cost of care.

10. The correct response is *b.* Consumers are increasingly using their home computers to access healthcare information through the Internet.

Bibliography

American Hospital Association. (2003). Fast facts on U.S. hospitals from *Hospital Statistics.* Available at http://www.hospitalconnect.com/aha/resource_center/fastfacts.

American Nurses Association. (2002). *Nursing's agenda for the future.* Washington, DC: Author.

American Nurses Association. (2003a). *Today's registered nurse—numbers and demographics.* Available at http://www.nursingworld.org/readroom.

American Nurses Association. (2003b). *Nursing profession unveils strategic plan to ensure safe, quality patient care and address root causes of growing shortage.* Available at http://www.nursingworld.org.

American Public Health Association. (2000). *Healthy People 2010: National health promotion and disease prevention objectives.* Washington, DC: Author.

Centers for Medicare & Medicaid Services. (2003). *Medicare information; Medicaid information.* Available at http://cms.hhs.gov.

Ellis, J., & Hartley, C. (2003). *Nursing in today's world: Trends, issues, and management* (8th ed.). Philadelphia: Lippincott Williams & Wilkins.

Frey, L. (2002). The changing face of health care. *Registered Nurse Journal, 14*(6), 4.

Maier, F., & Hart, A. (2003). Bookmark this site: A guide to home care & hospice websites. *Caring, 22*(3), 12–14, 16.

National Center for Health Statistics. (2002). *National home and hospice care survey Description.* Available at http://www.cdc.gov/nchs/about/major/nhhcsd/nhhcsd.htm.

Odom, J. (2003). Disparity of health care. *Journal of Perianesthesia Nursing, 18*(1), 72–74.

Pew Health Professions Commission. (1991). *Healthy America: Practitioners for 2005.* Durham, NC: Author.

Pew Health Professions Commission. (1998). *Twenty-one competencies for the twenty-first century.* Durham, NC: Author.

Pew Health Professions Commission. (1998). *Chapter IV: Recreating health professional practice for a new century.* Durham, NC: Author.

Rossi, P. (1999). *Case management in health care: A practical guide.* Philadelphia: W. B. Saunders.

Wakefield, M. K. (2003). Health care policy or politics—which prevails in 2003? *Nursing Economics, 21*(1), 47–48.

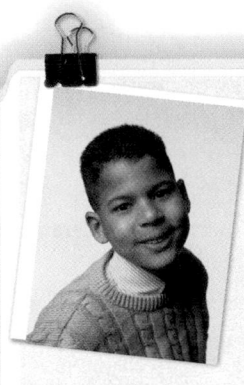

Jeff Hart is a 9-year-old with severe mental retardation. He is transferred from the state home for children to the hospital for respiratory complications.

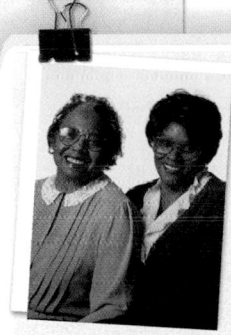

Laura Degas, a 78-year-old woman, has been caring for her sister, Ellen, at home. She says, "She was diagnosed with Alzheimer's disease 2 years ago. This surgery to fix her broken hip has really been tough. I want to take her home, but I'm not sure if I can give her the care that she needs now."

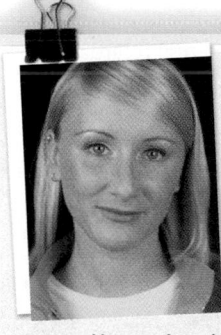

Jennifer Lenner, a 20-year-old woman diagnosed with a seizure disorder, had surgery 3 days ago. She says, "My doctor says that I'm going home today. I can't wait! My parents are coming to pick me up later this morning." Review of her medical record indicates that the attending physician had not written discharge orders.

Focusing on Blended Skills

The types of blended skills you'll need to respond to the case scenarios include:

Cognitive Skills

- Knowledge of mental retardation, Alzheimer's disease, and seizure disorders
- Knowledge of the services and settings available to meet the needs of a patient with profound mental retardation and physical complications, the sister of a woman who has Alzheimer's disease and who has recently undergone repair of a fractured hip, and a young adult with a seizure disorder who has undergone surgery
- Knowledge of measures associated with patient transfer, home care, and discharge planning
- Knowledge of patient needs and the resources available to meet these needs in the patient's home and in different practice settings
- Knowledge of how to communicate effectively patient priorities and the related plan of care as a patient is transferred between different practice settings
- Ability to incorporate knowledge of the healthcare delivery system to meet the needs of patients with different needs, such as a child with mental retardation, an older woman caring for her sister at home, and a young woman at risk for postoperative complications secondary to a seizure disorder

Technical Skills

- Strong assessment skills for children and adults related to mental retardation and physical complications, needs of an older woman caring for her sister at home, and teaching needs for a young woman with a seizure disorder who is at risk for postoperative complications
- Ability to provide the technical nursing assistance necessary to meet the needs of patients across the life span and their families in different practice settings
- Ability to adapt interventions to meet the needs of patients at different developmental stages with multiple needs
- Ability to demonstrate competence in skills, such as communicating with a child who is profoundly mentally retarded, with an older woman who appears overwhelmed with the care needed by her sister, and with a young adult at risk for postoperative complications who is eager to go home

Interpersonal Skills

- Ability to establish trusting professional relationships with patients, family caregivers, and healthcare professionals in different practice settings to ensure continuity of care
- Ability to work with the different resources available to ensure safe, quality care
- Ability to demonstrate respect for a patient's human dignity and autonomy throughout the patient's care
- Special interpersonal competence to interact and collaborate with other healthcare personnel, seeking assistance and information when needed
- Ability to communicate effectively with healthcare team members in other settings to ensure safe, effective continuity of care

Ethical and Legal Skills

- Commitment to preparing patients and their families and professional caregivers to continue the plan of care when a patient is transferred or discharged
- Commitment to securing the best setting for care for patients and the best coordination of resources to support the level of care needed
- Ability to participate as a trusted and effective patient advocate
- Knowledge of the nurse's legal and ethical obligations as patients are transferred between home and different practice settings
- Ability to practice in an ethically and legally defensible manner, including knowledge of the policies of different settings and role responsibilities related to transfers between agencies, referrals to home care, and discharge planning
- Strong sense of accountability for the health and well-being of patients, which translates into a commitment to getting them the help they need within the scope of nursing responsibilities and available resources
- Willingness to hold oneself accountable for safe, high-quality continuity of care
- Ability to work collaboratively with other members of the healthcare team to ensure continuity of care for a child with profound mental retardation experiencing medical complications, an older woman caring for her sister at home, and a young adult woman with a seizure disorder being discharged after surgery

Learning Outcomes

After completing the chapter, the learner should be able to accomplish the following:
1. Describe the role of the nurse in ensuring continuity of care between and among healthcare settings in the community.
2. Discuss considerations for establishing an effective nurse–patient relationship when admitting a patient to a healthcare setting.
3. Compare and contrast admission of a patient to an ambulatory care setting and a hospital setting.
4. Discuss transfer of patients within and among healthcare settings.
5. Explain how nurses use the components of discharge planning to provide continuity of care.

Key Terms

community-based care
continuity of care
discharge planning

People enter healthcare settings and become consumers of healthcare services (patients) for many different reasons. Consider the following examples:

- Joe Sol, aged 5 years, has been having an increasing number of throat infections, and his tonsils are badly infected. Mrs. Sol takes Joe for a checkup at his pediatrician's office. Joe's pediatrician decides that Joe must have a tonsillectomy (removal of tonsils). The procedure will be a same-day surgery at his local hospital; Joe will enter the morning of surgery and go home that afternoon.
- Tom Valiz, aged 28 years, injured his back while working at his construction job. After undergoing diagnostic studies as an outpatient in his local hospital, he has been going to a community health center each day for heat therapy and exercises.
- Sadie Aird, aged 78 years, has had congestive heart failure for the past 10 years. Her daughter, with the help of a home health nurse and aide, cares for her at home.
- Jim Zamba, aged 28 years, suffered severe head injuries in a motorcycle accident. He was admitted to the hospital through the emergency room, sent to surgery, and then admitted to the intensive care unit. After recovery from the acute phase of care, Jim will be transferred to a special rehabilitation center.

Although all of these individuals require care, they do not all have the same kinds of needs, nor are they alike as patients. Some of them will be admitted and discharged on the same day; some of them will remain in the acute care setting only as long as acute care is needed; and some will require long-term care.

Entering and leaving a healthcare setting, as well as receiving care at home, are experiences that produce anxiety for both patients and family members. The nurse is often the person who helps the patient make a smooth transition from one type of care setting to another. (See the accompanying Reflective Practice box for an example.) This chapter discusses continuity of care, community-based nursing practice, admission and discharge from a healthcare setting, transfer from one type of setting to another, and discharge planning in preparation for home healthcare. It focuses on the patient's needs and the nurse's role in providing continuity of care.

ESSENTIAL CONCEPTS

Two concepts essential to nursing care of patients within and across healthcare settings are continuity of care and community-based care. Planning for and providing nursing interventions that promote health, prevent illness, and support coping with disability are critical in today's culturally diverse society. It is no longer enough only to consider the patient's needs within the hospital setting; nurses must also consider how those needs will be met as the patient makes the transition from the acute care setting to care at home with support and services from his or her community.

Consider Laura Degas, the sister of the woman with Alzheimer's disease who had undergone a

hip repair. Due to her sister's increased complexity of care, Ms. Degas is unsure if she can continue to care for her sister at home. The nurse would work with Ms. Degas to determine her needs and possibly enlist the aid of social services for assistance with a referral to home care and appropriate resources and community services.

Continuity of Care

Continuity of care is a process by which healthcare providers give appropriate, uninterrupted care and facilitate the patient's transition between different settings and levels of care. Continuity of care ensures a smooth transition between ambulatory or acute care and home healthcare or other types of healthcare settings in the patient's community. Coordination helps ensure a patient-focused and individualized continuum of healthcare so that the patient may attain maximum recovery and health.

Most people are born in a hospital, thus becoming consumers of healthcare from the first day of life. Over their lifetime, most people continue to require services of some type, in a variety of healthcare settings. Although a patient's healthcare may involve many different providers and settings (discussed in Chap. 8), the nurse is often the primary person responsible for communicating the patient's needs, teaching self-care, and, in many instances, providing care. As a result, one of the primary responsibilities of the nurse as caregiver is ensuring continuity of care.

Continuity of care is essential in the current healthcare system. The emphasis on health promotion and the prevention of illness makes teaching individuals of all ages a crucial component of patient care. To provide continuity of care, nurses must consider teaching and referrals in the care of any person admitted to any type of healthcare setting and must also involve the patient and family in the planning process. The nurse must also collaborate with other members of the healthcare team in meeting the physical, psychological, sociocultural, and spiritual needs of the patient and family in all settings and at all levels of health or illness.

Think back to Jennifer Lenner, the young adult woman with a seizure disorder who had undergone surgery. The nurse would need to collaborate with the attending physician and resident to ensure that all of the patient's needs are addressed. Also, since the patient lives with her parents, the nurse would need to include the parents in any discharge teaching.

Community-Based Care

Community-based care is healthcare provided to people who live within a defined geographic area. That geographic area might be a small neighborhood in a large urban area or a large area of rural residents. Each community is unique and is defined

Reflective Practice
Challenge to Interpersonal Skills

Last week in clinical, I was assigned to care for four patients. Although the care for the patients did not appear to be incredibly complex, this was my first time having four patients at once. Needless to say, I was slightly nervous. In report, I was told that one of the patients, Jennifer Lenner, a 20-year-old woman with a seizure disorder who had had surgery 3 days ago, was going to be discharged sometime today. Therefore, we needed to do discharge planning as well as get her ready to go home. Although the unit nurse was very helpful, she had been feeling sick all morning and at some point needed to go down to Employee Health.

While I was completing my morning assessment of Jennifer, she told me how eager she was to get home. Her parents had been told to come to the hospital sometime in the morning to bring her home. However, when reviewing Jennifer's chart for discharge orders, I noted that no orders had been written. The nurse and I made a call to the resident to ask about Jennifer's status, because she had been told by the attending physician that she was going home today. The resident responded that that was not the case and that she was going to have to wait until tomorrow to go home per the order of the attending physician. The resident reported that they were concerned about postoperative complications. However, the patient was already 3 days postsurgery. In the meantime, the nurse with whom I was working had gone down to Employee Health. The charge nurse as well as my clinical instructor were still with me, but they had not been dealing with the situation the whole morning. So I was left with two options: I could listen to what the resident said and tell the patient that the plans had changed and we were going to continue with her daily care, or I could call the attending and see if that was indeed what he had in mind for Jennifer.

Thinking Outside the Box: Possible Courses of Action

- Simply take what the resident said and continue with Jennifer's care. Although she would be very disappointed, I would just tell her that this is what her doctor wanted and there is nothing I can do.

- Look in the chart for a means of contacting the attending physician and ask him if these were the plans he had in mind for Jennifer.

Evaluating a Good Outcome: How Do I Define Success?

- The patient is first of all healthy enough to be discharged home without fear of any complications.
- The patient's interests are taken into account because she had already been told that she would be going home that day.

- I stand up and advocate for my patient when she cannot do so herself.

Personal Learning: Here's to the Future!

I paged the attending physician with the charge nurse by my side. I was very nervous because I was worried he wasn't going to want to listen to what I, a nursing student, had to say. He called back and I explained the situation to him. He replied that indeed he had intended for Jennifer to go home today, and he even thanked me for calling to check! He sent a resident up to write discharge orders, and we took out her intravenous catheter and reviewed her discharge instructions. Jennifer was happy to go home, and I was comfortable with the fact that she was healthy enough to be sent home.

Reflection

How do you think you would respond in a similar situation? Why? What does this tell you about yourself and about the adequacy of your skills for professional practice? How might the nursing student's patient assignment have affected the actions taken? What questions could the nursing student and/or charge nurse have posed to the resident to determine the resident's knowledge of the situation? Can you think of other ways to respond? What other skills (cognitive, interpersonal, technical, ethical/legal) would you need to respond well in this situation? How did the nursing student ensure continuity of care? Suppose the attending physician had said that the patient's discharge had to wait one more day. How would you respond to the situation and then inform the patient of this decision? Do you agree with the criteria to evaluate a successful outcome? Did the nursing student meet the criteria? Please explain your answer.

Kathryn Southerton, Georgetown University

---

by the people, area, social interactions, and common ties within that community.

In contrast to community health and public health nursing (which are population based and focus on the health of the community), community-based care is centered on individual and family healthcare needs. It emphasizes the provision of comprehensive, coordinated, and continuous services for patients with acute or chronic health problems (Stanhope & Lancaster, 2004). Within a framework of community-based care, nurses help people wherever they are, including where they live, work, play, worship, and go to school.

The nurse practicing community-based care considers the continuity of the care the patient requires when moving from one level or setting of care to another, providing interventions to promote health, manage acute or chronic illnesses, and promote self-care. Community-based care is designed to meet the needs of people as they move into, between, and among different healthcare settings within the overall healthcare system.

ADMISSION TO A HEALTHCARE SETTING

As a result of increasing costs and of healthcare cost reimbursement programs that are prospective more often than retrospective (meaning that costs are often predetermined for specific illnesses or treatments), hospital admissions and lengths of hospital stay have decreased. Increasing numbers of patients are having surgery, diagnostic tests, and emergency care in ambulatory care settings or on an outpatient basis. Even patients who are admitted may stay for less than 24 hours, may be admitted the morning of the surgery, or may go home during an interim period between diagnosis and care.

All people who enter a healthcare setting take on a new role. They must add to their already established roles (e.g., spouse, parent, sibling, student) the role of patient. They also enter an environment in which they are surrounded by strangers and in which they encounter different sounds, sights, and smells.

To meet patients' healthcare needs during the admission process, nurses provide holistic care and establish the basis for how patients will respond to and evaluate the remainder of their stay. Box 9-1 describes guidelines for establishing an effective nurse–patient relationship to ensure that each patient is considered as an individual in any setting.

BOX 9-1 Establishing an Effective Nurse–Patient Relationship on Admission

- Recognize and take steps to reduce the patient's anxiety. Anxiety is a natural reaction to the unknown, but it can be reduced by therapeutic communication, teaching, and acceptance. Some common concerns that cause anxiety are: *Will I have pain? Who will take care of my family if I die? Will strangers be looking at my body? How much will this cost? What if I can't keep my job?*
- Remember that the medical or surgical condition for which the patient is being treated is only one part of the patient's life. Although it may be the primary concern for the patient, other concerns include family needs, financial status, and the future.
- Communicate with the patient as an individual so that he or she can maintain his or her own identity. Ask patients how you should address them—some people prefer Mr., Mrs., Miss, or Ms. [last name]; others would rather be called by their first name. Do not call all older adults "Grandma" or "Grandpa." Do not refer to Mr. Jones, admitted to room 2218 for treatment of a ruptured appendix, as "the appendix in 2218."
- Take time to learn who the patient being admitted is, including his or her cultural and religious background. Respect the patient's values and beliefs even though they may differ from yours.
- Encourage the patient's family to participate in and make decisions about all aspects of care.

During admission, the nurse acts not only as a practitioner but also as an advocate concerned about the welfare of the patient and family. The admission period corresponds to the orientation phase of the helping relationship described in Chapter 21. In addition, regulatory guidelines direct both the continuity and the quality of care. For example, the Joint Commission on Accreditation of Healthcare Organizations has established standards for admission to a hospital. These standards assert that each patient's need for nursing care related to admission should be assessed by a registered nurse; this assessment includes consideration of biophysical, psychosocial, environmental, self-care, educational, and discharge planning factors. In addition, nurses collaborate, as appropriate, with physicians and members of other clinical disciplines to make decisions regarding the patient's need for nursing care.

Remember Jeff Hart, the 9-year-old boy with respiratory complications who is profoundly retarded. The nurse would need to communicate closely with the healthcare team at the state facility to determine the child's plan of care. Also, the nurse would need to perform a complete assessment of the child upon admission to the current facility to determine the child's priority needs.

Admission to an Ambulatory Care Facility

Ambulatory care facilities, described in Chapter 8, are those in which the patient receives healthcare services but does not remain overnight. An individual may receive care in many different kinds of ambulatory facilities, including physician offices, clinics, outpatient services, emergency rooms, and same-day surgery centers. The goal of these facilities is to provide patients who are able to provide self-care at home with assistance as necessary from healthcare providers. Individuals go to ambulatory settings for health promotion, health maintenance, or medical or surgical treatment.

In most office and clinic facilities, patients enter a reception area, where they are asked to complete a short health history unless they have already done so during a previous visit. They then go to an examination room where a physical assessment (often specific to the reason for the visit) is completed. Depending on their needs, patients may be given diagnostic tests, may be immunized, may be prescribed medications, or may undergo minor surgery. All patients require teaching, which should include written instructions about care at home, health promotion activities, and how to contact someone for further questions. Referrals to community agencies, support groups, or other types of healthcare settings might also be necessary.

Admission to ambulatory or same-day surgery facilities is somewhat different. Screening tests, teaching, and admission procedures are usually completed before patients enter the setting. They arrive at the setting, have the procedure, and go home when recovery is satisfactory (see Chap. 30). If patients have outpatient or short-stay surgery in the hospital setting, the regular admission procedures are completed on arrival; in most instances, screening tests and teaching are done before the day of surgery. It is the nurse's responsibility to assess what has been done and tailor the care plan to the patient's needs.

Admission to the Hospital

In most hospitals, admission begins in the admitting office. Staff obtain information about the patient and print that information on an admission sheet. This admission sheet, which includes the information listed in Box 9-2, becomes part of the patient's permanent record.

The identification number, as well as the patient's name and physician's name (and any other information required by the particular institution), is printed on the identification bracelet that is placed on the patient's wrist. This bracelet is an important safety component during the patient's stay because it accurately identifies the individual for procedures and treatments, including medication administration, diagnostic tests, and surgery. The bracelet is worn by all patients but is especially important as a means of identifying patients who are irrational, comatose, or young.

During the initial interview, the nurse provides other information about legal and ethical components of care. The patient is asked to sign forms that give consent to treatment and allow the hospital to contact healthcare insurance companies or public agencies (eg, Medicare) for reimbursement of services. Patients are asked if they have established advance directives, such as a living will or durable power of attorney, to indicate their treatment preferences about prolonging life. If they have, a copy is placed in their hospital record. If they have not, the purpose is explained and they are given a form to complete if they wish to do so. Chapter 33 discusses advance directives and provides a sample form. With the federal mandate to protect patient privacy rights under the 1996 Health Insurance Portability and Accountability Act (HIPAA), providers must give patients a clear written explanation of how health infor-

mation will be used and disclosed (Chap. 7 discusses the privacy of information). Patients may also be asked to provide the names of family or friends to whom health status information may be given. Lastly, almost all hospitals have some form of a Patient Bill of Rights that is given to the patient. Discussed further in Chapter 6, this document includes rights to obtain information about one's illness or injury, to refuse medication or treatment, to receive considerate and respectful care, to have every consideration of privacy, and to expect reasonable continuity of care when appropriate (American Hospital Association, 1992).

After the necessary forms have been completed in the admitting office, a nurse who works in that area might complete the admission health history and physical assessment, or patients may also be taken to an assigned unit for these admission procedures. Laboratory studies and x-rays, as well as the admitting office procedures, are usually completed on an outpatient basis before or on the day of admission. If the patient has an unscheduled admission or is going to have only a limited stay (eg, those who are admitted the morning of a diagnostic examination and then go home later in the day), admission procedures and assessments may be completed on the unit.

Preparing the Room for Admission

The admitting office notifies the unit to which the patient is to be admitted before the patient arrives so that the room can be prepared. Although the nurse might delegate most of the activities in preparing the room for an admission, it is a nursing responsibility to ensure that other personnel do them. Guidelines for Nursing Care 9-1 outlines the activities carried out in anticipation of the patient's arrival (Fig. 9-1).

Welcoming the Patient to the Unit

Although other members of the healthcare team may assist in the admitting procedure, the nurse is responsible for ensuring the comfort and well-being of the patient upon arrival in the unit. The nurse completes the admission assessment and documents the information on the admission database (Fig. 9-2). The sample form in Figure 9-3 illustrates typical information that is collected and documented. The information on the form is used to develop the nursing care plan for the patient and also is used as a database for discharge planning and home care. In addition, an inventory of personal belongings is often completed to ensure these are returned to the patient on discharge or transferred with the patient if he or she moves to another unit or facility.

The patient should be welcomed to the unit in the same courteous manner that would be used in welcoming a guest into one's own home. In most instances, the patient is accompanied by family members who may either remain with the patient to provide support and information or who may be asked to wait in the waiting room during the admission procedure. The nurse needs to assess the needs of the patient and family, and they should mutually agree about whether family should be present during admission.

BOX 9-2 Information Collected During Admission to a Hospital

Full name
Address
Date of birth
Name of admitting physician
Gender
Marital status
Nearest relative
Occupation and employer
Financial status for healthcare payment
Religious preference
Date and time of admission
Identification number
Admitting diagnosis

TRANSFERRING WITHIN AND BETWEEN HEALTHCARE SETTINGS

It is common for some type of move to be made within settings as well as between settings. Examples of transferring within and between settings include the following:

- Patients often are moved within the hospital, such as from the emergency room to a hospital room, from an intensive care unit (ICU) to a hospital room (and vice versa), from one floor to another, or from one room to another room on the same floor.
- Patients are transferred to and from acute care settings and long-term settings.
- Patients are transferred from acute care settings to their homes.
- Patients are transferred from ambulatory care settings to acute care settings.

When a transfer occurs, the patient must readjust to new surroundings, new roommates, new routines, and new people providing care. If the transfer is to a higher level of care, as in a move to the ICU, the patient experiences unfamiliar sights and sounds. A transfer to a long-term facility may not be desired by the patient or family but may be necessary if family members cannot provide care at home or if no other support people are available. All of these factors cause stress and anxiety.

> *Recall Laura Degas, the woman who is not sure if she will be able to care for her sister at home. If it is determined that Ms. Degas cannot care for her sister at home, she may decide to have her sister transferred to a long-term care facility. In this case, the nurse must provide Ms. Degas with support and guidance to ease the transition and help minimize the stress and anxiety of this move.*

The nurse may not be responsible for the actual physical move but is responsible for ensuring that the comfort, safety, and teaching needs of the patient and family are met. Although documentation and procedures differ depending on the institution and type of transfer, patient needs are always a priority in ensuring a smooth transition and continuity of care.

Transfer Within the Hospital

When a patient is transferred within the hospital, his or her personal belongings must be moved and put in the new room.

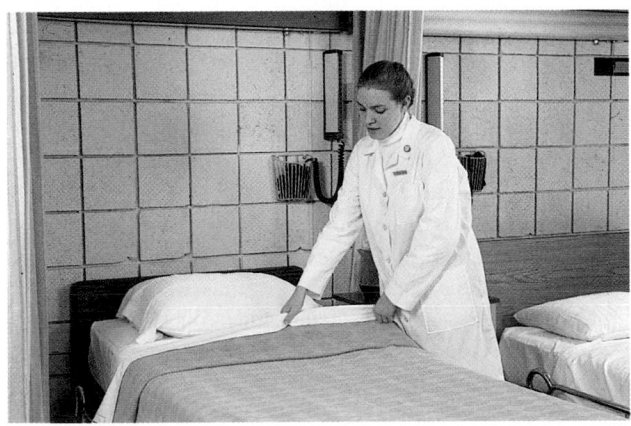
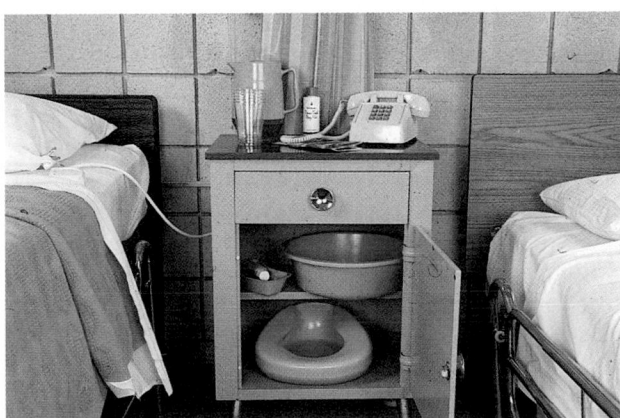

FIGURE 9-1 In anticipation of the patient's arrival on the hospital unit, the bed should be opened and positioned correctly, and necessary supplies and equipment should be available.

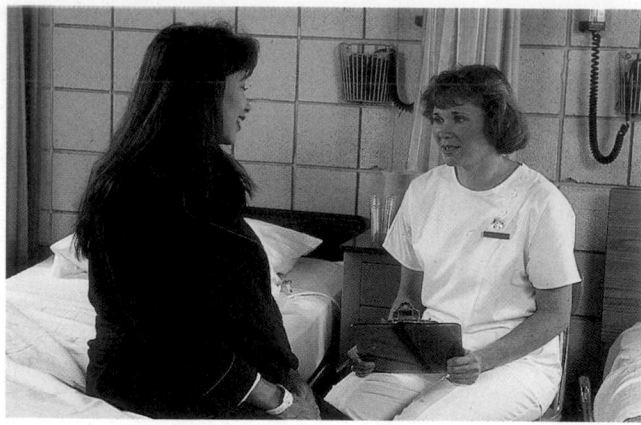

FIGURE 9-2 When a patient is admitted to a healthcare setting, the nurse is responsible for collecting information to complete the health history.

Every effort must be made to ensure that belongings are not misplaced or lost. The patient's chart, Kardex, care plan, and medications must be correctly labeled for the new room, and other hospital departments (eg, dietary, pharmacy, or physical therapy) must be notified. If the patient is moved to the ICU, family members may need to take personal belongings and flowers home.

When a patient is transferred to another unit, the nurse in the original area gives a verbal report about the patient to the nurse in the new area. The report should include the patient's name, age, physicians, admitting diagnosis, surgical procedure (if applicable), current condition and manifestations, allergies, medications and treatments, laboratory data, and any special equipment that will be needed to provide care. Nursing care priorities are identified, and the existence of advance directives is noted. Accurate, concise, and complete verbal communication is essential.

Transfer to a Long-Term Care Facility

When a patient is transferred from the hospital to a long-term care facility, he or she is discharged from the hospital setting but a copy of the chart may be sent to the long-term care facility (depending on the physician's preference and the agency's protocol). The original chart, which is a legal document, remains at the hospital. All of the patient's belongings are carefully packed and sent to the facility with the patient. Prescriptions and appointment cards for return visits to the physician's office may also be sent with the patient.

In most instances, a detailed assessment and care plan is sent from the hospital to the long-term care facility. In addition, the nurse at the hospital often provides a verbal report to the nurse at the long-term care facility.

Remember Jeff Hart, the 9-year-old boy transferred from the state facility to the hospital due to respiratory complications. Once the child's problems have been resolved, the nurse would prepare Jeff to be transferred back to the state facility. Information about the events of the hospitalization would be recorded and reported. In addition, communication between healthcare team members at the hospital and those at the state facility is essential to ensure continuity of care for Jeff.

DISCHARGE FROM A HEALTHCARE SETTING

In meeting the needs of the patient being discharged from a healthcare setting, nurses consider that the person may be expecting a change from a dependent role to a more independent (self-care) role. Patients are discharged from a healthcare facility when the expected outcomes of care are met and the patient or caregiver has the necessary knowledge and skills to provide care. Although discharge is almost always a welcome event, it also can be stressful.

Discharge Planning

The purpose of planning for continuity of care, which is more commonly referred to in hospital-based settings as **discharge planning,** is to ensure that patient and family needs are consistently met as the patient moves from the acute care setting to care at home. Essential components of discharge planning include assessing the strengths and limitations of the patient, the family or support person, and the environment; implementing and coordinating the plan of care; considering individual, family, and community resources; and evaluating the effectiveness of care.

Planning for discharge actually begins on admission, when information about the patient is collected and documented. The key to successful discharge planning is an exchange of information among the patient, the caregivers, and those responsible for care, while the patient is in the acute care setting and after the patient returns home. This coordination of care is usually the nurse's responsibility.

With earlier hospital discharges, patients often are still acutely ill when they go home, and many require complicated treatment and care by family members. It is no longer unusual for family members to change sterile dressings, monitor intravenous medications, manage high-technology equipment, give complete physical care, and prepare special diets. If they are unprepared or unable to carry out these interventions correctly, the patient may have an exacerbation of the illness or experience complications that could require readmission or additional treatment. The nurse must ensure that family members are taught the necessary knowledge and skills (Fig. 9-4) and that referrals are made to agencies such as home healthcare or social services to provide support and assistance during the recovery period. (Home care is discussed in Chap. 10.)

Initiating the process involves identifying which patients will need which level of discharge planning. All patients need

Admission Database

NURSING ADMISSION DATA

CURRENT MEDICATIONS, SUPPLEMENTS, NON-PRESCRIPTION DRUGS:

NAME	DOSE/FREQUENCY	LAST DOSE
Aspirin	2 prn	1 month
Maalox	prn	this Am

☐ MEDICATION TO PHARMACY ☐ MEDICATION SENT HOME

ALLERGEN: (DRUGS, FOOD, TAPES, DYES, OTHERS)

ALLERGEN	SYMPTOMS
Penicillin	rash

DATE __1-16-04__ TIME __0900__

ADMISSION   ☐ **OBSERVATION**

☒ AMBULATORY ☐ WHEELCHAIR ☐ STRETCHER
☐ CORRECT INDENTIFICATION BAND
ADMITTED FROM: ☒ HOME ☐ NURSING FACILITY
☐ EMERGENCY ROOM ☐ OTHER_____
INFORMATION GIVEN BY: ☐ FAMILY MEMBER ☐ FRIEND ☒ PATIENT
☐ UNABLE TO TAKE HISTORY - PATIENT UNRESPONSIVE/CONFUSED
NOT ACCOMPANIED BY FAMILY OR FRIEND
☐ PREVIOUS MEDICAL RECORD

ORIENTATION TO ROOM
☒ VISITING HOURS ☒ CALL LIGHT IN REACH: ☒ EXPLAINED
☒ OPERATION OF BED AND SIDE RAILS ☒ USE OF PHONE
☒ VALUABLES SENT HOME ☐ IN SAFE ☐ IN POSSESSION
SPECIFY _____
☒ PATIENT HANDBOOK   ☒ INTRODUCED TO ROOMMATE

MEDICAL HISTORY
ADMITTED MEDICAL DIAGNOSIS __Peptic Ulcer__

PAST HOSPITALIZATIONS AND/OR ILLNESS: (MEDICAL, SURGICAL, EMOTIONAL PROBLEMS) __1999 - Appendectomy__

WHAT IS REASON FOR ADMISSION? (PATIENT'S OWN WORDS)_____
"My doctor says I have An ulcer"

LEGAL GUARDIAN (NAME/PHONE)_____
CONTACT PERSON (NAME/PHONE)__Mrs. Dolle, 335-4001__
PHYSICIAN NOTIFIED __✓__ TIME __0830__
PRIMARY CARE PHYSICIAN __Dr. Wills__

*OBJECTIVE DATA:
1. CLINICAL DATA
AGE __36__ HEIGHT __5'6"__
WEIGHT __122__ ☒ BEDSCALE ☐ STANDING APPROXIMATE__
TEMP: __98.4__ PULSE: __118__ RESPIRATIONS __16__
BLOOD PRESSURE (RIGHT ARM) __120/68__ (LEFT ARM) __122/70__
☒ SITTING ☐ LYING
N.T./N.A. INITIALS __O.B.__

2. NUTRITIONAL/METABOLIC PATTERN
ORAL MUCOSA: ☒ HEALTHY COLOR_____
☐ MOIST ☐ DRY ☐ LESIONS_____
TEETH: ☒ NO PROBLEM CONDITION:_____
☐ DENTURES ☐ UPPER ☐ LOWER ☐ PARTIAL
☐ MISSING TEETH ☐ CAPS/CROWNS
☒ WELL NOURISHED ☐ OBESE ☐ EMACIATED
SKIN: ☒ TURGOR NORMAL ☐ OTHER_____
☒ INTACT ☐ OTHER_____
TEMP __Warm__ COLOR __brown__ ☐ DIAPHORESIS
☐ TUBES_____

3. RESPIRATION/CIRCULATION PATTERN
BREATH SOUNDS __Clear__
LIP COLOR __Pink__ ☐ USE OF ACCESSORY MUSCLES
COUGH: ☐ NON-PRODUCTIVE ☐ PRODUCTIVE SPUTUM COLOR_____
APICAL RATE __120__ RHYTHM: ☒ REGULAR ☐ IRREGULAR
ABNORMAL HEART SOUNDS NOTED __No__
NECK VEIN DISTENTION AT 45 DEGREES: ☐ PRESENT ☒ ABSENT
☐ EDEMA: LOCATION_____
RIGHT DORSALIS PEDAL PULSE: ☒ STRONG ☐ WEAK ☐ ABSENT
LEFT DORSALIS PEDAL PULSE: ☒ STRONG ☐ WEAK ☐ ABSENT
CALF TENDERNESS ☒ NO ☐ YES ☐ N/A
EXTREMITIES COLOR __brown__
TEMP __Warm__

4. ELIMINATION PATTERN
ABDOMEN: ☒ SOFT   ☐ FIRM
☐ NON-TENDER   ☐ TENDER
☐ NON-DISTENDED ☐ DISTENDED _____Girth
☐ OSTOMIES/TUBES: TYPE_____
☐ NORMAL BOWEL SOUNDS ☐ HYPOACTIVE ☒ HYPERACTIVE ☐ ABSENT

*SUBJECTIVE DATA:
1. HEALTH PERCEPTIONS/HEALTH MANAGEMENT PATTERN
GENERAL HEALTH __Excellent__
USE OF: ☐ TOBACCO: HOW MUCH/HOW LONG? __No__
☐ ALCOHOL: HOW MUCH/HOW LONG? __No__
☐ OTHER DRUGS TYPE(s) __None__

2. NUTRITIONAL/METABOLIC PATTERN
DIET/RESTRICTIONS/SUPPLEMENTS: __Regular diet__

☐ INSTRUCTED IN DIET PREVIOUSLY BY:_____
TIME OF LAST P.O. INTAKE: __0700__
FLUID INTAKE (AMOUNT/DAY) __5-6 glasses__
WEIGHT: ☐ NO PROBLEMS_____
☐ GAIN_____ ☒ LOSS/HOW MUCH/HOW LONG __10 lbs / 1 month__
☒ SKIN NORMAL ☐ HEALING PROBLEMS
☐ COLOR CHANGE OF SKIN
☐ SKIN LESIONS/RASH

3. RESPIRATION/CIRCULATION PATTERN
HISTORY OF: ☐ COUGH ☐ SPUTUM_____
☐ SHORTNESS OF BREATH ☐ WITHOUT EXERCISE ☐ WITH EXERCISE

HISTORY OF: ☐ PACEMAKER ☐ RATE_____
☐ BLOOD CLOTS ☐ CHEST PAIN ☐ PEDAL EDEMA

☒ CHECK BOX IF DATA IS PERTINENT
*SEE NURSES NOTES FOR FURTHER NOTATIONS OR ANY CHANGES.

(Courtesy of Southeast Missouri Hospital, Cape Girardeau, Missouri.)

FIGURE 9-3 Admission database sample. (*continued*)

Admission Database   *(continued)*

*SUBJECTIVE DATA (Cont'd) LBM_____

4. ELIMINATION PATTERN
BOWEL HABITS: STOOLS/DAY __2__ COLOR _dk. brown_ ☒ SOFT/FORMED
      ☐ CONSTIPATION: ☐ LAXATIVE ☐ ENEMA
      ☐ DIARRHEA   ☐ INCONTINENCE
BLADDER HABITS: URINATES/DAY _5-6_ ☒NO PROBLEM ☐ SELF-CATH
      ☐ URGENCY . FREQUENCY ☐ NOCTURIA
      ☐ DYSURIA . HEMATURIA ☐ INCONTINENCE

5. SEXUALITY/REPRODUCTIVE PATTERN (IF APPROPRIATE)
LAST MENSTRUAL PERIOD _1-10-04_ MENSTRUAL PROBLEMS ☐ YES ☒ NO
BIRTH CONTROL MEASURES _None_ # PREGNANCIES _2_
COMPLICATIONS OF PREGNANCIES _None_
HX VENEREAL DISEASE _No_
SEXUAL CONCERNS: _None_

6. ACTIVITY/EXERCISE PATTERN
ENERGY LEVEL: ☐ TIRES EASILY ☐ AVERAGE ☒ HIGH/ENERGY
ABLE TO: ☒ FEED SELF ☒ BATHE SELF
    ☐ BATHE/FEED SELF WITH ASSISTANCE
    ☒ AMBULATE ☒ CLIMB STAIRS
    ☒ CAN DO HOUSEHOLD CHORES
AIDS: ☐ CANE ☐ WALKER ☐ WHEELCHAIR ☐ OTHER _____
GAIT: ☐ STEADY ☐ UNSTEADY ☐ LIMP ☐ UNABLE TO WALK
PROTHESIS_____

7. SLEEP/REST PATTERN
DO YOU FEEL RESTED AFTER SLEEP? ☒ YES ☐ NO ☐ NO PROBLEM
SLEEP PROBLEMS: ☐ TROUBLE FALLING ASLEEP ☐ EARLY AM WAKING
    ☐ OTHER_____

8. COGNITIVE/PERCEPTUAL PATTERN
HEARING: ☒ NORMAL ☐ IMPAIRED: ☐ LEFT EAR ☐ RIGHT EAR ☐ AID
VISION: ☐ NORMAL ☐ IMPAIRED ☒ GLASSES ☐ PROTHESIS
    ☐ FARSIGHTED ☐ NEARSIGHTED
OTHER PROBLEMS_____
COMMUNICATION: LANGUAGE SPOKEN _English_
UNDERSTANDS_____ UNABLE TO: ☐ READ ☐ WRITE
ABLE TO: ☒ READ ☒ WRITE ☐ LIP READ
COGNITION: ☒ NO PROBLEMS ☐ RECENT MEMORY CHANGE
    ☐ DIFFICULTY LEARNING
DISCOMFORT/PAIN: ☐ NO ☒ YES DESCRIBE _Epigastric_
HOW DO YOU MANAGE YOUR PAIN? _Bland food, Maalox_

9. COPING/STRESS TOLERANCE PATTERN
SPECIAL CONCERNS REGARDING HOSPITALIZATION? ☐ NO ☒ YES
Care of Children

10. SELF-PERCEPTION/SELF-CONCEPT PATTERN
CONCERNS ABOUT HOW YOUR ILLNESS AFFECTS YOU? ☐ NO ☒ YES
Concerned about health

11. ROLE/RELATIONSHIP PATTERN
MARITAL STATUS: ☐ MARRIED ☐ SINGLE ☐ WIDOWED ☒ DIVORCED
CHILDREN (#) _2_ OTHER DEPENDENT(S) _0_
OCCUPATION _Secretary_
RESIDENCY (TYPE) _apartment_
WHO LIVES AT HOME WITH YOU? _Children_
SUPPORT SYSTEM (CLOSE FRIEND/FAMILY MEMBER) _Yes_
FAMILY CONCERNS ABOUT HOSPITALIZATION? _Yes_

12. VALUE/BELIEF PATTERN
RELIGIOUS AFFILIATION _Baptist_
RELIGIOUS RESTRICTIONS _0_
☐ WOULD LIKE CHAPLAIN TO VISIT (IF YES, NOTIFY CHAPLAIN)

☒ WOULD LIKE FAMILY MINISTER TO VISIT
NAME _Mr. Ame_ PHONE _314-6000_
RELIGIOUS ACTIVITIES IMPORTANT TO YOU _Bible_
SUBJECTIVE DATA SIGNATURE _P. LeMone, RN_ (Nurse)

6. ACTIVITY/EXERCISE PATTERN
ROM: ☒ FULL ☐ OTHER_____
BALANCE AND GAIT: ☒ STEADY ☐ UNSTEADY ☐ LIMP_____
HAND GRASPS: ☒ EQUAL ☒ STRONG
    ☐ WEAKNESS/PARALYSIS ☐ RIGHT ☐ LEFT
LEG MUSCLES: ☒ EQUAL ☒ STRONG
    WEAKNESS/PARALYSIS ☐ RIGHT ☐ LEFT

8. COGNITIVE/PERCEPTUAL PATTERN
LEVEL OF CONSCIOUSNESS: ☒ ALERT ☒ RESPONDS TO PAIN
ORIENTED TO: ☒ TIME ☒ PLACE ☒ PERSON
MOOD: ☒ CALM ☐ SAD ☐ ANGRY
    ☐ WITHDRAWN ☐ OTHER_____
PUPILS: ☒ EQUAL ☒ REACTIVE ☐ OTHER_____
COGNITION: ☒ ABLE TO FOLLOW SIMPLE COMMANDS
    ☒ RESPONDS APPROPRIATELY TO QUESTIONS
    ☐ UNABLE TO FOLLOW COMMANDS
    ☐ OTHER_____
HEARING: ☒ NORMAL ☐ OTHER_____
VISION: ☒ NORMAL ☐ OTHER_____
MANIFESTATIONS OF PAIN_____

10. SELF-PERCEPTION/SELF-CONCEPT PATTERN
EYE CONTACT: ☒ APPROPRIATE ☐ DOWNCAST ☐ STARING
BODY POSTURE: ☒ RELAXED ☐ STOOPED ☐ RIGID
BEHAVIOR: 1   ②   3   4   5 (CIRCLE)
    RELAXED   NERVOUS
OTHER_____

11. ROLE/RELATIONSHIP PATTERN
BEHAVIOR: ①   2   3   4   5 (CIRCLE)
    PASSIVE   ASSERTIVE   AGGRESSIVE
INTERACTION WITH FAMILY/SIGNIFICANT OTHER: ☐ N/A
☒ RELAXED ☐ TENSE ☐ ANGRY ☐ WITHDRAWN ☐ OTHER_____

COMMENTS: _____

Worried about effect of illness and possible surgery on care of children, job, and income. Has strong support of family.

SIGNATURE _P. LeMone, RN_ (Nurse)

FIGURE 9-3 Continued

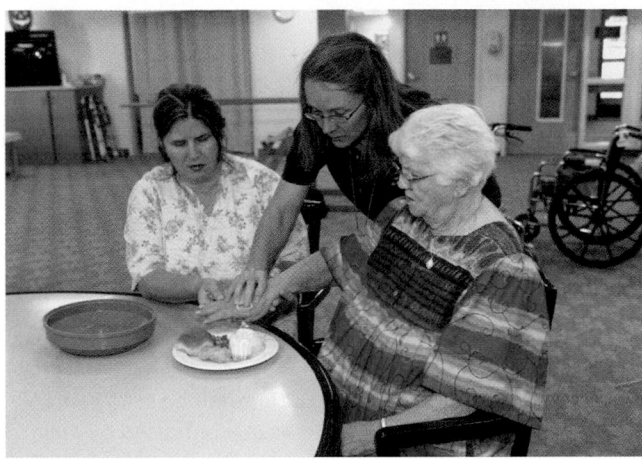

FIGURE 9-4 Patients or caregivers must be taught special skills, such as medication administration, diet planning, or feeding, so that they can care for themselves when nursing services are no longer provided. (Photo by Rick Brady.)

discharge planning in general, but certain patients have more comprehensive needs for specific services. The nurse who conducts the initial nursing assessment is in the best position to determine these special needs.

> *Recall Jennifer Lenner, the young woman with a seizure disorder at risk for postoperative complications. Information about Jennifer's underlying neurologic problem would have been obtained when Jennifer was admitted. From that information, the nurse would develop a discharge plan that addresses the patient's specific postoperative risks. Since Jennifer lives with her parents, a referral for home care may or may not be appropriate, depending on further assessment of Jennifer's parents and the home situation.*

Patients who meet any of the following criteria need a formal discharge plan and referral to another agency:

- Lack of knowledge of the treatment plan
- Social isolation
- Recently diagnosed chronic disease
- Major surgery
- Prolonged recuperation from major surgery or illness
- Emotional or mental instability
- Complex home care regimen
- Financial difficulties
- Lack of available or appropriate referral sources
- Terminal illness

Guidelines for Discharge Planning

For a patient hospitalized with a serious illness or injury, discharge planning may be done over time; for a patient treated in an ambulatory facility, it may be completed relatively quickly. A nursing case manager or discharge planner is often responsible for discharge planning for patients in acute care settings and may follow a plan of care or a critical path established for the patient. No matter what organizing plan is used, the nurse assesses the patient's needs and identifies problems, develops goals with the patient, carries out teaching, and makes referrals. An example of discharge planning is provided in Box 9-3.

Assessing and Identifying Healthcare Needs

The first step in discharge planning involves collecting and organizing data about the patient. (Assessment and interviewing are covered in detail in Chaps. 25 and 12, respectively.) When assessing the patient for discharge, the nurse includes the family because both the patient and family must be actively involved if the transition from the healthcare setting to home is to be effective. Factors to assess in discharge planning are listed in the accompanying Focused Assessment Guide 9-1. Other assessment formats may be used, depending on institutional procedures, to evaluate the patient's ability to carry out activities of daily living (bathing, dressing, toileting, transferring, continence, and feeding) and instrumental activities of daily living (using the telephone, shopping, preparing food, doing housekeeping and laundry, taking medications, accessing transportation). The medical record and physician orders must also be consulted for the exact medication and treatment plan before the nursing care plan is developed.

Nursing diagnoses, developed from the discharge planning assessment, identify the needs of both the patient and the family. Examples of nursing diagnoses for a patient being discharged are listed in the Examples of NANDA Nursing Diagnoses box. It is important to determine whether problems are present now or are potential problems. For example, a patient with chronic respiratory problems may have assistance from a member of the family who has come to stay for 1 month, but after that the patient will be alone at home. In this case, the problem is not an actual problem now but could become one unless planning is done to meet needs when there is no longer a family caregiver.

Setting Goals With the Patient

The expected goals of the discharge plan are set mutually and must be realistic if they are to be met. If the patient is involved in establishing goals, it is more likely that the expected outcomes of the plan of care will be met. The patient may fail to follow the plan if the goals that are not mutually agreed on or are not based on a complete assessment of the patient's needs. For example, the nurse or another healthcare provider may do a thorough job of teaching a patient about a special diet, but the patient may not actually follow the diet after discharge because he may not be able to afford the special food, he may not be able to get to the grocery store, or he may not have a refrigerator at home for food storage.

Teaching

Important teaching topics about self-care at home must be covered before discharge. These topics include medications, procedures and treatments, diet, referrals, and health status.

The patient needs to understand the drug name, dosage, purpose, effects, times to be taken, and possible side effects. Information about medications should be given both verbally

BOX 9-3 **A Discharge Planning Example**

Mr. Smith is a 55-year-old married man, admitted to the hospital with a diagnosis of stroke. He now has left-side weakness and difficulty communicating verbally. He has had a history of high blood pressure for 10 years. If his blood pressure remains stable, Mr. Smith is to be discharged from the hospital in 3 days. He will be going home with four new medications and an indwelling urinary catheter. A low-sodium diet is prescribed.

After reviewing the medical record, the nurse interviews Mr. and Mrs. Smith. The assessment reveals that Mr. Smith has a limited ability to transfer from bed to chair. Both Mr. and Mrs. Smith are fearful of discharge. Mr. Smith believes he will be able to return to work as an accountant in 3 weeks and hates the thought of being an invalid at his age, but Mrs. Smith thinks he will never work again. They have never faced a life-threatening or disabling illness in the past. They have no strong cultural preferences for diet. They have two adult children who live out of state with their own families. Mrs. Smith has a younger sister who lives nearby. They are both college educated. The Smiths live in a suburban area in a two-story home with narrow stairs leading to the second floor's two baths and three bedrooms. They have adequate plumbing. Their doctor's office is about 1 mile away, and shopping is nearby.

Mrs. Smith is worried about managing care of the catheter and moving Mr. Smith in and out of bed. She needs instruction in the new medications and diet regimen. She is terrified that she may be unable to handle an emergency in the middle of the night. Financially, this two-income family has abruptly become a one-income family. Mr. Smith is not 65 years old and thus is not yet eligible for Medicare, although he does have disability insurance that will cover a portion of his salary.

Planning

How would the nurse coordinate this discharge plan? The physician must be consulted for diet, medication, other treatments, and home health orders. The dietitian needs to counsel the Smiths on a low-sodium diet and on creative ways to prepare low-salt meals. Physical therapy has already been initiated at the hospital and will continue through home healthcare. An occupational therapist will visit to provide teaching about strengthening exercises and assistive devices, such as a walker. The social worker has been called for financial assessment to determine exactly what services the Smiths can expect to have reimbursed by their insurance plan and how they will manage their out-of-pocket expenses.

The nurse discusses Mr. and Mrs. Smith's healthcare needs with the home health agency. A teaching plan for medications and care of the urinary catheter is implemented. Mrs. Smith demonstrates how to care for the catheter. The physical therapist teaches Mrs. Smith how to transfer Mr. Smith into and out of the bed and assures her that he will help her practice at home. Written information about high blood pressure, stroke, low-sodium diet, and prescribed medications is given to the Smiths, along with the telephone number of a local support group for people who have had strokes. Although Mrs. Smith still verbalizes concern about providing care at home, she says she feels more in control now. Mr. Smith is beginning to realize that recovery may take longer than he anticipated. At the time of discharge, the nurse tells the Smiths that someone from the hospital will call them the next day and that the home health nurse will visit them that afternoon.

and in writing. Patients often find it helpful when the nurse draws a clock face and write the names of the medications in the correct time slots.

All steps of a procedure (eg, dressing changes) should be demonstrated, practiced, and provided in writing. The patient or caregiver should then perform the procedure or treatment in the presence of the nurse to demonstrate his or her understanding. The caregiver should know the purpose of what is being done and how to get supplies.

The purpose of the diet and its expected outcomes should be clearly described. Patients find examples of written diet plans and meals helpful. If the patient has been in the hospital, it also is helpful to save menu or meal forms to use as a reference at home.

Appointments for the first visit to a physician or agency are often made before discharge. Whether or not this is done, the patient and family members should know how to contact the providers of follow-up care and should know whom to call if they have questions or problems. This referral information takes into account the patient's economic situation, access to transportation, support systems, and home environment.

All aspects of the illness or effects of treatment should be clearly described, both verbally and in written materials. Many forms of written information are available to give to patients,

ranging from printed literature (eg, from the American Heart Association) to teaching materials developed by the healthcare facility. Written instructions are given to the patient (Fig. 9-5). The patient should be able to talk about the anticipated physical and emotional effects of the illness and also describe what will be done to achieve the highest level of health possible. All teaching should be documented in the patient's record and the discharge summary. The patient's or family member's demonstrations of care procedures must be satisfactory, and the patient and caregiver must have exposure to and practice with the equipment they will be using at home.

Think back to Jennifer Lenner, the young woman who is to be discharged after surgery. The nurse would include teaching about any antiseizure medications ordered, wound care or dressing changes needed secondary to the surgery, diet and activity level allowed and restricted, and follow-up with the surgeon and her regular physician.

Providing Home Healthcare Referrals

For home healthcare visits to be reimbursed, the physician must write an order for all services and the patient must meet the eligibility criteria. As much information as possible

Focused Assessment Guide 9-1

Discharge Planning

Factors to Assess	Questions and Approaches
Health data	Establish a database that includes age, gender, height and weight, medical diagnoses, past medical history, current health problems, surgery, functional limitations (eg, impaired sight or hearing, amputation, use of wheelchair or walker).
Personal data	Ask the patient: *"What language do you prefer to use?"* *"How do you feel about being discharged?"* *"What are your expectations for recovery?"* *"What do you do to help you cope with stress? Are these things helpful?"*
Caregivers	Establish the caregiver's age, gender, relationship to the patient, past experiences with this illness or treatment, values and beliefs, and cultural practices that might affect prescribed care. Ask the caregiver: *"Do you live with the patient?"* *"What are your expectations about providing care at home?"* *"What are your fears about providing care at home?"*
Environment	Assess the home, noting if there will be barriers to using prescribed assistive devices (eg, wheelchairs or walkers), if the patient will be able to use bathroom facilities safely, and if hot water, heat, and room for supplies are available. Assess the community, noting location (such as rural or urban), whether healthcare is available and accessible, whether transportation is available, and any known environmental hazards.
Financial and support resources	Discuss expenses of prescribed care, including dressing supplies, medications, equipment, and special foods. Discuss available resources, including Medicare and Medicaid, parish nursing, and meal services to the home. Discuss, especially if the patient will be living alone, support services and resources and how they can be accessed. Include friends, church groups, and support groups specific to the patient's age and healthcare needs.

Examples of NANDA Nursing Diagnoses | Discharge from a Healthcare Setting

Nursing Diagnoses	Related Factors
Anxiety	Concern about uncertain future following radiation treatment for breast cancer
Risk for Caregiver Role Strain	Care of 75-year-old wife with dementia from Alzheimer's disease
Readiness for Enhanced Coping	Attendance at support group meetings and verbally defining stressors as manageable
Delayed Surgical Recovery	Infection of large abdominal wound and needed help to complete self-care
Readiness for Enhanced Therapeutic Regimen Management	Demonstrates accurate dressing change and verbalizes confidence in managing recovery and preventing complications

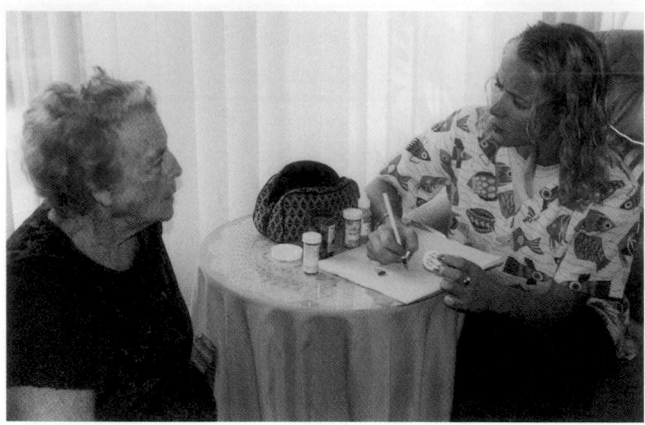

FIGURE 9-5 Written instructions for continuing self-care at home should be given to the patient. In addition, the nurse reviews the instructions with the patient to ensure that the patient understands. (Smeltzer, S. C., & Bare, B. G. [2004]. *Brunner & Suddarth's textbook of medical-surgical nursing* [10th ed., p. 47]. Philadelphia: Lippincott Williams & Wilkins.)

about the patient should be given to the home health agency. Such information includes the kind of surgery or injury, medications, the patient's physical and mental status, significant social factors (eg, frail caregiver with health problems, or no caregiver), and the family's expected needs.

Evaluating Discharge Planning Effectiveness

Evaluating the discharge plan is crucial to ensure that the discharge planning works. Planning and referrals must be scrutinized to ensure the quality and appropriateness of services. Evaluation is ongoing, and care plans may need to be changed. Further evaluation of the discharge process is usually conducted a few weeks after the patient goes home. It may be carried out by way of a telephone call, a questionnaire, or a home visit.

Leaving the Hospital Against Medical Advice

A patient sometimes decides to leave the hospital against medical advice (AMA). Although the patient is legally free to do so, this choice carries a risk for increased illness or complications. A patient who decides to leave AMA must sign a form that releases the physician and healthcare institution from any legal responsibility for his or her health status. The patient is informed of any possible risk before signing the form. The patient's signature must be witnessed, and the form becomes part of the patient's record.

■ Developing Critical Thinking Skills

1. Interview a classmate or family member who has been admitted to a hospital. What were his or her concerns on admission? How did those concerns differ from those experienced on discharge?

2. Compare and contrast the needs of the following patients and their families:
   - A 2-year-old who is admitted to an ambulatory surgery center for minor surgery
   - A 34-year-old woman who is discharged home after treatment for a fractured arm in the emergency room
   - A 50-year-old woman who is returning to a clinic to learn the results of her mammogram
   - A 78-year-old man who is being transferred from the hospital to a nursing home

■ Practicing for NCLEX

1. Jane Wye, RN, is the discharge planner at a large metropolitan hospital. What activity would she do to ensure continuity of care as patients move from acute care to home care?
   a. Perform an admission health assessment
   b. Participate in the transfer of patients to the ICU
   c. Make referrals to appropriate agencies
   d. Maintain records of patient satisfaction with services

2. Which of the following phrases best describes the philosophy of community-based care?
   a. It considers the healthcare needs of the community as a whole.
   b. It centers on individuals and families with acute and chronic illness needs.
   c. It has a population-based focus, with an emphasis on illness prevention.
   d. It provides direction for the roles of the nurse in the acute care setting.

3. When admitting a patient to the hospital, the nurse may delegate some activities to other members of the healthcare team. Which activity would be appropriate to delegate?
   a. Collecting information for a health history
   b. Performing a physical assessment
   c. Contacting the physician for medical orders
   d. Preparing the bed and collecting needed supplies

4. Based on the Health Insurance Portability and Accountability Act (HIPAA), a patient admitted to a healthcare facility must be provided with a written explanation of:
   a. The names and addresses of responsible providers
   b. The Patient's Bill of Rights
   c. How health information will be used and disclosed
   d. How often family members or friends may visit or call

5. A patient is being transferred from the ICU to a regular hospital room. As the ICU nurse, what must you be prepared to do as part of this transfer?
   a. Provide a verbal report to the nurse on the new unit

b. Provide a detailed written report to the unit secretary
c. Delegate the responsibility for providing information
d. Make a copy of the patient's medical record

6. At what point during a hospital stay should discharge planning be initiated?
   a. After surgery and successful recovery
   b. After the patient is less anxious
   c. Immediately before discharge
   d. On admission to the acute care setting

7. Which of the following statements or questions would be appropriate in establishing a discharge plan for a patient who has had major abdominal surgery?
   a. "I'll bet you will be so glad to be home in your own bed."
   b. "What are your expectations for recovery from your surgery?"
   c. "Be sure and take your pain medications and change your dressing."
   d. "You will just be fine! Please stop worrying."

8. A patient who decides to leave the hospital against medical advice (AMA) must sign a form. What is the purpose of this form?
   a. To indicate the patient's wishes
   b. To use in the event of readmission
   c. To release the physician and hospital from legal responsibility for the patient's health status
   d. To ethically illustrate that the patient has control of his or her own care and treatment

■ Answers With Rationale

1. The correct answer is *c*. Making appropriate referrals for patients as they move from acute care to home care is an essential component of discharge planning for continuity of care.
2. The correct answer is *b*. Community-based care centers on individuals and families with acute and chronic healthcare needs.
3. The correct answer is *d*. The nurse may delegate preparation of the bed and collection of needed supplies to unlicensed personnel but would perform the other activities listed.
4. The correct answer is *c*. HIPAA ensures privacy of information use and disclosure.
5. The correct answer is *a*. The ICU nurse gives a verbal report about the patient's condition and nursing care needs to the nurse on the new unit. This information is not given to a unit secretary, nor is it delegated to others. The medical record is transferred with the patient; a copy is not made.
6. The correct answer is *d*. Effective discharge planning begins on admission.

7. The correct answer is *b*. It is important to assess the expectations of the patient (and family) when assessing healthcare needs for discharge planning.
8. The correct answer is *c*. Patients who leave the hospital AMA sign a form releasing the physician and hospital from legal responsibility for their health status. This signed form becomes part of the medical record.

Bibliography

American Hospital Association. (1992). A patient's bill of rights. Available at: http://www.hospitalconnect.com/aha/about/pbillofrights.html.

Chaboyer, W., Foster, M., Kendall, E., & James, H. (2002). ICU nurses' perceptions of discharge planning: A preliminary study. *Intensive Critical Care Nursing, 18*(2), 90–95.

Christakis, D., Wright, J., Zimmerman, F., Bassett, A., & Conell, F. (2002). Continuity of care is associated with high-quality care by parental report. *Pediatrics, 109*(4), e54 6p.

Department of Health and Human Services. (2001). HIPAA fact sheet. Available at: http://www.aspe.hhs.gov/admnsimp.

Haines, S., Crocker, C., & Leducq, M. (2001). Providing continuity of care for patients transferred from ICU. *Professional Nurse, 17*(1), 17–21.

Kovner, C., & Harrington, C. (2001). Counting nurses: What is community health-public health nursing? *American Journal of Nursing, 101*(1), 59–60.

Kumehawa, J. (2001). Health information privacy protection: Crisis or common sense? *Online Journal of Issues in Nursing, 6*(3), Manuscript 2. Available at: http://www.nursingworld.org/ojin/topic16/tpc16_2.htm.

Mainous, A., & Gill, J. (1998). The importance of continuity of care in the likelihood of future hospitalization. *American Journal of Public Health, 88*(10), 1539–1541.

Mancini, A., & White, A. (2001). Discharge planning from a neonatal unit: An exploratory study of parents' views. *Journal of Neonatal Nursing, 7*(2), 59–62.

NANDA International. (2003). *Nursing diagnoses: Definitions & classification 2003–2004*. Philadelphia: NANDA International.

Naylor, M., & Buhler-Wilkerson, K. (1999). Creating community-based care for the new millennium. *Nursing Outlook, 47*(3), 120–127.

Parkes, J., & Shepperd, S. (2003). Discharge planning from hospital to home. (Cochrane Review). In: *The Cochrane Library,* Issue 2, 2003. Oxford: Update Software.

Rudd, C., & Smith, J. (2002). Discharge planning. *Nursing Standard, 17*(5), 33–37.

Smeltzer, S. C., & Bare, B. G. (2004). *Brunner & Suddarth's textbook of medical-surgical nursing* (10th ed., p. 47). Philadelphia: Lippincott Williams & Wilkins.

Stanhope, M., & Lancaster, J. (2004). *Community & public health nursing* (6th ed.). St. Louis: Mosby.

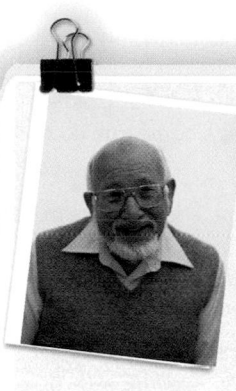

Alphonse Califano, a widower who lives alone, is receiving weekly visits from the home healthcare nurse. He has a history of diabetes, hypertension, and renal disease.

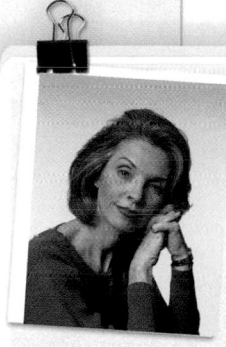

Jane Friel, a single woman with end-stage breast cancer, lives with a friend who provides most of her care. She is receiving hospice care with weekly visits unless complications require additional visits.

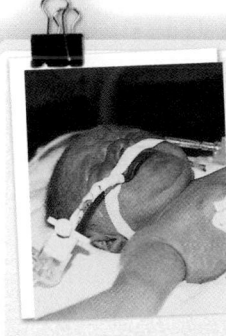

Joey Marshall, an extremely low-birthweight baby (1,100 g) has spent 7 months in the hospital before being discharged home. His mother is now at home full time caring for him, his twin (who is healthier), and their 3-year-old sister. Joey is still being fed artificially, is on a ventilator, and needs care round the clock.

Focusing on Blended Skills

The types of blended skills you'll need to respond to the case scenarios include:

Cognitive Skills

- Knowledge of home healthcare
- Ability to incorporate knowledge of the healthcare delivery system to meet the needs of patients receiving care in the home
- Knowledge of patient needs and the resources to meet those needs in the patient's home
- Knowledge of care for a high-risk infant; nursing care related to diabetes, high blood pressure, and renal disease; and care of a terminally ill patient with breast cancer, all in the home
- Knowledge of how to coordinate the home care that patients receive, drawing on family caregivers, visiting nurse assistants, and other resources
- Knowledge of the resources available within the community to meet the needs of homebound patients

Technical Skills

- Ability to provide technical nursing assistance to meet the nursing needs of patients at different developmental stages and their caregivers
- Ability to adapt technical nursing assistance as necessary for a high-risk newborn, an older adult with numerous health concerns, and a woman with a terminal illness
- Ability to use equipment correctly, competently, and safely to meet the needs of a high-risk infant and a terminally ill patient
- Ability to ask for assistance as necessary when performing technologically complex procedures or when faced with new situations

Interpersonal Skills

- Ability to establish trusting professional relationships with homebound patients, their family caregivers, and others within the community
- Ability to demonstrate professional care and compassion for homebound patients and their caregivers
- Ability to work with different resources to ensure safe, quality home care
- Demonstration of respect for a patient's human dignity and autonomy throughout the patient's home care course

Ethical and Legal Skills

- Commitment to providing safe and effective care in home settings
- Ability to practice in an ethically and legally defensible manner in home settings
- Knowledge of the ethical and legal obligations related to care of high-risk infants and terminally ill patients in the home
- Commitment to securing the best coordination of resources to support the level of care needed by a high-risk infant, an older man, or a terminally ill woman
- Ability to participate as a trusted and effective patient advocate for patients at different developmental stages, such as a high-risk infant, a widowed man, and a terminally ill woman

Learning Outcomes

After completing the chapter, the learner should be able to accomplish the following:

1. Discuss the types and funding of home healthcare services.
2. Describe the characteristics and roles of the home health nurse.
3. Explain the essential components of the pre-entry and entry phases of the home visit.
4. Compare and contrast the role of the family in home healthcare to that in hospital-based care.

Key Terms

advocacy
home healthcare

In the past decade, many changes have occurred in the healthcare system and in the settings where nurses provide care. A major and important change is an ever-increasing shift from hospital-based settings to community-based home healthcare. Home healthcare has experienced an unprecedented rate of growth. In its effort to decrease costs, managed care has had a major effect on the move from hospital to home care, and this trend is expected to continue. Home healthcare is one of the fastest-growing areas of healthcare today; the National Association for Home Care (2001) estimated that more than 20,000 providers deliver home healthcare services to 7.6 million people. (See the accompanying Reflective Practice box for an example.)

Chapters 8 and 9 discussed the facilities providing community-based care and continuity of care between settings. This chapter defines home healthcare and discusses how nurses provide care in the patient's home.

HOME HEALTHCARE SERVICES

Home healthcare is care provided in a patient's place of residence, such as in a private home, an apartment, a homeless shelter, a boarding house, a dormitory, a nursing home, a group home, or older adult housing. It can involve patients of all ages with both chronic and acute healthcare needs, disabilities, and terminal illnesses.

> *Think back to Joey Marshall, the high-risk infant being discharged home with tube feedings and mechanical ventilation. Joey has both acute and chronic healthcare needs. As part of his plan of care, the nurse addresses not just Joey's needs but those of his family, too, to ensure holistic continuity of care.*

Home healthcare services include high-technology pharmacy services, skilled professional and paraprofessional services, custodial care, medical equipment services, hospice services (discussed in Chap. 8), and community support services. Examples of each area, with related services, are listed in Table 10-1.

There are two types of home healthcare agencies: those that are certified by Medicare and those that are not. An agency must be certified by Medicare to receive reimbursement for services from Medicare. Agencies that are not certified by Medicare are

Reflective Practice
Challenge to Technical Skills

Joey Marshall, an extremely low-birthweight baby (1,100 g) spent 7 months in the hospital before being discharged home. His mother is now at home full time caring for him, his twin (who is healthier), and their 3-year-old sister. Joey is still being fed via tube feedings, is on a ventilator, and needs care around the clock. When I first visited Joey on the day he was discharged home, I was frightened at the sight of such a small baby surrounded by beeping machines and tubes. While this was not a new sight for Joey's mom, she seemed very uncomfortable being his primary caregiver. She said she had lots of practice taking care of him in the hospital, but nothing had prepared her for the reality of his coming home and needing help around the clock.

Thinking Outside the Box: Possible Courses of Action

- Take a "pass" on this family and tell my instructor that this family's needs exceed my capacity to care; an adult with a lot of tubes is one thing, but a BABY!
- Ask for an experienced mentor to guide me through a comprehensive family assessment and planning to meet every-

one's needs; use this as a challenge but ask for help until I feel competent and confident.
- Act like I know what I'm doing and pray I don't make mistakes!

Evaluating a Good Outcome: How Do I Define Success?

- Joey's mother develops the competence and confidence she needs to provide Joey's care at home.
- I am honest about my ability and seek help when I need it.

- I learn something from each situation that will prepare me to meet the next clinical challenge.
- I don't let my fear interfere with my learning.

Personal Learning: Here's to the Future!

I decided that options one (taking a pass) and three (acting like I knew what I was doing) weren't really options, although they seemed tempting. An experienced home health nurse who once worked in the neonatal intensive care unit (NICU) agreed to visit this family with me, and she talked me through a comprehensive assessment. I was able to use MY fear to identify with how Joey's mom was feeling, and I believe I was able to make her feel com-

fortable. I told her that we would learn how to do everything together! By the end of this rotation we were both comfortable with Joey's care. I learned a valuable lesson: to seek help when I am in over my head and to relish a challenge. I hope I will remember this experience as I grow more confident so that I never forget how overwhelmed many families feel when they first bring a loved one home!

Reflection

How do you think you would respond in a similar situation? Why? What does this tell you about yourself and about the adequacy of your skills for professional practice? Can you think of other ways to respond? What technical skills were needed in this situation? What other skills (cognitive, interpersonal, technical, ethical/legal)

would you need to respond well in this situation? What factors do you think may have influenced how Joey's mother was feeling? How the nursing student was feeling? Do you agree with the criteria to evaluate a successful outcome? Did the nursing student meet the criteria? Please explain why or why not.

TABLE 10-1 Examples of Home Healthcare Services

Area of Service	Type of Service Provided
High-technology pharmacy services	Intravenous therapy Home uterine monitoring Ventilator management Chemotherapy
Skilled professional/paraprofessional services	Nursing care (provided by a licensed practical nurse, a registered nurse, or a nurse practitioner) Care by home health aides Personal care Physical therapy Occupational therapy Speech therapy Medical social work Respiratory therapy
Custodial services	Homemaking and housekeeping Hourly or shift coverage Live-in services Companionship
Home medical services	Providing durable medical equipment, such as beds, braces, canes, crutches, wheelchairs, commodes, and oxygen
Hospice services	Pain management Physician services Spiritual support Respite care Bereavement counseling
Community support services	Meals on Wheels Transportation Friendly visitor Delivery services Emergency answering services

not certified for many reasons; for example, home care agencies that do not provide skilled nursing care are not eligible to participate in Medicare. Medicare is the largest single payer of home care services. It provides payment for services through a prospective payment plan based on an "episode of care" (usually considered a 60-day period). All patients receiving home healthcare services must have a physician's order. The requirements for eligibility for Medicare-covered home care are listed in Box 10-1.

When providing home healthcare, nurses focus on community-based care, taking into account the environmental, socioeconomic, cultural, and personal factors that affect the patient's and family's health. The essential components of home healthcare include the patient, the family, healthcare professionals from various disciplines, and the goals of helping the patient reach maximum independence and health. The role of each member of the healthcare team is outlined in Table 10-2.

Care of the patient in the home is different from care in the hospital. Hospitalized patients conform to the hospital routine and follow the hospital's schedule for eating, bathing, taking medications, and visiting with their families. But when

BOX 10-1 Eligibility Requirements for Medicare-Covered Home Healthcare

- A physician must decide that medical care is needed at home and make a plan of care for care at home.
- At least one of the following must be needed:
   Intermittent skilled nursing care
   Physical therapy
   Speech/language therapy
   Occupational therapy
- The patient must be homebound, or normally unable to leave the home unassisted. Although a patient may leave home for medical treatment or short infrequent trips for nonmedical reasons (such as to the barbershop or to attend religious services), leaving the home must require considerable and taxing effort.
- The home health agency must be Medicare certified.

(Source: Centers for Medicare & Medicaid Services. [2003]. Medicare and home health care. Available at: http://www.cms.hhs.gov/quality/hhqi/hhbenefits.pdf.)

TABLE 10-2 Collaborative Roles of Members of the Home Healthcare Team

Member	Role
Physician	Certifies that the patient has a health problem to receive home healthcare. Prescribes and certifies a plan of care for treatment for the patient receiving home healthcare.
Nurse	Provides direct care to patients and families. Teaches patient and family self-care. Conducts research to ensure cost-effectiveness and quality of care. May be administrator of home health agency and serve as consultant to staff. Coordinates services of other healthcare providers.
Physical therapist	Provides direct care, such as muscle-strengthening exercises, gait training, and massage. Teaches patient and family to promote self-care.
Occupational therapist	Evaluates the patient's functional level and teaching activities to promote self-care in activities of daily living. Assesses the home for safety and provides adaptive equipment as necessary.
Speech pathologist	Provides direct care services to patients with speech, language, or hearing needs. Teaches patient and family to facilitate speech and language ability as well as eating and swallowing.
Social worker	Assists patient and family in dealing with the social, emotional, and environmental factors that affect their well-being. Makes referrals to appropriate community resources. Provides assistance with securing equipment and supplies, and with healthcare finances.
Home health aide	Implements the plan of care designed by the nurse. Assists patients with hygiene. May carry out light housekeeping.

entering the patient's home, the nurse must adapt care to the patient's schedules, customs, and needs. The hallmark of a quality home healthcare nurse is the ability to blend clinical skills with flexibility.

Consider Alphonse Califano, the older man with several health problems. The nurse providing home care to Mr. Califano needs to adapt to his schedule. For example, the nurse might want to visit around breakfast time to evaluate his meal pattern and his diabetes. However, the patient says that he likes to take his time in the morning and doesn't want the nurse to visit until the afternoon. Even after the nurse explains the rationale for wanting to visit earlier in the day, the patient insists that the nurse visit in mid-afternoon. The nurse must abide by the patient's request.

BRIEF HISTORY OF HOME HEALTHCARE NURSING

In the late 1800s, America experienced a large influx of immigrants, and most cities grew rapidly. Home nursing agencies were started in New York, Boston, and Philadelphia to meet residents' health needs. Lillian Wald and Mary Brewster opened the Henry Street Settlement House in New York City in 1893. Visiting nurses from this agency cared for poor residents living in tenements. Eventually, these providers of home healthcare became known as Visiting Nurse Associations (VNAs), which focused on providing personal care to the sick and teaching about health to families.

Before World War II, physicians often made house calls to treat the sick. During the war, physicians shifted their practice setting from the home to the hospital and office, and nurses began to provide most of the home healthcare visits. VNAs were started in most major cities throughout the country. Hospital-based home care agencies were also formed as hospitals looked for ways to expand services to their communities.

In the mid-1960s, home healthcare services expanded to include the older population. The 1965 Social Security Act provided coverage for home healthcare to older persons participating in Medicare. Not long after, Medicaid home healthcare benefits were initiated. The Medicare and Medicaid programs (discussed in Chap. 8) provide the structure for most home healthcare agencies today.

There are many reasons for the expansion in home healthcare. The need for home healthcare services is increasing as the population ages. Fewer people live in the same community as their parents do; thus, home healthcare providers may be needed to care for ill parents if the children live far away. Because patients are being discharged from the hospital earlier in their recovery, many will need skilled professional care after they return home. In addition, third-party payers have sought a way to reduce the escalating costs of healthcare through the use of managed care programs that include home healthcare.

THE HOME HEALTHCARE NURSE

Until about 1990, home healthcare nurses were considered generalists, but recently many home healthcare nurses have gained advanced skills to meet the growing demands of acutely ill patients being cared for at home. These specialties include enterostomal therapy, cardiac care, mental health, and maternal and child health. Specialized nursing knowledge and skills and sophisticated technology allow many patients with acute and chronic healthcare needs to be treated safely and effectively in the home.

Think back to Joey Marshall, the infant discharged home after 7 months in the neonatal intensive care unit. Joey still requires high-tech, specialized skills associated with tube feedings and ventilator care.

The nursing profession has its roots in home healthcare, although in the past several decades most nurses practiced in hospitals. As the home healthcare industry continues to grow, nursing practice is coming full circle and moving back to the home.

Home healthcare nursing is unique in that the care is provided in a setting that is unfamiliar to the nurse but familiar and comfortable to the patient. For most people, the home is a place of safety and security and has meaning and value, rooted in ownership, family relationships and memories, and independence. Home healthcare is provided to the patient in a setting that is controlled by the patient and family. Instead of the patient coming to the nurse, the nurse goes to the patient. Patients or their caregivers must give permission for the nurse to enter the practice setting because the nurse is a guest in their home. The nurse cannot regulate the setting where care is provided but rather must adapt to the patient's environment (instead of the patient adapting to the hospital environment) (Fig. 10-1).

Defining Characteristics

Nurses choose to practice home healthcare nursing for various reasons. Many nurses enjoy practicing in an autonomous setting where they can use their expertise in an expanded role. Others enjoy managing their time independently and like the satisfaction they derive from patients welcoming them into their home and life. Home healthcare nurses find satisfaction

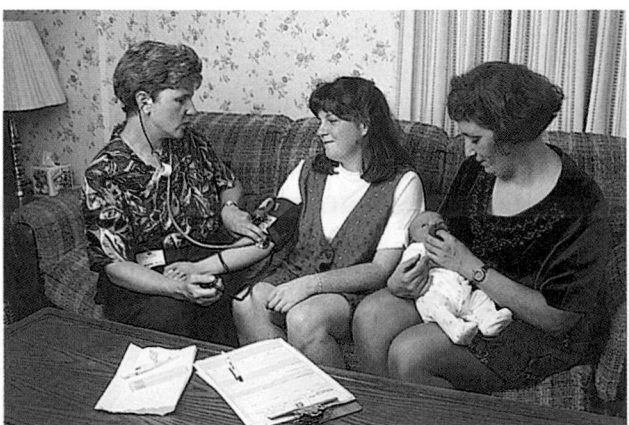

FIGURE 10-1 The nurse providing care in the home integrates knowledge and skills to implement family-centered specialized care.

in networking with community agencies to provide individualized care. Home healthcare provides an opportunity for nurses to be creative in delivering care. Home healthcare nurses must possess several key qualities: they must be knowledgeable and skilled in their practice, must be able to make decisions independently, and must remain accountable.

Knowledgeable and Skilled

Nurses who provide care in the home must have the knowledge and skills needed to provide appropriate care. Effective communication is essential, and clinical skills are important (Fig. 10-2). In fact, many home healthcare agencies require a minimum of one year of clinical practice as a prerequisite for employment. Physical assessment skills are necessary to identify positive and negative changes in a patient's health status. Procedures such as administering intravenous fluids, changing complex wound dressings, caring for ostomies, and providing ventilator care are often required. Home healthcare nurses have identified the following areas of knowledge as most important in home care: legal regulations, physical assessment, body mechanics, nursing diagnoses, and infection control.

Independent in Making Decisions

Nurses providing care in the home make independent decisions and assume responsibility for decision making. They are generally alone when providing care and thus cannot consult with other healthcare professionals. Therefore, they must be able to make patient care decisions independently. The combination of a sound theoretical foundation, proficiency in clinical skills, and ability to solve problems creatively enables the nurse to make appropriate patient care decisions.

Think back to Jane Friel, the woman who is terminally ill with breast cancer. The nurse has been visiting once a week but would increase the frequency of visits if needed based on the patient's condition. This decision requires the nurse to have a solid foundation of knowledge about the disease and its complications.

Accountable

Accountability is another important characteristic of home healthcare nurses. In a hospital, the nurse generally works a shift and reports to the next shift nurse, who then continues to care for the patient. The home healthcare nurse generally does not have a next shift to report to but must rely on family or other caregivers to continue the care. If there is no caregiver in the home, the nurse returns to face the same issues at the next visit. The nurse is accountable to the patient, the family, and the primary healthcare provider. This increased autonomy may increase the nurse's legal risk (see Chap. 7). Home healthcare nurses must consider questions such as the following:

• Whom do I call if the patient's physician is not available?
• What should I do if a family member becomes acutely ill?
• How do I learn to perform advanced procedures?
• How do I document the patient's decisions about treatment?
• How do I ensure that other providers know about and document the plan of care?

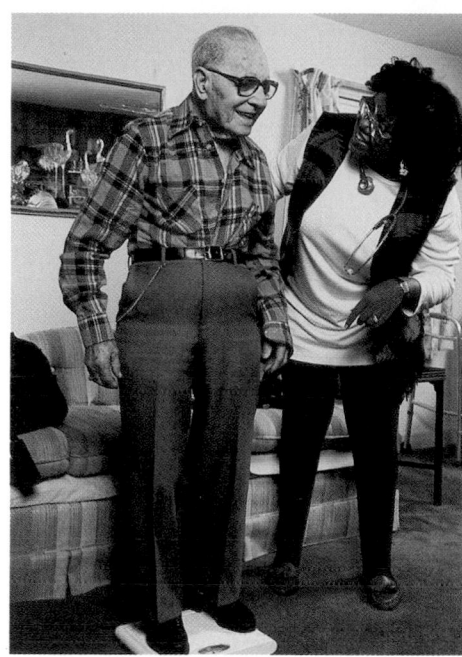
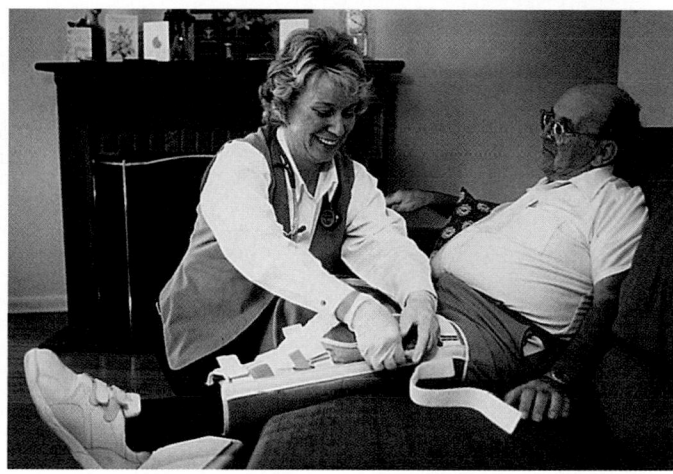

FIGURE 10-2 Home health nurses combine effective communication skills with a sound clinical knowledge base when caring for patients.

Roles

In addition to having caregiving skills, the nurse providing care in the home is a patient advocate, coordinator of services, and patient and family educator. These roles are briefly described here; further information is found in Unit V.

Patient Advocate

Advocacy—the protection and support of another's rights—is an important role of the home healthcare nurse. Patients often need help understanding the complex healthcare system, handling insurance problems, or dealing with state and federal regulations affecting their care and their environment. For example, the nurse may have to convince the patient's insurance carrier of the need for continued home health services. Patients might need help understanding complex billing issues related to their care. Home healthcare nurses can often mobilize services needed to improve the patient's environment.

The nurse acts as an advocate when communicating with the patient's primary healthcare provider. The physician may not be aware of the home environment and may order a treatment that cannot be accomplished in this patient's home setting. Communicating the patient's needs to the physician enables the nurse to implement appropriate treatments that fit into the patient's lifestyle.

Coordinator of Services

The home healthcare nurse is generally the coordinator of all other healthcare providers visiting the patient, including physical therapists, occupational therapists, speech therapists, medical social workers, and home health aides. The nurse is the primary source of communication and coordination of the patient's care with the primary healthcare provider. He or she must use effective communication skills with other healthcare providers while coordinating services for the patient. The sample forms shown in Figures 10-3 and 10-4 illustrate how the home healthcare nurse coordinates services among other healthcare providers and teaches the patient's caregiver to assist in or provide care.

The home healthcare nurse is also responsible for coordinating community resources needed by the patient. A sound knowledge of community resources enables the nurse to provide comprehensive services to the patient. For example, the nurse must understand the role of a social worker or physical therapist to determine a need for these services. The nurse should know about available community resources, such as Meals on Wheels, the American Cancer Society, services for patients who are visually or hearing impaired, and local services for the aging. As the coordinator of care, the nurse directs the various services toward a common goal of improving the patient's health and promoting independence.

Educator

Nurses providing home healthcare find that they spend most of their time teaching patients and families about the disease process, nutrition, medications, or treatment and care of wounds. The nurse identifies learning needs; then the nurse, patient, and family mutually develop goals for teaching information necessary to promote health. Family members or other caregivers may be taught any skill that they are able and willing to perform.

The nurse provides the information necessary to keep the patient safe until the next visit, using methods that work best in the home. The goal is to increase the patient's ability to provide self-care and the caregiver's ability to care for the patient.

HOME HEALTH CERTIFICATION AND PLAN OF TREATMENT

1. Patient's HI Claim No.	2. Start Of Care Date	3. Certification Period		4. Medical Record No.	5. Provider No.
777-88-7788A	100303	From: 100303	To: 120303	S2521	78-9999

6. Patient's Name and Address
Smythe, Samuel A.
25952 North Hawthorne Lane
Sky City, WI 50000

7. Provider's Name, Address and Telephone Number
BHC Home Care
2001 Oak Lane
Sky City, WI 50000

8. Date of Birth 021730

9. Sex [X] M [ ] F

10. Medications: Dose/Frequency/Route (N)ew (C)hanged
Cephradine 250 mg. Q 6 hrs. PO x 21 days
DC p̄ 10 AM dose 102400 (N)
Tolectin 400 mg. TID (C)
Furosemide 20 mg. Q AM PO (C)
KCl 10 mEq. Q AM PO (C)
Digoxin 0.125 mg. Q AM PO
Vitamin-mineral supplement 1 cap. QD PO
Acetaminophen tabs. 2 Q 4 hrs. PRN PO - pain

11. ICD-9-CM	Principal Diagnosis	Date
890.1	Open wound, left hip	100103
12. ICD-9-CM	**Surgical Procedure**	**Date**
79.35	Open reduction, left femur	092703
13. ICD-9-CM	**Other Pertinent Diagnoses**	**Date**
820.9	Fracture, left femur	092603
428.0	Congestive heart failure	090503
715.09	Osteoarthritis	030003
250.00	NIDDM	010094

14. DME and Supplies: Wheelchair, walker

15. Safety Measures: Proper footwear, clear pathways when ambulating. O_2 precautions.

16. Nutritional Req. 1800 calorie ADA, 2 gm. Na

17. Allergies: No known allergies

18.A. Functional Limitations
1 [ ] Amputation
2 [ ] Bowel/Bladder (Incontinence)
3 [ ] Contracture
4 [ ] Hearing
5 [ ] Paralysis
6 [X] Endurance
7 [X] Ambulation
8 [ ] Speech
9 [ ] Legally Blind
A [ ] Dyspnea With Minimal Exertion
B [X] Other (Specify) Occasional orthopnea

18.B. Activities Permitted
1 [ ] Complete Bedrest
2 [ ] Bedrest BRP
3 [ ] Up As Tolerated
4 [X] Transfer Bed/Chair
5 [X] Exercises Prescribed
6 [ ] Partial Weight Bearing
7 [ ] Independent At Home
8 [ ] Crutches
9 [ ] Cane
A [X] Wheelchair
B [X] Walker
C [ ] No Restrictions
D [ ] Other (Specify)

19. Mental Status: 1 [X] Oriented 2 [ ] Comatose 3 [ ] Forgetful 4 [ ] Depressed 5 [ ] Disoriented 6 [ ] Lethargic 7 [ ] Agitated 8 [ ] Other

20. Prognosis: 1 [ ] Poor 2 [ ] Guarded 3 [X] Fair 4 [ ] Good 5 [ ] Excellent

21. Orders for Discipline and Treatments (Specify Amount/Frequency/Duration)

Wound care Ⓛ hip daily: Irrigate with 1:1 H_2O_2/water, rinse with normal saline, pack with saline-soaked 4x4s, dress with gauze. O_2 2L PRN HS per cannula - orthopnea.

Skilled Nursing: Daily for 62 days. Assess wound, S/S fluid retention. Perform wound care. Teach diet, O_2 precautions; new/changed medications.

Physical Therapy: One visit first week, 3 times a week for 8 weeks. Evaluation, therapeutic exercises, gait training. Teach use of walker, transfer technique. Establish home program.

Home Health Aide: 3 times a week for 9 weeks. Personal care. Assist with transfers, home exercise program.

22. Goals/Rehabilitation Potential/Discharge Plans

Anticipate daily visits to end 010303. Rehab potential good for patient to ambulate independently with walker by 120303. Will be compliant with diet, medications, therapeutic regimen. Plan discharge to care of wife when wound complications resolved.

23. Nurse's Signature and Date of Verbal SOC Where Applicable: Jane Dayes, RN 100303

25. Date HHA Received Signed POT: OCT 13 2003

24. Physician's Name and Address
Albert Richard, MD
1641 Pine Circle
Sky City, WI 50000

26. I certify/recertify that this patient is confined to his/her home and needs intermittent skilled nursing care, physical therapy and/or speech therapy or continues to need occupational therapy. The patient is under my care, and I have authorized the services on this plan of care and will periodically review the plan.

27. Attending Physician's Signature and Date Signed: Albert Richard MD 10/10/03

28. Anyone who misrepresents, falsifies, or conceals essential information required for payment of Federal funds may be subject to fine, imprisonment, or civil penalty under applicable Federal laws.

Form HCFA-485 (U-4) (02-94)

SAMPLE

(Sample data © 1995 Beacon Health Corporation, Mequon WI. Used with permission.)

FIGURE 10-3 Example of home health plan of care.

The teaching and learning process is fully described in Chapter 22.

Remember Joey Marshall, the high-risk infant coming home after 7 months in the neonatal intensive care unit. In this situation the home healthcare nurse will fill many roles; one of the major roles will be that of educator, with the goal of teaching Joey's mother so that she can ultimately care for Joey independently.

SKILLED NURSING VISIT NOTE

Patient ___Samuel Smythe___

DATE 061303 TIME 11:00–11:45	No S/S fluid retention. Wound measures
VISIT FREQUENCY **Daily** ☐ Change ☐ Patient informed	9x5x3 cm. Small amount of purulent drainage.
BP 140/86 Standing (Sitting) Lying	Wound bed 70% slough, 30% granulation tissue.
TEMPERATURE 98.2°	Wound care performed: irrigated with normal
PULSE 80, regular (Apical) Radial	saline, covered with ABD. Surrounding skin
RESPIRATIONS 26	intact. Expresses discomfort during procedure
LUNG SOUNDS Clear	Taught use of pain med 1 hr. before
DIET/ 1800 cal. APPETITE Taught fiber sources.	procedure. Reports occasional constipation.
ACTIVITY Weak. Transfers with 1. LEVEL	Observed aide transfer patient. Uses safe
AIDE Observed SUPERVISION K. Jackson	technique. Patient satisfied with care. Can
PHYSICIAN Appt. 061503 CONTACT/APPT.	demonstrate exercises but reluctant to do
CARE Reviewed PT program COORDINATION with aide.	alone. Taught wife how to assist.
CONFERENCE	
☐ PROGRESS NOTE	SIGNATURE *Susan Jackson RN*

SKILLED NURSING VISIT NOTE

Patient ___Samuel Smythe___

DATE 091903 TIME 7:30–8:20	Venipuncture for FBS – (L) antecubital.
VISIT FREQUENCY Weekly.Aide dc'd0913 ☐ Change ☒ Patient informed	Verbalizes routine for blood, urine
BP 132/76 Standing (Sitting) Lying	testing. Still has difficulty performing
TEMPERATURE 97.6°	finger stick. Does not get enough blood on
PULSE 70, regular (Apical) Radial	strip for accurate reading. Demonstrated
RESPIRATIONS 22	procedure for finger stick.
LUNG SOUNDS Clear	
DIET/ 1800 cal. ADA APPETITE "Good appetite"	Blood sugar 175–225.
ACTIVITY Ambulates 30' – walker LEVEL No longer uses wheelchair.	Feeling more comfortable about performing
AIDE SUPERVISION	care.
PHYSICIAN Appt. 092303 CONTACT/APPT.	
CARE COORDINATION	
CONFERENCE	
☒ PROGRESS NOTE 091903	SIGNATURE *Susan Jackson RN*

FIGURE 10-4 Example of home health nursing progress note.

THE HOME VISIT

As described by Stulginsky (1993, p. 477), "few families understand why people are sent home from the hospital 'still sick.' Even fewer understand what home healthcare is. All they know is that the nurse is coming to help." Home healthcare patients often feel frightened, in pain, and abandoned, and family members often feel nervous about their new roles as care-

givers. The home healthcare nurse must keep these concerns and needs in mind when planning and carrying out care.

The Pre-entry Phase of the Home Visit

In the referral process, the physician or discharge planner of a hospital contacts the home care agency and provides them with a brief medical history, along with indications for home health services. During this pre-entry phase, the referral nurse at the home care agency collects as much information as possible about the patient's diagnoses, surgical experience, socioeconomic status, and treatments ordered. This phase of the home care visit is called the pre-entry phase. Once assigned the case, the nurse reviews the information and calls the patient to make initial contact and schedule a visit. During this conversation, the nurse can determine whether the patient's caregiver can answer questions related to the patient's and family's needs and can also learn about the patient's cognitive abilities, orientation, and caregiver status. This information is important to the nurse planning the first visit.

In the pre-entry phase, the nurse gathers the supplies that will be needed for the first visit, such as wound care products, dressings, and educational materials. The nurse organizes and takes to the first visit a field chart to document the assessment and care provided to the patient. This chart accompanies the nurse on subsequent visits.

The nurse should evaluate safety issues before making the first home visit; this includes the safety of the neighborhood where the patient lives. The nurse may need to arrange the visit at a time when it is safe to be in that area and should always know the exact destination before arriving for the visit. In some unsafe areas, police or security officers may accompany the nurse. Other guidelines for safety include carrying a cellular phone programmed with emergency numbers, making sure someone from the agency knows the nurse's itinerary, and being continuously alert to the environment.

The Entry Phase of the Home Visit

The second phase of the visit is the entry phase. In the entry phase, the nurse develops a rapport with the patient and family, makes assessments, determines nursing diagnoses, establishes desired outcomes (along with the patient and family), plans and implements prescribed care, and provides teaching. The nurse must remember that he or she is a guest in the patient's home and is offering services that the patient may accept or reject. Important considerations include negotiating and honoring visit times, establishing a rapport with the patient and family, defining what nursing care will be provided, and teaching to promote independence in self-care.

The nurse must gain the trust of the patient and family and must recognize and respect their values. Accepting the patient's living conditions is necessary even when they differ from those of the nurse. The nurse must ask permission before using the patient's home for activities such as handwashing. The nurse might believe the furniture in the patient's home or sick room needs to be rearranged to allow the use of equipment and to remove safety hazards, but the patient should give permission before any changes are made.

Nurses who provide home healthcare interventions do so based on an individualized plan of care for each patient, based initially on identifying his or her healthcare needs. In identifying the patient's needs and determining the interventions, the nurse fulfills the roles discussed earlier in the chapter.

Identifying Needs
Patient Needs

The ability to assess patients accurately is an important skill for home care nurses. Most of the initial assessment takes place during the first home visit, although ongoing focused assessment occurs during subsequent visits. The nurse must be skilled not only in physical assessment but also in psychological, socioeconomic, environmental, spiritual, and cultural assessment. Skilled assessment allows the nurse to make appropriate diagnoses. Examples of appropriate home care nursing diagnoses are found in the accompanying box. In addition, the nurse must determine and provide culturally sensitive care (see Chap. 3); although important for inpatients, this is even more important in the patient's home. Factors to consider include the following:

- What are the roles and responsibilities of family members? Who makes the decisions?
- What type of personal space is customary?
- How are important events celebrated?
- Are there cultural or ethnic influences on the family's usual diet?
- What cultural beliefs and taboos are followed?

Examples of NANDA Nursing Diagnoses | Home Healthcare

Nursing Diagnoses	Related Factors
Risk for Infection	Presence of large draining wound and unclean living environment
Impaired Home Maintenance	Fatigue and pain during recovery from injuries in automobile crash
Caregiver Role Strain	Requirement for 24-hour attention to needs and safety of husband with Alzheimer's disease
Readiness for Enhanced Knowledge	Requests from family members for increased information about providing care and using community resources and support services
Readiness for Enhanced Parenting	Children express satisfaction with home environment.

- What do the patient and family believe to be the cause of this illness? The treatment of this illness?
- Are traditional medical practices followed?

Recall Alphonse Califano, the widowed man with several health problems. Since he is a widower, the nurse would need to identify his primary caregiver or responsible party. The nurse also would need to determine the amount of support, if any, the patient has from his family. This information would provide a basis for possible referrals to community services.

Family caregivers must also be considered, taking into account the various roles that each family member plays and how they contribute to the patient's health status.

Family/Caregiver Needs

Traditionally, when a patient enters the hospital, the family plays a minor role in actual care. Families and friends visit with the patient and sometimes stay overnight, but they are generally not involved in the direct care of the patient. Hospital staff provide personal care for the patient and administer medications and treatments. After the patient is discharged, the responsibility for care is shifted to family caregivers, who may or may not be physically or mentally able to handle this responsibility.

Today's emphasis on home healthcare means that family caregivers must carry increased responsibilities. Patients are being discharged "quicker and sicker." Chronically ill patients may need long-term care at home that may not be covered by Medicare, and changes in Medicare funding may mean that fewer home visits will be covered. The financial burden associated with care is more than many families can afford, and home healthcare nurses must be alert for signs of such financial problems (eg, no food in the refrigerator or kitchen cupboards). A referral for services such as Meals on Wheels may be necessary to provide adequate nutrition for the patient.

In addition to the financial burden, family members face the challenges of handling equipment, providing new types of care to loved ones, and dealing with unfamiliar and often terrifying sounds, odors, and substances. Most caregivers are women, and many of them are older than 65 years of age. Older women may themselves have health problems or may not have the physical strength or energy to care for their husband. Even family members who are themselves nurses may find that providing care at home is very different from providing care in the hospital. The accompanying box, Through the Eyes of the Family Caregiver, describes one such experience.

The home healthcare nurse must identify the needs of the family and caregiver. The nurse can help the patient and family identify and use community resources to meet various needs. If a caregiver is becoming overwhelmed, the nurse can provide resources to relieve the stress. The nurse also supports family decisions about complex treatments or end-of-life care. The following questions may be used for discussion:

- What is most important to you?
- What do you want for your life and that of your family?
- How do you want to spend the rest of your life?

Through the Eyes of the Family Caregiver

"I'm So Glad to Have You Home, But What Do I Do Now?" (and this is just the first day. . . .)

I am a nurse, and have been a nurse for 30 years. I have a diploma in nursing, a baccalaureate in nursing, a master's in counseling, and a doctorate in nursing. I have taught others how to be nurses for more than 25 years. Nothing in all my educational and practice experiences prepared me to care for the complex needs of my husband, Jacque, when he had surgery 2 years ago. Following diagnosis of metastatic thyroid cancer, a large lower thoracic spinal cord tumor (which put pressure on the spinal nerves, causing leg weakness and bladder malfunction) and the thyroid gland were removed surgically, and steel rods were implanted almost the entire length of the spine. After 30 days in the hospital for diagnosis, surgery, and recovery, Jacque came home—unable to do more than move from the bed to a chair, and with a catheter in his bladder that was attached to a drainage bag.

Before he came home, I got a hospital bed with electric controls, a bedside commode, and a bedside table. I cleared out the family room furniture, got a friend to put the television up on a table (so it could be seen from the hospital bed), and thought I was all ready to give my husband expert care. The first challenge came when he got up in a chair to eat his dinner—we had no chairs with a high enough seat or a straight enough back to allow use of the bedside table. I ran up and down stairs to look at chairs, and finally decided the antique arm chair in the living room would work, and it did. Now another problem—where to hang the catheter drainage bag? And how best to move so it didn't pull when he moved? And remember to empty the bag before he gets up!

I fixed a wonderful homecoming meal for this man I love, and he could only eat a few bites. Now back to bed and a new problem. He got out of the bed and into the chair just fine, but now he can't get out of the chair and into the bed because his legs are still so weak. What did I do wrong—it worked in the hospital. It took me 2 days to realize that I forgot to lower the bed height so Jacque wouldn't have to push up so hard to get his bottom on the bed.

Then, after finally literally hauling him back in bed, I realized that I did not know how to move him up in bed. The physical therapist had taught him how to get up in a chair, but not how to move himself up in bed (they always did it for him in the hospital). This is a 250-pound man we are talking about. I could turn him from side to side, but I couldn't physically move him up in bed and he couldn't stay where he was. After a lot of trials, we figured out that he could wiggle one side of his body at a time and slowly inch up in bed. Now he was exhausted and in pain, and I felt totally incompetent. Thank goodness the home health nurse is coming to visit tomorrow.

If I felt this way, how must family members feel who know nothing about caring for someone who is sick or in pain? I have such respect for all those family members who provide such wonderful care and for the nurses who provide home care that calms the fears and answers the questions.

—Priscilla LeMone

- How is this technology supporting or not supporting what you want?

> *Remember Jane Friel, the terminally ill woman being cared for by a close friend. The nurse would need to ask both Jane and her caregiver the above questions to help address the terminal nature of the patient's illness and plan for future care.*

The nurse assesses whether the patient and family understand and are agreeable with the plan of care and determines if the caregivers understand the instructions provided and are capable of providing care. The nurse must assess the family unit overall and how the patient fits into this unit.

The nurse also assesses the physical environment of the home. Safety hazards, such as throw rugs or clutter, could easily cause falls. The home may be unsanitary, with rodent or insect infestations, or it may lack running water. Caregivers may have an alcohol or drug problem that impairs their ability to care for the patient. All of these factors must be considered because they could interfere with the patient's health and safety. Assessing the family helps the nurse to plan appropriate interventions and care for the patient.

Determining Interventions

Specific interventions are based on the patient's needs, but controlling infection and teaching the patient and caregiver are part of all home visits.

Controlling Infection

The nurse's use of infection control techniques is important to avoid spreading infection from one patient to the next. To prevent the spread of infection, nurses should use appropriate technique when handling their equipment bags, including the following:

- Perform hand hygiene before reaching into the bag for supplies.
- Clean any equipment removed from the bag before returning it to the bag.
- Place the bag on a liner when setting it down in the patient's home.

Of all the methods used to prevent infection, hand hygiene is the most important and is necessary before and after treating the patient. Nurses use standard precautions during home care visits, including wearing gloves when contacting blood, body fluids, secretions, excretions, and contaminated items. Clean gloves should be put on just before touching areas of broken skin or mucous membranes.

Teaching the Patient and Caregivers

Because home healthcare is meant to be short term and intermittent, the nurse includes the family and friends in the teaching process so they can learn how to care for the patient after the nurse's home care is no longer needed. The nurse designs and implements the teaching plan based on the patient's and caregiver's readiness to learn. It must be adapted to the patient's

and caregiver's physical and emotional status and must be understandable and "doable."

> *Consider Joey Marshall, the infant discharged home after 7 months. Because of the complex technology associated with his care and because his mother feels anxious and afraid, the nurse would need to provide the necessary teaching about his care, but in small sessions to avoid overwhelming the mother.*

Teaching should identify both the positive outcomes of following instruction and the serious consequences of failing to do so. The nurse points out the major problem areas specific to care in the home, focusing on the information needed to keep the patient safe until the nurse's next home visit.

Documenting Care Given in the Home

Documenting care given in the home is mandated by regulatory and federal agencies (see Chap. 17). The nurse may document the visit on preprinted forms or checklists or may use a computer.

The documented plan of care, the visit plan, and progress notes are routinely used by regulatory agencies and payer sources (eg, private insurance or Medicare) to determine whether various state and federal regulations are being met and if payment is warranted. Figures 10-3 and 10-4 illustrate such documentation.

During the initial visit, the nurse should assess the patient's healthcare needs, establish a plan of care that includes all the information needed to meet agency policy, regulatory requirements, and payer source needs, and set up a schedule for subsequent visits. The plan of care accurately reflects the condition of the patient, the need for skilled care, specific physician orders, anticipated progress, the criteria for discharge, the supplies needed, a visit schedule for all healthcare providers, and a list of support systems available. The plan of care includes the patient's functional limitations and safety needs; it establishes specific measurable goals and specifies a time frame for reaching the goals.

Progress notes are made to document each visit made by the nurse. These notes must accurately describe the patient's condition, the skilled care provided, the patient's response, the patient's progress toward discharge, and an ongoing plan for continued care. They also include the nurse's plan for the next visit. To meet reimbursement requirements, each progress note must indicate that the care provided requires the knowledge and skills of a professional nurse.

THE FUTURE OF HOME HEALTHCARE

The 1990s were a time of transition, growth, and specialization for the home care industry. In the new century, more complex services are being provided at home. Increasing numbers of surgical procedures are being performed on an outpatient or short-stay basis; thus, families and friends have more responsibility for providing care at home. Specialization will continue to expand in the areas of cardiac care, wound care, and high-technology services. The role of prevention will continue to grow in home healthcare through the use of health screening, immunization, and community education programs. Keeping people healthy in the home will be a goal to prevent illnesses resulting in hospitalization. Home healthcare nurses will need to expand their knowledge and skills continually to meet the challenges of providing preventive, acute, chronic, and end-of-life care to patients in their homes.

◼ Developing Critical Thinking Skills

1. Interview a nurse employed in a hospital setting and a nurse employed by a home healthcare agency. How are their roles and responsibilities alike? How do they differ?

2. Consider what you would do in the following home healthcare situations:
   - An 85-year-old patient cannot move by himself and refuses to eat. His 83-year-old wife tries to care for him, but she is under a great deal of stress and begins to cry when you enter their apartment.
   - A 43-year-old woman is receiving home care after surgery to repair a herniated vertebral disk ("slipped disk"). When you arrive for the scheduled visit, you find that her speech is slurred and she does not remember how much pain medication she has taken.
   - A 2-year-old has a malignant brain tumor. He is not expected to live more than 1 week and is receiving hospice care.

◼ Practicing for NCLEX

1. Which one of the following statements is a requirement for Medicare home healthcare reimbursement?
   a. The patient must be essentially homebound.
   b. The patient must require intravenous therapy.
   c. The caregiver must be able to provide all physical care.
   d. The caregiver must live with the patient.

2. In general, how does home care nursing compare with hospital-based nursing?
   a. Nursing care provided in the home is no different than hospital-based nursing care.
   b. Home care patients do not have the same basic needs as those in the hospital.
   c. In the home, care must be adapted to the patient's schedules and customs.
   d. The family or caregiver's role is less important in home care nursing.

3. Although the home care nurse follows an established plan of care, he or she is more independent in what role?

   a. Deciding which physician orders can be followed
   b. Assuming responsibility for decision making
   c. Shifting accountability for care to family caregivers
   d. Delegating advanced clinical skills to unlicensed personnel

4. Although all of the following skills are important, what would be the *most* important to effective coordination of care and services?
   a. Physical assessment
   b. Knowledge of the law
   c. How to use equipment
   d. Effective communication

5. Which of the following activities would the nurse do in the pre-entry phase of the home visit?
   a. Call the physician for a referral order
   b. Conduct a health history and physical assessment
   c. Collect information and schedule a visit
   d. Establish mutually acceptable goals for care

6. Before washing her hands, what might a home health nurse ask or say to the patient?
   a. "I need to wash my hands. May I use your bathroom?"
   b. "I'm going to wash my hands in your bathroom."
   c. "I will wash my hands after I leave so I don't bother you."
   d. "How often do you wash your hands?"

7. What one activity is most important in preventing infection when providing home care?
   a. Wearing gloves whenever touching the patient
   b. Following proper procedures for sterile dressing changes
   c. Asking the caregiver to step out of the room during visits
   d. Performing hand hygiene before and after care

8. How often must a home care nurse document progress notes?
   a. Once a week
   b. At the initial visit
   c. At each visit
   d. At the final visit

◼ Answers With Rationale

1. The correct answer is *a*. To be eligible for Medicare reimbursement, the patient must be essentially homebound, or normally unable to leave the home unassisted. The other answers are not requirements.

2. The correct answer is *c*. In the hospital, patients must conform to established schedules for treatments, medications, meals, and visitors. In contrast, in the home it is the patient or caregiver who establishes the schedule and controls the environment.

3. The correct answer is *b*. The home healthcare nurse is more independent and assumes responsibility for

decision making. None of the other answers is legally or ethically correct.

4. The correct answer is *d*. The home healthcare nurse must use effective communication skills with other healthcare providers while coordinating services for the patient.

5. The correct answer is *c*. During the pre-entry phase of the home visit, the nurse collects information and schedules the first visit.

6. The correct answer is *a*. The nurse must ask permission before rearranging furniture or using facilities for handwashing.

7. The correct answer is *d*. Performing hand hygiene before and after caring for the patient is critical in preventing infection.

8. The correct answer is *c*. The home health nurse must document progress notes at each visit.

Bibliography

CareScout. (2003). What is home health care? Available at: http://www.carescout.com/resources/home_health/definition.htm.

Centers for Medicare & Medicaid Services. (2003). Medicare and home health care. Available at: http://www.cms.hhs.gov/quality/hhqi/hhbenefits.pdf.

Centers for Medicare & Medicaid Services. (2003). Medicare hospice services. Available at: http://www.cms.hhs.gov/medlearn/nefhospice.asp-33k.

Marrelli, T. (2003). Home health care. A home care update. *Geriatric Nursing, 24*(1), 60–61.

Moll, J., & Tripp, E. (2002). Nursing delegation: Implications for home care. *Caring, 21*(9), 24–26, 28, 30.

NANDA International. (2003). *Nursing diagnoses: Definitions and classification 2003–2004*. Philadelphia: NANDA International.

Narayan, M. (2002). Data collection: The basics. *Home Healthcare Nurse, 20*(8), 503–505, 531–532.

National Association for Home Care. (2001). *Basic statistics about home care*. Washington, DC: National Association for Home Care.

National Center for Health Statistics. (2003). Home health & hospice care. Available at: http://www.cde.gov/nchs/fastats/homehosp.htm.

Roush, C., & Cox, J. (2000). The meaning of home: How it shapes the practice of home and hospice care. *Home Healthcare Nurse, 18*(6), 384–394.

Stanhope, M., & Lancaster, J. (2004). *Community & public health nursing* (6th ed.). St. Louis: Mosby.

Stulginsky, M. (1993). Nurses' home health experience. II. The unique demands of home visits. *Nursing & Healthcare, 14*(9), 476–485.

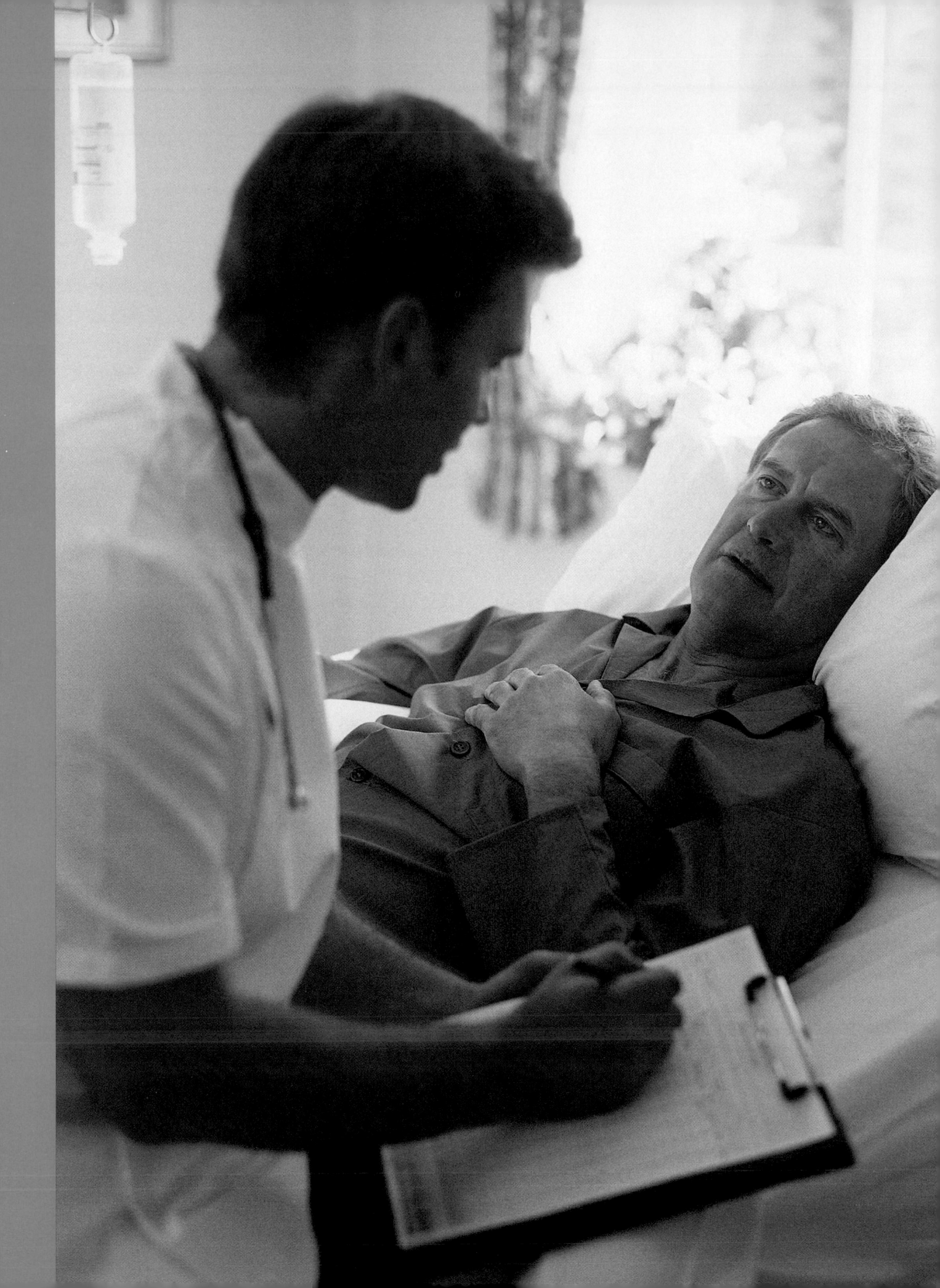

The Nursing Process

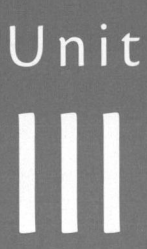

". . . the nursing process is educative and therapeutic when nurse and patient can come to know and to respect each other, as persons who are alike, and yet different, as persons who share in the solution of problems."

Hildegard Peplau (1909–   )
has been an active participant in ANA and NLN, and a leader in recognizing the significance of interpersonal relationships in psychiatric nursing. Her landmark book integrated theory into her model at a time when nursing theory was in its infancy.

The nursing process is a systematic, patient-centered, goal-oriented method of caring that provides a framework for nursing practice. Unit III discusses each of the five steps of the nursing process—assessing, diagnosing, planning, implementing, and evaluating. It also describes the blended skills nurses need to use the process for promoting patient well-being, and concludes with a chapter on documentation, reporting, and conferring.

The steps of the nursing process are not actually separate items but, rather, are parts of a whole, used to identify needs, to establish priorities of care, to maximize strengths, and to resolve actual or potential alterations in human responses to health and illness, thereby promoting health to the highest level possible for each patient.

Assessment, the systematic and continuous collection and communication of data, allows analysis of data to identify problems and strengths of patients. During planning, the nurse and patient mutually identify expected outcomes and agree on nursing interventions necessary to meet these outcomes. The nurse implements the plan of care, adapting it to each individual, and documents nursing actions and patient responses. After implementation, the nurse and patient evaluate the effectiveness of the plan, based on achievement of outcomes, and determine if the plan should be continued, modified, or terminated.

The nursing process is nursing practice in action. Unit III provides the information necessary to begin to apply the nursing process. As blended skills are learned and practiced (both by students and by nurses), the process becomes an integral component of each nurse–patient interaction. The outcome is comprehensive and individualized nursing care.

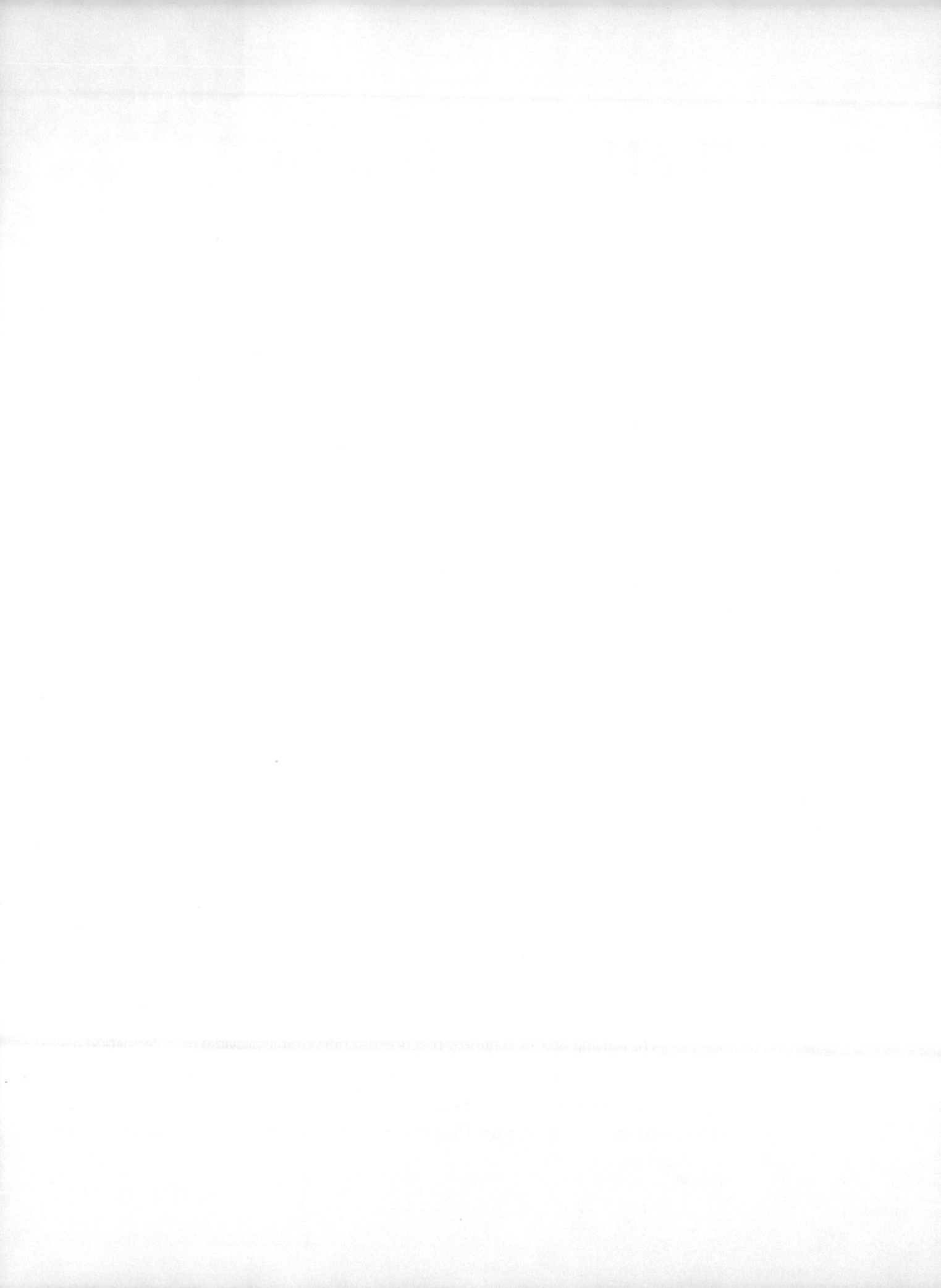

Blended Skills and Critical Thinking Throughout the Nursing Process

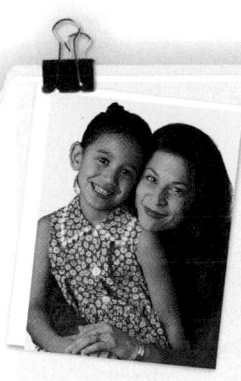

Charlotte Horvath is a single mother whose 5-year-old daughter is to be discharged soon. Ms. Horvath is to learn how to perform wound care for her daughter at home. However, she has missed every planned teaching session thus far.

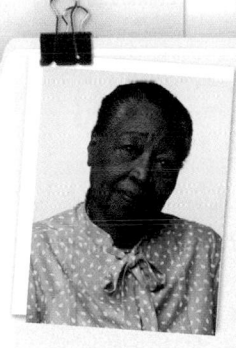

Addie Warner is an elderly African American woman who had suffered a cerebrovascular accident (CVA). She is currently being cared for in a neurologic step-down unit. The patient frequently uses her call light and is called "demanding" by the staff.

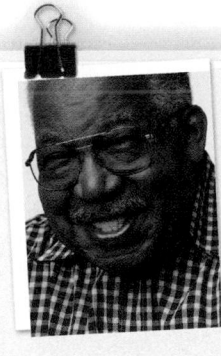

Jermaine Byrd is a 58-year-old man who has just returned to the medical-surgical unit after undergoing vascular surgery on the femoral artery. Orders include assessing the distal pulses to ensure adequate blood flow. However, when assessing the patient, the posterior tibial pulse is not palpable.

Focusing on Blended Skills

The types of blended skills you'll need to respond to the case scenarios here include:

Cognitive Skills

- Knowledge of the science of nursing care related to wound care, pulse assessment, and cerebrovascular accident
- Ability to integrate knowledge of how to assess, diagnose, and then plan, implement, and evaluate nursing care for patients with different needs, such as a patient requiring teaching, postoperative care, and assistance after a CVA
- Knowledge of teaching and learning principles, including factors affecting teaching and learning, and compliance with the plan
- Knowledge of postoperative care priorities, including assessment techniques
- Ability to demonstrate understanding of the needs of a patient after a CVA, incorporating these needs into the plan of care
- Knowledge of the nurse–patient relationship

Technical Skills

- Ability to provide the technical nursing assistance necessary to implement the plan of care safely and effectively for the patient requiring teaching, postoperative assessment, and assistance after a CVA
- Strong assessment skills to determine a patient's needs, such as reasons for not attending planned teaching sessions, lack of a palpable pulse (actual deficit or lack of skill), and frequent use of call light
- Ability to ask for assistance and know one's own limitations when performing new or technologically complex procedures or in interpreting findings

Interpersonal Skills

- Ability to establish trusting professional relationships with vulnerable patients across the lifespan
- Ability to counsel the woman who is finding it difficult to respond to the challenge of caring for her daughter at home
- Ability to communicate and interact effectively with patients who have different needs, such as the single mother, a postoperative patient, and an elderly woman after suffering a CVA
- Ability to demonstrate respect for a patient's human dignity throughout the patient's care

Ethical and Legal Skills

- Ability and willingness to master the knowledge and skills needed to meet the nursing needs of patients and families safely and effectively in new practice areas
- Demonstration of a strong sense of personal responsibility and accountability for the health and well-being of patients at various developmental stages with different needs
- Ability to integrate knowledge of the ethical and legal guidelines to perform care safely
- Ability to practice nursing in an ethically and legally defensible manner, consistent with the nursing code of ethics and within the scope of nursing practice
- Commitment to patient safety and quality care, including the ability to report problem situations immediately
- Ability to participate as a trusted and effective patient advocate; for example, advocating for the patient who is considered to be demanding

Learning Outcomes

After completing the chapter, the learner should be able to accomplish the following:

1. Describe the historic evolution of the nursing process.
2. Describe the nursing process and each of its five steps.
3. List five characteristics of the nursing process.
4. List three patient benefits and three nursing benefits of using the nursing process correctly.
5. Describe the four blended skills essential to nursing practice.
6. Use a model of critical thinking when making clinical judgments and decisions.
7. Identify four habits that assist in the development of technical skills.
8. Describe a personal plan to develop the interpersonal skills essential to quality care.
9. Explain the relationship between a nurse's sense of accountability and the patient's well-being.
10. Identify personal strengths and weaknesses in light of nursing's essential knowledge and skills.

Key Terms

assess
cognitively skilled
critical thinking indicators
ethically and legally skilled
evaluate
expected outcomes
implement
interpersonally skilled
intuitive thinking
nursing diagnoses
nursing process
plan
scientific problem-solving
standards for critical thinking
technically skilled
trial-and-error problem
whistle-blowing

Traditionally, nurses prided themselves on comforting those who were ill and on executing with precision such tasks as dressing wounds, administering medications, and bathing, feeding, and ambulating patients. Physicians ordered many of these tasks, and few nurses in the past would have characterized their "work" as being independent, evidence-based, or creative.

But as society and the healthcare delivery system change, so does nursing. Nurses now work with healthy and ill patients in both private and institutional settings. In addition to their role as caregivers, nurses fill specialized roles as care managers/coordinators, teachers, counselors, advocates, and researchers. Nurses are responsible for a unique dimension of healthcare—"the diagnosis and treatment of human responses to actual or potential health problems" (American Nurses Association, 1980) and, as such, are knowledgeable, competent, and independent professionals who work collaboratively with other healthcare professionals to design and to deliver holistic care.

As the practice of nursing became more complex, nurses began to study the process of nursing to both understand and improve the means nurses use to accomplish their aims. (See the accompanying Reflective Practice display for an example of this process.) This chapter begins with an overview of the nursing process and ends with a description of the blended skills needed to successfully use the nursing process.

THE NURSING PROCESS

Historical Perspective

Since Hall first used the term nursing process in 1955, many nurses have struggled to define exactly what constitutes the "work of nursing" and what makes nurses successful. In the 1960s, nursing theorists began to describe nursing as a distinct entity among the healthcare professions and also delineated specific steps in a process approach to nursing practice. In 1967, Yura and Walsh published the first comprehensive book on nursing process, in which they described four steps in the nursing process: assessment, planning, intervention, and evaluation. They viewed the element of nursing diagnosis as the logical conclusion of the assessment phase, whereas Gebbie and Lavin (1974) made nursing diagnosis a separate step in the process. These and other studies led to the development of the five-step nursing process commonly used today: assessment, diagnosis, outcome identification and planning, implementation, and evaluation.

Reflective Practice
Challenge to Ethical and Legal Skills

Recently I spent time working as a pediatric nurse technician. My job was to provide basic care to patients, such giving bed baths, assisting with meals, and changing linens. One of the nicest parts of my job was that I was able to spend more time than most nurses are able to, talking with my patients and getting to know them, and hopefully making a positive difference in their days. One day I was assigned to float to the neurologic step-down unit. Here, I met Addie Warner, an elderly African American woman who had suffered a cerebrovascular accident (CVA). Because of what happened that day, I became responsible for her care for the rest of the day.

When I arrived on the unit that morning, the nurses told me what a "pain" Mrs. Warner was, describing how she kept demanding that the nurse come into her room and help her with this or that. They told me I should "ignore her," and they told me I didn't need to listen to her. I was immediately appalled. So, the very next thing I did, after witnessing yet another nurse stand outside her door and condescendingly tell her in an annoyed voice, "I'll be with you when I have time," was to go into her room and ask how I could help her. Mrs. Warner had been trying unsuccessfully to get someone's attention for quite a while because she needed to go to the bathroom. Unfortunately, no one spoke to her long enough to find out what sort of help she needed. Ultimately, she urinated on herself in bed. She was humiliated, furious, scared, and angry. I proceeded to help her with her current problem, as well as to check in with her regularly throughout the rest of my shift to make sure all her additional needs were met.

Thinking Outside the Box: Possible Courses of Action

- Listen to all the nurses out of personal ignorance, out of fear for being reprimanded by them, or out of selfishness, and continuing to ignore this patient and her needs just like everyone else was doing.
- Ask one of the nurses to go into the room with me to determine what the patient's needs were and to help me meet them, despite the nurses' obvious dislike of the patient and obvious lack of desire to help her.
- Go into the patient's room by myself, assess her needs for the simple purpose of relaying them to the nurse, and then not do anything to meet any of her needs myself.
- Enter the patient's room by myself, assess her needs, assure her I would try to help her meet her needs once the nurse be-
came available, and then drop the ball in the end, not helping her much myself or with the nurse.
- Go into her room by myself, assess her needs, assure her I would help her meet her needs, and take the steps to meet them later in the shift when I had more time.
- Proceed into her room by myself, assess her needs, assure her I would help her meet them, and take the steps to meet them immediately and throughout the whole shift.
- Ignore the patient, stating that meeting her needs was not my job, but encourage the nurses to go into the room to assess and meet her needs.

(continued)

Reflective Practice
Challenge to Ethical and Legal Skills (Continued)

Evaluating a Good Outcome: How Do I Define Success?

- The patient's needs are assessed and met by the most compassionate and most qualified professional possible.
- The patient feels heard and respected.
- I feel respected, feeling that I used my professional patient-care skills to the best of my ability to facilitate resolution of the patient's situation.
- The patient's inherent dignity, worth, and uniqueness is respected by everyone who comes into contact with her.

- The patient remains the primary commitment for me and the nurses.
- The patient feels that she is the primary commitment for the nurse and me.
- The health, safety, and rights of the patient are promoted, advocated for, and protected.
- The integrity of my patient, myself, and my fellow nurses is preserved.

Personal Learning: Here's to the Future!

Immediately upon starting my shift, I went into Ms. Warner's room to see what the problem was. She told me, in tears, that she's had to go to the bathroom for the past 2 hours, and that no one would help her. As a result, she ended up urinating on herself in bed. I immediately helped her out of bed into a chair, gave her soap and towels to start washing herself, and set about changing her linens. All the while, I listened to her talk about how humiliated and upset she was about having been forced to "wet the bed." She also was upset that she'd ruined the only pair of underwear she had with her in the hospital. So I washed the underwear in the sink for her. I asked her questions about what had happened that morning and validated her feelings. I helped her finish bathing, set her up to be sitting comfortably in the chair, and got her lunch tray, which I then set up for her. Although, for the most part, she could feed herself, her CVA had left her with some residual weakness, necessitating some help with opening containers, cutting foods, and placing items within her reach on the tray. She also wanted me to bring her the phone and help her dial, which I did. I let her eat and talk on the phone alone, promising I would come back to check on her soon.

Throughout the rest of the shift, I peeked my head into her room every half hour or so, eventually helping her back into her

bed after she was comfortable, fed, and less upset. Probably the most important thing I did for her, besides resolving the wet bed situation, was to listen to her as she purged her feelings. I validated her feelings and did everything in my power to make sure that she experienced no further episodes of disrespect. Unfortunately, while the patient's needs were met by the most compassionate professional possible (me), they were not met by the most qualified professional possible (the nurse). I believe the patient did feel heard and respected after our interactions. However, she stated that she felt ignored after her interactions with the nurses and physicians.

I felt that my actions were respected because none of the nurses gave me a difficult time or made fun of me for taking the extra time to soothe this patient. I did feel that I provided professional patient care to this patient in the best manner I knew. I respected her inherent dignity, worth, and uniqueness, and I believe the patient felt my primary commitment was to her. Unfortunately, this only highlighted the fact that no one else's primary commitment had been to her. I certainly promoted, advocated for, and strove to protect this patient's health, safety, and rights. However, it seemed the nurses went out of their way not to do that for this patient.

Reflection

How do you think you would respond in a similar situation? Why? What does this tell you about yourself and about the adequacy of your skills for professional practice? What reasons can you postulate to account for the nursing staff's actions? Would these reasons be justified? Can you think of other ways to respond? What other skills (cognitive, interpersonal, technical, ethical/legal) would you need to respond well in this situation? Do you think the nursing student should have approached the nursing staff about what she

had found? Did the nursing student violate any ethical or legal principles based on her position as a nursing technician? Please explain. Do you agree with the criteria to evaluate a successful outcome? Did the nursing student meet the criteria. Please support your response.

Tracey Sara Miller, Georgetown University

The steps of the nursing process were legitimized in 1973, when the ANA Congress for Nursing Practice developed Standards of Practice to guide nursing performance. These standards, which were revised in 1991, 1998, and 2003 appear in Chapter 1. In the latest edition of the standards of practice, the ANA lists six separate steps of the nursing process: assessment, diagnosis, outcome identification, planning, implementation and evaluation. Although the ANA refers to a six-step nursing process, many practitioners still commonly refer to a five-step nursing process in which outcome identification and

planning are combined into one step. The five-step nursing process is presented throughout this textbook.

The Canadian Nurses Association (1987) also has a standard noting that nursing practice requires the effective use of the nursing process. The standards for nursing practice were quickly reflected in revised nurse practice acts in many states and provinces.

The Joint Commission on Accreditation of Healthcare Organizations requires that care be documented according to the nursing process, and the National League for Nursing has recommended that educational programs incorporate the nursing process as their intellectual process. In 1982, the state board examinations for professional nursing practice underwent major revisions and began to use the nursing process as an organizing concept. The revised examinations are structured to test the practitioner's ability to assess patients; to diagnose health problems amenable to nursing therapy; and to plan, implement, and evaluate nursing care. The examinations had previously organized content on a medical model, structured according to medical specialties—medicine, surgery, maternity, pediatrics, and psychiatry.

Description of the Nursing Process

The **nursing process** is a systematic method that directs the nurse and patient as together they accomplish the following: (1) **assess** the patient to determine the need for nursing care; (2) determine **nursing diagnoses** for actual and potential health problems; (3) identify **expected outcomes** and **plan** care; (4) **implement** the care; and (5) **evaluate** the results. The steps in this patient-centered, outcome-oriented process are interrelated; each step depends on the accuracy of the steps preceding it. The process provides a framework that enables the nurse and patient to accomplish the following:

- Systematically collect patient data (assessing)
- Clearly identify patient strengths and actual and potential problems (diagnosing)
- Develop a holistic plan of individualized care that specifies the desired patient goals and related outcomes and the nursing interventions most likely to assist the patient to meet those expected outcomes (planning)
- Execute the plan of care (implementing)
- Evaluate the effectiveness of the plan of care in terms of patient goal achievement (evaluating)

Consider Addie Warner, the elderly patient who had suffered a CVA and is considered "demanding" by the staff. The nurse integrates the use of this framework to determine the patient's presenting problem, that is, the reason for using the call light. By systematically collecting information, determining the patient's strengths and needs, quickly developing a plan for these needs, executing it, and then determining the effectiveness of the plan, the nurse provides the patient with safe, quality effective care.

The five steps of the nursing process are shown in Figure 11-1 and described in Table 11-1. In each step of the process, the nurse and patient work together as partners (Fig. 11-2); the patient's health state and resources influence the patient's level of participation. When the patient is an infant or is unconscious or uncooperative, the steps of the process are worked through with the help of a family member or support person whenever possible.

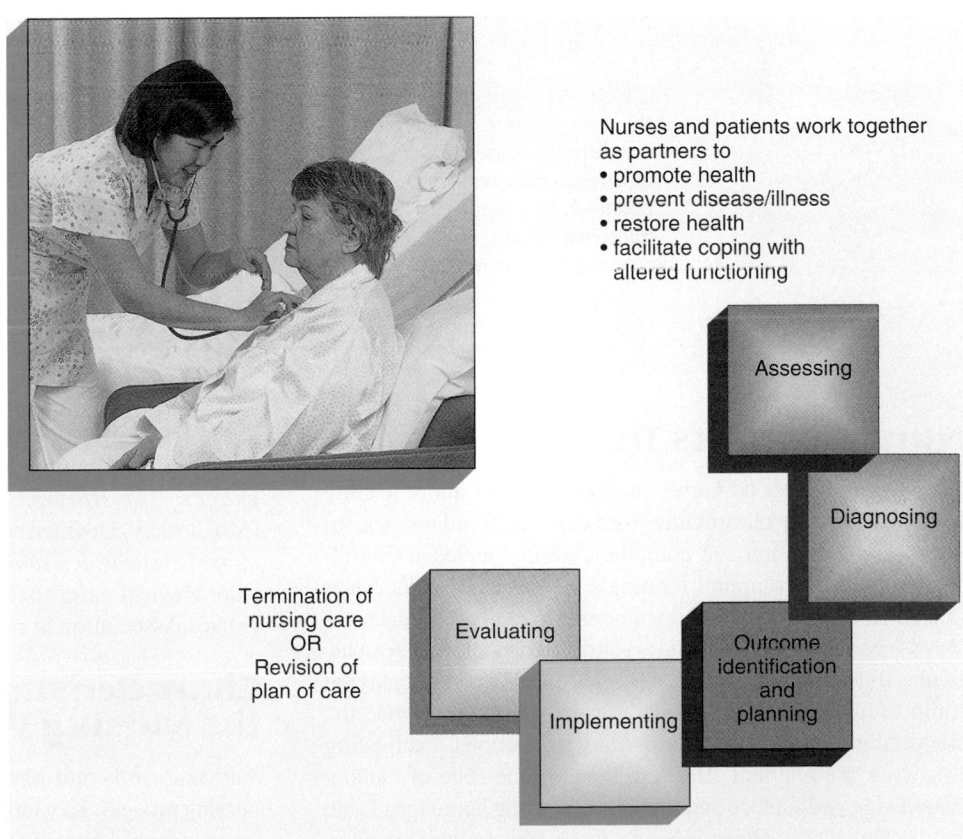

Nurses and patients work together as partners to
- promote health
- prevent disease/illness
- restore health
- facilitate coping with altered functioning

Assessing

Diagnosing

Outcome identification and planning

Implementing

Evaluating

Termination of nursing care OR Revision of plan of care

FIGURE 11-1 The steps in the patient-centered, outcome-oriented nursing process are dynamic and interrelated. Each of the five steps depends on the accuracy of the preceding step. (Photo © B. Proud.)

TABLE 11-1 Overview of the Nursing Process

Component	Description	Purpose	Activities
Assessing	Collection, validation, and communication of patient data	Make a judgment about the patient's health status, ability to manage his or her own healthcare, and need for nursing. Plan individualized holistic care that draws on patient strengths and is responsive to changes in the patient's conditions.	1. Establish the database: • Nursing history • Physical assessment • Review of patient record and nursing literature • Consultation with patient's support people and healthcare professionals 2. Continuously update the database. 3. Validate data. 4. Communicate data.
Diagnosing	Analysis of patient data to identify patient strengths and health problems that independent nursing intervention can prevent or resolve	Develop a prioritized list of nursing diagnoses.	1. Interpret and analyze patient data. 2. Identify patient strengths and health problems. 3. Formulate and validate nursing diagnoses. 4. Develop prioritized list of nursing diagnoses.
Outcome identification and planning	Specification of (1) patient outcomes to prevent, reduce, or resolve the problems identified in the nursing diagnoses; and (2) related nursing interventions	Develop an individualized plan of nursing care.	1. Establish priorities. 2. Write outcomes, and develop an evaluative strategy. 3. Select nursing interventions. 4. Communicate plan of nursing care.
Implementing	Carrying out the plan of care	Assist patients to achieve desired outcomes—promote wellness, prevent disease and illness, restore health, facilitate coping with altered functioning.	1. Carry out the plan of care. 2. Continue data collection, and modify the plan of care as needed. 3. Document care.
Evaluating	Measuring the extent to which the patient has achieved the outcomes specified in the plan of care; identifying factors that positively or negatively influenced outcome achievement; revising the plan of care if necessary	Continue, modify, or terminate nursing care.	1. Measure how well the patient has achieved desired outcomes. 2. Identify factors that contribute to the patient's success or failure. 3. Modify the plan of care (if indicated.)

Nursing Process Trends

Although experienced nurses might tell stories about lengthy handwritten plans of individualized care, the trend today is toward standardization and computerization. Nurses at centralized or bedside computer terminals have access to databases that allow them to plan and document care easily. Critical pathways (see Chap. 14), which target desired outcomes for particular illnesses, procedures, or conditions and accompanying multidisciplinary staff actions along a timeline, provide the standard guidelines for care in many institutions. Facilitating this work are national efforts to develop the state of nursing knowledge and science and a standard nursing language (Table 11-2). This work is described in subsequent chapters on diag-

nosis, planning, and implementation. Two recent milestone monographs in nursing science are *Unifying Nursing Languages: The Harmonization of NANDA, NIC, and NOC* (McCloskey, Dochterman, & Jones, 2003) and *Clinical Information Systems: A Framework for Reaching the Vision* (American Medical Informatics Association Staff with American Nurses Association Staff, 2002).

Characteristics of the Nursing Process

Various words and phrases have been used to describe the nursing process. Key descriptors include systematic, dynamic, interpersonal, outcome oriented, and universally applicable.

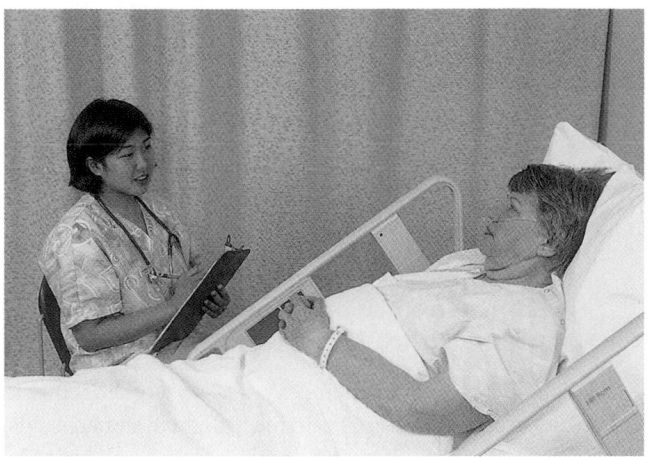

FIGURE 11-2 Nurses work collaboratively with patients when using the nursing process to plan and deliver care.   (Photo © B. Proud.)

tivity that precedes it and influences the actions that follow it. Without a complete and accurate database, the nurse cannot identify patient strengths and problems. Lacking knowledge of these, it is impossible for the nurse and patient to develop a plan of care based on realistic and valued patient goals. Unless the goals and outcomes are well written, nursing actions and evaluation lack focus and might be ineffective. The nursing process directs each step of nursing care in a sequential, ordered manner.

Dynamic

Although the nursing process is presented as an orderly progression of steps, in reality, there is great interaction and overlapping among the five steps. No one step in the nursing process is a one-time phenomenon; each step flows into the next step. In some nursing situations, all five stages occur almost simultaneously.

Systematic

Each nursing activity is part of an ordered sequence of activities. Moreover, each activity depends on the accuracy of the ac-

Interpersonal

Always at the heart of nursing is the human being. Read one student's account of this truth in the accompanying box, Through

---

TABLE 11-2 Examples of Groups Developing Standard Nursing Language*

Group Name	Focus	Purpose
North American Nursing Diagnosis Association (NANDA)	Diagnoses	Identify, label, validate, and classify health problems that nurses diagnose and treat (for listing, see Nursing Diagnosis Quick Reference Section). (NANDA, 2001). **Website:** http://www.nanda.org/html/about.html
Nursing Interventions Classification (NIC)	Interventions	Identify, label, validate, and classify actions nurses perform, including interventions directly with patients (eg, teaching) and those done indirectly (eg, obtaining laboratory studies) (McCloskey & Bulechek, 2000). **Website:** http://www.nursing.uiowa.edu/centers/cncce/nic/NIC%203%20Label%20Definitions.pdf
Nursing-Sensitive Outcomes Classification (NOC)	Outcomes	Identify, label, validate, and classify nursing-sensitive patient outcomes and indicators to evaluate the validity and usefulness of the classification, and define and test measurement procedures for the outcomes and indicators (Johnson, Maas, & Moorhead, 2000). **Website:** http://coninfo.nursing.uiowa.edu/noc/index.htm
Omaha Nursing Classification System for Community Health	Diagnoses, Interventions, Outcomes	Facilitate practice, documentation, and information management in home care and community health nursing by describing and measuring health-related problems, interventions, and outcomes of care. (Martin & Scheet, 1992). **Website:** http://con.ufl.edu/omaha/omahas.htm
Perioperative Nursing Data Set (PNDS)	Diagnoses, Interventions, Outcomes	Develop, refine, and validate a structured nursing vocabulary that reflects nursing responsibilities and patient outcomes related to perioperative patients' experience from preadmission until discharge. (Beyea, 2000). **Website:** http://www.aorn.org/research/pnds.htm
Home Health Care Classification (HHCC)	Diagnoses, Interventions, Outcomes	Provide a structure for documenting and classifying home health and ambulatory care. **Website:** http://www.sabacare.com
International Classification for Nursing Practice (ICNP®)	Diagnoses, Interventions, Outcomes	Capture nursing's contributions to health and provide a framework into which existing vocabularies and classifications can be cross-mapped, enabling comparison of nursing data from various countries throughout the world. **Website:** http://www.icn.ch/icnp.htm

*The terms *uniform nursing language*, *standard nursing language*, and *structured nursing vocabularies* often are used interchangeably.
Used with permission. Alfaro-LeFevre, R. (2002). *Applying nursing process* (5th ed.). Philadelphia: Lippincott Williams & Wilkins, p. 85.

Through the Eyes of a Student

My first experience with an open wound was with a woman who had a stage IV sacral decubitus. I needed to do a dressing change with packing. I was fearful of what the wound would look like. I thought for sure I was going to be "grossed out," and I was—not by the appearance of the wound, but by the odor. The stench was awful! I started to feel queasy, and I began to sweat, and I thought I was going to pass out and fall right over on the patient. While I was packing the wound, I kept thinking that I was never going to get out of that room. I looked over at my clinical instructor and searched her face for approval of my technique, and I wondered if she also smelled anything and if it was making her feel sick too!

After the procedure was over and I left the room, I asked my instructor if all wounds smell that awful and would the smell always make me feel sick. Her response was that sometimes an odor will be really bad, and it might make me feel sick. With this kind of reassurance, I thought this is it—I never want to smell that again, and no way do I want to be a nurse.

Later I realized that I had forgotten there was someone else in that room: the patient. She had to stay in there with that wound and its odor. It was for this reason I changed my mind about leaving nursing. I remembered that it was wanting to help patients to deal with their wounds that made me decide to be a nurse in the first place.

—Barbara L. Dlugosz
Holy Family College, Philadelphia, PA

the Eyes of a Student. The nursing process ensures that nurses are patient centered rather than task centered (Fig. 11-3). Rather than simply approaching a patient to take vital signs, the nurse might ask "How are you today, Mr. Byrd? Are our nursing actions helping you to achieve your goals? What are the most important things you'd like me to do?" The nurse might also consider any new data that indicate a need to modify the patient's plan of care.

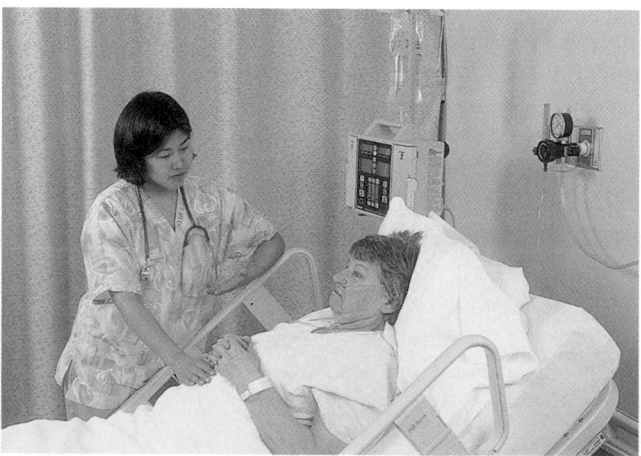

FIGURE 11-3 Nurses focus on people, not problems or tasks. The nursing process is patient-centered, not task-centered.   (Photo © B. Proud.)

Consider Charlotte Horvath, the single mother who requires wound care teaching but has failed to attend any scheduled teaching sessions. Incorporating the interpersonal aspect, the nurse would investigate with Ms. Horvath the reasons underlying her inability to make the teaching sessions. This investigation may reveal many reasons, possibly inability to get away from work, fear, feelings of being overwhelmed, or lack of awareness about the importance of the wound care.

The nursing process encourages nurses to work together to help patients use their strengths to meet all their human needs. This is different from viewing the patient as a "problem to be solved" and interacting mechanically to provide the solution. Working intimately with patients helps nurses to explore their own strengths and limitations and to develop themselves personally and professionally.

Outcome Oriented

The nursing process offers a means for nurses and patients to work together to identify specific outcomes related to health promotion, disease and illness prevention, health restoration, and coping with altered functioning; to determine which outcomes are most important to the patient; and to match them with the appropriate nursing actions. When these are recorded in the plan of care, each nurse can quickly determine the patient's priorities and begin nursing with a clear sense of how to proceed. The patient benefits from continuity of care, and each nurse's care moves the patient closer to outcome achievement.

Universally Applicable in Nursing Situations

The one constant in healthcare is change. When nurses have a working knowledge of the nursing process, they find that they can practice nursing with well or ill people, young or old, in any type of practice setting. The student's efforts to master the nursing process result in possession of a valuable tool that can be used with ease in any nursing situation.

It should be clear from the preceding discussion that the nursing process provides a framework for all the nurse's activities. In each nurse–patient interaction, it is important to assess the patient, note any significant alterations in health status, determine whether the nursing action is helping the patient achieve his or her goals, and modify the plan of care as necessary. Thus, the nurse who feeds a child through a special tube as ordered by a physician continually assesses how the child is responding to the feeding and whether the child or family will be able to manage the feedings independently when the child is discharged. Depending on the results of the nursing assessment, new nursing diagnoses might be needed, along with related additions to the plan of care. The nursing process offers direction for all the activities carried out by the nurse when caring for patients.

Problem-Solving and the Nursing Process

One of the strengths of the nursing process is that it is based on a methodology that is familiar to most nursing students—problem-solving. Problem-solving is a basic life skill; identifying a problem and then taking steps to resolve it are a matter of common sense. However, different approaches to problem-solving yield different results, some of which are more successful than others.

Trial-and-Error Problem-Solving

Trial-and-error problem-solving involves testing any number of solutions until one is found that works for that particular problem. This method is not efficient for the nurse and can be dangerous to the patient; it is, therefore, not recommended as a guide for nursing practice. For example, although you might enjoy experimenting with different types of ethnic food as you discover and develop personal food preferences, you would not want to use the trial-and-error method of determining food preferences for a dehydrated and malnourished patient. You want to know, based on clinical research, exactly what food and fluid supplements are most likely to reverse his or her deficiencies.

Consider Jermaine Byrd, the patient who has returned from vascular surgery and whose posterior tibial pulse cannot be palpated. The nurse might use trial-and-error to determine if the pulse is indeed absent or just difficult to palpate or locate. For example, the nurse might try to reposition the fingers for palpation or apply less pressure during palpation to determine if the pulse can be palpated.

Scientific Problem-Solving

Scientific problem-solving is a systematic, seven-step, problem-solving process that involves (1) problem identification, (2) data collection, (3) hypothesis formulation, (4) plan of action, (5) hypothesis testing, (6) interpretation of results, and (7) evaluation, resulting in conclusion or revision of the study. This method is used most correctly in a controlled laboratory setting but is closely related to the more general problem-solving processes commonly used by healthcare professionals as they work with patients, such as the nursing process.

Again, think back to Jermaine Byrd, the postoperative patient with a nonpalpable pulse. The nurse would use scientific problem-solving to investigate the situation. For example, after attempts at repositioning yield no change, the nurse would collect more data, such as the temperature and the color of the patient's extremity when compared with the opposite leg, existence of pulses above and below the posterior tibial pulse, complaints of pain, numbness or tingling in the extremity, and the patient's overall condition. These findings would lead the nurse to identify if the patient was experiencing vascular compromise, the pulse was difficult to palpate, or the nurse needed more skill in palpation. In addition, the nurse could summon the assistance of another nurse to negate or validate the findings. Once the problem is identified, the nurse would then be able to plan care appropriately to meet the patient's need.

Intuitive Thinking

For years, nurse theorists and educators argued that clinical judgments should be based on data alone (the logical, scientific, evidence-based method), in an attempt to establish nursing as a science, worthy of the respect of other professions. Today, nurses acknowledge the role of **intuitive thinking** in clinical decision making. Many veteran nurses can describe situations in which an "inner prompting" led to a quick nursing intervention that saved a patient's life. When they directly apprehend a situation based on its similarity or dissimilarity to other situations, they use intuitive problem-solving. A recovery room nurse who realizes that a postoperative patient is "going bad" before there are measurable signs to suggest trouble is using intuitive problem-solving, as is an oncology nurse who somehow senses the right moment to teach, offer encouragement, affirm, or simply listen.

Advocates of intuition recommend the following:

- Welcoming flashes of intuition as additions to logical reasoning, rather than as disruptions
- Validating intuitions: when an intuition cannot be validated (eg, when the nurse senses that something is wrong with the patient, although there are no clinical signs), careful monitoring of the patient should be initiated
- Furthering nursing research to help find ways to (1) cultivate intuition and its typical results (accurate and early diagnosis, vigilant monitoring, better patient care), and (2) document the information intuition supplies (Rew, 1987)

Beginning nurses must use nursing knowledge and scientific problem-solving as the basis of care they give; intuitive problem-solving comes with years of practice and observation. If the beginning nurse has an intuition about a patient, that information should be discussed with the supervisor.

Critical Thinking: Intuitive, Logical, or Both

While this text makes a strong case for clinical reasoning that is logical, scientific, and evidence-based, it also promotes clinical reasoning that is creative and intuitive. Alfaro-LeFevre, an expert in critical thinking, is quick to note that critical thinking is contextual and changes depending on the circumstances. As examples, she cites brainstorming sessions as a good method for nurturing intuition because logical thinking might constrain and block ideas. On the other hand, developing policies, procedures, and plans of care requires more logical, evidence-based thought. In summary, when intuition is used alone, there are increased risks and fewer benefits. Intuition often moves problem-solving forward quickly, but it might result in a lot of trial-and-error approaches. Logic is the safest approach, but it doesn't foster out-of-the-box ideas and might inhibit right-brain thinkers from getting started. Pairing intuitive and logical thinkers who have learned specific strategies to promote reasoning (eg, mind mapping) can bring great results (Alfaro-LeFevre, 2004).

Documenting the Nursing Process

The ability to communicate clearly is a critical nursing skill. Accurate, concise, timely, and relevant documentation provides all the members of the caregiving team with a picture of the patient. The patient record is the chief means of communication among members of the interdisciplinary team. Legally speaking, a nursing action not documented is a nursing action not performed. If accused of negligent care, a nurse might tell the court that she faithfully assessed the patient's needs, diagnosed problems, and implemented and evaluated an effective plan of care. Unless the patient's health records contain documentation supporting her claims, however, the court has no reason to accept her word rather than that of the patient or family who are claiming that such care was not given. Each chapter in this unit offers specific documentation guidelines for nursing process activities; Chapter 17 discusses documentation in general. It is helpful to practice documentation while learning any given nursing activity; like any other nursing skill, documentation improves with practice. Examples of nursing documentation, nursing assessments, plans of care, and notes are provided throughout this text.

Benefits of the Nursing Process

When used well, the nursing process achieves for the patient scientifically based, holistic, individualized care; the opportunity to work collaboratively with nurses; and continuity of care. Nurses who use the nursing process in a thoughtful and systematic way achieve a clear, efficient, and cost-effective plan of action by which the entire nursing team can achieve the best results for patients; the satisfaction that they are making an important "difference" in the lives of their patients; and the opportunity to grow professionally as they evaluate the effectiveness of interventions and variables that contribute positively or negatively to the patient's achievement of valued outcomes. See Box 11-1 for an example of the nursing process in action.

Evaluating the Use of the Nursing Process

The chapters that follow describe each step of the nursing process in detail. Student nurses beginning to use the nursing process should evaluate their growing skill in using the nursing process correctly. Box 11-2 presents a checklist to help evaluate this personal skill in using the nursing process.

BOX 11-1 Example of the Nursing Process in Action

Assessing
You are checking on a patient who had abdominal surgery yesterday and hear that the patient has considerable pain. "It kept me up all night." The patient has been reluctant to ask for any pain medication, fearing effect of the drug. "I don't want to become a junkie." The patient's blood pressure and pulse rate are slightly elevated.

Diagnosing
You analyze the data above and write the nursing diagnosis: *Unrelieved pain related to a fear of taking pain-relieving medications.* The patient agrees that this is becoming a problem.

Outcome Identification and Planning
You decide to work with the patient to achieve the outcome: *By 3:00 p.m. patient reports sufficient relief of pain to enable him to rest and to get out of bed to go to the bathroom.* The patient wants to accomplish the outcome. You identify teaching as the primary nursing intervention.

Implementing
After asking the patient about his experiences with pain-relieving medications, you explain that although many of these drugs are addictive when abused, there is no harm if they are taken as prescribed postoperatively. You also explain that it is important for him to experience enough pain relief to be able to cough and deep breathe, ambulate, and do other things important to his recovery. You suggest that the medication will be most effective if taken before his pain peaks and becomes intense. You administer the prescribed medication for pain when the patient indicates that he is willing to give it a try.

Evaluating
After enough time has elapsed for the medication to take effect, you check back with the patient to evaluate whether he has obtained relief and met his outcome. If the patient is satisfied and you both feel comfort is no longer a problem, you terminate the plan of care for this diagnosis. If the patient still feels pain or is dissatisfied with the medication, each of the preceding steps of the nursing process is reevaluated, and necessary changes are made in the plan of care.

BLENDED SKILLS AND CRITICAL THINKING

The primary purpose of the nursing process is to help nurses manage each patient's care scientifically, holistically, and creatively. To do this successfully, the nurse needs many cognitive, technical, interpersonal, and ethical/legal skills, along with the willingness to use them creatively and critically when working with patients to promote or restore health, to

---

BOX 11-2 Checklist for Evaluating Your Use of the Nursing Process

Assessing

- [ ] The initial database is obtained by means of a nursing history and nursing examination.
- [ ] Assessment data are documented:
  - [ ] Accurately—Questionable data are validated.
  - [ ] Completely—Use of a systematic guide ensures that recorded data describe (1) the patient's functional ability to meet each basic human need, and (2) responses to health and illness.
  - [ ] Concisely—Irrelevant data and meaningless generalizations are avoided.
  - [ ] Factuality—Patient behaviors are recorded rather than the nurse's interpretation of these behaviors.
- [ ] The initial database communicates a "real sense" of the patient that makes possible individualized care.
- [ ] Focused assessment data are recorded for each patient problem.
- [ ] Data collection and documentation are ongoing and responsive to changes in the patient's condition.

Diagnosing

- [ ] A prioritized list of nursing diagnoses is on the plan of care.
- [ ] Each nursing diagnosis describes an actual or potential patient health problem that independent nursing intervention can prevent or resolve. Each nursing diagnosis:
  - [ ] Is derived from an accurate and validated interpretation of a cluster of significant patient data or "cues"
  - [ ] Contains a precise problem statement describing what is unhealthy about the patient and what needs to change—suggests patient goals
  - [ ] Identifies factors that contribute to the problem (etiology)—these suggest nursing interventions
  - [ ] Uses nonjudgmental language and is written using legally advisable terms
- [ ] Old nursing diagnoses are deleted from the plan of care once resolved, and new diagnoses are added as soon as identified.

Outcome Identification and Planning

- [ ] A comprehensive, individualized, and up-to-date plan of care that specifies patient outcomes and nursing orders for each nursing diagnosis is developed with the assistance of the patient and family.

- [ ] Planning is comprehensive:
  - [ ] Initial
  - [ ] Ongoing
  - [ ] Discharge
- [ ] Long-term goals alert the entire nursing team to realistic patient expectations after discharge.
- [ ] Short-term outcomes:
  - [ ] When achieved, demonstrate a resolution of the problem specified in the nursing diagnosis
  - [ ] Describe a single, observable, and measurable patient behavior
  - [ ] Are valued by the patient and family
  - [ ] Are realistic in terms of the resources of the patient and the nurse
- [ ] Nursing orders:
  - [ ] Clearly and concisely describe the nursing intervention to be performed (ongoing assessment; nursing treatments and procedures; teaching, counseling, advocacy)
  - [ ] Are individualized to the patient
  - [ ] Are consistent with standards of care and supportive of other therapies
  - [ ] Are effective in accomplishing the desired patient outcomes
- [ ] The plan of care encourages patient and family participation.

Implementing

- [ ] The patient record contains daily documentation of the nursing measures used to (1) assist the patient to meet basic human needs, (2) resolve health problems, and (3) implement select aspects of the medical plan of care.
- [ ] The plan of care is implemented:
  - [ ] Competently
  - [ ] Confidently
  - [ ] Caringly
  - [ ] Creatively

Evaluating

- [ ] Evaluative statements are recorded on the plan of care to document the patient's level of outcome achievement at targeted times.
- [ ] Ongoing evaluation of the patient's responses to the plan of care are used to make decisions about terminating, continuing, or modifying nursing care.

---

prevent disease or illness, and to facilitate coping with altered functioning.

Defining the Four Blended Skills

Before studying each step of the nursing process in more depth, it is useful to look at the skills essential to nursing practice. Understanding their importance helps the student work consciously to develop them while beginning to master the nursing process. Cognitive and technical skills equip nurses to manage the clinical problems stemming from the patient's changing health or illness state. Interpersonal and ethical skills

are essential, however, for nurses concerned about the patient's broader well-being.

Few nurses excel naturally in all four of these skills, and even experienced nurses continue working on becoming more proficient in the skills that lead to excellence. The remainder of this chapter discusses the blended skills that are essential to professional caregiving and successful use of the nursing process. Please note that each chapter in this text opens with a feature entitled *Focusing on Blended Skills*. Each chapter also contains a feature entitled *Reflective Practice: Developing Blended Skills*. These displays are written by nursing students.

Cognitive Skills

Cognitively skilled nurses think about the nature of things sufficiently to "make sense" of their world and to grasp conceptually what is necessary to achieve valued goals. Cognitively skilled nurses are able to accomplish the following:

- Offer a scientific rationale for the patient's plan of care (prerequisite sciences include nursing and medical science as well as basic sciences, such as chemistry, microbiology, anatomy, physiology, psychology, sociology, and anthropology)
- Select those nursing interventions that are most likely to yield the desired outcomes
- Use critical thinking to solve problems creatively

Cognitively skilled nurses are critical thinkers. **Critical thinking** is defined as "a systematic way to form and shape one's thinking. It functions purposefully and exactingly. It is thought that is disciplined, comprehensive, based on intellectual standards, and, as a result, well-reasoned" (Paul, 1993, p. 20). Paul's four domains of critical thinking (Box 11-3) include elements of thought (the basic building blocks of thinking), abilities (the skills essential to higher-order thinking), affective dimensions, and intellectual standards. Central to Paul's work are carefully delineated standards, potential problems, and principles.

Technical Skills

Technically skilled nurses manipulate equipment skillfully to produce a desired outcome or result. Technical competence involves everything from manual dexterity and good eye–hand coordination to an ability to troubleshoot when equipment malfunctions, based on an understanding of the technical workings of the equipment. Technically skilled nurses are able to accomplish the following:

- Use technical equipment with sufficient competence and ease to achieve goals with minimal distress to participants involved
- Creatively adapt equipment and technical procedures to the needs of particular patients in diverse circumstances

Interpersonal Skills

Interpersonally skilled nurses establish and maintain caring relationships that facilitate the achievement of valued goals while simultaneously affirming the worth of those in the relationship. Nurses skilled in interpersonal relations are able to accomplish the following:

- Use interactions with patients, their significant others, and colleagues to affirm their worth
- Elicit the personal strengths and abilities of patients and their significant others to achieve valued health goals
- Provide the healthcare team with knowledge about the patient's valued goals and expectations
- Work collaboratively with the healthcare team as a respected and credible colleague to reach valued goals

Ethical/Legal Skills

Ethically and legally skilled nurses conduct themselves in a manner consistent with their personal moral code and professional role responsibilities. Nurses skilled in ethical/legal competence are able to accomplish the following:

- Be trusted to act in ways that advance the interests of patients
- Be accountable for their practice to themselves, the patients they serve, the caregiving team, and society
- Act as effective patient advocates
- Mediate ethical conflicts among the patient, significant others, healthcare team, and other interested parties
- Practice nursing faithful to the tenets of professional codes of ethics and appropriate standards of practice
- Use legal safeguards that reduce the risk of litigation

> *Recall Addie Warner, the elderly patient described in the Reflective Practice display? By responding to the patient's needs, the nurse was able to develop a trusting relationship with the patient, thereby allowing the patient to verbalize her frustrations.*

Developing Cognitive Skills

The exercises below should help you to develop the ability to think critically in professional practice.

Developing the Method of Critical Thinking

Nurses who wish to develop the critical thinking skills essential to quality nursing practice will find it helpful when posed with a thinking challenge to work methodically through a set of five types of considerations. These are the purpose of thinking, adequacy of knowledge, potential problems, helpful resources, and critique of judgment/decision.

Purpose of Thinking

The first step when thinking critically about a situation is to identify the purpose or goal of your thinking. This helps to discipline your thinking by directing all thoughts toward the goal. The purpose of critical thinking might be to make a judgment about a particular patient or situation or to make a decision about how best to intervene.

Adequacy of Knowledge

At the outset of critical thinking, it is important for you to judge whether the knowledge you have is accurate, complete, and relevant. If you reason with false information or a lack of important data, it is impossible to draw a sound conclusion. You also want to be sure that you understand all the details relevant to the issue. What is at stake? How much time do you have to make a decision? How much room is there for error?

> *Consider Addie Warner, the patient described as "demanding" by the nursing staff. Rather than accept the staff's description, the nurse answers the patient's call light, thereby obtaining information from which to make an informed decision.*

BOX 11-3 **The Four Domains of Critical Thinking**

I. Elements of Thought: The Basic Building Blocks of Thinking

Element	Fundamental Standard	Potential Problems	Principle
Purpose	1. Clarity of purpose 2. Significance of purpose 3. Achievability of purpose 4. Consistency of purpose	1. Unclear purpose 2. Trivial purpose 3. Unrealistic purpose 4. Contradictory purposes	All reasoning has a purpose.
Question at issue or central problem	1. Clarity of question 2. Significance of question 3. Answerability 4. Relevance	1. Unclear 2. Insignificant 3. Not answerable 4. Irrelevant	To settle a question, you must understand what it requires.
Point of view	1. Flexibility in point of view 2. Fairness of point of view 3. Clarity of point of view 4. Breadth of point of view	1. Restricted 2. Biased 3. Unclear 4. Narrow	Reasoning is better when multiple, relevant points of view are sought out, articulated clearly, empathized with fairly and logically, applied consistently and dispassionately.
Empirical dimension	1. Clear evidence 2. Relevant information 3. Fairly gathered and reported evidence 4. Accurate data 5. Adequate evidence 6. Consistently applied data	1. Unclear 2. Unfairly or self-servingly gathered 3. Inaccurate 4. Insufficient	Reasoning can only be as sound as the evidence it is based on.
Concepts and ideas	1. Clarity of concepts 2. Relevance of concepts 3. Depth of concepts 4. Neutrality of concepts	1. Unclear 2. Irrelevant 3. Superficial 4. Biased	Reasoning can only be as clear, relevant, and deep as the concepts that shape it.
Assumptions	1. Clarity of assumptions 2. Justifiability of assumptions 3. Consistency of assumptions	1. Unclear 2. Unjustified 3. Contradictory	Reasoning can only be as sound as the assumptions it makes.
Implications and consequences	1. Significance of implications 2. Realistic nature of implications 3. Clarity of articulated implications 4. Precision of articulated implications 5. Completeness of articulated implications	1. Unimportant 2. Unrealistic 3. Unclear 4. Imprecise 5. Incomplete	To reason through an issue or decision, you must understand the implications and consequences that follow from it.

II. Abilities: The Skills Essential to Higher-Order Thinking

- Ability to evaluate the credibility of sources of information
- Ability to analyze arguments, interpretations, beliefs, or theories
- Ability to clarify the meaning of words and phrases
- Ability to transfer insights into new contexts
- Ability to generate and assess possible solutions
- Ability to develop criteria for evaluation: clarify values and standards
- Ability to read, listen, write, and speak critically

III. Affective Dimensions: The Attitudes, Dispositions, Passions, and Traits of Mind Essential to Higher-Order Thinking in Real Settings

- Thinking independently
- Exercising fair-mindedness
- Developing insight into egocentricity and sociocentricity
- Developing intellectual humility and suspending judgment
- Developing intellectual courage
- Developing intellectual good faith and integrity
- Developing intellectual perseverance
- Developing confidence in reason
- Developing intellectual curiosity

IV. Intellectual Standards: The Standards Used to Critique Higher-Order Thinking

Clear	Precise
Specific	Accurate
Relevant	Plausible
Consistent	Logical
Deep	Broad
Complete	Significant
Adequate (for purpose)	Fair

Content from Paul, R. W. (1993). *Critical thinking: How to prepare students for a rapidly changing world*. Santa Rosa, CA: Foundation for Critical Thinking, pp. 123–132. Used with permission.

Potential Problems

As you become skilled in critical thinking, you will learn to "flag" and remedy the pitfalls to sound reasoning. Common problems include working with untested or faulty assumptions, accepting an unproven claim or line of argument, allowing bias to color your thinking, and reasoning illogically, such as making a generalization on the basis of a single experience or case, or allowing emotion to rule reason. The more familiar you are with these common impediments to critical thinking, the easier it is to detect them in your own thinking.

Helpful Resources

Wise professionals are quick to recognize their limits and to seek help in remedying their deficiencies. Experienced clinicians know that learning is continuous and expect their practice to present challenges that demand new knowledge. Critical thinkers know what help they need to assist their reasoning and what resources to tap. Key resources include experienced clinicians, texts and journals, institutional policies and procedures, and professional groups and writings.

Critique of Judgment/Decision

Ultimately, you must identify alternative judgments or decisions, weigh the merits of each, and reach a conclusion. It is helpful to try to predict the consequences of your major options before concluding your reasoning. You will also want to evaluate the alternative you selected as your decision begins to influence your actions.

After using this method to work through an intellectually challenging situation, critique your use of the method in light of the **standards for critical thinking:** clear, precise, specific, accurate, relevant, plausible, consistent, logical, deep, broad, complete, significant, adequate (for the purpose), and fair.

Focused Critical Thinking Guides

Focused Critical Thinking Guide 11-1 illustrates the use of these five considerations to facilitate critical thinking about a care dilemma experienced by a nursing student. The merits of thinking critically about which of the options is most likely to meet that patient's needs are readily apparent. Because nurses are accountable for the well-being of their patients, sloppy reasoning is both dangerous and inexcusable—even for someone new to nursing and clinical practice. Other examples of this method are found throughout the book.

Developing the Attitudes and Dispositions to Think Critically

Certain habitual dispositions are needed by anyone who wants to be a critical thinker. Some of the most important of these are described below. Review this list, and assess the degree to which the dispositions characterize your thinking.

Thinking Independently

Nurses who are independent thinkers are careful not to allow the status quo or a persuasive individual to control their thinking.

Remember Addie Warner, the elderly woman who was considered to be demanding by the staff? The nurse demonstrated independent thinking by not accepting the staff's description of the patient. Rather, the nurse confronted the situation, obtained information and then acted based on this information.

When confronted with an intellectual challenge, such as "Why is this patient so resistant to change?," they proceed cautiously, consulting with the patient and respected colleagues and reviewing the literature. Only then do they reach a clinical judgment. Compare this with a nurse who makes a snap judgment that a patient is "unreasonable" based on the comments of one nurse—even if this nurse is the nurse manager.

Recall Charlotte Horvath, the single mother needing wound care teaching? A nurse who is not an independent thinker might quickly assume that Ms. Horvath just wasn't interested in caring for her child at home. Conversely, the nurse who is an independent thinker would investigate the situation further before making a decision.

Being Fair-Minded

Nurses who are fair-minded are open to different points of view and hear all sides of an argument before making a judgment. When a patient complains about another nurse or a physician, a fair-minded nurse seeks to validate the complaint and talks with the person being complained about before reaching a decision. A fair-minded thinker recognizes the limits of being egocentric ("It's right because this is what I think!") and sociocentric ("It's right because this is the way Americans—or Philadelphians—think!").

Being Intellectually Humble

One can easily differentiate between nurses who are convinced that "they know it all" and those who are open and willing to learn. Intellectually humble nurses are learning all the time, often from patients and their nonprofessional caregivers, other colleagues, and the media. Never be afraid to say "I don't know the answer to that question, but I'll be happy to talk with you after I've had time to research the topic."

Being Intellectually Courageous

Nurses who are intellectually courageous are not afraid to challenge the status quo and "go against the flow." They resist the comment "But we've always done it that way here . . ." when their experience or intuition suggests that another way might be better. They are not afraid to ask "Is there something we might be able to do differently that would help this patient or situation?"

Demonstrating Good Faith and Integrity

Commitment to integrity helps nurses who are critical thinkers remain sensitive to discrepancies in the way one reasons in different situations and with different people. This sensitivity, for example, might result in our mind "throwing out a red flag" when it catches us reasoning unfairly.

Focused Critical Thinking Guide 11-1

Western vs. Alternative Medicine

You are a nursing student. Your friend, Amy Chang, confides to you that she is very worried about her grandmother. When you meet Mrs. Chang, she demonstrates many of the assessment findings related to congestive heart failure. Although her family has entreated her to seek medical attention, Mrs. Chang insists on relying on herbal teas and traditional Chinese remedies. Now 88 years old, Mrs. Chang came to America from mainland China when she was 14. Although she raised a family that is now thoroughly "Americanized," Mrs. Chang has resisted embracing her new culture and now wants nothing to do with "American medicine." Amy, who is also a nursing student, loves her grandmother dearly and is frustrated by her stubborn refusal to see an internist. Both of you have reason to believe that she could be helped by medical attention. What do you do?

1. **Identify Goal of Thinking**

   Clarify your thinking about alternative medicine so that you can decide how you ought to respond to Mrs. Chang's worsening physical condition.

2. **Assess Adequacy of Knowledge**

   Pertinent circumstances: Although you have strong reason to believe that Mrs. Chang is suffering from congestive heart failure, she has not been medically diagnosed, and you lack definitive knowledge about her medical condition and the likelihood that she would respond to treatment. You do know that she places a high value on traditional Chinese culture and strongly believes that if she is to be healed, the healing will result from herbal teas and traditional Chinese remedies. She has no confidence in American medicine. Her family describe her as being extremely strong-willed and very lovable. You do not know if she has the benefit of seeing a competent practitioner of Chinese medicine.

   Prerequisite knowledge: To decide how you should respond in this situation, you need to know that traditional Western medicine is not the only beneficial system of medicine. It would be helpful for you and Mrs. Chang's family to learn more about Chinese medicine and the probability of its benefiting her (as well as the possibility of its harming her) in her present condition. You will also need to learn more about what is essential to Mrs. Chang's well-being. How much value does she place on physical health? How important is it for her to live (and possibly die) within the familiar and comforting boundaries of her culture? You will want to assess what teaching, counseling, and support Mrs. Chang needs to reach an informed and voluntary decision that is right for her.

   Room for error: Because Mrs. Chang's life may literally be at stake, there is not much room for error in the manner you and her family choose to respond. Even if her condition is not life-threatening, her sense of well-being may be severely threatened if she feels forced to pursue treatment that is alien and frightening.

   Time constraints: Although you are uncertain about the seriousness of her condition, you understand that the sooner Mrs. Chang receives effective therapy, the better. Unless her condition suddenly deteriorates, this is not a decision that needs to be made within the next 24 hours.

3. **Address Potential Problems**

   The most serious obstacle to critical thinking in this situation would be an inability to weigh the respective merits of alternative healing systems. Cultural bias may result in the untested assumption that American medicine is necessarily superior to all other systems of healing and that it would be morally wrong to support a choice of anything else. The love of Mrs. Chang's family and their desire to do everything possible to keep her well may interfere with their ability to allow her the freedom to make the choice that is right for her.

4. **Consult Helpful Resources**

   Your first challenge will be to learn more about traditional Chinese medicine, and you will want to consult with local authorities as well as available literature. The National Institutes of Health have now established an Office of Alternative Medicine, which may provide helpful information and which is easily accessed through their web site. Your most important resource may be Mrs. Chang herself, and it will be important to try to learn from her as much as you can about what she values and what her goals are at this point in her life. You will also want to be sure that Mrs. Chang has the benefits of a competent practitioner of Chinese medicine.

5. **Critique Judgment/Decision**

   After getting to know Mrs. Chang better, you realize that she is firmly committed to her ways and adamant about not going to an American doctor or into a hospital at this point of her life. You (with her family) thus have only two options: to force her to see an internist against her will, possibly deceiving her to get her to the internist's office, or to support her choice to rely on familiar remedies, which may or may not successfully resolve her problems. The first alternative may save her life, and her family can see no other choice. You realize that by making this choice, the family is imposing its values on Mrs. Chang and violating her autonomy, her right to determine the course of her life. You decide to support her and to try to explain to her family the importance of doing this. You understand that if her condition is serious and her traditional remedies prove ineffective, her death may be hastened, but she accepts this consequence and prefers it to embracing an alien and frightening culture.

Being Curious and Persevering

Nurses who persevere intellectually resist "easy answers." When the answer to "Why is this patient so resistant to change?" comes back "Oh, that's just the way he is," the persevering nurse keeps questioning: "But why is he that way? What experiences, values, or beliefs have made him so resistant? Until we understand these things we won't be able to help him!"

Being Disciplined

Nurses who are disciplined are thorough and take the time necessary to reach well-reasoned conclusions. When an initial conclusion or judgment does not "feel right," they are willing to go back to try to reason out a better judgment. They consult wise colleagues and are not afraid of doing the hard work of critical thinking.

Being Creative

Thinking critically might mean "thinking outside the box." The solution to a challenge might involve resources as yet untapped, effective and cost-saving interventions as yet undiscovered and untried. The process of brainstorming might bring out, along with unworkable options, one or two realistic suggestions that would not have surfaced otherwise.

Demonstrating Confidence

Nurses who routinely think critically develop confidence in their judgments and are not afraid to take and defend a position. When challenged by a patient or colleague to defend a course of action, they can reply with confidence "I am doing it this way because research (or reason) convinced me that this is the best course of action."

Developing Technical Skills

Some people are naturally "good with their hands" and quickly master intricate procedures that involve working with technical equipment. Others have to practice procedures many times before they feel competent handling the equipment and performing clinical activities independently. Whatever your natural technical skill, you can help master the manual skills essential in the nursing process by developing the following habits:

- When a procedure demands manual dexterity, practice the necessary skill until you feel confident in its execution before attempting to perform it with a patient.
- Take time to familiarize yourself with new equipment before using it in a clinical procedure. Understand how it works and what supplies are needed to ensure optimal functioning. If possible, anticipate problems and know how to remedy them.
- Identify nurses who are technical experts, and ask them to share their secrets. Many experienced clinicians have developed quality, time-saving techniques they are willing to share.
- Never be ashamed to ask for help when feeling unsure of how to perform a procedure or manage equipment. Never

forget that the patient's well-being and sometimes the patient's life depend on your technical competence.

Many nursing procedures are described in the clinical chapters in this text. Performance checklists break each procedure down into its component parts, allowing you to evaluate your performance of each step of the procedure. This type of self-knowledge enables you to identify quickly and remedy recurrent deficiencies in technical skills.

Developing Interpersonal Skills

Characteristics of interpersonal caring that are essential to the practice of nursing include the following:
- Promotion of the dignity and respect of patients as people
- Centrality of the caring relationship
- Mutual enrichment of both participants in the nurse–patient relationship

Promoting Human Dignity and Respect

Nurses committed to respecting the human dignity of patients find it helpful to reflect on the following questions:
- What obligates me to respect patients' human dignity? Must all patients be respected equally? Are some patients more deserving of respect? Can a patient ever forfeit the right to be respected?
- What does it mean to respect the dignity of patients? What are five concrete ways I can demonstrate respect?
- What are my strengths and deficiencies when it comes to respecting patients?
- In what ways (if any) must I change to be faithful to the duty of respecting the dignity of patients?
- What patients most challenge my ability to give care respectfully? How do I respond to this challenge? What does this teach me for the future?

Nurses often underestimate their power to help a patient heal simply through their respectful and caring presence. Each time a nurse walks into a room, he or she communicates one of two messages: (1) "You are a job to be done. You mean nothing to me." or (2) "You are a person of worth, and I care about you." Even a 60-second nurse–patient interaction can enhance or jeopardize human well-being. It is important for nurses to be sensitive to what their looks, speech, and touch communicate to patients and colleagues. The more vulnerable the patient and the more threatened the patient's sense of self, the more powerful effect the nurse's message has on the recipient's sense of worth and well-being.

> *Consider Addie Warner, the patient described in the Reflective Practice display. Imagine the message that she received from the staff when she used her call light to ask for help. Most likely the message conveyed was negative. Compare this to the message communicated by the nursing student who helped get her out of bed and get washed, a more positive message supporting the patient's self-worth.*

The learning activity in Box 11-4 was developed for nurses caring for older patients in a nursing home. To help develop

BOX 11-4 **Developing Interpersonal Skills**

Human Dignity: How Who I Am as a Caregiver Affects Others

Description

The purpose of this exercise is to explore the notion of "therapeutic use of self." You will be challenged to reflect on the effect your looks, speech, and touch have on other people. Role play and guided discovery will be used to enable you to experience the affirming and negating influences of different means of human relating.

Objectives

Upon conclusion of this exercise, you will be able to:

1. Demonstrate how looks, words, and touch can be used to harm or benefit others
2. Describe how the way you approach others enhances or diminishes their well-being
3. Identify one care behavior you plan to modify to improve your nursing practice

Learning Activities

Invite an experienced nurse to demonstrate how looks, words, and touch can be used to communicate two different messages to others: "You are a job to be done; you mean nothing to me"; and "You are precious, and I care about you." After the demonstration, team up with another student, and experience giving and receiving these messages. Share the feelings you both experienced. After these preliminary exercises, role play the suggested nursing situations (or others of your choosing), and once again process the experience. Talk about the relevance of this experience to human interaction in general, and conclude the exercise by writing a goal for your practice.

Worksheet

A. Practice looking at a colleague two different ways:
   1. "You are a job to be done; you mean nothing to me" look
   2. "You are precious, and I care about you" look

B. Practice speaking to a colleague in two different ways:
   1. Indifferent: "Your resident, your light."
   2. Helpful: "I think Mrs. Jones' light is on again. Do you need help?"
C. Practice touching a colleague in two different ways:
   1. Indifferent: Pick up your colleague's wrist and feel for a pulse.
   2. Using warm lotion, massage your colleague's hands.
D. Talk about how each of the above looks, words, and touches made you feel. Talk about how you think they make patients or residents feel.
E. Role play each of the situations below in two different ways, trying to incorporate looks, words, and touches that communicate:
   First time: You are a job to be done; you mean nothing to me.
   Second time: You are precious, and I care about you.
   1. Student feels overwhelmed by patient care assignment and approaches clinical instructor to discuss her options.
   2. Student walks into patient's room to begin morning care.
   3. Student assists elderly patient to stand and ambulate around room.
   4. Student brings medication to patient.
   5. Student approaches another student and asks for help changing the bed linens of an obese patient who is on complete bed rest.
F. Name one thing you have decided to try to do differently when you take care of your patients as a result of this session.
G. Does what you experienced today have any implications for who you are when you are not nursing?

---

interpersonal skills, try these activities with a friend. Take turns being both the nurse and the older adult, and talk about how different types of nursing presence makes you feel.

Establishing Caring Relationships

Increasingly, nurses are reporting that new systems of care and the demand to work "harder, faster, and smarter" to keep up in today's competitive healthcare arena are making traditional nurse–patient relationships difficult to attain. As you begin your nursing practice, ask yourself what priority you assign to caring. Nurses who accept that there can be no excellence in nursing in the absence of this relationship commit themselves to finding creative means to establish caring relationships. Obviously, many variables influence the quality of relationships that are possible, not the least of which is the acuity level of the patient and the patient's length of stay. Helpful reflection questions include the following:

• Do I know my patients well enough to promote anything more than the well-being of their body?

• If asked to describe a patient, would I be able to report on anything other than the patient's physical condition?
• Is the care I routinely provide really holistic, individualized, prioritized according to medical need and the patient's interests, and continuous? Do my care plans reflect this?
• What does the content of the patient report and nursing documentation communicate about nursing priorities in my practice setting?
• What are my strengths and deficiencies in creating caring relationships?
• In what ways (if any) must I change to establish better caring relationships?

Nurses committed to caring relationships routinely use opportunities for conversation to communicate genuine interest in who the patient is and what the patient is experiencing to provide meaningful nursing assistance. For example, rather than just "chattering" aimlessly with a talkative older adult, a nurse skilled in developing caring relationships will direct the conversation. Leading statements or questions that are often successful in eliciting useful information from older patients include the following:

- "Tell me something about your life at home. What do you miss most now that you are here?"
- "What family members and friends do you see most often? Who do you think knows you best and you would trust to speak for you if you were ever unable to speak for yourself?"
- "Most of us have some goal or dream that keeps us going. It might be owning our own home, seeing some relationship patched up, or being able to celebrate the birth of a grandchild. What is your dream?"
- "When you've had troubles in the past, what did you draw on for strength? What keeps you going?"
- "Looks like you've got a lot of time for thinking these days . . . would you like to share what's been on your mind?"
- "Looks like we'll be spending some time together . . . what would you like to do with this time? How may I help you?"

Nurses who are sensitive to the well-being of their patients can find many ways to communicate caring. Happily, most caring is mutually enriching, and nurses who care find themselves re-energized for the more demanding aspects of their practice. Read one patient's account of the importance to her of nurse caring in the accompanying box, Through the Eyes of a Patient.

Enjoying the Rewards of Mutual Interchange

In any helping profession, but especially in nursing, countless opportunities exist to interact with others. Those committed to interpersonal caring enrich everyday interactions by investing them with something of themselves and, in return, receiving something of the other, as shown in Figure 11-4. Think of your last encounter with a patient. Whether you were administering a medication, checking vital signs, or preparing the patient for discharge, you had the choice of merely accomplishing the given task or accomplishing the task while simultaneously communicating a personal gift of support, caring, strength, and peacefulness. Frequently overlooked, these interpersonal gifts might contribute to a patient's healing as significantly as medical interventions. Rather than deplete their giver, these interpersonal gifts invite similar gifts from the recipient, which in return enrich the caregiver. Nothing causes burnout faster than a practice that is reduced to the performance of multiple tasks stripped of their human significance. When a patient is given care in a way that "makes a difference" in terms of his or her well-being, the patient's gratitude, even when unspoken, helps renew the nurse's energy. Too seldom do we stop our busy practices long enough to reflect on how who we are that day is influencing the well-being of those receiving our care. It is helpful to question:

- How conscious am I of how my mood influences the well-being of others?
- Have I ever consciously tried to transmit strength, peace, support, or joy to another? What were the results?
- Am I aware of any situation in which my fatigue, anxiety, frustration, or negativity was communicated to a patient

Through the Eyes of a Patient

I recently spent 2 months in a university teaching hospital while doctors tried to find a way to regulate my heart beats. Many of the days were filled with tests, some of which were frightening. I was given many drugs—most of which turned out not to be helpful. I was a 2-hour car ride away from my home, family, and friends—which meant there wasn't always a familiar face at my bedside.

I quickly learned I could judge what kind of day I was going to have as soon as I saw my nurse each morning.

All of them brought my medicines and helped with the treatment plan. With some nurses, however, I also experienced the comfort and security of knowing that my expressed needs would be promptly and respectfully tended to. If I needed help getting up to the bathroom or asked for something for pain, I could count on help coming quickly. And finally there were those few with whom I knew I was going to have a great day because they would "make it happen" no matter how sick I was feeling. These were the nurses who offered a hug with their medicines, who had a moment to sit and listen, who teased about the "fashion statements" I was making with my nightgowns, and who "walked me through" new tests so that at least I felt better prepared to face the unknown. Most often, it wasn't what they did but how they did it.

I wish all nurses understood the power they have to influence a patient's basic sense of well-being. A hospital can be a pretty scary, lonely place. Nurses can make all the difference!

—Mildred Taylor, Pine Grove, PA

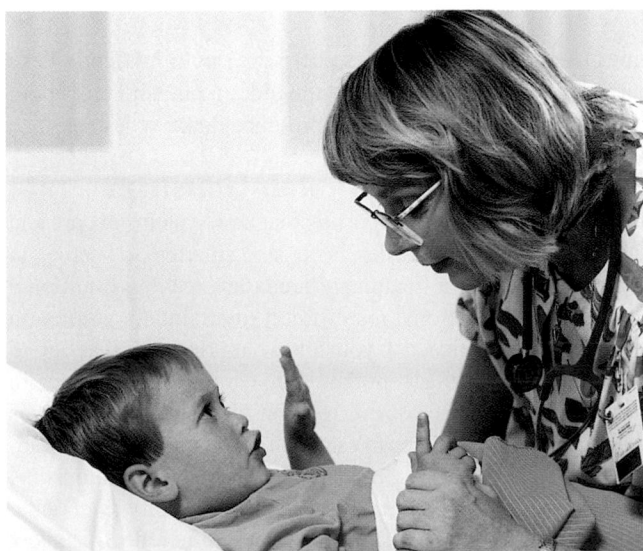

FIGURE 11-4 Interpersonal caring enriches the lives of everyone participating, providing a mutual exchange of giving and receiving. (Photo by Einrosia, courtesy of Shore Memorial Hospital and Nursing Spectrum.)

in a manner that negatively influenced his or her well-being?

- Am I conscious of ways in which patients enrich me personally or enrich my practice?
- In what ways is my practice different when I am attuned to the interpersonal dimensions of nurse–patient interactions?
- In what ways must my practice change if I am to facilitate healing by willing something of my essence to patients?

Developing Ethical/Legal Skills

Nurses who prize their role in securing patient well-being are sensitive to the ethical and legal implications of nursing practice. Chapters 6 and 7 describe essential components of ethical and legal competence for nurses. Although it can take years to master effective patient advocacy skills and to become proficient in mediating ethical conflict, even beginning nurses are responsible for certain basic ethical skills. For example, one of the greatest challenges nursing students face is balancing the competing demands of home life, school, and the hospital or practice setting. Learning to be true to oneself, to the patients for whom one is responsible, to the caregiving team, and to the profession and society is an ongoing struggle. Examining one's sense of accountability is crucial as one assumes professional responsibilities.

Developing Accountability

Nurses committed to interpersonal caring hold themselves accountable for the human well-being of patients entrusted to their care. Being accountable means being attentive and responsive to the healthcare needs of individual patients. It means that my concern for the patient transcends whatever happens during my shift, and that I ensure continuity of care when I leave a patient. In today's system of increasingly fragmented care, patients often find themselves unable to point to any one caregiver who knows their overall situation and is capable and willing to coordinate the efforts of the healthcare team. Being responsive and responsible earns a patient's trust that "all will be well" as healthcare needs are addressed. Nurses committed to responsible caring reflect on the following:

- To what extent does my commitment to securing the human well-being of those in my care dictate my work priorities?
- How comfortable am I voicing unmet patient needs to other members of the healthcare team?
- Do other caregivers listen when I present patient concerns because of my successful record of patient advocacy?
- What system variables (eg, nurse–patient ratios, skill mix, availability of resources) need to change for us to meet the human needs of our patients adequately?
- In what ways must I change for my patients to be able to count on me to respond in a responsible way to their needs?

Nurses who are sensitive to the legal dimensions of practice are careful to develop a strong sense of both ethical and legal accountability. Competent practice is a nurse's best legal

safeguard. Nurses seeking to develop legal competence might find it helpful to ask the following questions:

- Do I know the legal boundaries of my practice?
- Am I familiar with pertinent institutional procedures and policies?
- Do I "own" my personal strengths and weaknesses and seek assistance as needed?
- Am I careful never to accept responsibility for an assignment for which I am unprepared?
- Am I knowledgeable about, and respectful of, patient rights?
- Does my documentation provide a legally defensible account of my practice?

When working to develop ethical and legal accountability, nurses must recognize that both deficiencies and excesses of responsible caring are problematic. Although it is reasonable to hold oneself accountable for promoting the human well-being of patients, nurses can err by setting unrealistic standards of responsiveness and responsibility for themselves. Prudence is always necessary to balance responsible self-care with care of others. Inexperienced nurses might feel totally responsible for effecting patient outcomes beyond their control and become frustrated and sad when unable to produce the desired outcome. Conversations about what is reasonable to hold ourselves and others accountable for are always helpful. The sample learning activity in Box 11-5 was designed to explore such accountability issues.

Reporting Incompetent, Unethical, or Illegal Practices

Each employing institution or agency providing nursing services has an obligation to establish a process for the reporting and handling of practices by individuals or by healthcare systems that jeopardize a patient's health or safety. The ANA Code for Ethics obligates nurses to report professional conduct that is incompetent, unethical, or illegal. For nurses, incompetent practice is measured by nursing standards, unethical practice is evaluated in light of professional codes of ethics, and illegal practice is identified in terms of violations of law. Parameters for evaluating each follow:

- Parameters of competent nursing practice: State Nurse Practice Acts and Regulations, the Scope of Practice, Professional Standards of Nursing Practice, and other practice guidelines and protocols
- Parameters of ethical nursing practice: Professional codes of ethics
- Parameters of legal nursing practice: Federal and State health regulations, pharmacy laws, Occupational Safety and Health Administration standards and regulations, medical records and communicable disease laws, environmental laws, Centers for Disease Control and Prevention guidelines, antidiscrimination laws, service facility regulations, Clinical Improvement Act, and JCAHO regulations (ANA, 1994)

Whistle-blowing refers to employees who report their employer's violation of the law to appropriate law enforcement agencies outside the employer's facilities. Citing the inade-

BOX 11-5 **Developing Ethical/Legal Skills**

Accountability

Description
The purpose of this exercise is to explore the issue of accountability. You will be challenged to reflect on whether your everyday nursing practice demonstrates a commitment to ensuring the human well-being of those in your care. Individual patterns of responding to human need and responsible caring will be critiqued. Role playing and guided discovery will be used to invite you to experience the effects of both responsible caring and the indifferent provision of services.

Objectives
Upon conclusion of this exercise, you will be able to:

1. Describe how the way you respond (or fail to respond) to the needs of patients influences their general sense of well-being.
2. Critique the amount of responsibility you and other nurses accept for the well-being of individual patients.

Worksheet

Objective
To critique our responsiveness to patient need and the amount of responsibility we each assume to secure patient well-being

Exercise One
Take a moment to reflect on a recent experience when you felt vulnerable (eg, new role responsibilities: first clinical rotation, new job, new spouse, new parent; car breaks down; major purchase). Share with a colleague how the conduct of the one(s) you expected to be sensitive and responsive to your need influenced your overall sense of well-being. Draw parallels to nursing.

Exercise Two
List all the *personal* variables that enable you to care for your patients responsibly (eg, coming to work rested, honestly caring about patients) and that impede your ability to do this (eg, you come to work but are mentally and emotionally back home with some other problem, such as difficulties with spouse, sick child).

Positive Personal Variables	Negative Personal Variables

Next, list all the *system* variables that enable you to care for your patients responsibly (eg, patient assignments are matched to your developing level of expertise, good team spirit among caregivers and their willingness to work together to meet complex patient needs) and that impede your doing this (eg, student assignments are unrealistic, chronic understaffing results in staff being unavailable to direct students, sense in the healthcare institution that management has "given up" and is

3. Describe one way your practice will change in order for you to be more accountable to yourself, your patients, the nursing profession, and society.

Learning Activities
Choose another student, and work through exercises 1 to 4. Begin by describing your own positive and negative experiences of being cared for, and draw parallels to how patients feel when they believe they can count on their caregivers to recognize and respond to their needs. Then develop and discuss a list of personal, patient, and system variables that either facilitate or impede responsible caring. Finally, role play the given scenarios, and focus discussion on how different nursing responses influence patient well-being. End the discussion by developing a goal for your practice that will help you to be accountable to yourself, patients, the nursing profession, and society.

no longer concerned about the quality; that the bottom line is always money).

Positive System Variables	Negative System Variables

Finally, list *patient* variables that positively and negatively influence your ability/willingness to care for your patients responsibly (eg, patient looks like me, patient is pleasant and makes few demands, patient has strong potential for complete recovery, or patient is homeless, has a history of self-abuse).

Positive Patient Variables	Negative Patient Variables

Talk about how you plan to address the negative variables that interfere with your ability to care for patients responsibly. What does it mean to be accountable to yourself, your patients, the nursing profession, and society?

Exercise Three
Role play each of the scenarios below, and discuss how the nurse responds (or fails to respond) is likely to influence the patient. It would be helpful to discuss how you think nurses

---

BOX 11-5 (Continued)

on your unit *would* respond to this type of situation and how you think they *should* respond. If these differ, discuss why.

1. You suspect from the blood pressure reading you just obtained that the elderly clinic patient you are examining is not taking his medication or complying with other aspects of the treatment plan. "I try to take 'em but sometimes I forgets." The clinic is understaffed, and you have many more patients to see, some of whom have waited for more than an hour.
2. You tell the resident that you don't think the pain medication one woman with metastatic cancer is receiving is adequate, and the resident tells you that it's a more than adequate dose.
3. Another nurse tells you that he's utterly frustrated because Dr. Braxton refuses to talk with a patient about ad-

vance directives because "it might depress her." You share this nurse's belief that the patient wants to participate in decision making and that it is very possible that she will lose the ability to do this soon.

4. You are making a home visit to a 32-year-old man with end-stage AIDS. He tells you that he is tired of fighting, has no money, and no longer wants to be a bother to his friends. He asks you what he can do to end his life.

Exercise Four
Review each of the above four situations, and discuss with your colleague the legal implications of being accountable. What legal safeguards would you recommend?

Exercise Five
Name one thing about your practice that you have decided to change as a result of this session.

---

quacies of current laws to protect whistle-blowers, the ANA offers the following caution: "because of the limits of current law, nurses should be advised that they might not be protected against retaliation for reporting the incompetent, unethical or illegal practices of their employers" (ANA, 1994, p. 12). Many individual nurses and nursing organizations are working to secure state and federal legislation to protect whistle-blowers.

CRITICAL THINKING AND CLINICAL REASONING

People use critical thinking skills whenever they want to use clear, focused thinking to achieve a result. I can think critically about how to survive the day's challenges, find a partner for life, pass a licensing exam, or become president! Critical thinking applied to clinical reasoning and judgment in nursing practice:

- Entails purposeful, informed, outcome-focused (results-oriented) thinking that requires careful identification of key problems, issues, and risks involved
- Is driven by patient, family, and community needs
- Is based on principles of nursing process and scientific method (eg, making judgments based on evidence rather than guesswork)
- Use both intuition and logic, based on knowledge, skills, and experience
- Is guided by professional standards and ethics codes
- Requires strategies that make the most of human potential (eg, using individual strengths) and compensate for problems created by human nature (eg, overcoming the powerful influence of personal views)
- Is constantly reevaluating, self-correcting, and striving to improve (Alfaro-LeFevre, 2004, p. 57)

Each of the nursing process chapters that follow have a section highlighting the type of critical thinking necessary to successfully implement that step of the nursing process.

Critical Thinking Indicators™

Alfaro-LeFevre (2004) has carefully developed a list of **critical thinking indicators** (CTIs™), that is, evidence-based descriptions of behaviors that demonstrate the knowledge, characteristics, and skills that promote critical thinking in clinical practice. See Boxes 11-6 and 11-7. If you are serious about developing the critical thinking skills needed for professional practice, now would be a good time to sit down with someone who knows you well to see which critical thinking characteristics you possess and which need work. One way to do this is to ask with each characteristic:

1. On a scale of 1 to 7 (with 1 almost never and 7 always), to what degree do I demonstrate this characteristic that promotes critical thinking?
2. Think of examples of times when you both demonstrated and failed to demonstrate these characteristics. What were the consequences in these situations?

It can be helpful to see if you and others you invite to evaluate your characteristics reach the same conclusions about your strengths and areas for improvement.

Another way to use this list is to try to determine as a class which characteristics accurately describe your class! Alternatively, you can compare groups. For example, as a rule, which characteristics do nurses as a group and physicians as a group demonstrate.

As you begin clinical practice, you can also use the Critical Thinking Indicators™ Behaviors Demonstrating Knowledge and Intellectual Skills list to critique your competence for professional practice.

Concept Mapping

Concept mapping is an instructional strategy that requires learners to identify, graphically display, and link key concepts. Concept maps, also called cognitive maps, mind maps, and meta cognitive tools for learning, are a proven means to promote

BOX 11-6 Critical Thinking Indicators™: Behaviors Demonstrating Knowledge and Intellectual Skills

Knowledge
Requirements vary, depending on context (eg, specialty practice):

Clarifies:
- ☐ Nursing and medical terminology
- ☐ Nursing vs. medical and other models, roles, and responsibilities
- ☐ Signs and symptoms of common problems and complications
- ☐ Related anatomy, physiology, pathophysiology
- ☐ Normal and abnormal function (bio-psycho-social-cultural-spiritual)
- ☐ Factors that promote or inhibit normal function (bio-psycho-social-cultural-spiritual)
- ☐ Related pharmacology (actions, indications, side effects, nursing implications)
- ☐ Reasons behind interventions and diagnostic studies
- ☐ Normal and abnormal growth and development
- ☐ Nursing process, nursing theories, and research principles
- ☐ Applicable standards, laws, practice acts
- ☐ Policies and procedures and the reasons behind them
- ☐ Ethical and legal principles
- ☐ Spiritual, social, and cultural concepts
- ☐ Where information resources can be found

Demonstrates:
- ☐ Focused nursing assessment skills (eg, breath-sounds or IV site assessment)
- ☐ Related technical skills (eg, n/g tube or other equipment management)

Clarifies:
- ☐ Personal values, beliefs, needs
- ☐ How own thinking, personality, and learning style preferences may differ from others' preferences
- ☐ Organizational mission and values

Intellectual Skills/Competencies
Nursing Process and Decision-making Skills:
- ☐ Applies standards and principles when planning, giving, and adapting care
- ☐ Assesses systematically and comprehensively; uses a nursing framework to identify nursing concerns, uses a body systems framework to identify medical concerns
- ☐ Detects bias; determines credibility of information sources
- ☐ Distinguishes normal from abnormal; identifies risks for abnormal
- ☐ Determines significance of data; distinguishes relevant from irrelevant; clusters relevant data together
- ☐ Identifies assumptions and inconsistencies; checks accuracy and reliability; recognizes missing information; focuses assessment as indicated
- ☐ Concludes what's known and unknown; makes reasonable inferences (conclusions) and judgments—gives evidence to support them
- ☐ Identifies both problems and their underlying cause(s) and related factors; includes patient and family perspectives
- ☐ Considers multiple explanations and solutions
- ☐ Determines individualized outcomes; focuses on results
- ☐ Manages risks, predicts complications, promotes health, function, and well-being; anticipates consequences and implications—plans ahead accordingly
- ☐ Sets priorities and makes decisions in a timely way; includes key stakeholders in making decisions
- ☐ Weighs risks and benefits; individualizes interventions
- ☐ Reassesses to check responses and monitor results (outcomes)
- ☐ Communicates effectively orally and in writing
- ☐ Identifies ethical issues and takes appropriate action
- ☐ Identifies and uses technologic, information, and human resources

Additional Related Skills:
- ☐ Establishes empowered partnerships with patients, families, peers, and coworkers
- ☐ Teaches patients, self, and others
- ☐ Addresses conflicts fairly; fosters positive interpersonal relationships
- ☐ Facilitates and navigates change
- ☐ Organizes and manages time and environment
- ☐ Facilitates teamwork (focuses on common goals; helps and encourages others to contribute in their own way)
- ☐ Gives and takes constructive criticism
- ☐ Delegates appropriately; leads, inspires, and motivates others
- ☐ Demonstrates systems thinking (shows awareness of the interrelationships existing within and across healthcare systems)

BOX 11-7 **Critical Thinking Indicators™: Behaviors Demonstrating CT Characteristics/Attitudes**

Critical Thinking Indicators™ (CTIs™) are brief descriptions of behaviors that demonstrate characteristics that promote critical thinking. Indicators are listed in context of clinical practice.

☐ **Self-aware:** Clarifies biases, inclinations, strengths, and limitations; acknowledges when thinking may be influenced by emotions or self-interest

☐ **Genuine:** Shows authentic self; demonstrates behaviors that indicate stated values

☐ **Self disciplined:** Stays on task as needed; manages time to focus on priorities

☐ **Healthy:** Promotes a healthy lifestyle; uses healthy behaviors to manage stress

☐ **Autonomous and responsible:** Shows independent thinking and actions; begins and completes tasks without prodding; expresses ownership of accountability

☐ **Careful and prudent:** Seeks help when needed; suspends or revises judgment as indicated by new or incomplete data

☐ **Confident and resilient:** Expresses faith in ability to reason and learn; overcomes disappointments

☐ **Honest and upright:** Seeks the truth, even if it sheds unwanted light; upholds standards; admits flaws in thinking

☐ **Curious and inquisitive:** Looks for reasons, explanations, and meaning; seeks new information to broaden understanding

☐ **Alert to context:** Looks for changes in circumstances that warrant a need to modify thinking or approaches

☐ **Analytical and insightful:** Identifies relationships; expresses deep understanding

☐ **Logical and intuitive:** Draws reasonable conclusions (if this is so, then it follows that . . . because . . .); uses intu-ition as a guide to search for evidence; acts on intuition only with knowledge of risks involved

☐ **Open and fair-minded:** Shows tolerance for different viewpoints; questions how own viewpoints are influencing thinking

☐ **Sensitive to diversity:** Expresses appreciation of human differences related to values, culture, personality, or learning style preferences; adapts to preferences when feasible

☐ **Creative:** Offers alternative solutions and approaches; comes up with useful ideas

☐ **Realistic and practical:** Admits when things aren't feasible; looks for user-friendly solutions

☐ **Reflective and self-corrective:** Carefully considers meaning of data and interpersonal interactions, asks for feedback; corrects own thinking, alert to potential errors by self and others, finds ways to avoid future mistakes

☐ **Proactive:** Anticipates consequences, plans ahead, acts on opportunities

☐ **Courageous:** Stands up for beliefs, advocates for others, doesn't hide from challenges

☐ **Patient and persistent:** Waits for right moment; perseveres to achieve best results

☐ **Flexible:** Changes approaches as needed to get the best results

☐ **Empathetic:** Listens well; shows ability to imagine others' feelings and difficulties

☐ **Improvement-oriented (self, patients, systems):** *Self—*Identifies learning needs; finds ways to overcome limitations, seeks out new knowledge. *Patients—*Promotes health; maximizes function, comfort, and convenience. *Systems—*Identifies risks and problems with healthcare systems; promotes safety, quality, satisfaction, and cost containment

Note: The above is the ideal—no one is perfect. Even the best thinkers' characteristics vary depending on circumstances, such as comfort and familiarity with the people and situations at hand. What matters is *patterns* of behavior over time (is the behavior usually evident?). If you're a critical thinker, you can probably easily pick three or more of the above characteristics that you'd like to improve (critical thinkers are naturally focused on self-improvement).

Used with permission

critical thinking and self-directed learning. McHugh Schuster (2002), who recommends concept mapping as a "critical-thinking approach to care planning," writes:

The important ideas that must be linked together during clinical care planning are the medical and nursing diagnoses, along with all pertinent clinical data. Concept map care planning can be used to promote critical thinking about patient problems and treatment of problems. Through concept mapping of diagnoses and clinical data, you can evaluate what you know about the care of a patient and what further information you need to provide safe and effective nursing care. The visual map of relationships among diagnoses allows you and your clinical faculty to exchange views on why relationships exist among diagnoses. It also allows you to recognize missing diagnoses and linkages, thus suggesting further learning (p. 3).

Steps in concept map care planning are:

1. Develop a basic skeleton diagram.
2. Analyze and categorize data.
3. Analyze nursing diagnoses relationships.
4. Identify goals, outcomes, and interventions.
5. Evaluate patient's responses.

Examples of concept maps prepared by a student at Delaware County Community College with the related patient database problem list forms are illustrated in Figure 11-5.

(*text continues on page 223*)

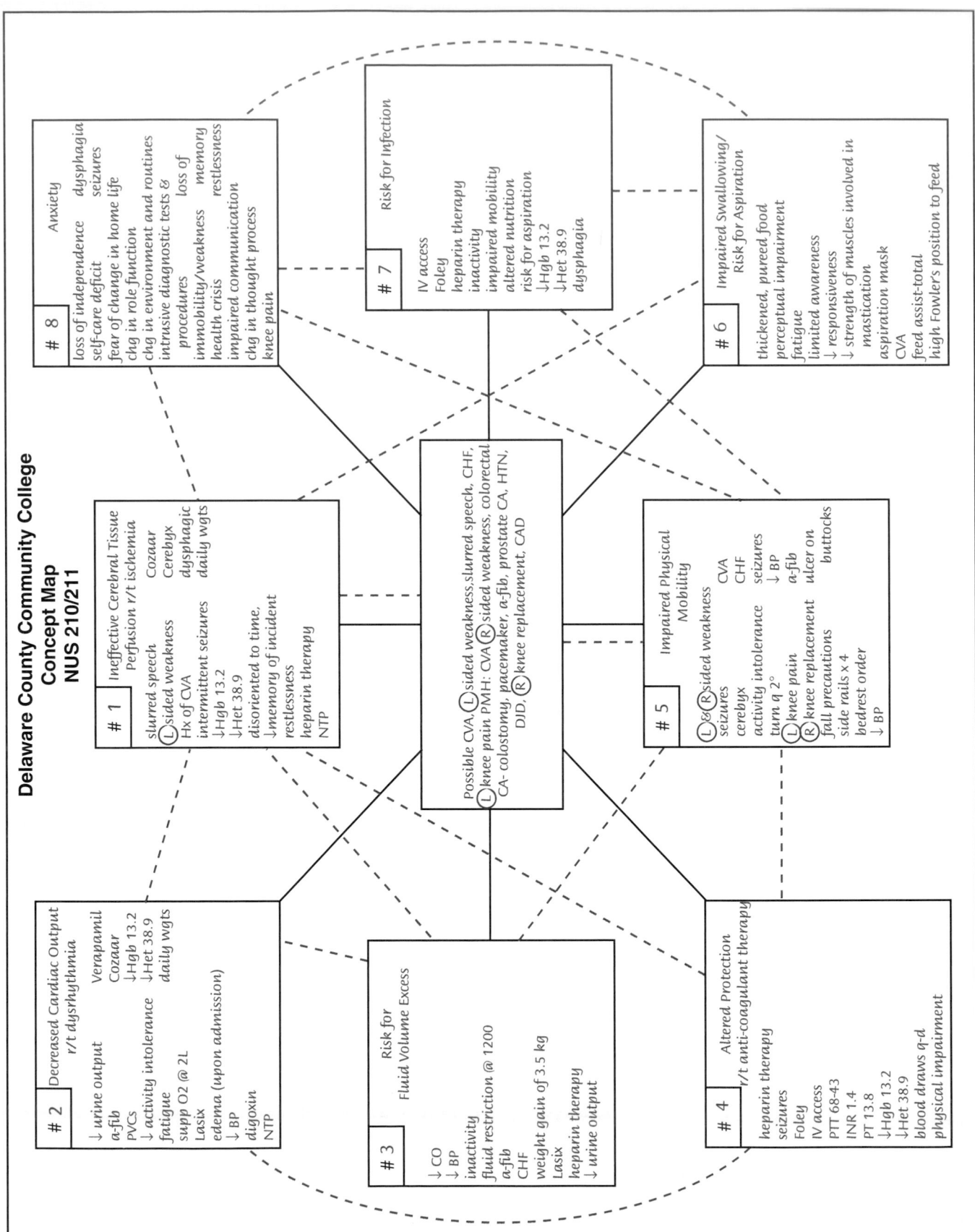

FIGURE 11-5 Sample concept map and supporting data. (Adapted from Schuster, P. M. [2002]. *Concept mapping: A critical-thinking approach to care planning*. Philadelphia: F. A. Davis. Completed forms used with permission from Janet Heck, Delaware County Community College.)

Delaware County Community College
NUS 210/211
Patient Database

Admission Information			Student Name: JANET HECK		

Date of Care	Patient Initials	Age	Growth & Development	Sex	Adm date
2—27—06	DR	79	Ego Integrity vs Despair	M	2—24—06

Medical Diagnosis/Surgical Procedure:
Possible CVA, (L) sided weakness, slurred speech, CHF, (L) knee pain

Past Medical History: CVA (R) sided weakness, colorectal CA—colostomy, pacemaker, A-fib, prostate CA, HTN, DJD, (R) knee replacement, CAD

Psychosocial History	Smoking yes (no)	Alcohol yes (no)
Religious Preference: Protestant	**Marital Status:** Widower	
Health Care Insurance: Keystone 65	**Occupation:** Retired	

Advanced Directives	Living Will yes (no)	Do Not Rescucitate yes (no)

Medications:	Allergies: NKA

Name of Medication	Why is patient taking this medication?
IV Heparin 24 cc/hr /raised to 28 cc/hr per PTT protocol	anti-coagulant -prevention of thrombi (a-fib)
K-DUR 20 meQ qd	potassium supplement (K 3.5)
Lasix 40 mg po qd	diuretic - treat CHF/edema upon admission
Digoxin 0.25 mg po qd	to treat a-fib, ↑ CO
Verapamil SR 120 mg qd	calcum channel blocker, treat dysrhythmia (a-fib)
NTP 1" q 6° to chest wall	coronary dilator, ↑ blood flow, treat CHF ↓ BP
Protonix 40 mg qd	suppress gastric acid
Cozaar 50 mg & Het 212.5 mg qd	blocks angiotension II, acts to vasodilate & ↓ BP
Cerebyx 1000 mg IV @ 10 cc/hr	anti-convulsant; treat seizures

Laboratory Data							
Lab Value	**On adm**	**Current**	**Why abnormal**	**Lab Value**	**On adm**	**Current**	**Why abnormal**
WBS	8.6	9.2	WNL	Na	128	NOT DONE	WNL
Hemoglobin	14.1	13.2↓	heparin; ↓nutrition	K	3.5	"	WNL (but K supp administered)
Hematocrit	42.2	38.9↓	heparin; ↓nutrition	Cr	1.2	"	WNL
Platelets	233	232	WNL	BUN	11	"	WNL
PT	13.8	—	WNL	Blood Glucose	114	"	WNL
INR	1.4	—		ABG		NOT DONE	
PTT	68	43↓	heparin therapy	Other Mg	1.9	"	WNL
Troponin	<0.5	—	WNL	Other CA	8.5	"	WNL
CPK	47	—	WNL	Other Dig	1.4	"	WNL

Diagnostic Tests		
CXR ✓ shows CHF	EKG ✓ A-fib	Echocardiogram —
Other CT-scan ⊝ No △; bleed (x2)	Other	

FIGURE 11-5 Continued

Treatments:	Daily wgts
	Pulse Ox q shift – > 90% (on 2L NC)
	No neuro checks ordered
	Turn q 2•

Diet

Type: Pureed, ↓NA 2 gm	Restrictions: thickened only 1200cc po fluid	Appetite: Good
Difficulty Swallowing: (yes) no		Assist with Feeds: (yes) no

Fluid Status

IV solution & rate: Heparin 28cc/hr	Type of IV access: Peri	Site condition: Ø swelling, Ø redness
24 hr intake: 1460	24 hr output: 1000	Balance: +460
5 hr intake: 480	5 hr output: 250	Balance: +230
Weight: 86.2 kg admin; 89.7 kg	Amount of gain or loss: +3.5 kg	

Elimination

Continent:	Bladder: (yes) no	Bowel: (yes) no
Foley: (yes) no	Urine color: dark amber	Last BM: 2/27/06

Activity

Activity Order:	Gait:	Use of Assistive Devices:
Bedrest	N/A	N/A
Risk for Falls: (yes) no	Weakness: (yes) no	Restraints: yes (no)

Vital Signs 8 am	BP 112/60	P 66	R 16	T 97° SAO2 99%
Any additional vs 1200	94/60	70	18	97° (AX) SAO2 99%

Narrative Assessment Notes for Clinical Day:

2/27/06 0800. Rec'd pt sleeping– responsive to verbal stimuli. Pt is oriented to person, place only. Responds slowly c̄ one word answers or head motion. Heparin infusion running at 24 cc/hr s̄ incident IV site #11 shows ↓ swelling and ↓ redness. Pt denies pain. VS BP 112/60, T 97+(0); P66, R16, Pt on 2L O₂ via nc, SAO₂ @ 99%. Pt has colostomy bag - no BM present. Foley draining c̄ dark amber urine. Pt's lungs are clear but decreased in bases. BS⊕, Radial and DI pulses palpable +2. Skin warm and dry. Rash evident on face– pt picks and scratches at face especially nose and mouth frequently. Inspected nose and mouth, both clear c̄ no evidence of inflammation or sores. Pt weak in both LE and upper extremities, limited mvmt. Pt grimaces upon manipulation or mvmt of (L) knee. (R) arm spasms frequently– subsides c̄ touch. Pt dozes on & off but responsive to verbal stimuli. Pt has duoderm on (L) buttock - unable to inspect wound. Complete bed bath given c̄ mouthcare, pt tolerated well. Capillary refill brisk. ↓ edema present. PEARL; heart sounds S, S₂ c̄ murmur ——————————————— JM DCCCSN

FIGURE 11-5 Continued

Delaware County Community College Concept Map Care Plan

Problem #1 Ineffective Cerebral Tissue Perfusion r/t ischemia (thrombosis)
Short-term Goal: Cerebral perfusion pressure will be maintained during hospital stay.
Long-term Goal: Pt will participate in rehabilitation exercises to regain optimal strength in (L) extremities.

Nursing Interventions:	Patient's Response:
1. Monitor VS q 4°, check pupils	1. BP 112/60, T97°, P66, RR16, PEARL @ 0800
2. Monitor I & O strict q shift.	2. BP 94/60, T97°, P70, RR18, PEARL @ 1200
3. Monitor pulse Ox q shift	3. Pt on restricted 1200cc fluids po, 5 hr intake=480, SAO_2 99% on 2L NC.
4. Keep head of bed 30° or lower (except when feeding)	4. Pt responsive to verbal stimuli, oriented to person & place.
5. Cluster activities to ↓ ICP.	5. Pt tolerated assessment, bath and feeding before tiring.
6. Administer heparin infusion.	6. Pts PTT 68 to 43.

Summarize your impressions of patient progress towards goals Pt displays Ø worsening of symptoms of reduced of cerebral perfusion. Continue interventions.

Problem #2 Decreased Cardiac Output r/t dysrhythmia
Short-term Goal: Pt will maintain optimally compensated cardiac output evidenced by clear lung sounds, Ø SOB, increased urine output on ↑activity tolerance while hospitalized.
Long-term Goal: Pt will comply c̄ medication regimen to maintain optimal cardiac output after discharge.

Nursing Interventions:	Patient's Response:
1. Assess rate & quality of apical & peripheral pulses.	1. Pulses palpable +2, apical rate S_1S_2 c̄ murmur; Ø pulse deficit.
2. Assess BP q 4°	2. BP 112/60 @ 0800, 94/80 @ 1200.
3. Assess lung sounds q 2°	3. Lungs clear but decreased in bases bilaterally.
4. Assess urine output.	4. Urine output 50 cc/hr (250 in 5 hrs)
5. Assess SAO_2.	5. Pt SAO_2 99% c̄ 2l O_2 via nc.
6. Weigh pt daily.	6. Pt has gained 3.5 kg from 2/24 to 2/27.

Summarize your impressions of patient progress towards goals Pt is maintaining good cardiac output as evidenced by ↑ urine output, clear lung sounds and ↓ edema. Continue interventions.

Problem #3 Risk for Fluid Volume Excess
Short-term Goal: Pt will maintain optimal fluid balance as evidenced by stable wgt, clear lung sounds, Ø edema and adequate urine output.
Long-term Goal: Pt will maintain fluid balance upon discharge by compliance c̄ medication regimen and fluid intake.

Nursing Interventions:	Patient's Response:
1. Weigh pt daily.	1. Pt gained 3.5 kg since admission.
2. Monitor strict I & O (1200 cc/24 hr)	2. Pt's intake was 480, output 250 in 5 hrs.
3. Evaluate urine output.	3. Urine output is 50 cc/hr for 5 hrs (0800—1300)
4. Administer Lasix as ordered.	4. Lasix given @ 1000 40 mg po.
5. Monitor electrolytes (side effect of diuretic)	5. All electrolytes WNL.
6. Assess for edema.	6. Ø edema present.

Summarize your impressions of patient progress towards goals Pt is maintaining optimum fluid balance presently c̄ exception of wgt gain. Continue interventions.

Problem #4 Altered Protection r/t anticoagulant therapy
Short-term Goal: Pt will maintain therapeutic blood level of anticoagulant as evidenced by PTT, PT and INR WNL.
Long-term Goal: Pt will set up schedule for bloodwork to be drawn after discharge to maintain therapeutic levels.

Nursing Interventions:	Patient's Response:
1. Monitor pt for adverse effects to anti-coagulant.	1. Pt shows Ø signs of unexplained bleeding– Ø bruising, Ø petechic.
2. Monitor vs q 4°.	2. Pts BP 112/60, T978, P66, RR16 @ 0800, 94/60, T974, P20, RR18@1200.
3. Ensure IV infusion & site is uninterrupted.	3. Heparin infusing s̄ incident, IV site shows Ø signs of inflammation or bleeding.
4. Monitor lab results of PTT, PT, INR and intact.	4. Pts PTT 68 to 43, PT 13.8, INR 1.4.
5. Monitor Hgb & Hct for internal bleeding.	5. Hgb ↓ 13.2, Hct 38.9 ↓

Summarize your impressions of patient progress towards goals Pt currently shows Ø signs of bleeding caused by anti-coagulant therapy. Continue to monitor –check H&H to see if continues downward trend. Continue interventions.

FIGURE 11-5 *Continued*

Delaware County Community College Concept Map Care Plan

Problem #5 Impaired Physical Mobility
Short-term Goal: Pt will maintain maximum level of function and risk of complications will be reduced while hospitalized.
Long-term Goal: Pt will regain optimal level of functioning as dictated by severity of CVA.

Nursing Interventions:	Patient's Response:
1. Assess pt's degree of weakness in both upper & lower extremities.	1. Pt's (L) side shows ↑ weakness to (R) side.
2. Determine active & passive ROM capabilities.	2. Pt can move (R) arm independently, other extremities require passive ROM.
3. Monitor skin integrity for potential breakdown.	3. Pt's skin intact c̄ exception of (L) buttock -opaque dsg- cannot assess.
4. Change pt's position q 2°.	4. Pt appears comfortable, Ø breakdown present.
5. Use pressure relieving devices to ↓ stress.	5. Placed pillows under legs to elevate heels, pillow under (R) or (L) side to ↓ pressure on sacrum.
6. Implement fall precautions for pt safety.	6. Side rails x 4, bed in low, locked position.

Summarize your impressions of patient progress towards goals   Pt has Ø falls. Pt shows Ø skin breakdown and passive ROM performed on lower extremities & (L) arm. Continue interventions.

Problem #6 Impaired Swallowing/Risk for Aspiration
Short-term Goal: Pt will not experience aspiration while hospitalized.
Long-term Goal: Pt will maintain adequate nutrition, as evidenced by stable wgt and albumin WNL.

Nursing Interventions:	Patient's Response:
1. Before mealtime, provide adequate rest periods.	1. Pt was able to stay alert through meal.
2. Provide oral care before feeding.	2. Pt's mouth moistened, displayed good appetite.
3. Place pt in high Fowler's position for feeding.	3. Pt swallowed and chewed well.
4. Prompt pt to chew/swallow.	4. Pt responsive to prompts.
5. Identity food given to pt before each mouthful.	5. Pt nodded recognition- frowned to display distaste.
6. Crush pills and place in pureed food.	6. Pt took all medications s̄ incident

Summarize your impressions of patient progress towards goals   Pt did not aspirate and completed 75% of meals. Continue interventions.

Problem #7 Risk for Infection
Short-term Goal: Pt will remain free of infection as evidenced by VS WNL, Ø purulent drainage from tubes.
Long-term Goal: Pt will remain free of infection post discharge.

Nursing Interventions:	Patient's Response:
1. Monitor VS q 4°.	1. VS WNL: Temp 97°, HR66
2. Monitor WBC.	2. WBC WNL - 9.2.
3. Monitor pt for S & S of infection.	3. Pt shows Ø S & S of inflammation, swelling, drainage at any IV site.
4. Practice aseptic technique at all times.	4. Pt remains free of infection.
5. Monitor appearance of urine.	5. Pt's urine is dark, amber color. MD notified. Culture ordered.
6. Encourage intake of protein & calorie rich foods.	6. Pt completes app. 75% of food offered.

Summarize your impressions of patient progress towards goals   Pt has remained free of S/S of infection—awaiting results of urine culture. Continue interventions.

Problem #8 Anxiety
Short-term Goal: Pt will demonstrate a reduced level of anxiety evidenced by ↓ seizures, ↓ restlessness.
Long-term Goal: Pt will demonstrate positive coping mechanisms.

Nursing Interventions:	Patient's Response:
1. Acknowledge awareness of pt's anxiety.	1. Pt appeared grateful, nodded affirmatively.
2. Maintain a calm manner c̄ pt.	2. Pt appears calm and responsive.
3. Maintain frequent contact c̄ pt.	3. Pt demonstrates recognition when I appear.
4. Use simple language & brief statements to explain procedures & tasks.	4. Pt followed commands appropriately.
5. Reduce sensory stimuli.	5. Pt appears calm and resting comfortably.

Summarize your impressions of patient progress towards goals   Pt is experiencing less restlessness and appears more comfortable c̄ environment. Continue interventions.

FIGURE 11-5 *Continued*

BOX 11-8 **Take the Challenge**

Read the professional behaviors below, and circle the number that best reflects the proficiency you now have in each of these essential nursing competencies.

1 = no skills	3 – moderately skilled	5 = excellent skills
2 = somewhat skilled	4 = well skilled	

Cognitive Competencies

1	2	3	4	5	• Offer a scientific rationale for the plan of care.
1	2	3	4	5	• Select those nursing interventions that are most likely to yield desired outcomes.
1	2	3	4	5	• Use critical thinking to problem-solve creatively.

Technical Competencies

1	2	3	4	5	• Use technical equipment with sufficient competence and ease to achieve goal with a minimum of distress to involved participants.
1	2	3	4	5	• Creatively adapt equipment and technical procedures to the needs of particular patients in diverse circumstances.

Interpersonal Competencies

1	2	3	4	5	• Creative use of look, speech, and touch to communicate respect and to enhance sense of worth
1	2	3	4	5	• Skilled use of presence and conversation to demonstrate empathy and to obtain sufficient knowledge about the patient to personalize care and serve as an effective advocate
1	2	3	4	5	• Responsible, competent attentiveness to the holistic needs of patients such that trust is built and patients experience comfort of security
1	2	3	4	5	• Value mutual enrichment of both participants in the nurse–patient relationship

Ethical/Legal Competencies

1	2	3	4	5	• Self-motivated to act in ways that advance the interests of patients (consistently trustworthy)
1	2	3	4	5	• Accountable for practice to self, patients served, the caregiving team, and society
1	2	3	4	5	• Consistently serve as effective patient advocate
1	2	3	4	5	• Skilled in mediating ethical conflict among the patient, significant others, healthcare team, and other interested parties
1	2	3	4	5	• Practice nursing faithful to the tenets of professional codes of ethics
1	2	3	4	5	• Use legal safeguards that reduce the risk of litigation

---

ASSESSING BLENDED SKILLS AND CRITICAL THINKING

Nurses who are sincerely committed to quality care learn early to make self-evaluation an integral part of their nursing practice. Self-evaluation skills promote professional development, enhance self-esteem, and help one develop self-awareness. The Reflective Practice exercises in each chapter illustrate this practice. Each exercise describes a particular challenge to the student's competence, a range of possible responses, the criteria the student used to evaluate a good response, and a brief statement about what the student learned from this experience.

The nurse who is just beginning to develop in the caregiver role might find it helpful to conclude each caregiving experience with a brief moment of reflection that identifies and celebrates the nursing skills used and targets skills that need to be developed. This practice can keep one from feeling overwhelmed by everything that remains to be mastered and yet strongly motivated to learn new skills.

This chapter concludes with an assessment tool you can use to assess your proficiency in the skills essential for competent use of the nursing process (see Box 11-8). After completing the exercise, share your self-evaluation with a trusted colleague or clinical instructor and see whether your assessments of your abilities agree. Celebrate your natural and developed strengths. Begin now to plan a strategy to boost those skills in which you are deficient. This might sound trite, but it is true: your patients will be grateful you cared enough to be your best.

Identified in the patient care studies that conclude the clinical chapters in this text are the specialized knowledge and skills that the nurse needs to implement the plan of care. It is helpful when planning care to identify what nursing resources are needed to ensure that you meet each challenge. Nurses sensitive to mastering both the art and the science of nursing care evaluate whether they have the prerequisite skills for each nurse–patient encounter, as well as the skills needed to perceive, respond to, and appreciate the uniqueness of each patient. Quality care is each nurse's responsibility.

■ Developing Critical Thinking Skills

1. A nursing student realizes that her college roommate's behavior has changed dramatically during the past month. Once outgoing and funny, she is now withdrawn and moody, rebuffing efforts to discuss the change. Compare and contrast the processes and likely outcomes of using different methods of problem-solving (trial-and-error, scientific, intuitive) and the nursing process to address the roommate's needs.

2. The nursing process is an interpersonal process that is always patient centered rather than task centered. Discuss with other students the meaning of this claim. Think through (and discuss) the implications of approaching patients as "problems to be solved."

3. Describe how you would structure an assessment of the situation described below, using critical thinking considerations: purpose of thinking, adequacy of knowledge, potential problems, helpful resources, and critique of judgment/decision.
   - A 28-year-old woman is admitted to a hospital for multiple contusions and a hairline fracture of the skull. She claims that she "fell down the steps," but on examination, it appears that several of the injuries are inconsistent with a fall. The woman sticks to her story that her fall was an accident. You are her nurse.
   - Assess whether your attitudes and dispositions would help or hinder the task of critical thinking if you were the nurse in this situation. Share your self-evaluation with another student and compare your responses.

4. Using the above scenario, identify the cognitive, technical, interpersonal, and ethical/legal skills you would need to meet the nursing needs of this woman. If possible, compare your list with that of an experienced nurse and discuss the differences.

■ Practicing for NCLEX

Read the patient scenario below and then match each numbered and boldfaced nursing activity with the correct step of the nursing process.

*Annie seeks your help in the student health clinic because she suspects that her roommate Angela suffered date-rape. She is concerned because Angela chose not to report the rape and does not seem to be coping well. (1) **After talking with Annie you learn that although Angela blurted out that she had been raped when she first came home, since then she has refused verbalization about the rape ("I don't want to think or talk***

*about it"), has stopped attending all college social activities (a marked change in behavior), and seems to be having nightmares. After analyzing the data, you believe that Angela might be experiencing (2) **rape-trauma syndrome: silent reaction.** Fortunately, Angela trusts Annie and is willing to come to the student health center for help. After a conversation with Angela confirms your suspicions and problem identification, you talk with Angela (3) **to develop some treatment goals that you formulate as outcomes, and begin to think about the types of nursing interventions most likely to yield the outcomes you both seek.** In your initial meeting with Angela, (4) **you encourage her expression of feelings and help her to identify personal coping strategies and strengths.** You and Angela decide to meet in 1 week (5) **to assess her progress toward achieving targeted outcomes.** If she is not making progress, you might need to modify the plan of care.*

1. The nursing activity represented as (1) is an example of which step of the nursing process?
   a. Assessing
   b. Diagnosing
   c. Evaluating
   d. Implementing
   e. Planning

2. The nursing activity represented as (2) is an example of which step of the nursing process?
   a. Assessing
   b. Diagnosing
   c. Evaluating
   d. Implementing
   e. Planning

3. The nursing activity represented as (3) is an example of which step of the nursing process?
   a. Assessing
   b. Diagnosing
   c. Evaluating
   d. Implementing
   e. Planning

4. The nursing activity represented as (4) is an example of which step of the nursing process?
   a. Assessing
   b. Diagnosing
   c. Evaluating
   d. Implementing
   e. Planning

5. The nursing activity represented as (5) is an example of which step of the nursing process?
   a. Assessing
   b. Diagnosing
   c. Evaluating
   d. Implementing
   e. Planning

6. Which of the following statements about the nursing process is most accurate?
   a. The nursing process is a four-step procedure for identifying and resolving patient problems.

b. Beginning in Florence Nightingale's days, nursing students learned and practiced the nursing process.

c. Use of the nursing process is optional for nurses, since there are many ways to accomplish the work of nursing.

d. The state board examinations for professional nursing practice now use the nursing process rather than medical specialties as an organizing concept.

7. The nursing process ensures that nurses are patient centered rather than task centered. Rather than simply approaching a patient to take vital signs, the nurse thinks "How is Mrs. Barclay today? Are our nursing actions helping her to achieve her goals? How can we better help her?" This demonstrates which characteristic of the nursing process?

a. Systematic
b. Interpersonal
c. Dynamic
d. Universally applicable in nursing situations

8. An experienced nurse tells you not to bother studying too hard, since most clinical reasoning becomes "second nature" and "intuitive" once you start practicing. What thinking below should underlie your response?

a. When intuition is used alone, there are increased risks and fewer benefits. Intuition often moves problem-solving forward quickly, but it might result in a lot of trial-and-error approaches.

b. For nursing to remain a science, nurses must continue to be vigilant about stamping out intuitive reasoning.

c. The emphasis on logical, scientific, evidence-based reasoning has held nursing back for years. It's time to champion intuitive, creative thinking!

d. It's simply a matter of preference. Some of us are logical, scientific thinkers, and some are intuitive, creative thinkers.

9. This text is based upon a notion of blended skills. Simply described, this means:

a. Nursing works best when nurses competently use the intellectual and technical skills that achieve patient outcomes. Nursing has been held back by outdated notions of care and compassion (interpersonal skills), which can be done by anyone.

b. Nursing works best when each nurse competently uses the intellectual, interpersonal, technical, and ethical/legal skills demanded by each situation.

c. All of the blended skills are important, but not every nurse has to be skilled in each area. We benefit patients by knowing what we do best. I might be utterly deficient in interpersonal skills but excellent in intellectual skills.

d. Every nursing situation demands the same blend of basic nursing skills, intellectual, technical, interpersonal, and ethical/legal.

10. The best description of critical thinking indicators (CTIs™) is which of the following:

a. Evidence-based descriptions of behaviors that demonstrate the knowledge that promotes critical thinking in clinical practice

b. Evidence-based descriptions of behaviors that demonstrate the knowledge and skills that promote critical thinking in clinical practice

c. Evidence-based descriptions of behaviors that demonstrate the knowledge, characteristics, and skills that promote critical thinking in clinical practice

d. Evidence-based descriptions of behaviors that demonstrate the knowledge, characteristics, standards, and skills that promote critical thinking in clinical practice

■ Answers With Rationale

1. The correct answer is *a*.
2. The correct answer is *b*.
3. The correct answer is *e*.
4. The correct answer is *d*.
5. The correct answer is *c*.
6. The correct answer is *d*. The nursing process is a five-step process (*a*); the term nursing process was first used by Hall in 1955 (*b*); and standards demand the use of the nursing process (*c*), so it is not optional.
7. The correct answer is *b*, interpersonal. Each of the other options are characteristics of the nursing process, but the conversation and thinking quoted best illustrates the interpersonal dimension of the nursing process.
8. The correct answer is *a*. When intuition is used alone, there are increased risks and fewer benefits. Intuition often moves problem-solving forward quickly, but it might result in a lot of trial-and-error approaches. (*b*) is incorrect because there is a place for intuitive reasoning in nursing, but it will never replace logical, scientific reasoning (*c*). Critical thinking is contextual and changes depending on the circumstances, not on personal preference (*d*).
9. The correct answer is *b*. Every nurse must be competent in all four basic skill areas and judge what skills each situation needs. Each situation is unique and might call for a different "blend" of basic skills.
10. The correct answer is *c*, evidence-based descriptions of behaviors that demonstrate the knowledge, characteristics, and skills that promote critical thinking in clinical practice.

Bibliography

Aiken, T. D., & Catalano, J. T. (1994). *Legal, ethical, and political issues in nursing*. Philadelphia: F. A. Davis.

Alfaro, R. (2002). *Applying nursing process: Promoting collaborative care* (5th ed.). Philadelphia: Lippincott Williams & Wilkins.

Alfaro-LeFevre, R. (2004). *Critical thinking and clinical judgment: A practical approach.* Philadelphia: W. B. Saunders.

American Association of Colleges of Nursing. (1998). *Essentials of baccalaureate education for professional nursing.* Washington, DC: Author.

American Nurses Association. (1980, 1995). *Nursing: A social policy statement.* Washington, DC: Author

American Nurses Association. (2001). *Code for nurses with interpretive statements.* Washington, DC: Author.

American Nurses Association. (1994). *Guidelines on reporting incompetent, unethical or illegal practices.* Washington, DC: Author.

American Nurses Association Congress for Nursing Practice. (1973; revised 1991, 1998, 2003). *Standards of practice.* Washington, DC: Author.

Aroskar, M. A. (1993). Incompetent, unethical or illegal practice—teaching students to cope. *Journal of Professional Nursing, 9*(3), 130.

Benner, P. (1984, 2001). *From novice to expert.* Menlo Park, CA: Addison-Wesley.

Benner, P., & Wrubel, J. (1989). *The primacy of caring in health and illness.* Menlo Park, CA: Addison-Wesley.

Canadian Nurses Association. (1987). *Standards of nursing practice.* Ottawa, Ontario: Author

Chafree, J. (1990). *Thinking critically* (3rd ed.). Boston: Houghton Mifflin.

Christensen, P. J., & Kenney, J. W. (1994). *Nursing process: Application of conceptual models* (4th ed.). St. Louis: C. V. Mosby.

Craft-Rosenberg, M., & Delaney M. (1997). Nursing diagnosis extension and classification (NDEC). In M. J. Rantz & D. LeMone (Eds.) *Classification of Nursing Diagnoses: Proceedings of the Twelfth Conference North American Nursing Diagnosis* (pp. 26–31). Glendale, CA: CINAHL Information Services.

Daley, B. J. (1996). Concept maps: Linking nursing theory to clinical nursing practice. *Journal of Continuing Education in Nursing, 27*(1), 17–27.

Davies, E. (1995). Reflective practice: A focus for caring. *Journal of Nursing Education, 34*(4), 167–174.

DiVito-Thomas, P. (2000). Identifying critical thinking behaviors in clinical judgments. *Journal of Nursing Staff Development, 16*(3), 174–180.

Ennis, R. H. (1996). *Critical thinking.* Upper Saddle River, NJ: Prentice-Hall.

Facione, P., & Facione, N. (1992). *California critical thinking disposition inventory.* Millbrae, CA: California Academic Press.

Facione, P., Facione, N., & Sanchez, C. (1994). Critical thinking disposition as a measure of competent clinical judgment: The development of the California Critical Thinking Disposition Inventory. *Journal of Nursing Education, 33*(8), 345–351.

Fonteyn, M. E., & Cooper, L. F. (1994). The written nursing process: Is it still useful to nursing education? *Journal of Advanced Nursing, 19*(2), 315–319.

Gebbie, K., & Lavin, M. A. (1974). Classification of nursing diagnosis. *American Journal of Nursing, 74,* 250–253.

Hall, L. E. (1955). Quality of nursing care. Address given at the Department of Baccalaureate and Higher Degree Programs of the New Jersey League for Nursing. *Public Health News (June).* New Jersey: New Jersey State Department of Health.

Hansten, R., & Washburn, M. (2001). Intuition in professional practice: Executive and staff perceptions. *Journal of Nursing Administration, 30*(4), 185–188.

Heinrich, K., & Killeen, M. E. (1993). The gentle art of nurturing yourself. *American Journal of Nursing, 93*(10), 41–44.

Iowa Intervention Project. (1997). Nursing interventions classification (NIC): An overview. In M. J. Rantz & P. LeMone (Eds.), *Classification of Nursing Diagnoses: Proceedings of the Twelfth Conference, North American Nursing Diagnosis* (pp. 32–39). Glendale, CA: CINAHL Information Systems.

Irvine, L. (1995). Can concept mapping be used to promote meaningful learning in nurse education. *Journal of Advanced Nursing, 21,* 1175–1179.

Jacono, B. J., & Jacono, J. K. (1995). A holistic approach to teaching responsibility and accountability. *Nurse Educator, 20*(1), 20–23.

Johnson, J. (1994). A dialectical examination of the nursing art. *Advances in Nursing Science, 17*(1), 1–14.

Johnson, M., & Mass, M. L. (Eds.) (1997). *Nursing outcomes classification (NOC).* St. Louis: Mosby–Year Book.

Joint Commission on Accreditation of Healthcare Organizations. (2003). *Accreditation manual for hospitals.* Oakbrook Terrace, IL: Author.

Kataoka-Yahiro, M. (1994). A critical thinking model for nursing judgment. *Journal of Nursing Education, 33*(8), 351–356.

Kolcaba, K. Y. (1995). The art of comfort care. *Image—The Journal of Nursing Scholarship, 27*(4), 287–289.

Lamond, D., & Thompson, C. (2000). Intuition and analysis in decision making and choice. *Journal of Nursing Scholarship, 32*(3), 411–414.

Locsin, R. C. (1995). Machine technologies and caring in nursing. *Image—The Journal of Nursing Scholarship, 27*(3), 201–203.

McCloskey, J. C., & Bulechek, G. M. (Eds.) (2000). *Nursing intervention classification (NIC)* (3rd ed.). St. Louis: Mosby–Year Book.

Miller, M. A., & Babcock, D. E. (1996). *Critical thinking applied to nursing.* St. Louis: C. V. Mosby.

Paul, R. W. (1993). *Critical thinking: How to prepare students for a rapidly changing world.* Santa Rosa, CA: Foundation for Critical Thinking.

Renz, M. C. (1993). Learning from intuition. *Nursing, 23*(7), 44–45.

Rew, L. (1987). Nursing intuition: Too powerful—and too valuable—to ignore. *Nursing, 17*(7), 43–45.

Rubenfeld, M. G., & Scheffer, B. K. (1999). *Critical thinking in nursing: An interactive approach* (2nd ed.). Philadelphia: Lippincott Williams & Wilkins.

Schraeder, B. D., & Fischer, D. K. (1986). Using knowledge to make clinical decisions. *MCN, 11,* 161–163.

Scheffer, B., & Rubenfeld, M. (2000). A consensus statement on critical thinking in nursing. *Journal of Nursing Education, 39*(8), 352–359.

Schuster, P. M. (2002). *Concept mapping: A critical-thinking approach to care planning.* Philadelphia: F. A. Davis.

Stark, J. (1995). Critical thinking: Taking the road less traveled. *Nursing, 25*(11), 53–56.

Taylor, C. (1995). Rethinking nursing's basic competencies. *Journal of Nursing Care Quality, 9*(4), 1–13.

Wilkinson, J. (2001). *Nursing process and critical thinking* (3rd ed.). Redwood City, CA: Addison-Wesley Nursing.

Yura, H., & Walsh, M. B. (1967, 1988). *The nursing process: Assessing, planning, implementing, evaluating* (5th ed.). Norwalk, CT: Appleton-Century-Crofts.

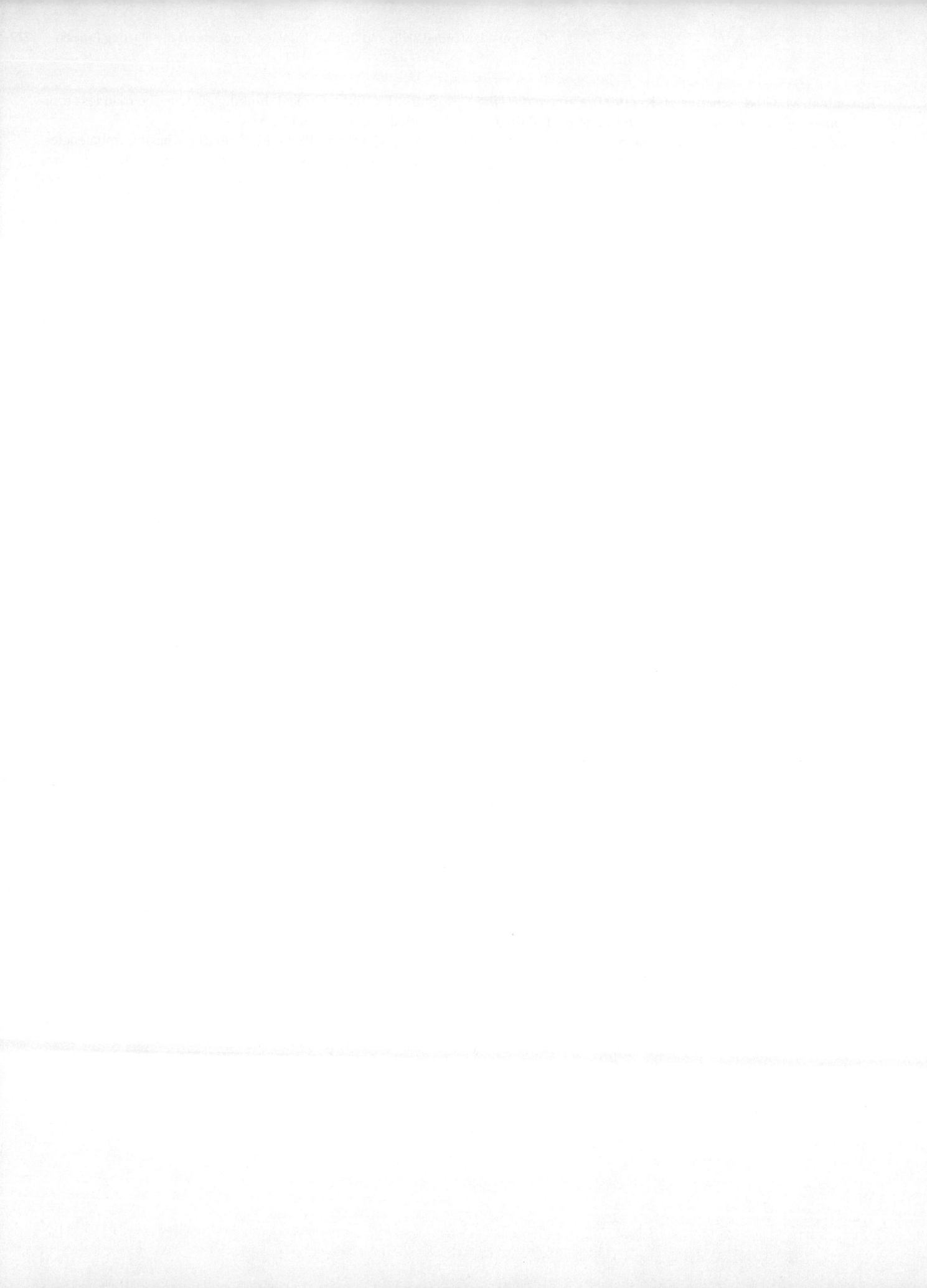

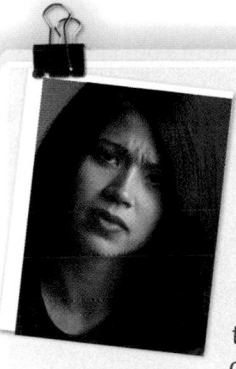

Susan Morgan is a 34-year-old woman newly diagnosed with multiple sclerosis (MS). She says "How am I going to tell my husband? We were just married last year and planned to do lots of hiking and outdoor sports. It's not fair for him to be tied down to me if I can't be the wife and partner that he thought he had married."

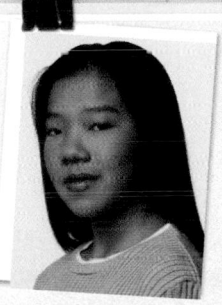

Sylvia Wu, a 17-year-old woman has just arrived back in the United States after a visit to her family in mainland China. She comes to the emergency department because she woke up that morning with flu-like symptoms (cough, sore throat, fever, muscle aches, fatigue). "I'm scared because of everything I've seen on television and read in the newspapers about that new virus, SARS."

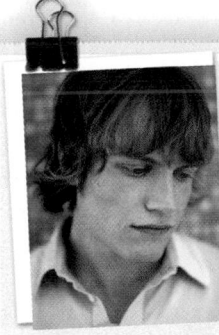

James Farren is a college junior who comes to the student health center complaining of difficulty sleeping, eating, and studying. He reveals that his mother died when he was 8 years old, and last semester his father died suddenly, a victim of a fatal car crash. "Ever since my dad died, nothing seems to mean anything anymore. All I see is gray."

Focusing on Blended Skills

The types of blended skills you'll need to respond to the case scenarios include:

Cognitive Skills

- Knowledge of the signs and symptoms of MS, depression, and SARS
- Ability to integrate knowledge of underlying pathophysiology to guide assessment
- Ability to differentiate relevant subjective and objective data, focusing on appropriate patient priorities
- Ability to identify factually pertinent information related to the specific patient situation, such as MS, depression, or SARS
- Knowledge of appropriate sources for additional information and supportive services

Technical Skills

- Ability to use appropriate patient-focused questions during the nursing history to elicit information related to MS, depression, and SARS
- Ability to demonstrate strong physical assessment skills to diagnose health problems related to MS, depression, and SARS
- Ability to ask for assistance when necessary when obtaining the nursing history or completing the physical examination
- Ability to incorporate appropriate assessment tools and techniques based on patient needs
- Demonstration of competency in data communication

Interpersonal Skills

- Ability to establish a trusting nurse–patient relationship with any patient, regardless of the patient's complaints or problems
- Demonstration of strong people skills for dealing with individuals experiencing alterations in health
- Ability to communicate concern about patient, patient's complaints, and situation
- Demonstration of respect for patient's human dignity to promote patient's self-esteem
- Interpersonal competence to mobilize patients experiencing physiologic and psychologic threats to body integrity

Ethical and Legal Skills

- Strong sense of accountability for the health and well-being of individuals
- Commitment to assisting patients obtain the necessary help for achieving health goals within the scope of nursing responsibilities and available resources
- Strong advocacy skills and a willingness to use them for patients needing assistance
- Ability to integrate ethical and legal principles into patient assessments, both documenting and communicating pertinent data to appropriate healthcare providers

Learning Outcomes

After completing the chapter, the learner should be able to accomplish the following:

1. Define and describe the purpose of four types of nursing assessments.
2. Explain the relationship between nursing assessment and medical assessment.
3. Differentiate objective and subjective data.
4. Describe the purpose of nursing observation, interview, and physical assessment.
5. Obtain a nursing history using effective interviewing techniques.
6. Identify five sources of patient data useful to the nurse.
7. Plan patient assessments by identifying assessment priorities and structuring the data to be collected systematically.
8. Identify common problems encountered in data collection, noting their possible cause.
9. Explain when data need to be validated and several ways to accomplish this.
10. Describe the importance of knowing when to report significant patient data and of proper documentation.
11. Obtain and document complete, accurate, factual, and relevant patient data.

Key Terms

assessing
cue
data
database
emergency assessment
focused assessment
inference
initial assessment
interview
minimum data set
nursing history
objective data
observation
physical assessment
subjective data
time-lapsed assessment
validation

Assessing is the systematic and continuous collection, validation, and communication of patient data; these **data** reflect how health functioning is enhanced by health promotion or compromised by illness and injury. A **database** includes all the pertinent patient information collected by the nurse and other healthcare professionals. The database enables a comprehensive and effective plan of care to be designed and implemented for the patient. The collection of patient data is a vital step in the nursing process because the remaining steps depend on complete, accurate, factual, and relevant data.

Refer to the Reflective Practice box regarding Sylvia Wu, a patient who fears that she has SARS. The nurse's assessment would reveal possible factors that increase her risk for developing SARS. Additionally, the patient's statements about her fears provide further data on which to develop a plan of care.

The initial comprehensive nursing assessment results in baseline data that enable the nurse to:

- Make a judgment about a patient's health status, the ability to manage his or her own healthcare, and the need for nursing
- Refer the patient to a physician or other healthcare professional, if indicated
- Plan and deliver individualized, holistic nursing care that draws on the patient's strengths

In addition to an initial assessment of the patient, the nurse makes ongoing assessments. These assessments alert the nurse to changes in the patient's responses to health and illness, and suggest necessary changes in the plan of nursing care or care offered by other healthcare professionals. Ongoing nursing assessments may be problem focused, time lapsed, or emergency based.

During the assessment step of the nursing process, the nurse establishes the database by interviewing the patient to obtain a nursing history. The nurse may also perform a nursing examination to collect data. Other sources of patient information used by the nurse include the patient's family and significant others, the patient record, the patient's healthcare profession-

Reflective Practice
Challenge to Intellectual Skills

While on a clinical rotation in the emergency department, I met Sylvia Wu, a 17-year-old young woman who had just arrived back in the United States after a visit to her family in mainland China. She came to emergency department because she woke up that morning with flu-like symptoms (cough, sore throat, fever, muscle aches, fatigue) and was terrified because of everything she had seen on television and read in the newspapers about the latest new virus, SARS (severe acute respiratory syndrome). Although 64 people have died already, she knows that most of the cases are in Asia. She came to the emergency room, begging to be told that she doesn't have SARS, but, rather, that most likely her symptoms are due to fatigue or a cold. I want to calm her, but I honestly don't know what she has. Besides, I am starting to feel a bit anxious myself because the one thing everyone knows about SARS is the fact that it is extremely "contagious." I could feel myself recoil when Sylvia sneezed.

Thinking Outside the Box: Possible Courses of Action

- Reassure Sylvia and tell her not to worry because the overwhelming probability is that her symptoms aren't anything serious.
- Quickly get someone with more experience to care for Sylvia because I don't want to be anywhere near her if she does have SARS.

- Document and report her concerns, trying to keep her isolated and away from other patients, while trying to find more information about SARS quickly, since I'm not sure about its signs and symptoms.

Evaluating a Good Outcome: How Do I Define Success?

- Sylvia gets the medical treatment she needs, and her fears are appropriately addressed.
- In the event that Sylvia does have a highly communicable disease, the risk for disease transmission to others is reduced.

- I manage to control my fears, being able to respond to Sylvia's concerns appropriately.
- I learn something about my immediate response to feeling at risk and my commitment to professionalism.

Personal Learning: Here's to the Future!

Although I am not proud of my response, I falsely reassured Sylvia that this was probably nothing. As a result, I did not report or document her fears. Unfortunately, Sylvia was diagnosed with SARS and several others in our emergency department at that time became infected. For some reason, I escaped. In the future, I hope I'll never be so insensitive to a patient's concerns or insights again.

Reflection

How do you think you would respond in a similar situation? Why? What does this tell you about yourself and about the adequacy of your skills for professional practice? What factors might have influenced this nursing student's actions? What types of data could have led the nursing student to a different course of action? How might the nursing student assessed the patient differently? Can you think of other ways to respond? What other skills (cognitive, interpersonal, technical, ethical/legal) would you need to respond well in this situation? Do you agree with the criteria to evaluate a successful outcome? Did the nursing student meet the criteria? If not, what else might the nursing student have done to ensure a successful outcome?

als, and nursing and other healthcare literature. After the nurse has established the database, data about the patient are collected continuously because the patient's health status can change quickly. Questionable data are verified (validated) as part of the assessment step of the nursing process. All pertinent data are recorded and, when appropriate, communicated to other healthcare professionals so that the data can best benefit the patient (Fig. 12-1). In addition to collecting data, nurses might use intuition to assess patients (see Chap. 11).

UNIQUE FOCUS OF NURSING ASSESSMENT

When nurses make nursing assessments, they do not duplicate medical assessments. Medical assessments target data pointing to pathologic conditions, whereas nursing assessments focus on the patient's responses to health problems. For example, is there interference with the patient's ability to meet basic human needs? Can the patient perform the activities of daily living? Although the findings from a nursing assessment may contribute to the identification of a medical diagnosis, the unique focus of nursing assessments is on the patient's responses to actual or potential health problems.

Remember Susan Morgan, a patient recently diagnosed with MS? By looking at the data supplied by the patient, the nurse would be

able to determine that the patient's new diagnosis of MS is affecting her body image and self esteem. The nurse then would use this information to focus assessment questions to obtain additional information to be included in the database, from which a plan of care specific to Susan's needs can be developed.

TYPES OF NURSING ASSESSMENTS

Nursing assessments include the comprehensive initial assessment, the focused assessment, the emergency assessment, and the time-lapsed assessment. In this chapter we will focus on assessing the health status of an individual. As you develop expertise in nursing assessments, you will be able to assess communities and special populations, such as school children or people with AIDS or other infectious diseases.

Initial Assessment

The **initial assessment** is performed shortly after the patient is admitted to a healthcare agency or service. Most institutions have policies specifying the time interval within which the assessment must be completed. The purpose of this assessment is to establish a complete database for problem identification

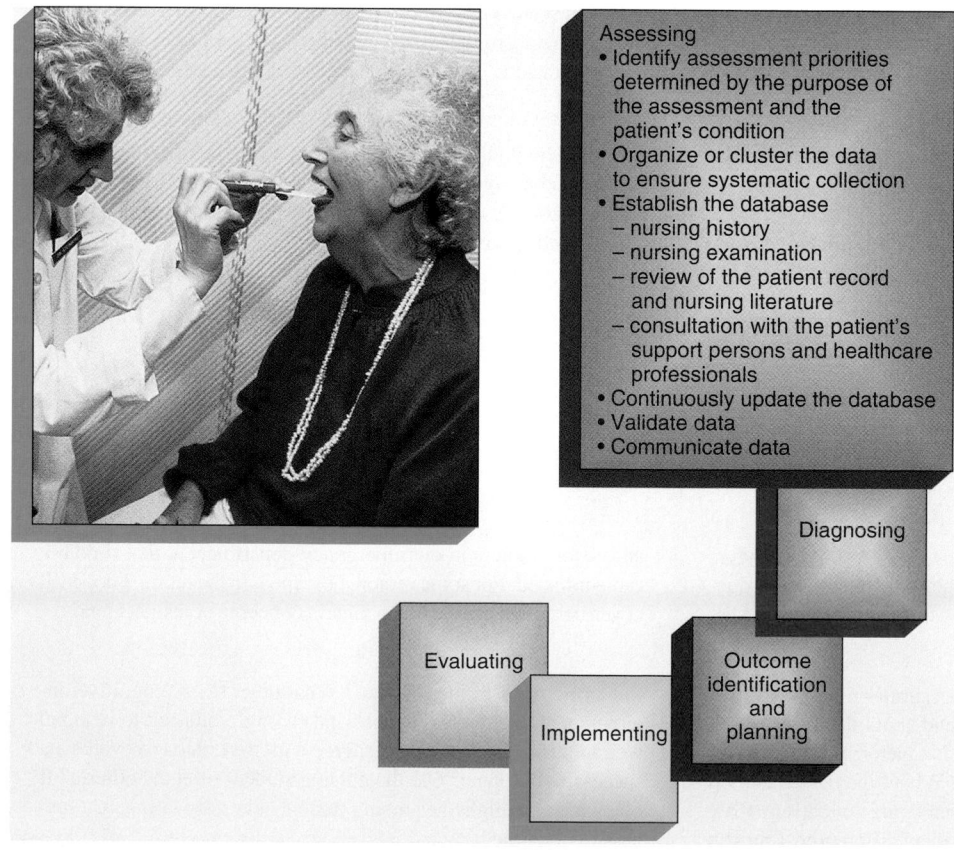

Assessing
- Identify assessment priorities determined by the purpose of the assessment and the patient's condition
- Organize or cluster the data to ensure systematic collection
- Establish the database
  – nursing history
  – nursing examination
  – review of the patient record and nursing literature
  – consultation with the patient's support persons and healthcare professionals
- Continuously update the database
- Validate data
- Communicate data

Diagnosing

Evaluating

Implementing

Outcome identification and planning

FIGURE 12-1 Assessing. The primary source of patient information is the patient. Resources include the patient's support people, the patient record, information from other healthcare professionals, and information from nursing and healthcare literature.

and care planning. The nurse collects data concerning all aspects of the patient's health, establishing priorities for ongoing focused assessments and creating a reference for future comparison. See Figure 12-2 for a sample of an initial assessment.

Focused Assessment

In a **focused assessment,** the nurse gathers data about a specific problem that has already been identified. A focused assessment may be done during the initial assessment if patient health problems surface, but it is routinely part of ongoing data collection. Another purpose of the focused assessment is to identify new or overlooked problems.

> Remember Sylvia Wu, the 17-year-old who comes to the emergency department because she thinks that she might have SARS? The nurse would use a focused assessment to evaluate her complaints that is specifically related to her respiratory status. This information would be supplemented by additional data about the patient's recent travel to mainland China.

Emergency Assessment

When a physiologic or psychological crisis presents, the nurse performs an **emergency assessment** to identify life-threatening problems. A nursing-home resident who begins choking in the dining room, a bleeding patient brought to the emergency room with a stab wound, an unresponsive patient in the rehabilitation unit, and a factory worker threatening violence are all candidates for an emergency assessment.

Time-Lapsed Assessment

The **time-lapsed assessment** is scheduled to compare a patient's current status to baseline data obtained earlier. Most patients in residential settings and those receiving nursing care over longer periods of time, such as homebound patients with visiting nurses, are scheduled for periodic time-lapsed assessments to reassess health status and to make necessary revisions in the plan of care.

PREPARING FOR DATA COLLECTION

Establishing assessment priorities and systematically structuring data collection are two important considerations when preparing for data collection.

Establishing Assessment Priorities

Before beginning to collect data on any patient, the nurse should have a good sense of the type of data needed to develop a satisfactory plan of care. Nurses spend more or less time on different components of the nursing history depending on the patient's reason for needing nursing assistance. For example, pediatric nurses are careful to establish the developmental age and milestones obtained by children admitted to a pediatric unit so that they can respect and promote these achievements. A school nurse who suspects child abuse pays careful attention to the child's statements about living conditions at home and relationships with family members and caregivers. A nurse preparing to discharge a patient from same-day surgery makes sure that the patient has the human and physical resources needed to supply appropriate postoperative care.

The purpose for which the assessment is being performed offers the best guideline about what type and how much data to collect. Assessment priorities are influenced by the patient's health orientation, developmental stage, and need for nursing.

Health Orientation

Health assessments, such as *Health-Style: A Self-Test* in Chapter 4, and the Promoting Health displays in each clinical chapter, may be used by nurses to help patients identify potential and actual health risks, and to explore their habits, behaviors, beliefs, attitudes, and values that influence levels of wellness. The literature abounds in specialized assessment tools that focus on relationships; psychological, environmental, and physical self-care; relaxation; spirituality; humor and play; movement and exercise; sleep and dreams; nutrition; and sexuality. In terms of the type of patient data gathered, these assessments are different from the assessments of patients being hospitalized for disease-related treatment.

Developmental Stage

Nursing assessments are modified according to the developmental needs of patients. For example, when assessing an infant, special attention is given to weight gain and physical growth, feeding and elimination problems, sleep–activity cycles, and the parenting skills of caregivers. When children are hospitalized, it is important to note how independent the child is with basic care measures (toileting, hygiene, dressing, eating), what words the child uses to indicate the need to void and defecate, play preferences, and so forth.

Need for Nursing

Whether nurses will be interacting with the patient for a short or a long period (eg, same-day surgery versus surgery that necessitates a long recovery in an intensive care unit) and the nature of nursing care needed by the patient (eg, assistance with the birth of a baby versus support and home care throughout a terminal illness), both powerfully influence the type of data the nurse collects. A general guideline when assessing patients is to gather only data that are helpful when planning and delivering care. It would be inappropriate, for example, to collect a detailed sexual history on a patient admitted to the hospital overnight after a slight concussion. Conversely, a nurse should not fail to ask a pregnant woman admitted to the hospital for observation because of bleeding during her first trimester whether she has any questions about resuming sexual activity after she gets home.

(text continues on page 238)

NAZARETH HOSPITAL

NURSING ADMISSION HISTORY

I. GENERAL INFORMATION

ARRIVAL: Date: _9/2/06_   Time: _2:00 PM_

Transportation Method: ☐ Ambulatory   ☐ Stretcher   ☑ W/C

Admitted Via: ☑ ED   ☐ Direct Admission   ☐ PACU   ☐ SDS**
☐ Other:_____

Accompanied By: ☐ Self ☐ Spouse ☑ Daughter ☐ Son
☐ Mother ☐ Father ☐ Friend ☐ Other:_____

Correct Name On Identiband?   ☑ YES   ☐ NO

PATIENT/SIGNIFICANT OTHER ORIENTED TO:
Call Light at Bedside/in BR :   ☑ YES ☐ NO ☐ N/A
Operation of Bed/Siderails: ☑ YES ☐ NO ☐ N/A
Phone/TV: ☑ YES ☐ NO ☐ N/A

PATIENT ADVISED HOSPITAL NOT RESPONSIBLE FOR VALUABLES:
☑ YES ☐ NO

Does Patient Have Any Valuables?   ☑ YES* ☐ NO
If Yes*, Disposition of Valuables?   ☐ Sent Home
☐ Security - Envelope #_____
☑ Patient Refused Security - Valuables kept with Patient

LIST & DESCRIBE PATIENT'S VALUABLES
eyeglasses @ bedside
yellow metal watch on patient
yellow metal wedding ring on pt.
sent purse home with daughter

MEDICATION BROUGHT TO HOSPITAL: ☐ YES ☑ NO
If YES, :   ☐ Home   ☐ Pharmacy

_____ Date: _____ Time: _____
STAFF SIGNATURE REQUIRED FOR ALL SDS** PATIENTS

INFORMATION GIVEN BY PATIENT: ☑ YES ☐ NO
IF NO:Name: _____
Number: _____
Relationship: _____
☐ Unable to obtain history - REASON

REASON FOR ADMISSION ACCORDING TO PATIENT:
"I fell at home this a.m. Couldn't move
(L) leg for awhile; headaches

PATIENT AWARE OF DIAGNOSIS: ☐ YES ☑ NO
FAMILY AWARE OF DIAGNOSIS: ☐ YES ☑ NO
DOES PATIENT HAVE AN ORGAN DONOR CARD? ☐ YES ☑ NO
If no, & the patient requests further information,   provide
KIDNEY-1 Number.   1-800-KIDNEY-1
ALLERGIES:
  ***** ALLERGY DOCUMENTATION MUST BE COMPLETED AT
  TIME OF ADMISSION ON THE ALLERGY FORM*****
CURRENT MEDICATIONS   ☑ NONE
(INCLUDE RX, INHALERS, OVER-THE-COUNTER)

NAME	DOSE	FREQUENCY	LAST DOSE
REASON			
hydralazine	dose ?	OD	yesterday am
for high blood pressure			
aspirin	X 2	prn	noon today- headache
metamucil	1 Tbsp	prn	this am for constipation

HOSPITALIZATIONS/SURGICAL HISTORY   ☐ NONE
DIAGNOSIS/REASON

gallbladder surgery 1985

hospitalized for ↑BP 2002

FAMILY HISTORY: ☐ NONE
☐ Diabetes   ☐ Pulmonary   ☑ Heart Disease   ☑ CA
☐ Anesthesia   ☐ Other:
Complication

II. PAST MEDICAL HISTORY

SKIN: ☑ NEGATIVE HISTORY
☐ Scars   ☐ Eczema   ☐ Psoriasis   ☐ Cancer
☐ Other: _____

NEUROLOGICAL: ☐ NEGATIVE HISTORY
☐ TIA ?   ☐ Anxiety   ☐ Dementia   ☐ Syncope
☐ H/A   ☐ Tremors   ☐ Parkinson's   ☐ Depression

FIGURE 12-2 Sample nursing admission assessment form from Nazareth Hospital.   (Courtesy of Nazareth Hospital, Philadelphia, PA.)

NAZARETH HOSPITAL

NURSING ADMISSION HISTORY

☑ Falls	☐ Seizures	☐ Alzheimer's	☑ Vertigo
☐ CVA	☐ Tumor	☐ Migraines	☐ Mood
☐ R Hemiplagia	☐ Benign	☐ Vertigo	Changes
☐ L Hemiplagia	☐ Malignant	☑ Other: _"slightly dizzy"_	

Memory Impairment: ☑ NONE
☐ Acute → ☐ Short Term ☐ Long Term ☐ Chronic → ☐ Short Term ☐ Long Term

MUSCULOSKELETAL: ☐ NEGATIVE HISTORY
- ☐ Fractures: _____
- ☐ Arthritis: _____
- ☐ Amputation: _____
- ☐ Prosthesis: **TYPE:** _____ ☐ R ☐ L ☐ WITH PATIENT
- ☑ Other: ✓ _movement & strength (L) leg_ _____

If **with patient, remind patient hospital not responsible for article.

EENT   _"pins & needles in (L) leg"_
VISION: ☐ NEGATIVE HISTORY

☑ Glasses ☑ WITH PT	☐ Contacts ☐ WITH PT	☐ Prosthesis ☐ WITH PT
☐ Nearsighted	☐ R ☐ L	☐ R ☐ L
☐ Farsighted	☑ Blurred Vision	☐ Blind
☐ Glaucoma	☐ R ☐ L	☐ R ☐ L
☐ R ☐ L	☐ Double Vision	☐ Implants
☐ Cataract	☐ R ☐ L	☐ R ☐ L
☐ R ☐ L		

HEARING: ☐ NEGATIVE
HISTORY

☑ HOH	☐ Deaf	☐ Earache
☐ R ☑ L	☐ R ☐ L	☐ R ☐ L
☐ Tinnitus	☐ Hearing Aid ☐ WITH PT	
☐ R ☐ L	☐ R ☐ L	

If with Patient, remind patient hospital not responsible for article.

THYROID: ☑ NEGATIVE HISTORY
- ☐ Hypothyroid   ☐ Hyperthyroid   ☐ Surgery
- ☐ Radiation   → Have large doses of radioactive material been used within the last week?   ☐ YES* ☐ NO
  If YES*, notify Nuclear Medicine Department.

Speech Impairment: ☐ NONE   ☐ New*   ☐ Old
  If NEW*, notify Coordinated Care.

CARDIOVASCULAR: ☐ NEGATIVE HISTORY

☐ MI	☐ PVD	☐ Anemia	☐ Rheumatic H D
☑ HTN	☐ CHF	☐ Phlebitis	☐ Syncope Fainting
☐ CP/Angina		☐ Palpitations	☐ Bleeding Problems
☐ Hypotension		☐ Murmur	☐ Arrhythmia
☐ Pacemaker		☐ Internal	_____
Date:_____		Defibrillator	☐ Other:
Plutonium Operated		Date:_____	_____

☐ YES* ☐ NO
If YES*, notify Nuclear Medicine Department.

PULMONARY: ☑ NEGATIVE HISTORY

☐ TB	☐ Hemoptysis	☐ Cancer
☐ Asthma	☐ Emphysema	_____
☐ Bronchitis	☐ Asbestos Exposure	☐ Other
☐ Pneumonia		_____
☐ Trach	☐ Exposure to	
☐ Old ☐ New	Fumes/Smoke	
☐ Closed		

Dyspnea: ☑ NONE ☐ Activity ☐ Walking Stairs ☐ #pillows/sleep___
Home O2: ☑ NONE ☐ Activity ☐ Night ☐ Day ☐ PRN FlowRate____
GASTROINTESTINAL: ☐ NEGATIVE HISTORY

☐ Colitis	☐ Hepatitis	☐ Diabetes
☐ Ulcers	☐ Heart Burn	☐ Diet
☐ Reflux	☐ Hiatal Hernia	☐ Insulin
☐ Jaundice	☑ Hemorrhoids	☐ PO Meds
☐ Nausea	☐ Hematemesis	☐ Vomiting within
☐ Cirrhosis	☐ Diverticulosis	last 24 - 48 hrs
☐ Cancer	_____	_____/day
☐ Other:	_____	

Bowel Pattern:
Last BM: _9/1/06_   ☐ Daily ☐ QOD ☐ Q3Day ☑ Other: _Q2-3 day_
Bowel Problem: ☐ NONE ☑ Constipation ☐ Incontinence
☐ Diarrhea within last 24 - 48 hours _____/day

NUTRITION:

☑ Regular Diet	☐ ↑ Fiber	☐ _____ Calorie ADA
☐ ↓ Fat	☐ Bland	☐ Fluid Restriction
☐ ↓ Chol	☐ Gluten Free	_____cc
☐ ↓ Sodium	☐ Kosher	
☐ Other	_____	

Food Intolerances: ☑ NONE ☐ Type: _____
Supplements: ☑ NONE ☐ Type: _____
Weight Change: ☑ NONE ☐ Gain ☐ Loss
Amount: _____   Time Period: _____ ☐ Intentional ☐ Unintentional*
Intake < 50% in 3 Days. ☐ YES↓ ☑ NO
Chewing Difficulties: ☐ YES* ☑ NO
If any * above, notify Nutrition Services.

DENTURES: ☑ YES* ☐ NO		*BROUGHT TO HOSPITAL: ☑ YES ☐ NO		
☐ Partial ☐ ↑	☐ With Pt	FIT: ☐ Loose	☐ Good	☐ Not Worn
☐ ↓	☐ With Pt	FIT: ☐ Loose	☐ Good	☐ Not Worn
☐ Full ☑ ↑	☐ With Pt	FIT: ☐ Loose	☑ Good	☐ Not Worn
☑ ↓	☐ With Pt	FIT: ☐ Loose	☑ Good	☐ Not Worn

If with Patient, remind patient hospital not responsible for article

Swallowing Difficulties: ☑ NONE ☐ Recent* ☐ Long Term
                             ☐ Solids ☐ Liquids
Coughing During Or After Meals: ☑ YES* ☐ NO
If any * above, notify Coordinated Care.

GENITOURINARY: ☑ NEGATIVE HISTORY
☐ Renal Disease   ☐ Kidney Stones   ☐ Prostate Problems
☐ Cancer _____ ☐ Other: _____

PROBLEMS URINATING: ☑ NONE

☐ Anuria	☐ Nocturia	☐ Dialysis
☐ Hesitancy	_____/night	☐ Peritoneal
☐ Dysuria	☐ Self	☐ Hemo
☐ Urgency	Catheterization	Site _____
☐ Incontinence	Frequency____	Schedule____
☐ Frequency		☐ Other: _____
	☐ Hematria	

GENITALIA PROBLEMS: ☑ NONE
☐ Discharge   ☐ Burning   ☐ Abnormal Bleeding ☐ STD
☐ **Other:** _____

FIGURE 12-2 Continued

NAZARETH HOSPITAL

NURSING ADMISSION
HISTORY

Date of LMP: ___N/A___

FUNCTIONAL STATUS PRIOR TO ADMISSION

I - Independent   A - Assistance Required   D - Dependent

FEED SELF	☑ I	☐ A*	☐ D*
BATHE SELF	☑ I	☐ A*	☐ D*
DRESS SELF	☐ I	☐ A*	☐ D*
HOUSE CHORES	☐ I	☐ A*	☐ D*
AMBULATE	☐ I	☐ A**	☐ D**
CLIMB STAIRS	☑ I	☐ A**	☐ D**
CHAIR BOUND	☐ I	☐ A**	☐ D**
BED BOUND	☐ I	☐ A**	☐ D**

If * or ** circled, were changes made within past 6 months? ☐ YES* ☐ NO
If YES*, Notify Coordinated Care

III.   PSYCHO-SOCIAL ASSESSMENT

Occupation: _homemaker_   ☑ RETIRED
Marital Status: ☐ Married   ☐ Single   ☐ Separated
    ☐ Divorced   ☑ Widowed ☐ Common Law *husband died this year
Residential Information: ☐ Home   ☐ ECF   ☑ Other *Just moved
Usual Living Arrangement: ☐ Alone   ☐ Child   ☐ Spouse *in with*
    ☑ Other Family   ☐ Parent   ☐ Friend   ☐ S.O.   ☐ ECF *daughter*
Contact Person #1: _Barbara Tembra_

Relationship: _daughter_   H#: _215-634-5221_   W#: _____

PRIMARY LANGUAGE:
☑ English   ☐ Polish   ☐ Russian   ☐ German   ☐ Ukrainian
☐ Italian   ☐ Spanish   ☐ Indian   ☐ Korean   ☐ Chinese
☐ Japanese   ☐ Other _____
Does Patient understand English?   ☑ YES   ☐ NO*
    *Contact Person for Translation: _____
    Relationship: _____   H#: _____   W#: _____

ASSISTIVE DEVICES/DURABLE MEDICAL EQUIPMENT: ☑ NONE
☐ Cane ☐ w/pt   ☐ Crutches ☐ w/pt   ☐ Walker ☐ w/pt   ☐ Wheelchair ☐ w/pt
☐ Tub Seat   ☐ Commode   ☐ Grab Bars   ☐ Hospital Bed
☐ Stair Glide   ☐ Other: _____

SPIRITUAL/CULTURAL ASSESSMENT:
Does patient express any spiritual, cultural, or emotional concerns which
may impact on this hospitalization?   ☐ YES*   ☑ NO
    Explain: _____
Does patient express a desire to meet with a Spiritual Care member?
    her own minister   ☑ YES*   ☐ NO
    Priest?   ☐ YES*   ☑ NO   If YES*, notify Spiritual Care.
Coping Mechanisms (How does patient deal with stress?)   ☐ NONE
    Type: _talk with friends, pray * misses husband_
Support Groups   ☑ NONE
    Type: _____
Sleep: _8_ hrs/night   Up at night: _1-2_ times/night
Tobacco: ☐ YES   ☑ NO Amount/day: _____ How Long: _____ ☐
Quit
ETOH: ☐ YES   ☑ NO
Substance Abuse: ☐ YES* ☐ NO   *Type _____
    Has patient been in treatment?   ☐ YES ☐ NO

IV.   EDUCATIONAL ASSESSMENT
Patient Assessed: ☑ YES ☐ NO **Family Assessed:** ☐ YES ☐ NO
Patient Responsible for Learning Anticipated Needs: ☑ YES ☐ NO*
    *OTHER: _____   #: _____
Patient's Preferred Method of Learning: ☑ No Preference Stated
    ☐ Hearing ☐ Seeing ☐ Reading ☐ Hands-on

What does patient want to learn about? ☐ Unidentified At This Time
☑ Disease Process   ☐ Diet & Nutrition   ☐ Community Resources
☐ Medication   ☐ Medical Equipment   ☑ Follow-up Care
☐ Pain Management   ☐ Rehab Techniques   ☐ Other: _____

ANTICIPATED EDUCATIONAL NEEDS IDENTIFIED BY STAFF:
☑ Disease Process   ☐ Diet & Nutrition   ☑ Community Resources
☑ Medication   ☐ Medical Equipment   ☑ Follow-up Care
☐ Pain Management   ☐ Rehab Techniques   ☐ Other: _____

ASSESSMENT OF PATIENT'S BARRIERS TO LEARNING:
Motivation: ☑ Good   ☐ Fair   ☐ Poor
Learning Ability: ☑ Good   ☐ Fair   ☐ Poor
Emotional/Mental Factors: ☐ NONE
☑ Anxious   ☐ Confused   ☐ Depressed
☐ Agitated   ☐ Combative   ☐ Does Not Follow Command
Physical Factors: ☐ NONE
☐ Pain   ☑ Age Related   ☐ Language Barrier
☐ Fatigue   ☐ Medication Effect   ☐ Limitation of Illness

V.   ADVANCE DIRECTIVE
Patient has an advance directive? ☐ YES ☑ NO
Patient would like help to prepare an advance directive? ☑ YES ☐ NO

VI.   DISCHARGE PLANNING
Return: ☐ Home ☑ Family ☐ Rehab ☐ ECF ☐ Unknown
Is Patient currently receiving Home Care Services? ☐ YES* ☑ NO
    *Agency: _____

Were any needs identified requiring notification of Coordinated Care?
            ☐ YES   ☑ NO

VII. PHYSICIAN NOTIFICATION
ATTENDING: _Dr. Skomar_

9/26/06	2:30 PM	C Tayn RN
DATE	TIME	NOTIFIED BY

HOUSE OFFICER: _____

DATE	TIME	NOTIFIED BY

NURSING ASSESSMENT COMPLETED BY:

9/2/06	2:35 PM	C Tayn
DATE	TIME	RN SIGNATURE

FIGURE 12-2 Continued

NAZARETH HOSPITAL
NURSING ADMISSION
PHYSICAL

V S

BP 184/120 P 88   R I R   18   T 98.2 O R A T

HT 5'2"   Actual   Estimated   **WT** _____ (Actual)   Estimated

P A I N

Current Pain Intensity(0-10): 3

Scale Used: (Numeric Scale)   Faces Scale   FLACC Scale

Has Patient had pain in the last week? (Yes)   No   H/A

Unable to obtain information

Complete Initial Pain Assessment Form if Pain Intensity is >5 or if patient has had pain in the last week.

S K I N

Turgor: (Normal)   Tenting

Color: Normal   (Pale)   Flushed   Mottled

    Jaundiced   Dusky   Cyanotic

Temperature: (Cool)   Warm   Clammy   Hot   Wet

Integrity: (Normal)

   Abrasion _____   Burn _____

   Ecchymosis _____   Scar _____

   Laceration _____   Wound _____

   Rash →   Macule _____   Papule _____

Are Multiple Alterations in Skin Integrity or Pressure Ulcers Present? ☐YES* ☑NO   If YES*, Complete Skin Integrity Assessment

Norton Risk Assessment Scale

Circle 1 item for each area, add up total score. Range is 5 - 20. The Lower the total score the greater the risk of developing a pressure ulcer

Physical		Mental		Activity		Mobility		Incontinent	
Good	4	(Alert)	4	(Ambulant)	4	(Full)	4	(Almost never)	4
(Fair)	3	Apathetic	3	Walk/help	3	Sl. limited	3	Occasionally	3
Poor	2	Confused	2	(Chairbound)	2	V. limited	2	Usually UA	2
V.Poor	1	Stupor	1	Bed	1	Immobile	1	Both UA/BM	1

Total Score: 19

If <15, implement Potential Risk For Impaired Skin Integrity Care Plan.

N E U R O M U S C U L A R

LOC: (Alert)   Lethargic   Unresponsive

Mental Status: Pleasant   (Cooperative)   (Anxious)   Agitated

   Follows Command   Depressed   Confused   Combative

Oriented: (Person)   (Place)   (Time)

Pupils: Right (/mm)   Left (/mm)

Reaction: (Brisk)   (Brisk)

     Sluggish   Sluggish

     Non-reactive   Non-reactive

Appearance: (Normal)   (Normal)

     Dilated   Dilated

     Constricted   Constricted

     Fixed   Fixed

Speech: (Clear)   Slurred   Garbled   Stuttering

   Aphasic →   Receptive   Expressive

Gait: Steady   (Unsteady)   Shuffling   Limping

   Bedbound

Extremities: (Well Developed)   Hypertrophied

   Atrophied   Contracted

Tone: (Normal)   Rigid   Flaccid   Spastic

Strength: Strong   (Weak)   Left leg

E E N T

Eyes: Normal R: (Normal)   Red   Jaundiced   Discharge

         L: (Normal)   Red   Jaundiced   Discharge

Ears: Normal R: (Normal)   Discharge   Other: _____

         L: (Normal)   Discharge   Other: _____

Nose: Normal R Nare: (Normal)   Discharge/Drainage

         L Nare: (Normal)   Discharge/Drainage

Oral Cavity: (Normal)   Bleeding   Lesions   Other: _____

Teeth: Normal   (Missing)   Dentures

C A R D I A C

Edema: None

   Arm: RU: +1 +2 +3 +4   LU: +1 +2 +3 +4

         RL: +1 +2 +3 +4   LL: +1 +2 +3 +4

   Leg: RU: +1 +2 +3 +4   LU: +1 +2 +3 +4

         RL: (+1) +2 +3 +4   LL: (+1) +2 +3 +4

   Sacral   Anasarca   Other: _____

Apical Rate: 90   Regular   Irregular

Radial Pulse: R: (Strong)   Weak   Absent   Doppler

        L: Strong   Weak   Absent   Doppler

Pedal Pulse: R: (Strong)   Weak   Absent   Doppler

        L: (Strong)   Weak   Absent   Doppler

Vascular Dialysis Access: None   R   L

   Type: _____   **Bruit:** Present   Absent   N/A

P U L M O N A R Y

Cough: (None)   Non-Productive   Productive

   Clear   White   Green   Yellow   Tan

   Hemoptysis   Thick   Thin

Breathing Pattern: (Normal)   Dyspnea   Kussmaul

   Labored   Periodic Apnea   Cheyne-Stokes   Agonal

Breath Sounds: (Clear)   **Right Lung**   **Left Lung**

   Absent _____ _____

   Diminished _____ _____

   Rhonchi _____ _____

   Rales/Crackles _____ _____

   Insp. Wheeze _____ _____

   Exp. Wheeze _____ _____

G A S T R O

Bowel Sounds:

RUQ:	(Normal)	Increased	Decreased	Absent
LUQ:	(Normal)	Increased	Decreased	Absent
RLQ:	(Normal)	Increased	Decreased	Absent
LLQ:	(Normal)	Increased	Decreased	Absent

Abdomen: (Soft)   Firm   Tender   Non-tender

Abdominal Tubes/Ostomies: (None)   Peg   Gastro

   Biliary   Jejunostomy   Colostomy   Ileostomy

APPLIANCE:

G U

Urinary Device: ☑None   ☐ Catheter-TYPE _____

                               LAST CHANGED _____

Urostomy - APPLIANCE _____

Nephrostomy Tube: ☑None   Right   Left

Flank Tenderness: ☑None   Right   Left

Urine Appearance: ☑Not Visualized

   Clear   Cloudy   Pale   Straw   Sediment

   Sediment   Hematuria   Concentrated

Genitalia Appearance: ☑Not Visualized   Normal

   Other: _____

Does any of the physical assessment findings reflect suspected elder, domestic or child abuse?

☐ YES* ☑ NO

If YES, notify Social Worker by consult.*

RN Signature: Carol Tayn

Date: 9/2/06   **Time:** 2:35 PM

FIGURE 12-2 *Continued*

Think back to James Farren, the college junior who was described at the beginning of the chapter. The nurse would assess his sleeping, eating, and activity habits as well as his emotional status to gain further insight into his possible problems. However, a detailed assessment of his elimination habits would probably be inappropriate at the present time.

Practical Considerations

Data already collected from the patient and in the patient record should not be repeatedly sought from the patient unless there is a need to validate them. Repetitious questioning can be annoying to a patient and may cause the patient to wonder about the lack of communication among healthcare professionals. A careful review of the patient record before interviewing the patient helps prevent this problem.

Before meeting a new patient, it is helpful to take a minute to think carefully about the type of data needed to plan quality care. After the comprehensive nursing assessment has been completed, patient health problems dictate assessment priorities for future nurse–patient interactions.

Structuring the Assessment

Because many different types of data are collected about patients, there is a need to structure data collection systematically. Using systematic guidelines specifically developed for a nursing assessment ensures that comprehensive, holistic data are collected for each patient and lead easily to formulating nursing diagnoses. When the nurse internalizes such assessment guidelines, it is easier to focus on the patient during the assessment rather than to worry about what to assess next.

Most schools of nursing and healthcare institutions establish a **minimum data set** that specifies the information that must be collected from every patient and use a structured assessment form to organize or cluster this data. Many nursing assessment guides are based on holistic models rather than medical models. Gordon's (1994) framework identifies 11 functional health patterns and organizes patient data into these patterns. Maslow uses a hierarchy of five sets of human needs. A medical model used to organize data collection with which all nurses are familiar is the body systems model. This method organizes data collection according to organ and tissue function in various body systems. Although it is helpful in formulating diagnoses related to physiologic problems, it neglects patient problems and strengths in psychosocial and spiritual dimensions of health and well-being. See Box 12-1.

DATA COLLECTION

Types of Data: Subjective and Objective

There are two types of data: subjective and objective. **Subjective data** are information perceived only by the affected person; these data cannot be perceived or verified by another person. Examples of subjective data are feeling nervous, nauseated, or chilly and experiencing pain. Subjective data also are called symptoms or covert data.

Objective data are observable and measurable data that can be seen, heard, or felt by someone other than the person experiencing them. Objective data observed by one person can be verified by another person observing the same patient. Examples of objective data are an elevated temperature reading (eg, 101°F), skin that is moist, and refusal to look at or eat food. Objective data also are called signs or overt data. Table 12-1 compares subjective and objective data.

Paying attention to both subjective and objective data promotes critical thinking because the two types of data complement and clarify one another.

Review the data provided in the scenario for Sylvia Wu in the Reflective Practice display. Her complaints of flu-like symptoms provide the nurse with subjective data. Hearing her cough, noting any sputum produced, inspecting her throat for redness and irritation, and checking her temperature would provide the nurse with objective data that help to clarify and substantiate the patient's complaints.

Characteristics of Data

When collecting and recording patient data, nurses should be complete, accurate, factual, and relevant.

Complete

As much as possible, all the patient data needed to understand a patient health problem and develop a plan of care to maximize health and well-being should be identified. For example, knowing that a patient has lost weight is not fully meaningful until the nurse discovers (1) if the weight loss was intentional or unintentional, (2) if it was related to a change in eating or exercise patterns or to some underlying pathologic condition, and (3) how the patient views and is responding to the weight loss.

Factual and Accurate

Both the patient and the nurse may intentionally or unintentionally misrepresent or distort patient information. For example, a patient who values being thin may describe a weight gain of several pounds as the onset of obesity. Nurses concerned with accuracy and fact continually verify what they hear with what they observe, using other senses and validating all questionable data. At the outset of data collection, it is crucial to determine whether the patient or caregiver who is supplying the data is reliable. When nurses suspect that their own personal bias or stereotyping is influencing their data collection, they should consult with another nurse. It is also best to describe observed behavior rather than to interpret the behavior. Such a description may read: "Patient frequently is observed lying with his face to the wall. Attempts to engage him in conversation fail. He refused lunch today and ate only soup for dinner."

BOX 12-1 Models for Organizing or Clustering Data

Holistic			Medical
Human Needs (Maslow)	**Functional Health Patterns (Gordon)**	**Human Response Patterns (Unitary Person)**	**Body System Model**
Physiologic (Survival) Needs: Food, fluids, oxygen, elimination, warmth, physical comfort	*Health Perception/Health Management:* Perception of general health status and well-being. Adherence to preventive health practices	*Exchanging:* Nutritional status, temperature, elimination, oxygenation, circulation, fluid balance, skin, and mucous membranes, risk for injury	Neurologic Cardiovascular Respiratory Gastrointestinal Musculoskeletal Genitourinary Psychosocial
Safety and Security Needs: Things necessary for physical safety (eg, a cane) and psychological security (eg, a child's favorite toy)	*Nutritional–Metabolic:* Patterns of food and fluid intake, fluid and electrolyte balance, general ability to heal	*Communicating:* Ability to express thoughts verbally; orientation, speech impairments, language barriers	
Love and Belonging Needs: Family and significant others	*Elimination:* Patterns of excretory function (bowel, bladder, skin) and client's perception	*Relating:* Establishing bonds, social interaction, support systems, role performance (including parenting, occupation, and sexual role)	
Self-esteem Needs: Things that make people feel good about themselves and confident in their abilities (eg, being well groomed, having accomplishments recognized)	*Activity/Exercise:* Pattern of exercise, activity, leisure, recreation, and ADL; factors that interfere with desired to expected individual pattern	*Valuing:* Religious and cultural preference and practices, relationship with deity, perception of suffering; acceptance of illness	
Self-actualization Needs: Need to grow, change, and accomplish goals	*Cognitive–Perceptual:* Adequacy of sensory modes, such as vision, hearing, taste, touch, smell, pain perception, cognitive functional abilities	*Choosing:* Ability to accept help and make decisions, adjustment to health status, desire for independence/dependence, denial of problem, adherence to therapies	
	Sleep/Rest: Patterns of sleep and rest-relaxation periods during 24-hour day, as well as quality and quantity	*Moving:* Activity tolerance, ability for self-care, sleep patterns, diversional activities, disability history, safety needs, breastfeeding	
	Self-Perception/Self-Concept: Attitudes about self, perception of abilities, body image, identity, general sense of worth and emotional patterns	*Perceiving:* Body image, self-esteem, ability to use all five senses, amount of hopefulness, perception of ability to control current situation	
	Role/Relationship: Perception of major roles and responsibilities in current life situation	*Knowing:* Knowledge about current illness or therapies; previous illnesses; risk factors, expectations of therapy, cognitive abilities; readiness to learn, orientation, memory	
	Sexuality and Reproductive: Perceived satisfaction or dissatisfaction with sexuality. Reproductive state and pattern	*Feeling:* Pain, grieving, risk for violence, anxiety level, emotional integrity	
	Coping/Stress Tolerance: General coping pattern, stress tolerance, support systems, and perceived ability to control and manage situations		
	Value-Belief: Values, goals, or beliefs that guide choices or decisions		

Adapted from Alfaro-LeFevre, R. (2002). *Applying nursing process* (p. 67). Philadelphia: Lippincott Williams & Wilkins.

On the other hand, the statement "Patient is depressed" is the nurse's interpretation of the patient's behavior; it is not a factual statement. Recording the patient's behaviors factually allows other healthcare professionals to explore causes of the behavior with the patient.

Relevant

Because recording comprehensive data can become an endless task, one challenge facing nurses is to determine what type of data and how much data to collect for each patient. This chapter describes ways to do this. The aim is to record concisely all pertinent data. Often, only experience teaches nurses what data are needed in specific cases.

Learning how to collect, validate, and communicate data that are complete, accurate, factual, and relevant is the focus of the remainder of this chapter.

Sources of Data

Patient

The patient is the primary and usually the best source of information. Unless specified otherwise, it is assumed that the

TABLE 12-1 Comparison of Objective and Subjective Data

Objective Data	Subjective Data
32-year-old man Height: 5'8" Weight: 9/18/05—224 lb 2/4/06—202 lb	"I'm beginning to feel better about myself now that I'm losing weight and I seem to have more energy."
Posterior, left midcalf is warm and red.	"My leg hurts when I walk."
Patient observed fidgeting with bed covers; facial features are tightly drawn.	"I'm so afraid of what they might find when they cut me open tomorrow."

Through the Eyes of a Student

During my chronic medical–surgical rotation, my clinical group was placed on an oncology floor. My first thought was "Oh no, not the cancer floor!" The word *fear* didn't even begin to describe how I felt. These patients had enough problems without some "green" nursing student aggravating them all day. I kept thinking these people are extremely ill and won't want to be bothered by my intruding questions.

Nonetheless, I knew I had to do it. Not only did I have to take care of this patient all day, I had to develop a database and plan of care. I knew I would have to do a lot more than give him his morning care and leave him alone. I would have to carry on an extended conversation with this patient to get all the information I needed.

As if all of this wasn't enough to make me throw in the white flag, when my patient assignment was given, I discovered my patient was a man only 1 year older than me. A 28-year-old man with terminal cancer—this was too scary!

Clinical day came, as I knew it would, and I was shaking. I walked in that room and together the patient and I planned his care. I explained to him the things I needed to talk about with him and I couldn't believe it—he didn't tell me to go away! We talked at length about his disease process and how it had affected his plans and goals. He opened up to me about his spirituality, his relationships with friends and family, and other personal subjects. Periodically, he would cringe, and I could tell it was time for a break. He was hurting too badly to go on at that time.

At the end of that day, my viewpoint was totally different than it had been that morning. I walked away from that room and off that floor feeling like I had made a difference for this person. We had shared a lot and he seemed so appreciative for the time I took to talk with him. The information he shared helped me to develop a better plan of care that was more responsive to his particular needs. The amazing part was that all I had to do was just be myself and allow him to do the same and our day flowed smoothly. The lesson I learned here was important for me: Keep calm and hold on to compassion, and nursing offers many rewards!

—Nancy E. Driskill,
Southeast Missouri State University,
Cape Girardeau, Missouri

data recorded in the nursing history were collected from the patient. Most patients are willing to share information when they know it is helpful for planning their care. See Through the Eyes of a Student. Although data collected from the patient are usually accurate, the nurse should be alert for certain difficulties. For example, a patient who is acutely ill may not be able to communicate adequately if the pain is severe or consciousness is altered in any way. An emotionally upset patient may distort information; for example, patients who are fearful because they think their illness may threaten their work or life may deny certain symptoms or deliberately give misleading facts. If the nurse becomes aware that a patient's report of symptoms differs from physical findings or data obtained from other sources, it is important to note this and to explore the cause of the discrepancy. Patients with limited mental or communication capacity, such as young children and older adults with dementia, cannot be relied on to report accurately. Children and people with decreased mental capacity or impaired verbal ability should, however, be encouraged to respond to interview questions as best they can. Bypassing these patients and automatically turning to a family member, friend, or caregiver for information communicates powerfully that the nurse either has no time for the patient to express his or her needs or mistakenly doubts the patient's ability to communicate these needs.

Family and Significant Others

Family members, friends, and caregivers are especially helpful sources of data when the patient is a child or has limited capacity to share information with the nurse. Husbands and wives can supply information concerning their spouses. Friends often accompany a patient to a health agency and can supply useful information. Care must be taken to determine that the patient does not object to data being gathered from friends and that the friends want to participate. Also, there should be a clear understanding by the patient, family, and friends of the confidentiality of the data collected. Whenever data are

gathered from support people, this should be indicated in the nursing history.

When patients do not speak English, the services of a translator are needed. It is important not to assume that a family member is accurately translating what you are trying to communicate to the patient. The general rule of thumb is to use a medical translator first, since family members might misinterpret medical content, paraphrase the patient's response incorrectly, or the patient might be uncomfortable sharing certain information with the family translator.

Patient Record

Records prepared by different members of the healthcare team provide information essential to comprehensive nursing care. The nurse should review records early when gathering data—in some instances, before the first contact with the patient. Such a review helps to focus the nursing assessment and to confirm and amplify information obtained from other sources.

The patient's health record or chart, which lists such information as age, sex, occupation, religious preference, next of kin, and financial status, is one type of record. The health record includes information entered by various healthcare professionals, such as physicians, social workers, dietitians, physiotherapists, and laboratory technicians.

> *For Susan Morgan, the 34-year-old patient recently diagnosed with MS, the nurse would review her medical record for information related to her diagnosis, treatment plans, including specialized consultations and therapy, as well as her current home situation. This information would be important in determining the nurse's approach to the nursing history and physical examination and in planning the patient's care.*

Nurses who want their care to be supportive of the patient as he or she responds to changes in health status must be familiar with the many sections of the patient record, in addition to the documentation of the nursing plan of care and nursing notes. The following are important sources of data for the nurse.

Medical History, Physical Examination, and Progress Notes

These sources record the findings of physicians as they assess and treat the patient; they focus on identifying pathologic conditions and their causes and on determining the medical regimen for treatment.

Consultations

The patient's physicians may invite specialists to assess and to work with the patient. Their focus is on identifying findings that help to establish a medical diagnosis or on planning and executing the treatment regimen.

Reports of Laboratory and Other Diagnostic Studies

Reports of laboratory studies and other diagnostic tests, such as radiographs, offer the nurse objective data that can either confirm or conflict with data collected during the nursing history or examination. Results of diagnostic studies are helpful to physicians for establishing a diagnosis and monitoring the patient's response to treatment. The results of these same studies may also be helpful to nurses in evaluating the success of nursing interventions.

Reports of Therapies by Other Healthcare Professionals

Other healthcare professionals who interact with the patient also record their findings and note any progress the patient is making in their specific areas—for example, nutrition, physical therapy, or speech therapy. These reports help the nurse to assess the patient's progress and are useful when determining the patient's ability to return home and manage care independently.

Records of previous admissions for healthcare and records from other health agencies, such as a social service agency or a home healthcare agency, are also valuable sources of data. They contain information about the patient's previous medical or surgical problems and response patterns, which may be important determinants of the current plan of care.

Other Healthcare Professionals

Nurses can learn a great deal about a patient's normal health habits and patterns and response to illness by talking with other nurses, physicians, social workers, and others on the healthcare team (Fig. 12-3). Although such communication is always important, it can be crucial when patients are transferred from home to an institution or from one hospital or institution to another. The only way to ensure continuity of care is to make special efforts to share pertinent information.

Nursing and Other Healthcare Literature

To obtain a comprehensive patient database, it may be necessary to consult the nursing and related literature on specific health problems. For example, if a nurse has not cared for a patient with Paget's disease before, it is important for him or her to read about the clinical manifestations of the disease and its usual progression to know what to look for when assessing the patient. In addition to information concerning the medical diagnoses, treatment, and prognosis, a literature review offers nurses important information about nursing diagnoses, developmental norms, and psychosocial and spiritual practices that is helpful when assessing and caring for patients.

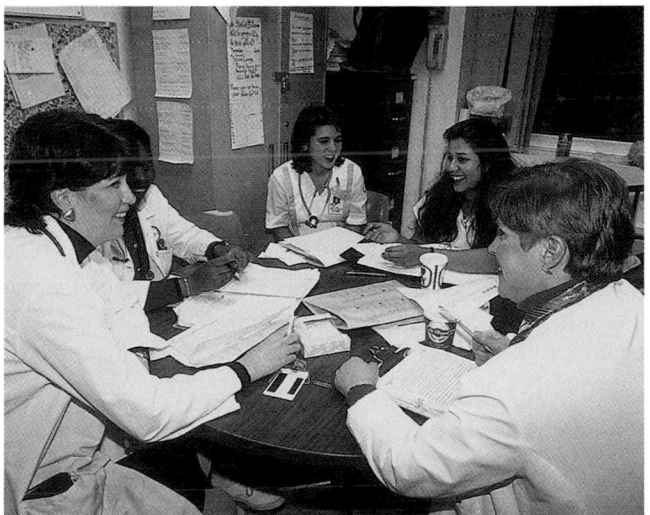

FIGURE 12-3 Nurses can learn a great deal about a patient's health habits and patterns and responses to illness by talking with other nurses, physicians, social workers, and other members of the healthcare team. This exchange of information is particularly important when patients transfer from one healthcare setting to another, or to home.

For Sylvia Wu, the possible diagnosis of SARS can be extremely frightening. To provide the most appropriate care, the nurse would need to know as much as possible about the disease. In doing so, the nurse would be better able to act as an advocate for the patient.

Components of Data Collection

Components of data collection include the nursing history and the nursing physical assessment. These data may be documented on a separate assessment tools or incorporated into a combined database assessment form, as shown in Figure 12-2.

Observation is a key nursing skill, whether gathering the nursing history or performing the physical examination. Observation is the conscious and deliberate use of the five senses to gather data. Skilled nurses use each nurse–patient interaction to observe and to interpret meaningful stimuli (data). Student nurses can develop such observation skills by training themselves to observe carefully the following each time they encounter a patient:

- What are the patient's current responses (physical and emotional) to his or her situation? Be alert to signs of distress— difficulty breathing, bleeding, pain, heightened anxiety— as well as anything out of the ordinary, such as sudden eruption of rash or changes in level of consciousness.
- What is the patient's current ability to manage his or her care (need for additional information or nursing assistance)?
- What is the immediate environment? Consider the safety of the environment as well as the functioning of equipment (intravenous therapy, oxygen, drains). Who are the people in the room and home? What are the temperature and odor of the room?
- What is the larger environment (hospital or community)?

Nursing History

Ideally, the nursing history captures and records the uniqueness of the patient, so that care planning may be patterned to meet the patient's individual needs. The nursing history should therefore be obtained as soon as possible after a patient presents for care and should be followed by the nursing physical assessment. The nursing history should clearly identify the patient's strengths and weaknesses, health risks, such as hereditary and environmental factors, and potential and existing health problems. The nursing history focuses on getting to know the person.

When obtaining the nursing history from Sylvia Wu, it would be important for the nurse to ascertain when the patient had traveled in China, how long she had been there, how long she had been home, and with whom she may have been in contact, and if these individuals exhibited any signs and symptoms. This information would be important in determining the patient's actual risk for developing SARS.

Components of a Nursing History

Components of a nursing history include:

- Profile: name, age, sex, marital status, religion, occupation, education
- Reason for seeking healthcare
- Normal health habits and patterns and related needs for nursing assistance
- Cultural considerations in relation to diet, decision-making, and activities
- Current state of health, functioning of body systems, degree of pain, and past medical and surgical history
- Current medications, allergies, and record of immunizations and exposure to communicable diseases
- Perception of health status and the meaning the patient attributes to health and illness, and characteristic response or coping patterns
- Developmental history, family history, environmental history, and psychosocial history
- Patient's and family's expectations of nursing and of the healthcare team
- Patient's and family's educational needs and ability and willingness to learn
- Patient's and family's ability and willingness to participate in the plan of care
- Whether or not an advance directive exists, or if the patient wants help to prepare an advance directive
- Patient's personal resources (strengths) and deficits
- Patient's potential for injury

Interview

An **interview** is a planned communication. The nurse interviews the patient to obtain a nursing history. Strong interviewing skills are needed to establish a successful working partnership with the patient, to communicate care and concern for the patient, and to obtain the necessary patient data. The interview can be understood in terms of its four phases, which include the preparatory phase, introduction, working phase, and termination. More detailed information on interviewing techniques is provided in Chapter 21.

Preparatory Phase

Before initiating the interview, the nurse prepares to meet the patient by reading current and past records and reports, when available. During this phase, it is important not to let one's stereotypes and prejudices affect the nurse–patient relationship. Nurses who are aware of their own prejudices can deal with them constructively. Professional nurses learn to approach patients with open minds and to be sensitive to the human needs that underlie diverse behaviors.

During the preparatory phase, the nurse should ensure that the environment in which the interview is to be conducted is private and relaxed. Unless the patient wants family members or friends present during the interview, the nurse should interview the patient alone, either in the patient's room or in a quiet office.

Both the seating arrangement and the distance between nurse and patient are important (Fig. 12-4). Chairs placed at

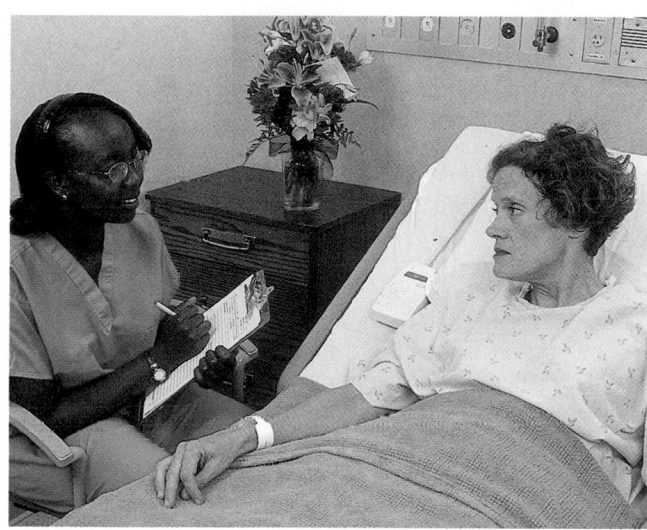

FIGURE 12-4 In the interview, both the seating arrangement and the distance from the patient are important in establishing a relaxed and comfortable environment for data collection. (Photo © B. Proud)

right angles to each other and about 3 to 4 feet (0.9–1.2 m) apart facilitate an easy exchange of information. If the patient is in bed, placing a chair at a 45-degree angle to the bed is helpful. If the nurse stands at the foot or side of the patient's bed and physically talks or looks down at the patient, a superior–inferior relationship is communicated and can negatively affect the interview. Whenever possible, it is best to communicate with patients at eye level.

The interview should be scheduled when both the nurse and the patient are free of concerns and distractions, so that they can concentrate on the task. Ten to 15 minutes may be all that is necessary in some circumstances, whereas an hour or more may be required in others. Information can be gathered in several meetings, especially if the nurse notices that the patient is tiring or is in pain.

Introduction

The interview's introduction is crucial because it sets the tone not only for the remainder of the interview but also for every following nurse–patient interaction. At the end of this phase of the interview, the patient should know the name of the primary nurse and what he or she can expect of nursing care, should sense that the nurse is competent and cares about him or her, and should know what is expected of him or her in terms of developing the plan of care and participating in its execution.

The nurse initiates the interview by stating his or her name and status, identifying the purpose of the interview, and clarifying the roles of nurse and patient. A typical introduction might run like this: "Good afternoon, Miss LeBon. My name is Lisa Gray and I'll be your student nurse. Right now I'd like to ask you a few questions about yourself so that we can plan your nursing care together. Feel free to respond only to those questions you feel comfortable answering, and know that your responses will be treated confidentially by the staff. This will take about 20 minutes. Is this time convenient for you? Do you need anything before we start?"

The initial impression the nurse creates is crucial, especially with patients who are new to the healthcare environment. All nurses whom the patient encounters in the future may be judged in light of this first impression. When the nurse communicates respect and genuine concern for the patient, the patient is then encouraged to discuss health concerns and problems freely. The interpersonal qualities of a respectful presence, professionalism, and caring invite the patient's confidence and ensure the patient that help is available.

During the introduction, the nurse should assess the patient's comfort and ability to participate in the interview. It is also appropriate to assure the patient of confidentiality. The patient should know where the data being recorded are stored, how they will be used, and who has access to them. Some nurses record data on the appropriate form while with the patient, whereas other nurses take notes and complete the form later. Bedside computers are facilitating quick documentation. However, documenting data should not interfere with the sharing of information during the interview. In unusual situations in which a contractual agreement that clearly identifies the responsibilities of both patient and nurse is indicated (eg, a gerontologic nurse entrepreneur), terms are discussed at this time.

Working Phase

During the working phase of the interview, the nurse gathers all the information needed to form the subjective database. The accuracy, completeness, and relevance of the database depend on the nurse's use of the interviewing and basic communication techniques discussed in Chapter 21. The communication techniques highlighted in Box 12-2 are important guidelines for a successful interview.

Many patient variables can positively or negatively affect the outcome of an interview. Table 12-2 identifies patient variables that can negatively influence an interview unless the nurse responds appropriately.

Termination

The successful interview is concluded carefully. A patient should be advised that the interview is coming to an end. It is helpful to recapitulate the interview, highlighting key points. Both the patient and the nurse should be satisfied that the important data are recorded. A helpful strategy is to ask the patient after the summary: "Is there anything else you would like us to know that will help us plan your care?" This gives the patient an opportunity to add data the nurse did not think to include.

Before leaving the patient, it is helpful to alert the patient as to what he or she can expect. The patient should also know when the nurse will reestablish contact; for example, "Thank you for answering these questions, Miss LeBon. Please feel free to keep us informed of anything you think we should know. I'll be leaving soon, but when I return tomorrow morning, I'll discuss your plan of care. This afternoon will be busy for you—some blood tests and a chest x-ray have been ordered. Your evening will probably be quiet. Do you have any questions? Is there anything else I can do for you before I leave?"

BOX 12-2 Communication Techniques for a Successful Interview

- Focus on the patient during the interview, demonstrating interest and concern: use the patient's name of choice, use eye contact appropriately, and avoid rushing the patient.
- Listen to the patient attentively; use reflection and paraphrase to communicate to the patient that you understand him or her.
- Ask about the patient's main problem first, using terminology the patient understands; save personal or delicate questions for later, when a rapport has been established. Defer less important questions until a later interview if the patient is too ill or upset to communicate easily.
- Pose questions and comments to the patient in the manner best suited to produce the desired communication (see Chap. 21):

Closed questions elicit specific information.
Open-ended questions allow the patient to verbalize freely.
Reflective questions encourage the patient to elaborate on thoughts and feelings.
Direct questions can validate information, clarify information, or place events into a meaningful sequence.
- Avoid comments and questions that impede communication (see Chap. 21)—clichés, questions that require a "yes" or "no" answer only, intimidating "why" or "how" questions, probing questions, giving advice, using judgmental comments, changing the subject, and giving false assurance.
- Use silence and touch appropriately.

TABLE 12-2 Patient Variables That Can Negatively Influence an Interview and Suggested Nursing Responses

Patient Variables	Effect on Interview	Nursing Response
High anxiety	Patient may speak rapidly or incoherently and may jump from one topic to another; patient may deny or misrepresent what he or she is experiencing.	Normalize anxiety: "Many people find it difficult to talk about their health and become anxious"; approach patient gently, speak slowly and softly; underscore importance of the patient sharing what he or she is experiencing so nurses can help.
Pain	Patient offers clipped responses and "yes" or "no" answers whenever possible; overriding concern is pain relief.	Do everything possible to make patient comfortable before the interview, including obtaining an order for and administering pain medication; if pain persists, obtain only vital data and defer remainder of interview until patient is more comfortable.
Language difficulty (patient not fluent in nurse's language because patient speaks a different language, has a limited education, or fears saying the "wrong thing")	Vital patient data will not be communicated; patient may mistakenly be labeled "indifferent" or "noncommunicative."	Speak clearly (do not raise voice) using simple language; whenever possible, obtain the assistance of an interpreter (family member may help, but if patient data are confidential, a stranger may be preferable).
Previous negative experience with nurses or healthcare delivery system	Patient is aloof, unwilling to participate in interview; general attitude: "Why should I waste my time telling you anything . . . it won't do me any good."	"I know other people who have had a tough time with nurses or the system . . . life isn't perfect . . . but how about giving us a chance this time to show you what nurses can do?" Communicate respect for the patient and competence.
Unrealistic expectations of healthcare professionals	Patient expects nurses and other healthcare professionals magically to know everything about him or her and to "take care" of him or her; "surrenders" himself or herself to the system—"you know best" attitude.	Communicate clearly that no one knows or understands the patient like the patient does, and invite him or her to become involved in his or her care; "No two persons are alike, and unless you tell me a little more about yourself and how you are feeling, there is no way we'll be able to plan good care."

Nursing Physical Assessment

Physical assessment is the examination of the patient for objective data that may better define the patient's condition and help the nurse in planning care. The physical assessment normally follows the nursing history and interview, and may verify data gathered during the history or yield new data. There has been a great deal of controversy about nursing's role in the physical assessment of the patient, caused by concern that this is a duplication of medicine's role. Physicians traditionally have performed the intake physical assessment, which commonly is the mechanism of entry into the healthcare delivery system as well as the basis for medical treatment. Some nurses in advanced practice roles perform comprehensive intake physical assessments similar to their physician colleagues, which identify health and illness states, and then recommend or prescribe appropriate follow-up care. In any case, all nurses conduct selected aspects of physical assessment for nursing purposes.

Unlike the physical assessment performed by the physician to identify pathologic conditions and their causes, the nursing physical assessment focuses primarily on the patient's functional abilities. If a neurologic deficit is present, the nurse is concerned with identifying how this deficit affects the patient's reasoning and sensorimotor abilities. For example, a patient who has had a cerebrovascular accident (brain attack or stroke) is examined to determine ability to comprehend and communicate information and execute the tasks of everyday life.

The physical assessment for Susan Morgan, the young woman newly diagnosed with MS described at the beginning of the chapter, would include investigation of the patient's muscle strength, endurance level, the effects of MS on the patient's ability to perform daily activities. Also as part of the physical examination, the nurse would be alert to indications of fatigue or inability to complete specific activities. This information would help the nurse to respond appropriately to her concerns about her marriage.

Purposes of the nursing physical assessment include the appraisal of health status, the identification of health problems, and the establishment of a database for nursing intervention. See Through the Eyes of a Student and Figure 12-5. See Chapter 25 for a detailed description of physical assessment skills.

Nurses practicing in different settings may use different physical assessment techniques for different purposes. Nurses in the coronary care unit use sophisticated, high-technology assessment techniques, whereas nurses in a rehabilitation center use a wide range of physical assessment skills that focus on identifying functional and nonfunctional response patterns to disabilities.

The nursing physical assessment involves the examination of all body systems in a systematic manner, commonly using a head-to-toe format. Four methods are used to collect data dur-

Through the Eyes of a Student

As a first-year nursing student, I often questioned myself on my technique in assessing a patient. Sure, I understood what my instructors taught me, but was I doing it right? So I find my patient has an elevated temperature, or perhaps urinary output is scanty—but what does it all mean? I often wondered if I would be able to make sense of all this information, and would I *really* be able to detect a problem should one develop. Well, it works! Keep assessing, recording, and reporting.

During my 2nd year (first semester), I realized how an assessment can aid in saving your patient's life. A continuous assessment for 2 days saved my 91-year-old patient. I detected early signs of pulmonary edema and congestive heart failure and was able to notify appropriate medical personnel and immediately implement life-saving procedures. Sure it was scary, but how proud I felt when the nursing staff congratulated me on a job well done! I realized how significant my assessment was for my patient, when, as I stood with her in the radiology department, she looked up at me from her stretcher and thanked me for taking good care of her. Knowing my patient was aware of what I had done for her meant the world to me, and at this point, I realized why I had chosen the nursing profession.

—Delores (Dee) C. Pascale,
Delaware County Community College,
Media, Pennsylvania

ing a physical assessment: inspection, palpation, percussion, and auscultation. Nurses may also use physical assessment skills to evaluate selected body systems. These techniques and the basic skills for physical assessment are described in Chapter 25.

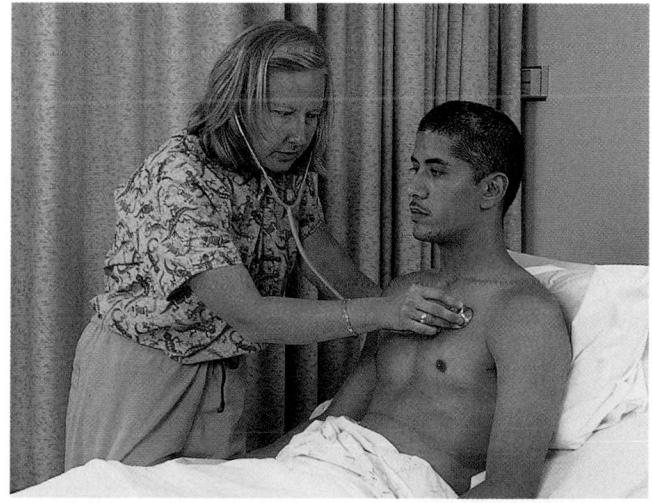

FIGURE 12-5 The nurse provides a physical examination. No matter what the setting or the age of the patient, the physical examination should include appraisal of health status, identification of health problems, and establishment of a database for nursing intervention. (Photo © B. Proud)

Problems Related to Data Collection

Common problems encountered during data collection include inappropriate organization of the database, omission of pertinent data, inclusion of irrelevant or duplicate data, erroneous or misinterpreted data, failure to establish rapport and partnership, recording an interpretation of data rather than observed behavior, and failure to update the database. Table 12-3 describes possible causes and remedies for such problems.

DATA VALIDATION

Validation is the act of confirming or verifying. The purpose of validating is to keep data as free from error, bias, and misinterpretation as possible. Validation is an important part of assessment because invalid information can lead to inappropriate nursing care.

Identifying Data To Be Validated

Because validation of all data is neither possible nor necessary, nurses need to decide which items need verification. For example, data need to be verified when there are discrepancies: a patient tells the nurse he is fine and has no concerns, but the nurse notes that he demonstrates tense body musculature and seems curt in his responses. When there is a discrepancy between what the person is saying and what the nurse is observing, validation is necessary to determine accuracy. Validation in this instance may take the form of the nurse saying "You tell me you feel fine, but right now your body and behaviors are telling me something else. Tell me more about this."

Data also need verification when they lack objectivity. For example, a nurse suspects that the patient hears in one ear but does not seem to hear well in the other. The nurse should validate the data before proceeding and should determine whether the patient does indeed have a hearing problem. Suspicions are not objective. In this instance, the nurse needs to test the patient's hearing in both ears. Speaking toward the suspected better ear, the nurse explains "It seems to me that you hear better

TABLE 12-3 Common Problems of Data Collection, Possible Causes, and Suggested Remedies

Problem	Possible Causes	Suggested Remedies
Database inappropriately organized	Failure to plan for the assessment by identifying needed data; use of inappropriate tools for data collection	Review the guidelines for specifying pertinent data. Consider modifying tool for data collection or select an alternative tool.
Pertinent data omitted	Not following up on cues during data collection; inappropriate guidelines	Identify potentially relevant factors in advance of collection. Practice interview strategies.
Irrelevant or duplicate data collected	Failure to identify specific purpose of data collection; failure to review available patient records; use of inappropriate tools for data collection	Determine specific purpose of data collection for each patient. Consider existing data before initiating collection. Consider modifying data collection tool or selecting alternative.
Erroneous or misinterpreted data collection	Failure to observe carefully or validate during data collection; interviewer prejudices or stereotypes	Sharpen observation skills by independently observing the same situation with a peer and comparing notes afterward. Role play several validation techniques.
Failure to establish rapport	Failure to establish sufficient rapport or use appropriate communication techniques with patient; failure to know what information is wanted	Review and practice communication techniques discussed in Chapter 21. Role play several explanations of purpose of data collection. Identify general data desired before collection.
Interpretation of data is recorded rather than the observed behavior	Nurse jumps to hasty conclusion about patient's behavior and deprives others of exploring with the patient possible causes of the behavior; deficient validation	Review the distinction between data and interpretation of data. Practice documenting observed patient behavior concisely.
Failure to update the database	Erroneous belief that assessment is concluded after the initial database is recorded; low priority attached to ongoing data collection	Recollect that it is impossible to give quality, individualized care without knowledge of changes in the patient's status. Ongoing data collection is critical to the deletion or modification of old problems and the identification of new problems.

out of one ear than the other. I would like to test this. I'll bring a watch slowly toward your right ear first and then toward your left. Please look straight ahead and tell me when you first hear the watch ticking." The nurse then records how far the watch was from each ear when the patient first heard it ticking.

Identifying Cues and Making Inferences

Nurses now use the language of cues and inferences to describe the process of validation. The subjective and objective data you identify (patient does not respond when I speak to him on his left side) is a **cue** that something may be wrong. The judgment you reach about the cue (the patient's hearing may be impaired on his left side) is an **inference.** Until you check the patient's hearing you cannot be sure that your inference is correct. Inferences may be validated in multiple ways:

- Physical examination, using the proper equipment and procedure (you may need to have an expert confirm your findings)
- Clarifying statements ("You said this is not a problem, but I sense you may still be worried.")
- Sharing your inferences with other respected members of the team
- Checking your findings with research reports

See Figure 12-6 for an illustration of validating inferences.

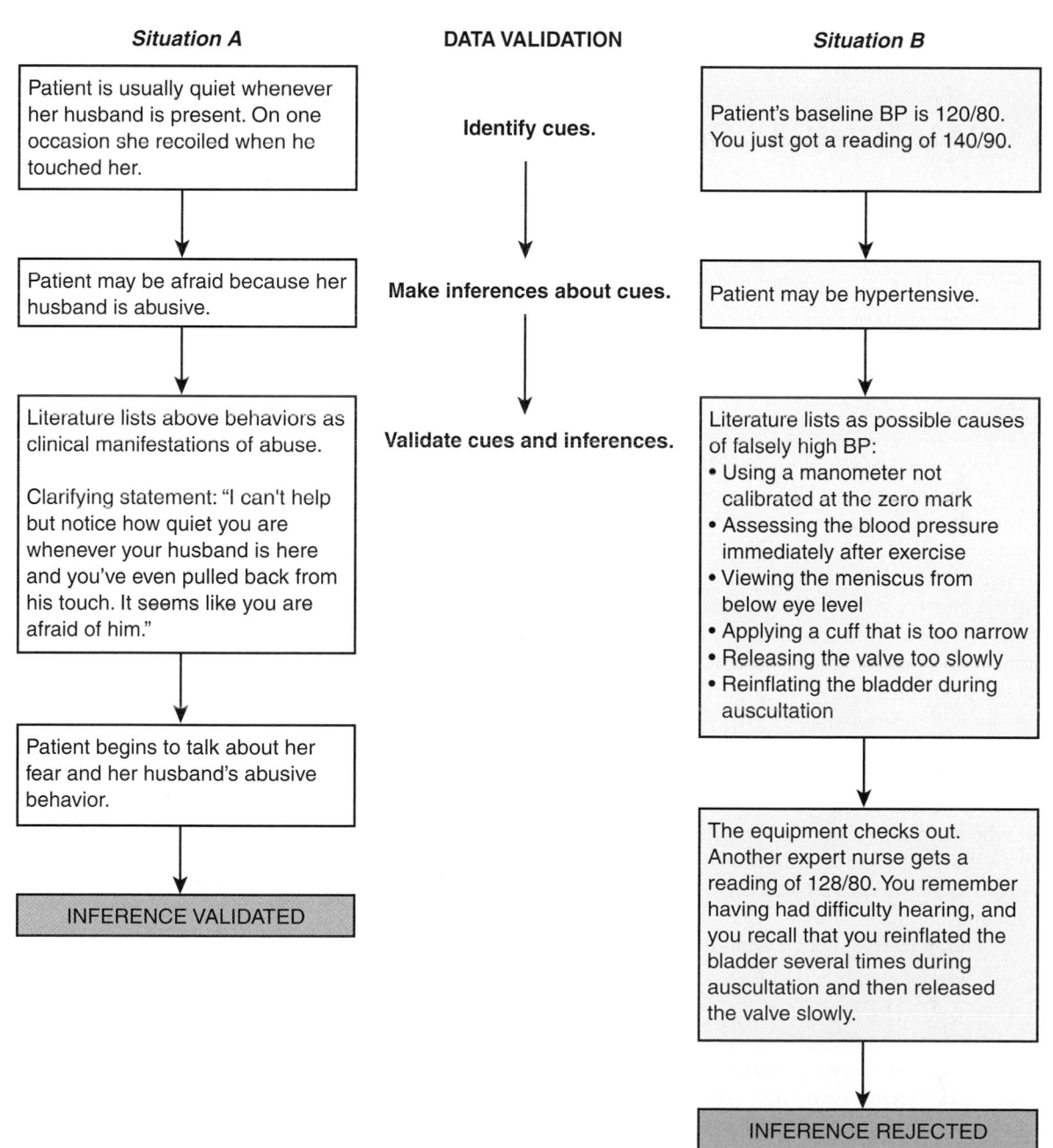

FIGURE 12-6 An illustration of the process used to validate cues and inferences.

The nurse may validate data as they are collected or at the end of the data-gathering process. When it is clear that the data are correct, the nurse is ready to analyze the data and formulate nursing diagnoses—the next step of the nursing process.

DATA COMMUNICATION

The patient data collected by the nurse, both initially and as patient contact continues, are of no benefit to the patient and the healthcare team unless they are appropriately communicated. See Box 12-3: Legal Alert. Appropriate communication involves correct timing and proper documentation.

Timing

Immediate verbal communication of data is indicated whenever assessment findings reveal a critical change in the patient's health status that necessitates the involvement of other nurses or healthcare professionals. The nurse who observes an elevated temperature of 103.2°F (39.5°C) in a patient scheduled for surgery that morning must report this to the charge nurse and to the surgeon, who might then cancel surgery. Failure to communicate this finding could result in the patient's receiving preoperative sedation, being taken to the operating room, and even having the surgery performed under less than optimal conditions. Similarly, a nurse who hears a patient making suicidal remarks must communicate this information to the healthcare team, so that all are alerted to the patient's danger and that suicide precautions may be taken immediately.

A nurse who is unsure of the significance of a particular finding is well advised to consult with another nurse. In some situations, years of experience are needed to distinguish significant from nonsignificant findings. Neither ignorance nor the fear of appearing less than competent justifies failure to report critical data.

The nurse would need to report Sylvia Wu's complaints along with the underlying history of travel to China immediately to the appropriate healthcare personnel. Doing so ensures that the necessary precautions are taken to reduce the risk of infection transmission, should the patient actually have SARS.

Documentation

The initial database should be entered into the computer or recorded in ink, using the designated agency forms, the same day the patient is admitted to the agency. If, for any reason, important data cannot be obtained during the initial assessment, this needs to be documented so that they are obtained as soon as possible. Objective and subjective patient data should be summarized and written, so that data communicate a unique sense of the patient and are comprehensive, concise, and easily retrievable. The data should be written legibly, and good grammar and only standard medical abbreviations should be used. To facilitate quick data retrieval, data should be presented under clearly marked headings.

Whenever possible, subjective data should be recorded using the patient's own words. Quotation marks should be used: "I feel tired from the moment I first get up in the morning. Any more it seems I have no energy at all." Patient reports may also be paraphrased: Patient reports feeling dyspneic, has difficulty catching breath when walking one flight of stairs.

The tendency to record data using nonspecific terms that are subject to individual definition or interpretation—words like adequate, good, average, normal, poor, small, large—should be avoided. One nurse's sense of what constitutes an average fluid intake may be very different from that of another nurse. It is important to be specific. Chapter 20 offers general documentation guidelines.

■ Developing Critical Thinking Skills

1. Working with another student, interview patients in both home and institutional settings, and record your findings separately. Make a list of the objective and subjective data you gather on each patient interviewed and the inferences you make from these cues. Compare your data lists and inferences. Describe to one another how you plan to validate your inferences. Explore possible reasons for the differences you discover.

2. Allow another student to perform a comprehensive nursing assessment (interview and physical assessment) on you. Reflect on what you experienced. Offer the student feedback about which of her or his behaviors were helpful, comforting, or distressing. Change roles and talk about what you learned from this experience.

3. Collect several different forms for recording the initial comprehensive nursing assessment (hospital, nursing home, home care, and school of nursing forms). Identify and explain the differences you see. Experiment with using the different forms, and make a list of features that help you get all the data you need in the easiest way possible.

■ Practicing for NCLEX

1. Although the nursing process is presented as an orderly progression of steps, in reality there is great in-

teraction and overlapping among the five steps. This characteristic of the nursing process is described as:
a. Systematic
b. Dynamic
c. Interpersonal
d. Outcome oriented

2. While administering a medication to relieve a patient's pain, you wonder if there are some non-pharmacologic interventions that would enhance relief by complementing the pain medication. When you discuss this with your instructor you are most likely to hear:
   a. "You should wait until after you evaluate the effect of the medication you just administered before planning a different intervention."
   b. "One step at a time, dear. Don't start planning a new intervention until you evaluate the old."
   c. "Let's talk about this . . . we often get new information that we can incorporate successfully into the plan of care. Sometimes the steps of the process interact or overlap."
   d. "Think about this patient. Nonpharmacologic interventions wouldn't be effective with her."

3. When a patient you are admitting to the unit asks you why you are doing a history and exam since the doctor just did one, your best reply is:
   a. "In addition to providing us with valuable information about your health status, the nursing assessment will allow us to plan and deliver individualized, holistic nursing care that draws on your strengths."
   b. "It's hospital policy. I know it must be tiresome, but I will try to make this quick!"
   c. "I'm a student nurse and need to develop the skill of assessing your health status and need for nursing care. This information will help me develop a plan of care individualized to your unique needs."
   d. "We want to make sure that your responses are consistent and that all our data are accurate."

4. When you receive shift report, you learn that your patient has no special skin care needs. You are surprised during the bath to observe reddened areas over bony prominences. You should:
   a. Correct the initial assessment form.
   b. Redo the initial assessment and document current findings.
   c. Conduct and document an emergency assessment.
   d. Perform and document a focused assessment on skin integrity.

5. Fearful of attempting your first nursing history, you ask your instructor how anyone ever learns everything you have to ask to get good baseline data. You are most likely to hear:
   a. "There's a lot to learn at first, but once it becomes part of you, you just keep asking the same questions over and over in each situation until you can do it in your sleep!"

   b. "You make the basic questions a part of you and then learn to modify them for each unique situation, asking yourself how much you need to know to plan good care."
   c. "No one ever really learns how to do this well because each history is different! I often feel like I'm starting afresh with each new patient."
   d. "Don't worry about learning all of the questions to ask. Every agency has its own assessment form you must use."

6. A patient complains about feeling nauseated after lunch. This is an example of what type of data?
   a. Subjective
   b. Objective
   c. Signs and symptoms
   d. Overt

7. When you enter the patient's room to begin your nursing history, the patient's wife is there. You should:
   a. Introduce yourself to both and thank the wife for being present.
   b. Introduce yourself to both and ask the wife if she wants to remain.
   c. Introduce yourself to both and ask the wife to leave.
   d. Introduce yourself and ask the patient if he would like the wife to stay.

8. The patient is Vietnamese and does not speak English. Her son is with her and does speak English. How should you respond?
   a. Ask the son if he is willing to translate and be sure to thank him if he says yes.
   b. Determine if the son can translate medical information and if so, begin.
   c. After determining that the son can translate, evaluate if he can do so objectively and if the patient wants him to serve in this capacity.
   d. Explain to the son that hospital policy forbids using family members as translators and find a hospital-approved translator.

9. You are surprised to detect an elevated temperature (102°F) in a patient scheduled for surgery. The patient has been afebrile and shows no other signs of being febrile The first thing you do is to:
   a. Inform the charge nurse
   b. Inform the surgeon
   c. Validate your finding
   d. Document your finding

10. You tell your instructor that your patient is fine and has "no complaints." You are likely to hear:
    a. "You made an inference that she is fine because she has no complaints. How did you validate this?"
    b. "She probably just doesn't trust you enough to share what she is feeling. I'd work on developing a trusting relationship."
    c. "Sometimes everyone gets lucky. Why don't you try to help another patient?"
    d. "Maybe you should reassess the patient. He has to have a problem—why else would he be here?"

Answers With Rationale

1. The correct answer is *b*. The term dynamic is used to describe the fact that there is much interaction and overlap among the steps of the nursing process. In some situations, all five steps may occur almost simultaneously.

2. The correct answer is *c*. There may be much interaction and overlap among the steps of the nursing process. In this case, though you want to evaluate the effect of the medication you administered (options *a* and *b*), there is no reason to wait for this to happen before exploring other valid options. (*d*) is incorrect because it is not possible to judge the effectiveness of nonpharmacologic methods before their use, and the instructor's response possibly indicates a prejudice toward complementary and alternative modalities.

3. The correct answer is *a*. Though it may be true that you need to develop assessment skills (*c*), the chief reason you are doing a nursing history and exam is because there needs to be a documented nursing admission assessment to serve as a basis for nursing care. The fact that this is also hospital policy (*b*) is a secondary reason.

4. The correct answer is *d*. Perform and document a focused assessment on skin integrity since this is a newly identified problem. The initial assessment stands as is and cannot be redone (*b*) or corrected (*a*). This is not a life threatening event, and thus there is no need for an emergency assessment (*c*).

5. The correct answer is *b*. Once you learn what constitutes the minimum data set, you can adapt this to any patient situation. It is not true that each assessment is the same even when you are using the same minimum data set (*a*), or is it true that each assessment is uniquely different (*c*). (*d*) is incorrect because relying solely on standard agency assessment tools does not allow for individualized patient care or critical thinking.

6. The correct answer is *a*. A patient report of "feeling nauseated" cannot be perceived or validated by the nurse, and this is subjective data, not objective (*b*) or overt (*d*), which are observable and measurable. (*c*) is wrong since signs are examples of objective data.

7. The correct answer is *d* since the patient has the right to indicate who he would like to be present for the nursing history and exam. You should neither presume that he wants his wife there (*a*), nor that he does not want her there (*c*). Similarly, the choice belongs to the patient, not the wife (*b*).

8. The correct answer is *c*. This is difficult, but it is important to evaluate whether or not the son can adequately translate medical information, can be trusted to translate what is said without introducing his bias, and if the patient wants him to serve in this capacity. The choice belongs to the patient, not the son (*a*) and there is no policy that prohibits family members from translating (*d*). (*b*) is incomplete.

9. The correct answer is *c*. You should first validate your finding if it is unusual, deviates from normal, and is unsupported by other data. Should your initial recording prove to be in error, it would have been premature to notify the charge nurse (*a*) or the surgeon (*b*). You want to be sure that all data you record is accurate, so it should be validated before documentation if you have doubts (*d*).

10. The correct answer is *a*. Your instructor is most likely to challenge your inference that the patient is "fine" simply because he is telling you that he has no problems. It is appropriate for her to ask how you validated this inference. Jumping to the conclusion that the patient does not trust you (*b*) is premature and is an invalidated inference. (*c*) is wrong because it accepts your invalidated inference. (*d*) is wrong because it is possible that the condition is resolving.

Bibliography

Alfaro-Lefevre, R. (2002). *Applying nursing process: Promoting collaborative care* (5th ed.). Philadelphia: Lippincott Williams & Wilkins.

American Nurses Association. (1980/1995). *Nursing: A social policy statement.* Washington, DC: Author.

Bickley, L. (2003). *Bates' Guide to physical examination* (8th ed.). Philadelphia: Lippincott Williams & Wilkins.

Braverman, B. G. (1990). Eliciting data from the patient who is difficult to interview. *Nursing Clinics of North America, 25*(4), 743–750.

Catherman, A. (1990). Biopsychosocial nursing assessment: A way to enhance care plans. *Journal of Psychosocial Nursing, 28*(6), 31–33.

Domarad, B. R., & Buschmann, M. T. (1995). Interviewing older adults: Increasing the credibility of interview data. *Journal of Gerontological Nursing, 21*(9), 14–20.

Fields, S. (1991). History-taking in the elderly: Obtaining useful information. *Geriatrics, 46*(8), 26–34.

Gordon, M. (1994). *Nursing diagnosis: Process and application* (3rd ed.). St. Louis. MO: Mosby–Year Book.

Laschinger, H. S. (1990). Helping students apply a nursing conceptual framework in the clinical setting. *Nurse Educator, 15*(3), 20–24.

McPhetridge, L. M. (1968). Nursing history: One means to personalize care. *American Journal of Nursing, 68*(1), 68–75.

Milholland, D. K. (1994). Privacy and confidentiality of patient information: Challenges for nursing. *JONA, 24*(2), 19–24.

Simonsen, S. M. (2001). *Telephone health assessment: Guidelines for practice* (2nd ed.). St. Louis: C. V. Mosby.

Stewart, C. J., & Cash, W. B. (1991). *Interviewing principles and practice* (6th ed.). Dubuque, IA: Brown.

Vessey, J. A., & Richardson, B. L. (1993). A holistic approach to symptom assessment and intervention. *Holistic Nursing Practice, 7*(2), 13–21.

Diagnosing

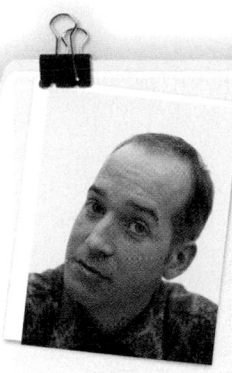

Martin Prescott, a 46-year-old man, comes to the health clinic for a routine physical examination. During the assessment, he states "I've had problems with constipation and have seen some blood when I wipe myself after a bowel movement. It's just hemorrhoids, right? Nothing to worry about?"

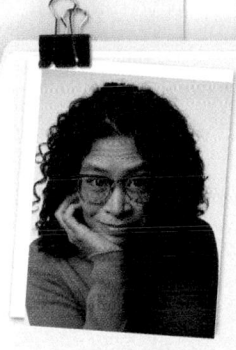

Antonia Zuccarelli is a middle-aged woman newly diagnosed with cancer that is treatable. However, she continually fails to show up for follow-up appointments for both diagnosis and treatment.

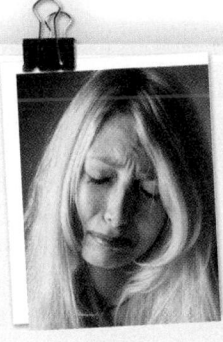

Angie Clarkson, a college sophomore, tearfully reports that she believes she was a victim of date-rape. She had too much to drink at a party and can only remember waking up in a strange room with a guy she just met, unsure if she passed out because of the alcohol or date-rape drugs. A virgin, Angie was sure there was penetration because of blood and semen stains she discovered upon waking. It is now a month later and she has not been able to "get her life together" and move on.

Focusing on Blended Skills

The types of blended skills you'll need to respond to the case scenarios include:

Cognitive Skills
- Ability to think critically and to engage in diagnostic reasoning
- Ability to develop nursing diagnoses that are responsive to the patient's health problems: bowel elimination, cancer treatment and follow-up, and rape
- Knowledge of pertinent standards and agency or institutional policies related to diagnoses
- Knowledge of gastrointestinal elimination, including hemorrhoids and risks factors for possible colon cancer, psychosocial responses and required treatment and follow-up for cancer, and rape trauma and responses to it
- Knowledge of resources available for support and guidance related to cancer and rape
- Ability to incorporate knowledge of key assessment areas for patients with varying needs

Technical Skills
- Ability to research the literature to obtain the knowledge necessary for developing the list of nursing diagnoses
- Ability to use a documentation system competently to communicate the list of nursing diagnoses
- Ability to ask for assistance as necessary when developing nursing diagnoses for patients with different needs

Interpersonal Skills
- Ability to establish trusting nurse–patient relationships that yield knowledge of the individual needs and strengths of patients and their families

- Ability to communicate to the patient concern about the patient, his or her priorities, and his or her well-being
- Ability to identify and respond to the needs of patients experiencing different stressors, such as a patient with a problem involving gastrointestinal function, a woman who fails to maintain follow-up for cancer, and a young woman who was a victim of date-rape
- Ability to work collaboratively with other members of the healthcare team to meet the needs of patients

Ethical and Legal Skills
- Demonstration of a strong sense of accountability for the health and well-being of individuals based on identified needs and nursing diagnoses
- Commitment to developing and communicating a list of nursing diagnoses that are responsive to the patient's individualized needs
- Ability to demonstrate a commitment to assisting patients in getting the help they need to achieve their health goals, within the scope of nursing practice
- Ability to incorporate knowledge of the ethical and legal principles that guide decision making and the development and documentation of nursing diagnoses
- Ability to serve as a trusted and effective patient advocate, including advocating for both the patient who fails to participate in follow-up treatment for cancer and the young woman who was a victim of date-rape

Learning Objectives

After completing the chapter, the learner should be able to accomplish the following:

1. Describe the term nursing diagnosis, distinguishing it from a collaborative problem and a medical diagnosis.
2. Describe the four steps involved in data interpretation and analysis.
3. Use the guidelines for writing nursing diagnoses when developing diagnostic statements.
4. Describe means to validate nursing diagnoses.
5. Describe the benefits and limitations of nursing diagnoses.

Key Terms

actual nursing diagnoses
collaborative problems
cue
data cluster
diagnosing
diagnostic error
health problem
medical diagnoses
nursing diagnoses
possible nursing diagnoses
risk/high-risk nursing diagnoses
standard
syndrome nursing diagnoses
wellness diagnoses

After the nurse has collected and recorded the patient data, the work of **diagnosing** begins—the second step in the nursing process. The purpose of diagnosing is to (1) identify how an individual, group, or community responds to actual or potential health and life processes; (2) identify factors that contribute to or cause health problems (etiologies); and (3) identify resources or strengths the individual, group, or community can draw on to prevent or resolve problems.

In the diagnosing step of the nursing process, the nurse interprets and analyzes data gathered from the nursing assessment (Fig. 13-1). The data help the nurse identify patient strengths and health problems. A **health problem** is a condition that necessitates intervention to prevent or resolve disease or illness or to promote coping and wellness. See the accompanying Reflective Practice display for an example.

Alfaro-LeFevre (2004) counsels nurses to understand the types of problems they should focus on to better understand their responsibilities relating to diagnosis and management of health problems. She lists the following as the types of nursing concerns that are clearly nursing responsibilities:
- Monitoring for changes in health status
- Promoting safety and preventing harm; detecting and controlling risks
- Identifying and meeting learning needs
- Tailoring treatment and medication regimens for each individual
- Promoting comfort and managing pain.
- Promoting health and a sense of well-being
- Recognizing and addressing problems that impede the ability to be independent and live a healthy lifestyle
- Determining human responses (how individuals, families, or groups respond to health problems or life changes) (pp. 77–78)

When a health problem is identified, the nurse must decide which healthcare professional can best treat the problem. Actual or potential health problems that can be prevented or resolved by independent nursing intervention are termed **nursing diagnoses.** The nurse formulates, validates, and lists nursing diagnoses for each patient (Fig. 13-2). Nursing diagnoses provide the basis for selecting nursing interventions that will achieve valued patient outcomes for which the nurse is responsible (Fig. 13-3). See Box 13-1 for Alfaro's rule about the legal implications of diagnoses.

Alfaro recommends using both a nursing model and a body systems approach (see Chap. 12) to organize assessment data to detect both nursing and medical problems.

EVOLUTION OF NURSING DIAGNOSES

The term *nursing diagnosis* first appeared in the literature in the 1950s. As early as 1966, Hammond wrote that nurses need to be competent in information-seeking strategies and should have a good background of theoretical knowledge to search for cues and evaluate evidence. These skills and knowledge result in accurate diagnosing. Key elements in the evolution of nursing diagnosis as an integral component of nursing process include the following:
- In 1953, the term nursing diagnosis was introduced by V. Fry (1953) to describe a step necessary in developing a care plan.
- In 1972, the New York State Nurse Practice Act identified diagnosing as part of the legal domain of professional nursing; practice acts in many other states have been revised similarly since then.
- In 1973, the American Nurses Association's Standards of Practice included diagnosing as a function of professional nursing.
- Also in 1973, Gebbie and Lavin, of St. Louis University, called the First National Conference on Classification of Nursing Diagnoses, beginning a national effort to identify, standardize, and classify health problems treated by nurses. At this first meeting, the National Group, since renamed the North American Nursing Diagnosis Association (NANDA), appointed a task force to accomplish the following goals:
  - Gather information and disseminate it through the Clearinghouse for Nursing Diagnosis.
  - Encourage educational activities at regional and state levels to promote the implementation of nursing diagnoses. These activities include conferences to organize nurses to identify additional diagnostic labels and workshops to teach nurses about nursing diagnoses.
  - Promote and organize activities to continue the development, classification, and scientific testing of nursing diagnoses. These activities include planning national conferences, identifying criteria for accepting diagnoses, surveying current research activities, and exploring varied methods for classification.
- In 1980, the ANA Social Policy Statement defined nursing as "the diagnosis and treatment of human response to actual or potential health problems" (ANA, 1980).
- In March 1990, at the Ninth Conference of NANDA, the General Assembly approved an official definition of nursing diagnosis:

  Nursing diagnosis is a clinical judgment about individual, family, or community responses to actual or potential health problems/life processes. Nursing diagnosis provides the basis for selection of nursing interventions to achieve outcomes for which the nurse is accountable (NANDA, 1990).
- NANDA conferences are held every 2 years, and much progress continues to be made in defining, classifying, and describing nursing diagnoses.

Now an accepted and essential step in the nursing process, nursing diagnosis was initially confused with medical diagnosis, sparking controversy. Although this confusion has been resolved, many nurses have been slow to understand and to accept the "work" of diagnosing.

The most recent change in the way nurses understand the diagnosing step in the nursing process is the change in focus from nurses only diagnosing and treating nursing diagnoses, to

The following diagram shows how the activities of *Assessment* lead to what many consider to be a pivotal point in the nursing process: *Diagnosis*.

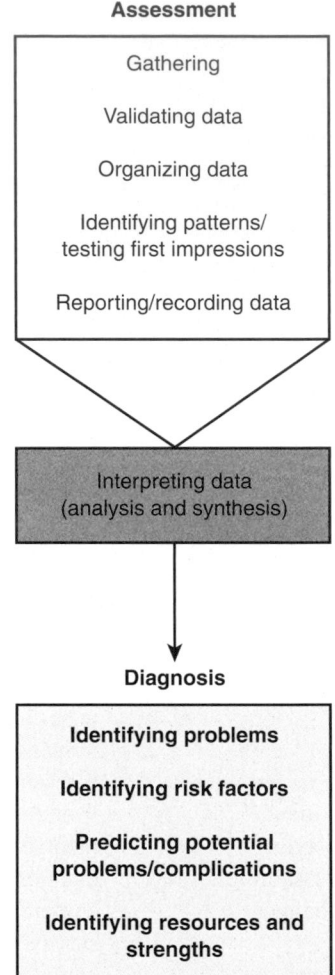

Assessment

Gathering

Validating data

Organizing data

Identifying patterns/
testing first impressions

Reporting/recording data

Interpreting data
(analysis and synthesis)

Diagnosis

Identifying problems

Identifying risk factors

**Predicting potential
problems/complications**

**Identifying resources and
strengths**

Diagnosis is a pivotal point for three reasons:

1. **The accuracy and relevancy of the entire plan depends on your ability to clearly and specifically identify both the problems and what's causing them.** Incorrectly diagnosing the problems or what's causing them is likely to send you and everyone else in the wrong direction, resulting in inefficient, perhaps even dangerous care. For example, imagine what could happen if you decide someone's left shoulder pain is related to his arthritis when the pain is actually related to cardiac problems.

2. **Creating a proactive plan that promotes health and prevents problems *before they begin* depends on your ability to recognize risk factors (things that we know cause problems, such as sedentary lifestyle).** Even when there are *no* problems, you must ask, "Are there risk factors that need to be addressed?" For example, you assess an overweight businessman and learn that both of his parents had hypertension. Knowing that obesity and family history of hypertension are risk factors for hypertension, you stress the importance of preventing hypertension through exercise, weight control, and decreased salt intake.

3. **The resources and strengths you identify are the key to reducing costs and maximizing efficiency.** Be sure you identify and use one of your most valuable resources: the person requiring care and his or her network of support. For example, in the case of a diabetic individual, you may have time only to do the minimally acceptable amount of teaching and follow-up. But if you take a few moments to motivate the person to get involved with the local Diabetes Association to learn more and give him the appropriate phone numbers to call, he's likely to expand and re-enforce what he learns from you.

FIGURE 13-1 From assessment to diagnosis: a pivotal point. (Used with permission from Alfaro-LeFevre, R. [2002]. *Applying nursing process* [5th ed., pp. 80–81]. Philadelphia: Lippincott Williams & Wilkins.)

Reflective Practice
Challenge to Cognitive and Interpersonal Skills

Angie Clarkson, a college sophomore, told me tearfully that she believes she was a victim of date-rape her first week in school. She knows she had too much to drink at a party and can only remember waking up in a strange room with a guy she met at the party. She is not sure if she passed out because of the alcohol or if one of the date-rape drugs was involved. A virgin, Angie was sure there had been penetration because of the blood and semen stains she discovered upon waking. It is now a month later and she has not been able to "get her life together" and move on. Angie told me that I am the first person she has told because she feels "so ashamed" and can't believe she let this happen to her. This is my first encounter with an experience like this. I don't do drugs or alcohol and am not sexually active.

Thinking Outside the Box: Possible Courses of Action

- Try to be a good friend and simply suggest she get professional help.
- Advocate for Angie by finding out what resources exist on campus.
- Inform Angie that everything she is describing sounds like the defining characteristics of rape-trauma syndrome and explain how to get professional help and why getting help is so important.

Evaluating a Good Outcome: How Do I Define Success?

- Angie gets the professional help she needs to survive this well.
- I prove worthy of her trust in me.
- I use this experience to learn more about a common problem on campus and the adequacy of existing resources.
- I learn something about my ability to diagnose a health problem and plan accordingly.

Personal Learning: Here's to the Future!

Responding to Angie's clear cry for help certainly moved me out of my comfort zone and made me aware of how my newly developing clinical skills will at times complicate something as simple as being a friend. I felt somewhat responsible for Angie's ability to cope with being raped and believed that I had to do more that simply provide a listening ear. I was pleasantly surprised to discover all the resources that exist on campus. I guess I wasn't surprised that it took a quite a bit of coaxing to get Angie to seek professional help. When I showed her some of what is written about the diagnosis of rape-trauma syndrome, she seemed to find her experience validated and finally agreed to try the student health service counseling center. I felt positive about my role in helping to make this happen.

Reflection

How do you think you would respond in a similar situation? Why? What does this tell you about yourself and about the adequacy of your skills for professional practice? Can you think of other ways to respond? What if the person was a patient for whom you were providing care? Would your response be any different? Should it be? Explain your answer. What other skills (cognitive, interpersonal, technical, ethical/legal) would you need to respond well in this situation? What resources would be appropriate? Do you agree with the criteria to evaluate a successful outcome? Did the nursing student meet the criteria? Please support your response.

---

nurses diagnosing and managing the varieties of health problems described above.

UNIQUE FOCUS OF NURSING DIAGNOSIS

In the diagnosing step of the nursing process, the nurse identifies nursing's unique concern for a patient (ie, what it is about the patient that gives rise to the need for nursing, as opposed to the need for medicine or for physical therapy). Nursing diagnoses are written to describe patient problems that nurses can treat independently.

Consider Antonia Zuccarelli, the middle-aged woman recently diagnosed with cancer but failing to maintain follow-up. Although the patient's diagnosis of cancer is important, the nurse would focus on the patient's lack of follow-up and the possible underlying reasons.

For example, the patient may not realize the importance of the follow-up, thereby indicating a lack of knowledge. Or the patient may be too overwhelmed with the diagnosis, possibly denying its existence, and being unable to cope.

As nurses interpret and analyze patient data, they may identify health problems that are better treated by physicians (medical diagnoses) or by nurses working with other healthcare professionals (collaborative problems). In such a case, the nurse reports the findings to the physician or other appropriate healthcare professionals and works collaboratively with them to resolve the problem.

Nursing Diagnosis Versus Medical Diagnosis

Medical diagnoses identify diseases, whereas nursing diagnoses focus on unhealthy responses to health and illness. Medical diagnoses describe problems for which the physician

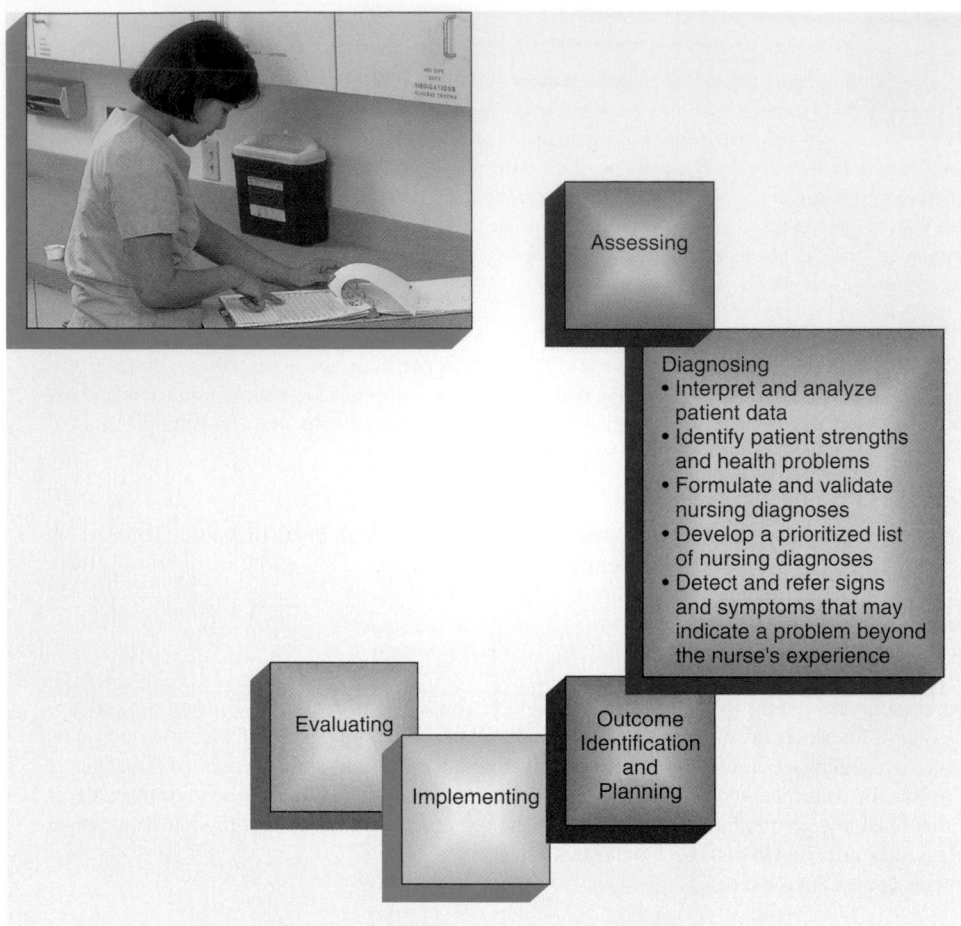

FIGURE 13-2 Diagnosing is the interpretation and analysis of patient data to identify patient strengths and health problems that nursing intervention can prevent or resolve. Nursing diagnoses may change from day to day as the patient's responses to health and illness change.   (Photo © B. Proud.)

directs the primary treatment, whereas nursing diagnoses describe problems treated by nurses within the scope of independent nursing practice. A medical diagnosis remains the same for as long as the disease is present, whereas a nursing diagnosis may change from day to day as the patient's responses change. These distinctions reflect key differences in medical and nursing practices.

Myocardial infarction (heart attack) is a medical diagnosis. Examples of nursing diagnoses for a person with myocardial infarction include Fear, Altered Health Maintenance, Knowledge Deficit, Pain, and Altered Tissue Perfusion.

Think back to Angie Clarkson, the college sophomore who was a victim of date-rape. Possible nursing diagnoses might include Ineffec- *tive Coping, Rape Trauma Syndrome, Post-Trauma Syndrome, Risk for Situational Low Self-Esteem, and Risk for Infection.*

Nursing Diagnosis Versus Collaborative Problems

Nursing diagnoses are also different from collaborative problems. Together, nursing diagnoses and collaborative problems constitute the range of responses that nurses treat, and as such they define the unique nature of nursing. Carpenito defines **collaborative problems** as "certain physiologic complications that nurses monitor to detect onset or changes in status. Nurses manage collaborative problems using physician-prescribed

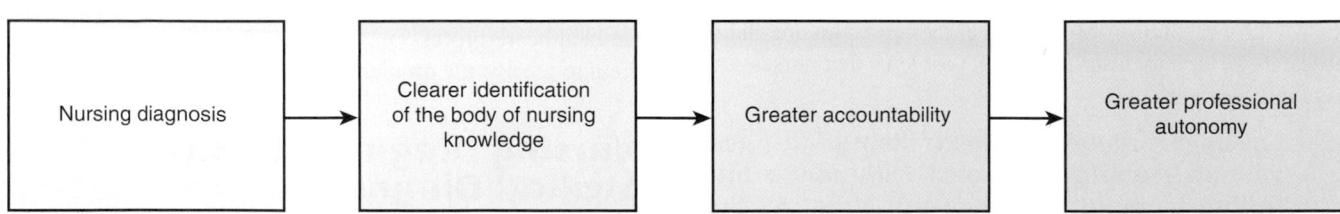

FIGURE 13-3 The relationship of nursing diagnosis to accountability and autonomy. (Used with permission from Carpenito-Moyet, L. J. [2004]. *Nursing diagnosis: Application to clinical practice* [10th ed.]. Philadelphia: Lippincott, Williams & Wilkins.)

BOX 13-1 Legal Alert: Alfaro's Rule

The terms *diagnose* and *diagnosis* have legal implications. They imply that there is a specific problem that requires management by a qualified expert.

- If you make a diagnosis, it means that you accept accountability for accurately naming and managing the problem.
- If you treat a problem or allow a problem to persist without ensuring that the correct diagnosis has been made, you may cause harm and be accused of negligence.
- You are accountable for detecting, identifying, or recognizing signs and symptoms that might indicate problems beyond your expertise. *Example:* Staff nurses are not qualified to diagnose and manage pneumonia independently.

However, they are accountable for:

1. Detecting and reporting signs and symptoms of pneumonia (for example, fever, productive cough, malaise)
2. Diagnosing and managing risk factors for pneumonia (for example, weak breathing efforts due to surgical pain, spinal cord injury, or disease; in complicated cases, these risk factors may require medical management)
3. Diagnosing and managing human responses to pneumonia (for example, fatigue and problems with airway clearance related to pneumonia)
4. Ensuring that the medical treatment plan is implemented as prescribed (Alfaro-LeFevre, 2004, p. 77).

and nursing-prescribed interventions to minimize the complications of the event" (2004, p. 19).

Unlike medical diagnoses, collaborative problems are the primary responsibility of nurses. Unlike nursing diagnoses, with collaborative problems, the prescription for treatment comes from nursing, medicine, and other disciplines. When the

nurse writes patient outcomes that require delegated medical orders for goal achievement, the situation is not a nursing diagnosis, but a collaborative problem. Because collaborative problems involve potential complications, they must be identified early so that preventive nursing care can be instituted early. Figure 13-4 shows collaborative problems identified by a nurse caring for a patient with ovarian cancer. These problems are related to a medical disease, a medical treatment, and a diagnostic study. To write a diagnostic statement for a collaborative problem, follow Alfaro's rule:

If you need to write a diagnostic statement for a collaborative problem, focus on the potential complications of the problem. Use "PC" (for potential complication), followed by a colon, and list the complications that might occur. For clarity, link the potential complications and the collaborative problem by using "related to." Example: PC: pneumothorax related to fractured ribs. (1998, p. 115)

Table 13-1 shows how nurses successfully interpret different clusters of data to identify a nursing diagnosis, collaborative problem, and medical diagnosis. In the first example, a nursing diagnosis is identified and successfully treated. In the next example, the nurse identifies a collaborative problem and initiates intervention within the scope of nursing practice. When this fails to resolve the problem, a physician is contacted to order medication or a catheterization. In this example, the nurse's early detection and reporting of the problem to the physician lead to the physician's prompt medical diagnosis of cystitis and successful antibiotic therapy.

DIAGNOSTIC REASONING AND CRITICAL THINKING

Successful implementation of each step of the nursing process requires high level skills in critical thinking. To correctly diagnose health problems:

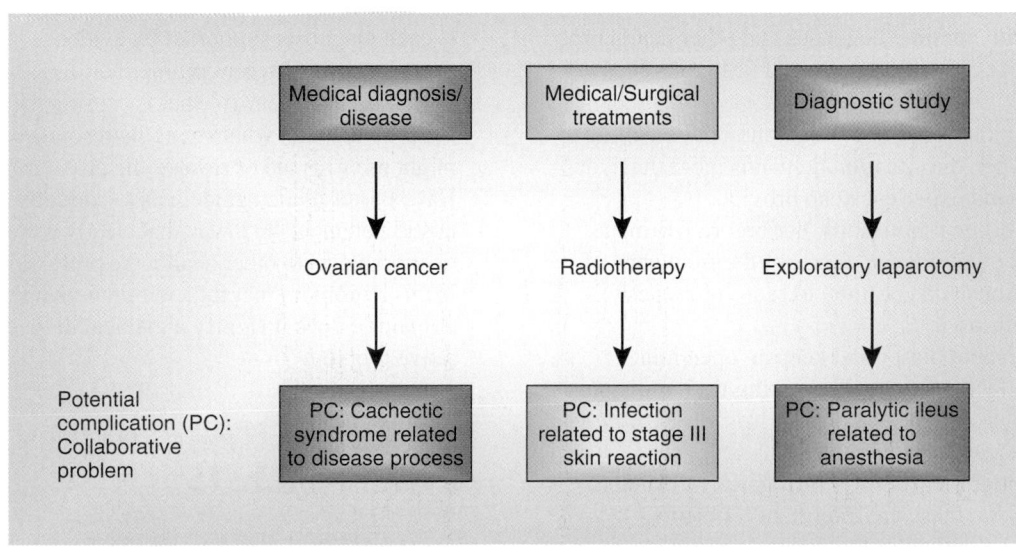

FIGURE 13-4 Collaborative problems.

TABLE 13-1 A Comparison: Nursing Diagnosis, Collaborative Problem, Medical Diagnosis

	Nursing Diagnosis	Collaborative Problem	Medical Diagnosis
Definition	A nursing diagnosis is a clinical judgment about individual, family, or community responses to actual or potential health problems or life processes. Nursing diagnosis provides the basis for selection of nursing interventions to achieve outcomes for which the nurse is accountable (NANDA).	Certain physiologic complications that nurses monitor to detect onset of changes in status (Carpenito)	Traumatic or disease condition or syndrome validated by medical diagnostic studies
Focus	Monitoring human responses to actual and potential health problems	Monitoring pathophysiologic responses of body organs or systems	Correcting or preventing pathology of specific organs or body systems
Sample data cluster	56-year-old mother of seven; 5'4", 167 lb; "Whenever I sneeze lately, I dribble urine. This is embarrassing."	42-year-old woman; 1 hour after delivery; spinal anesthesia; 1500 mL fluid infused in past 4 hours without patient voiding; unable to void	"Whenever I have to urinate it burns terribly. I also feel like I have to go all the time—real bad." Small, frequent voidings, cloudy urine; T—100.8°F
Diagnostic statement	Stress Urinary Incontinence related to degenerative changes in pelvic muscles and structural supports associated with advanced age, obesity, gravid uterus	Potential complication: Urinary Retention related to fluid overload and effects of anesthesia	Cystitis
Select nursing responses	Teach Kegel exercises to increase muscle tone; explore patient's willingness and motivation to pursue weight reduction and exercise program; evaluate need for bladder-training program.	Monitor for signs of increasing urine retention; offer bedpan, and encourage voiding with running water, warm water dripped over perineum, and so forth; if no result, administer physician-prescribed medication; if no result, perform physician-prescribed catheterization.	Report signs and symptoms to physician; obtain urine culture; report results to physician; administer appropriate physician-prescribed antibiotic.

- Be familiar with nursing diagnoses and other health problems; read professional literature and keep reference guides handy.
- Trust clinical experience and judgment, but be willing to ask for help when the situation demands more than your qualifications and experience can provide.
- Respect your clinical intuitions, but before writing a diagnosis without evidence, increase the frequency of your observations and continue to search for cues to verify your intuition.
- Recognize personal biases and keep an open mind.
   Questions to facilitate critical thinking during diagnostic reasoning include:
- Are my data accurate and complete?
- Has the patient or the patient's surrogates validated (if able to do so) that these are important problems?
- Have I given the patient or the patient's surrogate an opportunity to identify problems that I may have missed?

- Is each diagnosis supported by evidence? Might these cues signify a different problem or diagnosis?
- Have I tried to identify what is causing the actual or potential problem, and what strengths/resources the patient might use to avoid or resolve the problem?
- Have I used agency guidelines to correctly document diagnostic statements in a way that clearly communicates patient problems to other healthcare professionals?
- Is this a problem that falls within nursing's independent domain or does it signify a medical diagnosis or collaborative problem?

DATA INTERPRETATION AND ANALYSIS

Most experienced nurses begin the work of interpreting and analyzing data while they are still collecting (assessing) it. The term **cue** is often used to denote significant data or data that influence this analysis. Significant data should "raise a red flag" for the nurse, who then looks for patterns or clusters of data that signal an actual, potential, or possible nursing diagnosis.

> *Remember Martin Prescott, the 46-year-old man with bleeding associated with bowel movements? The report of bleeding accompanied by the patient's complaint of constipation should alert the nurse to a potential problem involving the patient's bowel elimination.*

Recognizing Significant Data

Sorting out healthy patient responses from those that are not healthy is not as clear-cut as it may seem. To avoid erroneously labeling selected patient health patterns as unhealthy (**diagnostic error**) while failing to detect an actual unhealthy behavior, nurses must be familiar with comparative standards to be used in data interpretation and analysis.

A **standard,** or a norm, is a generally accepted rule, measure, pattern, or model to which data can be compared in the same class or category. For example, when determining the significance of a patient's blood-pressure reading, appropriate standards include normative values for the patient's age group, race, and illness category. The patient's own normal range, if known, is an important standard. A pressure of 150/90 mm Hg may be high for someone whose pressure normally is 120/70 mm Hg, but it may be normal for a person with hypertension. Examples of how standards can be used to identify significant cues include the following (Gordon, 1994):

1. Changes in a patient's usual health patterns that are unexplained by expected norms for growth and development: *Example*—An infant who took to breastfeeding easily as a newborn suddenly stops sucking when put to the breast and begins to lose weight.
2. Deviation from an appropriate population norm: *Example*—A first-year college student begins to accelerate her exercise habits dramatically and starts inducing vomiting after binge eating. She rapidly loses weight.
3. Behavior that is nonproductive in the whole-person context: *Example*—A college student breaks up with her boyfriend and begins to believe that she is "unfit" for any other relationship, withdrawing from her friends and social activities.
4. Behavior that indicates a developmental lag or evolving dysfunctional pattern: *Example*—A 16-year-old single mother with a 6-month-old infant continues to "party hard" with her friends, hangs out at the mall, and shows no interest in caring for her son, who is repeatedly left with concerned family members.

Recognizing Patterns or Clusters

A **data cluster** is a grouping of patient data or cues that points to the existence of a patient health problem. Nursing diagnoses should always be derived from clusters of significant data

rather than from a single cue. The danger of deriving a nursing diagnosis from a single cue is illustrated in the following example. Diagnosing a woman recovering from gallbladder surgery with Ineffective Coping solely on the basis of tears may misinterpret the patient's crying, which may be a healthy release of emotion. If the same patient begins to exhibit a cluster of significant cues, such as refusing to eat, preferring bed rest to scheduled ambulation, and reporting increasing discomfort, an unhealthy pattern is emerging.

> *Think back to Angie Clarkson, the college sophomore. Verbalization of the rape trauma is significant. However, even more significant is Angie's report that the event happened more than 1 month ago and she is having difficulty "getting her life together" and moving on.*

Table 13-2 offers examples of how clusters of significant data lead to formulation of accurate nursing diagnoses.

Identifying Strengths and Problems

The next step in analyzing data is to determine the patient's strengths and problems. When determining a patient's strengths and problems, it is helpful to determine whether the patient agrees with the nurse's identification of strengths and problems and is motivated to work toward their resolution.

Determining the Patient's Strengths

If a patient appears to meet a standard, the nurse concludes that the patient has a strength in that particular area, and that this strength contributes to the patient's level of wellness. For example, a person with a history of maintaining a well-balanced diet is usually better able to cope with illness than a person who has a history of eating poorly.

Patient strengths might include healthy physiologic functioning, emotional health, cognitive abilities, coping skills, interpersonal strengths, and spiritual strengths. Resources such as the presence of support people, adequate finances, and a healthy environment may all contribute to patient strengths. Many people take their strengths for granted and might not know how to use them effectively when responding to illness. Discussing observed strengths with patients and counseling patients about ways to develop and use their strengths are important nursing measures.

Determining the Patient's Problem Areas

A person who does not meet a certain health standard probably has a limitation in this aspect of health status and may benefit from professional care. For example, a person with a long history of constipation probably needs care to help overcome this problem. As stated previously, the nurse decides whether the data represent a nursing diagnosis or a collaborative problem, or whether the data should be reported to the physician because they might lead to a medical diagnosis.

TABLE 13-2 Formulating Accurate Nursing Diagnosis Based on Data Clusters

Data Interpretation and Analysis		Formulation of Tentative Nursing Diagnosis	Validation of Nursing Diagnosis
Significant Cues	Sample Data Clusters		
Change in a patient's usual health patterns that is unexplained by expected norms for growth and development	• "I guess I lost about 20 to 30 pounds over the last 6 months—I think I've just been too busy to eat." • Height: 5'8" • Weight: 102 lb • 35-year-old mother of 4-year-old twin boys; returned to work (executive secretary) for first time since delivery of twins 7 months ago	Imbalanced Nutrition: Less Than Body Requirements, related to stress of new job; role conflict and demands	Accurate diagnosis: Patient validates this diagnosis, agreeing with contributing factors
Deviation from an appropriate population norm	• Teacher notices and reports frequency of bruises on third-grade boy who is repeatedly observed alone during recess periods and who is withdrawn in classroom. • In conversation with the school nurse, one parent remarks: "That boy brings out the worst in me! I don't know why, but I often have to smack him hard to make him listen."	Risk for Other-Directed Violence (Child Abuse) related to ? etiology (deficient parenting skills?)	Incomplete diagnosis: Additional data collection yields new information: • Father out of work for past 18 months • Father was abused as a child Diagnosis restated: Risk For Other-Directed Violence (Child Abuse) related to increased family stress and father's history of being abused
Behavior that is non-productive in the whole-person context	• Fiancé abruptly terminated relationship 3 months before established wedding date • Noticeable change in physical appearance; frequently wears same clothes; makeup, jewelry, hair-styling are absent; strong body odors present • No desire to be with others; goes home (lives alone) immediately after work • Stopped attending aerobics classes	Risk for Situational Low Self-esteem related to feeling rejected by fiancé	Premature diagnosis resulting from incomplete data collection. Patient has a long history of major depressive states, one of which may have resulted in the breakup of this relationship. Medical diagnosis and treatment indicated. Changes in appearance are indicative of depressive state. Need to explore related nursing diagnoses.
Behavior indicating developmental lags or evolving dysfunctional patterns	• Admitted to nursing home 2 months ago • "I have nothing to live for anymore . . . why don't I die?" • Wishes to remain in room seated in chair—will only ambulate with great urging • Anything requiring movement has become "too much bother." • Decreased muscle mass, tone, and strength, reduced joint mobility	Impaired Physical Mobility related to difficult transition to nursing home	Accurate but routinized diagnosis that may result in staff's acceptance of status quo unless a more specific cause is identified

Determining Problems the Patient Is Likely to Experience

It is important for nurses to identify potential health problems. For example, a nurse notes that a patient has signs of a wound infection, but laboratory test results show that the patient's white blood cell count has not increased, as is usual when such an infection is present. The nurse concludes that the body apparently is not building up normal defenses to combat the infection. The nurse then predicts the problems this patient is likely to encounter, such as a longer-than-normal healing period. Possible nursing diagnoses alert other caregivers to problems the patient may experience if the certain trends in the patient's condition continue unreversed. This prediction has implications for nursing care, such as measures related to the patient's diet, fluid intake, urine output, and mobility.

Reaching Conclusions

The nurse reaches one of four basic conclusions after interpreting and analyzing the patient data. Different nursing responses are possible for each conclusion:

NO PROBLEM

- No nursing response is indicated.
- Reinforce patient's health habits and patterns.
- Initiate health-promotion activities to prevent disease or illness or to promote a higher level of wellness.
- Wellness diagnosis might be indicated.

POSSIBLE PROBLEM

- Collect more data to confirm or disprove suspected problem.

ACTUAL OR POTENTIAL NURSING DIAGNOSIS

- Begin planning, implementing, and evaluating care designed to prevent, reduce, or resolve the problem.

If unable to treat problem because patient denies problem and refuses treatment, make sure patient understands possible outcomes of this stance.

CLINICAL PROBLEM OTHER THAN NURSING DIAGNOSIS

- Consult with appropriate healthcare professional and work collaboratively on problem.
- Refer to medicine or other services as indicated.

FORMULATING AND VALIDATING NURSING DIAGNOSES

Writing Nursing Diagnoses

When the nurse recognizes a cluster of significant patient data indicating a health problem that can be treated by independent nursing intervention, a nursing diagnosis should be written. Most nursing diagnoses are written either as two-part statements listing the patient's problem and its cause or as three part statements that also include the problem's defining characteristics (Table 13-3).

Those just beginning to write nursing diagnoses might find it helpful to consult the list of health problems accepted by NANDA for testing and study (Box 13-2). The NANDA list is a beginning list of suggested terms for health problems that might be identified and treated by nurses. Each of the

(text continues on page 264)

TABLE 13-3 Formulation of Nursing Diagnosis Statements

	Definition	Purpose	Example
Problem	Identifies what is unhealthy about the patient, indicating the need for change (clear, concise statement of the patient's health problem)	Suggests the patient outcomes (expectations for change)	Bathing/Hygiene Self-Care Deficit ↓ related to ↓
Etiology	Identifies the factors that are maintaining the unhealthy state or response (contributing or causative factors)	Suggests the appropriate nursing measures	Fear of falling in the tub and obesity ↓ as manifested by ↓
Defining characteristics	Identify the subjective and objective data that signal the existence of the problem (cues that reflect the existence of a problem)	Suggest evaluative criteria	Strong body and urine odor, unclean hair: "I'm afraid I'll fall in the tub and break something." (5'4", 170 lb)

Examples:
Two-part diagnostic statement: Bathing/Hygiene Self-Care Deficit related to fear of falling in tub and obesity
Three-part diagnostic statement: Bathing/Hygiene Self-Care Deficit related to fear of falling in tub and obesity, as manifested by strong body and urine odor, unclean hair, statement of fearing fall in tub, and height and weight: 5'4", 170 lb

BOX 13-2 NANDA-Approved Nursing Diagnoses

This list represents the NANDA-approved nursing diagnoses for clinical use and testing.

Domain 1: Health Promotion
Description
The awareness of well-being or normality of function and the strategies used to maintain control of and enhance that well-being or normality of function
Approved Diagnoses
Effective Therapeutic Regimen Management
Ineffective Therapeutic Regimen Management
Ineffective Family Therapeutic Regimen Management
Ineffective Community Therapeutic Regimen Management
Health-Seeking Behaviors (specify)
Ineffective Health Maintenance
Impaired Home Maintenance
Readiness for Enhanced Management of Therapeutic Regimen
Readiness for Enhanced Nutrition

Domain 2: Nutrition
Description
The activities of taking in, assimilating, and using nutrients for the purpose of tissue maintenance, tissue repair, and the production of energy
Approved Diagnoses
Ineffective Infant Feeding Pattern
Impaired Swallowing
Imbalanced Nutrition: Less Than Body Requirements
Imbalanced Nutrition: More Than Body Requirements
Risk for Imbalanced Nutrition: More Than Body Requirements
Deficient Fluid Volume
Risk for Deficient Fluid Volume
Excess Fluid Volume
Risk for Imbalanced Fluid Volume
Readiness for Enhanced Fluid Balance

Domain 3: Elimination
Description
Secretion and excretion of waste products from the body
Approved Diagnoses
Impaired Urinary Elimination
Urinary Retention
Total Urinary Incontinence
Functional Urinary Incontinence
Stress Urinary Incontinence
Urge Urinary Incontinence
Reflex Urinary Incontinence
Risk for Urge Urinary Incontinence
Readiness for Enhanced Urinary Elimination
Bowel Incontinence
Diarrhea
Constipation
Risk for Constipation
Perceived Constipation
Impaired Gas Exchange

Domain 4: Activity/Rest
Description
The production, conservation, expenditure, or balance of energy resources
Approved Diagnoses
Disturbed Sleep Pattern
Sleep Deprivation
Readiness for Enhanced Sleep
Risk for Disuse Syndrome
Impaired Physical Mobility
Impaired Bed Mobility
Impaired Wheelchair Mobility
Impaired Transfer Ability
Impaired Walking
Deficient Diversional Activity
Dressing/Grooming Self-Care Deficit
Bathing/Hygiene Self-Care Deficit
Feeding Self-Care Deficit
Toileting Self-Care Deficit
Delayed Surgical Recovery
Disturbed Energy Field
Fatigue
Decreased Cardiac Output
Impaired Spontaneous Ventilation
Ineffective Breathing Pattern
Activity Intolerance
Risk for Activity Intolerance
Dysfunctional Ventilatory Weaning Response
Ineffective Tissue Perfusion (specify type: Renal, Cerebral, Cardiopulmonary, Gastrointestinal, Peripheral)

Domain 5: Perception/Cognition
Description
The human information-processing system, including attention, orientation, sensation, perception, cognition, and communication
Approved Diagnoses
Unilateral Neglect
Impaired Environmental Interpretation Syndrome
Wandering
Disturbed Sensory Perception (specify: Visual, Auditory, Kinesthetic, Gustatory, Tactile, Olfactory)
Deficient Knowledge (specify)
Readiness for Enhanced Knowledge
Acute Confusion
Chronic Confusion
Impaired Memory
Disturbed Thought Processes
Impaired Verbal Communication
Readiness for Enhanced Communication

Domain 6: Self-Perception
Description
Awareness about the self

BOX 13-2 (Continued)

Approved Diagnoses
Disturbed Personal Identity
Powerlessness
Risk for Powerlessness
Hopelessness
Risk for Loneliness
Readiness for Enhanced Self-Concept
Chronic Low Self-Esteem
Situational Low Self-Esteem
Risk for Situational Low Self-Esteem
Disturbed Body Image

Domain 7: Role Relationships
Description
The positive and negative connections or associations between persons or groups of persons and the means by which those connections are demonstrated
Approved Diagnoses
Caregiver Role Strain
Risk for Caregiver Role Strain
Impaired Parenting
Risk for Impaired Parenting
Readiness for Enhanced Parenting
Interrupted Family Processes
Readiness for Enhanced Family Processes
Dysfunctional Family Processes: Alcoholism
Risk for Impaired Parent/Infant/Child Attachment
Effective Breastfeeding
Ineffective Breastfeeding
Interrupted Breastfeeding
Ineffective Role Performance
Parental Role Conflict
Impaired Social Interaction

Domain 8: Sexuality
Description
Sexual identity, sexual function, and reproduction
Approved Diagnoses
Sexual Dysfunction
Ineffective Sexuality Patterns

Domain 9: Coping/Stress Tolerance
Description
Contending with life events/life processes
Approved Diagnoses
Relocation Stress Syndrome
Risk for Relocation Stress Syndrome
Rape-Trauma Syndrome
Rape-Trauma Syndrome: Silent Reaction
Rape-Trauma Syndrome: Compound Reaction
Post-Trauma Syndrome
Risk for Post-Trauma Syndrome
Fear
Anxiety
Death Anxiety
Chronic Sorrow
Ineffective Denial
Anticipatory Grieving
Dysfunctional Grieving
Impaired Adjustment

Ineffective Coping
Disabled Family Coping
Compromised Family Coping
Defensive Coping
Ineffective Community Coping
Readiness for Enhanced Coping
Readiness for Enhanced Family Coping
Readiness for Enhanced Community Coping
Autonomic Dysreflexia
Risk for Autonomic Dysreflexia
Disorganized Infant Behavior
Risk for Disorganized Infant Behavior
Readiness for Enhanced Organized Infant Behavior
Decreased Intracranial Adaptive Capacity

Domain 10: Life Principles
Description
Principles underlying conduct, thought, and behavior about acts, customs, or institutions as being true or having intrinsic worth
Approved Diagnoses
Readiness for Enhanced Spiritual Well-Being
Spiritual Distress
Risk for Spiritual Distress
Decisional Conflict (specify)
Noncompliance (specify)

Domain 11: Safety/Protection
Description
Freedom from danger, physical injury, or immune-system damage, preservation from loss, and protection of safety and security
Approved Diagnoses
Risk for Infection
Impaired Oral Mucous Membrane
Risk for Injury
Risk for Perioperative Positioning Injury
Risk for Falls
Risk for Trauma
Impaired Skin Integrity
Risk for Impaired Skin Integrity
Impaired Tissue Integrity
Impaired Dentition
Risk for Suffocation
Risk for Aspiration
Ineffective Airway Clearance
Risk for Peripheral Neurovascular Dysfunction
Ineffective Protection
Risk for Sudden Infant Death Syndrome
Risk for Self-Mutilation
Self-Mutilation
Risk for Other-Directed Violence
Risk for Self-Directed Violence
Risk for Suicide
Risk for Poisoning
Latex Allergy Response
Risk for Latex Allergy Response
Risk for Imbalanced Body Temperature
Ineffective Thermoregulation

(continued)

BOX 13-2 (Continued)

Hypothermia
Hyperthermia

Domain 12: Comfort
Description
Sense of mental, physical, or social well-being or ease
Approved Diagnoses
Acute Pain
Chronic Pain
Nausea
Social Isolation

Domain 13: Growth/Development
Description
Age-appropriate increase in physical dimension, organ systems, and/or attainment of developmental milestones
Approved Diagnoses
Risk for Disproportionate Growth
Adult Failure to Thrive
Delayed Growth and Development
Risk for Delayed Development

Used with permission: North American Nursing Diagnosis Association. (2003). *NANDA nursing diagnoses: Definitions and classification, 2003–2004*. Philadelphia: Author.

---

diagnoses in *Nursing Diagnoses: Definitions and Classification, 2003–2004* is presented in taxonomic order and includes the basic components of a nursing diagnosis: definition, defining characteristics, and related factors or risk factors (Box 13-3). This structure has recently been simplified to facilitate the parallel development of an electronic database for nursing diagnoses. There are distinct advantages to nurses' use of common terminology when formulating nursing diagnoses. These range from communication advantages (everyone uses the same words to describe common problems) to promoting the development of nursing science by facilitating

research and the dissemination of research findings. The 5-digit code structure provides for the growth and development of the classification structure without having to change codes when new diagnoses, refinements, and revisions are added. The code structure is compliant with recommendations from the National Library of Medicine concerning healthcare terminology codes.

Pocket-sized handbooks of NANDA-approved nursing diagnoses are available and help students unfamiliar with this grouping of problem statements. Nurses who encounter different health problems within the scope of their practice that they believe to be nursing diagnoses may submit these to the NANDA Diagnosis Review Committee.

BOX 13-3 Components of a NANDA Nursing Diagnosis

Label
Imbalanced Nutrition: More Than Body Requirements (1975).

Definition
Intake of nutrients that exceeds metabolic needs.

Defining Characteristics
- Triceps skin fold greater than 25 mm in women, greater than 15 mm in men
- Weight 20% over ideal for height and frame
- Eating in response to external cues, such as time of day, social situation
- Eating in response to internal cues other than hunger (eg, anxiety)
- Reported or observed dysfunctional eating pattern (eg, pairing food with other activities)
- Sedentary activity level
- Concentrating food intake at the end of the day

Related Factors
Excessive intake in relation to metabolic need.

North American Nursing Diagnosis Association. (2003). *NANDA nursing diagnoses: Definitions and classification, 2003–2004*. Philadelphia: Author.

Types of Nursing Diagnoses

NANDA describes five types of nursing diagnoses: Actual, risk, possible, wellness, and syndrome.

Actual Nursing Diagnoses

Actual nursing diagnoses represent a problem that has been validated by the presence of major defining characteristics. This type of nursing diagnosis has four components: label, definition, defining characteristics, and related factor (see Box 13-3).

Risk Nursing Diagnoses

Risk nursing diagnoses are clinical judgments that an individual, family, or community is more vulnerable to develop the problem than others in the same or similar situation.

Possible Nursing Diagnoses

Possible nursing diagnoses are statements describing a suspected problem for which additional data are needed. Additional data are used to confirm or rule out the suspected problem.

An actual nursing diagnosis for a patient who has experienced vomiting, diarrhea, and excessive diaphoresis for 3 days is Deficient Fluid Volume related to abnormal fluid loss. If the diarrhea persists and weakness interferes with the patient's normal perineal hygiene, he might be at risk for skin breakdown. This is written as the potential diagnosis, Risk for Impaired Skin Integrity. If the nurse suspects that a disturbance of self-concept is also present but lacks the necessary data (defining characteristics) to confirm this, it can be written as a possible diagnosis: Possible Chronic Low Self-Esteem. This alerts other nurses to the need to collect more data about the patient's self-esteem.

Wellness Diagnoses

Wellness diagnoses are clinical judgments about an individual, group, or community in transition from a specific level of wellness to a higher level of wellness. Two cues must be present for a valid wellness diagnosis:

- A desire for a higher level of wellness
- An effective present status or function

A persistent critique of nursing diagnoses that focuses exclusively on patient health problems is their limited applicability in nursing settings that deal primarily with healthy patients. To remedy this concern, wellness diagnoses were proposed and are now readily accepted. For an individual or group to have a wellness diagnosis, two cues should be present: (1) a desire for increased wellness, and (2) effective present state or function (Carpenito, 2004, p. 12). The diagnostic statement for wellness diagnoses is a one-part statement that contains the label Readiness for Enhanced, followed by the desired higher-level wellness. Related factors are not included. Examples include Readiness for Enhanced Family Coping, Readiness for Enhanced Health Maintenance, Readiness for Enhanced Parenting, and Readiness for Enhanced Self-Esteem.

Syndrome Nursing Diagnoses

Syndrome nursing diagnoses comprise a cluster of actual or risk nursing diagnoses that are predicted to be present because of a certain event or situation; for example, Rape Trauma Syndrome or Post-Trauma Syndrome.

Parts of Nursing Diagnoses

Problem

The purpose of the problem statement is to describe the health state or health problem of the patient as clearly and concisely as possible. Because this section of the nursing diagnosis identifies what is unhealthy about the patient and what the patient would like to change in his or her health status, it suggests patient outcomes. NANDA recommends use of the following quantifiers when writing the problem statement: ability, anticipatory, balance, compromised, decreased, deficient, defensive, delayed, depleted, disproportionate, disabling, disorganized, disturbed, dysfunctional, effective, excessive, functional, imbalanced, impaired, inability, increased, ineffective, interrupted, low, organized, perceived, and readiness for enhanced.

Etiology

The etiology identifies the physiologic, psychological, sociologic, spiritual, and environmental factors believed to be re-

lated to the problem as either a cause or a contributing factor. Because the etiology identifies the factors that maintain the unhealthy patient state and prevent the desired change, the etiology directs nursing intervention. Unless the etiology is correctly identified, nursing actions might be inefficient and ineffective. For example, a diabetic patient who is frequently admitted to the hospital with hyperglycemia and who has a poor history of dietary and pharmacologic management is diagnosed to be noncompliant. Assuming that the noncompliance is related to a knowledge deficit and then channeling all nursing activities and energies into teaching the patient how to manage the diabetes is useless if the noncompliance is actually a result of the patient's decreased will to live, which would necessitate a different group of nursing interventions.

Recall Antonia Zuccarelli, the middle-aged woman recently diagnosed with cancer who fails to maintain follow-up? A nursing diagnosis that might be appropriate would be "Noncompliance related to repeated failure to maintain appointments for follow-up treatment and diagnostic testing."

Defining Characteristics

The subjective and objective data that signal the existence of the actual or potential health problem are the third component of the nursing diagnosis. NANDA has identified defining characteristics for each accepted nursing diagnosis, and familiarity with these characteristics helps nurses recognize clusters of significant data. Table 13-3 defines the three components of a nursing diagnosis statement and shows how they affect patient outcomes, nursing measures, and evaluation. Other examples of nursing diagnosis statements are found throughout the book.

Guidelines for Writing Nursing Diagnoses

Remember the following to ensure that your diagnostic statements are correctly written.

1. Phrase the nursing diagnosis as a patient problem or alteration in health state rather than as a patient need.
2. Check to make sure that the patient problem precedes the etiology and that the two are linked by the phrase "related to."
3. Defining characteristics, when included in the nursing diagnosis, should follow the etiology and be linked by the phrase "as manifested by" or "as evidenced by."
4. Write in legally advisable terms.
5. Use nonjudgmental language.
6. Be sure the problem statement indicates what is unhealthy about the patient or what the patient wants to change (enhance).
7. Avoid using defining characteristics, medical diagnoses, or something that cannot be changed in the problem statement.
8. Reread the diagnosis to make sure the problem statement suggests patient outcomes and that the etiology will direct the selection of nursing measures.

Remember Angie Clarkson, the college sopho-more who was a victim of date-rape? An appropriate nursing diagnosis could be "Rape-Trauma Syndrome related to feelings of em-barrassment and shame as manifested by the patient's reporting of event 1 month after it happened, and by patient's statements of in-ability to get life together and move on."

Common errors in writing nursing diagnoses are shown in Table 13-4, along with suggestions for correcting them.

What Is Not a Nursing Diagnosis

The nursing diagnosis statement is written in terms of a patient problem, alteration in health state, or patient strength for which nursing provides the primary therapy. Table 13-5 uses

TABLE 13-4 Common Errors in Writing Nursing Diagnoses and Recommended Corrections

Error	Example	Correction	Example
Writing the diagnosis in terms of needs and not response	Needs assistance with bathing related to bed rest	Write the diagnosis in terms of response rather than need	Bathing/Hygiene Self-Care Deficit related to immobility
Making legally inadvisable statements	Noncompliance due to hostility toward nursing staff (the words *due to* imply a direct cause-and-effect relationship)	Use "related to" rather than "due to" or "caused by" to link the etiology to the problem statement	Noncompliance related to hostility toward nursing staff (denotes a relation between the problem and etiology but not necessarily a causal relation)
	Spouse Abuse related to husband's immaturity and violent temper	Write diagnosis in legally advisable terms: statements that may be interpreted as libel or that imply nursing negligence are legally hazardous to all the nurses caring for the patient	High Risk for Violence: Spouse Abuse related to husband's reported inability to control behavior
	Impaired Skin Integrity related to patient's lying on back all night		Impaired Skin Integrity related to mobility deficit
Identifying as a problem a patient response that is not necessarily unhealthy	Mild Anxiety related to impending surgery	Include in the problem statement of the nursing diagnosis only patient responses that are unhealthy or that the patient wants to change	No need for nursing diagnosis: mild anxiety before surgery is a healthy response that motivates preoperative self-care behavior
Identifying as a problem signs and symptoms of illness	Cough related to long history of smoking	Avoid including signs and symptoms of illness in the problem statement of the nursing diagnosis	Ineffective Airway Clearance related to 20-year history of smoking
Identifying as a patient problem or etiology what cannot be changed	Alterations in Bowel Elimination: Permanent Colostomy related to cancer of bowel	Express the problem statement and etiologic factors in terms that can be changed; otherwise, nursing energies are being directed to a hopeless task	Self-Care Deficit: Care of Colostomy, related to severe anxiety about cancer and feelings of powerlessness
	Grieving related to death of spouse		Dysfunctional Grieving related to inability to accept death of spouse
Identifying environmental factors rather than patient factors as a problem	Cluttered Home related to inability to discard anything	Express the problem statement in terms of unhealthy patient responses rather than environmental conditions	Risk for Injury related to cluttered home (inability to discard anything)

(continued)

TABLE 13-4 (Continued)

Error	Example	Correction	Example
Reversing clauses	Deficient Knowledge related to alteration in parenting	Avoid reversing the problem statement and etiologic statement	Impaired Parenting related to knowledge deficit: child growth and development, discipline
Having both clauses say the same thing	Impaired Comfort related to pain (pain is the comfort alteration—what is contributing to the pain?)	Be sure that the two parts of the diagnosis do not mean the same thing	Unrelieved Incisional Pain related to fear of addiction
Including value judgments in the nursing diagnosis	Poor Home Maintenance related to laziness	Write the diagnosis without value judgments; avoid words such as *poor, inadequate, abnormal, unhealthy*	Impaired Home Maintenance related to low value ascribed to home safety and cleanliness
Including the medical diagnosis in the diagnostic statement	Impaired Home Maintenance related to arthritis	Do not include the medical diagnosis in the nursing diagnosis statement	Impaired Home Maintenance related to mobility, endurance, and comfort alterations

Common errors adapted from Mundinger, M. O., & Jauron, G. D. (1975). Developing a nursing diagnosis. *Nursing Outlook, 23*(2), 94–98. Guidelines for writing nursing diagnoses adapted from Iyer, P., Taptich, B., & Bernocchi-Losey, D. (1991). *Nursing process and nursing diagnoses* (2nd ed.). Philadelphia: W. B. Saunders.

TABLE 13-5 What a Nursing Diagnosis Is *Not*, and Why

What a Nursing Diagnosis Is Not	Example	Rationale
Medical diagnosis	Diabetes mellitus	Although there is nursing care associated with medical illnesses, the illness is not primarily amenable to nursing intervention. Nursing's concern is the *person* who has the illness and the effect of the illness on human functioning.
Medical pathology	Hypoglycemia	Nurses need to understand the pathology underlying disease states to plan appropriate nursing care, but once again, nursing's focus is the person, not the pathology. The person's response to hypoglycemia, how hypoglycemia affects human functioning—these are the domain of *nursing* diagnoses.
Diagnostic tests, treatments, equipment	Fasting blood glucose Insulin therapy Insulin syringe Infusion pump	Nursing's concern is the person's response to the diagnostic study, treatment, or equipment. If the need for insulin therapy reveals a deficient knowledge or self-care deficit, this becomes the nursing diagnosis, not insulin therapy in and of itself.
Therapeutic patient needs	Needs to learn the relation among diet, exercise, and insulin	The diagnosis should be written as a patient health problem rather than a patient need. *Example:* Impaired Health Maintenance (Diabetic Care) related to lack of knowledge of relation among diet, exercise, and insulin.
Therapeutic nursing goals	To develop therapeutic diabetic self-care behaviors	The diagnosis should be written from the patient perspective rather than the nursing perspective and phrased as a patient health problem. *Example:* Self-Care Deficit: Diabetic Self-Care Behaviors, related to decreased value on life and decreased motivation to learn.
A single sign or symptom	After successfully administering own insulin for 3 days, patient tells nurse, "You give me my shot today."	A nursing diagnosis is not developed until a pattern or cluster of significant cues is detected. The signs and symptoms lead to the identification of the problem statement but are not the problem statement. In this situation, no nursing diagnosis is indicated until further data collection, interpretation, and analysis take place.
An *unvalidated* nursing inference	Above incident leads to the nursing inference: Noncompliance related to depression	This is a premature nursing diagnosis that may not accurately reflect a patient problem. More data and the validation of the tentative nursing diagnosis (nursing inference) are needed before the diagnoses can be recorded.

a patient with diabetes mellitus to illustrate what nursing diagnoses are not. For example, nursing diagnoses are not medical diagnoses or statements of patient need.

Validating Nursing Diagnoses

After a tentative nursing diagnosis is formulated, it should be validated. An affirmative response to each of the following questions validates a tentative diagnosis:
* Is my database sufficient, accurate, and supported by nursing research?
* Does my synthesis of data (significant cues) demonstrate the existence of a pattern?
* Are the subjective and objective data I used to determine the existence of a pattern characteristic of the health problem I defined?
* Is my tentative nursing diagnosis based on scientific nursing knowledge and clinical expertise?
* Is my tentative nursing diagnosis able to be prevented, reduced, or resolved by independent nursing action?
* Is my degree of confidence above 50% that other qualified practitioners would formulate the same nursing diagnosis based on my data?

In addition, patients who are able to participate in decision making should be encouraged to validate the diagnosis. "It seems to me that bathing has become a problem now that you are afraid of falling in the tub. What's your sense of this?" Table 13-2 lists possible outcomes of validating tentative nursing diagnoses.

DOCUMENTING NURSING DIAGNOSES

The nurse documents validated nursing diagnoses in the patient record. Depending on the documentation system in use, nursing diagnoses might be recorded in the nursing plan of care and on the multidisciplinary problem list at the front of the patient record. Tables 13-3 and 13-4 illustrate how to document nursing diagnoses using both two- and three-part diagnostic statements.

NURSING DIAGNOSIS: A CRITIQUE

The current nursing diagnosis literature contains many examples of nurses writing about how using nursing diagnoses has improved their clinical practice; articles also detail the many benefits nursing diagnosis brings to the profession. Conversely, other articles point out the limitations of nursing diagnosis and urge nurses to be cautious so that an uncritical use of nursing diagnosis does not restrict their practices.

The primary benefit that nursing diagnosis offers the patient is the individualization of patient care. For example, nurses might be caring simultaneously for three women who have had a modified radical mastectomy because of breast cancer. Although the postoperative nursing management of these women is similar, priorities of care may differ. A prioritized list of nursing diagnoses enables nurses to direct their energies toward these differing patient priorities.

PATIENT A
* Disturbed Body Image
* Ineffective Coping

PATIENT B
* Pain
* Bathing/Hygiene Self-Care Deficit

PATIENT C
* Sexual Dysfunction
* Powerlessness

The use of nursing diagnoses also allows patients to be informed and willing participants in their care as they validate their diagnoses and assist in prioritizing them. The process of prioritizing nursing diagnoses is the first step in planning care and is addressed in Chapter 14.

Improved communication among nurses and other healthcare professionals is probably the most important benefit that accurate, up-to-date diagnoses—expressed in well-defined and standardized terminology—offer nurses. This communication aids in planning, charting, patient data retrieval, health team conferences, change-of-shift reports, and healthcare follow-up. It also promotes nursing accountability for the problems that nurses diagnose.

Among the other benefits of nursing diagnoses for the profession is help in defining the domain of nursing for healthcare administrators, legislators, and other healthcare providers; this is important when seeking funding for nursing and reimbursement for nursing services. Nursing diagnoses are also used to define curriculum content and to direct specialization and advancement in nursing and nursing research.

When the diagnostic process is used incorrectly, a patient might be "misdiagnosed."

COMMON SOURCES OF ERROR
* Premature diagnoses based on an incomplete database: *Example*—A diagnosis of Defensive Coping is made after the patient verbally attacks one nurse who was attempting to teach him self-care for his wound.
* Erroneous diagnoses resulting from an inaccurate database or a faulty data analysis: *Example*—A diagnosis of Dysfunctional Grieving is made in a patient observed crying after learning that her cancer had returned, before anyone had time to evaluate whether this was simply an appropriate response to bad news.
* Routine diagnoses resulting from the nurse's failure to tailor data collection and analysis to the unique needs of the patient: *Example*—A diagnosis of Deficient Knowledge is made in a diabetic patient who is frequently hospitalized with diabetes-related complications, when she actually has excellent knowledge of diabetes and related self-care

demands, but has lacked the motivation to care for herself appropriately.

- Errors of omission: Failure to modify diagnoses and to identify new diagnoses as the patient's status changes may also be problems. Failures in diagnosis lead to failures in nursing care.

Recall Martin Prescott, the 46-year-old man with rectal bleeding and constipation? Although an initial nursing diagnosis may involve Deficient Knowledge related to possible causes of rectal bleeding, further assessment may reveal that the patient's constipation resulting from a diet inadequate in fiber and fluids is the underlying cause of the bleeding. Thus, the nurse would need to revise the nursing diagnosis to focus on Constipation related to inadequate intake of high-fiber foods and fluids as manifested by hard stool and rectal bleeding, and Deficient Knowledge related to foods high in fiber.

These are not so much limitations of nursing diagnosis as they are problems of nurses diagnosing incorrectly. More serious criticisms of nursing diagnoses are raised by nurses who claim that a classification of standardized nursing diagnoses limits nursing, curbing nurses' originality and ability to think things through.

Although some nurses believe that diagnosis offers a valued shortcut to practice, critics find this attitude offensive and respond that rather than invest nursing's energies in perfecting a shortcut, nurses need to change the working conditions that interfere with in-depth problem solving and thoughtful nursing care.

Critics of diagnostic labeling point out that instead of identifying what is unique and positive about nursing, nursing diagnoses make a clear statement that nurses are concerned about what is deviant, wrong, or pathologic (Hagey & McDonough, 1984). The ever-changing and dynamic human person with a need for nursing care becomes objectified (Gebbie, 1984). The practice of many experienced nurses who find nursing diagnoses helpful in coordinating the care efforts of all involved in caring for unique patients with unique needs counters these concerns.

Nurses who are sensitive to transcultural issues raise important concerns about the cultural limitations of the NANDA diagnoses. Foremost among these concerns is that NANDA diagnoses and behaviors assume that the patient is "wrong" and the provider is "right" and deny the validity of cultural and healthcare beliefs and practices that are different from those of the nurse (Geissler, 1991). Examples of nursing diagnoses that often are misused in labeling such cultural deviations as abnormal include Impaired Verbal Communication, Impaired Social Interaction, and Noncompliance. Nurses who provide culturally sensitive care (see Chap. 3) and who work collaboratively with the patient as a partner avoid these problems.

In conclusion, nursing diagnosis has become a valued and essential step in the nursing process. Used correctly, it is a powerful tool for individualizing patient care and ensures that nurses' energies are being used in the most efficient way to meet patients' needs. Nurses who are as concerned about the art and spirit of nursing as they are about its science are careful to avoid labeling patients in a way that objectifies them or limits the potential range of nurse–patient interactions.

■ Developing Critical Thinking Skills

1. Find a patient with a well-established medical condition. List potential medical and nursing diagnoses and collaborative problems. Explain the differing purposes of medical and nursing diagnoses and collaborative problems. What is nursing's diagnostic contribution to the interdisciplinary team's effort to care for this patient?

2. Interview several experienced nurses, and find at least one nurse who is strongly committed to using nursing diagnoses and another who believes they are a waste of time. Interview both until you can explain their different experiences with nursing diagnoses. Try to identify different patient outcomes related to their use or nonuse of nursing diagnoses. List the benefits and limitations of using nursing diagnoses.

3. Interview two patients with the same medical diagnosis. Develop a prioritized list of nursing diagnoses for both, and reflect on the differences. Compare and contrast the strengths of both patients. If you can do this exercise with another student, it would be helpful to explore why there are differences in your lists of nursing diagnoses and patient strengths.

■ Practicing for NCLEX

1. Identify all of the following that are purposes of diagnosing. The purpose of diagnosing is to identify:
   (1) how an individual, group, or community responds to actual or potential health and life processes
   (2) factors that contribute to or cause health problems (etiologies)
   (3) strengths the patient can draw on to prevent or resolve problems
   (4) nursing interventions to resolve health problems
      a. (1) and (2)
      b. (3) and (4)
      c. (1), (2), and (3)
      d. All of the above

2. The terms *diagnose* and *diagnosis* have legal implications. They imply that there is a specific problem that requires management by a qualified expert. Which of the following statements is false?
   a. If you make a diagnosis, it means that you accept accountability for accurately naming and managing the problem.
   b. If you treat a problem or allow a problem to persist without ensuring that the correct diagnosis

has been made, you may cause harm and be accused of negligence.

c. You are accountable for detecting, identifying, or recognizing signs and symptoms that may indicate problems beyond your expertise

d. When nurses diagnose a medical problem, they are just as accountable as physicians for detecting, identifying, and managing the signs and symptoms of disease.

3. Which was the first state to identify diagnosing as part of the legal domain of professional nursing?
   a. New Jersey
   b. New York
   c. North Carolina
   d. North Dakota

4. Which group is responsible for the promotion and organization of activities to continue the development, classification, and scientific testing of nursing diagnoses?
   a. American Nurses Association
   b. National Nursing Diagnosis Association
   c. North American Nursing Diagnosis Association
   d. Clearinghouse for Nursing Diagnoses

5. Altered Health Maintenance is an example of:
   a. Collaborative problem
   b. Interdisciplinary problem
   c. Medical problem
   d. Nursing problem

6. To determine the significance of a blood-pressure reading of 148/100, it is first necessary to:
   a. Compare this data to standards.
   b. Check the taxonomy of nursing diagnoses for a pertinent label.
   c. Check a medical text for the signs and symptoms of high blood pressure.
   d. Consult with colleagues.

7. When the initial nursing assessment revealed that the patient had not had a bowel movement for 2 days, the student wrote the diagnostic label "constipation." Which of the following comments is she most likely to hear from her instructor?:
   a. "Hold on a minute . . . Nursing diagnoses should always be derived from clusters of significant data rather than from a single cue."
   b. "Job well done . . . You've identified this problem early and we can manage it before it becomes more acute."
   c. "Is this an actual or a possible diagnosis?"
   d. "This is a medical, not a nursing problem."

8. A clinical judgment that an individual, family, or community is more vulnerable to develop the problem than others in the same or similar situation is what type of nursing diagnosis?
   a. Actual
   b. Risk
   c. Possible
   d. Wellness
   e. Syndrome

9. Which of the following nursing diagnoses are correctly written as two-part nursing diagnoses?
   (1) Ineffective Coping related to inability to maintain marriage
   (2) Defensive Coping related to loss of job and economic security
   (3) Altered Thought Processes related to panic state
   (4) Decisional Conflict related to placement of parent in nursing home
   a. (1) and (2)
   b. (3) and (4)
   c. (1), (2), and (3)
   d. All of the above

10. Which of the following nursing diagnoses are correctly written as three-part nursing diagnoses?
    (1) Disabled Family Coping related to lack of knowledge about home care of child on ventilator
    (2) Imbalanced Nutrition: Less Than Body Requirements related to inadequate caloric intake while striving to excel in gymnastics as evidenced by 20-pound weight loss since beginning the gymnastic program, and greatly less than ideal body weight when compared to standard height weight charts
    (3) Need to learn how to care for child on ventilator at home related to unexpected discharge of daughter after 3-month hospital stay as evidenced by repeated comments "I cannot do this," "I know I'll harm her because I'm not a nurse," and "I can't do medical things."
    (4) Spiritual Distress related to inability to accept diagnosis of terminal illness as evidenced by multiple comments such as "How could God do this to me?," "I don't deserve this," "I don't understand. I've tried to live my life well," "How could God make me suffer this way?"
    (5) Caregiver Role Strain related to failure of home health aides to appropriately diagnose needs of family caregivers and initiate a plan to facilitate coping as evidenced by caregiver's loss of weight and clinical depression.
    a. (1) and (3)
    b. (2) and (4)
    c. (1), (2), and (3)
    d. All of the above

Answers With Rationale

1. The correct answer is *c*. Identifying nursing interventions to resolve health problems is done during the planning step of the nursing process.
2. The correct answer is *d*. While nurses are accountable to identify and document nursing diagnoses and the signs and symptoms suggestive of medical and collaborative problems, their responsibility for medical problems is related only to the scope of their

practice and they do not share the same responsibility as their physician colleagues.

3. The correct answer is *b*. New York was the first state to identify diagnosing as part of the legal domain of professional nursing.

4. The correct answer is *c*, North American Nursing Diagnosis Association.

5. The correct answer is *d*, Nursing Problem, because it describes a problem that can be treated by nurses within the scope of independent nursing practice.

6. The correct answer is *a*. A standard, or a norm, is a generally accepted rule, measure, pattern, or model to which can be compared data in the same class or category. For example, when determining the significance of a patient's blood-pressure reading, appropriate standards include normative values for the patient's age group, race, and illness category. Deviation from an appropriate norm may be the basis for writing a diagnosis.

7. The correct answer is *a*. A data cluster is a grouping of patient data or cues that points to the existence of a patient health problem. Nursing diagnoses should always be derived from clusters of significant data rather than from a single cue. There may be a reason for the lack of a bowel movement for 2 days, or it might be this individual's normal pattern.

8. The correct answer is *b*. A clinical judgment that an individual, family, or community is more vulnerable to develop the problem than others in the same or similar situation is a Risk nursing diagnosis.

9. The correct answer is *d*. Each of the four diagnoses is a correctly written two-part diagnostic statement that includes the problem or diagnostic label and the etiology or cause.

10. The correct answer is *a*. (2) is written in terms of needs and not unhealthy response and (4) is a legally inadvisable statement.

Bibliography

Ackley, B. J., & Ladwig, G. B. (2002). *Nursing diagnosis handbook: A guide to planning care*. St. Louis: Mosby.

Alfaro, R. (1998). *Applying nursing process: A step-by-step guide* (4th ed.). Philadelphia: Lippincott Williams & Wilkins.

Alfaro-LeFevre, R. (2002). *Applying nursing process: Promoting collaborative care* (5th ed.). Philadelphia: Lippincott Williams & Wilkins.

Alfaro-LeFevre, R. (2004). *Critical thinking and clinical judgment: A practical approach* (3rd ed.). Philadelphia: W. B. Saunders.

American Nurses Association. (1980, 1995). *Nursing: A social policy statement*. Washington, DC: Author.

Aspinall, M. J. (1976). Nursing diagnosis: The weak link. *Nursing Outlook, 24*(7), 433–436.

Atkinson, J., & Murray, M. E. (1990). *Understanding the nursing process* (4th ed.). New York: Macmillan.

Carnevali, D. L., Mitchell, P. H., Woods, N. F., & Tanner, C. A. (1984). *Diagnostic reasoning in nursing*. Philadelphia: J. B. Lippincott.

Carnevali, D. L., & Thomas, M. D. (1993). *Diagnostic reasoning and treatment decision making in nursing*. Philadelphia: J. B. Lippincott.

Carpenito, L. J. (1985). Diagnostics: Actual, potential, or possible? *American Journal of Nursing, 85*(4), 485.

Carpenito, L. J. (2004). *Nursing diagnosis: Application to clinical practice* (10th ed.). Philadelphia: Lippincott Williams & Wilkins.

Carroll-Johnson, R. M. (Ed.). (1991). *Classification in nursing diagnosis: Proceedings of the ninth national conference*. Philadelphia: J. B. Lippincott.

Dobrzyn, J. (1995). Components of written nursing diagnostic statements. *Nursing Diagnosis, 6*(1), 29–35.

Dossey, B., & Guzzetta, C. E. (1981). Nursing diagnosis. *Nursing, 11*(6), 34–38.

Dougherty, C. M., Jankin, J. J., Lunney, M. R., & Whitley, G. G. (1993). Conceptual and research-based validation of nursing diagnoses: 1950–1993. *Nursing Diagnosis, 4*(4), 156–165.

Fitzpatrick, J. J., Kerr, M. E., Saba, V. K., Hoskins, L. M., Hurley, M. E., Milles, W. C., Rottkamp, B. C., Warren, J. J., & Carpenito, L. J. (1989). Translating nursing diagnosis into ICD code. *American Journal of Nursing, 89*(4), 493–495.

Gebbie, K. M. (Ed.). (1975). *Summary of the second national conference*. St. Louis: Clearinghouse for Nursing Diagnoses.

Gebbie, K. M. (1984). Nursing diagnosis: What is it and why does it exist? *Topics in Clinical Nursing, 5*(4), 1–9.

Gebbie, K. M., & Lavin, M. A. (1973). *Summary of the first national conference*. St. Louis: C. V. Mosby.

Geissler, E. M. (1991). Transcultural nursing and nursing diagnosis. *Nursing and Health Care, 12*(4), 190–192, 203.

Gordon, M. (1976). Nursing diagnosis and the diagnostic process. *American Journal of Nursing, 76*(8), 1298–1300.

Gordon, M. (1994). *Nursing diagnosis: Process and application* (3rd ed.). St. Louis: C. V. Mosby.

Gordon, M. (1995). *Manual of nursing diagnosis: 1995–1996 edition*. St. Louis: Mosby–Year Book.

Hagey, R. S., & McDonough, P. (1984). The problem of professional labeling. *Nursing Outlook, 32*(3), 151–157.

Hammond, K. R. (1966). Clinical inference in nursing: A psychologist's view point. *Nursing Research, 15*(1), 27–38.

Hurley, M. (Ed.). (1986). *Classification of nursing diagnoses: Proceedings of the sixth conference*. St. Louis: C. V. Mosby.

Kerr, M., et al. (1993). Taxonomic validation: An overview. *Nursing Diagnosis, 4*(1), 6–14.

Kim, M. J., McFarland, G. K., & McLane, A. M. (Eds.). (1984). *Classification of nursing diagnosis: Proceedings of the fifth national conference*. St. Louis: C. V. Mosby.

Kim, M. J., & Moritz, D. A. (1982). *Classification of the third and fourth national conferences.* Hightstown, NJ: McGraw-Hill.

Kritek, P. B. (1985). Nursing diagnosis in perspective: Response to a critique. *Image—The Journal of Nursing Scholarship, 16*(1), 3–8.

Lindsey, A. M. (1990). Identification and labeling of human responses. *Journal of Professional Nursing, 6*(3), 143–150.

Lunney, M. (1982). Nursing diagnosis: Refining the system. *American Journal of Nursing, 82*(3), 456–459.

Martens, K. (1986). Let's diagnose strengths, not just problems. *American Journal of Nursing, 86*(2), 192–193.

McLane, A. M. (Ed.). (1987). *Classification of nursing diagnoses: Proceedings of the seventh conference.* St. Louis: C. V. Mosby.

Mitchell, G. J. (1991). Nursing diagnosis: An ethical analysis. *Image—The Journal of Nursing Scholarship, 23*(2), 99–103.

Mundinger, M. O., & Jauron, G. D. (1975). Developing a nursing diagnosis. *Nursing Outlook, 23,* 94–98.

North American Nursing Diagnosis Association. (1990). *Taxonomy I revised with official diagnostic categories.* St. Louis: Author.

North American Nursing Diagnosis Association. (2003). *NANDA nursing diagnoses: Definitions and classification, 2003–2004.* Philadelphia: Author.

Popkess, S. (1981). Diagnosing your patient's strengths. *Nursing, 11*(7), 34–37.

Popkess, S., & Vawter, S. (1991). Wellness nursing diagnosis: To be or not to be? *Nursing Diagnosis, 2*(1), 19–25.

Porter, E. J. (1986). Critical analysis of NANDA nursing diagnosis taxonomy I. *Image—The Journal of Nursing Scholarship, 18*(4), 136–139.

Price, M. R. (1980). Nursing diagnosis: Making a concept come alive. *American Journal of Nursing, 80*(4), 668–674.

Rasch, R. F. R. (1987). The nature of taxonomy. *Image—The Journal of Nursing Scholarship, 19*(3), 147–149.

Roberts, S. L. (1990). Achieving professional autonomy through nursing diagnosis and nursing DRGs. *Nursing Administration Quarterly, 14*(4), 54–60.

Rubenfeld, M. G., & Scheffer, B. K. (1995). *Critical thinking in nursing: An interactive approach.* Philadelphia: J. B. Lippincott.

Shamansky, S. L., & Yanni, C. R. (1983). In opposition to nursing diagnosis: A minority opinion. *Image—The Journal of Nursing Scholarship, 15*(2), 47–50.

Vincent, K. G., & Coler, M. S. (1990). A unified nursing diagnostic model. *Image—The Journal of Nursing Scholarship, 22*(2), 93–95.

Warren, J., & Hoskins, L. (1990). The development of NANDA's nursing diagnosis taxonomy. *Nursing Diagnosis, 1*(4), 162–168.

Weber, G. (1991). Making nursing diagnosis work for you and your patient: A step-by-step approach. *Nursing and Health Care, 12*(8), 424–430.

Wilkinson, J. M. (2000). *Nursing diagnosis handbook with NIC interventions and NOC outcomes* (7th ed.). Upper Saddle River, NJ: Prentice Hall Health.

Outcome Identification and Planning

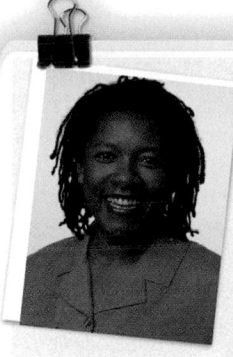

Glenda Kronk, a 35-year-old woman, comes to the health center for a routine checkup. During the visit, she expresses a strong motivation and desire to become physically fit, lose weight, increase her muscle tone, and improve her cardiorespiratory capacity. "I know it will involve some major lifestyle changes, including diet. What's with all these diets and diet supplements now?" she asks.

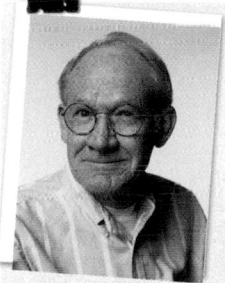

Elijah Wolinski is a thin, frail, 85-year-old man who is bed-bound due to severe degenerative joint disease. He is being cared for by his 56-year-old nephew at his home. Assessment on a home visit reveals Elijah lying on soiled linens with a large pressure ulcer on his sacrum, approximately 3" in diameter and about 1" deep with purulent drainage.

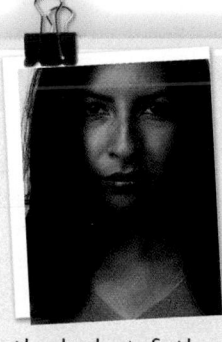

Darla Jefferson, a 29-year-old single woman, is about 14 weeks pregnant. She describes herself as a "hopeless addict" who has tried to stop "more times than I can remember." Although currently drug-free, she is not hopeful of preventing relapse. She does not know the baby's father and has mixed feelings about keeping the baby, saying, "On the one hand I want someone to love me, but I'm not sure I'd want me for a mother."

Focusing on Blended Skills

The types of blended skills you'll need to respond to the case scenarios include:

Cognitive Skills

- Knowledge of what information is needed to develop a plan of care that meets the nursing needs of a woman who wants to improve her fitness level, an frail, older adult with a pressure ulcer, and a single pregnant woman with a history of drug abuse: in other words, how to establish priorities, develop patient-centered outcomes and related evaluative strategies, select nursing interventions, and communicate the plan of nursing care
- Knowledge of pertinent standards of care and agency and institutional policies
- Ability to think critically about how best to respond to the patient's need for nursing
- Knowledge of important assessments related to the patient's status, such as healthy lifestyles, pressure ulcers, and drug abuse and pregnancy
- Knowledge of factors associated with skin breakdown and pressure ulcer formation, infection control measures, wound care, and personal care and hygiene

Technical Skills

- Ability to research the literature to obtain knowledge to develop the plan of care
- Ability to use a documentation system to communicate the plan of care
- Computer literacy
- Ability to identify areas of technical assistance to be implemented with the plan of care, such as patient teaching, wound care, infection control measures, and counseling for drug abstinence
- Competence in identifying appropriate interventions based on sound scientific rationales

Interpersonal Skills

- Ability to establish trusting nurse–patient relationships grounded in responsible caring with patients with special needs: woman wishing to lead a healthy lifestyle, frail, elderly man with a pressure ulcer, and a young pregnant woman with a history of drug abuse
- Ability to empathize with patients, sharing their struggles and celebrating their achievement of valued goals
- Ability to work collaboratively with members of the health-care team to develop the interdisciplinary plan of care
- Ability to demonstrate respect for the patient's human dignity as a key component of the plan of care
- Knowledge of personal values and morals, with demonstration of respect for individuals who believe, value, choose, or behave differently than you do

Ethical and Legal Skills

- Ability to communicate respect and to promote the patient's and family's sense of worth
- Demonstration of a strong sense of accountability for the health and well-being of patients, which translates into a commitment to developing a plan of care that allows patients to get the help they need to achieve their health goals
- Commitment to secure the patient's well-being within the bounds of your professional responsibilities and scope of practice
- Ability to serve as a trusted and effective patient advocate
- Consistent use of appropriate legal safeguards while developing and documenting the plan of care

Learning Objectives

After completing the chapter, the learner should be able to accomplish the following:

1. Describe the purpose and benefits of outcome identification and planning.
2. Identify three elements of comprehensive planning.
3. Prioritize patient health problems and nursing responses.
4. Describe how patient goals/expected outcomes and nursing orders are derived from nursing diagnoses.
5. Develop a plan of nursing care with properly constructed outcomes and related nursing interventions.
6. Differentiate nurse-initiated interventions, physician-initiated interventions, and collaborative interventions.
7. Use criteria to evaluate planning skills.
8. Describe five common problems related to planning, their possible causes, and remedies.

Key Terms

clinical pathways (critical pathways, CareMaps)
computerized plans of nursing care
consultation
criteria
discharge planning
expected outcome
goal
initial planning
Kardex care plan
nursing intervention
ongoing planning
outcome identification
patient outcome
plan of nursing care
planning
standardized care plans

After the nurse collects and interprets patient data, identifying patient strengths and health problems, it is time to plan for nursing action (see the accompanying Reflective Practice box for an example.) During the **outcome identification** and **planning** steps of the nursing process, the nurse works in partnership with the patient and family to:

- Establish priorities
- Identify and write expected patient outcomes
- Select evidence-based nursing interventions
- Communicate the plan of nursing care (Fig. 14-1)

A **goal** is an aim or an end. A **patient outcome** is an expected conclusion to a patient health problem, or in the event of a wellness diagnosis, an expected conclusion to a patient's health expectation. The words "goal," "objective," and "outcome" are often used interchangeably. In some practice settings, the term "goal" or "objective" is used to describe what is wanted and the term "outcome" is used to describe the results achieved. In nursing, the phrase **expected outcomes** is used to refer to the more specific, measurable **criteria** used to evaluate the extent to which a goal has been met. This chapter uses "outcome" to refer to expected patient outcomes.

The nurse, patient, and family should work together as much as possible in the outcome identification and planning stage. If the outcomes specified in the plan of care are not valued by the patient or do not contribute to the prevention, resolution, or reduction of the patient's problems or the achievement of the patient's health expectations, the plan of care may be meaningless. Outcome determination is, therefore, a critical skill for successfully intervening with patients.

This chapter describes outcome identification and planning as a formal process, a deliberate step in the nursing process. A formal plan of care allows nurses to:

- Individualize care that maximizes outcome achievement
- Set priorities
- Facilitate communication among nursing personnel and their colleagues
- Promote continuity of high-quality, cost-effective care
- Coordinate care
- Evaluate the patient's responses to nursing care
- Create a record that can be used for evaluation, research, reimbursement, and legal purposes
- Promote the nurse's professional development

Reflective Practice
Challenge to Ethical and Legal Skills

While working in a women's shelter, I met Darla Jefferson, a 29-year-old single woman who was about 14 weeks pregnant. Darla described herself as a "hopeless addict" who had tried to stop "more times than I can remember." She was drug-free at the moment but not hopeful of preventing relapse. She did not know the baby's father and had mixed feelings about keeping the baby. She said, "On the one hand I want someone to love me, but I'm not sure I'd want me for a mother." I knew I needed to explore her commitment to this pregnancy, but I am strongly opposed to abortion and did not think I could talk with her objectively about her decision. I needed to develop a plan for dealing with this topic.

Thinking Outside the Box: Possible Courses of Action

- Tell Darla that I believe it is her responsibility to have this baby and to then make a decision about whether to offer the baby for adoption based upon her assessment of her parenting readiness.
- Help Darla assess her readiness to become a parent, and in light of this explore all her options regarding continuing or terminating the pregnancy.
- Get someone else to talk with Darla so that she gets the counseling she needs and I am not morally compromised.

Evaluating a Good Outcome: How Do I Define Success?

- Darla gets the help she needs to make the decision that is right for her and her unborn baby.
- I am faithful to both my nursing responsibilities to counsel this patient and my duty to maintain my moral integrity.

Personal Learning: Here's to the Future!

Unfortunately, I overestimated my ability to counsel Darla without compromising myself, and as I result I don't think I was as helpful to her as I should have been. Ideally, I planned to objectively explore her readiness to be a mother and then have an open and unbiased discussion about her options. When she began to talk about getting an abortion, I found myself urging her to have the baby and then place the baby up for adoption if she still felt she couldn't care for him or her after delivery. Regrettably, I let my personal opinions come through in the discussion. Through my actions, I think she lost trust in me. I'm going to talk with other nurses to see how they handle this challenge.

Reflection

How would you respond in a similar situation? Why? What does this tell you about yourself and about the adequacy of your skills for professional practice? Can you think of other ways to respond? What actions might have proved more effective? What actions might be helpful for the nursing student so that when faced with similar situations in the future, the outcome would be more positive? What other skills (cognitive, interpersonal, technical, ethical/legal) would you need to respond well in this situation? Suggest an alternative course of action that might have been effective, and explain why. Do you agree with the criteria to evaluate a successful outcome? Did the nursing student meet the criteria? Support your response.

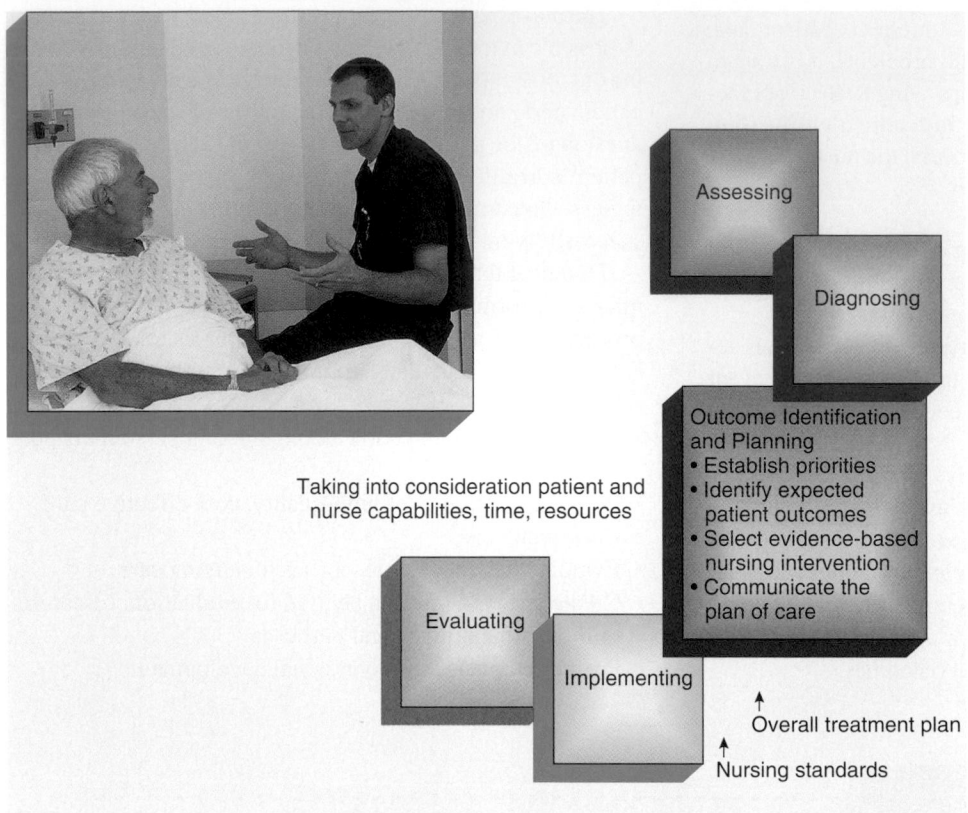

Taking into consideration patient and
nurse capabilities, time, resources

FIGURE 14-1 Outcome Identification and Planning. The nurse and patient work together to establish priorities, identify expected patient outcomes, and select the evidence-based nursing interventions. It is important for the plan of care to be consistent with nursing standards, congruent with other planned therapies, and realistic in terms of the patient's and nurse's abilities or resources. Ensuring that the plan of care is recorded is also an important nursing responsibility. (Photo © B. Proud.)

Informal planning is often also observed by students in practice settings. This is the link between identifying a patient's strength or problem and providing an appropriate nursing response. When a nurse on a busy surgical unit learns that a postoperative patient is complaining of incisional pain and quickly reshuffles priorities to allow time to assess the course and qualities of the pain and determine nursing measures to reduce discomfort, planning has occurred. When a postpartum nurse on the 3-to-11 shift realizes the evening before discharge that he or she has not seen a particular father hold his new daughter and makes a mental note to observe the father–daughter interactions that evening and facilitate their bonding, planning has occurred. When a nurse in a geriatric day-care center hears a patient choking and rushes to his side to perform the Heimlich maneuver if necessary, planning has occurred. Informal planning on a more conscious level is illustrated by a hospice nurse who drives home pondering how best to support a patient with terminal cancer who is gradually relinquishing her hold on life. She may elect to initiate a more formal process of planning the next day when she consults with colleagues who have cared for patients with similar health needs. In each of the above examples, the process of informal planning allowed an individual nurse to think about how best to help a particular patient—ideally, with good results. What is lacking is a coordinated plan known by everyone caring for the patient.

UNIQUE FOCUS OF NURSING OUTCOME IDENTIFICATION AND PLANNING

The primary purpose of the outcome identification and planning step of the nursing process is to design a plan of care for and with the patient that, once implemented, results in the prevention, reduction, or resolution of patient health problems and the attainment of the patient's health expectations, as identified in the patient outcomes.

Think back to Glenda Kronk, the woman verbalizing a need to improve her fitness level. Based on a comprehensive patient assessment, together the nurse and patient would develop an appropriate plan to achieve this improved level of health, such as planning for 20-minute walks three times a week, eating a nutritious diet, and making routine follow-ups to determine the patient's progress toward the ultimate outcome.

A comprehensive plan of care additionally specifies any routine nursing assistance the patient needs to meet basic human needs (eg, assistance with hygiene or nutrition) and describes appropriate nursing responsibilities for fulfilling the collaborative and medical plan of care. For example, physicians may delegate to nurses caring for a surgical patient the redressing of the surgical incision, the administration of prescribed medications and intravenous therapy, and responsibility for scheduling laboratory studies. Nurses design plans of care that incorporate both their independent and collaborative responsibilities. Because nursing is concerned with the patient's responses to health and illness, the plan of care is supportive of nursing's broad aims—to promote wellness, prevent disease and illness, promote recovery, and facilitate coping with altered functioning.

OUTCOME IDENTIFICATION, PLANNING, AND CRITICAL THINKING

Successful implementation of each step of the nursing process requires high-level skills in critical thinking. To plan healthcare correctly, the nurse must:

- Be familiar with standards and agency policies for setting priorities, identifying and recording expected patient outcomes, selecting evidence-based nursing interventions, and recording the plan of care
- Remember that the goal of patient-centered care is to keep the patient and the patient's interests and preferences central in every aspect of planning and outcome identification
- Keep the "big picture" in focus: What are the discharge goals for this patient, and how should this direct each shift's interventions?
- Trust clinical experience and judgment but be willing to ask for help when the situation demands more than your qualifications and experience can provide; value collaborative practice
- Respect your clinical intuitions but before establishing priorities, identifying outcomes, and selecting nursing interventions be sure that research supports your plan
- Recognize personal biases and keep an open mind

> *Remember Darla Jefferson, the pregnant woman with a history of drug abuse described in the Reflective Practice box. Although the nursing student planned to engage the patient in an unbiased discussion of her alternatives, unfortunately the student was unable to adhere to the plan, inserting personal opinions in the discussion. As a result, the plan of care was thwarted and the patient lost trust in the student.*

Questions to facilitate critical thinking during planning and outcome identification include:

- Setting priorities: Which problems require my immediate attention or that of the team? Which problems are my responsibility, and which should I refer to someone else? Which problems are most important to the patient?
- Identifying outcomes: What must I observe in the patient to demonstrate the resolution of the problems identified by the nursing diagnoses and general problem list? What is the time frame for accomplishing these outcomes? Do the outcomes need to be modified in light of the patient's response (or lack of response) to the planned interventions?
- Selecting evidence-based nursing interventions: What do nursing science and my clinical experience suggest is the likelihood that this particular nursing intervention will help the patient realize his or her expected outcomes? How can I tailor my interventions to increase the likelihood of patient benefit? What is the worst thing that might happen with this intervention, how likely is it to happen, and what can I do to minimize the possibility of this harm?
- Communicating the plan of care: Does the plan of care adequately address the patient's priorities today? If the plan of care is computerized or standardized, does it adequately address the specific needs of this particular patient? Can anyone reading the plan of care know how to intervene effectively with this patient?

COMPREHENSIVE PLANNING

In acute care settings, three basic stages of planning are critical to comprehensive nursing care: initial, ongoing, and discharge. In other settings such as long-term care, hospice care, or a community clinic, initial and ongoing planning may be the primary stages used. If a nurse develops a comprehensive plan of care on the patient's first day but fails to update the plan, the plan will not be effective or efficient. Failure to update the plan of care as needed is a common problem in all healthcare settings.

Initial Planning

Initial planning is developed by the nurse who performs the admission nursing history and the physical assessment. This comprehensive plan addresses each problem listed in the prioritized nursing diagnoses and identifies appropriate patient goals and the related nursing care. **Standardized care plans** are prepared plans of care that identify the nursing diagnoses, outcomes, and related nursing interventions common to a specific population or health problem. (An example of a standardized care plan is shown later in the chapter.) They can provide an excellent basis for the initial plan if the nurse individualizes them. Resources for standardized plans include computerized plans, textbooks with prepared care plans, and agency-developed plans/maps/critical pathways. By using such standardized plans, the nurse is free to direct time and expertise to individualizing the plan.

Ongoing Planning

Ongoing planning is carried out by any nurse who interacts with the patient. Its chief purpose is to keep the plan up to date to facilitate the resolution of health problems, manage risk factors, and promote function. The nurse caring for the patient uses new data as they are collected and analyzed to make the plan more specific and accurate and therefore more effective. The work of ongoing planning includes stating nursing diagnoses more clearly (both the problem statement and the cause), developing new diagnoses, making previously developed patient outcomes more realistic, developing new outcomes as needed, and identifying nursing interventions that will best accomplish the patient goals.

> *Consider Elijah Wolinski, the frail elderly man who developed a pressure ulcer. Ongoing planning is necessary because the patient's pressure ulcer would most likely take some time to heal or at least improve. In addition, other needs might become apparent during subsequent home visits, thereby requiring the nurse to update the plan of care.*

At this stage of planning, standardized plans based on medical conditions or procedures might be useful in developing new nursing diagnoses and related nursing interventions, but the emphasis is clearly on individualizing the plan to meet unique patient needs. For example, the standard nursing order "force fluids" would be rewritten as "offer 60 mL cranberry or orange juice between meals, and keep fresh water at bedside." A preliminary order such as "explore with the patient existing supports" might be replaced with "keep daughter Barbara informed of mother's progress and coach her in effective support strategies: Barbara Clems, (h) 448-3211, (w) 654-8999."

Discharge Planning

Discharge planning is best carried out by the nurse who has worked most closely with the patient and family, possibly in conjunction with a nurse or social worker with a broad knowledge of existing community resources. In acute care settings, comprehensive discharge planning begins when the patient is admitted for treatment. Careful planning ensures that the nurse uses teaching and counseling skills effectively to help the patient and family develop sufficient knowledge of the health problem and the therapeutic regimen to carry out necessary self-care behaviors at home competently. Discharge planning is further discussed in Chapter 9.

ESTABLISHING PRIORITIES

To develop a prioritized list of nursing diagnoses, the nurse needs guidelines for ranking diagnoses as high, medium, or low priority. High-priority diagnoses pose the greatest threat to the patient's well-being. Non–life-threatening diagnoses are ranked as medium priorities, and diagnoses that are not specifically related to the current health problem are of low priority. In all levels, psychosocial needs must be considered as well as physiologic needs.

In addition to developing a prioritized list of nursing diagnoses, nurses working within an interdisciplinary team need to set priorities for nursing care that take account of all the patient's health needs as recorded on the general problem list. This involves looking at all problems to determine the relationships among the problems (what's causing or contributing to what). Thus, it generally makes sense to deal with medical (or suspected medical) problems first. If these can be resolved, many human response problems are gone. If a nurse sees the classic signs and symptoms of appendicitis and tries to identify and manage a nursing diagnosis of pain without consulting a physician or nurse practitioner, the patient's appendix might rupture before even developing a nursing plan to relieve pain!

Three helpful guides to facilitate critical thinking when prioritizing patient problems include Maslow's hierarchy of human needs, patient preference, and anticipation of future problems.

Maslow's Hierarchy of Human Needs

Because basic needs must be met before a person can focus on higher ones, patient needs may be prioritized according to the following hierarchy:
1. Physiologic needs
2. Safety needs
3. Love and belonging needs
4. Self-esteem needs
5. Self-actualization needs

For example, a geriatric patient who is incontinent of urine and sitting in a wet disposable brief (physiologic need) will be unable to participate fully in a music therapy diversional activity (self-esteem need) until the more basic need is met.

Patient Preference

It is best to first meet the needs the patient thinks are most important, if this order does not interfere with other vital therapies. For example, a woman is admitted to an orthopedic unit with a fractured pelvis and multiple lacerations after an automobile accident. The morning after the accident, she complains of pain and needs assistance with bathing and attention to her lacerations, but she refuses to do anything until she calls home to find out who is caring for her 15-month-old twins. The nurse should help her to call home before beginning other care as long as it does not interfere with life-saving emergency care.

Anticipation of Future Problems

Nurses must tap their knowledge base to consider the potential effects of different nursing actions. Assigning low priority to a diagnosis that the patient wants to ignore but that can result in harmful future consequences for the patient might be nursing negligence. For example, an obese patient with multiple sclerosis and greatly decreased limb strength who spends most of her day in bed may see no value in diet modification and position changes. A nurse who is alert to the potentially serious problem of pressure ulcers would assign high priority to this diagnosis, nonetheless, and incorporate weight management and position changes into the plan of care despite the patient's reluctance.

Critical Thinking and Establishing Priorities

The work of setting priorities demands careful critical thinking. Alfaro (2002, p. 125) suggests that nurses ask:

1. What problems need immediate attention and which ones can wait?
2. Which problems are your responsibility, and which do you need to refer to someone else?
3. Which problems can be dealt with by using standard plans (eg, critical paths, standards of care)?
4. Which problems aren't covered by protocols or standard plans but must be addressed to ensure a safe hospital stay and timely discharge (or simply safe care of high quality)?

Think back to Darla Jefferson, the pregnant woman with a history of drug abuse. The nurse would incorporate critical thinking by asking these four questions, thereby ultimately arriving at the patient problems requiring the most immediate attention.

When planning nursing care for each day, it is helpful to consider the following:

- Have changes in the patient's health status influenced the priority of nursing diagnoses? For example, when a routine home visit to an older adult reveals evidence of possible elder abuse, a new set of priorities for care is needed, which may even result in a new diagnosis.
- Have changes in the way the patient is responding to health and illness or the plan of care affected those nursing diagnoses that can be realistically addressed? For example, a nurse might have identified Ineffective Coping as a high-priority diagnosis for the patient after the patient learned the medical diagnosis, and planned to initiate counseling. If the patient adamantly requests to be left alone for a day to think things through, however, the nurse has to modify priorities of care for that day.
- Are there relationships among diagnoses that require that one be worked on before another can be resolved?
- Can several patient problems be dealt with together?

After answering these questions, the nurse ranks the diagnoses in the order in which they should be addressed. Setting priorities enables the nurse to make sure that time and energy are being directed first to the patient's most important problems.

IDENTIFYING AND WRITING OUTCOMES

Learning to identify and write appropriate outcomes takes practice. The text that follows and the guidelines in Box 14-1 will help you to identify outcomes that will maximize your effectiveness when working with patients.

BOX 14-1 Guidelines for Writing Outcomes

Written outcomes can be evaluated by seeing if they conform to the following criteria:

- Each set of outcomes is derived from only one nursing diagnosis.
- At least one of the outcomes shows a direct resolution of the problem statement in the nursing diagnosis.
- Both long-term and short-term outcomes are identified as necessary.
- Cognitive, psychomotor, and affective outcomes appropriately signal the type of change needed by the patient.
- The patient and family value the outcomes.
- Each outcome is brief and specific (clearly describes one observable, measurable patient behavior/manifestation), is phrased positively, and specifies a time line.
- The outcomes are supportive of the total treatment plan.

Deriving Outcomes From Nursing Diagnoses

Outcomes are derived from the problem statement of the nursing diagnosis. For each nursing diagnosis in the plan of care, at least one outcome should be written that, if achieved, demonstrates a direct resolution of the problem statement (Table 14-1).

Other outcomes that contribute to the resolution of the problem may be written. For example, for the nursing diagnosis Imbalanced Nutrition: More Than Body Requirements related to excessive snacking and inactivity, in addition to the outcome "within 12 weeks (12/6/06), the patient will lose 20 pounds and reach target weight (122 lb)," the following goals are appropriate: "within 3 days of teaching: the patient will identify 10 low-calorie snack foods he is willing to try; the patient will have 3-day diet recall consistent with nutritionally balanced

TABLE 14-1 Examples of Goals/ Outcomes to Relieve Problems

Problem Statement of the Nursing Diagnosis	Related Patient Goal/Outcome
Pain	Within 8 hours, patient will report pain is absent or diminished
Imbalanced Nutrition: More Than Body Requirements	By 12/6/06, patient will reach target weight of 122 lb
Impaired Physical Mobility	Before discharge, patient will ambulate length of hallway independently

1,500-calorie diet; the patient will report incorporating three half-hour periods of walking at 5 miles per hour into each week." If the patient can identify low-calorie snack foods and adopt a more active lifestyle, there is a greater likelihood that he will reach his target weight, but it is entirely possible for a patient to achieve these secondary outcomes without resolving the chief problem. Remember, at least one outcome per nursing diagnosis must directly resolve the problem statement in the nursing diagnosis.

The Nursing Outcomes Classification (NOC) developed by the Iowa Outcomes Project presents the first comprehensive standardized language used to describe the patient outcomes that are responsive to nursing intervention (Johnson et al., 2000, 2001). Explicit linkages between the North American Nursing Diagnosis Association (NANDA) diagnoses and the NOC facilitate a comprehensive approach to care planning.

Establishing Long-Term Versus Short-Term Outcomes

Outcomes might be either long term or short term. Long-term outcomes require a longer period (usually more than a week) to be achieved than do short-term outcomes. They also may be used as discharge goals, in which case they are more broadly written and communicate to the entire nursing team the desired end results of nursing care for a particular patient. For example, two women, both 77 years of age, are on a nursing unit after undergoing similar operations for fractured left hips. One woman has spent the past 2 years in bed in a nursing home; the other woman fractured her hip at the YMCA, where she swims daily. Their nursing care should not be the same because it is directed toward different long-term goals, even though their short-term goals might be similar (see Box 14-2: Examples of Long-Term and Short-Term Outcomes).

Consider Elijah Wolinski, the frail elderly man with a pressure ulcer. The nurse might establish a long-term outcome such as, "The patient's sacral area will exhibit no evidence of a pressure ulcer." Short-term outcomes might include, "The patient's sacral pressure ulcer demonstrates an absence of purulent drainage within 1 week of initiating wound care. By week 2, the patient's pressure ulcer has decreased in size by a quarter-inch. By week 2, the patient's caregiver demonstrates measures to relieve pressure on the skin while the patient is in bed."

Cognitive, Psychomotor, and Affective Outcomes

Outcomes might be categorized according to the type of change they describe for the patient. Cognitive outcomes describe increases in patient knowledge or intellectual behaviors—for example: "Within 1 day after teaching, the patient will list three benefits of continuing to apply moist com-

---

BOX 14-2 Examples of Long-Term and Short-Term Outcomes

Patient on Bed Rest From Nursing Home
Long-Term Outcome
Mrs. Goldstein returns to the nursing home pain free with her incision healed and her left leg in good alignment.
Short-Term Outcomes
- Whenever observed, patient will be lying in bed with legs in correct alignment (abductor pillow in place if ordered).
- Before discharge, Mrs. Goldstein's hip incision will show signs of healing (skin surfaces approximate, free from signs of infection—redness, swelling, heat, purulent drainage).
- Whenever observed, patient will report that comfort measures and medication are satisfactorily managing pain.

Active Patient from Private Home
Long-Term Outcome
Mrs. Silverstein returns home to her husband pain free with incision healed, fully mobile (full weight bearing on left leg), and capable of independent activities of daily living.
Short-Term Outcomes
- By 1/28/06, the patient will verbalize willingness to participate in physical therapy program.
- By 2/4/06, the patient will ambulate (with nursing assistance and walker) to bathroom (full weight bearing).
- By 2/11/06, the patient will ambulate with nursing assistance only (no walker) in her room.
- Goals for incision and pain relief same as for Mrs. Goldstein.

---

presses to leg ulcer after discharge." Psychomotor outcomes describe the patient's achievement of new skills—for example, "By 6/12/06, the patient will correctly demonstrate application of wet-to-dry dressing on leg ulcer." Affective outcomes describe changes in patient values, beliefs, and attitudes. Difficult both to write and to evaluate, affective outcomes might be critical to the resolution of a complex patient problem—for example, "By 6/12/06, the patient will verbalize valuing health sufficiently to practice new health behaviors to prevent recurrence of leg ulcer." In this example, even if the patient intellectually grasps the reasons for taking care of her leg and can competently redress her ulcer, unless she is motivated to take care of herself, her knowledge and skills will not result in healthy outcomes. See Chapter 16 for other examples of these outcomes.

Involving Patient and Family in Outcome Development

One of the most important considerations in writing outcomes is to encourage the patient and family to be as involved in goal development as their abilities and interest permit. The more involved they are, the greater the probability that the goals will be achieved. When developing patient outcomes, the nurse and patient look at the problem statement of the nursing diagnosis and ask, "What patient changes or outcomes will result in the prevention or resolution of this problem?" The answer, when carefully worded, becomes the patient outcome.

Identifying Outcomes Supportive of the Total Treatment Plan

When identifying outcomes, it is always important to remember that nurses nurse people, not problems. This means that every outcome you write should support the overall treatment plan and "make sense" in terms of the overall goals for the patient. For example, identifying nutritional outcomes may be appropriate for a patient who is losing weight, but if this patient is in a hospice and dying, this may not be an appropriate outcome if it is incompatible with the overall goal of a peaceful death with dignity.

Writing Measurable Outcomes

To be measurable, outcomes should have the following:
- Subject: the patient or some part of the patient
- Verb: indicates the action the patient will perform
- Conditions: specifies the particular circumstances in or by which the outcome is to be achieved. Not every outcome specifies conditions.
- Performance criteria: describe in observable, measurable terms the expected patient behavior or other manifestation
- Target time: specifies when the patient is expected to be able to achieve the outcome

Verbs helpful in writing measurable outcomes include:
- Define
- Prepare
- Identify
- Design
- List
- Verbalize
- Describe
- Choose
- Explain
- Select
- Apply
- Demonstrate

The target time or time criterion may be a realistic, actual date or other statement indicating time, such as before discharge, after viewing film, whenever observed.

Following are examples of properly constructed measurable outcomes:
- During the next 24-hour period, the patient's fluid intake will total at least 2,000 mL.
- At the next visit, 12/23/06, the patient will correctly demonstrate relaxation exercises.

It might be helpful to include special conditions when writing an outcome if this information is important for other nurses (eg, "Before discharge, the patient will ambulate independently the length of hallway and back, using a Philadelphia collar to support cervical vertebrae").

Common Errors

Common errors when writing patient outcomes include the following:
- Expressing the patient outcome as a nursing intervention. Incorrect: "Offer Mr. Myer 60 mL fluid every 2 hours while awake." Correct: "Mr. Myer will drink 60 mL fluid every 2 hours while awake, beginning 2/24/06."
- Using verbs that are not observable and measurable. Incorrect: "Mrs. Gaston will know how to bathe her newborn." Correct: "After attending the infant care class, Mrs. Gaston will correctly demonstrate the procedure for bathing her newborn." Verbs to be avoided when writing goals include "know," "understand," "learn," and "become aware." These verbs are too general and cannot be measured. Verbs that are helpful when writing outcomes that are observable and measurable were listed previously.
- Including more than one patient behavior/manifestation in short-term outcomes. Incorrect: "Patient will list dangers of smoking and stop smoking." Correct: "By next meeting, 3/11/06, the patient will (1) identify three dangers of smoking and (2) describe a plan he is willing to try to stop smoking. By 6/20/06, the patient will report that he no longer smokes."
- Writing outcomes that are so vague that other nurses are unsure of the goal of nursing care. Incorrect: "Patient will cope better." Correct: "After teaching, 10/20/06, the patient will (1) describe two new coping strategies he is willing to try and (2) demonstrate decreased incidence of previously observed ineffective coping behaviors (chain smoking, withdrawal behavior, heavy alcohol consumption)."

DEVELOPING EVALUATIVE STRATEGIES

Well-written outcomes define the evaluative strategy to be used by the nurse. Patient outcomes are meaningless unless nurses evaluate the patient's progress toward their achievement. The nurse records the date the outcome was written and the date it is achieved. Evaluative statements (Box 14-3) include a statement about achievement of the desired outcome (met, partially met, not met) and list actual patient behavior as evidence supporting the statement. If the plan is not achieved, recommendations for revising the plan of care are included in the evaluative statement. Chapter 16 deals specifically with the evaluative component of the nursing process.

IDENTIFYING NURSING INTERVENTIONS

A **nursing intervention** is any treatment, based on clinical judgment and knowledge, that a nurse performs to enhance patient outcomes (McCloskey & Bulechek, 2000). There are nurse-initiated, physician-initiated, and collaborative interventions.

Nurse-Initiated Interventions

A nurse-initiated intervention is an autonomous action based on scientific rationale that a nurse executes to benefit the patient in a predictable way related to the nursing diagnosis and projected outcomes. Nursing interventions are actions performed by the nurse to:

1. Monitor health status
2. Reduce risks
3. Resolve, prevent, or manage a problem
4. Facilitate independence or assist with activities of daily living
5. Promote optimal sense of physical, psychological, and spiritual well-being (Alfaro, 2002, p. 142)

Nurse-initiated interventions do not require a physician's (or other team member's) order. Nurse-initiated interventions, like patient goals, are derived from the nursing diagnosis. But whereas the problem statement of the diagnosis suggests the patient goals, it is the cause of the problem (etiology) that suggests the nursing interventions (Fig. 14-2). Effective nurses select nursing interventions that specifically address factors that cause or contribute to the patient's problems. For example, many factors may contribute to obesity, such as deficient nutritional knowledge, convenience of high-calorie fast foods, lifetime snacking habits, limited food budget, little exercise, and low self-esteem. The nurse working with a patient who wants to lose weight could attempt to deal with all these factors, but this approach would be inefficient. When a carefully developed nursing diagnosis identifies the specific factors that contribute to a particular patient's weight problem, nursing interventions can be selected to deal directly with these factors.

Remember Glenda Kronk, the woman desiring to improve her fitness. Based on assessment, the nurse would determine the factors that have played a role in the patient's current status, developing appropriate nursing diagnoses and outcomes from which to establish appro-

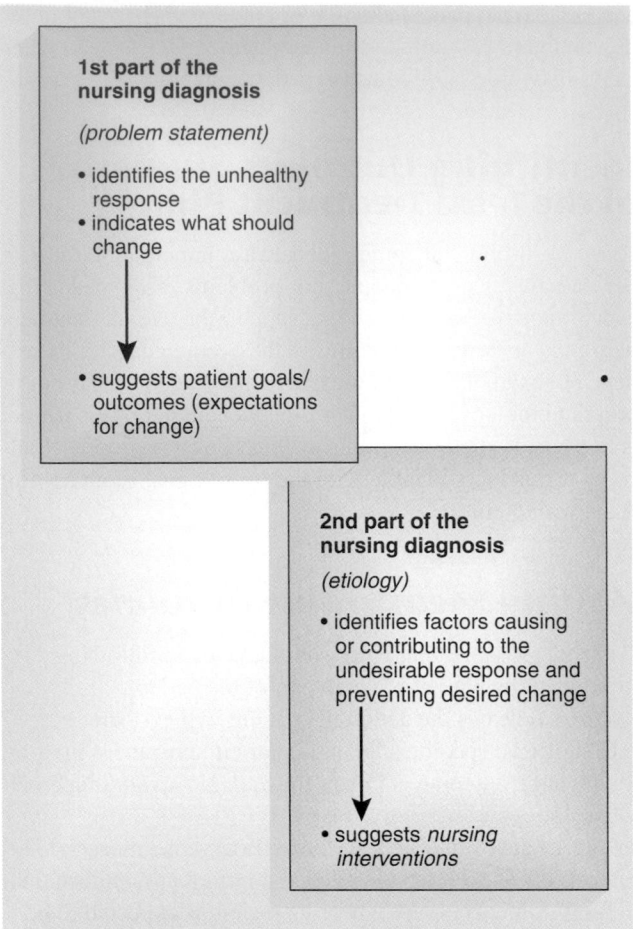

FIGURE 14-2 Deriving patient goals/outcomes and nursing orders from nursing diagnoses.

priate interventions. For example, if the patient has been sedentary over the past several years, interventions should focus on measures to increase the patient's activity level, thereby promoting improvement in her overall health and fitness.

Similarly, nursing interventions for the patient with the diagnosis Imbalanced Nutrition: More Than Body Requirements related to lifetime snacking habits and heavy reliance on high-calorie fast foods might include education about the fat content and calories in fast foods and an exploration of ways the patient could change her eating habits to eat more nutritionally balanced meals with fewer calories. Thus, the nursing approach is not the same for every patient with a weight problem. The art of nursing involves the careful identification of the specific nursing interventions needed by particular patients to meet their individual needs.

Identifying and Selecting Appropriate Nurse-Initiated Interventions

After writing the patient outcomes, the nurse identifies various nursing interventions to help the patient achieve the outcomes. The Nursing Intervention Classification System (NIC), the first comprehensive, validated list of nursing interventions applicable to all settings that can be used by nurses in multiple specialties, greatly facilitates the work of identifying appropriate interventions (McCloskey & Bulechek, 2000). Examples of using NIC to facilitate care planning for specific patient health problems may be found in each clinical chapter of this text.

The effectiveness of the nurse is directly proportional to his or her knowledge of varied nursing strategies. Consider these different nursing care options identified by three nurses when they are asked to describe nursing care for a woman 2 days after cesarean delivery who is complaining of pain in the incisional area.

NURSE A

- Check to see what type of pain medication is ordered, and give it if the time interval is sufficient.

NURSE B

- Assess the quality of the pain, and use this time to communicate support by means of expression and squeeze of hand.
- Administer analgesic if indicated.
- Assess effectiveness of the analgesic ordered.

NURSE C

- Assess quality of the pain, and explore the possibility of contributing factors such as the effects of increased gas in the abdominal area or concern about the newborn, herself, or other family members.
- Use empathic listening (possibly touch) to communicate support and to encourage the mother to share her concerns.
- Change the patient's position in bed.
- Offer a backrub.
- If appropriate, suggest activity that will distract attention from the pain (eg, watching a film about newborn care or listening to music).
- Give the prescribed medication for pain, and observe its effect.
- When administering the medication, use the power of positive suggestion to enhance its effectiveness: "This will start taking the pain away in about 10 minutes and will help you relax."

It is possible that the patient simply needs her prescribed analgesic to achieve the outcome: "Patient will report minimal to no pain at assessment every 2 hours." In that case, all three nurses would be effective in meeting the patient's need for nursing care. It is highly possible, however, that the prescribed medication is not working or the pain is compounded by the mother's fears about caring for her new baby or by her worries that the baby will ruin her relationship with her husband. Therefore, nurse C, whose knowledge level is more comprehensive, is most likely to be effective in resolving the patient's problem.

The more varied the options available to the nurse, the more effective the nursing response. In different situations, a skilled nursing procedure, the appropriate use of silence, respectful listening, humor, teaching, counseling, and touch can all be effective nursing strategies. Nurses who are merely task-oriented and satisfied to meet every patient problem with a mechanical procedure are limiting their effectiveness.

When selecting nursing interventions for individual patients, use the guidelines in Box 14-4. Use of these guidelines increases the chances that the patient will achieve the outcome. Ongoing evaluation enables the nurse to determine the effectiveness of the selected interventions.

Nurse researchers are attempting to establish a statistical pattern for predicting the probability of success of select nursing interventions. Competent nurses use research findings (science of nursing), experience, and knowledge of the patient (art of nursing) to aid in the selection of effective nursing interventions. Consultation with nurse colleagues and continuing education enable the nurse to develop effective nursing approaches to patients' problems.

Writing Nurse-Initiated Interventions in the Plan of Care

Nursing interventions describe in writing, and thus communicate to the entire nursing staff and healthcare team, the specific nursing care to be implemented for the patient. Well-written nursing interventions accomplish the following:

- Assist the patient to meet specific outcomes that are related directly to one outcome
- Clearly and concisely describe the nursing action to be performed (answer the questions who, what, where, when, and how)
- Are dated when written and when the plan of care is reviewed
- Are signed by the nurse prescribing the order or intervention
- Use only those abbreviations accepted in the institution (these are usually found in the agency's policy manual; a list of commonly accepted abbreviations appears in Chap. 17)
- Refer the nurse to the agency's procedure manual or other literature for the steps of routine, lengthy procedures

Following are examples of well-stated nursing interventions:

- Offer patient 60 mL water or juice (prefers orange or cranberry juice) every 2 hours while awake for a total minimum PO intake of 500 mL.

BOX 14-4 Guidelines for Selecting Nursing Interventions

Nursing interventions should be:

- Appropriate in terms of the nursing diagnosis and related patient outcomes
- Consistent with research findings and standards of care
- Realistic in terms of the abilities, time, and resources available to the nurse and patient
- Compatible with the patient's values, beliefs, and psychosocial background
- Valued, whenever possible, by the patient and family
- Compatible with other planned therapies

- Teach patient the necessity of carefully monitoring fluid intake and output; remind patient each shift to mark off fluid intake on record at bedside.
- Walk with patient to bathroom for toileting every 2 hours (on even hours) while patient is awake.

The set of nursing interventions written to assist a patient to meet an outcome must be comprehensive. Comprehensive nursing interventions specify what observations (assessments) need to be made and how often; what nursing interventions need to be done and when they must be done; and what teaching, counseling, and advocacy needs patients and families have.

Many sets of nursing interventions are inadequate because they fail to indicate the ongoing assessment priority needs for a specific problem or goal. Clearly stating assessment priorities helps all nurses to be more sensitive to important patient data.

> *Review the scenario at the beginning of the chapter for Glenda Kronk. The nurse would need to establish assessment priorities. For example, when assisting Glenda, who wants to lose weight to reach her target weight, appropriate nursing interventions might include the following: "6/17/06: Continue to assess (1) patient's motivation to participate in weight loss program, and (2) factors that positively or negatively influence weight loss."*

Similarly, it is often assumed that all patients have the same teaching needs. Nothing is farther from the truth. In fact, many patients have an excellent knowledge base (which might be greater than that of the nurse for a particular disease). Their need for nursing might be a need for counseling, instead of teaching, as they learn to live with a chronic illness. However, it is important to obtain proof of the patient's knowledge or competency before proceeding with the plan of care. For example, a diabetic patient would need to state the signs and symptoms of hypo- and hyperglycemia or to give a return demonstration of doing a fingerstick glucose.

Comprehensive nursing interventions relate to individual patient needs.

Physician-Initiated Interventions

A physician-initiated intervention is an intervention initiated by a physician in response to a medical diagnosis but carried out by a nurse in response to a doctor's order. For example, a physician examining a patient brought into the emergency room after a motor vehicle accident might ask the nurse to administer a medication to relieve pain and schedule the patient for radiographs and other diagnostic tests. The nurse who performs these interventions is implementing physician-initiated interventions. Both the physician and nurse are legally responsible for these interventions, and nurses are expected to be knowledgeable about how to execute these interventions safely and effectively. Nurses who question the appropriateness of physician-initiated interventions are legally responsible to seek clarification of the order with responsible parties. Under no circumstances should a nurse implement a questionable intervention, even at the urging of a physician or other professional. Chapter 7 addresses nurses' legal responsibility for their actions.

Collaborative Interventions

Nurses also carry out treatments initiated by other providers, such as pharmacists, respiratory therapists, or physician assistants. For example, nurses caring for a patient who was in a motor vehicle accident might eventually be implementing interventions written by a physical therapist, occupational therapist, or other member of the healthcare team.

Structured Care Methodologies

Efforts to standardize nursing care have taken different forms. Approaches popular during different decades include procedures (1960s), standards of care (1970s), algorithms (1980s), and clinical practice guidelines (1990s). Each of these aims to help the nurse identify and select interventions that produce optimal care, reduce legal risks, and lower healthcare costs. A description of each approach follows:

- Procedure: a set of how-to action steps for performing a clinical activity or task
- Standard of care: a description of an acceptable level of patient care or professional practice
- Algorithm: a set of steps that approximates the decision process of an expert clinician and is used to make a decision; these clinical rules are typically embedded in a branching flow chart
- Clinical practice guideline: a statement or series of statements outlining appropriate practice for a clinical condition or procedure

National guidelines such as those published by the U.S. Agency for Health Care Research and Quality (AHRQ; http://www.ahrq.gov) and the Cochrane Library (http://www.cochrane.org/cochrane/cc-broch.htm#CC and http://www.update-software.com/cochrane/) are generally based on the latest, most comprehensive scientific evidence and expert analysis. They provide standards for delivering and evaluating care for patients with the same diagnosis. Box 14-5 compares structured care methodologies. Additional examples may be found in Chapter 16.

Consulting

A nurse designing the plan of care might discover that more information is needed about the nature of the problems underlying the need for nursing or about specific interventions. **Consultation,** a process in which two or more individuals with varying degrees of experience and expertise discuss a problem and its solution, often proves helpful. Nurses might consult with nurse specialists and other members of the healthcare team, including physicians, nutritionists, social workers, therapists, pastoral caregivers, and ethicists (Fig. 14-3). Consultations are

---

BOX 14-5 **Structured Care Methodologies**

Algorithm
- Useful in management of high-risk subgroups within the cohort; may be "layered" on top of a pathway to control care practices that are used to manage a specific problem
- Binary decision trees that guide stepwise assessment and intervention
- Intense specificity; no provider flexibility
- May use analytical research methods to ensure cause and effect

Critical Pathway
- Represents a sequential, interdisciplinary, minimal practice standard for a specific patient population
- Provides flexibility to alter care to meet individualized patient needs
- Abbreviated format, broad perspective
- Phase or episode driven
- Ability to measure cause-and-effect relationship between pathway and patient outcomes prohibited by lack of control; changes in patient outcomes directly attributable to the efforts of the collaborative practice team

Guideline
- Broad, research-based practice recommendations
- May or may not have been tested in clinical practice

- Practice resources helpful in construction of structured care methodologies
- No mechanism for ensuring practice implementation

Order Set
- Preprinted provider orders used to expedite the order process after a practice standard has been validated through analytical research
- Complements and increases compliance with existing practice standards
- Can be used to represent the algorithm or protocol in order format

Protocol
- Prescribes specific therapeutic interventions for a clinical problem unique to a subgroup of patients within the cohort
- Multifaceted; may be used to drive practice for more than one discipline
- Broader specificity than an algorithm; allows for minimal provider flexibility by way of treatment options
- May be "layered" on top of a pathway

Agency for Health Care Policy and Research's (now Agency for Healthcare Research and Quality) Clinical Practice Guideline Development, AHCPR program note in Publication 93-0023, 1993.

---

a valuable means for nurses to expand their nursing knowledge and repertoire of effective strategies.

Review the Reflective Practice box describing Darla Jefferson. The nurse would consult other healthcare team members for assistance. For example, the nurse might consult social services for assistance with drug treatment and rehabilitation. Should the patient decide to keep her baby, social services also would be helpful, such as with obtaining food stamps and infant formula through government programs, appropriate housing, and follow-up in the community. A consultation with a nutritionist would be helpful prenatally to ensure that Darla meets the requirements for herself and her fetus, and also postpartum to ensure that the infant is receiving adequate nutrition to grow and develop.

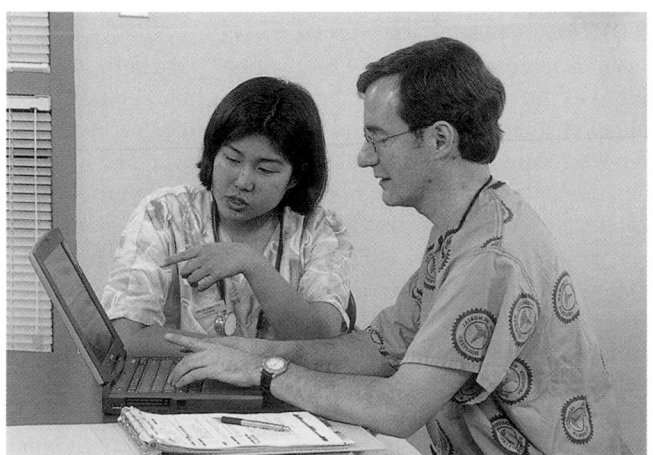

FIGURE 14-3 Consulting with a nursing colleague or other member of the healthcare team can assist the nurse in developing an effective nursing plan of care. (Photo © B. Proud.)

COMMUNICATING AND RECORDING THE PLAN OF NURSING CARE

The **plan of nursing care** (patient care plan) is the written guide that directs the efforts of the nursing team as nurses work with patients to meet their health goals. It specifies nursing diagnoses, outcomes, and associated nursing interventions. Well-written plans of care offer many benefits to the patient, nurse, nursing unit, nursing administration, and nursing profession. Primarily, plans of nursing care ensure that the nursing team works efficiently to deliver holistic, goal-oriented, individualized care to patients. A well-written plan of nursing care accomplishes the following:

- Represents an effective philosophy of nursing and advances nursing's four aims: promotes health, prevents disease and illness, promotes recovery, facilitates coping with altered functioning
- Is prepared by the nurse who best knows the patient and is recorded on the day the patient presents for treatment and care according to agency policy; modifications to the initial plan are signed and dated
- Is responsive to the individual characteristics and needs of the patient
- Clearly identifies the nursing assistance the patient needs and nursing's collaborative responsibilities for fulfilling the medical and interdisciplinary plan of care (clearly specifies nursing diagnoses, patient outcomes, nursing interventions, and evaluative strategies)
- Directs the nurse's assessment priorities, caregiving behaviors, and teaching, counseling, and advocacy behaviors
- Is based on scientific principles and incorporates findings of nursing research
- Meets the developmental, psychosocial, and spiritual needs of the patient, as well as his or her physiologic needs
- Is updated to reflect changes in the patient's status and related needs for nursing care
- Addresses the discharge needs of the patient and family
- Provides for as much patient and family participation as possible
- When appropriate, is compatible with the medical plan of care and that of the interdisciplinary team
- Creates a record that can be used for evaluation, research, reimbursement, and legal purposes

Many suggestions for plans of care appear in the nursing literature. Each school of nursing and each healthcare institution and agency has its own format, which may reflect a particular nursing theory. Common to all formats is a minimum of three columns for documenting nursing diagnoses, patient outcomes, and nursing interventions. Formats differ in the way assessment data and the nursing evaluation are addressed.

Institutional and Agency Plans of Care

The Joint Commission on Accreditation of Healthcare Organizations requires healthcare institutions and agencies to formulate, maintain, and support a patient-specific plan for care, treatment, and rehabilitation. A great variety of formats are used to communicate the plan of care. In most institutions and agencies, the plans of care, regardless of their format, communicate directions for three different types of nursing care: nursing care related to basic human needs, nursing care related to nursing diagnoses, and nursing care related to the medical and interdisciplinary plan of care.

Nursing Care Related to Basic Human Needs

The plan should concisely communicate to caregivers the data about the patient's usual health habits and patterns, obtained during the nursing history, that are needed to direct daily care.

For example, it is important to know whether a toddler is toilet-trained and what words he or she uses to indicate the need to void or defecate. Directives about the patient's usual health habits and patterns might be modified by current treatment orders, such as an order to fast for a diagnostic procedure or to limit or increase activity. This information is useful to caregivers only if it is kept current as the patient's condition changes. Any nurse should be able to find in the plan of care the instructions needed to provide competent care.

Nursing Care Related to Nursing Diagnoses

The plan contains outcomes and nursing interventions for every nursing diagnosis as well as a place to note the patient's responses to care. This section is the heart of the nursing care plan because it represents the independent component of nursing practice. If well developed, it demonstrates the nurse's clinical competence (knowledge of the science of nursing), sensitivity to the individual needs of the patient, and creativity in mobilizing the resources of the patient and the caregiving team to meet the patient's health needs.

Nursing Care Related to the Medical and Interdisciplinary Plan of Care

The plan of care also records current medical orders for diagnostic studies and treatment and specified related nursing care.

Kardex Plans of Care

Many healthcare institutions and agencies use a **Kardex care plan,** in which the plan of nursing care for each patient is concisely recorded on a folded card and placed in a central Kardex file, where it is easily accessible. The plan is eventually placed in the patient's health record. The outside of the card contains basic information, such as the patient's profile, admitting diagnosis, activity levels, diet, and routine treatments, medications, and procedures. The inside of the Kardex contains the nursing care plan specifying at the very minimum nursing diagnoses or health problems and related outcomes and nursing interventions.

Computerized Plans of Care

In an increasing number of settings, nurses use **computerized plans of nursing care.** The benefits of using computerized plans include ready access to a large knowledge base; improved record keeping, with resultant improvement in audits and quality assurance; documentation by all members of the healthcare team with printouts for the patient's record and for change-of-shift reports; and reduced time spent on paperwork. One nurse researcher, however, has studied the negative impact of computerized plans on the professionalization of staff nurses. Harris (1990) cautions that computerized systems for patient care planning and the larger systems in which they are embedded contribute to the loss of autonomy, loss of individualization of care, and loss of nursing expertise. Individual nurses, as well as researchers, need to respond to this challenge from Harris: "Does a lot of nursing time spent in procedural, rule-governed, step-by-step thinking processes destroy part of the nurse's ability to care, to empathize, to intuit, to gain insight, to function in the expert mode?" (1990, p. 73)

Case Management Plans of Care

Case management is a healthcare delivery system that has as its objective providing high-quality, cost-effective care for individuals, families, and groups. The emphasis is on clearly stating expected patient outcomes and the specific times within which it is reasonable to achieve these outcomes. **Clinical pathways (critical pathways, CareMaps)** are tools used to communicate the standardized, interdisciplinary plan of care for patients. Chapter 17 provides examples of how critical pathways are used with select documentation tools in a computerized system. Figure 14-4 illustrates a standardized plan of care for patients with congestive heart failure. Care guidelines and outcomes are specified for each day of the patient's stay. In this case, the patients receive a version of their own plan of care on admission, based on the rationale that knowing what to expect will result in less stress, quicker recovery, and earlier discharge.

Student Plans of Care

The care plans that students are required to develop are often more detailed than those found in practice settings. The aim is to assist students to assimilate each of the five steps of the nursing process. Although care plan formats vary among different nursing programs, most are designed so that the student systematically proceeds through the interrelated steps of the nursing process, and many use a five-column format.

The sample student plan of care shown in Box 14-6 demonstrates a plan developed for the patient whose admission assessment form is in Chapter 12. This 72-year-old woman was admitted to the hospital after experiencing a mini-stroke/brain attack (transient ischemic attack) at home. Her condition is stable, and the three prioritized diagnoses written in the plan address her inability to deal with this new medical diagnosis and to prevent a major stroke (high priority), ineffective coping (medium priority), and constipation (low priority).

Assessing

The student records the assessment data that led to the determination of each diagnosis in the assessment/diagnosis column. Recording these data helps to link specific defining characteristics with diagnostic problem statements.

Diagnosing

Nursing diagnoses are recorded in the assessment/diagnosis column in a prioritized list beginning with the top-priority diagnosis. For each diagnosis, a clear and concise problem statement is followed by an etiology statement that identifies specific contributing factors.

Outcome Identification and Planning

The outcome identification and planning column contains the expected changes in patient health status or in patient behaviors (ie, patient outcomes). If achieved, these resolve the problem statement in the nursing diagnosis.

Implementing

Sets of nursing orders that describe specific nursing interventions are written for each patient outcome. These specify what nursing interventions are to be performed, how they are to be performed, when they are to be performed, and who is to perform them. In many nursing programs, students are asked to document the source of the nursing interventions they propose. Although students might be able to "pull from their head" some nursing strategies, developing the practice of consulting the nursing literature is a sure means to increase nursing knowledge. Some programs also require students to provide a scientific rationale for the interventions they propose. A succinct rationale statement demonstrates that the student is deliberately choosing the nursing intervention because of its high probability to effect the desired change.

Evaluating

Incorporating evaluative statements in the plan of care clearly communicates the message that nursing care is never complete until achievement of patient outcomes is evaluated. Just as some say that teaching does not occur if learning does not take place, so nursing care is incomplete if the desired patient goals are not achieved.

Concept Map Care Plan

A concept map care plan is a diagram of patient problems and interventions. Your ideas about patient problems and treatments are the "concepts" that will be diagrammed. These maps are used to organize patient data, analyze relationships in the data, and enable you to take a holistic view of the patient's situation (Schuster, 2002). Examples of concept map care plans can be found in Chapter 11.

PROBLEMS RELATED TO OUTCOME IDENTIFICATION AND PLANNING

Problems commonly encountered while developing plans of nursing care include failure to involve the patient in the planning process, insufficient data collection, use of inaccurate or insufficient data to develop nursing diagnoses, outcomes that are stated too broadly, outcomes that are derived from poorly developed nursing diagnoses, failure to write nursing orders clearly, written nursing orders that do not resolve the problem, and failure to update the plan of care.

> *Recall Elijah Wolinski, the frail, elderly man with a pressure ulcer. Since the nurse is providing care in the patient's home, a written plan of care is extremely important because more than one caregiver may be involved in the patient's care. In addition, the nurse must update the plan regularly to ensure that regardless of who is providing the care, the correct care is given consistently.*

(text continues on page 293)

Chart 1
Sacred Heart—St. Mary's Hospitals, Inc.
PLAN OF CARE: CONGESTIVE HEART FAILURE
ESTIMATED LENGTH OF STAY: 4 Days
Supplies Given: Adm. Kit _PN 2-1-06_   **Urinal** _PN 2-1-06_   **Bedpan** _PN 2-1-06_   **Air Mattress** _PN 2-1-06_

FOCUS Date:	Day of Admission	Day 2	Day 3	Day 4
ACTIVITY	Activity Intolerance related to dyspnea • Restrict activity 30 min before and 60 min after meals _Expected outcome_ • Activity as tolerated _PN 2-1_	• Restrict activity 30 min before and 60 min after meals • Chair 30 min t.i.d. for meals • Ambulate 60 ft in hall w/ assist • Bathroom privileges _Expected outcome_ • Able to tolerate activity without distress _PN 2-2_	• Ambulate 100 ft t.i.d. _Expected outcome_ • Able to perform ADLs and ambulation without the use of O_2 ⎯⎯	• Prepare pt for discharge home _Expected outcome_ • Able to tolerate activity without distress ⎯⎯
NUTRITION Needs assist _no_ Consult needed? _no_	⟨NAS diet or⟩⎯⎯ _PN 2-1_	NAS diet or ⎯⎯	NAS diet or ⎯⎯	NAS diet or ⎯⎯
TREATMENTS Skin protocol _PN 2-1_ Fall protocol _PN 2-1_	Excess Fluid Volume related to compromised cardiac output • Vital signs q4h • I&O • Daily weight • Telemetry if ordered • Heparin lock • O_2 at _3 l/min_ • Assess lung and heart sounds q shift and p.r.n. • Assess pedal edema and pulses q shift	• Vital signs q4h • I&O • Daily weight • Telemetry if ordered • Heparin lock • O_2 at _3 l/min_ • Assess lung and heart sounds q shift and p.r.n. • Assess pedal edema and pulses q shift _Expected outcomes_ • Pt's foot edema is decreased or pt has lost weight (min 1 lb) _PN 2-2_ • Pt has improved breath sounds _PN 2-2_	• Vital signs q shift • I&O • Daily weight • Discontinue telemetry if previously ordered ⎯⎯ • Heparin lock • O_2 p.r.n. (If still needed, consult cardio-pulmonary services for need for home O_2.) • Assess lung and heart sounds q shift • Assess pedal edema and pulses q shift	• Vital signs q shift • I&O • Daily weight • Discontinue heparin lock ⎯⎯ • Discontinue O_2 ⎯⎯ • Assess lung and heart sounds q shift • Assess pedal edema and pulses q shifts _Expected outcomes_ • Feet/ankle edema resolved • Unlabored respirations ⎯⎯
TEACHING	• Review Plan of Care with pt • Explain medications to pt • Give copy of Plan of Care to pt • Give info sheet on congestive heart failure to pt • Home health referral needed _yes_ _PN 2-1-06_ • Home O_2 needed _possibly_ _PN 2-1-06_	_Expected outcomes_ • Pt can verbalize understanding of present medications _PN 2-2_	• Discharge medication sheets given ⎯⎯ • Home health referral arranged if needed ⎯⎯ • Home O_2 arranged if needed ⎯⎯	_Expected outcomes_ • Pt can verbalize understanding of present medications ⎯⎯ • Discharge medication sheet reviewed and pt can verbalize understanding ⎯⎯ • Discharge instructions reviewed and pt can verbalize understanding ⎯⎯ • Pt can verbalize understanding for need of follow-up visit and when to call doctor ⎯⎯

OTHER FOCAL AREAS
• Durable power of attorney _yes PN 2-1_
• Living will _yes PN 2-1_
• Code status _full PN 2-1_

FIGURE 14-4 Standardized plan of care for a patient with congestive heart failure. (Adapted from Rasmussen, N., & Gengler, T. [1994]. Clinical pathways of care: The route to better communication. *Nursing 94, 24*[2], 48–49. Used with permission.)

Chart 2
Sacred Heart—St. Mary's Hospitals, Inc.
PLAN OF CARE: CONGESTIVE HEART FAILURE PATIENT COPY
ESTIMATED LENGTH OF STAY: 4 Days

FOCUS Date:	Day of Admission	Day 2	Day 3	Day 4
ACTIVITY	You can move around as you are able. Avoid becoming overtired or short of breath. You should remain in bed 30 minutes before and after your meals.	You should increase your activity slowly. Start by sitting up in the chair for meals and walking short distances with the help of the nurses twice a day.	You should be starting to feel better and should be able to do mild activities without your oxygen.	You should be able to walk in the halls and take your own bath without trouble breathing. You'll go home today if your doctor feels you're ready.
NUTRITION	You'll be on a no-added-salt diet. The dietitian will come to talk to you about this if you don't understand. A salt substitute is available if you need it. (Salt causes your body to hold in extra fluids, making your swelling worse and causing your heart to work even harder.)	Low-salt diet.	Low-salt diet.	Low-salt diet. Ask your doctor or nurse if you should continue this diet at home.
TREATMENTS	The nurse will measure the amount of fluid you take in and put out. The nurse will listen to your heart and lungs to see if they are getting better. You may have to use oxygen for the first day or two to help you breathe easier. You'll be weighed daily. You'll have an intravenous needle placed in your hand or arm. This will be used to give you medication. You may have a telemetry heart monitor on. Nurses in the intensive care unit will monitor your heart's rhythm.	Treatments will remain the same.	Some treatments will remain the same. You'll use oxygen only when you feel you need it The heart monitor will be discontinued if previously ordered.	Some treatments will remain the same. Your oxygen may be discontinued. Your needle will be removed if you're going home.
TEACHING	You'll need to understand what is going on with your body. Please ask questions if you don't understand something. You'll be given a sheet to explain what congestive heart failure is. Ask about your medications if you're unfamiliar with them.		You'll be given information sheets that explain the medication you'll take at home. You should know about the right foods to eat and what types of food you should avoid. Your doctor may order a follow-up by a home health nurse.	You'll need to follow up with your doctor. Make sure you know when your appointment is. Know what problems may require medical attention.

FIGURE 14-4 *Continued*

BOX 14-6 **Student Plan of Care**

Assessment/Diagnosis

Subjective data: "Will I get a stroke now? I don't think I could handle that." "How can I help myself prevent it?"

Objective data: Admitting diagnosis:

TIA

BP: 184/120

Strengths: Past pattern of adhering to prescribed health behaviors.

Nursing diagnosis: Ineffective Health Maintenance Response to TIA and Stroke Prevention related to knowledge deficit

Goal/Outcome

Before discharge, the patient will:

- Describe the terms *TIA* and *stroke*, identifying the underlying disease process, causes, symptoms, and treatment

After discussion with the physician and nurse, the patient will:

- Correctly describe the treatment plan:
  - Medications (drugs, intended effect, dose, time, route)
  - Dietary modifications
  - Exercise prescription
  - Signs and symptoms to report
  - Follow-up appointment date

Subjective data: Husband died 8 months ago; moved in with daughter 6 months ago after selling family home

Daughter reports mother had been a very independent, strong woman in the past—seemed to "crumple" after husband's death.

History of headaches

Objective data: Clutches daughter's hand

Strengths: History of handling life stressors well

Limitations: In the past, her husband was her primary support

Nursing diagnosis: Ineffective Coping related to illness, recent death of husband, and relocation with daughter

Beginning 9/7/06, the patient will:

- Verbalize her feelings related to the loss of her husband, loss of family home, loss of health

- Identify coping patterns that have helped her in the past

- Identify three personal strengths and three outside supports that will help her now

Before discharge, the patient will:

- Verbalize that she feels "okay" (sufficiently in charge of her life) about returning home

BOX 14-6 (Continued)

Nursing Orders

Assess what the patient knows about TIA and stroke (correct any misinformation). Assess learning needs, readiness to learn, and factors that will influence learning.

Plan teaching and learning sessions to involve family members designated by patient

Include in the teaching plan a description of TIA and stroke and the underlying disease process, causes, symptoms, and treatment plan.

After the treatment plan has been developed, make sure the patient and family can restate it (teaching) and value the prescribed lifestyle modification (counseling).

Scientific Rationale

Each person's learning needs are different; each person learns in own unique way; learning is dependent on readiness.

The more support people knowledgeably committed to the plan of care, the greater the probability the patient will achieve goals.

New self-care behaviors are dependent on knowledge.

New self-care behaviors are dependent on motivation. Unless the patient is committed to stroke prevention and values this outcome, she will not follow the treatment plan.

Evaluation

9/10/06—Outcome not met. Patient says her head is "too old" to learn all this stuff. Equates stroke with death.

Revision: Reteach content in simpler terms. Reassess learning readiness.
                                   M. Foley, SN

9/10/06   Too early to evaluate.
                                   M. Foley, SN

Once during each shift, primary nurse should sit at patient's bedside for at least several minutes to communicate caring and to explore with the patient her current stressors and the adequacy of her coping response.

· Assess factors compounding her losses.
· Reinforce her personal strengths and support systems; counsel her to tap into these now.
· Suggest local support groups if indicated.

Primary nurse to explore with daughter, Lisa, how her mother's moving in with her has affected the family. Recommend support systems.

The nurse's unhurried, attentive, and caring presence communicates to the patient that she is important to the nurse and that the nurse values her well-being. It is an invitation to the patient to become actively involved in recovery. Also, it is logical to explore adequacy of past and current coping mechanisms before suggesting new approaches.

Adult children of aging parents frequently experience overwhelming stress as they try to deal with their own and their parents' problems. Supporting this family is supporting the patient indirectly.

9/10/06   Outcome partially met. Patient speaks freely about how much she misses her husband and how fearful this hospitalization makes her. When asked about living with her daughter, she becomes uncharacteristically quiet.
                                   M. Foley, SN

9/10/06   Outcome met. Patient talks about how everything seemed better in the past after she talked it over with her husband and God.
                                   M. Foley, SN

9/10/06   Outcome not met. Patient couldn't think of anything about herself that is healthy or strong. Says "maybe" her family can help her now.

Revision: Counsel regarding personal strengths. Help her to experience them.
                                   M. Foley, SN

9/11/06   Too early to evaluate.
                                   M. Foley, SN

(continued)

BOX 14-6 (Continued)

Assessment/Diagnosis

Subjective data: "I move my bowels every 2 or 3 days; get constipated at least once a week. Often Metamucil helps."

"I drink plenty of fluids and eat fruits and vegetables."

History of hemorrhoids secondary to straining

Objective data: No bowel movement in past 4 days

On bed rest since hospitalized

Nursing diagnosis: Constipation related to decreased physical activity and long-term laxative use (Metamucil)

Goal/Outcome

Beginning 9/7/06, the patient will:

• Pass soft, formed stool every 1 to 3 days without use of laxatives

By 9/10/06, the patient will:

• Verbalize the importance of the following natural aids to bowel elimination:
  • Daily intake of foods high in bulk
  • Daily fluid intake of 8 to 10 glasses
  • Regular time for elimination
  • Daily physical exercise: walking

Nursing Orders

Monitor bowel elimination patterns; identify causative factors of constipation and successful corrective measures.

Explain the importance of adhering to a regular time for defecation (patient suggests after breakfast)—adhere to this in the hospital.

When given medical clearance, assist patient with progressive ambulation. Recommend that she include brisk walking into daily health habits (build strength to 20- to 30-minute brisk walk daily).

Explain the long-term effects of laxative abuse on the bowel, and discourage their use.

Reinforce the patient's fluid intake and ingestion of high-bulk foods, such as fresh fruits and salad.

Scientific Rationale

This patient's elimination problems will not be resolved until all the specific causes of her constipation and successful corrective measures are identified. Needs to be an ongoing assessment priority.

This encourages positive use of circadian rhythms.

Peristalsis is stimulated by physical exercise.

Laxative abuse leads to decreased peristaltic response to food and loss of intestinal tone

Commenting on these positive self-care behaviors reinforces them.

Evaluation

9/10/06   Outcome partially met. Soft, formed stool passed every 2 to 3 days with aid of Colace.

M. Foley, SN

9/10/06   Outcome met. Patient correctly related value of four natural aids to elimination. Questions whether she will be strong enough to walk.

Revision: Encourage assisted ambulation.

M. Foley, SN

■ Developing Critical Thinking Skills

1. Write nursing diagnoses for three obese patients, and make sure that the etiologies for the problem statement (Imbalanced Nutrition: More Than Body Requirements) differ. Describe how these different etiologies result in different plans of care.

2. Use one of the nursing diagnoses from exercise 1 and write related cognitive, psychomotor, and affective goals. Explain the different purposes of each type of goal and why it may be necessary to include all three to resolve a patient problem successfully.

3. An alert 82-year-old widow who has a history of unsafe behaviors has recently been discharged from the hospital to her home. Caregivers attempted to secure her consent to be transferred to a nursing home, but she flatly refused. Responsible for her home care, you list Risk for Injury as a priority nursing diagnosis. Join several students and independently list the nursing measures that are most likely to achieve the outcome of preventing injury. Compare your lists of interventions and discuss how practicing nurses can be sure they select the best nursing interventions for each expected patient outcome.

■ Practicing for NCLEX

1. During the outcome identification and planning step of the nursing process, the nurse works in partnership with the patient and family to do which of the following?
   (1) Formulate and validate prioritized nursing diagnoses
   (2) Identify expected patient outcomes
   (3) Select evidence-based nursing interventions
   (4) Communicate the plan of nursing care
      a. 1 and 3
      b. 2 and 4
      c. 2, 3, and 4
      d. All of the above

2. Mr. Price tells the nurse he fears becoming "hooked on drugs" and consequently waits until his pain becomes unbearable before requesting his prn analgesic. The nurse plans to be more attentive to Mr. Price and to assess his needs for pain management more closely. Which of the following consequences of informal planning ought to be the major concern for this nurse?
   a. The lack of a coordinated plan known by everyone will result in uneven pain management.
   b. Faulty prioritization of patient needs
   c. Inability to evaluate the patient's responses to nursing care
   d. Lack of a record for reimbursement purposes

3. When helping Mr. Price turn in bed, the nurse notices that his heels are reddened and plans to place

him on precautions for skin breakdown. This is an example of:
   a. Initial planning
   b. Standardized planning
   c. Ongoing planning
   d. Discharge planning

4. Use Maslow's hierarchy of human needs to prioritize the following patient problems from highest priority (#1) to lowest priority (#4):
   (1) Disturbed Body Image
   (2) Ineffective Airway Clearance
   (3) Spiritual Distress
   (4) Impaired Social Interaction
      a. 2, 4, 1, 3
      b. 3, 1, 4, 2
      c. 1, 4, 3, 2
      d. 3, 2, 4, 1

5. From which of the following are outcomes derived?
   a. The problem statement of the nursing diagnosis
   b. The etiology of the problem of the nursing diagnosis
   c. The defining characteristics of the problem
   d. The evaluative statement

6. Which of the following is an example of an affective outcome?
   a. Within 1 day after teaching, the patient will list three benefits of continuing to apply moist compresses to leg ulcer after discharge.
   b. By 6/12/06, the patient will correctly demonstrate application of wet-to-dry dressing on leg ulcer.
   c. By 6/19/06, the patient's ulcer will begin to show signs of healing (eg, size shrinks from 3″ to 2.5″).
   d. By 6/12/06, the patient will verbalize valuing health sufficiently to practice new health behaviors to prevent recurrence of leg ulcer.

7. Which of the following is an optional element in a measurable outcome?
   a. Subject
   b. Verb
   c. Performance criteria
   d. Conditions
   e. Target time

8. Which of the following outcomes are correctly written?
   (1) Offer Mr. Myer 60 mL fluid every 2 hours while awake.
   (2) During the next 24-hour period, the patient's fluid intake will total at least 2,000 mL.
   (3) By discharge Mrs. Gaston will know how to bathe her newborn.
   (4) At the next visit, 12/23/06, the patient will correctly demonstrate relaxation exercises.
      a. (1) and (3)
      b. (2) and (4)
      c. (1), (2), (3)
      d. All of the above

9. Which of the following guidelines for outcome writing are correct?

(1) At least one of the outcomes shows a direct resolution of the problem statement in the nursing
diagnosis.
(2) The patient (and family) values the outcomes.
(3) The outcomes are supportive of the total treatment plan.
(4) Each outcome is brief and specific (clearly
describes one observable, measurable patient
behavior/manifestation), is phrased positively,
and specifies a time line.
  a. (2) and (4)
  b. (1) and (3)
  c. (1), (2), and (3)
  d. All of the above
10. Which of the following are examples of well-stated
nursing interventions?
(1) Offer patient 60 mL water or juice (prefers
orange or cranberry juice) every 2 hours while
awake for a total minimum PO intake of 500 mL.
(2) Teach patient the necessity of carefully monitoring fluid intake and output; remind patient each
shift to mark off fluid intake on record at bedside.
(3) Walk with patient to bathroom for toileting
every 2 hours (on even hours) while patient is
awake.
(4) Manage patient's pain.
  a. (1) and (3)
  b. (2) and (4)
  c. (1), (2), and (3)
  d. All of the above

Answers with Rationale

1. The correct answer is *c*. Formulating and validating
nursing diagnoses occur during the diagnosing step
of the nursing process.
2. The correct answer is *a*. If this nurse fails to incorporate this learning into the formal plan of care, other
professional caregivers will not be aware of the need
to monitor the patient's pain needs more closely.
(*b*), (*c*), and (*d*) may all be correct responses, but
they should not be the major concern of the nurse.
3. The correct answer is *c*. Ongoing planning is
problem-oriented and has as its purpose keeping the
plan up to date as new actual or potential problems
are identified.
4. The correct answer is *a*. Maslow's hierarchy is
(1) physiologic needs; (2) safety needs; (3) love and
belonging needs; (4) self-esteem needs; and (5) self-
actualization needs. (2) is an example of a physiologic need, (4) is an example of a love and belonging
need, (1) is an example of a self-esteem need, and
(3) is an example of a self-actualization need.
5. The correct answer is *a*. Outcomes are derived from
the problem statement of the nursing diagnosis. For
each nursing diagnosis in the plan of care, at least one

outcome should be written that, if achieved, demonstrates a direct resolution of the problem statement.
6. The correct answer is *d*. Affective outcomes describe
changes in patient values, beliefs, and attitudes.
Cognitive outcomes (*a*) describe increases in patient
knowledge or intellectual behaviors; psychomotor
outcomes (*b*) describe the patient's achievement of
new skills. (*c*) is an outcome describing a physical
change in the patient.
7. The correct answer is *d*. Conditions specify the particular circumstances in or by which the outcome is to
be achieved. Not every outcome specifies conditions.
8. The correct answer is *b*. Common errors when writing patient outcomes include the following:
(1) Expressing the patient goal as a nursing intervention. Incorrect: "Offer Mr. Myer 60 mL fluid
every 2 hours while awake." Correct: "Mr. Myer
will drink 60 mL fluid every 2 hours while
awake, beginning 2/24/06."
(3) Using verbs that are not observable and measurable. Incorrect: "Mrs. Gaston will know how to
bathe her newborn." Correct: "After attending
the infant care class, Mrs. Gaston will correctly
demonstrate the procedure for bathing her newborn." Verbs to be avoided when writing goals
include "know," "understand," "learn," and
"become aware."
9. The correct answer is *d*.
10. The correct answer is *c*. (4) lacks sufficient detail to
effectively guide nursing intervention. The set of
nursing interventions written to assist a patient to
meet an outcome must be comprehensive. Comprehensive nursing interventions specify what observations (assessments) need to be made and how often;
what nursing interventions need to be done and when
they must be done; and what teaching, counseling,
and advocacy needs patients and families have.

Bibliography

Ackley, B. J., & Ladwig, G. B. (2002). *Nursing diagnosis
handbook: A guide to planning care* (5th ed.). St. Louis:
C. V. Mosby.

Alfaro, R. (2002). *Applying nursing process: Promoting collaborative care* (5th ed.). Philadelphia: Lippincott Williams
& Wilkins.

Alfaro-LeFevre, R. (2004). *Critical thinking in nursing:
A practical approach.* Philadelphia: W. B. Saunders.

Atkinson, L. D., & Murray, M. E. (1990). *Understanding the
nursing process* (4th ed.). New York: Pergamon.

Carpenito, L. J. (1995). *Nursing care plans and documentation*
(2nd ed.). Philadelphia: Lippincott Williams & Wilkins.

Carpenito, L. J. (2004). *Nursing diagnosis: Application to clinical practice* (10th ed.). Philadelphia: Lippincott Williams
& Wilkins.

Gage, M. (1994). The patient-driven interdisciplinary care plan. *Journal of Nursing Administration, 24*(4), 26–38.

Harris, B. L. (1990). Becoming deprofessionalized: One aspect of the staff nurse's perspective on computer-mediated nursing care plans. *Advances in Nursing Science, 13*(2), 63–74.

Iowa Intervention Project. (1997). Nursing interventions classification (NIC): An overview. In M. J. Rantz & P. LeMone (Eds.), *Classification of Nursing Diagnoses: Proceedings of the Twelfth Conference, North American Nursing Diagnosis* (pp. 32–39). Glendale, CA: CINAHL Information Systems.

Johnson, M., Mass, M. L., & Moorhead, S. (Eds.). (2000). *Nursing outcomes classification* (2nd ed.). St. Louis: Mosby–Year Book.

Johnson, M., Bulechek, G., McCloskey Dochterman, J., Maas, M., & Moorhead, S. (2001). *Nursing diagnoses, outcomes and interventions: NANDA, NIC, NOC, linkages.* St. Louis, MO: Mosby.

Joint Commission on Accreditation of Healthcare Organizations. (2003). *2003 Accreditation manual for hospitals.* Oakbrook Terrace, IL: JCAHO.

McCloskey, J. C., & Bulechek, G. M. (Eds.). (2000). *Nursing intervention classification* (3rd ed.). St. Louis: Mosby–Year Book.

Raiwet, C., Halliwell, G., Andruski, L., & Wilson, D. (1997). Care maps across the continuum. *Canadian Nurse, 93*(1), 26–30.

Rasmussen, N., & Gengler, T. (1994). Clinical pathways of care: The route to better communication. *Nursing 94, 24*(2), 47–49.

Rubenfeld, M. G., & Scheffer, B. K. (1999). *Critical thinking in nursing: An interactive approach* (2nd ed.). Philadelphia: Lippincott Williams & Wilkins.

Schuster, D. M. (2002). Concept mapping: A critical thinking approach to care planning. Philadelphia: F. A. Davis.

Sparks, S. M. (1992). Computer consult: Exploring electronic support groups. *American Journal of Nursing 94, 92*(12), 62–65.

Ulrich, S. P., Canale, S. W., & Wendell, S. A. (1990). *Nursing care planning guides: A nursing diagnosis approach* (2nd ed.). Philadelphia: W. B. Saunders.

Vasey, E. K. (1979). Writing your patient's care plan . . . efficiently. *Nursing, 9*(4), 67–71.67–71.

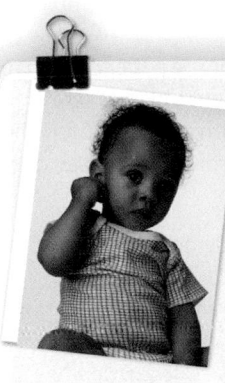

Antoinette Browne, a toddler, is brought to the well-child community clinic by her grandmother. The health history reveals recurrent nausea, vomiting, and diarrhea. Her physical examination reveals a negligible gain in height and weight, lethargy, and a delay in achieving developmental milestones.

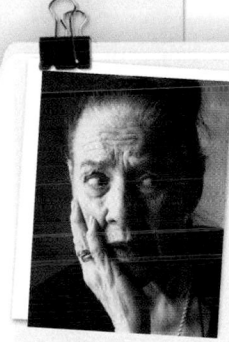

Estelle Morrissey is an 86-year-old woman who is in a nursing home because of multiple chronic health problems. She is alert and oriented to person, place, and time. She states "I'm all alone. There's no one left and I want to die. Can you help me?"

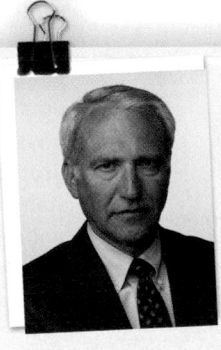

James McMahon, a 62-year-old man, is admitted to the intensive care unit in hepatic failure. He is critically ill, being monitored continuously, and is receiving intravenous fluids and medications via central and peripheral IV catheters.

Focusing on Blended Skills

The types of blended skills you'll need to respond to the case scenarios include:

Cognitive Skills

- Knowledge of appropriate information necessary to implement the nursing interventions that effectively meet the nursing needs of the toddler with physical and developmental delays, a nursing home resident with diminished will to live, and a patient who is critically ill with multiple needs
- Ability to carry out the plan of care, continue data collection, modify the plan as needed, and communicate care
- Ability to explain the principles for and reasons underlying necessary interventions
- Ability to incorporate knowledge of pertinent standards of care and agency and institutional policies when implementing care
- Ability to use critical thinking skills to intervene appropriately to meet patients' needs across the lifespan

Technical Skills

- Ability to competently use the equipment and techniques specified by the patient's plan of care
- Ability to ask for assistance as necessary when performing new or technologically complex procedures or working with unfamiliar equipment
- Ability to perform nursing care safely, based on sound scientific rationales
- Ability to adapt procedures and equipment to meet the needs of patients across the lifespan

Interpersonal Skills

- Ability to establish a trusting nurse–patient relationship grounded in responsible caring
- Ability to communicate to the patient that you are more concerned about the patient and his or her well-being than about rote implementation of the plan of care or accomplishment of discrete tasks
- Ability to demonstrate respect for the patient's human dignity when implementing the patient's plan of care
- Ability to work collaboratively with members of the healthcare team to implement the interdisciplinary plan of care

Ethical and Legal Skills

- Commitment to successfully implement the plan of care, within the scope of legal practice
- Ability to participate as a trusted and effective patient advocate
- Consistent use of appropriate legal safeguards while implementing the plan of care
- Demonstration of accountability for all actions performed

Learning Outcomes

After completing this chapter, the learner should be able to accomplish the following:

1. Distinguish nurse-initiated, physician-initiated, and collaborative nursing interventions.
2. List advantages of having a standard classification of nursing interventions and outcomes.
3. Use cognitive, interpersonal, technical, and ethical/legal skills to implement a plan of nursing care.
4. Describe six variables that influence the way a plan of care is implemented.
5. Use seven guidelines for implementation.
6. Use ongoing data collection to determine how to safely and effectively implement a plan of care.
7. Explain why reassessment after nursing intervention is important.

Key Terms

collaborative interventions
delegation
evidence-based practice
implementing
nurse-initiated intervention
nursing interventions
physician-initiated intervention
protocols
standing orders
unlicensed assistive personnel
  (UAP)

During the **implementing** step of the nursing process, nursing actions planned in the previous step are carried out. The purpose of implementation is to assist the patient in achieving valued health outcomes: promote health, prevent disease and illness, restore health, and facilitate coping with altered functioning. For an example, see the accompanying Reflective Practice box. The plan of care is best implemented when patients who are able and willing to participate have maximum opportunities to provide self-care. Family members and other support people, as well as other healthcare professionals, may also be involved in successfully implementing the plan of care (Table 15-1). During the implementation step, the nurse continues to collect data and to modify the plan of care as needed (Fig. 15-1). All activities are documented in the format used by the nurse's institution or agency.

UNIQUE FOCUS OF NURSING IMPLEMENTATION

In all nurse–patient interactions, the nurse is concerned with the patient's response to health and illness and their ability to meet basic human needs. Whereas other healthcare profes-

Reflective Practice
Challenge to Technical Skills

James McMahon, a 62-year-old man, is admitted to the intensive care unit (ICU) in hepatic failure. He is critically ill, being monitored continuously, and receiving intravenous (IV) fluids and medications via central and peripheral IV catheters. During a recent clinical rotation in an ICU, I followed an extremely busy nurse who was caring for Mr. McMahon. He had several IV infusion lines and required numerous technologic devices for monitoring and care. The nurse asked me to hang a new bag of IV medication. I found myself completely overwhelmed and confused by the myriad tangle of IV lines and knew that I wouldn't be able to determine how to run the medication without the guidance of the nurse. I became frustrated because I should have been able to perform this task quickly and correctly if I had been working independently. I didn't want to risk hanging the IV medication and infusing it into a line with another fluid that was possibly incompatible. Nor did I want to risk running the medication through the incorrect port. The nurse was extremely busy and I felt pressured to perform this task immediately.

Thinking Outside the Box: Possible Courses of Action

- Request that the nurse hang the medication once she was through with her other tasks.
- Hang the medication, hoping that it was compatible with the other fluids that were already infusing.
- Ask another nurse on the unit to hang the medication.

- Wait until the nurse was through with what she had to do, admit to her that I felt uncomfortable hanging the medication on my own, and then ask that she walk me through the process.

Evaluating a Successful Outcome: How Do I Define Success?

- The patient remains free from harm while receiving the necessary medication.
- The nurse recognizes the need to provide me with more guidance.

- I feel comfortable and competent in my skills.
- The patient receives efficient, safe care.

Personal Learning: Here's to the Future!

Luckily, there was a positive ending to this situation. I explained to the nurse that I was confused by the maze of IV lines and that I was uncomfortable administering the IV medication on my own. The nurse immediately recognized that the patient's lines were tangled and disorganized, some of which were unlabeled. With me at her side, she took the time to reorganize and label all of the lines, making it easier to visualize all of the medications and fluids the patient was receiving. We referenced a drug book to ensure that the medication was compatible with the other fluids that were running. She also walked me through the process of hanging the medication and connecting it to the appropriate port. The nurse appreciated the fact that I waited to ask her for help. As a result, the patient remained safe from injury. In addition, she realized that she shouldn't have asked me to perform this task independently. I benefited from the experience because I became more familiar with this particular skill. As of now, I still find myself feeling somewhat anxious and uncomfortable with certain technical skills. However, I am finding that with each new clinical experience, I become more comfortable and more independent in my practice.

Reflection

How do you think you would respond in a similar situation? Why? What does this tell you about yourself and about the adequacy of your skills for professional practice? Can you think of other ways to respond? What other skills (cognitive, interpersonal, technical, ethical/legal) would you need to respond well in this situation? What factors might have influenced the nurse in assigning this task to the student? Did the nurse effectively delegate this intervention?

Why or why not? Did the student adhere to ethical and legal guidelines with the response? If so, please explain how. If not, what issues were present? Do you agree with the criteria to evaluate a successful outcome? Were the criteria appropriate for the situation and skill?

Colleen Kilcullen, Georgetown University

TABLE 15-1 Professional Nursing Relationships: Role Responsibilities and Related Competencies

Relationship	Role Responsibilities	Related Competencies
Nurse–patient	• Communicate to the patient that someone is concerned about him or her (as well as the disease) and is interested in how this change in health state will affect his or her overall well-being. • Create an environment in which the patient can commit his or her energies to health promotion or restoration or peaceful dying, confident that basic human needs are being addressed. • Challenge the patient to develop self-care abilities that promote holistic health.	• Repertoire of therapeutic interpersonal behaviors—attending, listening, interviewing, nonverbal communication, touching, facilitating, coaching • Ability to establish trusting nurse–patient–family relationships • Demonstrated competence in the nursing roles of caregiver, teacher, counselor, advocate
Nurse–patient–family	• Develop in the patient and family the knowledge, attitude, and skills that will enable them to respond to the self-care challenge of their health or illness state. • Intervene as appropriate to promote healthy family functioning. • Educate the family to be wise and assertive healthcare consumers.	
Nurse–nurse	• Support one another's efforts to deliver quality nursing care; work collaboratively with nursing administration to improve quality care. • Provide creative leadership—formally or informally—to make the nursing unit a satisfying and challenging place to work. • Supervise the nursing care given by other nursing personnel; affirm the nursing strengths of others, and constructively address the nursing deficiencies encountered. • Enhance the professional development of self and other nurses through active participation in professional organizations.	Communication Teaching/counseling/ advocacy Assertiveness Collaboration Coordination Group process Organization Leadership Delegation Change strategies Problem solving Decision making Conflict resolution
Nurse–healthcare team	• Communicate clearly nursing's perspective regarding the patient and family to the healthcare team. • Coordinate the inputs of the multidisciplinary team into a comprehensive plan of care. • Serve as a liaison between the patient and family and the healthcare team, as necessary.	

sionals focus on selected aspects of the patient's treatment regimen, nurses are concerned with how the patient is responding to the plan of care in general.

The Nursing Interventions Taxonomy Structure

In 1992, McCloskey and Bulechek published *Nursing Interventions Classification* (NIC), a report of research to construct a taxonomy of nursing interventions. New editions appeared in 1996 and 2000. Each of the interventions listed has a label, a definition, a set of activities that a nurse performs to carry out the intervention, and a short list of background readings. See the box "Examples of Nursing Interventions Classification" in this chapter and in each clinical chapter. Advantages of having a standard classification of nursing interventions include the following:
• To standardize nomenclature
• To expand nursing knowledge
• To develop information systems

• To teach decision making
• To ensure appropriate reimbursement for nursing services
• To allocate nursing resources
• To communicate nursing to non-nurses
• To link nursing content: standardized nursing diagnoses, outcomes, and interventions (Iowa Intervention Project, 2000, pp. 16–19.)

Table 15-2 illustrates the NIC taxonomy structure designed to help clinicians locate and select interventions most helpful for patients.

The researchers involved in the development of NICs are also committed to developing a classification of patient outcomes for nursing interventions, called Nursing Outcomes Classifications (NOCs). This research aims to:
1. Identify, label, validate, and classify nursing-sensitive patient outcomes and indicators
2. Evaluate the validity and usefulness of the classification in clinical field testing
3. Define and test measurement procedures for the outcomes and indicators

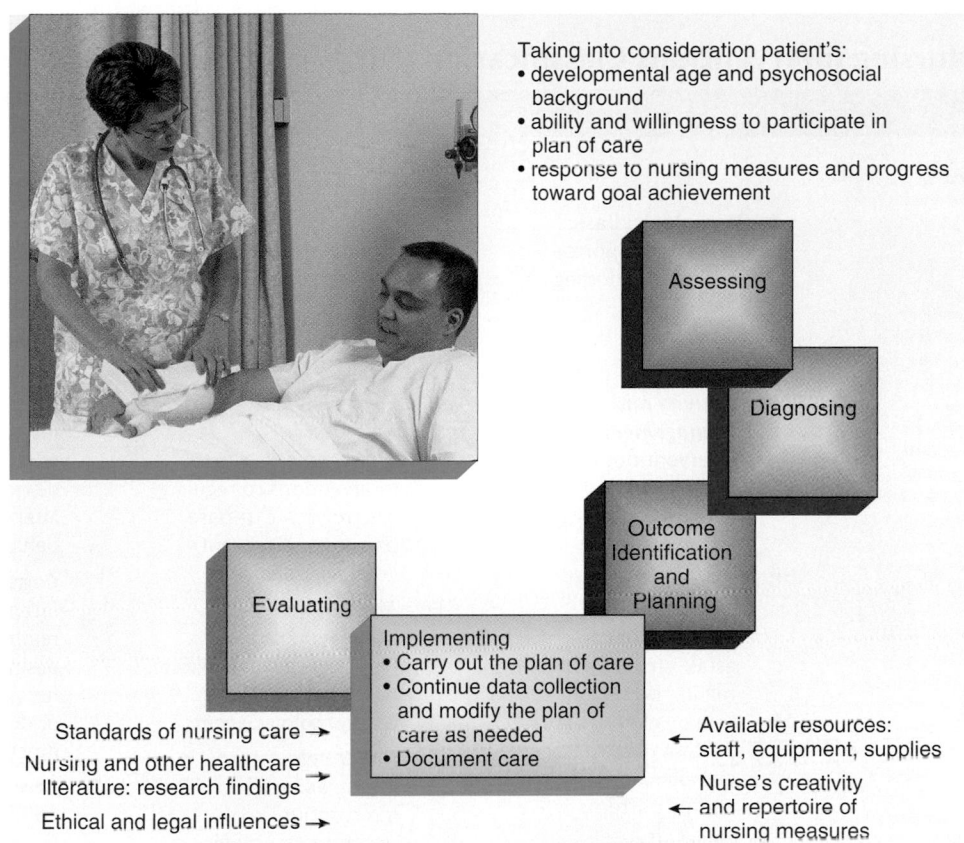

Taking into consideration patient's:
- developmental age and psychosocial background
- ability and willingness to participate in plan of care
- response to nursing measures and progress toward goal achievement

Assessing

Diagnosing

Outcome Identification and Planning

Evaluating

Implementing
- Carry out the plan of care
- Continue data collection and modify the plan of care as needed
- Document care

Standards of nursing care →

Nursing and other healthcare literature: research findings →

Ethical and legal influences →

← Available resources: staff, equipment, supplies

← Nurse's creativity and repertoire of nursing measures

FIGURE 15-1 Implementing involves carrying out the plan of care, which is modified in response to patient changes. Numerous variables influence the way the plan of care is implemented (*see arrows*).   (Photo © B. Proud.)

Examples of Nursing Interventions Classification (NIC)
Implementing Care for a Patient and Family Requiring Assistance With Home Maintenance

The Nursing Interventions Classification (NIC) can be used to implement care for a patient and family who require assistance to maintain the home as a clean, safe, and pleasant place. Based on the intervention *Home Maintenance Assistance*, representative nursing activities include the following:

- Determine patient's home maintenance requirements.
- Involve patient and family in deciding home maintenance requirements.
- Suggest necessary structural alterations to make the home accessible.
- Provide information on how to make the home environment safe and clean.
- Advise for the alleviation of all offensive odors.
- Suggest services for pest control, as needed.
- Offer solutions to financial difficulties.
- Order homemaker services, as appropriate.
- Provide information on respite care, as needed.

McCloskey, J., & Bulechek, G. (2000). *Nursing interventions classification (NIC)* (3rd ed., p. 378). St. Louis: Mosby–Year Book. (A full listing of nursing activities for each nursing intervention can be found in this book.)

Examples of proposed NOC indicators for the outcome "Caregiver Home Readiness" (caregiver's preparedness to assume responsibility for the healthcare of a family member or significant other in the home) include the following (Johnson & Mass, 1997, p. 103):

- Willingness to assume caregiving role
- Knowledge about caregiving role
- Demonstration of positive regard for care recipient
- Participation in home care decisions
- Confidence in ability to manage care at home
- Knowledge of where to obtain needed equipment

This research continues in an effort to develop a common nursing language to optimize the design and delivery of safe, high quality and cost-effective care.

The Nurse as Coordinator

One of nursing's major contributions to the healthcare team is the role of coordinator. Care can easily become fragmented when patients are seen by numerous specialists—each interested in a different aspect of the patient. At best, patients complain that no one person really knows them and can talk with them about what is going on and how it all may affect them in the future. At worst, the orders of different specialists may conflict with one another and be counterproductive. Therefore, it is important for nurses to make rounds with other healthcare

(text continues on page 304)

TABLE 15-2 Nursing Interventions Classification (NIC) Taxonomy

	Domain I	Domain II	Domain III
Level 1 Domains	1. **Physiologic: Basic** Care that supports physical functioning	2. **Physiologic: Complex** Care that supports homeostatic regulation	3. **Behavioral** Care that supports psychosocial functioning and facilitates lifestyle changes

Level 2 Classes

Domain I	Domain II	Domain III
A **Activity and Exercise Management:** Interventions to organize or assist with physical activity and energy expenditure	G **Electrolyte and Acid–Base Management:** Interventions to regulate electrolyte/acid–base balance and prevent complications	O **Behavior Therapy:** Interventions to reinforce or promote desirable behaviors or alter undesirable behaviors
B **Elimination Management:** Interventions to establish and maintain regular bowel and urinary elimination patterns and manage complications due to altered patterns	H **Medication Management:** Interventions to facilitate desired effects of pharmacologic agents	P **Cognitive Therapy:** Interventions to reinforce or promote desirable cognitive functioning or alter undesirable cognitive functioning
C **Immobility Management:** Interventions to manage restricted body movement and the sequelae	I **Neurologic Management:** Interventions to optimize neurologic function	Q **Communication Enhancement:** Interventions to facilitate delivering and receiving verbal or nonverbal messages
D **Nutrition Support:** Interventions to modify or maintain nutritional status	J **Perioperative Care:** Interventions to provide care before, during, and immediately after surgery	R **Coping Assistance:** Interventions to assist another to build on own strengths, to adapt to a change in function, or to achieve a higher level of function
E **Physical Comfort Promotion:** Interventions to promote comfort using physical techniques	K **Respiratory Management:** Interventions to promote airway patency and gas exchange	S **Patient Education:** Interventions to facilitate learning
F **Self-Care Facilitation:** Interventions to provide or assist with routine activities of daily living	L **Skin/Wound Management:** Interventions to maintain or restore tissue integrity	T **Psychological Comfort Promotion:** Interventions to promote comfort using psychological techniques
	M **Thermoregulation:** Interventions to maintain body temperature within a normal range	
	N **Tissue Perfusion Management:** Interventions to optimize circulation of blood and fluids to the tissue	

McCloskey, J. C., & Bulechek, G. M. (Eds.) (2000). *Iowa Interventions Project: Nursing interventions classification* (3rd ed., pp. 90–91). St. Louis: Mosby–Year Book. Used with permission.

Domain IV	Domain V	Domain VI	Domain VII
4. Safety Care that supports protection against harm	**5. Family** Care that supports the family unit	**6. Health System** Care that supports effective use of the healthcare delivery system	**7. Community** Care that supports the health of the community
U *Crisis Management:* Interventions to provide immediate short-term help in both psychological and physiologic crises V *Risk Management:* Interventions to initiate risk reduction activities and continue monitoring risk over time	W *Childbearing Care:* Interventions to assist in understanding and coping with the psychological and physiologic changes during the childbearing period Z *Childrearing Care:* Interventions to assist in raising children X *Lifespan Care:* Interventions to facilitate family unit functioning and promote the health and welfare of family members throughout the lifespan	Y *Health System Mediation:* Interventions to facilitate the interface between patient/family and the healthcare system *a. Health System Management:* Interventions to provide and enhance support services for the delivery of care *b. Information Management:* Interventions to facilitate communication among healthcare workers	*c. Community Health Promotion:* Interventions that promote the health of the whole community *d. Community Risk Management* Interventions that assist in detecting or preventing health risks to the whole community

professionals and to read the results of consultations patients have had with specialists. Nurses can then interpret the specialists' findings for patients and family members, prepare patients to participate maximally in the plan of care before and after discharge, and serve as a liaison among the members of the healthcare team. Nurse case managers are specialists in the role of care coordinator.

> Look back at Antoinette Browne, the toddler described at the beginning of the chapter. As a result of the child's delays, multiple disciplines would likely be involved in caring for the child. The nurse would play a major role as coordinator for the child's care, ensuring communication among all team members. Additionally, the nurse would act as the liaison between the other members of the team to ensure that the child's grandmother understands the plan of care.

TYPES OF NURSING INTERVENTIONS

When the nurse carries out the interventions identified in the plan of care, he or she is implementing the plan of care. When implementing the plan of care, nurses function independently, dependently, and collaboratively. These are the three types of **nursing interventions** described in the preceding chapter.

Independent Nursing Action

Nurse-initiated interventions, or independent nursing actions, involve carrying out nurse-prescribed interventions resulting from their assessment of patient needs written on the nursing plan of care, as well as any other actions that nurses initiate without the direction or supervision of another healthcare professional. Nurses are legally accountable for their assessments and their nursing responses.

Protocols and standing orders expand the scope of nursing practice in certain clearly defined situations. **Protocols** are written plans that detail the nursing activities to be executed in specific situations. Although some protocols specify routine aspects of nursing care (eg, protocols that describe nursing responsibilities when a patient is admitted to or discharged from the institution), other protocols include **standing orders** that empower the nurse to initiate actions that ordinarily require the order or supervision of a physician. Examples include admission protocols for obstetric and gynecology patients, protocols for bowel programs that allow the nurse to select and administer necessary bowel interventions, standard orders for narcotic overdoses that specify the agents the nurse is to administer to reverse respiratory depression in an emergency, and standard orders for pain management that enable the nurse to select the strength of the medication to be given within preset ranges.

Dependent and Collaborative Nursing Action

Physician-initiated interventions, or dependent nursing actions, involve carrying out physician-prescribed orders. State Nurse Practice Acts specify from whom nurses can receive orders. Nurses are still accountable for dependent orders they implement and are thus responsible for the clarification of any questionable order.

> Recall James McMahon, the critically ill patient in ICU? The nurse administers IV fluids and medications based on orders written by the physicians.

Collaborative interventions, or interdependent nursing actions, are those performed jointly by nurses and other members of the healthcare team. Because nurses are increasingly respected as professional colleagues with unique patient knowledge, they are increasingly involved in collaborative ventures with the healthcare team.

> The three types of nursing actions can be illustrated by the example of Antoinette Browne, the toddler with gastrointestinal symptoms and delays in growth and development. If the physician orders a series of gastrointestinal studies, it is the nurse's responsibility to prepare the patient by executing the physician's order for cleansing the bowel. This nursing action is a physician-initiated intervention. When the nurse senses that the grandmother seems unusually fearful of the outcome of the studies, and explores her fears and then follows up with appropriate teaching and counseling, the nurse is using nurse-initiated interventions. When a multidisciplinary team conference is held to discuss the patient's failure to progress, the nurse works collaboratively with the psychiatrist, gastroenterologist, social worker, and child development specialist to develop a comprehensive plan of care; this involves collaborative nursing interventions.

IMPLEMENTING THE PLAN OF CARE

When carrying out the plan of care, nurses use specialized abilities to (1) determine the patient's new or continuing need for nursing assistance, (2) promote self-care, and (3) assist the patient to achieve valued health outcomes.

Reassess the Patient and Review the Plan of Care

Since a patient's condition can change dramatically in a matter of minutes, it is critical to assess the patient carefully before initiating any nursing intervention to make sure that the plan of care is still responsive to the patient's needs and prioritized to the most pressing of those needs. It is also important for each nurse implementing the plan:

- To be sure that each nursing intervention is supported by a sound scientific rationale, as demanded by an **evidence-based practice**
- To be sure that each nursing intervention is consistent with professional standards of care and consistent with the protocols, policies, and procedures of the institution or agency
- To be sure that the nursing actions are safe for this particular patient and individualized to his or her preferences
- To clarify any questionable orders

Clarify Prerequisite Nursing Skills

To implement the plan of nursing care, nurses need blended intellectual, interpersonal, technical, and ethical/legal skills. Each nurse has a unique blend of these skills and can act effectively to the extent that her or his abilities match the patient's need for nursing care.

> Remember James McMahon, the critically ill patient in the intensive unit? Although technological skills are key in this area, the nurse also needs to implement care that integrates intellectual, interpersonal, and ethical and legal skills because of the patient's complex needs.

These blended skills are described in Chapter 11 and are illustrated in the opening of each chapter. Be sure to notify your nursing instructor or nurse mentor if you believe that you lack any skills needed to safely implement the plan of care.

Organize Resources

Successful implementation of the plan of care requires a high degree of organization and efficiency in today's hectic healthcare environments.

Patient and Patient Visitors

Make sure the patient is physically and psychologically prepared for what you are going to do! Many interventions are unsuccessful because a patient is in too much pain to cooperate, fails to understand what is being attempted and therefore does not cooperate, or is simply distracted (may want to talk with visitors or watch TV). If visitors are in the room, check with the patient to see if she or he wants the visitor(s) to stay during the procedure. If a family caregiver needs to learn new caregiving skills, try to schedule your interventions at a time both appropriate for the patient and convenient for the family caregiver.

Equipment

Anticipate all the equipment you will need to successfully carry out the intervention and arrange it so that it is easily accessible. Be sure to order sufficient supplies at the beginning of the shift for the care you expect to provide, and be thought-

ful of the nurse who will follow you by leaving adequate supplies. Follow agency policy when ordering supplies to ensure proper charges. Many nurses have been injured on the job because they failed to take the time to use proper assistive devices, such as lifts for heavy patients or transfer boards for patients with limited mobility.

Environment

Think through the proper environment for each intervention. Pay special attention to respecting the patient's dignity, privacy, and safety needs. Patient privacy is routinely violated in some care settings when measures as simple as closing a door or pulling drapes are neglected. These considerations are of special importance when patients or residents share rooms. For example, if an enema is being administered, it can be embarrassing for the patient and unpleasant for the patient's roommate. With some planning, the intervention can be scheduled in a private bathroom or at a time when the roommate is absent.

Personnel

Identify if you are able to carry out the planned intervention independently or if you are likely to need assistance. Both patients and professional caregivers can be harmed when interventions are attempted by the wrong person or by an insufficient number of people. It is easy for a student to underestimate the strength it takes to lift or support a large patient. Until experienced, it is always safer to err on the side of having too much help rather than not enough. One helpful tip for teams of student nurses is to begin each rotation by asking "Who thinks they might need help today?" The team can then plan to coordinate care so that help is available when needed.

Anticipate Unexpected Outcomes/Situations

When you learn about new nursing procedures and interventions, you often see a description of possible adverse effects listed. While everyone hopes never to encounter these complications, they do occur with some frequency. The skilled nurse knows what might happen if an intervention "goes wrong" and is prepared to deal with the new challenge. This may be as simple as accurately assessing how much support a patient will need to avoid a fall when ambulating for the first time after surgery, or being prepared to respond to complaints of burning at a new IV site. For further consideration of unexpected outcomes and situations, refer to *Taylor's Clinical Nursing Skills* by Pam Evans-Smith and *Taylor's Video Guide to Clinical Nursing Skills* by Lippincott Williams & Wilkins.

Promoting Self-Care: Teaching, Counseling, and Advocacy

Although most people can independently meet their basic human needs, illness and the stress of diagnostic and therapeutic measures may interfere with a person's usual practice of self-care. The nurse assesses the patient's abilities to meet his or her human needs independently. Nurses can fail patients by doing too much for them and by encouraging negative, sick-role behaviors, such as inappropriate dependence. Conversely, there is a time and a place for the "tender loving care" that says to a patient "I know you may be able to do this for yourself, but just this once, how about if I do it and we'll talk!" Balancing the need to encourage a patient's best self-care effort with the effort to make each patient feel cared for and loved is an important component of the art of nursing.

Recall Estelle Morrissey, the 86-year-old woman living in a nursing home, asking to die? The nurse's ability to apply knowledge of counseling and advocacy would be important in developing a plan of care that addresses the patient's needs.

The plan of nursing care should include specific instructions for any nursing assistance the patient needs to meet basic human needs, including the need for significant nursing encouragement to promote greater independence in functioning. When routines of self-care (or assisted self-care) are included (eg, colostomy management), instructions should include the time of the procedure, the equipment used, the process, and the level of patient involvement. Continuity of nursing care is essential to the patient's development of a comfortable routine.

If patients and their families want to participate actively in seeking wellness, preventing disease and illness, recovering health, and learning to cope with altered functioning, they need to possess effective self-care behaviors. Nurses sensitive to the importance of patients learning to direct and manage their own care use nurse–patient interactions for both planned and spontaneous teaching, counseling, and advocacy. These nursing roles are described in Chapter 6 (Values and Ethics in Nursing) and Chapter 22 (Teacher and Counselor). For example, while caring for a child recently diagnosed as having cystic fibrosis, the nurses work continuously with the parents and siblings, helping them to develop the knowledge and skills that will enable them to care for the child after discharge. Referring families such as this to a community support group or other resources further enhances the self-care behaviors being developed. See "Through the Eyes of the Family Caregiver" for a description of one wife's experiences when her husband was discharged home.

Assisting Patients to Meet Health Outcomes

In this phase of the implementation process, the nursing team carries out the nursing orders detailed in the nursing plan of care. If the plan of care is well constructed, carrying out its orders is the nurse's most important task and should receive top priority. The nursing actions planned to promote patient goal/outcome achievement and the resolution of health problems should be carefully executed. Implementation guidelines are listed in Box 15-1.

Because understaffing is a problem in many practice settings, nurses must learn to use their time wisely and to maximize each patient encounter. A patient bath can be simply that, or it can be an opportunity to gather additional focused data, to

Through the Eyes of the Family Caregiver

"The nurses never told me there'd be days like this." I wasn't prepared for a roller coaster ride when my husband became ill. My husband was admitted to the hospital in an emergency condition, became confused when his electrolytes were off balance, went into cardiac arrest and had CPR, was placed on a ventilator, and was sedated because he was too apprehensive about the ventilator. I had reached the lowest point as I sat by his bedside for days, talking to him and wondering if he heard me.

My spirits soared the day they brought him out of his sleep state and he recognized me and was hungry for real food. The next day when I went to the hospital I plummeted to the low point again when he was crumpled in bed like a confused rag doll with his hospital gown up to his chest and the sheet to his ankles. I started to cry, and the nurse came and put her arm around me. She said, "Don't think he's taken a turn for the worse. There will be good days and bad days as he recovers." No one had prepared me for that—and her arm around me and her words were so consoling.

When I brought him home after 6 weeks in the hospital, I was not prepared for his anger at being confined to the house (in a heat wave) and not being allowed to drive. His reasoning that he had to get a haircut because he hadn't had one in 2 months made sense to him. My saying that no one would care about the length of his hair did not soothe his anger.

He couldn't accept the fact that he was too weak to go up and down the steps more than once a day, so he insisted on going to the basement. Going down was simple; coming up wasn't. We forgot there was no railing (which he needed to haul himself up) on the last four steps. He solved the problem by sitting on the steps and lifting himself up a step at a time. Then he got to the floor at the top and couldn't stand up. I couldn't lift him. We were stuck. Again I took a nose dive.

I thought I understood how difficult it would be for him to readjust. I knew he would be depressed and expected him to lean on me. But I was not prepared for his frustration to come out as anger at me. It would have been helpful to have someone prepare me. Or it would be nice to have a nurse put her arm around me now when my roller coaster plummets.

—Eleanor Faven,
Philadelphia, Pennsylvania

communicate concern for what the patient is experiencing and offering support, and to teach and counsel as appropriate. How the nurse uses the 30 minutes that he or she is in the patient's room for the bath determines how effective the nurse is in helping the patient to achieve his or her goals/outcomes. See the accompanying "Through the Eyes of a Student" for one student's account of an important bath.

Variables That Influence Outcome Achievement

When working with patients to achieve the outcomes specified in the plan of care, remember that nothing about the plan of

BOX 15-1 Implementing Guidelines

- When implementing nursing care, remember to act in partnership with the patient/family.
- Before implementing any nursing action, reassess the patient to determine whether the action is still needed.
- Approach the patient competently. Know how to perform the nursing action, why the action is being performed, and potential adverse responses. Have all equipment and supplies ready.
- Approach the patient caringly. Explain the nursing action using language the patient understands. Communicate genuine concern for what the patient is experiencing.
- Modify nursing interventions according to the patient's (1) developmental and psychosocial background, (2) ability and willingness to participate in the plan of care, and (3) responses to previous nursing measures and progress toward goal/outcome achievement.
- Check to make sure that the nursing interventions selected are consistent with standards of care and within legal and ethical guides to practice.
- Always question that the nursing intervention selected is the best of all possible alternatives. Consult colleagues and the nursing and related literature to see if other approaches might be more successful. Evaluate the effectiveness of the intervention selected, noting any factors that positively or negatively influenced the outcome.
- Develop a repertoire of skilled nursing interventions. The more options one can choose from, the greater the likelihood of success.

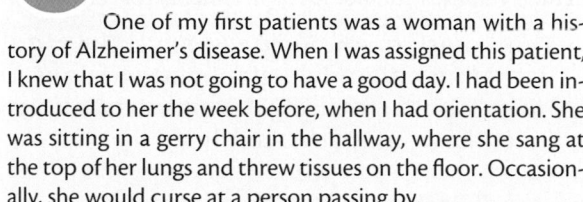

Through the Eyes of a Student

One of my first patients was a woman with a history of Alzheimer's disease. When I was assigned this patient, I knew that I was not going to have a good day. I had been introduced to her the week before, when I had orientation. She was sitting in a gerry chair in the hallway, where she sang at the top of her lungs and threw tissues on the floor. Occasionally, she would curse at a person passing by.

I took a deep breath and entered her room. At her bedside I introduced myself. With a few choice words, she told me to get out of her room. I tried to ignore her response and prepared her breakfast tray. She proceeded to throw her scrambled eggs around the room. After I took the tray away from her and finished cleaning up the mess, it was time for preconference. At preconference, my instructor told me that we were going to "tub" my patient. I had visions of a grand fiasco in the tub room, and I dreaded giving her the bath.

My instructor and I took her to the tub room by wheelchair. Once we convinced her to get in the tub, she did nothing but yell that it was cold. We started the water and she yelled even louder. I knew everyone could hear her in the hallway as she cursed and yelled, but as the bath proceeded, she quieted down and stopped fighting me. We completed the bath and wheeled her back down the hall to her room. I bundled her up in blankets and put her in the gerry chair in the hallway. She was so relaxed from the bath that she let me brush her hair and put it in a ponytail. While I was brushing her hair, she fell asleep. I did my chart until her lunch arrived. When I set her up for her lunch and told her I would be leaving, she thanked me, and it made my day. All the struggling I went through all day with her and she thanked me. When I went home I felt really good about helping her. During all my worrying about the day being a fiasco and the embarrassment of having a patient yell at me, I had lost sight of the patient herself and what she needed me to do for her. By her thanking me at the end of the day, I realized that when my clinical instructor forced me to do something for my patient that the regular staff of the hospital wouldn't do, I was meeting her basic needs, and my patient recognized that.

—Jeanene C. Smith,
Delaware County Community College,
Media, Pennsylvania

care is fixed. Some of the most important variables that influence how the plan of care is implemented follow.

Patient Variables

Ideally, the patient is primary in determining how nursing interventions are implemented. Successful nurses modify their nursing actions according to the patient's (1) changing ability and willingness to participate in the plan of care and (2) previous responses to nursing interventions and progress toward goal/outcome achievement. Other important patient variables are developmental stage and psychosocial background.

Developmental Stage

Addressing the developmental needs of a patient is much more than simply identifying the patient's developmental stage on the plan of care. The developmental tasks related to this stage and their relationship to nursing care seldom need to be considered. For example, the nurse may recommend that the parents of a premature infant make a tape of their voices to stimulate their infant in the neonatal intensive care unit. Nurses must be careful not to let stereotypes about developmental stages and tasks influence patient care. In nursing homes, for example, the developmental needs of older patients are ignored when a staff member selects a

radio station that plays rock music, makes humorous comments about "romances" among the residents, embarrasses some residents by calling them cute names or putting big, bright bows in their hair, or demeans some patients by planning childish group activities. Perhaps the worst stereotype is the belief that all older people have to do is wait to die, and that there are no developmental challenges for this age group.

Remember Estelle Morrissey, the nursing home resident who wants to die? Knowledge about this stereotype would be important for the nurse when implementing the patient's care.

To implement a comprehensive and holistic plan of care, nurses must find creative ways to meet developmental needs. This is of greatest importance when patients are separated from their families and home environments for long periods.

> *Think back to Antoinette Browne, the toddler with physical and developmental delays. The nurse would creatively adapt interventions to meet the needs of this toddler.*

Psychosocial Background

The same is true of the psychosocial needs of patients. Although few nurses would claim that people from all socio-economic groups and cultures are the same, some practice nursing as if this were so. When choosing nursing interventions, the nurse should consider and respect the patient's background. Confronted with a malnourished patient on a limited income who rents a single room in a boarding home, a nurse cannot simply teach the importance of including more protein in the diet. To be effective, the nurse must explore the realistic issue of whether the patient can afford and obtain foods rich in protein. Moreover, the nurse needs to assess whether the patient values this intervention and is willing to make the necessary changes.

Nurse Variables

Nurse variables that influence the implementation of the plan of care include levels of expertise, creativity (ability to match patient needs with specific nursing strategies), willingness to provide care, and available time. Focused Critical Thinking Guide 15-1 illustrates the importance of a nurse's ability to think critically about intervention strategies.

Resources

The most elaborately designed plan of care cannot be fully effective in a chronically understaffed or undersupplied nursing unit. Adequate staff, equipment, and supplies are all important determinants of patient care. The financial resources of the patient and adequacy of community-based resources also influence the plan of care.

Current Standards of Care

All nursing actions for implementing the plan of care must be consistent with standards of practice. See Chapter 16 for a discussion of these standards. All nurses are responsible for learning the standards that dictate practice in their specialty. Failure to practice according to these standards may result in a charge of negligence.

Research Findings

Nurses concerned about improving the quality of nursing care use research findings to enhance their nursing practice. Reading professional nursing journals and attending continuing education workshops and conferences are excellent ways to learn about new nursing strategies that have proved effective.

Research boxes throughout this text demonstrate the difference nursing research can make in improving patient outcomes.

Ethical and Legal Guides to Practice

Nurses cannot practice good nursing if they are ignorant of the laws and regulations that affect healthcare and the ethical dimensions of clinical practice. A sincere motivation to benefit the patient and a conscientious attempt to implement nursing orders are no longer sufficient. Each nurse is responsible for becoming sensitive to the ethical and legal dimensions of practice, and moral and legal accountability are inherent in the practice of professional nursing.

> *Look back on the scenario presented at the beginning of the chapter for Estelle Morrissey. Ethical and legal guidelines are crucial in determining how the nurse intervenes. Additionally, the nurse needs to evaluate the ethical and legal ramifications of his or her action in light of the patient's request to die.*

Chapters 6 and 7 discuss the ethical and legal dimensions of practice. Hospital risk managers and ethics committees are increasingly available as institutional resources for nurses.

CONTINUING DATA COLLECTION AND RISK MANAGEMENT

An important nursing intervention is ongoing data collection. In every patient encounter, the nurse needs to be sensitive to both subtle and dramatic changes in the patient's condition. Skilled nurses monitor the patient's responses to planned interventions to determine if the plan of care is working. These assessment findings are used to update and revise the plan of care. Sensitivity to how the patient is responding to nursing interventions and to the patient's progress toward outcome achievement allows the nurse to modify nursing interventions appropriately.

Another vital nursing intervention is ongoing risk management. While monitoring the patient's responses to the plan of care, nurses are also alert to the development of new problems that may result in the identification of new diagnoses or collaborative problems. As nurses get to know patients and recognize clusters of significant data, they can identify problems for which the patient is at risk and intervene appropriately to promote health and to prevent disease.

DOCUMENTING NURSING CARE

Remembering the legal truth "It wasn't done if it wasn't documented," each nurse carefully documents all nursing inter-

Focused Critical Thinking Guide 15-1

Situation

One of the nurses on the oncology unit where you have been working for 6 months since graduation wants to develop a "humor room" where patients, their families, and staff can "take a break" from the serious business of illness. Designed to lift the spirits, amuse, distract, and thus speed the healing process, humor rooms are gaining popularity as new therapeutic tools. Funny books, comic movies on a large-screen TV, games and puzzles—and ideally, even clowns, magicians, musicians, and stand-up comedians—are being envisaged (Buxman, 1991). Several nurses have vocally expressed their lack of support for the project and think the idea is "stupid" at best, and potentially a great waste of money, time, and energy that could be devoted to "tried and true" methods of healing. You have been asked to support the project and must decide how to respond.

1. Identify Goal of Thinking

Clarify your thinking about humor as a therapeutic measure so that you can decide whether to support this project.

2. Assess Adequacy of Knowledge

Pertinent circumstances: The nurse who wants to develop the humor room is more popular with patients than she is with her colleagues. Her nurse friends are quick to point out that while it's true that she is "a bit flaky" and unorthodox, she is an efficient nurse who is well-loved by her patients and their families. The hospital is in the midst of cutting expenses and has laid off both professional and nonprofessional employees.

Prerequisite knowledge: To decide how you should respond in this situation, you need to research the healing benefits of humor. Are there clinical studies demonstrating its effectiveness as a therapeutic measure? If studies point to humor's effectiveness, you will need to determine (1) what priority it should have among other treatment modalities and (2) the feasibility of creating a humor room in the current climate of cutting expenses. Is there a creative way to finance this venture?

Room for error: Since life and death do not hinge on how you elect to respond to this plea for support, there is a rela-

tively wide margin for error. Because personal energy and finances are limited, however, you do not want to involve your unit in a futile project.

Time constraints: There is no rush for an immediate decision on your part, which gives you adequate time to develop the knowledge base you need to make an informed decision.

3. Address Potential Problems

The most serious obstacle to critical thinking in this situation would be the lack of an open mind and refusal to weigh the merits of a new treatment modality. Complicating factors include divided loyalties among the nurses and the tendency to support or refuse support for the project on the basis of whether one likes the nurse advocating the project, rather than on the merits of the project. Finally, the lowered morale caused by lay-offs may squash all creativity and willingness to "dream new dreams."

4. Consult Helpful Resources

Your first challenge will be to learn more about humor as a healing measure. Ideally, you may be able to consult a local expert and invite her or him to meet with the staff. Alternately, you can research the literature, looking for clinical studies and reports of the first-person experiences of others.

5. Critical Judgment/Decision

After a search of the literature convinced you and some of the other nurses of the clinical benefits of humor, you decide to explore the feasibility of developing a humor room. Your options are to "play it safe" and not rock the boat during a difficult period in the hospital by trying something new, or to become an advocate for the project and commit your energies to making it happen. You decide that a creative project may be exactly what the staff needs to rediscover the "joy of nursing" and begin to explore means to fund the project. You plan to "start small" and to reassess the project every 6 months. Since your research educated you about the potential benefits *and harms* humor can create, you decide that your first objective must be to educate the staff.

---

ventions. See Chapter 17 for a description of guidelines for written documentation and see the plans of nursing care at the end of each clinical chapter for samples of documented nursing interventions.

WHEN A PATIENT FAILS TO COOPERATE WITH THE PLAN OF CARE

When a patient fails to follow the plan of care despite the nurse's best efforts, it is time to reassess strategy. The first ob-

jective is to identify why the patient is not following the therapy. One possibility is that the plan of care may not be right for this patient. In this event, what is needed is not a change in the patient but, rather, a change in the plan of care. If the nurse determines, however, that the plan of care is adequate, he or she must identify and remedy the factors contributing to the patient's noncompliance. Common reasons for a failure to cooperate include:

- Lack of family support
- Lack of understanding about the benefits of compliance
- Low value attached to outcomes or related interventions
- Adverse physical or emotional effects of treatment (such as pain and fatigue)

- Inability to afford treatment
- Limited access to treatment

DELEGATING NURSING CARE

Because of the pressure to reduce healthcare costs and the increasing demand for nursing services in the midst of a critical shortage of professional nurses, many employers of nurses have increased their use of unlicensed assistive personnel (UAP) or "nurse extenders." **Unlicensed assistive personnel** are individuals who are trained to function in an assistive role to the licensed registered nurse (RN) in the provision of patient activities as delegated by and under the supervision of the registered professional nurse. **Delegation** is the transfer of responsibility for the performance of an activity to another individual while retaining accountability for the outcome. In some cases, the new mix of professional and nonprofessional staff is threatening patient safety. Never has it been more important for nurses to critically identify which nursing interventions require professional nurses and which can be safely delegated. This can be especially challenging for new nurses.

> *Review the patient scenario for James McMahon, the critically ill patient described at the beginning of the chapter and in "Reflective Practice: Challenge to Technical Skills." The nurse's ability to delegate effectively would be important in providing safe, efficient care.*

Boucher aptly describes the dangers of fewer nurses caring for sicker patients while simultaneously supervising UAPs who are performing patient care that, until recently, was reserved for professional nurses.

> *Even when the delegation is appropriate (that is, the right task assigned to the right person using clear, concise communication) and the task is performed correctly, the nurse–patient dynamic is absent. It's this dynamic, or contextual presence—seeing the patient within the contexts of time, location, and physical and emotional conditions—that is the core of nursing. UAPs aren't trained to see a patient within a specific context, do a focused assessment, and know the significance of what the assessment reveals . . . UAPs are prepared to do many things, but they are not prepared to know (this is the absence of the critical thinking component)*
> (Boucher, 1998, p. 28).

See Box 15-2 for Boucher's list of "Essentials of Effective Delegation."

Guidelines for Delegating Nursing Care

Before delegating any nursing intervention, a number of factors should be considered: (1) the patient's condition, (2) the complexity of the activity, (3) the potential for harm, (4) the

---

BOX 15-2 Essentials of Effective Delegation

The following will help you with the essential responsibilities and techniques of delegating care tasks:

- Know your state and institutional policies on delegation (the policy and procedure manual is available on each unit; for state policies, contact the state nurse association).
- Be clear on the difference between nursing process and nursing tasks.
- Know the training and background of the unlicensed assistive personnel (UAP). (Administration must have a standard and process to validate the UAP's preparation.)
- Know the patient's needs and what he or she is at risk for.
- Know what clinical cues the UAP should be alert for and why.
- Assess which tasks can be safely delegated.
- Have the UAP repeat your instructions to be sure you have communicated them clearly.
- Make frequent walking rounds to assess patients.
- When talking with the patient, members of the patient's family, or UAPs, listen for cues that indicate changes in the patient's condition.
- Take frequent mini-reports for the UAP.
- Evaluate the UAP's performance and the patient's response.

Boucher, M. A. (1998). Delegation alert! *American Journal of Nursing, 98*(2), 26–32.

---

degree of problem-solving and innovation necessary, (5) the level of interaction required with the patient, (6) capabilities of the UAP, and (7) the availability of professional staff to accomplish the unit workload. The American Nurses Association, which is committed to monitoring the regulation, education, and use of UAP, recommends adherence to the following principles:

- It is the nursing profession that determines the scope of nursing practice.
- It is the nursing profession that defines and supervises the education, training, and use of any unlicensed assistant roles involved in providing direct nursing care.
- It is the registered nurse who is responsible and accountable for nursing practice.
- It is the registered nurse who supervises any assistant involved in providing direct patient care.
- It is the purpose of assistive personnel to work in a supportive role to the registered nurse, carrying out tasks to enable the professional nurse to concentrate on nursing care for the patient (Pennsylvania Nurses Association, 1992).

Nursing care or tasks that should never be delegated except to another RN include (Haas, 1999):

- The initial and ongoing nursing assessment of the patient and his or her nursing care needs
- The determination of the nursing diagnoses, nursing care plan, evaluation of the patient's progress in relation to

care plan, and evaluation of the nursing care delivered to the patient
- The supervision and education of nursing personnel; patient teaching that requires an assessment of the patient and his or her education needs
- Any other nursing intervention that requires professional nursing knowledge, judgment, and/or skill
  In conclusion, the *Five Rights of Delegation* are:
- *Right Task:* One that is delegable for a specific patient
- *Right Circumstances:* Appropriate patient setting, available resources, and other relevant factors considered
- *Right Person:* Right person is delegating the right task to the right person to be performed on the right person (patient)
- *Right Direction/Communication:* Clear, concise description of the task, including its objective, limits, and expectations

- *Right Supervision:* Appropriate monitoring, evaluation, intervention as needed, and feedback
  Helpful guides for nurses who are learning to delegate are the delegation decision trees developed by the Ohio Nurses Association (Fig. 15-2*A, B*).

Delegation and the Student Nurse

Student nurses may find themselves the recipient of delegated care that they cannot safely perform. Whenever you are asked by a staff nurse to perform an intervention for which you lack training, you should consult with your instructor to see if you can safely perform it with supervision. Under no circumstances should you attempt to perform interventions beyond your capacity without supervision, even if instructed to do so by a staff nurse. Students who work as nursing assistants while enrolled

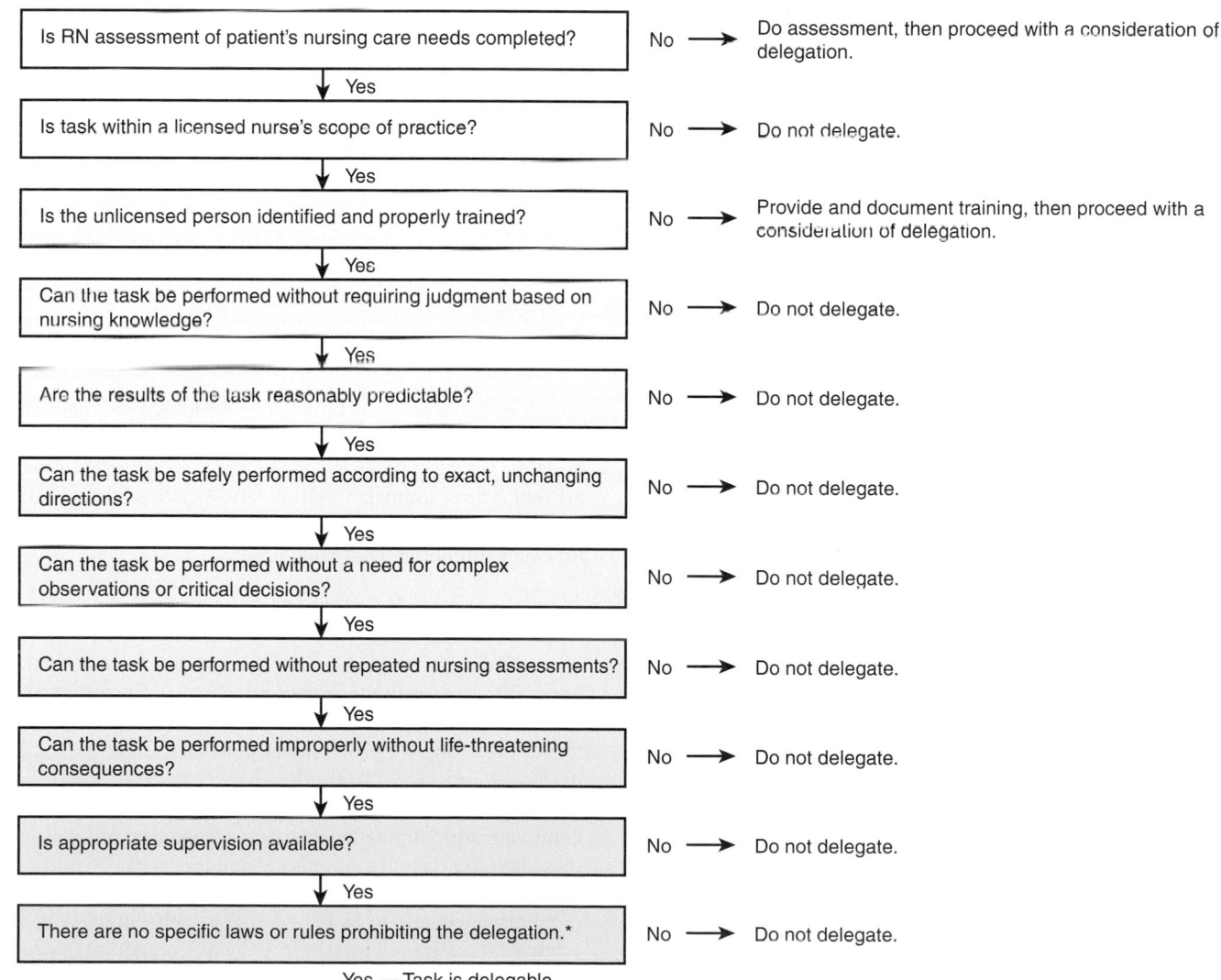

Is RN assessment of patient's nursing care needs completed? — No → Do assessment, then proceed with a consideration of delegation.

↓ Yes

Is task within a licensed nurse's scope of practice? — No → Do not delegate.

↓ Yes

Is the unlicensed person identified and properly trained? — No → Provide and document training, then proceed with a consideration of delegation.

↓ Yes

Can the task be performed without requiring judgment based on nursing knowledge? — No → Do not delegate.

↓ Yes

Are the results of the task reasonably predictable? — No → Do not delegate.

↓ Yes

Can the task be safely performed according to exact, unchanging directions? — No → Do not delegate.

↓ Yes

Can the task be performed without a need for complex observations or critical decisions? — No → Do not delegate.

↓ Yes

Can the task be performed without repeated nursing assessments? — No → Do not delegate.

↓ Yes

Can the task be performed improperly without life-threatening consequences? — No → Do not delegate.

↓ Yes

Is appropriate supervision available? — No → Do not delegate.

↓ Yes

There are no specific laws or rules prohibiting the delegation.* — No → Do not delegate.

Yes — Task is delegable.

A   *Medication administration can be delegated by a licensed nurse to a trained unlicensed person ONLY in an MR/DD County Board facility, or ICF/MR of fifteen beds or less, or when school policies have been developed in accordance with Ohio Board of Nursing rules on delegation and Ohio education law.*

FIGURE 15-2 (**A** and **B**) Sample delegation decision trees for delegated nursing responsibilities. (Figure continues on p. 312. Used with permission from the Ohio Nurses Association.)

in professional programs are especially likely to be asked to perform interventions beyond their mastery.

GUIDE FOR STUDENTS

Organizing Care

Student nurses trying in advance to organize their nursing care for a particular clinical day can use the guidelines for student clinical responsibilities in Box 15-3 to help identify nursing

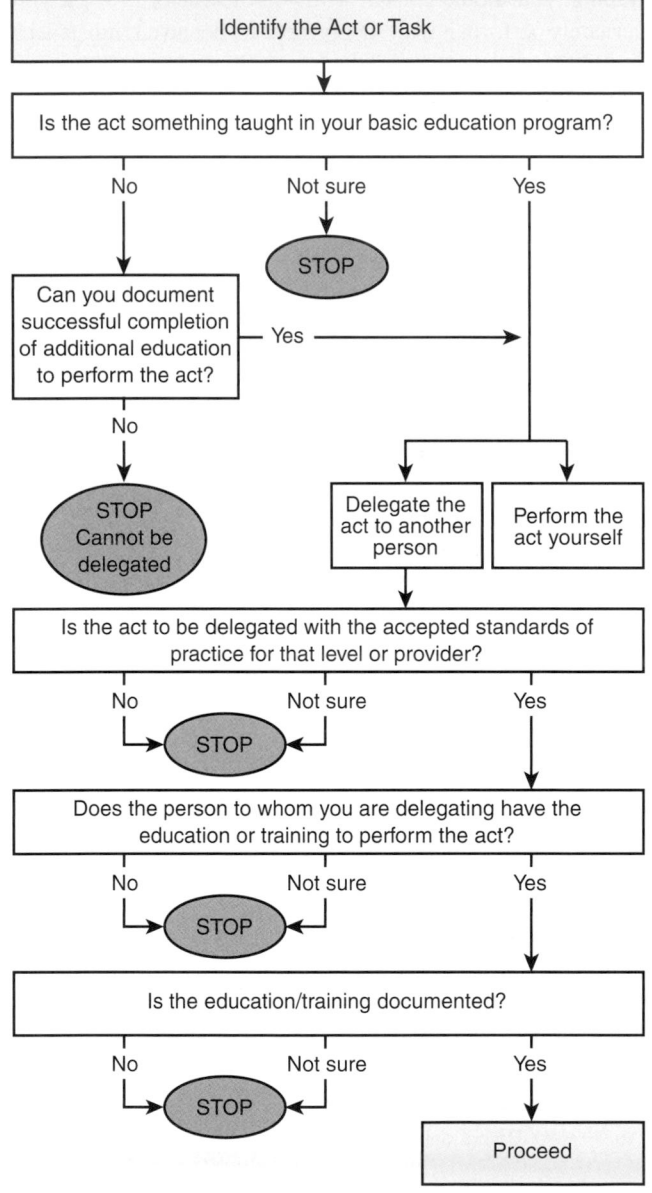

IMPORTANT NUMBERS

Ohio Nurses Association
800-430-0056

JCAHO
630-792-5642

Ohio Board of Nursing
614-466-3947

American Nurses Association
800-274-4262

Ohio Department of Health
Complaint Hotline
800-342-0553

Contact ONA if you have any questions.

B

FIGURE 15-2 *Continued*

> **BOX 15-3 Organizing Student Clinical Responsibilities**
>
> To organize clinical responsibilities, check:
> 1. Patient profile
> 2. Name by which patient wishes to be addressed
> 3. Patient's chief complaint and reason for admission
> 4. Patient's current health status
>   - Note any physical or emotional changes indicating the need to modify the plan of care.
> 5. Routine assistance patient needs to meet basic human needs
> 6. Priorities for nursing care:
>   - Priorities identified by the patient as "most important." The nurse might state "I'll be your nurse until 3 PM, and I'm interested in learning what you would most like to accomplish today."
>   - Prioritized nursing diagnoses, patient outcomes, and related nursing interventions
>   - Medical orders that need to be implemented
>   - Interdependent or collaborative nursing responsibilities
> 7. Special "events" of the day that may require special observation of the patient, teaching, preparation, or aftercare:
>   - Diagnostic tests
>   - Consultations with specialists
>   - New therapies (physical therapy, medications, surgery, radiotherapy, etc.)
> 8. Special teaching, counseling, or advocacy needs
> 9. Special needs of the family

measures for which they will be responsible. After these have been identified, working out a time schedule may provide clear direction for the clinical day and ensure that the patient's needs are met. The accompanying Reflective Practice box presents a scenario in which a nursing student learns to better manage her time and appropriately organize care.

Nursing Oneself

It is difficult for nurses to be sincerely attentive to patient needs if their own human needs are not met. Because no one is perfectly healthy or "whole" all the time, it is important that nurses preparing for professional practice spend time getting to know themselves. Activities that promote psychological health when practiced on a regular basis include self-awareness, communication, time management, preparation for crisis and loss, developing and maintaining support systems, and concurrent practice of self-care in all areas. The characteristics of emotional health include self-esteem, self-knowledge, satisfying interpersonal relationships, environmental mastery, stress management, a positive body image, a sense of humor, and the ability to experience pleasure.

Nurses who want to be competent practitioners learn early to nurse themselves and other nurses before attempting to nurse patients. Good personal health enables nurses not only to practice more efficiently but also to be a health model for

Reflective Practice
Challenge to Interpersonal Competence

For our complex care clinical we were assigned to the hospital's cardiac care unit. I missed orientation because I was instructed to attend my public health orientation and was told that it would be easy to make up. The first day of clinical we received report and were informed that the nurse assigned to our patient was not responsible for helping us with patient care, and that it was our clinical instructor's responsibility to assist all seven of us with patient care. My patient was a 53-year-old obese, diabetic African American man who came into the ER the previous day with shortness of breath and generally not feeling well. He was scheduled for a PICC line placement the day I was assigned to care for him, so I was instructed to complete his vital signs, give his 8 AM medications, take his blood glucose, and complete my head-to-toe assessment of him, all before he was scheduled to go down. Since this was my first time on the unit, I did not know where anything was and it took me a long time to find the necessary supplies. My nurse was of little help to me. By the time I got organized and was ready to start my care at 7:30 AM, a transporter was there to take my patient down for his procedures, and none of the tasks that I needed to complete were done. My nurse told me it was fine for him to go down without having his vitals or blood glucose taken. My patient had his PICC line put in, and then was sent for a foot x-ray, an echo, and a pressure test on his extremities. By the time I got back up to the unit with my patient 3 hours later, I was overwhelmed by the amount of care I needed to catch up on, and meanwhile my nurse was yelling at me about how I should have completed my care before leaving the unit.

Thinking Outside the Box: Possible Courses of Action

- I could have asked my clinical instructor or the nurse assigned to my patient to help me with the tasks I needed to carry out before my patient went down for his procedures.
- I could have asked a fellow classmate to help me collect the necessary supplies and to assist me in carrying out my care before leaving the floor.
- I could have organized and prioritized the care that needed to be delivered to my patient before his procedures. I could have carried out the most important tasks, such as taking his blood glucose and vital signs, in the short amount of time I

had before he went down, and then completed the rest of my care when we returned to the unit.
- I could have been more organized when I returned to the unit, asking for the necessary help to provide adequate care for my patient and catching up on the tasks that I missed while we were off the unit.
- I could have become flustered upon returning to the unit, since I was behind on my care and since the nurse was yelling at me about completing his care, when she initially said it was "ok" for it not to be done before leaving the unit.
- I gained skill in prioritizing care.

Evaluating a Good Outcome: How Do I Define Success?

- The patient's needs were addressed in a timely and compassionate manner.
- The patient was comfortable and content with the care provided.
- The patient was respected by all individuals who were responsible for his care.
- The patient recognized our commitment as healthcare professionals to provide the best quality of care possible to him.
- I advocated on behalf of my patient to protect his health and rights as an individual.
- The needs of the nurses were met as to provide the best patient care possible for the patient.

Personal Learning: Here's To The Future!

When I got back to the floor with my patient, I was overwhelmed by the amount of patient care that I needed to catch up on. I was having difficulty finding the blood glucose machine and the vitals machine. It was as if I were running around like a chicken with my head cut off and I was accomplishing nothing productive. Finally, my instructor pulled me aside because she could see that things were spiraling out of control. We sat down and prioritized from "most important" to "least important" the tasks I needed to do for my patient. First, I took his blood glucose, which was very low since he had not eaten all morning, and I ordered him a lunch tray. Next, I gave his morning medications that he missed. I then took his vital signs and completed my head-to-toe assessment and recorded my findings in his chart. I spent the rest of my day in clinical trying to make my patient comfortable and caring for his needs.

I think I became flustered when I returned to the floor because of the way the nurse treated me. She made me feel incompetent and stupid because I had not carried out all my care in the short

time I was allotted. However, she did nothing to help me or assist me in caring for our patient. Looking back, I learned a great deal from this clinical experience. I should have told my nurse that I needed help in caring for the patient because I was trying to catch up on what was missed during the morning. If she was unwilling to help me, I should have consulted my clinical instructor or classmates for their assistance. I also should have pulled my nurse aside and confronted her about how she contradicted herself, in that she initially told me that it was okay for my patient to go down to his procedures without his care being complete, and then later reprimanded me for not carrying out his care before we left. I do not think my reactions to this clinical situation were unusual, and I think most nursing students would have become frustrated and overwhelmed under similar circumstances. Although this situation tested my interpersonal skills in working with this nurse, I feel as though I was able put my frustrations aside and provide quality care in a professional manner to meet the needs of my patient.

Reflection

How do you think you would respond in a similar situation? Why? What does this tell you about yourself and about the adequacy of your skills for professional practice? Can you think of other ways to respond? How might the nursing student have approached the nurse assigned to the patient's care for assistance? What could the nursing student have done to prepare for this assignment? What other skills (cognitive, interpersonal, technical, ethical/legal) would

you need to respond well in this situation? What role do you think the clinical environment (a cardiac care unit) played in the nursing student's feelings of being overwhelmed? Do you agree with the criteria to evaluate a successful outcome? Were the criteria met? Please explain why or why not.

Kate Sullivan, Georgetown University

patients and their families. Nurses can help patients to imitate good health behaviors and eventually integrate them into their daily life through the process of identification.

Developing Critical Thinking Skills

1. Team up with another student and take turns role-playing a nurse visiting a homebound older man who needs his vital signs and nutritional status assessed. Discuss with each other the truth or falsity of the claim "Who the nurse is, is as important as, and sometimes more important than, what the nurse does."

2. Receive the same clinical assignment as another student, and independently outline your care priorities, specifying what you plan to accomplish during each of your clinical hours. Talk with the other student about the differences in what you both hope to accomplish and how you would do this. Try to imagine what these differences would mean to the patient.

3. You are the only RN on a 50-bed wing in a long-term care facility. You have one LPN working with you and two personal care assistants. Each of the 50 residents requires assistance with activities of daily living, all take at least some medications, and most require monitoring for multiple chronic (and sometimes acute) illnesses. How will you decide which interventions to delegate? When the home is short-staffed, you are sometimes the only RN covering two 50-bed units.

4. Describe how you would probably respond, and how you would like to respond (if these are different), to hearing another nurse in the shift report say that one of the patients you are assigned to was a real "PIB." ("pain in the butt") all day and "just impossible" to care for. Reflect on the importance of the language we use to report on a patient to one another.

Practicing for NCLEX

1. A school nurse notices that Jill is losing weight and wants to perform a focused assessment on Jill's nutritional status, fearing that she might have an eating disorder. How should the nurse proceed?
   a. Perform the focused assessment. This is an independent nurse-initiated intervention.
   b. Request an order from Jill's physician since this is a physician-initiated intervention.
   c. Request an order from Jill's physician since this is a collaborative intervention.
   d. Request an order from the nutritionist since this is a collaborative intervention.

2. Which of the following would you expect to find in the Nursing Interventions Classification Taxonomy?
   a. Case studies illustrating a complete set of activities that a nurse performs to carry out nursing interventions
   b. Nursing interventions, each with a label, a definition, and a set of activities that a nurse performs

to carry it out, with a short list of background readings
   c. A complete list of nursing diagnoses, outcomes, and related nursing activities for each nursing intervention
   d. A complete list of reimbursable charges for each nursing intervention

3. You are a brand new RN. When you orient to a new nursing unit that is currently understaffed, you are told that the UAPs have been trained to obtain the initial nursing assessment. What is the best response?
   a. Allow the UAPs to do the admission assessment and report the findings to you.
   b. Do your own admission assessments but don't interfere with the practice if other professional RNs seem comfortable with the practice.
   c. Tell the charge nurse that you are choosing not to delegate the admission assessment at this time until you can get further clarification from admission.
   d. Contact your labor representative and complain.

Answers With Rationale

1. The correct answer is *a;* this is an independent nurse-initiated intervention. The nurse therefore does not need an order from the physician (*b, c*) or the nutritionist (*d*).

2. The correct answer is *b.* The Nursing Interventions Classification Taxonomy lists 336 interventions, each with a label, a definition, a set of activities that a nurse performs to carry it out, and a short list of background readings. It does not contain case studies (*a*), diagnoses (*c*), or charges (*d*).

3. The correct answer is *c.* You do not delegate this nursing admission assessment because you learned that only nurses can perform this intervention. You should seek clarification for this policy from nursing administration.

Bibliography

Alfaro, R. (2002). *Applying nursing process: Promoting collaborative care* (5th ed.). Philadelphia: Lippincott Williams & Wilkins.

Alfaro-LeFevre, R. (2004). *Critical thinking and clinical judgment: A practical approach.* St. Louis: W. B. Saunders.

Benner, P. (1984). *From novice to expert: Excellence and power in clinical nursing practice.* Menlo Park, CA: Addison-Wesley.

Benner, P., & Wrubel, J. (1989). *The primary of caring: Stress and coping in health and illness.* Menlo Park, CA: Addison-Wesley.

Blegen, M. A., Gardner, D. I., & McCloskey, J. C. (1992). Who helps you with your work? *American Journal of Nursing, 92*(1), 26–31.

Boucher, M. A. (1998). Delegation alert! *American Journal of Nursing, 98*(2), 26–32.

Brider, P. (1992). The move to patient-focused care. *American Journal of Nursing, 92*(9), 26–33.

Bulechek, G. M., & McCloskey, J. C. (1987). Nursing interventions: What they are and how to choose them. *Holistic Nursing Practice, 1*(3), 36–44.

Buxman, K. (1991). Make room for laughter. *American Journal of Nursing, 91*(12), 46–51.

Dossey, B. (1991). Awakening the inner healer. *American Journal of Nursing, 91*(8), 31–34.

Eisenhauer, L. A. (1994). A typology of nursing therapeutics. *Image—The Journal of Nursing Scholarship, 26*(4), 261–264.

Ellis, J. R., & Hartley, C. L. (1995). *Managing and coordinating nursing care* (2nd ed.). Philadelphia: J. B. Lippincott.

Gibson, L. (1994). Healing with humor. *Nursing, 24*(9), 56–57.

Haas, M. (1999). Delegation and supervision of nursing care in Minnesota. *Minnesota Nursing Accent, 71*(7), 8–15.

Hansten, R., & Washburn, M. (1992a). Delegation: How to deliver care through others. *American Journal of Nursing, 92*(3), 87–90.

Hansten, R., & Washburn, M. (1992b). How to plan what to delegate. *American Journal of Nursing, 92*(4), 71–72.

Hill, L., & Smith, N. (1990). *Self-care nursing: Promotion of health* (2nd ed.). East Norwalk, CT: Appleton & Lange.

Iowa Intervention Project. (1993). The NIC taxonomy structure. *Image—The Journal of Nursing Scholarship, 25*(3), 187–192.

Iowa Intervention Project. (1995). McCloskey, J. C., & Bulechek, G. (Eds.). Validating and coding of the NIC taxonomy structure. *Image—The Journal of Nursing Scholarship, 27*(1), 43–49.

Iowa Intervention Project. (1997). Nursing interventions classification (NIC): An overview. In M. J. Rantz & P. LeMone (Eds.), *Classification of nursing diagnoses: Proceedings of the Twelfth Conference, North American Nursing Diagnosis* (pp. 32–39). Glendale, CA: CINAHL Information Systems.

Johnson, M., & Mass, M. L. (Eds.) (1997, 2000). *Nursing outcomes classification* (NOC). St. Louis: Mosby–Year Book.

Joint Commission on Accreditation of Healthcare Organizations. (2003). *2003 Accreditation manual for hospitals.* Oakbrook Terrace, IL: Author.

McCloskey, J. C., & Bulechek, G. M. (Eds.) (1992). *Nursing intervention classification (NIC).* St. Louis: Mosby–Year Book.

McCloskey, J. C., & Bulechek, G. M. (Eds.) (1996). *Nursing intervention classification (NIC)* (2nd ed.). St. Louis: Mosby–Year Book.

McCloskey, J. C., & Bulechek, G. M. (Eds.) (2000). *Nursing intervention classification (NIC)* (3rd ed.). St. Louis: Mosby–Year Book.

Neighbors, M., Eldred, E., & Sullivan, M. (1991). Nursing skills necessary for competing in the high-tech health care system. *Nursing and Health Care, 12*(2), 92–97.

Paris, L. L. (1994). Improving the process of communication at the bedside. *Journal of Nursing Care Quality, 9*(1), 10–15.

Pennsylvania Nurses Association. (1992, January). Perspectives in practice: RNs working with unlicensed assistive personnel. *Pennsylvania Nurse,* 7–8.

Prescott, P. A., Phillips, C. Y., Ryan, J. W., & Thompson, K. O. (1991). Changing how nurses spend their time. *Image—The Journal of Nursing Scholarship, 23*(1), 23–28.

Rubenfeld, M. G., & Scheffer, B. K. (1999). *Critical thinking in nursing: An interactive approach* (2nd ed.). Philadelphia: Lippincott Williams & Wilkins.

Seeger-Jablonski, R. A. (1992). Remember the person attached to the ventilator. *Nursing, 92*(4), 67–70.

Sundeen, S. J., Wiscarz, S., DeSalvo-Rankin, F. A., & Cohen, S. A. (1994). *Nurse–patient interaction: Implementing the nursing process* (5th ed.). St. Louis: C. V. Mosby.

Valega, T. M. (1984). It's time for nurses to begin nursing. *Nursing and Health Care, 5*(6), 331–335.

Wichowski, H. C., & Kubsch, S. (1995). Improving your patient's compliance. *Nursing, 25*(1), 66–68.

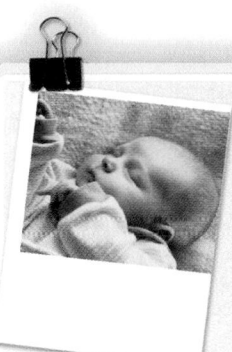

Tyler Jameson, a term neonate born 30 hours ago, has yet to pass stool. Follow-up assessment reveals that he does not have a patent anus, a finding that was not detected in the neonate's initial assessment.

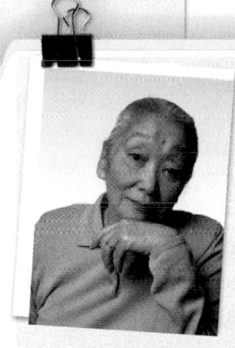

Mioshi Otsuki, an elderly woman with a history of heart failure being treated with diuretics, is receiving home care. Questioned about her prescribed drug-therapy regimen, the patient states "I take this one labeled 'furosemide' every day in the morning along with this other one labeled 'Lasix.'"

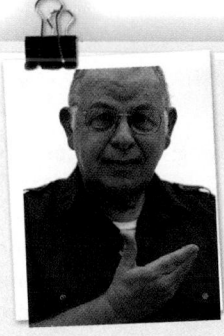

Nicholas Soros is a 68-year-old patient newly diagnosed with diabetes. His initial assessment revealed that he was about 50 pounds overweight due to poor diet and lack of exercise. A plan was developed to help Mr. Soros better manage his diabetes through planned weight reduction and regular exercise. At a follow-up visit, assessment reveals a weight gain of 5 pounds. He stated, "I'm too old to worry about diet and exercise. You can control my diabetes with medication, right?"

Focusing on Blended Skills

The types of blended skills you'll need to respond to the case scenarios include:

Cognitive Skills

- Knowledge of normal neonatal findings, diuretic therapy, and diabetes
- Knowledge of how to assess systematically and comprehensively to determine current health status
- Ability to incorporate knowledge of assessment, diagnosing, planning, and implementing nursing care when evaluating care for patients with different needs, such as neonate, elderly woman taking too much prescribed medication, or a newly diagnosed patient with diabetes having difficulty adapting to the treatment plan
- Knowledge of the principles of teaching and learning
- Knowledge of the nurse–patient relationship
- Knowledge of what information is needed to evaluate whether or not the plan of care is effectively meeting the patient's health needs (ability to measure how well the patient has achieved valued outcomes and to think critically about the factors contributing to patient success or failure)
- Knowledge of how to modify the plan of care, if indicated, or of how to remedy other variables interfering with the achievement of valued outcomes
- Knowledge of pertinent standards of care, and agency and institutional policies
- Ability to use critical thinking skills to evaluate a patient's plan of care effectively to meet the patient's needs
- Ability to identify factors affecting the adoption of healthy lifestyle practices, especially for the patient with diabetes

Technical Skills

- Ability to use diagnostic equipment to evaluate the patient's health status
- Ability to identify changes or adaptations in equipment and techniques necessary, based on the evaluation of outcome achievement for patients across the lifespan

- Ability to use a documentation system competently to record the patient's progress toward outcome achievement

Interpersonal Skills

- Ability to maintain a trusting nurse–patient relationship grounded in responsible caring with the neonate with a physical anomaly and his parents, an older adult woman taking too much prescribed medication, or a middle-aged man with diabetes and inadequate patterns of self-care
- Ability to communicate that you are more concerned about the patient's overall well-being than the isolated task of evaluating outcome achievement
- Demonstration of respect for a patient's human dignity when evaluating the plan of care
- Ability to work collaboratively with the healthcare team to address factors interfering with patient's ability to meet identified outcomes
- Ability to identify and to respond to the changing needs of patients experiencing different alterations in health status

Ethical and Legal Skills

- Ability to communicate respect for and to promote the patient's and family's sense of worth
- Commitment to evaluating patient achievement of outcomes in a timely fashion and to addressing whatever is interfering with outcome achievement within the scope of nursing practice
- Ability to serve as a trusted and effective patient advocate
- Demonstration of a strong sense of accountability to self, patient, the profession, and society
- Consistent use of appropriate legal safeguards when evaluating the plan of care, including documentation of the evaluation

Learning Objectives

After completing the chapter, the learner should be able to accomplish the following:

1. Describe evaluation, its purpose, and its relation to the other steps in the nursing process.
2. Evaluate the patient's achievement of outcomes specified in the plan of care.
3. Manipulate factors that contribute to the success or failure in outcome achievement.
4. Use the patient's response to the plan of care to modify the plan as needed.
5. Explain the relation between quality-assurance/quality-improvement programs and excellence in healthcare.
6. Value self-evaluation as a critical element in developing the ability to deliver quality nursing care.

Key Terms

concurrent evaluation
criteria
evaluating
evidence-based practice
nursing audit
outcome evaluation
peer review
performance improvement
process evaluation
quality-assurance program
quality improvement
retrospective evaluation
standards
structure evaluation

In the fifth step of the nursing process, **evaluating,** the nurse and patient together measure how well the patient has achieved the outcomes specified in the plan of care. When evaluating patient outcome achievement, the nurse identifies factors that contribute to the patient's ability to achieve expected outcomes and, when necessary, modifies the plan of care (Fig. 16-1). The purpose of evaluation is to allow the patient's achievement of expected outcomes to direct future nurse–patient interactions. Based on the patient's responses to the plan of care, the nurse decides to:

- Terminate the plan of care when each expected outcome is achieved
- Modify the plan of care if there are difficulties achieving the outcomes
- Continue the plan of care if more time is needed to achieve the outcomes

When evaluation points to the need to modify nursing care, the nurse reviews each preceding step of the nursing process (assessing, diagnosing, planning, and implementing). Successful evaluation enhances the public's image of nursing and helps ensure nursing's survival by promoting continued selection and funding of nursing services in the competitive healthcare market.

UNIQUE FOCUS OF NURSING EVALUATION

As members of the healthcare team, nurses are involved in many types of evaluation. Nurses measure patient outcome achievement; how effectively nurses help targeted groups of patients to achieve their specific outcomes; the competence of individual nurses; and the degree to which external factors, such as different types of healthcare services, specialized equipment or procedures, or socioeconomic factors, influence health and wellness. *The patient, however, is always the nurse's primary concern.* A nurse may perform a nursing procedure competently, creatively, and with care, but if this nursing intervention does not help the patient reach desired outcomes, it is not fully meaningful. Either directly or indirectly, the aim of all nursing evaluation is quality nursing care that aids patient outcome achievement. Therefore, the most important act of evaluation performed by nurses is evaluating outcome achievement with the patient (see the accompanying Reflective Practice box for an example).

The Institute of Medicine's Committee on Quality of Health Care in America is educating the public on what it is reasonable for patients to expect from their healthcare (Box 16-1). Even beginning nurses can use these guidelines to evaluate the care they are providing.

CRITICAL THINKING AND MEASURING PATIENT OUTCOME ACHIEVEMENT

The five classic elements of evaluation are (1) identifying evaluative criteria and standards (what you are looking for when you evaluate, eg, expected patient outcomes); (2) col

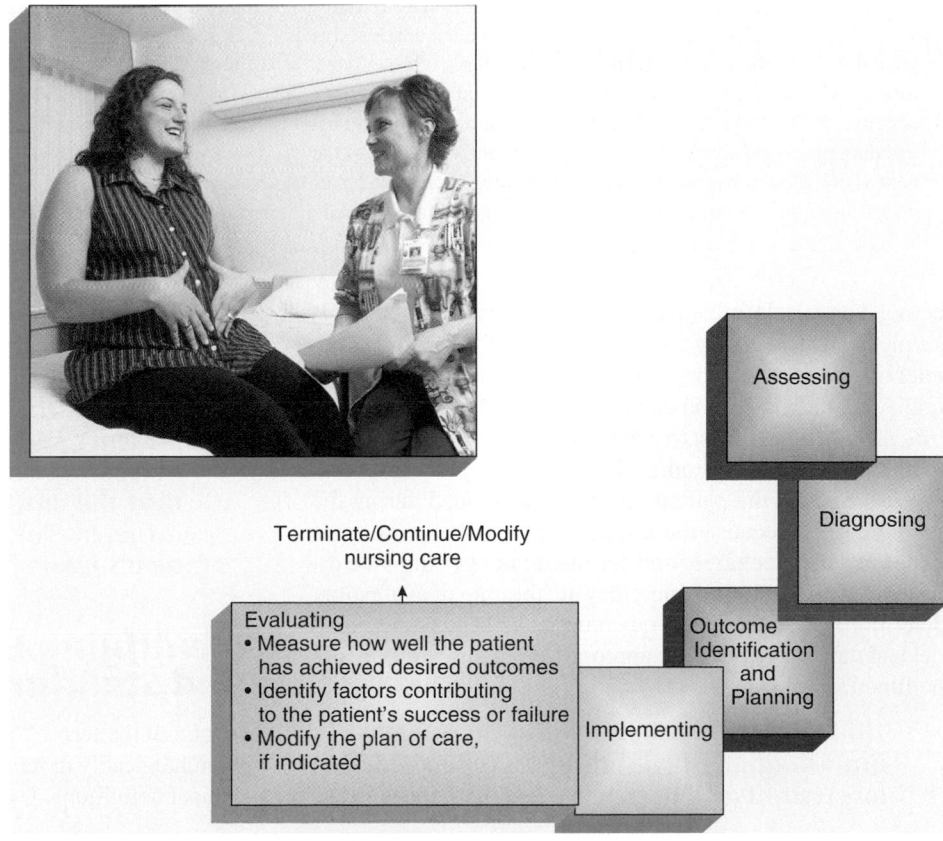

FIGURE 16-1 Evaluating. The nurse and patient together measure how well the patient has achieved the outcomes specified in the plan of care. Factors that contribute to the patient's success or failure are identified, and the plan of care is modified if necessary. Patient responses to the plan of care determine whether nursing care is to be continued as is, modified, or terminated. (Photo by Joe Mitchell.)

Terminate/Continue/Modify nursing care

Evaluating
- Measure how well the patient has achieved desired outcomes
- Identify factors contributing to the patient's success or failure
- Modify the plan of care, if indicated

Implementing

Outcome Identification and Planning

Diagnosing

Assessing

Reflective Practice
Challenge to Interpersonal Skills

I first met Mr. Nicholas Soros, a 68-year-old client newly diagnosed with diabetes, in the clinic. He was about 50 pounds overweight, and his health history revealed the need for major dietary changes and an exercise program. The interdisciplinary team devised a plan to help Mr. Soros better manage his diabetes through planned weight reduction and regular exercise, for which I did much of the initial teaching. Unfortunately, when Mr. Soros returned for his next check-up, he had gained 5 additional pounds and reported being "too old" to worry about diet and exercise. "You can control my diabetes with medication, right?" When I reported this to the nurse practitioner, he told me that Mr. Soros knows what to do and now it is his responsibility. I wasn't perfectly comfortable with this response and thought that Mr. Soros needed more than someone wagging a finger in his face.

Thinking Outside the Box: Alternate Courses of Action

- Remind Mr. Soros of what he needs to do and tell him that responsibility for this is his!
- After I make sure that he does indeed know what to do, spend time making sure that he values his health sufficiently to try these new behaviors.

- Make sure that Mr. Soros trusts us sufficiently to value working with us to achieve his health goals.

Evaluating a Good Outcome: How Do I Define Success?

- Mr. Soros achieves his target weight and is faithful to a program of regular exercise.
- Mr. Soros feels that his independence and ability to determine his own life plan are respected, at the same time feeling that we care about his health status.

- I learn more about developing a trusting nurse–patient relationship, exploring the relationship's role in helping patients to achieve valued health outcomes.

Personal Learning: Here's to the Future!

I learned something about myself and an important distinction between teaching and counseling. Clearly, just teaching Mr. Soros about diet and exercise wasn't sufficient. Mr. Soros was in no way going to change his lifestyle until he valued his health enough to make needed changes, including understanding why these changes were important. I also learned how important nurse–patient relationships are. When Mr. Soros came for his third visit, he asked the nurse who greeted him where I was, telling her "I want to see that nurse who cared about me!"—positive reinforcement for the relationship's importance.

Reflection

How do you think you would respond in a similar situation? Why? What does this tell you about yourself and about the adequacy of your skills for professional practice? Can you think of other ways to respond? Describe the type of teaching plan that the nursing student may have used at the initial teaching session. How might that teaching plan have changed based on the patient's response at the next visit? Would the outcomes identified initially need to be revised based on any changes in the teaching plan? Please explain why or why not. What other skills (cognitive, interpersonal, technical, ethical/legal) would you need to respond well in this situation? Classify these other skills as belonging to the cognitive, affective, or psychomotor domains. Do you agree with the criteria to evaluate a successful outcome?

Megan Kyle, Georgetown University

---

lecting data to determine whether these criteria and standards are met; (3) interpreting and summarizing findings; (4) documenting your judgment; and (5) terminating, continuing, or modifying the plan. Each element requires the nurse to *think critically* about how best to evaluate the patient's progress toward valued health outcomes. In the nursing process, evaluative criteria are the patient outcomes developed during the planning step. Because these reflect desired changes or outcomes in patient behavior and because nursing actions are directed toward these outcomes, they are the core of evaluation. Determining whether these outcomes have been or are being met and then identifying the appropriate nursing response are the functions of evaluation.

Think back to Nicholas Soros, the 68-year-old man diagnosed with diabetes who needed to lose weight and to exercise. The outcomes iden-

tified initially most likely focused on weight loss and adherence to an exercise program. Teaching at this initial visit also focused on ways to achieve these outcomes. However, the patient's statements and weight gain on his next clinic visit would lead the nurse to suspect that the outcomes identified were not being achieved. Therefore, some changes in the patient's plan of care are necessary.

Identifying Evaluative Criteria and Standards

Although the terms "criteria" and "standard" are often used interchangeably in reference to the evaluation step, they have distinct definitions. **Criteria** are measurable qualities, attrib-

BOX 16-1 What Patients Should Expect from Their Healthcare

1. **Beyond patient visits:** You will have the care you need when you need it . . . *whenever* you need it. You will find help in many forms, not just in face-to-face visits. You will find help on the internet, on the telephone, from many sources, by many routes, in the form you want it.

2. **Individualization:** You will be known and respected as an individual. Your choices and preferences will be sought and honored. The usual system of care will meet most of your needs. When your needs are special, the care will adapt to meet you on your own terms.

3. **Control:** The care system will take control only if and when you freely give permission.

4. **Information:** You can know what you wish to know, when you wish to know it. Your medical record is yours to keep, to read, and to understand. The rule is: "Nothing about you without you."

5. **Science:** You will have care based on the best available scientific knowledge. The system promises you excellence as its standard. Your care will not vary illogically from doctor to doctor or from place to place. The system will promise you all the care that can help you, and will help you avoid care that cannot help you.

6. **Safety:** Errors in care will not harm you. You will be safe in the care system.

7. **Transparency:** Your care will be confidential, but the care system will not keep secrets from you. You can know whatever you wish to know about the care that affects you and your loved ones.

8. **Anticipation:** Your care will anticipate your needs and will help you find the help you need. You will experience proactive help, not just reactions, to help you restore and maintain your health.

9. **Value:** Your care will not waste your time or money. You will benefit from constant innovations, which will increase the value of care to you.

10. **Cooperation:** Those who provide care will cooperate and coordinate their work fully with each other and with you. The walls between professions and institutions will crumble, so that your experiences will become seamless. You will never feel lost.

From The Institute of Medicine's Committee on Quality Health Care in America. (1999). *Measuring the quality of health care.* Washington, DC: National Academy Press.

BOX 16-2 Clinical Practice Guidelines and Evidence-Based Practice*

What are clinical practice guidelines (CPGs)? CPGs are recommendations for how care should be managed in specific diseases, problems, or situations (eg, how to best manage smoking cessation or neonate umbilical cord care). CPGs must be developed for specific use, and are best designed by a collaborative panel of clinical and scientific experts. When scientific evidence is sufficient, practice guidelines are obvious and clear. When scientific evidence is insufficient, other sources of knowledge—for example, wisdom gained from clinical experts or specific cases—must be brought to bear on the recommendations to fill in the gaps in the research evidence.

What are the best evidence-based practice (EBP) websites for updating practice standards?
The two best EBP resources are the Agency for Healthcare Research and Quality (AHRQ), found at http://www.ahrq.gov and the Cochrane Library, found at http://www.cochrane.org/resources/brochure.htm and http://www.update-software.com/cochrane/.

How do you best use the information on these websites?
AHRQ offers free access to evidence summaries and reports (on their home page, click on Evidence-Based Practice, then see listings under Evidence Reports). They also archive their old CPGs developed between 1992–1996. If you access archived CPGs, use the information only after updating them with the latest research on the topic.

The Cochrane Library produces systematic reviews, which give a single statement that summarizes the state of the science and draws on all research on a given topic. A systematic review is the strongest level of evidence for clinical decisions. Evidence summaries can be searched and located through the bibliographic database (such as CINAHL) by limiting results of the search to "publication type: systematic review." Full text summaries are available only through subscription (to subscribe, go to http://update-software.com/clibng/cliblogon.htm).

Evidence summaries and reports are the essence of EBP and hold promise for improving care, patient outcomes, and efficiency of healthcare. Moreover, EBP provides mechanisms for fulfilling our social responsibility to provide the best care in the most effective and affordable way.

*(Answers provided by Kathleen R. Stevens, RN, EdD, FAAN, Professor and Director, Academic Center for Evidence-Based Practice (ACE), The University of Texas Health Science Center at San Antonio. Phone 210-567-3135. Fax 210-567-5822. E-mail: acestar@uthscsa.edu).

Used with permission: Alfaro-LeFevre, R. (2004) *Critical thinking and clinical judgment: A practical approach* (3rd ed.). Philadelphia: W. B. Saunders.

utes, or characteristics that specify skills, knowledge, or health states. They describe acceptable levels of performance by stating the expected behaviors of the nurse or the patient. Chapter 14, Planning, describes how patient criteria are identified and formulated as patient outcomes.

Standards are the levels of performance accepted and expected by the nursing staff or other health-team members. They are established by authority, custom, or consent. A good ex-

ample of standards is the American Nurses Association's *Standards of Nursing Practice,* which are displayed in Chapter 1. Box 16-2 offers examples of websites to find clinical practice guidelines, a term used interchangeably with standards and protocols, all of which describe how care should be managed in certain situations. The goal is to design and deliver nursing care which evidence supports as likely to produce the expected patient outcomes, i.e., *evidence-based practice.*

Collecting Evaluative Data

The nurse collects evaluative data to determine whether or not the patient has met the desired outcomes. Whereas the nurse collects data in the nursing assessment to identify patient health problems, the data collected in the evaluation step are used to determine whether the identified health problems have been or are being resolved through outcome achievement.

> *Consider Mrs. Otsuki, the older adult woman who is inadvertently taking double the dose of prescribed diuretic. This initial assessment indicates a need for teaching. Thus, when evaluating outcome achievement for this patient, the nurse would determine whether the patient demonstrates understanding of her drug therapy regimen and is no longer taking two doses of the same drug.*

This section discusses (1) the different types of data collected to evaluate the achievement of different types of patient outcomes and (2) time criteria for data collection.

Types of Outcomes

The type of patient data collected to support the evaluation of outcome achievement is determined by the nature of the outcome. Samples of these outcomes are shown in Box 16-3: Evaluating Four Types of Outcomes in the Plan of Nursing Care. The data collected to determine the degree of outcome achievement are recorded in the corresponding evaluative statements.

Cognitive Outcomes

Cognitive outcomes involve increases in patient knowledge. These outcomes may be evaluated simply by asking patients to repeat information or, at a higher level of performance, by ask-

---

BOX 16-3 Evaluating Four Types of Outcomes in the Plan of Nursing Care

Nursing Diagnosis:

High Risk for Altered Parenting related to no previous experience in childrearing (fear)

Assessment Data:

Subjective: "My husband and I are both afraid we won't know what to do when we get the baby home."
Objective: Both parents are single children, report no childrearing experience; healthy newborn son delivered 2/4/06; first born

Strengths:

VIB (very important baby): parents are both 38; history of infertility with one miscarriage; strong motivation to learn and use good parenting skills; strong support network

Expected Outcomes	Nursing Interventions	Evaluative Statement (Actual Outcomes)
Psychomotor outcomes: Before discharge, parents will demonstrate confidence in: • Holding baby • Diapering, dressing baby • Bathing baby • Feeding baby	Assess both parents' knowledge of childrearing practices; identify and reinforce motivation to learn; correct any misinformation. Develop and implement at a time convenient for both parents a teaching plan to include: • The primary nurse role-modeling techniques for comfortably and safely holding, talking to, and dressing baby • Parents independently viewing videocassettes on: Baby care Baby bath Breastfeeding Followed by one-on-one discussion • Class for new parents: nurse to demonstrate baby bath and discuss general principles of care • Primary nurse observing mother and infant during initial feeding sessions and offering teaching and support as necessary	2/6/06 Outcome partially met. Both parents have correctly demonstrated safe techniques for holding, dressing, and bathing the baby. Mother is still concerned baby is not getting enough milk. *Revision:* Continue to spend time with mother and infant during feeding— provide positive reinforcement. *F. Morales, RN*

BOX 16-3 (Continued)

Expected Outcomes	Nursing Interventions	Evaluative Statement (Actual Outcomes)
Cognitive outcomes: By 2/6/06, parents will report appropriate action to be taken if questions or problems arise after discharge: • Name and number of primary nurse • Name and number of pediatrician • La Leche League contact and number	Answer parents' questions and address related concerns. Assess parents' knowledge of infant problems frequently encountered by new parents. Inform parents of available community resources and describe appropriate action to take if questions or problems arise.	2/6/06 Outcome met. Parents discussed some infant problems related to feeding, elimination, and illness and reported appropriate community resource to contact. *F. Morales, RN*
Affective outcome: Before discharge, parents will verbalize decreased anxiety in regard to caring for son.	Assess parents' level of anxiety and potential negative effects on child-rearing. Discuss this with parents. Explore adequacy of parents' coping strategies—increased knowledge, practice in supportive environment, community resources. Counsel as necessary. Compliment parents on new parenting skills. Allow for ventilation of anxiety or specific fears. Respond with teaching or emotional support as necessary.	2/6/06 Outcome partially met. Except for concern about breastfeeding, *both* parents expressed feeling comfortable and eager to care for their son at home. *F. Morales, RN*
Physiologic outcomes: At 1-month postpartal telephone interview, 3/4/06 (by parents' report), the baby will demonstrate adequate: • Weight gain (birth weight, 7 lb 6 oz) • Sleep–wakefulness patterns • Comfort level indicating adequate parenting.	Use a 1-month postdelivery telephone interview to assess the adequacy of parenting skills. With positive report of growth and development, compliment (reinforce) the parents. With negative report, teach or counsel and refer as appropriate.	3/4/06 Outcome met. Parents' report of baby's weight gain and behavior indicates good parenting skills. *F. Morales, RN*

ing patients to apply the new knowledge to their everyday situations. For example, asking patients to describe new dietary restrictions is different from asking them to plan a weekly menu compatible with these restrictions.

Psychomotor Outcomes
Psychomotor outcomes describe the patient's achievement of new skills; they are evaluated by asking the patient to demonstrate the new skill.

Affective Outcomes
Affective outcomes pertain to changes in patient values, beliefs, and attitudes and are more complex to evaluate. Observation of patient behavior and conversation can determine whether affective outcomes have been achieved.

Physiologic Outcomes
In the final type of outcome statement, physiologic outcomes, physical changes in the patient are the targeted outcome. To evaluate achievement of this type of outcome, the nurse uses physical assessment skills to collect relevant data and compares these with previous patient data.

Remember Tyler Jameson, the neonate who has not passed any stool due to the lack of a patent anus? The nurse would develop a physiologic outcome focusing on bowel elimination and the passage of stool.

Time Criteria
In addition to knowing what type of data to collect to determine outcome achievement, it is important to know when to collect the data. When the patient outcomes were developed, a time frame was established for determining whether the specified changes have been achieved. At the designated time, the nurse, in collaboration with the patient, the family, and other members of the nursing team, evaluates the patient's attainment of the outcome. If outcomes are developed in observable and measurable terms, the task of collecting data for evaluation is clearcut. Examples of three types of time criteria follow:
• By 7/8/06, the patient will walk the length of hallway with support of walker.

- Beginning 7/8/06, the patient will demonstrate a weight loss of 3 lb per month until target weight (135 lb) is achieved (6/8/06, weight: 151 lb).
- Before discharge, parents will correctly demonstrate chest physiotherapy procedures for patient.

It is important for nurses to evaluate patient outcome achievement as early as possible. Celebrating outcome attainment with the patient usually helps encourage the patient and leads to further outcome achievement. When failure to meet designated outcomes is detected early, the plan of care can be modified to remedy the failure.

> *Think back to Nicholas Soros, the 68-year-old patient with diabetes. By recognizing the lack of outcome achievement on the next visit, the nurse can gather additional data to revise the plan of care. For example, perhaps Mr. Soros did not completely understand the teaching that was presented. Or, he may have had difficulty accepting his diagnosis, thereby interfering with his ability to comply with the plan, ultimately leading to weight gain instead of a weight loss.*

The most common mistake nurses make when evaluating in acute care settings is waiting until the day the patient is to be discharged before evaluating outcome achievement. At that point, it is too late to revise the plan of care.

Interpreting and Summarizing Findings

Before the nurse can make a judgment about the patient's achievement of outcomes, it is necessary to study and interpret the data collected. Just as clusters of data are interpreted before the nurse identifies and validates a nursing diagnosis, so too does evaluative data need to be interpreted. For example, a patient who is expected to walk the length of the hallway with support of a walker asks to be taken back to her room because she feels weak. The nurse must gather more data and then determine if this is a one-time incident linked to medications or a temporary metabolic imbalance, or if it signals a consistent inability to achieve this behavior. Interpreting evaluative data requires critical thinking and is a skill that must be practiced.

When interpreting and summarizing findings, it is important to consider factors that influence outcome achievement. Numerous patient, nurse, and healthcare system variables contribute positively or negatively to patient outcome achievement. Identifying these variables allows the nurse to reinforce positive factors by drawing on them in the future, as well as to deal with other variables that are creating problems. The more sensitive and responsive nurses are to these variables, the more rewarding their practices will be.

Examples of positive factors include a patient's strong motivation to learn new health behaviors, a nurse who comes to work well rested and with a new care idea learned from a nursing journal, and a healthcare institution or agency that offers incentives for quality nursing and has an optimal nurse-to-patient ratio.

When the nurse understands what factors are helpful to the patient who is trying to reach desired outcomes, she or he can often manipulate these factors. For example, if a patient is learning to ambulate independently after hip surgery and you notice that he seems to make his best effort when his wife is present, mention this to her and plan to ambulate the patient at least once a day when she is present. Conversely, if a patient seems more fearful when his wife is present, note in the plan of care that ambulation is best attempted when the patient's wife is not on the unit. Ideally, this fear would be explored with the patient before discharge, so that he can continue to make progress when he is discharged home with his wife.

Table 16-1 presents common variables that can negatively influence patient outcome achievement. Tentative nursing approaches are suggested. Nurses need to think critically about the effects of these variables and respond creatively to them.

Documenting Your Judgment

After the data have been collected and interpreted to determine patient outcome achievement, the nurse makes and documents a judgment summarizing the findings. This is termed the evaluative statement. The two-part evaluative statement includes a decision about how well the outcome was met, along with patient data or behaviors that support this decision. The nurse has three decision options for how outcomes have been met: met, partially met, or not met.

- 1/21/06—Outcome met. Patient reports 1 week of no tobacco use. C. Taylor, RN
- 1/21/06—Outcome partially met. Patient reports decreasing tobacco use from one pack per day to 4 to 6 cigarettes per day. C. Taylor, RN
- 1/21/06—Outcome not met. Patient reports no change in tobacco use. Revision: Reexplore patient's commitment to try tobacco-use control strategies and adequacy of personal support systems to eliminate tobacco use. C. Taylor, RN

The nurse signs and dates the evaluative statement (see Box 16-3). Alternatively, the nurse follows the documentation guidelines for evaluating outcome achievement specified in the institution's computerized documentation systems.

Modifying the Plan of Care

When evaluation reveals that the patient has made little or no progress toward outcome achievement, the nurse needs to reevaluate each preceding step of the nursing process to try to identify the contributing factors pointing to problems with the plan of care. New assessment data might need to be collected, diagnoses may be added or altered, outcomes might need to be modified or rewritten, nursing orders may be changed, or evaluation may be targeted more frequently.

> *Remember Tyler Jameson, the neonate who has not passed any stool after 30 hours? The initial outcome may have stated that the neonate would pass stool within 18 to 24 hours after birth. However, this outcome was developed*

TABLE 16-1 Patient, Nurse, and Healthcare System Variables That May Detract From Quality Nursing Care

Variables	Possible Solution
Patient Variables	
Patient who is physically and cognitively capable of self-care gives up—refuses to cooperate with therapeutic regimen or thwarts the regimen	Identify one nurse who is able to develop a trusting relationship with the patient and determine the reason underlying the observed behavior: • No longer finds meaning and purpose in life • Overwhelming sense of powerlessness • Previous history of being "hurt," "exploited," "cheated" by the healthcare system • Inability to accept illness and related life-style changes Counsel appropriately. Use a team conference to develop a consistent plan of nursing care.
Patient who quietly accepts whatever is done or not done for him or her; seldom communicates needs or dissatisfaction	Note on the plan of care the need to assess this patient thoroughly because the patient will probably not advocate for himself or herself. Educate the patient to become a more assertive healthcare consumer.
Nurse Variables	
Nurse who sincerely desires to give 150% all the time and who becomes quickly frustrated when observing substandard care; may feel alienated from other staff; excellent candidate for burnout	Learn to give quality care during designated work period; leave on time; avoid the temptation to do the work of others; leave work concerns at work. After establishing a reputation for delivering quality nursing care, seek creative solutions for nursing problems (strategies to increase nursing resources, motivation, morale) and try them—hopefully with a support network. View concerns as challenges rather than overwhelming obstacles. Develop a realistic sense of how much nursing care and of what quality can be delivered with existing resources. If resources do not permit quality care, explore change strategies within the institution. If administration is not supportive, explore other practice settings.
Nurse with overwhelming outside concerns: • Preparation for marriage, childbirth, divorce • Illness (self or family members) • Role conflict (familial roles, school, work, and so forth) • New apartment, house	During periods of peak demand, may need to accept less than optimal performance at work. If this becomes the norm rather than the exception, carefully evaluate priorities. May need to cut work hours rather than "cheat" patients.
Nurse who is bored	After reflection, write down *personal* objectives related to work. Explore avenues within work setting for professional growth and development: initiate changes in nursing unit to improve patient care and to stimulate peer development; join institutional committees; participate actively in staff development programs; develop patient and family support groups. Look for new position that offers new challenges within or outside the institution. Join professional organizations and participate actively. Evaluate educational goals and explore possibilities—continuing education programs and degree work.
Healthcare System Variables	
Inadequate staffing	Develop and use a patient classification system that incorporates an identification of the kind and amount of nursing services required. Record staffing patterns and relate to needs for nursing care and patient outcomes. Clearly demonstrate and document that adequate staffing makes a difference. Present these data to nursing administration with the request for additional staff. If necessary, use professional bargaining unit.
Nursing administration has sold out nursing; insensitivity to nursing demands within the institution	It may be impossible to practice quality, progressive nursing in this environment. If there seems to be no hope for change after appropriate channels have been explored, look for a new practice setting. Evaluate the new setting on the basis of what experience has taught you.

based on data that was inaccurate. Therefore, the nurse, learning of the new data, would revise the outcome to correlate with the neonate's condition, dependent on the treatment to correct the anomaly.

Review the checklist for help in evaluating your use of the nursing process in Chapter 11. Table 16-2 suggests appropriate nursing responses to common problems encountered during evaluation.

When the nurse has identified the factors contributing to the outcomes not being achieved, the evaluative statement can be used to suggest the necessary revision in the plan of care: (1) delete or modify the nursing diagnosis, (2) make the outcome statement more realistic, (3) increase the complexity of the outcome statement, (4) adjust time criteria in outcome statement, or (5) change the nursing intervention. Increasing the complexity of a outcome after it has been achieved facilitates optimal function. For example, the initial outcome for a patient with the diagnosis "Impaired Physical Mobility" might be "patient transfers from the bed to the chair." After this is achieved, however, the outcome needs to be stepped up in complexity to "patient walks around room with support of walker."

TABLE 16-2 Common Problems Noted During Evaluation of the Nursing Process

Problem	Nursing Response
Assessing	
1. Inaccurate database → inaccurate nursing diagnoses and a distorted plan of care	1. a. Identify the patient or nurse variables responsible for inaccuracy. b. Revise the recorded database.
2. Database does not reflect changes in patient condition.	2. Review with the *entire* nursing staff the importance of making assessment a priority in every patient interaction as well as the recording of the new data obtained.
3. Database is superficial: · Fails to communicate uniqueness of patient · Lacks sufficient detail on major problems or developments	3. a. Rethink the critical relation between an adequate database and quality care. b. Develop interviewing and physical assessment skills. c. Begin to identify the key data that need to be collected for specific nursing diagnosis and medical diagnosis and to assess patient response to therapeutic regimen (use of a nursing diagnosis handbook may be helpful).
Diagnosing	
1. General sense that nursing diagnoses are "common sense" and therefore do not need to be put in writing → failure to address patient's real problems	1. Carefully develop and record priority nursing diagnoses for several patients and fairly evaluate whether this makes a difference in terms of the continuity of quality care.
2. General sense that nurses are too busy doing treatments, "passing meds," and doing paperwork to develop nursing diagnoses carefully → independent dimension of nursing remains underdeveloped	2. Examine practice and see whether *independent* nursing has a place; what percentage of every day is devoted to independent nursing functions? If this percentage is nonexistent or small, there understandably may be *no felt need* for nursing diagnoses—but a desperate need to revise practice priorities.
3. Nursing diagnoses are too vague to be helpful → routinized patient care	3. a. Revise the problem statement to describe more accurately what is *unhealthy* about the patient (the behavior that needs to be changed). b. Revise the etiology to more accurately identify what is making the problem a problem—this should be a guide to nursing intervention. c. Check NANDA lists.
4. Nursing diagnoses are not up to date → no one uses the plan of care	4. Have a process for periodically reviewing the plan of care to delete nursing diagnoses when problems have been resolved and to add a new diagnosis as needed.
Planning	
1. The plan of care contains only the standard knowledge most nurses would know without a written plan.	1. Make use of standardized (computerized) plans as a basis for care planning. Devote nursing energies to *individualizing* this plan.

TABLE 16-2 (Continued)

Problem	Nursing Response
2. The long-term goal is vague, standard; fails to make clear the discharge goal for this patient.	2. Practice writing specific long-term goals that clarify for all nurses the aim toward which all nursing care is directed (eg, patient returns home ambulatory with walker, right hip incision healing, able to manage activities of daily living with minimal assistance from spouse).
3. The nursing outcomes, even if met, do not necessarily guarantee a resolution of the patient problem.	3. When writing goals, it often is helpful to develop outcomes related to etiologic factors. Because the stated etiology may be incomplete or inaccurate, it is essential that at least *one outcome* be written so that if it is achieved, the problem in the nursing diagnosis is resolved.
4. The outcomes are incorrectly developed; progress toward goal achievement is difficult to evaluate	4. After writing outcomes, check them against the following criteria: • Subject is the patient or some part of the patient. • The patient behavior is stated in observable, measurable terms. • Criteria of acceptable performance are specified. • Time criteria are included in notes.
5. Nursing orders are superficial → patient receives routinized care	5. Review nursing orders to ensure that they indicate the *specific* nursing strategies or interventions most likely to result in successful outcome achievement *for this patient* (eg, particular comfort measures that are successful adjuncts to analgesic administration for a particular patient. In specifying the "who, what, when, where, how, and how much" of nursing interventions, be sure to list the type of equipment and supplies needed in various treatments. As new patient data are obtained, update nursing orders. Delete inappropriate or unnecessary orders.
6. The initial plan of care fails to be updated → plan of care will not be consulted by nurses—if used, it will be to patient's detriment	6. If personal accountability for updating plan fails, develop a process on the nursing unit to ensure care plan review and revision.
7. The plan of care addresses the immediate needs of the patient but fails to anticipate discharge needs → patient returns home unable to manage self-care activities	7. Work hard at developing the ability to project yourself into the patient's home after discharge. Learn to anticipate problems and concerns and prepare the patient and family for these. Use all discharge resources in the institution. Learn from patients what their needs were after previous discharge.

Implementing

Problem	Nursing Response
1. Nurses are not aware of patient priorities and the plan of care; lack of continuity; inefficient use of nursing resources → patient fails to achieve goals/outcomes	1. a. Use shift report to update staff on status of priority nursing diagnosis and concomitant nursing care. b. Review plan of care and nursing notes before beginning care.
2. Nursing care becomes routine and mechanized → patient never has the sense that he or she is personally known by nurses	2. Explore creative strategies to make quality nursing care on this particular unit a *challenge* rather than a *burden;* use ongoing education, problem-solving strategies by the nursing team, gaming, and other incentives.
3. Documentation is inadequate → because there is no complete written record of nursing care, *legally* this care was never provided.	3. a. Develop the philosophy that quality nursing care *deserves* to be documented. Review legal reasons for careful documentation. b. Become familiar with the flow sheets and note format used within the work setting so that charting can be done quickly and comprehensively.

Evaluating

Problem	Nursing Response
1. It is not done → mastery of nursing process is stunted; severely limits accomplishment of nursing aims.	1. Develop the belief that quality nursing care does not happen automatically and that only ongoing evaluation will identify needed areas of revision. Devise an evaluative strategy and carry it out. Study its effect on quality of care after 6 months' implementation.

The following evaluative statement might be noted, for example, if a patient did not meet the specified outcome: "Patient will participate in a minimum of two planned social activities per week beginning 9/16/06." "9/27/06—Outcome not met. Resident chose not to participate in any group activities this week." Many courses of action are then available to the nurse. Possible revisions to any plan of care include the following:

- *Delete or modify the nursing diagnosis.* This might not be a problem or concern for the resident. Evaluate and validate data pointing to the nursing diagnosis.
- *Make the outcome statement more realistic.* Carefully determine the resident's need for activities and ability or desire to participate in activities.
- *Adjust time criteria in outcome statement.* Reevaluate after 3 weeks; resident may need more time to adjust to being institutionalized and more encouragement.
- *Change nursing interventions.* Make a special effort to familiarize yourself with the resident's interests, and match these with available programs and activities.

Once the nurse, in partnership with the patient if possible, makes a decision about how to respond, this must be communicated to the patient or the patient's surrogate and to other members of the professional caregiving team via the patient's record.

> *Think back to Mioshi Otsuki, the elderly woman taking too much diuretic. The home care nurse would work with the patient to develop a teaching plan about her heart failure, specifically related to her drug-therapy regimen. This plan then would be documented on the patient's record and communicated to all individuals involved in the patient's care, such as other home care agency nurses who may be on-call or filling in to visit the patient or home health aides involved in providing personal care and hygiene for the patient.*

EVALUATING QUALITY NURSING CARE

In addition to each nurse's evaluation of patient outcome achievement and subsequent modifications to the plan of care, many informal and formal mechanisms are used to ensure quality nursing care.

Performance Improvement in Everyday Clinical Practice

It is not unusual for nurses to discover problems with the delivery of nursing care in their practice setting. The Institute of Medicine's Committee on Quality of Health Care in America (Kohn, Corrigan & Donaldson, 2003) suggests 10 new rules to redesign and improve care:

1. Care based on continuous healing relationships
2. Customization based on patient needs and values
3. The patient as the source of control
4. Shared knowledge and the free flow of information
5. Evidence-based decision making
6. Safety as a system property
7. The need for transparency
8. Anticipation of needs
9. Continuous decrease in waste
10. Cooperation among clinicians

Each nurse must decide how to respond when it is perceived that patient care is being compromised. Nurses committed to healthier patients, quality care, reduced costs, and the personal satisfaction of knowing that they *are actually making a difference* versus merely *wishing things were different* value **performance improvement.** The following four steps are crucial in improving performance (Haase & Miller, 1999):

- Discover a problem.
- Plan a strategy using indicators.
- Implement a change.
- Assess the change; if the outcome is not met, plan a new strategy.

See Box 16-4: Steps in Performance Improvement for an example of a performance-improvement strategy.

Peer review, the evaluation of one staff member by another staff member on the same level in the hierarchy of the organization, is an important mechanism nurses can use to improve their professional performance. This can be done formally or informally by inviting a peer you respect to give you feedback on nursing skills you are trying to develop. "How do you think that session went with the patient's daughter? She's been so critical of us and I'm trying to understand the situation from her point of view and respond appropriately."

Evaluative Programs

In the United States, regulatory agencies, such as state boards of nursing, the Joint Commission on Accreditation of Healthcare Organizations (JCAHO), the Professional Standards Review Organization, and the National Health Planning and Resources Development Act of 1975, require nurses to document that nursing standards are being implemented and maintained. Each of these agencies is concerned with quality care and quality control. The decreased availability of resources to treat patients in hospitals and the unavailability of sufficient alternative treatment settings pose a strong challenge to the nursing profession to find ways to avoid compromising quality of care. Numerous professional organizations are working to meet this challenge (Box 16-5: National Quality Initiatives; Box 16-6: Selected Web Resources for Patients and Families).

Quality Assurance

Specially designed programs that promote excellence in nursing are called **quality-assurance programs.** These range from small programs conducted by nurses on a small nursing unit to those developed for an entire institution, state, province, or country.

Quality-assurance programs enable nursing to be accountable to society for the quality of nursing care. Such programs

BOX 16-4 Steps in Performance Improvement

The following four steps are crucial in improving performance:

- **Discover a problem**

  Advance directives are a powerful legal tool for people to indicate their end-of-life care preferences. Nurses on an oncology unit are becoming frustrated because many of the patients on their unit lack advance directives. By the time decisions need to be made about ventilators, coding, dialysis, and so forth, patients are often no longer able to communicate their preferences. The hospital has a policy about advance directives, but no one seems to be taking responsibility for initiating discussions with patients when they are first admitted.

- **Plan a strategy using indicators**

  The nurses call an interdisciplinary meeting with the oncologists, social workers, and pastors, who decide that the nurse case manager will be responsible for working with patients on admission to see if they want help in preparing an advance

directive. Each case manager will be responsible for documenting within 48 hours of admission the patient's decision regarding an advance directive. Staff nurses will be able to direct patient and family requests to do advance planning to the case manager and appropriate team members. The ethics committee was asked to do an inservice on advance directives for the team.

- **Implement a change**

  Case managers begin assuming this responsibility, and one nurse volunteers to monitor progress at 3-month intervals by checking charts for advance directive content and by speaking with the staff nurses who voiced the initial frustration about decision making.

- **Assess the change;** if the goal is not met, plan a new strategy

  At the end of 6 months, everyone seems satisfied that the new plan is working, but a decision is made to a 6-month follow-up evaluation to prevent backsliding.

Four-step process from Haase, R., & Miller, K. (1999). Performance improvement in everyday clinical practice. *American Journal of Nursing, 99*(5), 52, 54.

BOX 16-5 National Quality Initiatives

Organization	Initiative	Description
JCAHO (Joint Commission on Accreditation of Healthcare Organizations) Regulatory accreditation (private) http://www.jcaho.org/pms/index.htm	ORYX	Integrates use of outcomes and performance measures into accreditation process; requires accredited hospitals and long-term care agencies to identify two clinical measures related to at least 20% of patient population; number of measures and percentage of patient population will increase each year.
NCQA (National Committee for Quality Assurance) Accrediting body for managed care http://www.ncqa.org	HEDIS (Health Plan Employer Data and Information Set)	HEDIS targets these areas: effectiveness of care, access and availability of care, patient satisfaction, health plan stability, use of services, costs, and health plan descriptive information. Quality Compass reports (available on CD-ROM/electronic data file) include performance data on managed care plans.
ANA (American Nurses Association) Voluntary http://www.nursingworld.org/readroom/fssafety.htm	Nursing Report Card for Acute Care Settings	Indicators and measurement tools for evaluating quality of nursing care in acute care settings. The three categories of indicators are structure, process, and outcomes. Outcome indicators include nosocomial infection rate; patient injury rate; and patient satisfaction with nursing care, pain management, educational information, and care during hospitalization.
Centers for Medicine and Medicaid Services http://www.cms.hhs.gov/oasis/default.asp	OASIS (Outcome and Assessment Information Set)	Set of assessment questions to collect clinical, financial, and administrative data in home health agencies. Goals of OASIS: to improve quality of care delivered to home health care patients and to provide data to HCFA.
FACCT (Foundation for Accountability) Voluntary http://www.facct.org		Aims to improve information available to consumers when choosing health plan, provider, hospital, and treatment. Has designed outcomes-based performance measures for a number of clinical conditions, such as asthma, breast cancer, diabetes, and major depressive disorder, and for health plan satisfaction.

Oermann, M. H., & Huber, D. (1999). Patient outcomes: A measure of nursing's value. *American Journal of Nursing, 99*(9), 40–48.

BOX 16-6 **Selected Web Resources for Patients and Families**

Organization	Internet Address	Available Information
Agency for Health Care Policy and Research (AHCPR)	http://www.ahcpr.gov	Website includes links to health information for consumers.
	http://www.ahcpr.gov/consumer	Healthfinder is a gateway for health information with many links. Consumer versions of clinical practice guidelines by condition available at site.
	http://www.ahcpr.gov/consumer/hlthpln1.htm	Consumer guide for choosing and using a health plan
	http://www.ahcpr.gov/consumer/qualguid.pdf	"Your Guide to Choosing Quality Health Care" is a comprehensive consumer reference for choosing health plans, physicians, treatments, hospitals, and long-term care (PDF file).
	http://www.ahcpr.gov/consumer/quick.htm	"Quick Checks for Quality" is a short guide for determining quality in health care.
Foundation for Accountability (FACCT)	http://www.facct.org	Foundation to help the public understand healthcare quality and make informed decisions about care
	http://www.facct.org/facct/site/facct/facct/measures/	Provides quality measures for selected clinical conditions, such as asthma, breast cancer, diabetes, and depression
Joint Commission on Accreditation of Healthcare Organizations (JCAHO)	http://www.jcaho.org	General public menu includes information about reporting a complaint about a healthcare organization, making healthcare choices, and performance measurement.
	http://www.jcaho.org/qualitycheck/directry/directry.asp	With Quality Check, consumers can retrieve information about how Joint Commission-accredited organizations have been rated in areas such as patient rights, infection control, and others.
National Committee for Quality Assurance (NCQA)	http://www.ncqa.org/programs/qsg/reportcards.htm	NCQA Consumer Page includes links to information on healthcare organizations. Consumers can search NCQA's accreditation status list and see if their health plan has an accreditation summary report.
	http://www.ncqa.org/pages/communications/publications/	Guide for consumers in choosing a health plan

Oermann, M. H., & Huber, D. (1999). Patient outcomes: A measure of nursing's value. *American Journal of Nursing, 99*(9), 40–48.

---

are also a response to the public mandate for professional accountability. They ensure survival of the profession, encourage nursing's fidelity to its moral and ethical responsibilities, and assist nursing to comply with other external pressures.

There are two different approaches to ensuring quality. *Quality by inspection* focuses on finding deficient workers and removing them. Nurses and others working in this type of setting may be afraid to admit a mistake or error and wrongly attempt to hide a problem. Such behavior is never acceptable and may result in serious harm to patients. *Quality as opportunity,* on the other hand, focuses on finding opportunities for improvement and fosters an environment that thrives on teamwork, with people sharing the skills and lessons they have learned. Mistakes are viewed not as being caused by a lack of motivation or lack of effort by a worker but rather as a result of a problem in the system. In this work environment, nurses respond with openness and a desire to learn because their in-

tegrity and self-worth are not threatened. Our outcome should be to work in an environment in which quality measurements encourage our best efforts.

The American Nurses Association (ANA) in 1975 developed a model quality-assurance program consisting of seven steps: (1) identify values; (2) identify structure, process, and outcome standards and criteria; (3) measure the degree of attainment of criteria and standards; (4) make interpretations about strengths and weaknesses based on such measurements; (5) identify possible courses of action; (6) choose a course of action; and (7) take action. The ANA hoped the model would be used to develop and implement quality-assurance programs within institutions.

The ANA model directs attention to three essential components of quality care: structure, process, and outcome. Other types of quality-assurance programs may focus only on one of these components or on a mixture of components.

Structure

A **structure evaluation** or audit focuses on the environment in which care is provided. Standards describe physical facilities and equipment; organizational characteristics, policies, and procedures; fiscal resources; and personnel resources.

Process

The focus of the **process evaluation** is the nature and sequence of activities carried out by nurses implementing the nursing process. Criteria make explicit acceptable levels of performance for nursing actions related to patient assessment, diagnosis, planning, implementation, and evaluation.

Outcome

Outcome evaluation focuses on measurable changes in the health status of the patient or the end results of nursing care. Whereas the proper environment for care and the right nursing actions are important aspects of quality care, the critical element in evaluating care is demonstrable changes in patient health status.

From Quality Assurance to Quality Improvement

Concern about the spiraling costs of healthcare, coupled with the success of industrial models for quality improvement, led to a strong commitment to quality improvement in the 1990s. **Quality improvement** (also known as continuous quality improvement [CQI] or total quality management [TQM]) is "the commitment and approach used to continuously improve every process in every part of an organization, with the intent of meeting and exceeding customer expectations and outcomes" (Schroeder, 1994, p. 3). Unlike quality assurance, quality improvement is internally driven, focuses on patient care rather than organizational structure, focuses on processes rather than individuals, and has no end points. Its outcome is *improving* quality rather than *assuring* quality. The major premises of quality improvement are as follows (Schroeder, 1994, pp. 5–8):

- Focus on organizational mission
- Continuous improvement
- Customer orientation
- Leadership commitment
- Empowerment
- Collaboration/crossing boundaries
- Focus on process
- Focus on data and statistical thinking

From the patient's point of view, one of the most important outcomes of quality improvement is the recognition that patient satisfaction is as important as customer satisfaction in retail business. With increased competition for the healthcare dollar, providers are learning that it is important to offer services that patients value and to offer them in a way that is valued by patients. By reemphasizing the critical nature of nursing's *person* versus *task* orientation, quality improvement underscores the need for nurses to blend cognitive, technical, interpersonal, and ethical/legal skills successfully.

Nursing Audit

A **nursing audit** is a method of evaluating nursing care that involves reviewing patient records to assess the outcomes of nursing care or the process by which these outcomes were achieved. Successful nursing audits depend on careful nursing documentation.

Concurrent Versus Retrospective

Nursing care and patient outcomes may be evaluated while the patient is receiving care (ie, a concurrent evaluation) or after the patient has been discharged (ie, a retrospective evaluation). **Concurrent evaluation** is conducted by using direct observation of nursing care, patient interviews, and chart review to determine whether the specified evaluative criteria are met.

Retrospective evaluation may use postdischarge questionnaires, patient interviews (by telephone or face to face), or chart review (nursing audit) to collect data. The type of retrospective audit most familiar to nurses working in hospitals is the JCAHO retrospective chart review. This accrediting body initially required hospitals to conduct a certain number of audits per year.

SUMMARY

The cultivation of evaluation as a critical component of the nursing process ensures nursing's continued success in achieving desired changes in patient health status.

> *Recall Nicholas Soros, the patient described in the Reflective Practice display. The nurse's commitment to teaching and follow-up demonstrates concern for the patient and his needs. Success would be possible only if the nurse modifies the plan, works with the patient, and realizes the need for the patient to value his own health while respecting his independence and individuality.*

Only a firm commitment to evaluation enables nurses to answer the following questions:

- What are the patient's outcomes?
- What are nursing's values?
- How can these values be formalized in standards and evaluative criteria?
- What data exist to determine whether the specified evaluative criteria are being met?
- How can these data best be collected, analyzed, and interpreted?
- To what courses of action do the findings lead?

Nursing actions are far too valuable and costly resources to be haphazardly implemented. Evaluation that is carefully planned and executed can direct and redirect these actions to maximize the patient's benefit. This is the outcome and challenge of nursing evaluation. Criteria that might be helpful in determining the adequacy of the evaluation step of the nursing process include the following:

- Evaluation of the patient's achievement of desired outcomes
- Review of how the process is used and revision of the plan of care if necessary
- Participation in quality-assurance programs

Developing Critical Thinking Skills

1. Interview five students who have personal fitness outcomes. Ask them to describe what personal factors have helped or hindered their achieving their outcomes. Note commonalities and differences. Reflect on how you can help patients tap their own personal strengths to achieve their outcomes more successfully.
2. Interview several patients and ask them what qualities in a nurse are most helpful as they try to achieve their health outcomes. Similarly, ask what nurse qualities are most problematic. Reflect on how you measure up in terms of both positive and negative nurse qualities.
3. Interview three or more experienced nurses in the same practice setting. Ask them what system variables (such as philosophy of care, nurse-to-patient ratio, professional and nonprofessional staff mix, nursing management, adequacy of resources) most influence their ability to deliver quality care. Identify variables you want to look for when you interview for a job.

Practicing for NCLEX

1. Jeanne is a college student who wants to lose 20 pounds. She meets with the student health nurse and develops a plan to increase her activity level and decrease the consumption of the wrong types of foods and excess calories. The nurse plans to evaluate her weight loss monthly. When Jeanne arrives for her first "weigh-in," the nurse discovers that instead of the projected weight loss of 5 pounds, Jeanne has only lost 1 pound. Which is the best nursing response?
   a. Congratulate Jeanne and continue the plan of care.
   b. Terminate the plan of care since it is not working.
   c. Try giving Jeanne more time to reach the targeted outcome.
   d. Modify the plan of care after discussing possible reasons for Jeanne's partial success.
2. The following are all classic elements of evaluation. Which item below places them in their correct sequence?
   (1) Interpreting and summarizing findings
   (2) Collecting data to determine whether evaluative criteria and standards are met
   (3) Documenting your judgment
   (4) Terminating, continuing, or modifying the plan
   (5) Identifying evaluative criteria and standards (what you are looking for when you evaluate, cg, expected patient outcomes)

a. (1), (2), (3), (4), (5)
b. (3), (2), (1), (4), (5)
c. (5), (2), (1), (3), (4)
d. (2), (3), (1), (4), (5)

3. When a new nurse is oriented to the subacute unit, she is told that each nurse is expected to observe her patients at least every hour, and more if their condition warrants extra monitoring. This expectation is best termed:
   a. Standard
   b. Criteria
   c. Custom
   d. Order
4. Remember Jeanne, the college student who wants to lose 20 pounds? When the nurse weighs her during the fifth step of the nursing process, what is she doing?
   a. Collecting assessment data to identify health problems
   b. Collecting assessment data to identify patient strengths
   c. Collecting evaluative data to justify terminating the plan of care
   d. Collecting evaluative data to measure outcome achievement
5. One of the outcomes Jeanne and the nurse planned is that Jeanne "appreciates or values a healthy body sufficiently to try to new behaviors." This outcome is best described as:
   a. Cognitive
   b. Psychomotor
   c. Affective
   d. Physical changes
6. Another of the outcomes Jeanne and the nurse planned is that Jeanne "can explain the relationship between weight loss, increased exercise, and decreased calorie intake." This outcome is best described as:
   a. Cognitive
   b. Psychomotor
   c. Affective
   d. Physical changes
7. Which of the following is the correct example of an evaluative statement?
   a. "Outcome not met."
   b. "1/21/06—Patient reports no change in tobacco use."
   c. "Outcome not met. Patient reports no change in tobacco use."
   d. "1/21/06—Outcome not met. Patient reports no change in tobacco use."
8. A quality-assurance program reveals a higher incidence of falls and other safety violations on a particular unit. A nurse manager states "We'd better find the folks responsible for these errors and see if we can't replace them." This is an example of:
   a. Quality by inspection
   b. Quality by punishment
   c. Quality by surveillance
   d. Quality by opportunity

9. One nursing unit with an excellent safety record meets to review the findings of the audit and the nurse manager states "We're doing well but we can do better! Who's got an idea to foster increased patient well-being and satisfaction?" This is an example of leadership that values:
   a. Quality assurance
   b. Quality improvement
   c. Process evaluation
   d. Outcome evaluation

Answers With Rationale

1. The correct answer is *d*. Since Jeanne has only partially met her outcome, the nurse should first explore the factors making it difficult for Jeanne to reach her outcome and then modify the plan of care. It would not be appropriate to continue the plan as it is since it is not working (*a*), and it is premature to terminate the plan of care (*b*) since Jeanne has not met her targeted outcome. Jeanne may need more than time to reach her outcome, which makes (*c*) the wrong response.

2. This is a sequenced list. The correct answer is *c*.

3. The correct answer is *a*, standard, the levels of performance accepted and expected by the nursing staff or other health team members. Criteria (*b*) are measurable qualities, attributes, or characteristics that specify skills, knowledge, or health states. Custom (*c*) sometimes establishes standards. Orders (*d*) are written to address the special needs of the patient.

4. The correct answer is *d*, collecting evaluative data to measure outcome achievement. While this may justify terminating the plan of care (*c*), that is not necessarily so. Assessment data (*a, c*) are collected during the first step of the nursing process.

5. The correct answer is *c*. Affective outcomes pertain to changes in patient values, beliefs, and attitudes. Cognitive outcomes (*a*) involve increases in patient knowledge; psychomotor outcomes (*b*) describe the patient's achievement of new skills; physical changes (*d*) are actually bodily changes in the patient (eg, weight loss, increased muscle tone).

6. The correct answer is *a*. Cognitive outcomes involve increases in patient knowledge; psychomotor outcomes (*b*) describe the patient's achievement of new skills; affective outcomes (*c*) pertain to changes in patient values, beliefs, and attitudes; physical changes (*d*) are actually bodily changes in the patient (eg, weight loss, increased muscle tone).

7. The correct answer is *d*. The evaluative statement contains a date; the words "outcome met," "outcome partially met," or "outcome not met," and the patient data or behaviors that support this decision. Answers (*a*), (*b*), and (*c*) are incomplete statements.

8. The correct answer is *a*. Quality by inspection focuses on finding deficient workers and removing them. Quality as opportunity (*d*) focuses on finding opportunities for improvement and fosters an environment that thrives on teamwork, with people sharing the skills and lessons they have learned. Answers (*b*) and (*c*) are distractors.

9. The correct answer is *b*. Unlike quality assurance (*a*), quality improvement is internally driven, focuses on patient care rather than organizational structure, focuses on processes rather than individuals, and has no end points. Its outcome is improving quality rather than assuring quality. Items (*c*) and (*d*) are types of quality-assurance programs.

Bibliography

Alfaro-LeFevre, R. (2002). *Applying nursing process: Promoting collaborative care.* (5th ed.). Philadelphia: Lippincott Williams & Wilkins.

Alfaro-LeFevre, R. (2004). *Critical thinking and clinical judgment: A practical approach* (3rd ed.). Philadelphia: W. B. Saunders.

American Nurses Association. (1975). *A plan for implementation of the standards of nursing practice.* Kansas City, MO: Author.

American Nurses Association. (1976). *ANA quality assurance workbook.* Kansas City, MO: Author.

American Nurses Association. (1991, 1998). *Standards of clinical nursing practice.* Washington, DC: Author.

American Nurses Association. (1999). *Nursing quality indicators: Guide for implementation* (2nd ed.). Washington, DC: Author.

Ardabell, T. R., Turjanica, M. A., Mastrovich, J., & Hirschman, V. (1995). Business process quality improvement: A step beyond continuous quality improvement. *MEDSURG Nursing, 4*(4), 279–288.

Bloch, D. (1975). Evaluation of nursing care in terms of process and outcome: Issues in research and quality assurance. *Nursing Research, 24,* 256–263.

Cassidy, C. A. (1999). Want to know how you're doing? *American Journal of Nursing, 99*(9), 51–58.

Committee on Quality of Health Care in America, Institute of Medicine. (1999). *Measuring the quality of health care.* Washington, DC: National Academy Press.

Committee on Quality of Health Care in America, Institute of Medicine. (2001). *Crossing the quality chasm: A new health system for the 21st century.* Washington, DC: National Academy Press.

Coulter, S. J., Atkins, P. M., Baily, D., Blatt, M. E., Blashford, L., & Shumway, S. (1994). Patient satisfaction: A QI pilot project. In P. Schroeder (Ed.), *Improving quality and performance.* St. Louis: C. V. Mosby.

Donabedian, A. (1980). *The definition of quality and its approaches.* Ann Arbor, MI: Health Administration Press.

Donabedian, A. (1982). *The criteria and standards of quality: Explorations in quality assessment and monitoring.* Ann Arbor, MI: Health Administration Press.

Haase, R., & Miller, K. (1999). Performance improvement in everyday clinical practice. *American Journal of Nursing 99*(5), 52, 54.

Hughes, S. J. (1995). Point-of-care information systems: State of the art. In M. J. Ball, K. J. Hannah, S. K. Newbold, & J. V. Douglas (Eds.), *Nursing informatics: Where caring and technology meet* (2nd ed.). New York: Springer-Verlag.

Joint Commission on Accreditation of Healthcare Organizations. (2003). *2003 Accreditation manual for hospitals.* Oakbrook Terrace, IL: Author.

Katz, J. M., & Green, E. (1996). *Managing quality: A guide to improving performance in health care.* St. Louis: Mosby–Year Book.

Koch, M. W., & Fairly, T. M. (1993). *Integrated quality management: The key to improving nursing care quality.* St. Louis: Mosby–Year Book.

Kohn, L. T., Corrigan, J. M., & Donaldson, M. S. (Eds.) (2003). Committee on Quality of Health Care in America, Institute of Medicine. *To err is human: Building a safer health system.* Washington, DC: National Academy Press.

LaRochelle, D. R., & Shahinpour, N. (Eds.) (1995). Staff nurse-initiated total quality management projects achieve quality nursing outcomes. *Nursing Clinics of North America, 30*(1), 1–162.

Ludwig-Beymer, P. (1993). Using patient perception to improve quality care. *Journal of Nursing Care Quality, 7*(2), 42–51.

Morin, G. D. (1995). A personal performance checklist. *Nursing Management, 26*(2), 325–326.

Oermann, M. H., & Huber, D. (1999). Patient outcomes: A measure of nursing's value. *American Journal of Nursing, 99*(9), 40–48.

Peters, D. (1991). Measuring quality: Inspection or opportunity? *Holistic Nursing Practice, 5*(3), 1–7.

Phaneuf, M. (1976a). *The nursing audit: Self regulation in nursing practice.* New York: Appleton-Century-Crofts.

Phaneuf, M. (1976b). Quality assurance: A nursing view. *New Zealand Nursing Journal, 69*(2), 9–11.

Rantz, M., Bostick, J., & Riggs, C. J. (2002). Nursing quality measurement: A review of nursing studies 1995–2000. Washington, DC: American Nurses Association.

Rubenfeld, M. G., & Scheffer, B. K. (1995). *Critical thinking in nursing: An interactive approach.* Philadelphia: J. B. Lippincott.

Schroeder, P. (1994). Improving quality and performance: Concepts, programs, and techniques. St. Louis: C. V. Mosby.

Western, P. (1994). QA/QI and nursing competence: A combined model. *Nursing Management, 25*(3), 44–46

Wright, D. (1984). An introduction to the evaluation of nursing care: A review of literature. *Journal of Advanced Nursing, 9*(5), 457–467.

Documenting, Reporting, and Conferring

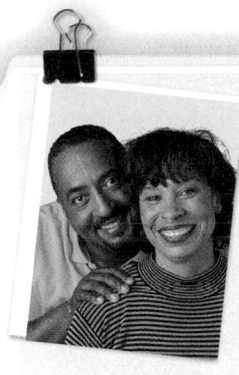

Phillippe Baron is a 52-year-old man being discharged from the outpatient surgery department after undergoing a colonoscopy for removal of three polyps. He will be going home with his wife, who is a nurse, and they both require discharge teaching.

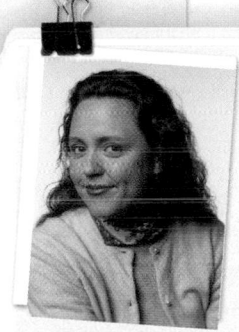

Millie Delong, a 44-year-old woman, develops a wound infection following abdominal surgery. Wound care with normal saline irrigations is ordered 4 times a day.

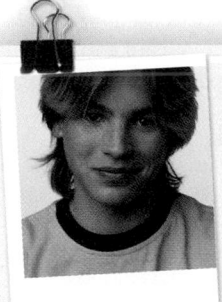

Jason Chandler, 15 years old and in police custody, is brought to the emergency department for treatment because he allegedly consumed a handful of individually wrapped crack rocks (estimated to be about 30 rocks) to avoid arrest. Treatment with insertion of nasogastric tube and bowel preparation solution is ordered. Jason is refusing treatment because he denies possession of drugs entirely.

Focusing on Blended Skills

The types of blended skills you'll need to respond to the case scenarios include:

Cognitive Skills

- Knowledge of colonoscopy as a diagnostic measure and need for follow-up
- Ability to incorporate knowledge of potential post-colonoscopy complications when developing a discharge teaching plan
- Knowledge of wound care and infection-control measures
- Knowledge of the legal principles involved when an adolescent patient refuses care that would prevent possible life-threatening complications
- Ability to communicate complete, accurate, concise, factual, organized, and timely data in writing
- Ability to incorporate knowledge needed to document nursing interventions that effectively meet the nursing needs of a patient requiring discharge teaching after a colonoscopy, a woman with a wound infection, and an adolescent who has allegedly swallowed drugs and is refusing treatment; this includes how to carry out the plan of care, continuation of data collection, modification of the plan as needed, and communication of care
- Knowledge of how different documentation systems work (such as outpatient surgery, hospital, and emergency department) and the purposes of documentation
- Knowledge of pertinent standards for documenting care, and agency and institutional policies
- Ability to think critically about how to best respond to the patient's need for nursing, and when and how to report and confer
- Knowledge of resources to contact when encountering questions about discharge teaching, wound care, and patient refusal of treatment

Technical Skills

- Strong assessment skills to identify potential risk factors that may affect a patient's care
- Ability to use agency- and department-specified documentation systems

- Demonstration of computer literacy
- Ability to document performance of technical nursing assistance, including any modifications necessary to meet the needs of patients with different conditions
- Ability to ask for assistance as necessary in situations involving new or technologically complex procedures or unfamiliar situations

Interpersonal Skills

- Strong interpersonal skills to establish a trusting nurse–patient relationship grounded in responsible caring
- Ability to communicate to patients, their families, and professional caregivers a greater concern about the patient and his or her well-being than about rote documentation of the plan of care
- Ability to demonstrate that what matters is communicating the plan of care so that coordination of care is achieved
- Ability to establish collaborative respectful relationships with health-team members to promote quality care
- Ability to demonstrate respect for the patient's human dignity and autonomy throughout the patient's care

Ethical and Legal Skills

- Commitment to honesty, integrity, and accountability in professional relationships
- Respect for the confidentiality of patient information
- Ability to document nursing interventions completely, accurately, concisely, and factually in a legally defensible manner
- Ability to incorporate ethical and legal principles that guide decision making related to a patient needing discharge teaching, a woman with a wound infection, and an adolescent in police custody who has allegedly swallowed drugs
- Ability to complete and correctly document events not consistent with the routine operation of a healthcare unit or routine patient care and that place a patient at risk of harm
- Ability to participate as a trusted and effective patient advocate

Learning Outcomes

After completing the chapter, the learner should be able to accomplish the following:

1. List guidelines for effective documentation.
2. Identify abbreviations and symbols commonly used for charting.
3. Describe the purposes of patient records.
4. Compare and contrast different methods of documentation: source-oriented record; problem-oriented record; PIE—problem, intervention, evaluation; focus charting; charting by exception; case management model; computerized records.
5. Describe the purpose and correct use of each of the following formats for nursing documentation: nursing assessment, nursing care plan, critical/collaborative pathways, progress notes, flow sheets, discharge summary, and home care documentation.
6. Document nursing interventions completely, accurately, concisely, and factually—avoiding legal problems.
7. Describe nursing's role in communicating with other healthcare professionals by reporting and conferring.

Key Terms

change-of-shift report
charting by exception
computer-based record
consultation
critical/collaborative pathway
discharge summary
documentation
flow sheet
focus charting
graphic sheet
incident report
Kardex care plan
medication record
minimum data set
narrative notes
nursing care conference
nursing care round
OASIS
patient record
PIE charting
problem-oriented medical record
progress notes
referral
reporting
SOAP format
source-oriented record
variance charting

Effective communication among healthcare professionals is essential to the coordination and continuity of care. Communicating effectively enables personnel to support and to complement one another's services and to avoid duplications and omissions in care. This chapter describes three methods of communication central to nursing's professional role: documenting, reporting, and conferring. The first day you care for patients, you will find yourself conferring with colleagues, recording your interventions, and reporting on your patient's progress toward valued goals and outcomes. As you develop these skills, you will quickly see a link between communicating information and critical thinking. As you document data, you are looking for relationships and patterns—things that might otherwise be overlooked. As you confer with the patient and the patient's family and professional caregivers, you might learn something about the patient that enhances your data set and clarifies the patient's health problem and related need for care (see the accompanying Reflective Practice box for an example). This chapter will help you assume these responsibilities with greater confidence and skill. The communication process itself and specific communication techniques are discussed in Chapter 21.

DOCUMENTING CARE

Documentation is the written, legal record of all pertinent interactions with the patient—assessing, diagnosing, planning, implementing, and evaluating. Increasingly sophisticated management information systems are being designed to manage patient-specific data and information. These data are used to facilitate patient care, serve as financial and legal records, help in clinical research, and support decision analysis. Information specialists aim to create an environment that supports timely, accurate, secure, and confidential recording and use of patient-specific information.

The **patient record** is a compilation of a patient's health information. Each healthcare institution or agency has policies that specify the nurse's documentation responsibilities. The Joint Commission on Accreditation of Healthcare Organizations (JCAHO, 2004) specifies that nursing care data related to patient assessments, nursing diagnoses or patient needs, nursing interventions, and patient outcomes are permanently integrated into the patient record. Each nurse is expected to practice according to local policies and professional standards.

Guidelines for Effective Documentation

The patient record is the only permanent legal document that details the nurse's interactions with the patient and is the nurse's best defense if a patient or patient surrogate alleges nursing negligence. Unfortunately, there are often crucial omissions in the nursing documentation, along with meaningless repetitious entries and inaccurate entries. Although these errors might go undetected and have no effect on the patient, they might also seriously affect the care the patient receives, undermine nursing's credibility as a professional discipline, and cause legal

Reflective Practice
Challenge to Ethical and Legal Skills

Working in the emergency department (ED) this summer never ceased to amaze me. Police brought Jason Chandler to the ED, a 15-year-old male who was in police custody for drug charges. Apparently, as police approached Jason, he consumed a handful of individually wrapped crack rocks (estimated to be about 30 rocks) to avoid arrest. He was brought to the ED as a precaution. If this bag broke inside his gastrointestinal tract, it would obviously have serious consequences. Jason was refusing treatment because he denied the possession of drugs entirely. The ED attending physician was unsure of his legal rights for treating the boy and called the hospital attorney. The attorney said the doctor could force treatment if there were probable signs that ingestion had occurred. However, the boy was not showing any clinical manifestations of chemical ingestion. This was a dilemma because if the bag of drugs burst open inside the boy, the physician stated that he most likely would not survive. The legal issue was whether or not the officer's statement of witnessing the ingestion was enough to constitute the need for treatment. The doctor was about to begin treating the patient when his mother arrived, threatening to sue anyone and everyone who "touched her little boy."

My preceptor and I were assigned to this patient and were given orders to insert a nasogastric (NG) tube so that a bowel preparation solution (GoLYTELY) could be used to flush out the drugs. The hospital attorney concluded that there was probable cause to justify forced treatment. However, the mother was furious and said she would sue under these circumstances, despite what the doctor or attorney said. As we entered the room to insert the NG tube and begin treatment, the boy, who was handcuffed to the bed, was screaming at us not to touch him.

Thinking Outside the Box: Possible Courses of Action

- Go with my preceptor and assist with the NG tube insertion.
- Refuse to treat the patient for fear of becoming part of a lawsuit.
- Allow my preceptor to sedate the patient against his will, to make the NG tube insertion easier.
- Inform the physician that I do not feel comfortable proceeding with treatment on a patient who refuses it and shows no clinical manifestations of drug toxicity.

Evaluating a Good Outcome: How Do I Define Success?

- The patient is benefited or, at the very least, not harmed by our actions.
- The hospital and its employees act in a legally defensible manner and (hopefully!) are not sued by the patient's family.
- The patient accepts treatment.
- The mother is able to realize the need for medical intervention.
- Hospital policy is maintained.
- I learn more about my legal and ethical responsibilities.

Personal Learning: Here's to the Future!

My preceptor and I went into the room and explained to the patient and his mother the procedure of NG tube insertion and what the bowel preparation solution was expected to do. I think the mother appreciated that we were not talking to them in a condescending fashion and, therefore, began to see us as trying to help her son, not harm him. She asked a couple of questions about side effects of the medication and how the NG tube worked. She began to show signs of calming down until the physician walked into the room. Then she started to show her frustration again. Therefore my preceptor politely asked the doctor to leave. Subsequently, we were able to insert the NG tube, despite some resistance from the patient. Several hours later, the patient passed a bag of crack rocks intact.

Obviously, this situation was very new to me. I had never dealt with a patient who was threatening to sue and who was clearly upset by what was happening. I was able to see the collaboration between the attending physician, the toxicologist, the hospital attorney, and the nurses and myself. This was an interesting case because the treatments were clearly necessary for the patient's well-being, but everyone wanted to make sure they were legally able to impose treatment. I learned that a hospital attorney is a good resource when legal questions or ambiguous situations arise.

I think that my professional legal skills need a fair amount of work. Unfortunately, I also believe that nurses violate the law more often than is recognized—for example, subtle breaches of the law such as failure to ensure patient safety and failure to follow agency policy. Although I feel that I understand many of the obvious legal violations, I think I have a lot to learn regarding legal issues in the nursing practice.

Reflection

How do you think you would respond in a similar situation? Why? What does this tell you about yourself and about the adequacy of your skills for professional practice? Can you think of other ways to respond? What legal and ethical principles were involved in this situation? Which ones had the potential to be violated? Did the preceptor and nursing student ensure the patient's rights? How might this situation have been different if the patient were over 18 years of age? What other skills (cognitive, interpersonal, technical, ethical/legal) would you need to respond well in this situation? Do you agree with the criteria to evaluate a successful outcome? Did the nursing student meet the criteria? Please explain your answer.

Julia Strobel, Georgetown University

problems for the nurses responsible. Adherence to the accompanying documentation guidelines shown in Box 17-1 helps to prevent errors. In brief, documentation should be consistent with professional and agency standards; complete, accurate, concise, factual, organized, and timely; legally prudent; and confidential.

Responding to the widespread nursing concern that the time spent documenting nursing care comes at the expense of providing safe, quality patient care, the American Nurses Associ-

ation (ANA) introduced a new tool to streamline the nursing documentation process in 2003. Available in a brochure format titled *Principles for Documentation*, this new guide includes policy statements, principles, and recommendations to assist nurses with documentation and to comply with institutional and regulatory requirements.

The policy statements and principles outlined in the guide are based on the *ANA Code of Ethics for Nurses With Interpretive Statements* (ANA, 2001) and *Standards of Clinical*

BOX 17-1 **Documentation Guidelines**

Aim: Complete, accurate, concise, factual, and organized data communicated in a timely and confidential manner to facilitate care coordination and serve as a legal document.

Content

- Enter information in a *complete, accurate, concise,* and *factual* manner.
- Record patient findings (observations of behavior) rather than your interpretation of these findings.
- Avoid words such as "good," "average," "normal," or "sufficient," which may mean different things to different readers.
- Avoid generalizations such as "seems comfortable today." A better entry would be "on a scale of 1 to 10, patient rates back pain 2 to 3 today as compared with 7 to 9 yesterday; vital signs returned to baseline."
- Note problems as they occur in an *orderly, sequential manner;* record the nursing intervention and the patient's response; update problems or delete as appropriate.
- Document all medical visits and consultations of which other nurses should be aware, either because of their impact on the patient or because of the nursing care the patient now requires.
- Document in a *legally prudent manner.* Know and adhere to professional standards and agency/institutional policy for documentation.
- Document the nursing response to questionable medical orders or treatment (or failure to treat). Factually record the date and time the physician was notified of the concern and the exact physician response. If this occurs by phone, have a second nurse listen to the conversation and cosign the note. If a nurse administrator was contacted, document this. Documentation should give legal protection to the nurse, other caregivers, the healthcare agency or institution, and the patient.
- Avoid the use of stereotypes or derogatory terms when charting.

Timing

- Chart in a *timely* manner. Follow agency policy regarding the frequency of documentation and *modify this if changes in the patient's status warrant more frequent documentation.*
- Indicate in each entry the date and both the time the entry was written and the time of pertinent observations and interventions. This is crucial when a case is being reconstructed for legal purposes.
- Document nursing interventions as closely as possible to the time of their execution. The more seriously ill the pa-

tient, the greater the need to keep documentation current. Never leave the unit for a break when caring for a seriously ill patient until all significant data are recorded.
- Never document interventions before carrying them out.

Format

- Chart on the proper form as designated by agency policy.
- Print or write legibly in *dark* ink to ensure permanence. Use correct grammar and spelling. Use **standard terminology**, only commonly accepted terms and abbreviations and symbols (see Table 17-1). Alternately, follow computer documentation guidelines.
- Date and time each entry.
- Chart nursing interventions chronologically on consecutive lines. Never skip lines. Draw a single line through blank spaces.

Accountability

- Sign your first initial, last name, and title to each entry. Do not sign notes describing interventions not performed by you that you have no way of verifying.
- Do not use dittos, erasures, or correcting fluids. A single line should be drawn through an incorrect entry and words "mistaken entry" or "error in charting" should be printed above or beside the entry and signed. The entry should then be rewritten correctly.
- Identify each page of the record with the patient's name and identification number.
- Recognize that the patient record is *permanent.* Follow agency policy pertaining to the color of ink and the type of pen or ink to be used. Ensure that the patient record is complete before sending it to medical records.

Confidentiality

- Patients have a moral and legal right to expect that the information contained in their patient health record will be kept private. Students should be familiar with agency policy and pertinent legislation about who has access to patient records, other than the immediate caregiving team, and the process used to obtain access (see HIPAA guidelines).
- Most agencies allow students access to patient records for educational reasons. Students using patient records are bound professionally and ethically to keep in strict confidence all the information they learn by reading patient records. Actual patient names and other identifiers should not be used in written or oral student reports.

Nursing Practice, 2nd edition (ANA, 1998). In addition, the formulated principles in many instances are based on standards set forth by state and federal regulatory agencies, the Centers for Medicare and Medicaid Services (CMS), and through accrediting organizations such as the Joint Commission on Accreditation of Healthcare Organizations (JCAHO) and the National Committee for Quality Assurance (NCQA).

A Word About Privacy and Confidentiality

Nurses and other professional caregivers learn and communicate private information about patients and their families every day.

What is Confidential?

All information about patients is considered private or confidential, whether written on paper, saved on a computer, or spoken aloud. This includes their name and all identifiers such as address, telephone and fax number, Social Security number, and any other personal information. It also includes the reason the patient is sick or in the hospital, office, or clinic, the treatments he or she receives, and information about past health conditions. Protected health information might be found in the patient medical record, computer systems, telephone calls, voice mails, fax transmissions, e-mails that contain patient information, and conversations about patients between clinical staff.

While most nurses are staunch advocates of a patient's right to privacy and confidentiality, many nurses thoughtlessly violate these rights every day. One nurse gives patient information over the phone to a patient's alleged spouse without knowing whether or not the patient wants his wife to know, another talks about a difficult patient in the elevator on the way to dinner, and another gives patient information to a professional caregiver who "knows" the patient but is not involved in the patient's care. Professional codes of ethics, agency policies, and state and federal privacy legislation dictate how patient information can be communicated (verbally and in writing), where and how it can be stored, the appropriate persons and entities to whom it may be divulged, and the purposes for which it may be divulged. It is essential for nurses to be familiar with these guidelines.

Health Insurance Portability and Accountability Act (HIPAA)

Congress passed the Health Insurance Portability and Accountability Act in 1996. The final regulations were published in December 2000, modified by the Bush administration, and released in August 2002. Most agencies now require workers to undergo HIPAA training and to review and to sign a confidentiality agreement when hired and at each performance review. As a student in a healthcare setting, it is important for you to discuss privacy guidelines with your instructor and nurse mentors. According to HIPAA, patients have a right to:

- See and copy their health record
- Update their health record
- Get a list of the disclosures a healthcare institution has made independent of disclosures made for the purposes of treatment, payment, and healthcare operations
- Request a restriction on certain uses or disclosures
- Choose how to receive health information

Consider Jason Chandler, the adolescent brought to the emergency department by the police. The nurse would need to be knowledgeable about HIPAA regulations to ensure Jason's confidentiality is maintained. In addition, the nurse would need to keep in mind that Jason is a minor, and any authorizations would probably require a parent's consent.

If a health institution wants to release a patient's health information for purposes other than treatment, payment, or routine healthcare operations, the patient must be asked to sign an authorization. See Box 17-2 for a list of permitted disclosures of patient health information and incidental disclosures.

ALERT!

The Health Insurance Portability and Accountability Act of 1996, or HIPAA for short, includes punishments for anyone caught violating patient privacy. Those who do so for financial gain can be fined as much as $250,000 or go to jail for as many as 10 years! Even accidentally breaking the rules can result in penalties—and embarrassment—for you and your organization.

Agency Policies

Most agencies have specific policies for patient records. Everyone who has access to the record (direct caregivers) is expected to maintain its confidentiality (see the discussion about privacy above). Most agencies grant student nurses access to patient records for education purposes. In this instance, the student assumes responsibility to hold patient information in confidence.

Agency policies also indicate which personnel are responsible for recording on each form in the record, and such policies might also describe the order in which the forms are to appear in the record. Additional policies might concern the frequency with which entries are to be made, whether routine care is recorded, the manner in which health personnel identify themselves after making an entry, which types of abbreviations are acceptable, and the manner in which recording errors are handled. Table 17-1 provides a list of commonly used abbreviations. One of the strategies the Joint Commission on Accreditation of Healthcare Organization (2004) is using to achieve National Patient Safety Goals is a list of "do not use" abbreviations, acronyms, and symbols. These may be found in Table 17-2. Be sure to know the latest JCAHO and agency policies regarding the use of abbreviations, acronyms and symbols in your practice setting. An issue of growing importance concerns documentation made by unlicensed personnel. Because professional nurses frequently supervise the care that unlicensed personnel give, it is essential to clarify which assessments and interventions may be charted by unlicensed personnel and which require documentation by a professional nurse.

BOX 17-2 The Health Insurance Portability and Accountability Act of 1996 Authorization Rule

If a health institution wants to release a patient's health information (PHI) for purposes other than treatment, payment, and routine health care operations, the patient must be asked to sign an authorization.

Permitted Disclosure of PHI

While the authorization rule covers most situations where we need to release patient information for purposes other than treatment, payment, and routine health care operations, there are some exceptions to the authorization rule for the good of the general population.

These three exceptions show situations where authorization is *not* required prior to releasing the patient's information:

Public health activities	• Tracking and notification of disease outbreaks • Infection control • Statistics related to dangerous problems with drugs or medical equipment
Law enforcement and judicial proceedings	• Medical records crucial to the investigation and prosecution of a crime • Medical records to identify victims of crime or disasters • Medical personnel reporting incidents of child abuse, neglect, or domestic violence • Medical records released according to a valid subpoena
Deceased individuals	• PHI needed by coroners, medical examiners, and funeral directors • PHI needed to facilitate organ donations • PHI provided to law enforcement in the case of a death from a potential crime

Incidental Disclosure of PHI

Incidental Disclosure of PHI is defined as a secondary disclosure that cannot reasonably be prevented, is limited in nature, and occurs as a byproduct of an otherwise permitted use or disclosure of PHI.

Examples of incidental disclosures that are permitted:

Permitted Disclosure	Necessary Conditions
• Use of sign-in sheets	• Provided that the sign-in sheet does not contain information on the reason for the patient's visit
• The possibility of a confidential conversation being overhead	• Provided that the surroundings are appropriate for a confidential conversation and voices are kept down
• Placing patient charts outside exam rooms	• Provided that unauthorized public traffic is not permitted in the area of the exam rooms and face sheets are turned towards the wall
• Use of white boards	• Provided that only the minimum information needed for the purpose of the white board is used
• X-ray light boards that can be seen by passers-by	• Provided that patient x-rays are not left unattended on the light board
• Calling out names in the waiting room	• Provided that the reason for the patient's visit is not mentioned
• Leaving appointment reminder voicemail messages	• Provided that the minimum amount of information is disclosed

Used with permission. MedStar Health. (2003). *Protecting patient privacy*, pp. 14–15. Columbia, MD: Author © 2003 MedStar Health, Inc. http://medstarhealth.org.

The storage of patient records when a patient is no longer receiving treatment is a function of the health agency's record department. Many patient records are microfilmed for compact storage or are entered into a computer to expedite accessibility of information.

Purposes of Patient Records

Patient records serve many purposes, such as communication with other healthcare professionals, recording of diagnostic and therapeutic orders, care planning, quality-of-care reviewing, research, decision analysis, education, legal documentation, reimbursement, and historical documentation.

Communication

The patient record helps healthcare professionals from different disciplines who interact with the patient at different times to communicate with one another. This is the primary purpose of the record. It is helpful to keep in mind that other healthcare professionals make judgments about nurses and nursing's contributions to the healthcare team partially on the basis of what is documented in the patient record.

Diagnostic and Therapeutic Orders

Patient records also include diagnostic and therapeutic orders. Nurses are responsible for insuring that these orders are entered in the patient record and implemented. It is the policy of

TABLE 17-1 Abbreviations and Symbols Commonly Used by Health Practitioners*

Activities

AMB	ambulatory
BRP	bathroom privileges
CBR	complete bed rest
OOB	out of bed
up ad lib	up as desired

Assessment Data

abd	abdomen
BP	blood pressure
bx	biopsy
C	Celsius (centigrade)
c/o	complains of
CTA	clear to auscultation
dx	diagnosis
F	Fahrenheit
FUO	fever of unknown origin
GI	gastrointestinal
GU	genitourinary
H/A	headache
h/o	history of
HPI	history of present illness
Imp	impressions
lt or Ⓛ	left
MAE	moves all extremities
NAD	no apparent distress
NKA	no known allergies
N/V	nausea and vomiting
neg	negative
P	pulse
PE	physical examination
PMH	past medical history
R	respirations
R/O	rule out
ROS	review of systems
rt or Ⓡ	right
SOB	short of breath
Sx	symptoms
T	temperature
⊕	positive
⊖	negative

Diseases

ASCVD	arteriosclerotic cardio-vascular disease
ASHD	arteriosclerotic heart disease
BPH	benign prostatic hypertrophy
CA	cancer
CAD	coronary artery disease
CHF	congestive heart failure
COPD	chronic obstructive pulmonary disease
CVA	cerebrovascular accident
DM	diabetes mellitus
HTN (↑ BP)	hypertension
MI	myocardial infarction
PE	pulmonary emboli
PVD	peripheral vascular disease
STD	sexually transmitted disease
URI	upper respiratory infection

Diagnostic Studies

ABG	arterial blood gases
BE	barium enema
CBC	complete blood count
CO_2	carbon dioxide
C&S	culture and sensitivity
CXR	chest x-ray
ECG (EKG)	cardiogram
lytes	electrolytes
RBC	red blood cells
UA	urinalysis
UGI	upper GI
WBC	white blood cells

Symbols

>	greater than
<	less than
↑	increase
↗	increasing
↓	decrease
↙	decreasing
2°	secondary to
=	equal to
≠	unequal
♀	female
♂	male
°	degree
▲	change
x̄	except

Miscellaneous

ā	before
ad lib	as desired
AMA	against medical advice
ASAP	as soon as possible
BM	bowel movement

BSD	bedside drainage
c̄ (C)	with
CABG	coronary artery bypass graft
CPR	cardiopulmonary resuscitation
dc (disc)	discontinue
DNR (no code)	do not resuscitate
Dsg	dressing
dx	diagnosis
FOB	foot of bed
Fx	fracture
GHWT	good handwashing technique
HOB	head of bed
hs	hour of sleep
Hx	history
I&O	intake and output
IV	intravenous
KVO	keep vein open
NG	nasogastric
noc	night
NPO (npo)	nothing by mouth
NS (NIS) (N/S)	normal saline
O_2	oxygen
OT	occupational therapy
p̄	after
postop	postoperative
preop	preoperative
prep	preparation
PRN (p.r.n.)	as needed
PT	physical therapy
pt	patient
q	every
ROM	range of motion
RX	treatment
s̄ (S)	without
SOB	side of bed
S/P	status post
STAT	immediately
TF	tube feeding
TPR	temperature, pulse, respirations
TURP	transurethral resection of prostate
TX	treatment
VS	vital signs
WA	while awake
×	times

* Use only those abbreviations and symbols accepted by your institution.

TABLE 17-2 JCAHO "Do Not Use" Abbreviations, Acronyms or Symbols

Abbreviation	Potential Problem	Preferred Term
Minimum Required List		
Beginning January 1, 2004, the following items must be included on each accredited organization's "Do Not Use" list:		
U (for unit)	Mistaken as 0 (zero), 4 (four), or cc	Write "unit."
IU (for international unit)	Mistaken as IV (intravenous) or 10 (ten)	Write "international unit."
Q.D., Q.O.D. (Latin abbreviation for once daily and every other day)	Mistaken for each other. The period after the Q can be mistaken for an "I" and the "O" can be mistaken for "I".	Write "daily" and "every other day."
Trailing zero (X.0 mg) Lack of leading zero (.X mg)	Decimal point is missed.	Never write a zero by itself after a decimal point (X mg), and always use a zero before a decimal point (0.X mg).
MS	Confused for one another.	Write "morphine sulfate" or "magnesium sulfate."
MSO4 MgSO4	Can mean morphine sulfate or magnesium sulfate.	
Additional Items		
Effective April 1, 2004, each organization must identify and apply at least another three "do not use" abbreviations, acronyms or symbols of its own choosing. The following items should also be considered when expanding the "Do Not Use" list:		
µg (for microgram)	Mistaken for mg (milligrams), resulting in one thousand-fold dosing overdose.	Write "mcg."
H.S. (for half-strength or Latin abbreviation for bedtime)	Mistaken for either half-strength or hour of sleep (at bedtime). q.H.S. mistaken for every hour. All can result in a dosing error.	Write out "half-strength" or "at bedtime."
T.I.W. (for 3 times a week)	Mistaken for 3 times a day or twice weekly, resulting in an overdose.	Write "3 times weekly" or "three times weekly."
D/C (for discharge)	Interpreted as "discontinue whatever medications follow" (typically discharge meds)	Write "discharge."
c.c. (for cubic centimeter)	Mistaken for U (units) when poorly written	Write "ml" for milliliters.
A.S., A.D., A.U. (Latin abbreviation for left, right, or both ears)	Mistaken for OS, OD, and OU, etc.	Write "left ear," "right ear" or "both ears"; "left eye," "right eye," or "both eyes."

From Joint Commission on Accreditation of Health Care Organizations. (2003, December 31). 2004 National Patient Safety Goals—FAQs. Retrieved January 23, 2004, from www.jcaho.org/accredited+organizations/patient+safety/04+npsg/04_faqs.htm

most agencies that diagnostic and therapeutic orders should be accepted and executed only when written and signed by the member of the house or professional staff who issued the orders, except in medical emergencies (verbal orders) or when the practitioner is unable to be present on the unit (telephone or faxed orders). Nurses may only take orders from physicians, dentists, psychologists, podiatrists, and advanced practice nurses who are licensed and have credentials. Medical students' orders may be executed only when countersigned by the attending physician, nurse practitioner, or a house officer assigned to the clinical department.

Remember Jason Chandler, the adolescent brought to the emergency department? The physician ordered insertion of a nasogastric tube and administration of a bowel preparation solution to evacuate the swallowed drugs from his gastrointestinal tract. These orders must be written and signed by the attending physician.

Verbal Orders

In most agencies, the only circumstance in which an attending physician, nurse practitioner, or house officer may issue orders verbally is in a medical emergency when the physician/nurse practitioner is present but finds it impossible, due to the emergency situation, to write the order. The order must be given directly by the physician or nurse practitioner to a registered professional nurse or registered professional pharmacist, who receives and executes the order. Verbal orders may not be given, received, or executed under any other circumstances. Sample policy follows:

A. The registered professional nurse or registered professional pharmacist who receives the verbal order will:
1. Record the orders in the patient's medical record.
2. Read back the order to verify accuracy of the order.

3. Date and note the time the orders were issued during the emergency.
4. Record V.O. (verbal orders), the name of the physician or nurse practitioner who issued the orders, followed by the nurse's own name and title.
B. Immediately after the conclusion of the emergency, it is the responsibility of the physician or nurse practitioner who has issued the verbal orders to:
1. Review the orders to ascertain whether they are correct.
2. Sign the orders with his or her name, title, and pager number.
3. Date and note the time he or she signs the orders.
C. It is the responsibility of the unit secretary and/or the registered professional nurse to see that the orders are transcribed according to procedure.

Telephone and Fax Orders

Agency policy must be followed regarding telephone orders. Every telephone order should be repeated back to the physician to ensure that the nurse correctly understands what was ordered. If the nurse is unsure of an order given by phone, he or she asks the physician to repeat it. Telephone orders must be transcribed on an order sheet; policy usually dictates that they be cosigned by the physician within a set time. If the nurse judges a telephone order to be inappropriate, another nurse should also listen to the order. Then, agency guidelines for questioning inappropriate orders are followed. Fax orders are acceptable as long as they are legible and issued from a credentialed and privileged individual. As always, if the nurse has any concerns, the ordering physician should be contacted. Sample policy:

A. An attending physician or nurse practitioner who finds it necessary to issue orders via telephone should be referred to a house officer or, in the absence of a house officer, to a registered professional nurse or a registered professional pharmacist.
B. If a registered professional nurse accepts the orders, he or she must:
1. Record the orders in the patient's medical record.
2. Read the order back to the ordering practitioner to verify accuracy.
3. Date and note the time the orders were issued.
4. Record T.O. (telephone orders), the full name and title of the physician or nurse practitioner who issued the orders.
5. Sign the orders with name and title (Example: "Demerol 100 mg IM now and q 4 hr p.r.n. for pain. T.O. James E. Walker, MD/Mary Pint, RN").

It is the responsibility of the physician or nurse practitioner dictating the orders to sign them as soon as practical, with the exception of orders for restraints, narcotics, anticoagulants, and antibiotics, which must be signed within 24 hours. He or she must also note the date and time the order is signed.

Care Planning

Each professional working with the patient has access to the patient's baseline and ongoing data and can see how the patient is responding to the treatment plan from day to day. Modifications of the plan of care are based on these data.

Think back to Phillippe Baron, the patient who had undergone a colonoscopy. The nurse would use the patient's chart to obtain information about the patient, including events of the colonoscopy and how the patient responded, so that an individualized discharge teaching plan could be developed.

Quality Review

Charts might be reviewed to evaluate the quality of care patients have received and the competence of the nurses providing that care. For example, in a nursing audit, a committee decides in advance certain standards of care it wants to evaluate (eg, pertaining to nursing assessment, nursing documentation, or safety measures). A number of charts are then randomly selected and reviewed for evidence that the nurses met the selected standards of care. If deficiencies are found, in-service training can be used to remedy the problem and to improve the quality of care. Accrediting agencies, such as JCAHO, might also use chart review to determine whether a particular agency or healthcare institution is meeting its standards.

Research

Researchers might study patient records, hoping to learn how best to recognize or treat identified health problems from the study of similar cases.

Decision Analysis

Information from record review often provides the data needed by administrative strategic planners to identify needs and the means and strategies most likely to address these needs. Record review might reveal both underused and overused services, patients with prolonged stays who require special assistance, and financial information about which services generate revenue compared with those that cost the institution or agency money.

Education

Healthcare professionals and students reading a patient's chart can learn a great deal about the clinical manifestations of particular health problems, effective treatment modalities, and factors that affect patient goal achievement.

Legal Documentation

Patient records are legal documents that might be used as evidence in court proceedings, and therefore they play an important role in implicating or absolving health practitioners charged with improper care. The record can also be used in accident or injury claims made by the patient.

Reimbursement

Patient records are also used to demonstrate to payers that patients received the care for which reimbursement is being sought.

Remember Millie Delong, with woman with a wound infection? The nurse would need to doc-

ument the patient's wound care thoroughly and specifically (eg, size, color, appearance, the need for wound care, and what specifically was done) to ensure that proper reimbursement is obtained for any supplies used for wound care and the nursing services provided.

Historical Documentation

Because the dates of entries on records are specified, the record has value as a historical document. Years later, information concerning a patient's past healthcare might be pertinent.

Methods of Documentation

While the different methods of documentation systems might initially seem confusing, each is designed to achieve certain aims. Familiarity with a variety of systems allows nurses to adapt quickly when in different practice settings.

Source-Oriented Records

A **source-oriented record** is one in which each healthcare group keeps data on its own separate form. Sections of the record are designated for nurses, physicians, laboratory, and x-ray personnel, and so on. Notations are entered chronologically, with the most recent entry being nearest the front of the record. An advantage of the source-oriented record is that each discipline can easily find and chart pertinent data. The main disadvantage is that data are fragmented, making it difficult to track problems chronologically with input from different groups of professionals.

Although the specifics vary among health agencies, the general characteristics of the source-oriented record have essentially remained the same. Types of forms typically used in a source-oriented patient record are presented in Table 17-3. Progress notes written by nurses in a source-oriented record are **narrative notes** that address routine care, normal findings, and patient problems identified in the plan of care. They include a

TABLE 17-3 Examples of Forms and Information in Source-Oriented Patient Records

Form	Typical Client Information
Admission sheet	Legal name, identification number
	Age, birthdate, sex
	Marital status
	Occupation and employer
	Religious preference
	Next of kin and person to notify in case of emergency
	Date, time, reason for admission
	Name of the attending physician
	Insurance information
	Discharge data
Admission nursing assessment	Results of nursing history and physical assessment
Graphic sheet (see Fig. 17-10)	Daily temperatures, pulse and respiratory rates, blood pressure (vital signs), pain level
	Daily weight
	Special measurements, such as the patient's fluid intake and output
Activity flow sheet (see Fig. 17-1)	Diet and how patient has eaten
	Bathing and skin care
	Activity level, safety measures
	Respiratory interventions
	Elimination
	Diagnostic measures, treatments
	Isolation
Narrative nurse's notes (see Fig. 17-1)	Descriptions of pertinent observations of patient
	Statements that specify the nursing care, including teaching, received by patient and his or her responses to nursing care
	Statements that describe patient's condition and progress, or lack of progress, toward recovery and goal achievement
	Descriptions of patient's complaints and how patient is coping, or failing to cope, with them and nursing's response
Medication sheet (see Chap. 29)	Name of prescribed medications administered on a regular or p.r.n. basis
	Dosage of medication administered
	Route by which medication was administered, unless given orally
	Time medication was administered
	Name or initials of person administering the medication

(continued)

TABLE 17-3 (Continued)

Form	Typical Client Information
Medical history and examination sheet	Results of physical examination performed by physician
	Current medical condition
	Health history, including previous illnesses
	Family medical history
	Confirmed or tentative diagnosis
	Plan of medical therapy
Physician's order sheet	Orders for medications
	Orders for treatments
	Other directives pertinent to a particular patient's care
Physician's progress notes	Interpretations of patient's pathology
	Responses of patient to medical therapy
Miscellaneous forms	Laboratory reports
	X-ray film reports
	Consultation reports
	Dietary requirements
	Results of social service consultations
	Types and results of physical, respiratory, and x-ray therapy

description of the status of the problem, related nursing interventions, patient responses, and needed revisions to the plan of care. Sample traditional narrative nursing notes are given in Figure 17-1. Traditional narrative nursing notes are also included in the nursing process patient care studies that conclude each clinical chapter.

Problem-Oriented Medical Records

Another type of record used in some health agencies is the **problem-oriented medical record** (POMR), or problem-oriented record, originated by Dr. Lawrence Weed in the 1960s. The POMR is organized around a patient's problems rather than around sources of information. An example is given in Figure 17-2. All healthcare professionals record information on the same forms. The advantages of this type of record are that the entire healthcare team works together in identifying a master list of patient problems and contributes collaboratively to the plan of care. Progress notes clearly focus on patient problems. Table 17-4 and Figure 17-2 describe and illustrate the major parts of the POMR: the defined database, problem list, care plans, and progress notes.

The acronym SOAP (**S**ubjective data, **O**bjective data, **A**ssessment [the caregiver's judgment about the situation], **P**lan) is used to organize data entries in the progress notes of the POMR. Caregivers select numbered problems from the master list on the front of the patient record and then work up the problem or "SOAP it" on the progress sheet. Some nurses believe that the SOAP method of charting focuses too narrowly on problems and advocate a return to the traditional narrative format. Variants of the **SOAP format** include SOAPE, SOAPIE, and SOAPIER (**I**ntervention, **E**valuation, and **R**esponse). Figure 17-2D incorporates a SOAP note.

PIE—Problem, Intervention, Evaluation

The **PIE charting** system is unique in that it does not develop a separate plan of care. The plan of care is incorporated into the progress notes in which problems are identified by number. In this documentation system, a complete patient assessment is performed and documented at the beginning of each shift using preprinted fill-in-the-blank assessment forms. Patient problems identified in these assessments are numbered, worked up using the **P**roblem, **I**ntervention, **E**valuation (PIE) format, and evaluated each shift. Figure 17-3 is an example. Continuing problems are documented and numbered each day. One advantage of this system is that it promotes continuity of care. It also saves time because there is no separate plan of care. The disadvantage of not having a formal care plan, however, is that nurses need to read all the nursing notes to determine problems and planned interventions before initiating care.

Focus Charting

The purpose of **focus charting** is to bring the focus of care back to the patient and the patient's concerns. Instead of a problem list or list of nursing or medical diagnoses, a focus column is used that incorporates many aspects of a patient and patient care. The focus might be a patient strength, problem, or need. Topics that may appear in the focus column include patient concerns and behaviors; therapies and responses; changes of condition; and significant events, such as teaching, consultations, monitoring, management of activities of daily living, or assessment of functional health patterns. The narrative portion of focus charting uses the **D**ata, **A**ction, **R**esponse (DAR) format (Fig. 17-4). The principal advantage of focus charting is the holistic emphasis on the patient and the patient's priorities. Ease of charting is also cited as an advantage of focus charting because it is not required that each note incorporate data, ac-

Shift	11-7:30 AM	7-3:30 PM	3-11:30 PM		Date	9/4/02 7 AM Pt. awake and
Diet or NPO	House = Soft	House = Soft	House = Soft		Time	alert. Awoke at 2 AM to void —
Nutrition		BR ☑ G ☐ F ☐ P LU ☐ G ☐ F ☐ P ☐ Feed ☑ Self	Di ☐ G ☑ F ☐ P HS Snack ☑ ☐ Feed ☑ Self			unable to fall back asleep. Refused sedative. Rested quietly. Speech clear, moving all extremities.—
Bathing Skin Care	☑ Mouth Care ☐ Skin Care Keri lotion	☐ S ☑ P ☐ C ☑ Mouth Care ☑ AM Care	☑ PM Care ☑ Mouth Care			— L. Gray. RN
Activity	☑ CBR ☑ Pos. q2° ☐ BRP ☐ BRP c̄ Asst. ☐ OOB Chair c̄ Asst. ☐ OOB Chair s̄ Asst. ☐ AMB c̄ Asst. ☐ AMB s̄ Asst.	☑ CBR ☑ Pos. q2° ☐ BRP ☐ BRP c̄ Asst. ☐ OOB Chair c̄ Asst. ☐ OOB Chair s̄ Asst. ☐ AMB c̄ Asst. ☐ AMB s̄ Asst.	☑ CBR ☑ Pos. q2° ☐ BRP ☐ BRP c̄ Asst. ☐ OOB Chair c̄ Asst. ☐ OOB Chair s̄ Asst. ☐ AMB c̄ Asst. ☐ AMB s̄ Asst.		9/4/06 10 AM	Prune juice & cup of hot water with breakfast resulted in soft formed BM - about 1 hour p̄ breakfast. No straining. Keri lotion to dry skin on legs and arms. Strength seems to be increasing in
Resp. Assessment	☑ Cough/D. Breathe q2° ☐ Trach Care ☐ Suction Freq ___	☑ Cough/D. Breathe q2° ☐ Trach Care ☐ Suction Freq ___	☑ Cough/D. Breathe q2° ☐ Trach Care ☐ Suction Freq ___			left arm & leg. Performs lt. leg exercises independently. During bath talked about how much she misses her husband and her house.
Treatments	Assisted ROM	P.T.	→			Explored feelings about participating in support group for widows - recommended by her friends. Feels
Protective Precautions	☐ Full ☑ Half	— ☐ Full ☐ Half	— ☐ Full ☐ Half			good about babysitting her 2 grandchildren.
Restraints	☐ Posey ☐ Wrist ☐ Ankle ☐ None ☑ q2° Check ☐ Other	☐ Posey ☐ Wrist ☐ Ankle ☑ None ☐ q2° Check ☐ Other	☐ Posey ☐ Wrist ☐ Ankle ☑ None ☐ q2° Check ☐ Other			— C. Taylor, RN
Elimination Bowel Bladder ☐ Foley	bedpan voiding q5 ☐ Commode	↑BM Voiding q5 bedpan ☐ Commode ☐ Foley Care	☐ Commode ☐ Foley Care		2 pm	Spent 30 min. teaching patient & daughter Lisa about T.I.A. and stroke. Strong family history of PVD, CVA and MI. Reviewed importance
Diagnostic Studies +/or Specimens Obtained	—	CAT Scan	—			of dietary modifications, regular exercise and taking prescribed medication. Excellent motivation for self-care — S Taylor RN
Isolation Type	—	—	—		9/4/06 8pm	VS 98.8 - 78 - 18 136/92 Quiet this evening. - Napping - Not hungry
Nursing Care Plan	☑ Reviewed ☐ Revised	☑ Reviewed ☐ Revised	☑ Reviewed ☐ Revised			at dinner: states "Busy day." Moving all extremities; alert.
Comments	awake @ 2am did not fall back to sleep	"when can I go home?" napped in pm	—			Daughter Barbara says her mother wants to do "too much." Still afraid
Signature	L. Gray RN	C Taylor RN	D. Kande RN			TIA automatically means stroke & death! — D. Kande RN.

Nazareth Hospital
Activity Flowsheet/Patient Care Notes

FIGURE 17-1 Sample of an activity flow sheet with narrative patient care notes.
(Courtesy of Nazareth Hospital, Philadelphia, PA.)

Summary of data base for client (17-2A)

---

72 year old, white, recently widowed female

brought to hospital after sudden fall caused by temporary paralysis of left leg; admitting diagnosis: transient ischemic attack (TIA), R/O cerebrovascular accident

treated for hypertension since 1990, otherwise in good health; history of headaches—once or twice a week (increasing in severity)—for last six months

ht 5′2″   wt 63.6 kg   98.2 F-88-18   BP L—184/120, R—180/120
↓ strength ↓ movement left lower extremity (LLE)

Problem List (17-2B)

XXXX Medical Center   4629F

Date	No.	Problem	Identified	Resolved
9/2/06	#1	transient ischemic attack (TIA) R/O cerebro-vascular accident	J. Gleer MD	
	#1A	impaired physical mobility related to weakness in left lower extremity	D. Kande RN	
9/4/06	#2	impaired adjustment related to major life stressors and decreased supports	D. Kande RN	

Plan of Care (17-2C)

Date	Problem
9/4/06 3 pm	#2 Impaired adjustment related to major life stressors (including illness) and decreased supports Goal: Prior to discharge patient reports feeling able to go home and take one day at a time Plan: *Diagnostic*: explore adequacy of patient's usual patterns of coping and motivation to learn new strategies *Therapeutic*: 1) explain all tests/ procedures to patient who wants to know and understand what is happening to her 2) create a restful environment 3) talk with patient's home minister (daughter will contact) *Educative*: Teach patient new coping skills, e.g., relaxation exercises. Refer to community support group for widows. _____ D. Kande RN

Progress Notes (17-2D)

Date	Problem-Oriented Progress Notes
9/6/06 10 am	Impaired mobility related to weakness left lower extremity (LLE) **S** "My left leg still feels queer, pins and needles—but I can move it alright." **O** Able to lift left leg off bed, positive flexion, positive extension; muscle strength in LLE 3/5 (normal movement against gravity) **A** recovering mobility as strength returns **P** *therapeutic*: consult with physician about complete bed rest order; *diagnostic*: continue to monitor muscle strength and movement at least once/shift; be alert for any signs of recurrent TIA; *educative*: instruct not to try to get out of bed without assistance until diagnostic work-up is complete; reinforce need for safety precautions._____ D. Kande RN

FIGURE 17-2 Sample of a problem-oriented medical record.

TABLE 17-4 Organization of the Problem-Oriented Medical Record

Part	Information

Database (see Fig. 17-2A)	The database is a compilation of all initial information about the patient and includes the following:
	  Health state profile prepared by the nurse
	  Medical history and the physical examination, prepared by the physician
	  Social history
	  Initial diagnostic test results

Problem list (see Fig.17-2B)	The multidisciplinary problem list itemizes major aspects of the patient's life that require health attention and includes the following:
	  Socioeconomic, demographic, psychological, and physiologic problems
	  Each problem is labeled, numbered, and categorized as active or inactive.

Plan of care (see Fig. 17-2C)	An initial plan is formulated for each specifically numbered problem on the problem list. The nursing plan, whether therapeutic, diagnostic, or educational, is expressed through nursing orders.

Progress notes (see Fig. 17-2D)
  Narrative progress notes
	Progress notes consist of narrative progress notes, flow sheets, and discharge notes, as follows: The narrative progress notes on the patient follow the SOAP format, as follows:
	  S—Subjective information reported by the patient
	  O—Objective observations made by health practitioners
	  A—Assessments drawn from new data
	  P—Plans or goals for action related to the patient's problems

Flow sheets	Flow sheets are used for recording information that is monitored over time. This information provides data for making comparisons of a patient's status at one time with that patient's status later.

Discharge notes	Discharge notes are the entries made at the time an episode of the patient's care is terminated and include the following information:
	  The date of the resolution of each problem, as had been described while using the SOAP format
	  Referrals made for the patient
	  Recommendations for unresolved or partially resolved problems

tion, and response. Some nurses report, however, that the DAR categories are artificial and not helpful when documenting care (Eggland, 1995).

For Mr. Baron, the nurse would use focus charting to document specific aspects of teaching related to the colonoscopy and postprocedural care. In addition, due to the effects of anesthe-

sia from the colonoscopy procedure, Mr. Baron might not completely remember all that is taught. Therefore, the nurse would document to include the patient's wife in the discharge teaching to ensure that the information presented was indeed understood. Remember that Mrs. Baron is a nurse. Her clinical knowledge and any necessary reinforcement of information would also be documented.

Charting by Exception

Charting by exception is a shorthand documentation method that makes use of well-defined standards of practice; only significant findings or "exceptions" to these standards are documented in narrative notes. Benefits of this approach include decreased charting time (freeing more time for direct patient care), a greater emphasis on significant data, easy retrieval of significant data, timely bedside charting, standardized assessment, greater interdisciplinary communication, better tracking of important patient responses, and lower costs. Widely billed as "a more efficient way to document," charting by exception is rapidly gaining advocates (Comstock & Moff, 1991; Murphy & Burke, 1990). A significant drawback to charting by exception is its limited usefulness when trying to prove high-quality safe care in response to a negligence claim made against nursing. Figure 17-5 shows one example of this type of charting.

P#1:
4/02/06
1300

Caregiver role strain related to patient's new safety needs and increased need for assistance with activities of daily living upon discharge.

I:

Sat with patient's daughter and made a list of patient's safety and basic needs upon discharge. Identified what patient already knows and feels comfortable providing and developed a teaching plan to address deficiencies. Patient is highly motivated. Explored community-based resources available to daughter and made referrals to support group for family members of persons with Alzheimer's disease. Social work will talk with daughter 4/03/06 to explore care options should it become impossible to continue providing care at home.

E:

Daughter verbalized feeling more in control and less anxious about her father's return home. —————— C. Taylor, RN

FIGURE 17-3 Sample PIE patient care note.

Date/Time	Focus	Patient Care Notes
7/11/06 9:15 am	High risk for trauma	**DATA:** *Patient crying when I entered room; confided that she is afraid to go home because her injuries are the result of husband's battery* **ACTION:** *Attending notified and discharge cancelled; Abuse network called with patient's permission and they are sending a counselor this afternoon to talk with her.* — *C. Taylor, RN*
10:00 am	Pain	**DATA:** *Patient complaining of pain in right rib area* **ACTION:** *Tylenol 3 administered as ordered.* — *C. Taylor, RN*
10:30 am	Pain	**RESPONSE:** *Patient reports relief from rib pain, still anxious about aftermath of discharge.* — *C. Taylor, RN*

FIGURE 17-4 Sample focus patient care notes.

Case Management Model

Managed care's emphasis on quality, cost-effective care delivered within a limited time frame has led to the development of interdisciplinary documentation tools that clearly identify those outcomes that select groups of patients are expected to achieve on each day of care. The case management model promotes collaboration, communication, and teamwork among caregivers; makes efficient use of time; and increases quality by focusing care on carefully developed outcomes. One limitation of this model, however, is that it works best for "typical" patients with few individualized needs. At present, there is little consensus about which documentation tools are best for recording routine aspects of care and avoiding repetition.

Collaborative Pathways

Collaborative pathways (may also be called a **critical pathway** or care map) are used in the case management model. A collaborative pathway for patients undergoing modified radical mastectomy is illustrated in Figures 17-6 through 17-8. In this particular documentation system, the collaborative pathway is part of a computerized documentation system that integrates the collaborative pathway and documentation flow sheets designed to match each day's expected outcomes. Developed at Vanderbilt University, this system has reduced charting time by 40% and increased staff satisfaction with the amount of paperwork from 0% to 85%. These gains were accomplished with no decrease in audited charting quality. More importantly, a time study demonstrated a directly proportional increase in time spent with the patient (Hatcher, 1995). Charting by exception is frequently used with collaborative pathway documentation systems.

Variance Charting

When a patient fails to meet an expected outcome or a planned intervention is not implemented in the case management model, this variance from the plan is documented. The usual format for **variance charting** is the unexpected event, the cause of the event, actions taken in response to the event, and discharge planning, when appropriate. The variances most likely to be documented are those that affect quality, cost, or length of stay.

Consider Millie Delong, the woman who developed a wound infection. Typically, after abdominal surgery, infection is a complication, not a normal or expected occurrence. Therefore, using the case management model, the nurse would need to document this unexpected outcome with variance charting.

Computerized Records

In an increasing number of healthcare institutions, comprehensive computer systems have revolutionized nursing documentation in the patient record (Fig. 17-9). In these settings, computer capacities exist in which the nurse:

1. Calls up the admission assessment tool on the computer screen and keys in patient data
2. Develops the plan of care using computerized care plans available for each North American Nursing Diagnosis Association (NANDA)-approved diagnosis
3. Adds to the patient database as new data are identified and modifies the plan of care accordingly
4. Receives a work list showing the treatments, procedures, and medications necessary for the patient throughout the shift
5. Documents care immediately using the computer terminal at the patient's bedside

The ANA has been instrumental in developing the Computer-Based Patient Record Institute (CPRI) in response to a recommendation by the Institute of Medicine that a computer-based patient record be adopted nationwide by all healthcare providers and systems.

As healthcare reform initiatives evolve, patient outcomes will become the primary focus when evaluating the effectiveness of care. This focus will intensify as the Health Care Financing Administration and other reimbursement-management sources develop standard outcome measurements for all healthcare organizations. Outcome evaluations will be an important part of the healthcare agency's report card for consumers buying healthcare in this managed-care environment. A key component to facilitate data and outcome comparisons will be the **minimum data sets.** These specific categories

(text continues on page 356)

THE WILLIAMSPORT HOSPITAL & MEDICAL CENTER
Williamsport, Pennsylvania 17701-3198
FLOW SHEET
Nursing Intervention

Abbreviation Key			
I = Independent	S = Sleeping	✓ = Within normal limits or performed	
AM = Morning	A = Assist	W = Awake	X = not within normal limits
PM = Evening	C = Complete	O = Patient off unit	
* Signature of assigned caregiver for shift			

Addressograph

Date: 7/10/06			Date: 7/11/06		
2400 - 0700	0800 - 1500	1600 - 2300	2400 - 0700	0800 - 1500	1600 - 2300
PM *. C. Taylor, RN	*	*	*	*	*

Dx #	Nursing Interventions						
	Personal Care	AM - A					
	Preops, preps & One-time Interventions	shave L groin					
	Activity	OOB + BRP					

		2400 0100 0200 0300 0400 0500 0600 0700 0800 0900 1000 1100 1200 1300 1400 1500 1600 1700 1800 1900 2000 2100 2200 2300	2400 0100 0200 0300 0400 0500 0600 0700 0800 0900 1000 1100 1200 1300 1400 1500 1600 1700 1800 1900 2000 2100 2200 2300
	Safety Precautions	✓ ✓ ✓ ✓	
	IV hourly check	✓ ✓ ✓ ✓ ✓	
	Patient Check	S S S W S S W W	
#3	skin care	✓ ✓	
#4	K- pad	✓ ✓ ✓ ✓ ✓ ✓ ✓	
	Frequent Interventions		

PAGE 2
MR - 6075 1/89

Nursing Diagnosis #	System	Date 7/10/06	7/10/06	7/10/06	7/10/06	7/11/06	
		Time 1200	1600	1800	2000	0200	
# 1	Resp	X SOB c exertion, lungs clear	→	Δ ↑SOB; see progress notes	✓	Δ less SOB	
# 2	Fluid Status	X IV @ KVO; ↑PO fluids		Δ IV to hep lock; ↑PO intake	✓	D/C →	→
# 3	Skin	X reddened area on coccyx			→	→	
# 4	musculoskeletal	X L calf edematous, red, warm	→	→	Δ ↑L calf pain - see progress notes	Δ K pad D/c'd per MD orders	
	Knowledge						
	Discharge Planning						
	Signature	CT	CT	CT	CT	CT	CT

THE WILLIAMSPORT HOSPITAL & MEDICAL CENTER
Williamsport, Pennsylvania 17701-3198
FLOW SHEET
Nursing Assessment

Please Do Not Write or Stamp Above Line

PAGE 3
MR - 6075 1/89

/ = Assessment not currently required.	Δ = Change in condition.	✓ = Assessment within normal limits.
D/C = System no longer requires assessment	X = New problem.	➡ = No change in condition since last assessment.

FIGURE 17-5 Sample documentation of nursing care using charting by exception.
(Courtesy of the Department of Nursing, Williamsport Hospital and Medical Center, Williamsport, PA.)

VANDERBILT UNIVERSITY MEDICAL CENTER

Mastectomy: Modified Radical

DRG Number: _____

ELOS: _____

	Pre Op (Outpatient)	Day of Operation (Holding Room) 1 hr	Day of Operation (OR → close) 2 hr 15 min	Day of Surgery PACU (2 hr)	Day of Operation (9 S)	POD 1 (9S)	POD 2 (9S/Day of Discharge)
Goals	Pre-op testing complete and data available for review 1-4 days pre-op / Pre-op testing results WNL for surgery / Pt/family teaching complete / Consent signed	Pre-op checklist completed / Support to family / Support to patient / Permit signed	Pt. safety maintained → / Sterile tech maintained → / Pt. positioned correctly → / Initial counts documented / Final counts correct	Pain controlled / VSS, Lung CTA / Normothermia achieved / SaO₂ ≥ 90%	Voids w/o difficulty / Temp < 100° / Drsg dry & intact / Incision w/o S/Sx infection / Drains patent & functioning / Tol reg diet w/o difficulty	Reach to Recovery referral made / Demonstrates drain care	Home care teaching complete / Drains patent and functioning till return to clinic / F/U appointment scheduled
Treatments		Shave/prep	Correct position / Pad extremities and bony prominence / Warm blanket / Pt. prep / Bovie pad / Counts x 3 if applicable	Standard PACU care / Monitor drainage in hemovac / Check dsg q 1 hr	No needle sticks, BP to arm / JP drains x 2		MD remove dressing / Till RTC
Activity	Ad lib	Bedrest	Check bony prominence	Progress as tolerated	OOB to chair in p.m.	OOB to chair / Ambulate halls TID	
Diet	NPO at MN night before surg	NPO		Sips and chips if tolerated	Clear liquids → advance to regular as tolerated		
Labs	SMA6 / SMA12 / CBC with plts / PT, PTT / UA	Pre-op value on charts	Specimen to Surgical Path.		PCV		
Tests	History & physical / CXR / EKG if > 50 yrs or indicated by history	Test results on chart					
Consults	Anesthesia	Surgical Resident / Anes. Resident / Circulator for the case	Core Staff / PCM (prn) / PACU Notified / Pathologist	Surgeon		Reach to Recovery (call early w/ bra size) / Assess need for HIR	
Meds/IV		IV access / Pre-op meds	Anesthesia drugs / Ancef 1 gm	Pain meds prn IV / Antibotic IV (if requested) / May D/C IV (if ordered)	Analgesic (IV, IM on PO)	PO analgesic	
Teaching/ D/C Plan	Procedure / Plan of care / VUMC orientation / Consent signed	Reinforce pre-op teaching / Support to family / • waiting room infor. / • update phone call / Support to pt. / • answer questions / • comfort		Volurex	TCDB / Request pain med if not PCA / Assess home situation/primary care giver	Drain care (empty, reactivate, record output & change dressing q d) / Request pain med	Post mastectomy teaching / Exercises / How to take care of arm / F/U Reach to Recovery / Review drain care, meds, activity, reportable S/Sx, precautions / Complete "patient discharge list" sheet
Patient Flow	H&P MD office / Labs: Pre adm testing / CXR: Radiology / EKG: Heart Station	HR	To OR suite	PACU	9S		
Equipment & Supplies		IV start kit / Anes. supplies / X-ray folder on bed	Case cart / Bovie / Padded armboard / OR supplies / JP drains x 2 / PACU stretcher	Respirator equipment	IMED		Schedule F/U 5-7 days post op to remove drains

Mastectomy Modified Radical
6/3/94
General Surgery 1

FIGURE 17-6 Sample collaborative pathway.

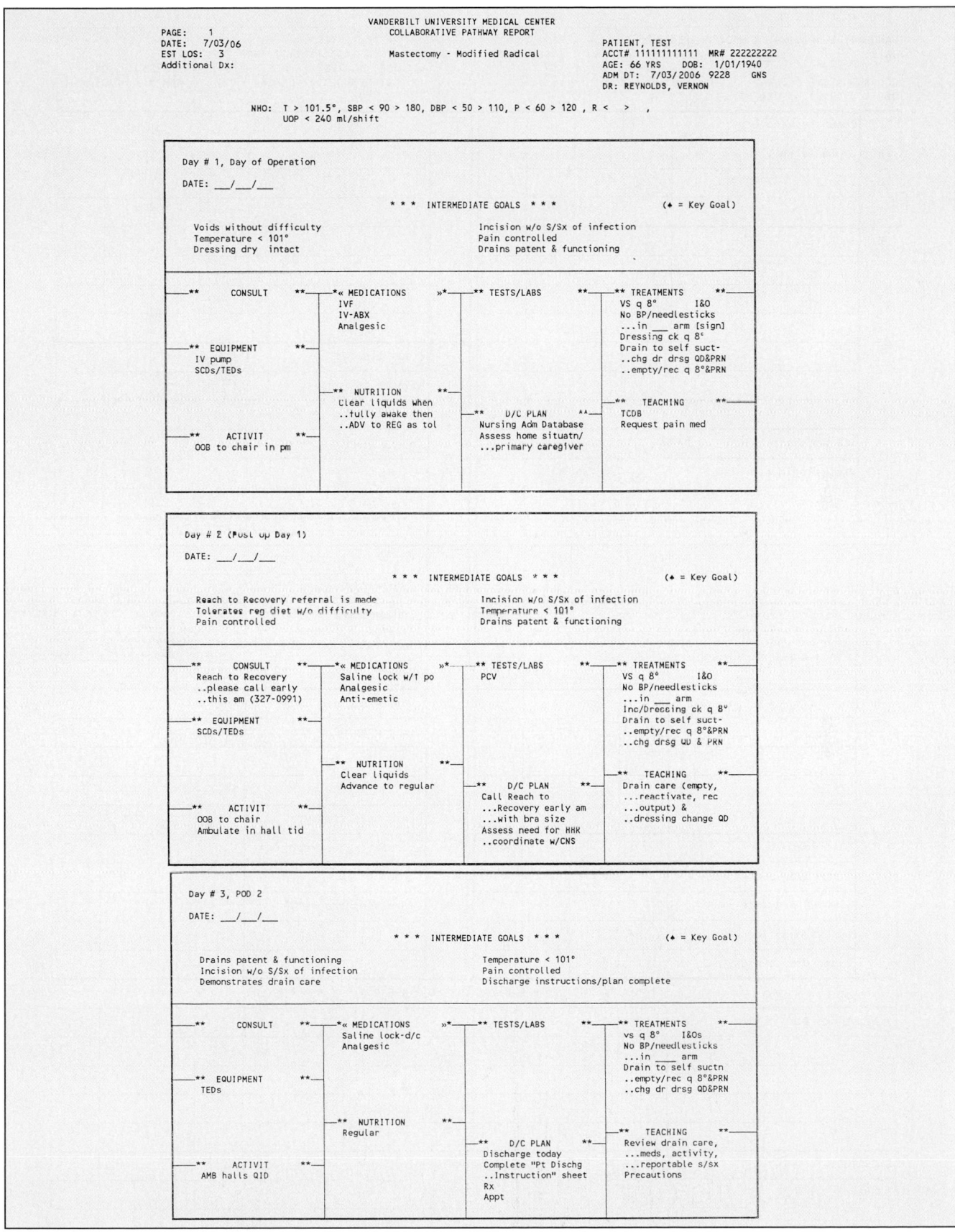

```
                              VANDERBILT UNIVERSITY MEDICAL CENTER
        PAGE:   1                 COLLABORATIVE PATHWAY REPORT
        DATE:   7/03/06                                              PATIENT, TEST
        EST LOS:  3              Mastectomy - Modified Radical       ACCT# 111111111111  MR# 222222222
        Additional Dx:                                              AGE: 66 YRS   DOB:  1/01/1940
                                                                    ADM DT:  7/03/2006  9228    GNS
                                                                    DR: REYNOLDS, VERNON

                 NHO:  T > 101.5°, SBP < 90 > 180, DBP < 50 > 110, P < 60 > 120 , R <    >  ,
                       UOP < 240 ml/shift
```

```
┌──────────────────────────────────────────────────────────────────────────────────────────┐
│  Day # 1, Day of Operation                                                                 │
│                                                                                            │
│  DATE: ___/___/___                                                                         │
│                                                                                            │
│                          * * * INTERMEDIATE GOALS * * *           (♠ = Key Goal)           │
│                                                                                            │
│     Voids without difficulty              Incision w/o S/Sx of infection                   │
│     Temperature < 101°                    Pain controlled                                  │
│     Dressing dry  intact                  Drains patent & functioning                      │
├──────────────────────────────────────────────────────────────────────────────────────────┤
│  __**     CONSULT     **__*« MEDICATIONS »*__** TESTS/LABS  **__** TREATMENTS      **__     │
│                           IVF                                  VS q 8°       I&O           │
│                           IV-ABX                               No BP/needlesticks          │
│                           Analgesic                            ...in ___ arm [sign]        │
│                                                                Dressing ck q 8°            │
│  __** EQUIPMENT     **__                                       Drain to self suct-         │
│     IV pump                                                    ..chg dr drsg QD&PRN        │
│     SCDs/TEDs                                                  ..empty/rec q 8°&PRN         │
│                                                                                            │
│                        __** NUTRITION  **__                                                │
│                           Clear liquids when   __** TEACHING    **__                       │
│                           ..fully awake then      TCDB                                     │
│                           ..ADV to REG as tol  __** D/C PLAN    **A__ Request pain med      │
│  __**    ACTIVIT    **__                          Nursing Adm Database                     │
│     OOB to chair in pm                            Assess home situatn/                     │
│                                                   ...primary caregiver                     │
└──────────────────────────────────────────────────────────────────────────────────────────┘
```

```
┌──────────────────────────────────────────────────────────────────────────────────────────┐
│  Day # 2 (Post op Day 1)                                                                   │
│                                                                                            │
│  DATE: ___/___/___                                                                         │
│                                                                                            │
│                          * * * INTERMEDIATE GOALS * * *           (♠ = Key Goal)           │
│                                                                                            │
│     Reach to Recovery referral is made    Incision w/o S/Sx of infection                   │
│     Tolerates reg diet w/o difficulty     Temperature < 101°                               │
│     Pain controlled                       Drains patent & functioning                      │
├──────────────────────────────────────────────────────────────────────────────────────────┤
│  __**    CONSULT    **__*« MEDICATIONS »*__** TESTS/LABS  **__** TREATMENTS      **__       │
│     Reach to Recovery     Saline lock w/T po   PCV            VS q 8°       I&O            │
│     ..please call early    Analgesic                          No BP/needlesticks           │
│     ..this am (327-0991)   Anti-emetic                        ...in ___ arm                │
│                                                               Inc/Dressing ck q 8°         │
│  __** EQUIPMENT     **__                                      Drain to self suct-          │
│     SCDs/TEDs                                                  ..empty/rec q 8°&PRN         │
│                                                               ..chg drsg QD & PRN          │
│                        __** NUTRITION  **__                                                │
│                           Clear liquids        __** TEACHING    **__                       │
│                           Advance to regular      Drain care (empty,                       │
│                                             __** D/C PLAN    **__ ...reactivate, rec        │
│                                                Call Reach to      ...output) &              │
│                                                ...Recovery early am  ..dressing change QD   │
│  __**    ACTIVIT    **__                       ...with bra size                            │
│     OOB to chair                               Assess need for HHK                         │
│     Ambulate in hall tid                       ..coordinate w/CNS                          │
└──────────────────────────────────────────────────────────────────────────────────────────┘
```

```
┌──────────────────────────────────────────────────────────────────────────────────────────┐
│  Day # 3, POD 2                                                                            │
│                                                                                            │
│  DATE: ___/___/___                                                                         │
│                                                                                            │
│                          * * * INTERMEDIATE GOALS * * *           (♠ = Key Goal)           │
│                                                                                            │
│     Drains patent & functioning           Temperature < 101°                               │
│     Incision w/o S/Sx of infection        Pain controlled                                  │
│     Demonstrates drain care               Discharge instructions/plan complete             │
├──────────────────────────────────────────────────────────────────────────────────────────┤
│  __**    CONSULT    **__*« MEDICATIONS »*__** TESTS/LABS  **__** TREATMENTS      **__       │
│                           Saline lock-d/c                     vs q 8°    I&Os              │
│                           Analgesic                           No BP/needlesticks           │
│                                                               ...in ___ arm                │
│                                                               Drain to self suctn          │
│  __** EQUIPMENT     **__                                      ..empty/rec q 8°&PRN         │
│     TEDs                                                       ..chg dr drsg QD&PRN         │
│                                                                                            │
│                        __** NUTRITION  **__                    __** TEACHING    **__        │
│                           Regular                                 Review drain care,       │
│                                             __** D/C PLAN    **__  ...meds, activity,       │
│                                                Discharge today    ...reportable s/sx       │
│  __**    ACTIVIT    **__                       Complete "Pt Dischg  Precautions            │
│     AMB halls QID                              ..Instruction" sheet                        │
│                                                Rx                                           │
│                                                Appt                                         │
└──────────────────────────────────────────────────────────────────────────────────────────┘
```

FIGURE 17-7 Sample collaborative pathway report.   (Courtesy of Vanderbilt University Medical Center, Nashville, TN.)

VANDERBILT UNIVERSITY MEDICAL CENTER
DATE: 7 / 5 /06   FLOWSHEET PAGE 2

PATIENT, TEST
ACCT# 111111111111   MR# 222222222
AGE: 66 YRS   DOB: 1/01/1940 9228   GNS
DR: REYNOLDS, VERNON   ADM DT: 7/03/06

COLLABORATIVE PATHWAY: Mastectomy - Modified Radical
Day # 2 (Post op Day 1)

CONSULT
- Reach to Recovery
- ..please call early
- ..this am (327-0991)   ✓ 8³⁰ AB

EQUIPMENT
- SCDs/TEDs   ✓ AB

NUTRITION
- Clear liquids   8 AB
- Advance to regular   12³⁰ AB   17³⁰ CD

ACTIVITY
- OOB to chair   8³⁰ AB
- Ambulate in hall tid   8⁴⁵ AB   16⁰⁰ CD   23⁰⁰ EF

TESTS/LABS
- PCV   7¹⁰ AB

TREATMENTS
- VS q 8°   I&O
- No BP/needlesticks   ✓ AB   ✓ CD   ✓ EF
- ...in rt_ arm
- Inc/Dressing ck q 8°   8 AB   16³⁰ CD   2200 EF
- Drain to self suct-
- ..empty/rec q 8°&PRN
- ..chg drsg QD & PRN   8⁵⁰ AB

TEACHING
- Drain care (empty,   8³⁰ AB   11³⁰ AB   20³⁰ CD
- ...reactivate, rec
- ...output) &
- ..dressing change QD

D/C PLAN
- Call Reach to   8³⁰ AB
- ...Recovery early am
- ...with bra size
- Assess need for HHR   8⁵⁰ AB
- ..coordinate w/CNS

** * * * * * INCIDENTAL ORDERS * * * * * **

chemsticks BID

| SIGNATURE | Alece Boyd RN | AB | SIGNATURE | Ellen Fisk RN | EF |
| SIGNATURE | Carol Dawn RN | CD | SIGNATURE | | |

FIGURE 17-8 Flow sheets that accompany the collaborative pathway on day 2, mastectomy—modified radical.   (Courtesy of Vanderbilt University Medical Center, Nashville, TN.)

VANDERBILT UNIVERSITY MEDICAL CENTER
DATE: 7/5/06   FLOWSHEET PAGE 3

PATIENT, TEST
ACCT# 111111111111   MR# 222222222
AGE: 66 YRS   DOB: 1/01/1940   9228   GNS
DR: REYNOLDS, VERNON   ADM DT: 7/03/06

COLLABORATIVE PATHWAY: Mastectomy - Modified Radical
Day # 2 (Post op Day 1)

ALLERGIES: penicillin

PREVIOUS DAY'S ACTIVE GOALS	Temperature < 101°

TODAY'S PATHWAY GOALS (✦ = Key Goal)	Reach to Recovery referral is made ✓AB Tolerates reg diet w/o difficulty ✓EF Pain controlled ✓EF	Incision w/o S/Sx of infection ✓EF Temperature < 101° EF Drains patent & functioning ✓EF

Time		8	10	12	14	16	18	20	22	24	2	4	6
Activity		bed	ch	ch	amb	bed	amb	bed	→	→	→	→	→
Comfort	Scale												
Sal lock	flush q8												
Trach	Care												
Saline	lavage												
Suction	trach												
Tubefeed	residual												
NGT pH													
Neuro	Pupils												
	React												
	EyesOpen												
Verbal	Response												
Motor	Response												
Strength	RUE/LUE												
Strength	RLE/LLE												
Linen o 8³⁰ BB	Bath	A 8³⁵ BB	Mouth	✓BB	Skin	✓BB	Perineal	✓BB					

* * * * * * S H I F T   A S S E S S M E N T S * * * * * *

** TIME/INITIALS **	8¹⁵ AB	1510 CD	2030 EF		** TIME/INITIALS **	8¹⁵ AB	1510 CD	2030 EF	
1. NEUROLOGICAL	✓	✓	✓		8. IV SITE	✓	✓	✓	
2. CARDIOVASCULAR	✓	✓	✓		9. INCISION	✓	✓	✓	
3. PULMONARY	✓	✱	✱		10. DRAINS	✓	✓	✓	
4. MUSCULOSKELETAL	✓	✓	✓		11. PSYCHOSOCIAL	✓	✱	→	
5. GASTROINTESTINAL	✓	✓	✓		12. SAFETY	✓	✓	✓	
6. GENITOURINARY	✓	✓	✓		13. COMFORT	✓	✓	✓	
7. INTEGUMENT	✓	✓	✓						

IV SITE: LOC/TYPE	RFA/PIV				COLLABORATIVE PATH REVIEW	EF

SIGNATURE	Alece Boyd, RN	AB	SIGNATURE	Betty Brown CP	BB	✓ = No significant finding
SIGNATURE	Carol Dawn, RN	CD	SIGNATURE			✱ = Significant finding see note
SIGNATURE	Ellen Fisk, RN	EF	SIGNATURE			-> = No change from last significant finding

FIGURE 17-8 *Continued*

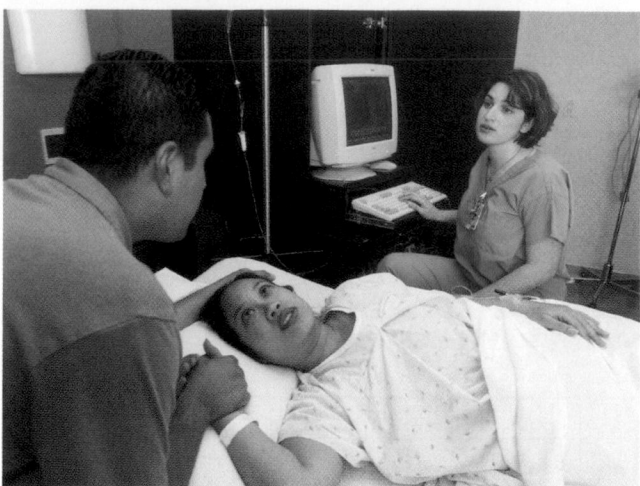

FIGURE 17-9 Computerized bedside charting allows the nurse to remain in contact with the data source while electronically documenting patient information. *(Photo by Joe Mitchell.)*

of information will use uniform definitions to create a common language among multiple healthcare data users.

The nursing minimum data set is organized into three categories:

• Nursing care elements (such as nursing diagnoses and interventions)
• Patient demographic elements (such as sex, date of birth, and ethnicity)
• Service elements (such as admission and discharge dates and expected payer for services)

With **computer-based records,** these data can be distributed among many caregivers in a standardized format, allowing them to compare and uniformly evaluate patient progress easily. Besides tracking the progress of individual patients, computerized outcome information can compare the progress of groups of patients with similar diagnoses. These results will contribute to research, education, and, ultimately, better and more efficient nursing practice (Eggland, 1995).

The increasing use of computerized patient information systems to store and analyze patient data has necessitated the development of policies and procedures to ensure the privacy and confidentiality of patient information. Policies should specify what types of patient information can be retrieved, by whom, and for what purpose. Patient consent is necessary for the use and release of any stored information that can be linked to the patient. Box 17-3 highlights guidelines for safe computer charting.

Formats for Nursing Documentation

When the nursing process is fully implemented, nursing documentation in the patient's permanent record includes information in the following areas:

Initial Nursing Assessment

A typical form used to record the initial database obtained from the nursing history and physical assessment is illustrated in

---

BOX 17-3 Safe Computer Charting

The American Nurses Association, the American Medical Record Association, and the Canadian Nurses Association offer the following guidelines and strategies for safe computer charting:

• Never give your personal password or computer signature to anyone—including another nurse in the unit, a float nurse, or a doctor.
• Don't leave a computer terminal unattended after you have logged on.
• Follow the correct protocol for correcting errors. To correct an error after storage, mark the entry "mistaken entry," add the correct information, and date and initial the entry. If you record information in the wrong chart, write "mistaken entry—wrong chart" and sign off.
• Never create, change, or delete records unless you have specific authority to do so.
• Make sure that stored records have back-up files—an important safety check. If you inadvertently delete part of the permanent record, type an explanation into the computer file with the date, time, and your initials and submit an explanation in writing to your manager.
• Don't leave information about a patient displayed on a monitor where others may see it. Keep a log that accounts for every copy of a computerized file that you've generated from the system.
• Never use e-mail to send protected health information unless it has been encrypted to protect it from unauthorized access.
• Follow the agency's confidentiality procedures for documenting sensitive material, such as a diagnosis of acquired immunodeficiency syndrome or human immunodeficiency virus infection.

Charting tips. Computer charting: Minimizing legal risks. (1993). *Nursing 93, 23*(5), 86.

Chapter 12. Accurate documentation of these data is important because it provides a baseline for later comparisons as a patient's condition changes.

Think back to Jason Chandler, the adolescent brought to the emergency department in police custody. Due to the nature of the admission, a complete nursing assessment would be inappropriate. However, the nurse would need to thoroughly assess the patient for signs and symptoms indicating problems associated with swallowing the bag of drugs. Later on, once the initial situation is resolved, an initial history and physical examination would be performed.

Kardex and Patient Care Summary

Many healthcare institutions and agencies use a **Kardex care plan** to communicate conveniently and concisely the plan of nursing care for each patient. The Kardex is recorded on a folded card and placed in a central Kardex file where it is easily accessible. The plan is eventually placed in the patient's health record. The outside of the card (activity and treatment section) contains basic information, such as the patient's profile, admitting diagnosis, and orders concerning activity levels, diet, vital signs, diagnostic tests, medications, and other treatments and procedures. The inside of the Kardex contains the nursing care plan specifying nursing diagnoses and health problems, related outcomes and nursing interventions, and special safety precautions. Some agencies now have computerized systems that are able to generate this same information in the form of a patient care summary for each shift.

Plan of Nursing Care

Patient records must communicate the patient's problems or diagnoses; related goals, outcomes, and interventions; and progress or resolution of the problems. The plan of nursing care may be written separately or incorporated into a multidisciplinary plan. In a traditional plan of nursing care, nursing diagnoses, goals and expected outcomes, and nursing interventions are written for each patient (see the sample student plan in Chapter 14 and the plans of care at the end of each clinical chapter). Standardized plans of care may also be used that identify common problems and related care for select patient cohorts. These generally incorporate standards of high-quality care, but unless such care plans are individualized, they might not sufficiently address individual patient needs. Formats for plans of care vary greatly.

Critical/Collaborative Pathways

The case management plan is a detailed, standardized plan of care that is developed for a patient population with a designated diagnosis or procedure. It includes expected outcomes, a list of interventions to be performed, and the sequence and timing of those interventions. The **critical/collaborative pathway,** illustrated in Figure 17-6 and in Chapter 14, is an abbreviated summary of key information taken from the more detailed case management plan.

Progress Notes

The purpose of **progress notes** is to inform caregivers of the progress a patient is making toward achieving expected outcomes. The method used to record the patient's progress depends on the documentation system being used. Common examples include narrative nursing notes, SOAP notes, PIE notes, focus charting, charting by exception, and flow sheets. The advantages and disadvantages of each are listed in Table 17-5.

Flow Sheets

Flow sheets are documentation tools used to record routine aspects of nursing care. Examples are shown in Figures 17-1 and 17-8.

Graphic (Clinical) Record

The **graphic sheet** is a form used to record specific patient variables such as pulse, respiratory rate, blood pressure readings, body temperature, weight, fluid intake and output, bowel movements, and other patient characteristics (Fig. 17-10).

A graphic record would be used for both Millie Delong and Phillippe Baron, described at the beginning of the chapter. Specifically for Millie Delong, documentation of vital signs would be significant because she has wound infection. Because Mr. Baron is post-colonoscopy, his vital signs also need to be assessed frequently. In addition, fluid intake and output are key postoperative assessment findings to document.

24-Hour Fluid Balance Record

Forms are available to document the 24-hour intake and output of fluids for patients with special needs. The forms include shift and daily fluid intake and output totals. A sample tool is shown in Chapter 46.

Medication Record

The patient's **medication record** must include documentation of all the medications administered to the patient (drug, dose, route, time), the nurse administering the drug, and, for some medications (eg, analgesics), the reason the drug was administered and its effectiveness. Sample medication records are shown in Chapter 29.

24-Hour Patient Care Records and Acuity Charting Forms

Flow sheets such as those illustrated in Figures 17-1 and 17-8 are often used to document routine aspects of nursing care efficiently throughout a 24-hour period. When well designed, they enable nurses to quickly document the routine aspects of care that promote patient goal achievement, safety, and well-being.

Twenty-four-hour reports are increasingly used in conjunction with acuity reports, which allow nurses to rank patients as high to low acuity in relation to both the patient's condition and need for nursing assistance or intervention. A trauma patient whose condition is changing rapidly and who requires intensive nurse monitoring and intervention will merit a higher acuity rank than a patient whose condition is stable. Acuity rankings are often used to determine staffing requirements. A nursing unit with patients with higher acuity rankings requires more professional nurses than a unit with the same number of patients but with lower acuity ranks.

Discharge and Transfer Summary

At the time a patient is discharged from care or transferred from one unit or institution or agency to another, a clinical report should be written that concisely summarizes the reason for treatment, significant findings, the procedures performed and treatment rendered, the patient's condition on discharge or transfer, and any specific pertinent instructions given to the patient and family.

Consider Phillippe Baron, the man who had undergone a colonoscopy. The nurse would be responsible for completing the discharge sum-

(text continues on page 361)

TABLE 17-5 Advantages and Disadvantages of Different Documentation Formats

Format	Advantages	Disadvantages
Narrative notes	Narrative notes allow nurses to describe a condition, situation, or response in their own terms, as they understand it.	It is time-consuming and difficult to read days and weeks of narrative notes to find a specific problem, its treatment, and patient response.
SOAP notes (subjective data, objective data, assessment–judgment, plan)	The location of the problem list at the front of the chart alerts all caregivers to patient priorities. Care and documentation of care is problem focused. Easy retrieval of information facilitates quality review and research. Healthcare professionals from different disciplines chart on same progress notes. SOAP format is consistent with nursing process.	The level of ability and consistency of caregivers in organizing data into the SOAP format may vary. Problem focus may reduce patients to "problems to be solved." Maintaining a neat, up-to-date problem list takes constant vigilance and routine review.
PIE (problem, intervention, evaluation)	Without a formal, separate care plan, the method saves time because a nurse does not have to create or update a plan. Consistent with nursing process	Because there is no formal care plan, the nurse preparing to provide care will need to read all the nursing notes to determine problems, planned interventions, and evaluations to see if those interventions are effective.
Focus charting	Ease of charting with DAR is an advantage because categories of data, action, and response are not required for each focus cited. Components of DAR can be cited alone or out of sequence.	Many nurses have difficulty documenting information by separating the data into DAR categories. The "result" portion of the note seems to be a particularly difficult area because some nurses relate this portion to the resulting problems identified from the assessment data rather than to the patient outcome of care after nursing intervention.
Charting by exception	Abnormal status can be seen immediately, with narrative easily retrieved. The flow-sheet format shows overall trends in the patient's condition. Guidelines provide specific but concise standard information regarding "normal" assessments and expected outcomes. Documentation time is decreased because standard care is not written in narrative and duplication of charting is eliminated. This results in charting being done in a more timely manner.	Preventive and wellness-promoting functions of nursing are not documented on this format because they do not address problems. The system requires predictable, defined patient outcomes, which are more difficult to predict for some patients and in some settings than in others. More difficult to computerize
Case management model	Makes efficient use of time because each day has planned interventions and patient expected outcomes written on the plan. Increases the probability that a patient will be discharged in a timely fashion. Care is goal focused, which potentially increases quality. Promotes collaboration, communication, and teamwork among caregivers	Effective for patients with one or two diagnoses and few complications; less helpful for patients with multiple variances Space to document is limited on critical pathways, and too much writing causes illegibility. Space for individualization is limited. Separate narrative notes must be used for documentation of care. The intervention flow sheet, nursing notes, and critical path must all be reviewed to get a picture of a patient's condition.

Data for this chart were adapted in part from Eggland, E. T., & Heinemann, D. S. (1995). *Nursing documentation: Charting, recording and reporting.* Philadelphia: J. B. Lippincott.

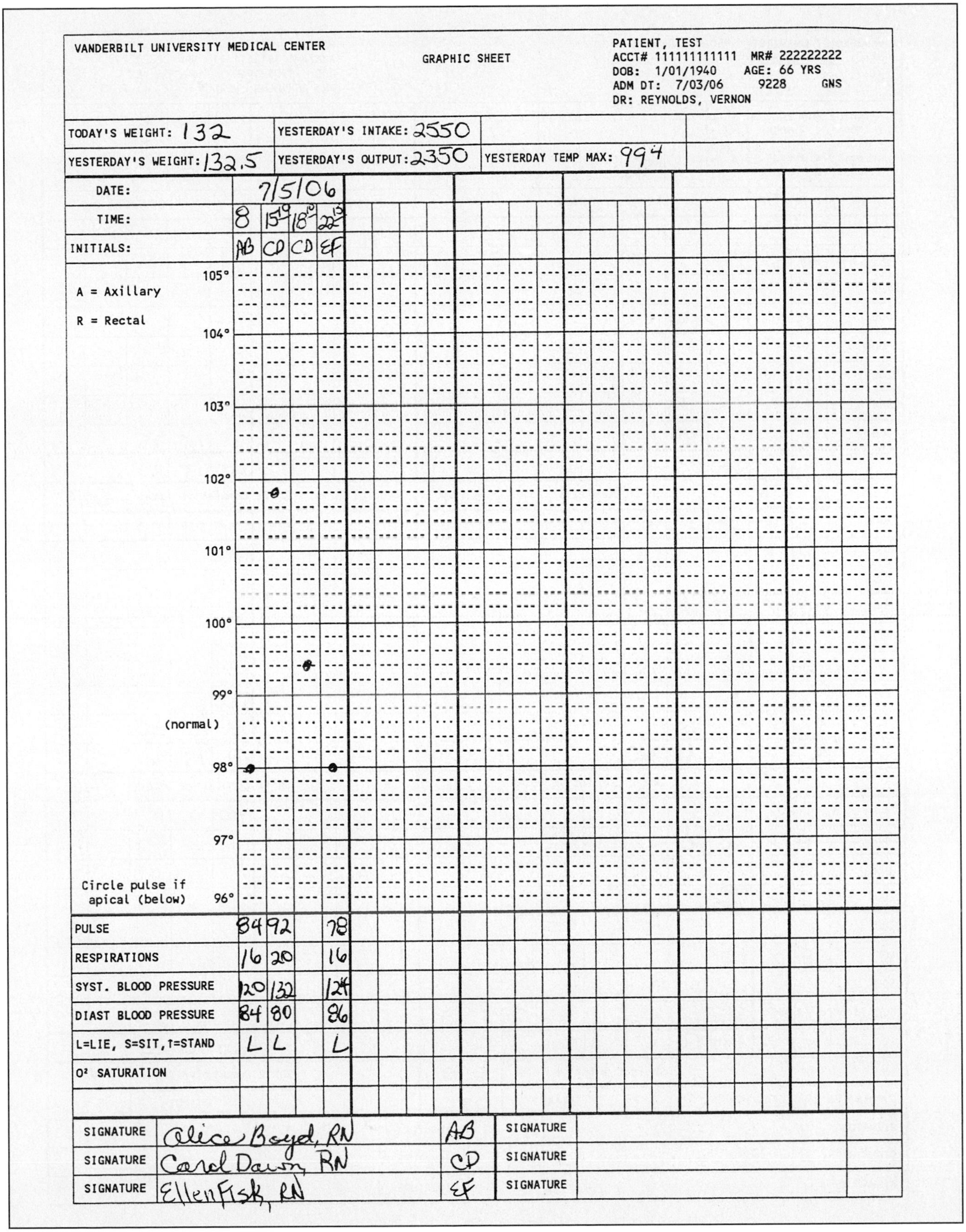

VANDERBILT UNIVERSITY MEDICAL CENTER	GRAPHIC SHEET	PATIENT, TEST ACCT# 111111111111 MR# 222222222 DOB: 1/01/1940 AGE: 66 YRS ADM DT: 7/03/06 9228 GNS DR: REYNOLDS, VERNON

TODAY'S WEIGHT: 132	YESTERDAY'S INTAKE: 2550	
YESTERDAY'S WEIGHT: 132.5	YESTERDAY'S OUTPUT: 2350	YESTERDAY TEMP MAX: 99⁴

DATE:	7/5/06				
TIME:	8 15⁰⁰ 18⁰⁰ 22⁰⁰				
INITIALS:	AB CD CD EF				

A = Axillary
R = Rectal

Temperature graph rows: 105° to 96°
(normal)
Circle pulse if apical (below)

Marked temperature points approximately at 102° (CD), 99° (CD), 98° (AB and EF).

PULSE	84 92 78				
RESPIRATIONS	16 20 16				
SYST. BLOOD PRESSURE	120 132 124				
DIAST BLOOD PRESSURE	84 80 86				
L=LIE, S=SIT, ↑=STAND	L L L				
O² SATURATION					

SIGNATURE	Alice Boyd, RN	AB	SIGNATURE
SIGNATURE	Carol Dawn, RN	CD	SIGNATURE
SIGNATURE	Ellen Fisk, RN	EF	SIGNATURE

FIGURE 17-10 Graphic record that accompanies the collaborative pathway in Figure 17-6. (*continued*)
(Courtesy of Vanderbilt University Medical Center, Nashville, TN.)

VANDERBILT UNIVERSITY MEDICAL CENTER
DATE: **7/5/06**

I & O SHEET

PATIENT, TEST   ADM: 7/03/06
ACCT# 111111111111   MR# 222222222
DOB: 1/01/1940   AGE: 66 YRS
DR: REYNOLDS, VERNON   9228   GNS

T = Tubing Change
▲ = Dressing Change
D = Diuretic
+ = Positive Blood
- = Negative Blood

TIME	INIT	SITE✓	D5½NS w/20K	Meds	PO					INTAKE OR OUTPUT				urine	JP#1	JP#2		BM
					INTAKE					INTAKE OR OUTPUT				OUTPUT				
0700																		
0800	AB	✓	240/60		400									200				
0900																		T
1000	AB	✓	180/60	50	100													
1100																		
1200	AB	✓	120/60		400													
1300														400				
1400	AB	✓	60/60	50											15	25		
			240	100	900									600	15	25		
					Shift Cumulative Total	1240					Shift Cumulative Total				640			
1500			T 1000/60															
1600	CD	✓												400				
1700																		
1800	CD	✓	930/70	T 100	240													
1900																		
2000	CD	✓	880/50		100													
2100														500				
2200	CD	✓	820/60	50											15	30		
			240	150	340									900	15	30		
					Shift Cumulative Total	730					Shift Cumulative Total				945			
2300														400				
2400	EF	✓	770/60	50														
0100																		
0200	EF	✓	705/65															
0300																		
0400	EF	✓	650/55															
0500																		
0600	EF	✓	580/80													10	25		
			240	50										400	10	25		
					Shift Cumulative Total	290					Shift Cumulative Total				440			
CUMULATIVE 24° TOTAL					INTAKE	2260						OUTPUT			2030			
SIGNATURE								SIGNATURE										
SIGNATURE								SIGNATURE										
SIGNATURE								SIGNATURE										

FIGURE 17-10 *Continued*

mary, making sure to include specific aspects of teaching and both the patient's and wife's understanding of the teaching.

Home Healthcare Documentation

Documentation of home care visits that reports the patient's progress serves multiple purposes. Sent to the attending physician with a request for signed medical orders to continue treatment, these records ensure continuity of care. Sent to third-party payers, they establish the need for continuing home care that results in continued reimbursement for necessary services. Medicare, for example, reviews progress summaries to determine whether a patient meets one of these Medicare requirements:

- The patient is homebound and still needs skilled nursing care.
- Rehabilitation potential is good (or the patient is dying).
- The patient's status is not stabilized.
- The patient is making progress in expected outcomes of care.

The **O**utcome and **A**ssessment **I**nformation **S**et (**OASIS**) is a group of data elements that:

- Represent core items of a comprehensive assessment for an adult home care patient
- Form the basis for measuring patient outcomes for purposes of outcome-based quality improvement (OBQI)

The OASIS is a key component of Medicare's partnership with the home care industry to foster and to monitor improved home healthcare outcomes. It is proposed to be an integral part of the revised *Conditions of Participation* for Medicare-certified home health agencies (HHAs). Overall, the OASIS items are useful for outcome monitoring, clinical assessment, care planning, and other internal agency-level applications. OASIS data items encompass sociodemographic, environmental, support system, health status, and functional status attributes of adult (nonmaternity) patients. In addition, selected attributes of health service use are included (see *http://cms.hhs.gov/oasis/oasisdat.asp*). Chapter 10 shows a sample home health certification and a skilled nursing note.

Long-Term Care Documentation

Documentation in long-term care settings is specified by the Resident Assessment Instrument (RAI), which helps staff gather definitive information on a resident's strengths and needs, and addresses these in an individualized plan of care. The RAI helps staff track changes in a resident's status by evaluating resident goal achievement and making appropriate revisions in the plan of care. The goal is to coordinate the efforts of the multidisciplinary team to ensure that residents achieve the highest level of functioning possible (Quality of Care) and maintain their sense of individuality (Quality of Life).

The RAI consists of four basic components:

- *Minimum data set*—a core set of screening, clinical, and functional status elements that forms the foundation of the comprehensive assessment of all residents in long-term care facilities certified to participate in Medicare or Medicaid. The items in the minimum data set stan-

dardize communication about resident problems and condition.

- *Triggers*—specific resident responses for one or a combination of minimum data set elements that identify residents who either have or are at risk for developing specific functional problems and who require further evaluation using resident assessment protocols.
- *Resident assessment protocols*—structured, problem-oriented frameworks for organizing minimum data set information and examining additional clinically relevant information about a resident. Resident assessment protocols help identify social, medical, nursing, and psychological problems and form the basis for individualized care planning.
- *Utilization guidelines*—specified in state operation manuals that instruct when and how to use the RAI.

Statutory law, federal regulations, and the Health Care Financing Administration specify how the RAI is implemented. An RAI must be completed for residents of Medicare skilled nursing facilities or Medicaid nursing facilities, hospice residents, and short-term stay or respite residents who are residing in a facility for longer than 14 days.

Benefits of using the RAI process according to Health Care Financing Administration (1998) include the following:

1. Residents respond to individualized care.
2. Staff communication becomes more effective.
3. Resident and family involvement increases.
4. Documentation becomes clearer.

Potential Legal Problems in Documentation

The results of one in four malpractice suits are determined on the basis of the patient's record. In Box 17-4, Potential Legal Problems in Documentation, Eggland and Heinemann (1995) outline documentation content and mechanics that increase a nurse's legal risk. No nurse can afford to be ignorant or careless with respect to agency policies and professional standards for documentation.

REPORTING CARE

To report is to give an account of something that has been seen, heard, done, or considered. **Reporting** is the oral, written, or computer-based communication of patient data to others. A laboratory report, for example, might communicate to the healthcare team that a patient's cardiac enzymes are normal or that a biopsy of breast tissue revealed malignant or atypical cells. A nurse's shift report or nursing note might communicate the progress a patient is making toward goal achievement. Common methods for reporting among health practitioners, in addition to the patient record, include face-to-face meetings, telephone conversations, messengers, written messages, audiotaped messages, and computer messages. Each of these methods has certain benefits and limitations, as detailed in Table 17-6.

Change-of-Shift Reports

A **change-of-shift report** is given by a primary nurse to the nurse replacing him or her or by the charge nurse to the nurse who assumes responsibility for continuing care of the patient. The change-of-shift report might be given in written form or orally in a meeting (Fig. 17-11), or it may be audiotaped. Many charge nurses find that taped reports decrease the amount of time spent reporting and allow more time for last-minute details.

Typical information shared among nurses in a change-of-shift report includes the following:

- Basic identifying information about each patient—name, room number, bed designation, and current diagnosis
- Current appraisal of each patient's health status:
  - Changes in medical condition (results of pertinent diagnostic studies) and the patient's response to medical therapy

  - Where the patient stands in relation to identified nursing diagnoses and goal achievement
- Current orders (especially any newly changed orders):
  - Nurse-prescribed orders
  - Physician-prescribed orders (changes in medications, intravenous fluids, diet, activity level)
- Summary of each newly admitted patient, including his or her medical diagnosis, age, plan of therapy, and general condition
- Report on patients who have been transferred or discharged

It is important to avoid unprofessional comments about patients that could predispose oncoming nurses to view and respond to patients negatively.

Telephone/Telemedicine Reports

Telephones and telemedicine equipment can link healthcare professionals immediately and enable nurses to receive and give critical information about patients in a timely fashion. For example, the hematology lab might call to report a dangerously low platelet count, and the nurse might in turn notify the attending physician to obtain new medical orders. When reporting significant changes in a patient's condition to physicians and other healthcare professionals, nurses should be prepared to do the following:

- Identify themselves and the patient, and state their relationship to the patient. ("Dr. Gomez-Lobo, this is Ellen McLouglin, and I'm calling about Mr. Clouser, a patient of yours who was just discharged home following a work-up for recurrent chest pain. I'm his new nurse case manager.")
- Report concisely and accurately the change in the patient's condition that is of concern and what has already been done in response to this condition. ("When I first arrived in his home, he was complaining of feeling dizzy, and his blood pressure was 190/110. Yesterday morning in the hospital it was 150/90. His wife appears very flustered and says she doesn't know how she is going to take care of him. I had him rest for 30 minutes, and when I checked his pressure at that time, it was still 186/110.")
- Report the patient's current vital signs and clinical manifestations.
- Have the patient's record at hand to make knowledgeable responses to any physician's inquiries. In this example, the physician will probably want to know all the vital signs and may ask questions about the treatment regimen both in the hospital and upon discharge.
- Concisely record the time and date of the call, what was communicated to the physician, and the physician's response.

Transfer and Discharge Reports

Nurses report a summary of a patient's condition and care when transferring patients from one unit or institution or agency to another (eg, from the postanesthesia care unit to a surgical floor) and when discharging patients. The nurse making the report should concisely summarize all the patient data that

TABLE 17-6 **Common Methods of Communication Among Healthcare Professionals**

Method	Advantages	Disadvantages
Face-to-face meeting	• Message can be delivered immediately. • Nonverbal messages are readily conveyed. • Message can be clarified; receiver's questions can be raised and answered.	• Both the communicating and the receiving people must be available at the same time, in the same place. • Ordinarily there is no permanent record for later use.
Telephone conversation	• Message can be delivered immediately. • Message can be clarified; receiver's questions can be raised and answered. • Two parties need not be present in same place.	• Only the tone of voice and voice inflections can be communicated—no nonverbal messages. • Ordinarily, there is no permanent record.
Written message	• Message can be exchanged at times convenient for the people involved. • Record is available. • Time-efficient if message is understood	• Message usually cannot be validated with the sender.
Audiotaped message	• Message can be exchanged at times convenient for the people involved. • Record is available. • Time-efficient if information communicated is complete	• Message usually cannot be validated with the sender.
Computer message	• Message can be delivered immediately—even to those at a great distance. • Parties need not be present in same place. • Two-way communication is possible by e-mail. • Record is available. • Many people can participate in exchange.	• No nonverbal messages can be communicated. • Privacy concerns remain an issue.

caregivers need to provide immediate care. See Chapter 9 for transfer and discharge reporting guidelines.

Reports to Family Members and Significant Others

Nurses play a crucial role in keeping the patient's family and significant others updated about the patient's condition and progress toward goal achievement. Nurses should clarify with the patient which visitors, if any, are entitled to progress reports. "Mrs. Neale, do you object to our disclosing your health information to family or friends?" Similarly, nurses need to clarify what types of information they are able to communicate. If the patient objects to disclosure, nurses are not permitted to discuss the patient's health condition with family or friends. If a patient is not able to communicate that he or she objects, such as in an emergency situation or when a patient is unconscious, professional caregivers must use their best professional judgment to decide whether to talk to family and friends.

For example, the nurse is generally not the caregiver who informs family members that a patient's biopsy has revealed a malignancy. The nurse does, however, often explain what this will mean for the patient after the family has this information. Information should be shared in a manner that is honest, compassionate, and respectful of the person's ability to understand medical concepts.

Incident Reports

An **incident report,** also termed a variance or occurrence report, is a tool used by healthcare agencies to document the occurrence of anything out of the ordinary that results in or has the potential to result in harm to a patient, employee, or visitor. These reports are used for quality improvement and should not be used for disciplinary action against staff members. They are

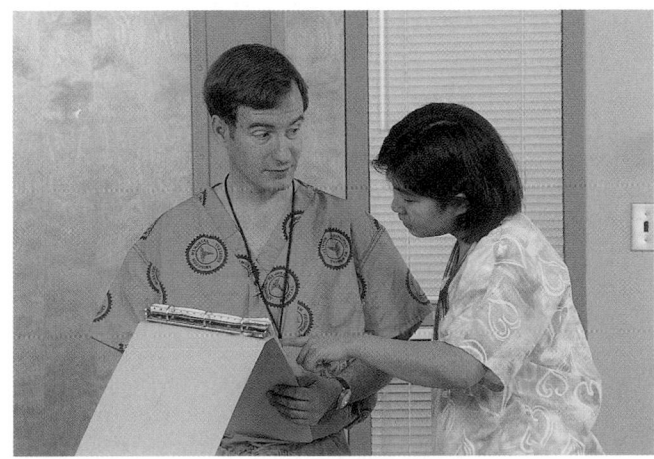

FIGURE 17-11 During a change-of-shift report, a nurse from the ending shift provides a summary of the patient's condition and current status of care to the nurse coming on duty.   (Photo © B. Proud)

a means of identifying risks. More harm than good results from ignoring mistakes. Incident reports improve the management and treatment of patients by identifying high-risk patterns and initiating in-service programs to prevent future problems. These forms also make all the facts about an incident available to the agency in case of litigation. It is important for nurses to be familiar with agency policy about their responsibilities and obligations if they are involved personally in an incident that results in or has the potential to result in harm to a patient, employee, or visitor, or if they witness such an incident. An example of an incident report form and a fuller discussion of this topic may be found in Chapter 7.

CONFERRING ABOUT CARE

To confer is to consult with someone to exchange ideas or to seek information, advice, or instructions. A nurse might consult with another nurse, such as when a primary care nurse consults with a nurse clinical specialist about a particular patient's care. A school nurse might confer with a child's teacher or a psychologist about a behavior problem. A community health nurse and a physician might confer about a patient's activity regimen. Health practitioners also confer with each other to validate information. Healthcare professionals increasingly use electronic support groups to consult with clinicians who share similar interests or who have expertise in other specialty areas.

> *Think back to Jason Chandler, the adolescent who was brought in to the emergency department by the police. He was refusing treatment. To determine the legal implications of administering to treatment to the patient, the physician consulted the hospital's attorney for legal guidance. Doing so helped to clarify what actions were and were not acceptable.*

Consultations and Referrals

When nurses detect problems they cannot resolve because they lie outside the scope of independent nursing practice or their expertise, they make consultations or referrals to other professionals. The process of inviting another professional to evaluate the patient and make recommendations to you about his or her treatment is called a **consultation.** The process of sending or guiding the patient to another source for assistance is called a **referral.** A patient might be referred by a hospital to a community health nursing service for assistance with home care. A school nurse might refer a student to a hospital emergency department. A community health nurse who learns that a patient with multiple sexual contacts is HIV positive will refer to the Department of Health for tracking of these contacts.

Most health agencies have policies for referrals. An agency may have a special form that personnel are to use when making referrals. Referral policies usually indicate who may initiate a referral, how it is to be done, and so on. Referrals are especially important in providing continuity of care for people who need a variety of services. It is essential that health practitioners to whom a patient is referred receive the information that is most useful to the continuity of care. The key question is "What would I want to know about this patient if I were the person who had to continue his or her care?" The patient must know and approve of a referral to another agency or to other health personnel.

Before requesting a consultation or making a referral, nurses should determine which profession has the needed expertise and which of its practitioners are appropriate for consultation or referral. A great disservice is done to patients when referrals are poorly made. Patients and family members also appreciate a phone number and practical tips about how to easily reach the referred practitioner.

> *Recall Millie Delong, the woman with the wound infection. Obtaining a consultation from a wound, continence, and ostomy nurse might be appropriate to assist with measures for wound care. Additionally, consultation with an infection-control nurse may be necessary if the patient's wound continues to remain infected or fails to heal.*

Nursing and Interdisciplinary Team Care Conferences

Nurses and other healthcare professionals frequently confer in groups to plan and coordinate patient care. Such conferences are also used for instructing students and practitioners. A **nursing care conference** is a meeting of nurses to discuss some aspect of a patient's care. For example, several nurses who are caring for a generally uncooperative patient might initiate a conference. This would allow each nurse an opportunity to offer his or her opinion about the patient's problem and its cause, and then together they could discuss possible solutions to the problem.

Nurses might invite other healthcare practitioners to a nursing care conference concerning a patient's care. For example, a clinical psychologist might be invited in the preceding example to address the possibility that a mental disorder is influencing this patient's behavior.

Nursing Care Rounds

Nursing care rounds are procedures in which a group of nurses visit selected patients individually at each patient's bedside. The primary purposes of nursing care rounds are to gather information to help plan nursing care, to evaluate the nursing care the patient has received, and to provide the patient with an opportunity to discuss his or her care with those administering it. As each patient is visited, the nurse assigned provides a short summary of the patient's nursing diagnoses and goals and the care being given. Nursing care rounds have two principal advantages over discussions in a meeting room: nursing personnel can actually see the patient as a report of care is given, and the patient can participate in discussions of his or her care.

Nurses should use language the patient can understand when holding discussions at the bedside. Otherwise, the patient is likely to feel excluded and cannot intelligently participate in the discussion. Nurses might also make rounds with physicians to share nursing's perspective with them.

Developing Critical Thinking Skills

1. Interview three practicing nurses and ask them to describe the documentation methods they have used in their practice. Which methods did they prefer? Which method was more effective, time efficient, and easiest to use?

2. A nurse overhears you complaining about writing narrative nursing notes and says to you "Don't sweat it. I never worry about documentation—it's a waste of time. I'd rather spend my time doing things for patients than writing up what I did." Think about what you would like to say to this nurse and your rationale for this. Ask other students for their response, and compare your answers.

3. Imagine that you are a nurse in a nursing home and that you and the home are being sued for negligence by the family of an elderly resident who fell and fractured her hip last year. You know the resident but do not remember much about the day she fell. What data do you hope to find recorded in her health record? Which documentation system would most likely provide the type of information you think you need to reconstruct the events surrounding her fall?

4. How would you respond to each of the following requests for patient information? Compare your responses with those of another student and talk about any differences.
   • The mayor of your town, who is up for reelection, was just admitted to your unit after an acute myocardial infarction. You receive a phone call from his office requesting information about his condition.
   • A woman you have never seen approaches you in the hallway, identifies herself as the sexual partner of a married male patient on your unit, and requests information about his condition.
   • A case manager from a managed care organization calls you to ask about the progress an elderly surgical patient is making postoperatively. You have heard that the organization is eager to discharge her quickly, and you feel uncomfortable reporting any information over the phone.

Practicing for NCLEX

1. Which of the following documentation guidelines are correct?
   a. Enter information in a complete, accurate, concise, factual, and organized manner.
   b. Use words such as "good," "average," "normal," or "sufficient" to communicate judgments about data.
   c. Wait until the end of the shift to document nursing interventions to ensure comprehensive charting.
   d. Date and time each entry.
      a. a, b, c, d
      b. a, c, d
      c. a, b, d
      d. a, d

2. Which of the following documentation guidelines are correct?
   a. Erase or use correcting fluid to completely delete mistaken entries.
   b. Document nursing interventions as closely as possible to the time of their execution.
   c. Note problems as they occur in an orderly, sequential manner.
   d. Carefully document all the factors that compromise patient safety and contribute to patient harm.
      a. a, c
      b. b, c
      c. b, c, d
      d. a, b, c, d

3. According to the Health Insurance Portability and Accountability Act of 1996, patients have a right to all of the following:
   a. To see and copy their health record
   b. To update their health record
   c. To get a list of the disclosures a healthcare institution has made independent of disclosures made for the purposes of treatment, payment, and healthcare operations
   d. To request a restriction on certain uses or disclosures
   e. To choose how to receive health information
      a. a, b, c
      b. b, d, e
      c. a, c, d, e
      d. a, b, c, d, e

4. According to the Health Insurance Portability and Accountability Act of 1996, if a health institution wants to release a patient's health information for purposes other than treatment, payment, and routine healthcare operations, the patient must be asked to sign an authorization. There are exceptions to this requirement. In which case below is an authorization needed?
   a. The patient is a public figure and the local news media are preparing a news report.
   b. Data are needed for the tracking and notification of disease outbreaks.
   c. Child abuse and neglect are suspected.
   d. Protected health information is needed to facilitate organ donations.

5. A friend of yours calls you and asks if you are still working at Memorial Hospital. You reply "yes." He tells you that his girlfriend's father was just admitted as a patient, and he wants you to find out how he

is. "Sue (his girlfriend) seems unusually worried about her dad, but she won't talk to me and I want to be able to help her." What is the best response you can make to your friend?

a. "Listen, you shouldn't be asking me to do this. I could be fined big bucks or even lose my job for disclosing this information."

b. "Sorry, but I'm not able to give information about patients to the public—even when my best friend or a family member asks."

c. "Because of the Health Insurance Portability and Accountability Act, you shouldn't be asking for this information unless the patient has authorized you to receive it! This could get you in trouble!"

d. "Why do you think Sue isn't talking about her worries?"

6. Your patient has an order for an analgesic medication to be given as needed. The correct abbreviation for "as needed" is:

a. TURP
b. PMH
c. PRN
d. TPR

7. If you were looking for trends in a patient's vital signs, what form should you consult first?

a. Admission sheet
b. Admission nursing assessment
c. Activity flow sheet
d. Graphic sheet

8. This method of documentation uses the categories data, action, and response (DAR) to facilitate charting.

a. Narrative notes
b. Focus charting
c. Charting by exception
d. Case management model

9. A resident called to see a patient in the middle of the night is leaving the unit and remembers that he forgot to write a new order for a pain medication you had requested for another patient. Tired and already being paged to another unit, he verbally tells you the order and asks you to document it on the physician's order sheet. Your best response is:

a. "Thank you!"

b. Get a second nurse to listen to the order, and after writing the order on the physician order sheet, have both nurses sign.

c. "I am sorry but verbal orders can only be given in an emergency situation that prevents us from writing them out. I'll bring the chart and we can do this quickly."

d. Try calling another resident for the order or wait until the next shift.

■ Answers With Rationale

1. The correct answer is *d.* Words such as "good" or "average" may mean different things to different readers and should not be used (*b*). Nursing interventions should be documented as closely as possible to the time of their execution (*c*).

2. The correct answer is *b.* Do not use dittos, erasures, or correcting fluids (*a*). Charting should always be done in a legally prudent manner according to agency policy (*d*).

3. The correct answer is *e.* Each item is correct.

4. The correct answer is *a.* Items (*b, c,* and *d*) are legitimate exceptions to the authorization rule. Under no circumstance, however, can a nurse provide information to a news reporter without the patient's express authorization.

5. The correct answer is *b.* You should immediately clarify what you can and cannot do. Since your primary reason for refusing to help is linked to your responsibility to protect patient privacy and confidentiality, you should not begin by mentioning the real penalties linked to abuses of privacy (*a, c*). Finally, it appropriate to ask about Sue and her worries, but this should be done after you clarify what you are able to do (*d*).

6. The correct answer is *c.* TURP (*a*) is transurethral resection of prostate; PMH (*b*) is past medical history; TPR (*d*) is temperature, pulse, respiration.

7. The correct answer is *d.* While one recording of vital signs should appear on the admission nursing assessment (*b*), the best place to find sequential recordings that show a pattern or trend is the graphic sheet. The admission sheet (*a*) does not include vital sign documentation and neither does the activity flow sheet (*c*).

8. The correct answer is *b,* focus charting, which is the only method of documentation that uses the categories data, action, and response (DAR) to facilitate charting.

9. The correct answer is *c.* In most agencies, the only circumstance in which an attending physician, nurse practitioner, or house officer may issue orders verbally is in a medical emergency, when the physician/nurse practitioner is present but finds it impossible, due to the emergency situation, to write the order.

Bibliography

American Nurses Association. (1998). *Standards of clinical nursing practice* (2nd ed.). Washington, DC: Author.

American Nurses Association. (2001). *Code of ethics for nurses with interpretive statements.* Washington, DC: Author.

American Nurses Association. (2003). *Principles for documentation.* Washington, DC: Author.

Barbera, M. L. (1994). Giving report: How to sidestep common pitfalls. *Nursing, 24*(9), 41.

Buckley-Womack, C., & Gidney, B. (1987). A new dimension in documentation: The PIE method. *Journal of Neuroscience Nursing, 19*(5), 256–260.

Bulechek, G. M., McCloskey, J. C., Titler, M. G., & Denehey, J. A. (1994). Nursing interventions' use in practice. *American Journal of Nursing, 94*(10), 59–62, 64.

Burke, L., & Murphy, J. (1988). *Charting by exception: A cost-effective quality approach.* Albany, NY: Delmar.

Calfee, B. (1994). 7 Things you should never chart. *Nursing, 24*(3), 43.

Capuano, T. A. (1995). Clinical pathways: Practical approaches, positive outcomes. *Nursing Management, 26*(1), 34–37.

Cohen, M. R. (1987). Play it safe: Don't use these abbreviations. *Nursing, 17*(7), 46–47.

Comstock, L. G., & Moff, T. E. (1991). Cost-effective, time-efficient charting. *Nursing Management, 22*(7), 44–48.

Cox, S. S. (1994). Taping report: Tips to record by. *Nursing, 24*(3), 64.

Eggland, E. T. (1995). Charting smarter. *Nursing, 25*(9), 35–41.

Eggland, E. T., & Heinemann, D. S. (1995). *Nursing documentation: Charting, recording, and reporting.* Philadelphia: J. B. Lippincott.

Ferraro-McDuffie, A. (1993). Documenting the primary nurse's summary note: A leap toward professionalism. *Pediatric Nursing, 19*(2), 189–193.

Hatcher, I. (1995). Personal communication.

Health Care Financing Administration. (Issued 1995, updated 1998). Long-term care facility resident assessment instrument (RAI) user's manual. Author.

The Health Insurance Portability and Accountability Act of 1996, Public Law, 104-191. http://www.hhs.gov/ocr/hipaa.

House, E. (1992). Resistance to documentation: A nursing research issue. *International Journal of Nursing Studies, 29*(4), 371–381.

Iyer, P. W., & Camp, N. (1995). *Nursing documentation: A nursing process approach* (2nd ed.). St. Louis: Mosby–Year Book.

Joint Commission on Accreditation of Healthcare Organizations. (2004). *Accreditation manual for hospitals.* Oakbrook Terrace, IL: Author.

Mandell, M. (1994). Not documented, not done. *Nursing, 24*(8), 62–63.

Marr, P. B. (1993). Bedside terminals and quality of nursing documentation. Part I. *Computers in Nursing, 11*(4), 176–182.

Marrelli, T. M. (1996). *Nursing documentation handbook* (2nd ed.). St. Louis: Mosby–Year Book.

Martin, F. (1994). Documentation tips to help you stay out of court. *Nursing, 24*(6), 63–64.

Meyer, C. (1992). Bedside computer charting: Inching toward tomorrow. *American Journal of Nursing, 92*(4), 38–44.

Murphy, J., & Burke, L. J. (1990). Charting by exception: A more efficient way to document. *Nursing, 20*(5), 65–69.

North American Nursing Diagnosis Association. (2003). *NANDA nursing diagnoses: Definitions and classification, 2003–2004.* Philadelphia: Author.

Rasmussen, N. (1994). Clinical pathways of care: The route to better communication. *Nursing, 24*(2), 47–49.

Rich, P. L. (1995). Protecting patient information. *Nursing, 25*(9), 32L.

Siegrist, L., Stocks, B., & Dettor, R. (1985). The PIE system: Complete planning and documentation of nursing care. *QRB, 11*(6), 186–189.

Simpson, R. L. (1994). Ensuring patient data privacy, confidentiality, and security. *Nursing Management, 25*(7), 18–20.

Staff, E. J. (1997). Privacy, confidentiality, and security in clinical information systems. *Nursing Administration Quarterly, 21*(3), 21–28.

Sullivan, G. H. (2000). Keep your charting on course. *RN, 63*(5), 75–79.

Windle, P. E. (1994). Critical pathways: An integrated documentation tool. *Nursing Management, 25*(9), 80F–L, 80P.

Wong, C. A., & Budgell, L. (1994). Documentation redesign. *Canadian Nurse, 90*(6), 38–41.

Zolot, J. S. (1999). Computer-based patient records. *American Journal of Nursing, 99*(12), 64–69.

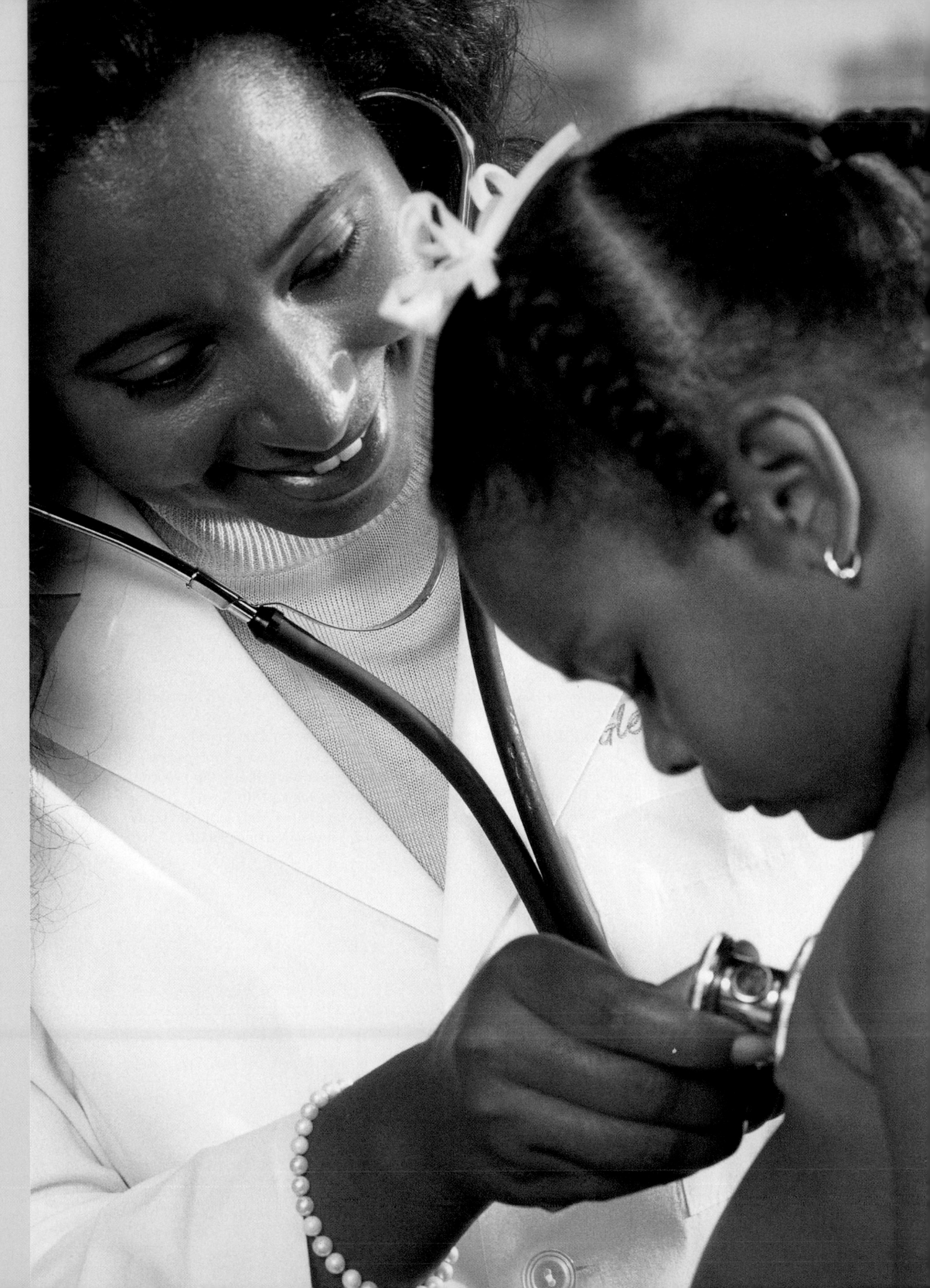

Promoting Health Across the Life Span

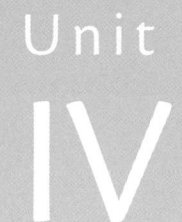

"The concern of nursing is with man in his entirety, his wholeness. Nursing's body of scientific knowledge seeks to describe, explain, and predict about human beings"

Martha Rogers (1914–1994)
a nationally renowned nurse theoretician, author, lecturer, and consultant, whose "theory of man" inspired tremendous creativity, research activity, and intellectual growth in the nursing profession

The chapters in Unit IV focus on growth and development through the life cycle. By considering all aspects of the individual, nurses provide healthcare oriented toward wellness and maximize the patient's strengths to reach his or her potential. Information specific to the influences of the family on growth and development is provided in Chapter 2.

Chapter 18 gives an overview of developmental concepts and theories necessary to understanding growth and development across the life span. Major theorists and their contributions to the understanding of psychosocial, physical, cognitive, moral, and faith development are described. Chapter 19 provides information about the individual from conception through young adulthood. Influences on growth and development, as well as physiologic, cognitive, psychosocial, moral, and spiritual development are discussed. Common health problems of each age group and the role of the nurse in health promotion and illness prevention for each age group are considered.

In Chapter 20, the adult years are divided into early, middle, and older-adult stages. Common health problems and the nurse's role in healthcare for the adult continue through older adulthood. The chapter ends with a look at the paradigm of aging and stereotypes common to the older adult. Gerontology and the healthcare system related to this field are discussed.

Developmental Concepts

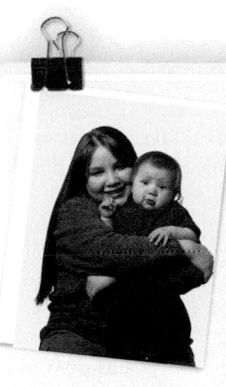

Melanie Kimber, a 24-year-old single mother, voices concerns about rearing her 12-month-old son by herself. "He is just so active, putting toys in his mouth, and getting into everything. I'm afraid to look away for even a second because he might get hurt. I don't know how other parents do it."

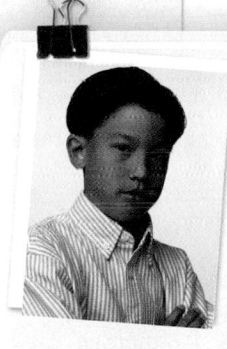

Juan Alvarez, an 8-year-old boy with encephalitis, becomes violent and combative at times, throwing himself against the bed and muttering words. He immediately calms down when an interpreter visits with him who speaks to him in Spanish, and when some of the nurses use Spanish words with him.

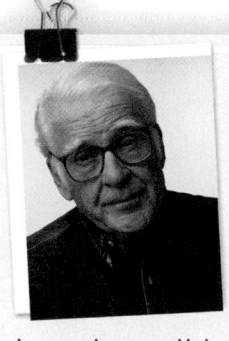

Joseph Logan, a 70-year-old man who fell and fractured his hip while repairing the exterior of his home, states "Go away and leave me alone. I'm a grown man, I can take care of myself . . . and get rid of this tray. I'm not hungry." Further investigation reveals that Mr. Logan has been the traditional head of his household and is now troubled by needing others, including his wife, to care for him.

Focusing on Blended Skills

The types of blended skills you'll need to respond to the case scenarios include:

Cognitive Skills

- Ability to evaluate factors influencing the growth and development of an individual, identifying how these factors may be interrelated and interdependent
- Knowledge of Freud's developmental stages as they relate to nursing care of an infant and school-aged child
- Ability to incorporate knowledge about Erikson's stages of psychosocial development and related challenges that require nursing assistance—for example, the crisis of intimacy versus isolation for the young adult or ego integrity versus despair experienced by older adults
- Knowledge of Piaget's theory of cognitive development related to sensorimotor and concrete operational stages and the implications for nurse–patient interaction and education
- Knowledge of Kohlberg's and Gilligan's theories on moral development and how these relate to the choices a single mother makes for herself and her child
- Knowledge of Fowler's theory of faith development as it relates to the changes experienced by older adults requiring assistance with their daily care
- Ability to apply theories of growth and development to nurse care planning

Technical Skills

- Ability to provide the technical nursing assistance necessary to meet the developmental needs of the patients entrusted to your care
- Ability to integrate developmental concepts into teaching plans appropriate for the patient's stage of growth and development
- Ability to use appropriate documentation systems and age-appropriate tools to record interventions

Interpersonal Skills

- Ability to establish trusting professional relationships with patients of different ages, to be sensitive to their developmental needs and challenges
- Ability to use therapeutic communication effectively to meet the needs of patients across the life span

Ethical and Legal Skills

- Value for the importance of incorporating theories of growth and development when assessing and planning nursing care for individuals and families
- Ability to view moral development as it relates to a person's acceptance or rejection of societal rules and regulations
- Ability to advocate for the unmet developmental needs of patients entrusted to your care

Learning Outcomes

After completing the chapter, the learner should be able to accomplish the following:

1. Summarize basic principles of growth and development.
2. Discuss the theories of Freud, Erikson, Havighurst, Gould, Piaget, Kohlberg, Gilligan, and Fowler.
3. Describe the importance of incorporating theories of growth and development in assessing and planning nursing care for individuals.
4. Explain implications for nursing practice based on an understanding of growth and development.

Key Terms

accommodation
assimilation
cognitive development
development
developmental task
faith
growth
moral development

Humans grow and develop throughout life. **Growth** is an increase in body size, or changes in body cell structure, function, and complexity. **Development** is an orderly pattern of changes in structure, thoughts, feelings, or behaviors resulting from maturation, experiences, and learning. Development is a dynamic and continuous process as one proceeds through life, characterized by a series of ascents, plateaus, and declines. The human processes of growth and development result from the interrelated effects of heredity and environment. Humans simultaneously grow and develop in physical, cognitive, psychosocial, moral, and spiritual dimensions, with each dimension being an essential part of the whole person.

Nurses promote health in people from birth to death. All people, regardless of age, have unique healthcare needs that result from their physical, intellectual, emotional, sociocultural, spiritual, and environmental dimensions at their developmental level. To plan and give holistic and individualized care, the nurse must understand typical growth and development characteristics, tasks, and needs of patients of all ages. (See the accompanying Reflective Practice box.)

This chapter presents theories and principles of growth and development across the life span that help us understand both healthy and ill people at various life stages. The major theories examining cognitive, psychosocial, spiritual, and moral development are discussed.

PRINCIPLES OF GROWTH AND DEVELOPMENT

Everyone's physical development has a predetermined genetic base because of inheritance patterns carried on the chromosomes. Thus, an unborn child begins life with specific physical attributes. Environmental factors from birth through the early years of growth provide initial psychological and social contact through positive or negative experiences with caregivers. As environmental influences expand beyond the immediate caregivers or family, development is influenced by a wide variety of psychosocial experiences. Cognitive, moral, and spiritual development are fostered through interactions within the family, school, and community. The nurse can better understand these interrelated variables at specific life stages through theories of human growth and development.

Growth and development are orderly and sequential as well as continuous and complex. All humans experience the same growth patterns and developmental levels, but, because these patterns and levels are individualized, a wide variation in biologic and behavioral changes is considered normal. Within each developmental level, certain milestones can be identified; for example, the time the infant rolls over, crawls, walks, or says his or her first words. Although growth and development occur in individual ways for different people, certain generalizations can be made about the nature of human development for everyone. These generalizations, outlined in Box 18-1, form the principles that help us understand growth and development.

FACTORS INFLUENCING GROWTH AND DEVELOPMENT

Many different factors influence both growth and development. One's growth and development might be facilitated or delayed by genetic heredity; prenatal, individual, and caregiver factors; and environment and nutrition. Other factors influencing growth and development are health–illness state (discussed in Chapters 2, 4, 19 and 20) and culture (discussed in Chapter 3).

> *Think back to Juan, the 8-year-old boy with encephalitis described in the case file at the beginning of the chapter. Although his behavior could be attributed to his infection, culture also may be a contributory factor for his behavior.*

Because of these often interrelated and interdependent factors, each person's growth and development is individualized.

Genetic Heredity

At conception, every human receives an equal number of chromosomes from each parent. The characteristics inherited from each parent are carried in gene pairs on the 23 pairs of chromosomes, which carry the genetic information that determine the person's cellular differentiation, growth, and function. As a result, physical characteristics such as height, bone size, and eye and hair color are inherited from our family of origin. Other characteristics, such as personality, are not as clearly identified with genetic heredity, but research is ongoing in this area. It is well known that genetic heredity influences the development of many diseases, such as cancer and diabetes. The Human Genome Project is a national and international project to map the estimated 35,000 to 140,000 genes in the human chromosomes. The purposes of this project are to identify the chemical basis for as many as 4,000 genetic diseases, and to provide tests to screen for, diagnose, and treat genetic disorders (Porth, 2002).

Prenatal, Individual, and Caregiver Factors

Prenatal, individual and caregiver factors influence development. Fetal development can be altered by maternal age (with risk greater in those younger than 15 years of age or older than 35 years of age), substance abuse, inadequate prenatal care, inadequate maternal nutrition, and maternal substance abuse. See the Research in Nursing box. Individual factors that might result in altered development from birth through adolescence include congenital or genetic disorders, brain damage from accidents or abuse, vision and hearing impairments, chronic illness, inadequate nutrition, chemotherapy or radiation therapy, lead poisoning, poverty, and substance abuse. Caregiver factors that negatively affect development are neglect and abuse, mental illness, mental retardation, or a severe learning disability.

Reflective Practice
Challenge to Ethical Skills

Two summers ago, while working in a nurse externship program, I worked with Juan, a Spanish-speaking 8-year-old boy diagnosed with encephalitis. The boy would become violent and combative at times, throwing himself against the bed and muttering words. Although his underlying disease was a likely cause of this behavior, he became calm when an interpreter was with him. The interpreter would speak to him in Spanish and he seemed to calm down. He also would appear calmer when nurses spoke Spanish words to him. Unfortunately, most nurses and physicians would ignore his screams in a language they did not understand, complaining about his behavior, and relying on medication to calm him. On one particular day, I was in the room with a physician who was writing an assessment note for Juan while I was getting his bath water ready for morning care. As usual, Juan, was muttering words and thrashing in the bed. I knew some measures to calm him; for example, speaking the few Spanish words I knew. The physician remained in her chair, looking at me and complaining about Juan's behavior, not making any effort to calm him. She said that she could not do anything to calm him down except prescribe sedative medications. I felt bad for the patient and knew he was frustrated. I knew that I could possibly help in this situation, but did not want to show disrespect to the physician.

Thinking Outside the Box: Possible Courses of Action

- I could nod in agreement with the physician. After all, I was only a nursing student and "didn't know better" than she did.

- I could tell her what measures I had used to help calm Juan.
- I could refrain from saying anything at all, wait until the physician had left, and then try to calm Juan.

Evaluating a Good Outcome: How Do I Define Success?

- Patient benefited from my actions.
- I did not disrespect the physician.
- I was able to use my intuition, authority, and common sense to the best of my ability.
  - Did I have the authority to jump in and give the physician advice on how to care for the patient?

- In this situation, my intuition and common sense told me to jump up and take action to calm down poor Juan, who was frustrated and upset.

Personal Learning: Here's to the Future!

Unfortunately, in this situation, I did not respond as I would have liked to. I did not say anything, but watched Juan become upset and mutter Spanish words. During this whole time, the physician shook her head, looked down on him, and told me she just "couldn't do anything about him" except to give him medications. I waited until the physician left, and then tried to calm Juan myself. In this situation, I should have let the physician know about the methods used to calm Juan previously, not just the simple use of drugs to sedate him. However, as a junior level nursing student, I did not feel comfortable enough to use this type of authority. I now see how important it is for nurses and all staff members to communicate their opinions, beliefs, and observations about patients for the benefit of the patient. These suggestions and opinions need to be heard so that patient receives the best possible care. In the future, as a practicing nurse, I will respect my fellow staff members, but always make sure that my voice is heard concerning a patient's needs.

Reflection

How do you think you would respond in a similar situation? Why? What do you think Juan might have been experiencing and why? What if the nursing student did approach the physician about using other methods to calm Juan? Would you consider this action to be disrespectful? How do you think the physician would have responded to the nursing student's feedback about the use of the Spanish language to calm Juan? What does this tell you about yourself and about the adequacy of your skills for professional practice? Do you think that you would act differently if the physician were male? At a different stage of development? For example, a 60-year-old physician instead of one that might be 45 years old? What would influence your actions in each of these situations? Can you think of other ways to respond or approach the situation? What other skills (cognitive, interpersonal, technical, ethical/legal) would you need to respond well in this situation? Would Juan's stage of growth and development influence your nursing care? Do you think that the nursing student's stage of growth and development may have played a role in the student's response? Why or why not? Do you agree with the criteria that the nursing student used to evaluate a successful outcome? Explain your answer.

Environment and Nutrition

Environment and nutrition influence all stages of development. Environmental factors that might alter development include poverty and violence. The effect of each can occur independently, but they are more likely to be interrelated, as seen in these examples:

- Infants who are malnourished in utero develop fewer brain cells than infants who have had adequate prenatal nutrition.
- Substance abuse by a pregnant woman increases the risk for congenital anomalies, low birthweight, and prematurity in her developing fetus.
- Federally sponsored school meal programs support enhanced learning with adequate nutrition.

BOX 18-1 Principles of Growth and Development

Growth and development are orderly and sequential as well as continuous and complex. All humans experience the same growth patterns and developmental levels. Because these patterns and levels are individualized, a wide variation in biologic and behavioral changes is considered normal. Within each developmental level, certain milestones can be identified; for example, the time the infant rolls over, crawls, walks, and says his or her first words.

Growth and development follow regular and predictable trends. Cephalocaudal (proceeding from head to tail) development is the first trend, with the head and brain developing first, followed by the trunk, legs, and feet. The second trend is proximodistal development, which means that growth progresses from gross motor movements (such as learning to lift one's head) to fine motor movements (such as learning to pick up a toy with the fingers). The last trend is symmetric development of the body, with both sides of the body developing equally.

Growth and development are both differentiated and integrated. As nerve pathways develop, they become more specialized, allowing the growing child to respond to different stimuli. Throughout the life span, each new learned ability builds on previously learned abilities, so that increasingly complex tasks can be accomplished. For example, the toddler learning to use a spoon combines motor skills, hand–eye coordination, cognitive patterning, and social imitation from watching others. As children grow and develop, the task of learning to use a spoon becomes basic, forming the foundation for learning skills requiring more manual dexterity.

Different aspects of growth and development occur at different stages and at different rates, and can be modified. For example, muscles and bones both grow most rapidly during the first year of life. During the toddler and preschool years, bone growth slows, but muscle fibers increase in size and strength. The most intense period of speech development is between 3 and 5 years of age. Sexual maturity begins during the preadolescent years and progresses into the adult years, but is based on gender and sex role identity established from birth. Many factors can modify growth and development, including nutrition, love and affection from caretakers, and illnesses.

The pace of growth and development is specific for each person. Both physical and psychological skills and maturation vary among people. For example, while learning to walk, a child may concentrate energies on the task and temporarily slow down in language development. Racial variations may also be seen; Asian children tend to be smaller than white children of the same age. In addition, one's genetic heredity places restrictions on the upper limits that can be achieved in growth and development.

Research in Nursing Making a Difference
Reducing Risk Factors for Altered Growth and Development

Pregnancy and parenthood in adolescent girls continue to be a major public concern. Risk behaviors are common in adolescence, but behaviors such as unsafe sex, poor nutrition, and experimentation with tobacco, alcohol, and drugs during pregnancy place the young mother and her child at high risk for pregnancy complications and poor birth outcomes. These risks are even greater for younger adolescents, whose diet may not meet the growth needs of their fetus in addition to their own.

Related Research
Koniak-Griffin, D., Mathenge, C., Anderson, N., & Verzemnieks, I. (1999). An early intervention program for adolescent mothers: A nursing demonstration project. *Journal of Obstetric, Gynecologic, and Neonatal Nursing, 28*(1), 51–59.

This is the report of a nursing intervention research project conducted to provide comprehensive public health nursing for pregnant adolescents. The nurses included four "preparation for motherhood" classes and up to 17 home visits during pregnancy and through the first year of the infant's life. In the home visits, interventions were provided in five major areas: health, sexuality and family planning, life skills, maternal role (including knowledge of fetal and infant growth and development), and social support systems. Telephone calls were made between visits to arrange and confirm home visits and provide follow-up information (such as referrals for healthcare). Early outcomes of this project support that home visitation by public health nurses positively affects the health of adolescent mothers and their babies.

Relevance to Nursing Practice
This study is one example of how nursing research is being used to facilitate normal growth and development—in this case, of both adolescent mothers and their infants. It supports developing and using nursing interventions to promote health in a high-risk vulnerable population and to reduce healthcare costs by preventing prematurity and reducing infant hospitalization days. Studies such as this one provide valuable information, demonstrating the effectiveness of nursing care in promoting positive health and social outcomes for pregnant adolescents. In addition, effective parenting behaviors by adolescent mothers help facilitate normal growth and development of their infants.

- Failure to thrive, a condition of early infancy, has been linked to both nutritional and emotional deprivation.
- Child abuse is an extreme example of physical and emotional harm or deprivation, leading to deficits in physical or psychosocial development, or both.
- Substance abuse by adolescents and young adults is associated with an increased incidence of teenage pregnancy, violence, accidents, and suicide. Abuse of alcohol and drugs is more prevalent in teenagers who have poor family relationships, low self-esteem, and poor social skills.

OVERVIEW OF DEVELOPMENTAL THEORIES

Human development and behavior have been studied since the beginning of the 20th century, and theories that explain human responses expected at certain ages during life have been developed. Although a psychological approach is common to all developmental theories, each theory has a different focus. The theories discussed in the following sections examine cognitive, social, and instinctual influences on human growth and development, and key points are summarized in Table 8-1.

Theory of Psychoanalytic Development: Sigmund Freud

Freud's (1923/1974) theory emphasizes the effect of instinctual human drives on behavior. Freud identified the underlying stimulus for human behavior as sexuality, which he called *libido*. Libido is defined as general pleasure-seeking instincts rather than purely genital gratification.

Four major components of Freud's theory are:
- the unconscious mind
- the id
- the ego
- the superego

The unconscious mind contains memories, motives, fantasies, and fears that are not accessible to recall but that directly affect behavior. The id is the part of the mind concerned with self-gratification by the easiest and quickest available means. Defense mechanisms are a means of unconscious coping to reduce stress in the conscious mind when the id's impulses cannot be satisfied. Defense mechanisms are discussed in Chapter 32.

The ego is the conscious part of the mind that serves as a mediator between the desires of the id and the constraints of reality so that one might live effectively within one's social, physical, and psychological environment. The ego includes one's intelligence, memory, problem solving, separation of reality from fantasy, and incorporation of experiences and learning into future behavior. Development of the ego allows the infant, by 6 months of age, to view self as separate from others and to begin to alter behaviors in response to cues. Ego development continues throughout life.

The superego is the part of the mind that represents one's conscience and develops from the ego during the first year of life, as the child learns praise versus punishment for actions. The superego represents the internalization of rules and values so that socially acceptable behavior is practiced.

In addition, Freud described a series of developmental stages through which all people must pass. The stages of development are based on sexual motivation. A discussion of the developmental stages follows.

Oral Stage (Ages 0 to 18 Months)
During the oral stage, the infant uses his or her mouth as the major source of gratification and exploration. Pleasure is experienced from eating, biting, chewing and sucking. The infant's primary need is for security. A major conflict occurs with weaning.

> Recall Ms. Kimber, the young, single, frustrated mother of a 12-month-old child. The nurse might apply the concepts of Freud's theory in the nursing care of Ms. Kimber and her child by explaining the oral behaviors typical of the stage of her child's development.

Anal Stage (Ages 8 Months to 4 Years)
This stage begins with the development of neuromuscular control to allow control of the anal sphincter. Toilet training is a crucial issue, requiring delayed gratification as the child compromises between enjoyment of bowel function and limits set by social expectations.

Phallic Stage (Ages 3 to 7 Years)
The child has increased interest in gender differences, his or her own gender (Fig. 18-1), and conflict and resolution of that conflict with the parent of the same sex (named the Oedipus complex in boys and the Electra complex in girls, based on feelings of intimate sexual possessiveness for the opposite-sex parent). Curiosity about the genitals and masturbation increase during this stage.

Latency Stage (Ages 7 to 12 Years)
This stage marks the transition to the genital stage during adolescence. Increasing sex-role identification with the parent of the same sex prepares the child for adult roles and relationships.

Genital Stage (Ages 12 to 20 Years)
At this stage, sexual interest can be expressed in overt sexual relationships. Sexual pressures and conflicts typically cause turmoil as the adolescent makes adjustments in relationships.

Theory of Cognitive Development: Jean Piaget

Piaget (1969) developed a theory of **cognitive development** from infancy through adolescence. Piaget believed that learning occurs as a result of the internal organization of an event, forming a mental schema (plan) and serving as a base for further schemata as one grows and develops. Intellectual growth

TABLE 18-1 Key Points of Developmental Theories

Theme	Freud	Erikson	Havighurst	Piaget	Fowler	Kohlberg
	Psychosexual	Psychosocial	Developmental	Cognitive	Faith	Moral
Infancy to toddlerhood	Oral stage; anal stage	Trust versus mistrust; autonomy versus shame and doubt	Learning to walk; learning to talk; learning to control body waste elimination	Basic reflexes; coordinates more than one thought at a time; begins to reason and anticipate events	Centers on relationship with primary caregiver	Oriented to obedience and punishment
Preschool to early school years	Phallic stage	Initiative versus guilt	Learning sex differences; forming concepts; getting ready to read	Increased language; increased understanding of life events and relationships	Imitates religious behaviors of others	Defines acts satisfying to self and some satisfying to others as right
School years	Latent stage	Industry versus inferiority	Learning physical skills; learning to get along with others; developing conscience and morality	Develops logical thinking; incorporates others' perspectives; uses abstract thinking and deductive reasoning; tests beliefs to establish values	Accepts existence of deity; stories define religious and moral beliefs	Morality of maintaining good relations and approval of others; aware of need to respect authority
Adolescent to adult years	Genital stage	Intimacy versus generation	Achieving gender-specific social role; achieving independence; acquiring a set of values and an ethical system to guide behavior	Adopts life-guiding values or religious practices	Selects principles to follow; concern for the rights and needs of others	
Middle adult years		Generativity versus stagnation	Achieving social and civic responsibility; accepting and adjusting to physical changes	Integrates others' viewpoints into own understanding of truth		
Later adult years		Ego integrity versus despair	Adjusting to decreasing physical status and health; adjusting to retirement	Values absolute love and justice of all; believes in the existence of the future		

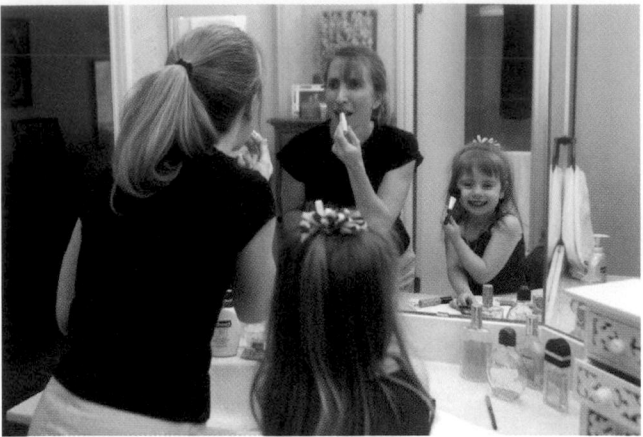

FIGURE 18-1 This preschool girl enjoys imitating her mother as she learns about the world around her. (Photo by Joe Mitchell.)

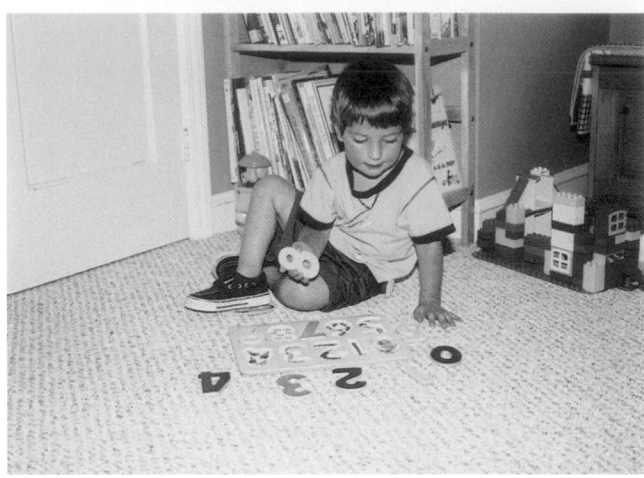

FIGURE 18-2 This child's cognitive development is characterized by the beginning use of symbols through language and pictures, an ability to learn simple sequences, and a basic ability to categorize objects.

is a continual restructuring of knowledge to progress to higher levels of problem solving and critical thinking. Two continual processes of assimilation and accommodation stimulate intellectual growth in the child. **Assimilation** is the process of integrating new experiences into existing schemata; **accommodation** is an alteration of existing thought processes to manage more complex information. Piaget described four stages of cognitive development, which are discussed here.

Sensorimotor Stage (Birth to 24 Months)

This stage is marked by progression through a series of developmental stages; for example:

- 0 to 1 month—Demonstrates basic reflexes, such as sucking
- 1 to 4 months—Discovers enjoyment of random behaviors (such as smiling or sucking thumb) and repeats them
- 4 to 8 months—Relates own behavior to a change in environment, such as shaking a rattle to hear the sound or manipulating a spoon to eat
- 8 to 12 months—Coordinates more than one thought pattern at a time to reach a goal, such as repeatedly throwing an object on the floor; only objects in sight are considered permanent
- 12 to 18 months—Recognizes the permanence of objects, even if out of sight; can understand simple commands
- 18 to 24 months—Begins to develop reasoning and can anticipate events

> *Recall Ms. Kimber, the single mother of a 12-month-old infant. Applying the knowledge of Piaget's theory, the nurse could develop a teaching plan for the mother that addresses appropriate anticipatory guidance to prevent injury while fostering the child's cognitive development.*

Preoperational Stage (Ages 2 to 7 Years)

This stage is characterized by the beginning use of symbols, through increased language skills and pictures, to represent the preschooler's world (Fig. 18-2). This stage is divided into two

parts: the preconceptual stage (ages 2 to 4 years) and the intuitive stage (ages 4 to 7 years). Play activities during this time help the child to understand life events and relationships.

Concrete Operational Stage (Ages 7 to 11 Years)

During this stage, children learn by manipulating concrete or tangible objects and can classify articles according to two or more characteristics. Logical thinking is developing, with an understanding of reversibility, relations between numbers, and loss of egocentricity, in addition to the ability to incorporate another's perspective.

Formal Operational Stage (Age 11 Years or Older)

This stage is characterized by the use of abstract thinking and deductive reasoning. General concepts are related to specific situations and alternatives are considered. The world is evaluated by testing beliefs in an attempt to establish values and meaning in life.

Theories of Psychosocial Development

Erik Erikson

Erikson's (1963) developmental theory was based on Freud's work but was expanded to include cultural and social influences in addition to biologic processes. His psychosocial theory is based on four major organizing concepts:

1. Stages of development
2. Developmental goals or tasks
3. Psychosocial crises
4. The process of coping

Erikson believed that development is a continuous process made up of distinct stages, characterized by the achievement of developmental goals that are affected by the social environment and significant others. He identified eight stages that progress from birth to old age and death. Each stage is characterized by a developmental crisis to be mastered, with possible successful or unsuccessful resolution of the crisis. Unsuccessful resolution at any one stage might delay progress through the next stage, but mastery can occur later. A discussion of the developmental stages follows.

Trust versus Mistrust (Infancy)

The infant learns to rely on caregivers to meet basic needs of warmth, food, and comfort, forming trust in others. Mistrust is the result of inconsistent, inadequate, or unsafe care (Fig. 18-3).

Autonomy versus Shame and Doubt (Toddler)

As motor and language skills develop, the toddler (ages 1 to 3 years) learns from the environment and gains independence through encouragement from caregivers to feed, dress, and toilet self. If the caregivers are overprotective or have expectations that are too high, shame and doubt, as well as feelings of inadequacy, might develop in the child.

Think back to Ms. Kimber, the single mother. The nurse could apply Erikson's theory to explain the child's "getting into everything" as his need for learning about the environment and gaining independence. Additionally, the mother's anxiety level and the child's attempts to investigate the environment through locomotion and oral exploration place the child at risk for injury from a fall or aspiration of a small object. With astute observation and knowledge of child development, the nurse

plays a primary role in prevention by educating the mother.

Initiative versus Guilt (Preschool)

Confidence gained as a toddler allows the preschooler (ages 4 to 6 years) to take the initiative in learning, so that the child actively seeks out new experiences and explores the how and why of activities. If the child experiences restrictions or reprimands for seeking new experiences and learning, guilt results, and the child hesitates to attempt more challenging skills in motor or language development.

Industry versus Inferiority (School-Aged Children)

Focusing on the end result of achievements, the school-aged child gains pleasure from finishing projects and receiving recognition for accomplishments (Fig. 18-4). If the child is not accepted by peers or cannot meet parental expectations, a feeling of inferiority and lack of self-worth might develop.

Think back to Juan, the 8-year-old boy described in the case file at the beginning of the chapter. The nurse could help to foster Juan's industry by offering positive reinforcement for his ability to calm down when spoken to in Spanish. The nurse also could incorporate activities into Juan's plan of care that would provide him with opportunities to succeed.

Identity versus Role Confusion (Adolescence)

With many physical changes occurring, the adolescent is in transition from childhood to adulthood. Hormonal changes produce secondary sex characteristics and mood swings. Trying on roles and even rebellion are considered normal behaviors as the adolescent acquires a sense of self and deciding what direction will be taken in life. Role confusion occurs when the adolescent is unable to establish identity and a sense of direction.

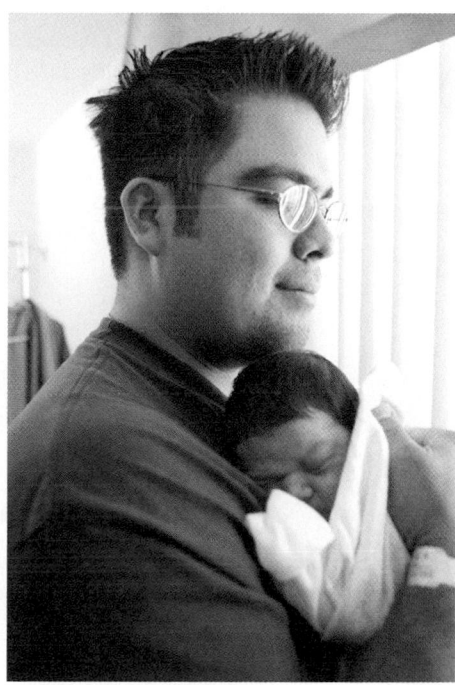

FIGURE 18-3 This caregiver provides comfort and affection to his daughter teaching her to trust in others.   (Photo by Joe Mitchell.)

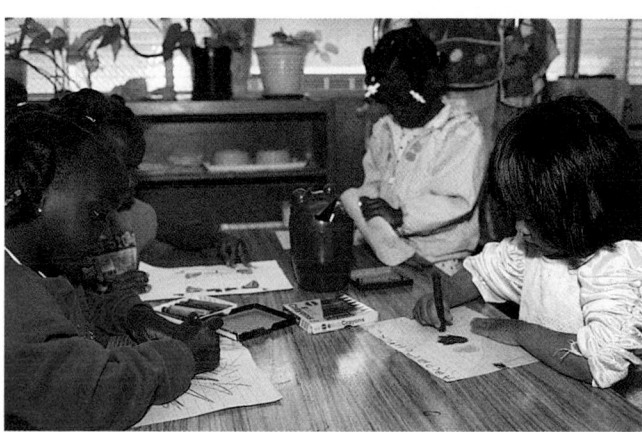

FIGURE 18-4 School-aged children focus on the end results of accomplishments—recognition and praise from family, teachers, and peers—in their development of a sense of competition and industry. (Photo © Kathy Sloane.)

Intimacy versus Isolation (Young Adulthood)

The tasks for the young adult are to unite self-identity with identities of friends and to make commitments to others. Fear of such commitments results in isolation and loneliness.

> *Remember Ms. Kimber, the single mother described at the beginning of the chapter. She appears to have a limited support system. Recognizing this, the nurse can assess further to identify the mother's potential problems with intimacy and subsequently, her progression toward generativity.*

Generativity versus Stagnation (Middle Adulthood)

The middle adult years are a time of concern for the next generation as well as involvement with family, friends, and community. There is a desire to make a contribution to the world. If this task is not met, stagnation results, and the person becomes self-absorbed and obsessed with her or his own needs or regresses to an earlier level of coping.

Ego Integrity versus Despair (Later Adulthood)

As one enters the older years, reminiscence about life events provides a sense of fulfillment and purpose. If one believes that one's life has been a series of failures or missed directions, a sense of despair might prevail.

> *Think back to Mr. Logan, the 70-year-old man who broke his hip. Applying Erikson's theory, the nurse could assess Mr. Logan for indications of despair due to his feelings of dependency on others, and plan appropriate interventions to foster a sense of fulfillment and purpose.*

Robert J. Havighurst

Havighurst (1972) believed that living and growing are based on learning, and that a person must continuously learn to adjust to changing societal conditions. He described learned behaviors as **developmental tasks** that occur at certain periods in life. Successful achievement leads to happiness and success in later tasks, whereas unsuccessful achievement leads to unhappiness, societal disapproval, and difficulty in later tasks. The developmental tasks arise from maturation, personal motives, and values that determine occupational and family choices, and civic responsibility. The developmental tasks, by age, follow.

Infancy and Early Childhood

Developmental tasks for infancy and early childhood include:
- Achieving physiologic stability
- Learning to eat solid foods
- Learning to walk and talk
- Forming simple concepts of social and physical reality
- Learning to relate emotionally to parents, siblings, and other people
- Learning to control the elimination of body wastes
- Learning to distinguish between right and wrong
- Learning sex differences and sexual modesty

Middle Childhood

Developmental tasks for middle childhood include:
- Learning physical skills necessary for games
- Learning to get along with age-mates
- Developing fundamental skills in reading, writing, and mathematics
- Developing a conscience, morality, and a scale of values
- Achieving personal independence

Adolescence

Developmental tasks for adolescence include:
- Accepting one's body and using it effectively
- Achieving a masculine or feminine gender role
- Achieving emotional independence from parents and other adults
- Preparing for a career
- Preparing for marriage and family life
- Desiring and achieving socially responsible behavior
- Acquiring an ethical system as a guide to behavior

Young Adulthood

Developmental tasks for young adulthood include:
- Selecting a mate (Fig. 18-5)
- Learning to live with a marriage partner
- Starting a family and rearing children
- Managing a home
- Getting started in an occupation
- Taking on civic responsibility
- Finding a congenial social group

Middle Adulthood

Developmental tasks for middle adulthood include:
- Accepting and adjusting to physical changes
- Attaining and maintaining a satisfactory occupational performance
- Assisting children to become responsible adults
- Relating to one's spouse as a person

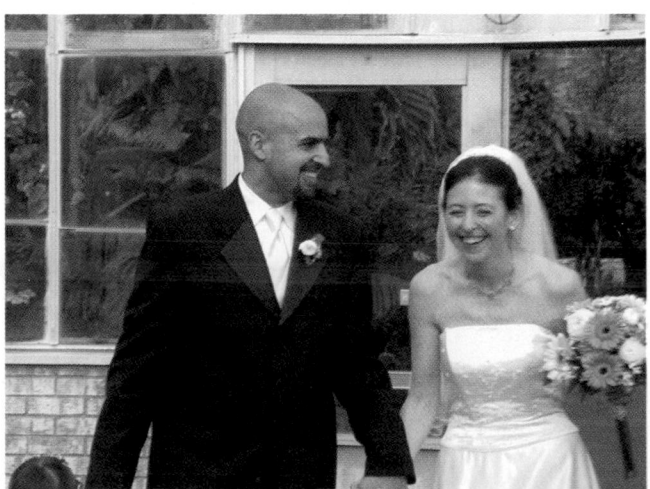

FIGURE 18-5 Choosing a life partner is often an important developmental task for young adults.

- Adjusting to aging parents
- Achieving adult social and civic responsibility

Later Maturity
Developmental tasks for later maturity include:
- Adjusting to decreasing physical strength and health
- Adjusting to retirement and reduced income
- Adjusting to death of a spouse
- Establishing an explicit affiliation with one's age group
- Adjusting and adapting social roles in a flexible way
- Establishing satisfactory physical living arrangements

> *Recall Mr. Logan, the older adult male with the fractured hip described at the beginning of the chapter. Based on his comments, the nurse could apply Havighurst's theory to conclude that Mr. Logan might be fluctuating between feelings of nonadjustment and feelings of acceptance of his declining health.*

Roger Gould
Gould (1978) studied men and women between the ages of 16 and 60 years, labeling the central theme for the adult years as "transformation," with specific beliefs and developmental phases.

Ages 18 to 22
During the young adult years, individuals typically struggle with leaving their parents' world and challenging false assumptions from their childlike consciousness (for example, "Only my parents can guarantee my safety."). However, these assumptions are replaced with new false assumptions, such as "Rewards will come automatically if we do what we are supposed to do."

Ages 22 to 28
Individuals in their 20s feel established as adults and separate from their families, but believe they must still demonstrate their competence as independent adults to their parents. They want to enjoy the present but build for the future.

Ages 29 to 34
Self-acceptance increases as the need to prove oneself disappears. Marriage and careers are well established, and young parents want to accept their own children for what they are becoming without imposing rules. Questions about life in general are still present.

Ages 35 to 43
Adults in this age group tend to continually look inward and question themselves, their values, and life. They see time as having an end and believe they have little time left to shape the behavior of their adolescent children (Fig. 18-6). They may be critical of their own parents, blaming them for many of their own problems.

Ages 43 to 50
At this phase, the adult accepts the reality of boundaries for the life span, and believes personalities are set. They are interested

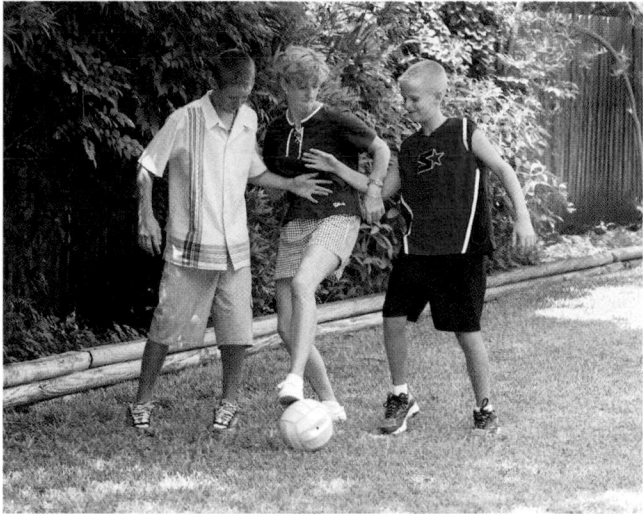

FIGURE 18-6 As her sons grow into young adults, this mom adapts to remain a positive influence in their lives.   (Photo by Joe Mitchell.)

in an active social life, church activities, community service, friends, and spouse. Life is viewed as neither simple nor controllable, which might result in periods of passivity, rage, depression, and despair.

Ages 50 to 60
Previous patterns of reflection and contemplation result in increased self-approval and self-acceptance. Increased marital happiness and contentment were associated with seeing spouse as a valued companion.

Daniel Levinson and Associates
Levinson and associates (1978) based their theory on the organizing concept of "individual life structure." The theory centered around the belief that the pattern of life at any point in time is formed by the interaction of three components: the self (values, motives), the social and cultural aspects of one's life (family, career, religion, ethnic background), and the particular set of roles in which one participates (husband, father, friend, student). When anything changes in one component, the whole life structure must then reorganize. According to Levinson and associates, the major phases in young and middle adult life are:
- Early adult transition
- Entering the adult world
- Settling down
- Midlife transition
- Pay-off years

Early Adult Transition
The major concerns of the young adult (age 18–22) are to break away from one's parents, to make initial career choices, and to establish intimate relationships. Many separations, losses, and transformations are necessary to terminate old relationships. This is also a time to begin to select personal values and establish goals, as one's life structure begins to be more integrated.

Entering the Adult World

The years of the middle to late 20s (age 22–28) are a time to build on previous decisions and choices, and to try different careers and lifestyles. By the late 20s, the young adult enters the age-30 transition period. The individual often feels uneasy that something is missing. During this transition, decisions are made either to find a new direction in life or to make a stronger commitment to previous choices.

Settling Down

In the settling-down phase (age 30–40), the adult invests energy into the areas of life that are most personally important. The areas of investment are primarily family, work, and community. The individual strives to gain respect, status, and a sense of authority.

Midlife Transition

Midlife transition (age 40–45) involves a reappraisal of one's goals and values. The established lifestyle may continue, or the individual may choose to reorganize and change careers. This is an unsettled time, with the individual often anxious and fearful.

The Pay-Off Years

The years from 45 to 65 are a time of maximum self-direction and self-approval. Physical and mental changes increase an awareness of one's aging and mortality.

Theories of Moral Development

Lawrence Kohlberg

Kohlberg (1969) developed a theory of **moral development** in levels that closely follow Piaget's theory of cognitive development. Kohlberg recognized that a person's moral development is influenced by cultural effects on one's perceptions of justice in interpersonal relationships. A child's beginnings of moral development result from caregiver and child communications during the early childhood years, as the young child tries to please his or her parents (Fig. 18-7). The concept of morality emerges as a subset of a person's beliefs or values and governs choices made throughout life. Rules and regulations established by society are eventually challenged and evaluated as a person either accepts societal rules into his or her own internal set of values or rejects them.

> *Remember Juan, the 8-year-old with encephalitis. Juan's language barrier and cultural heritage may be adding to the child's already heightened fears and anxieties due to hospitalization. Astute observation and knowledge of Kohlberg's theory by the nurse can help toward understanding the child's perceptions, beliefs, and, ultimately, his choices and actions.*

The levels of moral development include preconventional, conventional, and postconventional. Each level is further divided into separate stages.

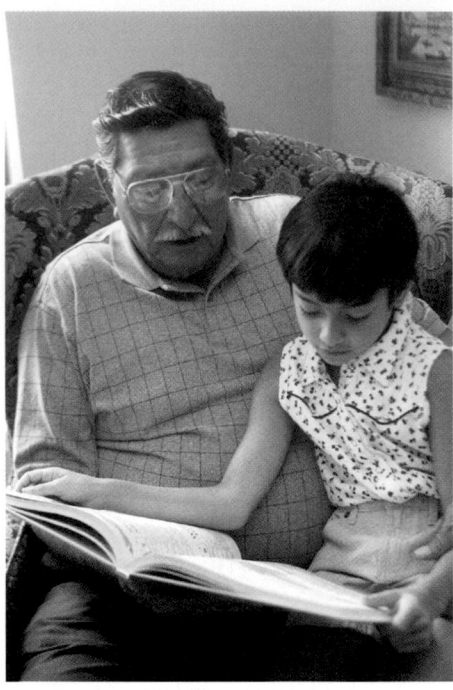

FIGURE 18-7 This grandfather reads traditional stories to his young granddaughter, teaching her important cultural values and beliefs and thereby influencing her moral development.   (Photo by Joe Mitchell.)

Preconventional Level

The preconventional level is based on external control as the child learns to conform to rules imposed by authority figures. At stage 1, punishment and obedience orientation, the motivation for choices of action is fear of physical consequences of authority's disapproval. As a result of the consequences, a perception of goodness or badness develops. At stage 2, instrumental relativist orientation, the thought of receiving a reward overcomes fear of punishment, so actions that satisfy this desire are selected.

Conventional Level

The conventional level involves identifying with significant others and conforming to their expectations. The person respects the values and ideals of family and friends, regardless of consequences. In stage 3, "good boy–good girl" orientation, the person strives for approval in an attempt to be viewed as "good." At stage 4, "law and order" orientation, behavior follows social or religious rules from a respect for authority. In his later work, Kohlberg maintained that many adults are at this stage because they think abstractly and view themselves as members of society.

Postconventional Level

The postconventional level involves moral judgment that is rational and internalized into one's standards or values. At stage 5, social contract and utilitarian orientation, correct behavior is defined in terms of society's laws. Laws can be changed, however, to meet society's needs, while maintaining respect for self and others. Stage 6, universal ethical principle orientation, represents the person's concern for equality for all human beings, guided by personal values and standards, regardless of those set by society or laws. Justice might be internalized at an even higher level than society. Few adults ever reach this stage of development.

Carol Gilligan

Gilligan (1977/1982) originally worked with Kohlberg. As she listened to women discuss their own real-life moral conflicts, she recognized that there was a conception of morality from the female viewpoint that was not represented in Kohlberg's work. Gilligan's theory views females as developing a morality of response and care, and males as developing a morality of justice.

In Gilligan's theory, males and females have different ways of looking at the world. Males are more likely to associate morality with obligations, rights, and justice. Females are more likely to see moral requirements emerging from the needs of others within the context of a relationship. This moral orientation of females is called the ethic of care, which develops through three levels. Each level ends with a transitional period—a time when the female considers new approaches to moral considerations and moves to a new level.

Level 1—Selfishness

In level 1, the focus is on one's own needs. "Should" and "would" are the same. Morality is seen in terms of sanctions by society. Relationships are often disappointing, and as a result, a woman might isolate herself to avoid getting hurt. The transition that follows this level is characterized by the move from selfishness to responsibility—a move that integrates the responsibility to care for oneself with the desire to care for others.

Level 2—Goodness

In level 2, moral judgment is based on shared norms and expectations, and societal values are adopted. Acceptance by others becomes critical, and the ability to protect and care for others is seen as the defining characteristic of female goodness. This characteristic is upheld through beliefs that one is responsible for the actions of others but that others are responsible for the choices they make. As a woman examines her self-sacrifice, the second transition occurs, with the woman asking if her own needs are not also important. A shift from goodness to truth (as well as a new conception of goodness) takes place.

> *Think back to Ms. Kimber, the single mother. The nurse could apply Gilligan's theory to assist Ms. Kimber in adjusting to her role as both a single parent caring for a child and as a woman with her own set of needs.*

Level 3—Nonviolence

In level 3, a changed understanding of self and a redefinition of morality allow reconciliation of selfishness and responsibility. Nonviolence (the injunction against hurting) governs all moral judgments and actions. Care becomes a universal obligation toward self and others. Moral problems are usually considered within the contexts of maintaining relationships and of promoting the welfare or preventing the harm of others.

Theory of Faith Development: James Fowler

Fowler (1981) postulated a developmental theory of the spiritual identity of humans, based on work by Piaget, Kohlberg, and Erikson. Fowler describes **faith** as follows:

"Faith is not always religious in its content or context. . . . Faith is a person's or group's way of moving into the force field of life. It is our way of finding coherence in and giving meaning to the multiple forces and relations that make up our lives. Faith is a person's way of seeing him or herself in relation to others against a background of shared meaning and purpose. Faith, therefore, is not necessarily religious, but it comprises the reasons one finds life worth living" (p.4).

Fowler's theory is composed of a prestage and six stages of faith development. The age when a certain stage occurs varies, but the sequence does not. Equilibrium, or a plateau in faith development, can occur at any stage from stage 2 and beyond.

In relation to the stages of faith development, Fowler explained a relationship among self, shared causes or values, and others that is the unifying factor in all stages and is based on trust. During the prestage, called undifferentiated faith, trust, courage, hope, and love compete with threats of abandonment and inconsistencies in the infant's environment. The strength of faith in this stage is based on the infant's relationship with the primary caregiver. The stages follow.

Stage 1—Intuitive–Projective Faith

Intuitive–projective faith is most typical of the 3- to 7-year-old child. Children imitate religious gestures and behaviors of others, primarily their parents. They take on their parents' attitudes toward religious or moral beliefs without a thorough understanding of them. Imagination in this stage leads to long-lived images and feelings that they must question and reintegrate in later stages.

Stage 2—Mythical–Literal Faith

Mythical–literal faith predominates in the school-aged child, who is having more social interaction. Stories represent religious and moral beliefs, and the child accepts the existence of a deity. The child can appreciate the perspectives of others as well as the concept of reciprocal fairness.

Stage 3—Synthetic–Conventional Faith

Synthetic–conventional faith is the characteristic stage for many adolescents. As the person experiences increasing demands from work, school, family, and peers, the basis for identity becomes more complex. The person has an emerging ideology but has not closely examined it until now. The person begins to question life-guiding values or religious practices in an attempt to stabilize his or her own identity.

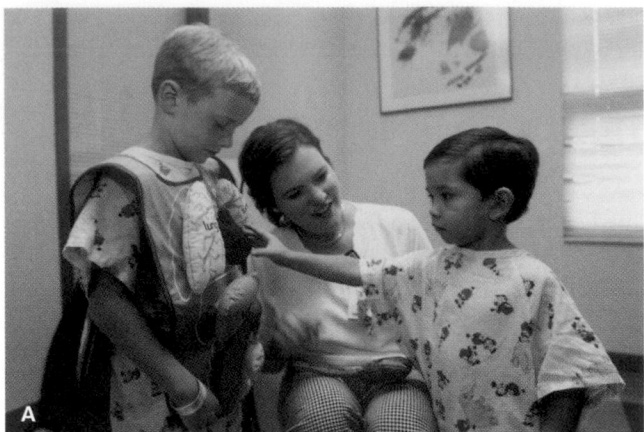
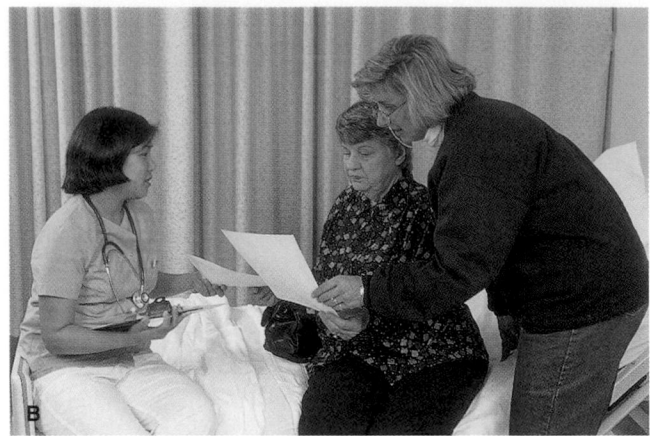

FIGURE 18-8 To provide holistic and individualized care, the nurse applies theories of growth and development. (**A**) The nurse caring for young children uses dramatic play to teach them about their hospital experience. (**B**) The nurse caring for an older adult includes the middle-aged daughter, with whom the patient now lives, in discharge teaching.   (A: Photo by Joe Mitchell. B: Photo © B. Proud.)

Stage 4—Individuative–Reflective Faith

Individuative–reflective faith is crucial for older adolescents and young adults because they become responsible for their own commitments, beliefs, and attitudes. Many adults do not develop to this stage, and for some people, it does not emerge until they are in their 30s or 40s. Searching for self-identity no longer defined by the faith compositions of significant others is a primary concern.

Stage 5—Conjunctive Faith

Conjunctive faith integrates other viewpoints about faith into one's understanding of truth. One is able to see the na-ture of the reality of one's own beliefs. Along with this realization, one observes the divisions of faith development among people.

Stage 6—Universalizing Faith

Universalizing faith involves making tangible the values of absolute love and justice for humankind. The faith relationship is characterized by total trust in the principle of actively "being-in-relation" to others in whom we invest commitment, belief, love, risk, and hope, and in the existence of the future, regardless of what religion or image of faith is involved.

BOX 18-2 Incorporating Principles and Theories of Growth and Development

General guidelines for incorporating principles and theories of growth and development and family dynamics into daily practice of nursing care are listed below. They are provided as suggestions for working with patients of all ages.

- Be knowledgeable about the various stages of cognitive, psychosocial, moral, and spiritual development and prepared to support developmental stages typical of certain ages.
- Maintain flexibility in assessing people, and respect the uniqueness of each person. Although the literature describes development typical of a particular age, not everyone fits into an exact mold.
- Anticipate possible regression during difficult periods or times of crisis, accepting and supporting a person's return to a forward progression in development.
- Become cognizant that environmental and cultural influences have a strong effect on development, especially psychosocial development. A deprived environment can be detrimental, whereas an enriched environment enhances development.

- Assess each person with an awareness that within each stage of development, a person may retain some behaviors of a previous stage, attain goals of the current stage, and begin to exhibit behaviors of the next stage. There is a time of transition to the next stage with no definite beginning or ending to the particular stage of development.
- Remember that patients are members of families and that the family unit can have both positive and negative influences on the development of individual members. Attempt to support good family relationships and healthy environments that assist members to reach their greatest potential for growth. Provide patient teaching to individuals and their families to aid in their understanding of periods of development.
- Be ready to provide healthcare to patients who are ill or who fail to meet developmental goals. Collaborate with other members of the healthcare team in providing care to prevent or minimize disruption of development and to promote optimal health throughout life.
- Provide environments and experiences that are developmentally challenging.

APPLYING THEORIES OF GROWTH AND DEVELOPMENT TO NURSING CARE

The complex and interrelated elements that contribute to human growth and development involve not only biophysical factors but also factors of personality development. The theories summarized in this chapter help us understand cognitive, psychosocial, moral, and spiritual development. To understand the whole person, nurses need to evaluate all the components of growth and development to understand certain life events or concerns (Fig. 18-8).

Although these theories offer a great deal of insight into the processes of human growth and development, they do have some limitations. When planning holistic nursing care for patients with diverse needs, backgrounds, and ages, nurses should therefore assess the patient as an individual and use interventions based on rationales from multiple developmental theories to provide comprehensive health promotion. Guidelines for incorporating the principles and theories of growth and development in nursing care are listed in Box 18-2.

Healthcare needs change quickly as a person grows and passes through life. These needs are unique for each person but include certain similarities at specific periods. The nurse must plan care based on the patient's general and unique health needs and must continually revise aspects of care as the growth process evolves or alterations in health status occur.

■ Developing Critical Thinking Skills

1. Identify developmental challenges for five of your family members or friends at different ages across the life span. Explain why meeting developmental needs is an essential role of nursing.
2. Compare and contrast the psychosocial theories of Erikson and Gould. Are the concepts in these theories relevant today? If your answer is no, what would you delete and what would you add?
3. Using Piaget's theory of cognitive development, describe how you would explain the death of a parent to children 4, 9, and 13 years of age.

■ Practicing for NCLEX

1. Sue has blue eyes and is 5 feet tall. Tom has brown eyes and is 6 feet tall. These physical characteristics are primarily determined by
   a. Socialization with caregivers
   b. Maternal nutrition during pregnancy
   c. Genetic information on chromosomes
   d. Meeting developmental tasks
2. The developing fetus exhibits a common trend in growth and development. Which of the following growth and development trends initially occurs?
   a. Symmetric
   b. Cephalocaudal
   c. Proximodistal
   d. Lateral
3. A 2-year-old grabs a handful of cake sitting on the table and stuffs it is his mouth. According to Freud, the child is satisfying his
   a. Id
   b. Superego
   c. Ego
   d. Unconscious mind
4. The primary developmental stage of the preschool age child, as described by Erikson, is
   a. Industry versus inferiority
   b. Autonomy versus shame and doubt
   c. Trust versus mistrust
   d. Initiative versus guilt
5. An older adult smiles as she talks about her life events. This, according to Erikson, is demonstrating
   a. Ego integrity
   b. Generativity
   c. Intimacy
   d. Identity
6. Havighurst defined a developmental task of the adolescent as
   a. Learning sex differences and sexual modesty
   b. Taking on civic responsibility
   c. Accepting one's body and using it effectively
   d. Taking on civic responsibility
7. Based on Piaget's theory, children between the ages of 2 and 7 years use play to
   a. Classify objects based on characteristics
   b. Understand life events and relationships
   c. Relate own enjoyment of random behaviors
   d. Incorporate the perspective of others
8. Moral development as defined in Kohlberg's theory is initially influenced by
   a. Parent–child communications
   b. Societal rules and regulations
   c. Social and religious rules
   d. One's beliefs and values
9. In Gilligan's theory, women develop morality differently than do men. She described this morality in women as one of
   a. Law and justice
   b. Obligations and rights
   c. Order and selfishness
   d. Response and care
10. During the development of faith, described by Fowler, the teenager commonly
    a. Accepts parental attitudes and beliefs
    b. Exhibits a value of justice for others
    c. Questions previously accepted values
    d. Demonstrates responsibility for own beliefs

■ Answers With Rationale

1. The correct response is *c*. Physical appearance and growth have a predetermined genetic base from inheritance patterns carried on the chromosomes.

2. The correct response is *b*. The head and brain (cephalocaudal) grow and develop first in the fetus.
3. The correct response is *a*. Freud defined the id as the part of the mind concerned with self-gratification by the easiest and quickest available means.
4. The correct response is *d*. The preschool child seeks new learning experiences (initiative); if restrictions or reprimands result the child feels guilty and is hesitant to try new skills.
5. The correct response is *a*. Reminiscence during the older years of one's life provides a sense of fulfillment and purpose (ego integrity).
6. The correct response is *c*. The adolescent must learn to accept his or her body and use it effectively.
7. The correct response is *b*. Children ages 2 to 7 years are in the preoperational stage, and use play to help understand life events and relationships.
8. The correct response is *a*. Moral development in the young child results from communications as the child tries to please his or her parents.
9. The correct response is *d*. Gilligan believed that, for women, response and care are a universal obligation toward self and others.
10. The correct response is *c*. Synthetic–conventional faith is characteristic of many adolescents, as they begin to question values in an attempt to stabilize their own identity.

Bibliography

Erikson, E. H. (1963). *Childhood and society* (2nd ed.). New York: Norton.

Fowler, J. W. (1981). *Stages of faith: The psychology of human development and the quest for meaning.* New York: Harper & Row.

Fowler, J. W. (1991). *Weaving the new creation: Stages of faith and the public church.* San Francisco: Harper Collins.

Freud, S. (1923/1974). *The ego and the id.* London: Hogarth.

Friedman, M. M., Bowden, V., & Jones, E. (2003). *Family nursing: Research, theory and practice* (5th ed.). Upper Saddle River, NJ: Prentice Hall.

Gilligan, C. (1977). In a different voice: Women's conceptions of the self and of morality. *Harvard Educational Review, 47,* 481–517.

Gilligan, C. (1982). *In a different voice.* Cambridge, MA: Harvard University Press.

Gould, R. (1978). *Transformations.* New York: Simon & Schuster.

Havighurst, R. J. (1972). *Developmental tasks and education.* New York: David McKay.

Kohlberg, L. (1969). Stage and sequence: The cognitive–developmental approach to socialization. In D. Gaslin (Ed.), *Handbook of socialization: Theory and research* (pp. 347–380). Chicago: Rand McNally.

Levinson, D., Darrow, C., Klein, E., et al. (1978) *The seasons of a man's life.* New York: Knopf.

Murray, R. B., & Zentner, J. P. (2001). *Health promotion strategies through the life span.* Upper Saddle River NJ: Prentice Hall.

North American Nursing Diagnosis Association (NANDA). (2001). *Nursing diagnoses: Definitions & classification 2001–2002.* Philadelphia: NANDA.

Piaget, J., & Inhelder, B. (1969). *The psychology of the child.* New York: Basic Books.

Porth, C. M. (2002). *Pathophysiology: Concepts of altered health states* (6th ed.). Philadelphia: Lippincott Williams & Wilkins.

Spahis, J. (2002). Human genetics: Constructing a family pedigree. *American Journal of Nursing, 102*(7), 44–50.

Thies, K., & Travers, J. (2001). *Human growth and development through the lifespan.* Thorofare, NJ: Slack Inc.

Conception Through Young Adult

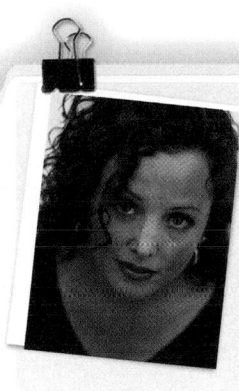

Patricia Lemming is a 26-year-old woman in the first trimester of her pregnancy. At a recent clinic visit, she states, "I've been trying to cut back on smoking and drinking alcohol, but I haven't had much success."

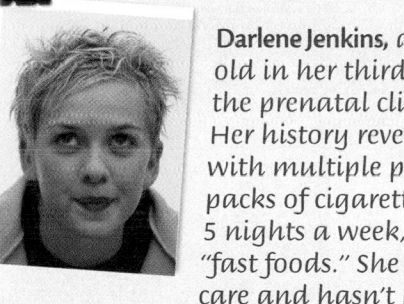

Darlene Jenkins, a pregnant 14-year-old in her third trimester, comes to the prenatal clinic for the first time. Her history reveals sexual activity with multiple partners, smoking two packs of cigarettes per day, beer "4 or 5 nights a week," and eating mostly "fast foods." She has had no prenatal care and hasn't been taking any prenatal vitamins. She is homeless but occasionally stays with an older girlfriend since her parents "threw her out of the house."

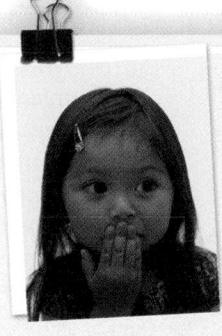

Hillarie Browning, who is 2 years old, is brought to the emergency room by her father, James Browning. She is unresponsive. Mr. Browning says that she "took a tumble" down the stairs, but assessment reveals that her injuries are inconsistent with this type of fall.

Focusing on Blended Skills

The types of blended skills you'll need to respond to the case scenarios include:

Cognitive Skills

- Knowledge of the developmental needs of fetuses, and the effects of maternal behaviors, such as smoking and alcohol consumption
- Knowledge of effective strategies to help pregnant women modify behaviors that harm fetuses
- Ability to recognize signs and symptoms of potential child abuse
- Knowledge of necessary obligations for reporting potential child abuse
- Ability to incorporate knowledge about child abuse to intervene effectively with potential abusers
- Knowledge of how to facilitate measures to meet the developmental needs of vulnerable populations, such those who live in poverty and the homeless.
- Knowledge of the common health concerns of adolescents, including adolescent pregnancy and effective intervention strategies

Technical Skills

- Ability to provide the technical nursing assistance necessary to assess and to meet the needs of patients from conception through young adult, such as the pregnant woman and her fetus, the potentially abused toddler, the potential child abuser, and the pregnant adolescent

- Ability to adapt technical assistance to meet the needs of the patient from conception through young adulthood
- Ability to incorporate developmentally age-appropriate assessment tools and techniques as part of effective nursing care

Interpersonal Skills

- Ability to establish trusting and respectful professional relationships with patients at different developmental stages
- Ability to demonstrate a nonjudgmental attitude when interacting in potentially emotionally charged situations, such as with potential child abuse and high-risk adolescent pregnancy
- Ability to use therapeutic communication effectively to meet the needs of patients across the life span
- Ability to mobilize necessary supportive resources to provide needed services

Ethical and Legal Skills

- Knowledge of the nurse's legal and ethical obligations in cases of maternal–fetal conflict, child abuse, and vulnerable populations
- Ability and willingness to advocate for vulnerable patients: fetuses, unresponsive children, and adolescents
- Ability to practice in an ethically and legally defensible manner, maintaining the rights of all persons involved

Learning Outcomes

After completing the chapter, the learner should be able to accomplish the following:

1. Summarize major physiologic, cognitive, psychosocial, moral, and spiritual developments from conception through the young adult.
2. List common health problems of each age period from conception through the young adult.
3. Describe nursing interventions to promote health in patients from conception through the young adult.

Key Terms

adolescence
attachment
bonding
child abuse
colic
failure to thrive (FTT)
infant
negativism
neonate
preschooler
puberty
regression
school-aged child
separation anxiety
sexually transmitted disease
   (STD)
sudden infant death syndrome
   (SIDS)
temperament
toddler
young adult

Growth and development occur throughout the life span. The nurse's knowledge of growth and developmental milestones provides a base for planning and implementing holistic, individualized nursing care. This chapter continues the discussion of developmental theories introduced in Chapter 18, with specific information related to the sequential stages of growth and development from conception through young adulthood.

Although divided into different stages, childhood encompasses the entire period before young adulthood. Included within this time span are the fetus, the neonate, the infant, the toddler, the preschooler, the school-aged child, and the adolescent. The discussion of each of these stages includes, as appropriate, physiologic, cognitive, psychosocial, and moral and spiritual development; health; and the nurse's role in promoting health. For an example addressing the adolescent, see the accompanying Reflective Practice box.

CONCEPTION AND PRENATAL DEVELOPMENT

Human growth and development begin at the moment the ovum is fertilized by the sperm. The fertilized ovum (zygote) contains the full complement of genetic information provided by each parent that determines gender and influences personality, intellect, and physical and psychological traits. The growth and development stages of the fetus are orderly and continuous, and proceed as follows:

Preembryonic Stage

The preembryonic stage lasts for about 3 weeks. The zygote, which implants in the uterine wall, has three distinct cell layers. The endoderm (inner layer) becomes the respiratory system, the digestive system, the liver, and the pancreas. The mesoderm (middle layer) becomes the skeleton, connective tissue, cartilage, muscles, and the circulatory, lymphoid, reproductive, and urinary systems. The ectoderm (outer layer) becomes the brain, spinal cord, nervous system, and outer body parts (skin, hair, and nails).

Embryonic Stage

The embryonic stage occurs from the 4th through the 8th week. Rapid growth and differentiation of the cell layers take place. By the end of this stage, all basic organs have been established, the bones have begun to ossify, and some human features are recognizable. Because this is a period of such rapid growth and change, the fetus is especially vulnerable to any factor that might cause congenital anomalies (such as maternal use of alcohol, nicotine, over-the-counter medications, or drugs).

Recall Patricia Lemming, the 26-year-old pregnant woman in her first trimester described at the beginning of the chapter. The nurse could incorporate knowledge about fetal growth during the embryonic stage when teaching her about the effects of alcohol and nicotine on the fetus, with the goal of fostering an even greater desire in the patient to stop using these substances.

Fetal Stage

The fetal stage lasts from 9 weeks to birth. All body organs and systems continue to grow and develop. At the end of the first trimester (12 weeks' gestation), some reflexes are present, kidney secretion begins, the heart beat can be heard by Doppler, and the sex of the infant is distinguishable by outward appearance. At the end of the second trimester (24 weeks' gestation), fetal heart tones are audible by stethoscope, the liver and pancreas are functioning, hair forms, sleep–wake patterns are established, lung surfactant is produced, and eyelids open. At the end of the third trimester (40 weeks' gestation), testes have descended, lung alveoli are formed, subcutaneous fat is deposited, and the fetus actively kicks. By birth, the average neonate weighs 7.5 lb (3.4 kg) and is 20 inches (50.8 cm) long.

During pregnancy, adequate maternal nutrition is essential for normal growth and development of the fetus. A fetus that does not have adequate nutrition might be small for gestational age, fail to have normal brain development, have learning disabilities as a child, and be at increased risk for chronic illnesses as an adult. Vitamin and mineral deficiencies can result in fetal megaloblastic anemia and neural tube defects (folic acid deficiency), inadequate bone calcification (vitamin D and calcium deficits), and hypothyroidism (iodine deficiency). Other health risks for the developing fetus are discussed later in this chapter.

NEONATE: BIRTH TO 28 DAYS

At birth, the **neonate** must adapt to extrauterine life through several significant physiologic adjustments. The most important occur in the respiratory and circulatory systems as the neonate begins breathing and becomes independent of the umbilical cord. The neonate is assessed immediately after birth. Of several existing measurement scales, the Apgar rating scale is the most commonly used. This scale is used to assess neonates 1 minute and 5 minutes after birth (Table 19-1).

Physiologic Development

The physical characteristics and behaviors of normal neonates follow:
- Reflexes include the Moro reflex, the stepping reflex, grasp reflex, hand-to-mouth activity, sucking, swallowing, blinking, sneezing, and yawning (Fig. 19-1a–d).
- Body temperature responds quickly to the environmental temperature.
- Senses are used to respond to the environment, see color and form, hear and turn toward sound, smell and taste, and feel touch and pain.

Reflective Practice
Challenge to Interpersonal Skills

I was admitting Darlene Jenkins, a pregnant, unmarried, 14-year-old to the prenatal clinic. This was her first visit and she was already in her third trimester. A quick history revealed multiple factors putting both her and her fetus at risk for health problems: lack of family (or other) support (homeless, occasionally staying with an older girlfriend); father of the baby unknown; multiple sexual partners; diet consisting mainly of fast food; no prenatal vitamins; little to no exercise; history of smoking (2 packs of cigarettes per day) and alcohol consumption ("beer 4 to 5 times a week"). When she was seen by the medical resident, he asked her quite curtly if she was trying to "kill her baby," telling her that it was probably too late for her to get the care she needed. "Why should we waste our time on you when other women here really want to be helped?" Although Darlene was acting "tough," I could tell from her expression that she was both angry and hurt. While I was upset by the choices that she had made so far and shared some of the resident's frustration, I knew we had to give her a reason to trust us if we wanted her to start taking better care of herself and her baby. I was also upset by the resident's lack of professionalism and wondered if I should say something to him.

Thinking Outside the Box: Possible Courses of Action

- Play the "good cop–bad cop" routine; after the resident finished his visit, I could try to be especially caring and explain why we were all concerned about her and her baby. Then I could talk to her about what she needed to do to maximize good outcomes.
- Challenge the resident in the patient's presence, thereby showing her that at least I honestly cared about her.
- Confront the resident later in a "cooler moment," hoping that this behavior doesn't repeat itself, while being prepared to report my concerns to a "higher authority" should this behavior occur again.
- Approach the resident outside the patient's presence and explain my concerns. Persuade the resident to apologize to Darlene in the interests of winning the patient's trust and compliance with prenatal care program.

Evaluating a Good Outcome: How Do I Define Success?

- The respect for each person's human dignity (Darlene, the resident, and myself) is affirmed.
- Each person feels empowered to make personal decisions that advance her/his interests and goals.
- The patient makes the needed lifestyle changes, with good outcomes for herself and her baby.
- Personal integrity is maintained; no one has to sacrifice her or his beliefs and values.
- Professional integrity is maintained.

Personal Learning: Here's to the Future!

In this situation, I don't think that I chose the best alternative because I tried to comfort Darlene and make "excuses" for the resident's behavior. I tried to explain that the resident was very busy and simply "out of sorts." I have to admit that, initially, I was probably just as shocked by the resident's response as Darlene. Personally, I knew that I'd die if someone said something like that to me. After I spoke with the resident, I realized there might be some value in shocking a patient into seeing the harm of her ways. However, in this encounter, Darlene had no way of knowing whether this response was well-intended (if indeed it was!) or not. While talking further with Darlene, I became convinced that she wouldn't start listening to us until she could trust us. I wish I had the courage to ask the resident to apologize to Darlene. His apology might have been exactly what was needed to get her to trust us. I'm learning that when patient welfare is at stake, I might have to sacrifice my own comfort level to challenge other professional caregivers. Hopefully I'll learn how to do this in a way that promotes respectful, collaborative relationships.

Reflection

How do you think you would respond in a similar situation? Why? What if the nurse confronted the resident in front of the patient? Would you consider this professional behavior? Do you feel that the resident acted in a professional manner? Could the resident's developmental stage have influenced his response to the patient? Please explain your answer. How might the nurse's developmental stage affect the actions taken toward the resident? Toward the patient? Do you agree with the nurse in the thinking that an apology from the resident would help in fostering trust? Why or why not? What does this tell you about yourself and about the adequacy of your skills for professional practice? Can you think of other ways to respond? What would the basis be for these other ways? What other skills (cognitive, interpersonal, technical, ethical/legal) would you need to respond well in this situation? Do you agree with the criteria proposed for use to evaluate a successful outcome?

TABLE 19-1 Apgar Scoring Chart

Category*	0	1	2
Heart rate	Absent	Slow (less than 100 beats/min)	More than 100 beats/min
Respiratory effort	Absent	Slow, irregular	Good, crying
Muscle tone	Flaccid	Some flexion of extremities	Active motion
Reflex irritability	No response	Weak cry or grimace	Vigorous cry
Color	Blue, pale	Body pink, extremities blue	Completely pink

* Each category is rated as 0, 1, or 2. The rating for each category is then totaled to a maximum score of 10. Normal neonates score between 7 and 10. Neonates who score between 4 and 6 require special assistance; those who score below 4 are in need of immediate life-saving support.

- Stool and urine are eliminated.
- Both an active crying state and a quiet alert state are exhibited (Fig. 19-1e, f).

The neonate inherits a transient immunity from infections as a result of immunoglobulins that cross the placenta. Breastfeeding provides further protection against bacterial and viral infections through antibodies, immunoglobulins, and leukocytes in breast milk. The high lactose content in breast milk, combined with limited protein, promotes an acid environment that is unsuitable for bacterial growth.

Health of the Neonate

Difficulties related to the birth process, the transition to extrauterine life, or congenital anomalies might require intervention by healthcare personnel.

Respiratory difficulties might occur, especially if drugs given to the mother during labor and delivery have sedated the neonate. Premature neonates are vulnerable to respiratory distress syndrome because of the relative immature lung function. Neonates delivered by cesarean birth are at risk for respiratory difficulties because of excess mucus in the lungs and might require frequent suctioning.

Incompatibility between the neonate's and mother's blood groups requires prompt care at birth. Congenital malformations, such as cleft palate and cleft lip, or neural tube defects (such as spina bifida) and hydrocephalus, might result in long-term health problems. Birth traumas that cause temporary symptoms are of concern because the parents need to be reassured that the symptoms will disappear. Examples include caput succedaneum (localized edema of the scalp), molding (elongation of the skull as the baby passes through the birth canal), and subconjunctival hemorrhage. The nonthreatening nature of physiologic jaundice, which commonly occurs in the neonate's first days, should also be explained to the parents.

Neonates born to mothers who smoke cigarettes, drink alcohol, or use drugs are at risk for developmental deficits as well as complications during birth. Smoking during pregnancy might cause low birthweight. Fetal alcohol syndrome caused by maternal drinking is believed to be a leading cause of birth defects, including growth retardation, developmental delay, and impaired intellectual ability.

> *Think back to Patricia Lemming, the 26-year-old mother in her first trimester. The nurse could integrate information about the typical effects occurring in neonates secondary to nicotine and alcohol use as a basis for planning care for Patricia as she progresses through her pregnancy.*

The maternal use of cocaine, crack-cocaine, and heroin increases the probability of congenital anomalies, prematurity, low birthweight, and drug withdrawal symptoms (Hockenberry, Wilson, Winkelstein, et al., 2003). Cocaine use in various forms, including crack, brings about abrupt changes in the mother's blood pressure, resulting in decreased fetal blood flow and oxygenation. "Crack babies" are jittery, hypersensitive to noise or stimuli, intolerant of cuddling, and feed poorly for 2 to 3 weeks after birth (Hockenberry et al., 2003).

INFANT: 1 MONTH TO 1 YEAR

The neonate becomes an **infant** at 1 month, a period lasting until the first birthday (Fig. 19-2).

Physiologic Development

The physical characteristics of the infant include the following:
- Brain grows to about half the adult size.
- Body temperature stabilizes.
- Motor abilities develop, allowing using building blocks, attempting to feed self, crawling, and walking.
- Eyes begin to focus and fixate.
- Heart doubles in weight, heart rate slows, and blood pressure rises.
- Deciduous teeth begin to erupt at 4 to 6 months.
- Birthweight usually triples by 1 year, when the average male infant weighs 22 lb (10 kg) and the average female infant weighs 21 lb (9.5 kg). Length increases by 50%.

Cognitive Development

Infants from birth to 1 year are in the sensorimotor stage of development described by Piaget. Language development is in the prelinguistic phase. Babies begin to coo and make sounds soon after birth, and by 12 months of age, they can convey their wishes through a few key words. Language development in infants has several consistent characteristics that occur with all languages:
- Use of syllable repetition (such as ma-ma, da-da, bye-bye)
- Universal early phonetic expressions (babbling sounds)
- Imitation of sounds and intonations spoken by caregivers

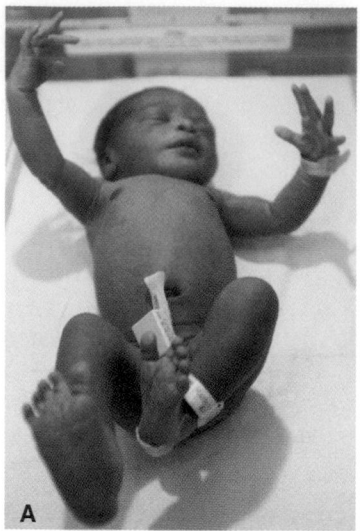

Moro reflex   (Photo by Joe Mitchell.)

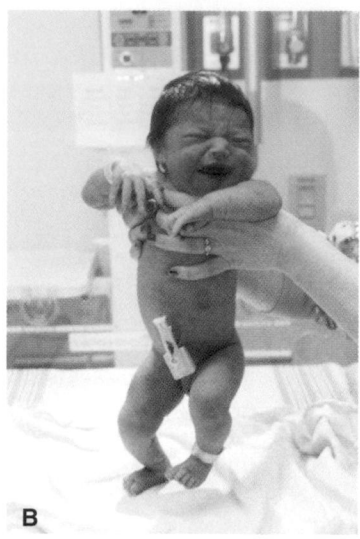

Stepping reflex   (Photo by Joe Mitchell.)

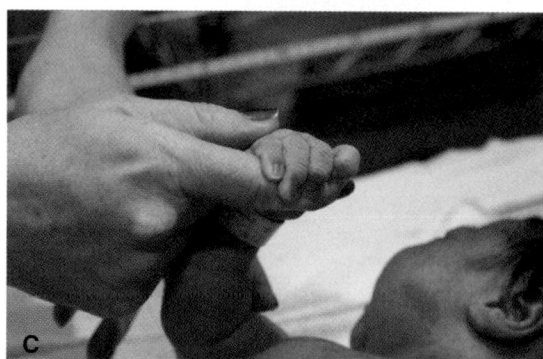

Grasp reflex   (Photo by Joe Mitchell.)

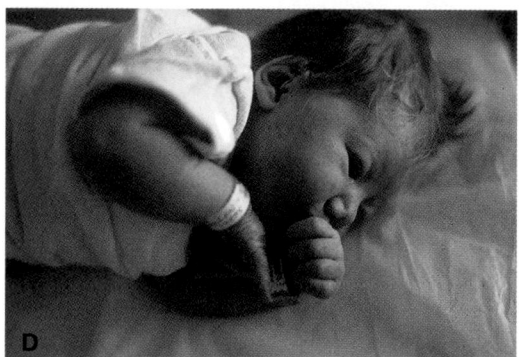

Hand to mouth and sucking activity

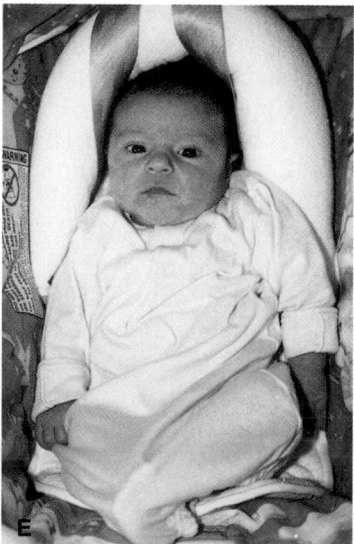

Quiet alert state

Active crying state   (Photo by Joe Mitchell.)

FIGURE 19-1 Reflexes and behaviors of the neonate.

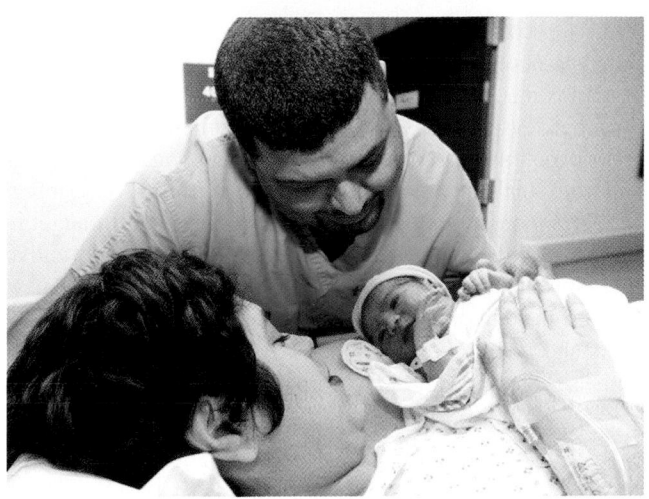

Bonding might occur in the first few hours after birth or later in the first few months and is necessary for later attachment.   (Photo by Joe Mitchell.)

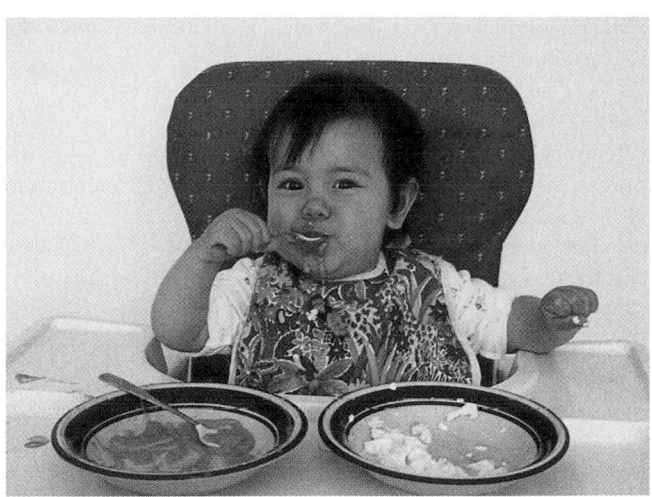

Developmental tasks of the first year include taking solid food.

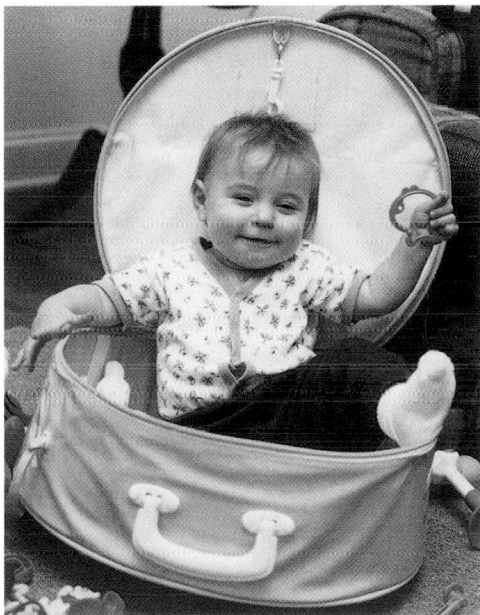

As the infant enters the second half of his first year, play will begin to involve manipulation of objects and the environment.

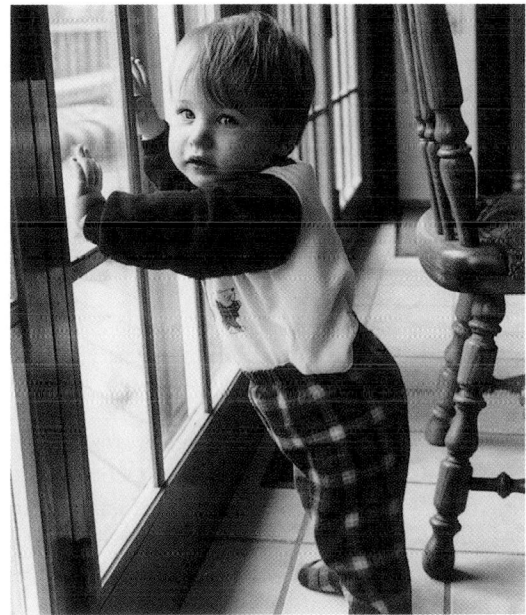

Later infancy is characterized by the ability to pull-to-stand, cruise, and often walk.

FIGURE 19-2 Development in the infant.

Psychosocial Development
Developmental Theories
In terms of the developmental theories discussed in Chapter 18, the infant has the following characteristics:
- Is in the oral stage (Freud), striving for immediate gratification of needs and having a strong sucking need
- Develops trust (Erikson) if the caregiver can be counted on to provide food when the infant is hungry; trust is also facilitated by diaper changing, warmth, and comforting
- Meets developmental tasks (Havighurst) by learning to take solid food, walk, and talk

Special Considerations
Other components of psychosocial development in the neonate and infant include attachment, bonding, play, and temperament.

Attachment and Bonding
Attachment is an active, affectionate, reciprocal relationship between two people, which is somewhat different from bonding. **Bonding,** described by Klaus and Kennell (1982), occurs during a sensitive period in the first few hours after birth (although bonding also might occur later in the first few months) and is necessary for later attachment. Bonding might be considered the emotional linkage of two people, and attachment the long-term maintenance and strengthening of the linked

state. Infants and children discover their environment and begin to learn how to control it through play.

Play

Beginning as soon as the baby is aware of sensations and the pleasure they produce, play progresses from self-pleasure to interaction with others. The two dimensions of play are social play and cognitive play. Social play, such as rolling a ball back and forth between two children, is motivated by a desire for fun, pleasure, and relationships with others. Cognitive play, as when a child puts a puzzle together, is motivated by the desire to learn.

Temperament

Temperament is primarily inborn, although it is influenced by environment. A baby or child might be said to be "easy," "slow to warm," or "difficult" (Thomas, Chess, & Birch, 1968). The "easy" infant sleeps, eats, and eliminates easily; smiles spontaneously; and cries in response to significant needs. The "slow-to-warm" infant is more passive and distant. The "difficult" infant has volatile and labile responses, often is a restless sleeper, is highly sensitive to noises, and eats poorly. These traits often remain fairly consistent throughout the individual's life. The behavior of caregivers as they care for the baby can influence either positively and negatively the degree to which temperament dictates behavioral style.

Health of the Infant

Various health problems in infancy might require the intervention of healthcare personnel. Gastroenteritis and food allergies are common. Skin disorders, such as diaper dermatitis (diaper rash), seborrheic dermatitis (infant dandruff), prickly heat rash, acute infantile eczema, and thrush (infection of the oral mucous membrane by the fungus *Candida albicans*), also often occur. Accidents, infant colic, failure to thrive, sudden infant death syndrome, and child maltreatment are of particular concern during infancy.

Accidental Injuries

Safety issues must be addressed during infancy. The swallowing reflex matures progressively from birth, but until it is fully developed, aspiration is a risk. Because infants put small objects in their mouths, choking is a risk. Choking might also result from small pieces of food, nuts, and popcorn. As the infant becomes more mobile, the risk for falls or for being caught in dangling cords (such as in miniblinds) increases. Preventive measures against such safety hazards must be taught to new parents. In addition, law mandates the use of special car safety seats and restraints for infants. See Examples of NANDA Nursing Diagnoses: Infancy Through School Age.

Infant Colic

Colic is uncontrollable, extended crying in an otherwise healthy and well-fed baby. Colic generally occurs during the first 3 months of life and has been referred to as the "100-day syndrome." This continuous crying can occur at any time but usually worsens in the evening. The infant cries loudly and draws the legs up to the abdomen. Despite the symptoms, the infant gains weight. Parents and other family members might experience stress and anxiety due to the constant crying (see Through the Eyes of a Caregiver).

The exact cause of colic is not known. One common belief is that an immature digestive system might be the cause. Swallowing excess air, feeding too rapidly or too much, improper feeding techniques, or allergies might lead to spasmodic contractions of the intestines, with acute abdominal pain. Another belief is that an immature nervous system might be the cause. Normal external stimulation might cause the baby to tense up.

Failure to Thrive

Failure to thrive (FTT) is a condition of inadequate growth in height and weight resulting from the infant's inability to obtain or use calories needed for growth. Infants with FTT have signs of malnutrition and delayed development. Causes and contributing factors might include physiologic causes, inadequate funds to buy sufficient food, the use of a fad diet, in-

---

Examples of NANDA Nursing Diagnoses — Infancy Through School Age

Nursing Diagnoses	Possible Related Factor
Risk for Infection	Exposure to other children in childcare and at school
Diarrhea	Milk intolerance
Deficient Fluid Volume	Severe case of vomiting and diarrhea
Risk for Suffocation	Caregiver's lack of knowledge of safety precautions
Disorganized Infant Behavior	Environmental overstimulation
Risk for Poisoning	Caregiver's lack of knowledge of proper storage of hazardous liquids
Risk for Injury	Lack of knowledge about proper use of skates, bicycles, roller blades, and trampolines
Low Self-Esteem	Physical abuse by caregiver

Through the Eyes of a Caregiver

When my son Luke was first born, he was an easy-going, pleasant baby. Then, when he was about 3 weeks old, it started. He cried inconsolably every night from 5 pm until 12 a.m. We could do nothing to comfort him. We took him to the pediatrician. The doctor said the word we already expected to hear: "colic." He gave us a prescription for an antacid and a muscle relaxant. He gave us some advice on how to comfort him . . . wrap him snugly, hold him like a football, eliminate milk and dairy from your diet (I was breast-feeding), put pressure on his belly. None of these things worked. Eventually we discovered that rocking him in our arms as we ran the shower seemed to calm him. Pink Floyd and Dark Side of the Moon also comforted him. We found this out quite accidentally when we played the CD in an attempt to drown out his crying. These methods somewhat helped with the crying, but little helped my anxiety. I was concerned for my little son, who was clearly upset or in pain. At the same time, I found it very difficult to bond with him. I'd find myself dreading the evening; dreading being with my baby. When I'd come home from work, I'd take a deep breath and stand paralyzed at the front door, wondering if I had to go in. I could hear his crying from the doorstep. I felt horrible about these feelings. I questioned my parenting skills. At one point, I spoke with a nurse whose daughter had colic. She said "My daughter's colic lasted 100 days, but it has taken me 14 years to forgive her!" This made me laugh for the first time in weeks. Then she asked how I was doing and if I wanted to talk about how I was feeling. I hadn't told anyone how I was feeling toward my son. How could I? I confided in her, though. I knew she wouldn't judge me. I knew she'd understand. After speaking with the nurse, I felt a lot better knowing that it was OK to feel the way I did. As time went on, Luke's crying spells got shorter and shorter, until the 99th day; then, miraculously, it ended. We had a party the next day, with a cake that said "Day 100. We made it." Today, he is a sweet, healthy child. He is no fussier than any other 3-year-old child. We have bonded exceptionally well. My husband and family were supportive and helped care for Luke when he had colic, but it was the nurse who helped care for me!

Dana Jameson
Philadelphia, PA

adequate nutritional knowledge, insufficient breast milk, and disturbances in maternal–child attachment. In most cases of FTT not caused by a physiologic problem, a team of healthcare providers is needed to meet the complex needs of the infant and caregivers.

Sudden Infant Death Syndrome

Sudden infant death syndrome (SIDS) is the sudden death of an infant under the age of 1 year, unexpected in light of the infant's history, in which a postmortem examination fails to reveal a cause of death. The incidence has decreased in the past decade, but is still the leading cause of death in infants ages 1 week to 1 year, with 90% of deaths occurring before 6 months of age (American Academy of Pediatrics, 2001) The exact cause is still unknown, but it is believed to be associated with neurologic regulation of cardiac and respiratory control. African American infants are at a greater risk for SIDS. Because sleep habits have been implicated with SIDS, it is recommended that healthy infants up to the age of 6 months sleep on their back (rather than the stomach) on a firm surface.

Child Abuse

Although child abuse may occur at any age, the greatest numbers of victims are from birth to age 3 years. Children younger than 1 year account for 44% of child fatalities from abuse (USDHHS, 2002). Forms of **child abuse** include intentional physical neglect or abuse, emotional neglect or abuse, and sexual abuse. Neglect, the failure of a caregiver to provide for the child's basic needs with an adequate level of care, is the most common form. Physical abuse, often referred to as the battered child syndrome, refers to deliberate physical abuse and is typically inflicted by a parent or caregiver. Sexual abuse includes incest, molestation, exhibitionism, child pornography, child prostitution, and pedophilia. These acts, when committed by a caregiver, such as a parent or babysitter, are considered sexual abuse. When a stranger commits such an act, it is considered sexual assault (a criminal act). Other forms of child maltreatment include violent shaking, called shaken baby syndrome, especially in infants younger than 6 months of age (resulting in brain trauma), and Munchausen syndrome by proxy, which is an illness fabricated or induced in another person. It is most often the mother who fabricates or causes an illness in a child to gain attention from healthcare providers.

Although child abuse occurs in all ethnic groups and at all levels of society, certain factors increase the risk, including the following:

- Parents experiencing stress from unemployment, depression, poor social and marital relationships, substance abuse, or health problems
- Children who cry frequently, have sleep difficulties, wet the bed, are hyperactive or aggressive, have difficult temperaments, or have physical, emotional, or cognitive disabilities
- Caregivers' lack of knowledge about parenting and the normal behaviors of children
- Lack of family and social support for caregivers

The number of reported cases of child abuse has increased dramatically and is a cause of national concern. Healthcare workers are in an excellent position to recognize families at risk and offer interventions, and they have a legal obligation to report suspected maltreatment (see Chapter 7). The long-term treatment of abused children and their families is complex and multidisciplinary.

Role of the Nurse in Promoting Health and Preventing Illness

The most essential role of the nurse in promoting health of the infant is teaching family members and caregivers. Teaching ranges from providing basic information about prevention of diaper rash to facilitating grieving in parents who have lost a baby to SIDS. Examples of specific areas of preventive teaching for parents of infants are shown in Teaching to Promote Health at Home 19-1. Immunization against contagious diseases begins during the first year of life and should follow a regular schedule, as outlined in Figure 19-3.

It is also important to assess the infant's growth and development. Growth rate is assessed in comparison with standardized growth charts developed for boys and girls, whose growth rates differ. Be careful when comparing an individual child's growth to standards on a chart for the following reasons:

- Every child has individual variations and short-term spurts and lags in growth.
- Atypical infants, such as those who are premature or have low birthweight, are not taken into account in such charts.
- Growth charts might be ethically and socioeconomically weighted in favor of white, middle-class children.

The Denver Developmental Screening Test (DDST) is commonly used to determine quickly and inexpensively atypical developmental patterns in infants and children. The crucial areas of development assessed in the DDST are gross motor behavior and skills, fine motor behavior and skills, language acquisition, and personal and social interaction. The test identifies problem areas that require more precise assessments. The DDST is described in more detail in most pediatric nursing texts.

When an infant in late infancy is hospitalized, **separation anxiety** behaviors are common. Separation anxiety occurs when a child is afraid of being sent away from loved ones who offer security. The infant might initially cry and scream in the phase of protest, but then stops crying and appears depressed (despair phase) (Hockenberry et al., 2003). Nurses should encourage parents to stay with the hospitalized infant and provide care, or if that is not possible, consistent healthcare providers are important to maintain the infant's trust in others.

TODDLER: 1 TO 3 YEARS

From 1 to 3 years of age, the child is considered a **toddler** (Fig. 19-4).

Physiologic Development

Physiologic development continues steadily through the toddler years, but the pace is considerably slower than that in infancy. Growth and development highlights include the following:

- Has rapid brain growth; increase in length of long bones of the arms and legs; growth of muscles
- Uses fingers to pick up small objects
- Walks forward and backward, runs, kicks, climbs stairs, and rides a tricycle
- Drinks from a cup and uses a spoon
- At 2 years of age, the toddler is typically four times the birthweight, averaging 30 to 35 lb (13.6 to 15.9 kg) and 23 to 37 inches (58.4 to 94 cm) in height.

- Has bladder control during the day and sometimes during the night (2.5–3 years of age)
- Turns pages in a book, and by 3 years of age, draws stick people

Cognitive Development

Toddlers are in Piaget's last two stages of sensorimotor development: beginning to understand object permanence, following simple commands, and anticipating events. Toddlers can understand self as separate from others and have a beginning perception of body image. Toddlers can identify and name several body parts and have a sense of gender identity. Language begins at about 1 year of age, with the use of single or bisyllable sounds. At about 2 years of age, children begin to use short sentences.

Psychosocial Development

Freud's Theory

The toddler is in Freud's anal stage. Increased muscle development and sphincter control encourage the child to focus on the pleasure of sphincter contraction and relaxation. Toilet training becomes a major focus during this period.

Erikson's Theory

The toddler enters Erikson's stage of autonomy versus shame and doubt. Autonomy is developing from independence in feeding, walking, dressing, and toileting, as well as the ability to express wishes verbally. Children who do not feel autonomous might be reluctant to explore and might be fearful of activities and people.

Negativism (characteristically expressed by saying no) and outbursts of temper result from the toddler's efforts at control over the environment. **Regression,** or behavior that is more characteristic of a younger age, can occur at any time in response to stressful circumstances. The most common regressive behaviors are excessive clinging to caregivers, loss of control over elimination, and the use of more infantile speech patterns.

Separation anxiety in response to separation from the mother figure intensifies at about 18 to 24 months, and can be as intense for the toddler as it was for the infant. The child might have feelings of anger, fear, grief and revenge (Murray & Zentner, 2001).

Havighurst's Theory

The toddler has the developmental task of learning to control the elimination of urine and feces; begins to learn sex differences, form concepts, learn language, and distinguish right from wrong.

Health of the Toddler

Accidents, such as motor vehicle crashes, poisonings, burns, drowning, choking and aspirations, and falls, are the major cause of death in toddlerhood. Dental problems can occur, *(text continues on page 400)*

Teaching to Promote Health at Home 19-1
Infants

Health Topic	Teaching Tip	Why is This Important?
Safety	• Feed the baby slowly and "burp" often. • Do not prop bottles and leave the baby unattended. • Use firmly attached bumper pads and keep the crib rails up at all times. Do not use pillows or fluffy covers in the crib. • Never leave unattended in or near water. • Use approved car seat. • Keep small objects out of reach. • Never leave the baby unattended on a table, chair, or regular bed. • Place the baby on his or her back for sleeping. • Keep plastic bags and miniblind cords out of reach. • Block stairs with gates. • Cover electrical outlets.	The leading causes of death in infants are drowning, suffocation, and falls. Infants wiggle, roll, creep, crawl, walk, and reach for objects. Placing babies on their back to sleep has significantly reduced the incidence of SIDS. Propping bottles, even in later infancy, might increase the risk of aspiration and tooth decay.
Nutrition	• How to breast feed, if chosen. • Preparing formula, information about positioning for feeding, and the importance of holding the baby for feeding, if this method is chosen. • Introducing solid foods, as prescribed by the healthcare provider. Do not add sugar, salt, or honey to foods. • Weaning is usually completed by the end of the first year.	Feeding is a time for the caregiver and baby to strengthen attachment and bonding. There is no one best time to introduce solid foods, but they should be started one at a time. Overfeeding or adding extra calories might cause obesity in the infant or in later life.
Hygiene	• Bathing the baby and caring for the umbilical cord. • Provide circumcision care for boys. • Keep the diaper area clean and dry.	Skin care, as well as care for the umbilical cord and circumcision site, are necessary in preventing infections and excoriations.
Elimination	• By 2 months, babies usually have 2 stools a day. • Breastfed babies vary more in bowel consistency, color, and times than do babies fed formula.	Renal and intestinal physiology develop throughout the first year of life.
Growth and Development	• Provide consistent care and love. • Growth and development differ for each infant, but there are some predicable milestones. • Provide educational toys appropriate to the age of the infant. • Talk and read to the baby. • Allow the baby to explore different shapes, sizes, tastes, and experiences.	The infant must be consistently loved and cared for in order to thrive, learn to trust, and achieve developmental tasks. Stimulation with age-appropriate toys and the freedom to explore influence intellectual development.
Promoting Health and Preventing Illness	• If a danger of lead ingestion exists, take appropriate measures and have the baby screened. • Maintain schedule of immunizations. • Contact healthcare provider for care of respiratory infections. • Stress importance of supplemental fluoride if water is not fluoridated. • Continue well-baby check-ups as recommended. • Do not smoke in the house or car with the baby.	Infants who ingest lead, as from eating peeling lead-based paint, are at risk for brain damage, behavioral problems, and mental deficiency. Immunizations are an essential part of healthcare. Upper respiratory infections may spread to involve the middle ear or lungs. Fluoride is necessary for tooth structure. Cigarette smoke of any type (active or passive) is dangerous, and might increase the risk of respiratory illnesses, asthma, and ear infections. Infants in day care have increased exposure to respiratory and skin infections and infestations.

Recommended Childhood and Adolescent Immunization Schedule
United States, 2003

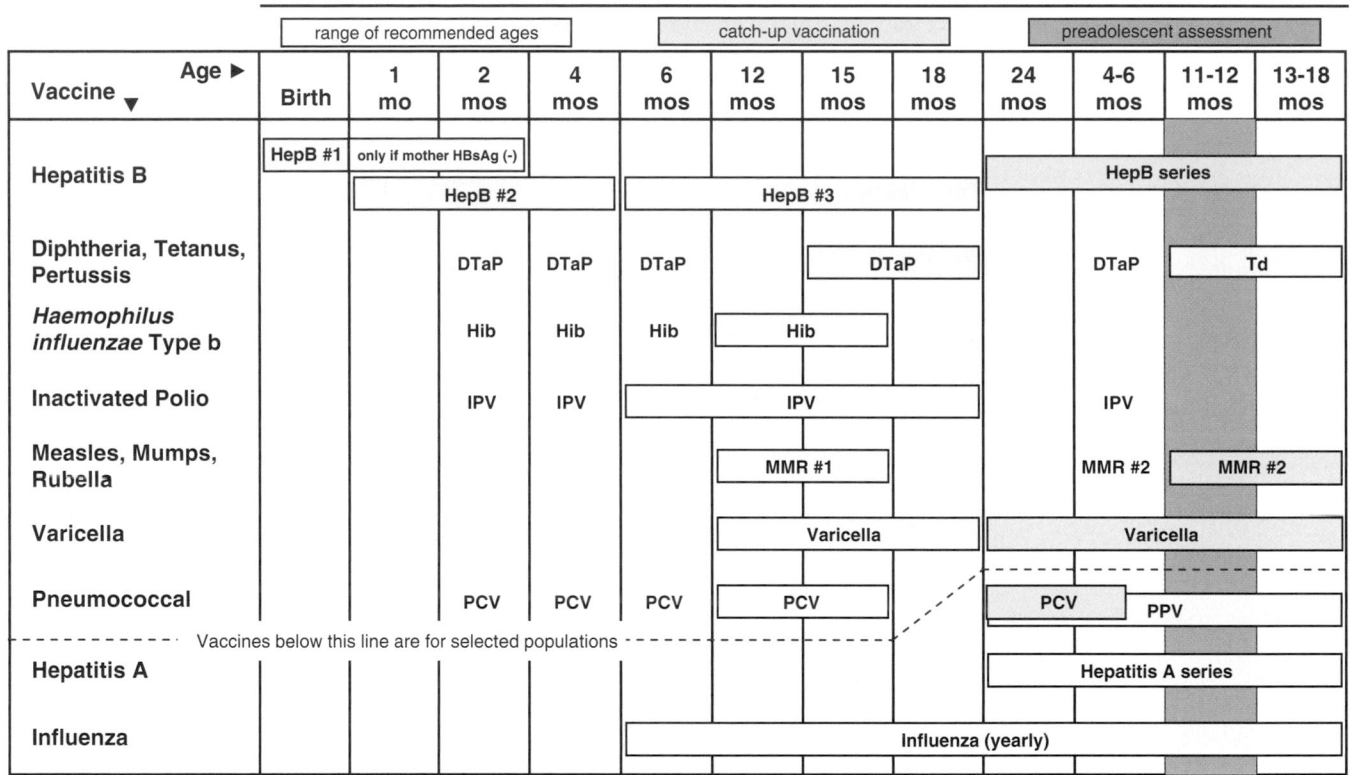

Vaccine ▼	Age ▶ Birth	1 mo	2 mos	4 mos	6 mos	12 mos	15 mos	18 mos	24 mos	4-6 mos	11-12 mos	13-18 mos
			range of recommended ages				catch-up vaccination			preadolescent assessment		
Hepatitis B	HepB #1	only if mother HBsAg (-)									HepB series	
		HepB #2			HepB #3							
Diphtheria, Tetanus, Pertussis			DTaP	DTaP	DTaP		DTaP		DTaP		Td	
Haemophilus influenzae Type b			Hib	Hib	Hib	Hib						
Inactivated Polio			IPV	IPV		IPV			IPV			
Measles, Mumps, Rubella						MMR #1			MMR #2		MMR #2	
Varicella						Varicella			Varicella			
Pneumococcal			PCV	PCV	PCV	PCV			PCV	PPV		
Hepatitis A									Hepatitis A series			
Influenza						Influenza (yearly)						

- - - - - - - - - - Vaccines below this line are for selected populations - - - - - - - - - -

This schedule indicates the recommended ages for routine administration of currently licensed childhood vaccines, as of December 1, 2002, for children through age 18 years. Any dose not given at the recommended age should be given at any subsequent visit when indicated and feasible. ▭ Indicates age groups that warrant special effort to administer those vaccines not previously given. Additional vaccines may be licensed and recommended during the year.

For additional information about vaccines, including precautions and contradictions for immunization and vaccine shortages, please visit the National Immunization Program Website at www.cdc.gov/nip or call the National Immunization Information Hotline at 800-232-2522 (English) or 800-232-0233 (Spanish).

Approved by the Advisory Committee on Immunization Practices (www.cdc.gov/nip/acip), the American Academy of Pediatrics (www.aap.org), and the American Academy of Family Physicians (www.aafp.org).

FIGURE 19-3 Recommended Childhood and Adolescent Immunization Schedule—United States, 2003.

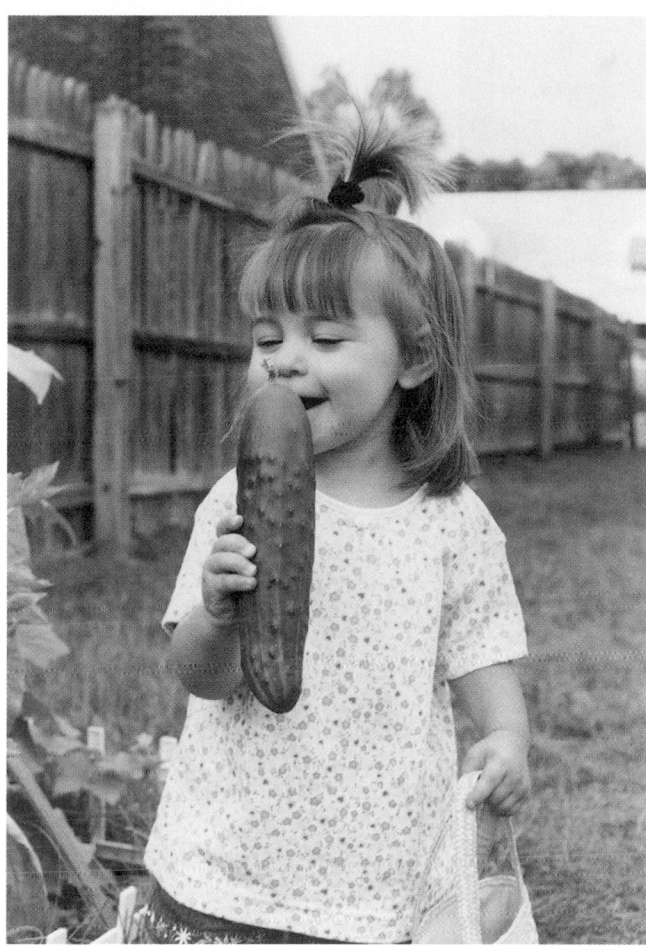

Toddlers enter a stage of autonomy, promoting exploration.

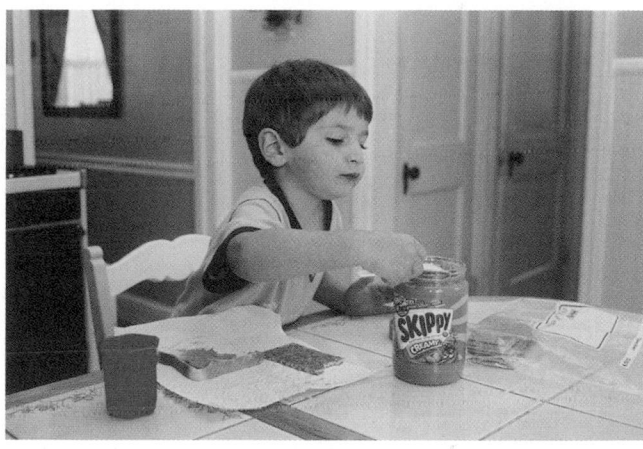

The curious and independent toddler often has a desire to do things by himself.

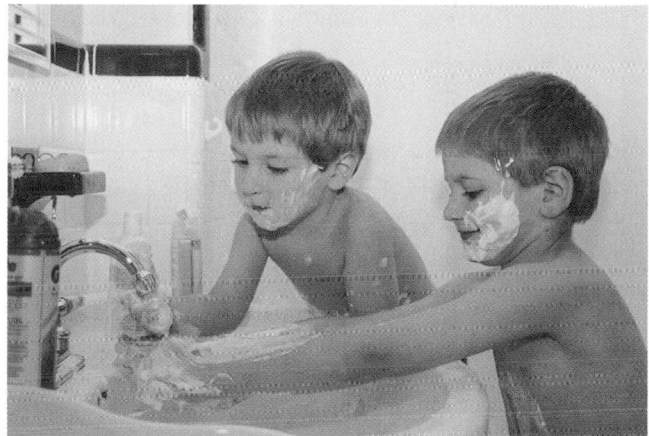

Cognitive development can be promoted by allowing the toddler the opportunity to observe and imitate. Younger siblings particularly enjoy mimicking older siblings.

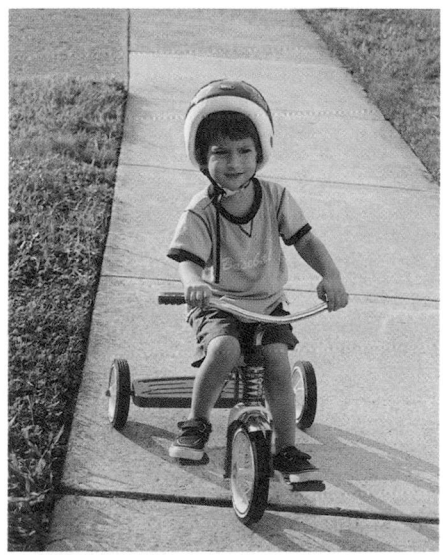

Safety is a common concern for caregivers.

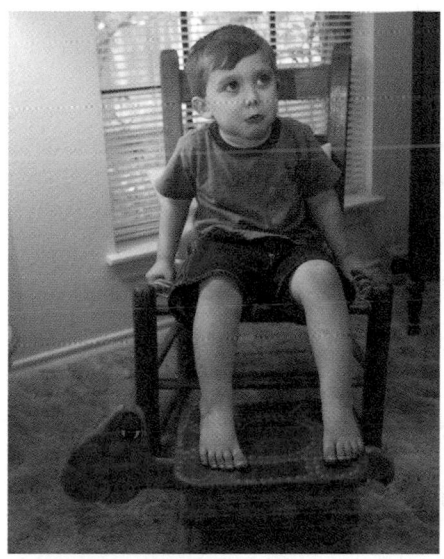

Discipline helps toddlers learn inner control and understand limits.   (Photo by Joe Mitchell.)

FIGURE 19-4 Development in the toddler. (*continued*)

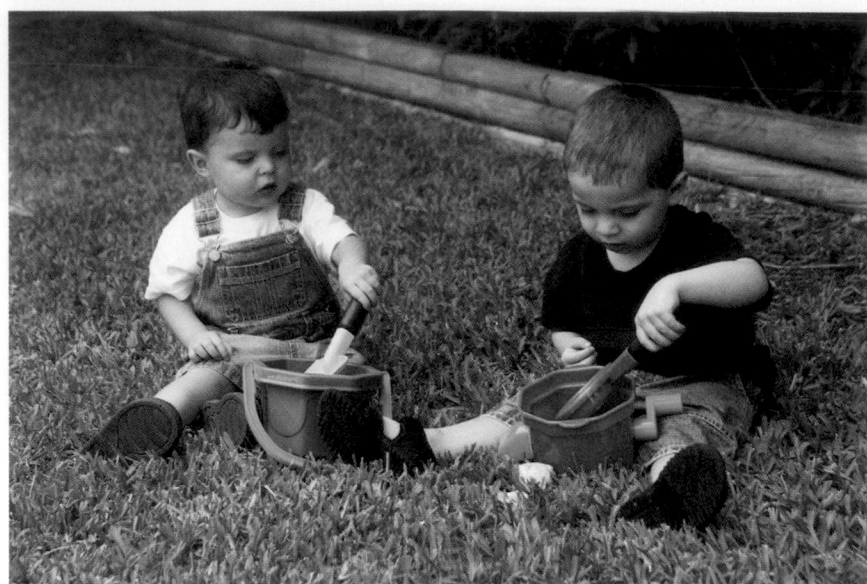

Play in toddlerhood might be solitary or parallel.
(Photo by Joe Mitchell.)

FIGURE 19-4 *Continued*

especially if the toddler is allowed to go to sleep while sucking on a bottle of milk or sweetened liquid. Respiratory tract and middle ear infections are common. Some surgeries, such as repair of a cleft lip and palate, might be done in the toddler years. Autistic disorder, with abnormal behavior, social interactions and communication, is usually diagnosed by the time the child is 3 years old.

Role of the Nurse in Promoting Health and Preventing Illness

The role of the nurse in promoting health in the toddler continues to be primarily teaching, as shown by the examples in Teaching to Promote Health at Home 19-2. An important part of teaching is helping caregivers encourage their toddler's independence while setting firm limits.

Toddlers who require care in the hospital setting experience stress and separation anxiety when parents are not present. To decrease stress from unfamiliar surroundings and caregivers, parents should be encouraged to provide care and remain with the toddler as much as possible. Every effort should be made to have consistency of healthcare providers and to maintain familiar routines and rituals. When they are ill or in pain, toddlers often regress to earlier behaviors, such as wanting a bottle to drink from.

Recall 2-year-old Hillarie Browning, who is unresponsive. The nurse could apply knowledge about the feelings of stress and separation for a hospitalized toddler when developing the plan of care for this child, especially in light of the possible child abuse. Consistency in staff members caring for the child and maintaining rituals would be helpful in fostering trust and minimizing upset.

PRESCHOOLER: 3 TO 6 YEARS

At around age 3, toddlers begin to move into the next stage: **preschooler.** Although growth and development are slower than in infancy and toddlerhood, they are still steady (Fig. 19-5).

Physiologic Development

The physical characteristics of the preschooler include the following:
- Head is close to adult size by 6 years of age.
- The body is less chubby and becomes leaner and more coordinated.
- Motor abilities include skipping, throwing and catching a ball, copying figures, and printing letters and numbers.
- Full set of 20 deciduous teeth is present; baby teeth begin to fall out and are replaced by permanent teeth.
- Average weight at 5 to 6 years of age is 45 lb (20.4 kg), with boys being slightly heavier than girls.

Cognitive Development

Preschoolers are in Piaget's preoperational stage of development. Passing through the preconceptual and the intuitive phases, preschoolers demonstrate the following transitional changes:
- Egocentrism decreases as socialization with other children increases, and the ability to express self verbally improves.
- Play is more related to real-life events (rather than fantasy).
- Basic curiosity results in constant questions and improved reasoning ability.

Language development is seen in more elaborate and grammatically correct sentences, with 6- to 18-word sentences be-

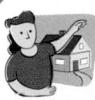

Teaching to Promote Health at Home 19-2
Toddlers

Health Topic	Teaching Tip	Why is This Important?
Safety	• Lock medicines, cleaning supplies, and yard-care products out of reach. • Use safety plugs in electrical outlets. • Block stairs with gates. • Use approved car seat. • Never leave unattended near water. • Do not give small hard foods, small toys or toy parts, or balloons. • Keep plastic bags and miniblind cords out of reach. • Teach danger in simple terms ("stove hot"). • Do not toss in the air or swing by the arms.	Accidents are a leading cause of injuries and death in toddlers. It is necessary to childproof the home to prevent injury, as the toddler moves quickly, lacks judgment, and explores his or her world by seeing, touching, and tasting. Small objects or balloons might be aspirated and cause suffocation. Joints might be dislocated by swinging the child.
Nutrition	• Do not scold for messiness while eating. • Provide finger foods. • Short periods of loss of appetite are normal. • Avoid foods that are high in fat, sugar, and salt content (often found in fast foods).	The toddler is growing less rapidly than the infant and does not require as many calories. Feeding self, even if messy, promotes independence. Giving too much food or food that is high in calories might result in obesity.
Hygiene	• Teach handwashing after eating and toileting. • Teach how to brush teeth. • Schedule dentist visit.	It is important to establish good hygiene and to serve as a role model. The first dentist visit might be just to become familiar with the office and provider.
Elimination	• Physical development is necessary for toilet training. • Begin training with bowel elimination. • Watch for signs of readiness (realizing wetness, staying dry for 2 or more hours). • Night dryness takes longer than day dryness.	The neuromuscular control necessary for elimination occurs between 1 and 3 years. Bowel training is a less complex task than bladder training.
Growth and Development	• Encourage independence in eating, dressing, and toileting. • Provide toys that emphasize gross motor skills and creativity. • Parallel play with other children is normal. • The concept of sharing is not yet developed. • Saying "no" to almost everything is normal.	The toddler gains a sense of security and control by being able to eat, dress, toilet self, and say "no."
Promoting Health and Preventing Illness	• If a danger of lead ingestion exists, take appropriate measures and have the toddler screened. • Complete immunizations. • See healthcare professionals for treatment of respiratory infections. • Do not smoke in the house or car with the child.	Toddlers who ingest lead, as from eating peeling lead-based paint, are at risk for brain damage, behavioral problems and mental deficiency. Immunizations are an essential part of healthcare. Respiratory infections might lead to ear infections. Avoid smoking to reduce risk of respiratory illness, asthma, and ear infections. Passive smoke is dangerous. Infants in day care have increased exposure to respiratory and skin infections and infestations.

coming common by 6 years of age. Incessantly asking "Why?" increases the child's knowledge, encourages further conversations, and helps develop language abilities.

Preschoolers clearly identify themselves as male or female, can understand basic body functions, and have a curiosity about sex differences. This curiosity often leads to "playing doctor," which is normal behavior at this stage. Many children in this age group want to look special or dressed up and gain increased self-esteem by receiving compliments about their appearance

Psychosocial Development
Freud's Theory
The preschooler is in Freud's phallic stage, with the biologic focus primarily genital. The child has a sexual desire for the

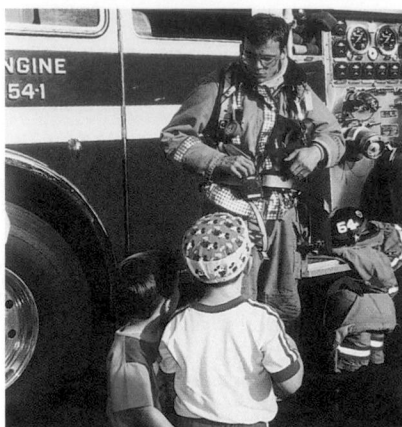

Basic curiosity results in questioning and an improved reasoning ability in the preschooler.

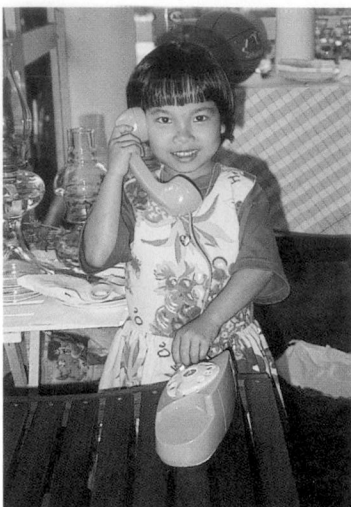

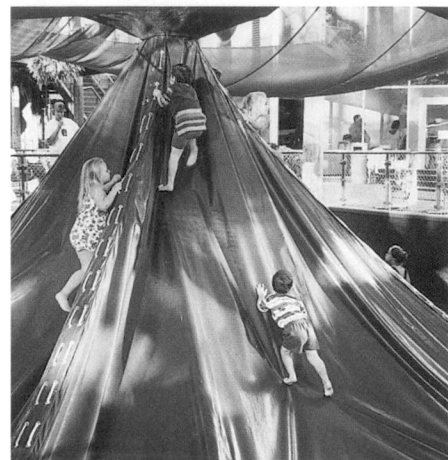

Preschooler play is associative and cooperative in its social dimension, and cognitive development is demonstrated in constructive and pretend play.

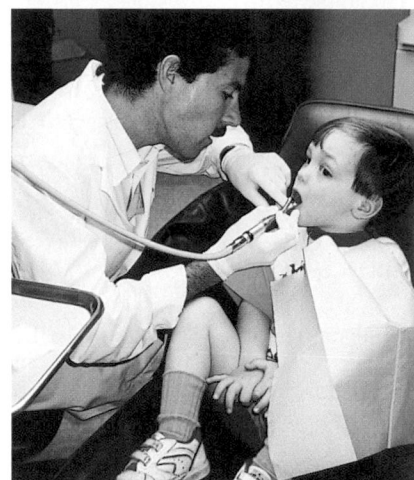

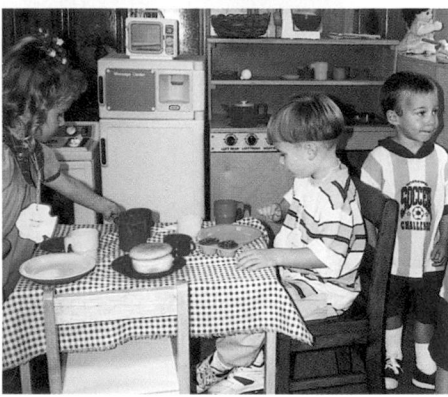

Symbolic play gradually becomes more related to real-life events.

A visit to the dentist is useful for teaching dental hygiene and helping the preschooler overcome fear of the unknown.

FIGURE 19-5 Development in the preschooler.

opposite-sex parent but, as a means of defense, strongly identifies with the same-sex parent; as a result of this conflict resolution, the superego and conscience begin to develop.

Erikson's Theory

The preschooler is in Erikson's stage of initiative versus guilt. Inner turmoil occurs when natural curiosity is pitted against a constant examination of the propriety of one's actions by a rigid conscience. Realistic self-limits are learned through social interactions.

Havighurst's Theory

According to Havighurst, the preschooler has four developmental tasks to accomplish: to learn sex differences and modesty, to describe social and physical reality through concept formation and language development, to get ready to read, and to learn to distinguish right from wrong.

Special Considerations

Preschoolers often have fears—most commonly fear of new places, fear of the dark, and fear during nightmares. These fears are often made worse by the child's own fertile imagination

and ability to fantasize. Support and validation of the preschooler's feelings by caregivers are essential.

Moral and Spiritual Development

Kohlberg's preconventional phase of moral reasoning dominates this age. The focus of this stage is obeying rules to avoid punishment or receive a reward. The cognitive, psychosocial, and moral developments of the preschooler provide a base for spiritual development, as described by Fowler. The preschooler might attend activities at church or synagogue with the family but does not understand religious concepts. The concept of a deity is literal, with God usually being viewed as a male human. Concepts such as heaven, hell, and holy spirits are incomprehensible and often frightening.

Health of the Preschooler

Preschoolers continue to have the health problems that are common in toddlerhood. Communicable diseases and respiratory tract infections are common, especially with increased interaction with other children at nursery schools and day care.

Preschoolers are prone to accidents because of their increased curiosity about the world. Some congenital disorders, such as hypospadias, inguinal hernias, and cardiac anomalies require surgery at this time. Dental caries become common if teeth are neglected. As language becomes more sophisticated, speech disorders might become apparent.

Role of the Nurse in Promoting Health and Preventing Illness

Teaching to Promote Health at Home 19-3 provides examples of teaching to promote health in preschoolers. When caring for a preschool-aged child who is scheduled for surgery or requires hospitalization, nurses must recognize the importance of the child's fear of pain as well as separation anxiety. The nurse can help decrease fears by explaining procedures in language the child can understand and by being honest about how much pain a procedure will cause. Many healthcare institutions and agencies have preprocedure visits so that the child having surgery becomes familiar with the setting and with the activities that will be done. Allowing the child to practice procedures on a doll and encouraging the child to express his or her feelings openly are also beneficial (Fig. 19-6). Encouraging caregivers to take an active role in the child's care helps to reduce fear and separation anxiety.

SCHOOL-AGED CHILD: 6 TO 12 YEARS

School-aged children, from 6 to 12 years of age, are typically sturdy and strong. Physical growth during this time is relatively

---

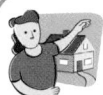

Teaching to Promote Health at Home 19-3
Preschoolers

Health Topic	Teaching Tip	Why is This Important?
Safety	• Lock medicines and cleaning and gardening supplies out of reach. • Use safety plugs in electrical outlets. • Teach child how to go up and down stairs. • Do not give small hard foods, small toys, or balloons. • Use approved car seat and bicycle helmets. • Teach simple traffic safety. • Teach to never talk to or get in the car with a stranger. Include information about inappropriate touching. • Never leave the child alone in public or unattended in a car. • Begin swimming lessons and teach water safety. • Teach danger of fire, and have a home fire safety plan.	Accidents are the leading cause of injury and death in preschoolers, most often from motor vehicles, drowning, burns, and poisoning. Even minor head trauma may cause hematoma formation. Children are at risk for harm from physical and sexual abuse and must be taught how to avoid situations that might increase that risk.
Nutrition	• A gradual increase in calories, with nutritious snacks, is necessary • Children who follow their own appetite patterns are less likely to be overweight. • Avoid foods that are high in fat, sugar, and salt (found in most fast foods). • Preschoolers like to eat one food at a time, and prefer those that are mildly flavored and lukewarm.	The preschool child needs the same food group nutrition as the adult, but in lesser amounts.
Hygiene	• Stress importance of handwashing before meals and after toileting. • Assist with brushing and flossing teeth after eating. • Teach disposal of used tissues. • Maintain regular dental checkups and care.	Preschoolers are able to carry out basic hygiene, but continue to need assistance and reminders. Dental caries often begins during this age.
Elimination	• Toilet training is completed, but night wetting may persist.	Recognizing the need to empty the bladder during sleep takes a longer time in some children. They should not be punished for wetting the bed.

(continued)

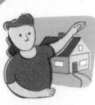

Teaching to Promote Health at Home 19-3
Preschoolers (Continued)

Health Topic	Teaching Tip	Why is This Important?
Growth and Development	• Night fears and bad dreams are common. • Make-believe play and imaginary friends are normal. • Although each child grows and develops differently, there are ranges of normal. • Play occupies most of the child's time; the child can play with others for periods of time. • Provide play materials that encourage physical activity, dramatic play, quiet play, and creativity. • Provide consistent, fair, and kind limits for behavior. • Masturbation is normal, although the child should learn that it is not acceptable in public.	Sleep problems usually resolve on their own; calm reassurance by parents is appropriate when they occur. Play is the work of the child; adults should provide time, space, equipment, and safety but should not structure the child's play.
Promoting Health and Preventing Illness	• If a danger of lead ingestion or poisoning exists, take appropriate measures and have the child screened. • Maintain immunizations. • Have vision tested. • Have hearing tested if necessary (eg, child does not seem to listen). • Maintain regular well-child checkups. • Preschoolers often fear dental and medical treatments. Avoid hospitalization if possible, but if necessary, prepare the child before the procedure.	Lead poisoning in preschoolers causes brain dysfunction. Immunizations and health-related checkups are essential in promoting health. Preschoolers often see dental or medical procedures as a punishment and fear damage to his or her body. Parents should set a good example, be honest with the child. Preparation for procedures and hospitalization can help decrease fear and separation anxiety.

slow but continues steadily, with both refinement and subtle changes taking place (Fig. 19-7).

Physiologic Development

Physiologic development of school-aged children includes the following:

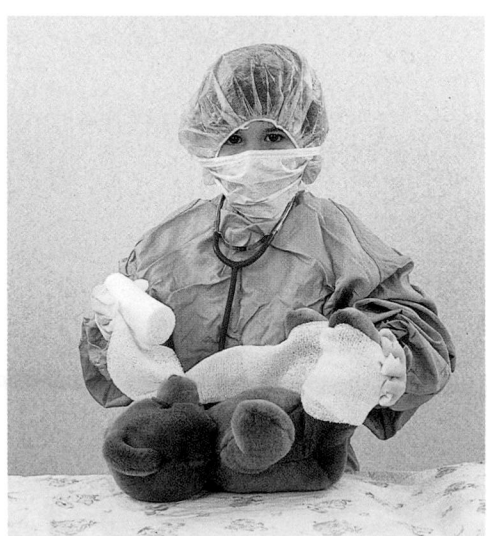

FIGURE 19-6 Abstract reasoning is necessary for children to understand that painful medical treatments given now will make them feel better later. Dramatic play may help the preschool child, who is not old enough to have developed abstract reasoning, to understand the uncomfortable experiences of the hospital stay.   (Photo © B. Proud.)

• The brain reaches 90% to 95% of adult size; by 12 years of age, the nervous system is almost completely matured, resulting in coordinated body movements.
• Motor abilities progress from the ability to hold a pencil and print words at 6 years of age to the ability to write in script and in sentences at 12 years of age.
• Sexual organs grow but are dormant until late in this period, when hormonal changes begin.
• All permanent teeth are present, except for the second and third molars, by 12 years of age.
• Height increases 2 to 3 inches (5.1 to 7.6 cm) and weight increases 3 to 6 lb (1.4 to 2.7 kg) a year.

Cognitive Development

The school-aged child is at Piaget's concrete operational stage of development, organizing facts about the environment to use for problem solving. In this period, the child has the following characteristics:
• Thinks logically and develops concepts of mass, volume, weight, and measurement
• Deals best with actual objects and people, but can relate concepts and compare events
• Uses inductive reasoning to solve new problems
• Generalizes about people, places, and things
• Develops classification systems
• Develops an awareness and understanding of other people's feelings and points of view
• Understands reversal of events

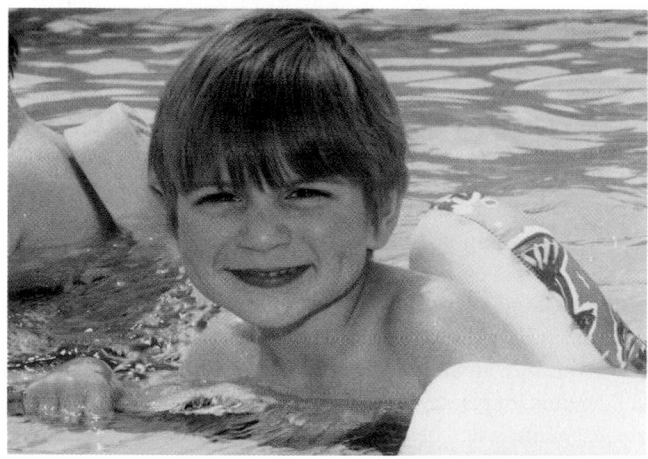

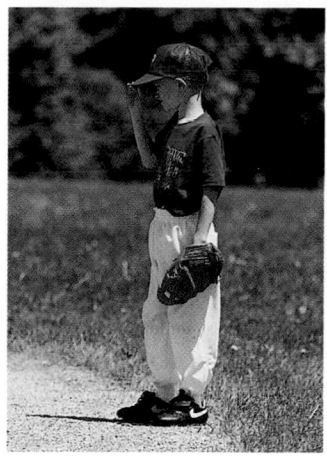

Play involves development of skill, games with rules, and competitive activities.

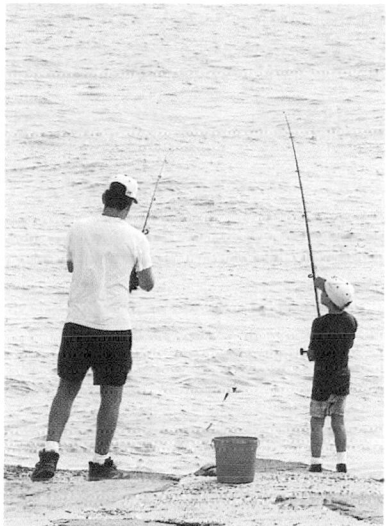

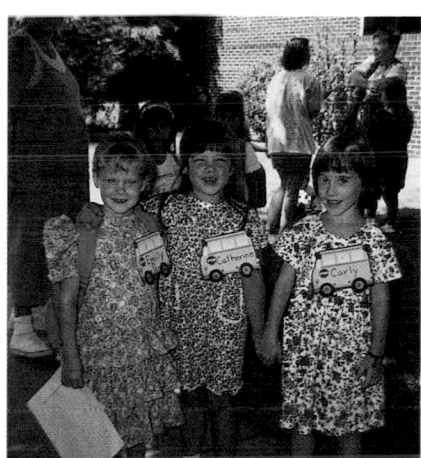

The school-aged child is aware of and understands a sequence of events.

Making friends is important to school-aged children.

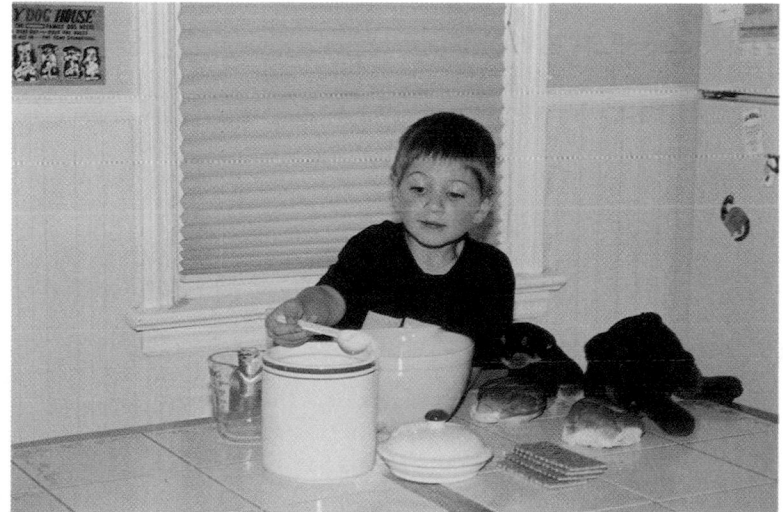

FIGURE 19-7 Development in the school-aged child.

School-aged children have well-developed language skills, using language in a more sophisticated manner. Their ability to store information in long-term memory and retrieve it in the remembering (recall) process is more efficient.

Psychosocial Development

Freud's Theory

The school-aged child is in the latency stage of Freud's theory, with psychosocial energies being channeled toward strong identification with one's own sex and creative activities. Privacy and understanding one's body are important at this age.

Erikson's Theory

The school-aged child is in the industry-versus-inferiority stage of Erikson's theory, with the child focused on learning useful skills and thereby developing positive self-esteem. A sense of identity begins to emerge, and values are integrated. The emphasis is on doing, succeeding, and accomplishing.

Havighurst's Theory

According to Havighurst, the school-aged child has the following developmental tasks:
- Learning physical game skills
- Learning appropriate masculine or feminine social role
- Developing fundamental skills in reading, writing, and calculating
- Developing concepts necessary for everyday living
- Achieving personal independence
- Developing conscience, morality, and a scale of values

Special Considerations

Peer relationships become the major gauge for determining status, skill, and personableness. Peer groups in middle childhood help prepare the child for getting along in the larger world and teach appropriate sex role behavior. They also act as transition modes for the child as he or she leaves the total caregiver influence and heads toward adult independence.

Body image, self-concept, and sexuality are interrelated. Sexual development results in a strong need to understand body function and to have accurate information about sexuality.

Moral Development

Most of middle childhood is spent in the conventional phase of moral development. Behavior is based on familial and peer group beliefs, and conformity to the norm is common. Following school regulations, respecting teachers, and viewing justice as a means of fair play are all important.

Spiritual Development

In Fowler's theory, school-aged children view religious faith as a relationship that involves reciprocal fairness. They take part in rituals of their faith, with a basic understanding of the ritual's significance. The importance of spiritual beliefs and the possibility of life after death is accepted, even if not totally understood.

Health of the School-Aged Child

Accidents continue to be common in school-aged children. With increased interactions with other children in school, communicable conditions, such as scabies, impetigo, and head lice are more prevalent. Other common health-related problems of the school-aged child include attention deficit hyperactivity disorder (ADHD) and learning disability (LD), and enuresis (bed wetting). In addition, chronic conditions such as sickle cell anemia, hyperactivity, seizure disorders, hypertension, diabetes mellitus, and obesity might affect the school-aged child. Scoliosis, an abnormal curvature of the spine, occurs most often in girls between the ages of 10 and 13 years.

ADHD and Learning Disabilities

ADHD is a developmentally inappropriate degree of inattention, impulsiveness, and hyperactivity. To be diagnosed with this disorder, the child must have manifested symptoms before 7 years of age, and they must be present in at least two settings. LD is a group of disorders in which the child has significant difficulty in listening, speaking, reading, writing, reasoning, mathematic abilities, or social skills (Hockenberry et al., 2003). Both of these conditions affect all areas of the life of the child, but they are most noticeable in the classroom. Multiple approaches are used in management, including medication, environmental strategies, and classroom education. Based on the Education for All Handicapped Children's Act, children with ADHD and LD must receive free public education in the least restrictive environment.

Enuresis

Enuresis is diagnosed when a child is at least 5 years of age and is still having involuntary urination, usually at night. Although this problem is significant to the child and his or her parents, it is defined as a benign and self-limiting disorder, usually ending between 6 and 8 years of age.

Role of the Nurse in Promoting Health and Preventing Illness

The nurse's role in promoting health for the school-aged child involves individual and family teaching, often conducted by school nurses. Because school violence has become more common, with school-aged children involved in mass shootings, school nurses must be prepared for a potential crisis. Teaching to Promote Health at Home 19-4 provides examples of nursing activities specific for this age group.

Because school-aged children are striving for independence and control, hospitalization might mean a loss of freedom of choice (eg, types of food, clothing, and activities). Children of this age should be allowed to have some measure of control over allowable activities and should be encouraged to do what they can, such as playing competitive games and making their own bed (Fig. 19-8).

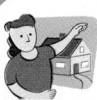

Teaching to Promote Health at Home 19-4
School-Aged Children

Health Topic	Teaching Tip	Why is This Important?
Safety	• Teach and require pedestrian traffic safety. • Wear seat belts and bicycle helmets. • Emphasize bicycle, scooter, skate, and skateboard safety. • Provide swimming lessons and water safety rules. • Rural children should be taught farm safety. • Teach how to "stop, drop, and roll" to extinguish clothing fire. • Teach the dangers of dangerous products and chemicals. • Keep guns locked up. Teach gun safety rules. • Teach use of proper equipment for contact sports.	Accidents are the leading cause of death in school-aged children, most often caused by motor vehicle crashes, fires, falls, drowning, and poisonings. Gun accidents to themselves and others occur in school-aged children. Accident prevention and safety education should be taught and reinforced both at home and at school.
Nutrition	• School-aged children need adequate calories, and might also require increased amounts of vitamin D and calcium. • Provide foods that meet nutritional needs and do not supply empty calories (as found in junk food and fast food). • Do not overemphasize table manners to keep meal times more pleasant.	Increased vitamin D and calcium are needed as bones enlarge, and for girls to prevent later osteoporosis. American children eat too much salt, sugar, and fats; nearly ¼ of all school-aged children have an elevated cholesterol level. Eating patterns for school age children will improve over time. Both undernutrition and overnutrition are seen in this age group.
Hygiene	• Teach girls how to wipe from front to back after urination. • Teach children not to share hats or combs.	Girls are prone to urinary infections because of their short urethra. Head lice and ringworm are common in school-aged children, and are easily spread to others.
Sexual Development	• Both girls and boys have characteristics of sexual maturity, including a growth spurt, growth of body hair, changes in body proportion, and the beginning of secondary physical sex changes. • Provide accurate information and answer questions honestly about sex, including anatomy, physiology, birth control, and STDs (including AIDS). • Monitor TV watching and computer use.	Girls have breast development, grow axillary and pubic hair, and may begin to menstruate. Boys have testicular growth, grow axillary and pubic hair, and the penis enlarges. Boys may also have temporary breast enlargement. School-aged children are curious, and if unsupervised, may watch pornographic television or computer material. In addition, the violence in television shows or video games may lead to aggressive behavior.
Growth and Development	• Best friends and groups of peer friends are important to the school-aged child. • Rules are rigidly followed during games with peers. • Encourage both quiet and active play activities. • Provide guidance and set limits for behavior, focusing on only one incident at a time. • Encourage feelings of industry by having realistic expectations and recognizing unique abilities and talents. • Provide positive statements that demonstrate the child is valued, loved, and important.	From ages 7 to 9, close friends are usually the same gender and age. This is not as important from ages 10 to 12. Unrealistic expectations or excessive discipline might result in stress and feelings of inferiority.
Promoting Health and Preventing Illness	• Maintain records of immunizations, and have boosters as recommended. • Promote regular physical activity and exercise. • Teach how to "just say no" to smoking, alcohol, and drugs. • Maintain dental examinations. • Maintain well-child checkups, and have screenings (if at risk or indicated by symptoms) and treatment for chronic conditions such as asthma, diabetes mellitus, sickle cell anemia, hypertension, seizure disorder, hyperactivity, and obesity. • Have vision tested if school problems with reading, coordination, or inability to see screen or monitor in front of the room occur.	Maintaining immunizations is essential to health; records are required for enrollment in school. Children need to know how to handle peer pressure to smoke, drink, and take drugs. Many school-aged children are at risk for and exhibit symptoms of chronic illnesses.

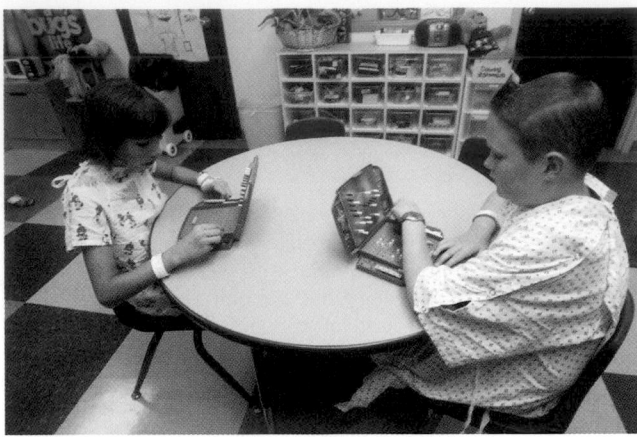

FIGURE 19-8 Allowing school-aged children to play competitive games promotes a positive hospital experience.   (Photo by Joe Mitchell.)

THE ADOLESCENT AND YOUNG ADULT

The adolescent and young adult years are a time of both change and stability. **Adolescence** begins with puberty and extends from 12 to 20 years of age; the **young adult** period is considered to be the 20s and 30s. However, these time periods are highly individualized. A person is defined as an adult when he or she is "physically and psychologically mature, ready to assume adult responsibilities and be self-sufficient" (Murray & Zentner, 2001, p. 525).

After experiencing rapid growth and development during adolescence, the young adult completes physical growth and develops internal and external controls and values acceptable to society. There are no specific measurements of maturity; each person is an individual and a wide range of normal values and behaviors are considered healthy (Fig. 19-9).

Physiologic Development

Changes in the adolescent's body transform him or her from a child to an adult in appearance. Physiologic development includes the following:

- The feet, hands, and long bones grow rapidly, accompanied by an increase in muscle mass (especially in boys).
- Primary and secondary sexual development occurs, with maturation of the genitalia; presence of body hair; breast development and menstruation in girls; facial hair growth, voice changes, and spermatogenesis in boys.
- **Puberty** (the time when the ability to reproduce begins) begins at 9 to 13 years of age in girls (with menstruation usually beginning between 10 and 14 years of age) and at 11 or 14 years of age in boys.
- Sebaceous and axillary sweat glands become active.
- Full adult size is reached, although some young men might continue to grow in their 20s.

Puberty can be divided into the following three stages (Table 19-2):

- Prepubescence: Secondary sex characteristics begin to develop, but the reproductive organs do not yet function.
- Pubescence: Secondary sex characteristics continue to develop, and ova and sperm begin to be produced by the reproductive organs.
- Postpubescence: Reproductive functioning and the development of secondary sex characteristics reach adult maturity.

Cognitive Development

According to Piaget, adolescence is the stage when the cognitive development of formal operations is developed. Deductive, reflective, and hypothetical reasoning are possible, and abstract concepts can be used. Long-term goals can be set as the concept of time, its passage, and the future become real. Challenging the decision making of adults is common. Egocentrism returns, and imaginary audiences and daydreaming are common.

Young adults, in comparison to the adolescent, are more creative in thought, are objective and realistic, and are less self-centered. Their learning is enhanced through educational and life experiences.

Psychosocial Development

Freud's Theory

The adolescent and young adult are in Freud's genital stage. The libido reemerges in a mature, adult form, and the individual is capable of full sexual function. There is a sense of self and others, extending to other adults and peers of the opposite gender. Creativity and pleasure are found in love and in work.

Erikson's Theory

Based on Erikson's theory, the adolescent tries out different roles, personal choices, and beliefs in the stage called identity versus role confusion. Self-concept is being stabilized, with the peer group acting as the greatest influence.

> *Think back to Darlene Jenkins, the 14-year-old pregnant teenager. The nurse could apply knowledge of Erikson's theory to foster a sense of identity in Darlene by explaining about important self-care measures and encouraging her participation in her pregnancy. In addition, establishing a trusting relationship with Darlene and subsequently with her and other members of the healthcare staff would help to further promote her identity.*

The young adult, in the intimacy-versus-isolation stage, needs to complete tasks such as achieving independence from parents, establishing intimate relationships, and choosing an occupation or career. If such developmental tasks are not accomplished, the young adult becomes isolated and self-absorbed.

Havighurst's Theory

According to Havighurst, more mature relationships with both boys and girls of the same age are achieved, a masculine or

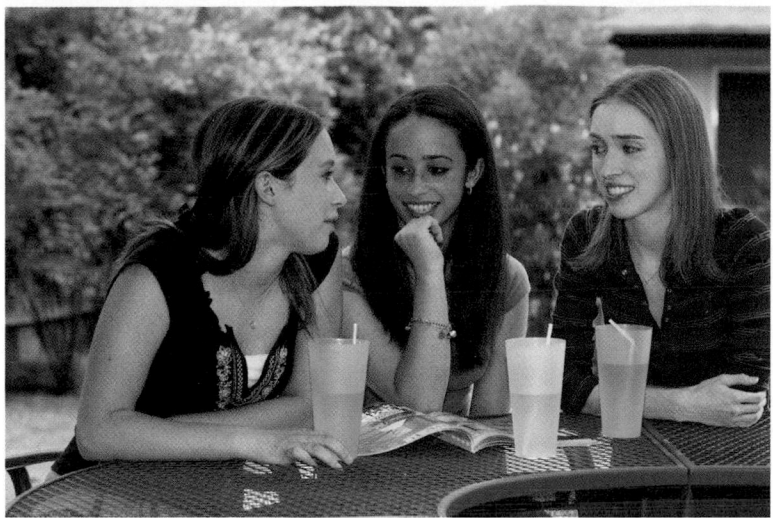

Peer relationships are particularly influential during adolescence. (Photo by Joe Mitchell.)

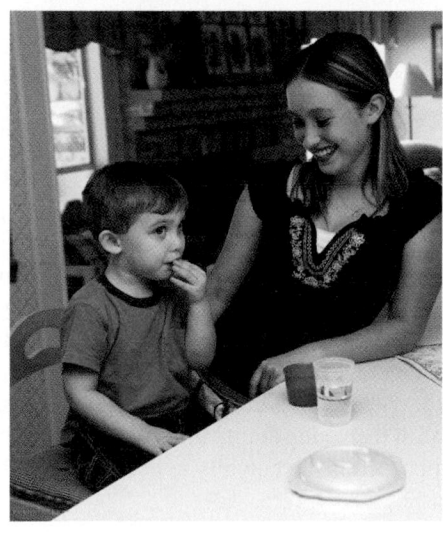

Babysitting offers an opportunity to practice formal adult skills. (Photo by Joe Mitchell.)

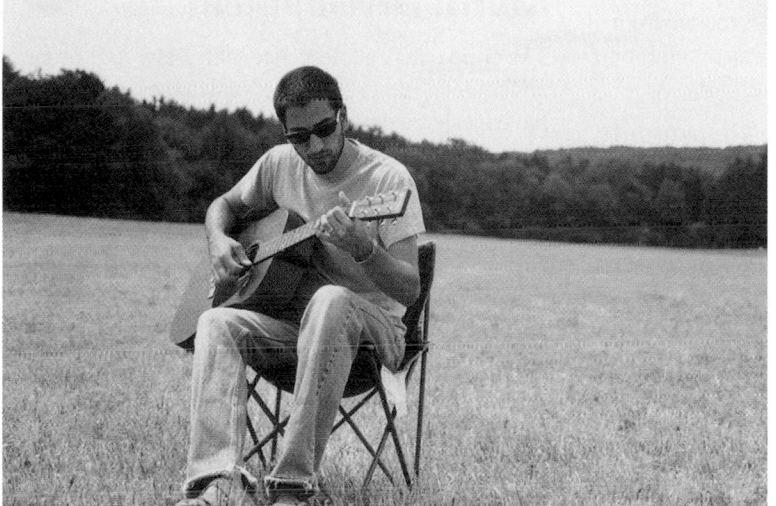

The development of self-identity in adolescence involves discovering talents and becoming emotionally independent.

FIGURE 19-9 Development in the adolescent.

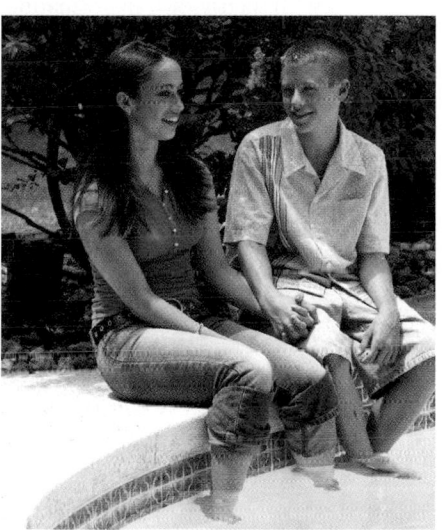

A primary developmental task of adolescence is to achieve new and more-mature relationships. (Photo by Joe Mitchell.)

TABLE 19-2 Adolescent Sexual Development

Stage	Males	Females
Prepubescence	• Progressive enlargement of testicles, seminal ducts, prostate gland • Enlargement and reddening of the scrotal sac • Increase in length and circumference of penis • Appearance of downy pubic hair	• Progressive enlargement of the ovaries • Ripening of graafian follicles • Rounding of the hips • Appearance of breast buds • Enlargement of the fallopian tubes, vagina, and uterus • Appearance of downy pubic hair
Pubescence	• Increase in amount, pigmentation, and curling of pubic hair • Growth spurt involving height and weight increase • Deepening of the voice due to growth of larynx • Enlargement of testicles • Increased pigmentation and growth of scrotum • Growth of penis in length and circumference • Beginning of spermatogenesis	• Increase in amount, pigmentation, and curling of pubic hair • Growth spurt involving height and weight increase • Menarche • Appearance of axillary hair • Enlargement of vulva and clitoris • Development of breast tissue • Ovulation
Postpubescence	• Completion of sexual growth and development • Fertility	• Completion of sexual growth and development • Fertility

feminine social role is developed, one's personal appearance is accepted, and a set of values and an ethical system as a guide to behavior are internalized.

Levinson's Theory

Based on Levinson's theory of individual life structure, the years from 18 to 22 are characterized by early adult transition (Levinson, Darrow, Klein, et al., 1978). This is a time of making initial career choices, establishing personal relationships, and selecting personal values and lifestyles. During the years from 22 to 28, the young adult builds on previous choices, but there might be a transient quality to occupational choices and friendships.

Gould's Theory

Gould's (1972) theory of transformation views young adults as having established their own control as adults separate from the family. They want to enjoy the present but also build for the future.

> Remember Patricia Lemming, the 26-year-old pregnant woman described at the beginning of the chapter. Applying Gould's theory, the nurse could interpret Patricia's desire to stop smoking and drinking as an example of her attempt to establish control as an adult, thus securing the future for herself and her baby. The nurse could build on this desire by teaching Patricia about appropriate and effective methods for smoking and drinking cessation.

Special Considerations
Choosing an Occupation or Career
A major psychosocial developmental requirement for the young adult is choosing a vocation. The decision to enter the world of work is strongly influenced initially by the need to become independent of one's family and to be self-sufficient. The choice of an occupation or a career is also guided by the factors such as the desire to get married, raise a family, and become part of the community (Fig. 19-10).

Occupational and career choices are largely tied to educational choices. Many careers require a college education. Adults learn from both informal and formal experiences and are largely goal-directed learners. If the person's identified goals are to increase career opportunities, maintain financial stability, and pursue upward mobility, the adult will be motivated to learn and change. The major factor in achieving satisfaction with one's vocational choice is the belief that one is functioning to capacity and making a contribution to society.

Establishing a Family
Establishing a family involves both parents, even though the physiologic changes of pregnancy take place in the woman. Pregnancy might be considered a period of developmental crisis, during which certain tasks must be completed for acceptance and coping by the expanding family. The cognitive, psychosocial, cultural, and educational dimensions of the prospective parents influence completion of the tasks.

The verification of pregnancy might raise conflicting emotions in the woman, influenced by such factors as whether the pregnancy was planned or unplanned and how the baby will affect career goals. As body changes occur and fetal movement is felt, the woman begins to visualize herself as a mother and normally assumes responsibility for the health of the growing baby. As the time for delivery becomes closer, the woman centers on maternal tasks (such as preparing the baby's room and having clothing ready), and prepares herself for labor and delivery. During the pregnancy, the expectant father needs to learn the normal physiologic and psychological changes of pregnancy, accept his supportive role in meeting maternal needs, and explore his feelings about the developing infant and the birth.

Moral Development

The child enters adolescence with a law-and-order orientation and might never progress beyond that point. Young adults who have mastered previous levels of moral development reach the conventional level and are concerned with maintaining expectations. They also value conformity, loyalty, and social order. Some people might enter the postconventional stage, in which they make moral judgments on the basis of universal beliefs.

Spiritual Development

Adolescents and young adults can think in the abstract and might question beliefs and practices that no longer serve to stabilize their identity or purpose. The individuating-reflective period in the young adult (defined by Fowler) brings discovery of the meaning of values as they relate to the achievement of social purposes and the acceptance of the value systems of others. Often, adolescents or young adults temporarily abandon traditional religious practices.

Health of the Adolescent and Young Adult

Although adolescence and young adulthood are times of maximum physiologic development and health, a wide variety of health problems can occur. Health promotion focuses on nutrition, relationships with self and others, and safety. Young adults should have a tetanus and diphtheria booster every 10 years, and it is recommended that college students receive the meningococcus vaccine (CDC, 2002c). See Examples of NANDA Nursing Diagnoses: Adolescence.

Injuries
Injuries are the leading cause of death for adolescents and young adults. Motor vehicle crashes are the most common cause of mortality, often associated with the use of alcohol or other drugs. One in every four deaths in adolescents age 15 to 19 years is caused by a firearm (CDC, 2002b).

Substance Abuse
Smoking and the use of illegal drugs (such as marijuana and cocaine) might be a problem, and the use of alcohol is sig-

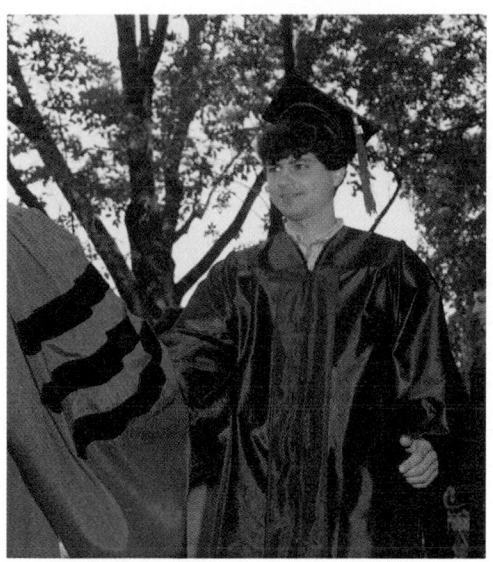

Graduating college or trade school is an important developmental milestone.

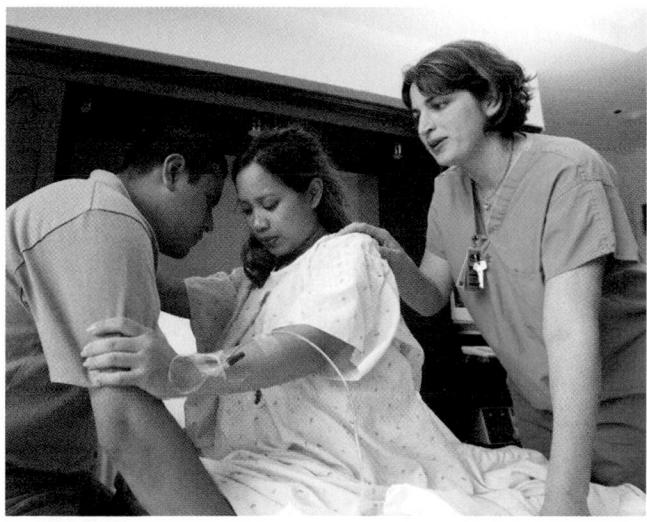

Choosing an occupation and starting a career are also important developmental milestones.

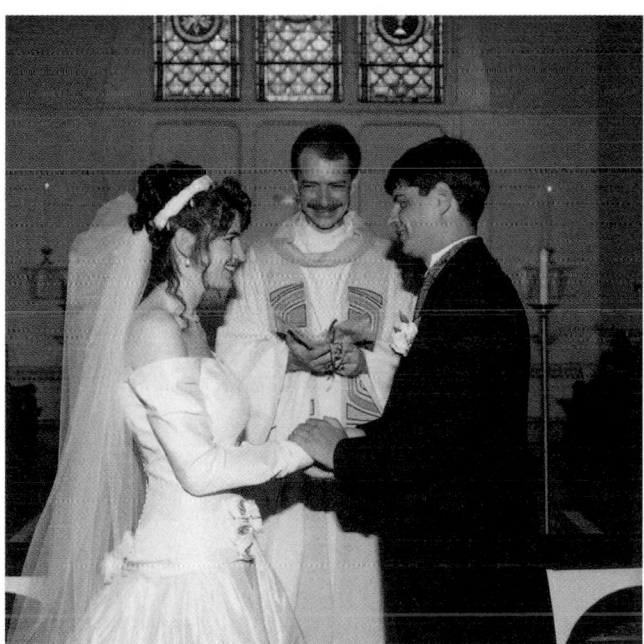

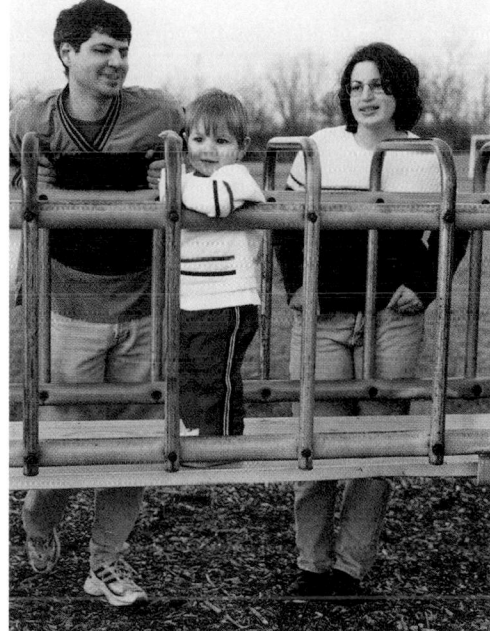

Developmental tasks of the young adult center on establishing intimate relationships, a home, and a family.

FIGURE 19-10 Development in the young adult.

nificantly related to risk-taking behavior. In addition, the use of crack-cocaine, as well as other relatively inexpensive and highly addictive drugs, has reached epidemic proportions in many areas of North America.

Suicide

The suicide rate of adolescents has increased drastically, with suicide being more prevalent in adolescents than in any other age group. Suicide is the third leading cause of death of adolescents and young adults (CDC, 2002a). Although females attempt suicide more often than males, males are more likely to

succeed. Depression is a possible contributing factor. Verbal or nonverbal indicators of suicide should not be ignored; rather, an immediate referral should be made to a professional trained in suicide intervention.

Pregnancy

The United States leads the developed countries in the number of pregnancies among adolescents 15 to 19 years old. These pregnancies are physically, psychologically, and economically costly for the adolescent mother, the infant, the family, and society. Many adolescent mothers are poor, do not complete

Examples of
NANDA
Nursing Diagnoses | Adolescence

Nursing Diagnoses	Possible Related Factor
Imbalanced Nutrition: More Than Body Requirements	Compulsive overeating
Imbalanced Nutrition: Less Than Body Requirements	Self-imposed dieting
Risk for Deficient Fluid Volume	Extended hours of football practice in heat
Risk for Injury	Risk-taking behavior while driving
Risk for Trauma	Lack of knowledge about water safety
Social Isolation	Perceived inability to be popular
Risk for Impaired Parenting	Teenage pregnancy
Disturbed Body Image	Obesity
Anxiety	Fear of failure in school
Ineffective Health Maintenance	Frequent use of alcohol and drugs

high school, and are at high risk for complications involving the pregnancy and the infant.

Nutritional Problems

Fad dieting and habitually eating fast foods are common among adolescents and young adults. For those obsessed with body image (particularly girls and young women), severe eating disorders can result. The most common are anorexia nervosa (compulsive dieting to the point of self-starvation) and bulimia (a destructive cycle of binge eating followed by self-induced vomiting in an effort to prevent weight gain). The psychodynamics of these conditions are complex but almost always involve a negative self-concept. Although these disorders were once considered uncommon, 1 of every 100 women and girls reports symptoms of anorexia, and bulimia appears to be even more prevalent. In the young adult years, fast foods and busy lifestyles might lead to increased caloric intake with minimal exercise. As a result, obesity can become a health problem.

Sexually Transmitted Diseases

Adolescents and young adults who engage in unprotected sexual intercourse are at a higher risk for contracting **sexually transmitted diseases (STDs)** and their complications than are adults. Lack of knowledge, lack of psychosocial maturity, embarrassment, and the denial of the need to plan ahead and use condoms are the most common reasons for this increased risk. Trichomonal and monilial infections, as well as human *Papillomavirus,* are common. Chlamydial infections occur in both genders, as do syphilis and herpes simplex type II (genital herpes). These STDs pose serious health threats.

Acquired immunodeficiency syndrome (AIDS) poses the greatest single threat to individuals and society as a whole. Although AIDS can be transmitted through means other than sexual contact, transmission is primarily through genital, oral, or anal sexual activities. AIDS is a major cause of death in the world, and its incidence is predicted to increase still further.

Developmental and Situational Stressors

Adolescents and young adults have to deal with many stressors as a result of their choices about lifestyle, occupation, and relationships. Family-centered stressors might be either positive or negative factors such as marriage, divorce, parenthood, and death of a parent. Stress might precipitate mental or physical health problems, aggravated by ineffective coping mechanisms, such as substance abuse, child abuse, spousal abuse, decreased nutrition and rest, and risk-taking behavior.

> *Consider Darlene Jenkins, the 14-year-old pregnant adolescent described in the case file at the beginning of the chapter. Analysis of this patient's assessment reveals multiple developmental and situational stressors affecting Darlene that place her and her fetus at high risk for problems. Using this information, the nurse could develop a highly individualized plan of care that focuses on these stressors (for example, her lack of adequate supports, multiple sexual partners, and poor nutritional habits), ultimately to the benefit of Darlene and her baby.*

An increasing number of men and women are remaining single, either by choice or situation. Singlehood status has advantages and disadvantages. Being single gives one the freedom to come and go as one chooses, to have more autonomy, and to spend money and time as one wishes. On the other hand, external pressures to marry and the desire for love, to belong, and to raise a family might make a young adult question his or her decision to remain single.

Couples might encounter difficulties conceiving, delay childbearing until their careers are established, or choose not to have children. If they want to have children, infertility

Teaching to Promote Health at Home 19-5
Adolescents and Young Adults

Health Topic	Teaching Tip	Why is This Important?
Safety	• Encourage drivers' education classes for adolescents, if available. • Discuss the relationship of alcohol and drug consumption to motor vehicle crashes. • Provide information about water safety, gun safety, and sports safety. • Provide information about emergency care measures.	Most deaths in people between the ages of 15 and 24 are the result of motor vehicle crashes, homicide, and suicide.
Nutrition	• Encourage a diet based on the food groups, with added calories during the adolescent growth spurt. • Refer for counseling for extremes in either underweight or overweight. • Discuss nutritional problems that may result from too much fast food and too many soft drinks. • A balance of food intake, exercise, and rest is important.	Nutritional needs increase to meet the accelerated physical growth and development during adolescence. Underweight may result from an inadequate intake of calories, or in extreme cases from anorexia nervosa or bulimia. Overweight results from an intake of calories in excess of metabolic needs
Sexual Development	• Secondary sex characteristics are fully developed. • Both males and females are physically capable of reproduction. • Discuss sexual behavior openly and honestly with adolescents.	The development of secondary sex characteristics that began in the school-aged child is completed during adolescence. Sexual behavior in adolescents and young adults might result in disease or pregnancy, as well as decreased self-esteem.
Growth and Development	• The adolescent is primarily influenced by the peer group. • Risk-taking behavior, especially in males, is common. • Maintaining open communications with teens is important. • Encourage increasing independence in the adolescent and young adult, but continue to provide love and support. • Assist with clarifying values and goals for future occupation.	Peer groups may have positive or negative effects. The rapid physical and emotional changes of adolescence require revising self-concept and body image. These should stabilize by late adolescence. The young adult is usually living independently and has an occupation of choice.
Promoting Health and Preventing Illness	• Have immunizations and boosters as recommended. • Have regular physical, vision and dental examinations. • Always have a physical examination before participating in sports activities. • Do a breast self-exam (females) and a testicular self-exam (males) each month. • Learn to say "no" to pressures to have sexual activity. • Practice safer sex practices if sexually active. • Have an annual Pap test and pelvic examination if sexually active. • Know the dangers of STDs (from genital, oral, and anal sex) and have HIV testing if safer sex is not practiced.	Immunizations and regular health-related examinations are essential to maintaining health. Chronic illnesses such as hypertension, cardiovascular disease, and diabetes mellitus might appear during adolescence and young adulthood. Sexual desires are high, and sexual activity is common. Sexually-transmitted diseases, including HIV and AIDS, are a major health problem, with more than two thirds of those infected younger than 25. Untreated STDs may result in sterility in females and males or infection of an unborn baby.

(defined as the inability to conceive after 1 year of coitus without contraception) might add even more stress. Women who have postponed having children might realize in their middle to late 30s that their so-called biologic clock is winding down; an increasing number of women in this age group are having their first child.

Divorce is common in our society, with rates being highest among those marrying young, having low income, and having low educational levels. It separates children from their families, has long-term emotional costs, and increases the number of single-parent families headed by women.

Role of the Nurse in Promoting Health and Preventing Illness

A true assessment of adolescent development must include the profound changes in reproductive functioning. Teaching activities to promote health for adolescents and young adults are listed in Teaching to Promote Health at Home 19-5 (previous page). Perhaps one of the more significant nursing activities for individuals in this stage is facilitating healthy family relationships. Mutual respect, open communications, and accurate information exchange among family members pave the road for a healthy transition from adolescence to adulthood.

Acute illness is often more of an annoyance than of serious consequence. If hospitalized, an adolescent's and young adult's motivation to recover and to resume normal activities is strong. Because independence and self-sufficiency are important to adolescents and young adults, they will not easily accept the dependent sick role.

Although chronic illnesses are less common, their occurrence can lead to delayed development, loss of independence, and permanent changes in personal and career goals. Prolonged hospitalization, long-term care, or home care increases the adolescent's feelings of isolation and may disrupt normal development. Educational and recreational activities should be provided if at all possible (Fig. 19-11).

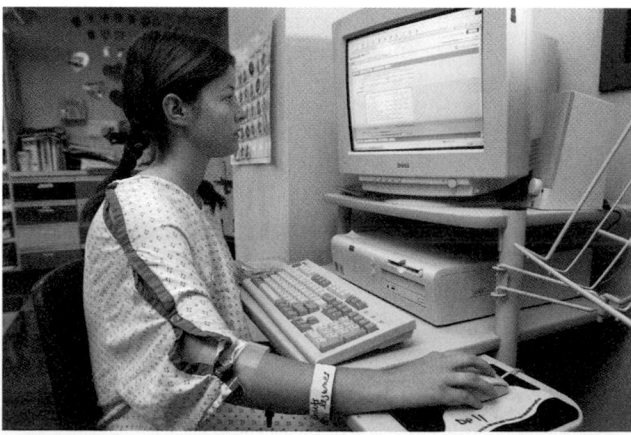

FIGURE 19-11 Allowing teens to "surf the net" and instant-message friends at home promotes a positive hospital experience. (Photo by Joe Mitchell.)

Developing Critical Thinking Skills

1. Based on the information presented in Chapters 18 and 19, describe nursing interventions to meet developmental needs for the following:
   - An infant hospitalized for treatment of a serious birth defect involving the heart and lungs
   - A toddler with a fracture of the left leg, treated in the emergency room and then sent home
   - A school-aged child, now in rehabilitation, with burns on both arms
   - A 20-year-old hospitalized for injuries resulting from an automobile accident after drinking alcohol
2. During your home visit for a 16-year-old with cancer, she says, "I don't believe in God." What would you reply? Why would you respond this way?
3. During a clinic visit, a 2-month-old appears listless and constantly cries. The mother tells you that he has colic, so she has been diluting his formula with water. What would you do now?

Practicing for NCLEX

1. Infections in the neonate are less likely in mothers who provided nutrition through
   a. Breast milk
   b. Water
   c. Formula
   d. Solid food
2. At what point during the first year of life would you normally expect bonding to occur?
   a. At 6 months
   b. At 3 weeks
   c. Soon after birth
   d. Not until 12 months
3. Parents of hospitalized infants should be encouraged to stay with their child to help decrease
   a. Problems with attachment
   b. Separation anxiety
   c. Risk for injury
   d. Failure to thrive
4. The toddler has the cognitive development necessary to
   a. Use fingers to pick up small objects
   b. Have bladder control during the day
   c. Develop independence in feeding self
   d. Identify and name body parts
5. Based on Freud' theory, the preschool-aged child is in the
   a. Phallic stage
   b. Anal stage
   c. Oral stage
   d. Latency stage
6. Which of the following best describes the moral and spiritual development of the school-aged child?
   a. Obeying rules to avoid punishment
   b. Valuing loyalty and social order

c. Accepting the value system of others
d. Faith involves reciprocal fairness
7. The ability to reproduce in the adolescent is defined as
  a. Maturation
  b. Adulthood
  c. Puberty
  d. Latency
8. A primary developmental task of the adolescent is to
  a. Succeed in school
  b. Achieve new and more mature relationships
  c. Develop athletic activities and skills
  d. Accept the decisions of parents
9. Which of the following nursing diagnoses should be considered for the obese adolescent?
  a. Risk for Injury
  b. Risk for Delayed Development
  c. Acute Confusion
  d. Disturbed Body Image
10. What is the leading cause of death in adolescents and young adults?
  a. Accidents
  b. Sexually transmitted diseases
  c. Substance abuse
  d. Unsound dieting

Answers With Rationale

1. The correct response is *a*. Breast milk contains antibodies, immunoglobulins, and leukocytes that provide protection against infections. It has a high lactose content, promoting an acid environment that hinders bacterial growth.
2. The correct response is *c*. Although bonding might occur later, it normally occurs during a sensitive period in the first few hours after birth.
3. The correct response is *b*. Separation anxiety, with crying initially and then appearing depressed, are common during late infancy in infants who are hospitalized.
4. The correct response is *d*. Both *a* and *b* are examples of physiologic development; *c* is an example of the development of autonomy. Toddlers can identify and name several body parts and are being to have a sense of gender identity.
5. The correct response is *a*. Preschoolers, according to Freud, have a biologic focus that is primarily genital, with a sexual desire for the opposite-sex parent.
6. The correct response is *d*. School-aged children view religious faith as involving reciprocal fairness and accept the importance of spiritual beliefs.
7. The correct response is *c*. Puberty is defined by reproductive function in the adolescent.
8. The correct response is *b*. Adolescence is a time to establish more mature relationships with both boys and girls of the same age.

9. The correct response is *d*. Adolescents who are obese are at high risk for an altered body image.
10. The correct response is *a*. Accidents are the leading cause of death in adolescents and young adults. They most often are the result of motor vehicle crashes and are frequently associated with an intake of alcohol or other drugs.

Bibliography

American Academy of Pediatrics Committee on Child Abuse and Neglect. (2001). Distinguishing sudden infant death syndrome from child abuse fatalities. *Pediatrics, 107*(2), 437–441.

Broadwater, H. (2002). Reshaping the future for overweight kids. *RN, 65*(11), 36–42.

Centers for Disease Control and Prevention (CDC). (2002a). National Center for Health Statistics. Suicide. Available at http://www.cdc.gov/nchs/fastats/suicide.htm.

Centers for Disease Control and Prevention (CDC). (2002b). National Center for Injury Prevention and Control. Facts on adolescent injury. Available at http://www.cdc.gov/ncipc/factsheets/adoles.htm.

Centers for Disease Control and Prevention (CDC). (2002c) National Immunization Program. Vaccines for teenagers. Available at http://www.cdc.gov/nip/recs/teen-schedule.htm.

Deering, C., & Cody, D. (2002). Communicating with children and adolescents. *American Journal of Nursing, 102*(3), 34–42.

Erikson, E. (1963). *Childhood and society.* New York: Norton.

Gould, R. (1972). The phases of adult life: A study in developmental psychology. *American Psychiatry, 129,* 33–43.

Hockenberry, M., Wilson, D., Winkelstein, M., et al. (2003). *Wong's Nursing care of infants and children* (7th ed.). St. Louis: Mosby.

Klaus, M. H., & Kennell, J. H. (1982). *Parent–infant bonding.* St. Louis: C. V. Mosby.

Levinson, D., Darrow, C., Klein, E., et al. (1978). *The seasons of a man's life.* New York: Knopf.

London, M., Ladewig, P., Ball, J., et al. (2003). *Maternal-newborn & child nursing: Family-centered care.* Upper Saddle River, NJ: Prentice Hall.

Murray, R., & Zentner, J. (2001). *Health promotion strategies through the life span* (7th ed.). Upper Saddle River, NJ: Prentice Hall.

Rew, L., Taylor-Seehafer, M., Thomas, N., et al. (2001). Correlates of resilience in homeless adolescents. *Journal of Nursing Scholarship, 33*(1), 40.

Thies, K., & Travers, J. (2001). *Growth and development through the lifespan.* Thorofare, NJ: Slack, Inc.

Thomas, A., Chess, S., & Birch, H. G. (1968). *Temperament and behavior discussed in children.* New York: New York University Press.

U.S. Department of Health & Human Services (USDHHS), National Child Abuse and Neglect Data System. (2002). Summary of key findings. Available at http://www.calib.com/nccanch/pubs/factsheet/canstats.

The Aging Adult

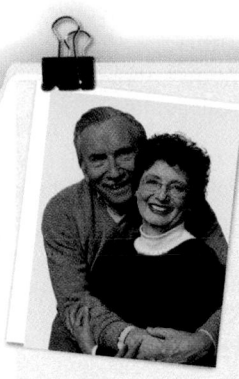

Rosemary Mason, a 59-year-old woman who comes to the clinic with her 64-year-old husband, confides that she wishes that Viagra had never been discovered. "I was happier when we just cuddled at night. Now he wants to try all sorts of things, and I'm just not ready for this!"

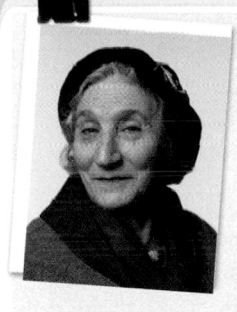

Ethel Peabody, an 88-year-old single woman with beginning dementia who was treated for cardiac problems, is being discharged. She has no family and lives in a small two-story house with her three cats. There is some concern about her safety at home. She depends on a neighbor for some help and refuses to consider moving to a retirement community or extended-care facility.

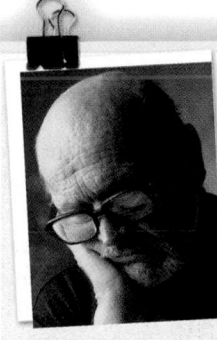

Larry Jenkins, a 67-year-old man with diabetes, states "Everything's gone downhill since I retired 5 months ago. The patient reports being "bored out of his mind" and drinking more alcohol simply because "there's nothing else to do!"

Focusing on Blended Skills

The types of blended skills you'll need to respond to the case scenarios include:

Cognitive Skills
- Knowledge of the theories of aging as they relate to the changes faced by the aging adult
- Ability to incorporate knowledge about developmental theories and related challenges affecting aging adults that require nursing assistance
- Knowledge of the developmental needs of early, middle, and older adults related to relationships, sexuality, family, meaningful work, and leisure
- Ability to identify the needs of an older adult patient based on physiologic and psychosocial changes
- Ability to incorporate knowledge of developmental needs of this population to plan effective nursing care

Technical Skills
- Ability to provide the technical nursing assistance necessary to assess and meet the nursing needs of adults facing developmental challenges
- Ability to use reminiscence as a means for fostering ego integrity
- Ability to adapt necessary skills and techniques to address the changes associated with the aging adult

Interpersonal Skills
- Ability to establish trusting professional relationships with adult patients of different ages, respecting their developmental needs

- Ability to intervene in a sensitive and nonjudgmental manner, demonstrating care and professional concern for developmental needs of the individuals involved
- Ability to consult with other members of the healthcare team to ensure the safety of aging adults
- Ability to use therapeutic communication effectively to meet the needs of aging adult patients
- Ability to mobilize necessary supportive resources to provide needed services for middle and older adults

Ethical and Legal Skills
- Ability and willingness to "get involved" with aging adults with problems and concerns associated with developmental needs
- Knowledge of the nurse's legal and ethical obligations in cases of safety issues for aging adults
- Value for the importance of incorporating theories of growth and development when assessing and planning nursing care for aging adults and their families
- Demonstration of a commitment to intervening with aging adults in a way that fosters achievement of developmental tasks
- Ability to practice in an ethically and legally defensible manner, maintaining the rights of the aging adult

Learning Outcomes

After completing the chapter, the learner should be able to accomplish the following:

1. Summarize major physiologic, cognitive, psychosocial, moral, and spiritual developments and tasks of middle and older adulthood.
2. Describe common health problems of middle and older adults.
3. Discuss physiologic and functional changes that occur with aging.
4. Describe common myths and stereotypes that perpetuate ageism.
5. Describe nursing interventions to promote health for middle and older adults.
6. Identify the healthcare needs of older adults in terms of chronic illnesses, accidental injuries, and acute care needs.

Key Terms

ageism
Alzheimer's disease
dementia
functional health
gerontologic nursing
gerontology
life review
middle adult
older adult
reality orientation
reminiscence
social isolation
sundowning syndrome

Aging is a gradual process, characterized by continued development and maturation. The changes of aging begin as one enters middle adulthood. The onset and the effect of those changes throughout the middle and older adult years are influenced by numerous biologic, psychosocial, and environmental factors (described in the subsequent Theories of Aging section). The physiologic changes of aging, first experienced in middle adulthood, become more obvious in older adults. Continued development throughout one's adult life depends to a great extent on a person's sense of self-concept and prior ability to adapt. For an example addressing the older adult, see the accompanying Reflective Practice box. This chapter continues the discussion of growth and development from previous chapters, focusing on the aging years.

THEORIES OF AGING

As one ages, changes in cells, tissues, organs, and organ systems occur. Scientists do not fully understand why some people, even within the same family or environment, age much more rapidly than others. Although internal processes may in part determine aging, other factors, such as nutrition and the environment, may also play a role. Numerous theories describe how and why aging occurs, but none is universally accepted. These theories focus on a variety of factors, including genetic inheritance, cell metabolism and function, and the immune system.

Genetic Theory of Aging

The genetic theory of aging holds that life span depends to a great extent on genetic factors. Genes within the organism control "genetic clocks," which determine the occurrence and rate of metabolic processes, including cell division. According to the wear-and-tear theory, organisms wear out from increased metabolic functioning, and cells become exhausted from continual energy depletion from adapting to stressors (Sorenson & Thorson, 1995).

Reflective Practice
Challenge to Ethical and Legal Skills

Mrs. Ethel Peabody is an 88-year-old single woman with beginning dementia hospitalized for cardiac problems. She has no family and her only visitor is a neighbor. She lives alone in a small two-story home with her three cats.

When the doctor ordered her discharge, I had grave worries about her ability to live safely on her own. When I asked her if she had ever thought about moving to a nursing home or retirement community, she said, "I'd rather die than go to one of those places!" When I told her I was worried about her safety, she told me her cats would take care of her! When I repeated this conversation to the charge nurse, she said "There is nothing we can do if the patient isn't willing to explore other options."

Thinking Outside the Box: Possible Courses of Action

- Feel satisfied that I had reported my concerns to the charge nurse and let whatever happens happen
- Explore hospital and other resources to determine realistic options for someone like Mrs. Peabody and the obligations of caregivers and the hospital

- Find my instructor and seek her counsel
- Seek out the unit's social worker, confide my worries, and see if she has other recommendations

Evaluating a Good Outcome: How Do I Define Success?

- Both Mrs. Peabody's safety and ability to make decisions (autonomy) are respected.
- I feel at peace with the decision that was made for the patient and the role I played in this decision.

- My personal and professional integrity are intact.
- My legal responsibilities and those of the institution are met.

Personal Learning: Here's to the Future!

Sadly, I must confess that I was invited to accompany another patient for a diagnostic study off the unit, so I never followed through on my concerns. Mrs. Peabody was discharged to her home, and I never learned what happened to her. However, I was troubled by my inaction and discussed this situation with my instructor. As a result, I am now aware of more options available that I can use when faced with similar situations in the future. The number of older adults will continue to grow, presenting many similar challenges in the future. I want to make sure I'm prepared for my next "Mrs. Peabody." Meanwhile, I will be talking with our patient-relations person, the social worker, hospital risk manager, and our office on aging to increase my knowledge of support services for older adults.

Reflection

How do you think you would respond in a similar situation? Why? What does this tell you about yourself and about the adequacy of your skills for professional practice? Can you think of other ways to respond? What could the nursing student have done differently? Imagine if the nursing student was a young adult. Do you think that the developmental stage would affect the student's action? What if the nursing student were a middle adult? How might this affect what was or was not done? What other skills (cognitive, interpersonal, technical, ethical/legal) would you need to respond well in this situation? What skills would be of particular importance when dealing with the charge nurse? Do you agree with the criteria to evaluate a successful outcome? What other criteria would you include and why?

Immunity Theory of Aging

The immunity theory of aging focuses on the functions of the immune system. This system, composed primarily of the bone marrow, thymus, spleen, and lymph nodes, seeks out and destroys foreign agents (such as viruses, bacteria, and perhaps cells undergoing neoplastic changes). The immune response declines steadily after younger adulthood as the thymus loses size and function. With decreasing T-cell differentiation production by the thymus, infections, immune disorders, and cancer increase as adults age. Some authorities believe that nutrition plays an important role in maintaining the immune response, and therefore there is much interest in vitamin supplements (such as vitamin E) to improve immune function.

Cross-Linkage Theory

Cross-linkage is a chemical reaction that produces damage to the DNA and cell death. As one ages, cross-links accumulate, leading to essential molecules in the cell binding together and interfering with normal cell function.

Free Radical Theory

Free radicals, formed during cellular metabolism, are molecules with separated high-energy electrons, which can have adverse effects on adjacent molecules. Lipids, found in cell membranes, as well as proteins and cell organelles, are affected. Over time, irreversible damage results from the accumulated effects of this damage.

THE MIDDLE ADULT

The **middle adult** years are generally considered to be ages 40 to 65. This is a period of gradual and individualized change in both physical and psychosocial dimensions. As the average life span increases, most people in this age group still consider themselves young compared with the older population. Visible signs of aging and a heightened awareness of the time left to live, however, lead middle adults to evaluate their achievement of goals and influence their adaptation to older age.

Physiologic Development

In the early years of this period of life, physical functions are usually still effective. As time passes, gradual internal and external physiologic changes occur. These are not pathologic changes but normal changes that result from aging. The person must modify his or her self-image and self-concept to adapt successfully to and to accept these normal changes. Physical changes of the middle adult are outlined in Box 20-1.

The hormonal changes that take place in midlife affect men and women differently. Women undergo menopause, a gradual decrease in ovarian function, with subsequent depletion of estrogen and progesterone. This change usually occurs between 40 and 55 years of age. With the cessation of ovulation,

---

BOX 20-1 Physical Changes in the Middle Adult

- Fatty tissue is redistributed; men tend to develop abdominal fat, women thicken through the middle.
- The skin is drier.
- Wrinkle lines appear on the face.
- Gray hair appears, and men may lose hair on the head.
- Cardiac output begins to decrease.
- Muscle mass, strength, and agility gradually decrease.
- There is a loss of calcium from bones, especially in perimenopausal women.
- Fatigue increases.
- Visual acuity diminishes, especially for near vision (presbyopia).
- Hearing acuity diminishes, especially for high-pitched sounds.
- Hormone production decreases, resulting in menopause or andropause.

---

menstrual periods stop either gradually or abruptly, and many women experience hot flashes, mood swings, and fatigue. The loss of estrogen also increases the risk for osteoporosis and heart disease. The process can last for several years, and afterward the woman can no longer become pregnant. Men do not experience physical symptoms from the decreased levels of hormones, called andropause. Androgen levels diminish slowly; the man may have some loss of sexual potency but is still capable of reproduction.

Remember Rosemary Mason, the 59-year-old woman described at the beginning of the chapter. The nurse could incorporate information about the differences in hormonal changes for men and women into a teaching plan to help Rosemary understand and adjust to the changes that are occurring.

Cognitive Development

Cognitive and intellectual abilities of middle adults change little from young adulthood. There often is increased motivation to learn, especially if the knowledge gained can be applied immediately and has personal relevance. Problem-solving abilities remain throughout adulthood, although response time may be slightly longer. This is due not to any decreased ability but, rather, to a longer search through more memories and to a desire to think a problem through before responding.

Psychosocial Development

The middle adult years often are a time of increased personal freedom, economic stability, and social relationships. This is also a time of increased responsibility and an awareness of one's own mortality (Fig. 20-1). One realizes that one's life may be half or more past and may feel many things are still un-

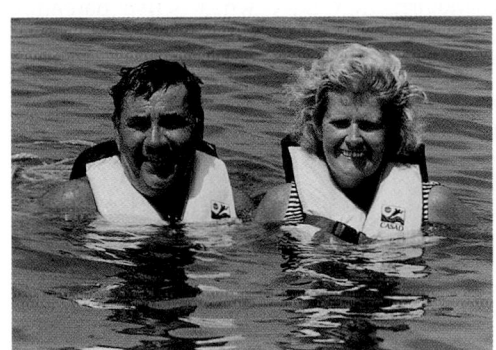
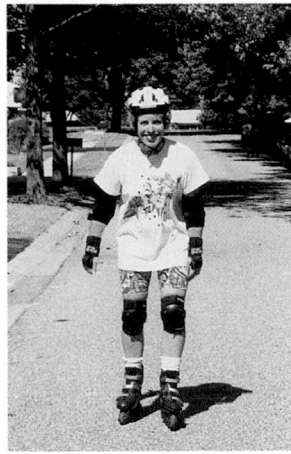
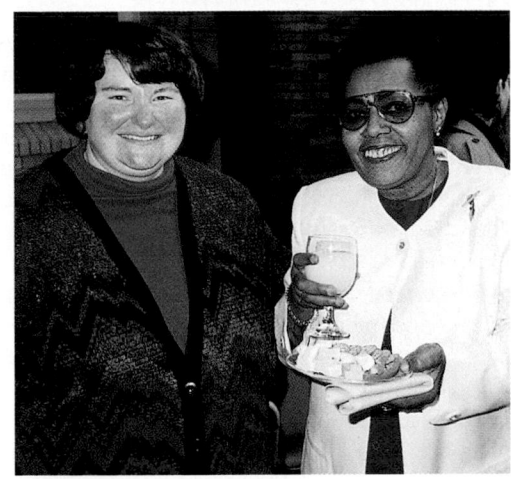
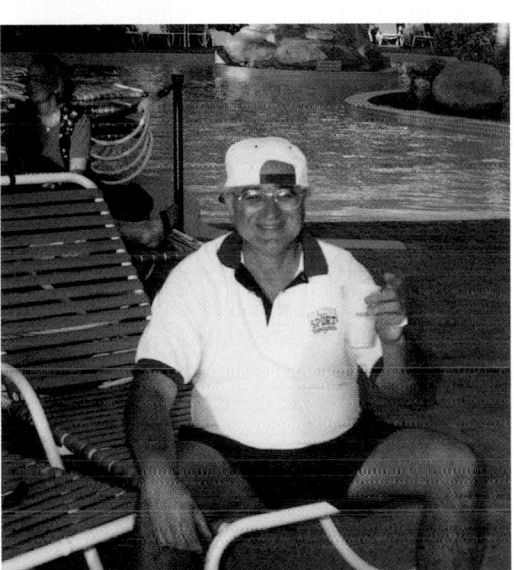
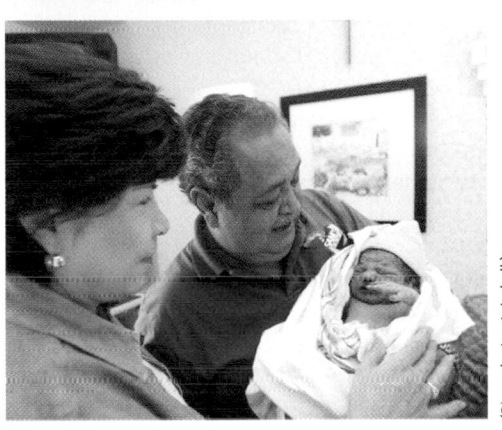

(Photo by Joe Mitchell.)

FIGURE 20-1 The middle adult years are characterized by greater expendable wealth, renewed relationship with one's spouse, and expanded social relationships and family roles.

done. This realization can lead to a developmental crisis and situational stressors. Several theorists describe developmental tasks of middle adulthood, as follows.

Erikson's Theory

According to Erikson's theory (1963), the middle adult is in a period of generativity versus stagnation. The tasks are to establish and guide the next generation, accept middle-age changes, adjust to the needs of aging parents, and reevaluate one's goals and accomplishments. Adults who do not achieve these tasks tend to focus on themselves, becoming overly concerned with their own physical and emotional health needs.

Havighurst's Theory

The developmental tasks of the middle adult described by Havighurst (1972) are learned behaviors arising from maturation, personal motives and values, and civic responsibility. To successfully master this developmental stage, the middle adult must accept and adjust to physical changes, maintain a satisfactory occupation, assist children to become responsible adults, adjust to aging parents, and relate to one's spouse or partner as a person.

Levinson's Theory

Levinson (Levinson, Darrow, Klein, Levinson, & McKee, 1978) theorized that the middle adult may choose either to continue an established lifestyle or to reorganize one's life in a period of midlife transition.

Gould's Theory

Gould (1972) viewed the middle years as a time when adults look inward (ages 35 to 43); accept their life span as having definite boundaries, and have a special interest in spouse, friends, and community (ages 43 to 50); and increase their feelings of self-satisfaction, value spouse as a companion, and become more concerned with health (ages 50 to 60).

Adjusting to the Changes of Middle Adulthood

Various changes can take place during the middle years. These changes include changes in employment; relationships with a spouse; relationships with children who are becoming adults; and relationships with aging parents. Midlife transition might occur in both men and women in their 40s. Although one does not feel that one is aging, realizing that others consider you older can be stressful.

Employment

Middle-aged adults might experience changes in employment. They may opt for a career change and return to school to obtain new knowledge and skills. These changes are often based on a need to have increased job satisfaction or to satisfy a life-long goal. Women who have been immersed in a career may decide to have children and either become "stay at home moms" or reduce their workload. Increasing numbers of middle-aged adults are self-employed, often working from home.

As the 50s approach, questions about retirement and economic security become more prevalent, with an increased interest in the benefits of financial and retirement plans.

Spousal Relationships

Relationships with one's spouse may change. Although for many this is a time of greater security and stability, with stronger emotional commitment and sharing, for some it is a time of disenchantment. A husband or wife may develop negative or critical feelings and attitudes as a result of changes in physical appearance, energy levels, or sexual needs and abilities.

> *Recall Rosemary Mason, the 59-year-old woman, voicing displeasure with her husband's desire to "try all sorts of things" sexually. The nurse could use this information about spousal relationships as a means to gather additional assessment data about the couple's relationship before Viagra was started. This would help develop an appropriate plan of care that addresses Rosemary's current displeasure.*

Dissatisfaction with not achieving career or family goals contributes to the stresses placed on the marriage. Extramarital affairs and divorce may result.

Widowhood is more likely to occur in the middle years. The loss of a spouse is a major crisis and a threat to one's self-concept as well as a major role change. A multitude of changes may occur, including a reduced income, changes in lifestyle and social relationships, and the need for help to work through the loss and grief (see Chapter 33 on Loss, Grief, and Dying).

Relationships With Children and Aging Family Members

Middle-aged adults may be caught in a "generation sandwich." Their children are often independent and married, with chil-

dren of their own. Although much has been written about the "empty-nest syndrome" that occurs when the last child leaves home, most middle-aged parents welcome the increased space, time, and independence they have when active parenting ceases. As their involvement with and responsibility for children decrease, they may have an increased need to help care for aging parents and other family members. The physical aging or death of a parent makes one's own aging and inevitable death a reality.

Moral Development

According to Kohlberg, a middle adult may either remain at the conventional level or move to the postconventional level of moral development, especially if he or she has had sustained responsibility for the welfare of others and has consistently applied ethical principles developed in adolescence. At this level, the adult believes that the rights of others take precedence and takes steps to support those rights.

Spiritual Development

As with moral development, not all adults progress to Fowler's (1991) paradoxical–consolidative state of spiritual development. Fowler believed that only some people reach this stage, and only after 30 years of age. Most middle adults are less rigid in their beliefs and have increased faith in a supreme being as well as trust in spiritual strength.

Health of the Middle Adult

Middle adults are subject to physical and emotional health problems associated with lifestyle behaviors, developmental or situational crises, family history, and the environment. Both acute and chronic illnesses are more likely to occur, and recovery takes longer. This is a result of slower and more prolonged responses to stressors, more pronounced reactions to an illness, and the possibility of more than one illness being present at a time.

The leading causes of death in the middle adult years are motor vehicle crashes, occupational accidents, suicide, and chronic diseases. The major health problems are cardiovascular and pulmonary diseases, cancer, rheumatoid arthritis, diabetes mellitus, obesity, alcoholism, and depression.

The risk for these common health problems often depends on a combination of lifestyle factors and aging. As one gets older, energy requirements decrease. Middle adults tend to maintain previous eating patterns and caloric intake while being less physically active. This trend can result in obesity and atherosclerosis, with an increased risk for high blood pressure, coronary artery disease, renal failure, and diabetes. Additionally, smoking and alcohol consumption put the person at greater risk for cancer, chronic respiratory diseases, and liver disease.

Chronic illness in middle adults has a major effect on self-concept and may precipitate changes in life structure. For example, after a serious heart attack, a man may face changes in his family role, his earning capacity, and his social relationships. Such changes usually cause great stress.

Middle age does not automatically result in physical or emotional health problems. Many men and women remain healthy throughout their lives, but knowing preventive health-care practices and their special needs at this age can help middle adults have improved quality and quantity of life.

Role of the Nurse in Promoting Health and Preventing Illness

The nurse has a major role in promoting health and preventing illness in middle adults by teaching, serving as a role model, and encouraging self-care responsibilities. See Examples of NANDA Nursing Diagnoses: The Middle Adult.

Health-related screenings, examinations, and immunizations for adults are outlined in Table 20-1. Additionally, the following health-promotion activities are recommended:

- Eat a diet low in fat and cholesterol, including fruits, vegetables, and fiber, and use sugar, salt, and sodium in moderation.
- Make regular exercise a part of life.
- Drink alcohol in moderation, if at all.
- Do not smoke.

The middle adult needs to know the dangers of substance abuse. Referrals to support groups and individual counseling may be necessary to strengthen a middle adult's coping mechanisms and promote acceptance of personal and family changes. Having successfully met developmental tasks, the middle adult is ready to enjoy the rest of life. A sense of continuity and adaptability from the early 20s through the 50s is essential to meeting the developmental tasks of aging satisfactorily and to enjoying one's remaining years.

THE OLDER ADULT

The U.S. population is growing older. Our society has arbitrarily labeled the **older adult** as one older than 65 years of age. The older adult period is often further divided into the young-old (ages 60 to 74 years), the middle-old (ages 75 to 84 years), and the old-old (ages 85 years and older). As reported by the Administration on Aging (USDHHS, 2002), the average life expectancy is 74.1 years for men and 79.5 years for women. There are 35 million older Americans, with the number estimated to more than double to about 70 million by 2030. By 2030, people ages 65 and older are predicted to comprise 20% of the population (as compared to 12.4% in 2000), with those 85 and older increased from 4.2 million to 8.9 million. Older women outnumber older men by a ratio of 3:2. The proportion of older people is higher in whites than in minority populations, although the number of minority older adults is projected to increase from 16% to 25% in 2030.

A Unique Population

The older adult population is the most unique group in today's society because its members have lived the longest and have participated in and adapted to complex societal changes. Within the life span of many older adults, society developed from a rural agricultural culture through industrialization to a service-oriented, high-technology culture. In the early 1900s, a 20-mile trip meant an all day undertaking in a horse-drawn wagon; today, a person can fly across the continent in less time and with considerably less effort. Lighting has progressed from kerosene and gas lamps to electricity. Information that once took weeks or months to be received now is instantaneous. Most older adults have lived through the trauma of world wars. Many had parents with strong ethnic ties to another country, and many were immigrants themselves. Older adults have lived through the Great Depression of the 1930s and developed self-sufficiency.

Further adaptations become necessary with advancing age because of physical or cognitive limitations, retirement, loss of a spouse or family members, or changing income. Older adults face numerous role changes related to their age or health status. Lost roles must be replaced with new roles and activities that are acceptable and satisfying to the person.

Examples of NANDA Nursing Diagnoses | The Middle Adult

Nursing Diagnoses	Possible Related Factor
Risk for Imbalanced Nutrition: More Than Body Requirements	High calorie diet and sedentary lifestyle
Constipation	Diet low in fiber and lack of exercise
Risk for Impaired Skin Integrity	Lifetime of sun exposure
Sexual Dysfunction	Alcohol abuse
Caregiver Role Strain	Long-term care of aging parents
Ineffective Denial	Continued smoking despite family history of lung cancer
Fear	Diagnosis of breast cancer

TABLE 20-1 Guidelines for Health-Related Screenings, Examinations, and Immunizations for the Aging Adult

Health-related Area	Recommendations
Physical examination	• Every 3 years to age 40 • Every year from age 40
Breast cancer (women)	• Breast self-examination each month • Breast clinical examination every 3 years to age 40, then every year • Mammogram every year beginning age 40
Cervical cancer (women)	• Pelvic examination with Papanicolaou (Pap) exam at least every 3 years • Women who have had a total hysterectomy (removal of the uterus and cervix) do not need cervical cancer screening, unless the surgery was for cervical precancer or cancer. • Women over age 65 to 70 with at least 3 normal Pap tests and no abnormal Pap tests in the last 10 years should consult with their healthcare provider about continuing cervical cancer screening.

Prostate (men, beginning age 50)	• Prostate-specific antigen (PSA) test every year
	• Digital rectal examination (DRE) every year
	  • Begin at age 45 if African American or a family history of prostate cancer.
	  • Screening is individualized based on healthcare provider and individual's concerns.

Testicular cancer (men)	• Testicular self-examination every month
Colorectal cancer (men and women, beginning age 50)	• Fecal occult blood test every year • Digital rectal examination (DRE) every year • Flexible sigmoidoscopy every 3–5 years, OR • Colonoscopy with follow-up every 3–5 years depending on size of polyps
Skin cancer (men and women)	• Self-examination every month • Clinical skin examination every year
Oral cancer (men and women)	• Every year as part of medical or dental checkups
Bone density	• Those at risk: postmenopausal women, maternal history of hip fracture, fracture after age 50, tall height at age 25
Vision	• Eye examination, with a test for glaucoma, every year
Immunizations	• Tetanus, diphtheria (Td): 1-dose booster every 10 years • Influenza: 1 dose every year • Pneumococcal polysaccharide vaccine (PPV): 1 dose every year up to age 64 for those with medical indications; 1 dose for those unvaccinated by age 65, or who received the first dose more than 5 years previously (before age 65)

Recall Larry Jenkins, the 67-year-old complaining of his life going downhill since he retired. The nurse could incorporate knowledge of role changes to develop an appropriate plan of care for the patient that fosters adjustment to his role changes.

Older people are thus living in a world that requires them to change and to adapt. It is a time to reach one's potential and to satisfy long-range goals that may have been delayed because of other responsibilities. It can also be a time for older adults to turn over to others tasks such as career or community leadership. Research has shown that most older adults do adjust and adapt to new roles, and most are satisfied with their lives and with what they have. Depending on the older adult's adaptability and supportive resources, older adulthood may be a time of happiness, peace, and understanding or of sorrow, conflict, and confusion.

Ageism and Common Stereotypes

Sometimes, older adults are a victim of ageism. **Ageism** is a form of prejudice, like racism, in which older adults are stereotyped by characteristics found in only a few members of their group. Fundamental to ageism is the view that older people are different and will remain different; therefore, they do not experience the same desires, needs, and concerns. Our industrial technologic world places a high priority on productivity, and some may think that retired people have "outlived their usefulness."

Think back to Larry Jenkins, the 67-year-old retiree. The nurse could incorporate knowledge of ageism as a basis for obtaining additional assessment data, examining possible factors contributing to the patient's feelings of boredom and uselessness.

As well, younger generations often have lost ties to the older generation because of increased mobility of the family, and thus many young adults lack experiences with older relatives and their friends.

Older people may be incorrectly depicted as being rigid or narrow-minded, unable to learn, unreliable because of memory loss, too old to enjoy sexual pleasure, or childlike and dependent. Many people fear advancing age because of pervasive views that older people are poor, lonely, in frail health, and headed for institutionalization in a nursing home. These descriptors are not true for most older adults (Fig. 20-2). Common myths are compared with the realities in Table 20-2.

Most older adults are satisfied with their lives, finding retirement and old age more enjoyable than they had anticipated. Three fourths live in their own homes, and one third of these live alone. Most older adults maintain close ties with their families and have incomes above the poverty level (USDHHS, 2002).

Physiologic Development

In older adults, all organ systems undergo some degree of decline in overall functioning, and the body becomes less efficient. Normal physiologic changes in structure and function of the body with aging are outlined in Box 20-2.

Body functions that require integrated activity of several organ systems are affected the most. For example, aging of the cardiac muscles causes fluid retention in both peripheral tissues and the lungs, causing swelling of the legs and making breathing more difficult. The most commonly encountered chronic disorders are cardiovascular diseases such as hypertension and strokes, cancers, and skeletal disorders such as arthritis and osteoporosis.

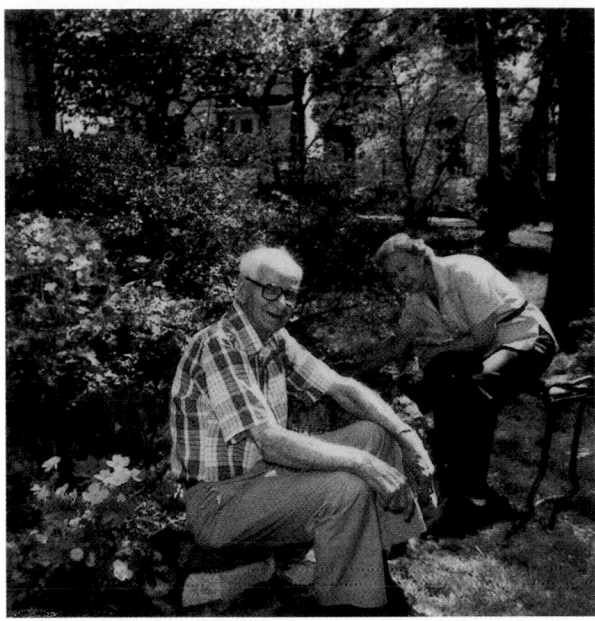

FIGURE 20-2 This couple, married 61 years, enjoys gardening together. They've found that they can continue most activities with only minor adjustments.

Recall Ethel Peabody, the 88-year-old woman with dementia and cardiac problems. Knowledge of physiologic changes associated with aging could help with developing an appropriate plan of care for this patient after discharge.

Most older adults regard themselves as healthy and deny they experience severe limitations in activities. Most are never

TABLE 20-2 Myths and Realities About Older Adults

Myth	Reality
Old age begins at 65 years of age.	Defining 65 years of age as "old age" happened arbitrarily when 65 years of age was set for Social Security payments in the 1930s, based on the labor market and the economy of that time.
Most older adults live in nursing homes.	Only about 5% of older adults live in nursing homes. Most older adults own their own homes; 31% live alone, 54% live with spouses, and the rest live with family or friends.
Most older adults are sick.	Fully 71% of all older adults rate their health as good or excellent.
Old age means mental deterioration.	Although response time may be prolonged from a longer processing time, neither intelligence nor personality normally decreases because of aging.
Older adults are not interested in sex.	Although sexual activity may be less frequent, the ability to perform and enjoy sexual activity lasts well into the 90s in healthy older adults.
Older adults don't care how they look.	Older adults want to be attractive to others.
Most older adults are isolated and lonely.	Loneliness results from death of loved ones or other losses, just as it does for people of all ages. Many older adults are active in social and community activities.
Bladder problems are a problem of aging.	Incontinence is not a part of aging; it requires medical attention.
Older adults do not deserve aggressive treatment for serious illnesses.	Older adults deserve aggressive treatment if they want aggressive treatment.

BOX 20-2 Normal Physiologic Changes of Older Adulthood

General Status
- Progressively decreasing efficiency of physiologic processes results in a fragile balance and hinders the body's ability to maintain homeostasis.
- Physical or emotional stressors cause the older adult to be more vulnerable because of decreased physiologic reserves.
- The older adult may continue to engage in all activities of middle age but intuitively adjusts to a modified pace and more frequent rest periods.

Integument
- Wrinkling and sagging of skin occur with decreased skin elasticity; dryness and scaling are common.
- Balding becomes common in men, and women also experience thinning of hair; hair loses pigmentation.
- Skin pigmentation and moles are common, although the skin may become pale because of loss of melanocytes.
- Nails typically thicken, becoming brittle and yellowed.

Musculoskeletal
- Decreases in subcutaneous tissue and weight commonly are found in the old-old.
- Muscle mass and strength decrease.
- Bone demineralization occurs, and bones become porous and brittle.
- Joints tend to stiffen and lose flexibility, and range of motion may decrease.
- Overall mobility commonly slows, and posture tends to stoop. Height decreases slightly.

Neurologic
- The central nervous system responds more slowly to multiple stimuli. Hence, the cognitive and behavioral response of the older adult may be delayed.
- Rate of reflex response decreases.
- Temperature regulation and pain/pressure perception become less efficient.
- The older adult may also experience difficulty with balance, coordination, fine movements, and spatial orientation, resulting in an increased risk for falls.
- Sleep at night typically shortens, and the older adult may awaken more easily. Cat-naps become common.

Special Senses
- Diminished visual acuity (presbyopia) occurs, with increased sensitivity to glare, decreased ability to adjust to darkness, decreased accommodation, decreased depth perception, and decreased color discrimination. Cataracts may further obscure vision. Difficulty reading small print might result. Daytime or night driving might be compromised.
- Diminished hearing acuity (presbyacusis) occurs, particularly diminished pitch discrimination in the presence of environmental noises. As a result of hearing problems, the older adult may withdraw from social events.
- The senses of taste and smell are decreased. Sensitivity to odors might be reduced. Problems with nutrition may result.

Cardiopulmonary
- Blood vessels become less elastic and often rigid and tortuous. Venous return becomes less efficient. Fatty plaque deposits continue to occur in the linings of the blood vessels. Lower-extremity edema and cooling may occur, particularly with decreased mobility.
- The body is less able to increase heart rate and cardiac output with activity.
- Pulmonary elasticity and ciliary action decrease, so that clearing of the lungs becomes less efficient. Respiratory rate may increase, accompanied by diminished depth.

Gastrointestinal
- Digestive juices continue to diminish, and nutrient absorption decreases.
- Malnutrition and anemia become more common.
- With reduced muscle tone and decreased peristalsis, constipation and indigestion are common complaints.

Dentition
- Tooth decay and loss continue for most older adults.
- Eating habits may change, particularly if the older adult lacks teeth or has ill-fitting dentures.

Genitourinary
- Blood flow to the kidneys decreases with diminished cardiac output.
- The number of functioning nephron units decreases by 50%; waste products may be filtered and excreted more slowly.
- Fluids and electrolytes remain within normal ranges, but the balance is fragile.
- Bladder capacity decreases by 50%. Voiding becomes more frequent; two or three times a night is usual. A decrease in bladder and sphincter muscle control may result in stress incontinence or incomplete bladder emptying.
- About 75% of men over 65 years of age experience hypertrophy of the prostate gland; surgery may be required if urinary retention occurs.
- There is atrophy, decrease of secretions, and thinning of the older woman's genital tract.

institutionalized nor do they suffer the effects of senility. Being healthy, however, does not necessarily mean without disease. More than four of five older adults suffer from at least one chronic illness. Like younger adults, they define their health in relation to how well they function. Functional health includes a person's ability to remain self-reliant, to "make do," and to maintain a sense of control and independence over self and environment. There is a trend in healthcare today toward fostering increasing independence and self-care in older adults.

Those who live alone are at greatest risk for loss of independence and increased need for assisted living or long-term care.

Remember Ethel Peabody, the woman described in the Reflective Practice box. The nurse can apply knowledge about functional health to determine the patient's needs for safety and independence while, at the same time, fostering the patient's view of herself.

There is growing evidence that aging is not synonymous with loss of function and disability. Although 90% of older adults have one or more chronic disorders, their ability to adapt determines whether they are ill or healthy. Most continue their activities from middle age and adapt intuitively to the gradual limitations of aging, although it may take longer to complete an activity or the activity may need to be modified. For example, an older adult with arthritis may need to use an electric can opener rather than a manual one, or a person with heart disease may need 3 hours to garden, resting several times, rather than the former 1 hour.

The greatest threat to the health of older adults is loss of the physiologic reserve of the various organ systems. When illness occurs, increased physical and emotional stress places an older adult at risk for complex reactions. An older adult is more likely to develop complications and to recover more slowly (Fig. 20-3). For instance, an older patient with a hip fracture is at high risk for pneumonia and skin breakdown because of immobility, a decreased ability to expel pulmonary secretions, and thinner, more fragile skin.

Cognitive Development

The term cognition indicates cerebral functioning, including the ability to perceive and understand one's world. Cognition does not change appreciably with aging. In fact, intelligence increases into the 60s, and learning continues through life. It is normal for an older adult to take longer to respond and react, however, particularly in new or unfamiliar surroundings. Knowing this, the nurse should slow the pace of care and allow older patients extra time to ask questions or complete activities. Mild short-term (recent) memory loss is common but can be remedied by an older adult using notes, schedules, and calendars. Long-term memory usually remains intact. Dementia, Alzheimer's disease, and confusion might occur and cause cognitive impairment. These are discussed later in relation to health of the older adult.

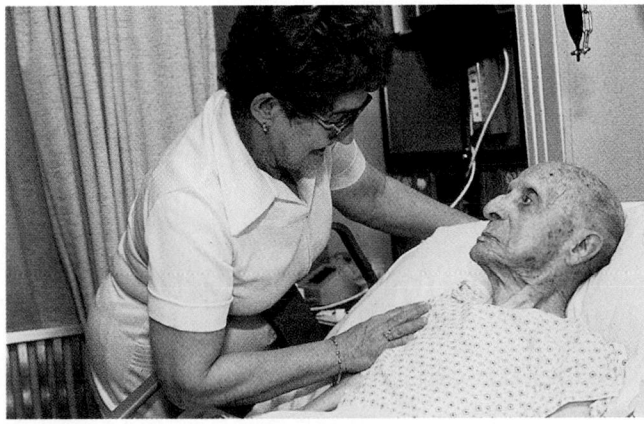

FIGURE 20-3 The hospitalized older adult requires nursing interventions to prevent complications.   (Photo © Kathy Sloane.)

Psychosocial Development

Most theorists agree that a person's self-concept is relatively stable throughout adult life. An older adult who has a strong sense of self-identity and has successfully met challenges earlier in life will probably continue to do so. This person substitutes new roles for old roles and perhaps continues former roles in a new context. For example, a business manager after retirement may continue to use his or her leadership talents in community or volunteer organizations. Older adults with a strong self-concept typically describe themselves as being healthier than others or "young for my years." On the other hand, events that may accompany aging can threaten a person's self-concept. Depending on the person's outlook on life and past ability to cope, events such as retirement, loss of health or income, and isolation can be devastating. For example, a retired teacher whose sense of identity was closely tied to career may suddenly find that he or she has lost friends, income, and sense of accomplishment and may consequently feel a great loss of control and self-identity.

Disengagement Theory

An early psychosocial theory, called the disengagement theory, maintained that older adults often withdraw from usual roles and become more introspective and self-focused. This withdrawal was theorized as intrinsic and inevitable, necessary for successful aging, and beneficial for both the person and for society. Later studies have shown that isolation is not desired or acceptable and that as societal interactions decrease, healthy older adults increase their close relationships with family and friends. According to the activity theory, successful aging involves the ability to maintain high levels of activity and functioning. An older adult may substitute activities but does not slow down or disengage from society. The identity-continuity theory assumes that healthy aging is related to the older adult's ability to continue similar patterns of behavior from young and middle adulthood.

Erikson's Theory

Erikson (1963) identified ego integrity versus despair and disgust as the last stage of human development, which begins at about 60 years of age. Older adults continue to look forward but now also look back and begin to reflect on their life. It is a time for realization of a "wholeness" perspective, with an inner search for meaning and order in the life cycle. Older adults search for emotional integration and acceptance of the past and present as well as acceptance of physiologic decline without fear of death. Older adults often like to tell stories of past events. This phenomenon is called **life review** or **reminiscence** and has been identified worldwide. In a sense, this is a way for an older adult to relive and restructure life experiences and is part of achieving ego integrity (Fig. 20-4). Nurses can also use reminiscence as a therapy to facilitate adaptation to present circumstances.

Think back to Larry Jenkins, the 67-year-old male described at the beginning of the chapter. The nurse could use life review to foster the patient's ego integrity.

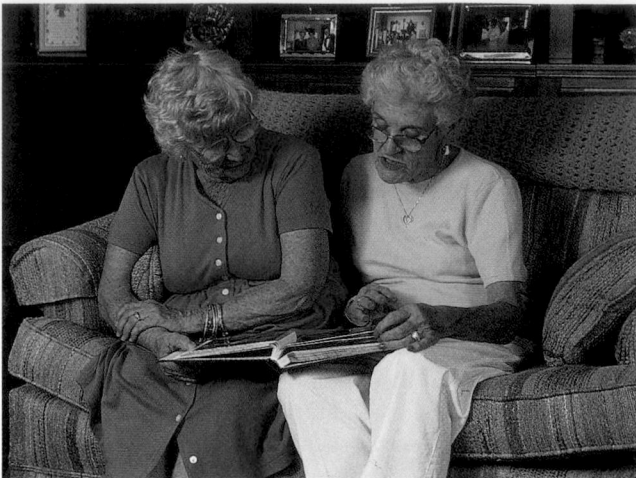

FIGURE 20-4 Reminiscing is a culturally universal phenomenon of aging. It is a way for the older adult to reassess life experiences and further develop a sense of accomplishment, fulfillment, and reward in life.   (Photo © B. Proud.)

See Examples of Nursing Interventions Classification (NIC): Selected Reminiscence Therapy Activities.

Ego integrity is facilitated when an older adult has successfully accomplished tasks earlier in life. Older adulthood can be a time for the person to look backward with pride and without regrets and forward with optimism and enthusiasm. A person who regrets the past and sees current problems as insurmountable, however, may despair. This person may view life as a series of unresolved problems and missed opportunities and feel worthless or hopeless. The despairing person may want to do things over but fears the lack of time before death.

The tasks of midlife continue or may resurface. Older adults still strive to guide the coming generations and to leave something behind (generativity versus stagnation). Their need for love and closeness continues (intimacy versus isolation), as does a strong sense of who one is in relation to family and community (identity versus role diffusion). Because of physical and social changes associated with aging, older adults are repeatedly faced with the need to adapt and to again face already completed tasks.

Havighurst's Theory

According to Havighurst (1972), the major tasks of old age are primarily concerned with the maintenance of social contacts and relationships. Successful aging depends on a person's ability to be flexible and adapt to new age-related roles. The person must find new and meaningful roles in old age while being reasonably comfortable with the social customs of the times.

Adjusting to the Changes of Older Adulthood

Older adults use their years of experience as a guide to adjusting to the changes that come with increasing age. These changes, based on Havighurst's tasks for later life, involve many areas of life, as described in the following sections.

> ### Examples of Nursing Interventions Classification (NIC)
> ### Selected Reminiscence Therapy Activities
>
> - Choose a comfortable setting.
> - Set aside adequate time.
> - Encourage verbal expression of both positive and negative feelings of past events.
> - Ask open-ended questions about past events.
> - Encourage writing of past events.
> - Tape the reminiscence, and play it back to the patient, as appropriate.
> - Ask the family to bring photo albums or scrapbooks.
> - Help the patient to begin a family tree.
> - Encourage the patient to write to old friends.
> - Encourage writing of past events (eg, culture, traditional values, wisdom, and lessons learned).
> - Inform family members about the benefits of reminiscence.
> - Gauge the length of the session by the patient's attention span.
> - Acknowledge previous coping skills.
> - Repeat session weekly or more often over prolonged period.
>
> From McCloskey, J., & Bulechek, G. (2000). *Nursing interventions classification (NIC)* (3rd ed.). (p. 554). St. Louis: C. V. Mosby. A full listing of nursing activities for each nursing intervention can be found in this book.

Physical Strength and Health

Most older adults gradually modify their lifestyle to accommodate for declining strength and health. They rest more frequently, although continued activity and exercise are important for maintaining all physiologic functions. An older adult is at high risk for accidents and falls and may need to curtail driving or use a cane or other aid to remain mobile. Diet modifications and prescribed medications may be necessary, and because of chronic illness, an older adult may need to adjust to living with some pain. With severe illness, loss of independence can occur. The loss of health is difficult to adjust to because it affects every aspect of life.

Retirement and Reduced Income

Retirement brings a change in a person's concept of time. Older adults must learn to occupy their leisure time in ways that maintain their self-esteem while being personally satisfying. Satisfaction with retirement is closely tied to income and the relationships one has outside of work. Many older adults have adequate retirement income, but a lack of adequate income can affect an older adult's ability to meet his or her needs, such as for medical care and housing or social and creative interests.

The Health of One's Spouse

When one's spouse becomes ill, numerous and difficult adjustments must be made. An older adult may face new roles for the first time. A husband may begin to cook meals; a wife may learn to handle family finances. These role changes come at a time when stress is already high. Giving physical care can be an overwhelming task if the other spouse is also frail or in poor health. Adaptations may be needed in living conditions and lifestyle, and the spouse may need to plan social and recreational events alone.

The need for love and belonging does not diminish with age and may become acute with the loss of one's spouse through illness or institutionalization. Humans are sexual beings, and sexual behavior does not necessarily stop in old age. Sexuality is part of who we are, and older adults are no exception. Like younger adults, older adults need to express their intimacy physically by touching and sexual activity and emotionally by sharing joys, sorrows, ideas, and values (Fig. 20-5).

Relating to One's Age Group

With an aging population, social organizations for older adults are becoming more numerous. For example, most communities have senior citizens' centers that offer meals, social and informational programs, and other activities for a nominal fee. Other organizations offer opportunities for travel, cultural events, and political involvement. Affiliation with others of the same age allows older adults to share common interests and concerns and to find status among their peers. It should not be assumed, however, that older adults want to associate only with others their age (Fig. 20-6).

Social Roles

Social roles change with the developmental tasks and adjustments of older adulthood, but the need to feel valued, useful, and productive continues. An older adult may develop new hobbies or increase his or her involvement in community, church, or family affairs. He or she may do volunteer work or even begin a new career. If an older adult cannot adjust and form new relationships, social isolation can become a problem. **Social isolation** is a sense of being alone and lonely as a

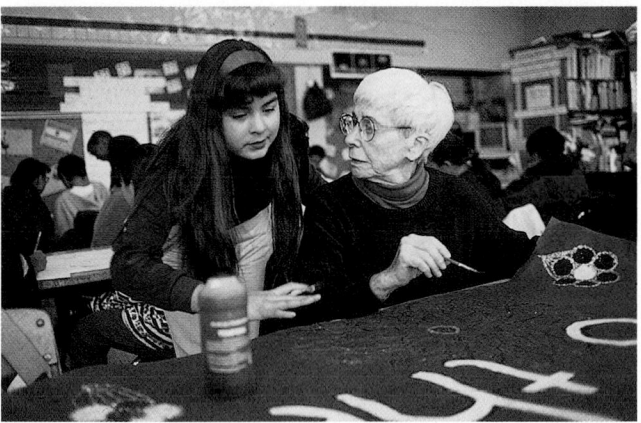

FIGURE 20-6 Social relationships and satisfying leisure activities remain important throughout life. This older adult volunteers in art class with 6th-grade Asian and Latina girls.   (Photo © Kathy Sloane.)

result of having fewer meaningful relationships. It may occur because of declining health or income, transportation problems, or ageism. Whatever the cause, prolonged social isolation has been associated with declining health and higher mortality rates.

Living Arrangements

Various types of housing options for older adults are outlined in Table 20-3. The ability to function safely and independently at home depends a great deal on one's functional health, transportation, income, and family. An older adult, for example, may need assistance with home repairs, house cleaning, or grocery shopping. Architectural barriers, such as steps, may need to be modified. Easy access to medical and recreational facilities and churches may become more important. Many older adults in poor health can continue living at home with some assistance from visiting nurses or with the aid of other services, such as home-delivered meals and senior transportation. Assisted-living housing is becoming more common, providing such requirements as meals, healthcare services, and housekeeping services.

Most older adults prefer to live in their own home and find it difficult to move. Moving in with adult children creates changes in roles and authority. If the older adult is chronically ill or cognitively impaired, the family caregivers face the need for daily caregiving, lack of freedom, and emotional stress. When one moves to an extended-care facility, such as a nursing home, the loss of one's home and possessions and the need to conform to the routines of institutional living can be traumatic for the person and family. Some people, however, choose to move for convenience, social relationships, or needed healthcare.

Retirement centers and senior citizens' housing have become common. For the family members of older adults who need healthcare, alternative methods of care have become available. Examples of alternative care are respite care facilities, which allow the family a needed rest by temporarily housing and caring for an ailing older family member, and day-care centers, which provide a safe, stimulating environment during

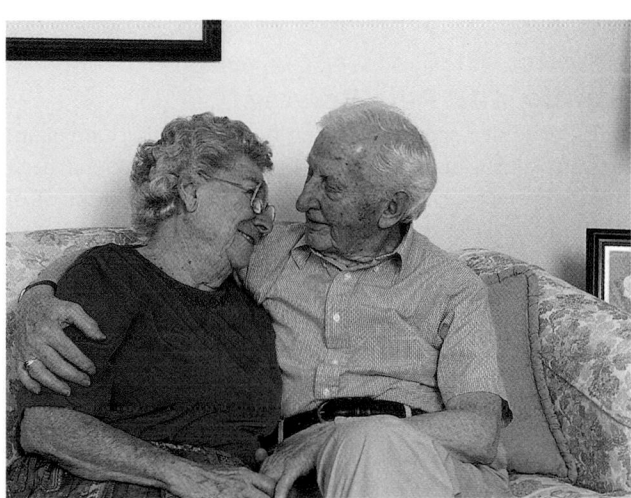

FIGURE 20-5 Stereotypical images of the older adult as narrow-minded, forgetful, sexless, and dependent are untrue for most of the older adult population. This couple exhibits the vitality, sensuality, joy, and playfulness of a young couple.   (Photo © B. Proud.)

TABLE 20-3 Housing Options for Older Adults

Type of Living Arrangement	Description
Home modification	By making changes, older adults may be able to stay in their own homes. Examples of modification are replacing door knobs with handles, replacing faucet handles with levers, and installing grab bars in bathtubs.
Homesharing	Two or more people may share an apartment or house. Each person usually has a private bedroom and shares the other living spaces. These homes may be sponsored by faith-based groups or community agencies.
Accessory apartments	A separate apartment is constructed in part of an existing house, such as a basement or attic. This allows older adults to live independently and privately, but they are not alone.
Elderly cottage housing opportunities (ECHO)	ECHO homes are small portable cottages that are placed (most often) in the yard of an adult child's home. These units typically cost $25,000 or more, but do allow living independently but close to support.
Senior retirement communities	A grouping of rental apartments or houses for residents who can take care of themselves and are mobile. Meals may be available in a central dining room, and housekeeping services may be offered (although there are additional costs for these services). Social and recreational activities are usually offered.
Continuing care retirement communities (CCRC)	This type of housing community offers several options and services, depending on the needs of the resident. Residents usually begin by living independently in apartments, then move to an assisted-living facility on the same grounds. A skilled nursing center is also part of the community and available when needed. Sometimes called "aging-in-place" models, this type of housing tends to be expensive.
Assisted living	These facilities generally provide housing, group meals, personal care and support services, and social activities in a social setting. There may be some healthcare provided. Costs vary from around $1,000 up to $3,000 or more a month. Some states pay for personal care services for those with limited incomes.
Board and care homes Adult family home Adult group homes	Smaller in scale than assisted-living facilities, these services provide a room, meals, and help with daily activities. They may be licensed or unlicensed. Costs range from $350 to $3,000 a month; Supplemental Security Income (SSI) will help pay for those with very limited incomes.
Nursing homes	Nursing homes provide skilled nursing care and/or long-term care, including meals, personal care, and medical care. Bedrooms and bathrooms may be shared. Costs average $56,000 per year, but many are more expensive. Medicare provides only short-term coverage following a hospitalization. Medicaid provides coverage for low-income, low-asset individuals.

Additional information about these housing options is provided by AARP at http://www.aarp.org/confacts/housing/housingoptions.html.

the day when family caregivers must work. Nurses should be knowledgeable about what healthcare and social services are available in the patient's community so that the patient and family can be referred.

The old-old have special significance for nursing care because they are more likely to need help with mobility and basic activities of daily living. They may need increasing assistance to maintain a safe and comfortable living environment. The older the person, the more likely that he or she needs family and community support to maintain functional health.

Remember Ethel Peabody, the 88-year-old woman with beginning dementia who lives alone. The nurse could work with social services to investigate possible community support resources available for the patient so that she can safely maintain her independence as much as possible.

Family and Role Reversal

An older adult's spouse and other family members are natural support systems that help the person maintain functional health and independence and meet the developmental tasks of old age. Supportive assistance may include providing transportation, food, shelter, social interactions, and even complex medical and nursing treatments. Significant others, such as close friends and neighbors, may also take on tasks formerly assumed to be the responsibilities of the traditional family.

Not all families can assist an aged member satisfactorily because of geographic distance, low income, poor health, strained marital relationships, or infringement on career or lifestyle. Adult children may feel "sandwiched" between responsibilities for their own children and careers and the needs of older parents. It can be a guilt-ridden and emotionally draining time for all involved when an older adult's physical or emotional illness reverses roles (with the child now assuming the role of parent, while the parent becomes dependent as the "child") and strains family resources.

The nurse must view the whole family as the recipient of care and assess the family for capabilities and limitations for assisting the aged member. The nurse can help ease the strain by listening to the patient's and family's concerns and by validating the importance of family needs. The nurse assists the patient and family to find workable solutions and may refer the family to community support services.

Moral and Spiritual Development

Older adults, according to Kohlberg (1969), have completed their moral development. Most are at the conventional level, following society's rules in response to others' expectations. Spiritually, an older adult may remain at an earlier level; often at the individuative-reflective level. Many older adults, however, demonstrate conjunctive faith, integrating faith and truth to see the reality of their own beliefs, or universalizing faith, in which they trust a greater power and believe in the future.

Self-transcendence is a characteristic of later life that helps one expand beyond personal limits to reach out to others and the environment and a greater awareness of others' beliefs and values. Integration of the past and future in the present facilitates acceptance of where one is in life without regretting past mistakes or fearing the future (Reed, 1996). As a person ages, spirituality and transcendence are a resource and a source of strength when faced with inevitable change and loss.

Health of the Older Adult

As the number of older adults increases, nurses will spend more time providing care for this population. Older adults who require care are in all types of healthcare settings, including hospitals, long-term care facilities, emergency departments, outpatient surgeries, and homes. Nursing care for older adults should be based on two principles:

- Most older people are not impaired but are functional in the community, thereby benefiting from health-oriented interventions.
- Older people are more vulnerable to physical, emotional, and socioeconomic problems than people in other age groups and may require special attention to health promotion and maintenance.

This section provides a broad introduction to the healthcare needs of the older adult in terms of chronic illness, accidental injuries, and acute illness.

Chronic Illness

The probability and incidence of a person becoming ill increase with age. The most common chronic illnesses in older adults are arthritis, hypertension, heart disease, hearing impairments, cataracts, bone disorders, sinusitis, and diabetes. Other causes of illness or disability include acute illnesses such as fractures, pneumonia, motor vehicle accidents, and falls. These acute illnesses or accidents may lead to chronic health

problems. The leading causes of death in the elderly are heart disease, cancer, and stroke.

Although illness affects all dimensions of a person regardless of age, older adults have to contend with a variety of problems as they live with chronic illness. Aging is a normal process, and chronic illness is a pathologic process, but both often occur at the same time. The changes of aging and the needs imposed by chronic illness interrelate to increase the risk for problems in all areas of life, including—but not limited to—self-care, lifestyle, economics, social factors, and living arrangements.

> *Think back to Ethel Peabody, the 87-year-old woman with beginning dementia and cardiac disease. The nurse could use the knowledge of chronic illness as a basis for a teaching plan that addresses the patient's increased needs for safety.*

Consider the following:

- Chronic illness limits activities in about 15% of the total population, but almost half of adults older than 65 years of age have limitations as a result of one or more chronic illnesses.
- Meeting the expenses of healthcare is often difficult for older adults and their families.
- Medication costs related to chronic illness continue for the rest of a person's life, with multiple medications being the rule rather than the exception.
- Hospitalization costs continue to rise, and the price of high-quality, long-term care may well be beyond the patient's or family members' ability to pay.
- Special diets, special equipment, and medical supplies increase economic difficulties.
- Family members must learn how to cope with the needs of the ill person. Included are personal hygiene, medication administration, special diets, elimination, activities of daily living, and recognition of symptoms that necessitate medical attention.
- Family members must also adapt to psychological stressors such as changes in communications, changes in roles (eg, an older mother becomes dependent), and changes in their own lifestyle as they become the caregivers.

Accidental Injuries

The older adult is at increased risk for accidental injury because of changes in vision and hearing, loss of mass and strength of muscles, slower reflexes and reaction time, and decreased sensory ability. In addition, the combined effects of chronic illness and medications may make an older adult more prone to accidents. Older adults with reduced income may live in inadequate housing in neighborhoods with heavy traffic and high crime rates. They may be isolated from family members, and many live alone. Combined with the normal changes of aging and the effects of any illness, older people not only are at increased risk but also have a more difficult time regaining health after an injury.

Research in Nursing Making a Difference
Living With Dementia: The Patient's Perspective

Dementia, most often due to Alzheimer's disease, is estimated to affect nearly 10% of the population. Although research has led to better ways of caring for people with dementia and meeting the needs of caregivers, not much has been done to understand the experience of what it is like to have mild to moderate dementia.

Related Research
Phinney, A. (1998). Living with dementia from the patient's perspective. *Journal of Gerontological Nursing, 24*(6), 8–15.

To discover how patients perceive dementia, five people with Alzheimer's disease and their spouses were interviewed during home visits. Two themes were revealed: being unsure and trying to be normal. Being unsure described how people no longer take themselves for granted in how they are. They experience gaps of

unawareness and memory loss that prevent them from self-trust, leading to embarrassment. Trying to be normal is an effort to decrease the effect of changes in daily activities, roles, and relationships. Patients tried to do this through self-monitoring, keeping an active mind, staying engaged with others, and downplaying the seriousness of their diagnosis.

Relevance to Nursing Practice
This study is an example of understanding illness from the perspective of the person who experiences it. By better understanding a "hidden" illness such as Alzheimer's disease, nurses can assess not only the patient's cognitive and functional status but also his or her coping strategies used in day-to-day life. Interventions can then be individualized to meet the special needs of each patient.

Dementia, Alzheimer's Disease, and Confusion

When a serious mental impairment occurs, the effect on the patient and family can be devastating. **Dementia** refers to various organic disorders that progressively affect cognitive functioning (see Research in Nursing: Making a Difference). Of the dementias that affect older adults, **Alzheimer's disease** (AD) is the most common degenerative neurologic illness and the most common cause of cognitive impairment (Porth, 2002). It accounts for about two thirds of cases of dementia in the United States, affecting adults in middle to late life. Scientists estimate that more than 4 million people have AD, and the number of people with AD doubles every 5 years beyond age 65. It affects brain cells and is characterized by patchy areas of the brain that degenerate. Alzheimer's disease is a progressively serious and ultimately fatal disorder. At first, forgetfulness and impaired judgment may be evident. Over a period of several years, the person becomes progressively more confused, forgetting family and becoming disoriented in familiar surroundings. When the ability to perform simple activities of daily living is lost, the person requires constant supervision and care, often in a nursing home. There is no effective medical treatment for AD at this time. Comprehensive and empathetic nursing care is important. Both the patient and family caregivers need emotional support and teaching and may benefit from community resources that can ease the family's burden.

Sometimes confusion and depression in an older adult are mistaken for true dementia. Drug interactions, circulatory or metabolic problems, or nutritional deficiencies are likely the real cause. An older adult may also become confused when too many changes or losses occur at one time or when moved to a different environment. A type of confusion called **sundowning syndrome** sometimes occurs, in which an older adult habitually becomes confused after dark.

The nurse can help other members of the health team determine the cause of a patient's confusion and help reorient

the patient. The nurse uses **reality orientation** interventions to redirect the patient's attention to what is real in the environment. See Examples of Nursing Interventions Classification (NIC): Reality Orientation I.

Older Adults and the Healthcare System

Our knowledge of aging has increased dramatically in the past 40 years. **Gerontology** is the scientific and behavioral study of all aspects of aging and its consequences. Normal changes that occur with aging are the result of complex interactions among genetics, biologic systems, and physical and social environments. Disease complicates a person's ability to adapt and maintain **functional health** (the ability to carry out usual and

---

Examples of Nursing Interventions Classification (NIC)
Reality Orientation I

- Inform patient of person, place, and time, as needed.
- Label items in environment to promote recognition.
- Provide a consistent physical environment and daily routine.
- Prepare patients for upcoming changes in usual routine and environment before their occurrence.
- Use environmental cues (eg, signs, pictures, clocks, calendars, and color coding of environment) to stimulate memory, reorient, and promote appropriate behavior.
- Address the patient by name when initiating interaction.
- Ask questions one at a time.
- Give one simple direction at a time.

McCloskey, J. C., & Bulechek, G. M. (Eds.). (2000). *Nursing interventions classification (NIC)* (3rd ed.), (pp. 547–548). St. Louis: Mosby. A full listing of nursing activities for each nursing intervention can be found in this book.

TABLE 20-4 Promoting Health in Older Adults

Area of Concern	Nursing Actions
Physiologic function	• Maintain physiologic reserves. Maintain ongoing assessments for early detection of problems. • Review perceptions of current health status, health problems, and prescribed or over-the-counter medications. • Include nursing care that maintains physical status, such as skin care and planned rest and activity.
Cognitive function	• Slow pace of activity and wait for responses. • Be sure eyeglasses and hearing aids are used; ensure lenses are clean and batteries are strong.
Psychosocial needs	• Be aware that illness, hospitalization, or changes in living arrangements are major stressors. • Assess and support sources of strength, including cultural and spiritual values and rituals. • Encourage use of support systems: family, friends, community resources, pets. • Set mutual goals and encourage the patient's role in making decisions about care. • Encourage life review and reminiscence. • Encourage self-care. • Consider the patient's background, interests, capabilities, values, culture, and lifestyle when planning care.
Nutrition	• Assess for lost or damaged teeth; ensure dentures fit properly. Provide foods appropriate to the patient's ability to chew. • Assess height, weight, eating patterns, and food choices. If weight is being lost, assess income, storage, and transportation. • Assess swallowing ability.
Sleep and rest	• Discourage excessive napping. • Assess normal bedtime, time for rising, bedtime rituals, effects of pain, medications, anxiety, and depression.
Elimination	• Assess frequency of bladder elimination as well as problems with incontinence. • Assess normal times for bowel movements, changes in activity, privacy, and medications. • Ensure that the floor is not cluttered, the toilet is easily accessible, lighting is adequate, and privacy is provided. • Suggest having safety bars installed in the bathroom. • Review diet for necessary fluid and fiber content.
Activity and exercise	• Assess ability to walk; ensure that assistive devices (such as a walker or cane) are available. • Consider effects of illness, surgery, medications, and changes in diet and fluid intake on strength and motor function. • Ensure an uncluttered environment with good lighting; suggest using a night light and removing throw rugs. • Slow the pace of care, allowing extra time to carry out activities.
Sexuality	• Assist as necessary with hygiene, hair care, oral care, clean clothing and bedding, makeup, and shaving. • Maintain a clean, odor-free environment. • Demonstrate genuine caring: ask preferred name, listen carefully, respect belongings. • Discuss safer sex if appropriate. • Discuss water-soluble lubricants with women; refer men for evaluation if erectile dysfunction is a concern.
Meeting developmental tasks	• Promote continued development and maintenance of functional health by identifying unmet tasks, feelings of isolation, and physical or sensory limitations. • Assist in finding creative solutions to developmental tasks. • Collaborate with other healthcare providers to provide information and referral to community resources for the patient and family.

desired daily activities). Mental or physical decline in older adults often may not be directly related to the aging process but may result from the absence of supportive care and services that could prevent disease and help maintain the older adult's ability to function.

The increasing aging population has greatly strained a healthcare system that has traditionally focused on cures and acute disease processes. For an older patient with chronic disorders, the focus of care should include the patient's and family's goals and promote functional health and independent living to the greatest extent possible. **Gerontologic nursing** combines the basic knowledge and skills of nursing with a specialized knowledge of aging in both illness and health.

Examples of
NANDA
Nursing Diagnoses

The Older Adult

Nursing Diagnoses	Possible Related Factor
Risk for Infection	Dry, thin skin
Risk for Imbalanced Body Temperature	Very high environmental temperatures and lack of air conditioning or fans
Risk for Injury	Unstable gait and decreased vision from cataracts
Risk for Loneliness	Death of spouse
Ineffective Coping	Diagnosis of chronic illness
Impaired Physical Mobility	Severe arthritic changes in legs
Impaired Home Maintenance Management	Recent surgery
Impaired Memory	Cognitive impairment from onset of Alzheimer's disease
Anxiety	Increase of crime and violence in neighborhood

Role of the Nurse in Promoting Health and Preventing Illness

The nurse should teach the patient and family general health-promotion activities. This is important because older people often believe themselves "too old" to worry about nutrition, exercise, health screenings, and immunizations. In addition to the recommended screenings, examinations, and immunizations outlined in Table 20-1, the following areas should be stressed:

- Eat a diet that includes all food groups; is low in fat, saturated fat, and cholesterol; balances calories with physical activity; has recommended amounts of fruits, vegetables, and grains; and uses sugar and salt in moderation.
- Make exercise a part of daily activities.
- Drink alcohol in moderation.
- Do not smoke.

An older adult who requires surgery or medical treatment for chronic or acute illness has special, age-related needs regardless of the setting for care. Nursing care to meet age-related needs in any setting are outlined in Table 20-4 (previous page).

Although nursing care adapted to the needs of older patients is described throughout this text, general principles for care are included here. Nurses must recognize physiologic and psychosocial interrelationships and view older patients holistically. See Examples of NANDA Nursing Diagnoses: The Older Adult.

Illness can severely disrupt an older adult's ability to function independently. The ill patient is under increased physical and emotional stress, which increases the risk for complications because of the lack of physiologic reserves. When a patient is hospitalized or institutionalized, family and community interactions are severely inhibited. The acute care environment itself adds new stressors, such as diagnostic tests, treatments, and surgery. In the face of new and unfamiliar routines and sensory stimulation, prior coping skills may not work, and an older patient may feel less able to understand and con-

trol the new environment. An older patient is more likely than a younger patient to suffer multisystem dysfunctions, iatrogenic complications (caused by medications or treatments), accidents such as falls, and increasing dependence and confusion.

The focus of nursing care is to assist older patients to function as independently as possible and to support their individual strengths. The nurse collaborates with the family and other disciplines to prevent complications of illness, to secure a safe and comfortable environment, and to promote the patient's return to health.

■ Developing Critical Thinking Skills

1. Complete the following sentences, and then analyze the reasons for your answers:
   a. When my parents can no longer care for themselves, I will _____.
   b. If my parents were living in a nursing home, I would want the nurses to _____.
   c. When I am old, I want my family to
      _____.

2. Consider your own family. Can you identify developmental tasks for family members who are middle adults and older adults? What factors in your family facilitate or are barriers to meeting these tasks?

■ Practicing for NCLEX

1. When assessing a 48-year-old woman, she tells you she is having hot flashes, fatigue, and mood swings. You recognize these manifestations as those of
   a. Andropause
   b. Puberty
   c. Menopause
   d. Senility

2. Based on Erikson's theory, middle adults who do not achieve their developmental tasks may be termed as being in stagnation. One example of this would be the following statement:
   a. "I am helping my parents move into an assisted-living facility."
   b. "I spend all of my time going to the doctor to be sure I am not sick."
   c. "I have enough money to help my son and his wife when they need it."
   d. "I earned this gray hair and I like it!"
3. Which of the following nursing diagnoses would be appropriate for the middle adult?
   a. Risk for Imbalanced Nutrition: More Than Body Requirements
   b. Delayed Growth and Development
   c. Self-Care Deficit
   d. Disturbed Thought Processes
4. Older adults may be stereotyped as different from other age groups and having outlived their usefulness. The term for this is
   a. Harassment
   b. World-view
   c. Racism
   d. Ageism
5. Which of the following statements is a myth about older adults?
   a. Most older adults live in their own homes.
   b. Healthy older adults enjoy sexual activity.
   c. Old age means mental deterioration.
   d. Older adults want to be attractive to others.
6. The leading cause of cognitive impairment in old age is
   a. Stroke
   b. Malnutrition
   c. Alzheimer's disease
   d. Loss of cardiac reserve
7. Which of the following questions would encourage reminiscence?
   a. "Tell me about how you celebrated Christmas when you were young."
   b. "Tell me how you plan to spend your time this weekend."
   c. "Did you enjoy your life when you were married?"
   d. "Why don't you want to talk about your feelings?"
8. A 90-year-old man who lives alone tells you he has no family or friends. Based on this information, what nursing diagnoses would be appropriate for him?
   a. Social Isolation
   b. Powerlessness
   c. Risk for Injury
   d. Risk for Falls
9. When teaching the older adult who is recovering from surgery, you remember to
   a. Talk in a much louder voice
   b. Repeat information as often as necessary
   c. Teach caregivers rather than the patient
   d. Provide information rapidly
10. Which statement by an 85-year-old woman would demonstrate that she has met an expected outcome of the plan of care for safety?
    a. "I only wear my glasses when I go to the store."
    b. "I am going to ask my daughter to come and give me a bath."
    c. "Would you please get me a drink of water for my pills."
    d. "I am going to take up all my little scatter rugs."

Answers With Rationale

1. The correct response is *c*. During menopause, the loss of estrogen often results in women experiencing hot flashes, fatigue, and changes in mood.
2. The correct response is *b*. Middle adults who do not reach generativity tend to become overly concerned about their own physical and emotional health needs.
3. The correct response is *a*. Middle adults tend to continue to maintain previous eating patterns while being less active, increasing the risk of obesity.
4. The correct response is *d*. Ageism is a form of prejudice in which older adults are stereotyped by characteristics found only in a few members of their age group.
5. The correct response is *c*. Although response time may be longer, intelligence does not normally decrease because of aging.
6. The correct response is *c*. Alzheimer's disease affect approximately 4 million older adults.
7. The correct response is *a*. Asking open-ended questions about events in the past can encourage the older adult to relive and restructure life experiences.
8. The correct response is *a*. Social isolation is a sense of being alone or lonely as a result of having few meaningful relationships.
9. The correct response is *b*. The stress of illness and hospitalization often makes the older patient feel less able to understand teaching. It is important to repeat the information as often as necessary.
10. The correct response is *d*. Removing throw rugs is one means of preventing falls and injury.

Bibliography

American Cancer Society. (2001). Prevention and early detection. Available at http://www.cancer.org.
Centers for Disease Control and Prevention. National Center for Health Statistics. (2002). Life expectancy. Available at http://www.cdc.gov/nchs/fastats/lifexpec.htm.

Department of Health and Human Services, Centers for Disease Control and Prevention. (2002). Recommended adult immunization schedule. Available at http://www.cdc.gov.

Erikson, E. (1963). *Childhood and society* (2nd ed.). New York: Norton.

Fowler, J. W. (1991). *Weaving the new creation: Stages of faith and the public church.* San Francisco: Harper Collins.

Gould, R. (1972). The phases of adult life: A study in developmental psychology. *American Psychiatry, 129,* 33–43.

Havighurst, R. J. (1972). *Developmental tasks and education* (3rd ed.). New York: David McKay.

Hayes, J. (1999). Respite for caregivers: A community-based model in a rural setting. *Journal of Gerontological Nursing, 25*(1), 22–26.

Hoban, S. (2000). Emergency: Elder abuse and neglect. *American Journal of Nursing, 100*(11). 49–50.

Hobbs, M., Teel, C., & Pendelton, M. (2002). Building a model of self-care for health promotion in aging. *Journal of Nursing Scholarship, 34*(4), 335–337.

Kohlberg, L. (1969). Stage and sequence: The cognitive–developmental approach to socialization. In D. Gaslin (Ed.), *Handbook of socialization: Theory and research* (pp. 347–380). Chicago: Rand McNally.

Levinson, D. J., Darrow, C. N., Klein, E. B., Levinson, M. H., & McKee, B. (1978). *The seasons of a man's life.* New York: Knopf.

Maas, M., Buckwalter, K., Hardy, M., et al. (2001). *Nursing care of older adults. Diagnoses, outcomes, & interventions.* St. Louis: Mosby.

McCloskey, J., & Bulechek, G. (Eds.). (2000). *Iowa intervention project: Nursing interventions classification* (3rd ed.). St. Louis: C. V. Mosby.

Murray, R., & Zentner, J. (2001). *Health promotion strategies through the life-span* (7th ed.). Upper Saddle River, NJ: Prentice Hall.

North American Nursing Diagnosis Association (NANDA). (2003). *Nursing diagnoses: Definitions & classification 2003–2004.* Philadelphia: Author.

Porth, C. M. (2002). *Pathophysiology: Concepts of altered health states* (6th ed.). Philadelphia: Lippincott Williams & Wilkins.

Reed, P. G. (1996). Transcendence: Formulating nursing perspectives. *Nursing Science Quarterly, 9*(1), 2–4.

Resnick, B. (2001). Question of practice: Acute illness in older adults. *American Journal of Nursing, 101*(8), 78.

Sorenson, H., & Thorson, J. (1995). Biological theories of aging. *Journal of Subacute Care, 1*(3), 35–39.

U.S. Department of Health and Human Services (USDHHS). Administration on Aging. (2002). *A profile of older Americans: 2001.* Washington, DC: Department of Health and Human Services.

Wold, G. H. (1999). *Basic geriatric nursing* (2nd ed.). St. Louis: C. V. Mosby.

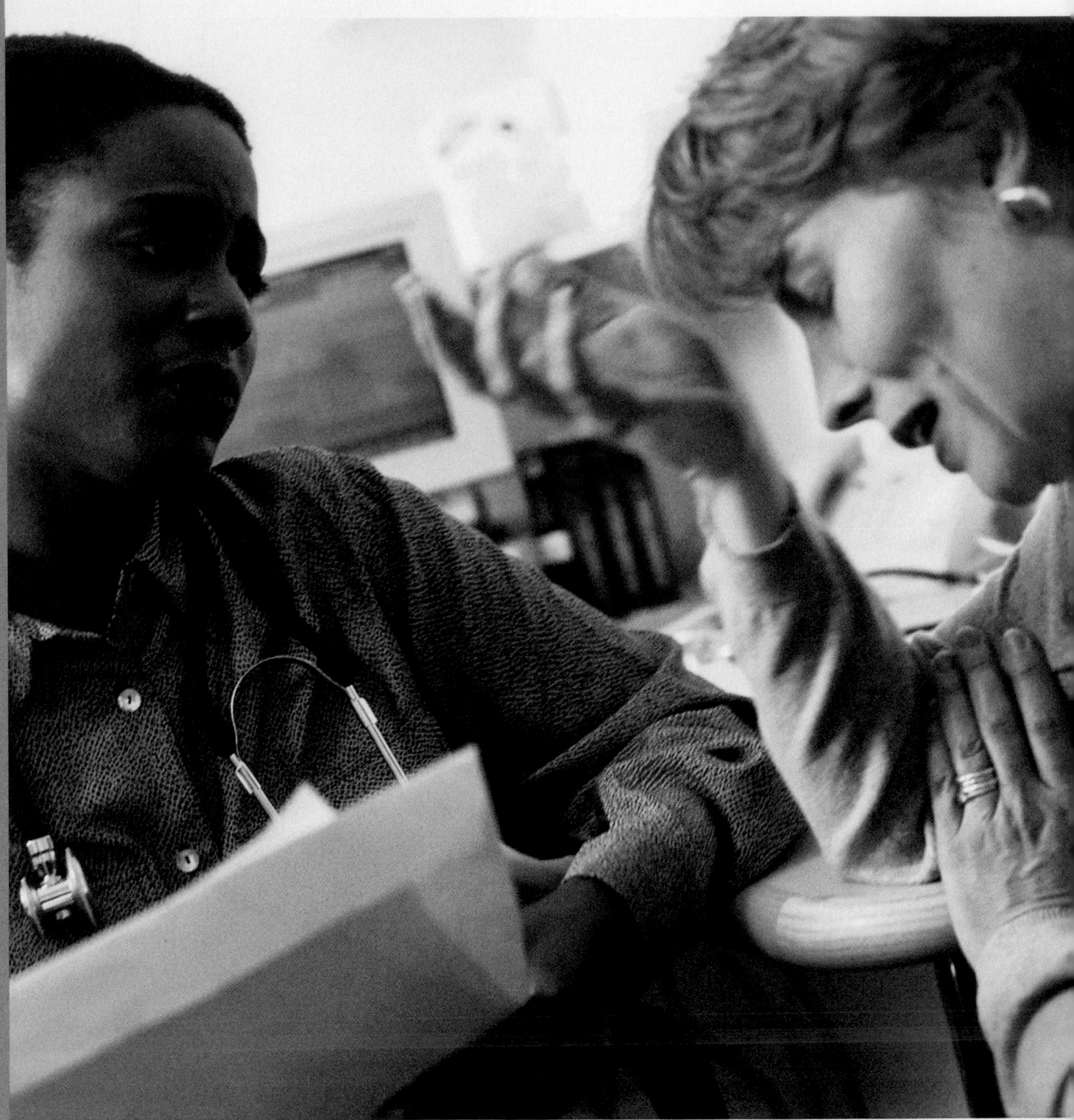

Roles Basic to Nursing Care

*"Clinical competence . . . has three dimensions. . . .
Care is the fundamental things we do to make
a patient comfortable. . . . curative nursing, . . .
the broader group of restorative and rehabilitative
activities . . . and counseling, . . . [providing]
emotional, intellectual, and psychological
support . . ."*

Frances Reiter (1904–1977)
the first chairperson of the American Nurses Association Committee on
Education, she coined the term "nurse clinician" and advocated advanced
preparation of nurse clinicians

Unit V discusses the nurse's professional roles of communicator, teacher, counselor, leader, and manager. These roles are interdependent, and each is an integral part of the broad nursing role of caregiver. The nurse in these roles helps patients of all ages to meet needs along the health continuum.

To be effective as a caregiver, the nurse must be proficient in both the art and the science of nursing. Communication is essential to each professional nursing role and is the heart of caring. Nursing is a person-centered service, based on relationships with patients, peers, and other members of the healthcare team. By developing effective interpersonal skills and using therapeutic communication skills, nurses can establish and maintain helping relationships.

As teacher, the nurse uses communication skills to teach individuals and families. Teaching, implemented throughout the nursing process, is used to meet learning needs. As counselor, the nurse provides information, makes appropriate referrals, and assists the patient in developing a systematic approach to problem solving and decision making. The nurse as a leader and/or manager practices assertive, self-directed nursing. Abilities to lead and to bring about change begin with the student nurse and progress as the nurse develops self-confidence and skill in interpersonal relationships and experience in healthcare settings. Unit V, therefore, enables beginning nurse caregivers to enrich their professional practice by integrating the professional nursing roles of communicator, teacher, counselor, leader, and manager. Nursing practice, as a specialized and unique service to others, is based on the application of knowledge and skills presented in this unit.

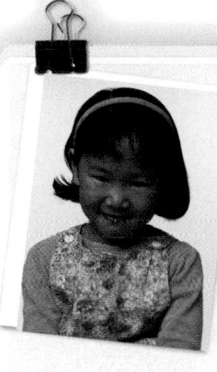

Susie Musashi is a 3-year-old patient with second-degree burns on both legs who currently is receiving débridement. Every time a health-care provider enters her room, she begins to cry, turning her body toward the wall and curling up with her knees to her chest. Her family lives approximately 1½ hours away and can only visit her about once or twice a week.

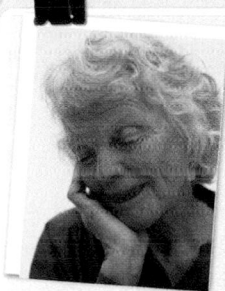

Irwina Russellinski, a 75-year-old woman transferred from the emergency department, is diagnosed with pneumonia. Her chart reveals that she is hard of hearing, "pleasantly confused" at times, and speaks "broken English." A nursing assessment is needed.

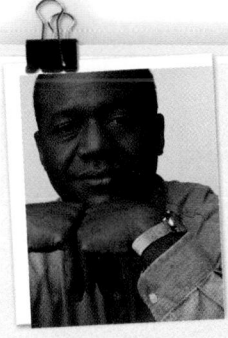

Randolph Gordon, a middle-aged man diagnosed with end-stage liver failure, is being cared for in the intensive care unit. He has been comatose for several weeks. He has numerous tubes and drainage devices in place and is receiving multiple therapies that require continuous electronic monitoring.

Focusing on Blended Skills

The types of blended skills you'll need to respond to the case scenarios include:

Cognitive Skills

- Knowledge of basic communication theory and factors that influence therapeutic communication, such as developmental level, sociocultural differences, and mental and emotional status
- Ability to incorporate knowledge of the goals and phases of helping relationships as a component of the patient's plan of care
- Knowledge about developmental stages, burn therapy, hearing disorders, and changes in mental status and their effect on patients and their ability to communicate
- Knowledge of effective communication strategies
- Knowledge of blocks to communication

Technical Skills

- Strong assessment skills to identify the factors influencing communication for patients across the lifespan
- Ability to integrate effective communication skills when correctly using the equipment and techniques necessary to meet the needs of patients
- Ability to adapt communication skills based on the needs of the patient when providing technical assistance

Interpersonal Skills

- Strong people skills, including the ability to communicate and interact effectively with patients across the lifespan, such as a 3-year-old child, an older adult woman with language and hearing problems, and a middle-aged man with a significant change in mental status
- Ability to establish trusting relationships with patients and other members of the healthcare team
- Ability to incorporate cultural influences to provide effective communication

- Demonstration of excellent therapeutic communication skills for interacting with patients and colleagues, including conversational skills, listening skills, silence, interviewing techniques, touch, humor, and assertiveness
- Ability to communicate to the patient a greater concern about the patient's status, such as a young child or a middle-aged man with end-stage liver disease
- Demonstration of respect for a patient's human dignity when implementing the plan of care, such as for a middle-aged man who is comatose
- Ability to establish good working relationships with colleagues—including the ability to confront other healthcare team members who fail to view the patient as a whole person

Ethical and Legal Skills

- Demonstration of a strong sense of accountability for the health and well-being of individuals of different age groups
- Ability to demonstrate respect, empathy, and honest caring in each professional encounter with both patients and colleagues
- Willingness to hold colleagues accountable for contributing to the team effort to provide care for the whole person, which is essential to quality care
- Ability to advocate for patients who are unable to do so themselves, such as a young child, an older adult patient with language and hearing problems, or a patient who is comatose
- Knowledge of the ethical and legal principles that guide professional relationships and behavior
- Ability to practice nursing, including the use of effective communication skills, in an ethically and legally defensible manner, consistent with the nursing code of ethics and within the scope of legal practice

Learning Outcomes

After completing the chapter, the learner should be able to accomplish the following:

1. Describe the communication process, identifying factors that influence communication.
2. List at least eight ways in which people communicate nonverbally.
3. Describe the interrelation between communication and the nursing process.
4. Identify patient goals for each phase of the helping relationship.
5. Use effective communication techniques when interacting with patients from different cultures.
6. Evaluate yourself in terms of the interpersonal competencies needed in nursing.
7. Describe how each type of the ineffective communication hinders communication.
8. Establish therapeutic relationships with patients assigned to your care and describe effective interventions for patients with impaired verbal communication.

Key Terms

assertive behaviors	group dynamics	noise	small-group
body language	helping relationship	nonverbal communication	communication
channel	interpersonal communication	organizational communication	source (encoder)
cliché	interviewing techniques	professionalism	stimulus
communication	intrapersonal communication	rapport	therapeutic touch
empathy	language	receiver (decoder)	verbal communication
feedback	message	semantics	

Any nurse who wishes to be an effective caregiver must first learn to communicate. Good communication skills enable nurses to get to know their patients and, ultimately, to diagnose and to meet their needs for nursing care. Nursing students who sit face to face with patients to obtain a comprehensive nursing history intuitively grasp the importance of the nurse's communicator role. To adequately document the patient's health history, the nursing student must understand and implement proper communication techniques. Communication skills are the building blocks of professional relationships between nurse and patient, nurse and nurse, and nurse and other health-team members. (See the accompanying Reflective Practice box for an example.)

Many experienced nurses identify the quality of their interpersonal relationships as the single most significant element in determining their helper effectiveness. Studies have shown that on nursing units where nurses freely exchange ideas and information, solve problems together when something goes wrong rather than assigning blame, compliment one another, and use humor creatively, staff morale is high, and there is a higher level of attainment of patient outcomes.

THE PROCESS OF COMMUNICATION

Communication is a the process of exchanging information and the process of generating and transmitting meanings between two or more individuals. It is the foundation of society and the most primary aspect of a nurse–patient interaction. Without communication, it would be impossible to share family experiences, gain knowledge, establish and maintain governmental agencies, and enhance entertainment. By nature, humans are social beings, and human needs are met in collaboration with other humans. Human relationships enable us to meet our physical and safety needs. Communication also assists in meeting our psychosocial needs of love, belonging, and self esteem. The ability to communicate is basic to human functioning and well-being.

David K. Berlo (1960) is credited with the classic description of the communication process, which involves a source (encoder), message, channel and receiver (decoder). The process is illustrated in Figure 21-1.

This communication process is initiated based on a **stimulus** or a patient need that must be addressed. The patient need might be due to a patient's discomfort, a need for information, or to address any uncertainty the patient might be experiencing. The sender or **source (encoder)** of the message is a person or group who initiates or begins the communication process.

The **message** is the actual physiologic product of the source. It might be a speech interview, telephone conversation, chart, conversation, gesture, memorandum, or nursing note. The **channel** of communication is the medium the sender has selected to send the message. The channel might target any of the receiver's senses. The message can be sent to the receiver through the following channels:

- Auditory—spoken words and cues
- Visual—sight, observations, and perception
- Kinesthetic—touch

Nurses use all three of these channels to communicate with patients. Test your knowledge of communication channels by reading the situation in Box 21-1.

The **receiver** or **decoder** must translate and interpret the message sent. Through the translation of the message the receiver must then make a decision about an accurate response. To be an effective communicator, the nurse needs to be considerate of the receiver. The nurse will need to select a message that appeals to the client's interests and that requires minimal effort and time to decode.

Recall Randolph Gordon, the middle-aged man who was comatose? When planning Mr. Gordon's care, the nurse would need to incorporate knowledge about changes in mental status and their effect on communication. The patient's current mental status mandates that the messages sent by the nurse and other healthcare providers be simple, clear, and easy to understand.

Confirmation of the message provides **feedback** (ie, evidence) that the receiver has understood the intended message. **Noise**—factors that distort the quality of a message—can interfere with communication at any point in the process. These

Reflective Practice
Challenge to Interpersonal Skills

Recently, I was accompanying a nurse in the intensive care unit (ICU) when I encountered some behaviors that I found to be unprofessional and lacking in interpersonal skills. We were caring for Mr. Randolph Gordon, a middle-aged patient who was in end-stage liver failure and had been comatose for several weeks. The extent of drains, tubes, and technologies being used to care for Mr. Gordon was overwhelming. It was almost difficult to recognize him as a human being. I was taken aback when the nurse and some residents entered the patient's room and immediately began to assess the technological equipment, without any regard for or recognition of the patient. They proceeded to have a conversation about the patient's poor condition, unsightly appearance, and foul smell at the bedside, in the direct presence of the patient. They did not speak to the patient and they made no attempt to interact with the patient, not even the slightest touch of a hand.

Thinking Outside the Box: Possible Courses of Action

- Ignore the conversation between the nurse and residents and acknowledge the patient through words or touch.
- Calmly ask the nurse and residents to leave the room before discussing the patient's condition.
- Confront the nurse and residents, stating that they need to pay attention to the patient and his psychosocial and emotional well-being.

Evaluating a Good Outcome: How Do I Define Success?

- The patient's healthcare team will act with professionalism.
- Healthcare team will demonstrate respect for the patient's human dignity.
- We will have regard for the whole patient, with attention to spiritual, emotional, and social issues.
- We will set a good example for others in our expression of caring.

Personal Learning: Here's to the Future!

I was somewhat disappointed by my actions in this situation because I did not confront the nurse and the residents when they were acting unethically and unprofessionally. I did, however, ask the nurse if this was common behavior in ICU, that is, demonstrating little regard for the patient's holistic well-being. The nurse stated that unfortunately this was the case. The patients in the ICU are critically ill and many healthcare professionals become extremely focused on the physical and technological aspects of care. I was hesitant to interrupt the nurse and the residents because of my status as a nursing student. I feared that my opinion would not be respected. I know that I will not be able to change the actions of everyone. However, in the future, I will demonstrate my concern for the patient, hoping that those around me will follow my example. I think that I should have immediately gone to the patient and said hello or touched his hand, even if he was comatose. Maybe my actions would have reminded the nurse and residents that there was a person in that bed. Then, possibly, they might have followed my lead.

Reflection

How do you think you would respond in a similar situation? Why? What does this tell you about yourself and about the adequacy of your skills for professional practice? What reasons can you propose to suggest the rationale for the nurse's and residents' behavior? How do you think that the residents would have reacted had the nursing student approached them about their behavior? Can you think of other ways to respond? What other skills (cognitive, interpersonal, technical, ethical/legal) would you need to respond well in this situation? Describe a plan that the nursing student could use to go about changing the staff's behavior. Do you agree with the criteria to evaluate a successful outcome? Did the nursing student meet the criteria? Please explain why or why not.

Colleen Kilcullen, Georgetown University

---

distractors might be from the television, or from pain or discomfort experienced by the patient.

Communication is a reciprocal process in which both the sender and the receiver of messages participate simultaneously. Messages might be influenced on either end by the person's previous knowledge, past experiences, feelings, or sociocultural level.

LEVELS OF COMMUNICATION

Throughout our lives and the lives of our patients, communication occurs at varying levels. There are four levels of communication in which nurses engage during nursing practice: intrapersonal communication, interpersonal communication, small-group communication, and organizational communication.

Intrapersonal Communication

Intrapersonal communication, or self-talk, is the communication that happens within the individual. Nurses use self-talk to enhance positive interaction with the patient and family. This communication is crucial because it affects the nurse's behavior. Imagine two different nursing students preparing for the first nursing experience with a critically ill patient. Both are frightened. One tells herself "Calm down, you've been in challenging situations before and always survived. You can handle this." The other repeatedly tells himself "There's no way you can survive this experience. The instructor will be all over you,

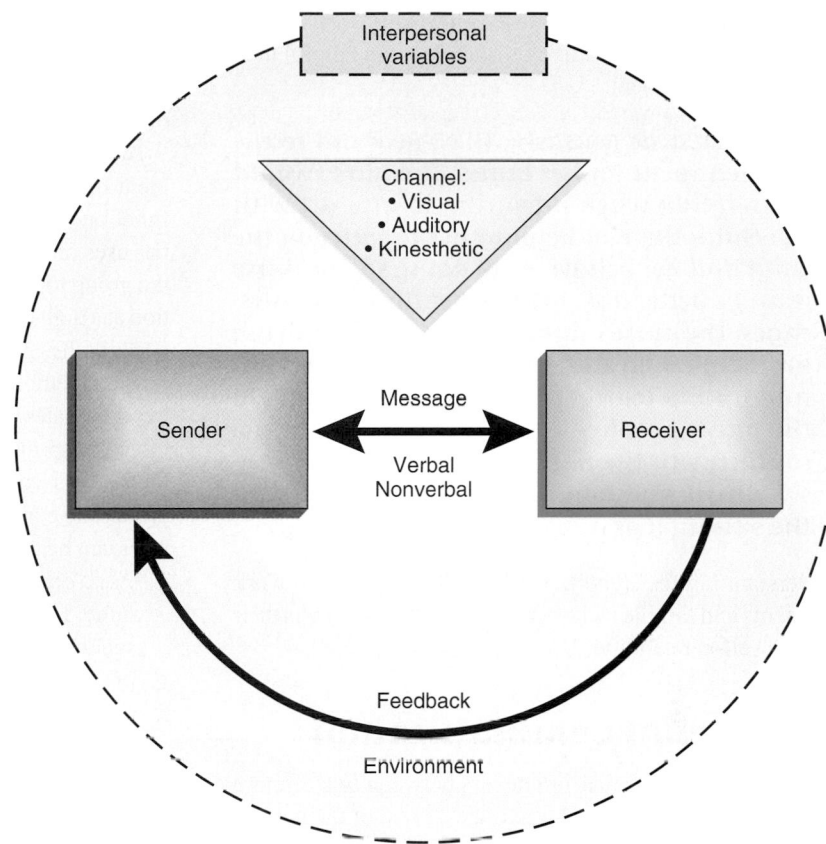

FIGURE 21-1 The various components in the process of communication.

BOX 21-1 Communication Challenges

Picture yourself walking into a patient's room to administer a pain medication by injection. What do you see yourself communicating through each of the three channels of communication?

Then read the scenario below and think about all the ways nurses might unintentionally communicate that they are not concerned about the patient or his pain. Use this exercise to guide both your verbal and nonverbal messages to patients.

Channel	Mode of Transmission	Outcome	Nursing Behavior
Visual	Sight	Receiving a visual stimulus	Patient sees nurse walking into the room holding desired medication.
	Observation	Interpreting a visual stimulation by making note of nonverbal enhancement	Patient makes note of the nurse's sense of competence, confidence, and sympathetic expression.
	Perception	Assigning meaning to a visual event	Patient concludes that the nurse is willing and able to help him and feels comforted.
Auditory	Hearing	Receiving an auditory stimulus	Patient hears the nurse say, "I understand your hip is hurting. This injection should help you to start feeling better within 15 minutes."
	Listening	Gaining awareness of underlying messages and feelings accompanying auditory events	Patient senses that the nurse said he should start feeling better soon and really wants this to happen because she cares about him.
Kinesthetic	Procedural touch	Performing nursing procedures and techniques	Patient feels the nurse touching him while administering injection in the left buttock.
	Caring touch	Conveying emotional support	Patient feels that the nurse cares about him as a person when she touches his shoulder upon first entering the room while asking about his pain.

and you might as well admit defeat before you start." Obviously, the first student's positive self-talk is more helpful than that of the second student.

> Consider Susie Musashi, the 3-year-old receiving treatment for her burns. The nurse would use self-talk when preparing to interact with the child, thereby helping her to focus on the child and her behaviors. In doing so, the nurse may be better able to interpret the child's messages. The nurse might say to herself "I will use broad opening statements to help the patient and family express their feelings. I will talk to the patient on her level. I must maintain eye contact with the patient and family and answer their questions. I will not make light of the situation or appear unconcerned."

Understanding the importance can also help you to work with patients and families whose negative self-talk affects their health and self-care abilities.

Interpersonal Communication

Interpersonal communication occurs between two or more people with a goal to exchange messages. Most of the nurse's day is spent communicating with patients, family members, and members of the healthcare team. The nurse's ability to communicate effectively at this level influences the nurse's interpersonal sharing, problem solving, goal attainment, team building, and effectiveness in critical nursing roles (eg, caregiver, teacher, counselor, leader, manager, and patient advocate).

Group Communication

Group communication includes small-group communication and organizational group communication. When making a determination about the effectiveness or ineffectiveness of a group, one studies the group dynamics.

Small-Group Communication

Small-group communication occurs when nurses interact with two or more individuals. To be functional, members of the small group must communicate to achieve their goal. Some examples of small-group communication include staff meetings, patient care conferences, teaching sessions, or support groups. The more people involved in the communication process, the more complex it becomes.

Organizational Communication

Organizational communication occurs when individuals and groups within an organization communicate to achieve established goals. Nurses on a practice council meeting to review unit policies or nurses working with interdisciplinary groups on strategic planning or quality assurance will use organizational communication to achieve their aims.

Group Dynamics

Group dynamics can be described most simply as how individual group members relate to one another during the process of working toward group goals.

Although effective leadership facilitates a group's achievement of its goals, the group's success or failure is largely a function of its members' behavior. Ideally, each group member uses his or her talents and interpersonal strengths to help the group to accomplish its goals. The group's ability to function at a high level depends on each member's sensitivity to the needs of the group and its individual members. Effective groups possess members who are mutually respectful. If a group member dominates or thwarts the group process, then the leader or other group members must confront the member to promote the needed collegial relationship. Effective and ineffective groups are contrasted in Table 21-1. Individual group-member roles can be categorized in one of three ways:

1. *Task-oriented roles*, focusing on the work to be done. For example, information giver, information seeker, clarifier, coordinator, delegator, energizer, or evaluator
2. *Group-building or maintenance roles*, focusing on the well-being of people doing the work. For example, active listener, harmonizer, trust builder, tension reliever, or supporter
3. *Self-serving roles*, which advance the needs of individual members at the group's expense. For example, attention seeker, dominator, blocker, special pleader, withdrawer, or aggressor

Think about groups in which you are a member and identify the roles that you and other members play.

An administrative team that recognized the crucial value of staff participation in designing and implementing a hospital restructuring project used a team approach to secure needed change. Their ground rules for team members follow (Scott & Rantz, 1994, p. 13):

- I know what I have to do, and the team's goals are clear.
- Everyone takes some responsibility for leadership.
- There is active participation by everyone.
- I feel appreciated and supported by others.
- Team members listen when I speak.
- Different opinions are respected.
- We enjoy working together and have fun.
- We are aiming for excellence, not perfection.
- Everyone on the team has an equal voice.
- We are always open to more education and information.
- Ask anything, challenge anything.
- We have a clean slate.
- We color outside the lines
- It is OK to take a risk and fail.

FORMS OF COMMUNICATION

Communication is the process of sending and receiving messages in the forms of verbal and nonverbal communication

TABLE 21-1 Characteristics of Effective and Ineffective Groups

Variable	Effective Group	Ineffective Group
Group identity	Members value and "own" the aims of the group; aims are clearly articulated	Group's aims are not of major importance to members
Cohesiveness	Members generally trust and like one another and are loyal to the group; high commitment; high degree of cooperation	Members often feel alienated from the group and from one another; low commitment; members tend to work better alone than with the group
Patterns of interaction	Honest, direct communication flows freely; members support, praise, and critique one another	Communication is sparing; little self-disclosure; self-serving roles (ie, dominator, blocker, or aggressor) may be unchecked
Decision making	Problems are identified, appropriate method of decision making is used (ie, individual, minority, majority, consensus, or unanimous); decision is implemented and followed through; group commitment to decision is high	Problems are allowed to build without resolution; little responsibility is shown for problem solving; group commitment to decision is low
Responsibility	Members feel strong sense of responsibility for group outcomes	Little responsibility for group felt by group members
Leadership	Effective style of leadership to meet desired aims	Ineffective leadership styles
Power	Sources of power are recognized and used appropriately; needs or interests of those with little power are considered	Power is used and abused to "fix" immediate problems; little attention to needs of powerless

techniques. Both verbal and nonverbal communication can occur separately or simultaneously.

Verbal Communication

Verbal communication is an exchange of information using words, including both the spoken and written word. Verbal communication depends on language. **Language** is a prescribed way of using words so that people can share information effectively. Language includes a common definition of words and a method of arranging the words in a certain order.

A person's use of written and spoken language forms reveals aspects of the person's intellectual development, educational level, and geographic and ethnic origin. Nurses must also consider if English is a second language for the patient. Language helps nurses assess what the patient knows and feels. In turn, nurses must develop their own language skills to assist in reciprocal responses in the communication process.

> *Think back to Irwina Russellinski, the older adult woman admitted with pneumonia. According to her medical record, the patient speaks "broken English." Therefore, the nurse must incorporate knowledge of this when attempting to communicate verbally with the patient, making adaptations during the interaction to ensure that messages are clear.*

Nurses use verbal communication extensively when providing patient care. Aspects of nursing in which verbal communication is imperative include verbal interactions with patients and family, giving oral reports to other nurses, writing care plans, and recording patient progress in the patient's chart. Other examples of verbal communication include public speaking, writing for publication, and composing signs and posters. Words and language in the previous examples communicate messages to others.

Nonverbal Communication

The transmission of information without the use of words is termed **nonverbal communication.** It is what is not said. Nonverbal communication is often termed **body language.** It often helps nurses to understand subtle and hidden meanings in what is being said verbally. For example, a nurse asks the patient "How do you feel today?" The patient responds "I feel all right." However, the nurse notes the patient does not maintain eye contact and his facial expression is tense. This would indicate that the nurse should investigate further because of the incongruence of the patient's verbal and nonverbal communication (Fig. 21-2).

> *Consider Susie Musashi, the 3-year-old described at the beginning of the chapter. Interpretation of her nonverbal behavior is essential to implementing an effective plan of care. For example, the nurse needs to interpret what her crying indicates, such as fear, pain, or loneliness. In addition, the nurse needs to examine the meaning of the child's turning away from the door. Does she want to be left alone? Is she frightened? Once this information is obtained and analyzed, the nurse is better equipped to develop a plan of care to meet the child's needs.*

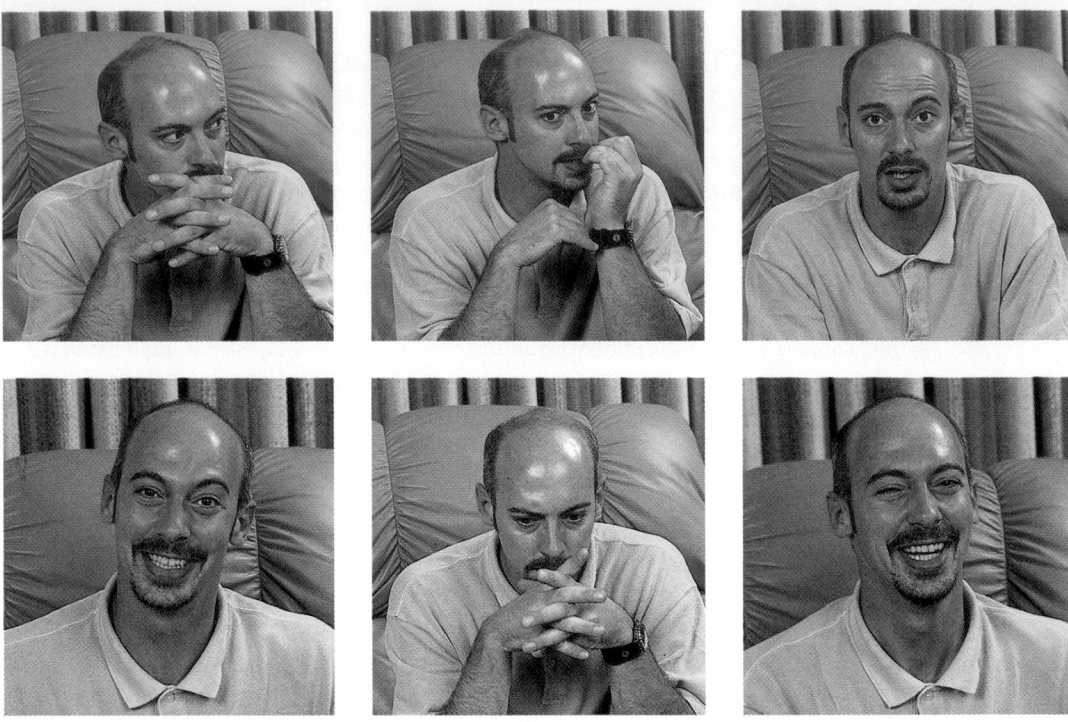

FIGURE 21-2 Eye contact, the lack of it, facial expression, posture, gesture, and silence send nonverbal messages to the receiver. What messages do you receive from each of these photographs?

Information is exchanged through nonverbal communication in various ways. It is generally accepted that nonverbal communication expresses more of the true meaning of a message than verbal communication. Therefore, nurses must be aware of both the nonverbal messages they send and the nonverbal messages they receive from patients. Nurses working with patients from diverse cultural backgrounds should attempt to understand cultural variations to avoid misunderstanding nonverbal communication. The various forms of nonverbal communication follow.

Touch

Tactile sense has been studied seriously as a form of nonverbal communication only since the 1960s. Touch is a personal behavior and means different things to different people. Familial, regional, class, and cultural influences largely shape tactile experiences. Factors such as age and sex also play a key role in meanings associated with touch. Despite its individuality, touch is viewed as one of the most effective nonverbal ways to express feelings of comfort, love, affection, security, anger, frustration, aggression, excitement, and many others.

Recall Mr. Gordon, the patient with end-stage liver disease who is in a coma? Although the patient may not respond verbally or be able to comprehend, the nurse could use touch to indicate concern and respect for the patient, thus sending a message that someone is there for him.

Eye Contact

Communication often begins with eye contact. A glance, for example, is often an attention-getting method to open conversation. Eye contact also suggests respect and a willingness to listen and to keep communication open. Its absence often indicates anxiety or defenselessness, or avoidance of communication. Americans view eye contact as the nonverbal communication that reveals a person's true nature. However, some Asian and Native American cultures view eye contact as an invasion of an individual's privacy. In some cultures, people are taught to avoid eye contact or, out of respect, not to make eye contact with a superior. In addition, the eyes themselves carry nonverbal messages. For example, the eyes fix in a stare during anger, tend to narrow in disgust, and ordinarily open wide in fear. Some individuals who experience fear might be unable to speak and only their eyes will send the message of anxiety. A blank stare can indicate daydreaming or inattentiveness.

Facial Expressions

The face is the most expressive part of the body. Examples of the various messages facial expressions convey are anger, joy, suspicion, sadness, fear, and contempt. Some people have extremely expressive faces, whereas others mask their feelings, making it more difficult to determine what the person is really thinking. Nurses need to learn to control their own facial expressions.

Take, for example, Susie Musashi, the 3-year-old with burns. Preschoolers are naturally curious. So she might watch the nurse's reaction when the nurse changes the burn dressings for the first time. Any sign of repulsion or disgust could greatly impact the child's self-image and recovery.

Posture

The way a person holds the body carries nonverbal messages. People in good health and with a positive attitude usually hold their bodies in good alignment. Depressed or tired people are more likely to slouch. Posture also often provides nonverbal clues concerning pain and physical limitations, for instance, a rigid, stiff appearance might be a good indicator of tension and pain.

Gait

A bouncy, purposeful walk usually carries a message of well-being. A less purposeful, shuffling gait often means the person is sad or discouraged. Certain gaits are associated with illness. For example, patients recovering from recent abdominal surgery usually walk slightly bent over and slowly and might need the assistance of handrails or a helping person.

Gestures

Gestures using various parts of the body can carry numerous messages—for example, thumbs up means victory, kicking an object often expresses anger, wringing the hands or tapping a foot usually indicates anxiety or anger, and a waving hand serves to beckon someone to come on, or if waved in another way, signifies that someone should leave. Gestures are often used extensively when two people speaking in different languages attempt to communicate with each other.

> *Remember Mrs. Russellinski, the 75-year-old with pneumonia? Gestures would be very helpful in communicating with the patient, especially in light of the patient's hearing and language deficits.*

General Physical Appearance

Most illnesses cause at least some alterations in general physical appearance. Observing for changes in appearance is an important nursing responsibility for detecting illness or evaluating the effectiveness of care and therapy. For example, a person with an insufficient intake of fluids has dry skin that wrinkles easily, eyes that might be sunken and dull in appearance, and poor muscle tone. On the other hand, the person in good health tends to radiate his or her healthy status through general appearance.

Mode of Dress and Grooming

A person's clothing and grooming practices carry significant nonverbal messages. For example, healthy people with high self-esteem tend to pay attention to details of dress and grooming, whereas, those with low self-esteem often show much less interest to them. People feeling ill often demonstrate little interest in personal appearance, and it is often a sign of returning health when interest in their physical appearance and mode of dress returns.

Sounds

Crying, moaning, gasping, and sighing are oral but nonverbal forms of communication. Such sounds can be interpreted in numerous ways. For example, a person might cry because of sadness or joy. Gasping often indicates fear, pain, or surprise. A sigh might be a sign of reluctant agreement to do something or of relief.

Silence

Periods of silence during a conversation often carry important nonverbal messages. A silence between two people might indicate complete understanding of each other, that the individuals are thinking, or it might mean that they are angry with each other. Silence and its possible uses and meanings are discussed later in this chapter.

FACTORS INFLUENCING COMMUNICATION

Factors influencing communication include level of development, gender, sociocultural differences, roles and responsibilities, space and territoriality, physical, mental, and emotional state, and environment.

Developmental Level

The rate of language development is directly correlated with the patient's neurologic competence and cognitive development. Thus, it is helpful for nurses to understand the process of language development and the stages of intellectual and psychosocial development. This understanding assists the nurse in the ability to communicate effectively with patients and family of all age ranges.

> *Remember Susie Musashi, the 3-year-old child with burns? The nurse would incorporate knowledge of the typical preschooler fears (such as fear of new places and fear of the dark) when developing the child's plan of care. Preschoolers gain self-esteem by receiving compliments about their appearance. The presence of the burns directly affects the child's appearance, possibly threatening self-esteem. Therefore, the nurse also needs to consider the child's current fears related to her burns and burn treatment and their effect on the child's self-esteem.*

The stages of development are presented in Chapter 18, 19, and 20. Knowing how each age group commonly perceives health, illness, and body functions guides nurses in their interactions with their patients. For instance, a 10-year-old child has limited understanding of what an infection is; therefore, the nurse must explain this in simple terms so that the child cooperates with the treatment without being frightened. Because adolescents are developing abstract thinking, more detailed and accurate explanations can be given to them. Being familiar with commonly used slang usually helps nurses when communicating with adolescents. Communicating with adults can be affected by years of positive or negative health-related experiences and by inaccurate information. Nurses communicating with older patients must assess for any problems with hearing or sight (discussed later in this chapter), confusion, or depression, any of which could affect nurse–patient interaction.

Gender

Men and women possess differing communication styles and might give different interpretations to the same conversation. Tannen (1990) believes that this is because girls and boys grow up communicating differently. Whereas girls generally play with "best friends" and use language to seek confirmation, minimize differences, and establish or reinforce intimacy, boys use language to establish their independence and to negotiate status activities in large groups. In contrast, Townsend (2000) states that gender roles are changing in American society because sexual roles are becoming less distinct. Factors contributing to this change are the use of the term "unisex" within our language and the fact women and men enter professions previously dominated by the other sex. It is necessary for nurses to be sensitive to the fact that men and women might communicate differently. As such, nurses working with patients of the opposite gender need to validate that both the nurse and patient are accurately receiving the message the other is trying to communicate.

Sociocultural Differences

Nurses need to develop skills in recognizing the ways in which culture, economic condition, and overall lifestyle influence a patient's preferred mode of communicating. This helps the nurse understand what the patient understands.

Culture refers to the common lifestyles, languages, behavior patterns, traditions, and beliefs that are learned and passed from one generation to the next. "Culture influences a person's world view (ie, philosophy of life) and relationships with the surrounding environment, religion, time, and others. Culture provides each person with specific rules for dealing with the universal events of life—birth, mating, childrearing, illness, pain, and death" (Luckman 1999, p. 22). Thus, understanding a patient's culture assists nurses in understanding nonverbal communication and enables the nurse to deliver accurate nursing care to the patient and family. For example, women in some cultures might speak of personal things only to their spouses. For this reason, a maternal care nurse might talk with the patient's husband about the woman's postdelivery care.

The healthcare system is a culture with its own customs, values, and language. Nurses must remain aware of these cultural variations and be careful to use lay terminology when speaking with patients, unless the patient is known to be a healthcare professional. Use of medical terminology (eg, myocardial infarction for heart attack, cerebrovascular accident for stroke [brain attack], or cholecystectomy for gall bladder operation) usually alienates patients and can inhibit further communication.

Roles and Responsibilities

A person's occupation might give the nurse a general supposition of his or her abilities, talents, interests, and economic status. Stereotyping a person according to occupation, however, can be misleading and should be avoided. This can be particularly dangerous when nurses assume that patients who are healthcare professionals know everything about their condition and need little nursing assistance, teaching, and counseling. The challenge for the nurse in the provision of care is to respect the patient's roles and responsibilities, especially because these influence their preferred manner of communicating, without denying the patient needed care. For example, a successful attorney might have a "take-charge" demeanor and seem utterly self-sufficient; a skilled nurse will note this but still provide an opening for the patient to verbalize his or her needs. "You seem well prepared for this procedure and in control, but I know that patients often have questions that never get answered or fears that remain unvoiced. Is there anything I can help you with while I'm here?" Similarly, nurses should be careful not to ignore an uncomplaining patient who never asks for anything, because the power differences in the healthcare professional–patient relationship make communication intimidating.

Space and Territoriality

Individuals are most comfortable in areas they consider their own. We generally feel relief when we come home, take our shoes and professionals clothes off, and relax. This urge to maintain an exclusive right to certain space is termed territoriality. You might have already noticed that patients behave differently when being interviewed in their homes, at a health fair in the mall, or in an institutional setting. Similarly, healthcare professionals might behave differently when they are "on their own turf" in a healthcare setting compared to when they enter a patient's home as a guest caregiver. It is important to understand how territoriality influences the nurse–patient relationship.

The actual physical difference between the nurse and patient during interaction is also important. Each person has a sense of how much personal or private space is needed and what distance between individuals is optimum. Some of this is dictated through culture and some is idiosyncratic. Anywhere from 18 inches to 4 feet might be optimal distance for a nurse to sit from a patient during an intake interview. It is best to take cues from patients, noting whether they are moving backward from you if you are too near or leaning forward to get closer to you. Because many nursing interventions place one in proximity to a patient and entail forced intimacy, it is crucial to develop sensitivity to how offensive this might be to certain patients who are accustomed to large areas of private space. Nurses should develop the habit of seeking the patient's permission before touching areas within a patient's private zones. Although most people consider their hands, arms, shoulders, and back within a social zone, increasing levels of privacy are accorded to (1) mouth and feet, (2) face, neck, and front of body; and (3) genitalia.

Physical, Mental, and Emotional State

The degree to which people are physically comfortable and mentally and emotionally free to engage in interactions also influences communication. A full bladder, a dull headache, crushing chest pain, anxiety about a pending diagnosis, or concern about what is happening at home or at work, and fear can all negatively influence communication. For example, a patient who thinks that a nurse wants to hurt him or her will be difficult to interview. Nurses, therefore, need to develop sensitivity to the physical, mental, and emotional barriers to effective communication.

Cognitively impaired patients present nurses with special communication challenges. For example, an elderly patient who has aphasia and is agitated due to pain from an abscessed tooth might be unable to communicate with the nurse.

The accompanying box, Examples of Nursing Interventions Classification, suggests helpful cognitive stimulation activities when communicating with these patients.

Remember Irwina Russellinski, the 75-year-old woman who was described as "being pleasantly confused" at times and requiring a nursing assessment? The patient's level of confusion would present challenges for the nurse when eliciting information for the nursing history. This challenge could be further complicated by the patient's difficulty speaking English. The nurse would need to speak clearly, distinctly and in terms that the patient would understand. In addition, the nurse would need to allow ample time for the patient to respond and explore other sources for needed information.

Examples of Nursing Interventions Classification (NIC)
Selected Cognitive Stimulation Activities

- Consult with family to establish patient's pre-injury cognitive baseline.
- Inform patient of nonthreatening news events.
- Offer environmental stimulation through contact with varied personnel.
- Provide a calendar.
- Orient to time, place, and person.
- Provide planned sensory stimulation.
- Use television, radio, or music as part of planned stimuli program.
- Reinforce or repeat information.
- Present information in small, concrete portions.

McCloskey, J., & Bulechek, G. (2000). *Nursing interventions classification (NIC)* (3rd ed). (p. 220). St. Louis: Mosby–Year Book. A full listing of nursing activities for each nursing intervention can be found in this book.

Values

Communication is influenced by the way people value themselves, one another, and the purpose of any human interaction. Nurses who believe that teaching is an important aspect of nursing and who value empowering patients will communicate this to patients. Conversely, a nurse who believes teaching is an unimportant chore is unlikely to be an effective teacher. Similarly, the patient's motivation (or lack of motivation) to develop new self-care behaviors cannot help but influence nurse–patient communication.

Environment

Communication happens best when the environment facilitates an easy exchange of needed information. The environment most conducive to communication is one which is calm and nonthreatening. The goal of the interaction is to minimize distractions and ensure privacy. The use of music, art, and interior design decorations might assist in placing the patient at ease. A patient newly diagnosed with human immunodeficiency virus (HIV) infection will find it difficult to discuss sexual history or genital warts in an area that lacks privacy. A toddler might find it easier to communicate with the nurse if a parent, favorite stuffed animal, or blanket is nearby.

USING THERAPEUTIC COMMUNICATION IN THE NURSING PROCESS

The nurse's ability to communicate with patients and with other nurses is essential for effective use of the nursing process. (See the accompanying Research in Nursing box.) Knowledge of the communication process and of effective communication techniques is fundamental to all steps of the nursing process. At the same time, the nursing process provides the nurse with the guidance and direction needed to communicate with patients effectively.

Assessing

The major focus of assessment is to gather information in both verbal and nonverbal communication forms. Nurses use the written word to obtain data concerning their patients. Nurses often read their patient's records or charts before meeting them. The spoken word is used to give and to receive reports to and from other health personnel. This is commonplace when admitting a patient to a hospital unit or before visiting the patient at home. Nurses use one-to-one communication with patients to obtain thorough nursing histories and physical examinations. Effective communication techniques, as well as observational skills, are used extensively during this phase. The data collected verbally and nonverbally are analyzed and then passed on to the appropriate people through oral and written communication.

Research in Nursing Making a Difference
Developing Communication Skills

Catherine Nuss Kotecki (2002). Baccalaureate nursing student's communication process in the clinical setting. *Journal of Nursing Education, 41*(2), 61–68

The application of communication theory in this research identified a personal communication repertoire for nursing students. According to King's General System Theory, communication is a key concept for the social system. Within King's theory there are three concepts of the interacting systems: personal, interpersonal, and social. Communication is a means "whereby social interaction and learning take place" (King, 1971, p. 101). Throughout nursing education the communications process is influenced by interrelationships of student goals, needs, and expectations.

Catherine Nuss Kotecki revealed that nursing students have a basic social psychological problem of "saying the right things to patients" in the clinical setting. She conducted qualitative interviews with 22 students and observed 14 students in various clinical settings. The findings of the study revealed that students progress through four stages in learning the communication process. Strategies identified in Stage I were "Affirming the Self." Students used self reflection, anticipation, and expectations. This stage involved intrapersonal communication or self talk. Stage II revealed the "Engaging of the Patient." During this stage, the students identified a sense of fear of intruding, particularly when entering the patient's home for a nursing visit. To gain confidence in this area the students understood the need to embrace

the role of the nurse. During the time the students engaged with the patient, they learned communication patterns of social, professional, and personal talk. The students' engagement with the patient contributed to building patient rapport. In Stage III, "Experiencing Communication Breakdown," students identified difficult patients, patients with language barriers, victims of trauma, and neurologic impairment as sources of difficulty in communication. Students learned to implement previous communication techniques with real nurse talk as noted when observing interactions with registered nurses. Stage IV involved "Refining the Repertoire." The students worked to resolve communication breakdown. The students would consider their individual personality strategies to communicate with the patient. In this stage, the students learned to be flexible and implement different strategies for communication, particularly if one failed, and then another would be implemented.

Relevance to Nursing Practice
This study allows students to understand the process of patient communication. Students use many behavior patterns when learning their roles as nurse and communicator. During the time they are students, periods of trial and error for communication techniques increase their ability to communicate therapeutically. The students also seek the input of skilled practitioners as role models for their own communication skills.

Diagnosing

Following the formulation of the nursing diagnoses, the nurse communicates them to other nursing professionals through the use of the written and spoken word. The written diagnosis becomes a permanent part of the patient's record.

Outcome Identification and Planning

The planning step requires communication among the patient, nurse, and other team members as mutually agreed-upon outcomes are developed and interventions are determined. Because a nurse is rarely able to implement all parts of a plan alone, oral and written communication is needed to inform others of what needs to be done to meet the set objectives or goals. The formal written plan of care is a form of communication. Without communication, the nurse's plan could not be implemented.

Implementing

Nurses assume many roles when they implement the plan of care. Verbal and nonverbal communication allows nurses to enhance basic caregiving measures and to teach, counsel, and support patients and their families during the implementation phase. Even a simple nursing order, such as "encourage patient

to drink 100 mL of fluid every hour while awake," requires countless messages to be sent and received between the patient and nurse. The nurse explains the importance of an adequate fluid intake, along with the amount and frequency of intake. The patient, in turn, informs the nurse of his or her ability or inability to meet targeted objectives. The patient's verbal and nonverbal messages are assessed during each nurse–patient interaction. The implementation of the plan of care is then documented in the patient's record.

Evaluating

Nurses often rely on the verbal and nonverbal cues they receive from their patients to verify whether patient objectives or goals have been achieved. Communication, through the exchange of positive and negative messages between the nurse and the patient, also facilitates the revision of parts of the care plan.

Documenting Communication

Continual assessment of the patient's needs and conditions requires accurate documentation in the appropriate place, unless the information is confidential. This documentation helps promote the continuity of care given by nurses and other healthcare providers. Because one nurse cannot provide 24-hour coverage for patients, significant information must be passed on to others through nursing progress notes and care plans. Documentation is discussed in Chapter 17.

USING THERAPEUTIC COMMUNICATION IN THE HELPING RELATIONSHIP

Nurses and other healthcare personnel enter healthcare in order to help people. Relationships between healthcare providers and patients are not accomplished randomly, but through purposeful relationships. A **helping relationship** exists among people who provide and receive assistance in meeting human needs. In this book, that term is used to refer to helping relationships between nurses and patients (Fig. 21-3). A helping relationship sets the climate for the participants to move toward common goals to meet human needs. Therefore, need gratification occurs as the result of a successful helping relationship.

When a nurse and patient are involved in a helping relationship, the nurse assists the patient to identify and achieve goals that allow the patient's human needs to be satisfied. The nurse is the helper, and the patient is the person being helped. The helping relationship between the nurse and patient is sometimes called the nurse–patient relationship.

The quality of one's relationship with another person is the most significant element in determining helping effectiveness. "Of all the problems that can arise in nursing care, perhaps the most common is failure to establish rapport and a helping–trust relationship with the other person" (Watson, 1985, p. 24). Communication is the means a nurse uses to establish rapport and helping–trust relationships.

A Helping Relationship Versus a Social Relationship

The difference between a helping relationship and a friendship is important. Helping relationships contain many of the qualities of a social relationship—they have in common the components of care, concern, trust, and growth. They are also very different:

- The helping relationship does not occur spontaneously, as do most social relationships. It occurs for a specific purpose with a specific person.

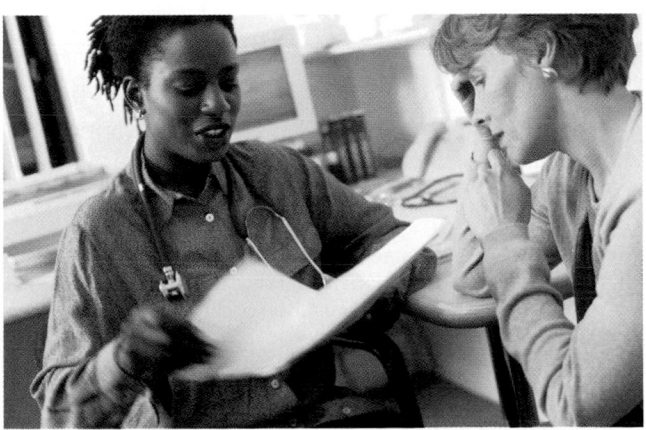

FIGURE 21-3 A helping relationship between the nurse and patient sets the climate for participants to move toward common goals. (Photo © B. Proud.)

- The helping relationship is characterized by an unequal sharing of information. The patient shares information related to personal health problems, whereas the nurse shares information in terms of a professional role. In a friendship, information sharing is more likely to be similar in quantity and type.
- The helping relationship is built on the patient's needs, not on those of the helping person. In a friendship, needs of both participants are generally considered. A friendship might grow out of helping relationship, but this is separate from the purposeful, time-limited interaction described as a helping relationship.

It is of great importance that nurses remember that helping relations are professional relationships. It can be helpful for nursing students and new nurses to identify nurses who communicate a clear sense of **professionalism** in their appearance, demeanor, and behavior. Patients and the public are more likely to trust and value nurses who appear competent and confident and who are focused on the patients entrusted to their care. Rudeness, sloppiness, inattention to person, sexually inappropriate behavior, and other breaches of professionalism undermine nursing's professional image and the effectiveness of individual nurses.

Think back to the Mr. Gordon, the patient described in the Reflective Practice display, and consider the behavior of the nurse and residents caring for the patient. Unfortunately, their focus was not on the patient as a whole, but, rather, on the patient's devices and technologic equipment. The nurse would need to keep in mind the highly technical nature of the intensive care unit and work to implement a plan of care that focuses on the "whole" patient.

Characteristics of the Helping Relationship

The helping relationship is intangible and therefore difficult to describe. Most authorities agree, however, that it has at least the following three basic characteristics:

- It is dynamic. Both the person providing the assistance and the person being helped are active participants to the extent each is able.
- It is purposeful and time limited. This means there are specific goals that are intended to be met within a certain period.
- Although both parties in the helping relationship have responsibilities, the person providing the assistance is professionally accountable for the outcomes of the relationship and the means used to attain them. The helping person should present his or her helping abilities as honestly as possible and not promise to provide more assistance than he or she can offer.

Goals of the Helping Relationship

The goals of a helping relationship between a nurse and a patient are determined cooperatively and are defined in terms of the patient's needs. Broadly speaking, common goals might include increased independence for the patient, greater feelings of worth, and improved health and well-being. Depending on the goals/outcomes, the nurse selects nursing interventions that will help the person move toward the goal. As the patient's needs and goals change, so do the nursing care interventions implemented to attain the patient's goals. The nurse might also have many needs to be met, but in the helping relationship between the nurse and the patient, the nurse's needs are temporarily set aside, and the focus is on the patient's needs.

Phases of the Helping Relationship

The helping relationship is ordinarily described as having three phases: (1) the orientation phase, (2) the working phase, and (3) the termination phase. In the helping relationship, the communication process follows the sequence of the nursing process. Both processes are continuous and reciprocal. Table 21-2 summarizes goals for patients during the three phases of an effective helping relationship. In some situations, one nurse initiates the helping relationship and works with the patient and family through to termination. More often (eg, in the hospital settings), there are different nurses at different times implementing different phases of the relationship. In preparation for the orientation phase, the nurse might use interpersonal communication to prepare for the data-gathering phase of the interaction with the patient.

Orientation Phase

The helping relationship ideally begins between the nurse and patient during the data-gathering part of the nursing process. It can also be initiated at other times during the nurse–patient relationship. In the orientation phase, the tone and guidelines for the relationship are established. The nurse and patient meet and learn to identify each other by name. It is especially important that the nurse introduce himself or herself to the patient; it might even be helpful for the nurse to write his or her name for the patient. Failure to do so might result in the patient becoming confused and mistrustful because of the number of caregivers with whom most patients come in contact.

The following activities generally occur during the orientation phase of the helping relationship:

- The roles of both people in the relationship are clarified. A successful relationship is more likely to occur when each participant's responsibilities are known and accepted and when the nurse, by virtue of role, generally assumes leadership. Leadership does not mean control in a restrictive or manipulative sense but, rather, involves taking the initiative to enlist the patient's point of view. When cooperative planning occurs with consideration for the patient's needs, the relationship between a nurse and a patient is more likely to be mutually satisfactory.
- An agreement or contract about the relationship is established. The agreement is usually a simple verbal exchange or, occasionally, a written document, especially if the relationship extends over a long period of time. Elements in the agreement include the goals of the relationship; location, frequency, and length of the contacts; and duration of the relationship. The agreement might also include the way in which personal information that the patient divulges will be handled.
- The nurse provides the patient with an orientation to the healthcare facility, its services, admission routines, and any pertinent information the patient requires to decrease anxiety. The nurse identifies this orientation as one of the goals in the nurse–patient helping relationship.

The development of a trusting relationship is critical to the development of the nurse–patient relationship. During the orientation phase, the patient might engage in behavior to test the nursing and healthcare staff. This might occur if the patient or family previously had negative healthcare experiences. The nurse's openness and interest in the concerns of the patient pave the way for development of trust and communicate care and respect.

Working Phase

The working phase is usually the longest phase of the helping relationship. During this phase, the nurse and patient work together to meet the patient's physical and psychosocial needs. Interaction is the essence of the working phase. Nurse–patient interactions that occur at this time are purposeful in that they

TABLE 21-2 Summary of Patient Goals for the Three Phases of the Helping Relationship

Orientation Phase	Working Phase	Termination
The patient will call the nurse by name. The patient will accurately describe the roles of the participants in the relationship. The patient and nurse will establish an agreement about: • Goals of the relationship • Location, frequency, and length of the contacts • Duration of the relationship	The patient will actively participate in the relationship. The patient will cooperate in activities that work toward achieving mutually acceptable goals. The patient will express feelings and concerns to the nurse.	The patient will participate in identifying the goals accomplished or the progress made toward goals. The patient will verbalize feelings about the termination of the relationship.

are designed to ensure achievement of health goals or objectives that were mutually agreed upon.

In the working phase, the nurse provides whatever assistance might be needed to achieve each goal. For example, if an older patient has a poor appetite and the goal is to increase food intake, the nurse discusses the idea of small, more frequent meals with the patient. With the patient's approval, the nurse makes the necessary arrangements. In another instance, a mother explains to a school nurse that she cannot afford the dental care recommended for her child, although she would like to have the work done. The nurse asks if a referral to a social agency for financial assistance would be acceptable. With the mother's permission, the nurse contacts the agency.

When sentiments and feelings between people are unsatisfactory, these people often cannot work cooperatively toward achieving a common goal. When sentiments and feelings are satisfactory, they can usually work together. In the preceding examples, satisfactory sentiments and feelings between the nurse and patients might be the key aspects. The older person's relationship with the nurse might allow a positive response to the small, more frequent meals. The mother's feelings about the nurse might allow her to accept financial assistance for dental care without feeling embarrassed.

In addition, the nurse as caregiver provides the patient with whatever assistance might be needed to perform activities of daily living. For example, if a patient with impaired mobility is unable to get out of bed except to use a bedside commode, the nurse needs to help with daily hygiene.

The nursing roles of teacher and counselor (see Chapter 22) are performed primarily during this phase. These roles involve motivating the patient to learn and to implement health promotion activities, to facilitate the patient's ability to execute the plan of care, and to express feelings about health problems, nursing care, any progress or setbacks, and any other areas of concern. This is where the nurse's interpersonal skills are used to their fullest (see the discussions of interpersonal skills and effective communication techniques later in this chapter). A breakdown of the helping relationship on one of these levels could result in serious consequences. For instance, a patient begins to break clinic appointments, although he previously seemed to be interested in his health when he visited the clinic. "The nurse at the clinic seems too busy; she doesn't seem to care if I come or go to that clinic." The lack of satisfactory interaction between the nurse and the patient discouraged him form continuing the relationship, even at the expense of his health. Had the nurse–patient interaction been satisfactory, the problem most likely would not have occurred.

Satisfactory interaction preserves people's integrity while promoting an atmosphere characterized by minimal fear, anxiety, distrust, and tension. People feel harmonious and contented with each other as they work cooperatively to reach common goals.

Termination Phase
The termination phase occurs when the conclusion of the initial agreement is acknowledged. This might happen at change-of-shift time, when the patient is discharged, or when a nurse leaves on vacation or for employment elsewhere. The patient and nurse examine the goals of the helping relationship for indications of their attainment or for evidence of progress toward them. If the goals/outcomes have been reached, this fact should be acknowledged. Such acknowledgment generally results in a feeling of satisfaction for the patient and nurse. If the goals/outcomes have not been reached, the progress can be acknowledged and either the patient or the nurse might make suggestions for future efforts.

Ordinarily, emotions are associated with the termination of a helping relationship. If the goals have been met, there is often regret about ending a satisfying relationship, even though a sense of accomplishment persists. If the goals have not been achieved, the patient might experience anxiety and fear about the future. Whatever the feelings, the patient should be encouraged to express his or her emotions about the termination.

The nurse can prepare for the termination of the helping relationship in various ways. The thoughtful nurse can set the stage for the patient to establish a helping relationship with another nurse, if appropriate. The nurse can assist the patient transferring from one agency to another or from one unit in an agency to another by offering explanations concerning the transfer. In some instances, the nurse might introduce the patient to personnel who will be giving care.

Occasionally, termination of the helping relationship causes a negative emotional reaction. The patient might feel angry, rejected by the nurse, or depressed and helpless, or might deny that a relationship ever really existed. If such a reaction occurs, the nurse should try to help and to support the patient rather than make him or her feel bad or guilty for having such a view. Emotional reactions of this sort are less likely to occur, however, if the patient has been involved in establishing goals and has been helped to anticipate termination of the helping relationship.

Interpersonal relations are discussed in greater detail in the classic works of nursing theorists Orlando (1961), Paterson and Zderad (1976), Peplau (1952), Travelbee (1971), and Watson (1985).

Factors Promoting Effective Communication Within the Helping Relationship
Dispositional Traits
A dispositional trait is a characteristic or customary way of behaving. Nurses who consistently demonstrate warmth and friendliness, openness and rapport, empathy, honesty, authenticity and trust, caring, and competence are well disposed to communicate effectively.

Warmth and Friendliness
The helping relationship depends on the nurse's ability to begin the orientation phase successfully. A pleasant greeting and friendly smile can facilitate this phase and place the patient at ease. By maintaining qualities of warmth and friendliness throughout the helping relationship, the nurse conveys contin-

uous acceptance of the patient and interest in discussing the patient's feelings and concern.

Openness and Respect

One key factor to effective communication is for the nurse to be open, accepting, frank, respectful, and without prejudice. When a patient feels that a nurse is being judgmental, he or she might withhold significant information. Nurses need to develop sensitivity to the unique challenges presented by each patient. Attention to patient variables that might influence the process of communicating (eg, gender, developmental level, culture, life experience) can make the difference between effective and ineffective interactions. Box 21-2 high-

lights guidelines for relating to patients from different cultures (see also Chap. 3).

Empathy

Empathy is identifying with the way another person feels. An empathetic nurse is sensitive to the patient's feelings and problems but remains objective enough to help the patient work to attain positive outcomes. A nurse who retains this quality can establish successful helping relationships without being a cold, stern figure, as is often portrayed in television or films. For example, although it is understandable for team members to become impatient with family members who never seem satisfied with the care their loved one is receiving, it is helpful if team

---

BOX 21-2 Relating to Patients From Different Cultures

Assess your personal beliefs surrounding people from different cultures.
- Review your personal beliefs and past experiences.
- Set aside any values, biases, ideas, and attitudes that are judgmental and may negatively affect care.

Assess communication variables from a cultural perspective.
- Determine the ethnic identity of the patient, including generation in America.
- Use the patient as a source of information when possible.
- Assess cultural factors that may affect your relationship with the patient and respond appropriately.

Plan care based on the communicated needs and cultural background.
- Learn as much as possible about the patient's cultural customs and beliefs.
- Encourage the patient to reveal cultural interpretation of health, illness, and healthcare.
- Be sensitive to the uniqueness of the patient
- Identify sources of discrepancy between the patient's and your own concepts of health and illness.
- Communicate at the patient's personal level of functioning.
- Evaluate effectiveness of nursing actions and modify nursing care plan when necessary.

Modify communication approaches to meet cultural needs.
- Be attentive to signs of fear, anxiety, and confusion in the patient.
- Respond in a reassuring manner in keeping with the patient's cultural orientation.
- Be aware that in some cultural groups, discussion concerning the patient with others may be offensive and may impede the nursing process.

Understand that respect for the patient and communicated needs is central to the therapeutic relationship.
- Communicate respect by using a kind and attentive approach.
- Learn how listening is communicated in the patient's culture.

- Use appropriate active listening techniques.
- Adopt an attitude of flexibility, respect, and interest to help bridge barriers imposed by culture.

Communicate in a nonthreatening manner.
- Conduct the interview in an unhurried manner.
- Follow acceptable social and cultural amenities.
- Ask general questions during the information-gathering stage.
- Be patient with a respondent who gives information that may seem unrelated to the patient's health problem.
- Develop a trusting relationship by listening carefully, allowing time, and giving the patient your full attention.

Use validating techniques in communication.
- Be alert for feedback that the patient is not understanding.
- Do not assume meaning is interpreted without distortion.

Be considerate of reluctance to talk when the subject involves sexual matters.
- Be aware that in some cultures, sexual matters are not discussed freely with members of the opposite sex.

Adopt special approaches when the patient speaks a different language.
- Use a caring tone of voice and facial expression to help alleviate the patient's fears.
- Speak slowly and distinctly, but not loudly.
- Use gestures, pictures, and play acting to help the patient understand.
- Repeat the message in different ways if necessary.
- Be alert to words the patient seems to understand and use them frequently.
- Keep messages simple and repeat them frequently.
- Avoid using medical terms and abbreviations that the patient may not understand.
- Use an appropriate language dictionary.

Use interpreters to improve communication.
- Ask the interpreter to translate the message, not just the individual words.
- Obtain feedback to confirm understanding.
- Use an interpreter who is culturally sensitive.

Used with permission from Gieger, J. N., & Davidhizar, R. E. (2004). *Transcultural nursing: Assessment and intervention* (4th ed.). St. Louis: Mosby.

members can empathize with the family who might be feeling frightened and helpless. "This must be a hard time for you . . . how are you coping?" "Is there any way I can be of help?" When the patient and family sense that the nurse has some idea of what they are experiencing and is committed to helping, the basis is set for a trusting therapeutic relationship.

Honesty, Authenticity, and Trust

Patients should be able to trust that nurses are who they say they are (professional helpers), and that they can be trusted to do everything within their level of expertise to secure the resources and to help meet the patient needs.

Caring

Patients quickly sense whether they are merely a "task to be performed" (task-centered caring), or a person of worth who is both cared about and cared for (relation-centered caring). Expert nurses know how to communicate genuine caring the minute they step into a patient's space by how they look at and touch the patient and what they say and do. Patients who feel cared for will feel accepted.

> Think back to Susie Musashi, the 3-year-old child with burns. How the nurse approaches the child will set the stage for the interaction. Consider how the child would respond to a nurse who enters the room and scolds the child for crying as compared to the nurse who enters the room and approaches the child's bed, touching the child's shoulder or hand gently and softly. The message conveyed by the second action would be much more caring.

Competence

Competent nurses are skilled in all aspects of basic nursing and can meet their patients' healthcare needs through their technical, cognitive, interpersonal, and ethical/legal skills. Nurses are responsible for evaluating their own strengths and weaknesses so that the patient will receive optimal care. Consequently, patients develop trust in and respect for their nurses, facilitating helping relationships and good communication.

Rapport Builders

Rapport, a feeling of mutual trust experienced by people in a satisfactory relationship (Fig. 21-4), can be achieved by paying attention to the following variables. Good rapport facilitates open communication.

Specific Objectives

Having a purpose for an interaction guides the nurse toward achieving a meaningful encounter with the patient. One objective might be to perform a head-to-toe physical assessment when greeting the patient and at the beginning of each shift. Another objective might the discussion of a patient's feelings about being newly diagnosed with diabetes. The shortest encounter with a patient can have an objective, even if it is as simple as conveying a feeling of friendliness. The nurse must be flexible at all times. The nurse should follow the patient's cues to work toward meeting all needs.

Comfortable Environment

A comfortable environment, in which both the patient and the nurse are at ease, helps to promote interactions. Suitable furniture, proper lighting, and a moderate temperature are important. Also, effective relationships are enhanced when the atmosphere is relaxed and unhurried. If the nurse seems preoccupied and on the run, or if the patient is ill at ease for fear of missing visitors or because of another commitment, communication is impaired.

Privacy

It might not always be possible to carry on conversations alone with the patient in a room, but every effort should be made to provide privacy and to prevent conversations from being overheard by others. Sometimes merely drawing the curtains around the bed in a hospital or nursing home or sitting in a corner of the waiting room or lounge can provide the sense of privacy that is so important in most interactions. Home visits might need to be timed to ensure the privacy the patient desires and needs.

Confidentiality

The confidentiality with which patient information is to be treated should be established with the patient. The nurse should indicate with whom the information that the patient gives will be shared. The patient should know about the right to specify who might have access to the information. Failure to consider this factor can be considered a breach of the patient's right to privacy. See Chapter 17 for guidelines concerning patient confidentiality.

Patient Versus Task Focus

Communication in the nurse–patient relationship should focus on the patient and patient needs, not on the nurse or an activity in which the nurse is engaged (see the accompanying box:

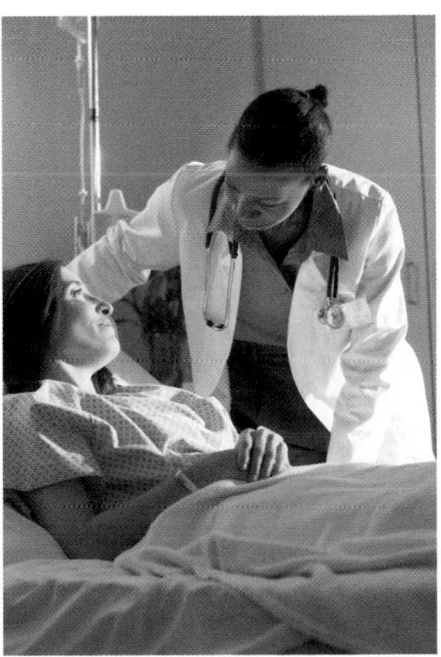

FIGURE 21-4 Rapport between the nurse and the patient/family is a necessary first step in planning care.

Through the Eyes of a Patient

I know you come to clinical every day with your head full of all the important things you need to do for me. Probably you worry about whether or not you will remember the steps to both simple and complex procedures and fear that you will never get everything done in the time allotted. I'm sure that there are many things that your clinical instructor will use as a basis for your evaluation and perhaps other things that are important to you for your self-evaluation. But I thought you might like to know what's important to me. Most of what I've listed are simple things that you can communicate each time you walk into my home or room.*

- Really listen to me.
- Ask me what I think.
- Don't dismiss my concerns.
- Don't treat me like a disease, treat me like a person.
- Talk *to* me, not *at* me.
- Respect my privacy.
- Don't keep me waiting.
- Don't tell me what to do without telling me how to do it.
- Keep me informed.
- Remember who I used to be.
- Let me know you care.

Thanks for giving me this chance to share with you what matters to me.

The list of nursing interventions that are valued highly by patients was compiled by Roberta Messner after a review of many patient satisfaction studies. These are cited in Messner, R. L. (1993). What patients really want from their nurses. American Journal of Nursing, 93(8), 38–41.

Through the Eyes of a Patient). Consider the following example, in which the nurse's comment focuses on the patient and the patient needs:

Patient: I don't know why these injections scare me, but they do.

Nurse: You are afraid of these injections?

In contrast, consider this example, in which the nurse's comment focuses instead on the nursing activity:

Patient: I don't know why these injections scare me, but they do.

Nurse: I give hundreds of injections. Don't be so immature.

Using Nursing Observations

Observations, which involves both seeing and interpreting, are especially useful for validating information. For example, a nurse suspects that a patient is afraid to hear the results of certain blood tests, but the patient insists that the results are unimportant. The nurse then observes the patient pacing in the corridor, apparently deep in thought. Observing the patient's behavior helps validate the nurse's suspicion that the patient is fearful, and the patient assertion that he or she is unconcerned appears to be a cover-up for truer feelings.

Observation serves several important purposes:

- It helps the nurse become aware of a patient's nonverbal messages.

- It is the primary source of information when a patient is unwilling or unable to communicate verbally.
- It demonstrates the nurse's caring and interest in the patient. (Patients often recognize when a nurse is unobservant and, rightly or wrongly, usually conclude that the nurse does not care.)

Optimal Pacing

A nurse must consider the pace of any conversation or encounter with a patient. For instance, it would be ineffective for the nurse to rush through a list of questions when obtaining a nursing history; it is more effective to let the patient set the pace. The nurse can let the patient know at the beginning of the interaction if time is limited so that the patient does not feel that the nurse is rushing because of a lack of concern or personal interest.

Respecting Personal Space

Perceptions of personal space vary. Nurses must try to determine each patient's perception of personal space because an invasion of this zone can evoke uncomfortable feelings. Nurses must assess a patient's personal space through careful observations of nonverbal communication. For example, when a person is speaking in close proximity, this might cause the person to back away because of feelings of discomfort in the close proximity. Other times the person speaking might touch the person during the conversation. This interaction of close proximity might be very comfortable for both individuals. It is important for nurses to be sensitive to personal space so that patients feel comfortable during interactions.

DEVELOPING THERAPEUTIC COMMUNICATION SKILLS

Although humans communicate during virtually all waking moments, the therapeutic use of communication requires training and practice. Box 21-3 contrasts therapeutic and nontherapeutic communication. Nursing students might feel awkward when first trying to develop therapeutic relationships. Practice makes perfect, however, and you will soon feel at ease if you work on developing the following communication skills.

Conversation Skills

Conversation, or the exchange of verbal communication, is a social interaction. As social beings, humans learn as children how to converse with others, and nursing students therefore have already had years of experience communicating verbally. However, nurses can improve their communications with patients and achieve a more effective helping relationship in the following ways:

- Control the tone of your voice so that you are conveying exactly what you mean to say and not a hidden message. The nurse's tone should indicate interest rather than boredom, patience rather than anger, acceptance rather than hostility, and so forth.

BOX 21-3 **Therapeutic Versus Nontherapeutic Communication**

Patient Scenario: Mr. Commens is a 65-year-old, divorced man who lives alone. His grown children are married and live out of town. He was recently diagnosed with cancer of the colon and underwent a colon resection. He is now home recuperating and has received a new diagnosis. The home health nurse is scheduled to visit Mr. Commens.

Nontherapeutic Communication

Nurse: Hello, Mr. Commens! I'm glad you're home. I only have 30 minutes to visit with you. It's been a very busy day.

Mr. Commens: I'm sorry you are having a bad day. I have been to the doctor and I'm very concerned about the report I received.

Nurse: Yes, I've had a busy day but not a bad day. I guess your day has been busy too. What report are you talking about?

Mr. Commens: Well, I need more tests because they think the cancer has spread.

Nurse: Now, who told you that? Maybe the test was wrong or you misunderstood the physician. Mr. Commens, I'll call your physician. Is there anything else bothering you?

Mr. Commens: No.

Nurse: I'll call your doctor and then call you tomorrow.

In this scenario the nurse seems unconcerned about Mr. Commens' test results and gives him the idea that he/she does not believe the information he has relayed. The nurse is more concerned about his/her busy day and less concerned about the patient.

Therapeutic Communication

Nurse: Hello, Mr. Commens! I'm sorry I am running a little behind schedule. Now that I'm here we will have as much time as we need to discuss how you're feeling and your visit to the physician. How are you feeling?

Mr. Commens: (His eyes are cast down to the floor and he is wringing his hands.) Well, I feel all right. I've had some pain in my right side.

Nurse: Mr. Commens, how would you rate your pain on a scale of 1 to 10?

Mr. Commens: About an 8.

Nurse: Mr. Commens, you seem concerned and a little preoccupied. Is there something bothering you?

Mr. Commens: Yes, I suppose there is. My doctor said my cancer has spread to my hip. I guess that's why I have pain in my right side. I have so many decisions to make and I'm very confused. The doctor said I need to start chemotherapy. I don't even know how I'll get there. My family is out of town.

Nurse: Mr. Commens, would it help if I spoke to your physician to obtain specific details about your treatment plan? This would then assist me in obtaining some help when you begin your chemotherapy.

Mr. Commens: That would be wonderful! If you call the doctor, then you can explain everything to me, and maybe it will help me to understand what I'll need to experience. Also, it might help me in making the decisions regarding my treatments.

Nurse: Mr. Commens, would you then like me to be here when you call your children about your diagnosis and treatment plan? I might be able to answer some of the questions they might have about your treatments.

Mr. Commens: That would be wonderful. I feel so much more relaxed knowing you are going to help me. Thank you so much.

Nurse: Mr. Commens, I'll call your physician and clarify the information you have received, and I'll be back at 5 p.m. Maybe at that time we can call your family.

Mr. Commens: That sounds like a good plan, but we might need to call my children at 6 p.m.

Nurse: That's just fine. I will be back at 5 p.m. to discuss the information I have, and we will call your children at 6 p.m.

Interpretation: The first scenario focuses on the nurse's needs, not the patient's needs. Most of the interaction in the first scenario blocks the communication process. The second scenario allows the patient to verbalize his concerns and his lack of decision making. The nurse provides the patient with broad opening statements and patient goals to assist in his planning and decision making.

- Be knowledgeable about the topic of conversation and have accurate information. When possible, a nurse should be familiar with the subject of conversation before discussing it with the patient. If the topic is an unfamiliar one (eg, the availability of community resources for family caregivers of patients with special needs), it is best to tell the patient and family so and to direct them to other resources. Convey confidence and honesty to the patient.
- Be flexible. A nurse might want to discuss a certain subject but learns that the patient wishes to discuss something else. It is better to follow the patient's lead whenever possible; in due time, the nurse can return to the subject. For example, a nurse arrives at the patient's bedside to administer a medication, but the patient begins to talk about his or her diet. It is better to take a little time to talk about the patient's interest than to insist on talking about only the procedure at hand, as long as there is enough time for the conversation.

- Be clear and concise, and make statements as simple as possible. Patients are often anxious and fail to understand the nurse's message unless the conversation is geared to a level the patient understands. Stay on one subject at a time. This will help decrease confusion.
- Avoid words that might have different interpretations. The study of the meaning of the words is called **semantics.** Even when two people speak the same language, some words—such as love, hate, freedom, and liberty—might have different meanings to different people.
- Be truthful. A patient who is given false information will soon distrust the nurse. If you're not sure about something, admit you don't know and seek an answer rather than make a comment that is likely to be an error.
- Keep an open mind. An attitude of "I know better than the patient" is quickly discerned by the patient. Patients can make valuable contributions to their own healthcare.

- Take advantage of available opportunities. During most caregiving situations, the nurse can facilitate conversation that makes even the most routine task meaningful. For instance, when giving a bed bath to a patient, a nurse can ask about the patient's employment. This would allow the patient to verbalize any positive or negative feelings about the job and his or her temporary absence from it, reducing the anxiety that often occurs with the loss of work. It is often comforting to know that someone understands and cares.

Listening Skills

Listening is a skill that involves both hearing and interpreting what the other says. It requires attention and concentration to sort out, evaluate, and validate clues to better understand the true meaning of what is being said (Fig. 21-5). The accompanying box, Through the Eyes of a Student, relates one student's experience with attentive listening. The following recommended techniques might help to improve listening skills:

- When possible, sit when communicating with a patient. Do not cross your arms or legs because that body language conveys a message of being closed to the patient's comments.
- Be alert and relaxed and take sufficient time so that the patient feels at ease during the conversation.
- Keep the conversation as natural as possible, and avoid sounding overly eager.
- If culturally appropriate, maintain eye contact with the patient, without staring, in a face-to-face pose. This technique conveys interest in the conversation and willingness to listen.
- Indicate that you are paying attention to what the patient is saying by using appropriate facial expressions and body gestures. Be attentive to both your own and the patient's verbal and nonverbal communication.
- Think before responding to the patient. Responding impulsively tends to disrupt communication and listening.
- Do not pretend to listen. Most patients are sensitive to an attitude of feigned attention or to boredom and apathy.

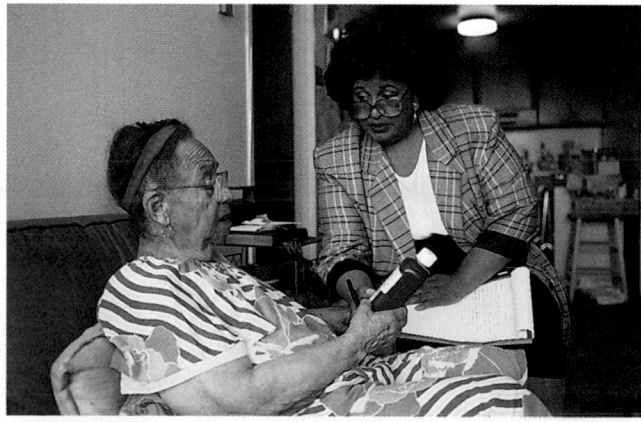

FIGURE 21-5 Listening attentively, with concentration and genuine concern, is key to productive communication.   (Photo © Kathy Sloane.)

Through the Eyes of a Student

It was my first day of clinical rotation and I was assigned to Mr. Anderson, who was in his early 90s. He was in the hospital because he had a second heart attack. Mr. Anderson had lived alone for 5 years after the death of his wife. He wanted to remain independent, but his daughter, who was herself in her late 60s, and his doctor believed that he would not be able to function well on his own any longer. Mr. Anderson was distressed about this belief.

Because it was my first day and, unlike some of my classmates, I had never worked in a hospital before, I felt insecure and nervous. There really wasn't a lot of work for us to do. We weren't allowed to give medication yet, and my patient was pretty self-sufficient. Because my skills were shaky, I took my time taking vital signs, assisted Mr. Anderson with his bath and toileting, and made his bed. After checking his chart, I began my nursing interview with him. I was overjoyed to discover that he was a real talker! His memory was tremendous—either that or he was a great improvisor! He recalled stories about his childhood and his wife with great detail and emotion. He smiled and laughed when he spoke of his daughter and grandchildren. He told me about his daughter's childhood illnesses as well as his own. We talked about the Depression and world wars and about music and art and education. He asked me about my family, and I felt like I had made a friend.

The next day Mr. Anderson told me about his fears. He talked about losing his wife, about his health and body deteriorating, and about losing his independence and home. He despised having to be sent to a nursing home and having to depend on others. It hurt him a lot and made me sad. Mr. Anderson left on my second day, and as I said goodbye I wished I could do something for him.

I thought about him a lot since then, and I've come to realize that in those 2 days that I knew Mr. Anderson, I did do something for him besides washing him and changing his sheets. I listened to him. Although his family had little time for him and the doctors quickly flew in and out of the room, I let him talk and heard all he said, both in words and in his eyes. He will always be a good memory for me—and I think I'll be a good memory for him.

—*Kristina Hofmeister, Holy Family College,*
Philadelphia, PA

- Listen for themes in the patient's comments. What are the repeated themes in the person's speech and behavior? What topics does the patient tend to avoid? What subjects tend to make the patient shift the conversation to other subjects? What inconsistencies and gaps appear in the patient's conversations?

Silence

The nurse can use silence appropriately by taking the time to wait for the patient to initiate or to continue speaking. During periods of silence, the nurse can reflect on what has already been shared and observe the patient without having to concentrate simultaneously on the spoken word. Periods of silence during communication can carry a variety of meanings, including the following:

- The patient might be comfortable and content in the nurse–patient relationship. Continuous talking is unnecessary.
- The patient might be trying to demonstrate stoicism and the ability to cope without help.
- The patient might be exploring his or her inner thoughts or feelings, and conversation would disrupt this. In effect, the patient is really saying "I need some time to think."
- The patient might be fearful and use silence as an escape from a threat.
- The patient might be angry and use silence to display this emotion.

In due time, the nurse might discuss the silence with the patient, especially if the nurse wishes to understand its meaning. Fear of silence sometimes leads to too much talking by the nurse. Also, excessive talking tends to place the focus on the nurse rather than on the patient.

Touch

Touch is a powerful means of communication with multiple meanings. It can connect people, provide affirmation, reassurance and stimulation, decrease loneliness, increase self esteem, and share warmth, intimacy, approval, and emotional support. It can also communicate frustration, anger, aggression, and punishment, invade personal space and privacy, and convey a negative (eg, subservient) type of relationship with another (Gieger & Davidhizar, 2004). Because of the personal nature of touching, a nurse needs to weigh the benefit of touch against the detrimental use of touch for each patient. Touch can be a powerful therapeutic tool when used at the right time. Anxiety or discomfort might result, however, when a patient does not understand the meaning of a tactile gesture or when the patient simply dislikes being touched.

Touch is the most highly developed sense at birth. Tactile experiences of infants and young children appear essential for the normal development of self and awareness of others. It has also been found that many elderly people long for touch, especially when isolated from loved ones because of hospitalization or nursing home care. Many older people have no living family to provide them with the caring touch so necessary for the sense of well-being. In such an instance, a nurse can provide some special care by holding the patient's hand (Fig. 21-6).

Many situations require the nurse to touch the patient while implementing nursing care. Physical closeness between the patient and the nurse is essential and inevitable. Therefore, every nurse needs to become comfortable with the judicious use of this nonverbal communication technique so that a sense of security, rather than anxiety, results. As well, dexterity and sureness in the use of the hands help to assure the patient of the nurse's expertise when measuring blood pressure or giving an injection.

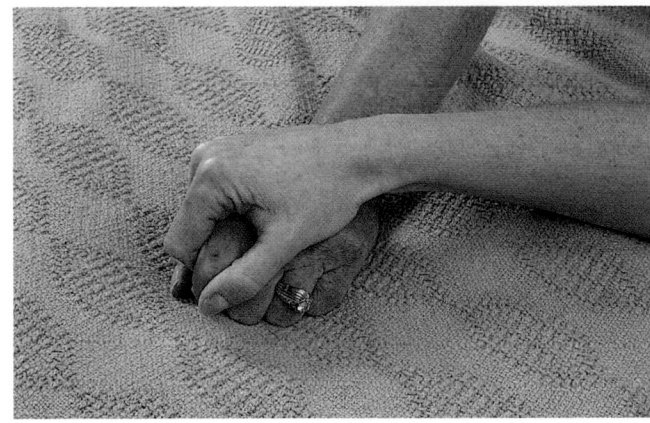

FIGURE 21-6 A reassuring handclasp uses touch to convey a message. Sometimes touch can be a more effective way of expressing concern and interest than verbal communication.   (Photo © B. Proud.)

Interest has been growing in the phenomenon known as **therapeutic touch.** Therapeutic touch involves "unruffling," or unblocking, congested areas of energy in the body and redirecting this energy. After assessing a patient's "energy field," the nurse uses therapeutic touch to promote comfort, relaxation, healing, and a sense of well-being. Many nurses are studying therapeutic touch in nursing educational programs and through special courses or workshops. It is becoming a widely accepted form of therapy as well as a subject for nursing research (Hutchison, 1999).

Humor

Humor is increasingly valued as both an interpersonal skill for the nurse and a healing strategy for patients. Nurses have a valuable tool when they can use humor effectively to maintain a balanced perspective in their work and to encourage patients to do the same. Nurses with a sense of humor are able to laugh at themselves and accept their failures, confront the absurdities of everyday practice without falling apart, and challenge patients to situate their current dilemma within the context of their larger life experiences. Laughter releases excess physical and psychological energy and reduces stress, anxiety, worry, and frustration. Humor, like other interpersonal competencies, is a learned skill. When used inappropriately, however, it can be destructive. Inexperienced nurses might find it helpful to identify nurses who use humor well and to "try on" behaviors they observe.

Interviewing Techniques

The purpose of the interview is to obtain accurate and thorough information. In nursing, the interview is a major tool for collecting data during the assessment step of the nursing process (see Chap. 12). Consequently, every nurse needs to become proficient in the use of the communication techniques described previously as well as interviewing techniques designed to gather and validate information.

All interviews should begin with an explanation of the purpose of the interview. During the interview, the nurse uses **interviewing techniques** to obtain needed information while remaining flexible in approach. The interview itself is a therapeutic interaction and might be an essential part of the orientation phase of the helping relationship. At the end of the interview, plans for further interactions can be made. The following interviewing techniques are useful in nearly all nurse–patient interactions, especially the interview.

Open-Ended Question or Comment

When obtaining a nursing history, the nurse uses the open-ended question technique to allow the patient a wide range of possible responses. It encourages free verbalization. The greatest advantage of this technique is that it prevents the patient from answering with a simple yes or no. Consider the following example of an open-ended question and the response:

Nurse: What did your physician tell you about your need for this hospitalization?

Patient: He told me that my blood pressure is dangerously high and that I need some special tests done while I am here.

The open-ended question by the nurse allows the patient to express what he or she understands to be true, yet is specific enough to prevent digressing from the issue at hand—the patient's hospital admission. The nurse could continue with an open-ended question such as the following:

Nurse: How did this news make you feel?

Patient: Well, it shocked and scared me because I thought my pressure was OK, and I know what happened to my dad as a result of his high blood pressure.

Now the nurse has even more information from the patient and can continue to seek additional information. This should be done in a way that does not make the patient feel as though the nurse is prying or probing.

Closed Question or Comment

The closed question provides the receiver with limited choices of possible responses and might often be answered by one or two words, "yes" or "no." Closed questions are used to gather specific information from a patient and to allow the nurse and patient to focus on a particular area. When not used appropriately, closed questions are a barrier to effective communication. The following is an example of an appropriate use of a closed question:

Nurse: What medicines have you been taking at home?

Patient: Let me see, my doctor gave me a water pill and a blood pressure pill to take every day.

This technique gives the nurse the exact information that is being sought. Closed questions should not be overused, because of their limiting effects on the patient's responses.

Validating Question or Comment

This type of question or comment serves to validate what the nurse believes is heard or observed. To continue the example used in the previous technique, the nurse could validate the patient's reply as follows:

Nurse: At home you have been taking both a water pill and a blood pressure pill every day. Did you take them today?

Patient: Yes, I took one of each with my breakfast.

The nurse is able to ascertain that the patient has been taking the medication regularly, as well as the correct dosage that day. However, overusing validating questions and comments might lead the patient to think the nurse is not listening.

Clarifying Question or Comment

The use of the clarifying question or comment allows the nurse to gain an understanding of a patient's comment.

Patient: I have never needed to take medicine before in my life.

Nurse: Is this the first health problem you have had?

Patient: Yes, I've always been healthy.

Overuse of clarifying questions or comments can lead the patient to believe that the nurse is not listening or might be unknowledgeable. When used properly, however, this technique can avert possible misconceptions that could lead to an inappropriate nursing diagnosis. In the above example, clarification of the patient's health allows the nurse to assess the patient's knowledge of the blood pressure problem and plan the necessary health teaching (see Chap. 22).

Reflective Question or Comment

The reflective question technique involves repeating what the person has said or describing the person's feelings. It encourages the patient to elaborate on his or her thoughts and feelings. An example of this technique follows:

Patient: I've been really upset about my blood pressure and have to take these pills.

Nurse: You've been upset . . .

Patient: I guess I'm worried about what could happen if my blood pressure gets too bad.

By saying this, the nurse has encouraged the patient to expand on this topic and express a more specific concern. Again, overusing this technique or using it mechanically might lead the patient to believe that the nurse is not listening or is uninterested.

Sequencing Question or Comment

Sequencing is used to place events in a chronologic order or to investigate a possible cause-and-effect relationship between events. This technique is evident in the following example:

Patient: I don't feel like myself anymore since I've been taking my blood pressure medicine. I'm tired and don't have any energy.

Nurse: Your tiredness began after you started taking your medicine?

This type of question could lead to possible discovery of a contributing factor to the patient's problem. Nursing assessment is facilitated when events leading to a problem are placed in sequence.

Directing Question or Comment

It might become necessary at times to obtain more information about a topic brought up earlier in the interview or to introduce a new aspect of the current topic. In such an instance, the nurse can attempt to direct the patient to that topic with a technique similar to the following:

Nurse: You mentioned your dad earlier. Did he develop complications related to high blood pressure?

Patient: Yes.

Nurse: What sort of complications?

Patient: Kidney failure. He was on dialysis for years before getting a transplant.

Nurse: Are you afraid this might happen to you?

In this way, the nurse has gained valuable information to consider in assessing the patient's health status and educational or counseling needs.

Assertiveness Skills

When interacting with patients, family members, other nurses, physicians, and other members of the healthcare team, nurses should communicate in a way that demonstrates respect for all parties. **Assertive behaviors,** which are one hallmark of professional nursing relationships, need to be distinguished from aggressive (ie, harsh, injurious, or destructive) behaviors, which are very different from assertive behaviors, and from avoidance or acquiescent behaviors. The key to assertiveness is open, honest, and direct communication. "I" statements— "I feel . . ." and "I think . . ."—play an important role in assertive statements. Table 21-3 gives examples of assertive and nonassertive speech.

Four basic components of the assertive response or approach are as follows: (1) having empathy, (2) describing one's feelings or the situation, (3) clarifying one's expectations, and (4) anticipating consequences (Angel & Petronko, 1983). For example, a student who is feeling overwhelmed by her weekly clinical assignments might communicate the following to her instructor:

Empathy: "I guess it must be hard for you to make our clinical assignments each week and to know what each one of us needs."

Description: "I have to share with you that right now I feel so overwhelmed that I go home from clinical in tears each week."

Expectation: "I am wondering if we could talk about this. I am willing to work hard, but I seem to need some help pulling everything together."

Consequences: "I expect to do well in clinical but I am afraid that if things continue the way they are right now, I might not last the semester. I would appreciate any help you can give me."

Characteristics of the assertive nurse's self-presentation include a confident, open body posture; eye contact; use of clear, concise "I" statements; and the ability to share honestly one's thoughts, feelings, and emotions. The assertive nurse's attitude toward work is characterized by working to capacity with or without supervision, the ability to remain calm under supervision, the freedom to ask for help when necessary, the ability to give and accept compliments, and honesty in admitting mistakes and taking responsibility for them.

BLOCKS TO COMMUNICATION

Failure to Perceive the Patient as a Human Being

It is of primary importance that the nurse focuses on the whole patient and not merely the patient's diagnosis. Patients report that nothing is more discomforting than to be treated as merely an object of care rather than a patient. It is also of primary importance that the patient is addressed by a formal name such as Mr., Mrs., Ms., or Dr. rather than slang terminology such as "honey" or "sweetie." What distinguishes nursing from other health professions is its focus on the whole person, not simply the illness or dysfunction.

Think back to Mr. Gordon, the patient with end-stage liver disease. In the scenario, the nurs-

---

TABLE 21-3 **Examples of Assertive and Nonassertive Speech**

	Assertive	Nonassertive
Nurse to Nurse	"I know we all lose track of time occasionally but I'm finding it harder and harder to cover for you when you take extra time for lunch. I don't think it's fair for your patient and I to have to wait an extra 30 minutes every day for you to come back from lunch. Can we talk about this?"	"Huh? No, I didn't really mind. Luckily I wasn't too busy today." Thought: "What a sucker I am. Now I'll have to grab a quick bite so that I can get back to the unit in time to do 2 p.m. treatments."
Nurse to Physician	"I know we talked about Mr. Esposito's pain medication before but I've collected some new data. Even with the change in dosage, he is only getting 1 to 1½ hours of relief. I believe a different analgesic agent might work better for him."	"Um . . . yes I know you already changed the dosage. It's just that I thought it still wasn't working. Maybe I didn't give it enough time. Thanks for listening to me anyway. I'm sorry to bother you with this."
Student Nurse to Preceptor	"Miss Cheng has a new order to be straight cathed. I reviewed the procedure but I'd sure appreciate your talking me through this because I've never done it before and I'm terrified."	"Uh . . . I'm sorry to be such a pain again. I have to do this cath and don't know where to begin. I know you must be busy, but, uh, is there any way you might have time for me?"

ing student voiced concerns about the staff nurse and residents focusing only on the technical aspects of the patient's care. To effectively communicate this concern to these individuals, the nurse would incorporate the four components of the assertive approach when speaking with them, stressing the need for providing care to the whole patient.

Failure to Listen

Patients might or might not feel able to speak freely to the nurse. Often, the signals indicating their readiness to talk are subtle. Nurses might miss valuable opportunities for important communication if they approach patients with closed minds or focus on their own needs rather than on the patient's needs. Nurses who lack confidence in their own ability to meet the challenges a patient presents might become defensive in response to a patient's comments. Nurse defensiveness is a huge barrier to open and trusting communication.

Inappropriate Comments and Questions

Certain types of comments and questions should be avoided in most situations because they tend to impede effective communications. A description of each type follows.

Using Clichés

A **cliché** is a stereotyped, trite, or pat answer. Most healthcare clichés suggest that there is no cause for anxiety or concern, or they offer false assurance. Their use tends to be interpreted as a lack of real interest in what has been said. For example, even though the common question "How are you?" could start a conversation, it can cause a problem if the patient hearing this suspects that the nurse is not sincerely interested in how he or she feels. Following are some common clichés that are best not said because they tend to impede effective communications:
"Everything will be all right."
"Don't worry. You will be just fine in another day or two."
"Your doctor knows best."
"Cheer up. Tomorrow is another day."

Another type of cliché makes a sweeping generalization that does not necessarily apply to a specific patient. It also tends to cut off communications and makes the person feel as though he or she is just another insignificant being. Consider the following examples:
"Men tolerate pain poorly. That must be why you are complaining of severe pain."
"Everybody is afraid of surgery. Why should you be any different?"
"You teenagers are all alike. You aren't cooperative because you deny authority."

Such comments rarely promote communication with patient whom they are addressed.

Using Questions Requiring Only a Yes or No Answer

Questions that can be answered by simply saying yes or no tend to cut off discussion, even when the person might wish to continue. Consider the following question:
Nurse: Did you have a good day?

The question begs for a noncommittal answer, which tells the nurse little. A better comment is as follows:
Nurse: Tell me about how your sessions in therapy, how did you feel they went today?

Another pitfall is to pose a question to which the patient can say no when that answer could present a problem. Consider the following question that a nurse asks a postoperative patient:
Nurse: Are you ready to get out of bed?

By offering the patient the chance to say no, the nurse might have created difficulties if the patient is to be out of bed.

There are times when questions that can be answered with yes or no are legitimate. Following are examples:
Nurse: Did you take your insulin before breakfast this morning?
Nurse: Do you have pain when I move your arm this way?

The problem with yes or no questions arises when the nurse is seeking more detailed information or when the question might create difficulty.

Using Questions Containing the Words Why and How

Questions using why and how are intimidating to many patients. Consider the following questions:
Nurse: Why were you not tired enough to sleep?
Nurse: How did you ever decide to go on a crash diet?

These two questions would be better stated as follows:
Nurse: What were you doing while you were unable to sleep?
Nurse: What things prompted you to decide to go on a crash diet?

Using Questions That Probe for Information

Questions that too obviously probe for information might cut off communication. Patients who are made to feel as though they are receiving the "third degree" become resentful and usually stop talking and try to avoid further conversation. Although the nurse might feel more information is needed, it is better to follow the patient's lead. Letting the patient take the initiative allows the nurse to delve more deeply at a time when the patient is ready. A nurse who says "Let's get to the bottom of this" is likely to destroy conversation, unless the patient is ready to face the real cause of the problem.

Using Leading Questions

A leading question suggests what response the speaker wishes to hear. Leading questions tend to produce answers that might please the nurse but are unlikely to encourage the patient to respond honestly without feeling intimidated. Consider the following examples:
Nurse: You aren't going to smoke that cigarette, are you?

Nurse: You have been well cared for by your nurses, haven't you?

These questions direct the patient to give an answer that pleases the nurse rather than to express his or her own thoughts.

Using Comments That Give Advice

Giving advice often implies that the nurse knows what is best for the patient and denies him or her the right to make decisions and have feelings. It also tends to increase the patient's dependence on caregivers. However, advice does have a rightful place when it requested and when the person giving the advice has expert knowledge that the patient does not.

Using Judgmental Comments

Using judgmental comments tends to impose the nurse's standards on the patient. Consider the comment of a nurse who notes that a young woman is crying:

Nurse: You aren't acting very grown up. How do you think your husband would feel if he saw you crying like this?

The nurse judges the patient as being immature, and the nurse's apparent hostility could end effective communication. A better comment in this situation might be as follows:

Nurse: I would like to help. Tell me, what is making you cry?

Consider the following exchange between a nurse and a patient about to have surgery:

Patient: I think I have a right to be afraid of this operation.

Nurse: Tell me what makes you feel afraid.

This patient is likely to feel safe when allowed to express his or her feelings without being judged.

> Remember Susie Musashi, the 3 year old with burns who is crying? Using a response such as "You're acting like a baby. You're a big girl now" would be intimidating, especially to a young child who is striving for acceptance. Instead, a response such as "Can you tell me what is making you cry or feel so sad?" would allow the child to verbalize her concerns without feeling intimidated or scolded. This response also would help in establishing a trusting nurse–patient relationship.

Changing the Subject

A quick way to stop conversation is to change the subject. The patient might be at a point of readiness to discuss something and can be expected to feel frustrated if put off by a change in the topic of conversation. The following example illustrates this:

Patient: When can I expect to be told about my insulin?

Nurse: Let's discuss your diet now so that you will know what to eat when you get home. We can discuss your insulin some other time.

A nurse might also change the subject when feeling uncomfortable about the topic of conversation. For example, the patient's needs are being met when the nurse allows the patient to speak of impending death, thoughts of suicide, or contemplated abortion. The nurse is ignoring the patient, however, when the subject is changed because the nurse feels uncomfortable talking about it.

Giving False Assurance

It is easier and more pleasant to deal with positive outcomes than negative outcomes. As such, nurses might try to convince the patient that things are going to turn out well even when knowing the chances are not good. False assurance might give patients the impression that the nurse is not interested in their problems. The use of clichés gives a patient false assurance. Communication might be impeded when providing the patient and family with false assurance. If the nurse inadvertently does use false assurance, then the nurse should explain with an apology and implement effective communication techniques.

Gossip and Rumor

Gossip and rumor are common forms of communication, particularly in healthcare settings. This can also be referred to as communication via the grapevine. Gossip and rumor can produce detrimental effects on relationships and group building. Gossiping might be used to inform, influence others, entertain, or ventilate. It can be harmless but could also damage the reputation of others. Rumors serve similar functions but tend to

Examples of **NANDA** Nursing Diagnoses	Communication	
Nursing Diagnoses	**Related Factors**	**Sample Defining Characteristics**
Impaired Verbal Communication	Decrease in circulation to the brain; brain tumor; physical barrier (tracheostomy, intubation); anatomic defect, cleft palate; psychological barriers (psychosis, lack of stimuli); cultural differences; developmental or age related	Individual is able to speak dominant language; speaks or verbalizes with difficulty; does not or cannot speak; stutters; slurs; has difficulty forming words or sentences; has difficulty expressing thought verbally; uses inappropriate verbalization; has dyspnea; is disoriented

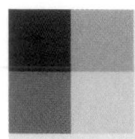

Focus on the Older Adult
What Are the Disorders of Communication That Most Frequently Affect Older People?

Our communication system, which involves speaking, hearing and understanding the speech of others, reading, and writing, is a unique human achievement. It plays a vital role in all aspects of everyday life—in our jobs, our families, and our recreation. When communication processes are damaged by disorders of speech, language, or hearing, the effects are always serious.

Disorders of speech, language, and hearing are frequently found among older adults. These individuals often find themselves at a distinct disadvantage on social, economic, and personal levels. With the number of older adults growing rapidly, and with the increased numbers of survivors of illnesses and accidents that can result in speech, language, or hearing disorders, more and more older adults with communication problems will be encountered. They require the understanding of family and friends as well as services from professionals in communication disorders.

Disorders of communication that affect older people may result from hearing impairment, stroke, cancer or other disease of the larynx, parkinsonism, or other neurologic disorders. The communication disorders vary widely and include difficulty with speaking and with understanding verbal messages. The effects of these disorders may be frustrating and bewildering and may lead to withdrawal and isolation. Participation on any social or economic level may become difficult or impossible either because of the disorder itself or the emotional consequences.

SPEECH, LANGUAGE, AND HEARING DISORDERS

APHASIA: Aphasia is a complex problem which may result, in varying degrees, in a reduced ability to understand what others are saying, to express oneself, or to be understood. Some individuals with this disorder may have no speech, while others may have only mild difficulties recalling names or words. Others may have problems putting words in their proper order in a sentence. The ability to understand oral directions, to read, to write, and to deal with numbers may also be disturbed. Strokes are the major cause of aphasia in the older population. It has been estimated that there are over one million adults with aphasia in the United States today. Many can be helped to communicate more effectively.

DYSARTHRIA: Dysarthria interferes with normal control of the speech mechanism. Speech may be slurred or otherwise difficult to understand due to lack of ability to produce speech sounds correctly, maintain good breath control, and coordinate the movements of the lips, tongue, palate, and larynx. Diseases such as parkinsonism, multiple sclerosis, and bulbar palsy, as well as strokes and accidents, can cause dysarthria. Many individuals with dysarthria are over 65. Their communication skills often may be improved by appropriate treatment.

HEARING PROBLEMS: It is estimated that of the approximately 27 million Americans over the age of 65, as many as 50 percent may be affected by hearing impairment. The hearing loss observed as a part of the aging process is called "presbycusis." Many of those with presbycusis describe the problem as being able to "hear" what others are saying, but being unable to understand what is being said. This condition can lead to withdrawal from personal interactions of all types. Family or friends may confuse the disorder with "forgetfulness" or "senility." A hearing aid can often improve communication for older people with hearing loss.

VOICE PROBLEMS: Laryngectomy, the surgical removal of the larynx (voice box) due to cancer, affects approximately 9,000 individuals each year, most of whom are older. They can usually learn to speak again by learning esophageal speech, by using an electronic device or by surgical implant of voice prosthesis. Other forms of disease may result in complete or partial loss of the voice. Most of these problems can be treated.

OTHER COMMUNICATION PROBLEMS: Brain diseases that result in progressive loss of mental faculties may affect memory, orientation to time, place and people, and organization of thought processes, all of which may result in reduced ability to communicate.

From *Communication Disorders and Aging.* American Speech-Language-Hearing Association, Rockville, Md. Reprinted with permission.

BOX 21-4 Communicating With Patients Who Have Special Needs

Patients Who Are Visually Impaired
- Acknowledge your presence in the patient's room.
- Identify yourself by name.
- Remember that the visually impaired patient will be unable to pick up most nonverbal cues during communication. Speak in a normal tone of voice.
- Explain the reason for touching the patient before doing so.
- Indicate to the patient when the conversation has ended and when you are leaving the room.
- Keep a call light or bell within easy reach of the patient.
- Orient the patient to the sounds in the environment and to the arrangement of the room and its furnishings.
- Be sure eyeglasses are clean and intact or that contacts are in place.

Patients Who Are Hearing Impaired
- Orient the patient to your presence before initiating conversation. This may be done by gently touching the patient or moving so you can be seen.
- Talk directly to the patient while facing him or her. If the patient is able to lip read, use simple sentences and speak in a quiet, natural manner and pace. Be aware of nonverbal communication.
- Do not chew gum or cover your mouth when talking with the patient.
- Demonstrate or pantomime ideas you wish to express, as appropriate.
- Use sign language or finger spelling, as appropriate.
- Write any ideas that you cannot convey to the patient in another manner.
- Be sure that hearing aids are clean, functioning, and inserted properly.

Patients With a Physical Barrier (Laryngectomy or Endotracheal Tube)
- Select one or more simple means of communication that the patient is physically able to use. Options include eye blinks or hand squeezes to communicate yes or no; writing pads or magic slates; communication boards with words, letters, or pictures; flash cards; sign language.
- Be sure that everyone communicating with the patient—family, friends, and caregivers—understands and is able to use the communication devices selected.
- Demonstrate patience with the time needed to communicate effectively, and reinforce the efforts made by the patient.

- Ensure that the patient has an effective means of signaling need for assistance, such as call bells or alarms.

Patients Who Are Cognitively Impaired
- Establish and maintain eye contact with the patient to hold attention.
- Communicate important information in a quiet environment where there is little to distract the patient's attention.
- Keep communication simple and concrete. Break down instructions into simple tasks and avoid lengthy explanations. Do not use pronouns or abstract terms. Use pictures or drawings when appropriate.
- Whenever possible, avoid open-ended questions. Ask "Would you like to wear the brown pants or the gray pants?" instead of "What would you like to wear?"
- Be patient and give the patient time to respond. If the patient does not respond after 2 minutes, repeat what you said. If there is still no response, take a break before continuing the conversation so that neither you nor the patient becomes frustrated.

An Unconscious Patient
- Be careful of what is said in the patient's presence. Hearing is believed to be the last sense lost, and therefore the unconscious patient is often likely to hear even though there is no apparent response.
- Assume the patient can hear you. Talk in a normal tone of voice about things you would ordinarily discuss.
- Speak with the patient before touching. Remember that touch can be an effective means of communication with the unconscious patient.
- Keep environment noises at as low a level as possible. This helps the patient focus on the communication.

Patients Who Do Not Speak English
- Use an interpreter whenever possible.
- Use a dictionary that translates words from one language to another so that you can speak at least some words in the patient's language.
- Speak in simple sentences and in a normal tone of voice.
- Demonstrate or pantomime ideas you wish to convey, as appropriate.
- Be aware of nonverbal communication. Remember that many nonverbal communication cues are universal.

---

be widespread. It is important to understand that rumors and gossip might cause blocks to team building and damage the reputations of the individuals who are the subject of the information.

IMPAIRED VERBAL COMMUNICATION

The ability to communicate is our most human characteristic. Human communication is essential for learning, working, and

social interaction. Impaired communication can affect every aspect of a person's life. Impaired Verbal Communication is an approved North American Nursing Diagnosis Association (NANDA) nursing diagnosis. According to NANDA, Impaired Verbal Communication is defined as the state in which an individual experiences a decreased or absent ability to use or understand language in human interaction. (See Examples of NANDA Nursing Diagnoses: Communication, p. 465.)

The Focus on the Older Adult box describes speech, language, and hearing disorders that most frequently affect older people. Box 21-4 offers guidelines for communicating with patients with special needs. The causes of hearing loss include chronic ear infections, heredity, birth defects, health problems at home, certain drugs, head injury, viral or bacterial infection, exposure to loud noise, aging, and tumors. Causes of speech and language disorders are related to hearing loss, cerebral palsy, and other nerve and muscle disorders, severe head injury, stroke, viral diseases, mental retardation, certain drugs, physical impairments such as cleft lip or palate, vocal abuse or misuse, and inadequate speech and language.

For Irwina Russellinski, the older adult woman admitted with pneumonia, the nurse would need to investigate the cause and degree of the patient's hearing loss and what, if any, treatments or measures have been used to manage the problem. The nurse would also need to gather additional data about the patient's confusion and her cultural background. Based on this information, the nurse would be able to develop a plan of care that addresses Mrs. Russellinski's needs.

A nurse who suspects a speech, language, or hearing problem should refer the patient to a speech-language pathologist or audiologist. A speech-language pathologist is a professional educated in the study of human communication, its development, and its disorders. An audiologist is a professional educated in the study of normal and impaired hearing.

Developing Critical Thinking Skills

1. Think about your class as a group and evaluate how effectively it is functioning (fair, average, good, exceptional). Identify positive and negative factors influencing your effectiveness. Talk with your classmates and see if they agree or disagree with your evaluation. Talk about how your class compares with classes of other years. What roles do you see yourself playing in your class group? Do others agree with your self-assessment?

2. Working with another student, attempt to express the following without using any form of verbal communication:
   - I am in pain.
   - I am genuinely concerned about your well-being.
   - I couldn't care less that you are my patient, and I wish I were anywhere else but here caring for you.
   - I am afraid that you will hurt me.

   Try to put into words what this exercise can teach you about the importance of nonverbal communication. Explain how this understanding will influence your nursing practice.

3. Conversation is both an art and an essential nursing tool. If you had 30 minutes to spend with each of the following patients while doing a procedure that allows you to communicate, what would you talk

about (communicate) and why? Compare your answers with another student's, and explore what your conversations would communicate to the patients involved.
   - An older adult, recently admitted to a nursing home
   - A 6-year-old boy newly admitted to a hospital for asthma
   - An HIV-positive 33-year-old man who has just been given the news that he has acquired immunodeficiency syndrome (AIDS)
   - A 45-year-old amputee who has been in a rehabilitation hospital for 3 weeks after a motorcycle accident
   - A 19-year-old woman who has just had an elective abortion and is in the recovery unit
   - An unconscious patient in a critical care unit

4. An experienced nurse observes your distress after leaving the room of a patient who has just told her family that her cancer has recurred and is in an advanced state. She tells you that you better "toughen up" if you want to survive in nursing. She counsels not getting emotionally involved with patients and families: "Become a rock." How do you respond to this nurse and why? Of what value, if any, is empathy?

Practicing for NCLEX

1. You are the charge nurse responsible for the evening shift. During rounds you hear the patient care technician yelling loudly to a patient regarding his transfer from the bed to chair. When entering the room your best response is:
   a. "You need to speak to the patient quietly. You are disturbing the patient."
   b. "Let me help you with your transfer technique."
   c. "When you are finished, be sure to apologize for your rough demeanor."
   d. "When your patient is safe and comfortable, meet me at the desk."

2. The public health nurse is leaving the home of a young mother who has a special needs baby. The neighbor states "How is she doing, since the baby's father is no help?" The nurse's best response to the neighbor is:
   a. "New mothers need support."
   b. "The lack of a father is difficult."
   c. "How are you today?"
   d. "It is a very sad situation."

3. A 3-year-old child is being admitted to the medical division for vomiting, diarrhea, and dehydration. During the admission interview, the nurse should implement which of the following communication techniques to elicit the most information from the parents?
   a. The use of statements that indicate the patient will be all right
   b. The use of questions that contain the word how

c. The use of a leading question and those involving yes or no
d. The use of questions that direct comments to clarify

4. The nurse enters the patient's room and examines the patient's IV fluids and cardiac monitor. The patient states "Well, I haven't seen you before. Who are you?" The nurse's best response is:
   a. "I'm just the IV therapist checking your IV."
   b. "I've been transferred to this division and will be caring for you."
   c. "I'm sorry, my name is John Smith. I'm responsible for your IV."
   d. "My name is John Smith. I'll be caring for you until 11 p.m."

5. The nurse enters the room of a patient with cancer. He is crying and states "I feel so alone." Of the following statements, which is the most therapeutic?
   a. The nurse stands at the patient's bedside and states "I understand how you feel. My mother said the same thing when she was ill."
   b. The nurse places a hand on the patient's arm and states "You feel so alone."
   c. The nurse stands in the patient's room and asks "Why do you feel so alone? Your wife has been here every day."
   d. The nurse holds the patient's hand and asks "What makes you feel so alone?"

6. During discharge teaching the nurse should:
   a. Determine the progress made in established goals
   b. Clarify when the patient should take medications
   c. Report the progress made in teaching to the staff
   d. Include all family members in the teaching session

7. The nursing student is nervous and concerned about the work she is about to do at the clinical facility. To allay anxiety and be successful in her provision of care it is important for her to:
   a. Determine the established goals of the institution
   b. Be sure her verbal and nonverbal communication is congruent
   c. Engage in self talk to plan her day and decrease her fear
   d. Speak with her fellow colleagues about how they feel

8. A nurse on the rehabilitation division states to her head nurse "I need the day off and you didn't give it to me!" The head nurse replies "Well, I wasn't aware you needed the day off, and it isn't possible since staffing is so inadequate." In the act of sending the message, which statement would be considered more effective?
   a. "Mr. Tyler, I placed a request to have August 8th off, but I'm working and I have a doctor's appointment."
   b. "Mr. Tyler, I would like to discuss my schedule with you. I requested the 8th of August off for a doctor's appointment. Could I make an appointment?"
   c. "Mr. Tyler, I will need to call in on the 8th of August because I have a doctor's appointment."
   d. "Mr. Tyler, since you didn't give me the 8th of August off, will I need to find someone to work for me?"

9. During a nursing staff meeting, the nurses determine that they will make sure all vital signs are reported and charted within 15 minutes following assessment. This is an example of:
   a. Group Decision Making
   b. Group Leadership
   c. Group Identity
   d. Group Patterns of Interaction

10. A patient walking to the bathroom with a stooped gait is noted with facial grimacing. It is important that the nurse assess the patient for:
    a. Pain
    b. Anxiety
    c. Depression
    d. Fluid Volume Deficit

11. A nursing student is preparing to administer morning care to the patient. The most important question that the nursing student should ask the patient is:
    a. "Would you prefer a bath or a shower?"
    b. "May I help you with a bed bath now or later this morning?"
    c. "I will be giving you your bath. Do you use soap or shower gel?"
    d. "I prefer a shower in the evening. When would you like your bath?"

12. A nurse is providing instruction to the patient regarding the procedure to change his colostomy bag. During the teaching session he asks "What type of foods should I avoid to prevent gas?" The question the patient has asked allows for:
    a. A closed-ended answer
    b. Information clarification
    c. The nurse to give advice
    d. A yes or no answer

13. When interacting with a patient, the nurse answers "I am sure everything will be fine. You have nothing to worry about." This is an example of an inappropriate communication technique known as a:
    a. Cliché
    b. Giving advice
    c. Being judgmental
    d. Changing the subject

14. A 76-year-old patient states "I have been experiencing complications of diabetes." The nurse needs to direct the patient to gain more information. What is the most appropriate comment or question to elicit additional information?

a. "Do you take two injections of insulin to decrease the complications?"

b. "Most physicians recommend diet and exercise to regulate blood sugar."

c. "Most complications of diabetes are related to neuropathy."

d. "What specific complications have you experienced?"

15. During an interaction with a critically ill patient's family, the nurse uses the communication technique of silence. This technique assists the family to:
a. Communicate with the patient
b. Plan for discharge
c. Organize their thoughts
d. Decrease anxiety

■ Answers With Rationale

1. The correct answer is *d*. The charge nurse should direct the patient care technician to determine the patient's safety. Then she or he should address any concerns regarding the patient care technician's communication techniques privately. It is important that the nurse directs the patient care technician on aspects of therapeutic communication.

2. The correct answer is *a*. It is important that the nurse maintain confidentiality when providing care. The statement of "New mothers need support" is a general statement that all new parents need help. The statement is not judgmental of the family's roles.

3. The correct answer is *d*. Direct comments which clarify will assist the nurse in obtaining adequate information.

4. The correct answer is *d*. The nurse should identify himself, be sure the patient knows what will be happening, and the time period he will be with his patient.

5. The correct answer is *d*. The use of therapeutic touch conveys acceptance, and the implementation of an open-ended question allows the patient time to verbalize freely.

6. The correct answer is *a*. The discharge planning phase coordinates with the termination phase of a helping relationship. It is important that the nurse determine the progress made in achieving the goals related to the patient's care.

7. The correct answer is *c*. By engaging in self talk, or intrapersonal communication, the nursing student can plan her day and enhance her clinical performance to decrease fear and anxiety.

8. The correct answer is *b*. Effective communication by the sender involves the implementation of non-threatening information by showing respect to the receiver. The nurse should identify the subject of the meeting and be sure it occurs at a mutually agreed-upon time.

9. The correct answer is *c*. Ascertaining that the staff completes a task on time and that all members agree the task is important is a characteristic of group identity.

10. The correct answer is *a*. A patient who presents with nonverbal communication of a stooped gait and facial grimacing is most likely experiencing pain. It is important that the nurse clarify this nonverbal behavior.

11. The correct answer is *b*. It is important that the nurse asks permission to assist the patient with a bath. This allows for consent to assist the patient with care that invades the patient's private zones.

12. The correct answer is *b*. The patient's question allows the nurse to clarify information that is new to the patient or that requires further explanation.

13. The correct answer is *a*. Telling a patient that everything is going to be all right is a cliché. The use of this statement is giving false assurance. The use of clichés gives the patient the impression that the nurse is not interested in the patient's condition.

14. The correct answer is *d*. Requesting specific information regarding complications of diabetes will elicit specific information to guide the nurse in further interview questions and specific assessment techniques.

15. The correct answer is *c*. Silence allows the family to organize their thoughts and develop any questions specific to understanding the patient's care.

Bibliography

Allen, L. J., & Van Ess Coeling, H. (1995). Quality of life: Its meaning to the long-term care resident. *Journal of Gerontological Nursing, 21*(2), 20–25.

Angel, G., & Petronko, D. K. (1983). *Developing the new assertive nurse: Essentials for advancement.* New York: Springer-Verlag.

Armstrong, J. (1996). Too close for comfort. *Nursing, 26*(4), 44–47.

Bergbom-Engberg, I. (1993). The communication process with ventilator patients in the ICU as perceived by the nursing staff. *Intensive Critical Care Nursing, 9*(1), 40–47.

Berlo, D. (1960). *The process of communication: An introduction to theory and practice.* New York: Holt, Rinehart & Winston.

Bottorff, J. L., & Morse, J. M. (1994). Identifying patterns of attending: Patterns of nurse's work. *Image—The Journal of Nursing Scholarship, 26*(1), 53–60.

Bower, F. L. (2000). *Nurses taking the lead: personal qualities of effective leadership.* Philadelphia: W. B. Saunders.

Chenevert, M. (1994). *STAT: Special techniques in assertiveness training for women in the health professions* (4th ed.). St. Louis: Mosby–Year Book.

Clark, C. C. (1978). *Assertive skills for nurses.* Wakefield, MA: Contemporary Publishing.

Crellin, K. (1998). 11 Easy ways to build rapport. *Nursing 98, 28*(11), 48.

Deering, C. G. (1993). Working with people: Giving and taking criticism. *American Journal of Nursing, 93*(12), 56–60.

Fine, J. I., & Rouse-Bane, S. (1995). Using validation techniques to improve communication with cognitively impaired older adults. *Journal of Gerontological Nursing, 21*(6), 39–45.

Gieger, J. N., & Davidhizar, R. E. (2004). *Transcultural nursing: Assessment and intervention* (4th ed.). St. Louis: Mosby.

Grossman, D., & Taylor, R. (1995). Working with people: Cultural diversity on the unit. *American Journal of Nursing, 95*(2), 64–67.

Hagerty, B. M. K., Lynch-Sauer, J., Patusky, K. L., & Bouwsema, M. (1993). An emerging theory of human relatedness. *Image—The Journal of Nursing Scholarship, 25*(4), 291–296.

Harvey, C., Dixon, M., & Padberg, N. (1995). Support group for families of trauma patients. *Critical Care Nurse, 15*(4), 59–63.

Heidt, P. R. (1990). Openness: A qualitative analysis of nurses' and patients' experience of touch. *Image—The Journal of Nursing Research, 21*(3), 180–186.

Hermann, J. F., Cella, D. F., & Robinovitch, A. (1995). Guidelines for support group programs. *Cancer Practice, 3*(2), 111–113.

Huber, D. (2000). *Leadership and nursing care management.* Philadelphia: W. B. Saunders.

Hutchison, C. P. (1999). Healing touch: An energetic approach. *American Journal of Nursing, 99*(4), 43–48.

King, I. M. (1971). *Toward a theory for nursing: General concepts of human behavior.* New York: John Wiley & Sons

Kotecki, C. N. (2002). Baccalaureate nursing student's communication process in the clinical setting. *Journal of Nursing Education, 41*(2), 61–69.

Laing, M. (1993). Gossip: Does it play a role in the socialization of nurses? *Image—The Journal of Nursing Scholarship, 25*(1), 37–43.

Luckman, J. (1999). *Transcultural communication in nursing.* Albany, NY: Delmar Publishers.

MacKay, M. (1990). *Empathy in helping relationship.* New York: Springer-Verlag.

Mackey, R. B. (1995). Discover the healing power of therapeutic touch. *American Journal of Nursing, 95*(4), 26–33.

Messner, R. L. (1993). What patients really want from their nurses. *American Journal of Nursing, 93*(8), 38–41.

Montagu, A. (1986). *Touching: The human significance of the skin* (3rd ed.). New York: Harper & Row.

Moore, J. R., & Gilbert, D. A. (1995). Elderly residents' perceptions of nurses' comforting touch. *Journal of Gerontological Nursing, 21*(1), 6–13.

Nance, T. A. (1995). Intercultural communication: Finding common ground. *Journal of Obstetric, Gynecologic, and Neonatal Nursing, 24*(3), 249–255.

Norris, R. M. (1989). Commonsense tips for working with blind patients. *American Journal of Nursing, 89*(3), 360–361.

North American Nursing Diagnosis Association. (2004). *NANDA nursing diagnoses: Definitions and classification, 2003–2004.* Philadelphia: Author.

Orlando, I. J. (1961). *The dynamic nurse–patient relationship.* New York: G. P. Putnam's Sons.

Paterson, J., & Zderad, L. (1976). *Humanistic nursing.* New York: Wiley.

Peplau, H. (1952). *Interpersonal relations in nursing.* New York: Putnam.

Quinn, J. F. (1988). Building a body of knowledge: Research on therapeutic touch. *Journal of Holistic Nursing, 6*(1), 37–45.

Ribeiro, V. F., & Blakeley, J. A. (1995). The proactive management of rumor and gossip. *JONA, 25*(6), 43–50.

Scott, J., & Rantz, M. (1994). Change champions at the grass roots level: Practice innovation using team process. *Nursing Administration Quarterly, 18*(3), 13.

Seldon, B. (1994). Communicating with Alzheimer's patients. *Journal of Gerontological Nursing, 20*(10), 51–53.

Sundeen, S. J., Stuart, G. W., Rankin, E. D., & Cohen, S. A. (1989). *Nurse–patient interaction* (4th ed.). St. Louis: C. V. Mosby.

Tannen, D. (1990). *You just don't understand: Women and men in conversation.* New York: Morrow.

Tennant, K. F. (1990). Laugh it off: The effect of humor on the well-being of the older adult. *Journal of Gerontological Nursing, 16*(12), 11–17.

Thompson, S. (1999). *The group context.* London: Jessica Kingsley Publishers.

Townsend, M. C. (2000). *Psychiatric mental health nursing concepts of care* (3rd ed.). Philadelphia, PA: F. A. Davis Publishers.

Travelbee, J. (1971). *Interpersonal aspects of nursing* (2nd ed.). Philadelphia: F. A. Davis.

Vanore-Black, N. (1990). Maintaining healthy relationships. *Holistic Nursing Practice, 4*(4), 39–45.

Watson, J. (1985). *Nursing: The philosophy and science of caring.* Boulder: Colorado Associated University Press.

White, C., & Howse, E. (1993). Managing humor: When is it funny—and when is it not? *Nursing Management, 24*(4), 80, 84, 86–96.

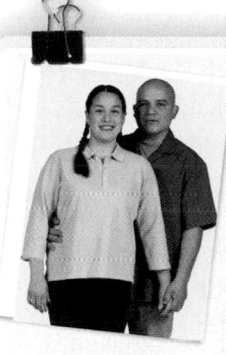

Marco García Ramírez accompanies his wife, Claudia, to the antepartal clinic for a routine visit. They are expecting their first child in 5 months. He reports that they are happy and excited but also scared and very nervous. They are planning for a home birth, asking lots of questions about childbirth and their new responsibilities as parents: "We're both wondering if we'll be good parents."

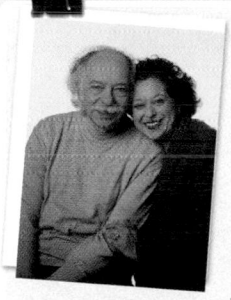

Rachel Blumenthal, age 40, is the second wife of a 57-year-old man who has suffered a serious myocardial infarction. They have been married for only 1 year. She says, "I'm a little embarrassed to talk with the cardiologist, but I have lots of questions about what my husband will be able to do after he gets home. I'm also wondering about resuming sexual activity."

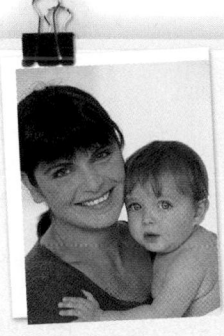

Alicia Bonet is the young mother of a baby boy; the baby's physician is recommending that he start long-term aspirin therapy. Ms. Bonet is quite concerned about agreeing to long-term aspirin therapy and asks, "I've heard so much about Reye's syndrome and aspirin. What should I do? What would you recommend?"

Focusing on Blended Skills

The types of blended skills you'll need to respond to the case scenarios include:

Cognitive Skills
- Knowledge of the process of teaching–learning
- Knowledge of the counseling process, including the types of counseling
- Knowledge of how to design an appropriate teaching program for childbirth and parenting, activity following a myocardial infarction (including information about sexual activity), and long-term aspirin therapy and Reye's syndrome
- Ability to interpret data to develop an effective teaching program for patients with differing needs

Technical Skills
- Strong assessment skills to identify factors influencing teaching and learning
- Ability to demonstrate childbirth and parenting psychomotor skills
- Ability to use effective communication skills when providing teaching and counseling interventions
- Ability to incorporate teaching and learning principles and counseling techniques with technical nursing assistance as necessary to meet the needs of patients
- Competence in adapting teaching techniques when providing instruction related to interventions
- Ability to ask for assistance as necessary when developing and implementing a teaching plan

Interpersonal Skills
- Strong people skills, including the ability to communicate and interact effectively with patients with complex learning and counseling needs and different levels of learning readiness and abilities to learn
- Excellent therapeutic communication skills, including conversational skills, listening skills, silence, interviewing techniques, touch, humor, and assertiveness for interacting with patients, such as anxious parents-to-be, the frightened spouse, and the overwhelmed young mother
- Ability to establish trusting relationships with patients to foster teaching and learning

Ethical and Legal Skills
- Ability to demonstrate respect, empathy, and honest caring in each professional encounter with patients
- Strong sense of accountability for the health and well-being of patients that translates into a commitment to getting patients the information they need
- Knowledge of the ethical principles that guide professional relationships and behavior in teaching and counseling situations
- Knowledge of the legal responsibilities for patient teaching as outlined by each state's Nurse Practice Act
- Ability to document teaching and counseling interventions in a legally prudent manner

Learning Outcomes

After completing the chapter, the learner should be able to accomplish the following:

1. Describe the teaching–learning process, including domains, developmental concerns, and specific principles.
2. Describe the factors that should be assessed in the learning process.
3. Describe the factors that influence patient compliance with the therapeutic plan.
4. Formulate diagnoses for identified learning needs.
5. Explain how to create and implement a culturally competent, age-specific teaching plan for a patient.
6. Name three methods for evaluating learning.
7. Explain what should be included in the documentation of the teaching–learning process.
8. Discuss the nurse's role as a counselor.
9. Summarize how the nursing process is used to help patients solve problems.
10. Describe how to use the counseling role to motivate a patient toward health promotion.

Key Terms

affective learning
andragogy
cognitive learning
contractual agreement
counseling
developmental crisis
formal teaching
informal teaching
learning
learning readiness
literacy
negative reinforcement
patient education
pedagogy
positive reinforcement
psychomotor learning
situational crisis
teaching–learning process

Helping patients and their families learn how to respond to their healthcare problems and how to protect their health is one of the most important nursing functions. Many patients lack the knowledge and self-care abilities they need to achieve their health goals. To work effectively with these patients, nurses must be skilled teachers and counselors. Both roles require strong communication skills. Current trends toward shorter hospital stays and decreased time for interactions between healthcare professionals and patient; dependence on complex technologies; evidence of health promotion/consumer empowerment; cost containment; and an increase in chronic illnesses have increased the need for effective teaching and counseling. Nurses are challenged with the task of teaching copious amounts of information, with limited time and resources, to patients who might or might not be ready, willing, or able to learn. (See the accompanying Reflective Practice box for an example.)

Never has the demand for quality education and counseling been greater. Nurses who are skilled educators and counselors can improve patients' health and well-being and reduce the demand for professional services. The Joint Commission

on Accreditation of Healthcare Organizations, an agency that evaluates the quality of patient care provided by hospitals, has identified several goals and standards for patient and family teaching (Box 22-1). These standards ensure that the patient and family receive the information they need to maintain optimal health.

AIMS OF TEACHING AND COUNSELING

Patient education is the process of influencing the patient's behavior to effect changes in knowledge, attitudes, and skills needed to maintain and improve health. Research supports the fact that educated patients experience better health and have fewer complications. This results in fewer hospitalizations and emergency department, clinic, and physician visits. To be successful, patient education must be ongoing and interactive. It must also take into account the patient's plan of care, educational level, and need for care across the continuum from the

Reflective Practice
Challenge to Intellectual Skills

It was during my senior practicum in pediatrics last spring that I met Alicia Bonet, the young mother of a baby boy for whom I was caring. The baby's physician was recommending long-term aspirin therapy (unfortunately, I cannot remember what condition the child had for which long-term aspirin therapy was being recommended). Ms. Bonet was quite concerned about agreeing to aspirin therapy, asking me if I knew much about Reye's syndrome. Then she asked me what I would recommend about whether or not to agree to long-term aspirin therapy. Not really understanding the risks versus the benefits of aspirin therapy or how it actually ties into Reye's syndrome, I did not feel competent to answer Ms. Bonet's questions, let alone make an educated recommendation to her.

Thinking Outside the Box: Possible Courses of Action

- Tell the mother that I could not be of help to her in making this decision because of my lack of knowledge about either topic.
- Inform her that I would have to ask other nurses and physicians to explain both topics to me (due to my lack of knowledge) before I could give her my opinion.
- Tell her that because I didn't know very much about either aspirin therapy or Reye's syndrome, I would research the topics in books and on the Internet when I had time and would get back to her with a recommendation based on my research.
- Be honest with the mother about my lack of knowledge about either aspirin therapy or Reye's syndrome and offer to

gather information from reputable sources for both of us so that we could discuss the topics.
- Provide her with information from the hospital library or the Internet so that she could educate herself (but not for my education so that I could assist her in making her decision).
- Lie to the mother (or withhold the fact that I did not know much about aspirin therapy or Reye's syndrome) and make an uneducated recommendation simply because I had the "authority" to do so.
- Ignore the mother's request, pretending not to have time to discuss her questions, rather than admitting my own ignorance or taking the time to educate myself.

Evaluating a Good Outcome: How Do I Define Success?

- The mother's needs are met. Not only does she receive a professional, educated, and competent recommendation, but she also is given the opportunity to make her own educated decisions by being given the information she needs.
- My intellectual competence is challenged and improved. I am able to admit a deficit in my knowledge and embrace the opportunity to improve it.
- The mother and patient benefit from my actions (or at least are not harmed) by the mother's informed choice.

- The mother's autonomy is encouraged—by providing her with all the necessary information, I enable her to make a healthy, educated decision.
- Quality care is provided to the patient and his family by competent professionals.
- The mother expresses an understanding of the information presented to her, feels comfortable asking additional questions, and makes an educated decision with which she is comfortable.

(continued)

Reflective Practice
Challenge to Intellectual Skills (Continued)

Personal Learning: Here's to the Future!

After explaining to the mother that I was not very familiar with aspirin therapy or Reye's syndrome, I first attempted to gather research information off the Internet for her. However, because I did not have a password to access the Internet from the nurse's station, I could not obtain the research I needed on my own. My next step was to ask my preceptor how to gather data for the mother if I could not get it off the Internet. She suggested calling down to the hospital library and asking them to put together an information packet that could be easily understood by a patient. I did this, and several hours later the packet arrived on the floor. After flipping through it briefly, I was satisfied with its contents and delivered it to Ms. Bonet. While I wished I had had the time to read all the information myself so that I could sit down with the mother and discuss it in detail, the day had been particularly busy. The best I could do was to pass the information on to the mother and hope she would read it herself. She was very grateful that I went to the trouble of gathering so much information for her, and she did not seem at all annoyed or disappointed that I did not have time to sit down with her to review the material. I did let her know that she could feel free to ask me any questions after she read the material, but she never got a chance to read the packet before my shift ended (because her son had visitors). As a result, we never got around to discussing her concerns.

Reflection

How do you think you would respond in a similar situation? Why? What does this tell you about yourself and about the adequacy of your skills for professional practice? Imagine if the nursing student had not informed Ms. Bonet about her lack of knowledge. Would the student's actions have been ethical? Legal? Professional? Please explain. Can you think of other ways to respond? What other skills (cognitive, interpersonal, technical, ethical/legal) would you need to respond well in this situation? How did the

One of the things that I learned from this experience is that it is okay to admit to a patient that you do not have all the answers. Moreover, admitting this helps to allay any doubt that he or she may have about my intellect or abilities as a nurse. Admitting a lack of knowledge is not a weakness, but a strength, for half the battle is knowing what you do not know. If anything, my willingness to admit my lack of knowledge and eagerness to educate both myself and my patient (by doing research) helped inspire trust and faith in me by my patient. I also learned that sometimes doing the best we can is better than doing nothing at all, even if the best we can do is not very much. Although I really needed to be able to sit down with Ms. Bonet and review the research with her, simply providing her with the material was enough to enable her to make an informed decision on her own. That simple act most likely empowered her to be much more comfortable with her decision in the end.

Although this occurred only a few months ago, I feel safe saying that my professional intellectual skills are quite adequate now—actually, they were quite adequate back then, too. Not knowing everything in nursing is not a reflection of inadequate professional intellectual skills, because it is impossible to know everything in this field. The fact that I knew that my knowledge was lacking, but that I knew where to go to find an answer, tells me my professional intellectual skills are more than adequate.

nursing student's communication skills improve the nurse–patient relationship? What, if any, teaching and learning principles did the nursing student use? Would any referrals be appropriate in this situation? If so, please describe. Do you agree with the criteria to evaluate a successful outcome? Did the nursing student meet the criteria? Please explain your answer.

Tracey Sara Miller, Georgetown University

BOX 22-1 Joint Commission on Accreditation of Healthcare Organization's Goals and Standards for Patient and Family Education

Goals
- Patient participation in and decision making about health-care options
- Increased potential to follow the healthcare plan
- Development of self-care skills
- Improved patient/family coping
- Increased participation in continuing care
- Adoption of a healthy lifestyle

Standards
- The client/family are provided with education that can enhance knowledge, skills, and behaviors that are necessary to benefit fully from the healthcare interventions provided by the organization.
- The organization plans and supports the provision and coordination of client/family education activities and resources.
- The client/family educational process is interdisciplinary as appropriate to the plan of care.
- The client/family receive education specific to the client's assessed needs, capabilities, and readiness.
- Information about any discharge instructions given to the client/family is provided to the organization or individual responsible for the continuing care of the client.

hospital to home care to long-term care. Patient education plans should be developed in collaboration with the entire healthcare team, including members of the hospital team (eg, dietitians, respiratory therapists, social workers, pharmacists) as well as home care agencies, wellness facilities, and long-term care agencies.

The basic purpose of teaching and counseling is to help patients and families develop the self-care abilities (knowledge, attitude, and skills) they need to maximize their functioning and quality of life (or to have a dignified death). For example, a patient newly diagnosed with diabetes must: (1) acquire knowledge about diabetes as a disease process and related medical management and self-care, (2) value health sufficiently to make certain lifestyle modifications (attitude), and (3) master certain skills, such as insulin injection. When used effectively by nurses, teaching and counseling are powerful tools for helping patients achieve health goals. Teaching provides the knowledge patients need to make informed healthcare decisions and to implement a plan of care.

> *Remember Alicia Bonet, the young mother worried about long-term aspirin therapy and Reye's syndrome. By providing Ms. Bonet with information, the nurse enables her to reach a decision that is based on sound knowledge and one with which she is comfortable.*

Counseling provides the resources and support patients need to participate actively in self-care and to facilitate their coping with what cannot be changed.

Maintaining and Promoting Health

Nurses can help patients to value health and develop specific health practices that promote wellness. Health teaching is varied and ranges from teaching passive exercises to a patient with left-sided paralysis to designing a safe exercise program for a young athlete.

Preventing Illness

Illness prevention, a major theme in health teaching and counseling, takes many forms. Nurses can counsel women of childbearing age about health practices that promote optimal fetal development, teach parents how to make their home safe for a toddler, or counsel individuals at high risk for heart disease, cancer, or communicable diseases.

Restoring Health

Once a patient is ill, teaching and counseling focus on developing self-care practices that promote recovery. Preoperative and postoperative teaching, sexual counseling for a patient recovering from a myocardial infarction, and lifestyle counseling for a patient with an ostomy are all examples of teaching and counseling directed at restoring health.

> *Consider Rachel Blumenthal, the wife of the patient who had suffered a myocardial in-farction. She is concerned about his activity level. When developing an appropriate teaching plan, the nurse would need to assess Mrs. Blumenthal's knowledge base before determining her actual teaching needs. In addition, the nurse would need to consult with the patient's cardiologist to determine what the patient's status is and what he will be allowed to do. These actions help to ensure that the teaching plan includes accurate information and is individualized to Mrs. Blumenthal's needs.*

Facilitating Coping

Developmental lifestyle changes and acute, chronic, and terminal illness all place demands on patients and families that may become overwhelming. Nurses work not only with patients but also with their families and friends to help them to come to terms with illness and whatever lifestyle modifications it entails. Not all patients fully recover from their illness or injury; many patients will need to learn to cope with permanent health alterations.

Summary

Nurse caregivers who are skilled teachers and counselors can promote the following outcomes:
- High-level wellness and related self-care practices
- Disease prevention or early detection
- Quick recovery from trauma or illness with minimal or no complications
- Enhanced ability to adjust to developmental lifestyle changes and acute, chronic, and terminal illness
- Family acceptance of the lifestyle changes necessitated by illness or disability

> *Remember Marco García Ramírez, the father-to-be described in the beginning of the chapter. Pregnancy and childbirth are considered developmental lifestyle changes. The nurse would need to incorporate knowledge of these changes when preparing an appropriate teaching plan for Mr. García Ramírez and his wife. The goal of teaching would be a positive adaptation to their new role as parents.*

General topics for health teaching are highlighted in Box 22-2.

THE NURSE AS TEACHER

Teaching is a planned method or series of methods used to help someone learn. The person using these methods is the teacher. **Learning** is the process by which a person acquires or increases knowledge or changes behavior in a measurable way as a result of the experience. Nurses assume the role of teacher and patients assume the role of learner when patients have identifiable learning needs. This teacher–learner relationship is

BOX 22-2 Topics for Health Teaching and Counseling

Promoting Health
- Developmental and maturational issues
- Normal childbearing
- Hygiene
- Nutrition
- Exercise
- Mental health
- Spiritual health

Preventing Illness
- First aid
- Safety
- Immunizations
- Screening
- Identification and management of risk factors

Restoring Health
- Orientation to treatment center and staff
- Patients' and nurses' expectations of one another
- The illness and physical condition: anatomy and physiology, etiology of problem, significance of symptoms, prognosis
- The medical and nursing regimens and how the patient can participate in care
- Self-care practices the patient and family need to manage the patient's condition independently

Facilitating Coping
- How the patient's physical and mental condition affects other areas of functioning; lifestyle counseling
- Measures that maximize independence and enhance self-concept
- Stress management
- Environmental alterations
- Community resources
- Appropriate referrals (eg, physical therapy, occupational therapy, self-help groups, psychiatric–mental health counselor)
- Grief and bereavement counseling

enhanced by the helping relationship (see Chap. 21) in which mutual respect and trust are established. The nurse builds on this trust by sharing information that the nurse and patient have mutually identified as important.

> Think back to Alicia Bonet, the young mother with questions about long-term aspirin therapy. The nurse was able to develop trust with Ms. Bonet by honestly admitting that she lacked the necessary knowledge about the therapy. The nurse was able to promote an ongoing therapeutic relationship by seeking the information, thereby solidifying the trust.

The patient may ask for this information, or the nurse may initiate teaching after assessing and diagnosing a learning need. Much patient education focuses on three critical areas:

- Preparation for receiving care
- Preparation before discharge from a healthcare facility
- Documentation of patient education activity

As with other clinical interventions, effective patient teaching demands analytic and problem-solving skills. To maximize the effectiveness of patient teaching, remember the acronym TEACH:

T: tune into the patient
E: edit patient information
A: act on every teaching moment
C: clarify often
H: honor the patient as a partner in the education process

Learning to be an effective teacher is a critical component of professional development. A basic understanding of the **teaching–learning process** aids nurses in developing their own teaching and learning skills. The process of patient teaching, which resembles the nursing process, consists of several steps that are necessary to provide teaching and to measure learning (Box 22-3). This process is often condensed because of limited time or resources, but the basic principles apply each time teaching–learning occurs.

To be a successful teacher, the nurse must have excellent communication skills and must be sensitive to all the factors that affect the patient's ability to learn (Fig. 22-1).

Factors Affecting Patient Learning

By taking into consideration the patient's age and developmental level, culture, family support networks and financial resources, language deficits, and literacy level, the nurse can individualize the teaching plan and maximize learning. This will support the nurse's goal of helping the patient to manage his or her own healthcare needs.

Age and Developmental Level

People learn throughout life, although what they learn and how learning occurs change according to developmental stages. Three critical developmental areas to consider when developing a teaching plan are the patient's physical maturation and abilities, psychosocial development, and cognitive capacity. Other concerns related to the teaching–learning process include the patient's emotional maturity and moral and spiritual development.

Child and Adolescent Learners

Piaget's theory of intellectual development is a major learning theory (see Chap. 18, Developmental Concepts). A nurse who understands how children and adolescents develop learning abilities can use this knowledge when teaching patients. When the patient is an infant, teaching is directed toward the parents. Toddlers and preschoolers may have some degree of understanding about medical tests or procedures, but health teaching continues to be directed toward the parents. For patients of this age, it is helpful for one nurse to establish a relationship with the patient and family and to be consistently involved in patient teaching activities. For example, if a 4-year-old girl must begin

---

BOX 22-3 **Steps of the Teaching–Learning Process**

Assess Learning Needs and Learning Readiness
1. Use all appropriate sources of information.
2. Identify the knowledge, attitudes, or skills needed by the patient and family.
3. Assess the patient's emotional and experiential readiness to learn.
4. Assess factors affecting the patient's ability to learn, including age and development level, family support networks and financial resources, cultural influences, literacy, and language barriers.
5. Develop critical pathways or teaching plans that span care delivery settings from hospital to home to take advantage of optimal learning readiness.
6. Identify the patient's strengths.
7. Use anticipatory guidance.

Diagnose the Patient's Learning Needs
1. Be realistic.
2. Validate with patient or family through conversations, questionnaires, and checklists.

Develop Learning Outcomes
1. Identify specific, attainable, measurable, and short-term outcomes for patient learning.
2. Make sure that proposed behavioral changes are realistic and explored in the context of the patient's resources and lifestyle.
3. Decide which domain of learning is involved (cognitive, psychomotor, affective).
4. Prioritize.
5. Include the patient and family. Unless the patient values these outcomes, little learning is likely to occur.

Develop a Teaching Plan
1. Select content, content sequencing, and appropriate teaching strategies/activities.
2. Relate the teaching content to the patient's learning style, interests, resources, and patterns of everyday living.
3. Pay careful attention to time constraints, scheduling, and the physical environment.
4. Decide on group versus individual teaching and formal versus informal methodologies.
5. Formulate a verbal or written contract with the patient.

Implement Teaching Plan and Strategies
1. Prepare the physical environment, with attention to comfort and privacy.
2. Communicate effectively with individuals, small groups, and, in some instances, large groups.
3. Gather all audiovisual materials and equipment.
4. Deliver the content in an organized manner using the selected teaching strategies.
5. Be flexible.
6. Keep teaching sessions short.
7. Vary strategies for sensory stimulation, which promotes learning.
8. Relate the material to the patients' life experiences, which will help them assimilate new knowledge.
9. Plan how you will evaluate learning.
10. Assess verbal and nonverbal feedback.

Evaluate Learning
1. Evaluate whether the learner outcomes were met:
   · Observe a return demonstration.
   · Ask the patient to restate the instructions.
   · Ask the patient questions to determine whether teaching reinforcement is needed.
   · Use written test or questionnaires.
   · Consult with the patient's family.
   · Consider patient feedback and comments.
2. Reinforce and celebrate learning.
3. Evaluate teaching:
   · Self-evaluation
   · Patient questionnaires
4. Revise the plan if the learner outcome is not met:
   · Alter content and teaching strategies.
   · Use motivational counseling.
   · Reschedule teaching sessions.
5. Document the teaching–learning process:
   · Patient and family learning needs and identified barriers to learning
   · Mechanisms used to overcome learning barriers
   · Patient and family readiness to learn
   · Current knowledge regarding the patient's condition and health status
   · Learning outcomes agreed on by the nurse, patient, and family
   · Identification of learning outcomes
   · Information and skills taught
   · Teaching methods used
   · Patient and family response
   · Evaluation of what patient and family learned and need for follow-up

---

to take insulin every day, the nurses who are caring for her must recognize her limitations in understanding diabetes. Information should be simplified to include only the most basic facts, with concrete examples or demonstrations; a detailed discussion of the pathophysiology of diabetes would not be appropriate. The girl could be told that she needs a shot every day to keep her from getting sick or feeling "funny." She could be allowed to play with the syringes and to give shots to a doll. Compared to adults, children have shorter attention spans,

combined with a great need for nurturing, support, and creative participation in learning activities.

School-age children are capable of logical reasoning and should be included in the teaching–learning process whenever possible. Teaching strategies that include clear explanations and reasons for procedures, stated in a simple and logical manner, are most successful.

The cognitive processes of adolescents are similar to those of adults, so the content and strategies of patient teaching

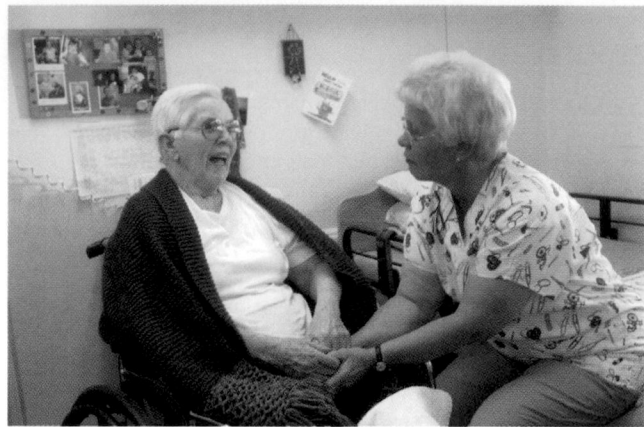

FIGURE 22-1 Effective communication is essential in the teaching–learning process.   (Photo by Rick Brady.)

resemble those used for teaching adults. A nurse who is teaching a sexually active 16-year-old girl about contraceptive methods needs to assess whether the young patient has reached the stage Piaget refers to as formal operations (the ability to use logical reasoning to solve hypothetical problems). If the patient's intellectual development is delayed and she is still in the period of concrete operations (use of logical reasoning to solve concrete problems), she may be unable to think abstractly—that is, she may not perceive pregnancy as a real possibility and therefore may not understand the need for contraception. If so, the nurse can alter the teaching plan to include audiovisual (AV) teaching aids that explain the topic in concrete terms. Peer group acceptance is a critical issue for adolescents. Teaching strategies designed for an adolescent patient should recognize the adolescent's need for independence as well as the need to establish a trusting relationship that demonstrates respect for the adolescent's opinions.

Motor development is also a concern in the teaching–learning process. The 4-year-old girl diagnosed with diabetes may not be able to give her own insulin shots if she lacks the fine motor skills needed to manipulate the equipment, but a 13-year-old patient could probably master the technique quickly.

Adult Learners

Many of the developmental concerns related to teaching and learning are affected by the patient's age. As people age, their personalities and learning abilities change. Most psychologists who have studied the teaching–learning process base their work on children and adolescents because a large amount of learning occurs early in life. The science of teaching (called **pedagogy**) generally refers to the teaching of children and adolescents. In recent years, the study of teaching adults (**andragogy**) has gained more attention.

Adults need to be taught differently. Knowles (1990) listed the following four assumptions about adult learners:

1. As a person matures, his or her self-concept is likely to move from dependence to independence.
2. The previous experience of the adult is a rich resource for learning.

3. An adult's readiness to learn is often related to a developmental task or a social role.
4. Most adults' orientation to learning is that material should be useful immediately, rather than at some time in the future.

Thus, andragogy focuses on a specific problem or need and on the immediate application of new material. In general, adult learners must believe that they need to learn before they are willing to learn. Nurses often must use their counseling skills (discussed later) to motivate patients to participate in the teaching–learning process. Adults may need to be shown the importance of learning new information, health practices, or skills.

Health promotion and injury avoidance are important activities throughout the life span, and teaching is often necessary for older patients. When developing a teaching plan for older adults, identify any learning barriers, such as sensory loss, limited physical mobility, or inability to comply with the recommended therapeutic regimen. Successful teaching plans for older adults incorporate extra time, short teaching sessions, accommodation for sensory deficits, and reduction of environmental distractions.

Family Support Networks and Financial Resources

No matter what the patient's age, working with the patient's family can be a great help in patient teaching. Assess the family's function and style by talking with them and observing how the patient and family interact. This assessment will yield information about family function, stress, transitions, and expectations. Informal conversations with both the patient and family can provide data that will help the nurse develop the teaching plan. The COPE model described in Box 22-4 is one method of helping family members to become effective problem solvers and support the nurse's teaching efforts.

BOX 22-4 **The COPE Model**

C: Creativity
Help the family to overcome obstacles to carrying out healthcare management and learning how to generate alternatives.

O: Optimism
Help the family caregivers learn how to view the caregiving situation with confidence.

P: Planning
Help the family learn how to plan for future problems and how to develop contingency plans that reduce uncertainty.

E: Expert Information
Help the family learn how to obtain expert information from healthcare providers about what to do in specific situations. This information empowers caregivers by encouraging them to develop plans for solving caregiving problems.

When teaching long-term family caregivers, include information about the disease process and resources available in the community that can help them with disease management and education, with a focus on planning, caregiving, decision making, and problem solving. Nurses need to view the family caregiver as a partner in providing care and to view themselves as health educators who teach families how to solve problems, rather than as experts who solve problems for them.

Evaluate the family's financial resources, because the patient may be unable to afford to follow a new treatment regimen. Nurses can often refer patients and families to community-based support groups and funding sources.

Cultural Influences

As our society becomes more ethnically diverse, nurses are continuously faced with the challenge of providing care and education to patients from many different cultural and ethnic backgrounds. To do so successfully, you may need to seek information from a variety of sources, such as the nursing literature and textbooks that describe the health practices and values of other cultures. Box 22-5 outlines strategies for providing patient education in a culturally competent manner.

One of the strategies is to develop written materials in the native language of the patient. Identify language deficits or barriers and develop strategies to address them, clearly communicating this in the plan of care. Do not assume that a family member is adequately translating information critical to the patient's learning.

Literacy

According to the National Institute for Literacy (2003), 46% to 51% of adults lack the basic literacy skills needed to function successfully in our society. Many have learned to compensate for this disability and may fool even experienced nurses. Never assume **literacy** (the ability to read and write) in a patient you are attempting to teach. By asking the patient to read a sheet of printed material aloud, you can assess his or her ability to understand printed material. For an illiterate patient, suggest non-print sources of information, such as videos or individual or group teaching sessions. This might also be an excellent time to suggest a community-based reading program for adults.

BOX 22-5 Culturally Competent Patient Teaching

- Develop an understanding of the patient's culture.
- Work with a multicultural team in developing educational programs.
- Be aware of personal assumptions, biases, and prejudices.
- Understand the core cultural values of the patient or group.
- Develop written materials in the patient's native language.
- Use testimonials of persons with the same cultural background as the patient

---

Learning Domains

Patients learn in three domains: cognitive, affective, and psychomotor (Bloom, 1956). The ability of patients to manage their daily life and resume their former roles depends on the degree to which cognitive, affective, and psychomotor learning results in behavioral changes. These domains influence the teaching and evaluation strategies the nurse selects. Effective teaching often involves the promotion of behaviors in all three domains.

Cognitive learning involves the storing and recalling of new knowledge in the brain (eg, the patient describes how salt intake affects blood pressure). Cognitive learning includes intellectual behaviors, such as the acquisition of knowledge, comprehension, application (using abstract ideas in concrete situations), analysis (relating ideas in an organized way), synthesis (assimilating parts of information as a whole), and evaluation (judging the worth of a body of information).

Learning a physical skill involving the integration of mental and muscular activity is called **psychomotor learning** (eg, the patient demonstrates how to change dressings using clean technique).

Affective learning includes changes in attitudes, values, and feelings (eg, the patient expresses renewed self-confidence after physical therapy).

Recall Marco García Ramírez, the father-to-be with concerns about his new role. The nurse would develop a teaching plan that focuses on the three domains of learning. The nurse would address the cognitive domain by teaching Mr. García Ramírez and his wife about labor and delivery, including the labor process and what events will occur. Teaching the couple about newborn care and breathing techniques to use during labor would address the psychomotor domain. Learning in the affective domain would be demonstrated if Mr. García Ramírez reports that the couple do not fear labor and feel comfortable handling a newborn.

Effective Communication Techniques

A critical component of effective patient education is the nurse's ability to be an effective communicator. Key points of effective communication associated with patient teaching include the following:

- Be sincere and honest; show genuine interest.
- Avoid giving too much detail; stick to the basics.
- Ask if the patient has any questions.
- Be a "cheerleader" for the patient. Avoid lecturing.
- Use simple words.
- Vary your tone of voice.
- Keep the content clear.
- Listen and do not interrupt when the patient speaks.

NURSING PROCESS FOR PATIENT AND CAREGIVER TEACHING

Patient teaching is approached most effectively using the steps of the nursing process. The teaching–learning process and the nursing process are interdependent.

Assessing

Sources of Information

Usually, patients themselves are the best source of assessment information. Patients are considered primary sources of information. By using effective interviewing techniques (see Chap. 21, Communicator), the nurse can obtain the data needed to identify the patient's learning needs. Relevant information can be obtained before actually meeting the patient by reviewing the patient's past and current medical records. These records are considered secondary sources of information and can provide a history of medical problems as well as documentation of the nursing assessments, nursing diagnoses, nursing physical examinations, and nursing interventions that have been performed.

The patient's family and significant others are also valuable sources of assessment data. Family members or significant others are sometimes needed to provide assessment data when the patient cannot communicate with the nurse because of health problems, language barriers, or impaired sensory functions. At other times, family members or significant others might be the most appropriate source of certain information; for example, if seeking information about how much salt is used in the family's cooking, the nurse could speak with the person who prepares the meals at home and could include that person in any teaching about food preparation. The patient's permission is needed before the nurse involves family members in the teaching–learning process.

Assessment Parameters

Four elements should be considered in each assessment of patient learning needs (Box 22-6). The nurse first identifies what new knowledge, attitudes, or skills are necessary for patients and families to learn in order to manage their healthcare. Second, assessment focuses on **learning readiness,** the patient's willingness to engage in the teaching–learning process (emotional readiness) and to begin the challenge of learning. Barriers to learning readiness include a patient's denial of his or her illness, lack of physical endurance, lack of human or financial resources, perceived benefit to continue in the sick role, and disparity of values between the patient and the healthcare provider. Readiness is distinguished from the patient's actual ability to learn, which is the third element. The fourth element of assessment is on the patient's strengths, the personal resources that the nurse can help the patient to tap.

Motivation

When assessing a patient's learning readiness, it is important to consider his or her motivation. Patients who are ready to

---

BOX 22-6 Assessment Parameters: Factors That Affect Learning

1. **Knowledge, attitudes, and skills needed for the patient and family to manage healthcare independently**

2. **Readiness to learn**
   - Emotional readiness
     Emotional health
     Motivation for learning
     Self-concept and body image
     Sense of responsibility for self
   - Experiential readiness
     Social and economic stability
     Past experiences with learning
     Attitude toward learning
     Culture

3. **Ability to learn**
   - Physical condition
   - Cognitive ability to learn
   - Acuity of senses
   - Developmental considerations
   - Level of education
   - Literacy
   - Communication skills
   - Primary language

4. **Learning strengths**
   - Successful learning in the past
   - Above-average comprehension, reasoning, memory, or psychomotor skills
   - High motivation
   - Strong network
   - Adequate financing

---

learn are able and motivated to process new information, develop new skills, and explore new attitudes and behaviors. Motivation is an internal impulse (such as emotion or physical pain) that encourages the patient to take action or change behavior.

Think back to Rachel Blumenthal, the wife of the patient who had a myocardial infarction. Although further assessment is necessary, analysis of Ms. Blumenthal's questions would lead the nurse to suspect that she is interested in finding out information, showing motivation and a beginning readiness to learn.

A patient's health beliefs can have great influence on motivation. The health belief model identifies several health beliefs as critical for patient motivation (Rosenstock, 1974). Motivation is enhanced when:

- Patients view themselves as susceptible to the disease in question
- Patients view the disease as a serious threat
- Patients believe there are actions they can take to reduce the probability of contracting the disease

- Patients believe the threat of taking these actions is not as great as the disease itself

The health belief model was designed to explain why persons are willing to take actions to support their health, but it evolved into a strategy for predicting the likelihood that patients would comply with therapies. Motivation plays a key role in the health belief model because it spurs the client to adopt health promotion and disease protection actions. Examples of motivational triggers include personal crisis and loss of social role due to disease symptoms. Nurses can use the health belief model when developing teaching plans, evaluating the ideas or beliefs that motivate a patient and applying these to the teaching plan. For example, if the nurse modifies a patient's perception of disease susceptibility, the patient might become more receptive to learning.

Compliance

Nursing assessment of the patient's learning needs is vital to developing a plan of care with which the patient can comply. Patients are considered compliant when they follow the treatment plan and use the information they have been taught. Noncompliance occurs when patients ignore instructions or do not follow them appropriately. Noncompliance can be associated with a lack of learning readiness and motivation, confusion, disappointment, misunderstanding, fear, inability to learn, or inadequate finances. When patients understand their diagnosis, treatment rationale, medication regimen, and the benefits of compliance, they are more likely to comply. Noncompliance can hurt the patient's health. Patients control the choices they make about following the plan of care and using what they have been taught, but it is the nurse's responsibility to help patients improve their health by sharing knowledge, solving problems, and providing support while the patient integrates the new knowledge and practices the new skills. Increased patient compliance is a direct outcome of effective patient teaching. Box 22-7 lists ways to help patients and families become compliant with the plan of care.

Diagnosing

If the patient lacks the required knowledge, attitudes, or skills to support health promotion, the nurse diagnoses the deficit.

BOX 22-7 Promoting Patient and Family Compliance

- Be certain that healthcare instructions are understandable and designed to support patient goals.
- Include the patient and family as partners in the teaching–learning process.
- Use interactive teaching strategies.
- Remember that teaching and learning are processes that rely on strong interpersonal relationships with patients and their families.

The nurse can use diagnoses or problem statements approved by the North American Nursing Diagnosis Association (NANDA) as a guide when diagnosing learning needs (see Chap. 13, Diagnosing). If the nurse believes that a patient's knowledge deficit is the primary problem, he or she can write a diagnosis identifying a specific knowledge deficit as the problem, followed by its etiology and the related signs and symptoms. For example: Deficient Knowledge: Breastfeeding related to inexperience, as manifested by anxiety and multiple questions.

More often, a knowledge deficit results in an actual or potential problem; therefore, the knowledge deficit is written as the etiology (second part of the diagnostic statement): for example, Imbalanced Nutrition: Less Than Body Requirements related to mother's lack of knowledge about infant feeding and deficient learning readiness (as manifested by mother's quick frustration when breastfeeding, refusal to engage in learning process, and infant's weight loss).

If the nurse learns that a pregnant woman plans to breastfeed and knows nothing about breastfeeding, "Deficient Knowledge: Breastfeeding" is the problem statement. The goal is to increase the mother's knowledge. If, on the other hand, a nurse observes a newborn failing to gain weight appropriately, and it is reasonable to suspect that the mother's lack of knowledge about how to breastfeed is interfering with the infant's nutritional intake, "Deficient Knowledge: Breastfeeding" is the etiology. The goal is to ensure the infant's proper nutrition.

Related nursing diagnoses include the following:
Impaired Health Maintenance
Ineffective Therapeutic Regimen Management
Noncompliance
Self-Care Deficit (specify)

Wellness diagnoses, such as Readiness for Enhanced Parenting or Readiness for Enhanced Self-Esteem, are written as one-part statements. Teaching and counseling are the primary nursing interventions used to achieve related outcome criteria.

In addition to identifying the patient's learning needs, nurses need to assess their own knowledge base and teaching skills. Nurses cannot teach information and skills to patients if they themselves lack the information and skills to be taught. Often, knowing where to find information or an appropriate resource person is the first step in correcting one's own knowledge deficits.

Outcome Identification and Planning

Planning for learning involves the development of a teaching plan. Teaching plans are similar to nursing care plans—both follow the steps of the nursing process. One type of teaching plan is presented in Box 22-8. It is directed toward teaching appropriate nipple care to reduce the likelihood of nipple cracking and redness in breastfeeding women.

Standardized teaching plans (some computerized) are available for major topics of health teaching. Such plans

BOX 22-8 Sample Teaching Plan

Diagnosis: Risk for Impaired Skin Integrity: Nipples related to knowledge and skill deficit (nipple care)
Signs and Symptoms: complaints of sore nipples, redness, cracking
Long-term Outcome: woman will be able to breastfeed as long as desired without nipple problems

Learner Outcome	Met	Content	Teaching Strategy	Learner Activity
Woman describes measures to prevent nipple cracking (cognitive)	8/10/06 L.I.	Protective measures: • Avoid soap • Avoid exposure to air and sunlight	Lecture with discussion Audiovisual: flip chart on breastfeeding	Read handout: Nipple care
Woman begins protective measures immediately (psychomotor)	8/10/06 L.I.	• Apply lanolin or vegetable oil • Avoid plastic liners in bra or bra pads		
Woman describes the correct procedure for breastfeeding (cognitive)	8/10/06 L.I.	Preparation for breastfeeding • Nipple roll before the feeding	Discussion Audiovisual: flip chart on breastfeeding	Read handout: Sore nipples
Woman explains why feedings should be shorter and more frequent (cognitive)	8/10/06 L.I.	Breastfeeding the baby • Feed baby every 2 hours during the day • Start baby on less sore side	Discovery: guide through each step; assist as necessary Return demonstration	Read handout: Positioning baby for breastfeeding Borrow books on breastfeeding from reference library
Woman demonstrates correct procedure for breastfeeding (psychomotor)	8/10/06 L.I.	• Get baby onto areolar area • Position properly • Change position for each feeding		
Display increasing confidence in breastfeeding skills and self-care (affective)	8/10/06 L.I.	• Remove baby from breast		
Value good nutrition and rest at home (affective)	8/10/06 L.I.	After feeding • Air dry the nipples • Inspect for open or cracked areas • Apply lanolin or vegetable oil	Discovery	
List the signs of thrush (cognitive)	8/10/06 L.I.			
		Home considerations • Maintain "demand feedings" • Ensure good nutrition • Get adequate rest • Know the signs and symptoms of thrush	Lecture with discussion Audiovisual: poster	Refer to handouts at home as needed; call maternity department's information number for any questions

must be tailored to the patient's learning needs and abilities. Remember that factors such as age, developmental level, family support networks, financial resources, cultural influences, literacy, and language barriers affect the patient's ability to learn; consider them when individualizing the teaching plan. Examples of teaching plans that are incorporated into critical path documentation systems are featured in Chapter 14, Outcome Identification and Planning, and Chapter 17, Documenting, Reporting, and Conferring.

Thoughtful planning of patient teaching maximizes the patient's learning while ensuring the most efficient use of the nurse's time and talents. Learner outcomes are developed for each diagnosis of a learning need. The nursing orders become

the content, teaching strategy, and learner activity columns of the written plan. This phase requires thought and creativity. The nurse's efforts are rewarded when the patient meets the outcomes at the end of the implementation phase.

When planning for learning, the nurse and patient together must decide who should be included in the learning sessions. When the patient is a young child, one or both parents may be the primary learners. For an adult patient, a spouse or close friend who will be giving the care that is to be learned may be included. For instance, the person who does the household's cooking is usually asked to be present for nutritional teaching. Teaching plans are developed according to the needs of the individuals being taught.

One nurse or several nurses can prepare and use a teaching plan. When two or more nurses plan and coordinate the implementation of the plan, this is called team teaching. An advantage of team teaching is that it takes advantage of the talents of more than one nurse.

Duplicating teaching that has already been completed by other members of the healthcare team wastes time and causes frustration. Accurate and thorough documentation of all patient teaching, along with review of the medical record before teaching sessions and effective communication with members of the interdisciplinary team, can eliminate this problem.

Several factors should be considered while formulating any teaching plan, as discussed in the next sections.

Patient Learning Outcomes

Learner outcomes are written in the same manner as the patient outcomes in the nursing process (see Chap. 14). When planning for the patient's learning, the nurse first determines which of the three learning domains (cognitive, psychomotor, or affective) will be the focus of teaching. The nurse can then write learning outcomes that reflect what learning is to occur. A well-constructed learning outcome serves as a guide for planning evaluation methods.

Choosing the verb for a learning outcome is probably the most difficult part of writing outcomes (Box 22-9). But a careful choice makes it easier to plan the content, teaching strategies, learner activities, and evaluation.

BOX 22-9 Verbs That Can Be Used When Writing Learner Outcomes

Cognitive Domain	Psychomotor Domain
compares	adapts
defines	arranges
describes	assembles
designs	begins
differentiates	changes
explains	constructs
gives examples	creates
identifies	demonstrates
names	manipulates
prepares	moves
plans	organizes
solves	rearranges
states	shows
summarizes	starts
	works

Affective Domain

chooses	justifies
defends	relates
displays	revises
forms	selects
gives	shares
helps	uses
initiates	values

The number of outcomes needed for each diagnosis varies. It is better to have several specific outcomes than to try to cover everything with only one or two broad outcomes. Many nurses write one long-term, general outcome for each diagnosis, followed by several short-term, specific outcomes. For example, a long-term outcome for the sample teaching plan could be: "The patient will be able to breastfeed her infant as long as desired without sore nipples." This outcome could be met in 2 weeks or 2 years, depending on how long the woman decides to breastfeed. Long-term outcomes are general statements. On the other hand, the outcomes written in the learner outcome column of the sample teaching plan are short-term, specific behaviors to be accomplished within a specified time.

Patients and appropriate family members or significant others should be included in planning the outcomes. When patients value the learning outcomes, their readiness to learn is enhanced, increasing the likelihood that they will achieve the goals.

Content

After writing the learner outcomes, the nurse must decide what information the patient needs to complete them. This information is the content of the teaching plan. The most effective teaching plans address the most important topics relevant to the patient's care. New nurses usually need to research the subject to be taught to determine what information exists about the topic. Books, journal articles, and manuals are available in many nursing units. Current nursing literature and research materials are available through several web-based databases. The most complete database of nursing journals is "The Cumulative Index to Nursing and Allied Health Literature" (CINAHL). This listing, published bimonthly, lists over 300 English-language nursing and allied health journals, as well as the publications of the American Nurses Association (ANA) and National League for Nursing (NLN). Content supported by nursing research is called evidence-based and reflects the most accurate and clinically supported information.

Nurses are often concerned about just how much patients should learn about topics such as illness, procedures, medications, and surgeries. Patients have been found to benefit from explanations of the physical sensations they will experience during a procedure. They appreciate knowing in advance what they will feel, taste, hear, see, and smell.

Content explaining why certain treatments and medications are needed is included in a teaching plan. Information on the prevention of illness or its complications should also be covered. Again, patients are more likely to implement a plan that they understand and value.

Teaching Strategies

The techniques used by a teacher to promote learning are called teaching strategies. Teaching strategies are planned before the actual teaching sessions so that every content area and learner outcome can be matched with an effective teaching technique. The strategies chosen depend on the teacher's familiarity with the method, the availability of educational resources and teaching aids, and factors affecting the patient's learning, such as educational level and cultural background. The nurse must also use age-appropriate methods; for example, a 10-year-old will be receptive to a comic book on personal safety, whereas an adult could learn similar material by discussing safety measures with the nurse.

Education experts generally agree that using a variety of teaching strategies enhances learning. In addition, some methods are better suited for certain learning outcomes. Box 22-10 gives suggested teaching strategies for the three learning domains. The sample teaching plan shows how teaching strategies vary according to the learner outcomes and content of that particular plan. Again, the nurse can be creative in choosing the methods. The nurse should try to stimulate as many of the patient's senses as possible when teaching. Seeing, hearing, and touching are superior to reading or hearing alone. We reportedly remember 10% of what we read, 20% of what we hear, 30% of what we see, 50% of what we see and hear, and 80% of what we say and do. Descriptions of common teaching strategies follow.

Role Modeling

The old saying "actions speak louder than words" explains why role modeling is effective. Patients watch their nurses closely; the nurse can use this opportunity to improve a patient's behavior. For example, nurses who formerly smoked can be role models for patients who are trying to quit smoking.

Consider Marco García Ramírez, the father-to-be concerned about his role as a parent. The

---

BOX 22-10 Suggested Teaching Strategies for the Three Learning Domains

Cognitive Domain
Lecture or discussion
Panel discussion
Discovery
Audiovisual materials
Printed materials
Programmed instruction
Computer-assisted instruction programs

Affective Domain
Role modeling
Discussion
Panel discussion
Audiovisual materials
Role playing
Printed materials

Psychomotor Domain
Demonstration
Discovery
Audiovisual materials
Printed materials

---

nurse would act as a role model to the couple when demonstrating newborn care.

Lecture

The term "lecture" means a presentation of information by a teacher to a learner. To be more effective, lectures usually include question-and-answer periods. This strategy is often used to deliver information to a large group of patients; it is rarely used for individual instruction except in combination with other strategies.

Discussion

Discussion involves a two-way exchange of information, ideas, and feelings between the teacher and the learners. It is an effective method when used by a nurse who is comfortable with leading a group and knowledgeable about group process (see Chap. 21, Communicator). It can also be an effective method for one-on-one instruction.

Remember Alicia Bonet, the young mother who had to make a decision about long-term aspirin therapy for her baby. The nurse could use a discussion to present information to Ms. Bonet about aspirin therapy, its risks and benefits, and Reye's syndrome. The nurse would also provide time for Ms. Bonet to ask questions and think about the information presented.

Panel Discussion

A panel discussion involves a presentation of information by two or more people. Panel discussions can be used to impart factual material but are also effective for sharing experiences and emotions. Debates are a form of panel discussion that include multiple sides of a controversial topic.

Demonstration

Demonstration of techniques, procedures, exercises, and the use of special equipment, combined with a lecture and discussion, is an effective strategy. The patient's learning can be evaluated by a return demonstration. Practice sessions are often included for the learner. Models of body parts or practice models, such as a resuscitation model, are frequently used. When teaching breast self-examinations, the use of a breast model allows the learner to feel different types of lumps commonly found in breast tissue. Childbirth educators usually demonstrate the birth of a baby by using a pelvic model, knitted uterus, and baby doll.

Discovery

In discovery learning, the nurse presents a problem or situation to the patient or group of patients and then guides the patients to discover the solution or approach. Discussion of other possible approaches and solutions can follow the patient's own solutions. This is a good method for teaching problem-solving techniques and independent thinking. For instance, a nurse could give a group of diabetic patients a short description of a situation that includes signs and symptoms. The group would decide whether the signs and symptoms indicate hypoglycemia (low blood sugar) or hyperglycemia (high blood sugar) and would choose what measures to take. Next, the nurse could discuss the group's decision as a further learning experience. Even if the patients chose a poor solution, the nurse can turn it into an effective learning experience.

> *Recall Rachel Blumenthal, the wife of the patient who had a myocardial infarction. The nurse could present Mrs. Blumenthal with a "what-if" situation: for example, What if your husband started to have chest pain while you were cuddling and kissing? How would you handle the situation? From her answer, the nurse would be able to tell how well she understands her husband's condition. The nurse would also have an opportunity for reinstruction, reinforcement, and validation of learning.*

Role Playing

Role playing gives the learner a chance to experience, relive, or anticipate an event. The nurse explains the scenario and then allows the patient to play out the scene with the teacher or with one or more other learners. Role playing can be used to work through emotional traumas or to plan for possible traumas. For example, a nurse could help a teenaged girl prepare herself to tell her mother about her pregnancy by letting the girl play herself while the nurse plays the girl's mother. This would help the patient rehearse what she wanted to say and anticipate the emotional atmosphere that she will experience. Role playing is a good strategy for adults as well as children. Puppets and dolls can help young children express negative feelings about hospitalization and traumatic procedures (Fig. 22-2).

Audiovisual Materials

AV materials such as computer programs, web-based course work, films, slides, television programs, videotapes, overhead transparencies, flip charts, posters, and diagrams are a popular

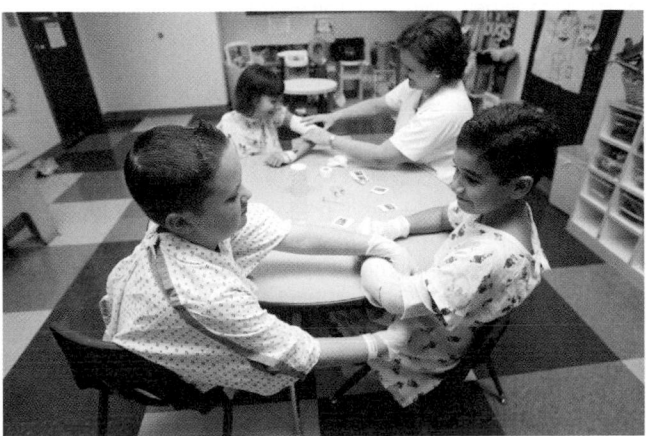

FIGURE 22-2 Role playing can help children learn and express negative feelings resulting from hospitalization and traumatic procedures. (Photo by Joe Mitchell.)

and effective teaching strategy when combined with a lecture or discussion. As noted above, the nurse should never assume the patient is literate. AV materials should never be the sole source of learning for a patient. The patient may view the AV material alone, but it should be preceded and followed with a discussion of the material.

Printed Material

The use of printed material depends on its availability. Many nurses have written materials for distribution to patients. Writing pamphlets, instruction sheets, books, and comic books for health teaching can be rewarding as well as useful. As with AV materials, printed materials are generally used in conjunction with other strategies. Specially prepared games, which are relatively easy to make, are a popular and fun way for patients to learn. For instance, cards with pictures of foods can be used to create a nutritional instruction game.

Print materials should be selected carefully based on how well they present the needed content in a format that is attractive, understandable, and helpful. Two samples of patient education materials appear in Boxes 22-11 and 22-12.

> *Consider how the nurse handled the situation of Alicia Bonet, the young mother described in the Reflective Practice box. The nurse provided Ms. Bonet with written materials that were at a level she could understand, thereby helping her make her decision.*

Programmed Instruction

Most programmed instruction books or booklets are prepared so that learners can use them independently of a teacher. However, educators generally agree that the teacher needs to spend time with the learner before and after the program to clarify the information, answer questions, and provide the personal touch necessary for a learner's motivation. Because this is a self-paced strategy, it can be beneficial for many learners.

Web-Based Instruction

Web sites appropriate to the patient's disease process, wellness interests, or health promotion focus can be valuable teaching and learning resources. These sites provide consumer information that is formatted for easy reading and access. The nurse should evaluate the web site chosen by the patient and advise him or her about its suitability and accuracy because some information found on the Internet is not grounded in scientific, medical, or nursing research.

Contractual Agreements

A **contractual agreement** is a pact between two people setting out mutually agreed-on goals. Contracts between nurses and patients are becoming a common practice in many healthcare settings. The contracts are usually informal and not legally binding. When the nurse is teaching a patient, such an agreement can serve to motivate both the patient and the nurse to do what is necessary to meet the patient's learning outcomes. The agreement notes the responsibilities of both the teacher

---

BOX 22-11 Sample Patient Education Materials for Managing Cancer Pain: Pain Control Plan

---

<u>Pain Control Plan</u>

Pain control plan for

_____

At home, I will take the following medicines for pain control:

Medicine	How to take	How many	How often	Comments
_____	_____	_____	_____	_____
_____	_____	_____	_____	_____
_____	_____	_____	_____	_____

Medicines that you may take to help treat side effects:

Side effect	Medicine	How to take	How many	How often	Comments
_____	_____	_____	_____	_____	_____
_____	_____	_____	_____	_____	_____
_____	_____	_____	_____	_____	_____

Constipation is a very common problem when taking opioid medications. When this happens, do the following:
- Increase fluid intake (8 to 10 glasses of fluid per day).
- Exercise regularly.
- Increase fiber in the diet (bran, fresh fruits, vegetables).
- Use a mild laxative, such as milk of magnesia, if no bowel movement in 3 days.
- Take _____

  every day at _____ (time) with a full glass of water.
- Use a glycerin suppository every morning (this may help make a bowel movement less painful).

Nondrug pain control methods:

_____

_____

_____

Additional instructions:

_____

_____

_____

Important phone numbers:

Your doctor _____

Your nurse _____

Your pharmacy _____

Emergencies _____
Call your doctor or nurse immediately if your pain increases or if you have new pain. Also call your doctor early for a refill of pain medicines. Do not let your medicines get below 3 or 4 days' supply.

Cancer Pain Management Guidelines Panel. (1994). *Managing cancer pain: Patient guide.* AHCPR Pub. 94-0595. Rockville, MD: Agency for Health Care Policy and Research. Public Health Service, US Department of Health and Human Services.

---

and the learner, emphasizing the importance of the mutual commitment (Box 22-13). If the contracted outcomes are achieved, the nurse can boost the patient's self-esteem with rewards; if the outcomes are not achieved, the nurse can try different teaching techniques.

Learning Activities

While planning teaching strategies, the nurse also decides what learning activities the patient will be doing independently. There are many ways that the patient can preview new material or reinforce what has already been taught. Printed materials, AV materials, and programmed instruction materials are often

assigned in the learning activity column of the teaching plan. This column is used to guide the patient in learning activities that can be done before, between, and after planned learning sessions. The accompanying Research in Nursing box describes the success of a project to prepare older patients to become more active in their care by learning to search for health information on the Internet. Practical considerations for planning learning activities are discussed below.

Time Constraints

Time constraints must be considered when planning for the patient's learning. Nurses often have a problem finding time

BOX 22-12 What to Do if You Have One or More Heart Attack Warning Signs

Patient's Name: _____

Physicians now have treatments that can stop heart attacks and lessen damage to the heart. To make sure you can benefit from these treatments, you need to act promptly if you begin to experience symptoms that might signal a heart attack.

1. This is what you may feel:
- Chest pain, discomfort, or pressure
- Left arm pain or discomfort
- Pain radiating to your neck or jaw
- Shortness of breath
- Sweating
- Upset stomach
- Discomfort in the area between your breastbone and navel
- A sense of dread
- Other: _____

2. Medication instructions:
- Chew one 325-mg tablet of uncoated adult aspirin.
- Place one tablet of nitroglycerin under your tongue as soon as you feel discomfort. Take a second tablet if the discomfort does not go away in 5 minutes. Take a third tablet after 5 more minutes if the discomfort does not go away.
- Other: _____

3. If the symptoms stop, call your physician at:_____

4. If symptoms continue for more than 15 minutes, call the emergency medical services phone number below immediately. (Often this is 9-1-1, but you should check to make sure.) Never wait longer than 15 minutes.

At home, the emergency phone number is: _____

At work, the emergency phone number is: _____

At _____ , the emergency phone number is: _____

_____

5. Know the location of the nearest 24-hour emergency department.

At home, the closest emergency department is: _____

At work, the closest emergency department is _____

At _____ , the closest emergency department is: _____

_____

Place this form next to the phone, near your other emergency numbers!

Signed: _____ MD/RN

Adapted with permission from the US Department of Health and Human Services, the Public Health Service, the National Institutes of Health, and the National Heart, Lung, and Blood Institute.

BOX 22-13 Example of a Contractual Agreement Between a Nurse and a Client

I will participate in the learning activities needed to help me learn about my low-salt diet. During my hospital stay, I will attend the class on low-salt diets, read the materials given to me, and ask questions as I need to. I will work with S. Moore, RN, to plan my meals and food preparation at home. If I need help when I get home, I will contact S. Moore.

Jim Mall

I will provide Jim Mall with the experiences needed for him to follow his low-salt diet accurately.

S. Moore RN

---

to meet patients' learning needs. Priorities must be set so that essential content is taught thoroughly. Less important content is taught last so that the more important learner outcomes can be met within the time available. If time permits, the remaining content can be addressed. Note that in the sample teaching plan, women are taught measures to use immediately.

To meet time constraints, nurses often plan together. Teamwork and cooperation allow nurses to meet deadlines. If teaching must continue beyond the hospitalization, home visit, or clinic visit, the nurse can schedule additional learning opportunities through outpatient programs or referrals to community-based programs. Home healthcare nurses often receive referrals from hospital nurses to continue the teaching begun during a patient's hospitalization. Discharge planning must be started early to ensure continuity of teaching.

Scheduling

It is better to plan for shorter, more frequent teaching sessions than for one or two longer sessions. Short sessions allow patients to digest the new material and prevent them from becoming too tired or uncomfortable because of a health problem. Sessions of 15 to 30 minutes are generally well tol-

erated. Usually, more formal classroom programs last for more than 1 hour. In such cases, the nurse should provide breaks after every 50 minutes of class time. The patient should be included in planning for the time and frequency of lessons. Scheduling teaching sessions when the patient is least stressed will enhance teaching.

Group Versus Individual Teaching

The nurse must consider several factors when choosing the teaching setting. Some learner outcomes are met more readily in a one-to-one encounter (Fig. 22-3), whereas others are achieved more easily in a group. For example, the outcome "The patient will change the dressing using sterile technique" would be taught and evaluated during a private session with the nurse. The outcome "The patient will discuss feelings about returning home after a heart attack" might be met more easily in a group discussion with other patients.

Formal Versus Informal Teaching

Most nurse–patient interactions can include **informal teaching** by the nurse. These unplanned teaching sessions are often effective because they deal with the patient's immediate learning needs and concerns. Informal teaching might also lead to additional planned, formal sessions. **Formal teaching** is the planned teaching done to fulfill learner outcomes. Both forms are effective when used appropriately.

Implementing

Implementing the teaching plan requires use of interpersonal skills and effective communication techniques. Teaching the patient can be a major part of the working phase of the helping relationship (see Chap. 21). The nurse must continually observe the patient for additional assessment data that could alter the original teaching plan. This requires skill in adapting and reorganizing the teaching plan.

The nurse can promote patient learning by using a warm and accepting approach. The nurse's attitude has more effect on the patient than any other factor (Fig. 22-4). The nurse must avoid taking a condescending attitude and should not use technical and medical terms (unless the patient has a background

---

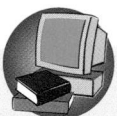

Research in Nursing Making a Difference
Promoting Active Roles in Health Education

Advances in scientific knowledge and related health information and sharp decreases in the amount of time available for one-on-one health education are making it imperative for patients and the public to assume more independent and active roles in health education.

Related Research

Leaffer, T., & Gonda, B. (2000). The Internet: An underutilized tool in patient education. *Computers in Nursing, 18*(1), 47–52.

   This two-stage pilot study involved 100 senior citizens who received instruction on how to conduct health information searches

on the Internet. The goals were to enable the seniors to assume an active role in their healthcare and to share their information with family and friends. The study results reveal a positive effect of the training on senior trainee confidence in using the computer and the Internet, conducting health information searches online, and sharing information with their physicians, families, and friends. Two thirds of the research subjects who searched for health information on the Internet talked about it with their physicians, with more than half reporting that they were more satisfied with treatment as a result of their searches and subsequent discussion with their physicians.

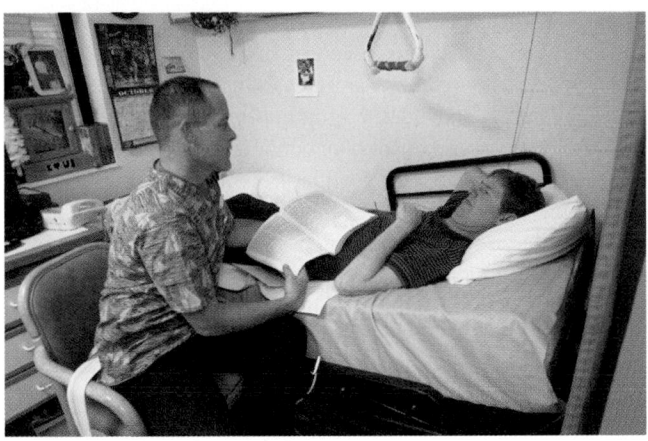

FIGURE 22-3 One-to-one teaching is used in many patient–nurse situations. The nurse must be able to assess whether individual teaching is needed or whether learning can occur in a group.   (Photo by Rick Brady.)

in this area). A nonthreatening teaching–learning atmosphere allows learning to occur.

The physical environment is another important consideration when implementing the teaching plan. Some planning may be needed to ensure adequate space and lighting, comfortable chairs, and good ventilation. Privacy is also important, as is freedom from distractions and interruptions.

In the implementation phase, the patient as a learner has certain role functions. To avoid any misunderstandings, it is helpful to review the contractual agreement before implementing the teaching plan. The patient is expected to listen, observe, and attempt to understand what is being taught.

Some people are uncomfortable in the role of learner; the nurse must assess this problem so that the patient can be assisted to assume the role more easily. If special techniques or procedures must be learned (eg, colostomy care, self-injections, or eye medication instillation), the nurse can assure the patient that it takes time and practice before anyone can perform new skills confidently.

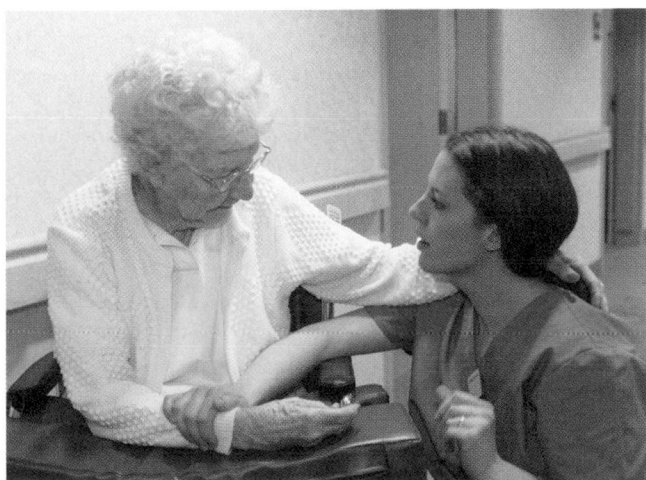

FIGURE 22-4 The nurse's warm approach is an important factor in interpersonal relationships.   (Photo by Rick Brady.)

The nurse must be prepared and organized before implementing the teaching plan. All teaching aids (eg, posters, films, or printed materials) should be gathered and organized before the teaching session. A disorganized teacher distracts the learner and hinders learning. Also, a procedure or skill must be taught in the correct sequence so that the patient does not become confused.

An important nursing responsibility is to make each learning session interesting and enjoyable for the patient. This nurse should have an enthusiastic and positive attitude and can make learning fun by creative use of planned teaching strategies. When the nurse approaches teaching positively, the patient is more likely to approach learning in a similar way.

Evaluating

Evaluating Learning

Nurses cannot be sure that patients have actually learned the content without some type of proof or feedback. The key to evaluation is the learner outcomes in the teaching plan, which describe what behaviors to measure. Methods for obtaining feedback about learning are discussed in the following section.

Methods of Evaluation

There are several methods of evaluation. For instance, cognitive domain learning may be evaluated through oral questioning; affective domain learning through the patient's response; and psychomotor domain learning by a return demonstration. Consider the following learner outcome in the cognitive domain: "The patient will be able to describe what a blood pressure reading represents." To evaluate this, the nurse could say to the patient, "Tell me what this blood pressure reading means to you." The patient then has a chance to talk about the reading while the nurse evaluates the patient's understanding of it.

Sometimes the nurse can use observational skills to determine whether the patient is using the material learned. For example, observing what the patient has ordered for lunch shows the nurse whether dietary lessons are being put into practice. The nurse depends on observation when evaluating the patient's psychomotor skills. The nurse observes the patient's demonstration of any new technique or skill to determine whether it is performed correctly.

The nurse can also use the patient's comments to decide whether learner outcomes have been met. The patient may verbalize his or her understanding of the information while avoiding further discussion of the topic. In such instances, using effective communication techniques when reintroducing the topic at a later time might provide the evaluation data needed.

Asking direct questions is often an efficient method of evaluating learner outcomes. The nurse simply asks the patient a question, and the answer reflects the patient's level of knowledge about a topic. Direct questions can also be used to evaluate the patient's affective learning.

A return demonstration is an excellent way of evaluating psychomotor domain learning (Fig. 22-5). Letting the patient change his or her own dressing, for example, provides the nurse with concrete evidence of satisfactory or unsatisfactory performance of the procedure. However, the nurse must take care to promote a nonstressful environment when the time comes for the patient's return demonstration.

Timing of Evaluation

Evaluation of learning is ongoing. If the nurse merely evaluates learning as soon as teaching is completed, the results may be misleading. Home healthcare nurses may evaluate what the patient learned in the hospital as well as what is being taught during home visits. Hospital nurses often check with family members or significant others after discharge to evaluate whether learner outcomes have been met.

Reinforcing and Celebrating Learning

Most people feel encouraged and supported when their efforts are acknowledged by another person, especially when they trust and value the other person. This is especially true in healthcare, where patients often feel overwhelmed by their illness. Nurses who recognize this dynamic can use **positive reinforcement** to affirm the efforts of patients who have mastered new knowledge, attitudes, or skills. Reinforcement may be as simple as a few words of acknowledgment ("You've mastered this diet quickly"), as spontaneous as a warm hug, or as planned as the entire staff joining to celebrate a patient's independent ambulation. **Negative reinforcement**—criticism or punishment—is generally ineffective; undesirable behavior is usually best ignored. Behavior modification programs that reward desired behaviors and ignore undesired behaviors might be designed for some patients.

Evaluating Teaching

Nurses need to evaluate their teaching to capitalize on their strengths and work on improving weaknesses. Like all nursing roles, effective teaching requires practice and experience. Even nurse educators agree that they are always learning better ways to promote learning. It is important to avoid becoming discouraged when evaluations of one's teaching are less than perfect.

It is best to evaluate one's own teaching effectiveness immediately after a teaching session. This involves a quick review of how well the nurse-teacher feels the plan was implemented. Mentally noting both the strengths and weaknesses of the teaching session helps the nurse plan better for subsequent sessions.

Nurses can also seek feedback from patients. A simple questionnaire can be used at the end of a teaching session or after discharge to gain the patient's perception of the nurse's teaching effectiveness. The questionnaire may be a standardized form used throughout the hospital or agency or one prepared by the nurse-teacher. When using an outcome format that requires only circles or checkmarks as answers, space should be provided for comments.

Revising the Plan

During evaluation, nurses and patients might decide that revisions are needed in the teaching plan. When revising the plan, it is important to identify teaching factors that might have reduced teaching effectiveness (Box 22-14). A reassessment might indicate that some patient factors were not considered in the original plan, and adjustments might be made accordingly to meet the patient's needs. Often, the use of a different teaching strategy is all that is needed for a patient to achieve the learner outcomes.

Revision is a natural part of the teaching–learning process and should not be viewed negatively. Neither the nurse nor the patient has "failed" when an outcome is not met. Most outcomes can be met with a change in approach, although sometimes the learner outcomes are unrealistic. Further assessment by the nurse might reveal that the content might be too complex or the time too short for successful achievement.

Documenting

The nurse is legally responsible for documenting teaching in the patient's record. Documentation of the teaching–learning process includes a summary of the learning need, the plan, the implementation of the plan, and the evaluation results. The

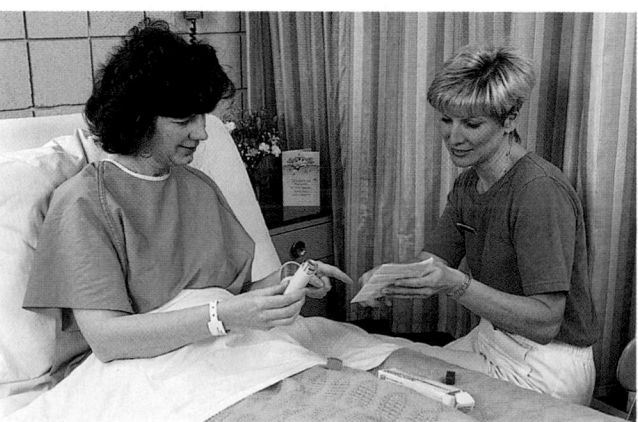

FIGURE 22-5 If the patient can correctly demonstrate what you've taught, you know learning has occurred.   (Photo © B. Proud)

> ### BOX 22-14 **Common Teaching Mistakes**
>
> - Ignoring the restrictions of the patient's environment
> - Failing to accept that patients have the right to change their mind
> - Using medical jargon
> - Failing to negotiate goals
> - Duplicating teaching that other team members have done
> - Overloading the patient with information
> - Choosing the wrong time for teaching
> - Not evaluating what the patient has learned
> - Not reviewing educational media, or relying exclusively on media
> - Failing to document patient teaching and plan for follow-up or teaching reinforcement

evaluative statement is crucial and must show the concrete evidence that demonstrates that learning has occurred. If the desired learning has not occurred, the nurse's notes should indicate how the problem was resolved. It is insufficient to document only what was taught; the charting must show evidence that the patient or significant other has actually learned the material taught. Box 22-15 gives an example of documentation.

THE NURSE AS COUNSELOR

Counseling is the interpersonal process of helping patients to make decisions that promote their overall well-being. Family members or significant others are often included in counseling sessions. Everyone participating must feel comfortable in the situation and surroundings. Like teaching, counseling may be formal or informal.

The interpersonal skills of warmth, friendliness, openness, and empathy are necessary for successful counseling. An effective counselor needs to be a caring individual. Caring is based on a humanistic philosophy (Watson, 1985), which is the core of nursing practice. A humanistic approach to counseling rooted in professional caring helps the patient strive toward the greatest health potential. Caring is important in all nursing roles but is fundamental in the counseling role.

Some advanced-practice psychiatric mental health nurses specialize in counseling, and this form of counseling has an important professional role. The focus in this chapter, however,

is on the everyday counseling that is a basic component of all nurses' practice. This counseling involves listening carefully to the patient's or family's questions, concerns, demands, and complaints and then responding in an effective manner.

> *Consider Rachel Blumenthal, the wife of the patient who had a myocardial infarction. By carefully listening to Mrs. Blumenthal's concerns, including her comment about being embarrassed to ask her husband's cardiologist, the nurse helps to establish a trusting relationship that forms the basis for counseling.*

Appropriate responses might be difficult for the nurse at first, but practice helps develop this skill. Each nurse–patient (or nurse–family) interaction is unique; a nursing response that works well with one patient might intimidate or anger another. Sensitivity to the unique needs of each patient and a willingness to get involved and make a difference are essential for effective counseling.

Table 22-1 presents typical counseling situations you might experience in your first year of nursing and analyzes both effective and ineffective nursing responses. You might want to role-play these situations with a friend. Nurses who wish to succeed as caregivers and counselors need to master the communication techniques described in Chapter 21.

In counseling situations, the nurse does not tell the patient what to do to solve the problem but instead assists and guides to solve problems and make decisions. If the patient lacks the knowledge and skills to approach a problem systematically, the nurse combines the teaching and counseling roles to help the patient solve the dilemma successfully. Box 22-16 highlights an award-winning patient education program for reducing cardiovascular risk and notes the counseling steps that the interdisciplinary team takes when promoting these lifestyle changes (Chu Lai & Cohen, 1999).

The nursing process is an essential tool for the nurse when guiding and teaching patients. Nurses are educated to approach all nursing situations in a logical, systematic way. In a crisis situation, whether minor or major, nurses can share their problem-solving abilities with patients. The nursing process is used to organize the nurse–patient counseling situation described in Box 22-17. Examples of NANDA-approved nursing diagnoses for which counseling may be indicated are included in the accompanying box.

Types of Counseling

Counseling may be situational, developmental, or motivational, and short term or long term.

Short-Term Counseling

Short-term counseling focuses on the immediate problem or concern of the patient or family. It can be a relatively minor concern or a major crisis, but in any case, it needs immediate attention (Fig. 22-6). Short-term counseling might be used dur-

---

BOX 22-15 Documentation Using a Problem-Oriented Progress Note to Meet a Learning Need

1/3/06   #2   **New Problem—High Risk for Impaired Skin Integrity: Nipples**

S Patient stated that her nipples were sore during and after her newborn's first feeding

O First day postpartum; patient is fair skinned with freckles; no reddened areas, no cracking yet; no nipple preparation before delivery

A At high risk for cracked, open areas; patient lacks experience and knowledge of preventive measures

P Reinforce teaching plan for nipple care

I Teaching plan implemented

E Patient able to meet all of the objectives satisfactorily as recorded on the teaching plan; she is currently doing protective and preparatory care for her nipples; when breastfeeding, she uses the correct feeding technique with good aftercare; she states that her nipples are no longer sore, and she is able to explain what she should do when she goes home

R None needed, but reinforcement of content will be continued

—*L. Sweeney, RN*

TABLE 22-1 Analysis of Nursing Responses in Common Counseling Situations

Ineffective Response	Analysis	Effective Response	Analysis
Situation A: You walk into the room of Ms. Goldstein, who learned earlier in the day that her tumor is malignant. She is crying.			
"Oh cheer up! Tomorrow's got to be a brighter day."	Provides false reassurance; communicates insensitivity to patient's feelings	Touch forearm and sit next to her quietly. After several minutes, say, "I can't even begin to imagine how difficult this must be for you. Please let me know if there is anything I can do to help."	Uses touch, silence, and caring appropriately
Situation B: You have been teaching 60-year-old Mr. Hyong diabetic self-care for 4 days, and he is still asking the same questions and refusing to administer his own insulin or check his blood sugar.			
"Well, I guess we are getting nowhere here. Is there anyone else who might be able to do this for you?"	Rejects patient without first evaluating the teaching plan and exploring patient variables that might be hindering learning	"We may have a bit of a problem here. . . . I hear you asking the same questions every day. Let's see if together we can figure out why this isn't making sense to you."	Enlists patient in problem solving
Situation C: One morning you walk into the room of an older resident who had withdrawn and become totally dependent on the nurses for basic care on her transfer into the nursing home. You are surprised to discover that she has washed and dressed herself—for the first time.			
"Well, I'm happy to see that you have rejoined the ranks of the living. Did you wash off your glasses?"	Misses opportunity to celebrate the resident's achievement of an important goal	Hugs resident warmly, looks her in the eye, and exclaims, "Don't you look wonderful today? What are you celebrating?" Defers an assessment of how thorough the morning care has been until later.	Rejoices spontaneously in the resident's achievement and reinforces this behavior. Gives the resident a reason to continue to make progress. Uses touch appropriately
Situation D: You are helping Mr. Stein out of bed; he has been on bed rest for 2 weeks because of a painful and debilitating illness. A fiercely independent man, he is embarrassed to need your support and looks disgusted with himself when he steps on your foot.			
"What's the problem, Honey? Haven't been eating your Wheaties?"	Uses terms of endearment, which often denote disrespect and condescension to patients, no matter in what spirit they are uttered	"No problem, Mr. Stein, my husband steps on my toes all the time when we go dancing!" After a few minutes . . . "It must be hard when you are used to doing everything for yourself to all of the sudden find yourself needing others for simple things . . . ?"	Uses humor and empathy appropriately; invites the patient to share his feelings
Situation E: Ms. Berretta recently underwent surgery resulting in a urinary diversion. She should be able to change her own ostomy bag by this time, but she is still unwilling to look at the stoma, and participate alone in her care. The nurses are getting impatient with her "childish" refusals to learn.			
"Really Helen, I'll do it myself but you'll be the loser once you get home with this thing and there's no one around to help."	Uses a threat in an attempt to coerce learning (negative reinforcement). Displays unwillingness to explore what is blocking Ms. Berretta's readiness to learn	Before beginning Ms. Berretta's care: "I think we need to talk before your treatment today. You will be discharged soon, and I want you to feel confident about caring for your stoma. I understand that until you can accept it, you don't want to learn anything about it. Would you like to talk about this with me, or would you prefer me to make a referral to someone else?"	Communicates respect for patient and sensitivity to her needs, without ignoring what is a real problem. Offers the possibility of a referral to another healthcare professional if the patient so wishes

---

BOX 22-16 **Promoting Lifestyle Changes**

Helping Patients Through the Stages of Change
Matching behavior-modification strategies to the stage of behavior change can facilitate patients' progress from one stage to the next and enhance long-term maintenance of new, healthier behaviors.

Stage: Precontemplation
Counseling Steps:
• Recommend lifestyle change; for example, walking 30 minutes daily as a goal.
• Provide personalized information, focusing on the patient's condition.

Stage: Contemplation
Counseling Steps:
• Identify patient willingness to change within the next 6 months.
• Discuss risks and benefits of behavior change to health. For example, patients may view possible weight gain with smoking cessation as a risk of behavior change.
• Examine barriers to change and past attempts to modify behavior.
• Explore the motivations that would keep the patient focused on changing behavior.
• Explain alternative means of achieving the behavioral goal; for example, using relaxation breathing rather than walking to help lower blood pressure.
• Provide self-help information materials, such as lists of low-fat foods.
• Refer to other resources for help, such as social support groups, psychiatric counseling, or a social worker.

Stage: Action
Counseling Steps:
• Set a date to start behavior modification.
• Outline concrete plans and develop strategies to integrate new behavior into current activities of daily living.
• Discuss potential problems and barriers based on past experiences or current obstacles.
• Investigate strategies to overcome barriers.
• Negotiate an achievable plan, allowing patients to set small intermediate goals.
• Review how to use social and professional support systems.
• Discuss potential for behavior relapse, emphasizing that it is not a personal failure, but a learning experience.

Stage: Maintenance
Counseling Steps:
• Examine parts of the plan that were helpful; identify potential and current problems.
• Revise plans and reset goals if necessary.
• Establish a schedule for periodic contact and follow-up.

Stage: Relapse
Counseling Steps:
• Identify triggers for relapse and barriers that prevented behavior maintenance.
• Discuss and reevaluate motivation to change behaviors, allowing patients to redevelop strategies to overcome barriers.
• Revisit counseling steps for precontemplation and contemplation stages, including additional referrals.

From Chu Lai, S., & Cohen, M. N. (1999). Promoting lifestyle changes. *American Journal of Nursing 99*(4), 66.

---

ing a **situational crisis,** which occurs when a patient faces an event or situation that causes a disruption in life. For example, a male patient in the hospital finds out that his wife has been involved in a car accident; she received only a few scratches, but their only car was demolished. The nurse is in an excellent position to help the patient decide what can be done to solve this situational crisis. The nurse can guide the patient to resources to help solve the travel, financial, and emotional difficulties that arise as a result of the accident. This holistic approach is especially important because the crisis could hinder the patient's recovery.

Long-Term Counseling

Long-term counseling extends over a prolonged period. A patient might need the counsel of the nurse at daily, weekly, or monthly intervals. A patient experiencing a developmental crisis, for example, might need long-term counseling. A **developmental crisis** can occur when a person is going through a developmental stage or passage. For example, many women going through menopause need the assistance of a nurse when adjusting to the changes they experience. Nurses may also lead support groups for group counseling.

Motivational Counseling

Motivational counseling involves discussing feelings and incentives with the patient. Nurses often become frustrated because their patients do not seem to want to get better or to learn how to care for themselves. Perhaps some patients do not have the inner drive or motivation to cooperate in their own healthcare. Some patients say, "I have nothing to live for." A nurse who has established a helping relationship with the patient can help him or her work through these feelings of despair. The nurse might be able to get the patient to talk about what is generating his or her lack of interest in recovery. If a problem is identified, the nurse and patient can use the problem-solving technique to work toward an acceptable solution.

If a patient is unwilling to participate in learning activities, the nurse can assess any factors from the past or present that might be decreasing his or her motivation for learning. Sometimes, if the nurse explains the need for certain knowledge and the consequences of not learning the material, the patient will become more receptive to the teaching–learning process. A trial learning session can be suggested to allow the patient to see what the sessions will be like. If the nurse uses the nursing process approach for counseling, the patient might become more motivated.

BOX 22-17 An Example of Problem Solving That Follows the Nursing Process

Situation

Monday, 7:30 p.m., Amy Purcell has been admitted to the children's unit with dehydration resulting from diarrhea. Amy is responding well to intravenous (IV) fluids. Her mother is visibly distraught.

Assessing

Amy is doing well but will need 24 hours of IV therapy.

Amy and her twin sister Susan have never been separated from their parents or each other. They are 2 years old.

Ms. Purcell has no idea who will care for Susan when Mr. Purcell goes to work in the morning.

The Purcells have no regular childcare arrangements and have no family members in the area.

Ms. Purcell wants to stay with Amy during her hospitalization.

The Purcells' neighbor is home during the day. Sometimes Amy and Susan play at her house.

There is a day care center near their home, but Susan might be upset about going there. It's also expensive.

Mr. Purcell cannot afford to take Tuesday off but will take Wednesday morning off.

Insurance does not cover a private room, which would allow Susan to come to stay in the hospital too.

Diagnosing

Anxiety related to stress of daughter's hospitalization, need for childcare for Susan, and uncertain resources.

Planning Goal

Ms. Purcell will demonstrate decreased anxiety over the care of Susan during Amy's hospitalization.

Together, Ms. Purcell and the nurse have planned the following:

- The neighbor will come to the Purcell home to care for Susan when Mr. Purcell leaves for work on Tuesday morning.
- The neighbor will bring Susan to the hospital for the afternoon visiting hours to be with Ms. Purcell and Amy.
- Mr. Purcell will come to the hospital after work to have dinner with the family.
- Mr. Purcell will take Susan home for bedtime.
- On Wednesday morning, Mr. Purcell will take off work in the morning. He and Susan will go to the hospital to pick up Ms. Purcell and Amy.

Implementing

Plan implemented by the Purcells with support of the nursing staff.

Evaluating

Ms. Purcell told the nurse that she feels that both Amy and Susan did well with the care they received from their parents. The family's stress was minimized, and she is relieved that everything went so well. The nurse decides that the goals were met.

Examples of NANDA Nursing Diagnoses | Counseling Needs

Nursing Diagnoses	Related Factors
Anxiety	Change in health status
Compromised Family Coping	Prolonged disability progression that is exhausting the caregiving capacity of family members
Decisional Conflict	Inability to authorize withdrawal of life-sustaining treatment in spite of believing this to be in the patient's best interests
Disturbed Body Image	Amputation of left leg
Dysfunctional Grieving	Inability to accept child's impending death
Fear	Strangeness of modern US hospital environment and language barrier
Health Seeking Behavior (specify)	Developmental challenge (menopause)
Hopelessness	Progression of debilitating symptoms and belief that "even God has abandoned me"
Impaired Adjustment	Absence of social support for new lifestyle changes
Impaired Parenting	High number of closely spaced pregnancies and absent social supports
Impaired Social Interaction	Communication barriers
Ineffective Role Performance	History of substance abuse and mental illness
Ineffective Denial	Refusal to acknowledge substance abuse problems
Ineffective Coping	High degree of threat and poor concentration, fatigue
Situational Low Self-Esteem	Recent lay-off and divorce
Powerlessness	Lifestyle of helplessness
Social Isolation	Inability to engage in satisfying personal relationships
Spiritual Distress	Challenged belief and value system

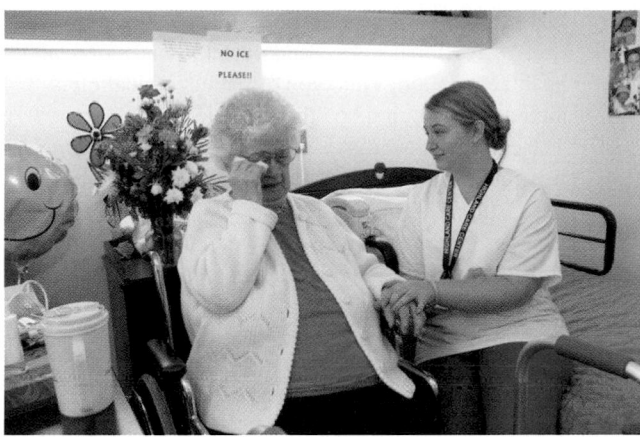

FIGURE 22-6 Counseling may involve a concern that needs immediate attention.   (Photo by Rick Brady.)

When assessing a motivational problem, the nurse must consider the patient's cultural values. Often the way a person feels about something is strongly influenced by his or her cultural background. For instance, if a person has grown up in a family in which illness is perceived as an inevitable result of aging, it will be difficult to motivate that person to practice preventive measures for health (see Chap. 3, Culture and Ethnicity). These problems seem insurmountable, yet a caring nurse can work toward helping the patient become interested in promoting his or her own health. When discouraged, the nurse can confer with a colleague to help solve patient-centered problems.

Referrals

Sometimes a patient needs specialized counseling by nurses with advanced training or by other healthcare professionals. In these cases, the nurse should offer to refer the patient to the appropriate professional (eg, psychiatric or mental health nurse, psychologist or psychiatrist, social worker, clergy, financial counselor, sex therapist, or occupational therapist). In other cases, a simple referral to a community resource, such as a neighborhood support group, may be all the patient needs. When making a referral, be sure to address any barriers that might prevent the patient from acting on the referral. Patients might fail to follow up with a referral for financial reasons, because they do not understand the reason for or value the referral, because they lack transportation, or because the agency is not open at times when they are free.

■ Developing Critical Thinking Skills

1. Explain what is meant by the following statement: "It is as important for patients to understand and value the proposed treatment regimen as it is for them to understand how to implement the proposed regimen." What are the implications of this for teaching and counseling?
2. A patient your age has just learned that she has tested positive for the human immunodeficiency virus. Make a list of some of the learning (cognitive, psychomotor, and affective) that you think should take place. What sorts of things might affect her readiness to learn? How would you tailor your nursing in response to these variables?
3. Mrs. Riley is being readmitted to your hospital unit with complications related to her diabetes. A coworker voices her frustrations and says, "We've taught her everything she needs to know to do a better job of managing her diabetes. I don't know what more we can do." How do you respond?

■ Practicing for NCLEX

1. Noncompliance with a therapeutic regimen can be a significant problem for elderly people. One of the common reasons for noncompliance in the elderly is:
   a. Lack of time
   b. Religious practice
   c. Childlike behavior
   d. Inadequate financial resources
2. A nurse is preparing to teach a 45-year-old patient with asthma how to use his inhaler. One of the best methods to teach the patient this skill is by:
   a. Demonstration
   b. Lecture
   c. Discussion
   d. Panel session
3. A nurse has taught a diabetic patient how to administer his daily insulin. The nurse should evaluate the teaching learning process by:
   a. Determining the patient's motivation to learn
   b. Deciding if the learning outcomes have been achieved
   c. Allowing the patient to practice the skill he has just learned
   d. Documenting the teaching session in the patient's medical record
4. A nurse is using the health belief model to assess a patient. Using this model, the nurse should begin to understand:
   a. Which clinical and financial resources the patient requires to improve his lifestyle
   b. What motivates the patient to learn new behaviors
   c. The effects the health delivery system has on the patient's health patterns
   d. Whether the patient is willing to take actions to support health
5. Nurses play a vital role in patient teaching because of their:
   a. Need for self-actualization
   b. Expertise in healthcare
   c. Desire to help others
   d. Ability to provide illness care
6. A nurse instructs a group of parents about how to make their home safe for their toddlers. This is an example of teaching aimed toward:
   a. Restoring health
   b. Facilitating coping

c. Preventing illness

d. Promoting health

7. When preparing a health promotion program for patients in an adult day care center, the first step the nurse must take is to:

a. Develop learning outcomes

b. Develop a teaching plan

c. Assess the patients' learning needs and learning readiness

d. Diagnose the patients' learning needs

8. When using facts from the patient's medical record as part of the necessary information to assess learning needs, the nurse is using which type of data source?

a. Primary

b. Historic

c. Secondary

d. Hospital-owned

9. The primary purpose of a contractual agreement between nurses and patients when beginning a teaching plan is to:

a. Create a formal and legal bond between the nurse and patient

b. Motivate both the patient and nurse to do what is necessary to meet the patient's learning outcomes

c. Outline the patient's learning outcomes

d. Limit the scope of the teaching session

10. One of the best ways to affirm the efforts of patients who master new knowledge, attitudes, or skills is through:

a. Dialog and discussion

b. A grading scale

c. Positive reinforcement

d. Encouraging the family to learn with the patient

■ Answers with Rationale

1. The correct answer is *d*. Noncompliance is often associated with patient confusion, disappointment, misunderstanding, fear, or inadequate finances.

2. The correct answer is *a*. Demonstration of techniques, procedures, exercises, and the use of special equipment is an effective patient teaching strategy.

3. The correct answer is *b*. The nurse cannot assume that the patient has actually learned the content unless there is some type of proof of learning. The key to evaluation is meeting the learner outcomes stated in the teaching plan.

4. The correct answer is *d*. The health belief model is designed to explain why persons are willing to take action to support their health.

5. The correct answer is *b*. Nurses who are skilled educators and counselors can improve patients' health and well-being. This is a function of their education and experience and their use of cognitive, technical, interpersonal, and ethical/legal skills.

6. The correct answer is *c*. Thorough assessment of the patients' learning needs may reveal the need for vehic-

ular safety, home safety, domestic-violence recognition, recreational safety, and occupational safety and health education. This type of patient education is aimed at enhancing health-protecting behaviors.

7. The correct answer is *c*. The first step of the teaching–learning process is to assess the patient's learning needs and learning readiness.

8. The correct answer is *c*. Past and current patient medical records are considered secondary sources of information and can provide a history of medical problems as well as documentation of nursing assessments, diagnoses, and interventions.

9. The correct answer is *b*. A contractual agreement is a pact two people make setting out mutually agreed-on goals.

10. The correct answer is *c*. People feel encouraged and supported when their efforts are acknowledged by another person, especially when they trust and value that other person.

Bibliography

Abbott, S. (1998). The benefits of patient education. *Gastroenterology Nursing, 21*(5), 207–209.

American Nurses Association. (1994). *The scope of practice for nursing informatics.* Washington, DC: Author.

Aquilera, D. C. (1994). *Crisis intervention: Theory and methodology* (7th ed.). St. Louis: Mosby–Year Book.

Archbold, P. G., et al. (1995). The PREP system of nursing intervention: A pilot test with families caring for older members. *Research in Nursing and Health, 18*(1), 3–16.

Armstrong, M. (1989). Orchestrating the process of patient education: Methods and approaches. *Nursing Clinics of North America, 24*(3), 597–604.

Babcock, D. E., & Miller, M. A. (1994). *Patient education: Theory and practice.* St. Louis: C. V. Mosby.

Bailey, K., Hoeppner, M., Jeska, S., Schneller, S., & Wolohan, C. (1995). The nurse as an educator. *Journal of Nursing Staff Development, 11*(4), 205–209.

Barnes, L. P. (1994). Useful tools in patient teaching: Interviewing skills. *MCN, 19*(5), 289.

Black, K. (1983). *Short-term counseling: A humanistic approach for the helping professions.* Menlo Park, CA: Addison-Wesley.

Bloom, B. S. (1956). *Taxonomy of educational objectives: The classification of educational goals.* New York: David McKay.

Bolwell, C. (1993). *Directory of education software for nursing* (5th ed.). New York: National League for Nursing; Athens, OH: Fuld Institute for Technology in Nursing Education.

Brazen, L., & Roth, R. A. (1995). Using learning style preferences for perioperative clinical education. *AORN Journal, 61*(1), 189, 191–195.

Canobbio, M. M. (1996). *Mosby's handbook of patient teaching.* St. Louis: C. V. Mosby.

Chu Lai, S., & Cohen, M. N. (1999). Promoting lifestyle changes. *American Journal of Nursing, 99*(4), 63–67.

Cordell, B., & Smith-Blair, N. (1994). Streamlined charting for patient education. *Nursing, 24*(1), 57–59.

Dellasega, C., Clark, D., McCreary, D., Schan, P., & Helmuth, A. (1994). Nursing process: Teaching elderly patients. *Journal of Gerontological Nursing, 20*(1), 31–41.

Doak, C. C., Doak, L. G., & Root, J. H. (1995). *Teaching patients with low literacy skills.* Philadelphia: J. B. Lippincott.

Elliot, L., & Kulwicki, G. (1993). Improving patient education documentation. *Nursing Management, 24*(10), 61–62.

Farthing, M. (1994). Health education needs of a Hutterite colony. *The Canadian Nurse, 90*(7), 20–26.

Freda, M. (1997). Cultural competence in patient education. *American Journal of Maternal/Child Nursing, 22*(4), 219–220.

Funnell, M. (2000, March). Helping patients take charge of their chronic illnesses. *Family Practice Management* (Electronic version). Available at: http://www.aafp.org.

Griffiths, M. (1995). Patient education needs: Opinions of oncology nurses and their patients. *Oncology Nursing Forum, 22*(1), 139–144.

Habel, M. (2002, July). *Patient education: Helping families take charge of their health.* Available at: http://www.nurseweek.com.

Hannah, K. J., Ball, M. J., & Edwards, M. J. A. (1994). *Introduction to nursing informatics.* New York: Springer-Verlag.

Hansen, M., & Fisher, J. (1998). Patient-centered teaching from theory to practice. *American Journal of Nursing, 98*(1), 56–60.

Harvey, C., Dixon, M., & Padberg, N. (1995). Support group for families of trauma patients: A unique approach. *Critical Care Nurse, 15*(4), 59–63.

Hussey, L. C. (1994). Minimizing effects of low literacy on medication knowledge and compliance among the elderly. *Clinical Nursing Research, 3*(2), 132–145.

Jabeck, M. E. (1994). Teaching the elderly: A commonsense approach. *Nursing, 24*(5), 70–71.

Jacono, B., & Jacono, J. (1995). The impact of teacher characteristics on teaching. *Journal of Nursing Staff Development, 11*(3), 146–149.

Katz, J. (1997). Back to basics: Providing effective patient teaching. *American Journal of Nursing, 97*(5), 33–36.

Kelly, P. (1992). Counseling patients with HIV. *RN, 55*(2), 54–58.

Knowles, M. S. (1990). *The adult learner: A neglected species* (4th ed.). Houston: Gulf Publishing.

Leaffer, T., & Gonda, B. (2000). The Internet: An underutilized tool in patient education. *Computers in Nursing, 18*(1), 47–52.

Lindberg, C. E. (1995). Perinatal transmission of HIV: How to counsel women. *MCN, 20*(4), 207–212.

Lorig, K. (1992). *Patient education: A practical approach.* St. Louis: Mosby–Year Book.

Melnyle, B. M. (1994). Coping with unplanned childhood hospitalization: Effects of informational intervention on mother and children. *Nursing Research, 43*(1), 50–55.

Miller, B. (1994). Determination of reading comprehension level for effective patient health education materials. *Nursing Research, 43*(2), 118–119.

National Institute for Literacy. 2003. Available at: http://www.nifl.gov.

Newbold, S. K. (1996). Maximizing technology for cost effective staff education and training. In B. R. Heller, M. E. Mills, & C. A. Romano (Eds.), *Information management in nursing and health care.* Springhouse, PA: Springhouse.

Nobel, C. (1991). Are nurses good patient educators? *Journal of Advanced Nursing, 16*(10), 1185–1189.

Price, J. L., & Cordell, B. (1994). Cultural diversity and patient teaching. *Journal of Continuing Education in Nursing, 25*(4), 163–166.

Rankin, S. H., & Stallings, K. D. (1990). *Patient education* (2nd ed.). Philadelphia: J. B. Lippincott.

Redman, B. K. (1992). *The process of patient education* (7th ed.). St. Louis: C. V. Mosby.

Reele, B. L. (1994). Effect of counseling on quality of life for individuals with cancer and their families. *Cancer Nursing, 17*(2), 101–112.

Rosenstock, I. (1974). Historical origins of the health belief model. *Health Education Monograph, 2,* 354.

Ruppert, R. A. (1996). Caring for the lay caregiver. *American Journal of Nursing, 96*(3), 40–45.

Schoenly, L. (1994). Teaching in the affective domain. *Journal of Continuing Education in Nursing, 25*(5), 209–212.

Sciartelli, C. H. (1995). Using a clinical pathway approach to document patient teaching for breast cancer surgical procedures. *Oncology Nursing Forum, 22*(1), 139–144.

Seley, J. (1994). Ten strategies for successful patient teaching. *American Journal of Nursing, 94*(11), 63–65.

Sitzer, C. R. (1995). A community-based breast cancer education and screening program for elderly women. *Geriatric Nursing, 16*(4), 151–154.

Vanetzian, E. (1997). Learning readiness for patient teaching in stroke rehabilitation. *Journal of Advanced Nursing, 26*(3), 589–594.

Wagner, J. (2003). Patient education: Teaching older adults. *Advance News Magazine.* Available at: http://www.advancesfornurses.com.

Wally, B. (1994). Reading, writing and health. *Canadian Nurse, 90*(2), 29–32.

Watson, J. (1985). *Nursing: The philosophy and science of caring.* Denver: Colorado University Press.

Weaver, J. (1995). Patient education: An innovative computer approach. *Nursing Management, 26*(7), 78–83.

Weinrich, S. P., & Boyd, M. (1992). Education in the elderly: Adapting and evaluating teaching tools. *Journal of Gerontological Nursing, 18*(1), 15–20.

Wong, M. (1992). Self-care instructions: Do patients understand educational materials? *Focus on Critical Care, 19*(2), 47–49.

Leader and Manager

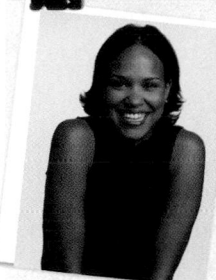

Rehema Kohls is a college sophomore who comes to the healthcare center requesting information about sexually transmitted diseases (STDs). During the visit, she says, "So many of my friends are concerned about STDs. They all say we should start a group on campus to discuss this problem, and they want me to set it up and be the leader. But I wouldn't know where to start or what to do!"

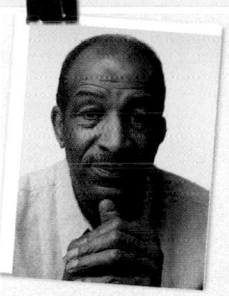

Stephen Wall, a 65-year-old widower who lives alone, is admitted to the intensive care unit after an automobile accident in which he sustained trauma to the head, chest, abdomen, and lower extremities. He is being monitored continuously via numerous invasive devices and requires complex care. His closest family member, a 40-year-old son, lives approximately 75 miles away.

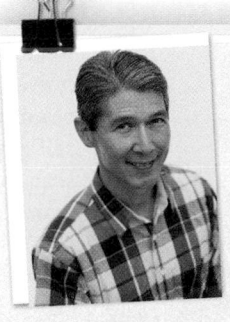

Jack Camp, a middle-aged single man with a history of diabetes mellitus, is receiving care for a compound fracture of his left lower extremity being treated with an external fixator. Compliance with his diabetic therapy regimen is questionable; he states, "I really love my sweets!" The patient frequently voices loud complaints about his room, the food, and the hospital routine. He also uses his call light very frequently, stating, "I just want to see if it's working and if the nurses will come check on me."

Focusing on Blended Skills

The types of blended skills you'll need to respond to the case scenarios include:

Cognitive Skills

- Basic knowledge of leadership and management theory
- Knowledge of leadership dynamics, including the types of power and ability to apply power appropriately
- Knowledge of leadership qualities
- Ability to identify personal leadership skills appropriately and apply personal leadership skills to a variety of patient situations
- Knowledge of leadership styles
- Knowledge of the culture and authority relationships in the hospital, on the unit, and in other patient care settings
- Knowledge of change theory and who can be of assistance when a workplace issue arises
- Knowledge of oneself

Technical Skills

- Ability to demonstrate appropriate leadership styles in different patient situations, such as with a college student, a critically ill older adult, and a demanding, boisterous patient
- Ability to implement activities and procedures to effect change
- Demonstration of effective time management skills

Interpersonal Skills

- Strong people skills; ability to communicate and interact effectively with nurse managers, coworkers, other members of the healthcare team, and the public
- Confidence in personal abilities, with the willingness to seek help when needed
- Knowledge of, and respect for, the challenge of both managers and clinicians in complex, contemporary healthcare organizations
- Ability to work as part of a multidisciplinary team

Ethical and Legal Skills

- Strong sense of responsibility and accountability for personal professional maturation
- Knowledge of and respect for your rights as a worker
- Ability to document leadership and management interventions in a legally prudent and defensible manner
- Ability to provide leadership and management based on sound ethical principles

Learning Outcomes

After completing this chapter, the learner should be able to accomplish the following:

1. Identify the qualities, four skills, and differing styles of leaders.
2. List the four managerial functions.
3. Summarize the steps in the process of change.
4. Describe areas in which beginning nurses can develop leadership skills that enhance the caregiver role.

Key Terms

autocratic leadership
change
decentralized decision-making process
democratic leadership
explicit power
implied power
laissez-faire leadership
leadership
management
planned change
power
quantum leadership
self-governance
situational leadership
transformational leadership

Many changes in society are affecting the provision of healthcare services to populations of varying needs. Currently healthcare providers are experiencing changes such as fiscal constraints, workforce shortages, sophisticated healthcare consumers, and technological/pharmacological advances. Never before has there been such a need for nurses to work competently and collaboratively with other healthcare professionals to secure cost-effective, high-quality healthcare for all. Never before has it been more important for nursing as a profession to be self-directed as it charts its future. To do all this successfully, nurses must be familiar with the healthcare organization in which they are employed, as well as the healthcare system at large. Although nurses might assume leadership roles by virtue of their positions, they become effective leaders by understanding the complexities of coordinating care, remaining open to differing points of view, and understanding the interdependency of the entire healthcare team. (See the accompanying Reflective Practice box for an example.)

This chapter explores the concept of leadership. It takes time and experience to develop leadership skills, but beginning nurses can begin developing leadership skills and monitoring their progress.

LEADERSHIP DYNAMICS

The concept of leadership is one of the most researched, studied, and debated fields of inquiry. Paradoxically, it is at the same time clear and vivid, and elusive and subtle. **Leadership** has been described as the ability to direct or motivate an individual or group to achieve set goals. Effective leaders in groups or systems do this by encouraging others to be their best selves as they work collaboratively in the pursuit of common organizational or unit goals. Leaders have power, whether it is explicit or implied. For example, an elected class leader has **explicit power** by virtue of his or her position. However, a stu-

Reflective Practice
Challenge to Ethical Skills

While in a clinical rotation my junior year, I was assigned the dreaded Jack Camp (I still remember his name). He was a middle-aged single man receiving care for a compound fracture of his left lower extremity being treated with an external fixator. He had a bad case of diabetes, and an even worse sweet tooth. Before I even met him, the nurses on the floor were saying things like "good luck," which made this junior nursing student extra paranoid (although I was grateful for the warning). The patient was known for voicing loud complaints about his room, the food, and the hospital routine. He also was using his call light very frequently. The nurses called him names and discussed their dislike of him in the nurses' station, which was in the center of the unit.

As the day progressed, I found out that all this patient wanted was some attention, because he was used to running things in his business. I actually found him entertaining.

Thinking Outside the Box: Possible Courses of Action

- Ignore the comments of the other nurses on the floor, hoping that no one else heard them.
- Report the nurses to my clinical instructor, possibly causing tension on the floor.
- Politely tell the nurses to keep it down and refrain from talking about the patient, risking my own comfort level; after all, I am only a visiting student—what do I know?

Evaluating a Good Outcome: How Do I Define Success?

- Act as a patient advocate despite my limited power, which means correcting unethical behaviors as cordially as possible.
- Have the courage to go to the next level if the nurses' behavior is not corrected.
- Inform the patient politely to modify his behavior.

Personal Learning: Here's to the Future!

My response was to ignore the nurses' comments and hope no one else heard them either. I was not courageous enough to be the patient advocate that we had been taught to be. I knew my response should have been to ask them to keep it down, which would allow them to maintain their personal opinions while at the same time keeping the comments from jeopardizing patient confidentiality. From this experience, I learned that you have to be a leader, speak up, and take the risk. Part of that means being able to go against the group, risking being ostracized. In doing so, others may follow your lead, but if they choose not to follow, at least you know you advocated for your patient. Since this experience, I have not been in a situation that has challenged my personal ethics, but I have the self-confidence to believe that I can be the leader that I spoke so passionately about.

Reflection

How do you think you would respond in a similar situation? Why? What does this tell you about yourself and about the adequacy of your skills for professional practice? Can you think of other ways to respond? What do you think the outcome might have been if the nursing student did speak up for the patient? Which type of leadership style might have been most effective with this group? What other skills (cognitive, interpersonal, technical, ethical/legal) would you need to respond well in this situation? Propose a plan that might effect a change in this situation. Do you agree with the criteria to evaluate a successful outcome? Would any other criteria be appropriate? If so, please explain.

Kim Gray, Georgetown University

dent in the class who has no designated leadership position might, by force of his or her personality, have more power to influence the class than the designated leader. This is **implied power.**

> *Consider Jack Camp, the patient described in the Reflective Practice scenario. The patient assumed a position of "running things in his business," thus having the explicit power of his position. Based on this, the patient used "implied power" while hospitalized to exert control over his situation. The nurse's understanding of power would be important in developing a plan to deal with the patient's behavior.*

Power to influence a group depends on the person's leadership style and how the person fulfills leadership responsibilities. The dynamics of leadership involve applying that power for personal or organizational growth or change. Nurses who use leadership skills can become proficient in effecting desired changes in many areas, including their patients' health patterns, the healthcare agency, the community, the nursing profession, and the healthcare system in general.

LEADERSHIP QUALITIES

Most people admire a charismatic, dynamic, enthusiastic, visionary leader who is poised, confident, and self-directed. These characteristics define leaders such as Mother Teresa, John Kennedy, Martin Luther King, Gandhi, and others. Not everyone can be as dynamic and inspirational as these individuals were. Yet leaders do need to be comfortable with themselves (ie, have a positive self-image) and present themselves as role models for followers. Ideally, they also have a vision that energizes the group and brings forth the best efforts of members. Critical thinkers and responsible decision makers, they commit high energy to achieving goals and are skilled in enlisting support and cooperation.

Leaders value learning and must be knowledgeable. Nurse leaders and managers cannot be knowledgeable about all aspects of the profession, although we desire this and may place unrealistic expectations upon them. They must be creative in the development and use of scarce resources. They use one another and other healthcare workers as resources, respecting each other's expertise. Contemporary nurse managers draw upon their own staff for clinical and organizational knowledge.

It is increasingly difficult for the nurse manager to be both a clinical and a managerial expert. The explosion of clinical knowledge and expectations for managerial expertise place unrealistic demands on this role. Typical nurse managers are expected to manage their unit budget within prescribed constraints; deliver a high level of quality care to patients on the unit; develop and serve as mentors for junior staff; comply with regulatory requirements, and be experts at human resource management. These are just a few of the responsibilities and demands that our healthcare system has placed upon these individuals. Although the role might seem overwhelming, it can also be quite satisfying to the manager, the staff, and the organization.

Political awareness is also important for nurse leaders. Knowing how to map the political terrain of the workplace is just as valuable as knowing how legislation at the local, state, and national levels affects the healthcare delivery system.

Flexibility is a must for all nursing leaders. All nursing functions and roles require flexibility. The needs of patients, families, and the nursing team can change from minute to minute. A nurse coordinator might plan to involve staff in a discussion about how best to distribute new work responsibilities, but if there are three unexpected new admissions to the unit, the discussion may need to be postponed to a quieter time. Similarly, a visiting nurse might plan to dedicate more time to a dying patient and his wife, but another patient on that day's caseload develops complications that require a longer visit. Flexible, responsive, and caring nurses are welcome leaders and team members.

Leadership potential is present in all nurses.

> *Recall Rehema Kohls, the college sophomore considering starting a campus group on STDs. The nurse would apply knowledge of leadership qualities when helping Rehema to decide about leading the group. In addition, the nurse would demonstrate these qualities when interacting with Rehema.*

With education and practice, these qualities can be developed to the point at which a nurse is skilled in the many behaviors necessary for leadership. A full discussion of all these qualities is beyond the scope of this text, but Box 23-1 summarizes how one might approach the role of leader. Beginning nurses can monitor their progress by periodically reviewing the checklist provided.

PERSONAL LEADERSHIP SKILLS

Four basic skills are needed for nursing leadership. Those listed below are not meant to be all-inclusive, but instead to serve as a basis for development:

- *Communication skills:* the ability to establish trusting interpersonal relationships with patients, peers, subordinates, and superiors to maximize goal achievement and enhance the personal growth of all participants
- *Problem-solving skills:* the ability to analyze all sides of a problem, to suspend judgment, to explore multiple options, and to work toward a creative solution
- *Management skills:* the ability to direct others toward goal achievement; this ability involves the recognition and fostering of unique talents and skills of others and the ability to match these with necessary tasks; organizational skills; financial skills; and the ability to generate and use resources wisely
- *Self-evaluation skills:* the ability to assess honestly one's effectiveness and to accept both praise and criticism; the ability to direct personal professional growth and development

BOX 23-1 Checklist for the Beginning Nurse Who Wishes to Develop Leadership Skills

Basic Attitudes and Skills

Read the statements on the right and circle the appropriate response: (1) rarely characterizes me, (2) sometimes characterizes me, and (3) often characterizes me.

1 2 3   1. I am self-directed. I know what I want and take the necessary steps to get it.

1 2 3   2. I know my strengths and limitations and feel confident with who I am and who I am becoming.

1 2 3   3. I get an idea ("vision") and energize others to help me "make it happen."

1 2 3   4. I coordinate or direct the activities of others, matching their abilities to the necessary task.

1 2 3   5. I think critically about a situation without letting my feelings or those of others bias my analysis.

1 2 3   6. Once I have identified a problem, I work at it until I resolve it—to the extent that this is within my power.

1 2 3   7. When I need help, I know where to find it and ask for it.

1 2 3   8. I recognize and encourage the talents of others and offer sincere compliments.

1 2 3   9. I accept responsibility for my decisions and behavior.

1 2 3   10. I accept compliments and enjoy my success.

1 2 3   11. I confront individuals who are abusing my rights or those of others in my group.

1 2 3   12. I use assertiveness techniques when defending rights.

1 2 3   13. I am flexible and can change direction once I see the value of another course of action.

1 2 3   14. I follow an appropriate chain of command when problem solving.

1 2 3   15. I question how nursing interventions might be improved.

The higher your score the better. Reread the statements where you checked "1" and see how you might plan to improve in these areas.

Beginning Execution of Leadership Role Responsibilities

Read the list of behaviors on the right and check the appropriate box—met or not met.

Met   Not Met

_____ _____ 1. Recognize some personal need you have been ignoring and take steps to ensure that it is met.

_____ _____ 2. Think of some group you belong to (eg, school, work, church, or social) whose members' needs are not being met and plan with other members to tackle the problem.

_____ _____ 3. Recognize the special advocacy needs of a patient you believe is being underserved by the healthcare system. Become an advocate for this patient.

_____ _____ 4. Find a nursing research study that recommends a specific type of care for one of your patients. Implement the recommendation and compare your findings with those of the researchers. Work collaboratively with the interdisciplinary team to implement needed changes.

_____ _____ 5. Join a professional nursing organization and become an active member.

_____ _____ 6. Analyze the media's portrayal of nurses in a specific television program, film, or book. Talk with a friend about how this portrayal of nursing influences your profession. Share your comments with the producer or author.

_____ _____ 7. Contact your legislator to share your views about pending legislation.

_____ _____ 8. Think about leaders you admire and respect; interview current nursing leaders; develop a plan for personal professional growth and development.

_____ _____ 9. Develop a mentoring relationship with a nursing leader.

The last skill is critical, especially as you begin professional practice. The ability to know oneself is the cornerstone of success in either implicit or explicit leadership roles. In a *Harvard Business Review* article, Peter Drucker (1999), a scholar of leadership, wrote that to be successful in our current knowledge culture (of which nursing is a part), one must possess self-knowledge; by so doing, we can place ourselves in positions where we can make the greatest contribution. In terms of nursing leadership roles, this translates into formal authority of position, such as a unit coordinator or director, or a clinical leader without a formal title.

Drucker advocated the personal inquiries described in Box 23-2. The answers to these questions will direct a nurse toward the correct leadership role, the correct organization, or the correct unit.

> *Think back to Rehema Kohls, the college sophomore who is thinking about starting a campus discussion group on STDs. The nurse would incorporate knowledge of Drucker's identified need for self-knowledge and personal inquiries when helping Rehema in making her decision about starting and leading the group.*

LEADERSHIP STYLES

Many different styles of leadership are present in contemporary healthcare settings. The complexity and persistent, rapid change drive many of the leadership styles that you will observe. It is helpful to think of leadership as a behavior, as something one individual does to influence another. This influence takes many forms and requires much creativity, intellect, and savvy. Different styles are applicable in different contexts and with different levels of employees. A few of those styles are explained in the next section. New graduates should carefully choose organizations that match their preferred leadership and management styles.

BOX 23-2 Personal Inquiries for Determining Complementary Leadership Roles and Working Environments

Identify your strengths: Continually improve the things you do best; discover your "intellectual arrogance" (being bright is no substitute for knowledge); work on acquiring the skills and knowledge you need to fully realize your strengths; remedy your bad habits.

Evaluate how you accomplish work: We all work in ways that yield the best results for us. Are you a visual or auditory learner? Do you learn best by reading or writing? Do you work more productively in teams or alone? Are you more productive as a decision maker or as an advisor?

Clarify your values: Working in an organization or on a unit whose value system is unacceptable or incompatible with yours will lead to frustration and poor performance. Identify your values and seek a work environment that is complementary, not adversarial.

Determine where you belong and what you can contribute: In small or large organizations, as a decision maker or as an advisor, prepare for opportunities that emerge in response to these queries. In this dynamic industry, set reasonable short- to medium-range goals.

Assume responsibility for relationships: Cultivate relationships and analyze the differences you may have with others. Know and understand the strengths, performance modes, and values of your coworkers and managers.

Autocratic Leadership

Autocratic leadership, also called directive leadership, involves the leader assuming complete control over the decisions and activities of the group. A nurse with an autocratic personality can be described as "firm, insistent, self-assured, and dominating with or without intent, and keeps at the center of attention" (Douglass, 1995). An extremely autocratic leader might make all decisions for workers or followers without considering the followers' ideas or feelings.

> *Consider Stephen Wall, the 65-year-old patient in the intensive care unit. The nurse would demonstrate autocratic leadership to perform specific care activities and to delegate responsibilities to appropriate personnel.*

Many nurses are used to working under autocratic leaders because this approach has been used in most hospitals until recently. It might have evolved from nursing's historical military and religious past, or from the industrial model of command and control prevalent in many organizations. This style of leadership is gradually being replaced by the democratic style of leadership as nurses demand and receive more say in decision making. However, there are many disciplines and many different levels of professional maturity present in any situation. Some healthcare workers respond best to the directive approach.

Example of Autocratic Leadership

Nurse A discovers that one of her patients is bleeding excessively from his surgical incision. She knows that he needs immediate attention, so she gives specific orders to another team member to attend to the other patients. She tells the registered nurse on her team to call the surgical resident to come as soon as possible. She implements a nursing plan of care to prevent further blood loss or complications. Nurse A assumed the autocratic style of leadership in this situation so that all of the necessary tasks would be accomplished immediately. Although she rarely uses this style, she implemented it effectively in this emergency situation. This example supports the premise that leadership is context dependent.

Democratic Leadership

Democratic leadership, also called participative leadership, is characterized by a sense of equality among the leader and other participants. Decisions and activities are shared. Participants are encouraged to develop their skills and strengths within the group. The group and leader work together to accomplish mutually set goals and outcomes.

> *Recall Stephen Wall, the patient in the intensive care unit. The nurse would use democratic leadership to work collaboratively with other healthcare disciplines to plan the most effective care for the patient. For example, the nurse might need to work with the surgical and neurologic staff, respiratory therapy, physical*

therapy, and social services in developing the patient's plan of care.

Most nurses currently use a democratic style of leadership. As professionals, nurses generally respond well to this style of leadership when they are the followers and feel more comfortable when they are the leaders of democratic groups. Group satisfaction and motivation are excellent benefits of this style.

In 1982, the American Academy of Nursing's Task Force on Nursing Practice in Hospitals conducted a study of 41 hospitals to identify and describe variables that created an environment that attracted and retained well-qualified nurses who promoted quality patient care through providing excellence in nursing services. These institutions were called "magnet" hospitals because they attracted and retained professional nurses who experienced a high degree of professional and personal satisfaction through their practice. These institutions used a decentralized decision-making process, **self-governance** at the unit level, and respect for and acknowledgment of professional autonomy. In 1990 the American Nurses Credentialing Center developed a formal process to recognize excellence in nursing service and to confer "magnet" status (Table 23-1). Research supports that magnet hospitals have better patient outcomes, shorter lengths of stay, higher patient satisfaction, and higher nurse job satisfaction and nurse retention than hospitals without this governance style of leadership (Aiken, 2001). Working in a magnet hospital can maximize the potential of new graduates who prefer democratic leadership.

Example of Democratic Leadership

Nurse B, a head nurse, observes that staff members have not been documenting patient teaching and learning in their progress notes. Nurse B is not sure why this has occurred but believes that this problem must be solved. He calls a staff meeting and leads a discussion to seek information on possible causes and solutions. Nurse B has decided that staff members need to be included in the problem-solving approach. He thinks the staff will be more motivated to document their teaching and the patients' learning if they have a say in what changes in practice are necessary and how the changes will be implemented. Nurse B has used the democratic style of leadership and **decentralized decision-making process** to resolve this issue.

Laissez-Faire Leadership

In **laissez-faire leadership,** also called nondirective leadership, the leader relinquishes power to the group, such that an outsider could not identify the leader in the group. This approach encourages independent activity by group members. This style depends on the strengths of followers to direct the group activities. It is most effective when all staff are clinical experts with a deep understanding of both clinical and administrative processes. This style is rarely useful because task achievement is difficult when each nurse is working independently, and the staff on most units and departments have varying levels of clinical maturity.

> *Consider Stephen Wall, the patient with multiple trauma who is in the intensive care unit. The patient has multiple priority needs, requiring interdependent actions of many individuals. Use of laissez-faire leadership would not be effective in this situation.*

However, it can be used effectively when the leader wants a problem to be solved completely by expert staff group members.

Example of Laissez-Faire Leadership

Nurse C, a clinical coordinator, has read an interesting research study that supports a change in the current instructions being given to new mothers who are breastfeeding. She posts the article with a summary of findings in all the nurses' stations in the maternity unit.

Nurse C is using a laissez-faire leadership style. She is confident that individual staff members are capable professionals who are concerned with keeping up with current research findings that they will use to improve their nursing care.

Transformational Leadership

Transformational leadership can create revolutionary change. Often described as charismatic, these leaders are unique in their ability to inspire and motivate others. They create intellectually stimulating practice environments and challenge themselves and others to grow personally and professionally and to learn. Gifted in creating a common vision, they demonstrate passion for their vision and keep others similarly focused. One

TABLE 23-1 Magnet versus Non-Magnet Hospitals

Magnet Hospitals	Non-Magnet Hospitals
• Self-scheduling	• Centralized decision making
• Autonomous, accountable professional nursing practice	• Practice dominated, and in some instances controlled, by physicians and others
• Healthy, collaborative relationships with physicians	• Higher staff vacancy rates
• Adequate numbers of competent, clinically expert peers	• Higher staff turnover
• Supportive nurse managers	• Higher levels of staff burnout and exodus from the bedside
• Control over practice environment	
• Support and provision for education	

of the unique qualities of transformational leaders is their vulnerability. They communicate honestly and openly and can express emotions as well as ideas as they share themselves with others. They show concern and care for others and are willing to take risks. They pay attention to process as well as outcomes.

Example of Transformational Leadership

Nurse D is troubled by the plight of women and children in the inner city where she lives. She unites with other nurses and healthcare professionals to design and implement strategies to meet their needs. Within 18 months, a nursing center is funded and running, improving maternal-child outcomes in the area. The founding group of healthcare professionals continues to meet monthly to dream about future strategies and to support each other in their work. They are proudest of the improved self-esteem and independence in many of the women they serve.

Situational Leadership

Generally speaking, nurses do best to use the leadership style with which they are most comfortable, if that style is effective for the task at hand and those they lead. The nurse's own personality, the group's personality, and the tasks or objectives to be accomplished should be considered in each leadership situation. **Situational leadership** theory considers the leader's style, the work group's maturity, and the situation at hand to form a comprehensive approach to management style.

For example, although all nurse managers in a healthcare agency might be charged with cutting costs, both the outcomes they target and the processes they use to achieve these outcomes might vary. The unique situations in each unit influence the management style used.

These leadership styles and their related similarities and differences have been used as models of skill development and maturation for most of the past century. Unfortunately, even the most creative of nursing leaders, who combine each of these styles to fit particular scenarios, frequently find they are lacking in depth and unresponsive to contemporary challenges.

Quantum Leadership

Porter-O'Grady and Malloch (2003), in *Quantum Leadership: A Textbook of New Leadership,* argued that leaders must move beyond the traditional modes used by all levels of workers. He, like Drucker (1999) and others, have begun to clarify the impact of the information age, identified at the turn of the last century, upon work and the worker. Vertical command and control structures that generated the leadership styles previously mentioned are no longer useful for managers and workers, nor are they able to yield productivity for organizations. The explosion of information and technology in healthcare, as in other industries, has spawned, by necessity, the "knowledge worker." This social transformation is affecting parts of all of our lives; perhaps most importantly, it is affecting how we lead and manage our organizations.

We are in a difficult transition period between the old and the new. In the old, change was viewed as an entity to be planned, carefully managed, and accepted. In the new "quantum age," change is conceived as dynamic, ever-present, and continually unfolding. We are forced to experience the change at the same time as we perceive it, with little or no opportunity to definitively and laboriously plan and manage it.

Porter-O'Grady and Malloch (2003, p. 11) identified the following characteristics of **quantum leadership** and behaviors of healthcare leaders who must confront this dramatic social transformation:

1. Healthcare leaders must be able to communicate to others their vision of the future and bring energy and commitment to the reformation of the system.
2. They must be relentless communicators, challenging current ways of thinking and doing.
3. They must openly seek critiques of their work.
4. They must encourage all stakeholders to continually examine the appropriateness of current work rituals and routines and determine what should be retained and what should be left behind as no longer relevant.
5. They must raise questions about the efficacy and effectiveness of current work routines and whether they meet new and emerging expectations and reality.

Leaders must model these new behaviors, particularly nursing leaders, who must combine these new attributes with the requisite technical skills.

LEADERSHIP AND MANAGEMENT

All nurses, to the extent that they work with others and influence others to be their best, can become leaders. Some nurses hold positions in the healthcare system that also make them managers. The role of **management** is to plan, organize, direct, and control available human, material, and financial resources to deliver quality care to patients and families. The managerial role is frequently conceptualized as the technical dimension of formal leadership roles. These technical areas of expertise, particularly in the financial or clinical resource management dimension, are mandatory for contemporary nurse managers. A few of their direct responsibilities, identified in a previous section, can be conceptualized into these four traditionally broad areas:

- Planning: identifying problems and developing goals, objectives, and related strategies to meet the demands of the clinical arena
- Organizing: acquiring, managing, and mobilizing resources to meet both clinical and financial objectives
- Directing: leading others in achieving goals within the constraints of the current fiscal and workforce shortage scenarios. This is a demanding task for managers and staff alike.
- Controlling: implementing mechanisms for ongoing evaluation, particularly in areas of clinical quality and financial accountability

Remember Jack Camp, the patient with diabetes and an external fixator. One possible solution to the problem would be to enlist the aid of the nurse manager for this unit to address the problem of the staff's overt criticism of the patient. Using planning, organizing, directing, and controlling, the nurse manager could ultimately create an environment that is conducive to the patient's recovery and health and satisfying to staff caring for this patient.

Nurse managers must be effective leaders to be successful. Nurse managers who cannot create a healthy group environment; who fail to resolve interpersonal issues that lower morale and result in numerous complaints from patients, nurses, and physicians; and who cannot develop a plan to resolve detrimental interpersonal issues lack leadership skills.

Centralized and Decentralized Decision Making

In a centralized management structure, decisions are generally made by senior managers. Those further down in the hierarchy of the organization are often responsible for implementing decisions into which they had little input. In a decentralized management structure, on the other hand, decisions are made by those who are most knowledgeable about the issues being decided. Nurses are thus intimately involved in decisions concerning patient care. Nurse managers are accountable for what happens on their nursing unit, including patient census, staffing, supplies, and budget. A decentralized system invites greater accountability and responsibility because most nurses feel more

responsible for decisions they have made themselves. However, you will most likely experience both modes of decision making, centralization and decentralization, in nursing units. Financial targets and other broad strategic directions are frequently established at executive levels of the organization. Clinical issues, processes of care delivery, clinical outcomes, and unit governance are usually resolved at the unit or department level.

Nursing Care Delivery Models

Models of nursing care delivery systems are highlighted in Box 23-3. Over time, these have evolved from highly technical, industrial-based, assembly-line models to more professional, self-managed, cross-functional methods. According to Kerfoot (1995, p. 41), "As nurses have moved to accept more professional status and the responsibility of delegating and working through others, they have moved into advanced practice models in which there is less supervision, more opportunity for independent thought and creativity, and more accountability." The evolving models of patient care delivery demonstrate that professional nurses will increasingly be expected to have significant managerial competence. For certain, other models will evolve in this quantum age. Perhaps you will be the creator!

Conflict Management

Nurse managers frequently encounter conflict between employees and between themselves and employees. Unresolved conflict can lower morale and threaten quality care. Clements (2003) described five styles for dealing with conflict—avoiding,

---

BOX 23-3 Evolving Models of Nursing Care Delivery . . . Evolving Accountability

Functional nursing	Nurses and other staff are assigned to specific tasks for a group of patients. Based on the assembly-line concept found in industry; specializing tasks increases efficiency but results in impersonal care.
Team nursing	A team made up of a registered nurse and other caregivers provides care to a designated group of patients on a given shift. Modified the depersonalized approach of functional nursing and focused on individual patient care.
Total care or case nursing	A nurse as caregiver provides total care to a group of patients for a designated shift. A patient-centered model; suffers from a lack of continuity between shifts and is expensive because highly paid nurses provide all aspects of care.
Primary nursing	A nurse is accountable for planning, evaluating, and directing the care of a patient 24 hours a day throughout the patient's stay. A method of providing comprehensive, individualized, and consistent care; expensive.
Case management	One nurse is responsible for overseeing the quality and financial outcomes of patient care; the nurse works collegially with physicians and other caregivers as well as with payers to manage patients along an agreed-on clinical pathway.
Patient-centered or patient-focused care	Cross-functional teams consisting of groups of professionals and assistive personnel from patient-nursing and other departments work together as a unit-based team to provide care to a given group of patients. Care is designed around the needs of the patients and not the needs of the departments or professionals.
Collaborative practice model	Nurses and physicians work together in collaborative practice models.

accommodating, competing, compromising, and collaborating—and noted that none of the five styles is bad. The problem is falling into a habitual style of conflict resolution that might not be the best for a particular situation. Effective nurses try out each style and learn to use the style best suited for each situation. Box 23-4 identifies 12 poor management practices that can lead to conflict.

EFFECTING AND EXPERIENCING CHANGE THROUGH LEADERSHIP

Change is the process of transforming or modifying something. It might be planned, unplanned, developmental, or, as Porter-O'Grady and Malloch suggested, quantum and ever-present. Nursing and the healthcare system are continually changing and evolving, and that momentum will only escalate in the years to come. Factors such as the increasing number of chronically ill and older people, the increasing role of government and industry in healthcare, the rising cost of healthcare, and the changing patterns of healthcare delivery have produced a need for innovation and change in healthcare.

There are many theories of change, most based on the classic theory of change proposed by Kurt Lewin (1951). Lewin posited the following three stages of change:
- Unfreezing: The need for change is recognized.
- Moving: Change is initiated after a careful process of planning.
- Refreezing: Change becomes operational.

These three rather simplistic stages do not fully reveal the very dynamic and personal nature of change of any kind. In healthcare we can find numerous examples of using change

theory to transform practice. Not so long ago, childbirth in the United States was routinely "medicalized." Women came to the hospital to deliver their babies; pain medications that interfered with the natural process of labor were routinely administered, necessitating forceps and assisted deliveries; and husbands, partners, and siblings were banished from the delivery room. Nurse midwives and others recognized the need for change (*unfreezing*) and set about researching childbirth and ways to improve infant and family outcomes. After a careful process of planning (*moving*), multiple natural childbirth options were made available to women and couples, and today they represent mainstream care (*refreezing*).

Similarly, someone who takes good health for granted might fail to develop healthy lifestyle practices until illness results in recognition of the need for change (*unfreezing*). A careful process of consultation and study might lead to the development of a well-developed fitness plan (*moving*), which ideally becomes part of the person's everyday life (*refreezing*). Effective nurses pay attention to their ability to influence the person's thinking and behavior in each stage of change.

Planned Change

Planned change is a purposeful, systematic effort to bring about change. Nurses most often implement planned change. The eight steps in the process of change, which are somewhat similar to the steps of the nursing process, are shown in Box 23-5. Before planning to make a change, a nurse should consider the following:
- What is amenable to change? Considering this question might reveal a behavior not amenable to change.
- How does the group function as a unit? Certain forces within a group may favor change, whereas other forces may resist it.

BOX 23-4 The Dirty Dozen: Management That Leads to Conflict

Below are 12 poor management practices that can destroy the communication climate and breed defensiveness, conflict, and/or violence among your employees. Work hard at avoiding them.

Dirty Dozen Description	Definition
1. Isolation (Ignoring)	Not paying attention to what's going on with staff. Apathy.
2. No Feedback or Recognition	Another example of not paying attention.
3. Only Negative Feedback	Making employees feel like all they can do is fail.
4. Favoritism	Sets up unhealthy competition amongst employees.
5. Mixed Messages	Giving conflicting messages to employees about their duties and responsibilities.
6. Lecturing/Talking Down	Treating employees like children. Being dictatorial.
7. Unrealistic Deadlines "Drive-by-Management"	Offloading your pressure on to your staff. Giving irrational orders and then disappearing.
8. Passive Aggression	Pretending to support employees but actually working against them.
9. Personal Put Downs	Making harsh negative personal criticisms. Acting superior, insulting, or sarcastic.
10. Breaking Promises	Making promises and then forgetting about them.
11. Threatening	Promising negative action if something is or is not done.
12. Attacking	Verbally and/or physically attacking.

As manager, you set the tone for your employees.

(Used with permission from Clements, J. [2003]. Judi Clements Training & Development. Clifton Park, NY: Speaker@nycap.rr.com.)

BOX 23-5 Planned Change: An Eight-Step Process

Planned change is a purposeful, systematic effort to alter or bring about change through the intervention of a change agent. The same steps apply whether dealing with individuals or groups.

1. *Recognize symptoms that indicate a change is needed and collect data.*
2. *Identify a problem to be solved through change.* Analyze the symptoms and reach a conclusion. Note resistance or barriers to change and factors that promote the desired change.
3. *Determine and analyze alternative solutions to the problem.* Consider the advantages, disadvantages, and consequences of each alternative. An analysis of various proposed solutions to a problem may result in using a combination of alternatives.
4. *Select a course of action from possible alternatives.* It is best to avoid initiating too many courses of action and thereby dissipating resources and energy.
5. *Plan for making a change.* This step is crucial to effect change successfully. Start by stating specific objectives, designing a

plan for change, developing timetables, selecting people to assist with making the change, and anticipating how to stabilize change and deal with resistance to change. Unless a plan is clearly designed, effecting change is likely to be a chaotic experience.
6. *Implement the selected course of action to effect change.* The plan for change is then put into effect. During this period, flexibility is important to adapt to unforeseen problems.
7. *Evaluate the effects of change by comparing them with objectives stated in the plan for change.* Adjustments can be made in the plan as necessary after evaluation. If the results of evaluation indicate that the course of action selected to solve a problem has been unsuccessful, an adjustment should be made or another course of action selected.
8. *Stabilize the change.* When a solution has been found, take measures to make the change permanent. Continue follow-up until the change is firmly established.

- Is the person or group ready for change and, if so, at what rate can that change be expected to be accepted? The pace of change must be consistent with the person's or group's readiness to assimilate change. Readiness involves both the ability and willingness to change. In contemporary healthcare organizations, change is dynamic, persistent, and very challenging. The concept of flexibility previously mentioned is put to a real test in any clinical or managerial arena.
- Are the changes major or minor? A series of small changes might be more easily accomplished than one large, dramatic change. The nursing leader/manager must support the staff during the difficult task of acquiring new skills and frequently new professional identities.

Resistance to Change

People might resist change for various reasons. The leader must identify whether any resistance is present, because this will determine the techniques that will be needed to overcome it.

Threat to Self

People generally view change in terms of how they are affected personally. Personal threats might include a loss of self-esteem, a belief that more work will be required, or a belief that social relationships will be disrupted. For example, when hospitals began to use more unlicensed assistive personnel for routine nursing care, many nurses resisted not only because of quality concerns but also because they found themselves legally and professionally responsible for supervising the care given by these new aides. There was also concern that some professional nurses would be replaced by unlicensed assistive personnel.

Lack of Understanding

Someone who does not understand the nature of change is likely to resist. The people who will be affected by the change must become involved and educated if resistance is to be overcome. For example, nurses who do not realize the effectiveness of using plans of care tend to resist preparing them because they believe they are not beneficial for providing patient care.

Limited Tolerance for Change

Some people simply do not like to function in a state of flux or disequilibrium. A person might understand the need for change but might be unable to cope emotionally with it. For example, a nurse might resist change because of the temporary confusion the change is likely to cause.

Disagreements About the Benefits of Change

Resistance might occur when the change agent and those resisting change have different information. If the information known by the people resisting change is more accurate and relevant than the change agent's information, their resistance might be beneficial. For example, the supervisor of community health services proposes to implement, in a low-income neighborhood, a home healthcare plan that has been effective in a middle-class section of the city. The nurse in charge of the health program in the low-income area resists, believing that the plan will not be successful in a financially and educationally disadvantaged neighborhood.

Fear of Increased Responsibility

Many people are worried about having to take on more complex responsibilities, especially if they feel unprepared for the planned changes. The changes might seem overwhelming, so they naturally resist them.

Overcoming Resistance to Change

Resistance can be subtle or distinct, gentle or aggressive. Responding to resistance is a both a leadership responsibility and a challenge in which the leader uses leadership qualities, leadership style, and knowledge of group dynamics to influence others toward a desired outcome. Nurses acting as change agents find the following guidelines helpful for overcoming resistance to change:

- Explain the proposed change to all affected people in simple, concise language.
- List the advantages of the proposed change, both for the individual and for members of the group.
- Relate the proposed change to the person's or group's existing beliefs and values.
- Help overcome resistance by providing opportunities for open communication and feedback.
- Indicate clearly how the change will be evaluated.
- If possible, introduce change gradually. Involve everyone affected by the change in the design and implementation of the process.
- Provide incentives for commitment to change, such as money, status, time off, or a better working environment.

> *Think back to Jack Camp, the patient described in the Reflective Practice display. The nurse could apply these guidelines when attempting to change staff behavior and the patient's behavior. Ultimately, a positive outcome for both could be achieved.*

Power

Nurses in leadership and managerial roles who wish to be effective change agents are sensitive to both the uses and abuses of power. **Power,** the ability to influence others to achieve a desired effect, has many sources. Nurses in management positions within an institution (eg, director of nursing or nursing coordinator) have ascribed power associated with the role. A group might attribute power to different individuals because of their expertise, leadership, or charisma. When introducing change, it is helpful to recognize and enlist the support of key power players who can then encourage others to become involved. You can probably think of people in the groups to which you belong (school, church, civic groups) who are "natural leaders" because of their demonstrated ability to influence others. These are the "key power players" whose support is essential to effecting change. Nursing leaders recognize the strengths and limitations of their own power and encourage others to develop and use power constructively. This is done as part of "mapping the political terrain" of the unit or organization. Most change requires identification of the power brokers who will support the initiative.

> *Recall Rehema Kohls, the college sophomore considering starting a campus discussion group about STDs. The nurse at the healthcare center would identify that Rehema is considered by her peers to have power and to be a*

leader. The nurse would integrate this information in helping Rehema develop the group.

THE NURSE CAREGIVER'S LEADERSHIP SKILLS

No one is born a leader. People develop leadership qualities through observation, knowledge, and experience. Nurses develop their leadership qualities in the same way, although they might enter nursing with some leadership experience. Nursing students and beginning practicing nurses have some leadership responsibilities, as described in the following sections, but they are still working at developing leadership skills and learning where and how to apply them. Fortunately, they have support systems for guidance.

Areas of Leadership

Leadership should be approached like any other new role or skill: slowly and carefully. Nursing students and beginning nurses should be prepared with all of the necessary tools or skills before attempting the new role. Initially, nurses develop leadership skills in well-defined clinical situations. With each experience, growth occurs and leadership is strengthened. It helps to remember that all nurse managers, nurse administrators, and nursing leaders also began as inexperienced nurses.

Patient Care Coordination

Even new graduate nurses have leadership responsibilities when they begin nursing. Nursing leadership begins with nursing care of the individual patient. Although patients are partners in their care planning, most do not have the knowledge base and skills to direct the plan. Through interpersonal skills and effective communication techniques, nurses lead their patients in acquiring new knowledge, solving problems, and changing behaviors. Managing care for even one patient can be an overwhelming responsibility for those new to nursing and its challenges. The student guide to organizing clinical responsibilities in Chapter 15, Implementing, offers practical help.

An ongoing leadership challenge for all nurses is time management. Following are helpful steps for using your time effectively:

- Establish goals and priorities for each day. Identify what you need to accomplish each day, differentiating "need to do" from "nice to do" tasks. Be sure to include the patient and/or the patient's family in establishing these priorities. Ask, "What is it important for you to accomplish today?"
- Evaluate your goals in term of their ability to meet the needs of the patients entrusted to your care as well as your duties to yourself and your colleagues (other students and members of the team). If one student has a patient whose care requires assistance, other students can plan their day so that they will be able to help at a particular time. This sort of teamwork is an important element of care coordination.

- Establish a time line. Allocate priorities to hours in your workday so that you will recognize when you are falling behind schedule in time to correct it before the day is lost.
- Evaluate your success or failure in managing time. If you fail to accomplish your goals in the time at hand, you will need to determine whether your goals were overambitious, whether things happened beyond your control (eg, your patient's condition worsened. requiring more care, or another student required your assistance), or whether you wasted time that could have been better spent (Fig. 23-1).
- Use the results of this evaluation to direct your next day's priorities and time line.

> *Remember Stephen Wall, the 65-year-old patient in the intensive care unit with multiple injuries. Due to his multiple and complex needs, time management for the nurse is crucial. Applying the steps identified above in this situation would be very helpful when planning and providing care.*

Employee Responsibilities

Nurses have specific tasks or duties to perform. These tasks are determined by the plan and objective of the healthcare agency. It is important to read your job description carefully and to continue to evaluate how institutional factors influence your own practice of nursing. Factors that compromise quality care should be noted and addressed in consultation with experienced nurses.

Managerial Responsibilities and Delegation

New graduate nurses use leadership techniques when they direct the work of nonprofessional staff and volunteers. Guidelines for delegating tasks to nonprofessional staff may be found in Chapter 15, Implementing. Gradually, new nurses assume increased leadership responsibilities as they become primary nurses, case managers, or unit coordinators.

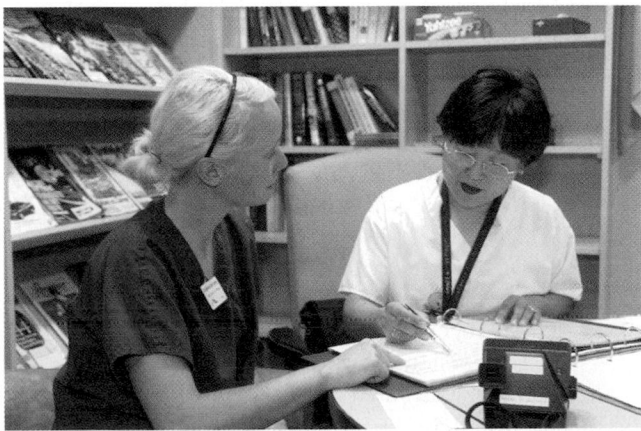

FIGURE 23-1 A student reviews her success in managing time with her clinical instructor. (Photo by Joe Mitchell.)

Nursing Department

The nursing team can also be viewed in the broader context of the entire nursing department of a healthcare institution or agency. Nurses should have an interest in the functioning of the department. Using this knowledge, nurses can seek information or change through appropriate channels. The more nurses understand how the nursing department runs, the better able they are to work constructively to meet the department's objectives.

Employing Institution or Agency

Nurses at all levels need to be knowledgeable about the administrative structure and functions of their employing institution or agency. When problems arise concerning professional, unit, departmental, or institutional or agency objectives, nurses must be able to use the proper channels of communication. For example, if a nurse believes that work assignments are routinely incompatible with basic patient safety and quality and gets no response after discussing this with an immediate nursing supervisor, he or she should take those complaints to the director of nursing. If the director of nursing fails to respond adequately, the nurse should determine to whom the director of nursing reports and should approach that individual. Similarly, a nurse concerned about medical care should first approach the medical attending; if he or she fails to respond, the nurse must then contact the nursing coordinator and in consult with him or her approach the medical director. The structure of these channels is shown in the agency's organization chart, which details the relationships among the various administrative positions, departments, and job titles. Sometimes the nurse is referred to committees that deal with specific issues.

Support for Leadership Training

Nurses intent on developing their leadership ability have multiple resources available to them: mentorship, preceptorship, participation in professional organizations, and continuing education.

Mentorship

Mentorship is a relationship in which an experienced individual (the mentor) advises and assists a less experienced individual (protégé). This is an effective way of easing a new nurse into leadership responsibilities. Mentors link with protégés by common interest and provide support, information, and network links. The relationship does not include financial reward. The advantages of having an effective mentor are highlighted in Box 23-6.

Mentorship is valuable in all types of nursing positions. As a nurse climbs the ladder of leadership responsibility, a mentor who is experienced in management and administrative functions might be of great assistance. A mentor can be key in helping a less experienced nurse assume added responsibilities and position changes. Many mentorship relationships also become lasting friendships.

BOX 23-6 Advantages of Having an Effective Mentor

- Gives upward mobility to your career
- Boosts self-esteem by believing in you
- Shares your dreams
- Provides advice, counsel, and support
- Teaches by example
- Introduces you to the corporate structure, players, and politics
- Imparts valuable information
- Gives feedback on your progress

Heidman, M., & Cobbold, D. (1995). Mentoring and career development revisited. *Registered Nurse*, 7(1), 29–30.

Preceptorship

An alternative model is preceptorship. The preceptor (experienced nurse) is selected (and generally paid) to introduce an employee to new responsibilities through teaching and guidance. The relationship is limited by the new employee's needs (Fig. 23-2).

Nursing and Other Professional Organizations

The many nursing organizations at the international, national, state, district, and local levels were discussed in Chapter 1, Introduction to Nursing. They are major forces for nursing leadership and have active groups throughout the United States and abroad. Participation in nursing and other professional organizations provides important opportunities for nurses to develop and exhibit leadership.

Continuing Education

Many programs for developing leadership, managerial, and administrative skills are available to nurses. Courses can also be taken by correspondence or over the Internet. Periodicals and books also provide continuing education for emerging leaders.

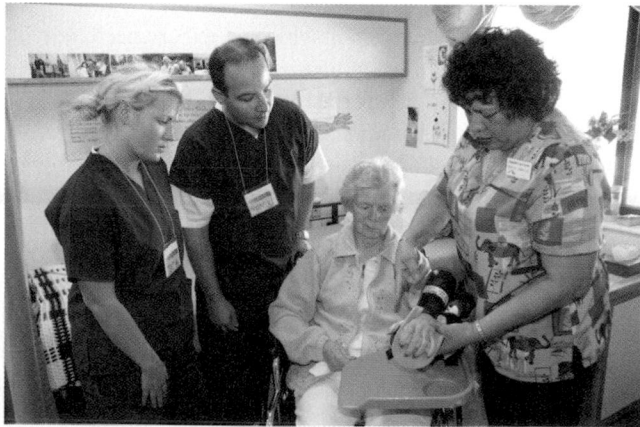

FIGURE 23-2 The nurse preceptor advises and teaches nursing students by example.   (Photo by Joe Mitchell.)

Many continuing education programs are available to prepare nurses before they assume higher levels of leadership; some are geared to nurses already in such positions. Nurses should choose a program that matches their learning needs.

Developing Critical Thinking Skills

1. Interview several experienced nurses and ask them what qualities make for the best nursing leaders. Reflect on your personal experience in groups (eg, within your family, church, school, and community). Identify the roles you characteristically assume and what qualities you bring to the group (eg, enthusiasm, positive thinking, vision, self-direction). Consider whether those qualities will serve you well in professional nursing groups and situations. Are there new qualities you need to develop if you want to become an effective nurse leader? Why?
2. Identify a situation in your class or school that "cried out for change." Discuss with your classmates which students emerged as leaders to address the need for change. Review and critique the steps they engaged in to bring about change. See if your group can reach consensus about the adequacy of their leadership behaviors.

Practicing for NCLEX

1. When evaluating the leadership style of a particular nursing unit, which characteristic would lead the nurse to determine that an autocratic leadership style is being used?
    a. One person is responsible for all decision making.
    b. Activities are shared among all participants.
    c. Each staff member works independently of others.
    d. The leader shows concern for others, taking risks as necessary.
2. When developing a presentation about magnet hospitals, which characteristics would you include? (Choose all options that apply.)
    a. Are located in large, progressive, tertiary centers
    b. Demonstrate a decentralized operational structure with self-governance
    c. Exhibit better patient outcomes and staff retention
    d. Promote control of practice by medical personnel
    e. Allow staff self-scheduling
3. Which phrase best describes transformational leaders?
    a. Drive rapid organization-wide change
    b. Are frequently seen at senior or executive levels
    c. Are focused exclusively on outcomes
    d. Lack vision and vulnerability
4. When teaching a group of students about quantum leadership, which information would be most appropriate for the instructor to include? (Choose all that apply.)

a. Involves rapid leaps or departures from command-and-control structures
b. Views change as something that is planned
c. Requires openness to continual and consistent feedback
d. Is responsive to persistent, unrelenting environmental change

5. A teaching plan about the differences between leadership and management would be considered effective if the students identified which as a difference?
a. Formal titles differentiate the two constructs.
b. Leadership is less tangible that management.
c. Managerial skills are the technical side of leadership.
d. Leadership and management are mutually exclusive.

6. There is evidence that planning for change can be beneficial for all. Which sequence would be best for the nurse to use when planning change?
a. Planning, checking, implementing, evaluating
b. Determining what to change, evaluating possible resistance, determining the appropriate rate and degree of change
c. Unfreezing, freezing and refreezing
d. Communicating, problem solving, managing, and self-evaluating

7. Resistance to change is a part of organizational life. Which action(s) would be most effective in approaching this resistance? (Choose all that apply.)
a. Containing the anxiety in a small group and moving forward with the initiative
b. Being sensitive to the personal dimensions that the change might affect
c. Explaining the change and listing the advantages to the individual and the organization
d. Reprimanding those that oppose the new initiative
e. Seeking guidance from staff

8. A nurse is asked to act as a mentor. The nurse interprets this position as:
a. A formal process for professional growth
b. A paid responsibility of all nurses
c. Limited to those with professional titles and rank
d. A means for participation in a professional organization

Answers With Rationale

1. The correct answer is *a*. Autocratic leadership in traditionally viewed as one or a few individuals exercising decision-making power and control over others.
2. The correct answers are *b, c,* and *e*. Magnet hospitals offer shared decision making via self-governance structures and autonomous, accountable professional practice with nurses exerting control over the practice environment and participating in staff self-scheduling. Better patient outcomes in magnet hospitals have been empirically documented. Size and patient population characteristics have no relevance to magnet status. In non-magnet hospitals, practice is dominated and in some instances controlled by physicians and others.

3. The correct answer is *a*. Transformational leaders might emerge from any level within the organization. Their focus is on both process and outcome. They are highly charismatic, are able to create a common vision, and take risks, thereby being vulnerable.
4. The correct answers are *a, c,* and *d*. Quantum leadership is dynamic and not dependent upon structured planned change.
5. The correct answer is *c*. Managerial skills are frequently defined as those relating to budgeting, the planning process, interviewing, adherence to employment law, and so forth, the technical side of leadership.
6. The correct answer is *b*. Planning for change involves a deliberate organizational assessment of what to change, how the change will be received, and the organization's ability to move forward with the change.
7. The correct answers are *b, c,* and *e*. Change is perceived to be ubiquitous, and so too is resistance to change. Individuals vary in their ability to understand and incorporate new learning and practice. In democratic, self-governance structures, staff can be instrumental in assisting with the process.
8. The correct answer is *a*. Mentoring is a deliberate, focused process leading to both personal and professional growth.

Bibliography

Aiken, L. (2001). Evidence-based management: key to hospital workforce stability. *The Journal of Health Administration Education* (special issue), pp. 117–124.

Benne, K. D., & Sheats, P. (1948). Functional roles of group members. *Journal of Social Issues, 4*(2), 41.

Bennis, W. G., Benne, K. D., Chin, R., & Corey, K. E. (1976). *The planning of change* (3rd ed.). New York: Holt, Rinehart & Winston.

Bernhard, L. A., & Walsh, M. (1994). *Leadership: The key to the professionalization of nursing* (3rd ed.). St. Louis: C. V. Mosby.

Brown, B. J., & Sample, S. (Eds.). (1994). Change: The challenge for nursing. *Nursing Administration Quarterly, 18*(3), entire issue.

Chenevert, M. (1997). *Pro-nurse handbook: Designed for the nurse who wants to thrive professionally* (3rd ed.). St. Louis: C. V. Mosby.

Clements, J. (2003). Judi Clements training and development. Clifton Park, NY (speaker@nycap.rr.com).

Douglass, L. M. (1995). *The effective nurse: Leader and manager* (5th ed.). St. Louis: Mosby–Year Book.

Drucker, P. (1999). Managing oneself. *Harvard Business Review,* March–April, 65–74.

Dunn, R. (2002). *Haimann's healthcare management* (7th ed.). Chicago: Health Administration Press.

Grensing-Pophal, L. (1998). Resolving conflicts: It's as easy as 1-2-3. *Nursing, 28*(9), 63.

Grohar-Murray, M. E., & DiCroce, H. R. (1996). *Leadership and management in nursing.* Englewood Cliffs, NJ: Prentice-Hall.

Gurka, A. M. (1995). Transformational leadership: Qualities and strategies for the CNS. *Journal for Advanced Nursing Practice, 9*(3), 169–174.

Hagenow, N. R., & McCrea, M. A. (1994). A mentoring relationship: Two viewpoints. *Nursing Management, 25*(12), 42–43.

Heidman, M., & Cobbold, D. (1995). Mentoring and career development revisited. *Registered Nurse, 7*(1), 29–30.

Hersey, P., & Blanchard, K. (1977). *Management of organizational behavior: Utilizing human resources* (3rd ed.). Englewood Cliffs, NJ: Prentice-Hall.

Hostutler, J., Kennedy, M. S., Mason, D., & Schorr, T. M. (1999). Then and now: Nurses as leaders. *American Journal of Nursing, 99*(10), 36–38.

Kerfoot, K. (1995). Models of patient care delivery. In K. W. Vestal (Ed.). *Nursing management: Concepts and issues* (2nd ed., pp. 37–47). Philadelphia: J. B. Lippincott.

Lewin, K. (1951). *Field theory in social science.* New York: Harper & Row.

Manfredi, C. M., & Valiga, T. M. (1994). Leadership in nursing. *Holistic Nursing Practice, 9*(1), entire issue.

Manion, J. (1995). Understanding the seven stages of change. *American Journal of Nursing, 95*(4), 41–43.

Marriner-Tomey, A. (1996). *Guide to nursing management and leadership.* St. Louis: Mosby–Year Book.

Porter-O'Grady, T., & Malloch, K. (2003). *Quantum leadership: a textbook of new leadership.* Boston: Jones & Bartlett.

Tiffany, C. R., Cheatham, A. B., Doornbos, D., Loudermelt, L., & Momadi, G. G. (1994). Planned change theory: Survey of nursing periodical literature. *Nursing Management, 25*(7), 54–59.

Tiffany, C. R. (1994). Analysis of planned change theories. *Nursing Management, 25*(2), 60–62.

Trofino, J. (Ed.) (1992). Transformational leadership. *Nursing Administration Quarterly, 17*(1), entire issue.

Wolf, G. A., Boland, S., & Aukerman, M. (1994). A transformational model for the practice of professional nursing. Part I: The model. *Journal of Nursing Administration, 23*(4), 51–57.

Wolf, G. A., Boland, S., & Aukerman, M. (1994). A transformational model for the practice of professional nursing. Part II: Implementation of the model. *Journal of Nursing Administration, 23*(5), 38–46.

Wolf, P. (1998). Guide to nursing organizations. *Nursing, 28*(12), 53–55.

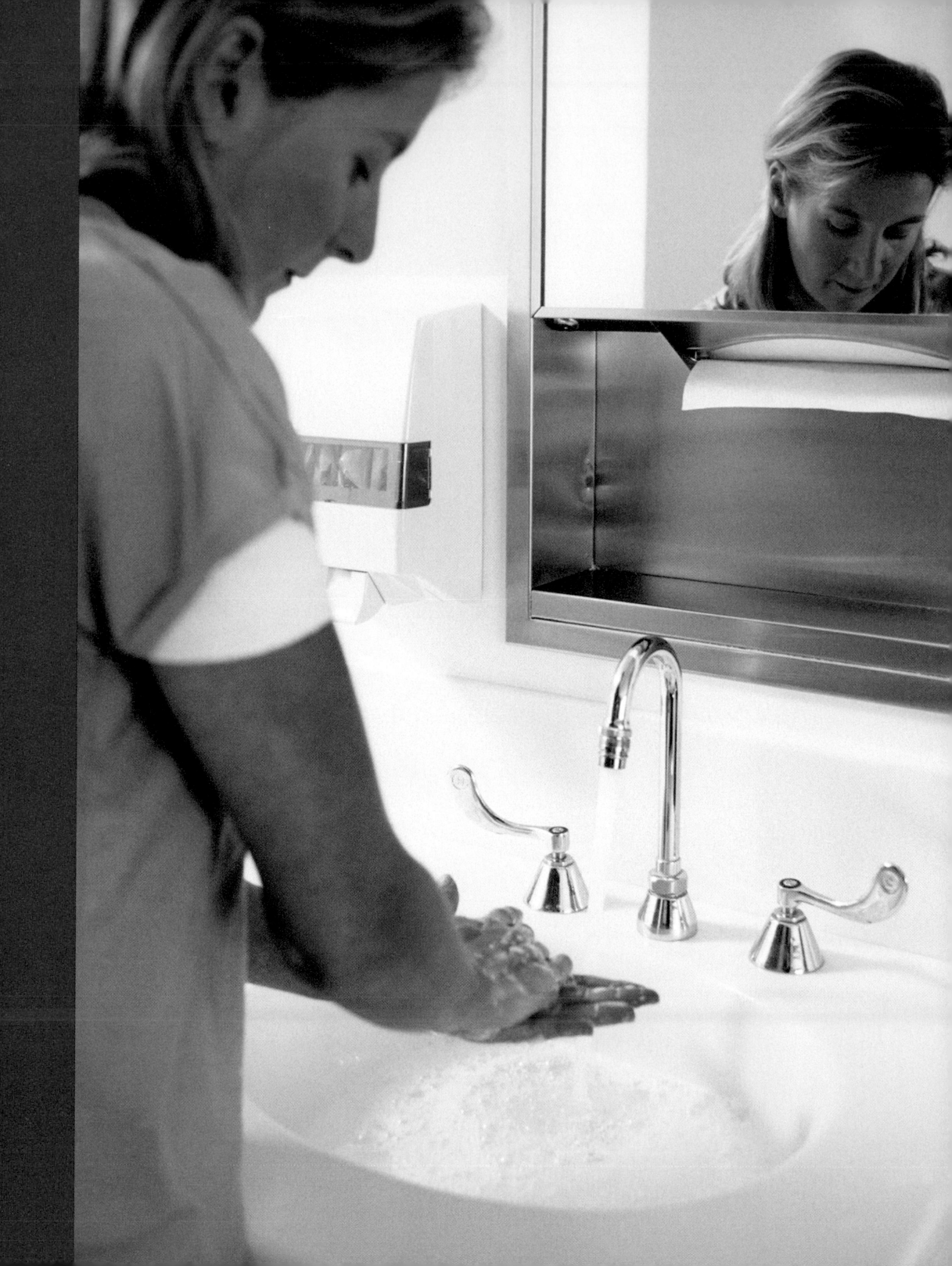

Actions Basic to Nursing Care

"Our intent when we lay hands on the patient in bodily care is to comfort."

Lydia Hall (1906–1969)
an innovator in nursing practice, she developed the theory that the direct nurse-to-patient relationship is itself therapeutic and that nursing care is the chief therapy for critically ill patients.

Unit VI focuses on the actions basic to nursing practice—those commonly planned, implemented, and evaluated to meet the healthcare needs of patients at any age, at any point along the health–illness continuum, and in all settings. The nursing actions discussed in this unit include taking vital signs, conducting a health history and assessment, maintaining safety, administering medications, and providing perioperative care.

Chapter 24 describes nursing responsibilities related to the assessment of vital signs, and Chapter 25 discusses conducting a health history and assessment. Nursing assessment is both an art and a science. The art of performing a skill is integrated into the science of nursing so that variations from normal are identified and evaluated and necessary nursing actions are implemented. The findings from assessments provide a database necessary to maintain or restore health and promote wellness.

Nurses are responsible for meeting basic human needs for physical safety and security. Chapter 26 discusses environmental safety, including threats from bioterrorism, plus nursing actions necessary for identifying risk factors for patients at any age and for implementing teaching and other nursing actions to prevent accidents. Chapter 27 explains medical and surgical aseptic techniques to prevent and to control the spread of microorganisms. Chapter 28 discusses complementary and alternative therapies, an ever-increasing component of healthcare.

Chapters 29 and 30 focus on collaborative and independent nursing actions necessary when administering medications and providing perioperative care. In most instances, the physician prescribes the medications and performs the surgery while the nurse orders and implements nursing interventions to promote patient safety and knowledge and to facilitate optimal function or recovery in both hospital and home settings. Although procedures and protocols are often used in these situations, nursing actions are individualized to the unique needs of each person requiring care.

Unit VI introduces the learner to the knowledge and skills basic to nursing practice in any setting. Using the nursing process, nurses make accurate assessments, ensure safety, prevent and control the spread of microorganisms, administer medications knowledgeably and safely, and provide perioperative care for patients in the hospital, home, and community.

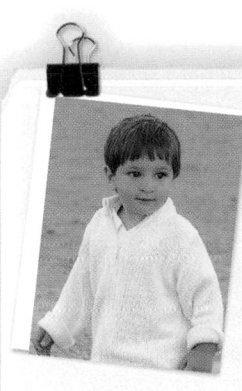

Noah Shoolin is a 2-year-old who is brought to the emergency department by his mother. When the nurse attempts to obtain a tympanic temperature, the child begins to scream uncontrollably, crying and pushing the device away from his ear.

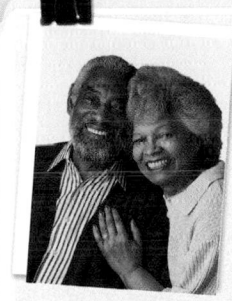

Doretha Renfrow brings her 65-year-old hypertensive husband to the clinic for evaluation. He is 5'10 and overweight. Mrs. Renfrow states "I really would like to learn how to take my husband's blood pressure so that I can keep track of his progress. Can you teach me how to do it?"

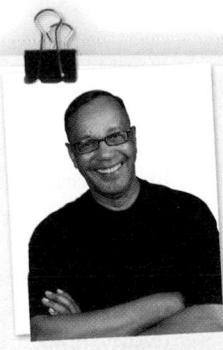

Tomas Esposito is a middle-aged man admitted to the hospital. He is placed in a private room with specialized infection-control precautions, requiring staff to don a gown and gloves when entering the room each time. A morning assessment, including vital signs, is needed.

Focusing on Blended Skills

The types of blended skills you'll need to respond to the case scenarios include:

Cognitive Skills

- Knowledge of the anatomy and physiology underlying vital signs and the significance of normal and abnormal findings
- Knowledge of nursing responsibilities in assessing temperature, pulse, respirations, and blood pressure
- Knowledge of how to tailor vital-signs technology to meet the individualized needs of patients (eg, best means to assess the temperature of a 2-year-old, the fact that a larger cuff is needed to accurately assess the blood pressure of the overweight man)
- Knowledge of how to teach patients and their family caregivers how to assess vital signs and how to respond to significant findings
- Ability to incorporate factors affecting vital signs into a patient's plan of care
- Ability to use critical-thinking skills to intervene appropriately in situations involving an upset toddler, an inquiring daughter, and an middle-aged man requiring infection-control precautions

Technical Skills

- Ability to correctly use the equipment necessary to assess and to document vital signs
- Ability to adapt techniques to meet the needs of patients, such as the toddler and an overweight man with hypertension
- Ability to identify limitations in performance of skills, asking for assistance as necessary when performing them
- Ability to maintain infection-control measures when encountering difficulties in a patient's care
- Ability to integrate time-management and organizational skills when caring for multiple patients, including a patient with an infection requiring vital-sign assessment

Interpersonal Skills

- Strong people skills to establish a trusting relationship with a toddler, a daughter seeking information, and a middle-aged man who is irritable and requires infection-control measures
- Ability to communicate and interact effectively with patients and their caregivers while assessing vital signs and teaching others how to assess vital signs accurately
- Confidence in own abilities and interpersonal competence to interact with other healthcare personnel, confronting the appropriate persons when help is needed
- Ability to demonstrate respect for the patient's human dignity throughout the patient's care

Ethical and Legal Skills

- Commitment to safety and quality nursing care
- Strong sense of responsibility and accountability
- Ability to put the need for accurate assessment over own discomfort about your questionable ability to auscultate heart and lung sounds
- Knowledge of ethical and legal principles related to assessing and to documenting vital signs in patients of varying ages and with differing needs
- Ability to document temperature, pulse, respirations, and blood-pressure findings accurately and according to agency policy

Learning Outcomes

After completing the chapter, the learner should be able to accomplish the following:

1. Explain the physiologic processes involved in homeostatic regulation of temperature, pulse, respirations, and blood pressure.
2. Discuss factors that may increase or decrease body temperature, pulse, respirations, and blood pressure.
3. Identify sites for assessing temperature, pulse, and blood pressure.
4. Accurately assess temperature, pulse, respirations, and blood pressure.
5. Know the normal ranges for body temperature, pulse, respirations, and blood pressure.
6. Provide information to patients about taking temperature, pulse, and blood pressure at home.

Key Terms

afebrile
apnea
blood pressure
bradycardia
bradypnea
diastolic pressure
dyspnea
dysrhythmia
eupnea
febrile
hypertension
hypotension
hyperthermia
hypothermia

Korotkoff sounds
orthopnea
orthostatic
    hypotension
pulse
pulse deficit
pulse pressure
pyrexia
respiration
systolic pressure
tachycardia
tachypnea
temperature
vital signs

Vital signs are a person's temperature, pulse, respiration, and blood pressure (abbreviated as T, P, R, and BP).

Health status is reflected in these indicators of vital body function, regulated through homeostatic mechanisms and falling within certain normal ranges. A change in vital signs might indicate a change in health.

Assessing vital signs is part of nursing care in any setting. Institutional and agency policies govern when and how frequently vital signs are to be assessed routinely. Vital signs are assessed at least every 4 hours in hospitalized patients with elevated temperatures, with high or low blood pressures, with changes in pulse rate or rhythm, or with respiratory difficulty, as well as in patients who are taking medications that affect cardiovascular or respiratory function or who have had surgery. Severely ill patients may have vital signs taken more frequently. In critical care settings, technologically advanced devices are often used for continual monitoring of patients' vital signs. In the home and in some self-care and psychiatric units, assessments are made as frequently as the nurse judges necessary.

Although vital sign assessment may be delegated to other healthcare personnel, it is the nurse's responsibility to ensure accuracy of data and to report abnormal findings. (See the accompanying Reflective Practice box for an example.) If a patient has untoward symptoms (eg, chest pain or dizziness) or has unexpected changes in vital signs, the nurse should double-check the findings and further assess the patient.

> *Recall Tomas Esposito, the patient requiring initial assessment described in the Reflective Practice display? The nurse's inability to auscultate heart and lung sounds would be an important finding that requires additional assessment. The nurse would need to evaluate these findings in conjunction with the patient's vital signs.*

The nurse should also know the normal variations in vital signs that occur at various ages (Table 24-1).

Vital signs are taken and compared with accepted normal values and the patient's usual patterns in a wide variety of instances, including screenings at health fairs and clinics, in the home, upon admission to a healthcare setting, when certain medications are given, before and after diagnostic and surgical procedures, before and after certain nursing interventions, and in emergency situations (Box 24-1). Nurses take vital signs as often as a patient's condition requires such assessment. How to assess each of the vital signs, with a discussion of normal and abnormal findings, is presented in this chapter. See Chapter 25 for additional information about health assessment.

TEMPERATURE

Body **temperature** is the heat of the body measured in degrees. Body temperature indicates the difference between production of heat and loss of heat. Heat is generated by metabolic processes in the core tissues of the body, transferred to the skin surface by the circulating blood, and then dissipated to the environment. Core body temperature is normally maintained within a range of 36.0°C (97.0°F) to 37.5°C (99.5°F). There are individual variations of these temperatures as well as normal changes during the day, with core body temperatures being lowest in the early morning and highest in the late afternoon (Porth, 2002).

Temperatures differ in various parts of the body, with core body temperatures being higher than surface body temperatures. Core temperatures are measured at tympanic or rectal sites, but they may also be measured in the esophagus, pulmonary artery, or bladder by invasive monitoring devices. Surface body temperatures are measured at oral (sublingual) and axillary sites.

Body Temperature Physiology

The core body temperature of a healthy person is maintained within a fairly constant range by the thermoregulatory center in the hypothalamus. This center receives messages from cold and warm thermal receptors located throughout the body and, in turn, initiates responses to either produce or conserve body heat or to increase heat loss.

Heat Production

The primary source of heat in the body is metabolism, with heat produced as a byproduct of metabolic activities that generate energy for cellular functions. Various mechanisms increase body metabolism, including hormones, muscle movements, and exercise. When additional heat is required to maintain balance, epinephrine and norepinephrine (sympathetic neurotransmitters) are released and alter metabolism so that energy production decreases and heat production increases. Thyroid hormone, produced by the thyroid gland, also increases metabolism and heat production, but over a much longer time period. Shivering, a response that increases the production of heat, is initiated by the hypothalamus and results in muscular tremors. The contraction of pilomotor muscles of the skin, causing piloerection, or "goose bumps," reduces the size of the surface to minimize heat loss. Exercise increases heat production through muscular activity.

Heat Loss

The skin is the primary site of heat loss. The circulating blood brings heat to the skin's surface, where small connections between the arterioles and the venules lie directly below the surface. These connections, called arteriovenous shunts, may remain open to allow heat to dissipate to the skin and thus to the external environment, or they may close and retain heat in the body. The sympathetic nervous system controls the opening and closing of the shunts in response to changes in core body temperature and in environmental temperature (Porth, 2002).

Other heat losses occur through evaporation of sweat, through warming and humidifying of inspired air, and through eliminating urine and feces. Heat is transferred to the external environment through the physical processes of radiation, con-

Reflective Practice
Challenge to Ethical and Legal Skills

At clinical 2 weeks ago, I had four patients for the first time and I was very busy. One of my patients, Tomas Esposito, required specialized infection-control precautions, so every time I entered his room, I had to put on a gown and gloves. It was getting to be late in the morning and I still had not completed this patient's full assessment, including his vital signs. Upon entering the patient's room, I discovered that the separate stethoscope usually found in isolation rooms was not there. As a result, I had to remove my gown and gloves and go find the nurse to help me locate the stethoscope. Ultimately, the nurse had to get me a new isolation stethoscope set and put it together for me. Unfortunately, these stethoscopes are poor in quality.

I went back to the patient's room and put on a new gown and gloves. By this time, Mr. Esposito was very irritable and just wanted me to do the assessment quickly and leave him alone. I attempted to listen to his heart sounds but I couldn't hear them. I played with the stethoscope for a few minutes and tried again, but I still couldn't hear his heart or lung sounds. My patient kept telling me to leave him alone. Being a 4th-year nursing student and self sufficient in doing the basic patient assessment, I felt stupid going to get the nurse or my instructor and telling her I couldn't hear anything. I was really pressed for time and now was faced with a critical decision.

Thinking Outside the Box: Possible Courses of Action

- Remove my gown and gloves, get my instructor and the nurse and tell them that I was unable to hear heart and lung sounds, and request their assistance.
- Leave the patient alone as he requested, saving precious time, pretending that I completed the assessment, and charting the same findings as the previous shift's assessment.
- Explain to the nurse that the patient wasn't cooperating and ask her to do the assessment without my instructor knowing about it.
- Try to complete the assessment using my own stethoscope and risk passing the patient's infections on to my other patients.

Evaluating a Good Outcome: How Do I Define Success?

- Patient receives the highest quality of care.
- Professional integrity of all healthcare team members involved is maintained.
- All information charted is accurate.
- Ethical and legal principles are maintained.

Personal Learning: Here's to the Future!

Luckily my conscience and my desire to always give the best care to my patients pushed me to the right decision. I took the time to remove my gown and gloves and went to find my instructor and the nurse. I told the nurse that I was having trouble hearing the patient's heart and lung sounds. She was very understanding and came to the room with me and tried herself. Upon further investigation, we found that the problem was a broken stethoscope, not my incompetence to complete an assessment. After assessing the patient with a properly functioning stethoscope, I found expira- tory wheezing and documented it. This finding also provided a clue that I should probably keep a very close eye on this patient. Mr. Esposito ended up experiencing increasing difficulty breathing and his oxygen saturation levels began to drop into the 80% range. As a result, I realized just how important the initial assessment is when caring for a patient throughout the day. Hopefully, the lesson about how important it is to do the "right" thing for the patient will stick with me forever.

Reflection

How do you think you would respond in a similar situation? Why? What does this tell you about yourself and about the adequacy of your skills for professional practice? Can you think of other ways to respond? What might the nursing student have done to prevent the numerous trips in and out of the patient's room? To determine whether the stethoscope was functioning properly? How do you think the nursing student's time management and organizational skills affected the situation? What other skills (cognitive, inter- personal, technical, ethical/legal) would you need to respond well in this situation? What ethical principles did the nursing student incorporate into the response to the situation? What responses related to the patient's irritability would have been appropriate by the nursing student? Do you agree with the criteria to evaluate a successful outcome? Did the nursing student meet these criteria? Please explain.

Catherine Barrell, Georgetown University

vection, evaporation, and conduction. These processes are defined and illustrated in Table 24-2.

Variations in Body Temperature

Body temperature may be within the normal range for one's age, or it may be increased or decreased from the normal range. Figure 24-1 illustrates the usual ranges of human body temperature.

Factors Affecting Body Temperature

A variety of different factors affect body temperature. These factors include circadian rhythms, age, gender, stress, and environmental temperatures.

Circadian Rhythms

Many environmental and physiologic processes occur in repeated cycles of time. Some events in humans recur at 24-hour intervals, referred to as circadian (meaning nearly

TABLE 24-1 Age-Related Variations in Normal Vital Signs

Age	Temperature (°C)	Pulse (beats/min)	Respirations (breaths/min)	Blood Pressure (mm Hg)
Newborn	36.8 (Axillary)	80–180	30–80	73/55
1–3 yr	37.7 (Rectal)	80–140	20–40	90/55
6–8 yr	37 (Oral)	75–120	15–25	95/75
10 yr	37 (Oral)	75–110	15–25	102/62
Teens	37 (Oral)	60–100	15–20	102/80
Adults	37 (Oral)	60–100	12–20	120/80
>70 yr	36 (Oral)	60–100	15–20	120/80 (May normally be up to 160/95)

every 24 hours) rhythm. Predictable fluctuations in measurements of body temperature and blood pressure are examples of functions that have a circadian rhythm. For instance, body temperature is usually about 0.6°C (1°–2°F) lower in the early morning than in the late afternoon and early evening. This variation tends to be somewhat greater in infants and children. Research indicates that the peak elevation of a person's temperature occurs in late afternoon, between 4 and 7 p.m.

Age and Sex

Both the very young and the very old are more sensitive to changes in environmental temperature. The body temperature of infants and children changes more rapidly in response to both heat and cold air temperatures.

> Consider Noah Shoolin, the 2-year-old brought to the emergency department by his mother. The nurse assessing the child's temperature would need to keep in mind the effect of environmental temperature changes on the child's temperature. Efforts to prevent chilling and overheating would be incorporated into the child's plan of care.

Older adults lose some thermoregulatory control and are at risk for harm from extremes of temperature.

BOX 24-1 When to Assess Vital Signs

- On admission to any healthcare agency or institution
- Based on agency or institutional policy and procedures
- Any time there is a change in the patient's condition
- Any time there is a loss of consciousness
- Before and after any surgical or invasive diagnostic procedure
- Before and after activity that may increase risk, such as ambulation after surgery
- Before administering medications that affect cardiovascular and respiratory function

Women tend to have more fluctuations in body temperature than men, probably the result of changes in hormones. The increase in progesterone secretion at ovulation increases body temperature as much as one-half to one degree.

Environmental Temperature

Most of us respond to changes in environmental temperature by wearing clothing that either allows increased heat loss when it is hot or retains heat when it is cold. When one is exposed to extreme cold without adequate protective clothing, however, heat loss may be increased to the point of **hypothermia** (low body temperature). Similarly, if one is exposed to extremes of heat for long periods of time, **hyperthermia** (high body temperature) may result. Both hypothermia and hyperthermia may cause serious illness or death.

Normal Body Temperature

Body temperature varies among individuals, with a range of 0.3° to 0.6°C (0.5°–1.0°F) from the average temperature considered to be within normal limits. Even wider variations from the average temperature have been found to be normal for certain people. A person with a normal body temperature is referred to as **afebrile**. Table 24-3 shows the average normal temperature standards for healthy adults at various body sites.

Increased Body Temperature

Pyrexia (fever) is an increase in body temperature caused by an upward displacement of the hypothalamic thermoregulatory center set point (Porth, 2002). A person with an increased body temperature is said to be **febrile**. Pyrexia results from a response to bacterial or viral infections. It also occurs in response to tissue injury, such as from myocardial infarction, pulmonary emboli, cancer, trauma, and surgery. In children, this response is often seen quickly. However, a mild elevation in temperature (such as a rectal temperature of 38°C (100.4°F) might indicate a serious infection in infants younger than 3 months of age who do not have well-developed temperature-control mechanisms. In older adults, who often have a lower baseline body temperature, pyrexia may be one of the later signs of illness, and the

TABLE 24-2 **Mechanisms of Heat Transfer**

	Radiation	Convection	Evaporation	Conduction
Definition	The diffusion or dissemination of heat by electromagnetic waves	The dissemination of heat by motion between areas of unequal density	The conversion of a liquid to a vapor	The transfer of heat to another object during direct contact
Example	The body gives off waves of heat from uncovered surfaces.	An oscillating fan blows currents of cool air across the surface of a warm body.	Body fluid in the form of perspiration and insensible loss is vaporized from the skin.	The body transfers heat to an ice pack, causing the ice to melt.
Illustration	Radiation	Convection	Evaporation	Conduction

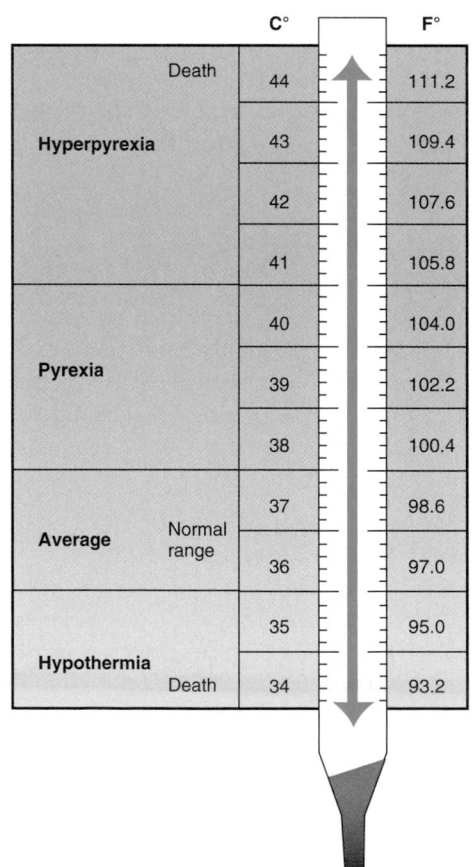

	C°		F°
Death	44		111.2
Hyperpyrexia	43		109.4
	42		107.6
	41		105.8
	40		104.0
Pyrexia	39		102.2
	38		100.4
	37		98.6
Average Normal range	36		97.0
	35		95.0
Hypothermia Death	34		93.2

FIGURE 24-1 The range of human body temperature, as measured orally.

temperature may be elevated only 1°F or 2°F above normal, even when pathologic processes are extensive.

When the set point is increased, the hypothalamus initiates shivering and vasoconstriction. After the body temperature rises to the new set point, heat-loss mechanisms again keep the body temperature from rising to dangerous levels. Most fevers are self-limiting, and the temperature returns to normal range after the factors causing it are controlled. The onset of an elevated body temperature may be sudden or gradual. Terms used to describe types of fever are listed in Box 24-2. Hyperpyrexia is a high fever, usually above 41°C (105.8°F).

Other types of increased body temperature are hyperthermia, neurogenic fever, and fever of unknown origin. Hyperthermia

TABLE 24-3 **Average Normal Temperatures for Healthy Adults at Various Sites**

Oral	Rectal	Axillary	Tympanic	Forehead
37.0°C	37.5°C	36.5°C	37.5°C*	34.4°C†
98.6°F	99.5°F	97.6°F	99.5°F	94.0°F

* The average normal tympanic temperature depends on the calibration and mode setting of the tympanic membrane thermometer.
† The manufacturer of Digitemp forehead thermometer (Hallcrest Products, 1820 Pickwick Lane, Glenview, IL 60025) says, "Most older children and adults have normal forehead temperatures between 93 and 95 degrees F."

differs from pyrexia in that the hypothalamic set point is not changed, but in situations of extreme heat exposure or excessive heat production (for example, during strenuous exercise), the mechanisms that control body temperature are ineffective. Neurogenic fever is usually the result of damage to the hypothalamus from intracranial trauma, intracranial bleeding, or increased intracranial pressure. Neurogenic fever does not respond to antipyretic medications (Porth, 2002). If it is difficult to determine the cause of pyrexia, it is often diagnosed as a fever of unknown origin (FUO).

Physical Effects of Increased Body Temperature

Patients with pyrexia usually experience loss of appetite, headache, hot, dry skin, flushed face, thirst, and general malaise. Young children or other people with high fevers may experience periods of delirium or seizures. Observing for other potentially dangerous manifestations of a fever, such as dehydration, decreased urinary output, and rapid heart rate, is an important nursing assessment.

Methods of Reducing Increased Body Temperature

Nursing interventions for the patient with a fever are outlined in Examples of Nursing Interventions Classification. Antipyretic (fever-reducing) drugs, such as aspirin or acetaminophen, may be administered in certain circumstances. These drugs are believed to lower the elevated set point regulated by the hypothalamus. They do not affect body temperature when it is within normal range. Aspirin should not be given to children under 2 years of age unless prescribed and medical supervision is available. Aspirin also should not be given to children and teenagers with chickenpox or influenza because of a possible association with Reye's syndrome. If the pyrexia is the result of a bacterial infection, an appropriate antibiotic is administered. Body temperature may also be lowered through other interventions, including cool sponge baths, cool packs, and cooling blankets (discussed in Chap. 38).

Decreased Body Temperature

Hypothermia is a body temperature below the lower limit of normal. Death may occur when the temperature falls below about 34°C (93.2°F), but survival has been reported in isolated cases when body temperatures have fallen in the range of severe hypothermia (28°C, or 82.4°F). This may happen to a person drowning in cold water or buried by snow. Rates of chemical reactions in the body are slowed, thereby decreasing the metabolic demands for oxygen.

Assessing Temperature

To accurately assess body temperature, the nurse must know what equipment to use, which site to choose, and what method is appropriate.

Equipment

Body temperature may be assessed with a variety of devices—electronic and digital thermometers, tympanic membrane thermometers, glass thermometers, disposable single-use thermometers, temporal artery thermometers, and automated monitoring devices.

Think back to Tomas Esposito, the patient requiring infection-control precautions and assessment. Because the patient required infection-control measures and a special "isolation stethoscope," the nurse should anticipate the need for using a thermometer designed for individual patient use, such as a disposable one.

Electronic and Digital Thermometers

Electronic and digital thermometers measure oral, rectal, or axillary body temperature in 4 to 60 seconds, depending on the site and product used. These battery-operated devices provide an LCD or LED temperature display and disposable probe covers. Some models also provide the last measurement, a full 60-second pulse timer, and automatic conversion from the Fahrenheit to the Celsius scale. Assessing body temperature with an electronic thermometer is described in Skill 24-1.

Tympanic Membrane Thermometer

Tympanic membrane thermometers use infrared sensors to detect heat given off by the tympanic membrane. The probe is covered with a probe cover and inserted into the ear canal tightly enough to seal the opening (see Skill 24-1). The reading takes from 1 to 3 seconds, depending on the product. Although tympanic temperatures are commonly taken in children, there is some question about the accuracy of the reading assessed with these thermometers, especially in children younger than 6 years of age (Lanham, Walker, Klocke, & Jennings, 1999).

(*text continues on page 534*)

SKILL 24-1   Assessing Body Temperature

EQUIPMENT

Digital, electronic, or glass thermometer
Probe covers for electronic thermometer
Water-soluble lubricant (for rectal thermometers)

Disposable gloves (as appropriate or indicated)

Soft tissues
Pencil or pen, paper, or flow sheet

FOR ALL TEMPERATURE ASSESSMENTS REGARDLESS OF ROUTE

ACTION	RATIONALE
1. Check physician's order or nursing care plan for frequency and route.	Provides for patient safety
2. Identify the patient.	Provides for patient safety
3. Explain the procedure to the patient.	Reduces patient apprehension and encourages patient cooperation
4. Gather equipment.	Provides organized approach to task
5. Make sure the electronic or digital thermometer is in operating condition.	An improperly functioning thermometer may not give accurate readings.
6. Perform hand hygiene and don gloves if appropriate or indicated.	Hand hygiene deters the spread of microorganisms.
7. Select the appropriate site.	Assess the patient's age, mental, and physical condition to ensure safety and accuracy of measurement.
8. Follow the steps as outlined below for the appropriate type of thermometer.	
9. Perform hand hygiene. If gloves are worn, discard them in the proper receptacle.	Deters the spread of microorganisms
10. Record temperature on paper, flow sheet, or computerized record. Report abnormal findings to the appropriate person. Identify site of assessment if other than oral.	Provides accurate documentation and reporting

ASSESSING TYMPANIC MEMBRANE TEMPERATURE

ACTION	RATIONALE
1. If necessary, push the "on" button and wait for the "ready" signal on the unit.	Thermometer will function improperly if not allowed to warm up appropriately.
2. Attach tympanic probe cover.	Deters the spread of microorganisms
3. Insert the probe snugly into the external ear, using gentle but firm pressure, angling the thermometer toward the patient's jaw line.	If the probe is not inserted correctly, the patient's temperature will be noted as lower than normal.

(*continued*)

SKILL 24-1 Assessing Body Temperature (continued)

ACTION	RATIONALE

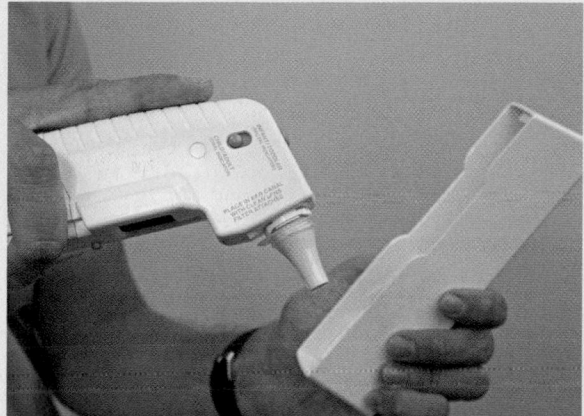

Action 1: Turning unit on and awaiting ready signal.
(Photo by Rick Brady.)

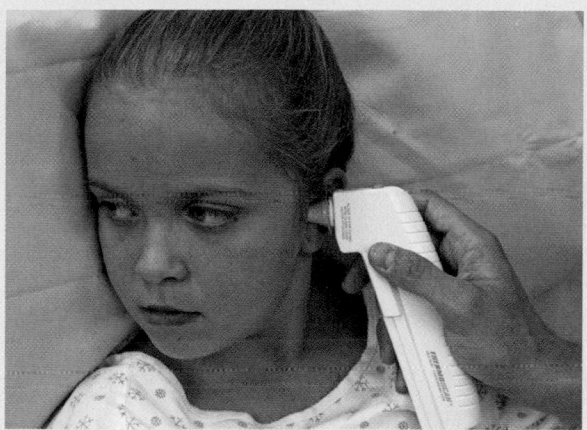

Action 3: Inserting tympanic membrane thermometer into the patient's ear.   (Photo by Rick Brady.)

4. Activate the unit by pushing the trigger button. The reading is immediate (usually within 2 seconds). Note the temperature reading.

The digital thermometer must be on to begin reading the temperature.

5. Discard the probe cover in an appropriate receptacle by pushing the probe release button, and replace the thermometer in its charger or holder.

Discarding the probe cover ensures that it will not be accidentally reused on another patient. The thermometer must stay on the charger so that it is ready to go at all times.

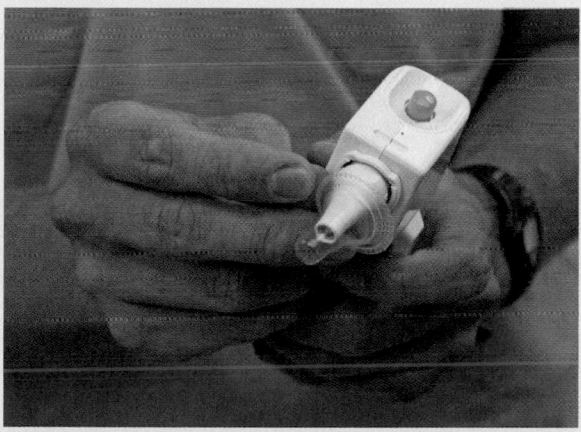

Action 5: Disposing of the probe cover.   (Photo by Rick Brady.)

ASSESSING ORAL TEMPERATURE WITH AN ELECTRONIC OR DIGITAL THERMOMETER

ACTION	RATIONALE

1. Release the electronic unit from the charging unit and remove the probe from within the recording unit.

Electronic unit must be taken into patient's room to assess the patient's temperature. On some models, removing the probe turns on the machine.

2. Cover thermometer probe with disposable probe cover and slide it until it snaps into place.

Prevents contamination of the thermometer probe

3. Place the probe beneath the patient's tongue in the posterior sublingual pocket. Ask the patient to close his or her lips around the probe.

When the probe rests deeply in the posterior sublingual pocket, it is in contact with blood vessels lying close to the surface.

(continued)

ACTION	RATIONALE

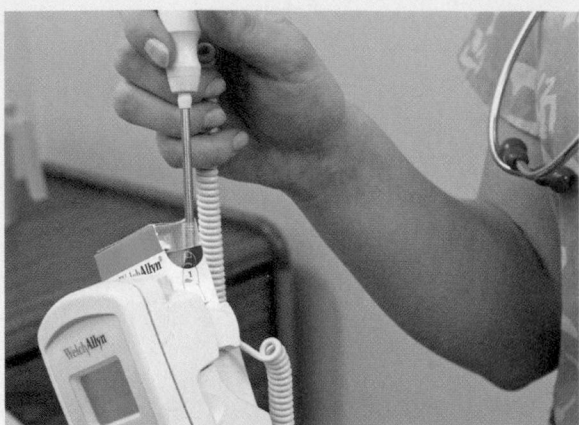

Action 2: Placing probe cover on thermometer.   (Photo by Rick Brady.)

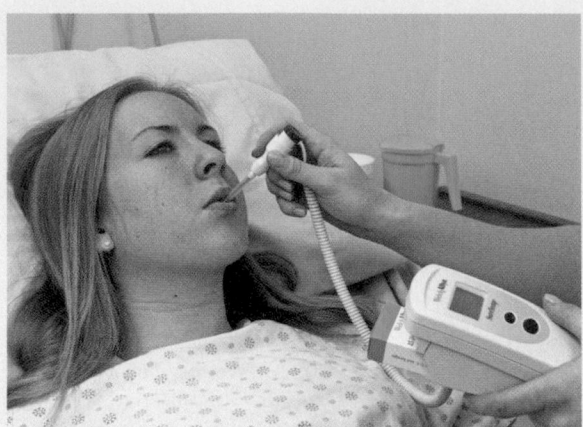

Action 3: Thermometer being placed under patient's tongue.
(Photo by Rick Brady.)

4. Continue to hold the probe until you hear a beep, letting you know that the reading is completed. Note the temperature reading.

If left unsupported, the weight of the probe tends to pull it away from the correct location. The signal indicates the measurement is completed. The electronic thermometer provides a digital display of the measured temperature.

5. Remove the probe from the patient's mouth and dispose of the probe cover by holding the probe over an appropriate receptacle and pressing the probe-release button.

Disposing of the probe cover ensures that it will not be accidentally reused on another patient.

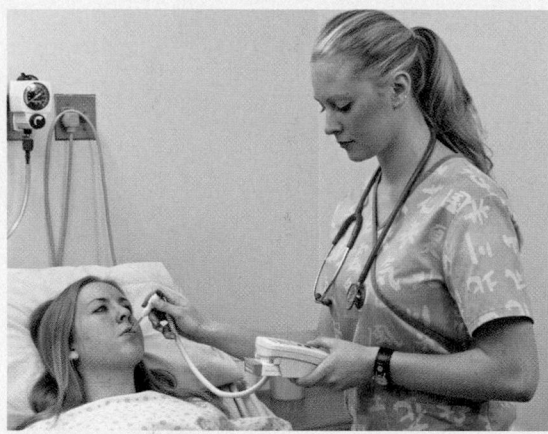

Action 4: Holding probe in place.   (Photo by Rick Brady.)

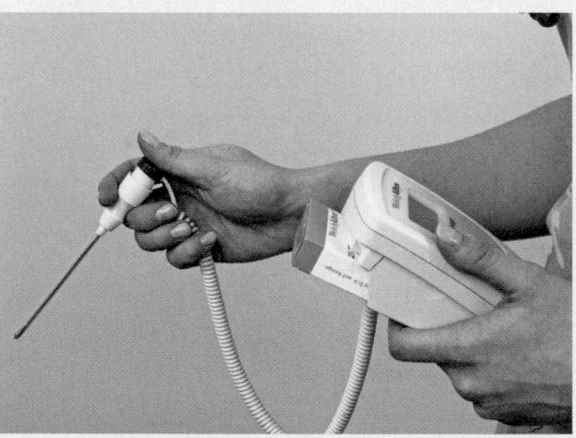

Action 5: Disposing of the probe cover.   (Photo by Rick Brady.)

6. Return the thermometer probe to the storage place within the unit and return the electronic unit to the charging unit to make sure it is fully charged.

Recharges the thermometer for future use

ASSESSING RECTAL TEMPERATURE WITH AN ELECTRONIC OR DIGITAL THERMOMETER

ACTION	RATIONALE
1. Put on gloves.	Protects nurse from microorganisms in the feces
2. Provide privacy for the patient by closing the door or curtain.	Ensures that patient's dignity is kept intact
3. Place the bed at an appropriate working height to reduce back strain during the procedure.	Reduces strain on the nurse's back

(continued)

SKILL
24-1   **Assessing Body Temperature** (continued)

ACTION	RATIONALE

4. Assist the patient onto a side-lying position. Pull back the covers enough to expose only the buttocks.

   The side-lying position allows the nurse to see the buttocks. By only exposing the buttocks, the nurse retains the patient's dignity and ensures that the patient remains warm.

5. Remove the probe from within the recording unit of the electronic thermometer. Cover the probe with a disposable probe cover and slide it until it snaps into place.

   Prevents contamination of the thermometer probe

6. Lubricate about 1 inch of the probe with a water-soluble lubricant.

   Lubrication reduces friction and facilitates insertion, minimizing irritation or injury to the rectal mucous membranes.

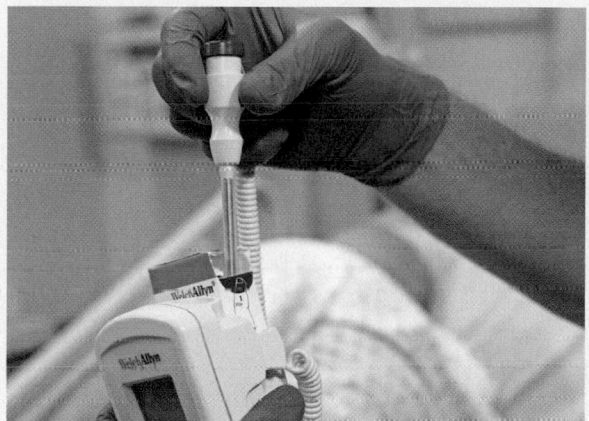

Action 5: Removing probe and attaching disposable probe cover.
(Photo by Rick Brady.)

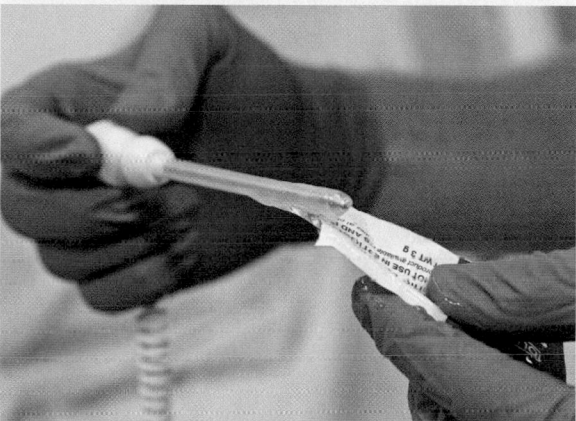

Action 6: Lubricating probe with water-soluble lubricant.
(Photo by Rick Brady.)

7. Reassure the patient. Separate the buttocks until the anal sphincter is clearly visible.

   If not placed directly into the anal opening, the thermometer probe may injure adjacent tissue or cause discomfort.

8. Insert the thermometer probe into the anus about 1½ inch in an adult or 1 inch in a child.

   Insertion length must be adjusted to the anatomic size of the rectum based on the patient's age; rectal temperatures are not normally taken in an infant.

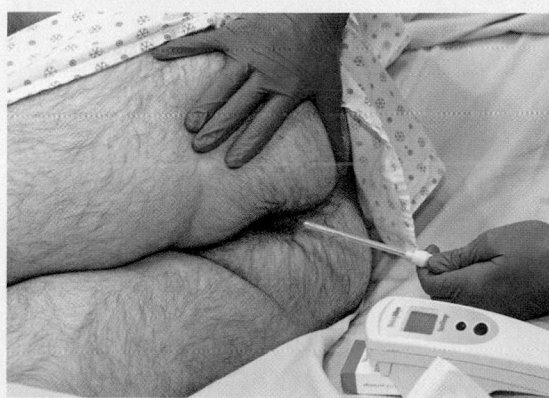

Action 8: Inserting thermometer into the anus.
(Photo by Rick Brady.)

9. Hold the probe in place until you hear a beep, then carefully remove the probe. Note the temperature reading on the display.

   If left unsupported, the weight of the probe tends to pull it away from the correct location. The signal indicates the measurement is completed. The electronic thermometer provides a digital display of the measured temperature.

10. Using toilet tissue, wipe the anus clean of any feces or excess lubricant.

   Promotes cleanliness

(continued)

SKILL 24-1 Assessing Body Temperature (continued)

ACTION	RATIONALE
11. Dispose of the toilet tissue. Dispose of the probe cover by holding the probe over an appropriate waste receptacle and pressing the release button.	Avoids transmission of microorganisms
12. Remove your gloves and discard. Perform hand hygiene.	
13. Cover the patient and help him or her to a comfortable position. Place the bed in the lowest position; elevate rails as needed.	Makes the patient comfortable. Provides for the patient's safety.
14. Return the thermometer to the charging unit.	Recharges the thermometer for future use

ASSESSING AXILLARY TEMPERATURE WITH AN ELECTRONIC OR DIGITAL THERMOMETER

ACTION	RATIONALE
1. Ensure privacy by closing the door or curtains.	Ensures that the patient's dignity is kept intact
2. Place the bed at an appropriate working height to reduce back strain during the procedure.	Reduces the strain on the nurse's back
3. Move the patient's clothing to expose only the axilla.	Ensures accurate placement of the thermometer
4. Remove the probe from the recording unit of the electronic thermometer. Place a disposable probe cover by sliding it on and snapping it securely.	Prevents contamination of the thermometer probe
5. Place the end of the probe in the center of the axilla. Have the patient bring his or her arm down and close to the body.	The deepest area of the axilla provides the most accurate measurement; surrounding the bulb with skin surface ensures a more reliable measurement.

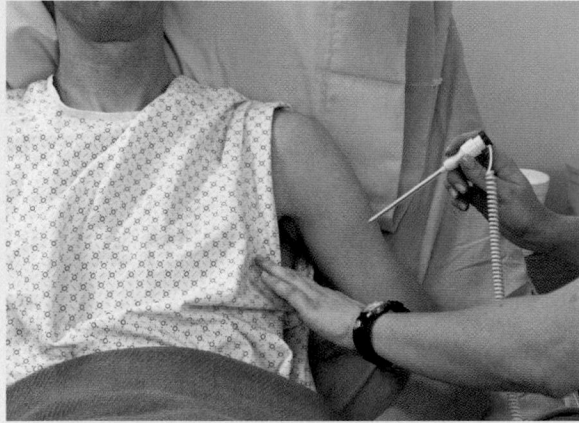

Action 3: Exposing axilla to assess temperature.   (Photo by Rick Brady.)

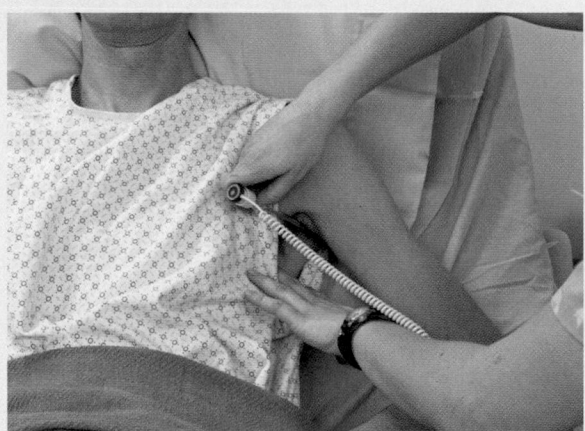

Action 5: Placing thermometer in center of axilla.   (Photo by Rick Brady.)

6. Hold the probe in place until you hear a beep, and then carefully remove the probe. Note the temperature reading.	Axilla thermometers must be held in place to receive an accurate temperature.
7. Dispose of the probe cover by holding the probe over an appropriate waste receptacle and pushing the release button.	Discarding the probe cover ensures that it will not be accidentally reused on another patient.
8. Place the bed in the lowest position and elevate rails as needed. Leave the patient clean and comfortable.	Provides for the patient's safety
9. Return the electronic thermometer to the charging unit.	Recharges the thermometer for future use

ASSESSING TEMPERATURE WITH A GLASS THERMOMETER

ACTION	RATIONALE
1. If stored in a chemical solution, wipe the thermometer dry with a soft tissue, using a firm, twisting motion. Wipe from the bulb toward the fingers.	Chemical solutions may irritate mucous membranes and have an objectionable taste. Twisting helps cover the entire surface. Wiping from an area of few or no organisms to an area where organisms might be present minimizes spread to a cleaner area.

(continued)

SKILL
24-1   Assessing Body Temperature (continued)

ACTION	RATIONALE
2. Grasp the thermometer firmly with the thumb and forefinger and, using strong wrist movements, shake it until the mercury line reaches at least 36°C (97°F).	Moves the chemical back into the bulb below the previous measurement
3. Read thermometer by holding it horizontally at eye level, and rotate it between the fingers until the mercury line can be visualized clearly.	Facilitates reading the chemical line
4. Place the mercury bulb of the thermometer within the back of the right or left pocket under the patient's tongue, and tell the patient to close the lips around the thermometer (oral); in the rectum, as described when using an electronic thermometer (rectal); or in the center of the axilla, with arm against chest wall (axillary).	The probe must be inserted correctly for an accurate reading.

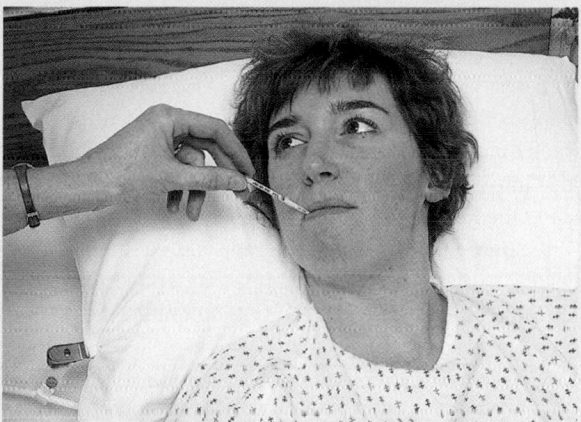

Action 4: Placing the thermometer.   (Photo © Ken Kasper.)

5. Leave the thermometer in place for 3 minutes, or according to agency protocol (oral); 2 to 3 minutes (rectal); and 10 minutes (axillary).	Allows time for the chemical to expand and accurately measure temperature. Axillary measurement requires a longer time for the chemical to expand. Staying with the patient ensures that the thermometer remains in the correct position and prevents breakage.
6. Remove the thermometer, and wipe it once from the fingers down to the mercury bulb, using a firm, twisting motion.	Minimizes spread of organisms from an area of higher concentration to a cleaner area; friction helps loosen material from the thermometer surface.
7. Read the thermometer to the nearest tenth.	Chemical may rise a bit above or below the calibration lines.

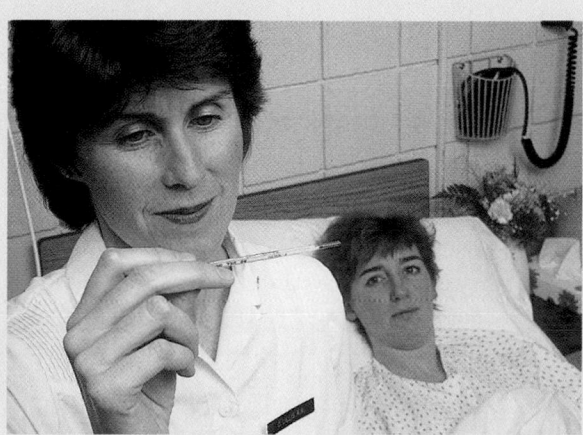

Action 7: Reading the temperature.   (Photo © Ken Kasper.)

(continued)

ACTION	RATIONALE
8. Dispose of the tissues in a receptacle for contaminated items.	Confining contaminated articles helps reduce the spread of pathogens.
9. Wash thermometer in lukewarm soapy water. Rinse it in cool water. Dry and replace the thermometer in its container.	Mechanical washing action removes organic material and organisms.

INFANT AND CHILD CONSIDERATIONS

The axillary, a temperature-sensitive tape, or the tympanic membrane is the preferred method of evaluating the body temperature of a child younger than 6 years of age (even though research is ongoing to determine accuracy of the measurement).

HOME CARE CONSIDERATIONS

The axillary or tympanic site should be used for a confused, disoriented, or comatose adult.

Reinforce differences in temperature reading depending on site used. Axillary temperatures are generally about 1°F lower than oral temperatures; rectal temperatures are generally about 1°F higher.

Remember Noah Shoolin, the toddler described at the beginning of the chapter? Although this type of thermometer yields a quick reading, the nurse would need to verify the accuracy of the reading, especially in light of the child's current upset, possibly by asking the mother if she had taken the child's temperature before coming to the emergency department or by using an alternative method.

Glass Thermometer

Although a glass thermometer with a mercury bulb has traditionally been used to measure body temperature, the danger of mercury poisoning has made this type almost obsolete. Many healthcare institutions no longer use or are phasing out mercury in any type of equipment, based on federal safety recommendations. However, many people still have mercury thermometers at home and might be continuing to use them. In some instances, glass thermometers might be used for patients in critical care units or on isolation. Information about the dangers of mercury, as well as how to handle a broken mercury thermometer, are important for nurses to know and teach. See Teaching to Promote Health at Home 24-1 for suggested teaching content.

Non-mercury glass thermometers are available. Non-mercury thermometers may be either spirit-filled (using a petroleum-based liquid) or alcohol-based. Thermometers with a red or blue liquid do not contain mercury (mercury is a silver liquid). This type of thermometer has a bulb at the end of a stem. The bulb contains a liquid that expands with heat and rises within the stem. Most commonly, a long, thin bulb is found on glass thermometers used to take oral temperatures, and a blunt bulb is found on glass thermometers used to take rectal temperatures.

Glass thermometers are generally calibrated in degrees of either centigrade (Celsius, C) or Fahrenheit (F) (see Fig. 24-1)

in a range of about 34°C (94°F) to about 42.2°C (108°F). The degrees on a thermometer using the Celsius scale are subdivided into gradients of 0.1°; the subdivisions on a thermometer using the Fahrenheit scale are the equivalent of 0.2°. Table 24-4 illustrates comparable centigrade and Fahrenheit temperatures and explains how temperatures are converted from one scale to the other. Assessing body temperature using a glass thermometer is described in Skill 24-1.

If glass thermometers are used within a healthcare institution, each patient has his or her own thermometer for the duration of inpatient care. The thermometer is kept in the patient's room, usually in a container of liquid disinfectant. It is recommended that glass thermometers used for patients with hepatitis (an infectious disease of the liver) and acquired immune deficiency syndrome (AIDS) be discarded when the patient is discharged.

In the home, clean thermometers in lukewarm soapy water, rinse in cool water, and then store for reuse. If the thermometer is to be used by more than one person or if the person has a known or suspected infection transmitted by oral secretions, disinfect the thermometer with an appropriate solution (such as alcohol) after cleaning. Follow the manufacturer's recommendations for the care and disposal of electronic and other types of thermometers and their probe covers.

Disposable Single-Use Thermometers

Disposable single-use thermometers, such as NexTemp, register within seconds and are nonbreakable. Because they are used only once, they eliminate the danger of cross-infection.

Temperature-sensitive patches or tape, commonly applied to the abdomen or forehead, change color at different temperature ranges. These devices may be used to check the temperature of a toddler or young child. A thermometer should be used to reassess the temperature if the color on the tape or patch indicates that the temperature is out of the normal average range.

Teaching to Promote Health at Home 24-1
Mercury Thermometers

Health Topic	Teaching Tip	Why is This Important?
What is mercury?	• Mercury is a heavy, odorless, silver liquid. • Glass thermometers containing mercury are easily broken.	Mercury is a toxic and hazardous material that affects the central nervous system. The liquid and the vapors from the liquid are both considered dangerous. Mercury not only is hazardous to people, but also pollutes the environment (especially if it gets into water). Mercury poisoning can lead to problems with mental development and learning disabilities.
What to do if a mercury thermometer breaks	**What Not to Do** • Sweep the area. • Vacuum the area. • Pour mercury down the drain. • Wash mercury-contaminated clothes. • Use household cleaning agents to clean the spill. **What to Do** • Open windows and close off the room from the rest of the house. Use fans for at least an hour if possible. • Use an eyedropper, a piece of heavy paper, or duct tape to scoop up the broken glass and beads of mercury. • Put the mercury, broken glass, and any materials used to scoop them up in a plastic zipper bag, and seal tightly with tape. Place this bag into a second bag and seal with tape, and then the second bag into a third bag, sealed with tape. Place the bags in a plastic wide-mouth sealable container. • Throw everything away that was exposed to the mercury (including linens, clothing, and towels). • Call your local health department to find out an approved disposal site. • Wash your hands with soap and water. Take a shower if you think any mercury touched other parts of the skin.	Sweeping breaks the mercury into smaller droplets. Mercury contaminates the vacuum. Mercury contaminates the washing machine and stays in the plumbing. Cleansing agents react with mercury, releasing a toxic gas.

TABLE 24-4 Equivalent Centigrade and Fahrenheit Temperatures*

Centigrade	Fahrenheit	Centigrade	Fahrenheit
34.0	93.2	38.5	101.3
35.0	95.0	39.0	102.2
36.0	96.8	40.0	104.0
36.5	97.6	41.0	105.8
37.0	98.6	42.0	107.6
37.5	99.5	43.0	109.4
38.0	100.4	44.0	111.2

* To convert centigrade to Fahrenheit, multiply by $9/5$ and add 32. To change Fahrenheit to centigrade, subtract 32 and multiply by $5/9$.

Temporal Artery Thermometer

Temporal artery thermometers measure body temperature by capturing the heat emitted from the skin over the temporal artery. These devices are battery operated, have an LED display, and can provide 1,000 readings per second (Bauer, 2003).

Automated Monitoring Devices

Automated monitoring devices are used in various healthcare settings to measure body temperature, pulse, and blood pressure simultaneously. They require less of the nurse's time, especially when these assessments are conducted frequently.

Sites and Methods of Assessing Body Temperature

Health agency policies and procedures often specify the site to be used for assessing patients' temperatures; however, the nurse is expected to select and to use alternative sites when appropriate. Factors affecting the site selection include the patient's age, state of consciousness, amount of pain, and other care being provided. It is customary to indicate the site used to assess the temperature when recording the measurement. Those sites most commonly used are discussed here.

An electronic probe or thermometer is placed under the tongue (sublingual area) of a person's mouth to assess an oral temperature, in the anal canal to assess a rectal temperature, or in an axilla (armpit) to assess an axillary temperature. A probe is placed in the ear to assess a tympanic temperature. For most clinical purposes, it would appear equally satisfactory to assess an oral, a rectal, a tympanic, or an axillary temperature, provided proper technique is used and normal variations among the methods are considered. Comparing the recordings using two different sites is a method for double-checking the validity of an unusual measurement.

Assessing a Tympanic Membrane Temperature

The tympanic membrane temperature is considered a core body temperature. Infrared sensors in the thermometer sense heat from the body as it is given off by a heat source; in the ear canal, the primary heat source is the tympanic membrane. The thermometer does not touch the tympanic membrane (see Skill 24-1). This site allows easy and safe measurement of temperature and is readily accessible. It should not be used for clients who have drainage from the ear or scars on the tympanic membrane. Temperature readings are not significantly altered by the presence of cerumen (ear wax) or otitis media (infection of the middle ear).

Assessing an Oral Temperature

One crucial criterion for selecting the oral site is that the patient must be able to close his or her mouth around the thermometer or probe. Assessing an oral temperature using a glass thermometer is contraindicated in unconscious, irrational, and seizure-prone patients and in infants and young children because of the danger of breaking the glass thermometer in the mouth. Oral temperatures also are contraindicated in people with diseases of the oral cavity and in those who have had surgery of the nose or mouth. If a patient has had either hot or cold food or fluids or has been smoking or chewing gum, it is generally recommended to wait 15 to 30 minutes to allow the oral tissues to return to normal temperature. Traditionally, oral temperatures have not been assessed in patients receiving nasal oxygen because it was believed that the oxygen causes a falsely low reading. Research is challenging this opinion. Oral temperatures should not be assessed in patients receiving oxygen by mask, however, because the time it takes to assess a reading is likely to result in a serious drop in the patient's blood oxygen level. The procedure for assessing an oral temperature is given in Skill 24-1.

Assessing a Rectal Temperature

The rectal temperature, a core temperature, is considered to be one of the most accurate. The rectal site is an alternative when-

ever the oral site is contraindicated (see Skill 24-1). However, patients are typically uncomfortable having their temperature taken rectally, so avoid this site if possible. Measuring rectal temperature is contraindicated in newborns, small children, and in patients who have undergone rectal surgery or have diarrhea or disease of the rectum. Because the insertion of the thermometer can slow the heart rate by stimulating the vagus nerve, assessing a rectal temperature may not be allowed in some institutions for people with certain heart diseases or after cardiac surgery. In addition, assessing a rectal temperature is contraindicated in clients who are neutropenic (have low white blood cell counts, such as in leukemia) and in clients who have certain neurologic disorders (for example, spinal cord injuries).

Assessing an Axillary Temperature

The axillary site may be used when both oral and rectal sites are contraindicated or when these sites are inaccessible. Some hospitals assess axillary temperatures in healthy newborns to avoid the potential for perforating the wall of the rectum with the thermometer. If the axilla has just been washed, delay assessing the temperature 15 to 30 minutes. Most authorities believe that when proper procedure is used, axillary temperatures are as accurate as oral or rectal temperatures. The procedure for assessing an axillary temperature is described in Skill 24-1.

Nursing Diagnoses

Examples of NANDA nursing diagnoses for alterations in body temperature are listed in the accompanying box.

PULSE

The **pulse** is a throbbing sensation that can be palpated over a peripheral artery or auscultated (listened to) over the apex of the heart. It results as a wave of blood is pumped into the arterial circulation by the contraction of the left ventricle. Each time the left ventricle of the heart contracts to eject blood into an already full aorta, the arterial walls in the cardiovascular system expand to compensate for the increase in pressure of the blood. Characteristics of the pulse, including rate, quality, rhythm, and volume, provide information about the effectiveness of the heart as a pump and the adequacy of peripheral blood flow.

Pulse Physiology

The pulse is regulated by the autonomic nervous system through the cardiac sinoatrial node (often called the pacemaker). Parasympathetic stimulation via the vagus nerve decreases the heart rate, and sympathetic stimulation increases the heart rate and force of contraction. The pulse rate is the number of pulsations felt over a peripheral artery or heard over the apex of the heart in 1 minute. This rate normally corresponds to the same rate at which the heart is beating.

Examples of NANDA Nursing Diagnoses | Altered Body Temperature

Nursing Diagnoses	Related Factors
Hyperthermia	Streptococcal upper respiratory infection
	Exposure to environmental heat without adequate cooling
	Abdominal surgery with general anesthesia
Hypothermia	Exposure to below freezing environmental temperature without adequate clothing
Risk for Imbalanced Body Temperature	Age (92 years) and head injury causing loss of consciousness
Ineffective Thermoregulation	Premature infant delivered at 30 weeks gestation

---

Variations in Pulse Rate, Amplitude, Quality, and Rhythm

Many factors can affect both the heart rate and volume; however, compensatory mechanisms attempt to maintain a sufficient supply of blood to the cells at all times. For example, when the stroke volume decreases, such as when the blood volume is decreased because of hemorrhage, the heart rate increases to try to maintain the same cardiac output. Conversely, in a physically fit athlete whose heart pumps a maximum volume of blood per stroke, the heart rate may be at the low range or below the range of normal, yet the body cells remain adequately supplied.

Pulse Rate

The pulse rate increases and decreases in response to a variety of physiologic mechanisms. It also might be altered by activity, medications, emotions, pain, heat and cold, and disease processes. The normal pulse rate ranges from 60 to 100 beats per minute.

Increased Pulse Rate

As the heart rate increases, cardiac output tends to increase. However, a rapid rate (**tachycardia**) decreases cardiac filling time, which, in turn, decreases stroke volume and cardiac output. An adult has tachycardia when the pulse rate is 100 to 180 beats/min. The factors contributing to tachycardia are listed in Box 24-3.

Decreased Pulse Rate

Bradycardia is a pulse rate below 60 beats/min in an adult. The pulse rate is normally slower during sleep, in men, and in people who are thin. It slows during hypothermia as metabolic processes decrease. With aging, the pulse tends to become slower. Normal pulse rates change across the life span, gradually diminishing from birth to adulthood, as shown in Table 24-5. Some medications, such as cardiotonic glycosides, slow the heart rate while also strengthening the force of contraction to increase cardiac output.

Sinus bradycardia results from the sinus node creating a slower-than-normal impulse rate. This type of bradycardia occurs at times when metabolic needs are decreased (eg, during sleep, in hypothermia, and in trained athletes at rest); from certain medications, such as beta blockers; from vagal stimulation (eg, from bearing down to have a bowel movement), during suctioning, or with severe pain, and in increased intracranial pressure and myocardial infarction. The nurse should immediately report bradycardia associated with difficult breathing, changes in level of consciousness, decreased blood pressure, ECG changes, and angina (heart pain). Emergency treatment consists of administering atropine intravenously to block vagal stimulation and to restore normal heart rate.

Pulse Amplitude and Quality

The pulse amplitude describes the quality of the pulse in terms of its fullness and reflects the strength of left ventricular contraction. It is assessed by the feel of the blood flow through the vessel. The amplitude of each pulse beat is normally strong at

---

BOX 24-3 Factors Contributing to Tachycardia

- A decrease in blood pressure, such as occurs with blood loss, when the heart's compensatory mechanisms attempt to meet the need for increased cardiac output
- An elevated temperature, which usually causes an increase of about 7 to 10 beats/min for each 0.6°C (1°F) of elevation above normal
- Any condition resulting in poor oxygenation of blood, for example, chronic pulmonary disease or anemia
- Exercise, when the heart's compensatory ability attempts to meet the need for increased blood circulation
- Prolonged application of heat
- Pain
- Strong emotions, such as fear, anger, anxiety, and surprise
- Some medications (eg, epinephrine [Adrenalin])

TABLE 24-5 Normal Pulse Rates (Beats per Minute) at Various Ages

Age	Approximate Range	Approximate Average
Newborn to 1 mo	120–160	140
1 to 12 mo	80–140	120
12 mo to 2 yr	80–130	110
2 to 6 yr	75–120	100
6 to 12 yr	75–110	95
Adolescence to adult	60–100	80

all areas where an artery can be palpated. A strong pulse can be obliterated with relative ease by exerting pressure over the artery, but it remains perceptible with moderate pressure. Table 24-6 presents a scale often used to describe and document pulse amplitude. In addition, the peripheral pulse may be described as full and bounding when it is forceful or weak and thready when it is feeble.

Pulse Rhythm

The pulse rhythm is the pattern of the pulsations and the pauses between them. This pattern is normally regular. An irregular pattern of heartbeats is called a **dysrhythmia.** Any irregularity in the heartbeat should be reported immediately. Common pulse rhythms are described and illustrated in Box 24-4.

Assessing the Pulse

The pulse may be assessed by palpating peripheral arteries or by auscultating the apical pulse with a stethoscope. The nurse needs to know how to use a stethoscope and which site and method are appropriate.

Remember Tomas Esposito, the middle-aged man requiring infection-control measures and

BOX 24-4 Pulse Rhythms

Regular Rhythms
The pulse rhythms and the pauses occur similarly.

Normal

Weak

Bounding

Dysrhythmias
The pulsations or lengths of pauses occur with no pattern or predictability.

Bisferiens

Pulsus alternans

Bigeminal
Premature contractions

assessment? Although the nurse had difficulty auscultating his heart and lung sounds, the nurse would need to assess his pulse radially and apically. It is possible that by palpating his radial pulse and then attempting to auscultate his apical pulse and not hearing anything, the nurse might have gotten a clue leading her to suspect that the stethoscope was not functioning properly.

Equipment

Depending on the health status of the patient, various types of equipment may be used to assess the pulse. The stethoscope is used to auscultate the apical pulse in most healthcare settings. A cardiac monitor may be used to assess the apical pulse in critical care or emergency department care. The monitor produces a graph or digital reading of the pulse rate and amplitude.

Stethoscope

The acoustical stethoscope, the most common type used, has an amplifying mechanism connected to earpieces by tubing (Fig. 24-2). The most common amplifying devices are the diaphragm, which is a large, flat disk, and the bell, which has a hollowed, upright, curved appearance. The diaphragm is more

TABLE 24-6 Pulse Amplitude

Number	Definition	Description
0	Absent pulse	No pulsation is felt despite extreme pressure.
1+	Thready pulse	Pulsation is not easily felt, and slight pressure causes it to disappear.
2+	Weak pulse	Stronger than a thready pulse; light pressure causes it to disappear.
3+	Normal pulse	Pulsation is easily felt, takes moderate pressure to cause it to disappear.
4+	Bounding pulse	The pulsation is strong and does not disappear with moderate pressure.

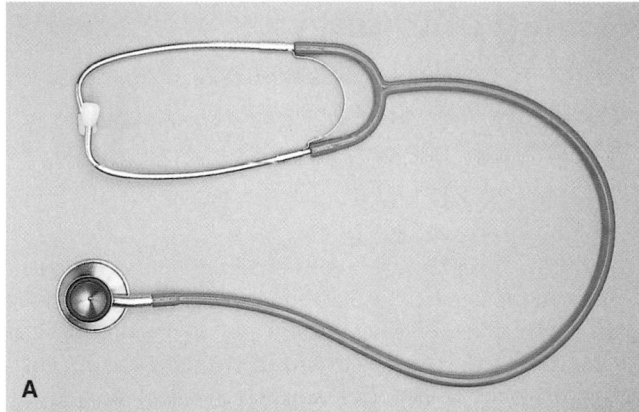

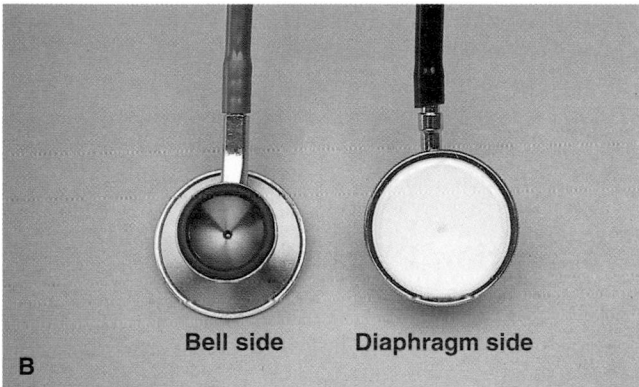

Bell side   Diaphragm side

FIGURE 24-2 (**A**) Stethoscope. (**B**) Two sides of stethoscope amplifier. (Photo © Ken Kasper.)

useful for hearing high-frequency sounds, such as respiratory sounds, because it screens out low-frequency sounds. The bell screens out high-frequency sounds and is more useful for hearing low-frequency sounds, such as those commonly made by the heart and the blood within the vessels.

The ear tips of the stethoscope should be selected to fit one's ear canals comfortably and snugly for the most effective auscultation. The tips should be large enough to block out extraneous noises in the environment when the stethoscope is being used. The tips should be directed into the ear canal, not against the ear itself.

Doppler Ultrasound Stethoscope

A Doppler ultrasound stethoscope may be used to assess pulses that are difficult to palpate or auscultate. The device has an earpiece connected to an audio unit with an ultrasound transducer. Techniques for assessing pulses with a Doppler ultrasound stethoscope are outlined in Guidelines for Nursing Care 24-1.

Sites and Methods of Assessing the Pulse

Nurses must know the correct site and method for assessing the pulse. Although peripheral pulses are most commonly assessed, an apical pulse or an apical-radial pulse should be assessed in certain situations, described below.

Guidelines for Nursing Care 24-1
Using a Doppler Ultrasound Stethoscope to Assess Pulse and Blood Pressure

A Doppler ultrasound stethoscope may be used to assess pulses or a blood pressure that are difficult to palpate or auscultate. This device has an ultrasound transducer and an audio unit and transmits the sounds of red blood cells moving through the blood vessel. The procedure for using this device is as follows:

- Perform hand hygiene.
- Collect the Doppler ultrasound stethoscope, the transducer in the Doppler probe (the probe looks like a small transistor radio), a stethoscope headset, and transmission gel.
- Plug the headset into one of the two output jacks next to the volume control.
- Apply a small amount of transmission gel to either the probe or to the patient's skin over the selected area.
- Use the "on" button to activate the transducer.
- Hold the probe at a 90-degree angle to the skin over the pulse site while maintaining contact with the skin and the transmission gel.
- Listen for pumping sounds, indicating arterial pulse.
- Count the rate of the pulse for 1 minute; when used for blood pressure, usually the only measurement that can be assessed is the systolic reading (first sound heard).
- Remove gel from the probe and the patient's skin; do not use alcohol to clean the transducer because it may damage the transducer covering.
- Perform hand hygiene, and document pulse rate by Doppler.

Assessing Peripheral Arterial Pulses

There are many peripheral artery sites that might be used to assess the pulse by palpation. Those most commonly used are illustrated in Figure 24-3. Of these sites, the radial pulse site is used most often in children and adults. Peripheral pulses are assessed by placing the middle three fingers over the artery and lightly compressing the artery so pulsations can be felt and counted. See Skill 24-2 for assessing the radial pulse.

Circulation to the legs and feet is assessed at the femoral, popliteal, posterior tibial, and dorsalis pedis sites. The carotid pulse site is used during emergency assessments, such as for patients who are in shock or have had a cardiac arrest. When taking a carotid pulse, lightly palpate only one side to prevent any decrease in cerebrovascular circulation. The brachial pulse site is used for infants who have had a cardiac arrest.

Assessing the Apical Pulse

If a peripheral pulse is difficult to assess accurately because it is irregular, feeble, or extremely rapid, the apical rate should be assessed. An apical pulse is also assessed when giving medications that alter heart rate and rhythm. In adults, the apical rate is counted for 1 full minute by listening with a stethoscope over the apex of the heart. The contraction of the heart can be heard in the space between the fifth and the sixth ribs, about

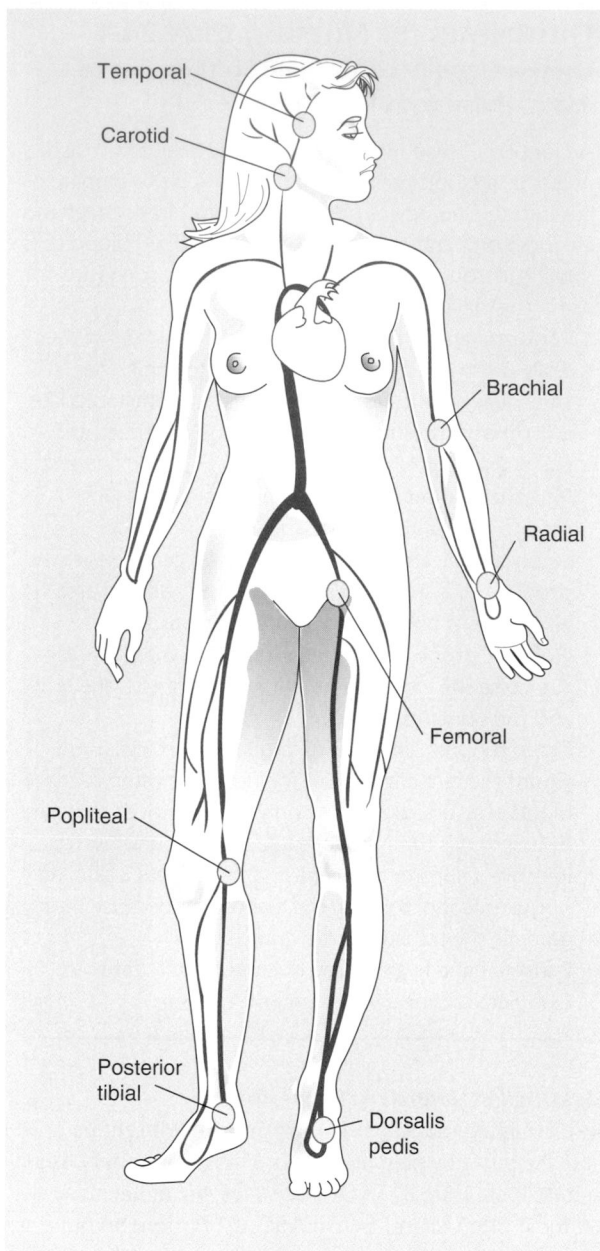

FIGURE 24-3 These arteries are located near the surface of the body. The pulse can be detected in any of these sites by light palpation.

Labels on figure: Temporal, Carotid, Brachial, Radial, Femoral, Popliteal, Posterior tibial, Dorsalis pedis

8 cm (3 inches) to the left of the median line and slightly below the nipple (see "Assessing the Apical Pulse" in Nursing Skill 24-2). The apical rate of an infant is easily palpated with the fingertips.

Assessing the Apical-Radial Pulse

When the radial pulse is irregular, counting the pulse at the apex of the heart and at the radial artery simultaneously is used to assess the apical-radial pulse rate. The techniques for taking an apical-radial pulse are outlined in Guidelines for Nursing Care 24-2. A difference between the apical and radial pulse rates is called the **pulse deficit,** and signals that all of the heartbeats are not reaching the peripheral arteries or are too weak to be palpated.

Nursing Diagnoses

Examples of NANDA nursing diagnoses for alterations in the pulse are listed in the accompanying box.

RESPIRATIONS

Respiration involves several physiologic events. Pulmonary ventilation (or breathing) is movement of air in and out of the lungs; inspiration (or inhalation) is the act of breathing in, and expiration (or exhalation) is the act of breathing out. External respiration is the exchange of oxygen and carbon dioxide between the alveoli of the lungs and the circulating blood through diffusion. Internal respiration is the exchange of oxygen and carbon dioxide between the circulating blood and tissue cells.

Although nurses assess the manifestations of changes in all of these respiratory events, the part that is measured as a vital sign is pulmonary ventilation, called respirations. Respiratory system assessment is described further in Chapter 25.

Respiration Physiology

The rate and depth of breathing can change in response to body demands. These changes are brought about by the inhibition or stimulation of the respiratory muscles by respiratory centers in the medulla and pons. The respiratory centers are activated by impulses from chemoreceptors located in the aortic arch and carotid arteries, from stretch and irritant receptors in the lungs, and from receptors in muscles and joints. An increase in carbon dioxide is the most powerful respiratory stimulant, causing an increase in respiratory depth and rate. The cerebral cortex of the brain allows voluntary control of breathing, such as when singing or playing a musical instrument. See Chapter 45 for a detailed discussion of respiratory physiology.

Variations in Respiratory Rate and Depth

The rate and depth of inhalation and exhalation are normally smooth, effortless, and without conscious effort. However, factors ranging from environmental changes to pathophysiologic alterations in various body systems many result in increases or decreases in respiratory rate and depth.

Factors Affecting Respiration

Many different factors may affect respiratory rate and depth. These factors include exercise, respiratory and cardiovascular disease, alterations in fluid, electrolyte, and acid–base balances, medications, trauma, infection, pain, and anxiety. Factors that affect respiratory rate, depth and movements are outlined in Box 24-5.

Respiratory Rate

Under normal conditions, healthy adults breathe about 12 to 20 times each minute, whereas infants and young children breathe more rapidly. Normal respiration is called **eupnea.**

SKILL 24-2   Assessing the Pulse

EQUIPMENT

Watch with second hand or digital readout   Pencil or pen, paper, or flow sheet   Alcohol swab (for stethoscope)
Stethoscope (for apical pulse)

Use guidelines outlined below for all sites and methods.

Guidelines for Assessing, Implementing, and Documenting Pulses

ACTION	RATIONALE
1. Identify the patient.	Provides patient safety
2. Explain the procedure to the patient.	Reduces patient apprehension and encourages patient cooperation
3. Gather equipment.	Provides organized approach to task
4. Perform hand hygiene and don gloves as appropriate.	Deters the spread of microorganisms
5. Select the appropriate site.	Different arteries may be used to assess the pulse; apical pulses are assessed if the peripheral pulse is rapid, irregular, or inaudible.
6. Follow the steps as outlined below for the appropriate pulse assessment.	
7. Perform hand hygiene.	Deters the spread of microorganisms
8. Record pulse rate and site on paper, flow sheet, or computerized record. Report abnormal findings to the appropriate person. Identify site of assessment if other than apical.	Provides accurate documentation and reporting

Assessing the Radial Pulse

1. The patient may either be supine with the arm alongside the body, wrist extended, and palms of the hand down or sitting with the forearm at a 90-degree angle to the body resting on a support with the wrist extended and the palm downward.

   These positions are comfortable for the patient and convenient for the nurse.

2. Place your first, second, and third fingers along the patient's radial artery, and press gently against the radius. Rest your thumb on the back of the patient's wrist.

   The sensitive fingertips can feel the pulsation of the artery.

3. Apply only enough pressure so that the artery can be felt distinctly.

   Moderate pressure facilitates palpation of the pulsations. Too much pressure obliterates the pulse, whereas the pulse is imperceptible with too little pressure.

4. Using a watch with a second hand, count the number of pulsations felt for 30 seconds. Multiply this number by 2 to have the rate for 1 minute. If the rate, rhythm, or amplitude of the pulse are abnormal in any way, palpate and count the pulse for 1 minute or longer.

   Sufficient time must be allowed to assess the rate, rhythm, and amplitude of the pulse. When pulse characteristics are abnormal, a longer time period is necessary for accurate assessment.

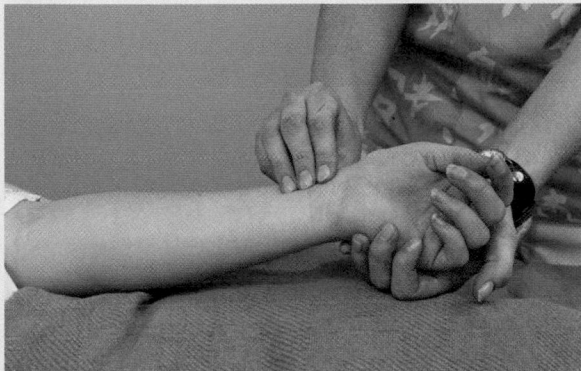

Action 2: Proper placement of the fingers along the radial artery.
(Photo by Rick Brady.)

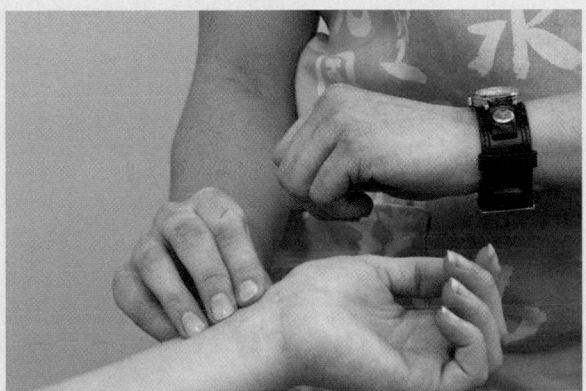

Action 4: Counting the pulsations felt for 30 seconds.
(Photo by Rick Brady.)

(continued)

ACTION	RATIONALE
Assessing the Apical Pulse	
1. Use alcohol swab to clean ear pieces and diaphragm of the stethoscope.	Deters transmission of microorganisms
2. Assist patient in sitting in a chair or sitting up in bed, and expose upper chest area.	This position facilitates identification of site for stethoscope placement.
3. Hold stethoscope diaphragm against the palm of your hand for a few seconds.	Warms diaphragm, promoting patient comfort
4. Palpate fifth intercostal space, and move to the left midclavicular line. Place the diaphragm over the apex of the heart.	This is the point of maximum impulse where the heartbeat is best heard.

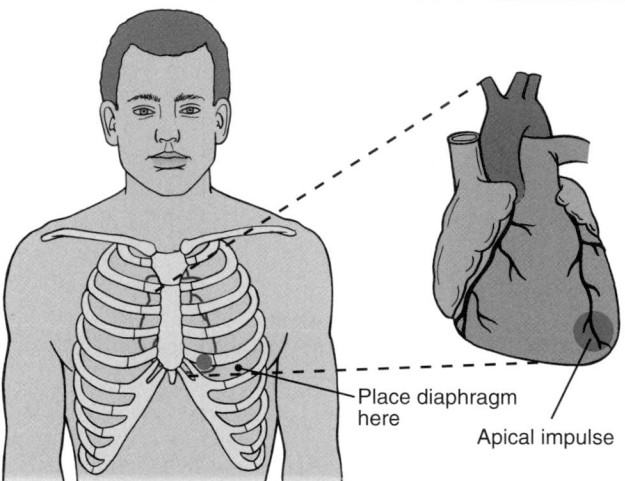

Place diaphragm here
Apical impulse

Schematic depiction of the thorax showing location of apical impulse.

5. Listen for heart sounds, identified as a "lub-dub" sound.	These sounds occur as the heart valves close.
6. Using a watch with a second hand, count the heartbeat for 1 minute.	A longer time period increases the accuracy of assessment.

Age Considerations	The normal heart rate varies by age.
Home Care Considerations	Teach the patient and family how to take own pulse.
	Inform the patient and family about digital pulse monitoring devices.
	Teach family members how to locate and monitor peripheral pulse sites.

Guidelines for Nursing Care 24-2
Taking an Apical-Radial Pulse

The following techniques are recommended to assess an apical-radial pulse rate:

- Two nurses are needed; one listens with a stethoscope over the apex of the heart for the heartbeat, and the other counts the rate at the radial artery.
- The patient's chest wall is exposed so that the stethoscope can be placed directly on the skin of the chest wall.

- One watch with a sweep second hand is placed, so that both nurses can read it simultaneously.
- The nurses determine where they can best hear and feel the pulse and decide on a time to start counting, such as when the second hand on the watch is at a specified place (such as the number 12).
- Both nurses count for 1 full minute and record their counts.

Examples of NANDA Nursing Diagnoses | Altered Pulse

Nursing Diagnoses	Related Factors
Decreased Cardiac Output	History of congestive heart failure and dysrhythmias Traumatic injury with extensive blood loss
Ineffective Tissue Perfusion: Peripheral	History of peripheral vascular disease with decreased popliteal pulses
Deficient Fluid Volume	Exposure to high environmental temperature, increased age, and tachycardia
Acute Pain	First postoperative day following major surgery, crying, and tachycardia

---

BOX 24-5 Factors Affecting Respiratory Rate, Depth, and Movements

- Age: The respiratory rate decreases with age, ranging from a normal range of 30–60 breaths/min in a newborn to 12–20 breaths/min in an adult.
- Gender: In males, respiratory movements are primarily diaphragmatic, whereas in women, there is greater intercostal muscle movement.
- Exercise: Exercise increases respiratory rate and depth.
- Acid–base balance: Alterations in acid–base balance (especially acidosis) commonly result in increased rate and depth of respirations (hyperventilation).
- Brain lesions: Lesions of the brain (such as hemorrhage or tumors) or brain stem can cause a change in both the depth and rate of respirations, most commonly manifested as Cheyne-Stokes respirations.
- Increased altitude: As an adaptation to higher altitudes, healthy people may exhibit Cheyne-Stokes respirations, especially when asleep. Higher altitudes also increase respiratory rate and depth prior to adaptation by increasing hemoglobin levels.
- Respiratory diseases: Any alterations in the normal respiratory structures may result in changes in respiratory rate, depth, and patterns, most often manifested as difficult breathing, using accessory muscles of respiration (such as the intercostal muscles), and increased rate. The depth may be shallower. Smoking can alter the pulmonary airways, resulting in an increase in respiratory rate at rest.
- Anemia: Anemia, a decrease in oxygen-carrying hemoglobin, may result in an increased rate of respirations.
- Anxiety: Anxiety can cause sighing type respirations (increased depth) and increased rate.
- Medications. Medications, such as narcotics, sedatives, and general anesthetics slow respiratory rate and depth. Other drugs, including amphetamines and cocaine, may increase rate and depth.
- Acute pain: Acute pain increases respiratory rate but may decrease respiratory depth.

The relationship of one respiration to four heartbeats is fairly consistent in healthy people. Respiratory rate increases in response to exercise, pain, and emotions.

> Think back to Noah Shoolin, the 2-year-old brought to the emergency department. The nurse would anticipate that the child's respiratory rate would be increased most likely as a result of his screaming and emotional upset.

Increased Respiratory Rate

Tachypnea, an increased respiratory rate, occurs in response to the increased metabolic rate during fever (pyrexia). Cells require more oxygen at this time and have more carbon dioxide that must be removed. The rate increases as much as 4 breaths/min with every 0.6°C (1°F) that the temperature rises above normal. Any condition causing an increase in carbon dioxide and a decrease in oxygen in the blood also tends to increase the rate and depth of respirations.

Decreased Respiratory Rate

Bradypnea, a decrease in respiratory rate, characteristically occurs in some pathologic conditions. An increase in intracranial pressure depresses the respiratory center, resulting in irregular or shallow breathing, slow breathing, or both. Certain drugs, such as narcotics (eg, morphine, meperidine [Demerol]), also depress the respiratory rate.

Respiratory Depth and Rhythm

The depth of respirations normally varies from shallow to deep. The depth of each respiration is about the same during rest. Periodically, each person automatically inhales deeply (sighs), filling the lungs with more air than with the usual depth of respiration.

Certain terms are used to describe the nature and depth of respirations. **Apnea** refers to periods during which there is no breathing. If apnea lasts longer than 4 to 6 minutes, brain damage and death might occur. **Dyspnea** is difficult or labored breathing. A dyspneic patient usually has rapid, shallow respirations and appears anxious. Dyspneic people can often breathe more easily in an upright position, a condition known as **orthopnea.** While sitting or standing, gravity lowers organs in the abdominal cavity away from the diaphragm. This gives more room for the lungs to expand within the chest, providing intake of more air with each breath. Table 24-7 describes and illustrates various respiratory patterns.

Assessing Respirations

The nurse assesses respiratory rate, depth, and rhythm by inspection (observing and listening) or by listening with the stethoscope. Other methods of assessing respiratory effectiveness include monitoring arterial blood gas results and using a pulse oximeter to determine oxygenation of blood. A description of a pulse oximeter and a procedure for using it are found in Chapter 45.

When assessing respirations while taking vital signs, the nurse counts the patient's respiratory rate. Skill 24-3 describes

how to assess the respiratory rate. Further assessments of respiratory structure and function are described in Chapter 25.

Nursing Diagnoses

Examples of NANDA nursing diagnoses for alterations in respirations are listed in the accompanying box.

BLOOD PRESSURE

Blood pressure refers to the force of the blood against arterial walls. Maximum blood pressure is exerted on the walls of arteries when the left ventricle of the heart pushes blood through the aortic valve into the aorta at the beginning of systole. The pressure rises as the ventricle contracts and falls as the heart relaxes. This continuous contraction and relaxation of the left ventricle creates a pressure wave that is transmitted through the arterial system (Porth, 2002). The highest pressure

TABLE 24-7 Patterns of Respiration

	Description	Pattern	Associated Features
Normal	12–20 breaths/min Regular		Normal pattern
Tachypnea	>24 breaths/min Shallow		Fever, anxiety, exercise, respiratory disorders
Bradypnea	<10 breaths/min Regular		Depression of the respiratory center by medications, brain damage
Hyperventilation	Increased rate and depth		Extreme exercise, fear, diabetic ketoacidosis (Kussmaul's respirations), overdose of aspirin
Hypoventilation	Decreased rate and depth; irregular		Overdose of narcotics or anesthetics
Cheyne-Stokes respirations	Alternating periods of deep, rapid breathing followed by periods of apnea; regular		Drug overdose, heart failure, increased intracranial pressure, renal failure
Biot's respirations	Varying depth and rate of breathing, followed by periods of apnea; irregular		Meningitis, severe brain damage

SKILL
24-3   **Assessing the Respiratory Rate**

EQUIPMENT

Watch with second hand or digital readout   Pencil or pen, paper or flow sheet

ACTION	RATIONALE
1. While your fingers are still in place after counting the pulse rate, observe the patient's respirations.	The patient may alter the rate of respirations if aware they are being counted.
2. Note the rise and fall of the patient's chest.	A complete cycle of an inspiration and an expiration composes one respiration.
3. Using a watch with a second hand, count the number of respirations for a minimum of 30 seconds. Multiply this number by 2 for the respiratory rate per minute.	Sufficient time is necessary to observe the rate, depth, and other characteristics.
4. If respirations are abnormal in any way, count the respirations for at least 1 full minute.	Increased time allows the detection of unequal timing between respirations.
5. Document respiratory rate on paper, the flow sheet, or the computerized record. Report any abnormal findings to the appropriate person.	Provides accurate documentation and reporting
6. Perform hand hygiene.	Deters the spread of microorganisms

is the **systolic pressure.** When the heart rests between beats during diastole, the pressure drops. The lowest pressure present on arterial walls at this time is the **diastolic pressure.** The difference between the two is called the **pulse pressure.**

Blood pressure is measured in millimeters of mercury (mm Hg) and is recorded as a fraction. The numerator is the systolic pressure; the denominator is the diastolic pressure. For example, if the blood pressure is 120/80 mm Hg, 120 is the systolic pressure and 80 is the diastolic pressure. The pulse pressure, in this case, is 40.

Blood Pressure Physiology

Blood pressure regulation is controlled by a variety of mechanisms to maintain adequate tissue perfusion. The arterial blood pressure has constant minor variations from activities of daily living, such as rising from a sitting to a standing position, exercise, or emotions (Porth, 2002).

Recall Doretha Renfrow, the wife of a man with hypertension? The nurse would need to integrate physiologic information about blood pressure regulation when developing the teaching plan for Mrs. Renfrow.

Peripheral Resistance and Compliance

Blood leaving the heart circulates through a continuous loop of blood vessels consisting of arteries, arterioles, capillaries, venules, and veins. Arterioles are very small elastic tubes that can contract or dilate to regulate the distribution of blood to various organs, tissues, or cells, depending on their moment-by-moment requirements. Normally, arterioles are in a state of partial contraction, resulting in peripheral resistance and creating a relatively constant level of restraint to blood flow. Peripheral resistance is one of the main factors affecting blood pressure.

Examples of
NANDA
Nursing Diagnoses | **Altered Respirations**

Nursing Diagnoses	Related Factors
Ineffective Breathing Pattern	Anxiety about diagnostic procedure for possible malignancy Increased intracranial pressure following head injury Infant delivered by cesarean delivery at 28 weeks gestation
Impaired Gas Exchange	Presence of acute respiratory distress following smoke inhalation
Risk for Activity Intolerance	History of smoking two packs of cigarettes a day for 20 years

Arteries have a considerable quantity of elastic tissue that allows them to stretch and distend (called compliance). When the heart rests between each beat, the walls of the arteries recoil, although pressure in them does not drop to zero. The state of pressure keeps the blood entering the capillaries in a continuous flow rather than in spurts. Simultaneously, the arterioles offer resistance. Therefore, the elasticity of the walls, in addition to the resistance of the arterioles, helps to maintain normal blood pressure. With age, the walls of arterioles become less elastic, which interferes with their ability to stretch and dilate. This can subsequently limit adequate blood flow and contribute to rising pressure within the vascular system.

Neural and Humoral Mechanisms

The autonomic nervous system mediates control mechanisms that function to maintain short-term regulation of blood pressure. These mechanisms include circulatory system baroreflex and chemoreceptor-mediated reflexes, as well as factors outside the circulatory system, such as pain and cold, that affect blood pressure responses. Blood pressure may change in response to central nervous system ischemia (decreased blood flow), mood, and emotion.

Many different hormones and humoral mechanisms also help regulate blood pressure. The renin-angiotensin-aldosterone system controls vasoconstriction to increase peripheral vascular resistance and also increases sodium and water retention by the kidneys to increase circulatory fluid volume and thus increase blood pressure. Antidiuretic hormone (ADH, vasopressin) is released from the posterior pituitary when stimulated by decreased blood volume and blood pressure, or by an increased osmolarity of the blood. As a result, water is retained to increase circulatory fluid volume and, in turn, increase blood pressure.

Cardiac Output

The quantity of blood forced out of the left ventricle with each contraction is called the stroke volume (SV). The cardiac output (CO) is the amount of blood pumped per minute, and aver-

ages from 3.5 L to 8.0 L/min in a healthy adult (Porth, 2002). This volume is determined by using the following formula: Cardiac Output = Stroke Volume × Heart Rate. Thus, the cardiac output of an adult with a stroke volume of 70 mL and a heart rate of 70 beats/min is 4.9 L/min. Cardiac output increases during exercise and decreases during sleep; it also varies depending on body size and metabolic needs. Trained athletes participating in maximal exercise may have a CO as great as 32 L/min (Porth, 2002).

When cardiac output is increased, the arteries distend more, resulting in increased blood pressure. When cardiac output is decreased, blood pressure falls. Hence, a weak pumping action results in a lower blood pressure than a strong pumping action. Cardiac output was described in relation to the pulse earlier in the chapter.

Variations in Blood Pressure

Studies of healthy people indicate that blood pressure can be within a wide range and still be normal. Because of considerable individual differences, it is important to know the normal blood pressure of a particular person. A rise or fall of 20 to 30 mm Hg in a person's blood pressure is significant, even if it is within the generally accepted normal range. Although blood pressure varies constantly, sustained long-term changes are not normal. Blood pressure categories for adults are found in Table 24-8.

Factors Affecting Blood Pressure

Those factors that commonly cause variations in blood pressure are listed in Box 24-6. Because of the many factors that influence blood pressure, a single blood pressure measurement is not necessarily significant. The American Heart Association recommends that blood pressure readings be averaged on two or more subsequent occasions before diagnosing high blood pressure. Measurements should be taken after the patient rests for at least 5 minutes and has not consumed caffeine or smoked for 30 minutes before the measurement.

TABLE 24-8 Categories for Blood Pressure Levels in Adults (Ages 18 and older)

Category	Blood Pressure Level (mm Hg)	
	Systolic	Diastolic
Normal (In regard to risk of heart disease, optimal is defined as less than 120/80 mm Hg.)	<120	<80
High Blood Pressure		
Prehypertension	120–139	80–89
Stage 1	140–159	90–99
Stage 2	≥160	≥100

These categories are from the National Heart, Lung, and Blood Institute, National Institutes of Health, new clinical guidelines, 2003, and are available from http://www.nhlbi.nih.gov/hbp/detect/categ.htm.

Factors Contributing to Blood Pressure Variations in Healthy People

- *Age:* The older adult has decreased elasticity of the arteries, which increases peripheral resistance and therefore increases blood pressure.
- *Circadian rhythm:* Normal fluctuations occur during the day. The blood pressure is usually lowest on arising in the morning. The blood pressure has been noted to rise as much as 5 to 10 mm Hg by late afternoon, and it gradually falls again during sleep.
- *Sex:* Women usually have lower blood pressure than men of the same age until menopause.
- *Food intake:* Blood pressure increases after eating food.
- *Exercise:* Systolic blood pressure rises during periods of exercise and strenuous activity.
- *Weight:* Blood pressure is usually higher in people who are obese than in those who are thin.
- *Emotional state:* Emotions, such as anger, fear, excitement, and pain, generally cause the blood pressure to rise, but the pressure falls to normal when the situation passes.
- *Body position:* A person's blood pressure tends to be lower in a prone or supine position than when sitting or standing.
- *Race:* Race is a factor in increased blood pressure (hypertension), which is more prevalent and more severe in African American men and women.
- *Drugs/Medications:* Oral contraceptives cause a mild increase in blood pressure in many women.

Increased Blood Pressure

Hypertension is blood pressure that is above normal for a sustained period. It is one of the most common health problems in adults and the leading cause of cardiovascular disorders. It is estimated that about 25% of all people older than age 18 years have hypertension (Porth, 2002). Primary or essential hypertension is hypertension without a known cause. When the hypertension is caused by a known pathology, it is called secondary hypertension. Hypertension is a major risk factor for heart disease and is the most important risk factor associated with stroke. It is often called "the silent killer" because there are few symptoms beyond the increased blood pressure; approximately 22 million Americans do not know they have hypertension (Ofili, 2003).

The basis for hypertension is dysfunction of the neurohormonal system. Overactivation of both angiotensin and aldosterone result in an increase in blood pressure. Over time, this sustained increase results in a permanent remodeling and thickening of the blood vessels. As a result, there is increased peripheral resistance, and a back-up of pressure to organs affected by the vascular system, such as the brain, heart, and kidneys. Disorders of these organs include thickening of the myocardium, enlargement of the ventricles, congestive heart failure, myocardial infarctions, stroke, and kidney damage.

There are many risk factors for the development of hypertension. Significant risks are a family history of hypertension, sedentary lifestyle, obesity, and continual stress. Other high-risk factors include cigarette smoking, alcohol consumption, high salt intake, and a high-fat, high-calorie diet. Although the exact reason has not been determined, hypertension is almost twice as common in African Americans as in Americans of European descent.

Remember Mrs. Renfrow, the wife of a man who is overweight and diagnosed with hypertension? The nurse would need to incorporate information about various risk factors for developing hypertension as well as information about risk related to hypertension in the teaching plan for Mrs. Renfrow.

Hypertension can be controlled by medications and lifestyle changes. The categories of antihypertensive medications include diuretics (to decrease fluid volume), beta-adrenergic blockers (to block sympathetic stimulation and decrease cardiac output), vasodilators and calcium channel blockers (to relax smooth muscles of arterioles and decrease peripheral vascular resistance), and ACE inhibitors (to prevent vasoconstriction by angiotensin II and decrease circulatory fluid volume by reducing aldosterone production). Lifestyle changes include following a low-calorie, low-fat diet; losing excess weight and maintaining weight loss; limiting alcohol intake; eliminating smoking; reducing salt intake; and having regular physical activity. Nurses can influence the health of the public through screenings, education, and referrals.

Decreased Blood Pressure

Hypotension is below-normal blood pressure. A consistently low blood pressure (eg, a systolic reading of 90–115 mm Hg) is normal in some adults, such as highly trained athletes. Most cases of hypotension are the result of pathology. Pathologic hypotension might result from vasodilation of the arterioles, failure of the heart to function as an effective pump, or loss of blood volume (such as with a hemorrhage). The nurse should immediately report assessments of hypotension, tachycardia, pallor, increased sweating, and confusion.

Orthostatic hypotension (postural hypotension) is a low blood pressure associated with weakness or fainting when one rises to an erect position (either supine to sitting, supine to standing, or sitting to standing). It is the result of peripheral vasodilation without a compensatory rise in cardiac output. Patients most at risk for postural hypotension are older adults, patients who have been on prolonged bed rest, and those who are dehydrated or have sustained a significant blood loss. Some drugs, such as meperidine hydrochloride (Demerol) cause hypotension.

Arising and moving about slowly, especially after a period of bed rest, might prevent this type of hypotension. When ambulating the postoperative patient, the nurse should first raise the head of the bed, then assist the client to a sitting position on the side of bed (often called "dangling") for a few minutes to assess for dizziness or faintness, and then assist to a standing position. If the patient becomes dizzy or feels faint, he or she should be returned to bed and placed in a supine position, which restores blood flow to the brain. See Guidelines for Nursing Care 24-3 for how to assess orthostatic hypotension.

Assessing Blood Pressure

To accurately assess blood pressure, the nurse must know the appropriate equipment to use, which site to choose, and how to describe the sounds that are heard.

Equipment

Blood pressure may be assessed with different types of devices. Most commonly, nurses assess blood pressure by using a stethoscope and sphygmomanometer. Blood pressure may also be estimated with a Doppler ultrasound stethoscope (described with the discussion of the pulse), estimated by palpation, and assessed with electronic or automated devices.

Equipment used to measure blood pressure must be in good repair and function properly to avoid inaccurate measurements. Any time the accuracy of the equipment is questionable, it should be checked and repaired or replaced, as indicated. If mercury leaks out of a manometer, it should be reported to the proper authorities as a hazardous waste spill.

Sphygmomanometer

A sphygmomanometer is used to assess blood pressure. The sphygmomanometer consists of a cuff and the manometer (Fig. 24-4). The cuff contains an airtight, flat rubber bladder covered with cloth. A cuff of the proper width (ranging from neonate to adult thigh) must be selected to obtain an accurate blood pressure reading. The width of the cuff should be about 40% of the circumference of the limb to be used. The bladder inside the cuff should enclose at least two thirds of the adult limb and all of a child's limb. If the cuff is too narrow, the reading could be erroneously high because the pressure is not evenly transmitted to the artery. This occurs, for example, when an average-sized cuff is used on an obese or overweight person.

Think back to Mrs. Renfrow, the wife of a patient with hypertension who is overweight. The nurse would need to caution Mrs. Renfrow to make sure that the device she uses to measure her husband's blood pressure is sized adequately. Otherwise, the readings may be erroneous, possibly leading to inappropriate management based on inaccurate readings or a false sense of security that the hypertension is being controlled.

If a cuff is too wide (eg, using an adult cuff on the arm of a child), the reading may be erroneously low because pressure is dispersed over a disproportionately large surface area. Recommendations for the selection of an appropriately sized cuff are given in Table 24-9.

Depending on the product, cuffs may be disposable or reusable. They are closed around the limb with contact closures, such as nylon fabric that can be fastened to itself with Velcro™ or hooks. Some long cuffs are applied by encircling the arm several times. Two tubes are attached to the bladder within the cuff. One is connected to a manometer and the other is attached to a bulb used to inflate the bladder. The bladder is inflated enough to obstruct the flow of blood through the artery. A needle valve on the bulb allows the cuff to be deflated while the pressure is being read.

A mercury manometer has a mercury-filled cylinder or tube calibrated in millimeters. When mercury rises in the

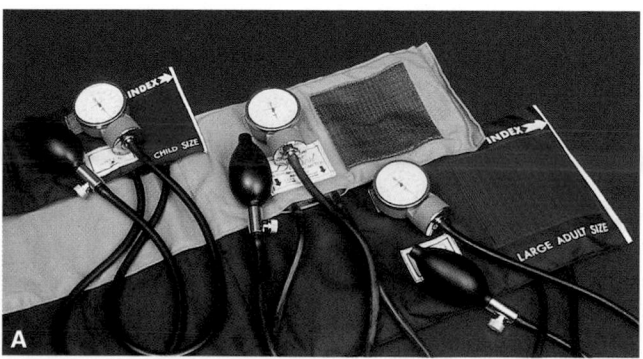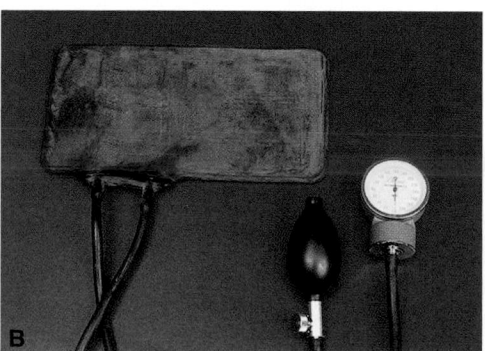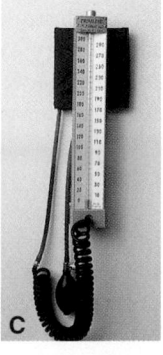

FIGURE 24-4 Parts of a sphygmomanometer. (**A**) Three cuff sizes: a small cuff for a child or a small or frail adult; a normal adult-sized cuff; and a large cuff, called a *leg cuff*, for measuring blood pressure on a leg, or for use on an obese adult. (**B**) An aneroid manometer. (**C**) A mercury manometer.

TABLE 24-9 Acceptable Bladder Dimensions (in cm) for Arms of Different Sizes*

Cuff	Bladder Width (cm)	Bladder Length (cm)	Arm Circumference Range at Midpoint (cm)
Newborn	3	6	<6
Infant	5	15	6–15†
Child	8	21	16–21†
Small adult	10	24	22–26
Adult	13	30	27–34
Large adult	16	38	35–44
Adult thigh	20	42	45–52

*There is some overlapping of the recommended range for arm circumferences to limit the number of cuffs; it is recommended that the larger cuff be used when available.
†To approximate the bladder width: arm circumference ratio of 0.40 more closely in infants and children, additional cuffs are available.
Circulation. 1993;88:2460–2467. Requests for reprints should be sent to the Office of Scientific Affairs, American Heart Association, 7272 Greenville Avenue, Dallas, TX 75231-4596.

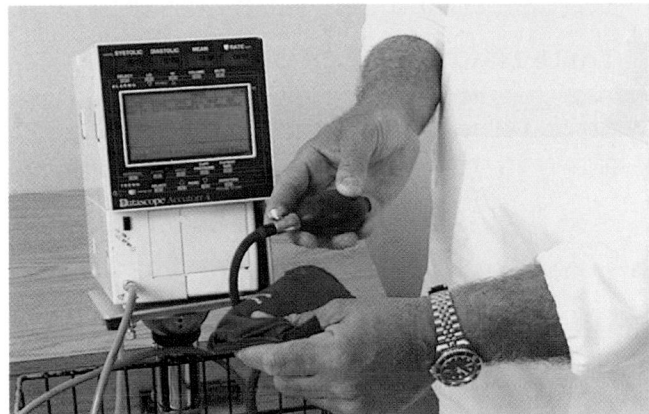

FIGURE 24-5 The automatic blood-pressure monitor reports systolic, diastolic, and mean blood pressure. (Photo © B. Proud.)

tube, the upper or top surface of the mercury forms a convex curve called the meniscus. When determining blood pressure with a mercury manometer, the top of the curve of the meniscus within the calibrated cylinder indicates the pressure. If the meniscus is observed above eye level, the pressure reading appears higher than it really is. If the meniscus is lower than eye level, it appears lower than it really is. Another type of manometer is called the aneroid manometer. It too has a cuff, but it is attached to a round, calibrated dial with a needle that indicates pressure.

Noninvasive Blood Pressure Monitors

Electronic blood pressure monitors sense vibrations within the artery wall, record the pressure readings, and display them in digital numbers (Fig. 24-5). They also may provide measurements of pulse rate, pulse oximetry, and/or temperature.

Doppler Ultrasound

The blood pressure may be taken with an ultrasound or Doppler apparatus, which amplifies sounds. This is especially useful if the sounds are indistinct or are inaudible with a regular stethoscope. See Guidelines for Nursing Care 24-1.

Direct Electronic Measurement

It is possible to measure blood pressure directly through the insertion of a thin catheter into an artery (an arterial line). The tip of the catheter senses the pressure and transmits this information to a machine that displays the systolic and diastolic pressure in a waveform. This technique is used primarily in intensive care areas.

Assessment Sites and Methods

The nurse assesses the blood pressure by listening for specific sounds, called Korotkoff sounds. Although various sites may be used to assess the blood pressure, the brachial artery and the popliteal artery are most commonly used.

Korotkoff Sounds

The series of sounds for which the nurse listens when measuring the blood pressure are called **Korotkoff sounds,** described and illustrated in Table 24-10. In some adults, each of these sounds is distinct, whereas in others only the beginning and ending sounds are heard. It is important to determine institutional policy for recording blood pressure sounds and to be consistent in taking and documenting the readings.

The first sound heard through the stethoscope, which is the onset of phase I, represents the systolic pressure. It is recorded as the first number in the fraction—for example, if the blood pressure reading is 120/80 mm Hg, 120 is the systolic pressure. The second number, which represents the diastolic pressure (in this case, 80), notes the level at which either a change in or a cessation of the loud, distinct sounds took place. This occurs in either phase IV or phase V.

The blood pressure is most commonly recorded with two numbers written as a fraction, with the bottom number indicating either the change of the sound or the last sound heard. However, the American Heart Association recommends that in instances when both a change in the sounds and a cessation of the sounds are heard, all numbers should be recorded. In this case, the blood pressure would be recorded as 120/80/64. If the sounds were heard all the way down to zero, the blood pressure recording would be 120/80/0. It is important to know the procedure for recording blood pressure at each agency or institution so that readings are consistent.

Assessing a Brachial Artery Blood Pressure

Skill 24-4 describes how to assess the blood pressure with a mercury manometer using the brachial artery. It is important to follow the recommended techniques to avoid the common errors identified in Table 24-11.

TABLE 24-10 Korotkoff Sounds

Phase	Description	Illustration
Phase I	Characterized by the first appearance of faint but clear tapping sounds that gradually increase in intensity; the first tapping sound is the systolic pressure	
Phase II	Characterized by muffled or swishing sounds; these sounds may temporarily disappear, especially in hypertensive people; the disappearance of the sound during the latter part of phase I and during phase II is called the *auscultatory gap* and may cover a range of as much as 40 mm Hg; failing to recognize this gap may cause serious errors of underestimating systolic pressure or overestimating diastolic pressure.	
Phase III	Characterized by distinct, loud sounds as the blood flows relatively freely through an increasingly open artery	
Phase IV	Characterized by a distinct, abrupt, muffling sound with a soft, blowing quality; in adults, the onset of this phase is considered to be the first diastolic figure	
Phase V	The last sound heard before a period of continuous silence; the pressure at which the last sound is heard is the second diastolic measurement	

A brachial artery blood-pressure assessment should not be taken on an arm with an intravenous line or with an arteriovenous fistula or shunt. Blood pressure should also be avoided in the arm on the side of an axillary node dissection or mastectomy, as the pressure might increase the risk of developing lymphedema in the affected arm.

Assessing a Popliteal Artery Blood Pressure

When the patient's brachial artery is inaccessible, the nurse can assess the blood pressure using the popliteal artery in the leg. The systolic pressure is normally 10 to 40 mm Hg higher at this site, although the diastolic pressure is the same. The technique for assessment is outlined in Guidelines for Nursing Care 24-4.

Palpating the Blood Pressure

Assessing the blood pressure through palpation is sometimes referred to as the sensory detection method. It requires only the use of the sphygmomanometer. The cuff is inflated 30 mm Hg above the point at which the pulsation in the artery disappears. As the air in the cuff is released, the nurse feels for the return of the pulse. Usually, no diastolic pressure is recorded because the artery continues to pulsate as long as blood flows through it. Some home patients assess their blood pressure this way. Instead of palpating the artery, however, the person notes the pressure on the manometer when experiencing the onset and disappearance of the throbbing sensation.

(text continues on page 554)

SKILL 24-4   Assessing the Blood Pressure

EQUIPMENT

Stethoscope
Sphygmomanometer

Blood pressure cuff of appropriate size
Pencil or pen, paper or flow sheet

Alcohol swab

Use guidelines outlined below.

Guidelines for Implementing and Documenting Blood Pressure

ACTION	RATIONALE
1. Identify the patient.	Provides patient safety
2. Explain the procedure to the patient.	Reduces patient apprehension and encourages patient cooperation
3. Gather equipment.	Provides organized approach to task
4. Perform hand hygiene.	Deters the spread of microorganisms
5. Follow procedure as outlined below.	
6. Perform hand hygiene. If gloves are worn, discard them in the proper receptacle.	Deters the spread of microorganisms
7. Record findings on paper, flow sheet, or computerized record. Report abnormal findings to the appropriate person. Identify site of assessment if other than brachial.	Provides accurate documentation and reporting

Guidelines for Assessing Blood Pressure

1. Delay obtaining the blood pressure if the patient is emotionally upset, is in pain, or has just exercised, unless it is urgent to obtain the blood pressure.	Factors such as emotional upset, exercise, and pain alter usual blood pressure measurements.
2. Select appropriate arm for application of cuff (no IV infusion, breast or axilla surgery on that side, cast, arteriovenous shunt, or injured or diseased limb).	Measurement of blood pressure may temporarily impede circulation to a diseased or compromised extremity.
3. Have the patient assume a comfortable lying or sitting position with the forearm supported at the level of the heart and the palm of the hand upward.	This position places the brachial artery on the inner aspect of the elbow, so that the bell or diaphragm of the stethoscope can rest on it easily.
4. Expose the area of the brachial artery by removing garments, or move a sleeve, if it is not too tight, above the area where the cuff will be placed.	Clothing over the artery interferes with the ability to hear sounds and may cause inaccurate blood pressure readings. Tight clothing on the arm causes congestion of blood and possibly inaccurate readings.
5. Center the bladder of the cuff over the brachial artery, about midway on the arm, so that the lower edge of the cuff is about 2.5 to 5 cm (1 to 2 inches) above the inner aspect of the elbow. The tubing should extend from the edge of the cuff nearer the patient's elbow.	Pressure in the cuff applied directly to the artery provides the most accurate readings. If the cuff gets in the way of the stethoscope, readings are likely to be inaccurate. A cuff placed upside down with the tubing toward the patient's head may give a false reading.
6. Wrap the cuff around the arm smoothly and snugly, and fasten it securely or tuck the end of the cuff well under the preceding wrapping. Do not allow any clothing to interfere with the proper placement of the cuff.	A smooth cuff and snug wrapping produce equal pressure and help promote an accurate measurement. A cuff too loosely wrapped results in an inaccurate reading.
7. Check that a mercury manometer is in a vertical position. The mercury must be within the zero area with the gauge at eye level. If an aneroid gauge is used, the needle should be within the zero mark.	Tilting a mercury manometer, inaccurate calibration, or improper height for reading the gauge can lead to errors in determining the pressure measurements.
8. Palpate the pulse at the brachial or radial artery by pressing gently with the fingertips.	Palpation allows for measurement of the approximate systolic reading.

(continued)

ACTION

RATIONALE

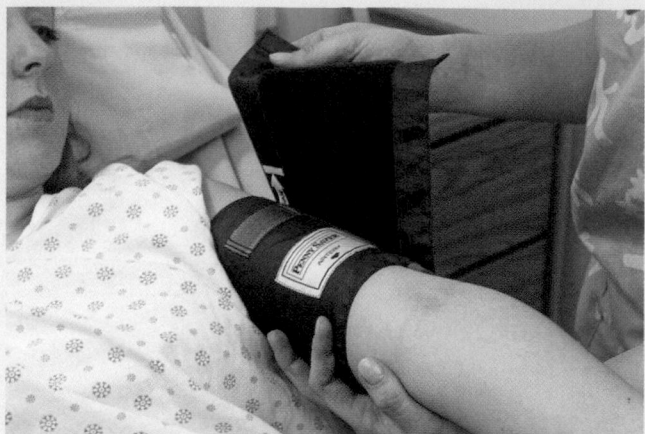

Actions 5 and 6: Centering the cuff over the brachial artery and wrapping smoothly and snugly.   (Photo by Rick Brady.)

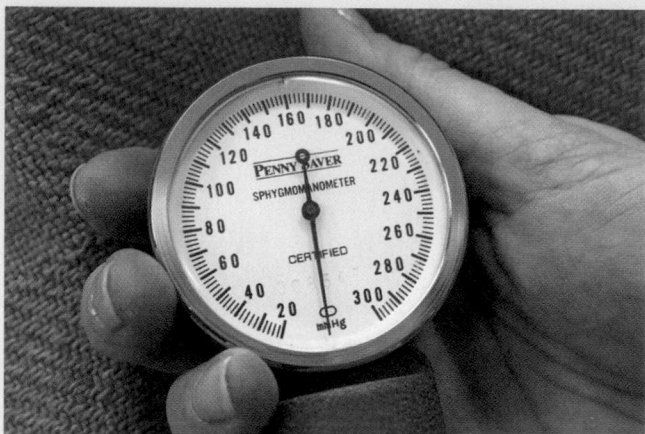

Action 7: Ensuring gauge starts at zero.   (Photo by Rick Brady.)

9. Tighten the screw valve on the air pump.

10. Inflate the cuff while continuing to palpate the artery. Note the point on the gauge where the pulse disappears.

The bladder within the cuff will not inflate with the valve open.

The point where the pulse disappears provides an estimate of the systolic pressure. To identify the first Korotkoff sound accurately, the cuff must be inflated to a pressure above the point at which the pulse can no longer be felt.

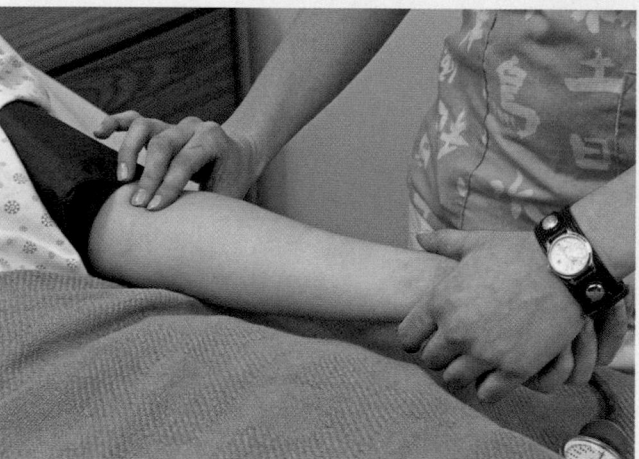

Action 8: Palpating the brachial artery.   (Photo by Rick Brady.)

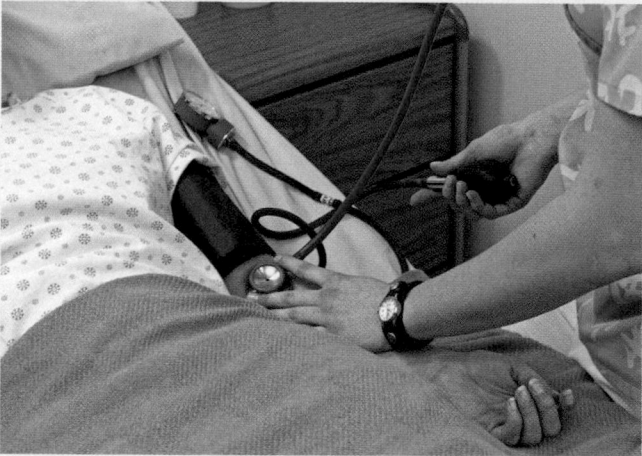

Action 14: Proper placement of diaphragm of stethoscope.   (Photo by Rick Brady.)

11. Deflate the cuff and wait 15 seconds.

12. Assume a position that is no more than 3 feet away from the gauge.

13. Place the stethoscope earpieces in the ears. Direct the eartips forward into the canal and not against the ear itself.

14. Place the bell or diaphragm of the stethoscope firmly but with as little pressure as possible over the brachial artery. Do not allow the stethoscope to touch clothing or the cuff.

Allowing a brief pause before continuing permits the blood to re-fill and circulate through the arm.

A distance of more than about 3 feet can interfere with accurate readings of the numbers on the gauge.

Proper placement blocks extraneous noise and allows sound to travel more clearly.

Having the bell or diaphragm directly over the artery makes more accurate readings possible. Heavy pressure on the brachial artery distorts the shape of the artery and the sound. Placing the bell or di-aphragm away from clothing and the cuff prevents noise, which will distract from the sounds made by blood flowing through the artery.

(continued)

SKILL
24-4   **Assessing the Blood Pressure** (continued)

ACTION	RATIONALE
15. Pump the pressure 30 mm Hg above the point at which the systolic pressure was palpated and estimated. Open the valve on the manometer and allow air to escape slowly (allowing the gauge to drop 2–3 mm per heartbeat).	Increasing the pressure above where the pulse disappeared ensures a period before hearing the first sound that corresponds with the systolic pressure. It prevents misinterpreting phase II sounds as phase I.
16. Note the point on the gauge at which there is an appearance of the first faint, but clear, sound that slowly increases in intensity. Note this number as the systolic pressure.	Systolic pressure is the point at which the blood in the artery is first able to force its way through the vessel at a similar pressure exerted by the air bladder in the cuff. The first sound is phase I of Korotkoff sounds.
17. Read the pressure to the closest even number.	It is common practice to read blood pressure to the closest even number.
18. Do not reinflate the cuff once the air is being released to recheck the systolic pressure reading.	Reinflating the cuff while obtaining the blood pressure is uncomfortable for the patient and may cause an inaccurate reading. Reinflating the cuff causes congestion of blood in the lower arm, which lessens the loudness of Korotkoff sounds.

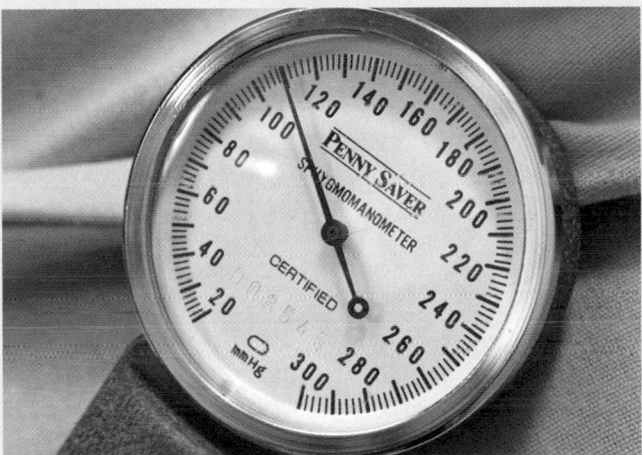

Action 16: Measuring systolic blood pressure.   (Photo by Rick Brady.)

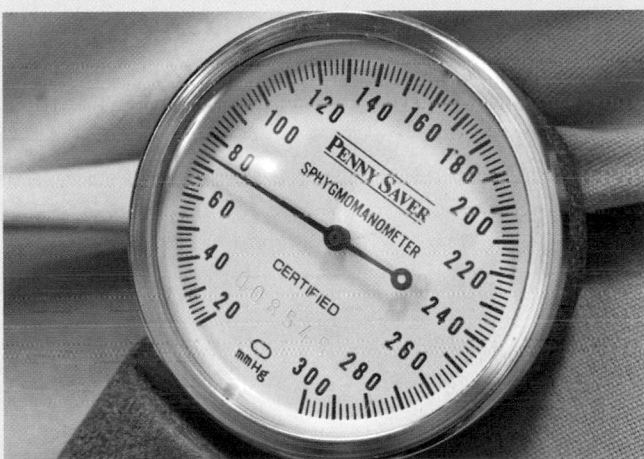

Action 19: Measuring diastolic blood pressure.   (Photo by Rick Brady.)

19. Note the pressure at which the sound first becomes muffled. Also, observe the point at which the sound completely disappears. These may occur separately or at the same point.	The point at which the sound changes corresponds to phase IV of Korotkoff sounds and is considered the first diastolic pressure reading. According to the American Heart Association, this is used as the diastolic pressure recording in children. The last sound heard is the beginning of phase V and is the second diastolic measurement.
20. Allow the remaining air to escape quickly. Repeat any suspicious reading, but wait 30 to 60 seconds between readings to allow normal circulation to return in the limb. Be sure to deflate the cuff completely between attempts to check the blood pressure.	False readings are likely to occur if there is congestion of blood in the limb while obtaining repeated readings.
21. Remove the cuff, and clean and store the equipment.	Equipment that must be shared among personnel should be left in a manner ready for use.

Special Considerations   If this is the initial nursing assessment of a patient, take the blood pressure on both arms. It is normal to have a 5- to 10-mm Hg difference in the systolic reading between arms. Use the arm with the higher reading for subsequent pressures.

(continued)

Special Considerations

When having difficulty hearing the blood pressure sounds, the following technique is recommended:

- Raise the patient's arm, with cuff in place, over his or her head for 15 seconds before rechecking the blood pressure.
- Inflate the cuff while the arm is elevated, and then gently lower the arm while continuing to support it.
- Position the stethoscope, and deflate the cuff at the usual rate while listening for Korotkoff sounds.

Raising the arm over the head helps relieve congestion of blood in the limb, increases pressure differences, and makes the sounds louder and more distinct when blood enters the lower arm.

Home Care Considerations

- Use cuff size appropriate for limb circumference. Inform patient that cuff sizes range from a pediatric cuff to a large thigh cuff and that a poorly fitting cuff may result in an inaccurate measurement.
- Inform patient about availability of digital blood pressure monitoring equipment. Though costly, most provide an easy-to-read recording of systolic and diastolic measurements.

TABLE 24-11 **Blood Pressure Assessment Errors and Contributing Causes**

Error	Contributing Causes	Error	Contributing Causes
Falsely low assessments	· Hearing deficit · Noise in the environment · Viewing the meniscus from above eye level · Applying too wide a cuff · Inserting eartips of stethoscope incorrectly · Using cracked or kinked tubing · Releasing the valve rapidly · Misplacing the bell beyond the direct area of the artery · Failing to pump the cuff 20 to 30 mm Hg above the disappearance of the pulse	Falsely high assessments	· Using a manometer not calibrated at the zero mark · Assessing the blood pressure immediately after exercise · Viewing the meniscus from below eye level · Applying a cuff that is too narrow · Releasing the valve too slowly · Reinflating the bladder during auscultation

---

Guidelines for Nursing Care 24-4
Assessing Blood Pressure in the Leg

- Place the patient in the prone position, if possible. If that position is not possible, place the patient in the supine position with the knee slightly flexed.
- Use a cuff that is specifically made for this assessment, or one that is large enough to make an accurate assessment.
- Place the cuff 2.5 cm (1 inch) above the popliteal artery, with the bladder over the posterior of the midthigh.
- Follow the same procedure for auscultation as for the brachial artery.

Nursing Diagnoses

Examples of NANDA nursing diagnoses for alterations in blood pressure are listed in the accompanying box.

TEACHING VITAL SIGNS FOR HOME CARE

Patients at home often need to check their own temperature, pulse, or blood pressure. Guidelines for teaching self-assessment and care of equipment are presented in the accompanying display, Teaching to Promote Health at Home 24-2.

Examples of NANDA Nursing Diagnoses | Altered Blood Pressure

Nursing Diagnoses	Related Factors
Decreased Cardiac Output	Serious blood loss with hypovolemia
	Myocardial infarction with damage to cardiac pacemaker
Ineffective Health Maintenance	Lack of financial resources to seek medical care for hypertension
Effective Therapeutic Regimen Management	Blood pressure remains within normal limits for six months
Risk for Falls	History of falls, age (86 years) and presence of orthostatic hypotension

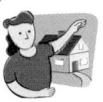

Teaching to Promote Health at Home 24-2
Self-Checking Temperature, Pulse, and Blood Pressure

Health Topic	Teaching Tip	Why is This Important
Taking the Temperature	• The temperature may be taken with a glass thermometer, a digital thermometer, a single-use disposable thermometer, or a temperature-sensitive tape. • Adults who use a glass thermometer usually take an oral temperature. It is important that the temperature be taken at least 30 minutes after eating or drinking hot or cold foods or fluids, or after smoking. Infants and small children should have their temperature taken either with a temperature-sensitive tape on the forehead or a single-use thermometer in the axilla (armpit). • Shake the liquid down into the bulb of the thermometer until the level of the liquid is below 98°F (36.5°C). To see the liquid level, hold the thermometer sideways at eye level and rotate it until the liquid can be seen. If the thermometer uses a Fahrenheit scale, each long mark is one degree and each short mark is two tenths of a degree; a centigrade scale uses long marks for one half of a degree and short marks for one tenth of a degree. • Place the glass thermometer as far back as possible under the side of the tongue and close the lips. Do not talk while the thermometer is in the mouth. • Leave the thermometer in place for 2 to 3 minutes. • Remove the thermometer and determine the point at which the liquid is level. This is the body temperature. Call your healthcare provider if the temperature is greater than 100°F (37.7°C), or if you are concerned. • Wash the thermometer with soap and warm water, rinse it with cold water, dry it well, and store it in a clean, dry area. Do not use the thermometer to take another person's temperature unless it has been cleaned. If several members of the household have an infection or illness, the thermometer should soak in 70% isopropyl alcohol between uses; be sure to rinse off the alcohol with cold water before using it again.	This will ensure an accurate temperature is assessed. Infants and small children should not have rectal temperatures taken because of the risk for damage to the rectal area. To ensure accuracy of the temperature when it is taken. Cleaning the thermometer is necessary to prevent transfer of illness from one family member to another.

(continued)

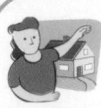

Teaching to Promote Health at Home 24-2
Self-Checking Temperature, Pulse, and Blood Pressure (Continued)

Health Topic	Teaching Tip	Why is This Important
Taking the Pulse	• The pulse is often taken before taking certain medications, such as those to make the heartbeat stronger. People who exercise and want to monitor the effect of the exercise on heart function also take their pulse. • It is necessary to be able to see a watch or a clock with a second hand when taking the pulse. • Place one arm on a firm surface so that the palm is upward. Using the middle three fingers of the other hand, gently feel the outside of the arm just below the wrist with the fingertips. Do not press hard. When pulsations are felt, watch the second hand of the watch or clock and begin to count when the second hand reaches 12 (any number is fine, but it is often easier to remember to always begin counting when the second hand is on 12). Count each pulsation (beat) for 1 minute (when the second hand again reaches 12), and write the number down.	If the pulse is very fast, very slow, or irregular, or if you have any concerns, contact your healthcare provider.
Taking the Blood Pressure	• The blood pressure is often taken to determine how well medications are working to control high blood pressure. The blood pressure is usually checked once a week. A record of blood-pressure readings over time is more important than one reading. • The blood pressure can be measured at home with a blood-pressure monitoring device or by using the mechanical devices found in many grocery or discount stores with a pharmacy. • If a home device is used, be sure the cuff is the proper size and that all parts of the device are working properly. The measurement should be taken while sitting comfortably, and the arm should be supported on a firm surface.	If the blood pressure numbers increase or decrease by more than 10, or if you have any concerns, contact your healthcare provider. It is important to use the same device or machine each time and to write down the numbers.

Developing Critical Thinking Skills

1. Take your own pulse several times a day, such as when you first get up, before and after meals, and before and after exercise. Write down the rate, rhythm, and quality of the pulse. What changes did you see? What are the physiologic rationales for these changes?

2. Describe differences you might expect to find in the vital signs of the following individuals, and include the physiologic reasons for these differences:
   • A teenager who has his first football practice in 95°F heat
   • An infant with a bacterial ear infection
   • A young woman arriving at the emergency department after an attempted assault
   • A middle-aged man who sustained serious trauma and bleeding in an automobile accident
   • A 92-year-old woman

Practicing for NCLEX

1. An elevation of the body temperature above normal is labeled
   a. Pyrexia
   b. Hypothermia
   c. Hypertension
   d. Afebrile

2. For which of the following patients would you use an oral thermometer?
   a. 6-month-old infant
   b. Patient receiving oxygen therapy
   c. 42-year-old healthy woman
   d. Unconscious patient

3. Insertion of a rectal thermometer may cause a potentially harmful condition. This condition is
   a. An increase in heart rate
   b. A decrease in heart rate

c. An involuntary loss of stool

d. An increase in respirations

4. While taking an adult patient's pulse, a student finds the rate to be 140 beats/min. What should the student do next?
   a. Check the pulse again in 2 hours.
   b. Check the blood pressure.
   c. Record the information.
   d. Report the rate.

5. A patient complains of severe abdominal pain. When assessing the vital signs, the nurse would not be surprised to find
   a. An increase in the pulse rate
   b. A decrease in body temperature
   c. A decrease in blood pressure
   d. An increase in body temperature

6. The apical pulse is assessed by using
   a. Sphygmomanometer
   b. Electronic thermometer
   c. Stethoscope
   d. Doppler apparatus

7. The difference between the apical and radial pulse rates is called the
   a. Pulse deficit
   b. Pulse amplitude
   c. Ventricular rhythm
   d. Heart arrhythmia

8. The normal respiratory rate in adults is considered to be
   a. 1 to 6 breaths/min
   b. 12 to 20 breaths/min
   c. 60 to 80 breaths/min
   d. 100 to 120 breaths/min

9. A patient is having dyspnea. To facilitate respirations, the nurse would
   a. Remove pillows from under the head
   b. Elevate the head of the bed
   c. Elevate the foot of the bed
   d. Take the blood pressure

10. Blood pressure is the measurement of the
    a. Flow of blood through the circulation
    b. Force of blood against arterial walls
    c. Force of blood against venous walls
    d. Flow of blood through the heart

11. With aging, blood pressure is often higher due to
    a. Loss of muscle mass
    b. Changes in exercise and diet
    c. Decreased peripheral resistance
    d. Decreased elasticity in arterial walls

12. A patient has a blood pressure reading of 130/90 mm Hg when visiting a clinic. The nurse would recommend
    a. Follow-up measurements of blood pressure
    b. Immediate treatment by a physician
    c. Nothing, because the nurse considers this reading is due to anxiety
    d. A change in diet and exercise

13. In recording a blood pressure of 120/80 mm Hg, the 120 represents the
    a. Pulse rate
    b. Diastolic pressure
    c. Systolic pressure
    d. Pulse deficit

14. It is important to have the appropriate cuff size when taking the blood pressure. A cuff that is too large or too small may result in
    a. An incorrect reading
    b. Injury to the patient
    c. Prolonged pressure on the arm
    d. Loss of Korotkoff sounds

15. A patient has intravenous fluids infusing in the right arm. When taking a blood pressure on this patient, the nurse would
    a. Take the blood pressure in the right arm
    b. Take the blood pressure in the left arm
    c. Use the smallest possible cuff
    d. Report inability to take the blood pressure

■ Answers With Rationale

1. The correct response is *a*. Pyrexia is an elevation of body temperature. Hypothermia (*b*) is low body temperature. Hypertension (*c*) is elevated blood pressure. Afebrile (*d*) means that there is not an elevation of body temperature.

2. The correct response is *c*. Use of oral thermometers is contraindicated in infants (*a*), patients receiving oxygen therapy (*b*), and unconscious patients (*d*).

3. The correct response is *b*. Insertion of a rectal thermometer may stimulate the vagus nerve, which, in turn, would decrease heart rate. This may potentially be harmful for patients with cardiac problems.

4. The correct response is *d*. A rate of 140 in an adult is an abnormal pulse, and should be reported to the instructor or the nurse in charge of the patient.

5. The correct response is *a*. The pulse often increases when an individual is experiencing pain. Pain does not affect body temperature and may increase (not decrease) blood pressure.

6. The correct response is *c*. The apical pulse can only be assessed by listening with a stethoscope.

7. The correct response is *a*. The difference between the apical and radial pulse rate is called the pulse deficit. The other responses are names given to volume and rhythm of the pulse.

8. The correct response is *b*. The normal respiratory rate for adults is 12 to 20 breaths/min.

9. The correct response is *b*. Dyspnea is difficult respirations. Elevating the head of the bed allows the abdominal organs to descend, giving the diaphragm greater room for expansion and facilitating lung expansion. Any other intervention would not facilitate respirations.

10. The correct response is *b*. Blood pressure is the measurement of the force of blood against arterial walls. Other responses are incorrect in describing blood pressure.

11. The correct response is *d*. With aging, elasticity in arterial walls is decreased, contributing to an elevated blood pressure reading. The other responses may contribute to changes in readings, but they are not the physiologic basis for blood pressure findings in the older adult.

12. The correct response is *a*. A single blood pressure reading that is mildly elevated is not significant, but the measurement should be taken again over time to determine if hypertension is a problem. The nurse would recommend a return visit to the clinic for a recheck.

13. The correct response is *c*—120 is the systolic pressure. The diastolic pressure is 80. The other responses relate to pulse rather than blood pressure.

14. The correct response is *a*. A blood pressure cuff that is not the right size may cause an incorrect reading. It will not cause injury (*b*) or loss of sounds (*d*).

15. The correct response is *b*. The blood pressure should be taken in the arm opposite the one with the infusion. Blood pressure should not be taken in the arm with an intravenous infusion because the pressure of inflating the cuff may allow the artery to clot.

Bibliography

Baue, W. (2003). Phase-out of mercury thermometers continues to rise. SocialFunds.com. Available at: http://www.socialfunds.com/news/article.cgi?sfArticleId=752.

Bauer, J. (2002a). Blood pressure cuffs. *RN, 65*(8), 61–62.

Bauer, J. (2002b). Vital signs monitors. *RN, 65*(7), 61–62.

Bauer, J. (2003). Thermometers. *RN, 66*(3), 53–64.

Boutain, D. (2001). Discourses of worry, stress, and high blood pressure in rural south Louisiana. *Journal of Nursing Scholarship, 33*(3), 225–230.

Faria, S. (1999). Assessment of peripheral arterial pulses. *Home Care Provider, 4*(4), 140–141.

Gall, G. (2002). A useful screening tool. *RN, 65*(9), 41–43.

Holtzclaw, B. (2001). Circadian rhythmicity and homeostatic stability in thermoregulation. *Biological Research for Nursing, 2*(4), 221–235.

Joint National Committee on Prevention, Detection, Evaluation, and Treatment of High Blood Pressure. (1997). *The sixth report of the Joint National Committee on Prevention, Detection, Evaluation, and Treatment of High Blood Pressure*. Bethesda, MD: National Institutes of Health.

Lanham, D., Walker, B., Klocke, E., & Jennings, M. (1999). Accuracy of tympanic temperature readings in children under 6 years of age. *Pediatric Nursing, 25*(1), 39–42.

McKenzie, N. (1998). Fever: Upping the body's thermostat. *Nursing, 28*(10), 41–45.

NANDA International. (2003). *Nursing diagnoses: Definitions & classification 2003–2004*. Philadelphia: Author.

National Heart, Lung, and Blood Institute. National Institutes of Health. (2003). *The seventh report of the Joint National Committee on Prevention, Detection, Evaluation, and Treatment of High Blood Pressure*. Available at: http://www.jama.com.

Nicoll, L. (2002). Heat in motion: Evaluating and managing temperature. *Nursing, 32*(5), 1–12.

Ofili, E. (2003). *Early detection and control of high blood pressure vital to the vascular system*. Available at: http://www.ama-assn.org/ama/pub.

Porth, C. (2002). *Pathophysiology: Concepts of altered health states* (6th ed.). Philadelphia: Lippincott Williams & Wilkins.

Ruffolo, D. (2002). Hypothermia in trauma: The cold, hard facts. *RN, 65*(2), 46–52.

Thomas, S., Liehr, P., DeKeyser, F., Frazier, L., & Friedmann, E. (2002). A review of nursing research on blood pressure. *Journal of Nursing Scholarship, 34*(4), 313–321.

Weber, J., & Kelley, J. (2003). *Health assessment in nursing.* (2nd ed.). Philadelphia: Lippincott Williams & Wilkins.

Health Assessment

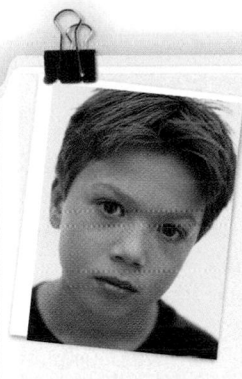

Billy Collins, a 9-year-old boy with a history of allergies, including an allergy to insect stings, is spending a week at summer camp. He reports to the camp counselor that he was just stung by a bee.

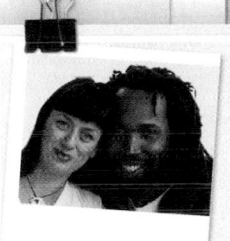

Tammy Browning, who is expecting her first child, has been on the antepartum unit for 1 week, and is about to be moved to the delivery room. She and her partner, both in their late 20s or early 30s, have a history of substance abuse, primarily alcohol and marijuana. A urine specimen is to be collected for routine evaluation and a drug screen. Tammy is unaware that drug testing will be done.

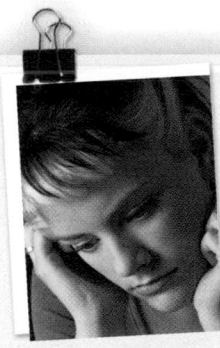

Ramona Lewis, a 19-year-old college student, comes to the emergency department. She is upset and crying and reports that she was date-raped.

Focusing on Blended Skills

The types of blended skills that you'll need to respond to the case scenarios include:

Cognitive Skills

- Knowledge of how to conduct and document a health assessment in a systematic manner, identifying normal and abnormal findings
- Ability to integrate knowledge of subjective and objective data into a health assessment
- Knowledge of how to individualize the basic health assessment to specific populations (a school-aged child with a bee sting, a young adult rape victim, and a pregnant woman with a history of drug abuse)
- Knowledge of the typical assessment findings associated with an allergic reaction, rape, and substance abuse

Technical Skills

- Ability to use the equipment and techniques necessary to assess health status
- Ability to position the patient correctly for each body system assessment
- Ability to adapt equipment and techniques for patients of different developmental stages
- Ability to document assessment findings accurately

Interpersonal Skills

- Strong people skills to develop a trusting nurse–patient relationship
- Ability to communicate and interact effectively with patients and their significant others, especially during times of stress,

such as a child with a bee sting, a woman who was raped, and a pregnant woman with a history of substance abuse
- Demonstration of self-confidence in own abilities and the willingness to get help when needed
- Ability to identify and respond to the needs of patients experiencing stress, such as a child with an allergic reaction and a young rape victim
- Ability to demonstrate respect for a patient's human dignity during a health assessment

Ethical and Legal Skills

- Knowledge of ethical and legal principles underlying patient care
- Commitment to safe, quality care, including ability to report problematic situations immediately
- A strong sense of responsibility and accountability
- Ability to participate as a trusted and effective patient advocate, including advocating for the pregnant patient and her fetus, a child, and a rape victim
- Ability to document health assessment findings according to agency policy
- Knowledge of special regulations and legislation detailing nursing responsibilities when assessing pregnancy, providing first aid in camp situations, and caring for a rape victim

Learning Outcomes

After completing the chapter, the learner should be able to accomplish the following:

1. Identify the purposes and types of health assessment.
2. Explain preparation of the patient and the environment for a health assessment.
3. Describe and use the techniques employed during a physical assessment.
4. Identify the equipment and positions used during a physical assessment.
5. Use appropriate questions to elicit information during a health history.
6. Conduct a physical assessment in a systematic manner.
7. Document significant health assessment findings in a concise, descriptive manner.
8. Describe nursing responsibilities before, during, and after diagnostic procedures.

Key Terms

adventitious breath sounds
auscultation
bronchial sounds
bronchovesicular sounds
bruits
cyanosis
ecchymosis
edema
erythema
inspection
jaundice
pallor
palpation
percussion
petechiae
precordium
turgor
vesicular breath sounds

Health assessment is an integral component of nursing care and is the basis of the nursing process. Assessments are used to plan, implement, and evaluate teaching and care in order to promote an optimal level of health through interventions to prevent illness, restore health, and facilitate coping with disabilities or death. Health assessments are a part of nursing care for patients across the life span and may be conducted in any setting. (See the accompanying Reflective Practice box for an example.) The two components of a health assessment are a heath history and a physical assessment.

CONDUCTING A HEALTH ASSESSMENT

The scope and type of assessment conducted vary based on the setting, the healthcare needs of the patient, and the acuity of the

Reflective Practice
Challenge to Ethical and Legal Skills

I have always been interested in labor and delivery, so I was very excited to have the opportunity to follow a nurse in labor and delivery and assist and witness the beginning of life. I had no idea that the whole process could be so complicated.

It was here that I met Tammy Browning, who was expecting her first child. She and her partner were, an interracial couple, in their late 20s or early 30s. They had been on the antepartum unit for approximately 1 week, and she was going to be moved to the delivery room shortly. The nurse gave me a brief rundown of what we were expected to do throughout the morning.

On entering the patient's room for the first time, I was shocked at what I saw. The room was dark and extremely cluttered with food, candy wrappers, and trash overflowing onto the floor. The patient's partner had been sleeping in the room and both of their belongings were all over the place. I could not believe it! When we left the room, the nurse told me that both the patient and her partner had a history of drug use, mainly alcohol and marijuana. We had to get a urine sample from her to do a dipstick test. The specimen was also going to be used for a drug screen, but the patient was not going to be told about this. I was shocked and confused by this action. I thought that we had to tell the patient everything we were going to do—right?

Thinking Outside the Box: Possible Courses of Action

- Go along with what the nurse decided to do, and when we got out of the patient's room, ask why she decided to take this course of action.
- Inform myself of the legality of taking this route of action.

- Inform my instructor and head nurse about the case, asking if this was a usual occurrence and requesting that they tell or educate me on what basis they were allowed to do this.

Evaluating a Good Outcome: How Do I Define Success?

- Safety of patient and neonate is ensured.
- Patient and baby benefit from the decided-on course of action.
- No breach of duty or harm is done.

- Patient receives proper care and treatment regardless of her past drug use and results of the drug tests.
- Respect for patient is maintained.

Personal Learning: Here's to the Future!

I really had no idea what to do. Because I did not feel legally competent to challenge the nurse and suggest a different course of action, I followed her and went along with her story. Afterwards I asked her if we were allowed to do this. Her answer was that she was doing it because the patient had a history of drug use and she suspected that she had been smoking marijuana throughout her stay. The test was not going to harm the baby or the mother; if anything, the test was going to be beneficial in providing the most adequate care for her and her baby. It was also going to assist in preparing for any complications that may arise during the delivery.

When she gave me this explanation, I figured that her reasons were valid and it was all right to do this since no one was going to get hurt and it would be beneficial. However, I was left with the thought that we were violating the patient's privacy. I also spoke with my clinical instructor about the situation. Through this experience, I realized that I need to educate myself more on the legal aspects of nursing. I had never paid much attention to the fact that I am exposed to many legal situations every day as a healthcare provider. Therefore, I must be prepared to confront them. I think that it is vital to be skilled as well as to be competent medically and legally. By having this knowledge, many difficult situations may be avoided and/or resolved. With this knowledge I will also be a better advocate for my patients.

Reflection

How would you respond in a similar situation? Why? What does this tell you about yourself and about the adequacy of your skills for professional practice? What do you think might have happened if the patient were told about the drug testing? Do you feel that the nurse's action of not telling the patient was based on appropriate ethical and legal principles? Why or why not? If so, what ethical and legal principles formed the basis for the action? If not, what ethical and legal principles were violated? Can you think of other ways to respond? What other skills (cognitive, interpersonal, technical, ethical/legal) would you need to respond well in this situation? Do you agree with the criteria to evaluate a successful outcome? Did the nursing student meet the criteria? Explain your answer.

Stephanie Cuellar, Georgetown University

health problem. The following sections discuss general guide-lines that apply to both the health history and physical assess-ment, including types of assessment, preparing the patient, preparing the environment, and cultural considerations. Also included in this section are guidelines specific to the health his-tory (eg, components of the history) and the physical assess-ment (eg, equipment, positioning, draping, and techniques).

Types of Assessment

A health assessment may be comprehensive, ongoing partial, focused, or emergency. A comprehensive assessment with a health history and complete physical examination is usually conducted when a patient enters a healthcare setting, with in-formation providing a baseline for comparing later assess-ment. An ongoing partial assessment is one that is conducted at regular intervals (eg, at the beginning of each home health visit or each hospital shift) during care of the patient. This type of assessment focuses on identified health problems to monitor positive or negative changes and evaluate the effec-tiveness of interventions. A focused assessment is conducted to assess a specific problem. For example, if the patient is having abdominal pain, the nurses asks questions about uri-nary problems, bowel problems, allergies, and menstrual his-tory (for women) during the health history and then assesses vital signs and abdominal structures during the physical assess-ment. An emergency assessment is a type of rapid focused as-sessment conducted to determine potentially fatal situations. For example, assessing the airway, breathing, and circulation before beginning cardiopulmonary resuscitation is part of an emergency assessment.

> *Consider Billy Collins, the 9-year-old who was stung by a bee. In this situation, the nurse would conduct an emergency assessment to de-termine the immediate effects of the bee sting, assessing for indications of an allergic reaction. Once this emergency assessment is completed, the nurse would perform a focused assessment to address the boy's history of allergies.*

Preparing the Patient

The patient's physiologic and psychological needs should be considered before and during the health assessment (Fig. 25-1). Explain that the first part of the assessment will involve ques-tions about the patient's health concerns, health habits, and lifestyle. After the health history is completed, body structures will be examined. Tell the patient that the assessments should not be painful. The patient may be anxious for various reasons. Explaining the assessment in general terms can help decrease the patient's embarrassment, fear of possible abnormal physi-cal findings, or fear of "failing" a test. Each assessment is then explained in greater detail as it is performed. Answer the pa-tient's questions directly and honestly.

> *Think back to Ramona Lewis, the college stu-dent who reported that she was a victim of*

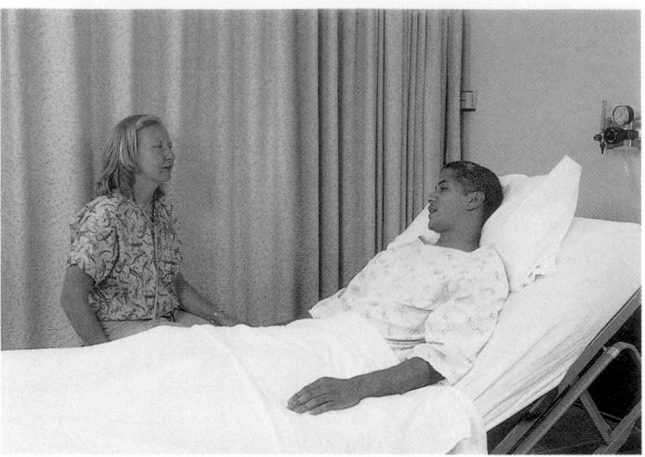

FIGURE 25-1 A brief explanation of the examination before begin-ning and just before each stage alleviates patient fear and anxiety. (Photo © B. Proud.)

> *date rape. The nurse would need to incorpo-rate knowledge of the emotional and physi-cal effects of rape when communicating with Ms. Lewis. In addition, the patient's anxiety is likely to be high; thus, using empathy and establishing a trusting nurse–patient rela-tionship are key.*

Direct the patient to a private dressing area or to a com-fortable area in the home and ask the patient to change into a gown. If necessary, assist the patient with undressing. Ask the patient to empty the bladder before the examination so that he or she will be more comfortable during the assessment and assessment of the abdomen will be easier.

Preparing the Environment

The environment needs to be prepared before the health as-sessment is conducted. The nurse and patient should agree on the time for the assessment. It should not interfere with meals or daily routines for patients in the home or with treatments or visiting hours for patients in acute care settings. A time should be chosen when the patient is as free of pain as possible.

Clinics, offices, and hospitals may have a special examina-tion room that provides a quiet, private space for assessment. If such a room is available, the examination table is prepared, a gown and drape for the patient are provided, and instruments and special supplies needed for the assessment are gathered. If the area is open to others, an enclosure with a curtain or screen is essential. The room should be warm enough to prevent chill-ing and the area or room should be adequately lighted, either by sunlight or overhead lighting.

Cultural Sensitivity

Each person is a unique individual. The patient's culture does not affect how a health assessment is conducted, but it is an in-tegral component of the interactions between the nurse and the patient. Nurses should know risk factors for alterations in health that are based on racial inheritance, as well as normal variations that occur within races. Nurses must consider their patients within the context of family, culture, and community (Weber & Kelley, 2003). Chapter 3 provides information about cultural diversity and the importance of providing culturally sensitive nursing care.

Health History Guidelines

A health history is a collection of subjective data that provides a detailed profile of the patient's health status. Nurses use therapeutic communication skills and interviewing techniques during the health history to establish an effective nurse–patient relationship and to gather data to identify actual and potential health problems as well as sources of strength.

> *Recall Tammy Browning, the pregnant woman with a history of substance abuse. Therapeutic communication skills would be key to establishing a trusting nurse–patient relationship, which is essential for gathering data about the patient's recent drug use.*

Information is collected during an interview with the patient, who is the primary source of data. Components of the health history, with examples of questions to ask, are outlined in the accompanying Focused Assessment Guide 25-1. Interviewing skills are described in Chapters 12 and 21. Nurses should be sensitive to cultural differences that influence how both verbal and nonverbal communications are interpreted.

Risk factors for alterations in health are another important part of the health history. Be sure to ask about the risk factors for and warning signs of cancer (Box 25-1). Risk factors often relate specifically to the body system being assessed. Therefore, in this chapter, questions to ask regarding risk factors for altered health are provided in the health history section of each body system under the heading "Components of the Health Assessment."

Physical Assessment Guidelines

A physical assessment is the systematic collection of objective information that is directly observed or is elicited through examination techniques. To perform a physical assessment, the nurse needs to be knowledgeable about the equipment

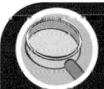 **Focused Assessment Guide 25-1**

Health History

Factors to Assess	Questions and Approaches
Biographical data	The following information is often collected during admission to a healthcare facility or agency and documented on a specific form. • Name, address, gender, marital status, occupation, religious preference, healthcare financing • Primary healthcare provider
Chief complaint	"Tell me why you are here today." (Document in the patient's own words.)
History of present illness	"When did you first begin having this problem?" "Did it happen suddenly or slowly?" "Show me exactly where you are having this problem." "What other symptoms have you had with this problem?" "How have you treated this problem?"
Past medical history	"Tell me about the childhood illnesses, such as measles or mumps, that you had." "What are you allergic to?" "Describe any accidents, injuries, and surgeries you have had." "What prescribed or over-the-counter medications do you use? Do you take any herbal or dietary supplements?"
Family history	"How old are the members of your family?" "If any members of your family are not living, what caused their death?" "Is there any history of this health problem you have in other family members?"
Lifestyle	"Do you smoke, drink, or use drugs? If so, for how long and how much?" "Describe the foods you eat during a typical day." "Tell me about how well you sleep." "How much exercise do you get each day?" "Who in your family or community is available to help you with health problems if you need it?"

BOX 25-1 American Cancer Society CAUTION Model

Change in bowel or bladder habits
A sore that does not heal
Unusual bleeding or discharge
Thickening or lump in the breast or elsewhere
Indigestion or difficulty in swallowing
Obvious change in wart or mole
Nagging cough or hoarseness

From the American Cancer Society.

being used, proper patient positioning and draping, and the techniques used. In this chapter, a complete physical assessment is detailed under the heading "Components of the Health Assessment."

Equipment

The equipment used in a physical assessment should be readily accessible, clean or sterile, in proper working order, and organized for the correct sequence of use (Fig. 25-2). Equipment that will touch the patient should be warmed (by the examiner's hands or warm water) before use. Although not all the instruments described below will be needed in every assessment, they are commonly used in a total assessment. Some equipment, such as a tongue blade and penlight, may be used in the physical assessment but are not included in this discussion. Beginning students will not conduct all elements of a complete physical assessment, but the instruments and techniques are discussed here so they can understand what is being done by more advanced practitioners.

Stethoscope and Sphygmomanometer

The stethoscope and sphygmomanometer are illustrated and described in Chapter 24. Further information about the stethoscope is provided here as it is used to listen to sounds of the heart, lungs, abdomen, and cardiovascular system. The bell and diaphragm are illustrated in Figure 25-3. The bell of the stethoscope is pressed lightly against the body part to listen to low-pitched sounds, such as abnormal cardiovascular sounds. The diaphragm of the stethoscope is pressed firmly against the body part to listen to high-pitched sounds, such as normal heart sounds, breath sounds, and bowel sounds. When using the stethoscope, the body part to be auscultated should be exposed and environmental noises should be minimized.

Ophthalmoscope

An ophthalmoscope is a lighted instrument used to visualize the interior structures of the eye. It consists of two parts: a body that contains the light source and a detachable head that contains lenses that magnify the internal eye structures. The head is secured in the body. The dial on the head, when de-

pressed and turned, turns on the illumination. Several lenses are arranged on a wheel that controls the focus on structures in the eye. Each lens is labeled with a positive (black) or negative (red) number, with units of strength called diopters. Red numbers are used for near-sighted (myopic) patients, black numbers for far-sighted (hyperopic) patients. The zero lens is used when either the examiner or the patient has refractive errors.

Otoscope

An otoscope is a lighted instrument used to examine the external ear canal and the tympanic membrane. The ophthalmoscope and otoscope heads are interchangeable on the same body. An attached speculum directs the light in a narrow beam to improve visualization of ear structures. The specula come in various sizes; the largest speculum that will extend into the patient's ear canal is used.

Snellen Chart

The Snellen chart, used as a screening test for distant vision, consists of characters in 11 lines of different-sized type; the line of largest characters is at the top of the chart and the line of smallest characters is at the bottom. Scores ranging from 20/10 (the smallest line of characters) to 20/200 (the largest line of characters) are shown in the left-hand column, and distances are in the right-hand column next to the numbers.

Nasal Speculum

A nasal speculum is used to visualize the lower and middle turbinates of the nose. A penlight or flashlight is used for illumination. The blades of the speculum are inserted about ½″ (1 cm) into each naris and opened so that they do not press on the septum. Alternatively, the otoscope can be used to visualize the internal nares. The light is provided by the scope, and the shortest, widest speculum that will fit into the naris is used.

Vaginal Speculum

A vaginal speculum is a two-bladed instrument used to examine the vaginal canal and cervix. The speculum is inserted into the vagina and the speculum blades are opened, allowing visualization and assessment of the vagina and cervix. The speculum must be warmed and lubricated with warm water or a water-soluble agent before insertion.

Remember Ramona Lewis, the college student who reported that she was a victim of date rape. A vaginal examination would be crucial for collecting data to confirm the rape. Warming and lubricating the speculum would be very important to provide patient comfort during this extremely upsetting time.

Tuning Fork

A tuning fork is a two-pronged metal instrument used to test auditory function and vibratory perception. The fork is activated to vibrate by gently tapping its prongs against the palm

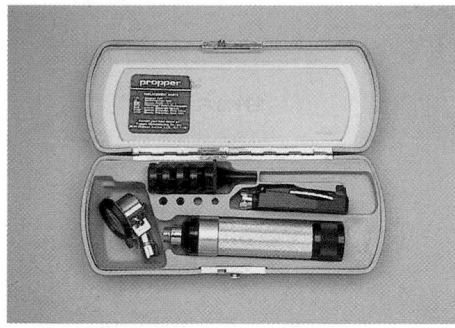

Ophthalmoscope and otoscope set

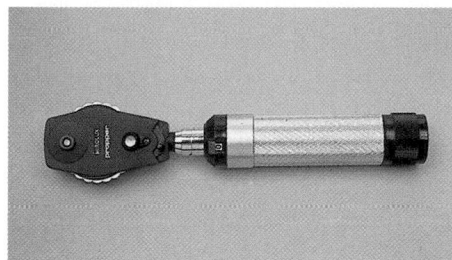

Ophthalmoscope

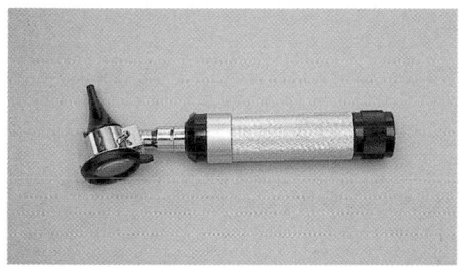

Otoscope

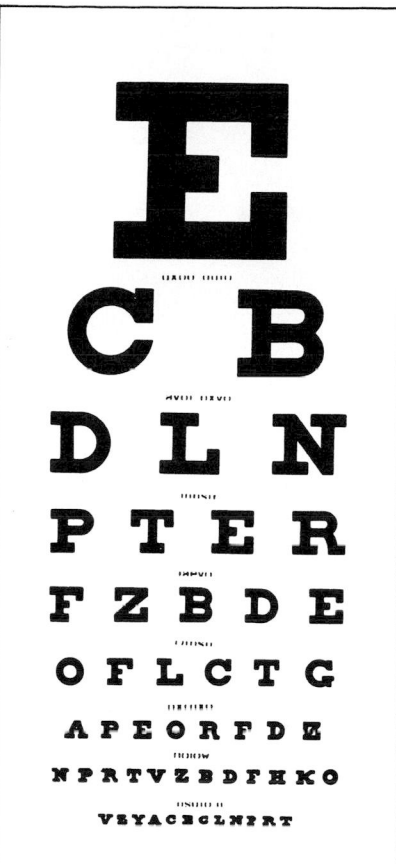

Snellen chart

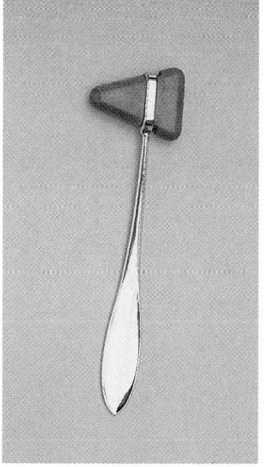

Percussion hammer

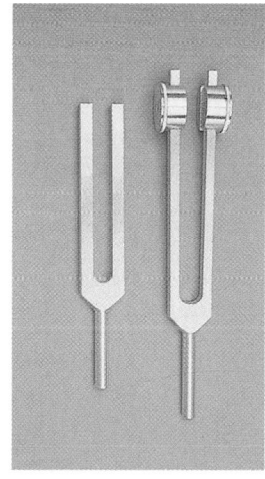

Tuning forks

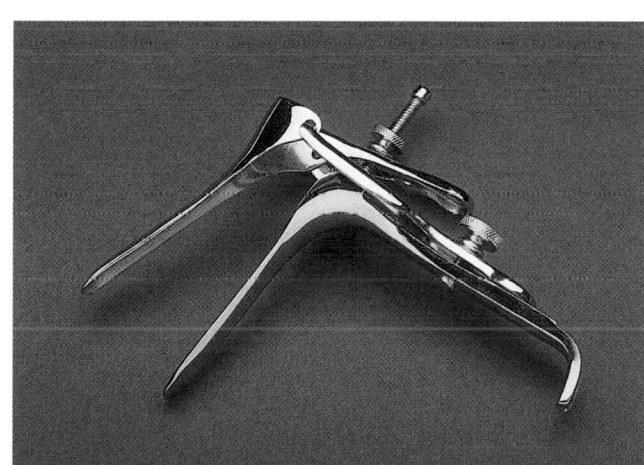

Vaginal speculum

FIGURE 25-2 Instruments used in the physical assessment. (Photos © Ken Kasper.)

of the hand. Once vibrating, the fork is held at the base to avoid diminishing the vibration of the prongs.

Percussion Hammer

A percussion hammer (also called a reflex hammer) is an instrument with a rubber head used to test deep tendon reflexes. The hammer is held between the thumb and index finger to direct a brisk tap on the selected body area. The quick, firm tap

is made with a rapid downward and backward wrist action. The pointed end of the hammer is used for smaller areas.

Positioning

A variety of positions are used during a physical assessment. During positioning, it is important to consider the patient's age, health status, mobility, physical condition, energy level, and privacy. Positioning patients who are weak may require assis-

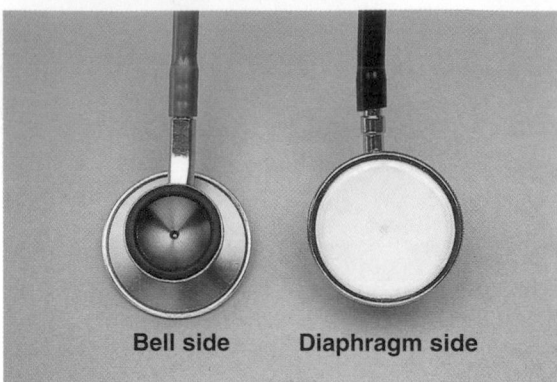

FIGURE 25-3 Stethoscope bell and diaphragm. Use the **diaphragm** of the stethoscope to detect high-pitched sounds. The diaphragm should be at least 1.5 inches wide for adults and smaller for children. Hold the diaphragm firmly against the body part being auscultated. Use the **bell** of the stethoscope to detect low-pitched sounds. The bell should be at least 1 inch wide. Hold the bell lightly against the body part being auscultated.

tance. Uncomfortable or embarrassing positions should not be maintained for long periods. The assessment should be organized so that several body systems can be assessed with the patient in one position, thus minimizing unneeded and possibly tiring movements. Positions that may be used during a physical assessment are illustrated and described in Table 25-1.

Draping

Draping prevents unnecessary exposure, provides privacy, and keeps the patient warm during the physical assessment. Drapes may be paper, cloth, or bed linens. Only the body parts being assessed are exposed as the assessment is conducted.

Techniques of Physical Assessment

The four primary assessment techniques are:

- Inspection
- Palpation
- Percussion
- Auscultation

These assessments are primarily used in the sequence listed; variations are noted in the discussion of specific body areas later in the chapter. Bilateral body parts are always compared; for example, the assessment findings of one leg are compared with those of the other leg. Bilateral body parts are normally symmetric; that is, they have the same size and shape as well as the same characteristics, such as movement or pulses.

Inspection

Inspection is the process of performing deliberate, purposeful observations in a systematic manner. The nurse observes visually but also uses hearing and smell to gather data throughout the assessment. Inspection begins with the initial patient contact and continues through the entire assessment. Adequate natural or artificial lighting is essential for distinguishing the color, texture, and moisture of body surfaces. A quiet environment allows sounds to be heard.

Inspect each area of the body for size, color, shape, position, and symmetry, noting normal findings and any deviations from normal. Inspection may be combined with

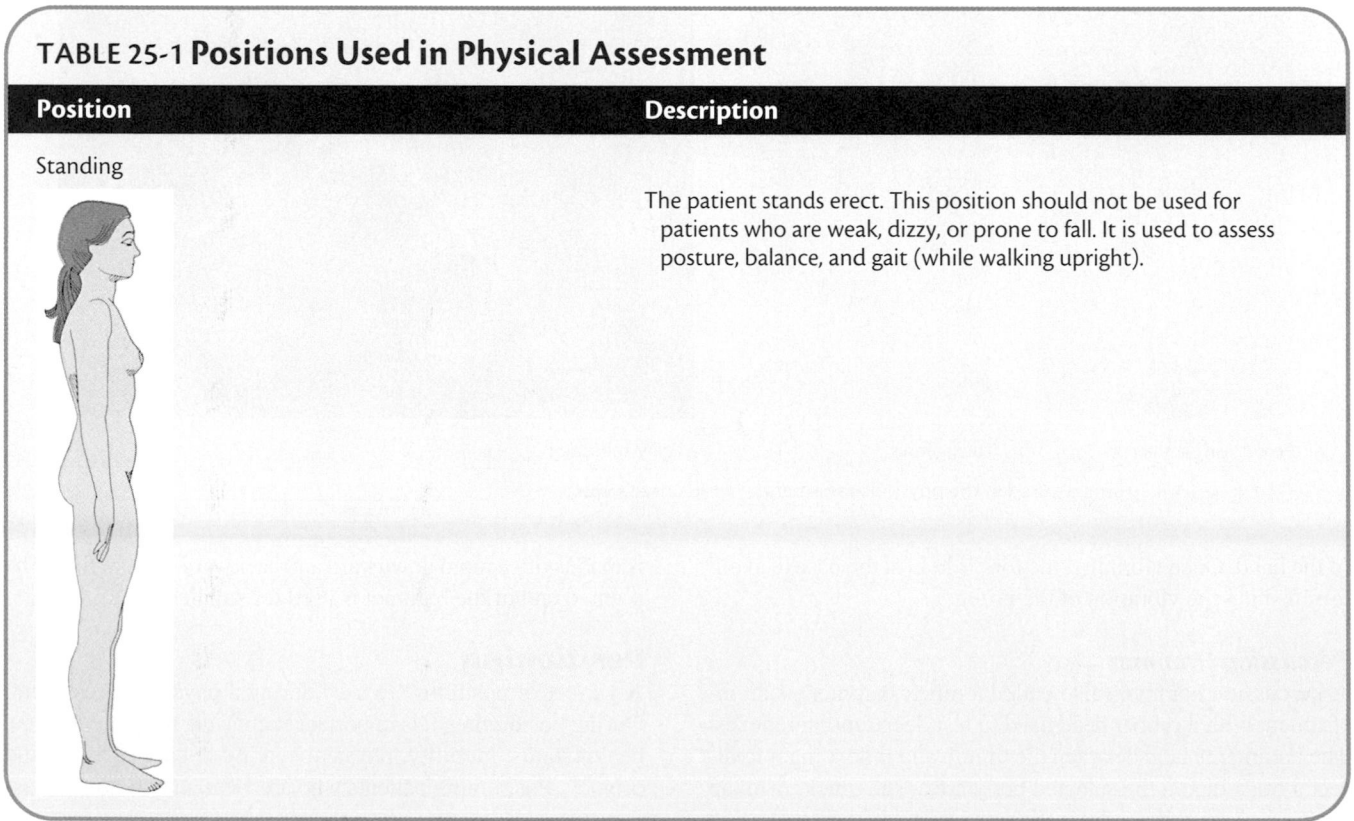

TABLE 25-1 Positions Used in Physical Assessment

Position	Description
Standing	The patient stands erect. This position should not be used for patients who are weak, dizzy, or prone to fall. It is used to assess posture, balance, and gait (while walking upright).

TABLE 25-1 (Continued)

Position	Description
Sitting 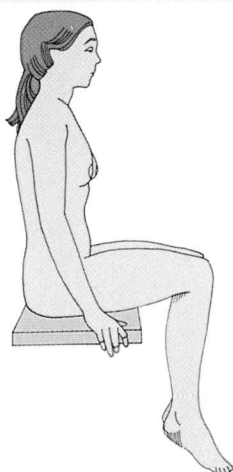	The patient may sit in a chair or on the side of the bed or examining table, or remain in bed with the head elevated. It allows visualization of the upper body and facilitates full lung expansion, and is used to assess vital signs and the head, neck, anterior and posterior thorax and lungs, heart, breasts, and upper extremities.
Supine 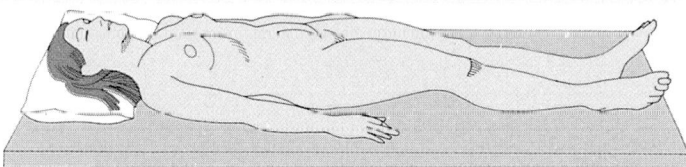	The patient lies flat on the back with legs extended and knees slightly flexed. It facilitates abdominal muscle relaxation and is used to assess vital signs and the head, neck, anterior thorax and lungs, heart, breasts, abdomen, extremities, and peripheral pulses.
Dorsal recumbent 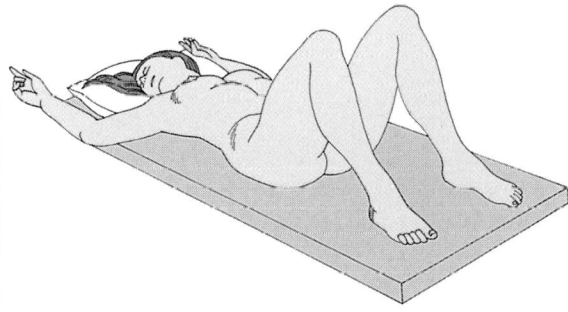	The patient lies on the back with legs separated, knees flexed, and soles of the feet on the bed. It should not be used for abdominal assessment as it causes contraction of the abdominal muscles. It is used to assess the head, neck, anterior thorax and lungs, heart, breasts, extremities, and peripheral pulses.
Sims' 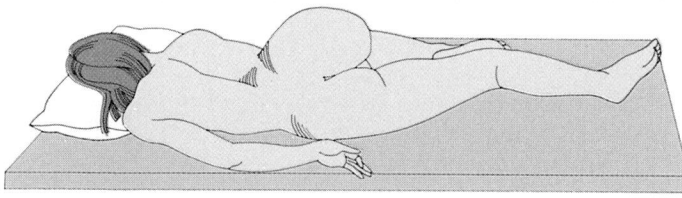	The patient lies on either side with the lower arm below the body and the upper arm flexed at the shoulder and elbow. Both knees are flexed, with the upper leg more acutely flexed. It is used to assess the rectum or vagina.
Prone 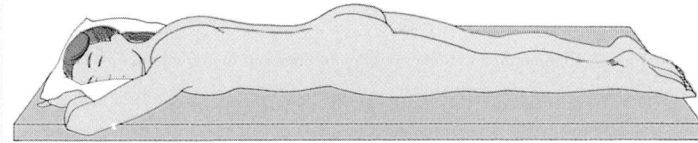	The patient lies flat on the abdomen with the head turned to one side. It is used to assess the hip joint and the posterior thorax.

(continued)

TABLE 25-1 (Continued)

Position	Description
Lithotomy 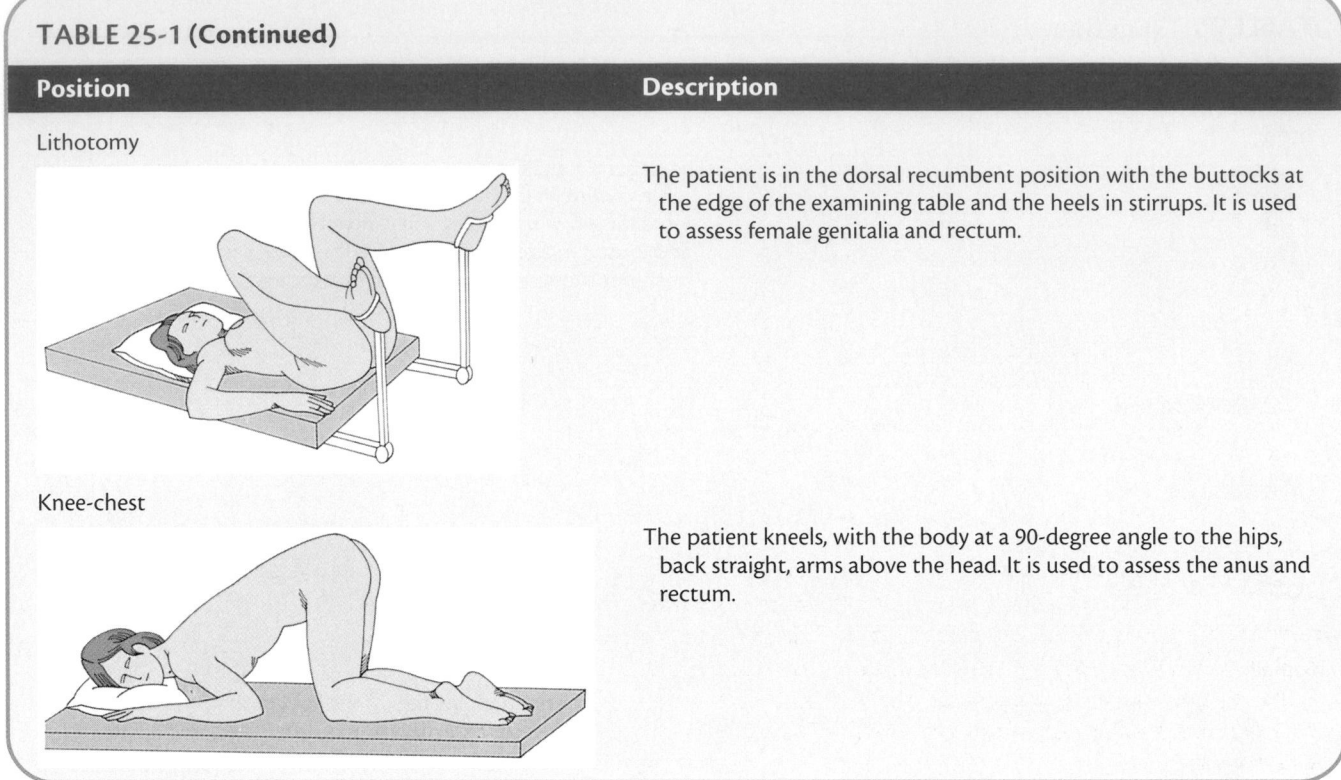	The patient is in the dorsal recumbent position with the buttocks at the edge of the examining table and the heels in stirrups. It is used to assess female genitalia and rectum.
Knee-chest	The patient kneels, with the body at a 90-degree angle to the hips, back straight, arms above the head. It is used to assess the anus and rectum.

the palpation phase of the assessment, with inspection preceding palpation.

Palpation

Palpation is an assessment technique that uses the sense of touch. The hands and fingers are sensitive tools and can assess temperature, turgor, texture, moisture, vibrations, and shape. The dorsum (back) surfaces of the hand and fingers are used for gross measure of temperature. The palmar (front) surfaces of the fingers and finger pads are used to assess texture, shape, fluid, size, consistency, and pulsation. Vibration is palpated best with the palm of the hand (Fig. 25-4).

The nurse's hands should be warm and the fingernails short. Any area of tenderness is palpated last. Light, moderate, or deep palpation may be used, the depth being controlled by the amount of pressure applied. For light palpation, apply light pressure with the fingers together depressing the skin and underlying structures less than 1 cm (0.5″) (Fig. 25-5A). Moderate palpation is conducted by depressing the skin surface 1 to 2 cm (0.5″ to 0.75″). For deep palpation, press inward about 2 cm (1″) (see Fig. 25-5B). Deep palpation, which carries a risk of internal injury, should be used cautiously and only after considerable practice.

Applying intermittent pressure to a specific area allows assessment of surface characteristics and underlying structures. Two hands are used for bimanual palpation (eg, palpating breast tissue); one hand applies pressure and the other hand feels the tissue or structure. Characteristics of masses, as determined by palpation, are described in Table 25-2.

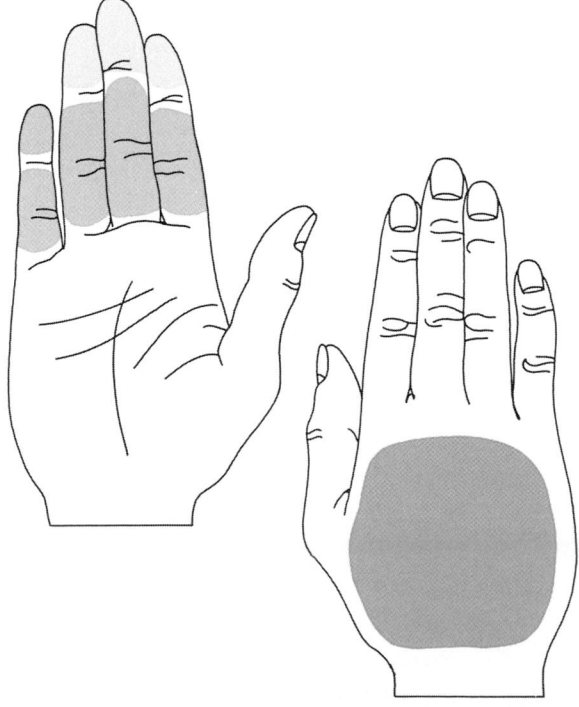

FIGURE 25-4 (*Left*) Palmar surfaces of the examiner's fingertips and finger pads are used for discriminatory sensation, such as texture, vibration, presence of fluid, or size and consistency of a mass. (*Right*) The dorsum, or back of the hand, is used to assess surface temperature.

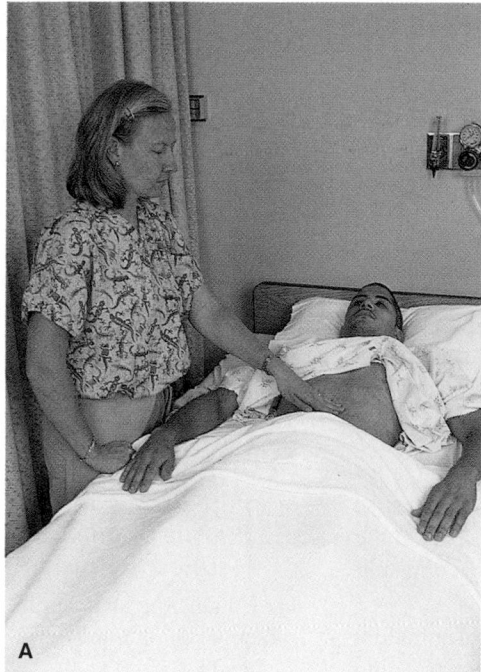 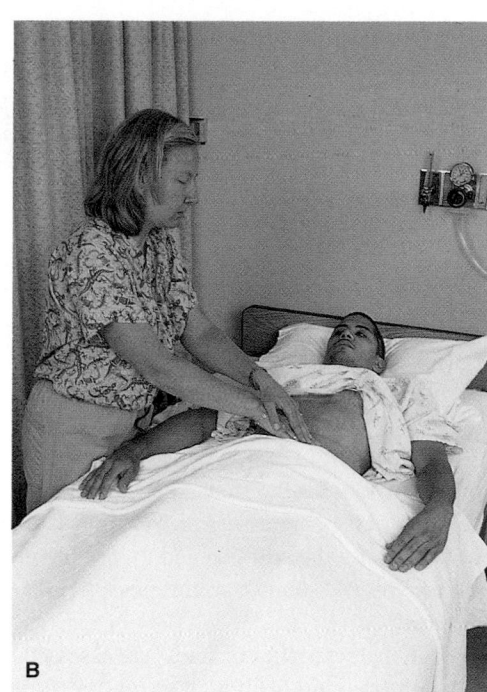

FIGURE 25-5 (**A**) In light palpation, light pressure is applied by placing the fingers together and depressing the skin and underlying structures about ¹/₂ inch (1 cm). (**B**) Deep palpation is used with caution. The skin and underlying structures are depressed about 1 inch (2 cm).   (Photos © B. Proud.)

Percussion

Percussion is the act of striking one object against another to produce sound. The sound waves produced by the striking action over body tissues are known as percussion tones. Percussion is used to assess the location, shape, size, and density of tissues.

Both hands are used to produce sound waves. The nondominant hand is placed directly on the area to be percussed, with the fingers slightly separated and the middle finger placed firmly on the body surface (Fig. 25-6, left). The other hand (dominant hand) provides the striking force, initiated by a sharp downward wrist movement with the forearm stationary and the wrist relaxed. The tip of the middle finger of the dominant hand strikes the middle finger of the opposing hand (see Fig. 25-6, right). This action produces a vibration that allows discrimination among five different tones, described in Table 25-3.

Auscultation

Auscultation is the act of listening with a stethoscope to sounds produced within the body. Auscultation is per-

TABLE 25-2 Characteristics of Masses Determined by Palpation

Quality	Characteristics to Determine
Shape	Round Ovoid Tubular Irregular
Size	Measured in centimeters
Consistency	Firm Edematous Spongy Cystic
Surface	Smooth Nodular Granular
Mobility	Fixed or nonmobile Mobile
Tenderness	Amount of tenderness to touch
Pulsatile	Pulsation can or cannot be felt in the mass

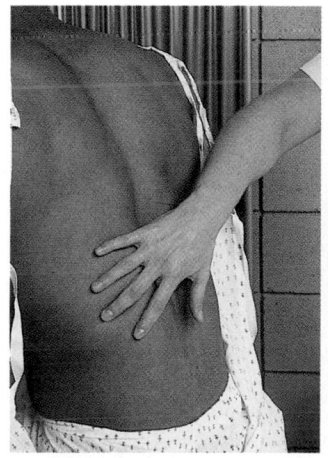 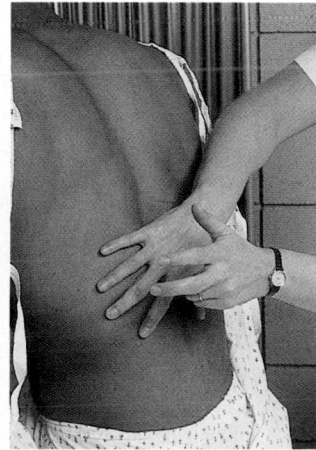

FIGURE 25-6 Percussion is used to access the location, shape, size, and density of tissues. (*Left*) The nondominant hand is placed directly on the area to be percussed, and the middle finger is placed firmly on the body surface. (*Right*) The tip of the middle finger of the dominant hand strikes the joint of the middle finger of the opposite hand. (Photos © Ken Kasper.)

TABLE 25-3 Percussion Tones

Tone	Relative Intensity	Sample Location
Flat	Soft	Thigh
Dull	Medium	Liver
Resonance	Loud	Normal lung
Hyperresonance	Very loud	Emphysematous lung
Tympany	Loud	Gastric air bubble or puffed-out cheek

formed by placing the stethoscope diaphragm or bell against the body part being assessed. When auscultating, the nurse should expose the part listened to, use the proper part of the bell for specific sounds, and (if possible) listen in a quiet environment.

Four characteristics of sound are assessed by auscultation: (1) pitch (ranging from high to low); (2) loudness (ranging from soft to loud); (3) quality (eg, gurgling or swishing); and (4) duration (short, medium, or long).

COMPONENTS OF THE HEALTH ASSESSMENT

The health assessment is usually conducted in a head-to-toe sequence or a system sequence but can be adapted to meet the needs of the patient. It is often necessary to modify the sequence, positions, and specific assessments based on the patient's age, energy level, and physical state, as well as time constraints. Even when modified, the health assessment should be conducted in an organized and knowledgeable manner.

Consider Billy Collins, the 9-year-old who was stung by a bee. The nurse would modify the health assessment by focusing on the immediate problem at hand: the bee sting and possible allergic reaction.

Conducting an accurate health assessment takes time and practice. Guidelines for physical assessment are provided in Table 25-4.

TABLE 25-4 Guidelines for Physical Assessment

Component and Equipment (as needed)	Sequence of Techniques	Assessment Parameters
General survey • Scales • Sphygmomanometer • Stethoscope	Inspection	• General appearance, hygiene, posture, gait, thought processes, speech patterns • Height and weight • Vital signs
Integument • Gloves	Inspection Palpation	• Skin: color, temperature, texture, moisture, lesions • Hair: texture, loss, unusual growth, infestations • Nails: condition
Head and neck • Gloves • Snellen chart • Ophthalmoscope • Otoscope • Tongue depressor	Inspection Palpation	• Skull and face: shape, symmetry • Neck: trachea, thyroid gland • Lymph nodes: size, shape, consistency, tenderness • Eyes visual acuity, extraocular movements, peripheral vision, discharge, alignment, internal structures • Ears: hearing acuity, position, external ear and tympanic membrane, cerumen • Nose, mouth, throat: color, consistency, condition of teeth, exudate, tonsils, tenderness
Thorax and lungs • Gloves • Stethoscope	Inspection Palpation Percussion Auscultation	• Thorax: posture, crepitus, expansion, respiratory rate, percussion tones, breath sounds • Breasts: size, shape, symmetry, color, areolas, nipple (discharge), retraction, dimpling, tenderness • Axillary lymph nodes: size, shape, consistency, tenderness
Cardiovascular • Stethoscope • Watch with a second hand	Inspection Palpation Percussion Auscultation	• Carotid arteries: bruit, pulse strength • Jugular vein: pulsations, distention • Precordium: pulsations, apical impulse, pulsations, heart rate and rhythm, heart sounds, murmurs
Peripheral vascular • Stethoscope	Inspection Palpation	• Peripheral pulses: symmetry, character, strength, rate, patency • Arms and legs: color, temperature, hair pattern, veins, lesions, edema

(continued)

TABLE 25-4 (Continued)

Component and Equipment (as needed)	Sequence of Techniques	Assessment Parameters
• Doppler (if needed)	Auscultation	
Abdomen • Stethoscope	Inspection Auscultation Percussion Palpation	• Abdomen: size, shape, contour, lesions, distention, hernia, tenderness, tones • Bowel sounds: intensity, frequency, pitch • Liver: location, consistency, tenderness • Aorta: bruits, pulsation
Male genitalia • Gloves	Inspection Palpation	• Inflammation, infestations, rashes, lesions, lumps, discharge
Female genitalia • Gloves • Speculum • Lubricant • Applicators • Culture tubes • Pap test supplies	Inspection Palpation	• Inflammation, infestations, rashes, lesions, lumps, discharge (color, odor, amount), swelling, bulging out of vagina • Uterus: size, position, shape and consistency • Ovaries: size, shape, mobility, and tenderness
Anus, rectum, prostate • Gloves • Lubricant • Occult blood test	Inspection Palpation	• Anus: hemorrhoids, lumps, ulcers, fissures • Stool: color, occult blood • Prostate: size, shape, consistency, tenderness
Musculoskeletal	Inspection Palpation	• Gait and posture • Joints and muscles: size, symmetry, color, edema, nodules, crepitus, strength • Joints: range of motion
Neurologic • Reflex hammer • Sharp/dull objects • Aromatic scents	Inspection	• Level of awareness • Level of consciousness • Dress, grooming, hygiene • Speech • Thought processes • Memory and abstract reasoning • Cranial nerves: ability to smell, see, clench teeth, move eyes, have facial expressions, hear, taste, feel touch, swallow, shrug shoulders against resistance, protrude tongue • Fine motor movement: ability to repeatedly touch nose with hand, pat knees with palms and backs of hands, run heel down opposite shin • Sensory: ability to distinguish between sharp and dull touch • Reflexes: degree of response

Not all assessments on this table are discussed in the narrative. Please consult an assessment textbook for further information.

General Survey

The general survey is the first component of the health assessment. Some information, such as the patient's appearance and behavior, is gathered when taking the health history. Measuring vital signs, height, and weight is also part of the general survey.

Appearance

Assessing appearance includes the following:
• Body build, posture, and gait (proportion of height to weight, erect or slumped posture, coordination of movements, pattern of gait)
• Hygiene, grooming (cleanliness, body odors)
• Signs of illness (posture, skin color, respirations, nonverbal communication of pain or distress, short attention span)
• Affect, attitude, mood (speech, facial expressions, ability to relax, eye contact, behavior)
• Cognitive processes (speech content and patterns, orientation, appropriate verbal responses)

Think back to Tammy Browning, the pregnant woman with a history of substance abuse. The nurse would perform a general survey of the patient to determine any findings suggestive of recent substance use.

Vital Signs

Vital signs are measured to establish a baseline for the database and to detect actual or potential health problems. Vital signs are discussed in Chapter 24.

Height and Weight

The ratio of height and weight is an assessment of overall health, hydration status, and nutrition. Height and weight should be measured using accurate scales and measuring devices. The patient should remove shoes and heavy clothing if the measurements are taken before undressing. If the patient cannot stand erect, weight can be obtained using a chair or bed scales. The patient's actual height and weight can be compared with recommended average weights on a standardized chart as a general guideline for assessing nutritional status and health (see the Guidelines for Nursing Care 25-1). Table 25-5 provides a height and weight table for use as a standard reference.

Children up to 2 years of age should have their height measured in the recumbent position with the legs fully extended. Infants should be weighed without any clothing, and children should be weighed in their underwear.

Guidelines for Nursing Care 25-1
Obtaining Height and Weight
With an Upright Balance Scale

Obtaining Height
- Ask the patient to remove shoes.
- Raise L-shaped sliding arm on the measuring device attached to the scale somewhat higher than the patient's approximate height.
- Ask the patient to step on the platform of the scale and stand erect with the back to the measuring device and the heels together.
- Lower the L-shaped sliding arm until it rests on top of the patient's head.
- Read the height in inches and record.
- Ask the patient to step down from the platform.

Obtaining Weight
- Balance the scale on zero.
- Ask the patient to remove shoes (and coat, if appropriate) and step onto the platform.
- Move the sliding indicator to the left until the scale balances.
- Read the weight in pounds and record.
- Ask the patient to step down from the platform.
- Return the scale weight indicator to zero.
- Considerations: Daily weights should be obtained at the same time each day (usually early morning), with the patient wearing the same clothing, and using the same scale.

Assessing the Integument

The integumentary structures assessed are the skin, nails, hair, and scalp.

Health History

Identify risk factors for altered health during the health history by asking about the following:
- History of rashes, lesions, change in color, or itching
- History of bruising or bleeding in the skin
- History of allergies to medications, plants, foods, or other substances
- Exposure to the sun and sunburn history
- Presence of wounds, bruises, abrasions, or burns
- Change in the color, size, or shape of a mole
- Recent chemotherapy or radiation therapy
- Exposure to chemicals that may be harmful to the skin, hair, or nails
- Degree of mobility
- Types of food eaten and liquids consumed each day

Physical Assessment

The skin, hair and nails are assessed by observation and palpation. Ask the patient to remove all clothing and put on an examination gown (if appropriate). The patient remains in the sitting position for most of the examination but will need to stand or lie on the side when the posterior part of the body is examined. Protect the patient's privacy by exposing only the body part being examined. If the patient has lesions, wear gloves during palpation.

Assessing the Skin
The skin is a general indicator of the patient's health status and provides information that might indicate an underlying disease. The assessment begins with an overall inspection of the skin's condition. Specific areas of the skin can be assessed during other body system assessments. Adequate lighting is essential for accurate assessments. The skin is inspected for color, vascularity, lesions (Fig. 25-7), and body odors and palpated for temperature, moisture, turgor, and texture.

Inspect Skin Color
Skin color varies among races and among individuals, ranging from a pinkish white to various shades of brown. Skin areas that are normally exposed, such as the face and hands, may have a somewhat different color from areas that are usually covered by clothing, but otherwise skin color is relatively constant. Special care must be taken to detect color changes in dark-skinned people, such as African Americans, Hispanics, Native Americans, people of Mediterranean descent, and whites who are deeply suntanned. Some body areas of dark-skinned people, such as the palms of the hands and the soles of the feet, normally have less pigmentation than other body areas. Terms used to describe abnormal appearance of the skin are summarized in Table 25-6.

TABLE 25-5 Height and Weight Table

	Weight (lb) Men*				Weight (lb) Woment		
Height	Small Frame	Medium Frame	Large Frame	Height	Small Frame	Medium Frame	Large Frame
5′ 2″	128–134	131–141	138–150	4′ 10″	102–111	109–121	118–131
5′ 3″	130–136	133–143	140–153	4′ 11″	103–113	111–123	120–134
5′ 4″	132–138	135–145	142–156	5′ 0″	104–115	113–126	122–137
5′ 5″	134–140	137–148	144–160	5′ 1″	106–118	115–129	125–140
5′ 6″	136–142	139–151	146–164	5′ 2″	108–121	118–132	128–143
5′ 7″	138–145	142–154	149–168	5′ 3″	111–124	121–135	131–147
5′ 8″	140–148	145–157	152–172	5′ 4″	114–127	124–138	134–151
5′ 9″	142–151	148–160	155–176	5′ 5″	117–130	127–141	137–155
5′ 10″	144–154	151–163	158–180	5′ 6″	120–133	130–144	140–159
5′ 11″	146–157	154–166	161–184	5′ 7″	123–136	133–147	143–163
6′ 0″	149–160	157–170	164–188	5′ 8″	126–139	136–150	146–167
6′ 1″	152–164	160–174	168–192	5′ 9″	129–142	139–153	149–170
6′ 2″	155–168	164–178	172–197	5′ 10″	132–145	142–156	152–173
6′ 3″	158–172	167–182	176–202	5′ 11″	135–148	145–159	155–176
6′ 4″	162–176	171–187	181–207	6′ 0″	138–151	148–162	158–179

* Weights at ages 25 to 59 yr are based on lowest mortality. Weight in pounds are according to frame (in indoor clothing weighing 5 lb, shoes with 1-inch heels).
† Weights at ages 25 to 59 yr are based on lowest mortality, Weight in pounds are according to frame (in indoor clothing weighing 3 lb, shoes with 1-inch heels).

Changes in skin color include erythema, cyanosis, jaundice, and pallor. These color changes are easier to assess in light-skinned people. **Erythema** (redness of the skin) is more often seen in the face and the neck. It is associated with sunburn, inflammation, fever, trauma, and allergic reactions.

> Think back to Billy Collins, the child who was stung by a bee. The nurse would use keen inspection skills to observe for erythema in the area of the sting.

Cyanosis is a bluish or grayish discoloration of the skin in response to inadequate oxygenation. Cyanosis is assessed as a blue tinge in patients with white skin and as dullness in patients with dark skin. **Jaundice** is a yellow color of the skin resulting from liver and gallbladder disease, some types of anemia, and hemolysis. It usually develops first in the sclera of the eyes and then in the skin and mucous membranes. Jaundice in dark-skinned people is more difficult to observe on the trunk of the body, but the sclera, oral mucous membranes, palms, and soles appear yellow to yellow-orange. **Pallor,** or paleness of the skin, often results from an inadequate amount of circulating blood or hemoglobin, causing inadequate oxygenation of the body tissues. Depending on severity, pallor may be visible over the entire skin surface or only in the lips, nailbeds, mucous membranes, and conjunctiva. Pallor in dark-skinned people is seen as an ashen gray or yellow tinge.

Inspect Skin Vascularity

Inspect the skin for vascularity, bleeding, or bruising; these signs might relate to a cardiovascular, hematologic, or liver dysfunction. **Ecchymosis** is a collection of blood in the subcutaneous tissues, causing purplish discoloration. **Petechiae** are small hemorrhagic spots caused by capillary bleeding. If they are present, assess their location, color, and size.

> Remember Ramona Lewis, the college student reporting a rape. The nurse would inspect the patient closely for signs and symptoms of trauma, including any bruising or petechiae. These findings would be important objective data to help substantiate the rape.

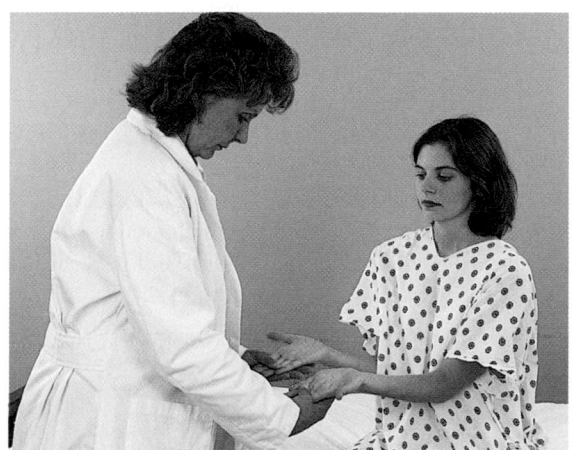

FIGURE 25-7 The skin is inspected for color, vascularity, and lesions. (Photo © B. Proud.)

TABLE 25-6 Skin Color Assessment

Color Variations	Assessment Areas	Possible Causes
Redness (erythema; flushing)	Facial area, localized area of skin on the body	Blushing, alcohol intake, fever, injury trauma, infection
Bluish (cyanosis)	Exposed areas, particularly the ears, lips, inside of the mouth, hands and feet, nailbeds	Cold environment, cardiac or respiratory disease (decreased oxygenation)
Yellowish (jaundice)	Overall skin areas, mucous membranes, and sclera	Liver disease (increase in bilirubin levels)
Paleness (pallor)	Exposed areas, particularly the face and lips, conjunctivae, and mucous membranes	Anemia (decreased hemoglobin) Shock (decreased blood volume)
Vitiligo	Overall skin areas, lips, nailbeds, conjunctivae Whitish patchy areas on the skin	Depigmentation (congenital or autoimmune conditions)
Tanned or brown	Sun-exposed areas	Overexposure (increased melanin production), pregnancy (brown spots)

Inspect Skin Lesions

Inspect the skin for lesions, which are areas of diseased or injured tissue (Table 25-7). Note bruises, scratches, cuts, insect bites, and wounds. Assess wounds (breaks in the continuity of the skin) for size, shape, depth, location, and presence of drainage or odor. Scars are healed wounds. (Wounds are discussed in Chap. 38.) Describe rashes (skin eruptions) in terms of their type, size, elevation, coloring, and presence of drainage or itching. Document the exact body surface areas involved.

Palpate Skin Temperature, Texture, Moisture, and Turgor

The skin is normally warm and dry. An increase in skin temperature and moisture can indicate an elevated body temperature. The texture of the skin may vary from smooth and soft to rough and dry. In the dehydrated patient, the texture is dry, loose and wrinkled and the mucous membranes are cracked and dry. An excessive amount of perspiration, such as when the entire skin is moist, is called diaphoresis.

Turgor (Fig. 25-8) is the fullness or elasticity of the skin and is usually assessed on the sternum or under the clavicle. Normal turgor results in elasticity of the skin; it can be picked up in a fold and returns to its shape when released. When the patient is dehydrated, the skin's elasticity is decreased, and the skin fold returns to normal slowly (however, this may be a normal finding in older patients).

Difficulty in lifting a skin fold may indicate **edema** (excess fluid in the tissues). Edema is characterized by swelling, with taut and shiny skin over the edematous area. If the area of edema is palpated with the fingers, an indentation may remain after the pressure is released; this is called pitting edema. Edema may be graded as 0 (none), +1 (trace, 2 mm), +2 (moderate, 4 mm), +3 (deep, 6 mm), or +4 (very deep, 8 mm). Edema may be the result of overhydration, heart failure, kidney failure, trauma, or peripheral vascular disease.

Assessing the Nails

The nails are inspected for shape, angle, texture, and color. The nails should be somewhat convex and should follow the natural curve of the finger. The angle between the nail and its base in the finger should be about 160 degrees. The nails should be smooth, and the nail base, when palpated, should be firm and nontender. Abnormal findings include indentations called Beau's lines (from acute illness); infection, painless separation of the nail plate from the nailbed (onycholysis) from infection or trauma; increased brittleness or thickness and angulation (from anemia or iron deficiency anemia); and clubbing (from long-term lack of oxygenation). Figure 25-9 illustrates nail abnormalities.

Assessing the Hair and Scalp

The hair is normally resilient, evenly distributed, and neither excessively dry nor oily. Hair is found on all body surfaces except the palms of the hands, the soles of the feet, and parts of the genitalia. Assess the hair for color, texture, and distribution. Abnormal findings include unusual balding (alopecia) and excessive amounts of hair on the face and body (hirsutism). Hair loss may be the result of chemotherapy, radiation therapy, infection, hormone disorders, or inadequate nutrition. Decreased oxygenation of peripheral tissues, especially of the lower extremities, may cause loss of hair. Excessive hair growth may occur in persons with hormone disorders.

Separate the hair to inspect the scalp for color, dryness, scaliness, lumps, lesions, or lice. Nits, which are the white eggs of lice, can be differentiated from dandruff or lint because they are attached to the hair shaft. If any lumps or masses are palpated, note their location, size, tenderness, and mobility.

Normal Age-Related Variations
Infant/Child

Common skin variations in newborns and children include:
• Jaundice and milia (whiteheads) in newborns
• Fine downy hair (lanugo) for the first 2 weeks of life

TABLE 25-7 Basic Types of Skin Lesions

Lesion Name	Description	Example
Primary Lesions*		
Circumscribed, Flat, Nonpalpable Change in Skin Color		
Macule	Lesion ≤1 cm	Petechiae, freckle
Patch	Lesion >1 cm	Vitiligo
Palpable, Elevated Solid Masses		
Papule	Mass ≤0.5 cm	Mole
Plaque	Mass >0.5 cm	Coalesced papules
Nodule	Mass 0.5–2 cm; firmer than a papule	Nevus (wart)
Tumor	Mass >2 cm	Lipoma
Wheal	Irregular, superficial area of localized skin edema	Hives, mosquito bite
Circumscribed, Superficial Skin Elevations Formed by Free Fluid in a Cavity Within the Skin Layers		
Vesicle	Filled with serous fluid, ≤0.5 cm	Herpes simplex
Bulla	Filled with serous fluid, >0.5 cm	2nd-degree burn
Pustule	Filled with pus	Acne, impetigo
Secondary Lesions†		
Loss of Skin Surface		
Erosion	Loss of superficial epidermis, moist, nonbleeding surface	Moist area after rupture of a vesicle, as in chickenpox
Ulcer	Loss of epidermis and dermis, may bleed and scar	Stasis ulcer
Fissure	Deep linear crack, extends into dermis	Athlete's foot
Material on the Skin Surface		
Crust	Dried residue of serum, pus, or blood	Impetigo
Scale	Thin flake of exfoliated dermis	Dandruff, dry skin
Miscellaneous Lesions		
Lichenification	Thickened and roughened epidermis, with increased visibility of skin furrows	Atrophic dermatitis
Atrophy	Thinning of the skin, loss of skin furrows, shiny appearance	Peripheral vascular disease
Excoriation	Scratch of the epidermis	
Scar	Fibrous tissue replaces tissue in the dermis or subcutaneous layer	
Keloid	Hypertrophied scar	
Other Common Skin Lesions, Not Technically Primary or Secondary		
Comedo	Plugged opening of a sebaceous gland, a hallmark of acne	Common blackhead
Telangiectasia	Small, dilated, red or bluish surface vessels; may be part of a basal cell carcinoma or skin injury from radiation	
Nevus	Flat to slightly elevated, round, evenly pigmented	Common mole

*May arise from previously normal skin.
†Result from changes in primary lesions.

- Smooth, thin skin at birth
- Pubic hair development at the onset of puberty

Older Adult
Common skin variations in the older adult include:
- Wrinkles, dryness, scaling, decreased turgor
- Raised dark areas (senile keratosis)
- Flat brown age spots (senile lentigines)
- Small round red spots (cherry angioma)
- Fine, brittle gray or white hair

- Hair loss
- Coarse facial hair in women, decreased body hair in men and women
- Thick, yellow toenails

Assessing the Head and Neck

Assessment of the head and neck includes the skull, face, eyes, ears, nose and sinuses, mouth and pharynx, trachea, thyroid gland, and lymph nodes.

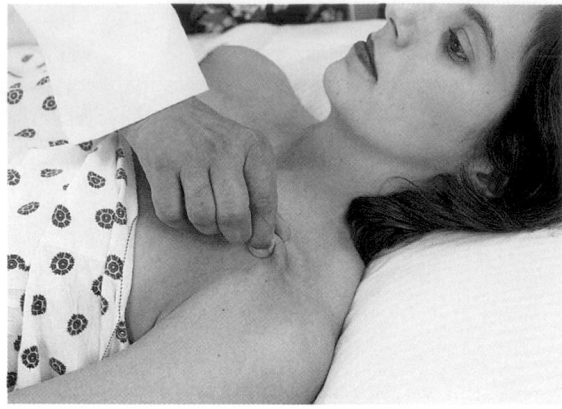

FIGURE 25-8 To assess skin turgor, a small fold of skin is picked up and then released to return to its normal shape. Difficulty in lifting a skin fold may indicate presence of edema.   (Photo © B. Proud.)

Health History

Identify risk factors for altered health during the health history by asking about the following:
- Changes with aging in vision or hearing
- History of use of corrective lenses or hearing aids
- Loss of an eye with insertion of artificial eye
- History of allergies
- History of disturbances in vision or hearing
- History of chronic illnesses, such as hypertension, diabetes mellitus, or thyroid disease
- Exposure to harmful substances or loud noises
- Exposure to ultraviolet light
- History of smoking, chewing tobacco, or cocaine use
- History of eye or ear infections
- History of head trauma
- History of persistent hoarseness

Physical Assessment

The structures of the head and neck are assessed with inspection and palpation, with the patient sitting.

Inspect and Palpate the Skull

Inspect and palpate the skull for size and shape. The parts of the head and face should be in proportion to each other and symmetric. Although the shape of the normal skull varies considerably, generally the shape is gently curved with prominences at the frontal and parietal bones. Abnormal findings include lack of symmetry or unusual size or contour of the skull (either may be the result of trauma or diseases affecting the growth of bone) and tenderness. If the skull appears disproportionately large or small, measure the circumference. Measuring head circumference is a normal part of infant assessment up to the age of 2 years and should be conducted at each visit.

Inspect the Face

Inspect the face for color, symmetry, and distribution of facial hair. The facial nerve and facial muscles are assessed by ask-

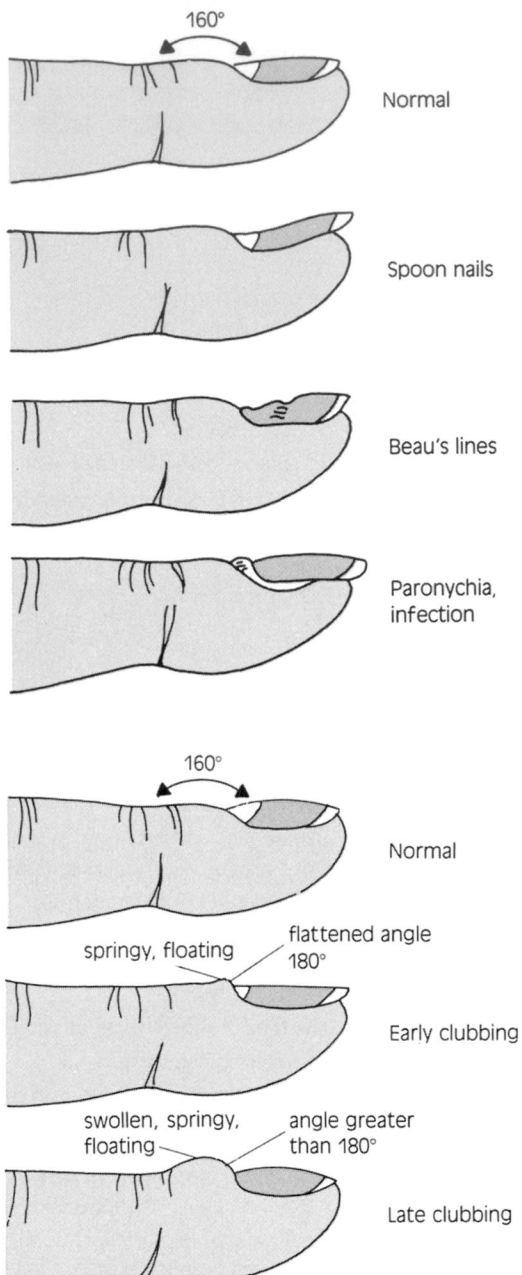

FIGURE 25-9 Examples of nail abnormalities.

ing the patient to raise the eyebrows, tightly close the eyes, puff out the cheeks, smile, and show the teeth. Edema of the face, especially around the eye (periorbital edema), and involuntary facial movements (eg, tics, fasciculations, and tremors) are abnormal findings. If abnormalities are noted, document their location, amount, and timing.

Assess the Eyes

Assess the structures and functions of the eyes using a penlight, an ophthalmoscope, and an eye chart. The eyes are assessed primarily by inspection. Assessments of the eye include external and internal eye structures (Fig. 25-10), visual acuity, extraocular movements, and peripheral vision.

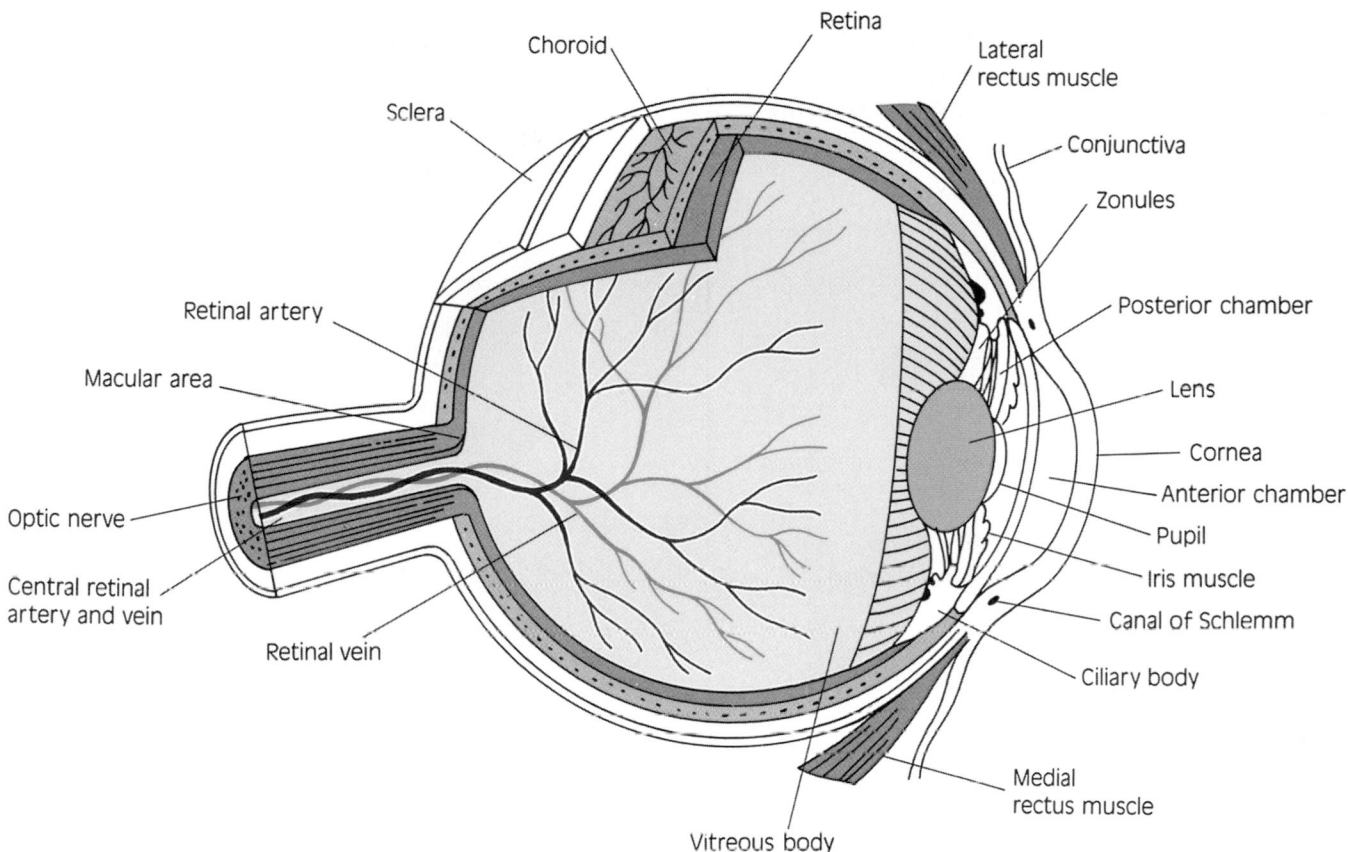

FIGURE 25-10 A cross-section of the eye.

Inspect External Eye Structures

Inspect the eyes, eyebrows, eyelids, eyelashes, lacrimal glands, and pupils and iris for position and alignment (Fig. 25-11). Inspect the eyes for symmetry and parallel alignment. The eyebrows should have equal distribution, and the eyelashes should

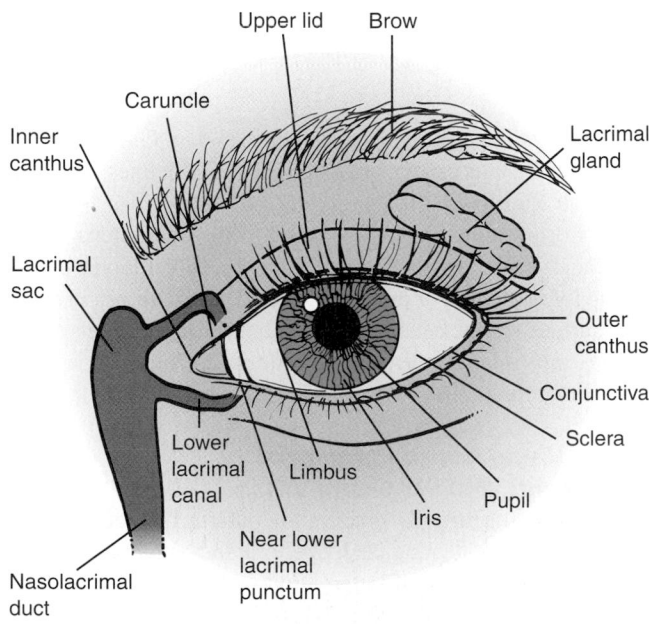

FIGURE 25-11 The eye and surrounding structures.

curl outward. Inspect the eyelids for color, edema, and equal coverage of the eyeball. Inspect and palpate the lacrimal glands for edema and pain.

The pupils are normally black, equal in size, round, and smooth. The pupils may be pale and cloudy if the patient has cataracts (loss of opacity of the lens). Injury to the eye, glaucoma, and certain medications may cause the pupil to dilate (mydriasis); certain drugs can cause constriction (miosis); and unequal pupils may result from central nervous system injury or illness.

Assess the pupils for their reaction to light and accommodation and for convergence (see Guidelines for Nursing Care 25-2). Figure 25-12 illustrates assessment of the pupillary reaction. Accommodation occurs when the patient moves the focus of vision from a distant point to a near point, causing the pupils to constrict (see Guidelines for Nursing Care 25-2 and Fig. 25-13). Move your finger toward the patient's nose to assess convergence. The patient's eyes should normally converge (assume a cross-eyed appearance), as illustrated in Figure 25-14.

Inspect Internal Eye Structures

The internal eye (Fig. 25-15) is examined with the ophthalmoscope to assess the fundus, including the retina, optic nerve disc, macula, fovea centralis, and retinal vessels. Using the ophthalmoscope takes practice. Normal findings are a uniform red reflex; a clear, yellow optic nerve disc; a reddish retina; and light-red arteries and dark-red veins, the veins being about

Guidelines for Nursing Care 25-2
Measuring Pupillary Reaction, Accommodation, Extraocular Movements, and Peripheral Vision

Pupillary Reaction
- Ask the patient to look straight ahead.
- Bring the penlight from the side of the patient's face and briefly shine the light on the pupil.
- Observe the pupil's reaction; it normally rapidly constricts (direct response).

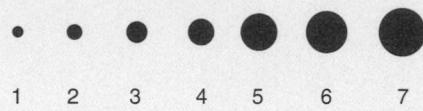

| 1 | 2 | 3 | 4 | 5 | 6 | 7 |

Pupillary gauge measures pupils (dilation or constriction) in millimeters (mm). (© B. Proud.)

- Repeat the procedure and observe the other eye; it too normally will constrict (consensual reflex).
- Repeat the procedure with the other eye.

Accommodation
- Hold the forefinger, a pencil, or other straight object about 10 to 15 cm (4″ to 6″) from the bridge of the patient's nose.
- Ask the patient to first look at the object, then at a distant object, then back to the object being held. The pupil normally constricts when looking at a near object and dilates when looking at a distant object.

Extraocular Movements
- Ask the patient to sit or stand about 2 feet away, facing you sitting or standing at eye level with the patient.
- Ask the patient to hold the head still and follow the movement of your forefinger or a penlight with the eyes.
- Keeping your finger or light about 1 foot from the patient's face, move it slowly through the cardinal positions: up and down, left and right, diagonally up and down to the left, diagonally up and down to the right.

Peripheral Vision
- Have the patient stand or sit about 2 feet away, facing you at eye level.
- Ask the patient to cover one eye with a hand or an index card.
- Ask the patient to look directly at your nose and fix his or her eyes on that spot.
- Cover your own eye opposite the patient's closed eye.
- Hold one arm outstretched to one side (right or left) equidistant from you and the patient, and move your fingers into the visual fields from various peripheral points.
- Ask the patient to tell you when the fingers are first seen (both you and the patient should see the fingers at the same time).
- Repeat the procedure for the other eye.

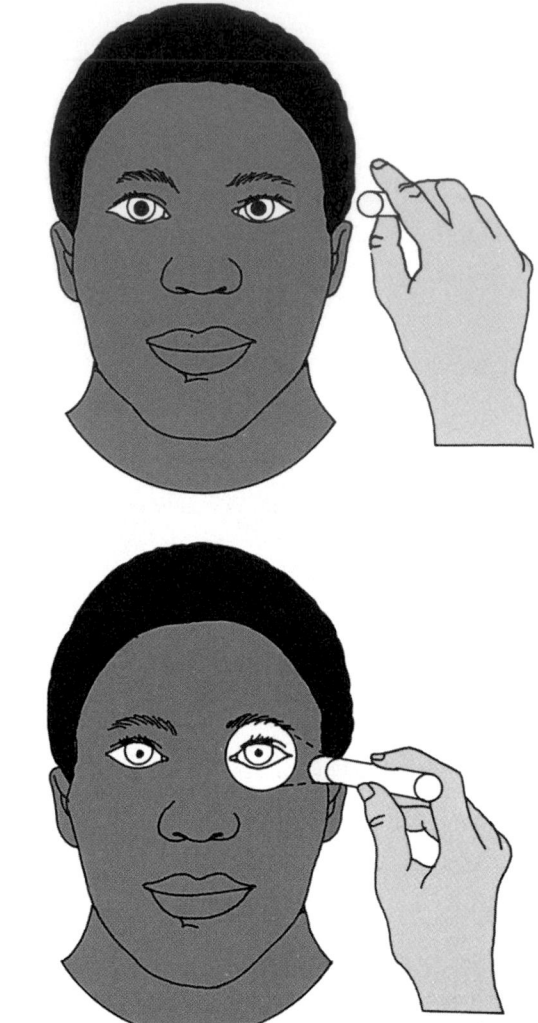

FIGURE 25-12 To test pupillary reaction to light, a penlight is moved from the side of the patient's face (*top*) to in front of the eye (*bottom*). The pupil should constrict when the light is present. The dilation or constriction shown is exaggerated for clarity.

1.5 times as large as the arteries (Fig. 25-16). Guidelines for assessing the internal eye are listed in the Guidelines for Nursing Care 25-3.

Abnormal findings include cloudiness of the lens (from cataracts), changes in the size and shape of blood vessels (from hypertension or arteriosclerosis), and changes in color and surface characteristics (from such health problems as diabetes mellitus, hypertension, trauma, inflammation, or a detached retina).

Assess Visual Acuity, Extraocular Movements, and Peripheral Vision

Assess visual acuity by placing the patient 20 feet from the Snellen chart and testing each eye. Ask the patient to read the smallest possible line of letters, first with both eyes and then with one eye at a time. Note whether the patient's vision is being tested with or without corrective lenses. Visual acuity is

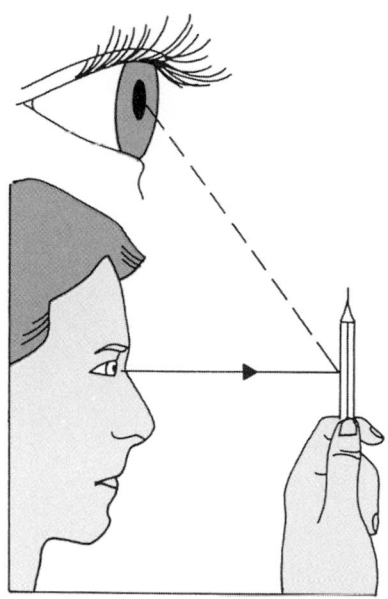

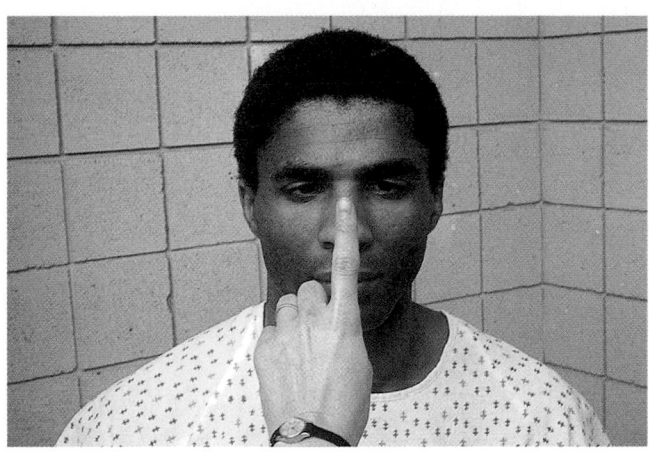

FIGURE 25-14 Convergence is assessed by moving the finger toward the patient's nose.   (Photo © Ken Kasper.)

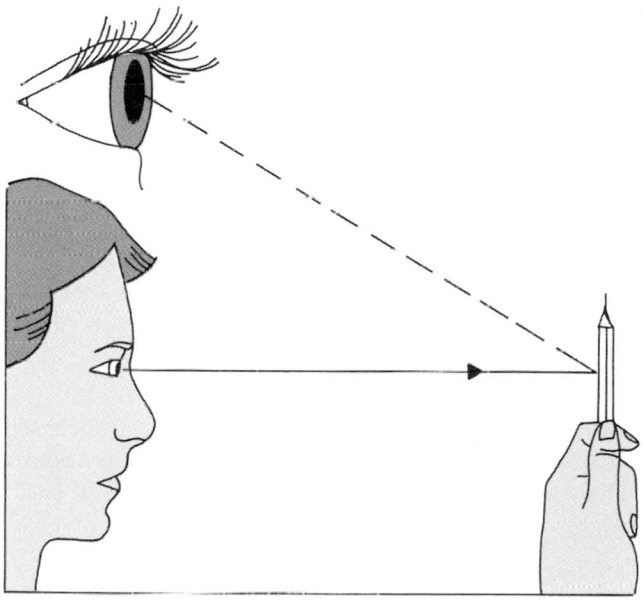

FIGURE 25-13 The normal pupil constricts when focused on a near object and dilates when focused on a far object. This is called *accommodation.*

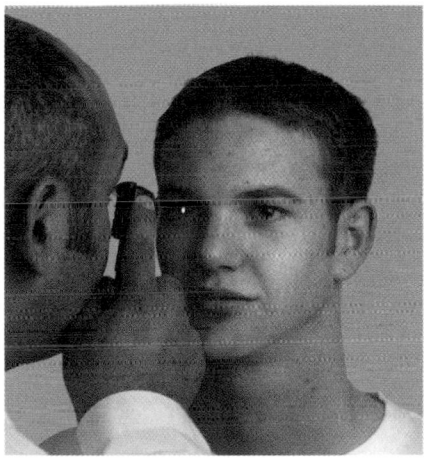

FIGURE 25-15 Examination of the internal structures of the eye, using an ophthalmoscope. (Used with permission from Bickley, L. S., & Szilagyi, P. G. [2003]. *Bates' guide to physical assessment and history taking* [8th ed., p. 152]. Philadelphia: Lippincott Williams & Wilkins.)

measured by standardized numbers listed on the side of the chart. The numerator is 20, representing the distance from which a person with normal vision (recorded as 20/20) can read the letters. The larger the denominator, the poorer the vision. Visual acuity is recorded as the smallest line of letters that can be read accurately with no more than two inaccurate readings (such as "20/30–2 with glasses").

Test extraocular movements by assessing the cardinal fields of vision for coordination and alignment (Fig. 25-17). Normally both eyes move together, are coordinated, and are parallel (see Guidelines for Nursing Care 25-2). Tests for peripheral vision (or visual fields) are used to assess retinal function and optic nerve function. Full peripheral vision is normal (see Guidelines for Nursing Care 25-2).

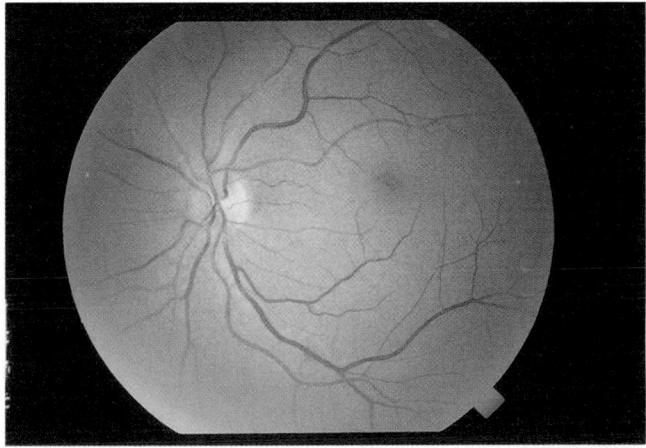

FIGURE 25-16 The normal fundus as seen through an ophthalmoscope.

Guidelines for Nursing Care 25-3
Assessing the Internal Eye

- Assemble the ophthalmoscope, beginning with the light setting at the large white light and the lens wheel at 0 setting.
- Darken the room and have the patient remove glasses. Allow time for the patient's pupils to dilate. The patient should be sitting.
- Sit facing the patient and ask him or her to look straight ahead during the examination.
- Keep both eyes open while looking through the ophthalmoscope viewer.
- Use your right hand and eye to examine the patient's right eye, and your left hand and eye for the patient's left eye.
- Shine the light on the pupil and observe the round red or orange glow (the red reflex).
- Focusing on the red reflex, slowly move the ophthalmoscope toward the patient's eye.
- Rotate the lens wheel until internal eye structures are sharp and clear.
- Follow blood vessels toward the midline to locate the optic disc; note color, size, shape, margins, and central area (physiologic cup).
- Follow blood vessels outward to each of the four quadrants, assessing color, size, and pattern.
- Ask the patient to look up, down, and from side to side, assessing the characteristics of the retina.
- Locate the macula by first locating the optic disc and then looking toward the patient's temple for a small circular structure near the disc; note color, characteristics, and area of reflected light (fovea centralis).

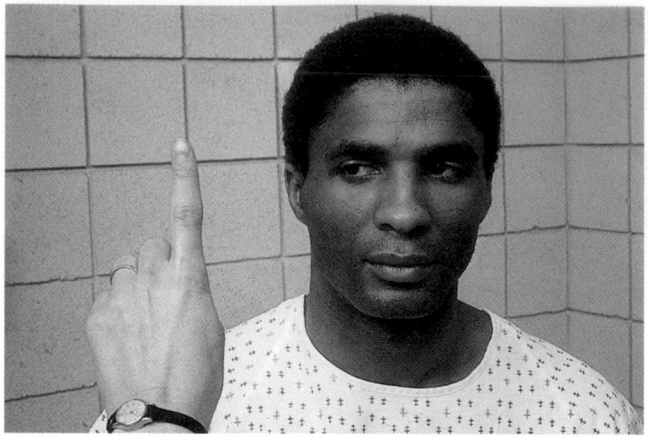
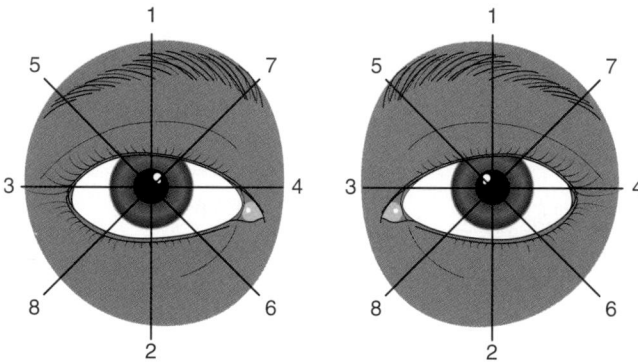

FIGURE 25-17 Test extraocular movement of the eye by asking the patient to hold his head still and follow the movement of your forefinger (*top*) through the cardinal positions of the eye (*bottom*). (Photo © Ken Kasper.)

Abnormalities of the external eye, pupil and iris, and visual assessment include asymmetry of position and alignment (may be due to muscle weakness or a congenital abnormality); drooping of the upper lids (ptosis) (may be due to damage to the oculomotor nerve, myasthenia gravis, or a congenital disorder); inward turning of the lower lid (entropion); outward turning of the lower lid (ectropion); redness or drainage (from infection of the lid margins, conjunctivae, or hair follicles); decreased or absent pupillary response (indicating blindness or serious brain damage); inability of the eyes to accommodate or converge; and alterations in the visual fields.

Assess the Ears

The external ear, the middle ear, and the inner ear (Fig. 25-18) are assessed. The patient remains sitting while the nurse assesses the function and structure of the ears by inspection and palpation. An otoscope with the correct size of ear speculum may be used to inspect the ear canal; a tuning fork and ticking watch are used to assess hearing acuity.

Inspect the External Ear

Inspect the external ear for shape, size, and lesions. The external surfaces of the ear should be smooth, and the shape and size of the ears should be symmetric and proportional to the head.

Inspect the Ear Canal and Tympanic Membrane

The otoscope is used to examine the ear canal and the tympanic membrane with the patient sitting. Attach the largest speculum that will fit comfortably into the patient's ear to the otoscope. Insert the otoscope speculum as the patient's head is slightly tilted away from the examiner. To achieve better visualization, straighten the ear canal of the adult by gently pulling the pinna up and back. In children younger than 3 years of age, straighten the ear canal by pulling the pinna down and back.

The ear canal should be smooth and pinkish. Examine for wax, discharge, and foreign bodies. The tympanic membrane should be intact, translucent, shiny, and gray (Fig. 25-19). There should be no redness or discharge.

Abnormal findings include pain when manipulating the pinna (a symptom of an infection of the external ear), redness of the canal (from inflammation or infection), mastoid tenderness (from infection), a red and swollen eardrum (symptoms of an infection in the middle ear), a perforated eardrum (from an infection causing rupture or trauma), wax plugs in the ear canal (from an accumulation of cerumen), and drainage (from an infection or foreign body in the ear canal).

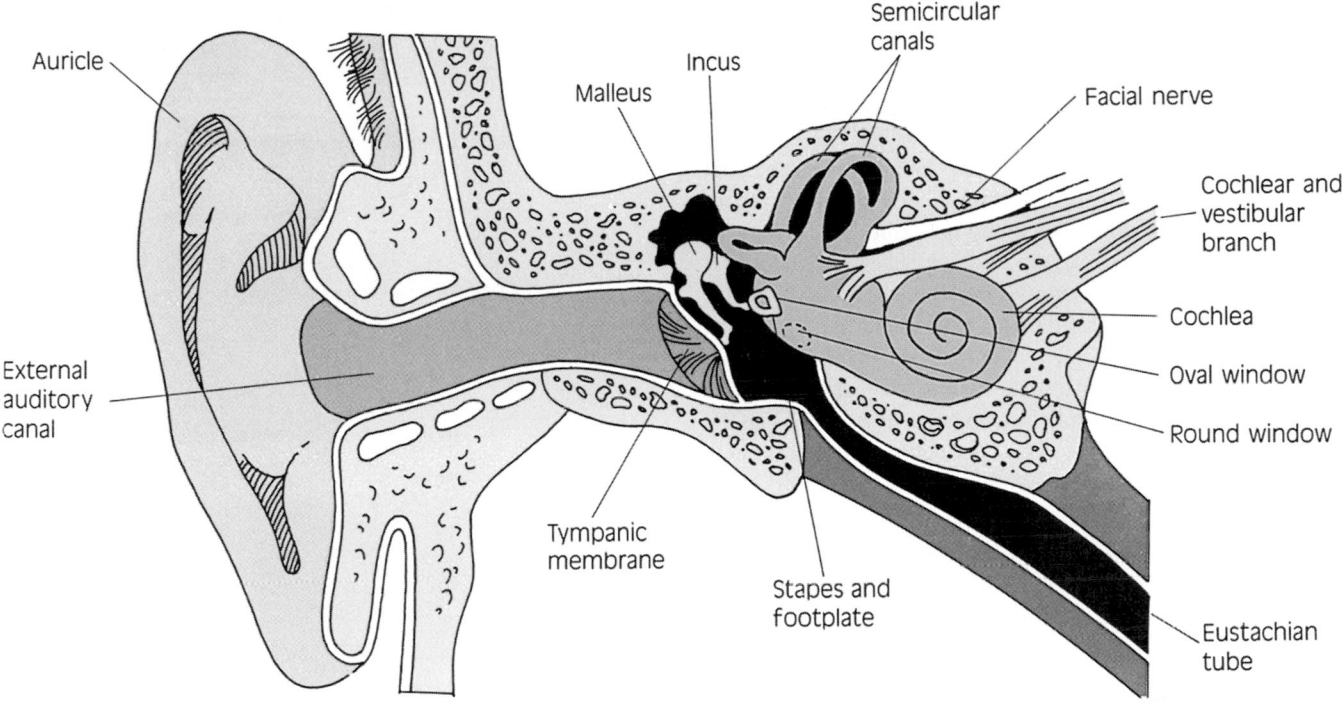

FIGURE 25-18 Internal structures of the ear.

Palpate the External Ear

Palpate the external ear gently for pain, edema, or presence of lesions (Fig. 25-20). Abnormal findings of the external ear include unequal height and size, uneven color, and lesions.

Assess Hearing and Sound Conduction

Hearing is assessed, one ear at a time, by determining whether the patient can hear a whispered voice or a ticking watch from a distance of 1 to 2 feet. Assess hearing acuity out of the patient's line of vision (to prevent lip-reading), with the opposite ear covered. When a hearing loss is found, a tuning fork or audiometer may be used for more precise assessment of hearing. Audiometry is not used generally in routine physical assessment.

Tuning fork tests are used to assess the type of hearing loss. Hearing loss may be conductive (the result of a problem with the transmission of sound waves through the outer and middle

FIGURE 25-19 Normal tympanic membrane, as seen through an otoscope.

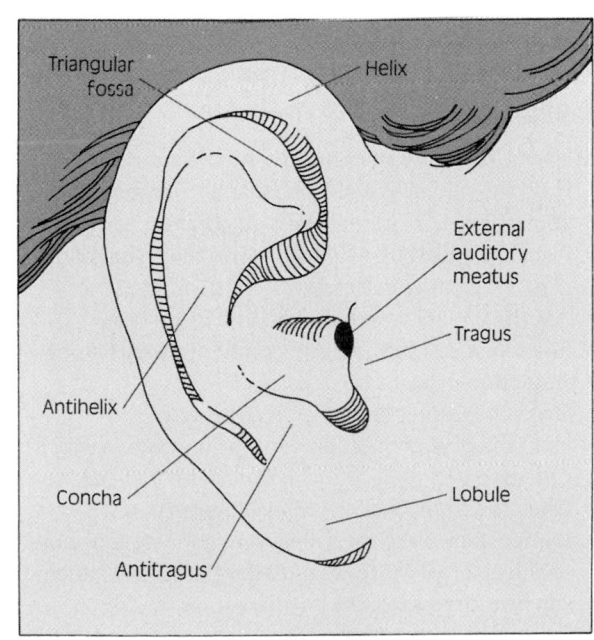

FIGURE 25-20 External structures of the ear.

ear); sensorineural (from inner ear damage); or mixed, a combination of both. Assess the patient for both bone conduction of sound and air conduction of sound with the Weber's test and the Rinne test. Guidelines for Nursing Care 25-4 discusses how to assess hearing with a tuning fork.

Normally, in the Weber's test, the sound is heard in both ears or is localized at the center of the head. Patients with conductive hearing loss hear the sound better in the affected ear because bone (in this case, the ossicles) transmits the sound directly to the ear. If the sound is heard better in the ear without a problem, it indicates damage to the inner ear or a nerve disorder.

Normally, in the Rinne test, air-conducted hearing is greater than bone-conducted hearing (documented as AC > BC). If the hearing loss is conductive, bone conduction will be the same or greater than air conduction.

Assess the Nose and Sinuses

Assess the nose by examining the external nose, the nares, and the turbinates (Fig. 25-21). The maxillary sinuses are located in the maxillary bone, the frontal sinuses in the frontal bone (Fig. 25-22). The nose is assessed by inspection and the sinuses by inspection and palpation. The patient sits with the head slightly tilted back.

Inspect the Nose

Test the nose for patency by occluding one nostril at a time and asking the patient to inhale and exhale through the nose. Inspect each nostril using an otoscope with a short, wide tip or using a nasal speculum and penlight (Fig. 25-23). Examine the mucous membranes for color and the presence of exudate or growths. Inspect the nasal septum for intactness and deviation. It is not necessary to use a nasal speculum with a child; push the tip of the nose upward with your thumb and shine a light into the nares. Normally, the nasal mucosa is moist and redder than the oral mucosa.

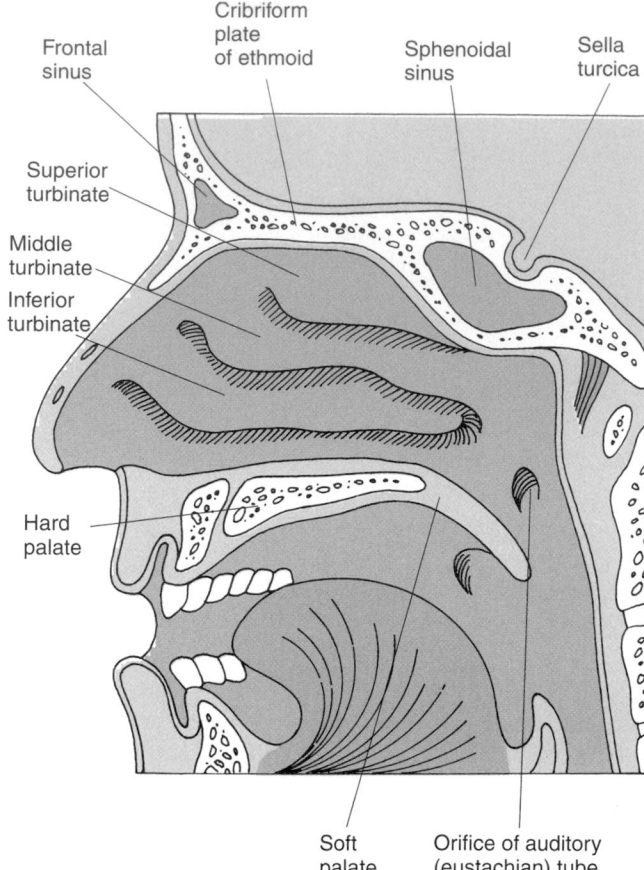

FIGURE 25-21 Cross-section of the nasal cavity.

Abnormal findings are swelling of the mucosa, bleeding or discharge (indicating allergies with inflammation or infection), perforation or deviation of the nasal septum (cocaine use may cause perforation; a deviated septum may be congenital or from trauma), and polyps (often seen with chronic allergies).

Guidelines for Nursing Care 25-4
Using a Tuning Fork to Assess Hearing

Weber's Test for Bone Conduction of Sound
- Hold the tuning fork at its base and strike it against your other palm so that the fork vibrates.
- Place the base of the tuning fork on the center of the top of the patient's head.
- Ask the patient where the sound is heard best.

Rinne's Test to Compare Air Conduction With Bone Conduction of Sound
- Strike the tuning fork as for Weber's test.
- Hold the base of the tuning fork against the mastoid process of the patient and ask the patient to tell you when the sound can no longer be heard.
- Immediately place the still-vibrating tuning fork close to the external ear canal and ask whether the patient can hear the sound; the normal ear will do so.
- Repeat the test with the other ear.

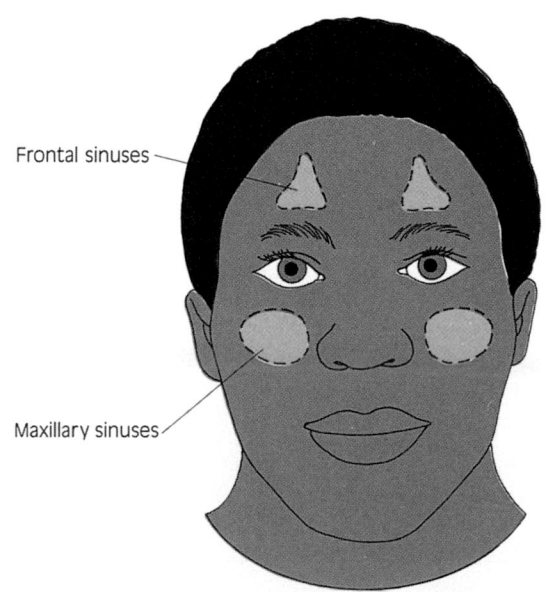

FIGURE 25-22 Location of the frontal and maxillary sinuses.

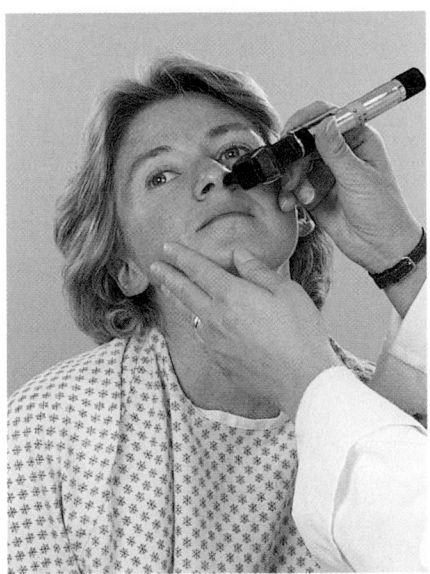

FIGURE 25-23 Examination of the nasal passages using an otoscope with a wide speculum.   (Photo © B. Proud.)

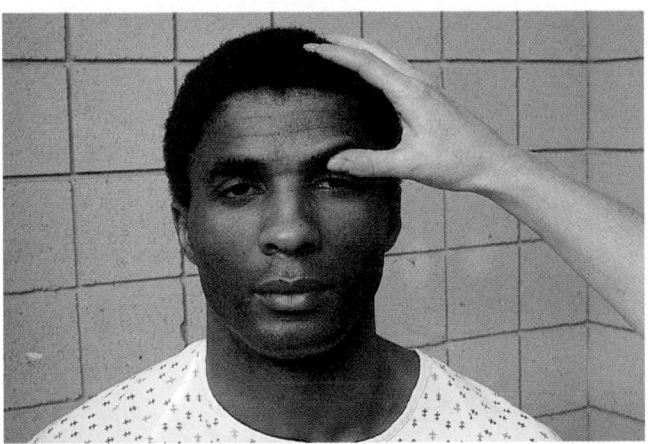

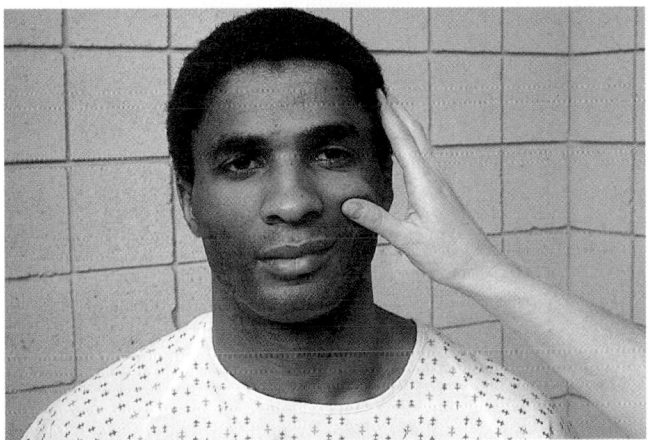

FIGURE 25-24 (*Top*) The frontal sinuses are palpated by gently pressing upward on the bony prominences above each eye. (*Bottom*) The maxillary sinuses are palpated by applying gentle pressure on the bony prominences of the upper cheek.   (Photos © Ken Kasper.)

Palpate the Sinuses

Palpate the frontal and maxillary sinuses for pain and edema. The frontal sinuses are palpated by gently pressing upward on the bony prominences located above each eye. The maxillary sinuses are palpated by gentle pressure on the bony prominences of the upper cheek (Fig. 25-24). Normally, the sinuses are not painful when palpated. Pain may be a finding if the sinuses are infected or obstructed.

Assess the Mouth and Pharynx

The mouth and pharynx are composed of the lips, tongue, teeth, gums, hard and soft palate, salivary gland, tonsillar pillars, and tonsils (Fig. 25-25).

Inspect the Mouth, Pharynx, and Neck

Equipment used to assess the mouth, pharynx, and neck includes a penlight, a tongue blade, a 4″ × 4″ gauze sponge, and gloves. The mouth and pharynx are assessed by inspecting the lips, gums and teeth, tongue, and hard and soft palates. Use palpation if any abnormalities are noted during inspection. The patient sits with the head tilted backward and the mouth opened wide. The nurse wears gloves when assessing a patient's mouth and may use 4 × 4 gauze to hold the tongue for palpation.

The lips should be pink, moist, and smooth. The tongue and mucous membranes are normally pink, moist, and free of swelling or lesions. If the patient wears dentures, they are removed for the inspection of the gums and roof of the mouth. The gums should be pink and smooth. With the tongue relaxed on the floor of the mouth, examine the mucous membrane of the oropharynx while depressing the base of the tongue with a tongue depressor. The uvula is normally centered and freely movable. The tonsils, if present, are small, pink, and symmetric in size. The teeth should be regular and free of cavities or have dental restoration.

Abnormal findings are pallor, cyanosis, or redness and swelling of the mucous membranes; lesions of the mucosa and lips; swollen, red tonsils (indicating infection); swollen, red, and bleeding gums (from nutritional deficits, inflammation or infection, poorly fitted dentures, or poor oral hygiene); poorly aligned, missing, or carious teeth; a white coating on the tongue (from poor oral hygiene, irritation, and smoking); a fissured tongue (from dehydration); a bright-red tongue (seen in deficiencies of iron, vitamin B_{12}, or niacin); or a black, hairy tongue (from antibiotic use).

Assess the neck (Fig. 25-26) with the patient sitting. The neck should be hyperextended slightly. Assess the neck for the size and position of the trachea and thyroid, range of motion, lymph nodes, and venous distention (Fig. 5-27). Ask the patient to tilt the head backward, forward, and side to side to assess range of motion. The neck should be symmetric, with full range of motion. No neck vein distention (indicating heart problems) should be visible.

Palpate the Trachea and Lymph Nodes

The trachea, normally midline at the suprasternal notch, is palpated for alignment and position. An unequal space between

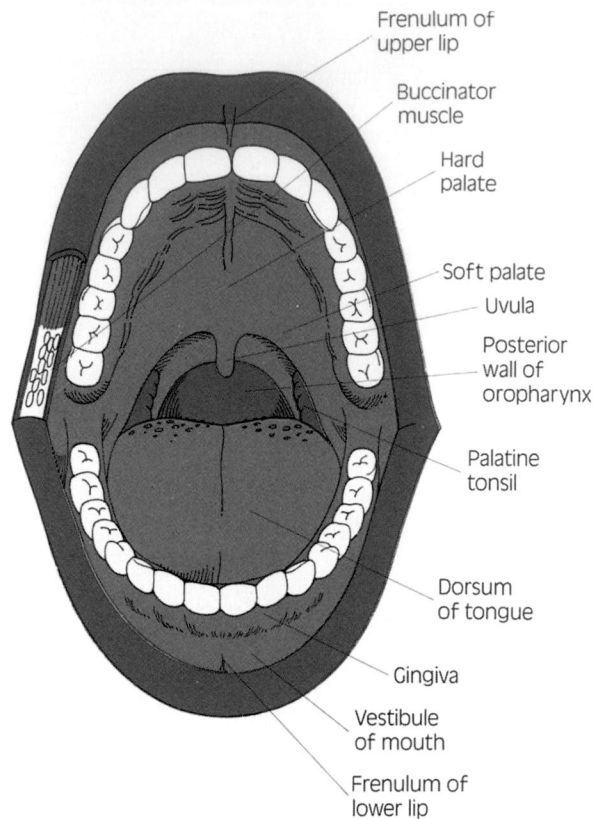

FIGURE 25-25 Structures of the mouth.

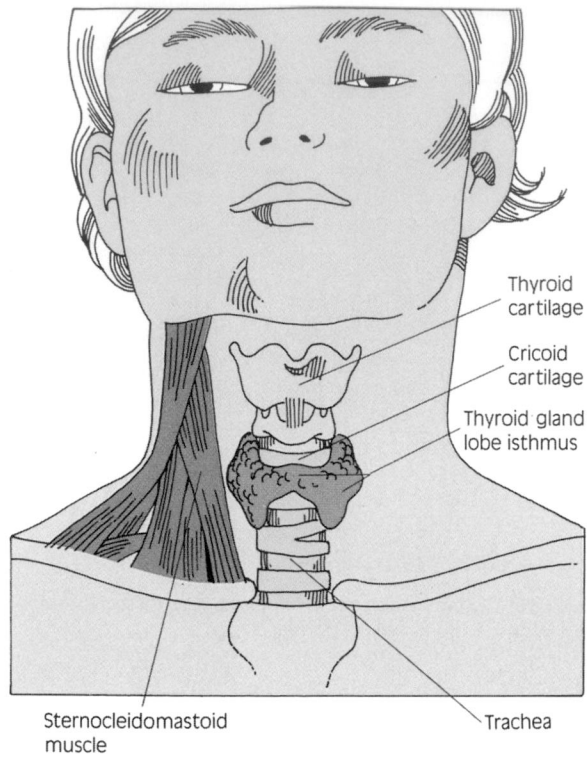

FIGURE 25-26 Structures of the neck.

the trachea and the sternocleidomastoid muscle on each side is an abnormal finding indicating tracheal displacement.

Palpate the lymph nodes (Fig. 25-28) with the pads of the fingers for enlargement, tenderness, and mobility. The nodes are generally not palpable; if palpable, they should be small, mobile, smooth, and nontender. If palpable, assess location, size, consistency, mobility, and tenderness. Enlarged lymph nodes (lymphadenopathy) may indicate infection, autoimmune disorders, or metastasis of cancer.

Palpate the Thyroid Gland

The thyroid gland is assessed by palpation, although it is normally not palpable in some patients. The patient is sitting, with the examiner using a posterior approach (Fig. 25-29). Palpate for size, shape, symmetry, tenderness, and presence of any nodules (see Guidelines for Nursing Care 25-5). If palpable, the thyroid gland should feel soft but elastic. It should be nontender and should have no enlargement, masses, or nodules (which may indicate thyroid gland disease, infection of the thyroid, or cancer).

Normal Age-Related Variations
Infant/Child

Common head and neck variations in newborns and children include:

- Closing of posterior fontanel at 8 weeks of age; soft anterior fontanel at about 18 months of age
- Gazing at and following bright objects by 1 month of age
- Focusing with both eyes by 6 months of age

- Pupils at the inner folds (pseudostrabismus)
- Startle reflex in newborns

Older Adult

Common head and neck variations in the older adult include:

- Impaired near vision (presbyopia)
- Decreased color vision and peripheral vision
- Decreased adaptation to light and dark
- A white ring around the cornea (arcus senilis)

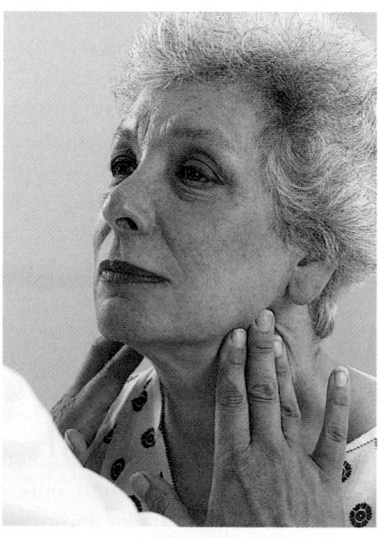

FIGURE 25-27 Palpating the neck.   (Photo © B. Proud.)

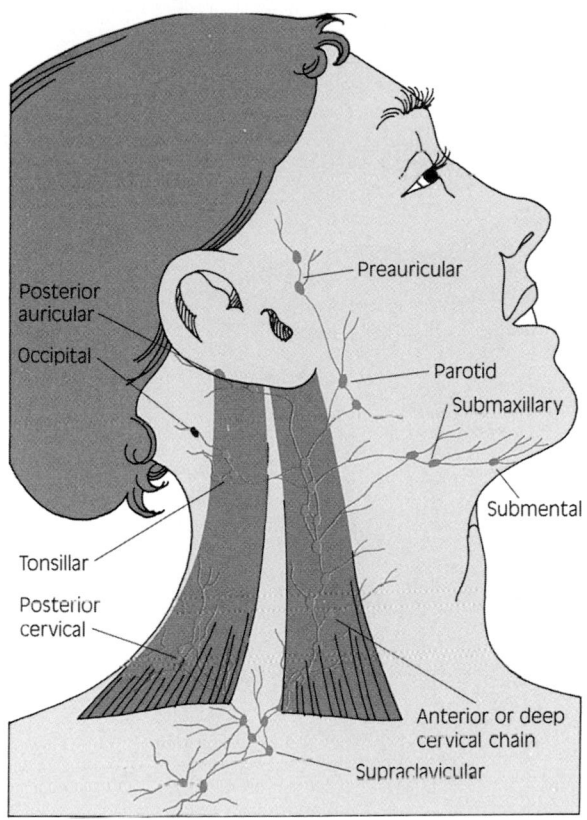

FIGURE 25-28 Location of the lymph nodes of the neck.

- Entropion and ectropion
- Hearing loss (presbycusis)
- Impaired conductive hearing
- Elongated ear lobes
- Prominent ear landmarks
- Decreased neck range of motion
- Nodular thyroid gland
- Smaller, more easily palpated lymph glands

Assessing the Thorax and Lungs

The thorax (Fig. 25-30) comprises the lungs, rib cage, cartilage, and intercostal muscles.

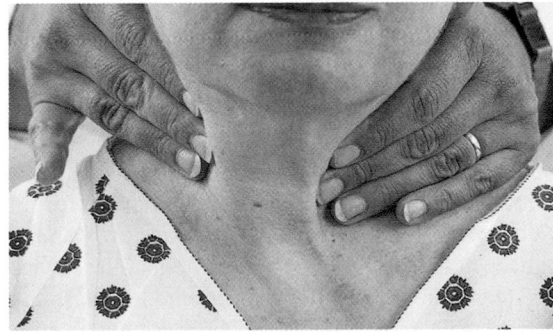

FIGURE 25-29 Assessing the thyroid. (Photo © B. Proud.)

> ## Guidelines for Nursing Care 25-5
> ### Palpating the Thyroid Gland
>
> - Standing behind the patient, place your hands around the patient's neck, with the fingertips over the lower half of the neck and trachea.
> - Ask the patient to swallow, and feel for enlargement of the gland as it rises.
> - Palpate each lobe of the thyroid by having the patient turn the head slightly toward the side to be examined; then gently displace the trachea with one hand.
> - Ask the patient to swallow, and palpate the thyroid with the other hand.
> - Repeat for the other side.

Health History

Identify risk factors for altered health during the health history by asking about the following:
- History of trauma to the ribs or lung surgery
- Having to use several pillows to breathe when sleeping
- History of chest pain with deep breathing
- History of persistent cough with or without producing sputum
- History of allergies
- Environmental exposure to chemicals, asbestos, or smoke
- History of smoking
- History of lung disease in family members or self
- History of frequent or chronic respiratory infections

Physical Assessment

Physical assessment of the thorax and lungs requires a stethoscope and a tape measure. The environment should be warm and adequately lit. The techniques for this assessment include inspection, palpation, percussion, and auscultation. The patient sits during the assessment.

Inspect the Thorax

Begin inspection by observing the patient's chest for color, shape or contour, breathing patterns, and muscle development. The color should be even and consistent with the color of the patient's face. The shape or contour should have a downward equal slope at the rib cage. The chest should be symmetric, with the transverse diameter greater than the anteroposterior diameter. An increased anteroposterior diameter, as seen in chronic lung diseases, is described as barrel-chest (Fig. 25-31). Respirations should be smooth and even, ranging from 12 to 20 breaths/min.

Abnormal findings include an increase in chest size and contour, abnormal breathing patterns with use of accessory muscles (symptoms of respiratory disease, such as chronic obstructive pulmonary disease or asthma), unequal chest expansion (may occur in chest trauma or pneumonia), and abnormal breath sounds (heard when the airways are obstructed by secretions or a foreign object).

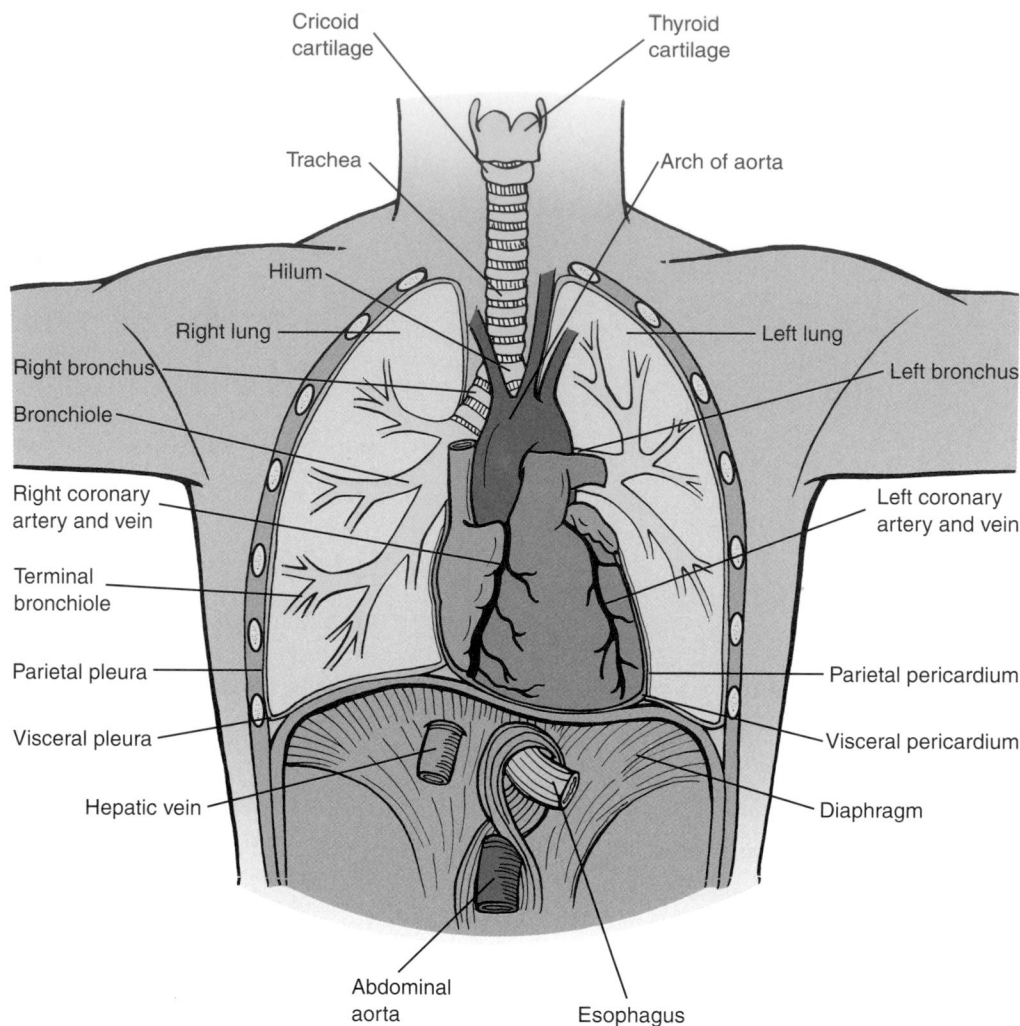

Cricoid cartilage

Thyroid cartilage

Trachea

Arch of aorta

Hilum

Right lung

Left lung

Right bronchus

Left bronchus

Bronchiole

Right coronary artery and vein

Left coronary artery and vein

Terminal bronchiole

Parietal pleura

Parietal pericardium

Visceral pleura

Visceral pericardium

Hepatic vein

Diaphragm

Abdominal aorta

Esophagus

FIGURE 25-30 Structures of the thorax.

Palpate the Thorax

Palpation is used to detect areas of sensitivity, chest expansion during respirations, and vibrations (fremitus). Use the palmar surface of the hands to palpate the anterior and posterior thoracic landmarks (Fig. 25-32) in a sequential pattern for temperature, moisture, muscular development, and any tenderness or masses. The same technique and sequence are used to test for tactile (vocal) fremitus, comparing bilateral sides. Normally, equal bilateral mild vibratory sensations are palpated. The skin should be warm and dry, with muscular development symmetric, and there should be no tenderness or masses.

Chest expansion is determined by placing the hands over the posterior chest wall, with the fingers at the level of T9 or T10. Ask the patient to take a deep breath, and observe the movement of your thumbs. The thorax should expand symmetrically (Fig. 25-33). Abnormal findings may be cool or excessively dry or moist skin; muscle asymmetry; tenderness; masses; increased or decreased vibratory sensation; asymmetric thoracic expansion; and abnormal breathing patterns (see Chap. 24).

Percuss the Thorax

Although not used frequently in assessing the lungs, percussion may be used to determine lung position and size and to detect the presence of air, liquids, or solids within the lungs. The shoulder area and anterior and posterior thorax are percussed in a systematic pattern (see Fig. 25-32). Note the intensity, pitch, duration, and quality of sounds produced. When a normal air-filled lung is percussed, the sound is hollow, loud, low in pitch, and of long duration. This percussion tone is known as resonance. A flat tone is heard over bony or well-developed muscle tissue. Abnormal percussion sounds are hyperresonance, heard over emphysematous lung tissue, and dullness, heard over fluid or a solid mass.

Auscultate Breath Sounds

Auscultation is used to detect airflow within the respiratory tract. The seated patient is asked to breathe slowly and deeply through the mouth. The warmed diaphragm of the stethoscope is placed over the thoracic landmarks, and breath sounds are auscultated in the same sequential pattern as used for palpation

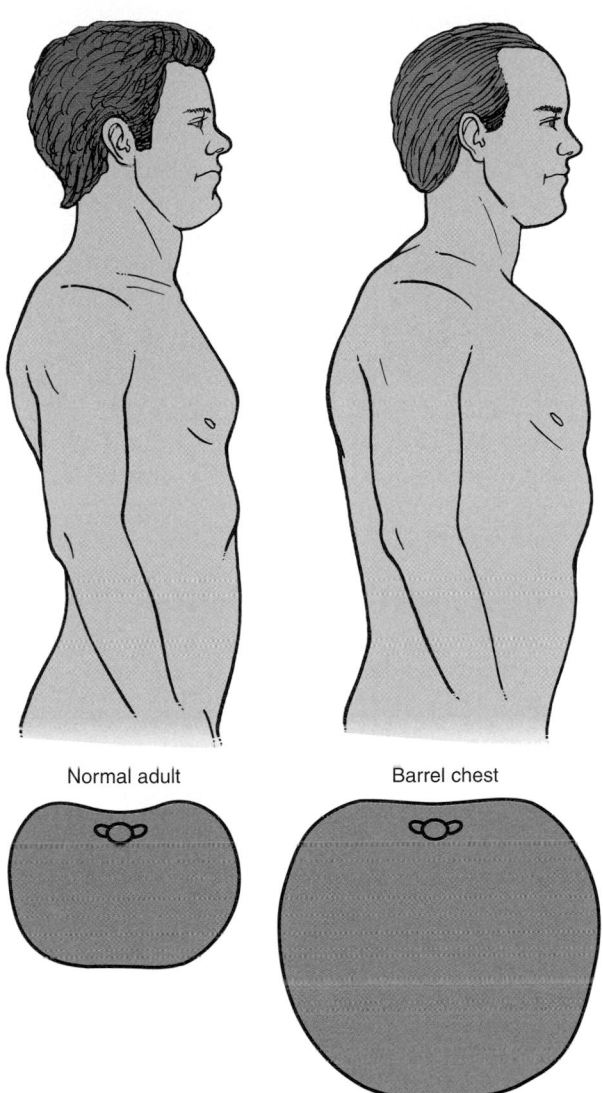

FIGURE 25-31 Profile and anteroposterior diameter of normal adult chest and barrel chest.

and percussion (see Fig. 25-32). Normally, breath sounds result from the free movement of air into and out of all parts of the bronchial tree. Listen for the duration, pitch, and intensity of the sounds, which normally vary over different parts of the lung.

Ordinarily, respirations are not audible without auscultation. **Bronchial sounds** heard over the trachea are high-pitched, harsh sounds, with expiration being longer than inspiration. **Bronchovesicular sounds** are heard over the mainstem bronchus and are moderate "blowing" sounds, with inspiration equal to expiration. **Vesicular breath sounds** are soft, low-pitched sounds, heard best over the base of the lungs during inspiration, which is longer than expiration. Terms used to describe the sounds that can be heard as the patient breathes are outlined and summarized in Fig. 25-34. **Adventitious breath sounds** are not normally heard in the lungs but, if present, may be auscultated along with normal breath sounds (Fig. 25-35).

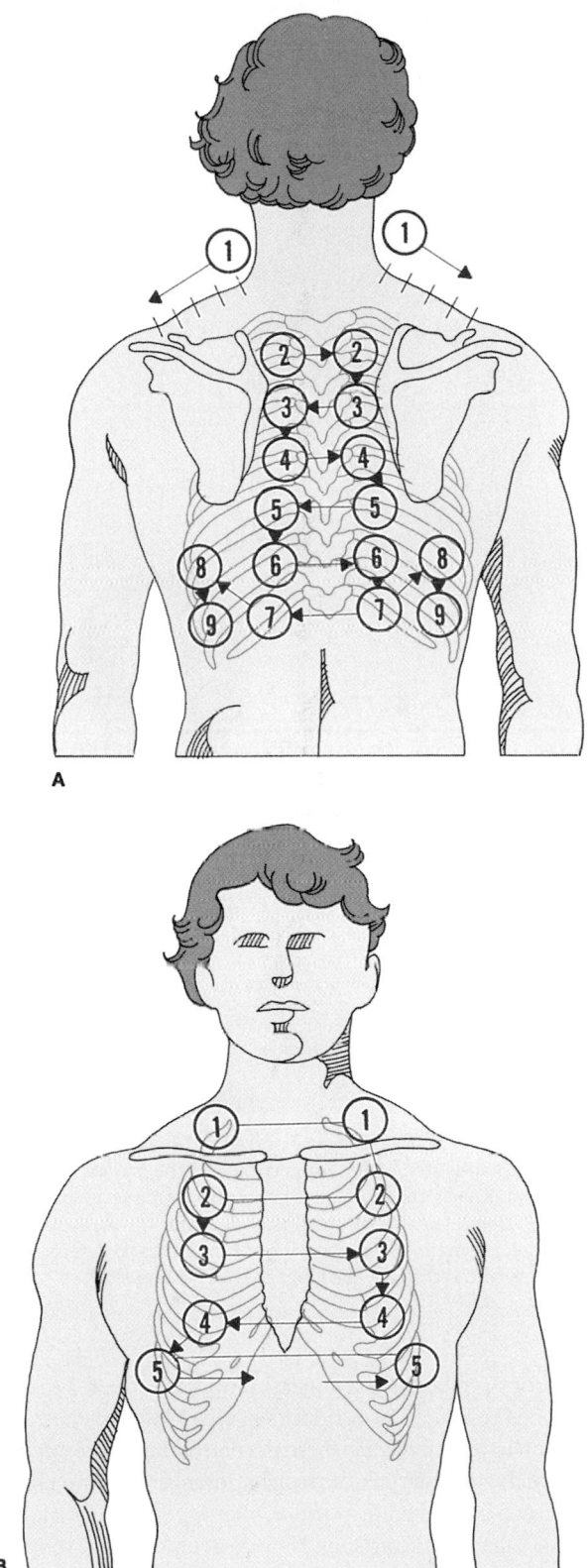

FIGURE 25-32 Posterior (**A**) and anterior (**B**) chest—landmarks and systematic sequence of assessment. The pattern is used for palpation, percussion, and auscultation of the chest.

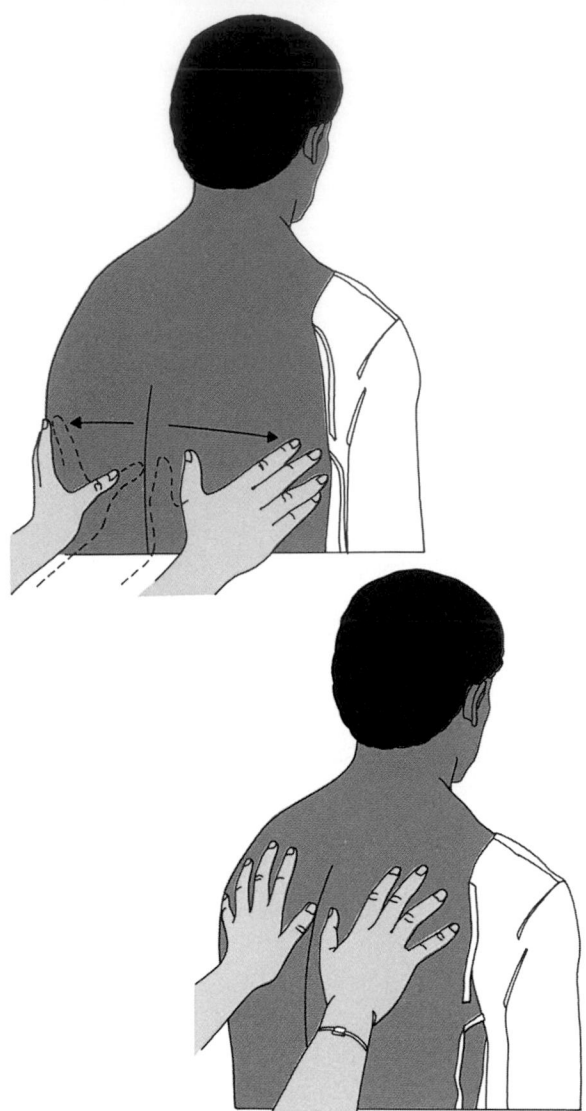

FIGURE 25-33 (*Top*) Palpating the posterior thorax excursion. The examiner's hands are placed symmetrically on the patient's back. As the patient inhales, the examiner's hands should move apart symmetrically. (*Bottom*) Palpation of the posterior thorax for vocal or tactile fremitus. The examiner uses the palms of the hands to detect vibrations transmitted through the lungs to the chest wall.

Stertorous breathing is a general term used to refer to noisy, strenuous respirations. Stridor is a harsh, high-pitched sound heard on inspiration when there is a narrowing of the upper airway, such as the larynx or trachea. Infants or young children with croup often manifest stridor when breathing. Crackles are fine to course crackling sounds made as air moves through wet secretions; they are most often heard on inspiration. Crackles are described as "fine" when they are made by air passing through moisture in small air passages and alveoli and as "coarse" when they are made by air passing through moisture in the bronchioles, bronchi, and trachea. Coarse crackles can also be documented as rhonchi. Wheezes are continuous sounds that originate in small air passages that are narrowed by secretions, swelling, or tumors. They may be inspiratory or expira-

tory and are high-pitched sounds. A pleural friction rub is a grating sound caused by an inflamed pleura rubbing against the chest wall.

> *Think back to Billy Collins, the 9-year-old who was stung by a bee. Incorporating knowledge of the signs and symptoms of an allergic reaction, the nurse would inspect Billy's chest for accessory muscle use and auscultate his lungs, noting any evidence of wheezing, which is commonly noted with allergic reactions.*

Although stertorous respirations, stridor, and wheezes can be heard without amplification, crackles and pleural friction rubs are usually heard only by auscultation with a stethoscope. If a productive cough occurs during assessment of the thorax and lungs, the sputum should be assessed for color, consistency, and amount.

Normal Age-Related Variations
Infant/Child
Common thorax and lung variations in newborns and children include:
- Louder auscultated breath sounds
- More rapid respiratory rate (until 8 to 10 years of age)
- Use of abdominal muscles during respiration

Older Adult
Common thorax and lung variations in older adults include:
- Increased anteroposterior chest diameter
- Increase in the dorsal spinal curve (kyphosis)
- Decreased thoracic expansion
- Use of accessory muscles to exhale

Assessing the Cardiovascular and Peripheral Vascular Systems

Cardiovascular and peripheral vascular assessment includes the heart and the extremities.

Health History

Identify risk factors for altered health during the health history by asking about the following:
- History of chest pain, palpitations, or dizziness
- Swelling in the ankles and feet
- Number of pillows used to sleep at night
- Type and amount of medications taken daily
- History of heart defect, rheumatic fever, or chest or heart surgery
- Family history of hypertension (high blood pressure), myocardial infarction (heart attack), coronary artery disease, high blood cholesterol levels, or diabetes mellitus
- History of smoking
- History of alcohol use
- Type and amount of exercise

Bronchial or Tubular

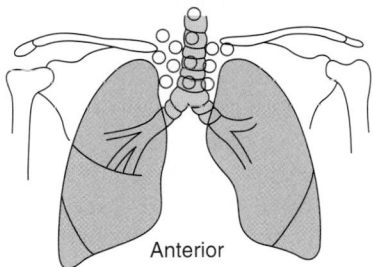

Anterior

Blowing, hollow sounds auscultated over the trachea

Ratio of inspiration to expiration

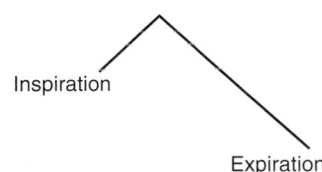

Inspiration

Expiration

Inspiration is shorter than expiration. Expiration is longer, lower, and higher-pitched than inspiration.

Bronchovesicular

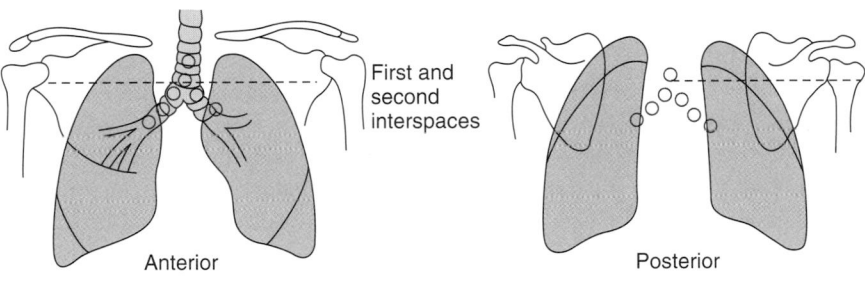

First and second interspaces

Anterior   Posterior

Medium-pitched, medium intensity, blowing sounds auscultated over the first and second interspaces anteriorly and the scapula posteriorly

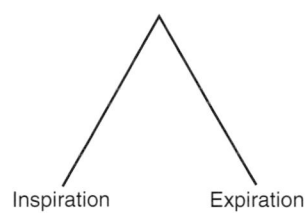

Inspiration   Expiration

Inspiration and expiration have similar pitch.

Vesicular

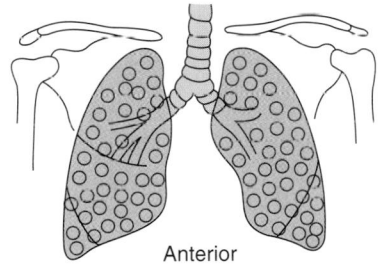

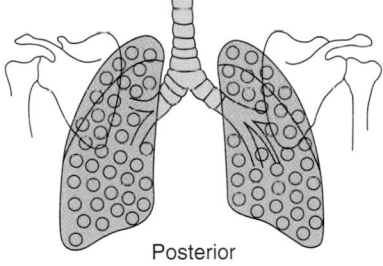

Anterior   Posterior

Soft, low-pitched sounds auscultated over the lung periphery

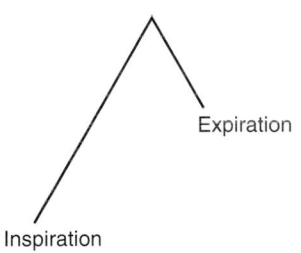

Expiration

Inspiration

Inspiration is longer, louder, and higher-pitched than expiration.

FIGURE 25-34 Normal breath sounds.

Breath Sounds	Characteristics	Breath Sounds	Characteristics
Wheeze 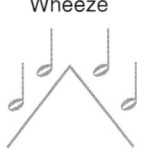	Musical or squeaking High-pitched and continuous sounds Auscultated during inspiration or expiration Occurs in small air passages	Crackles 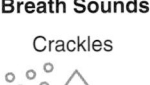	Bubbling, crackling, popping Low- to high-pitched, discontinuous sounds Auscultated during inspiration Occurs in small air passages, alveoli, bronchioles, bronchi, and trachea
Rhonchi 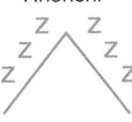	Sonorous or coarse Low-pitched and continuous sounds Auscultated during inspiration or expiration Occurs in large air passages (Coughing may clear the sound)	Friction Rub 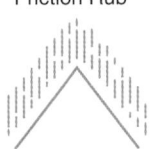	Rubbing or grating Loudest over lower lateral anterior surface Auscultated during inspiration and expiration

FIGURE 25-35 Abnormal breath sounds.

- Usual foods eaten each day
- Use of hormone replacement therapy (in postmenopausal women)
- Evidence of changes in color or temperature of the extremities
- History of pain in the legs when sleeping or pain that is worsened by walking
- History of blood clots or sores on the legs that do not heal
- History of edema of the lower extremities

Physical Assessment

Peripheral vascular assessment includes measuring the blood pressure and assessing peripheral pulses and perfusion. Assessments are done by inspection and palpation, with the patient sitting or supine. Peripheral vascular assessments may be combined with assessment of other body areas.

The techniques used for cardiovascular assessment include inspection, palpation, and auscultation. A stethoscope with a bell and diaphragm and a sphygmomanometer are used. The patient may be in a sitting position or in a supine position with the head raised about 30 degrees. Adequate lighting is essential for inspection of color and pulsations. A quiet environment is necessary for accurate auscultation of heart sounds. The nurse is usually positioned at the right side of the patient. Refer to Fig. 25-36 for a view of the heart, including the heart valves responsible for heart sounds.

Inspect the Neck and Precordium

Observe the neck and **precordium** (the aortic, pulmonic, tricuspid, and apical areas, and Erb's point; Fig. 25-37) for visible pulsations. There are usually no visible pulsations, except the apical impulse (or the point of maximal impulse [PMI]), located at about the fourth or fifth intercostal space at the left midclavicular line. Inspect the epigastric area at the tip of the sternum for pulsation of the abdominal aorta. Findings of neck vein distention (indicating heart disease) or visible pulsations in precordial areas other than the PMI (which may result from abnormalities of the ventricle) are considered abnormal.

Palpate the Precordium

The hands, which should be warm, are used to palpate the precordium gently for pulsations, using the palmar surface with the four fingers held together. Palpation proceeds in a systematic manner, with assessment of specific cardiac landmarks—the aortic, pulmonic, tricuspid, and mitral areas and Erb's point. Identify the PMI and record the apical impulse by interspace

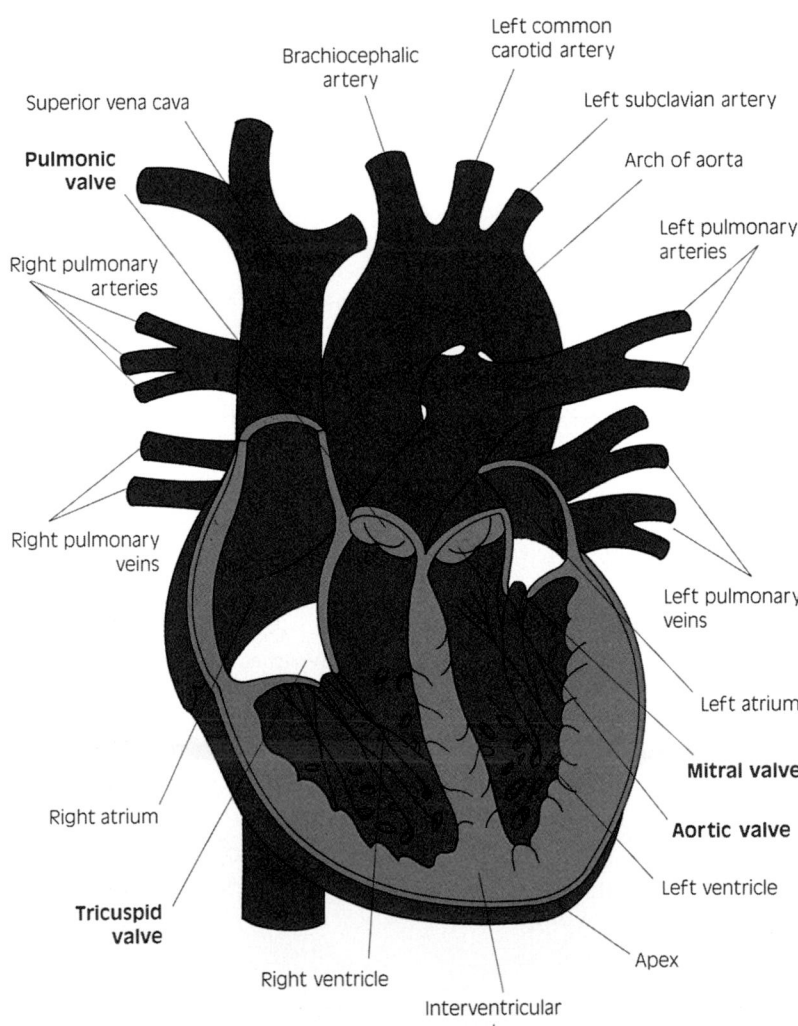

Superior vena cava

Brachiocephalic artery

Left common carotid artery

Left subclavian artery

Pulmonic valve

Arch of aorta

Left pulmonary arteries

Right pulmonary arteries

Right pulmonary veins

Left pulmonary veins

Left atrium

Mitral valve

Aortic valve

Left ventricle

Right atrium

Tricuspid valve

Apex

Right ventricle

Interventricular septum

FIGURE 25-36 View of the interior of the heart showing the atrioventricular and semilunar valves responsible for normal heart sounds.

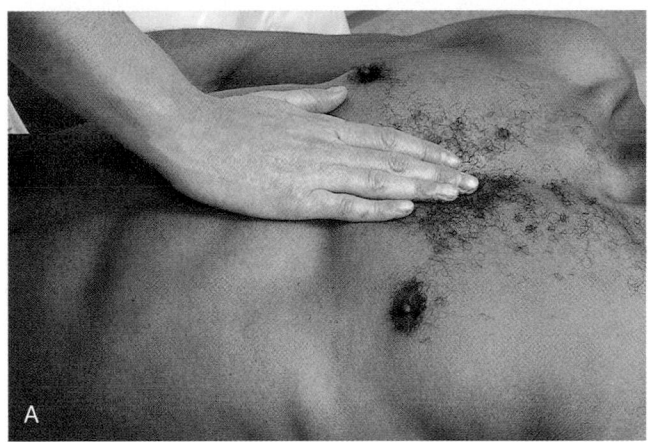

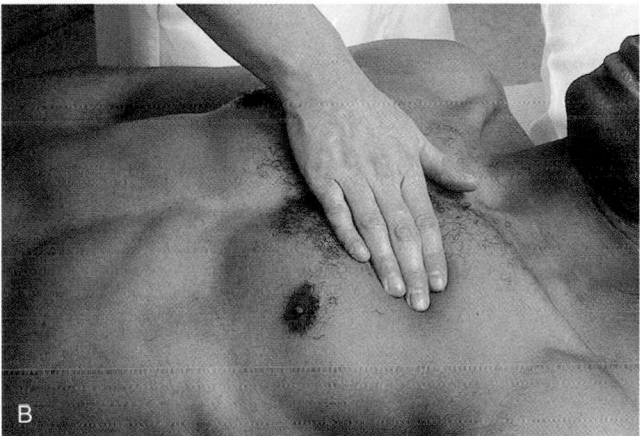

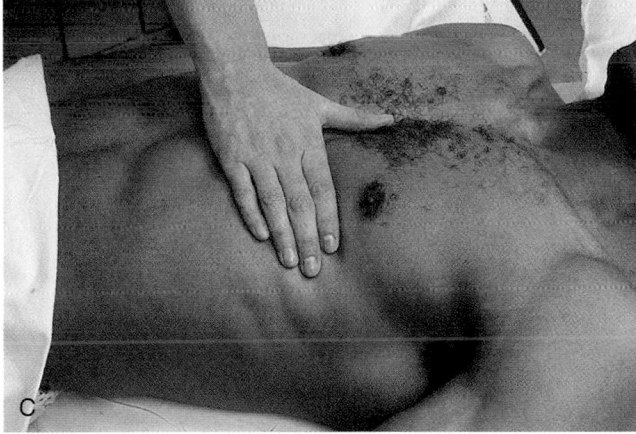

FIGURE 25-37 Palpating areas of the precordium: (**A**) aortic area, (**B**) pulmonic area, and (**C**) apical and tricuspid area.   (Photos © Ken Kasper.)

and relationship to the midsternal line or midclavicular line. Identify any precordial thrills, which are fine, palpable, rushing vibrations over the right or left second intercostal space, and any lifts or heaves, which involve a rise along the border of the sternum with each heartbeat. Normal findings include no pulsation palpable over the aortic and pulmonic areas, with a palpable pulsation at the PMI.

Auscultate Heart Sounds

Auscultation is used to determine the heart sounds caused by closure of the heart valves. A systematic approach is used to listen at all cardiac landmarks (Fig. 25-38): the aortic area, the pulmonic area, Erb's point, the tricuspid area, and the mitral (apical) area. Use systematic auscultation, beginning at the aortic area, moving to the pulmonic area, then to Erb's point, then to the tricuspid area, and finally to the mitral area. The patient should breathe normally. The stethoscope diaphragm is first used to listen to high-pitched sounds, followed by use of the bell to listen to low-pitched sounds. Focus on the overall rate and rhythm of the heart and the normal heart sounds (S_1 and S_2).

During auscultation, the first heart sound is heard as the "lub" of "lub-dub." This sound occurs when the mitral and tricuspid valves close and corresponds to the onset of ventricular contraction (Fig. 25-39). The sound, low-pitched and dull, is called S_1 and is heard best at the apical area. The second heart sound, S_2, occurs at the termination of systole and corresponds to the onset of ventricular diastole. The "dub" of "lub-dub," it represents the closure of the aortic and pulmonic valves. The sound of S_2 is higher pitched and shorter than S_1. The two sounds occur within 1 second or less, depending on the heart rate.

Consider Tammy Browning, the pregnant woman described in the Reflective Practice display. In addition to completing a health assessment for Tammy, the nurse would need to auscultate fetal heart sounds to assess fetal status.

Normal findings include S_1 that is louder at the tricuspid and apical areas, with S_2 louder at the aortic and pulmonic areas.

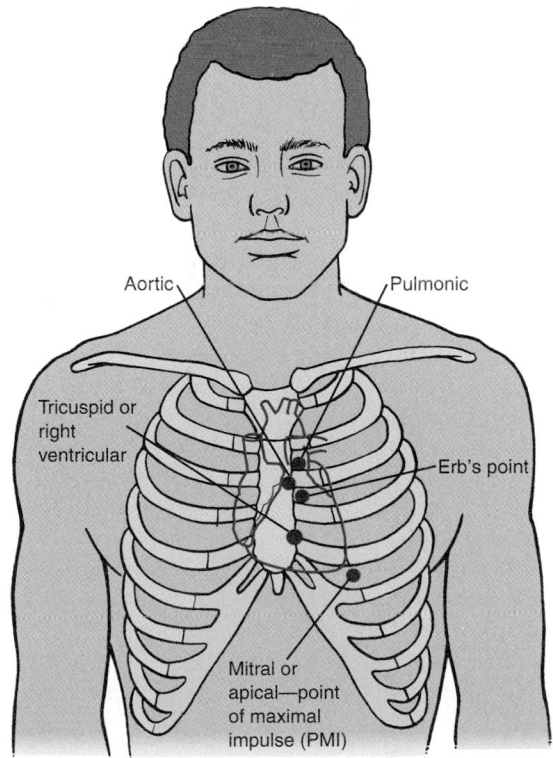

FIGURE 25-38 Cardiac landmarks and sequence of examination using auscultation.

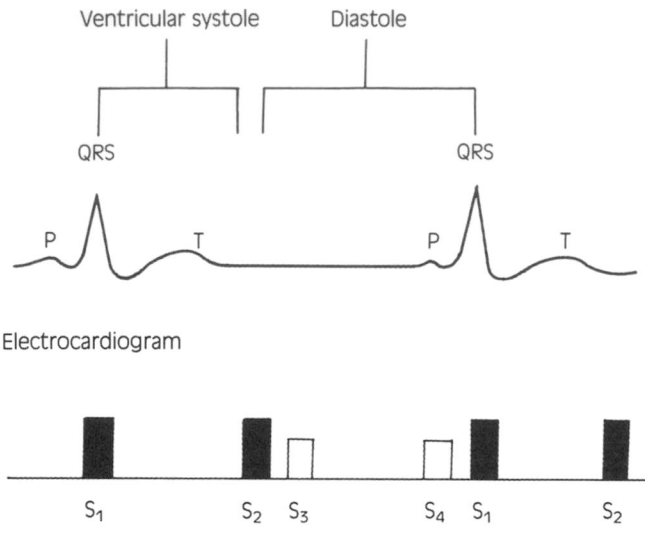

FIGURE 25-39 Heart sounds in relation to the cardiac cycle and an electrocardiogram.

Abnormal findings include extra heart sounds at any of the cardiac landmarks and abnormal rate or rhythm. Extra heart sounds are often heard when the patient has anemia or heart disease. A wide variety of conditions may alter the normal heart rate or rhythm, including serious infections, diseases of the heart muscle or conducting system, dehydration or overhydration, endocrine disorders, respiratory disorders, and head trauma.

Extra heart sounds may be S_3, S_4, murmurs, or bruits. S_3, known as the third heart sound, is often represented by a "lub-dub-dee" pattern ("dee" being S_3); this sound is best heard with the stethoscope bell at the mitral area, with the patient lying on the left side. S_3 is considered normal in children and young adults and abnormal in middle-aged and older adults. S_4 is the fourth heart sound, represented by "dee-lub-dub." S_4 is considered normal in older adults but abnormal in children and adults. Heart murmurs are extra heart sounds caused by some disruption of blood flow through the heart. The characteristics of a murmur depend on the adequacy of valve function, rate of blood flow, and size of the valve opening. Table 25-8 illustrates the grading of heart murmurs. **Bruits,** which are abnormal sounds, are "swooshing" sounds similar to murmurs and are heard over major blood vessels. The sound indicates a partially blocked or overextended artery, causing blood to swirl rather than flow normally. Bruits are most commonly heard over the carotid arteries, the abdominal aorta, and the femoral arteries.

Inspect the Extremities

Inspect the skin of the extremities for color, temperature, continuity, lesions (as described previously for assessment of the integument), venous patterns, and edema. There are normally no venous patterns, varicosities, rashes, ulcers, or edema on the lower extremities. The skin of the patient with peripheral vascular disease (resulting in decreased blood flow and oxygenation of tissues) is typically pale and cool, shiny with brown discolorations, and hairless. The toenails are thickened.

TABLE 25-8 Common Grading System for Heart Murmurs

Grade	Description
I	A murmur so faint that it can only be heard with great effort
II	A faint murmur but one that can be easily detected
III	A moderately loud murmur
IV	A very loud murmur that is usually associated with a thrill sound
V	An extremely loud murmur
VI	An exceptionally loud murmur that can be heard while the stethoscope is lifted off the skin

Palpate Peripheral Pulses

Use the pads of the index and middle fingers to palpate peripheral pulses for amplitude and symmetry. Palpate, one at a time and with caution, the carotid brachial, radial, femoral, popliteal, dorsalis pedis, and posterior tibial pulses (see Fig. 24-3 in Chap. 24). These should be strong and equal bilaterally. The amplitude of the pulses may be documented as 0 (absent), 1+ (weak), 2+ (normal), 3+ (increased), or 4+ (bounding).

Abnormal findings include an absent, weak, thready pulse (which may indicate a decreased cardiac output), a forceful or bounding pulse (seen in hypertension and circulatory overload), and an asymmetric pulse (related to impaired circulation). Phlebitis (inflammation of a vein) of the lower extremity is indicated by pain, redness, and swelling of the affected calf or thigh.

Other specific assessments to determine arterial blood flow include Allen's test, Buerger's test, and capillary refill (see Guidelines for Nursing Care 25-6).

Normal Age-Related Variations
Infant/Child

Common cardiovascular and peripheral vascular variations in newborns and children include:
- Visible pulsation if the chest wall is thin
- Sinus arrhythmia (the rate increases with inspiration and decreases with expiration)
- Presence of S_3 (in about one third of all children)
- More rapid heart rate (until about 8 years of age)

Older Adult

Common cardiovascular and peripheral vascular variations in older adults include:
- Difficult-to-palpate apical pulse
- Difficult-to-palpate distal arteries
- Dilated proximal arteries
- More prominent and tortuous blood vessels; varicosities common

Guidelines for Nursing Care 25-6
Assessing Peripheral Circulation

Allen's Test
- Ask the patient to rest his or her hand on the examining table with the palm up and to make a fist.
- Use your thumbs to occlude the radial and ulnar arteries and ask the patient to open his or her hand (the palm will be pale).
- Release your thumb pressure and observe the return of color to the palm (this should normally take 3 to 5 seconds).

Buerger's Test
- Ask the patient to assume a supine position and then raise one arm or one leg about 1 foot (30 cm) above the level of his or her heart.
- Ask the patient to briskly move the leg or arm up and down for 1 minute, then to sit up and dangle the arm or leg downward.
- Observe the time it takes for the original color of the patient's skin to return and for the veins to fill. Normally, color returns in 10 seconds, and veins fill in 15 seconds.

Capillary Refill
- Using your thumb and forefinger, squeeze the patient's fingernail or toenail until it appears white.
- Release the pressure and observe the time it takes for normal color to return. Normally, color returns immediately.
- Assess capillary refill in children by pressing the skin lightly over the forehead or top of the hand. Release the pressure; observe the time for return of color.

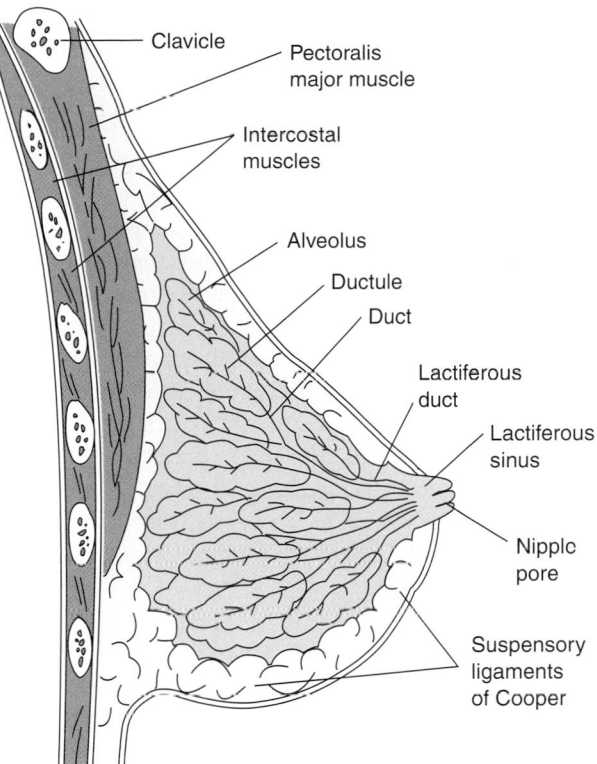

FIGURE 25-40 Lateral view of the female breast.

- Increased systolic and diastolic blood pressure
- Widening pulse pressure

Assessing the Breasts and Axillae

Although the assessments and disorders described here focus on the female breast, men also are at risk for breast disease. Each breast has a lymphatic network that drains into the underlying axilla (Fig. 25-40).

Health History

Identify risk factors for altered health during the health history by asking about the following:
- History of pain in one or both breasts, including relationship to menstrual period in women
- History of lumps or swelling, redness, change in size, or dimpling in the breasts
- History of discharge from the breast
- Family history of breast cancer
- History of breast disease, biopsy, or surgery
- Menstrual and pregnancy history
- Use of hormones, oral contraceptives, or antidepressants
- Exposure to radiation, benzene, or asbestos
- Usual dietary intake and alcohol consumption
- Knowledge and practice of breast self-examination (see Chap. 35)
- Most recent breast examination by a physician and mammogram

Physical Assessment

The breasts and axilla are assessed in both men and women by inspection and palpation. The patient is in the sitting or supine position. When sitting, the patient should sit erect, with arms at sides or raised overhead. When supine, the patient's hand on the side being examined is placed under the head.

Inspect the Breasts and Axillae

Inspect the breasts and axillae for size, shape, symmetry, color, texture, and skin lesions. The breasts should be relatively symmetric, although variations are normal. The size varies among individuals. The shape of the breasts is round and smooth, and there should be no skin depressions (retraction) or puckering (dimpling). The color should be consistent with the rest of the skin, and the texture of the skin should be soft.

Inspect the areola and nipples for size and shape and the nipples for discharge, crusting, and inversion. The areolar and nipple areas should be equal in size, round or oval, with a smooth surface. Montgomery's tubercles (sebaceous glands on the areolae of the breasts) are a normal component of the areola. The nipples are normally everted. Lesions and discharge from the nipples are abnormal findings except in pregnancy. Leaking is normal during pregnancy and breastfeeding.

Palpate the Breasts and Axillae

Palpate the breast to detect any abnormal masses or lumps. Palpate the nipple and areola and gently compress the nipple between the thumb and forefinger to assess for discharge. The breast is assessed in four quadrants: the upper outer quadrant, the lower outer quadrant, the upper inner quadrant, and the lower inner quadrant (Fig. 25-41). Using the pads of the first three fingers, palpate each quadrant of each breast in a systematic method as the breast tissue is gently compressed against the chest wall (Fig. 25-42). The breast tissue should be smooth and firm, with a granular consistency. If a mass is detected, carefully assess its location, size, shape, consistency, and tenderness. The breasts are normally tender during the week before menstruation.

Palpate the axillary areas for lymph nodes (Fig. 25-43), which normally are nonpalpable and nontender. If any nodes are palpable, assess their location, size, shape, consistency, tenderness, and mobility.

Abnormal findings include the presence of a lump, dimpling, nipple discharge, lesions, asymmetry, and palpable lymph nodes. An increase in the nodularity and tenderness of the breasts may be associated with the menstrual period or may indicate fibrocystic disease. Discharge, lumps, lesions,

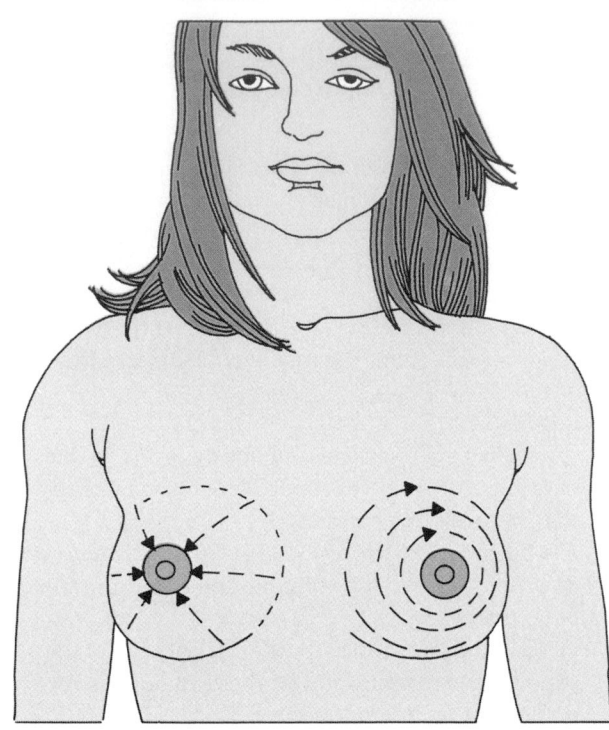

FIGURE 25-42 Two techniques for palpating the breast. (*Left*) Working in a clockwise direction, the examiner palpates the breast from the periphery toward the areola at "hour" positions. (*Right*) The breast is palpated from the outer periphery in smaller and smaller circles moving toward the areola.

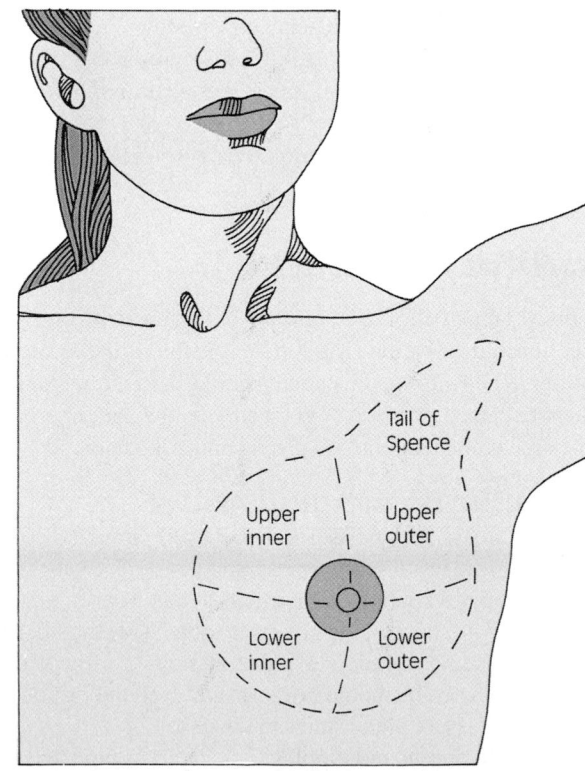

FIGURE 25-41 Location of assessment findings of the breast are identified by quadrant.

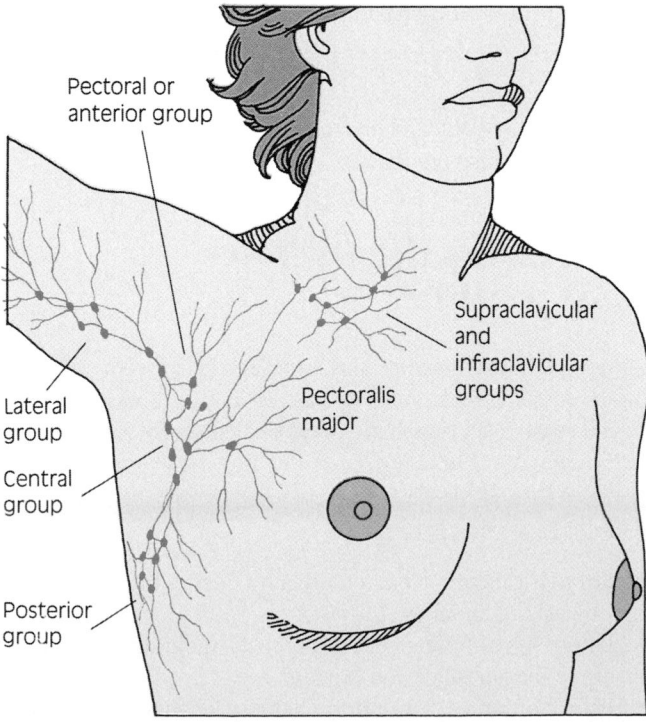

FIGURE 25-43 Location of the cervical, axillary, and mammary lymph nodes.

dimpling, asymmetry, and palpable lymph nodes may be indicative of breast cancer.

Normal Age-Related Variations
Infant/Child
Common breast and axillae variations in newborns and children include:
- Breast enlargement and a white discharge from the nipples (up to 2 weeks of age)
- Female breast growth beginning at 10 or 11 years of age
- Temporary enlargement of one or both breasts (gynecomastia) in pubescent boys

Older Adult
Common breast and axillae variations in older adults include:
- Granular, pendulous breasts

Assessing the Abdomen

The abdominal cavity (Fig. 25-44) contains several vital organs: the stomach, the small intestine, the large intestine, the liver, the gallbladder, the pancreas, the spleen, the kidneys, and the urinary bladder. Not all of these organs can be assessed. The abdominal cavity also contains the female reproductive organs, discussed in the following section.

Health History

Identify risk factors for altered health during the health history by asking about the following:
- History of abdominal pain
- History of indigestion, nausea or vomiting, constipation or diarrhea
- History of food allergies or lactose intolerance
- Appetite and usual food and fluid intake
- Usual bowel and bladder elimination patterns
- History of gastrointestinal disorders, such as peptic ulcer, bowel disease, gallbladder disease, liver disease, or appendicitis
- History of urinary tract disorders, such as infections, kidney stones, or kidney disease
- History of abdominal surgery
- Type and amount of prescribed and over-the-counter medications used
- History of abdominal surgery or trauma
- For women, menstrual history

Physical Assessment

A warm stethoscope, adequate lighting, and warm hands with short fingernails are needed to assess the abdomen. The

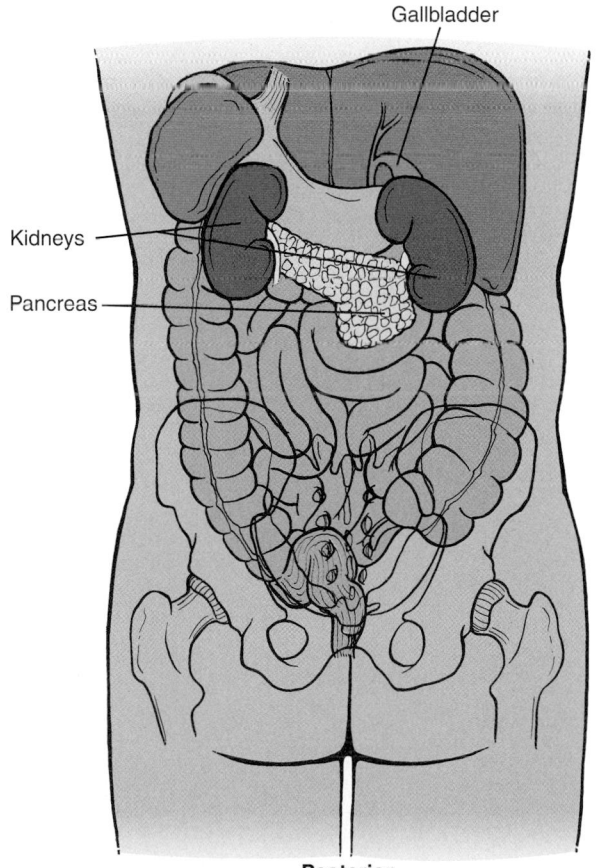

Liver
Stomach
Spleen
Transverse colon
Descending colon
Small intestine
Sigmoid colon
Cecum
Bladder
Ascending colon
Appendix
Anterior

Gallbladder
Kidneys
Pancreas
Posterior

FIGURE 25-44 Organs of the abdominal cavity.

patient lies supine with the head slightly elevated and arms at the sides. Small pillows may be placed under the head and knees. The patient should have an empty bladder and should be warm. These measures, as well as the position, help prevent contraction of the abdominal muscles, which makes palpation difficult.

To locate organs more easily and to make documentation more specific, the abdomen can be divided into four quadrants: right upper, right lower, left upper, and left lower (Fig. 25-45). The sequence of techniques used to assess the abdomen is inspection, auscultation, percussion, and palpation. Percussion and palpation stimulate bowel sounds and thus are done after auscultation of the abdomen.

Inspect the Abdomen

Sit at the side of the patient: a tangential view enhances shadows and contours. Inspect skin color and surface characteristics, including the umbilicus, contour, symmetry, peristalsis, pulsations, and masses. The skin color may be slightly lighter than exposed areas. Fine white or silver lines (striae) may be visible, often the result of skin stretching from weight gain or pregnancy. The umbilicus should be centrally located and may be flat, rounded, or concave. The abdomen should be evenly rounded or symmetric, without visible peristalsis. In

thin people, an upper midline pulsation may be visible (this is normal).

Auscultate Bowel Sounds and Vascular Sounds

Auscultation is used to assess bowel sounds and vascular sounds. Auscultation is performed in a systematic manner, using the four quadrants as a guide. The stethoscope is warmed, and the flat diaphragm is placed lightly on the abdomen in one of the selected quadrants. Listen carefully for bowel sounds, and note their frequency and character. They are heard as clicks and gurgles and usually occur every 5 to 20 seconds. Move the stethoscope in a clockwise manner, assessing all four quadrants systematically. Using the bell of the stethoscope, auscultate over the aorta, renal arteries, and iliac arteries for bruits.

Abnormal findings include increased bowel sounds (often heard when the patient has diarrhea or in early bowel obstruction), decreased bowel sounds (heard after abdominal surgery or late bowel obstruction), or absent bowel sounds (indicating peritonitis or paralytic ileus). Bowel sounds of high-pitched tinkling or rushes of high-pitched sounds indicate a bowel obstruction. A bruit is another abnormal sound that may be heard on auscultation. Bruits are low-pitched, murmur-like sounds that occur when blood flow in an artery is obstructed. These

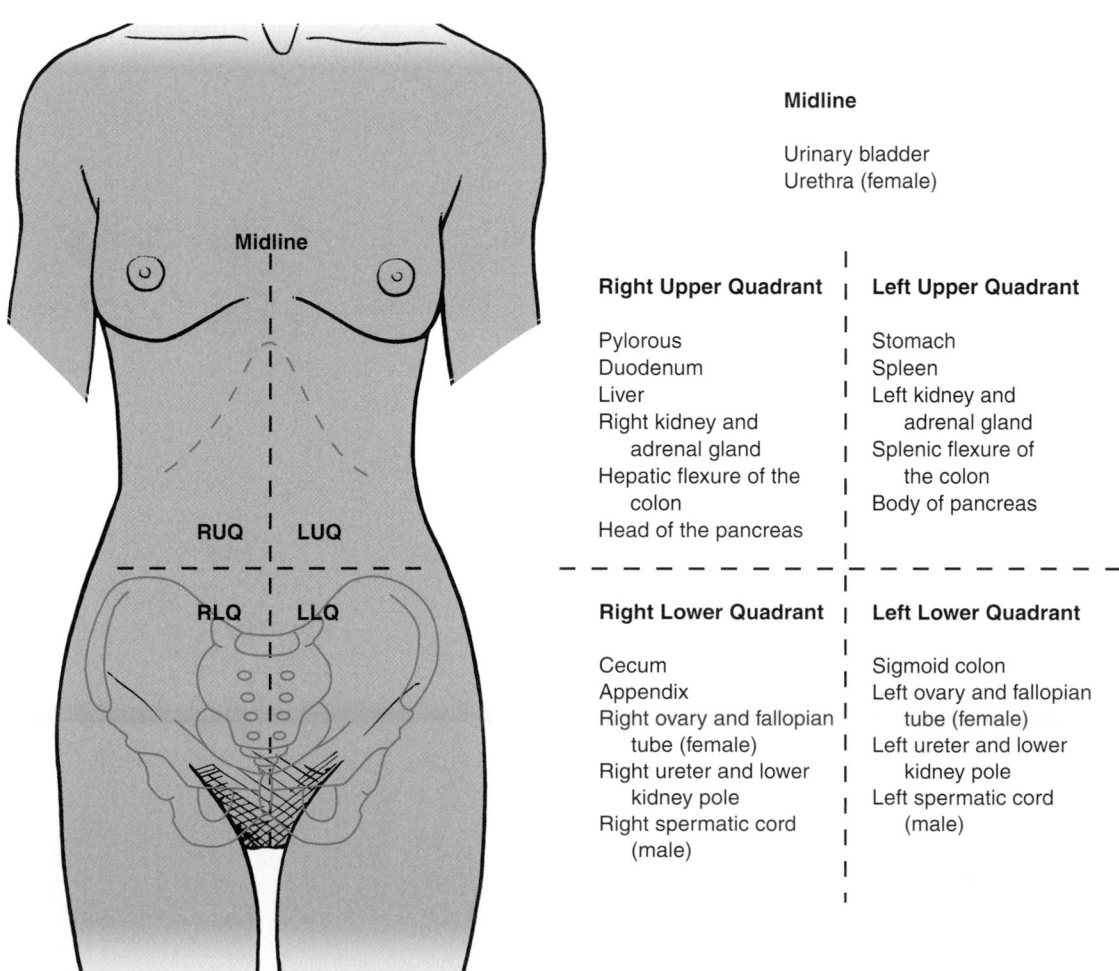

FIGURE 25-45 Diagram of abdominal quadrants and outline of underlying organs.

sounds may be heard if an aneurysm or stenosis is present in an abdominal artery. Report changes in or absence of bowel sounds.

Percuss the Abdomen

Percussion is useful in assessing a full bladder or changes in abdominal contents. All four quadrants are percussed in a systematic, clockwise manner to identify fluid, masses, or air. Note the distribution of sounds. Normal sounds are tympany over the abdomen and dullness over the liver and a full bladder. The dominant percussion note in abdominal assessment is tympany. Abnormal findings include decreased tympany and increased dullness, possibly caused by fluid or a mass.

Palpate the Abdomen

Use the pads of the fingers to palpate with a light, gentle, dipping motion. Watch the patient's face for nonverbal signs of pain during palpation. Palpate each quadrant in a systematic manner, noting muscular resistance, tenderness, enlargement of the organs, or masses. If the patient complains of abdominal pain, palpate the area of pain last. The abdomen should normally be soft, relaxed, and free of tenderness. Abnormal findings include involuntary rigidity, spasm, and pain (which may indicate trauma, peritonitis, infection, tumors, or enlarged or diseased abdominal organs).

Normal Age-Related Variations
Infant/Child

Common abdominal variations in newborns and children include:

- Umbilical cord in newborns; dries and falls off within the first few weeks of life
- A "pot-belly" (under 5 years of age)
- Visible peristaltic waves
- Easily palpated liver and spleen

Older Adult

Common abdominal variations in older adults include:

- Decreased bowel sounds
- Decreased abdominal tone
- Liver border palpated more easily

Assessing Female and Male Genitalia

The external female genitalia consist of the mons pubis, labia majora and minora, clitoris, vestibular glands, vaginal vestibule, vaginal orifice, and urethral opening (Fig. 25-46). The male genitalia (Fig. 25-47) include the penis, testicles, epididymis, scrotum, prostate gland, and seminal vesicles. The female and male rectum and anus may be assessed during part of this examination if a total health assessment is being performed.

Health History

Identify risk factors for altered female health during the health history by asking about the following:

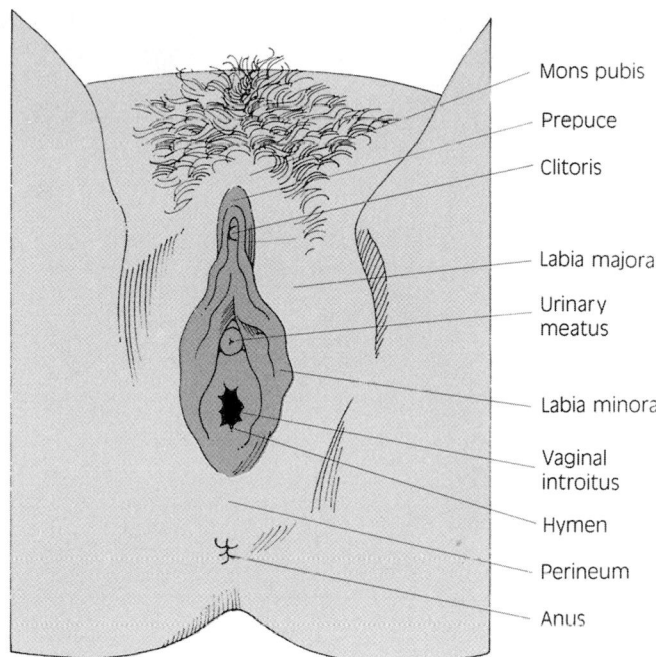

FIGURE 25-46 External female genitalia.

Labels: Mons pubis, Prepuce, Clitoris, Labia majora, Urinary meatus, Labia minora, Vaginal introitus, Hymen, Perineum, Anus

- Menstrual history (age of first or last period, length of flow, type of flow, pain)
- Sexual history
- Number of pregnancies
- History of sexually transmitted diseases
- Use of contraceptives
- Frequency of pelvic examinations and Pap smears
- History of vaginal discharge, itching, or pain on urination
- History of smoking
- Family history of reproductive or genital cancer

> Recall Ramona Lewis, the college student who reported that she was raped. As part of the focused assessment, the nurse would need to obtain a reproductive health history to provide a baseline for the patient's plan of care.

Identify risk factors for altered male health during the health history by asking about the following:

- Frequency of digital rectal examinations
- Frequency of testicular self-examination
- Use of contraceptives
- Occupational exposure to chemicals (tire and rubber manufacturing, farming, mechanics)
- History of sexually transmitted disease
- History of discharge from the penis
- Difficulty with urination (hesitancy, frequency, voiding at night)
- History of incontinence
- History of erectile dysfunction

Physical Assessment

The genitalia are assessed by inspection and palpation. A description of an internal pelvic assessment of women is included

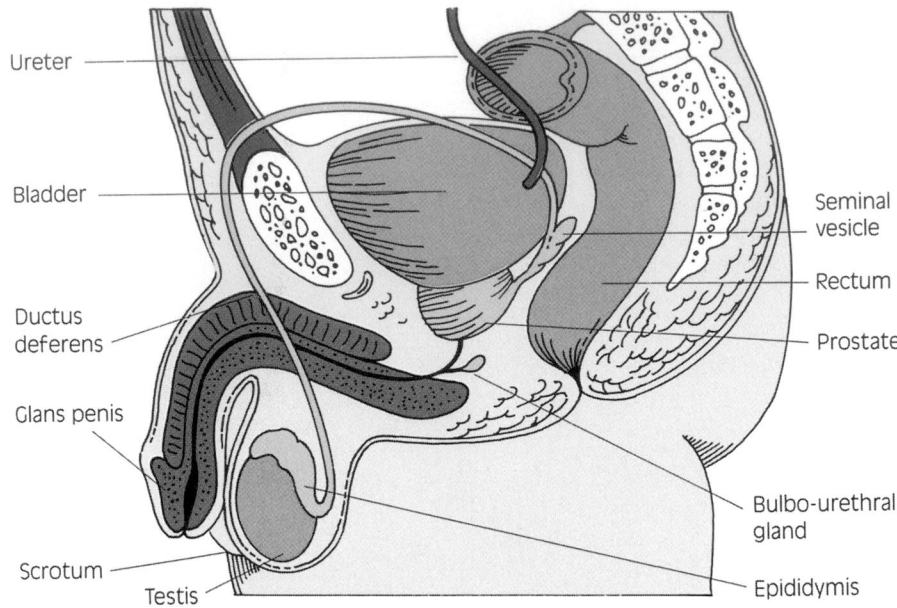

Ureter

Bladder

Ductus
deferens

Glans penis

Scrotum

Testis

Seminal
vesicle

Rectum

Prostate

Bulbo-urethral
gland

Epididymis

FIGURE 25-47 Organs of the male urogenital system.

in this chapter, although individual health agency policies vary on whether this is included as part of the health assessment. This is an advanced assessment technique, but nurses often assist in performing vaginal examinations and need to be familiar with the procedure. In many instances, male healthcare providers will ask that a female be present in the room as a chaperone during the examination. Equipment required includes a vaginal speculum (for the female examination), a good light source, and disposable gloves.

Inspect and Palpate the Female Genitalia

The bladder should be emptied before the examination. The woman is placed in the lithotomy position on the examination table, with the legs in stirrups, and draped so that only the genitalia are exposed. Explain the procedure to her and help her to relax as it is carried out. Gloves are worn during this assessment.

The external genitalia are inspected first. Inspect the pubic area for color, size, lesions, and discharge. The vulva normally has more pigmentation than other skin areas, and the mucous membranes are dark pink and moist. The skin and mucosa should be smooth, without lesions or swelling. There may be a small amount of clear or whitish vaginal discharge (this is normal). Guidelines for Nursing Care 25-7 lists the sequence of an internal vaginal examination with a speculum.

Think back to Ramona Lewis, the college student who arrived at the emergency department reporting that she was a victim of date rape. Examination of her external and internal genitalia is required to collect evidence indicating rape. The nurse would need to keep in mind the agency's policy and local and state legal requirements related to collection of rape evidence.

Abnormal findings include redness, swelling of glands, discharge, lesions, and pain, which may indicate infection, an abscess, a polyp, or cancer. For related assessments of the urinary tract and sexually transmitted diseases, see Chapters 43 and 35.

Guidelines for Nursing Care 25-7
Vaginal Examination

- Explain the procedure to the patient.
- Warm the speculum under warm running water; if cytologic specimens are to be taken, the water serves as the lubricant; if no specimens are needed, a water-soluble lubricant may be used.
- Don gloves.
- Using two fingers placed just inside the vagina, press down gently on the posterior vaginal wall.
- Insert the speculum blades vertically into the vagina, the posterior portion pointed at a 45-degree angle. Ensure that no pubic hair is caught in the speculum.
- Turn the speculum so that the handle is down and the blades are in a horizontal position.
- Open the blades and close the screw that locks the blades open.
- Inspect the cervix and os for size, color, shape, lesions, and discharge.
- Obtain specimens if needed.
- Withdraw the blades slowly, observing the vaginal walls.
- When the speculum blades are clear of the cervix, release the screw so that the blades close, and withdraw the speculum from the vagina.
- Provide the patient with tissues to remove the lubricating jelly (if used).

Inspect and Palpate the Male Genitalia

The patient may be standing or supine. Gloves are worn during this assessment. Inspect the external genitalia for size, placement, contour, appearance of the skin, redness, edema, and discharge. If the patient is uncircumcised, retract the foreskin for inspection of the glans penis. Assess the location of the urinary meatus. Inspect the scrotum for symmetry; it is not unusual for the left testicle to lie lower in the scrotal sac than the right testicle. The size, shape, and consistency of the scrotal contents should be similar bilaterally.

Abnormal findings are lesions, redness, edema, pain, discharge, fluid-filled masses in the scrotum (symptoms of a hydrocele or varicocele), and displacement of the urinary meatus or difficulties with voiding. Edema, redness, discharge, or pain may indicate an infection. Voiding difficulties may result from scarring due to infections or prostate enlargement. (See Chaps. 43 and 35 for further discussion of the male urinary tract and sexually transmitted diseases.)

Inspect and Palpate the Rectum and Anus

The rectum and anus are not assessed in all patients, but this is a part of a total health assessment. Techniques used to assess the rectum and anus include inspection and palpation. Necessary equipment includes lubricant and good lighting. Gloves are worn. The patient may be in the Sims', knee-chest, or lithotomy position or may be standing and leaning over the examination table.

Inspection is used to assess the anal area, which normally has increased pigmentation and some hair growth. Palpation is used to assess the rectum, using a well-lubricated, gloved index finger. Sphincter tone at the anus should be firm and the mucosal lining smooth. (Fecal specimens may be taken at this time, if necessary.) Abnormal findings include relaxed sphincter tone; skin cracks, nodules, or hemorrhoids at the anal sphincter; bleeding (which may indicate hemorrhoids or colorectal cancer); and hard or abnormally colored (such as clay-colored or dark-black) stools.

If a rectal assessment is conducted, the cervix in women may be felt as a small, round mass when palpating the anterior rectal wall. Abnormal findings include changes in consistency. The prostate gland in men can be assessed for size, shape, and consistency by palpation through the anterior rectal wall; the gland is normally smooth, firm, and about 1¾″ (4 cm) in size. Abnormal findings include enlargement or changes in consistency (which occur in benign prostatic enlargement or cancer).

Normal Age-Related Variations
Infant/Child
Common genitalia variations in newborns and children include:
- Enlarged labia and clitoris at birth

Older Adult
Common genitalia variations in older adults include:
- Decreased labia size
- Decreased vaginal secretions
- Shortened vaginal vault
- Decreased penis size
- Decreased pubic hair

Assessing the Musculoskeletal System

The primary structures of the musculoskeletal system are the bones, muscles, cartilage, ligaments, tendons, and joints. The muscles, bones, and joints are assessed.

Health History

Identify risk factors for altered health during the health history by asking about the following:
- History of trauma, arthritis, or neurologic disorder
- History of pain or swelling in the joints
- History of pain in the bones, muscles, or joints
- Frequency and type of usual exercise
- Dietary intake of calcium
- History of smoking
- History of alcohol intake
- Use of hormone replacement therapy in women

Physical Assessment

The patient assumes a variety of positions, including standing, sitting, and supine. Assessments of the musculoskeletal system can be integrated into the assessment of other body systems.

Inspect and Palpate the Muscles
Examine the muscles by inspection and palpation of muscle groups and by testing muscle tone and strength. Muscle groups are observed for bilateral symmetry and palpated for tenderness. Normally, they are symmetric and nontender. Evaluate muscle tone (the normal condition of a muscle at rest) by putting each joint and extremity through passive range of motion. Bilateral equal resistance should be present. Assess muscle strength by asking the patient to move against resistance. Observe muscle contraction and determine muscle strength exerted. An individual's dominant side is normally stronger than the nondominant side. Techniques for testing muscle strength are illustrated in Figure 25-48. Muscle strength should be bilaterally equal, with a slight increase on the dominant side.

Abnormal findings include atrophy (a decrease in size), tremors (involuntary movements), and flaccidity (weakness) of muscles. Other abnormal findings are loss of strength and tone, decreased range of motion, uncoordinated movements, swelling, and pain. Abnormal findings may indicate a musculoskeletal disease, trauma, or a neurologic disease.

Palpate the Bones
Palpate bones for normal contour and prominence as well as for bilateral symmetry. Abnormal findings include pain, enlargement, asymmetry, and changes in contour. Abnormal findings may indicate trauma, degenerative joint disease, musculoskeletal disease, or a neurologic disease.

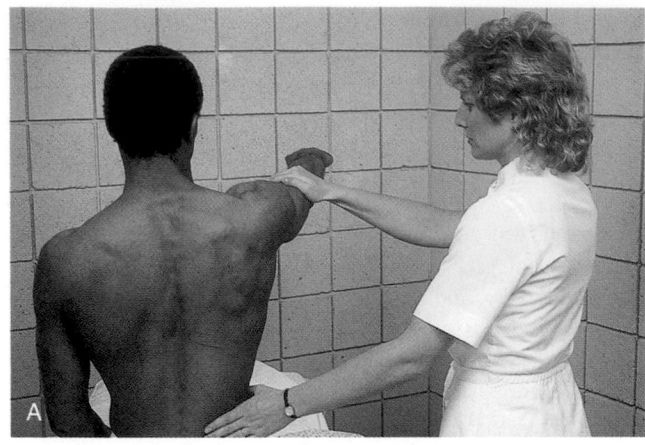

The patient flexes shoulder muscle against resistance of examiner's hand.

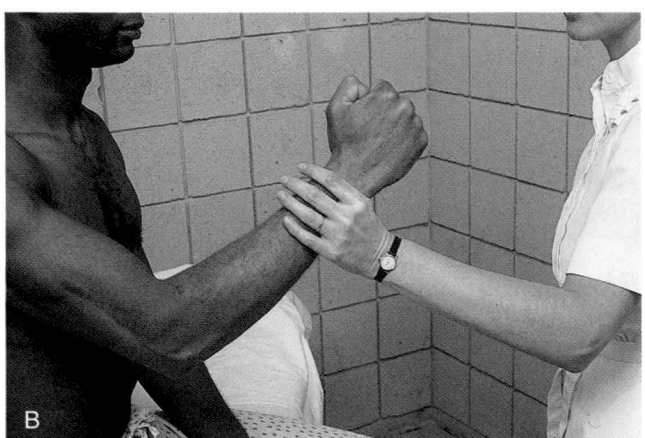

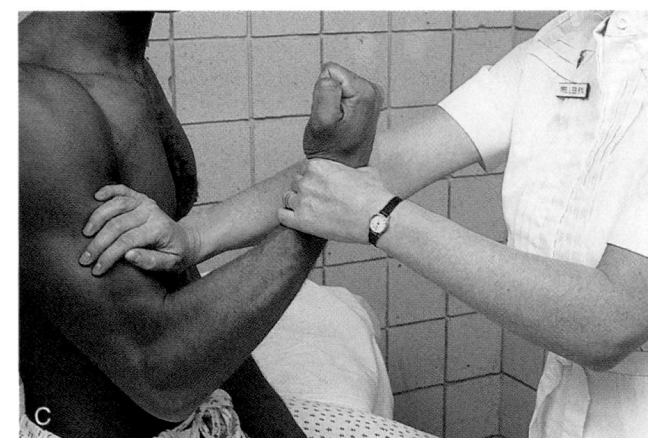

Elbow extension and flexion. The patient first extends elbow against resistance by the examiner, then flexes elbow against resistance.

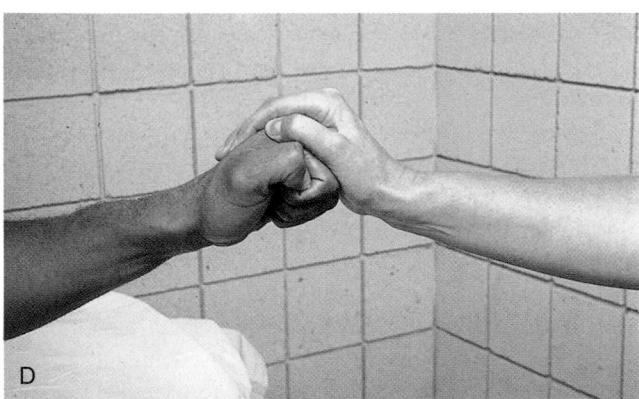

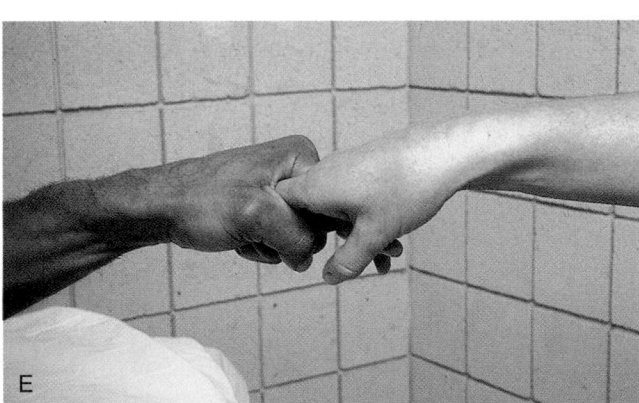

Wrist extension. The patient makes a fist and resists the examiner's attempts to pull wrist down.

Testing grip. Patient squeezes examiner's index and middle fingers.

FIGURE 25-48 Techniques for testing muscle strength.   (Photos © Ken Kasper.)

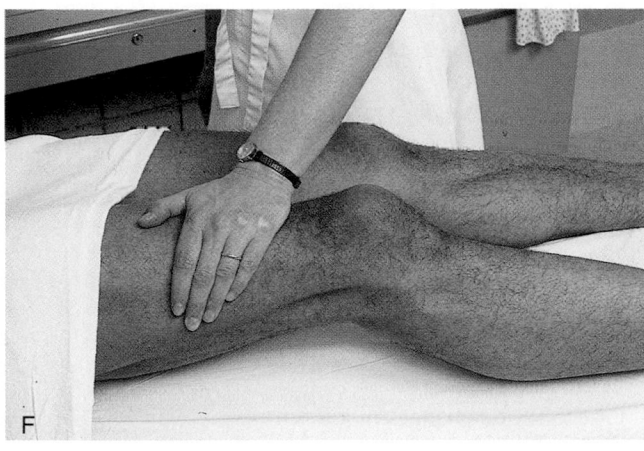

Hip flexion. Patient attempts to raise his thigh against examiner's resistance.

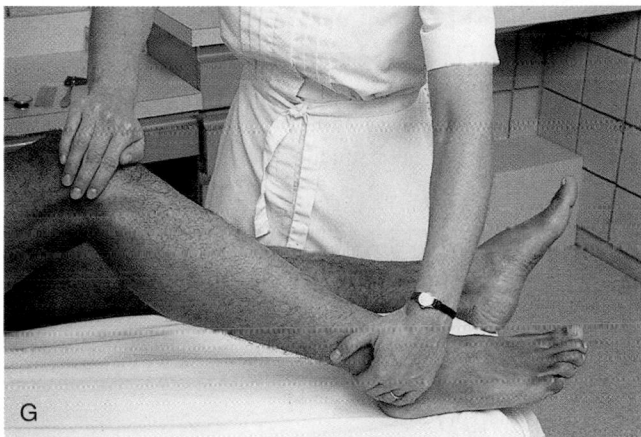

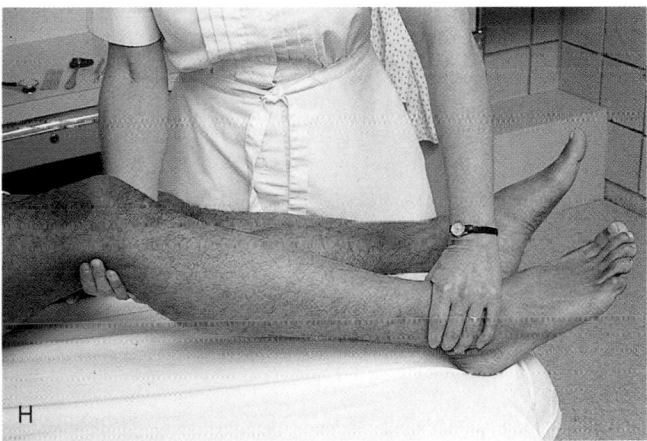

Knee flexion and extension. With the patient's knee bent and foot on the examining table, the patient attempts to keep foot down while examiner attempts to straighten the patient's leg to test flexion. To test extension, the examiner supports patient's knee, and the patient attempts to straighten his leg against examiner resistance at the ankle.

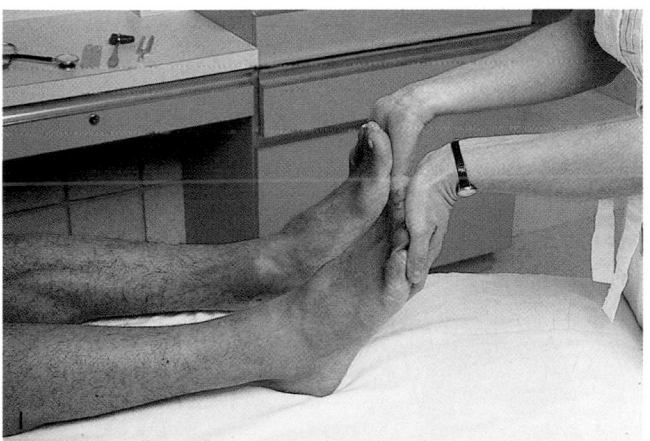

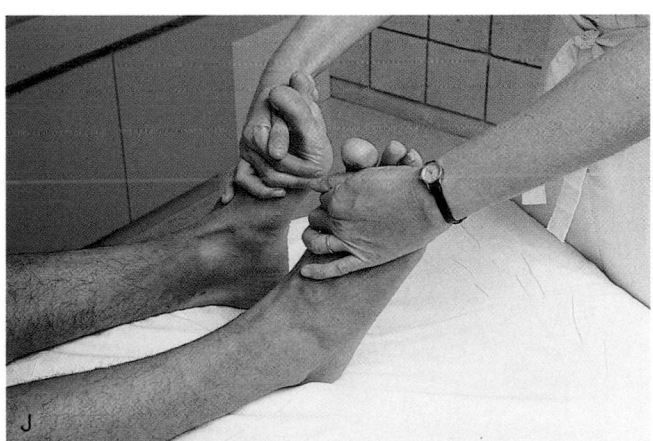

Ankle plantar flexion and dorsiflexion. The patient first pushes the balls of the feet against resistance of examiner's hands, then attempts to pull against examiner's resistance.

FIGURE 25-48 *Continued*

Inspect and Palpate the Joints

Each joint is put through its full range of motion to assess the degree of movement. Joint movements include flexion, extension, hyperextension, abduction, adduction, supination, and pronation. Normally, each joint has full range of motion, is nontender, and moves smoothly. Palpate joints for the abnormal findings of pain, swelling, nodules, and crepitation (a grating sound heard or felt on movement). See Chapter 39 for further discussion and illustration of joint mobility.

Inspect Spinal Curves

With the patient standing, inspect the spine from the back and from the side. The lumbar curve may be flattened with a herniated disk. Kyphosis (an increased thoracic spinal curve) is more often seen in older adults. An exaggerated lumbar curve (lordosis) is often seen during pregnancy or in obesity. Scoliosis is a lateral curvature of the spine with increased convexity on the side that is curved. School nurses often first identify scoliosis during screenings, which are recommended for girls in grades 5 and 7 and for boys in grades 8 or 9 (American Academy of Orthopedic Surgeons, 2001). Findings indicating scoliosis are illustrated in Figure 25-49.

Normal Age-Related Variations
Infant/Child

Common musculoskeletal variations in newborns and children include:

- C-shaped curve of spine at birth; the anterior cervical curve develops at about 3 to 4 months of age, and the anterior lumbar curve develops between 12 and 18 months of age
- Lordosis (an exaggerated lumbar curve)
- Pronation of the feet in children between 12 and 30 months of age
- Genu varum (bowleg) for 1 year after learning to walk

Older Adult

Common musculoskeletal variations seen in older adults include:

- Loss of muscle mass and strength
- Decreased range of motion
- Kyphosis
- Decreased height
- Osteoarthritic changes in joints

Assessing the Neurologic System

Neurologic assessment includes cerebral function, cranial nerve function, cerebellar function, motor and sensory function, and reflexes.

Health History

Identify risk factors for altered health during the health history by asking about the following:

- History of numbness, tingling, or tremors
- History of seizures
- History of headaches
- History of dizziness

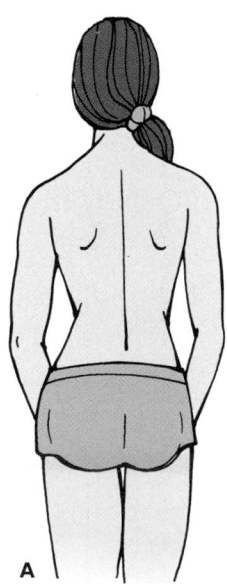 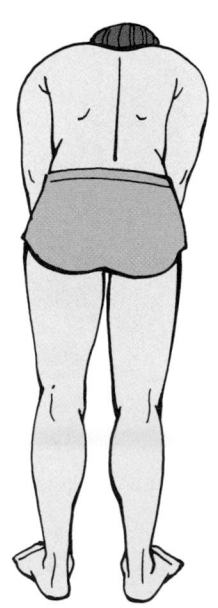 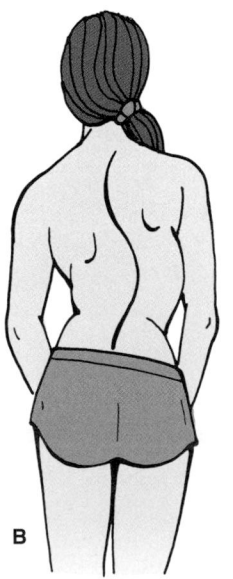 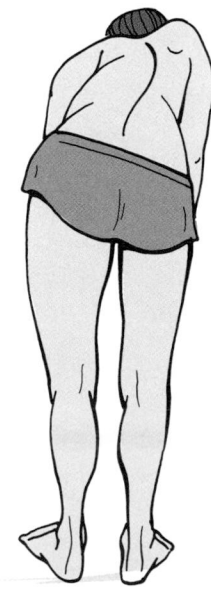

Is the head level and centered over the trunk? | Are the shoulders the same height? | Are the hips at the same level? | When bent forward with arms dropping towards feet, is rib cage level on both sides?

FIGURE 25-49 Screening for scoliosis. (**A**) Normal position and spinal curves. (**B**) Scoliosis indicators.

- History of trauma to the head or spine
- History of infections of the brain
- History of stroke
- Changes in the ability to hear, see, taste, or smell
- Loss of ability to control bladder and bowel
- History of high blood pressure
- History of smoking
- History of chronic alcohol use
- History of diabetes mellitus or heart disease
- Use of prescription and over-the-counter medications
- Family history of high blood pressure, Alzheimer's disease, epilepsy, cancer, or Huntington's chorea
- Frequency of blood cholesterol tests and results
- Exposure to environmental hazards (eg, lead, insecticides)

Physical Assessment

Assess cerebral function by observing the patient's behavior throughout the interview and physical assessment. Assess the patient's mental status, memory, emotional status, cognitive abilities, and behavior. Evaluate cerebellar function by assessing fine motor skills, coordination, and balance. Assess the sensory system by having the patient identify various sensory stimuli, and evaluate the reflexes by contraction of specific muscles.

Equipment includes vials of aromatic substances (eg, peppermint and vanilla), a visual acuity chart, a penlight, a sharp object (eg, a large safety pin), cotton balls, vials of solution to test taste (eg, salt or sugar), a tuning fork, a tongue depressor, a reflex hammer, and familiar objects such as a key or coin. The patient should be sitting, and the environment should be quiet.

Assess Mental Status

Mental status assessment includes level of awareness, level of consciousness, behavior and appearance, memory, abstract reasoning, and language. On initial contact, begin to evaluate the patient's orientation to person, place, and time as well as his or her cognitive abilities and affect (whether the patient knows who he or she is, where he or she is, and the day or month or year). Observe the patient's appearance, general behavior, and responses to questions. Note any variation in responses. Also assess the patient's ability to speak clearly.

The patient should have a clean, neat appearance with erect posture; should be oriented to person, place, and time; should have memory recall (both short-term and long-term memory); and should be able to demonstrate coherent and logical thought processes. Abnormal findings include poor hygiene, inappropriate dress, disorientation, absent memory recall, and incoherent or illogical thought processes. These abnormal findings may indicate a mental health disorder, mental retardation, organic brain disease, cerebrovascular disorder, alcohol or drug intoxication, or a tumor.

Think back to Tammy Browning, the pregnant woman with a history of substance abuse. The nurse would assess the patient's mental status for clues suggesting recent drug use, incorporating knowledge of abnormal findings into the assessment.

The following discussion of each of the mental status components includes sample questions or specific assessments to use during the assessment.

Level of Awareness

Evaluate orientation to time, place, and person to assess level of awareness. The following questions may be used:
- *Time*: What is today's date? What day of the week is it? What season of the year is this? What was the last holiday?
- *Place*: Where are you now? What is the name of this city? What state are we in?
- *Person*: What is your name? How old are you? Who came to visit you this morning?

Although exceptions may occur, individuals who have impaired awareness first lose time orientation, followed by place orientation, and then person orientation. Remember that it is often difficult to know the exact date when one is ill, in pain, or in unfamiliar surroundings.

Level of Consciousness

Consciousness is the degree of wakefulness or the ability of a person to be aroused. This is not the same as orientation; a patient may be conscious but not oriented. Level of consciousness is described as follows:
- Awake and alert: fully awake; oriented to person, place, and time; responds to all stimuli, including verbal commands
- Lethargic: appears drowsy or asleep most of the time but makes spontaneous movements; can be aroused by gentle shaking and saying patient's name
- Stuporous: unconscious most of the time; has no spontaneous movement; must be shaken or shouted at to arouse; can make verbal responses, but these are less likely to be appropriate; responds to painful stimuli with purposeful movements
- Comatose: cannot be aroused, even with use of painful stimuli; may have some reflex activity (such as gag reflex); if no reflexes present, is in a deep coma

The Glasgow Coma Scale (Table 25-9) is a standardized assessment tool that assesses level of consciousness. Three parameters are evaluated: eye opening, motor response, and verbal response. Scores are given in each category, and a total score is recorded, with higher scores indicating a more normal level of functioning. A score of 7 or less defines coma. This is a more accurate evaluation of mental status over time.

Memory

Assess memory by asking questions that call for answers demonstrating immediate recall and recall for past events. To

TABLE 25-9 Glasgow Coma Scale

Component	Response	Score
Eye opening	Spontaneous	4
	To verbal command	3
	To pain	2
	No response	1
Motor response	To verbal command	6
	To localized pain	5
	Flexes/withdraws	4
	Flexes abnormally	3
	Extends abnormally	2
	No response	1
Verbal response	Oriented/talks	5
	Disoriented/talks	4
	Inappropriate words	3
	Incomprehensible sounds	2
	No response	1

assess immediate memory, ask the patient to repeat a series of numbers forward or backward (eg, 3, 6, 9). Start with three numbers and gradually increase the digits until the patient cannot respond correctly. Most adults can repeat a series of five to eight numbers forward and four to six digits backward. You might also ask, "What did you eat for breakfast this morning?" To assess past memory, ask, "When is your birthday?" or "When is your wedding anniversary?"

Abstract Reasoning
Ask the patient to explain a proverb such as "the early bird catches the worm." If intellectual ability is impaired, the patient usually gives a literal explanation or repeats the phrase. Be sure that the phrase is not culture specific.

Language
The cerebral cortex controls the ability to express self through writing, words, or gestures and to understand the spoken and written word. Injury to the cortex can cause aphasia, which is a disorder of language ability. Aphasia may be expressive (the individual understands written and spoken words but cannot write or speak to communicate effectively) or receptive (the individual cannot understand written or spoken words). These aphasias may also be combined. Some simple methods of assessing language capabilities include asking the patient to name items in the room (eg, bed, flowers, gown, pajamas), to follow simple commands, such as "Point to your head," to read a short sentence aloud, or to match printed and spoken words with appropriate pictures.

Assess Cranial Nerve Function
The function of the 12 cranial nerves is assessed primarily during the neurologic assessment, although parts of cranial nerve function are assessed with other body systems (eg, pupillary response). The cranial nerves, with their function

and assessment methods, are outlined in Table 25-10. Each nerve has a specific function and is evaluated individually.

Assess Motor and Sensory Function
Evaluate motor ability by assessing balance, gait, and coordination. Assess sensory function by testing sensory discrimination of pain, light touch, and vibrations.

Balance and Gait
Evaluate balance and gait by having the patient walk across the room on the toes, on the heels, and heel to toe. Observe posture, balance, and arm and leg movements. The posture should be erect, with slight swaying in the standing position, and the gait even with simultaneous arm movements. Abnormal findings include loss of balance, shuffling, wide-based gait, and abnormal patterns of gait.

Motor Function and Coordination
Evaluate motor function and coordination by having the patient rapidly touch each finger with the thumb, rapidly pat the hand on the thigh, and tap the foot on the floor (or against your hand, if the patient is supine). Normally, the movements are coordinated.

Sensory Function
Test sensory perception by evaluating the patient's response to pain, light touch, and vibration. With the patient's eyes closed, use a sharp object and a soft object randomly to touch the upper and lower extremities to test sensation. The assessment proceeds from distal (hands, arms, feet, or legs) to proximal (the trunk). The patient should be able to distinguish between sharp (pain) and soft or dull touch. The same process is repeated by using the tuning fork to test for vibratory sensation and placing the fork on bony prominences. Abnormal findings include inability to perceive pain or light touch, inability to identify the location of touch, and absence of vibratory sensation.

Assess Reflex Function
Evaluate the deep tendon reflexes to determine the functional ability of specific spinal segment levels. Use the reflex hammer to elicit muscle contraction and reflexes. The patient may be either sitting or supine. Selected reflexes, with normal responses and methods of assessment, are illustrated in Table 25-11. They are usually graded on a scale of 0 to 4, as listed in Table 25-12. A grade of 2 is considered a normal or active response.

Normal Age-Related Variations
Infant/Child
Common neurologic variations for newborns and children include:
- Positive Babinski's reflex (normal in children between 12 and 24 months)
- Grasp reflex (present at birth)
- Motor control develops in head, neck, trunk, and extremities sequence

TABLE 25-10 Summary of Cranial Nerves

Nerve (Number)	Type	Functions	Methods for Examining Nerve
Olfactory (I)	Sensory	Sense of smell	Test each nostril for smell reception and interpretation.
Optic (II)	Sensory	Sense of vision	Test vision for acuity and visual fields.
Oculomotor (III)	Motor	Pupil constriction Raise eyelids	Test pupillary reaction to light and ability to open and close eyelids.
Trochlear (IV)	Motor/ Proprioceptor	Downward inward eye movement	Test for downward and inward movement of the eye.
Trigeminal (V)	Motor	Jaw movements—chewing and mastication	Ask patient to open and clench jaws while you palpate the jaw muscles.
	Sensory	Sensation on the face and neck	Test face and neck for pain sensations, light touch, temperature.
Abducens (VI)	Motor	Lateral movement of the eyes	Test ocular movement in all directions.
Facial (VII)	Motor	Muscles of the face	Ask the patient to raise eyebrows, smile, show teeth, puff out cheeks.
	Sensory	Sense of taste on the anterior two thirds of the tongue	Test for the taste sensation with various agents.
Acoustic (VIII)	Sensory	Sense of hearing	Test hearing ability.
Glossopharyngeal (IX)	Motor	Pharyngeal movement and swallowing	Ask the patient to say "ah," and have patient yawn to observe upward movement of the soft palate; elicit gag response; note ability to swallow.
	Sensory	Sense of taste on the posterior one third of the tongue	Test for taste with various agents.
Vagus (X)	Motor/ Sensory	Swallowing and speaking	Ask the patient to swallow and speak; note hoarseness.
Accessory (XI)	Motor/ Sensory	Movement of shoulder muscles	Ask the patient to shrug shoulders against your resistance.
Hypoglossal (XII)	Motor	Movement of the tongue; strength of the tongue	Ask the patient to protrude tongue; ask patient to push tongue against cheek.

Older Adult

Common neurologic variations for older adults include:

- Slower thought processes and verbal responses
- Decreased sensory ability (hearing, sight, smell, taste, temperature, and pain)
- Slower coordination and voluntary movements
- Decreased reflex responses
- May appear confused in unfamiliar surroundings
- Gait may be slower, with a wider base and flexed hips and knees.
- Decreased deep tendon reflexes

DOCUMENTING THE DATA

After completing the nursing history and assessment, organize all assessment data to identify actual and potential health problems, make nursing diagnoses, plan appropriate care, and evaluate the patient's responses to treatment. A pattern is often established that begins during the history and is confirmed during the physical assessment. Document the data, with each system recorded individually. A documentation example is illustrated in Box 25-2.

THE NURSE'S ROLE IN DIAGNOSTIC PROCEDURES

Nurses assist before, during, and after diagnostic tests. The nurse is also responsible for other activities associated with diagnostic tests, such as witnessing the patient's consent, scheduling the test, preparing the patient physically and emotionally for the test, providing care after the test, disposing of used equipment, and transporting specimens.

Think back to Tammy Browning, the pregnant woman with a history of substance abuse. A urine specimen was to be obtained for routine testing. In addition, the specimen was to be used for drug testing without the patient's

(text continues on page 608)

TABLE 25-11 **Normal Responses of Commonly Tested Reflexes**

How to Test Reflex	Normal Response
Biceps 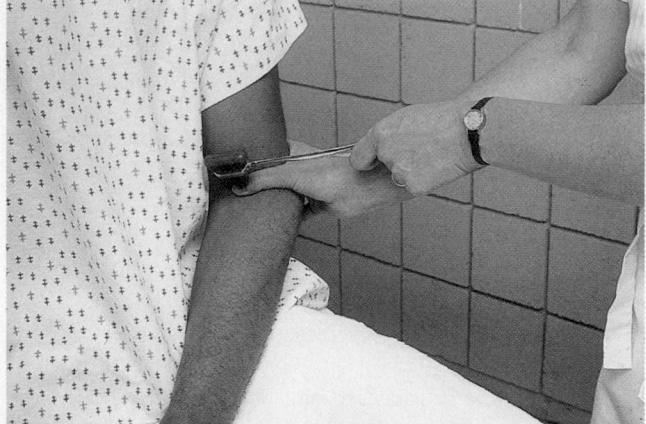	The contraction of the biceps can be seen and felt. To test the biceps reflex, the elbow is slightly bent, and the palm faces downward. The examiner's thumb is placed on the biceps tendon at the bend in the elbow. The percussion hammer strikes the examiner's thumb.
Triceps 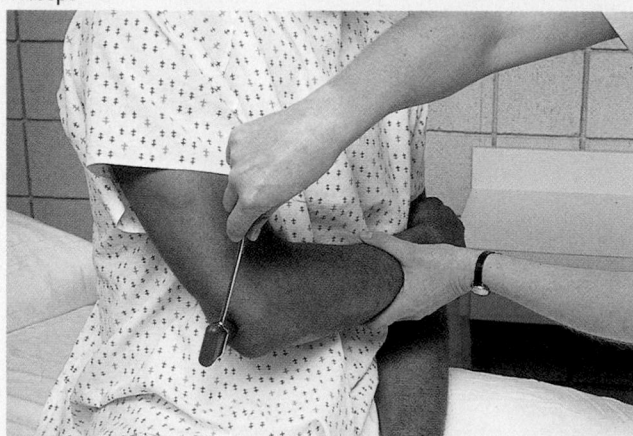	The contraction of the triceps can be seen as the elbow extends. To test the triceps reflex, the patient's elbow is sharply bent; the forearm is placed across the chest wall with the palm turned toward the body. The triceps tendon is struck with the percussion hammer just above the elbow.
Knee 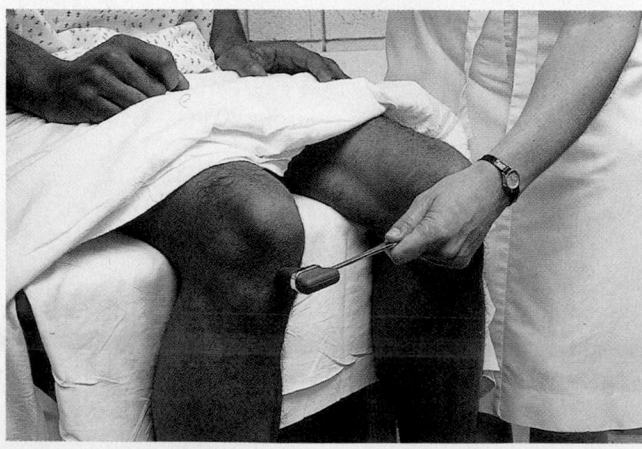	The contraction of the quadriceps causes the knee to extend. To test the knee reflex, the patient is in the sitting position. The patellar tendon just below the patella is struck with the percussion hammer. If the patient is lying down, the reflex is tested while the examiner's hands are placed under the knees to bend them.

(continued)

TABLE 25-11 (Continued)

How to Test Reflex	Normal Response

Ankle

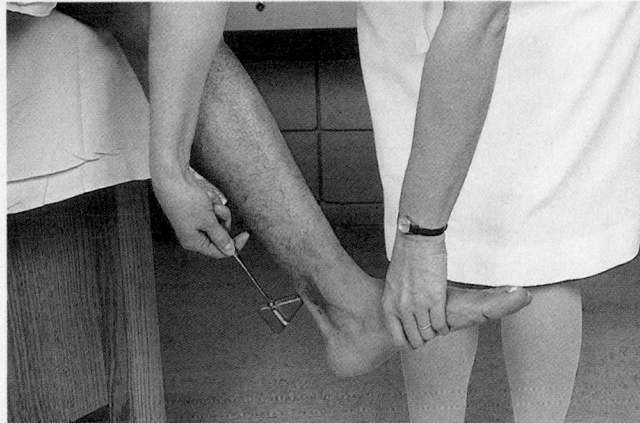

The foot jerks and moves downward.

To test the ankle reflex, the leg is bent at the knee and the foot is supported in a walking position. The Achilles tendon is struck with the percussion hammer.

Babinski

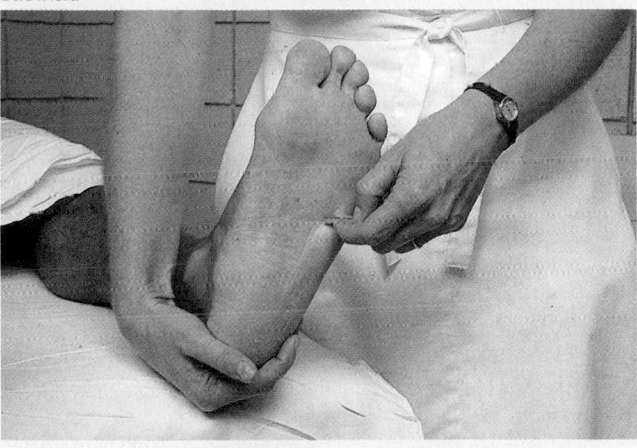

The toes bend or curl.

The lateral aspect of the sole of the foot is stroked with an object, such as a key or a thumbnail, from the heel to the ball of the foot.

Abdominal

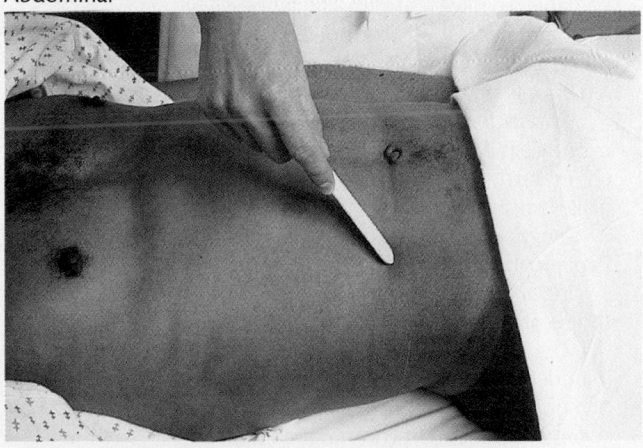

The contraction of abdominal musculature can be seen.

To test the abdominal reflex, with the patient lying on the back, each side of the abdomen is stroked from the sides toward the center with a tongue blade or key.

TABLE 25-12 Grading of Reflexes on a 0 to 4+ Scale

Grade	Description
4+	Very brisk, hyperactive; often indicative of disease; often associated with clonus (rhythmic oscillations between flexion and extension)
3+	Brisker than average; possibly but not necessarily indicative of disease
2+	Average; normal
1+	Somewhat diminished; low normal
0	No response

knowledge. Typically a signed consent form is not necessary for urine specimens. However, the nurse would need to know the agency's policy and legal statutes of the area regarding consent for drug testing before obtaining the specimen.

Diagnostic tests provide crucial information about a patient's health, and their results become a part of the total health assessment. Nurse practitioners and physicians make decisions concerning which diagnostic tests to schedule when problems are noted during the health history or physical assessment or because of a problem stated by the patient. Table 25-13 presents an overview of different types of diagnostic procedures.

BOX 25-2 Documenting a Health Assessment

Mrs. D. comes to a local community outpatient agency for her intolerance of eating fatty foods. She says, "I just started having a lot of gas and was sick to my stomach after eating fried foods." The nurse in charge of the agency makes the following assessments.

Health History

Mrs. D. is a 52-year-old woman who lives with her 54-year-old husband on a farm in a rural midwestern area. She graduated from high school and is employed as a secretary for a local insurance agency. Mrs. D. is well-groomed, alert, and oriented. She occasionally takes over-the-counter medications for constipation and colds. She takes a prescription medication twice a day for "high blood pressure." She says she has about two mixed drinks a week and does not smoke. She has had five pregnancies, resulting in five living children. She is postmenopausal (last period, 2 years ago) and takes hormone replacement therapy in a combination of estrogen and progesterone.

Mrs. D. had her tonsils removed at 5 years of age, had an appendectomy at 22 years of age, and is allergic to penicillin (causes rash and difficulty breathing). She has had all her immunizations, but her last tetanus shot was 10 years ago. Her family history of illness is as follows:

Maternal grandfather: died of heart problems at 77 years of age
Maternal grandmother, died of diabetes complications at 69 years of age
Paternal grandfather, died of stroke at 82 years of age
Paternal grandmother, died of unknown causes at 56 years of age
Sister, 49 years of age, healthy
Brother, died at 22 years of age in a car accident

Physical Assessment

Vital signs: T = 98.8°F (orally), P = 82 beats/min, R = 16 breaths/min, BP = 150/88 mm Hg
Height/weight: 5 feet, 4 inches tall, 178 pounds
Integument: Skin warm and dry, normal turgor. Numerous freckles over face and arms. Old scar, RLQ (appendectomy). Nails convex and smooth. Hair dark brown, shiny, normal distribution.
Head and neck: Skull size and shape normal. Facial features symmetric. Can raise eyebrows, close eyes, smile, puff out cheeks. External eye structures symmetric. Sclera white, con-

junctiva pink. Wears glasses to correct near-sightedness. Vision with glasses 20/30-2 on Snellen's chart. Pupils equal and react to light. Demonstrates accommodation, convergence, and peripheral vision. Lens clear. Hearing tested by use of a clock, which she heard clearly at 2 feet. External ears symmetric. Canals smooth and pink without excess cerumen. Tympanic membranes intact without redness or drainage. Right nostril clear, left nostril occluded with mucus. Left maxillary sinus slightly tender on palpation. Teeth in good repair with six fillings. Oral mucous membranes pink. Tonsils absent. Trachea midline, thyroid nonpalpable. No lymph nodes palpable.
Thorax/lungs/heart: Thorax symmetric with equal expansion. Respirations even and unlabored. Lung sounds clear. No visible pulsations noted in neck or precordium. S1 and S2 heard at pulmonic, aortic, tricuspid, and mitral areas. No extra heart sounds, murmurs, or bruits heard. Apical pulse 84 beats/min and regular.
Breasts and axilla: Skin pink. No dimpling or retraction noted. Areolae and nipples dark brown, no crusting or drainage. No masses palpated in breasts. Axillary lymph nodes are not palpable. To have mammogram at next visit.
Abdomen: Obese, rounded. Umbilicus midline. No pain on light palpation. Bowel sounds heard in all four quadrants. No bruits heard on auscultation.
Peripheral vascular: Pulses equal in both arms. Pulses equal in both legs. No edema present. Superficial varicose veins present on both lower extremities between ankle and knee. Toenails thick and yellow.
Genitalia: Will be assessed at next visit with pelvic and Papanicolaou's smear.
Rectum and anus: Inspected only. Small external hemorrhoids noted.
Musculoskeletal: Stands erect. Normal spinal curves. No joint deformities, tenderness, or crepitation. Full active range of motion in all joints. Muscle strength equal bilaterally, slightly stronger on the right (dominant side).
Neurologic: Alert and oriented to time, place, person. Facial expressions appropriate. Speech clear and appropriate. Demonstrates long-term and short-term memory. All cranial nerves tests were intact. Fine motor movements intact. Gait even. Perceives pain or light touch appropriately. All reflexes = 2.

TABLE 25-13 A Guide to Common Laboratory and Diagnostic Procedures

Procedure	Description	Examples
Aspiration procedures	Studies in which a needle or similar instrument is inserted into a body organ or cavity. Fluid or tissue is aspirated, prepared, labeled, and sent to the laboratory for examination.	Liver biopsy Lumbar puncture Paracentesis Thoracentesis
Electrical impulse procedures	Studies that use a machine with electrodes attached to the body to monitor electric activity. Electric impulses are recorded on a graph and displayed on paper or an oscilloscope screen.	Electrocardiogram (EKG) Electroencephalogram (EEG)
Endoscopic procedures	Studies that allow for direct visual examination of various body cavities and organs by means of a hollow, lighted tube called an endoscope. The tube may be flexible or rigid. May be used to obtain tissue specimens for biopsy or microscopic examination.	Bronchoscopy Colonoscopy Gastroscopy Sigmoidoscopy Laparoscopy
Laboratory procedures	Studies in which body fluids, secretions, or tissues are sent to the laboratory for analysis	Blood studies Urine studies Sputum studies Fecal studies Biopsies
Radiography procedures	Because of the ability of x-rays to penetrate human tissues, x-ray studies provide a picture of body structures that looks like a negative of a photograph.	Chest x-ray Dye-enhanced cardiac catheterization
Magnetic resonance imaging (MRI)	The computer-based procedure provides physiologic information and detailed views of fluid-filled soft tissues.	MRI of the brain, spine, extremities, joints, heart, pelvis, abdomen
Nuclear scanning	Studies that use the administration of a radionuclide and subsequent measurement of radiation from an organ to detect functional abnormalities	Brain scan Heart scan Lung scan Bone scan
Ultrasonography	Studies in which a harmless, high-frequency sound wave is emitted that penetrates the organ being studied. The sound waves bounce back to the sensor and are electronically converted into a picture of the organ or the contents of the organ.	Ultrasound of the pelvis, abdomen, heart, uterus

■ Developing Critical Thinking Skills

1. Describe how you would explain a cardiovascular assessment to the following patients:
   - A healthy 5-year-old
   - A college student who has never been ill
   - A 50-year-old man who has never had a physical assessment
   - An 85-year-old woman with heart problems
2. When you are conducting a health history, your patient gives you strange answers. Later, during the mental status assessment, she gives you the wrong answers for the date and place. She also cannot remember what medications she takes. How would you document this information? What would you do next?
3. When you make a home visit to conduct an initial health history and physical assessment, the patient refuses to let you do more than assess vital signs. What would you do?

■ Practicing for NCLEX

1. The internal structures of the eye can be visualized using which of the following instruments?
   a. Otoscope
   b. Ophthalmoscope
   c. Stethoscope
   d. Tuning fork
2. To make accurate assessments during inspection, the nurse must
   a. Compare bilateral body parts
   b. Have 20/20 vision
   c. Focus on selected body systems
   d. Use touch judiciously
3. Palpation is a physical assessment technique that uses the sense of:
   a. Intuition
   b. Vision
   c. Hearing
   d. Touch

4. When percussing over the stomach, the nurse notes a loud, drumlike sound. The term to document this percussion tone is:
   a. Dullness
   b. Flatness
   c. Tympany
   d. Resonance
5. The bell of the stethoscope is used to hear:
   a. Tympanic sounds
   b. Bowel sounds
   c. Lung sounds
   d. Heart sounds
6. Skin turgor may be assessed by which of the following techniques?
   a. Indenting with the fingertips
   b. Using special lighting
   c. Touching to detect moisture
   d. Lightly pinching a skin fold
7. Visual acuity may be assessed by using a Snellen chart. If a patient has acuity of 20/40 in both eyes, this means:
   a. The patient can see twice as well as normal
   b. The patient has double vision
   c. The patient has less than normal vision
   d. The patient has normal vision
8. When using an otoscope to assess the tympanic membrane of an adult, the ear canal is straightened by gently pulling the pinna:
   a. Up and back
   b. Down and forward
   c. Away from the examiner
   d. In any direction
9. When percussing the thorax and lungs, a dull sound indicates:
   a. An air-filled structure
   b. A bony structure
   c. Emphysematous tissue
   d. Fluid or a solid mass
10. When auscultating the thorax and lungs, coarse gurgling sounds are heard on expiration. These sounds can be broadly labeled as:
    a. Adventitious breath sounds
    b. Bronchovesicular breath sounds
    c. Vesicular breath sounds
    d. Bronchial sounds
11. Heart sounds are the result of:
    a. Blood flow through the heart
    b. Movement of blood into the heart from the aorta
    c. Closure of the heart valves
    d. Contraction of the cardiac muscle
12. When palpating the breast, the assessment should be conducted by which division of areas?
    a. Quadrants
    b. Halves
    c. Entire breast tissue
    d. Bilateral comparison

13. When assessing the abdomen, which assessment technique should be conducted after inspection?
    a. Percussion
    b. Palpation
    c. Auscultation
    d. Sequence does not matter
14. Which of the following assessments of mental status is *not* an assessment of orientation?
    a. Time
    b. Place
    c. Person
    d. Consciousness
15. As part of the assessment of the cranial nerves, the nurse asks the patient to raise the eyebrows, smile, and show the teeth. These actions provide information about which cranial nerve?
    a. Olfactory
    b. Optic
    c. Facial
    d. Vagus

Answers With Rationale

1. The correct answer is *b*. None of the other instruments can be used to visualize the internal eye.
2. The correct answer is *a*. A comparison of bilateral body parts is necessary for recognizing abnormal findings. Perfect vision is unnecessary; the nurse examines all body systems and uses touch during palpation.
3. The correct answer is *d*. Palpation is the technique that uses the sense of touch. The other answers are incorrect.
4. The correct answer is *c*. Tympany is a loud, drumlike sound, heard over an air-filled organ. Dullness has a thudlike quality. Flatness is a flat, high-pitched sound. Resonance is a hollow sound heard over lung tissue.
5. The correct answer is *d*. The bell of the stethoscope is used to hear low-pitched sounds, such as those produced by the heart and vascular system.
6. The correct answer is *d*. Skin turgor is assessed by lightly pinching a fold of skin and allowing it to return to its shape when released.
7. The correct answer is *c*. Normal vision is 20/20. A finding of 20/40 would mean that a patient has less than normal vision.
8. The correct answer is *a*. The ear canal of an adult is straightened by gently pulling the pinna of the ear up and back. In children younger than 3 years of age, the ear canal is straightened by pulling the pinna gently down and back.
9. The correct answer is *d*. A dull sound is heard when percussing over fluid or a solid mass.
10. The correct answer is *a*. Adventitious breath sounds are sounds not normally heard in the lungs. The other answers are normal breath sounds.

11. The correct answer is *c*. Heart sounds are the result of closure of the heart valves.

12. The correct answer is *a*. The breast is divided into four quadrants—outer upper quadrant, outer lower quadrant, inner upper quadrant, and inner lower quadrant. Each quadrant is systematically palpated in a clockwise direction.

13. The correct answer is *c*. When assessing the abdomen, the sequence is inspection, auscultation, percussion, and palpation. Auscultation follows inspection because percussion and palpation stimulate bowel sounds.

14. The correct answer is *d*. The other answers are assessments of orientation.

15. The correct answer is *c*. Motor function of the facial nerve (cranial nerve VII) is assessed by asking the patient to raise the eyebrow, smile, and show the teeth.

Bibliography

American Academy of Orthopedic Surgeons. (2001). School screening programs for the early detection of scoliosis. Available at http://www.aaos.org/wordhtml/papers/position/scolios.htm.

Andresen, G. (1998). Assessing the older patient. *RN, 61*(3), 46–56.

Bickley, L. (2002). *Bates guide to physical examination and history taking* (8th ed.). Philadelphia: Lippincott.

Darovic, G. (1997). Assessing pupillary answers. *Nursing, 27*(2), 49.

Faria, S. (1999). Assessment of peripheral arterial pulses. *Home Care Provider, 4*(4), 140–141.

Heath, H., & White, I. (2001). Sexuality and older people: An introduction to nursing assessment. *Nursing Older People, 13*(4), 29–31.

Incredibly easy! Interpreting abnormal abdominal sounds. (2000). *Nursing, 30*(6), 28.

Jackson, R., Alghareeb, M. Alaradi, I., & Tomi, Z. (1999). The diagnosis of skin disease. *Dermatology Nursing, 11*(4), 275–283.

Kirton, C. (1996a). Assessing breath sounds. *Nursing, 26*(6), 50–51.

Kirton, C. (1996b). Assessing normal heart sounds. *Nursing, 26*(2), 56–57.

Kirton, C. (1997). Assessing bowel sounds. *Nursing, 27*(3), 64.

Klingman, L. (1999). Assessing the female reproductive system: A guide through the gynecologic exam. *American Journal of Nursing, 99*(8), 37–43.

Lyneham, J. (2001). Physical examination (abdomen, thorax and lungs): A review. *Australian Journal of Advanced Nursing, 18*(3), 31.

Mangini, M. (1998). Physical assessment of the musculoskeletal system. *Nursing Clinics of North America, 33*(4), 643–652.

Sheppard, M. (2001). Assessing fluid balance. *Nursing Times, 97*(6 NTplus), 8–14.

Watson, R. (2001). Assessing the musculoskeletal system in older people. *Nursing Older People, 13*(5), 29–30.

Weber, K., & Kelley, J. (2003). *Health assessment in nursing* (2nd ed.). Philadelphia: Lippincott Williams & Wilkins.

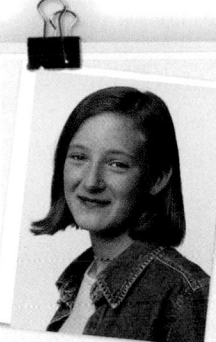

Kara Greenwood, a high school junior class representative and peer counselor, comes to the local community health center for a routine examination. During the interview, she says, "My guidance counselor has asked me and a few of my friends to develop a talk for our classmates on the dangers we face as adolescents. I know everybody is worried about terrorism, but I want to make sure that we talk about other safety issues, too."

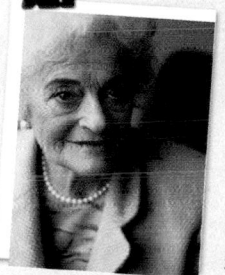

Bessie Washington, a 77-year-old woman, was recently discharged to her home after suffering a cerebrovascular accident (brain attack). She lives alone in a small one-bedroom apartment and uses a walker to ambulate. She says, "I have so much stuff crammed into this small apartment! I almost fell this morning going from my bedroom to the kitchen."

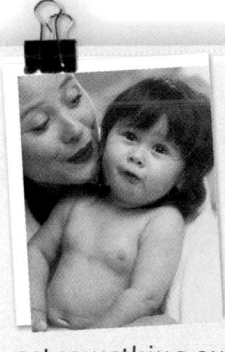

Juanita Flores is a young mother of a 1-year-old girl who has been diagnosed with failure to thrive and is being treated with a feeding program. While sitting on a cot with her daughter, whose legs are dangling at the edge of the cot about a foot above ground level, Juanita turns to get something out of her purse and the child falls to the floor and begins to cry loudly.

Focusing on Blended Skills

The types of blended skills you'll need to respond to the case scenarios include:

Cognitive Skills

- Knowledge of the safety and security needs of individuals of all ages, at different developmental stages, and with different health conditions and related nursing responsibilities and care
- Knowledge of the factors affecting an individual's safety and security
- Knowledge about safety issues for specific populations such as parents, adolescents, and the elderly and special circumstances (eg, adolescent dangers, cluttered home, and falls in healthcare institutions)
- Knowledge of available resources to meet safety, security, and emergency preparedness needs
- Knowledge of teaching and learning principles for different individuals, such as an adolescent, a woman with an infant, and an elderly woman with mobility problems

Technical Skills

- Ability to correctly use the equipment and techniques necessary to identify and respond to safety problems
- Ability to adapt techniques and procedures based on the developmental stage of the patient
- Ability to document information appropriately when safety is compromised

Interpersonal Skills

- Ability to communicate and interact effectively with members of the healthcare team, individuals, and groups to promote safety awareness and prevention
- Ability to create and sustain safe and secure working environments
- Ability to establish trusting relationships with patients, families, and public groups as a basis for counseling and education
- Ability to encourage individuals and groups to prepare for emergencies without causing undue alarm
- Knowledge of own limitations, with willingness to seek help when needed

Ethical and Legal Skills

- Knowledge of the ethical and legal principles underlying patient care
- Commitment to patient safety and quality care, including ability to report problem situations immediately
- Strong sense of personal responsibility and accountability for the health and well-being of patients at various developmental stages and with different needs
- Ability to document incidents according to agency policy (incident reports)
- Willingness to hold colleagues accountable for safe, quality practice

Learning Outcomes

After completing the chapter, the learner should be able to accomplish the following:

1. Identify factors that affect safety in an individual's environment.
2. Identify patients at risk for injury.
3. Describe specific safety risk factors for each developmental stage.
4. Select nursing diagnoses for patients in unsafe situations.
5. Describe basic first-aid measures.
6. Describe strategies to decrease the risk for injury in the home.
7. Describe health teaching interventions to promote safety for each developmental stage.
8. Describe nursing interventions to prevent injury to patients in healthcare settings.
9. Identify alternatives to using restraints.
10. Explore resources for developing and evaluating an emergency management plan.
11. Evaluate the effectiveness of safety interventions.

Key Terms

asphyxiation
bioterrorism
chemical terrorism
disaster
ground
incident report
nuclear terrorism
poison control center
restraint

Safety and security are basic human needs. Safety, or freedom from danger, harm, or risk, is a paramount concern that underlies all nursing care, and patient safety is a responsibility of all healthcare providers. Safety is a focus for all healthcare facilities as well as the home, workplace, and community. Many safety and security concerns are universal for all age groups, but there are unique considerations for each developmental stage.

Injuries and deaths from motor vehicle accidents, falls, fire, suffocation, and poisoning occur with alarming regularity across the life span. Violent behavior and its aftermath have also become a significant public safety concern. Many of these injuries and deaths can be prevented with appropriate safety awareness and precautions.

Ensuring that the environment is safe and secure requires an awareness of potential hazards for each developmental level. Studies have confirmed, for example, that pregnant women who use drugs, consume alcohol, or smoke expose their unborn children to substances that may adversely affect their normal growth and development. The nurse is often the initial healthcare provider in contact with an abused child or a battered woman. Prompt recognition of the potential or actual threat to safety is crucial, and the nursing assessment may play a vital role in identifying a harmful environment. For children, potential hazards multiply as their motor skills develop and their environment expands, yet many childhood accidents are preventable. Adolescents face great dangers when they abuse drugs or alcohol or engage in high-risk sexual activity. The increasing number of adolescents who become pregnant or who are victims of alcohol-related motor vehicle accidents, sexually transmitted diseases, and suicide is a devastating outcome of these unsafe behaviors. Abuse of the elderly has increased dramatically and affects approximately 5% of all older adults (Eliopoulos, 2003). Nurses have first-hand experience with the specific hazards confronting each age group and situation.

Since the mass casualties that occurred in the terrorist attacks of Sept. 11, 2001, the healthcare community has become increasingly aware of the need to be prepared should future incidents occur. Nurses are a vital part of any emergency response team and need knowledge about biological, chemical, and radioactive agents as well as the skills and competencies required to respond safely and effectively.

This chapter provides practical information on safety and security and introduces basic concepts of first aid and emergency preparedness. The nursing process facilitates the nurse's ability to recognize, assess, diagnose, and plan nursing interventions to ensure safety for all ages in all environments. (See the accompanying Reflective Practice box for an example.)

FACTORS AFFECTING SAFETY

Being aware of safety factors in the environment allows nurses to identify potential hazards and promote wellness. Table 26-1 lists the principal causes of accidental death in the United States.

Developmental Considerations

Each developmental level carries its own particular risks. Promoting safety and preventing injury are dual responsibilities of the nurse. Ideally, the nurse and the patient or family should work together to eliminate or reduce accident risks in the home, community, or healthcare setting. Nationally, emergency nurses are establishing partnerships and venturing into the community to offer injury prevention activities to children and families (Bernardo, 2002). Education to promote awareness of potentially dangerous situations must begin as early as possible and continue throughout the life span. Assessment of specific risks for each developmental level and appropriate nursing interventions are discussed later in this chapter.

Lifestyle

Certain occupations, recreational activities, and environments place people in more hazardous situations. A worker who operates industrial machinery or works in a perilous setting or with chemicals has a greater risk for accidental injury. Nurses are frequently exposed to needlestick injuries (Perry, Jagger & Parker, 2003). Nurses working in the operating room are regularly exposed to surgical smoke, a byproduct of laser and electrosurgery that contains chemicals that cause upper respiratory tract irritation (Rothrock, 2003). The Occupational Safety and Health Administration (OSHA) has determined that ladders are a major source of injuries and deaths among construction workers, and that older workers are at particular risk for sustaining a fatal injury (Partridge, Virk & Antosia, 1998).

Reproductive hazards may exist for women with long-term exposure to certain anesthetic agents, and an antiviral preparation (ribavirin) used for respiratory infections in infants and children may be harmful to a developing fetus (Pillitteri, 1999). Exposure to excessive noise (eg, a construction site, extremely loud music) may lead to hearing loss. OSHA identifies risks and develops standards to prevent serious injuries and illnesses due to work-related musculoskeletal disorders resulting from repetitive motions. Back pain and carpal tunnel syndrome may occur from work-related repetitive motion.

Some people by nature are more inclined to take risks and place themselves at jeopardy for injury. Failure to wear seat belts or to follow safety precautions is common behavior for some people. Stress may precipitate an unhealthful lifestyle that involves drug or alcohol abuse. Although much has been done to identify and control environmental pollutants, certain areas have proved to be more hazardous, and residents may be exposed to potentially unhealthy substances in the environment.

Living in an area where crime is prevalent can pose a threat to physical security and emotional well-being. Violence, acts of aggression, and terrorism are components of 21st-century life. Security measures such as locks, security systems, and exterior lighting can promote safety.

Mobility

Any limitation in mobility is potentially unsafe. An older patient with an unsteady gait is more prone to falling, and

Reflective Practice
Challenge to Ethical and Legal Skill

I first met Juanita Flores while working at a children's hospital two summers ago in a nurse externship program. Juanita was the mother of a 1-year-old girl diagnosed with failure to thrive who had been on the rehabilitation unit for some time. The child was very small and had a feeding program prescribed. One day while I was in the room, Juanita was sitting on the cot with her daughter, whose legs were dangling at the edge of the cot, about 1 foot above ground level. I was taking the child's vital signs. As the mother turned her back for a minute to grab something from her bag, I turned away to wash my hands in the sink. All of a sudden I heard a thud and crying as the child fell to the floor. Juanita tried to comfort here, picking her up and rocking and singing to her. Although I knew it was not completely my fault, I felt horrible about turning my back on the child for only the few seconds to wash my hands, the seconds that it took for the child to fall. Although Juanita was in the room, the child had been unsupervised for only a few seconds. However, I was not watching her at the moment the child fell. I wanted to tell my preceptor right away and knew I should in case anything had happened to the child, but I was nervous and afraid that I would get into trouble.

Thinking Outside the Box: Possible Courses of Action

- Tell my preceptor immediately that the child had fallen, and risk being asked why I had turned my back on the child.
- Report later that morning that the child had fallen earlier, and not make a big deal of it.
- Not mention it at all.

Evaluating a Good Outcome: How Do I Define Success?

- Patient is benefited by my actions, or at least is not harmed.
- My professional integrity is not compromised, nor is the personal integrity of the patient.
- A level of respect is maintained between the preceptor and student.
- Institutional policy for incident reporting is not violated.

Personal Learning: Here's to the Future!

Although I did tell my preceptor what had happened, I was not pleased by the way I handled the situation. Instead of reporting the incident right away, I waited until my preceptor was in the room with me, a half-hour or so later. I casually mentioned that the child had fallen earlier that morning but seemed to be fine. When my preceptor asked why I did not inform her earlier, I said that I couldn't find her and assumed that she was busy—plus, the child seemed fine and her mother was with her.

I was disappointed in how I dealt with this situation. Although I did not get reprimanded for the situation, an incident report was written documenting that the child had fallen. The physician also came to examine the child to ensure that the child was indeed okay. My preceptor stressed the importance of reporting incidents as soon as they happen, rather than delaying or ignoring them. This time the child was uninjured, but I learned that in the future I will report any problem immediately. A patient's fall could be detrimental. It is also very important to follow the institution's policy for reporting incidents to ensure both your professional integrity and the well-being of the patient.

Reflection

How do you think you would respond in a similar situation? Why? What does this tell you about yourself and about the adequacy of your skills for professional practice? Is the nurse extern's fear justification for the action? Please explain. What ethical and legal principles, if any, were violated in this situation? What liability would the nurse extern be required to assume? Can you think of other ways to respond? How might the nurse extern have interacted with the mother to promote the child's safety? What other skills (cognitive, interpersonal, technical, ethical/legal) would you need to respond well in this situation? Do you agree with the criteria to evaluate a successful outcome? How do you think this incident affected the relationship between the nurse extern and the preceptor? Please explain.

Anne Hrynko, Georgetown University

an unfamiliar setting, such as a healthcare facility, may aggravate the problem. Someone with paralysis or a spinal cord injury may require assistance with even simple movements. Supportive devices, such as canes, walkers, and wheelchairs, may facilitate movement, but they require careful patient instruction and preparation for safe use. Recent surgery or a prolonged illness can temporarily affect a patient's mobility and necessitate special precautions to prevent falls or injuries. Nurses must assess a patient's risk for injury with a view toward maintaining independence and fostering self-esteem while providing a safe and predictable environment.

Think back to Bessie Washington, the 77-year-old woman with a cerebrovascular accident (brain attack) who lives alone in a small apartment and requires a walker to ambulate. To ensure that the patient remains safe, the nurse needs to assess the patient's home environment closely for hazards, especially based on the patient's statement that she almost fell.

Sensory Perception

Alterations in sensory perception can have a devastating effect on safety. Any impairment in sight, hearing, smell, taste, or touch can reduce a person's sensitivity to the environment. Visual changes may cause a person to stumble, lose his or her

TABLE 26-1 Deaths and Death Rates From Accidents in the United States, 2000

Type of Accident	Total Deaths	Death Rate per 100,000 Population
Motor vehicle accidents	41,804	15.2
Firearms and handguns	808	0.3
Drowning	3,343	1.2
Fire and flames	3,265	1.2
Poisoning and exposure to noxious substances	9,893	3.6
Complications of medical-surgical care	2,886	1.0

Adapted from U.S. Census Bureau. (2002). *Statistical abstract of the United States, 2002* (122nd ed.). Washington, D.C.: U.S. Department of Commerce.

balance, and fall. A patient with a hearing deficit may not be able to hear safety alarms, automobile horns, and sirens and may not hear healthcare instructions. A patient with a reduced ability to distinguish odors may fail to detect leaking gas or smoke. A patient with a loss of taste may have unsafe eating habits or may eat tainted food. A patient whose tactile sense is impaired may not perceive temperature extremes that are a threat to safety.

Knowledge

An awareness of safety and security precautions is crucial for promoting and maintaining wellness. A patient needs instructions, for example, to adhere to a medical regimen or to follow safety precautions when oxygen is in use. He or she requires a certain amount of knowledge to manage new equipment and unfamiliar procedures. Nursing assessment includes identifying and recognizing potentially threatening circumstances.

Recall Juanita Flores, the young mother of a 1-year-old who fell from a cot. The nurse's knowledge of potential threats to safety for infants, in conjunction with providing anticipatory guidance to the mother about safety issues for infants, would be essential to prevent injury.

Recommendations for specific safety and security precautions are included throughout this chapter.

Ability to Communicate

The ability to communicate is basic to many safety practices. The nurse must assess any factor that influences the patient's ability to receive and send messages. Fatigue, stress, medication, aphasia, and language barriers are examples of factors that can affect personal communication and prevent the patient from accurately perceiving events. A valid assessment by the nurse not only identifies the patient's level of understanding but also facilitates a positive communication experience.

Physical Health State

Anything that affects the patient's health state potentially can affect the safety of the environment. When a person is chronically ill or in a weakened state, the focus of healthcare includes preventing accidents as well as promoting wellness and restoring the individual to a healthy state. The nurse caring for a patient who is recovering from a stroke or brain attack, for example, identifies the patient's neuromuscular impairment, pays particular attention to health teaching concerning the person's ability to maintain a sense of balance, and carefully assists the patient with ambulation to prevent falls. Many patients who fall have a primary or secondary diagnosis of cardiovascular disease, such as a stroke. Prevention of complications and return to the optimal level of functioning require attention to safety and become primary concerns in a stroke rehabilitation program. The nurse strives to maximize the patient's potential by considering safety factors in all phases of the illness and recovery experience.

Consider Bessie Washington, the woman who is now at home after having a cerebrovascular accident. The nurse would incorporate knowledge of safety factors along with knowledge of the patient's mobility limitations to develop a plan of care that maximizes the patient's potential while maintaining patient safety.

Psychosocial Health State

Stressful situations tend to narrow a person's attention span and make him or her more prone to accidents. Stress may occur over a long period, but the effects tend to be more devastating in the person's later years, when there is typically less adaptive and coping capacity. Depression may result in confusion and disorientation, accompanied by reduced awareness or concern about environmental hazards. Social isolation or lack of social contact may lead to a reduced level of concentration, errors in judgment, and a diminished awareness of external stimuli.

THE NURSING PROCESS FOR MAINTAINING SAFETY

Assessment

When performing a safety assessment, the nurse focuses on three categories: the individual, the environment, and specific risk factors.

Assessing the Individual

Assessment of the individual consists of a nursing history and a physical examination.

Nursing History

To help provide a safe environment, be alert to any history of falls or accidents, because a person with a history of falling is likely to fall again. Note any assistive devices that the patient uses (eg, a cane or walker). Be alert to any history of drug or alcohol abuse. Family members and significant others are often valuable resources. Knowledge of family support systems and the home environment is crucial for the nurse to plan protective health measures.

Some people seem more likely than others to have accidents. Some children, for example, are involved in multiple mishaps resulting in fractured bones or minor injuries requiring surgical repair. Adults at any age may also have this tendency. Experts disagree about the cause of accident-prone behavior, but most agree that a patient with a history of accidents is likely to have another one.

Physical Examination

Assess the patient's mobility status, ability to communicate, level of awareness or orientation, and sensory perception in the physical examination. Early identification of any potential safety hazards is essential. Recognize any manifestations that suggest domestic violence or neglect. Chapters 4, Health and Illness, and 19, Conception Through Young Adult, discuss families experiencing violence, neglect, or abuse.

Assessing the Environment

Assessment of the environment requires the same attention to safety. Risks in the home, community, and healthcare agency may cause injury.

Environmental safety hazards can result in falls, fires, poisoning, suffocation, and accidents involving motor vehicles, equipment, and procedures. Nursing assessment includes identifying individuals at risk and recognizing unsafe situations. This requires knowledge of the factors that influence safety and predispose people to accidents. Recognizing these factors helps the nurse develop an individualized plan of care and nursing interventions for protecting the patient. Assessment includes an awareness of risk factors in both the home and the healthcare agency, with the focus on the patient's developmental level and health status.

As student nurses become increasingly involved in community and home care settings, they need also to assess their own environmental safety when visiting unfamiliar areas. Carroll et al. (1999) suggest use of educational strategies and a questionnaire that can identify students' personal safety concerns in a community setting. Use the self-assessment checklist in the accompanying box, Promoting Health, to evaluate your own attention to your personal safety. Potential safety hazards in the patient's environment that require assessment and intervention are described in detail later in this chapter.

Performing a Specific Risk Factor Assessment

Be aware of the patients who are most at risk for injury as well as specific hazards.

Falls

Falls can occur at any age, but 35% to 40% of healthy adults 65 years or older living in the community fall at least once a year (Alexander & Edelberg, 2002). A large portion of healthcare for the elderly is used to care for fall-related injuries (Rawsky, 1998). Elderly people are at risk in all settings. Falls are responsible for most hospital incidents, and 45% to 75% of

---

Promoting Health 26-1 *Safety in the Community*

Use the following assessment checklist to determine how well you are meeting your need for maintaining personal safety as you assist with healthcare delivery in the community. Then develop a prescription for self-care by choosing appropriate behaviors from the list of suggestions.

ASSESSMENT CHECKLIST

(columns: almost always / sometimes / almost never)

1. I wear a badge or clothing that identifies me as a healthcare worker.
2. I dress in an unobtrusive, professional manner.
3. I keep my car in good working order.
4. I am aware of neighborhoods where personal safety and security may be a problem.
5. I confirm directions to the patient's residence before the visit.
6. I enter patients' homes only when invited in by responsible adult.

SELF-CARE BEHAVIORS

1. Call patients to schedule visits for an agreeable time.
2. Carry a map of the communities you plan to visit.
3. Avoid isolated areas.
4. Request that pets be secured before your visit.
5. Do not carry money, credit cards, or handbag on your person. If necessary, lock them in your trunk.
6. Avoid wearing expensive jewelry.
7. Consider the advantages of a cellular phone.
8. Request escort services as appropriate or make joint visits.
9. Keep your car locked when driving and when parked.
10. Make sure agency is aware of time/location of scheduled visits.

elderly adults in long-term care settings suffer a fall (Gentleman & Malozemoff, 2001). In general, 5% to 15% of these falls result in fractures or soft tissue injury (Dunn, 2001). Hip fractures are among the most serious fall-related injuries. Many falls at home go unreported because they do not cause injuries requiring medical attention. Also, the elderly fear activity restrictions, loss of independence, or placement in a nursing home. Fear of falling can also cause anxiety and panic and make an older adult more vulnerable to a fall.

Assessment of the risk for falling includes the use of nursing history and nursing examination. The nursing examination includes inspecting for factors that contribute to falls. An individual is considered at high risk for a fall if he or she has any of the following characteristics:

- Age older than 65 years
- Documented history of falls
- Impaired vision or sense of balance
- Altered gait or posture
- A medication regimen that includes diuretics, tranquilizers, sedatives, hypnotics, or analgesics
- Postural hypotension
- Slowed reaction time
- Confusion or disorientation
- Impaired mobility
- Weakness and physical frailty
- Unfamiliar environment

Falls in the elderly can be prevented if they can be predicted (Covinsky et al., 2001; Grenier-Sennlier et al., 2002), so surveillance must be continuous for environmental hazards in the healthcare facility and the home environment and of patients who are at risk for falls.

Remember Bessie Washington, the elderly woman described at the beginning of the chapter. Based on the assessment of the patient, the nurse would identify Mrs. Washington's risk for falls as high. It would be crucial to incorporate this information into the patient's plan of care to ensure her safety.

Most healthcare agencies have fall-prevention programs. Nurses have the responsibility to identify patients who are at high risk for falls, document pertinent assessments on the chart, and plan appropriate interventions to ensure their safety. A nurse whose behavior is reasonable and prudent and similar to the behavior that would be expected of another nurse in similar circumstances is unlikely to be found liable if a patient falls, even if an injury results (Sullivan, 1999). Checklists for preventing falls at home and in healthcare facilities appear later in the chapter.

Fires

Many home fires are started because someone smoked in bed or fell asleep while smoking on a sofa or chair. Most fatal home fires occur while people are sleeping, and most people who die in house fires die of smoke inhalation rather than burns. Kitchen stoves, candles, and electric heaters are other causes of home fires. Faulty wiring and unsafe electrical equipment

cause fires in homes and healthcare facilities. The risk for home fires can be determined by assessing the knowledge of family members.

People with limited financial resources should be asked about how they heat their house, because the electricity or gas may have been turned off and space or kerosene heaters, wood stoves, or a fireplace may be the sole source of heat. Fire safety recommendations for the home are included in the Home Safety Checklist in Box 26-4 later in this chapter.

Fire prevention and emergency response programs in healthcare facilities are sometimes viewed by staff as time-consuming or unnecessary exercises, but nurses must be prepared at all times to protect patients from injury. Hospitals are required by law to establish safety boards and to inspect the facility regularly for possible hazards. Equipment must be checked periodically, and escape routes must be kept open. Nurses, as part of their daily care procedures, must be aware of their agency's policies, review equipment and its proper functioning, and assess when and how often drills are performed.

Poisoning

Although the incidence of childhood poisoning has been reduced drastically in the past 10 years, accidental poisoning remains a concern. According to the latest government statistics, almost 10,000 deaths resulted from accidental poisoning in 2000, with many more people suffering nonfatal effects of poisons (U.S. Census Bureau, 2002). Causes of deaths from unintentional poisoning are listed in Table 26-2. Ingestion of analgesics and hydrocarbons are the most common causes of poisoning deaths in children (London et al., 2003). Annually, 1 million children under age 6 are exposed to a toxic substance (Crawley-Coha, 2002). In 2000, U.S. poison control centers handled one poison exposure every 15 seconds (Crawley-Coha, 2002). However, not all poisons cause death.

Consider the person's developmental stage when making a safety assessment. Younger children are more apt to ingest household chemicals, whereas older children may swallow medicines in a suicide attempt. Preschoolers are also at risk for ingestion of lead-containing substances in the home. Adolescents and young adults who experiment with drugs may suffer accidental poisoning and death. The ready availability of inhalants on store shelves and in the home may provide the opportunity for children to sniff or "huff" these dangerous substances.

Recall Kara Greenwood, the adolescent asking for information about adolescent dangers. An important area to include in the discussion would be drug experimentation.

An older person may inadvertently take an overdose of a medication because of confusion or forgetfulness. Poor vision is also a factor in accidental poisoning in older adults.

Most exposures to toxic fumes occur in the home. Poisoning may result from improper mixing of household substances, prolonged use of strong cleaning products, or malfunctioning household appliances (gas, oil, and kerosene

TABLE 26-2 Common Agents in Childhood Poisoning

Poisonous Agent	Source	Common Clinical Manifestations	Treatment
Salicylates	Products containing aspirin	Nausea, hyperpnea, dehydration, vomiting, confusion, fever, tinnitus, metabolic acidosis, respiratory alkalosis, seizures, coma	If clear history of intake is available and intake is 150–300 mg/kg,* use activated charcoal. Intake > 300 mg/kg, take child to ER.
Hydrocarbons	Gasoline Kerosene Furniture polish Lamp oil	Gagging, coughing, choking, dyspnea, grunting, nausea, chills, fever, lethargy	*Never induce vomiting!* Contact MD or PCC.
Caustics	Oven cleaner Drain openers Toilet bowl cleaners Battery contents Rust removers Hair perms	Burning pain in mouth and throat, drooling, edema of lips; oral, esophageal, gastric burns; vomiting, hemoptysis	*Never induce vomiting!* Never attempt to neutralize the caustic. Dilute with milk or water. Contact physician or PCC.
Iron	Vitamin preparations	Nausea, vomiting, diarrhea, abdominal pain, melena, hematemesis, lethargy, coma	If clear history of intake is available and exposure is 20–40 mg/kg,* use activated charcoal. Intake > 40 mg/kg, take child to ER.
Lead	Paint chips Paint dust	May be asymptomatic, anorexia, abdominal pain, anemia, encephalopathy, neurobehavioral deficits	Chelation therapy and monitor lead levels

*Clear history indicated knowledge of exact amount of drug ingested. Mg/kg can be calculated by dividing the total dose ingested into the weight in kg. If unclear, visit to emergency room (ER) may be recommended by poison control center (PCC).
Adapted from: Pillitteri, A. (1999). *Maternal & child health nursing* (3rd ed.). Philadelphia: Lippincott Williams & Wilkins.

heaters) that can release carbon monoxide. Carbon monoxide is a colorless, odorless, tasteless, and nonirritating gas, which makes it especially dangerous. Exposure can result in mild symptoms or progress to a life-threatening problem or long-term effects. Young children and older adults are more vulnerable to toxic fumes.

Poison control centers provide checklists for "poison-proofing" a home and provide lists of toxic household items. Such lists are helpful when assessing and teaching the family about poisonous materials. Refer to the Home Safety Checklist in Box 26-4 later in this chapter.

Suffocation and Choking

Suffocation, or **asphyxiation,** may occur at any age, but the incidence is greater in children. In suffocation, air does not reach the lungs and breathing stops. Common causes of suffocation are drowning, choking on a foreign substance inhaled into the trachea, and gas or smoke poisoning. An infant may suffocate when a pillow or a piece of plastic inadvertently covers the nose and mouth. A young child may be strangled accidentally by the shoulder harness of a seat belt or become trapped while playing in a discarded refrigerator and suffocate.

Drowning is a form of suffocation. Nearly half of all drowning victims are children younger than 5 years of age. Most drowning deaths in young children occur because of inadequate supervision of a bathtub or pool, even a small wading pool. Older children are more likely to drown while swimming or boating.

Educating the public about the causes of suffocation can save many lives. Assessing the knowledge level of individuals, especially parents, is vital. Hazards that might cause a child to asphyxiate or choke are included in the Home Safety Checklist later in the chapter.

Firearm Injuries

Preventing injuries caused by firearms has become a major concern for health professionals. Unintentional gunshot wounds are a leading cause of mortality and morbidity in children: in 1998, 121 children died of unintentional gunshot wounds, and 34% of children in the United States live in homes with at least one firearm (Crawley-Coha, 2002). Some people believe that keeping a gun in the home provides protection for family and property, but if not stored properly guns can be dangerous. Young children are curious and like to explore their surroundings, and when they encounter a loaded gun, the outcome is often tragic. Also, having a gun in the house increases the risk for domestic homicide threefold.

Gun ownership is a sensitive issue, and nurses need to approach this topic in a nonjudgmental manner with the focus on injury prevention. The intent is to inform families about the risks of firearm injury and discuss appropriate safety measures. Refer to the Home Safety Checklist later in the chapter.

Nursing Diagnoses

Unsafe situations and patients at risk are reflected in the nursing diagnosis and plan of care. The statement of the patient's actual or potential health status must be followed by the appropriate contributing factors or risk factors to individualize the nursing plan of care. Nursing diagnoses involving safety risks may include the following:

- Risk for Injury related to lack of awareness of environmental hazards; visual or auditory sensory deficits; history of falling; unsteady gait; substance abuse; refusal to use seat belt or child safety seat; effects of medication; age greater than 65 years; generalized weakness; biological, chemical, or nuclear exposure
- Risk for Poisoning related to impaired vision; medications stored in unlocked medicine cabinet that is accessible to a child; presence of poisonous plants; excess alcohol intake; use of illicit drugs; knowledge deficit; chemical contamination of food and water
- Risk for Suffocation related to a plastic bag that is accessible to a young child; child left unattended in bathtub; smoking in bed; placing an infant prone in a water bed; lack of safety precautions (door left on discarded refrigerator); unfamiliarity with fire prevention guidelines; household gas leaks
- Risk for Trauma related to history of previous falls; unsteady gait; presence of unsecured scatter rugs; smoking in bed; inoperable smoke detector; history of substance abuse; lack of experience operating an automobile; presence of unsecured loaded gun in the home; high-crime neighborhood
- Impaired Home Maintenance related to insufficient finances; substance abuse; physical disability; inadequate support systems; lack of knowledge
- Risk for Disuse Syndrome related to use of physical restraints

Outcome Identification and Planning

Many accidental injuries and deaths are preventable. Consider the various factors and the environment that affect the patient's safety and formulate expected outcomes uniquely suited to each situation and circumstance. Nursing interventions focus on meeting these safety needs. Some expected outcomes for patients that promote safety and prevent injury are as follows:

The patient will
- Identify unsafe situations in his or her environment
- Identify potential hazards in his or her environment
- Demonstrate safety measures to prevent falls and other accidents

- Establish safety priorities with family members or significant others
- Demonstrate familiarity with his or her environment
- Identify resources for safety information
- Remain free of injury during hospitalization

Implementation

Integral to the nursing plan of care is the patient's safety. It is important to intervene in order to control or modify the patient's environment. Safety recommendations in the following sections apply to health agency settings, the home, and the community. Nursing interventions are designed for each developmental level as well as for specific hazards in the environment. Developmentally disabled, demented, or delirious adults frequently need the same safety measures as those for children.

Acquiring First-Aid Knowledge

First aid is the immediate care given to an acutely injured or ill person. It is the temporary assistance that is rendered until competent, professional care, if required, arrives and takes over. It is very likely that friends and family will start asking your advice about sprains, bites, and heat and cold injuries as soon as they know you are studying nursing. While you always want to be sure to respect the limits of your professional knowledge and skill and refer people appropriately for professional services, you will find it extremely helpful to know basic first aid. Figure 26-1, an emergency first-aid chart from the American Safety and Health Institute, outlines how to respond to common problems. Absent from this list of emergencies is what to do if you are called to examine a student who fails to respond or awaken after consuming large amounts of alcohol or other drugs. Figure 26-2 describes emergency steps appropriate for this and other situations that require a prompt response.

Teaching to Prevent Accidents

Teaching is an important intervention for accident prevention and health promotion. Many teaching opportunities concerning safety measures arise while the nurse performs regular patient care, and many resources are available to supplement health teaching (Fig. 26-3). Careful assessment, diagnosis, and planning prepare nurses to use these opportunities wisely.

Assessment data and statistical information often prove helpful to healthcare personnel who are developing a safety program for patients at risk. Safety education classes, in addition to situational health teaching, can be worthwhile for hospitalized patients and their family members. Recent studies have demonstrated that early assessment of vulnerable patients and preventive education programs can decrease the incidence of falls (Alexander & Edelberg, 2002).

A school nurse has many opportunities and a ready audience for health teaching about safety, including screening programs (eg, vision and hearing), fire prevention sessions, drug and alcohol prevention programs, firearm safety, and classes on various accident prevention techniques. Managing

(text continues on page 625)

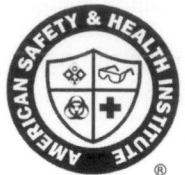

The American Safety & Health Institute
EMERGENCY FIRST AID

1-800-682-5067

Emergency Number _____

BLEEDING EMERGENCIES

First aid care for minor wound with minimal bleeding:

1. Clean wound with warm water and soap.
2. If worksite protocol allows apply antibiotic cream.
3. Dress wound with bandage to prevent infection. (You may leave wound uncovered if it is in a location that is not troublesome.)

The Bleeding Control Sequence Steps

1. Direct pressure
(At this time, a direct pressure bandage may be applied.)

2. Elevate
(Do no further harm.)

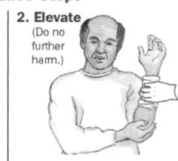

3. Pressure point
(If necessary.)

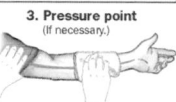
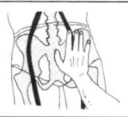

SHOCK

Signs of shock

- Anxiety, restlessness or irritability
- Altered consciousness
- Rapid pulse rate
- Rapid breathing
- Pale, cool, moist skin
- Eyes lackluster, dazed look
- Weak, helpless feeling
- Thirst
- Nausea

First aid care for shock

- Keep the victim lying down if possible.
- Try to make the victim comfortable.
- Speak in a comforting and reassuring tone to relieve stress or anxiety.
- Control any external bleeding if necessary.
- Elevate legs 10-12 inches, unless you suspect spinal damage or broken bones.
- Cover victim. Maintain body temperature.
- Do not give victim anything to eat or drink.
- Provide victim with plenty of fresh air.
- If victim is nauseous or begins to vomit, place the victim on his or her left side.
- Make sure a call is made to activate the EMS.

BURN CARE

1st & 2nd Degree Burns

A. Cool the burned area. Immerse in cold water or apply cold cloths.
B. Cover with clean, dry dressing.
C. Elevate burned limbs above heart level.
D. Treat for **SHOCK** if necessary.

3rd Degree Burns

A. Call EMS immediately. Do not apply water!
B. Cover with clean, dry dressing.
C. Elevate burned limbs above heart level.
D. Treat for **SHOCK**.

I - C - E
First Aid Care for Strains and Sprains

Ice Apply a cold pack. Do not place ice directly on skin.

Compress Use an elastic or conforming wrap, but not too tight.

Elevate Above heart level to control internal bleeding.

I - A - C - T
Dislocations and Fractures

1. **Immobilize area.**
   Use pillows, jackets, blankets, etc. Stop movement by supporting injured area.
2. **Activate EMS (911).**
   Or transport victim to a medical center.
3. **Care for shock.**
   See care for shock.
4. **Treat any additional secondary injuries.**

NECK OR BACK INJURIES

1. Stabilize head and neck. Stop movement.

2. Maintain an open airway.

3. Activate EMS.

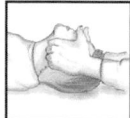
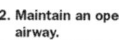
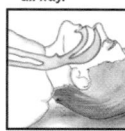
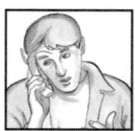

MEDICAL EMERGENCIES

Signs or symptoms

- Pale or flushed skin
- Cold sweats
- Dizzy, light-headed, weak, confused
- Nausea or vomiting
- Diarrhea
- Severe headache
- Paralysis
- Slurred speech
- Seizure
- Breathing difficulty
- Persistent pain or pressure
- Changes in consciousness

First aid care

- Help victim rest comfortably.
- Interview victim or bystanders. Ask:
  1. Are you allergic to anything?
  2. Are you on medication?
  3. When did you last eat?
  4. What led up to this problem?
- Look for medical alert tags.
- Reassure victim.
- Watch for signals/changes in breathing and consciousness.
- Don't give the victim anything to eat or drink (diabetic emergencies are an exception).
- Keep victim from getting chilled or overheated.
- Seek medical attention if appropriate.

SEVERE ALLERGIC REACTIONS

Signs and symptoms

- Rash, skin burning, itching and hives
- Noisy and/or difficult breathing
- Swelling of face, neck, lips, and/or tongue
- Confusion
- A feeling of tightness in the chest and throat
- Nausea
- Fainting, coma
- Dizziness

This is a true medical emergency! A severe allergic reaction can become life-threatening. Call EMS, provide prescribed medication if available, and monitor breathing and circulation. Provide necessary life support care until EMS arrives.

Causes of an allergic reaction include:
- An insect bite or sting.
- An ingested substance (foods such as spices, nuts, fish, shellfish, or medication such as penicillin).
- An inhaled substance (dust, pollen or chemicals).
- An injected substance (antitoxins or drugs such as penicillin).
- An absorbed substance (certain chemicals when in contact with skin can result in a severe allergic reaction).

POISONING

First aid care for poison emergencies

1. Assess the scene for clues and safety.
2. Get victim away from poison if necessary.
3. Assess victim response (level of consciousness, breathing and circulation).
4. Provide care for any life-threatening conditions.
5. If the victim is conscious, attempt to get more information.
6. Alert the Poison Control Center or your local emergency system. Bring any empty container, plant, etc., to the phone for verification purposes.

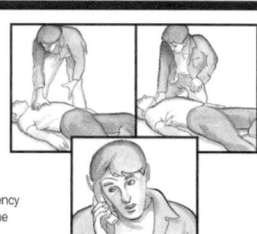

BITES & STINGS

First aid care for insect stings
- Wash site.
- Apply a cold pack.
- Monitor victim for allergic reaction. Seek medical assistance if appropriate.

Bees/Wasps/Hornets: Leave behind a stinger that may remain embedded in the skin. Do not pull the stinger out directly with fingers or tweezers. This will only inject additional poison into the body. Instead, use the edge of a credit card or something similar. The edge will snag the venom sack above the skin level and pull the embedded stinger out of the skin.
Spiders: Seek medical attention!
Ticks: Ticks must be removed with tweezers. Apply antiseptic ointment. If you are unable to remove head or if rash persists, obtain medical assistance.

First aid care for snake bites
- Call the Poison Control Center or EMS.
- Do not attempt to suck the venom out of the victim.
- Keep the affected limb below heart level.
- Calm and reassure victim.

HEAT & COLD

	HEAT CRAMPS	HEAT EXHAUSTION	HEAT STROKE	MILD HYPOTHERMIA	SEVERE HYPOTHERMIA	
SIGNS & SYMPTOMS	• Painful muscle cramps • Moist, cool skin • Heavy sweating	• Cold and clammy • Heavy sweating • Weak pulse • Shallow breathing • Nausea • Stomach cramps • Weakness, fatigue • Headache	• Hot, dry, red skin • Confusion or unconsciousness • Little or no sweating • Full, rapid pulse	• Shivering, slurred speech, stumbling or staggering (usually, victim is conscious and can talk)	• Body core temperature below 90°F • Shivering has stopped • Muscles have become stiff and rigid	• Skin has a bluish appearance • Skin does not react to pain • Pulse & respiration slow • Pupils dilated • Victim may appear dead
FIRST AID CARE	1. **Move** to cool place. 2. Give water or saline solution. 3. Massage muscle.	1. **Move** to cool place. 2. Elevate legs 3. Remove soaked clothing 4. Apply cool packs 5. Give water 6. Monitor!	1. **Move** to cool place. 2. Immediately cool victim by fanning and applying cool water. 3. Remove any excess clothing. 4. **Call EMS!** (Life threatening)	1. Remove from cold environment. 2. Provide a source of heat (warm water, fireplace). 3. Replace wet clothing with dry. 4. Provide a hat, blankets, coats. Insulate victim. 5. Seek medical attention.	1. Call EMS. 2. Keep victim warm. 3. Do not rewarm if victim can be transported within 12 hrs. 4. Take care when moving victim. Treat victim as if he/she could	break. 5. While checking vitals, make sure you perform a thorough pulse check before determining the need for CPR.

If the Victim

Faints
Position victim on back and then elevate legs 8-10 inches.
Do not elevate legs if you suspect a back or head injury.

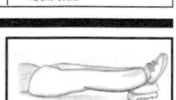

Vomits
Place victim in the recovery position (left side with head resting on arm).

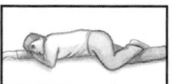

FIGURE 26-1 Emergency First Aid chart from The American Safety & Health Institute.   (Used with permission from The American Safety & Health Institute. [2003]. *Basic first aid for the community and workplace* [3rd ed.]. Holiday, FL: Author.)

Emergency Action Steps:
Assess – Alert – Attend

Assess the Scene for Safety

An emergency is an unforeseen event or condition that requires a prompt response. The emergency may be a result of an accident or sudden illness. As you approach, you must take care to *Assess* the emergency scene for safety. Ask yourself if it is safe to approach the victim(s).

Use all of your senses and look for danger (example, moving vehicles, downed power lines, broken glass, ice, etc.). Listen for crashing, screeching, hissing, or shattering noises. Smell the air. Can you detect traces of smoke or harmful gases? Be sure that you are not going to be injured while assisting the victim. Otherwise, if you feel that the danger level is high, immediately call EMS and notify other bystanders of the dangers present at the scene of the emergency. If the scene appears to be safe, approach victim and *Assess* victim for responsiveness.

Assess Victim

As you approach victim(s), look for additional bystanders for help. Having another bystander may be helpful if EMS must be called and also for assistance with victim, if necessary.

Gently tap victim and ask, "Are you alright?"

Alert

If victim is unresponsive or has an altered level of consciousness, EMS must be notified. If you are alone and the victim is an unresponsive adult, immediately locate phone and call EMS. Then go back and attend to the victim. If a bystander is nearby, send the bystander to notify EMS and immediately attend to the victim. If the victim is an unresponsive child and no one is available to call EMS for you, attend to victim and provide one minute of care, then call EMS.

Attend

Attend to victim and provide necessary care until EMS arrives and takes over care.

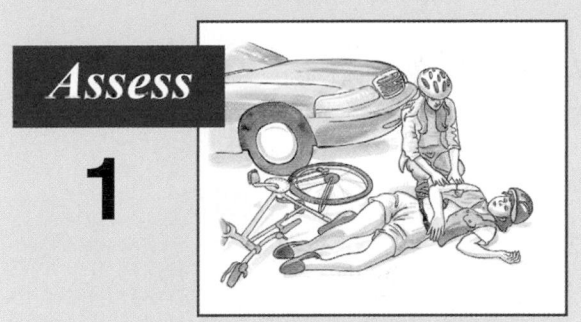

Whenever you recognize an emergency, you should:

1. **Assess** the scene for safety. Is it safe to approach the victim(s)? If the scene is not safe, alert EMS for help and make sure other bystanders are aware of existing danger.

2. **Assess** the victim(s) for life-threatening conditions and yell for help if necessary. For example, "I need help here!"

3. **Assess** and make a quick determination regarding the nature of the emergency and the approximate age of the victim (adult, child, or infant).

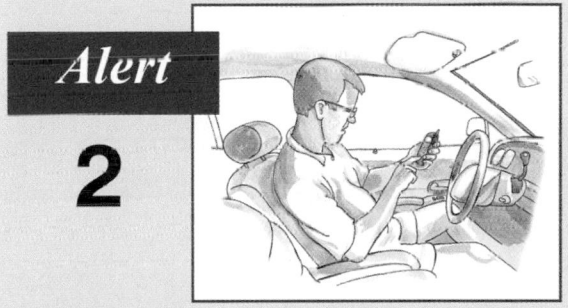

Alert EMS for medical assistance, if necessary. If you are alone, call EMS immediately as soon as you determine that an adult is unconscious. Assist a child for one minute and then call EMS.

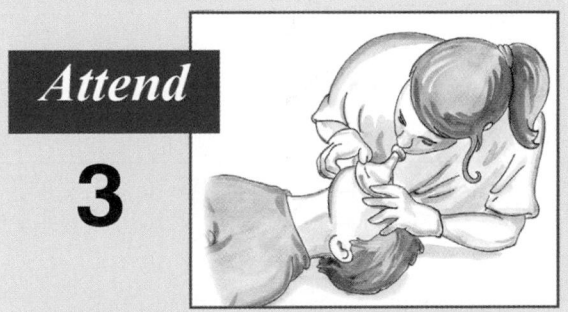

Attend to the victim(s) and provide necessary care until advanced medical help (EMS) arrives and takes over.

FIGURE 26-2 Emergency action steps. (*continued*)   (Used with permission from The American Safety & Health Institute. [2003]. *Essentials in basic emergency care* [pp. 5–9]. Holiday, FL: Author.)

How Is A Victim Assessment Performed?

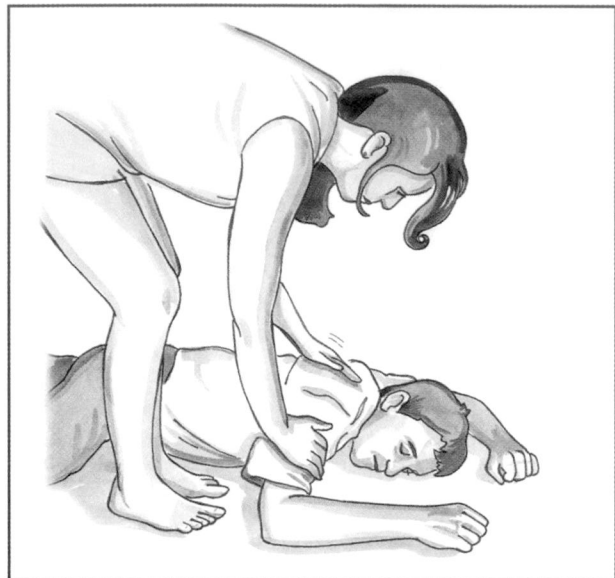

Gently tap the victim's shoulders and ask loudly, "Are you OK?"

CHECK FOR RESPONSIVENESS

No response (unconscious):

- Call 911.
- Open airway.
- Check for breathing/provide two (2) breaths, if needed.
- Check for signals of circulation/check pulse.
- Provide CPR or rescue breathing, if necessary.
- Control bleeding if necessary.
- Prevent/treat for shock.

Responsive (conscious):

- Introduction/request for consent.
- Control bleeding, if necessary.
- Complete a head-to-toe exam.
- Check for normal breathing and pulse.
- Provide first aid, if appropriate.
- Prevent/treat for shock.

EMS is required if victim:

- Has drowned/near drowned.
- Has altered consciousness.
- Is or becomes unconscious.
- Has chest pain or pressure.
- Has difficulty breathing (refer to the chart below, "Signs of Abnormal Breathing").
- Is bleeding severely.
- Has pain or pressure in the abdomen.
- Is passing blood or vomiting blood.
- Has slurred speech, a severe headache, or seizures.
- Has a head, neck, or back injury.
- Has possible broken bones.
- Has been poisoned.
- Has overdosed on drugs.
- Has been electrocuted.
- Has any suspected serious illness or injury.
- Has an altered mental state.

SIGNS OF ABNORMAL BREATHING

- Irregular breathing
- Wheezing, gurgling, or high-pitched noises when breathing
- Shortness of breath, often with dizziness, or light-headedness
- Flushed, bluish, or pale appearance

ACTION: Call EMS

- Provide rescue breathing, if needed.
- Provide emergency oxygen, if available.

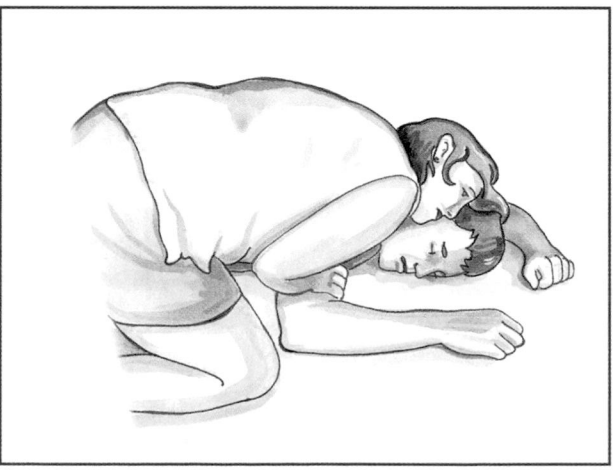

FIGURE 26-2 *Continued*

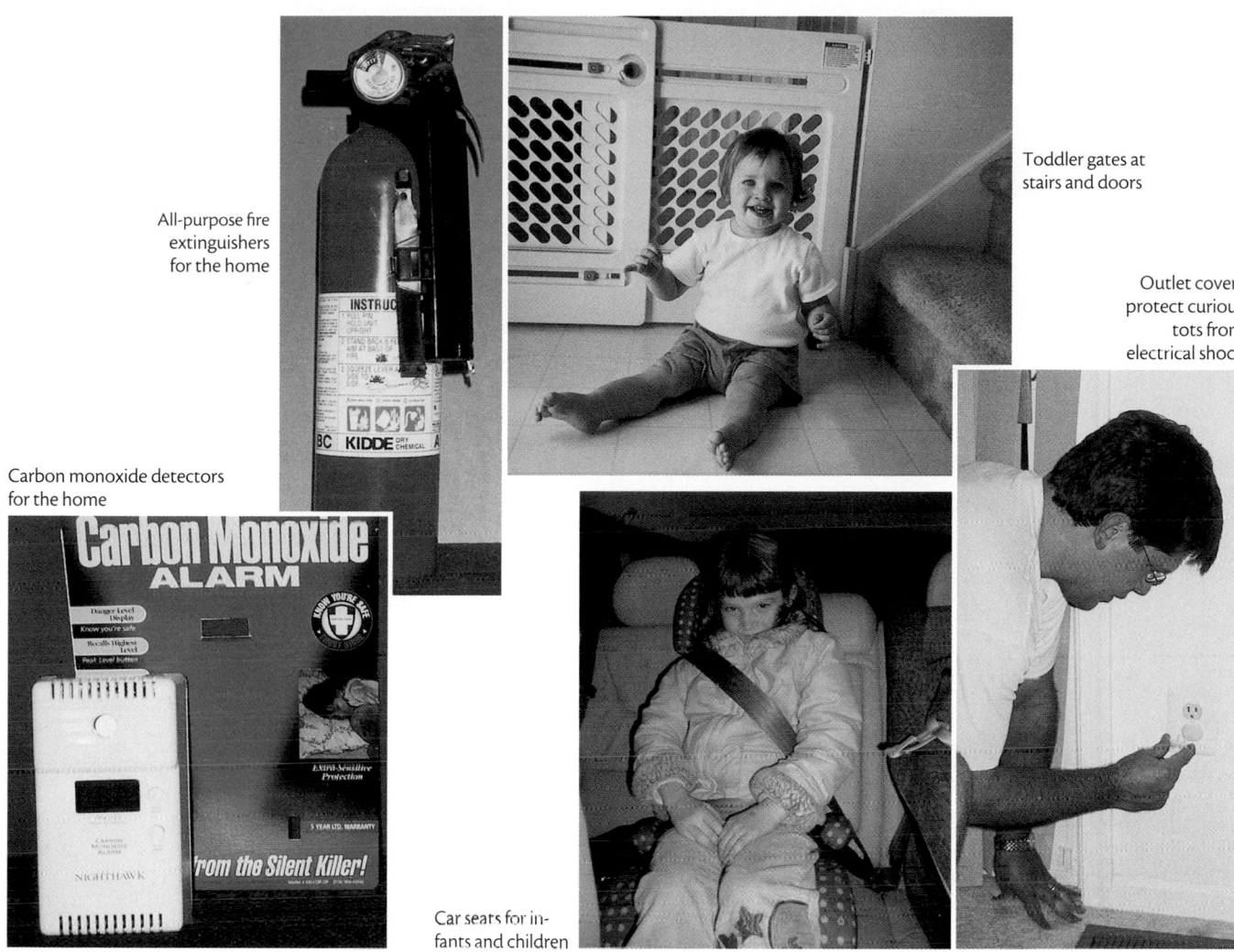

All-purpose fire extinguishers for the home

Carbon monoxide detectors for the home

Toddler gates at stairs and doors

Outlet covers protect curious tots from electrical shock

Car seats for infants and children

FIGURE 26-3 The nurse's responsibilities in home safety are primarily that of education and counseling, including providing information about home safety devices and sources for additional information. (Photos © B. Proud.)

minor accidents at school often provides an opportunity for additional preventive teaching. School nurses also interact with parents. In this setting, formal or informal health teaching can occur and should also include encouragement to do the following:

- Monitor the child's use of the Internet
- Get involved in school activities and ask pertinent questions
- Volunteer for safety committees that include staff and parents
- Ensure that the school's emergency preparedness plan is current

Preventing Injury

Injury control includes preventing injuries, providing acute care for injured patients, and rehabilitation services (Mace et al., 2001). Most importantly, injury prevention allows for the reduction of injuries through eliminating risky events, measuring the consequences of these events, and reducing the severity of injuries. There are many strategies for preventing injury. One method includes the four E's (Mace et al., 2001):

- Engineering: this can decrease or eliminate injuries by modifying the environment
- Enforcement: laws or regulations that can modify individual behavior
- Education: persuading individuals at risk to change their behavior
- Economics: create financial incentives for implementation of injury control measures

Addressing Developmental Considerations

Teaching to Promote Health at Home 26-1 lists common types of accidents according to developmental age, along with sample teaching tips that should be discussed with parents and in the school. The following discussions of developmental stages are also applicable to teaching.

Neonate and Infant

Safety considerations begin with an awareness of behaviors that may harm the developing fetus. Newborns of mothers

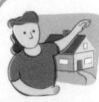

Teaching to Promote Health at Home 26-1
Preventing Accidents and Promoting Safety at Varying Developmental Stages

Developmental Stage/ Safety Risks	Sample Teaching Tip	Why is This Important?
Fetus Abnormal growth & development	• Abstain from alcohol and caffeine while pregnant. • Stop smoking or reduce the number of cigarettes smoked per day. • Avoid all drugs, including OTC drugs, unless prescribed by a physician or midwife. • Avoid exposure to pesticides and certain environmental chemicals. • Avoid exposure to radiation.	Any factors, chemical or physical, can adversely affect the fertilized ovum, embryo, and developing fetus. A fetus is extremely vulnerable to environmental hazards.
Neonate (first 28 days of life) Infection Falls SIDS	• Wash hands frequently. • Never leave infant unsupervised on a raised surface without side rails. • Use appropriate infant car seat that is secured in the back seat facing the rear of the car. • Handle infant securely while supporting the head. • Place infant on back to sleep.	Physical care for the newborn includes maintaining a patent airway, protecting the baby from infection and injury, and providing optimal nutrition.
Infant Falls Injuries from toys Burns Suffocation or drowning Inhalation or ingestion of foreign bodies	• Supervise child closely to prevent injury. • Select toys appropriate for developmental level. • Use appropriate safety equipment in the home (eg, locks for cabinets, gates, electrical outlet covers). • Never leave child alone in the bathtub. • Childproof the entire house.	Infants progress from rolling over to sitting, crawling, and pulling up to stand. They are very curious and will explore everything in their environment that they can.
Toddler Falls Cuts from sharp objects Burns Suffocation or drowning Inhalation or ingestion of foreign bodies/poisons	• Have poison control center phone number in readily accessible location. • Use appropriate car seat for toddler. • Supervise child closely to prevent injury. • Childproof house to ensure that poisonous products, drugs, and small objects are out of toddler's reach. • Never leave child alone and unsupervised outside. • Keep all hot items on stove out of child's reach.	Toddlers accomplish a wide variety of developmental tasks and progress to walking and talking. They become more independent and continue to explore their environment.
Preschooler Falls Cuts Burns Drowning Inhalation or ingestion Guns and weapons	• Teach child to wear proper safety equipment when riding bicycles or scooters. • Ensure that playing areas are safe. • Begin to teach safety measures to child. • Do not leave child alone in the bathtub or near water. • Practice emergency evacuation measures. • Teach about fire safety.	Though more independent, preschoolers still have an immature understanding of dangerous behavior. They may strive to imitate adults and thus attempt dangerous behavior.
School-aged child Burns Drowning Broken bones Inhalation or ingestion Guns and weapons Substance abuse	• Teach accident prevention at school and home. • Teach child to wear safety equipment when playing sports. • Continue immunizations as scheduled. • Provide drug, alcohol, and sexuality education. • Reinforce use of seat belts and pedestrian safety.	School-aged children have developed more refined muscular coordination, but increasing involvement in sports and play activities increases their risk for injury. Cognitive maturity improves their ability to understand safety instructions.

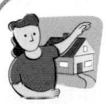

Teaching to Promote Health at Home 26-1
Preventing Accidents and Promoting Safety at Varying Developmental Stages

Developmental Stage/ Safety Risks	Sample Teaching Tip	Why is This Important?
Adolescent Drowning Motor vehicle accidents Guns and weapons Inhalation and ingestion	• Teach responsibilities of new freedoms that accompany being a teenager. • Enroll teen in safety courses (driver education, water safety, emergency care measures). • Emphasize gun safety. • Get physical examination before participating in sports. • Make time to listen to and talk with your adolescent (helps with stress reduction). • Follow healthy lifestyle (nutrition, rest, etc.). • Teach about sexuality, sexually transmitted diseases, and birth control. • Encourage child to report any sexual harassment or abuse of any kind.	Adolescence is a critical period in growth and development. The adolescent needs increasing freedom and responsibility to prepare for adulthood. During this time, the mind has a great ability to acquire and use knowledge. The teen's peer group is a greater influence than parents during this stage.

who smoke have a lower birthweight. Excessive alcohol consumption and use of drugs may cause adverse effects that are readily apparent at birth. Reinforce a pregnant woman's knowledge of the risks associated with excess alcohol consumption, smoking, drug use, and exposure to other dangers in the environment (see Teaching to Promote Health at Home 26-1).

The nurse has many opportunities to educate parents about safety and accident prevention for infants and young children. Young infants' lack of mobility limits opportunities for hazardous activity, but minimal safeguards are vital to prevent accidents. Safe care includes never leaving the infant unattended, using crib rails, and monitoring the setting for objects that the infant could place in the mouth and swallow. As the baby becomes more active, parents and caregivers must be alert to hazards that a curious, mobile child may encounter. All items within reach must be carefully inspected and, if dangerous, kept in a safe place. Because infants frequently climb or pull up on objects, hot liquids must be placed out of their reach.

All 50 states mandate the use of infant car seats and carriers when transporting a child in a motor vehicle. According to the Centers for Disease Control and Prevention, nearly 40% of all children still ride without seat belts or child safety seats (CDC, 2001). A rear-facing safety seat placed in the back seat is recommended for infants who are younger than 1 year old and weigh less than 20 lb (9.1 kg). The high force of sudden air bag inflation can cause injury to an infant in a safety seat or a child in the front seat. A recent study by the National Safe Kids Campaign found that 85% of parents use car seats incorrectly (Taft, Michalide & Taft, 1999). Most parents do not secure the car seat tightly enough with the seat belt or fail to tighten the car seat's harness straps. These seemingly small mistakes can lead to tragic consequences. Additional safety

counseling measures that focus on health teaching for this developmental level are included in Teaching to Promote Health at Home 26-1.

Toddler and Preschooler

To prevent accidental injury and death in toddlers and preschoolers, parents need to childproof the home environment. Play areas should allow for exploration but still provide for safety. Vigilant supervision by parents and guardians should anticipate hazards in the environment and protect the child with precautionary devices.

> *Remember Juanita Flores, the mother of the infant with failure to thrive who fell off a cot. As part of the plan of care, the nurse would review safe infant care with Juanita and also provide anticipatory guidance related to toddler safety in preparation for the child's discharge home.*

Childproofing products are available that help parents and children recognize dangerous items in the home.

Ingestion of poisons or medications is a major threat for preschoolers. Their overconfidence and initiative also make them more likely to dart into the street while chasing a ball, climb into a discarded refrigerator, or play with matches. A child who is older than 1 year of age and between 20 and 40 lb should be placed in a forward-facing safety seat in the back seat of the vehicle. An older child who must ride in the front seat should wear both shoulder and lap belts, and the seat should be moved as far back as possible to minimize danger from a deploying air bag.

Protecting a child also includes being alert to manifestations that indicate child abuse (see Box 26-1, Physical and Behavioral Manifestations of Child Abuse). In 1998, almost 1 million

BOX 26-1 Physical and Behavioral Manifestations of Child Abuse

History of similar injuries
Multiple or unexplained bruises
Multiple fractures
Thermal burns in a pattern
Scars or welts
Bite marks
Multiple fractures
Vaginal discharge
Urinary tract infection
Genital pain, itching, redness, or bruising
Sexually transmitted disease
Sleeping problems (nightmares)
Psychosomatic illnesses
Excessive sexual curiosity or play
Decreased attendance and performance in school
Fear of strangers
Suspicion of abuse

Adapted from Carlson, D. (1998). Uncovering the clues of child abuse. *Nursing, 28*(11), 32hn10–11; and Herendeen, P. (2002). Evaluation of physical abuse in children. Solid suspicion should be your guide. *Advance for Nurse Practitioners, 10*(8):32–37.

children in the United States were either at risk for child abuse or experienced it (CDC, 2001; Mulryan et al., 2000). Abuse can be physical, sexual, or emotional and may also be a result of neglect. All 50 states have laws that require healthcare personnel to report suspected child abuse. Health teaching topics that help safeguard toddlers and preschoolers are included in Teaching to Promote Health at Home 26-1.

School-Aged Child

As a child becomes more independent during the school years, accidents continue to be a leading cause of death. Although these children are increasingly independent, they still need help avoiding activities that are potentially dangerous. The nurse should counsel parents of school-aged children about specific interventions for safety at home, at school, and in the neighborhood.

Each year a significant number of children under the age of 10 are injured in bicycle accidents. Many of these injuries involve the head or face, and 10% of all pediatric trauma deaths are directly related to injuries sustained in a bicycle crash (Coffman, 2003). The protective effect of bicycle helmets among children is well documented, but their use is far from universal. Studies indicate that legislation and injury prevention strategies have had a positive impact on increasing helmet use and decreasing the number and severity of bicycle accidents that result in a head injury in this very vulnerable population. Because of their multiple experiences with children and parents, nurses have many opportunities for health teaching related to bicycle safety and helmet use. Points to include in any teaching session include the following:

- Children should wear helmets at all times when riding a bicycle.

- Young children who are secured in a child seat as a passenger on a bicycle should also wear a properly sized helmet.
- The helmet should rest flat on the top of the child's head (approximately 1″ above the eyebrows) and fit snugly.
- The chin strap on the helmet should be adjusted so that it fits securely. If you can slide two fingers under the strap, the helmet is too loose.
- Any helmet that is involved or damaged in a crash should be discarded and replaced.
- Parents are effective role models for their children when they also wear helmets when riding a bicycle.

Whether in the emergency department or a well-child setting, nurses are in a key position to promote strategies that prevent bicycle injuries.

The possibility of child abduction also needs to be addressed for this age group. Children may be kidnapped by unknown individuals or by someone they recognize. Some suffer sexual assault or are murdered by their captors. Adults who prey on children often take advantage of the innocence and trusting nature of children to persuade the child to accompany them. Even young children need basic instructions on how to recognize and respond to a potentially dangerous situation. Health teaching should also emphasize the need for parents to be alert and vigilant at all times regarding the whereabouts of their children.

Adolescent

Nurses and parents should collaborate to reinforce safety behaviors in adolescents. Much of the adolescent's time is spent away from home, with his or her peer group, or in automobiles. Adolescents are particularly at risk for motor vehicle accidents, and the U.S. Census Bureau (2002) lists motor vehicle accidents as the number-one cause of death for school-aged children, adolescents, and young adults. Adolescent drivers are less likely to drive after drinking but are more likely to have an accident when they do. Education should focus on safe driving skills and the importance of wearing a seat belt and should include discussions about drug and alcohol use.

Tobacco is an additional health problem for teenagers. More than 3 million children smoke almost 1 billion packs of cigarettes each year, a 16-year high point (Shahinian & Hawke, 1998). Half of the children who experiment with cigarettes become regular smokers, and at least one third of these children will die eventually of tobacco-related diseases. Federal law mandates a minimum age of 18 years to purchase tobacco products and bans billboard advertising within 1000 feet of schools and playgrounds. Research has indicated that educational programs and information can play a role in delaying or preventing smoking among young adults (Sarna & Lillington, 2002).

Body piercing has become increasingly popular with adolescents and young adults in recent years. Common sites include the ears, nose, eyebrows, lips, tongue, nipples, navel, and genitals. It is a quick procedure that does not require anesthesia, but the risk for infection is real. The U.S. and Canadian Red

Cross will not accept blood donations from anyone who has had a body piercing within the past year because of the risk for contracting hepatitis B virus from unsterile instruments or an unclean environment. Transmission of human immunodeficiency virus (HIV) is also possible, although less likely. Few states regulate body piercing. Meticulous post-piercing care reduces the risk for developing an infection. Nurses need to be informed about the health risks in order to be effective and well-informed health educators (Armstrong, 1998).

There are significant security issues related to adolescents and the use of guns. According to a recent CDC report (2001), in 1997, 85% of young homicide victims died of gunshot wounds. Teret et al. (1998) reported that 65% of adolescents who committed suicide used a gun. Adolescents need encouragement and education about ways to solve arguments without guns and violence and guidance and direction for developing a healthful lifestyle while coping with the stresses of daily living.

Think back to Kara Greenwood, the adolescent who is to present a discussion on adolescent dangers. Numerous issues face adolescents today, and providing safety information is crucial to help adolescents make mature decisions about health hazards they are likely to encounter.

Refer to Teaching to Promote Health at Home 26-1 for additional safety topics.

Adult

Young and middle-aged adults need to be reminded about the effects of stress on their lifestyle and health. Coping with the demands of raising a family and succeeding in a career may lead to unsafe health habits and a reliance on drugs or alcohol.

Domestic violence is widespread in the United States. Studies indicate that one in four women are victims of domestic violence at some point in their life (Gerard, 2000). Many men who batter their spouses also batter their children. Recent evidence suggests a relationship between childhood sexual abuse and certain physical symptoms in adulthood, such as gastrointestinal symptoms, eating disorders, and substance abuse. The nurse may be involved directly in health education and counseling measures or may suggest other resources to the family as additional support for safety and well-being and to interrupt the cycle of violence. The acronym RADAR has proved helpful in screening, assessment, and intervention in abuse cases:

- Routinely screen all female patients over age 14 for obvious signs of abuse as well as stress-related complaints and other physical symptoms.
- Ask simple, direct questions in a safe environment.
- Document your findings objectively and use direct quotes from the victim.
- Assess the safety of the victim and her children and determine the need for shelter and the person's willingness to go to one.

- Review options and referrals, including crisis hotlines, police phone numbers, and lists of available shelters (Gerard, 2000).

Older Adult

Most accidents that involve older adults are preventable. Falls, fires, and motor vehicle accidents are significant hazards for this age group. In 1998, falls were the leading cause of injury-related deaths in adults 65 years and older (CDC, 2001). Visual changes, slowed reaction time, and impaired thinking due to mental illness are realistic concerns that affect the older driver. Some become overly cautious, whereas others are prone to careless behavior. Interventions to help older adults drive safely include maintaining the automobile in optimal driving condition, scheduling regular eye examinations, wearing corrective lenses when necessary, and keeping noise from the radio and other equipment to a minimum. Some states require additional testing for older adults before they can renew their driver's license.

Older adults are at greater risk for suffering burn injuries. Confusion, forgetfulness, and diminished visual and olfactory senses are factors. Accidental overdosing on medications is also a safety risk, possibly related to poor eyesight or confusion. Special devices such as medication trays can be prefilled and help prevent older patients from taking additional doses. Additional health teaching interventions directed at helping to promote a safe environment for older patients at home are included in Teaching to Promote Health at Home 26-1.

Orienting the Person to Surroundings

A person who is familiar with his or her surroundings is less likely to suffer an accidental injury. As part of the hospital admission routine, orient the patient to the safety features and equipment in the room. An explanation and demonstration of the adjustable bed and side rails, call system, telephone, television, and bathroom help the patient adjust to the new environment. The patient identification bracelet and a discussion of agency routine further ensure safety and assist the patient to adapt to the unfamiliar setting. Similarly, teach the importance of orienting an older person to new surroundings when the older person moves in with a family member or other caregiver.

Preventing Falls
Preventing Falls in the Home

Major causes of falls in the home include slippery surfaces, poor lighting, clutter, and improperly fitting clothing or slippers. Common traffic pathways in the home, the bathroom, and access areas to and from the home are hazardous areas for older adults. Measures as simple as installing hand rails in bathrooms and on stairs, ensuring good lighting, and discarding or repairing broken equipment around the home help prevent accidents (see Box 26-4, Home Safety Checklist, later in this chapter). Safety assessments by the nurse can play a vital role in promoting safety in the home.

Consider Bessie Washington, the older woman who walks with a walker after suffering a cerebrovascular accident. Key to the patient's plan of care would be a thorough home safety assessment by the home care nurse. This assessment would be valuable in identifying areas that promote patient safety and hazards that need to be addressed.

One simple evaluation tool, the Get Up and Go test (Kimball, 2001), can help identify patients at risk for falling. A variety of factors such as poor vision, the effects of multiple medications, lower extremity weakness, or a gait disorder can reduce the patient's mobility. The test consists of the following:

- Have the patient sit in a straight-backed chair. Observe his posture while seated.
- Instruct the patient to stand. Can he stand in one fluid motion, or does he need the use of his hands to push up into a standing position? Does he require multiple attempts to stand?
- Once the patient is standing, ask him or her to keep his or her eyes open and stand as still as possible. Then ask him to close his eyes. Observe his stability.
- Ask him to open his eyes and walk 10 feet (3 meters). Once at that point, he should turn around and walk back to the chair.

During the test, assess the patient's stability, balance, gait, and lower body strength. Any limitations in any of these areas may indicate vulnerability for a fall. A timed Get Up and Go test involves getting up from a chair, walking 10 feet, and returning to the chair. A time of 9 seconds or less indicates full mobility; 10 to 19 seconds means the person is almost completely independent. Higher times can indicate impaired mobility status (Kimball, 2001).

Older adults can improve their balance and strengthen their lower extremities through regular physical activity. The martial art of tai chi is one exercise routine that has proved particularly effective. It involves slow, deliberate movements that can be practiced almost anywhere. Tai chi helps to prevent falls by developing balance control and stability in older adults.

Preventing Falls in the Healthcare Facility

Safety measures recommended to reduce the number of falls in acute and extended care facilities are given in Box 26-2, Nursing Interventions to Prevent Falls in a Healthcare Facility. Some common safety devices used in healthcare facilities are shown in Figure 26-4.

Using Restraints in Healthcare Facilities

Restraints are physical devices used to limit a patient's movement. Side rails, geriatric chairs with attached trays, and appliances tied at the wrist, ankle, or waist are types of physical restraints. Figure 26-5 shows examples of physical restraints that can be used for adults and children. Drugs that are used to

---

BOX 26-2 Nursing Interventions to Prevent Falls in a Healthcare Facility

- Complete a risk assessment.
- Indicate risk for falling on patient's door and chart.
- Keep bed in low position.
- Keep wheels on bed and wheelchair locked.
- Leave call bell within patient's reach.
- Instruct patient regarding use of call bell.
- Answer call bells promptly.
- Leave a night light on.
- Eliminate all physical hazards in the room (clutter, wet areas on the floor).
- Provide nonskid footwear.
- Leave water, tissues, bedpan/urinal within patient's reach.
- Document and report any changes in patient's cognitive status to the physician and other nurses at the change of shift.
- Use alternative strategies when necessary instead of restraints.
- As a last resort, use the least restrictive restraint according to agency policy.
- If restraint is applied, assess patient at the required intervals.

---

control behavior and are not included in the person's normal medical regimen can be considered chemical restraints. In the past, it was considered acceptable bedside care to restrain patients to protect them from harm, but recent studies have indicated that the use of restraints for this purpose is questionable.

Older patients are more likely to be restrained than younger patients. Older patients who are restrained are eight times more likely to die than those who are not restrained, and almost 50% of restrained elderly patients fall and sustain injuries while in the physical restraints (Napierkowski, 2002). The use of restraints is definitely on the decline as healthcare providers become more educated about the risks associated with their use. The physiological hazards associated with the use of restraints include the following:

- Danger of suffocation from entrapment in side rails or an improperly applied vest
- Impaired circulation
- Altered skin integrity (eg, abrasions, skin tears, bruises)
- Pressure ulcers and contractures
- Diminished muscle and bone mass
- Fractures
- Altered nutrition and hydration
- Aspiration and breathing difficulties
- Incontinence
- Changes in mental status (eg, combativeness, depression, anger)

Research has demonstrated that restraints do not guarantee safety and in fact are associated with more lethal injuries.

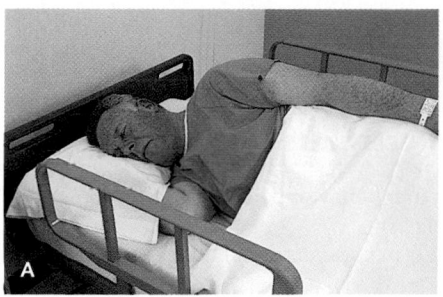 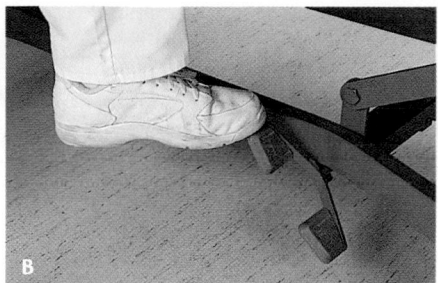 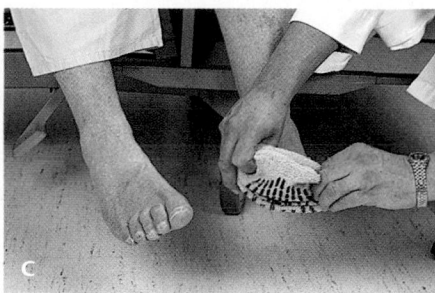

FIGURE 26-4 Some of the safety devices used in healthcare agencies and in the home to prevent falls. (**A**) Side rails on bed raised at patient's request; patient must be able to raise and lower the side rail himself. (**B**) Locking devices on wheeled equipment. (**C**) Nonskid slippers.   (Photos © B. Proud.)

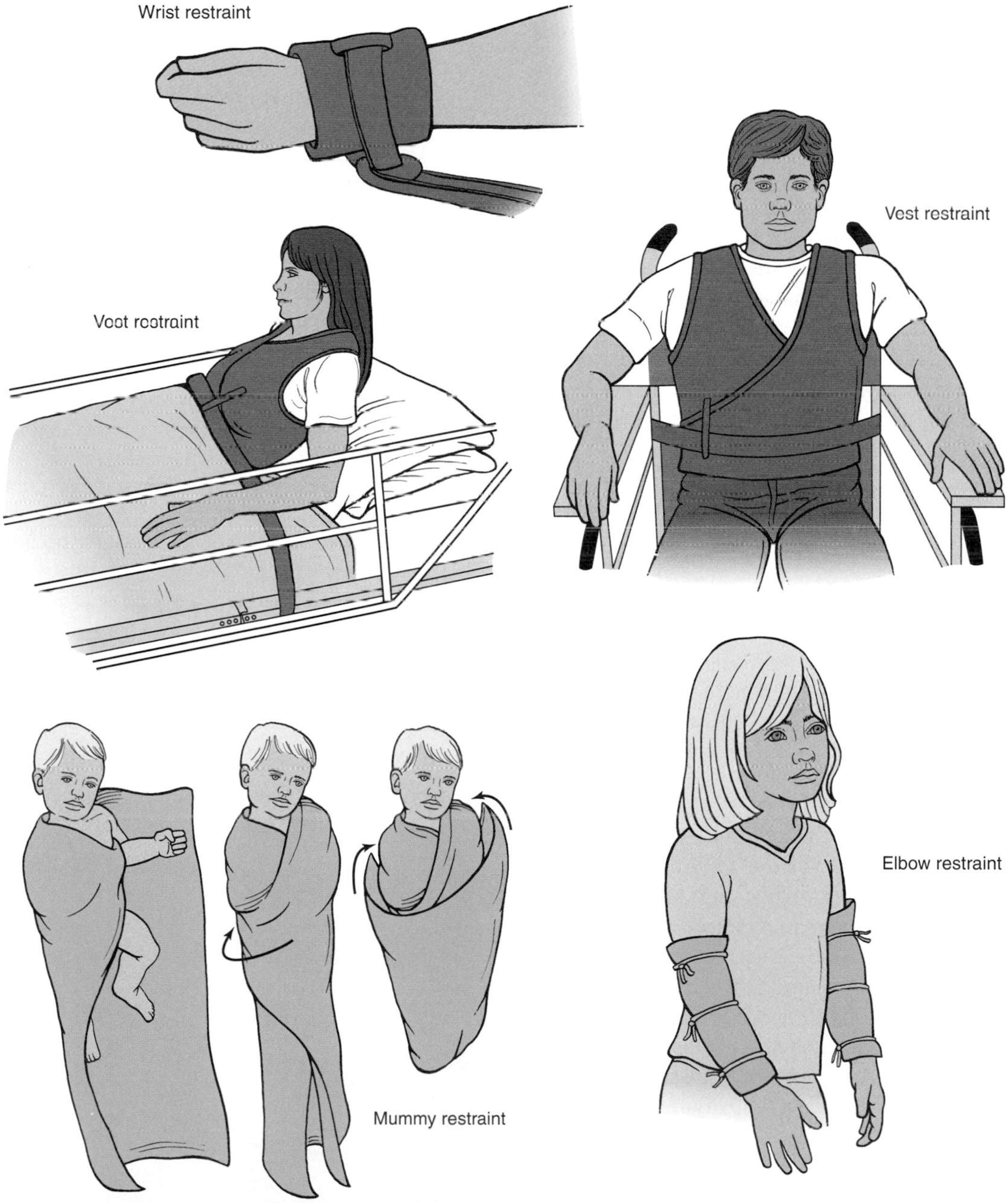

Wrist restraint

Vest restraint

Vest restraint

Mummy restraint

Elbow restraint

FIGURE 26-5 A variety of restraints used for adults and children. The purpose of restraints is to help prevent the patient from being harmed. Restraints should not interfere with physiologic functioning, such as impairing circulation, limiting muscular activity to the point of immobilization, or interfering with respiration. Restraints that can be adjusted to the desired activity limitation are most like to be accepted by the patient and family.

Since 1987, the federal government and accrediting agencies have worked to reduce or eliminate the use of restraints. Initial guidelines formulated by the Health Care Financing Administration as part of the 1987 Omnibus Budget Reconciliation Act encouraged the limited use of restraints in long-term settings. Federal and state mandates, as well as the Joint Commission on Accreditation of Healthcare Organizations (JCAHO), recommended that acute care agencies use restraints only as a last resort (Brenner & Duffy-Durnin, 1998). The JCAHO (1998), in an effort to reduce the use of restraints in all healthcare settings, stated that restraints can cause "physical and psychological harm, loss of dignity . . . and even death." Any healthcare facility that accepts Medicare and Medicaid reimbursement must abide by the federal guidelines for the use of restraints.

Using Side Rails as Restraints

In the past, side rails were used to provide support and aid equilibrium, but it is now recognized that they can pose serious risks for a confused or agitated patient. A person of small stature has a greater risk for entrapment or injury. Death from asphyxiation has occurred when patients have become wedged between the mattress and the bed frame or side rail. According to the U.S. Food and Drug Administration (FDA), between 1985 and 1999, 60% of the 371 patients who were entrapped by side rails died. Most of the victims of side rail fatalities were frail, elderly, or confused or had uncontrolled body movement (Todd, 2002). A 1995 FDA Safety Alert informed healthcare agencies of the hazards associated with side rail use.

A side rail is not considered a restraint if the patient requests that it be raised to aid in getting in or out of bed. Some patients may request that side rails be used at night while they are asleep to order to feel more secure (see Fig. 26-4a). The patient must be able to raise and lower the side rail himself or herself. If a family member requests the use of side rails for a patient, it is the nurse's responsibility to review benefits and risks associated with their use and periodically evaluate the reason for their use.

Using Alternatives to Restraints

Careful nursing assessment is the key to identifying appropriate alternatives to restraint use and finding an individualized solution (see Box 26-3, Choosing Alternatives to Restraints). Figure 26-6 shows an example of a position-sensitive electronic device (Ambularm) that is an alternative to using restraints. Nursing interventions may be used to reduce confusion or agitation and provide a safe environment. Using a restraint on an older patient who tends to wander is unjustified because a variety of alternative options can be used to keep such patients safe (see the accompanying Research in Nursing box).

Using Restraints as a Last Resort

Despite all efforts, restraints may be the only solution in some situations. The least restrictive restraint should be the first option. DiBartolo (1998) and Napierkowski (2002) recommend the following protocols when restraints are applied as a last resort:

BOX 26-3 Choosing Alternatives to Restraints

- Determine whether behavior pattern exists.
- Provide pain relief.
- Involve the family in patient's care.
- Reduce noise.
- Check environment for hazards.
- Use night light.
- Identify door of room (eg, use of balloon, sign, patient's picture, ribbon).
- Use an electronic alarm system (eg, bed or position-sensitive alarms).
- Allow restless patient to walk after ensuring that environment is safe.
- Use a large plant or piece of furniture as a barrier to limit wandering from designated area.
- Use low-height beds.
- Place floor mats on each side of the bed.
- Use therapeutic touch.
- Play music or video selections of the patient's choice.
- Use pillows wedged against the side of the chair to keep patient positioned safely.
- Use full-length body pillows.
- Assist with toileting at frequent intervals.
- Arrange for a bedside commode.
- Make the environment as homelike as possible.
- Provide a warm beverage.
- Provide comfortable rocking chairs.
- Allow the patient to assist the staff with simple tasks.
- Encourage daily exercise.
- Investigate possibility of discontinuing bothersome treatment devices (eg, intravenous line, catheter, feeding tube).

- The patient's current condition, not his or her past history, must determine the need for the restraints. They must never be applied for the convenience of the staff.
- Evaluate the potential for injury. Determine whether the patient is at increased risk for harming self or others.

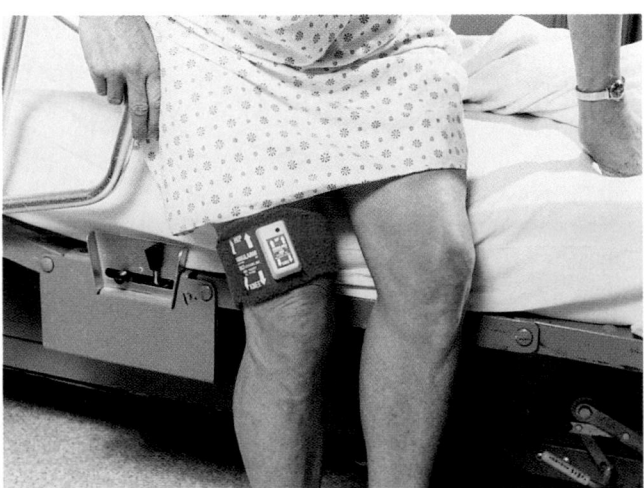

FIGURE 26-6 Ambularm device.   (Photo courtesy of AlertCare, Inc.)

Research in Nursing Making a Difference
Using Creative Alternatives to Reduce Restraint Use in a Large Medical Center

The Omnibus Budget Reconciliation Act reduced the use of restraints in long-term care centers, but this focus on restraint-free environments has not shifted to acute care facilities, even as studies continue to confirm the negative outcomes of using restraints. Acute care nurses are not as comfortable using alternatives to restraints because of their concern that critically ill patients, without restraints in place, may dislodge necessary medically invasive devices. Additional research findings and educational programs that explore alternative restraint strategies may encourage nurses in acute care settings to move toward restraint-free care.

Related Research
Coble, P., & Davis, J. (2001). Restraint reduction in a large tertiary medical center. *Journal of Nursing Administration, 31*(7/8), 344–345.

The goal of this research was to reduce restraint use in an 877-bed acute care facility and increase staff awareness of alternatives to restraints. A task force with representatives from all areas of the hospital developed a four-step approach. All types of restraints were reviewed and the vest restraint and limb holder were selected as the least restrictive, safest device; all staff received an in-service on these restraints. Additionally, a box containing various diverting activities was assembled for each nursing unit, and Activity Aprons featuring buttons, zippers, and Velcro closures were ordered and made available as needed. Finally, a 30-minute video that detailed policy revisions and demonstrated use of the diversionary box was produced and viewed by all staff members. The number of restraints purchased for an 8-month period before the interventions was compared to the 8-month period following full implementation of this program. Results indicated a 60% decrease in the number of limb holder restraints and a 13% decrease in the number of vest restraints purchased. Staff reported that the new restraint initiatives were most effective for patients with mild to moderate confusion and older postoperative patients. They were least effective for patients who were critically ill or very confused and disoriented elderly persons.

Relevance to Nursing Practice
Results of this study demonstrated that restraint use can be decreased in an acute care facility with use of creative diversionary activities. Staff also benefit from frequent updates that confirm the positive patient outcomes that result when restraints are used as a last resort. Additional research is needed to explore other innovative alternatives that can be used to distract severely confused and critically ill patients. Staffing rates and the mix of skilled workers employed in a facility might also affect restraint usage.

- The patient's family must be consulted and involved in the plan of care before applying restraints. They must be informed of the agency's policy regarding applying and removing restraints and may be asked to sign a release form to protect the agency from liability.
- Try using alternative measures first, and determine whether the alternatives are successful.
- Alert the physician if restraints are indicated. Agency policy, the JCAHO, and state and federal guidelines require an order from a physician or other healthcare professional licensed to prescribe in the state. The order should include the type of restraint, justification for the restraint, and criteria for removal. The order must never be written for p.r.n. use.
- In an emergency, the physical restraint can be applied, but a physician's order must be obtained within 1 hour. The order must state the intended duration of use.
- The patient must be monitored and assessed on a regular basis. Assessment must occur every 4 hours for an adult, at least every 2 hours for children ages 9 to 17, and at least once every hour for children under the age of 9.
- Documentation must reflect the date and time the restraint is applied, the type of restraint, alternatives that were attempted with their results, and notification of the patient's family and physician. Include the frequency of assessment, your findings, regular intervals when the restraint is removed, and nursing interventions.

Agency policies help nurses determine when to apply restraints as well as which type to use (see Focused Critical Thinking Guide 26-1). The policy reflects the institution's concern for patient safety as well as its respect for the quality of human life. Constant re-evaluation of the need for the restraint is vital. Chapter 7, Legal Implications, discusses the legal issues involved when restraints are used. Student nurses, from their earliest clinical experiences, need help to identify and assess the cause of a patient's behavior and not just the behavior itself. Careful patient assessment is needed to develop creative alternative strategies. Skill 26-1 demonstrates the proper method for applying restraints should they be necessary.

Preventing Fires and Maintaining Fire Safety

Careless smoking, faulty electrical equipment, and combustion of anesthetic agents are the most common causes of hospital fires. Orientations in healthcare agencies emphasize fire prevention information and the agency's smoking policy. Nurses are responsible for patients' safety and need to be familiar with the agency's fire safety plan, exits, the location and operation of fire extinguishers, and any special instructions for reporting a fire.

Most hospital procedures emphasize the following priorities and recommend that staff members remember the acronym RACE as a guide:

Focused Critical Thinking Guide 26-1

Restraints

You are a nursing student caring for Mrs. Mitchell, an 82-year-old nursing home resident who was admitted to a community hospital for treatment of dehydration secondary to pneumonia. Convalescing well, she is now allowed short periods of assisted ambulation and may sit up as tolerated. On the morning you first meet her, she is awake and demanding angrily to have her vest restraint removed so that she can walk independently to the bathroom. You remove her restraint, help her to the bathroom, and wonder whether or not to reapply the restraint as you get her back into bed. She seems clear-headed and tells you she has no idea why she is being tied to the bed since she knows enough to use her light to get help when she needs it. She demands you to take the restraint away and pulls back angrily when you attempt to place it over her head. You don't remember any mention of a restraint order when you read her chart the previous day and have not yet gotten report from the charge nurse. Your options are to leave her unrestrained while you clarify the need for the restraint or restrain her until you can ascertain the need. You like Mrs. Mitchell and feel sorry that anyone should have to be restrained and are reluctant to wrestle with an 82-year-old woman.

1. Goal of Thinking

Short term: Reach a prudent decision about the need to restrain Mrs. Mitchell until you can clarify the need for the restraint with the charge nurse.

Long term: Evaluate the implications of restraining patients in different types of situations to facilitate future decision making.

2. Adequacy of Knowledge

Pertinent circumstances: In her weakened condition, this patient may be at high risk for falls, and should she attempt to get out of bed unassisted, a fall is a real possibility. You feel sympathetic to her plight of being tied in bed against her will and wonder whether violating patient dignity and liberty is something nurses are routinely expected to do. You are unsure of your legal risk but feel fairly certain that you are responsible for keeping her safe and that not to do so could be grounds for negligence. No other students or staff nurses are in the room, and you cannot clarify the order without leaving the patient unattended.

Prerequisite knowledge: To make a decision in this situation, you need knowledge about the patient's need to be restrained and the benefits and risks of restraining and not restraining her. Given the situation of conflicting goods—preserving her dignity and liberty versus maintaining safety—you need to know how to determine which good ought to triumph in this situation. You should be familiar with the hospital's restraint policy and understand your moral and legal obligations. For example, failure to restrain her may be construed as negligence, whereas restraining her against her will may be assault and battery.

Room for error: Given the significant risks you are incurring by choosing either option—potential fall versus assault to

human dignity—there is little room for error. Until you know what her risk for fall is, you should err on the side of caution.

Time constraints: You may have time to wait with the patient until another nurse comes into the room who can stay with the patient until you clarify her need to be restrained. If this is not an option, you will need to decide quickly in order to be attentive to other priorities: getting report, beginning patient care, and so forth.

3. Potential Problems

- Sincere desire to do the right thing but great anxiety about not knowing what this is
- Untested, intuitive sense that restraining an alert, uncooperative patient is wrong under any circumstances
- Fear that if you don't restrain her and she falls, you will be legally responsible
- Fear of making a wrong clinical decision that will jeopardize your clinical grade
- Hope that your good interpersonal skills may save the day and buy you the time you need to get help

4. Helpful Resources

Key resources include experienced colleagues, nursing instructor, charge nurse, hospital policy, professional literature on restraint use, hospital risk manager, patient bill of rights.

5. Critique of Judgment/Decision

There are basically two options: to restrain or not restrain Mrs. Mitchell until you can clarify the need for a restraint. If you restrain her and there is no need, you run the risk of increasing her agitation and violating her dignity. If you fail to restrain her and the restraint is needed, she may fall and suffer a concussion or fractured hip. You decide to reapply the restraint carefully after explaining to Mrs. Mitchell that you are a student nurse and need to check the order for the restraint before leaving it off. Given all your uncertainties, you decide that maintaining the patient's safety ought to be your first priority until you determine whether there are overriding considerations. Mrs. Mitchell is not happy with your decision but seems to understand your reasoning and does not fight you when you reapply the vest restraint. You promise to return quickly and keep your promise.

When you talk with the charge nurse she tells you that there is no need for Mrs. Mitchell to be restrained and that she will investigate why the night nurse applied the restraint. You happily return to Mrs. Mitchell and remove the restraint. You later meet with your instructor to see what you can do to ensure that Mrs. Mitchell and other patients on the unit are not restrained for inappropriate reasons. Your instructor compliments you for reasoning well about what was in this patient's best interests. She remarks that had there been a need to restrain the patient you may have jeopardized her safety by unthinkingly following your sympathetic instinct to leave her unrestrained.

Applying Restraints

EQUIPMENT

Restraint   Padding, if necessary, for bony prominences

ACTION	RATIONALE
1. Determine the need for restraints. Assess patient's physical condition, behavior, and mental status.	Restraints should be used only as a last resort when alternative measures have failed, and the patient is at increased risk for harming himself or others.
2. Confirm agency policy for application of restraints. Secure a physician's order.	Policy protects the patient and the nurse and specifies guidelines for application as well as type of restraint and duration.
3. Explain reason for use to patient and family. Clarify how care will be given and needs will be met and that use of restraint is a temporary measure.	Explanation to patient and family may lessen confusion and anger and provide reassurance. A clearly stated agency policy on application of restraints should be available for patient and family to read. The family must give consent before a restraint is applied and be involved in the plan of care.
4. Perform hand hygiene.	Hand hygiene deters the spread of microorganisms.
5. Apply restraints according to manufacturer's direction:	Proper application ensures that there is no interference with patient's respiration and circulation. The U.S. Food and Drug Administration advises manufacturers to place "front" and "back" labels on vest restraints and that correct size be used.
a. Choose the least restrictive type of device that allows the greatest possible degree of mobility.	This provides minimal restriction.
b. Pad bony prominences.	Padding prevents skin breakdown.
c. For restraint applied to extremity, ensure that two fingers can be inserted between the restraint and patient's wrist or ankle.	This prevents impaired circulation to extremity.
d. Maintain restrained extremity in normal anatomic position.	This lessens possibility of contracture or musculoskeletal injury.
e. Use appropriate tie for all restraints.	A quick-release knot ensures that restraint will not tighten when pulled and can be removed quickly in an emergency.
f. Fasten restraint to the bedframe, *not the side rail*. Site should not be readily accessible to the patient.	Restraint secured to a side rail may injure the patient when side rail is lowered. Tying restraint out of patient's reach promotes security.

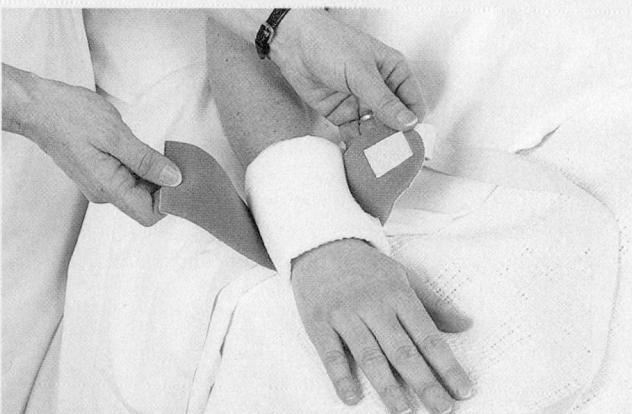

Action 5b: Applying restraint over padded bony prominences.

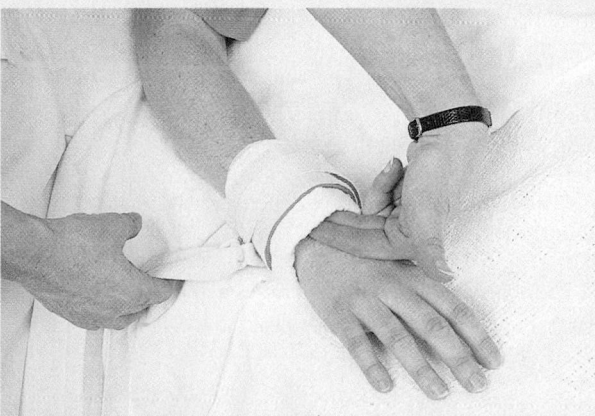

Action 5c: Ensuring that two fingers can be inserted between the restraint and the wrist.

(continued)

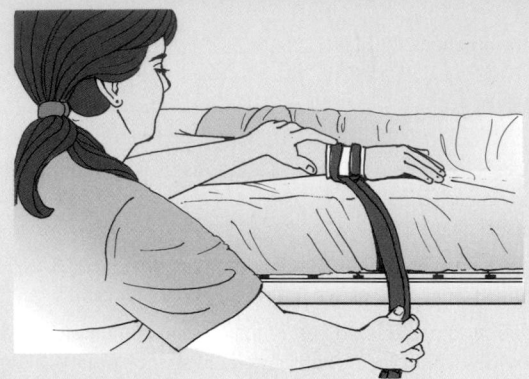

Action 5d: Keeping extremity in normal anatomic position.

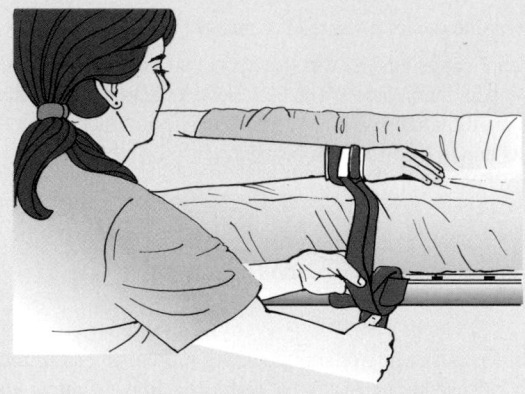

Action 5f: Fastening restraint to bed frame.

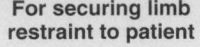

**For securing limb
restraint to patient**

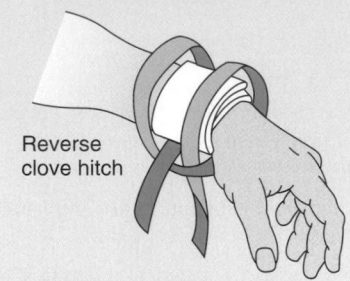

Reverse
clove hitch

**For securing restraint
to bedframe**

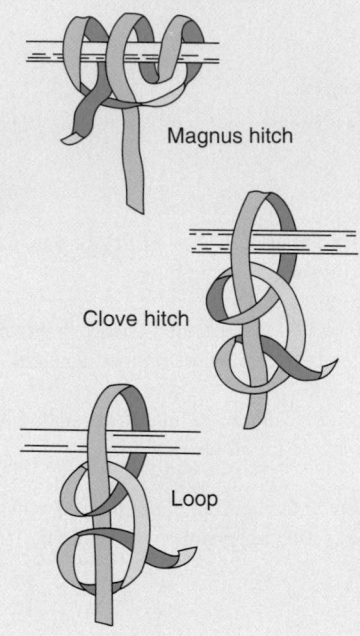

Magnus hitch

Clove hitch

Loop

Action 5e: Knots for restraints.

ACTION	RATIONALE
6. Remove restraint at least every 2 hours or according to agency policy and patient need.	Removal allows for assessment of patient and reevaluation of need for restraint. Assessment must be documented and occur on a regular basis.
a. Check for signs of decreased circulation or impaired skin integrity.	Improperly applied restraints may cause skin tears, abrasions, or bruises. Decreased circulation may result in paleness, coolness, decreased sensation, tingling, numbness, or pain in an extremity.
b. Perform range-of-motion exercises before reapplying.	Exercise increases circulation in the restrained extremity.
7. Reassure patient at regular intervals. Store call bell within easy reach.	Reassurance demonstrates caring and provides opportunity for sensory stimulation as well as ongoing assessment and evaluation. Call bell can summon assistance quickly.
8. Assess for signs of sensory deprivation, such as increased sleeping, day-dreaming, anxiety, panic, and hallucinations.	Use of restraints may decrease environmental stimulation and result in sensory deprivation.
9. Perform hand hygiene.	Handwashing deters the spread of microorganisms.
10. Document reason for restraining patient, alternative measures attempted before applying the restraint, date and time of application, type of restraint, times when removed, and result and frequency of nursing assessment every 2 hours. Obtain a new order after 24 hours if restraints are still necessary.	Careful documentation supports use of restraints, alternative measures to ensure safety, and assessment data. The Joint Commission on Accreditation of Healthcare Organizations recommends a 24-hour restraint limit for all nonpsychiatric patients.

- Rescue anyone in immediate danger.
- Activate the fire code system and notify the appropriate person.
- Confine the fire by closing doors and windows.
- Evacuate patients and other people to a safe area.

Type ABC fire extinguishers, the most common kind used in healthcare agencies, contain a material similar to baking soda that can be used on any type of fire.

In the home setting, cigarettes, grease, and electrical problems are most often responsible for fires. Educating parents

about home fire safety includes having a plan of action similar to that used in healthcare settings. Priorities and practical suggestions for fire and burn safety are included in Box 26-4, Home Safety Checklist.

Preventing Poisoning

Concerted efforts by individuals, communities, state governments, and the federal government have reduced the number of accidental deaths by poisoning. Childproof containers are primarily responsible for this reduction. Nursing interventions

---

BOX 26-4 Home Safety Checklist

Fire and Burn Safety

Have a list of emergency phone numbers posted near the phone.

Install smoke detectors in each room (or at a minimum, on each floor).

Replace smoke detector batteries when you reset your clock.

Have a fire extinguisher available on each floor, and know how to use it.

Practice a fire escape plan with your family.

Teach all family members to stop, drop, and roll if clothing catches on fire.

Keep matches and lighters out of reach of children.

Keep lighted candles out of children's reach.

Buy flame-resistant children's clothing, particularly sleepwear.

Keep bedroom doors closed while sleeping (use monitor to listen for a child).

Have ashtrays readily available if there is a smoker in the house.

Enforce a strict "no smoking in bed" policy.

After a party, check waste baskets, ashtrays, furniture, and carpets for carelessly discarded cigarettes.

Turn off a kerosene heater when no one is in the room and at bedtime.

Operate your fireplace or wood-burning stove safely (flue open, firescreen covering the opening, annual chimney cleaning, proper disposal of ashes).

Prevent trash or paint-saturated rags from accumulating in your garage.

Store oily rags, gasoline, or other flammables away from heating sources or open flames, such as the pilot light of the water heater.

Cook on back burners, and turn pot handles toward the back of the stove.

Keep hot dishes away from the edges of tables and counters.

Set water at a safe temperature (below 120°F).

Check bath water temperature with the back of your wrist before placing a child in bath.

Use sunscreen and protective clothing to minimize exposure to the sun and prevent sunburn.

Electrical Safety

Maintain electrical cords in good condition.

Protect unused electric outlets with safety covers.

Use the proper replacement for a blown fuse.

Keep an electric space heater away from curtains and flammable material.

Turn off appliances before going to bed or leaving the house.

Hire a professional to do electrical repairs.

Never overload wall outlets or extension cords.

Unplug appliances that are not in use.

Do not permit children to use the microwave.

Preventing Poisoning

Keep the phone number for the local poison control center next to the phone.

Color-code medication bottles for those who are visually impaired.

Keep the emergency drug syrup of ipecac in the home, but only administer when recommended by a physician or the Poison Control Center (1-800-222-1222).

Store all medicines in child-resistant containers in a locked medicine cabinet.

Destroy old medicines (flush down the toilet).

Keep all poisonous plants out of a child's reach.

Avoid eating any fresh or prepared foods that look or smell spoiled.

Store cleaning products, insecticides, and corrosives safely out of a child's reach.

Avoid mixing caustic products with any other household product (dangerous chemical reactions may occur).

Keep shampoos and cosmetics in a safe place.

Use safety latches on cabinets.

Store alcoholic beverages out of a child's reach.

Check that paint or finish on furniture and toys is nontoxic.

Install a carbon monoxide detector in your home.

Have your furnace professionally inspected each year.

Keep vents and chimneys clear of debris, and have them checked seasonally.

Don't operate cars, motorized equipment, or charcoal or gas grills in enclosed spaces.

Preventing Falls and Other Injuries

Keep stairways clear and uncluttered.

Maintain walkways, stairs, and railings in good repair.

Keep stairs, hallways, outside walkways, and working areas well lit.

Install safety gates at tops and bottoms of stairways.

Paint the bottom step of the stairs a different color.

Apply nonslip adhesive strips to the bottom surface of the tub or shower.

Have a raised toilet seat with support arms available if necessary.

Provide grab bars next to the toilet and in the tub or shower area.

(continued)

BOX 26-4 (Continued)

Use sturdy chairs that have armrests.

Eliminate scatter rugs, or secure them with adhesive strips on the underside.

Use a handheld device, such as pincers, when reaching for inaccessible items.

Buckle a child into an approved automobile safety seat even when making short trips.

Firearm Safety

Keep guns and ammunition stored separately and locked up.

Install trigger locks on all guns.

Make certain that the key to the locked gun storage area is not available to a child or young person.

Discuss the risk for injury from guns with your children.

Instruct your child never to touch a gun or remain in a friend's house where a gun is accessible.

Preventing Asphyxiation or Choking

Keep plastic bags out of a child's reach.

Check that crib slats are no more than $2\frac{3}{8}$ inches apart.

Ensure that the mattress fits the sides of the crib snugly.

Remove soft pillows or thick blankets from your infant's crib.

Never place an infant on a waterbed to sleep.

Cut food into small pieces before giving it to a young child.

Supervise young children when eating and drinking.

Avoid giving peanuts, hard candy, or other small treats to a young child.

Keep small objects, such as jewelry, buttons, and safety pins, out of a child's reach.

Use toys appropriate for the child's age.

Always watch a child who is in the tub.

Cover wading pools and sandboxes when not in use.

Check that nearby swimming pools are enclosed with a fence that your child cannot easily climb over.

Keep pool rescue equipment nearby.

Supervise your child closely when near water.

Know how to perform cardiopulmonary resuscitation and the Heimlich maneuver.

involve health education aimed at preventing accidental poisoning in the home. Every household must have the telephone number of the nearest poison control center readily available. Emphasize that parents should call the poison control center immediately, before attempting any home remedy. Parents may be instructed to bring the child immediately to an emergency facility for treatment. The focus of emergency treatment of poisoning is to stabilize vital body functions, prevent the absorption of the poison, and encourage excretion of the toxic substance.

Activated charcoal is considered the most effective agent for preventing absorption of the ingested toxin. It can bind with up to 60% of a toxin when given 30 to 60 minutes after the ingestion (Hayes, 2000). Syrup of ipecac is not used widely anymore because it may not remove all the poison with its emetic action. However, it still may be recommended for use with substances that are not highly toxic and when hospitalization is not required. Gastric lavage is no longer prescribed routinely for treatment of ingestion of a toxic substance because it may propel the poison into the small intestine, where absorption will occur. The amount of toxin removed by gastric lavage is relatively small.

Nursing education efforts can also change behaviors that place older adults at risk for poisoning. Although poisonings happen more frequently in children, poison control centers receive many calls from adults, particularly older adults, regarding accidental poisonings. Suggestions for preventing poisoning in older adults are included in the accompanying box, Focus on the Older Adult.

All healthcare providers should recommend that a carbon monoxide detector be installed to alert family members to toxic levels of the gas. Gas or oil companies and the local health authority can help identify and remove sources of contamination. Many communities are considering legislation requiring installation of carbon monoxide detectors by homeowners and landlords. Additional tips for preventing poisoning are provided in Box 26-4.

Preventing Suffocation

As a result of suffocation, unconsciousness, respiratory failure, and cardiac arrest can occur. Emergency measures must start without delay, beginning with the removal of any obstruction and administration of cardiopulmonary resuscitation. When teaching parents, the nurse should emphasize careful supervision of children and should outline specific situations that place children at risk for suffocation. Health education is a valuable preventive force. Refer to the Home Safety Checklist in Box 26-4 for specific interventions.

Preventing Injury From Firearms

Nurses are in a unique position to raise awareness and to help reduce high-risk behavior that may lead to firearm injuries and deaths. In homes, schools, and other healthcare settings, nurses can provide information on how parents can keep guns out of the hands of children. Parents may be unaware of how common gunshot injuries are or unaware of the dangers that can occur when a gun is accessible to children and young adults. As a prevention partner, the nurse can begin to have an impact on the epidemic of gun-related injuries and death. The Home Safety Checklist in Box 26-4 recommends measures to prevent injury from firearms.

Preventing Equipment-Related Accidents

With the marked increase in the use of highly sophisticated electronic equipment in healthcare settings, healthcare practitioners must learn to use the equipment properly and must recognize signs of malfunctioning equipment. Suction devices

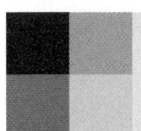

Focus on the Older Adult
Nursing Strategies to Prevent Poisoning

Age-Related Changes	Nursing Strategies
Confusion	• Do not hesitate to call the physician, nurse or pharmacist with any questions. • Develop good communication with your physician, nurse, and pharmacist. • Use a medication calendar or diary to keep track of your dosing schedule. • Use a pill dispenser as a reminder tool.
Reduced vision	• Request large-print labels from your pharmacist.
Polypharmacy	• Report side effects from medications to your healthcare provider. • Do not share medications with others or take their pills. • When a drug is discontinued, throw away any remaining medication.
Effect of drugs in the aging body	• Keep the telephone numbers for your healthcare providers and the poison control center in a readily accessible place. • Do not stop taking any prescription drug or change the dose without first consulting the physician or nurse. • Avoid doubling a dose if you forget a medication. Check with the physician or nurse first. • Avoid mixing alcohol with medicines without first checking with the pharmacist.

with inadequate vacuum and rate regulators or infusion equipment that delivers erratic amounts of solution have resulted in equipment-related accidents. Failure to use protective belts or side rails on stretchers and to lock wheelchair wheels can result in patient injury.

Electrical equipment can present a safety hazard to both the patient and healthcare practitioner when safety measures are ignored. Most electrical equipment used in hospitals is equipped with three-prong plugs. The third prong, when inserted into a properly wired wall outlet, provides a ground for the piece of equipment. A **ground** is a connection from an electricity source to the earth through which electric current leakage can be harmlessly conducted. Box 26-5 lists

guidelines to help reduce the number of equipment-related accidents.

Accidents in the home frequently result from careless use of equipment or from malfunctioning or poorly maintained equipment. Many injuries and deaths from electric shock can be prevented. Overloaded electric circuits, faulty appliances, frayed wires, careless use of electrical equipment, and handling of electrical devices and cords with wet shoes or hands can result in injury or death. Refer to the Home Safety Checklist in Box 26-4 for specific guidelines to prevent electrical injury.

Preventing Procedure-Related Accidents

The nurse must always be cautious and alert to prevent procedure-related accidents. Errors are possible when administering medications or intravenous solutions, transferring a patient, changing a dressing, or applying external heat to a patient's extremity. Therefore, nurses must follow correct procedures when administering care. Safeguards to prevent errors include making sure that the patient is identified correctly (Fig. 26-7). The nurse should use all available resources to answer any questions about correct procedure.

In an effort to promote a culture of safety, JCAHO (2003) has approved seven National Patient Safety Goals for 2004 (Box 26-6). Accreditation by JCAHO requires that a healthcare organization provide evidence that these goals have been addressed and requirements have been met. Effective alternatives may be acceptable depending on the services provided by the particular healthcare organization.

Filing an Incident Report

An accident in a healthcare agency requires filling out an **incident report,** a confidential document that objectively describes the circumstances of the accident. The report also details the

---

BOX 26-5 Decreasing Equipment-Related Accidents

• Use equipment only for the use for which it was intended.
• Do not operate equipment with which you are unfamiliar.
• Handle equipment with care to prevent damaging it.
• Use three-prong electric plugs whenever possible.
• Do not twist or bend electric cords. The wires inside the cord may break.
• Be alert to signs that indicate equipment is faulty, such as breaks in electric cords, sparks, smoke, electric shocks, loose or missing parts, and unusual noises or odors. Report signs of trouble immediately.
• Make certain that electric cords are not in a position to be trapped as beds are raised or lowered. This can strip insulation covering the electric wires.
• Be alert for wet surfaces on areas where electric cords or connections are present.

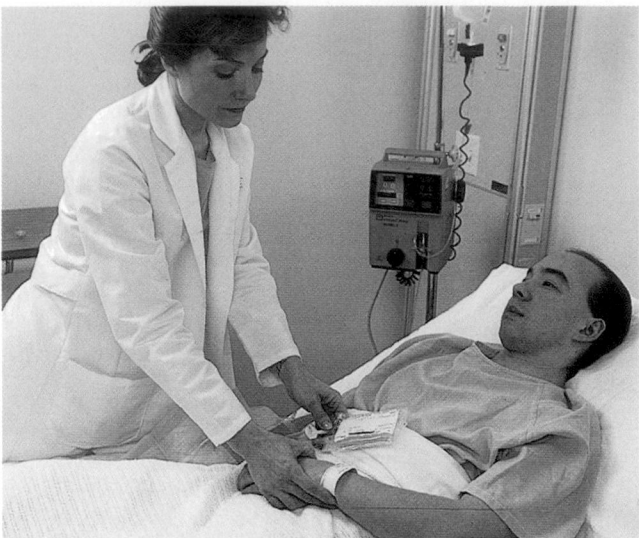

FIGURE 26-7 An essential nursing responsibility is checking the patient's identification bracelet before any procedure. Here, the nurse checks the patient's identification before administering medications.

patient's response and the examination and treatment of the patient after the incident. The nurse completes the incident report immediately after an accident and is responsible for recording the incident and its effect on the patient in the medical record. The incident report is not a part of the medical record and should not be mentioned in the documentation.

Since laws vary in different states, nurses must know their own state law regarding incident reports.

> *Recall Juanita Flores, the young mother whose child fell off the cot. As a result of the fall, an incident report was completed.*

All incident reports are reviewed carefully to detect any potentially threatening situation or pattern. Incident reports are discussed in more detail in Chapter 7.

When an incident results in a patient injury, the nurse has a responsibility to speak openly and honestly with the patient and family. The National Patient Safety Foundation (2001) provides guidelines for this type of discussion (Box 26-7).

Maintaining Emergency Preparedness

Emergency preparedness has always been a concern for healthcare workers. Nurses, as members of emergency response teams, need to be aware of their role when an emergency or disaster occurs. Existing community resources are usually sufficient to respond to an emergency situation, such as a multiple vehicle collision, a fire in an apartment complex involving a significant number of burn injuries, or an explosion or plane crash. Gebbie and Qureshi (2002) explained that a **disaster** is an event of greater magnitude that requires the response of people outside the involved community. Disasters can be categorized as natural (eg, a flood or an earthquake) or man-made (eg, a toxic spill, war, or a terrorist event). In any

---

BOX 26-6 JCAHO 2004 National Patient Safety Goals

1. Improve the accuracy of patient identification.
   a) Use at least two patient identifiers (neither to be the patient's room number) whenever taking blood samples or administering medications or blood products.
   b) Prior to the start of any surgical or invasive procedure, conduct a final verification process, such as a "time out" to confirm the correct patient, procedure, and site, using active, not passive, communication techniques.
2. Improve the effectiveness of communication among caregivers.
   a) Implement a process for taking verbal or telephone orders or critical test results that require a verification "read-back" of the complete order or test result by the person receiving the order or test result.
   b) Standardize the abbreviations, acronyms, and symbols used throughout the organization, including a list of abbreviations, acronyms, and symbols not to use.
3. Improve the safety of using high-alert medications.
   a) Remove concentrated electrolytes (including, but not limited to, potassium chloride, potassium phosphate, sodium chloride >0.9%) from patient care units.
   b) Standardize and limit the number of drug concentrations available in the organization.

4. Eliminate wrong-site, wrong-patient, wrong-procedure surgery.
   a) Create and use a preoperative verification process, such as a checklist, to confirm that appropriate documents (eg, medical records, imaging studies) are available.
   b) Implement a process to mark the surgical site and involve the patient in the marking process.
5. Improve the safety of using infusion pumps.
   a) Ensure free-flow protection on all general-use and PCA (patient-controlled analgesia) intravenous infusion pumps used in the organization.
6. Improve the effectiveness of clinical alarm systems.
   a) Implement regular preventive maintenance and testing of alarm systems.
   b) Ensure that alarms are activated with appropriate settings and are sufficiently audible with respect to distances and competing noise within the unit.
7. Reduce the risk of healthcare-acquired infections.
   a) Comply with current CDC hand hygiene guidelines.
   b) Manage as sentinel events all identified cases of unanticipated death or major permanent loss of function associated with a healthcare-acquired infection.

Source: Joint Commission on Accreditation of Healthcare Organizations. (2003). *2004 national patient safety goals.* Available at http://www.jcaho.org/accredited+organizations/patient+safety/04+npsg/04_npsg.htm.

BOX 26-7 Talking to Patients About Healthcare Injury

National Patient Safety Foundation Statement of Principle
When a healthcare injury occurs, the patient and the family or representative are entitled to a prompt explanation of how the injury occurred and its short- and long-term effects. When an error contributed to the injury, the patient and the family or representative should receive a truthful and compassionate explanation about the error and the remedies available to the patient. They should be informed that the factors involved in the injury will be investigated so that steps can be taken to reduce the likelihood of similar injury to other patients.

Healthcare professionals and institutions that accept this responsibility are acknowledging their ethical obligation to be forthcoming about healthcare injuries and errors.

The National Patient Safety Foundation urges all healthcare professionals and institutions to embrace the principle of dealing honestly with patients.

National Patient Safety Foundation. (2004). *Talking to patients about health care injury.* Available at http://www.npsf.org/html/statement.html.

disaster, the lives of the victims, their families, and the community are affected in incalculable ways.

The Sept. 11, 2001, terrorist attacks in New York, Washington, DC, and Pennsylvania served as a wake-up call to the American healthcare system. Though our ability to predict a disaster or public health emergency is limited, protocols must be in place to provide adequate healthcare whether the emergency is biological, chemical, nuclear, or a natural disaster.

Think back to Kara Greenwood, the adolescent described in the beginning of the chapter. Her statement revealed her peer group's awareness of terrorism. Kara would need to obtain additional information about terrorism from community sources when preparing the discussion.

JCAHO introduced new emergency preparedness standards for hospitals in 2001 that outline four phases of preparation for a disaster:
- Mitigation: identification of the types of emergencies that are most likely to occur and their probable impact
- Preparedness: development of a plan that includes a list of resources (supplies and staff), a primary and back-up communication system, and a schedule for practice drills
- Response: outline of all actions that must be taken in the event of an attack or disaster
- Recovery: plan for return to normal services and operation (JCAHO, 2001)

Communication is obviously an essential component of any disaster plan and must include a back-up communication system, external and internal communication processes, a media contact person, and a phone tree to contact family members of staff. JCAHO also requires that healthcare facilities maintain at least a 24-hour inventory of supplies and

pharmaceuticals. This can be supplemented by caches of medical and drug supplies that the CDC has stored in various locations throughout the United States for response to a terrorist attack.

Readiness initiatives must include awareness and education about the process of detection, identification of possible mass casualty threats (including biological, chemical, and nuclear agents), and the appropriate treatment and response.

Addressing Biological Threats

Bioterrorism involves the deliberate spread of pathogenic organisms into a community (Steinhauer, 2002). The organisms used in a mass attack may not be routine, and the clinical manifestations may be vague and nonspecific. Table 26-3 outlines some of the more common biological agents, including symptoms and interventions. If an unusual number of people suddenly develop similar signs and symptoms, healthcare personnel should consider whether they may have been exposed to a biological agent.

Healthcare personnel must adhere to the Standard Precautions recommended by the CDC. For certain diseases, additional safeguards may be necessary. If a contagious disease is suspected, the patient should be isolated accordingly. Though not usually required with biological agents, decontamination may be necessary if a patient's exposure status is uncertain. The patient may need to bathe or shower with soap and place his or her clothing in sealed plastic bags.

Addressing Chemical Threats

The use of chemical agents as a terrorist weapon is a growing concern. **Chemical terrorism** involves the deliberate release of a chemical compound for the purpose of causing mass destruction (Armstrong, 2002). The chemical would probably be dispersed in an enclosed space such as a subway or a closed sports arena to cause the maximum effect. Chemical agents act rapidly, and immediate decontamination is ideal before patients are transported to a hospital. Emergency preparedness requires the swift transfer of portable decontamination units, equipment, and trained personnel to the site of the chemical attack.

Several categories of chemicals can be used as weapons of mass destruction:
- Pulmonary agents
- Cyanide
- Vesicants
- Nerve agents
- Incapacitating agents

Box 26-8 summarizes the effects of the various chemical agents.

Addressing Nuclear Threats

Nuclear terrorism involves intentional dispersal of radioactive materials into the environment for the purpose of causing injury and death (Kilpatrick, 2002). The attack might involve use of a radiation dispersal device ("dirty bomb") or a planned assault at a nuclear power station or weapons facility.

TABLE 26-3 Biological Agents of Concern

Agents	Clinical Manifestations	Treatment/Protection
Anthrax (*Bacillus anthrax*)	Symptoms vary according to the form of anthrax: • Cutaneous: skin lesion with local edema that progresses, enlarges, ulcerates, and becomes necrotic • Gastrointestinal: nausea, vomiting, fever, abdominal pain, hematemesis, severe diarrhea • Inhalational: fever, fatigue, cough, dyspnea, pain, may progress to meningitis, septicemia, shock, and death	Standard barrier isolation precautions Decontamination may be required if there has been recent exposure. Rapid administration of antimicrobial therapy Supportive therapy for shock, fluid volume deficit, and airway management Vaccine is available but is currently recommended only for high-risk populations
Plague or "black death" (*Yersinia pestis*)	Expected attack would be airborne (inhalation of bacilli) with sudden appearance in ER of multiple patients with respiratory symptoms Symptoms similar to a severe respiratory infection Progresses rapidly to severe pneumonia, sepsis, and death	Standard Precautions with respiratory isolation during the first 48 hours of antibiotic therapy Antibiotic of choice is streptomycin (IM) or gentamicin sulfate (IM or IV). Oral antibiotics may also be effective when mass numbers of people are ill. Fatality rate is 100% for those who do not receive treatment within 24 hours of onset of symptoms.
Smallpox (*Variola major*, viral agent)	Spreads through direct contact or inhalation of respiratory droplets. Would most likely be spread via aerosol route. Flulike symptoms Characteristic rash that progresses to crusted scabs in 5 days, most prominent on face and extremities	Strict contact and airborne precautions—those exposed should be vaccinated. No proven treatment Supportive care may include antibiotics if secondary infections develop. Use of antiviral agents under investigation Vaccine is available but is currently recommended only for high-risk populations.
Botulism (*Clostridium botulinum*)	Could be released via airborne method, or food supplies could be contaminated Ocular symptoms such as blurred vision Skeletal muscle paralysis that progresses symmetrically and in a descending manner Muscle weakness that can result abruptly in respiratory failure	Standard Precautions Passive immunization with botulinum antitoxin Supportive respiratory care
Tularemia (*Francisella tularensis*)	Can be contacted via contaminated water, food, and soil but most likely use as a biological weapon would be aerosolization of bacteria Fever Nonproductive or productive cough May progress to respiratory failure	Standard Precautions Drug therapy includes streptomycin or gentamicin sulfate. Fluid and respiratory support measures Vaccine under investigation
Viral hemorrhagic fevers (eg. Lassa, Ebola, Marburg, yellow, and dengue fevers)	Could be spread via aerosol infection Fever Myalgias Conjunctival symptoms Mild hypotension Petechial hemorrhages Progresses to shock and hemorrhage	Various isolation precautions, including use of negative-pressure room Healthcare workers should use personal protective equipment. No proven treatment other than supportive care Avoid aspirin or other anticlotting drugs.

Adapted from Persell, D., et al. (2002). Preparing for bioterrorism. *Nursing. 32*(2), 37–43; and Steinhauer, R. (2002). A readied response: Bioterrorism. *RN, 65*(3), 48–54.

Even a small amount of radioactive material can have devastating effects.

Nurses serving on a radiological emergency response team must protect themselves and wear the necessary equipment, including a radiation detection device. They will assess patients in a Radiation Emergency Area (REA) designated by the hospital's emergency response plan. If patients have not been decontaminated at the scene of the attack, decontamination will occur at the medical facility.

Radiation burns occur as a result of exposure to a radioactive source. The severity of injury depends on a variety of factors, including the duration of the exposure and the distance

BOX 26-8 Categories of Chemical Agents

Pulmonary Agents
Examples: phosgene (CG), diphosgene (DP), chlorine (CL)
Effects: dyspnea, cough, pulmonary edema

Cyanide
Examples: hydrogen cyanide (AC), cyanogen chloride (CK)
Effects: loss of consciousness, convulsions, respiratory arrest

Vesicants
Examples: sulfur mustard (H or HD), lewisite (L)
Effects: skin erythema and blisters, eye irritation, progressively severe respiratory symptoms, damage to bone marrow

Nerve Agents
Examples: tabun (GA), sarin (GB), soman (GD)
Effects: constricted pupils, reddened eyes, loss of consciousness, convulsions, respiratory arrest

Incapacitating Agents
Examples: glycolate anticholinergic compound (BZ), Agent 15
Effects: hyperthermia, bizarre behavior, delirium

Adapted from Armstrong, J. [2002]. A readied response: Chemical warfare. *RN, 65*[4], 32–39

may be small, nurses need to be well informed, familiar with their agency's emergency response plan, and prepared to deal with a nuclear emergency.

Clarifying Disaster Resources

Each healthcare facility should determine in advance how to deliver care should an emergency or disaster occur. This involves collaboration with internal committees and external agencies. Organizations that serve as resources for recommendations and updated information are listed in Table 26-4.

The Federal Emergency Management Agency (FEMA) has published "Are You Ready? A Citizen's Guide to Emergency Preparedness" that can be accessed on the Internet at http://www.fema.gov/areyouready/. Revised in September 2002, "Are You Ready?" provides a step-by-step outline on how to prepare a disaster supply kit, emergency planning for people with disabilities, how to locate and evacuate to a shelter, and even contingency planning for family pets. Man-made threats from hazardous materials and terrorism are also discussed in detail.

Addressing Psychological Aspects of Disasters

Disasters affect the lives of victims, family members, and healthcare personnel in many ways. Fear and panic can be expected, as well as anger, horror, and real and exaggerated concerns about possible future events. Nurses and other healthcare providers, as first responders, rescue and recovery workers, or staff at a medical facility, can help to minimize panic by addressing risks and providing careful explanations. Anxiety can be treated with reassurance. The impact of a dis-

between the source and the person. A higher dose increases the likelihood of developing later effects such as bone marrow depression and cancer. Although the likelihood of a nuclear attack

TABLE 26-4 Emergency Preparedness Resources

Organization	Activities
National Disaster Medical System (NDMS) http://ndms.dhhs.gov	Has responsibility for managing and coordinating the federal medical response to major emergencies and federally declared disasters
Federal Emergency Management Agency (FEMA) http://www.fema.gov	Works to build and support the national emergency management system
Centers for Disease Control and Prevention (CDC) http://www.cdc.gov	The lead federal agency for disease prevention and control activities provides backup support to state and local health departments
Joint Commission on Accreditation of Healthcare Organizations (JCAHO) http://www.jcaho.org (For revised standards, see http://www.jcaho.org/accredited +organizations/hospitals/standards/hospital+faqs/management +of+env+of+care/emergency+management/	Accredits facilities according to established safety and quality standards, and revised the emergency management standards for healthcare facilities in 2001
American Red Cross http://www.redcross.org	Lead nongovernmental agency that provides safety information and disaster response
American Hospital Association http://www.aha.org (For disaster readiness, see http://www.hospitalconnect.com/ aha/key_issues/disaster_readiness/index.html	American Hospital Association connection to disaster readiness resources
Department of Homeland Security http://www.dhs.gov	Protects the nation against further terrorist attacks and coordinates the response for future emergencies

aster on each person varies, and it can have lingering effects. Most disaster survivors experience normal stress reactions, but one in three may exhibit acute stress disorder or posttraumatic stress disorders that require treatment (Bensing, 2003). Emergency preparedness education and planning must also address mental health issues.

Evaluating

Nurses must evaluate the effectiveness of their interventions to promote environmental safety, prevent injury, and promote emergency preparedness. If the expected patient outcomes have been met and evaluative criteria have been satisfied, the patient should be able to accomplish the following:

- Correctly identify real and potential unsafe environmental situations
- Implement safety measures in the environment
- Use available resources to obtain safety information
- Incorporate accident prevention practices into activities of daily living
- Remain free of injury

Developing Critical Thinking Skills

1. You are the visiting nurse for a frail older patient who lives alone in her own home and prizes her independence. You assess her to be at high risk for falls because of her general weakness, the medication she takes, and a long history of indifference to safety counseling. What nursing interventions are likely to be most effective in ensuring her safety?

2. Identify the safety hazards and threats to security for which you and family members of different ages are most at risk. What anticipatory planning and teaching could be done to prevent these hazards? Note your willingness and that of your family to make the necessary changes, and identify the nursing strategies that would be most likely to secure patient cooperation in making the needed changes.

Practicing for NCLEX

1. A school nurse reviewing healthcare topics for adolescents should be aware that:
   a. Tobacco use has decreased in this age group
   b. Most teenagers who commit suicide use a gun
   c. Teenagers are more likely to drink and drive
   d. Peer pressure is insignificant

2. When transporting a toddler in a motor vehicle, car seats are mandatory:
   a. In all 50 states
   b. In 36 of the 50 states
   c. If a seat belt is not available
   d. On interstate highways

3. Which child has the greatest risk for choking and suffocating?

   a. A toddler playing with his 9-year-old brother's construction set
   b. A 4-year-old eating yogurt for lunch
   c. An infant covered with a small blanket and asleep in the crib
   d. A 3-year-old drinking a glass of juice

4. Nursing consideration regarding the use of side rails for a confused patient is based on the knowledge that:
   a. They prevent confused patients from wandering
   b. A history of a previous fall from a bed with raised side rails is insignificant
   c. Alternative measures are ineffective to prevent wandering
   d. A person of small stature is at increased risk for injury from entrapment

5. The leading cause of accidental death for people 79 years of age and older is:
   a. Fires
   b. Exposure to temperature extremes
   c. Drug overdose
   d. Falls

6. Nursing education efforts that focus on prevention of firearm injuries are important because:
   a. The elderly population is particularly at risk
   b. Deaths among adolescents and children have increased sharply
   c. The National Safety Council recommends that every household have a gun to protect family members
   d. They have contributed to a decrease in injuries and deaths from guns

7. JCAHO standards for emergency preparedness require creation of a list of available staff and equipment resources. This should be done as part of the:
   a. Mitigation phase
   b. Preparedness phase
   c. Response phase
   d. Recovery phase

8. Mr. Kennedy is a disoriented older resident who likes to wander the halls of his long-term care facility. As an alternative to using restraints, the nurse might:
   a. Seat him in a geriatric chair
   b. Use the sheets to secure him snugly in his bed
   c. Keep the bed in the high position
   d. Identify his door with his picture and a balloon

9. While discussing home safety with the nurse, Mrs. Fuller admits that she always smokes a cigarette in bed before falling asleep at night. An appropriate nursing diagnosis would be:
   a. Impaired Gas Exchange related to cigarette smoking
   b. Anxiety related to inability to stop smoking
   c. Risk for Suffocation related to unfamiliarity with fire prevention guidelines
   d. Knowledge Deficit related to lack of follow-through of recommendation to stop smoking

10. Mr. D'Ambro has weakened knees due to arthritis. The home healthcare nurse is aware that he understands the need for safety modifications at home because he:
    a. Uses the towel bar for support to stand up from the commode
    b. Leans on the pedestal table in his bedroom when he dresses
    c. Sits only in chairs with armrests
    d. Uses a small stepladder to reach an item on an upper shelf

11. When a fire occurs in a patient's room, the nurse's priority should be to:
    a. Rescue the patient
    b. Extinguish the fire
    c. Sound the alarm
    d. Run for help

12. The nurse is planning a health teaching session for new parents about poisoning emergencies. She should tell the parents that their initial response should be to:
    a. Use salt water to induce vomiting
    b. Rush the child to the emergency department
    c. Call the poison control center
    d. Routinely administer syrup of ipecac for any poison ingestion

13. JCAHO guidelines regarding the use of restraints recommend that:
    a. Vest restraints be used, because they are the least restrictive type
    b. Restraints should be used only for 48 hours in nonpsychiatric patients
    c. Restraints should be applied to prevent wandering behavior
    d. Alternative measures must be attempted first

14. The nurse orients an older patient to the safety features in her hospital room. A vital component of this admission routine is to:
    a. Explain how to use the telephone
    b. Introduce the patient to her roommate
    c. Review the hospital policy on visiting hours
    d. Explain how to operate the call bell

15. When completing an incident report, the nurse should:
    a. Include suggestions on how to prevent the accident from recurring
    b. Provide minimal information about the incident
    c. Discuss the details with the patient before documenting them
    d. Objectively describe the incident in detail

■ Answers With Rationale

1. The correct answer is *b*. Ten percent of teenagers attempt suicide. Tobacco use in this age group has hit a 16-year high point, and half of those who experiment with cigarettes become regular smokers. Teenagers are less likely to drink and drive but more likely to have an accident if they do combine both behaviors. Much of adolescents' spare time is spent away from home and with peers, and peers are most influential in their decision making.

2. The correct answer is *a*. All 50 states require the use of safety seats for infants and toddlers at all times.

3. The correct answer is *a*. A young child may place small or loose parts in his or her mouth; a toy that is safe for a 9-year-old could kill a toddler. An infant sleeping in a crib without a pillow or large blanket and a 3-year-old and a 4-year-old drinking juice and eating yogurt are not particular safety risks.

4. The correct answer is *d*. Studies of restraint-related deaths have shown that people of small stature are more likely to slip through or between the side rails. The desire to prevent a patient from wandering is not sufficient reason for the use of side rails. Creative use of alternative measures indicates respect for the patient's dignity and may in fact prevent more serious fall-related injuries. A history of falls from a bed with raised side rails carries a significant risk for a future serious incident.

5. The correct answer is *d*. Falls are the leading cause of accidental death in the population 79 years of age and older. Fires, exposure to temperature extremes, and drug overdoses are significant causes of accidental death, but not in this age group.

6. The correct answer is *b*. The number of deaths among adolescents and children has increased sharply since 1990. Keeping a gun in the home can have dangerous consequences and increases the risk for domestic violence. Young children may also be unintentionally injured or killed. Recent efforts to prevent injuries from guns have become more serious because violent behavior has increased in our society.

7. The correct answer is *b*. The list of resources needed in an emergency response situation must be created during the preparedness phase. The other three phases are dedicated to assessment of hazards, the actual answer to the emergency, and the restoration of normal services.

8. The correct answer is *d*. Identifying his door with his picture and a balloon may work as an alternative to restraints. Using the geriatric chair and sheets are forms of physical restraint. Leaving the bed in the high position is a safety risk and would probably result in a fall.

9. The correct answer is *c*. Because Mrs. Fuller is not aware that smoking in bed is extremely dangerous, she is at risk for suffocation from fire. The other three nursing diagnoses are correctly stated but are not a priority in this situation.

10. The correct answer is *c*. Chairs with armrests can be used to increase the patient's leverage as he attempts

to rise. Towel bars are not designed to provide support, the pedestal table is unsteady and unsafe, and standing on a stool and reaching puts the patient at risk for falling.

11. The correct answer is *a.* The patient's safety is always the priority. Sounding the alarm and extinguishing the fire are important after the patient is safe. Calling for help, rather than running for assistance, allows you to remain with your patient and is more appropriate, if possible.

12. The correct answer is *c.* Always call the poison control center before attempting any home remedies. These answers may be dangerous for the victim. The poison control Center can supply the doctor or emergency department with specific information to assist in the victim's care.

13. The correct answer is *d.* Wandering behavior is not an indication for restraints. Careful assessment and attempts to find effective alternative measures are required before applying a restraint. Less restrictive restraints may include side rails, a geriatric chair, or wrist restraints instead of a vest. JCAHO recommends not using restraints for more than 24 hours on nonpsychiatric patients.

14. The correct answer is *d.* Knowing how to use the call bell is a safety priority; knowing how to use the phone, meeting the roommate, and knowledge of visiting hours will not necessarily prevent an accidental injury.

15. The correct answer is *d.* An incident report is a legal document and must be as objective and complete as possible. It is not a collaborative effort with the patient, and any suggestions to prevent this from happening again should be discussed at a postincident conference.

Bibliography

Alexander, N., & Edelberg, H. (2002). Assessing mobility and preventing falls in older patients. *Patient Care, 36*(2), 19–29.

American Safety and Health Institute (Feb. 2003). *Basic first aid for the community and workplace* (3rd ed.). Holiday, FL: Author.

American Safety and Health Institute (Feb. 2003). *Essentials in basic emergency care.* Holiday, FL: Author.

Armstrong, J. (2002). A readied response: Chemical warfare. *RN, 65*(4), 32–40.

Armstrong, M. (1998). A clinical look at body piercing. *RN, 61*(9), 26–30.

Bensing, K. (2003). Psychology of disaster. *Advance for Nurses, 5*(13), 17–21.

Bernardo, L. (2002). Emergency nurses' role in injury prevention. *Emergency Nursing, 37*(1), 135–142.

Brenner, Z., & Duffy-Durnin, K. (1998). Toward restraint-free care. *American Journal of Nursing, 98*(12), 16F–16I.

Carlson, D. (1998). Uncovering the clues of child abuse. *Nursing, 28*(11), 32hn10–11.

Carroll, M., Morin, K., Hayes, E., & Carter, S. (1999). Assessing students' perceived threats to safety in the community. *Nurse Educator, 24*(1), 31–35.

Centers for Disease Control and Prevention (2001). *Injury fact book: 2001–2002.* Atlanta: Author.

Centers for Disease Control and Prevention (2003). *Injury mortality reports, 1999–2000.* Available at: *http://webapp. cdc.gov/sasweb/ncipc/mortrate10.html*

Coffman, S. (2003). Bicycle injuries and safety helmets in children. *Orthopaedic Nursing, 22*(1), 9–15.

Covinsky, K. E., Kahana, E., Kahana, B, et al. (April 1, 2001). History and mobility exam index to identify community-dwelling elderly persons at risk of falling. *Journal of Gerontology, 56*(4), 253M–259.

Crawley-Coha, T. (2002). Childhood injury: a status report, part 2. *Journal of Pediatric Nursing, 17*(2), 133–136.

DiBartolo, V. (1998). 9 steps to effective restraint use. *RN, 61*(12), 23–24.

Dunn, K. (2001). The effect of physical restraints on fall rates in older adults who are institutionalized. *Journal of Gerontological Nursing, 27*(10), 40–48.

Eliopoulos, C. (2003). *Gerontological nursing* (5th ed.). Philadelphia: Lippincott Williams & Wilkins.

Gentleman, B., & Malozemoff, W. (2001). Falls and feelings: Description of a psychosocial group nursing intervention. *Journal of Gerontological Nursing, 27*(10), 35–39.

Gerard, M. (2000). Domestic violence: How to screen & intervene. *RN, 63*(12), 52–56.

Grenier-Sennlier, C., et al. (2002) Designing adverse event prevention programs using quality management methods: The case of falls in hospitals. *International Journal of Quality Health Care, 14*(5), 419–426.

Hayes, L. (2000). Poison emergency? *Nursing, 30*(9), 34–39.

Joint Commission on Accreditation of Healthcare Organizations. (1998). *1998 Hospital accreditation standards.* Oakbrook Terrace, IL: Author.

Joint Commission on Accreditation of Healthcare Organizations. (2001). *Emergency Management Standards.* Available at http://www.jcaho.org/accredited+organizations/hospitals/standards/hospital+faqs/management+of+end+of+care/emergency+management/.

Joint Commission on Accreditation of Healthcare Organizations. (2003). *2004 national patient safety goals.* Available at http://www.jcaho.org/accredited+organizations/patient+safety/04+npsg/04_npsg.htm. Accessed Oct. 2, 2003.

Kilpatrick, J. (2002). A readied answer: Nuclear attacks. *RN, 65*(5), 46–52.

Kimball, S. (2001). Before the fall. *Nursing, 31*(8), 44–45.

London, M., Ladewig, P., Ball, J., et al. (2003). *Maternal-newborn & child nursing.* Upper Saddle River, NJ: Prentice Hall.

Mace, S., Gerardi, M., Dietrick, A., et al. (2001). Injury prevention and control in children. *Annals of Emergency Medicine, 38*(4), 405–413.

Melillo, K., & Futrell, M. (1998). Wandering and technology devices. *Journal of Gerontological Nursing, 24*(8), 32–38.

Mulryan, K., Cathers, P., & Fagin, A. (2000). Protecting the child. *Nursing, 30*(7), 39–45.

Napierkowski, D. (2002). Using restraints with restraint. *Nursing, 32*(11), 58–62.

National Patient Safety Foundation. (2004). *Talking to patients about health care injury.* Available at http://www.npsf.org/html/statement.html.

North American Nursing Diagnosis Association. (2003). *NANDA nursing diagnoses: Definitions & classifications 2003–2004.* Philadelphia: Author.

Partridge, R., Virk, A., & Antosia, R. (1998). Causes and patterns of injury from ladder falls. *Academic Emergency Medicine, 5*(1), 31–34.

Perry, J., Jagger, J., & Parker, G. (2003). Nurses and needlesticks then and now. *Nursing. 33*(4), 22.

Persell, D., Arangie, P., Young, C., et al. (2002). Preparing for bioterrorism. *Nursing, 32*(2), 37–43.

Pillitteri, A. (1999). *Maternal & child health nursing* (3rd ed.). Philadelphia: Lippincott Williams & Wilkins.

Rawsky, E. (1998). Review of literature on falls among the elderly. *Image: The Journal of Nursing Scholarship, 30*(1), 47–52.

Rothrock, J. (2003). *Alexander's care of the patient in surgery.* St. Louis: Mosby.

Sarna, L., & Lillington, L. (2002). Tobacco: An emerging topic in nursing research. *Nursing Research, 51*(4), 245–253.

Shahinian, B., & Hawke, M. (1998). The terrible truth about teens and tobacco. *The Nursing Spectrum, 7*(18), 4–5.

Steinhauer, R. (2002). A readied response: Bioterrorism. *RN, 65*(3), 48–55.

Steinhauer, R., & Bauer, J. (2002). A readied answer: The emergency management plan. *RN, 65*(6), 40–46.

Sullivan, G. (1999). Minimizing your risk in patient falls. *RN, 62*(4), 69–72.

Taft, C., Michalide, A., & Taft, A. (Feb. 1999). *Child passengers at risk in America: A national study of car seat misuse.* Washington, DC: National SAFE KIDS Campaign.

Talerico, K., & Capezuti, E. (2001). Myths and facts about side rails. *American Journal of Nursing, 101*(7), 43–48.

Teret, S., et al. (1998). Making guns safer. *Issues in Science and Technology, 14*(4), 37–40.

Todd, J. (2002). When bed isn't a safe haven. *Nursing, 32*(12), 82.

U.S. Census Bureau (2002). *Statistical abstract of the United States, 2002* (122nd ed.). Washington, DC: Author.

Veenema, T. G. (2002). Chemical and biological terrorism: Current updates for nursing education. *Nursing Education Perspectives, 23*(2), 62–71.

Veenema, T. G. (2003). *Disaster nursing and emergency preparedness for chemical, biological, radiological terrorism, and other hazards.* New York: Springer Publishing Co.

Asepsis and Infection Control

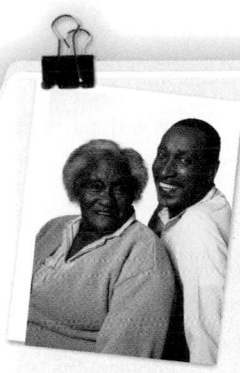

Jackson Ray Ivers comes to visit his mother, who has been hospitalized for tuberculosis. He notices a sign on the door to check at the nurse's desk before entering. He asks, "What's going on? Why do I have to wash my hands and wear a mask?"

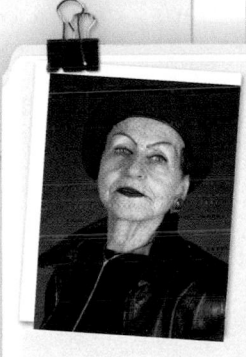

Esther Bailey, a 72-year-old female patient on the unit recovering from abdominal surgery and receiving antibiotic therapy for a wound infection, requires insertion of an indwelling urinary catheter due to development of postoperative urinary retention and inability to void.

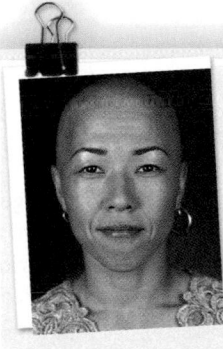

Giselle Turheis, a 38-year-old woman undergoing chemotherapy treatment for leukemia states "I know that my risk for infection is really high because of my poor immune status. But how do I respond to my Sunday school class, who are used to greeting me with a big hug. I want to be safe, but I know that I need these hugs too!"

Focusing on Blended Skills

The types of blended skills you'll need to respond to the case scenarios include:

Cognitive Skills
- Basic knowledge of the infection cycle and nursing interventions to break the chain of infection
- Ability to identify the principles of medical and surgical asepsis applicable to the care of patients to prevent and control infection
- Knowledge of factors that reduce the incidence of nosocomial infection
- Knowledge of Centers for Disease Control and Prevention guidelines for standard and transmission-based precautions

Technical Skills
- Demonstration of strong history and physical assessment techniques to determine a patient's risk for infection
- Ability to implement techniques correctly applying the principles of medical and surgical asepsis
- Ability to use the equipment and protocols necessary to conform to principles of medical and surgical asepsis
- Ability to use appropriate infection-control precautions and barrier techniques for infection prevention and control

- Ability to demonstrate competence in technical nursing assistance to meet the needs of patients who are at risk for or are experiencing an infection

Interpersonal Skills
- Strong people skills in conjunction with the ability to communicate and interact effectively with individuals and families
- Ability to communicate care and compassion to patients requiring infection-control precautions
- Ability to establish trusting relationships with patients and families as a basis for teaching, counseling, and securing compliance with infection-control measures

Ethical and Legal Skills
- Demonstration of a commitment to safety and quality; strong sense of responsibility, accountability; strong advocacy abilities
- Ability to identify breaches in infection-control measures that violate ethical and legal standards
- Knowledge of special regulations, legislation, and policy detailing nursing responsibilities related to asepsis and infection control

Learning Outcomes

After completing the chapter, the learner should be able to accomplish the following:

1. Explain the infection cycle.
2. Describe nursing interventions used to break the chain of infection.
3. List the stages of an infection.
4. Identify patients at risk for developing an infection.
5. Identify factors that reduce the incidence of nosocomial infection.
6. Identify situations in which hand hygiene is indicated.
7. Identify nursing diagnoses for a patient who has or is at risk for infection.
8. Describe strategies for implementing CDC guidelines for standard and transmission-based precautions when caring for patients.
9. Implement recommended techniques for medical and surgical asepsis.

Key Terms

aerobic
anaerobic
antibody
antigen
antimicrobial
asepsis
bacteria
disinfection
endogenous
exogenous
fungi
host
iatrogenic
infection
isolation
nosocomial
pathogens
reservoir
standard precautions
sterilization
transmission-based precautions
vector
virulence
virus

A major concern for health practitioners is the danger of spreading microorganisms from person to person and from place to place. Microorganisms are naturally present in almost all environments. Some are beneficial, but some are not. Some are harmless to most people, and others are harmful to many people. Still others are harmless except in certain circumstances.

Many groups are responsible for directing efforts toward a microorganism-safe environment, including government agencies at the international, national, state, and local levels; health personnel; and individuals. Such efforts include mass immu-

nization programs, laws concerning safe sewage disposal, regulations for the control of communicable diseases, and hospital infection-surveillance programs. Medical science continues to grapple with problems caused by increasingly virulent organisms that have become drug resistant and with problems related to patients who are immunologically compromised. Prevention of infection is a major focus for nurses. As primary caregivers, nurses are involved in identifying, preventing, controlling, and teaching the patient about infection (see the Reflective Practice box for an example). Use of the nursing process can prove critical in breaking the cycle of infection.

Reflective Practice
Challenge to Ethical and Legal Skills

This is my last clinical rotation before graduation and it has been a difficult year. My focus has been somewhat off for a while, and I haven't been as prepared as I should have been for my clinical and classroom experiences. My clinical instructor has been on my case for the last few weeks. I'm also realizing that in no time at all I will be out of school and on my own when it comes to patient care. So all of a sudden, I'm eager for as many clinical experiences as I can get. To make a long story short, I'm thrilled when offered the opportunity to catheterize Esther Bailey, a 72-year-old female patient on my unit. I quickly review the procedure and go to the patient's room, with the catheterization supplies in hand, feeling semiconfident. After introducing myself and my clinical instructor and explaining what I'm about to do, I open the sterile package, prepare the sterile field, and cleanse the meatus. In one quick moment, as the patient asks a question and diverts my instructor's gaze, I realize to my horror that I've contaminated the catheter. I've got a split second to decide what to do. I can tell my instructor what happened, obtain a new kit, and proceed anew, or pretend nothing happened and continue. I don't like that I'm even considering not admitting the mistake, after everything that has been drilled into us about the importance of sterility and the consequences of nosocomial infections. But I'm also prudent enough to realize that it is time to leave the unit because the rest of the group is waiting for postconference. Plus, after all, there are financial costs to ordering another tray. But what if I do not admit the error and by chance the instructor did see me contaminate the catheter? Then my goose is really cooked!

Thinking Outside the Box: Possible Courses of Action

- Obviously the simplest solution: admit my error and accept the consequences.
- Request a new catheter and inform my instructor later that the patient moved just as I was preparing to enter the meatus (a bit of deception but this makes the error not my fault).
- Alternatively, pretend that nothing happened and pray that no harm comes to the patient (after all, how much bacteria do

you need to contaminate a catheter? . . . and the patient is receiving antibiotic therapy anyway).
- Continue and not even be bothered by the contamination (Life is one big risk for everyone, right? All that matters is that you take care of #1).

Evaluating a Good Outcome: How Do I Define Success?

- Patient benefited from my actions or, at the very least, was not harmed.
- No one's integrity is compromised or sacrificed.

- No violations of the standards of practice or the American Nurses Association's Code of Ethics occurred.

Personal Learning: Here's to the Future!

At least I can say there was a happy ending to this story. I did stop, explain what happened, and waited while someone ran for a new catheterization tray. Amazingly my instructor told me later that she valued my maturity and honesty and ability to put the needs of

the patient ahead of my own needs, stating that I "might just have what it takes after all!" I'm not sure how often I'll be called upon to put the needs of a patient ahead of my own needs but hopefully I'll be ready to respond selflessly each time.

Reflection:

How do you think you would respond in a similar situation? Why? What does this tell you about yourself and about the adequacy of your skills for professional practice? Can you think of other ways to respond? Did the nursing student perform legally, adhering to the standards of practice? If not, what violations occurred? What ethical principles might have been violated had the nursing student not reported the catheter contamination? How did

the nursing student adhere to principles of medical and surgical asepsis? What other skills (cognitive, interpersonal, technical, ethical/legal) would you need to respond well in this situation? Do you agree with the criteria to evaluate a successful outcome? Were the criteria met? If not, what else might the nursing student have done to ensure a successful outcome?

PROCESS OF INFECTION

Infection Cycle

An **infection** is a disease state that results from the presence of **pathogens** (disease-producing microorganisms) in or on the body. An infection occurs as a result of a cyclic process, consisting of six components, as shown in Figure 27-1. These components are:

- Infectious agent
- Reservoir
- Portal of exit
- Means of transmission
- Portal of entry
- Susceptible host

Infectious Agent

Some of the more prevalent agents that cause infection are bacteria, viruses, and fungi. **Bacteria,** the most significant and most commonly observed infection-causing agents in healthcare institutions, can be categorized in various ways. They are categorized by shape as spherical (cocci), rod shaped (bacilli), or corkscrew shaped (spirochetes). Bacteria are either gram positive or gram negative, based on their reaction to the Gram stain. For example, gram-positive bacteria have a thick cell wall that resists decolorization (loss of color) and are stained violet. However, gram-negative bacteria have chemically more complex cell walls and can be decolorized by alcohol. Thus, gram-negative bacteria do not stain. This information is crucial for physicians when prescribing the most appropriate antibiotic therapy because antibiotics are classified as specifically effec-

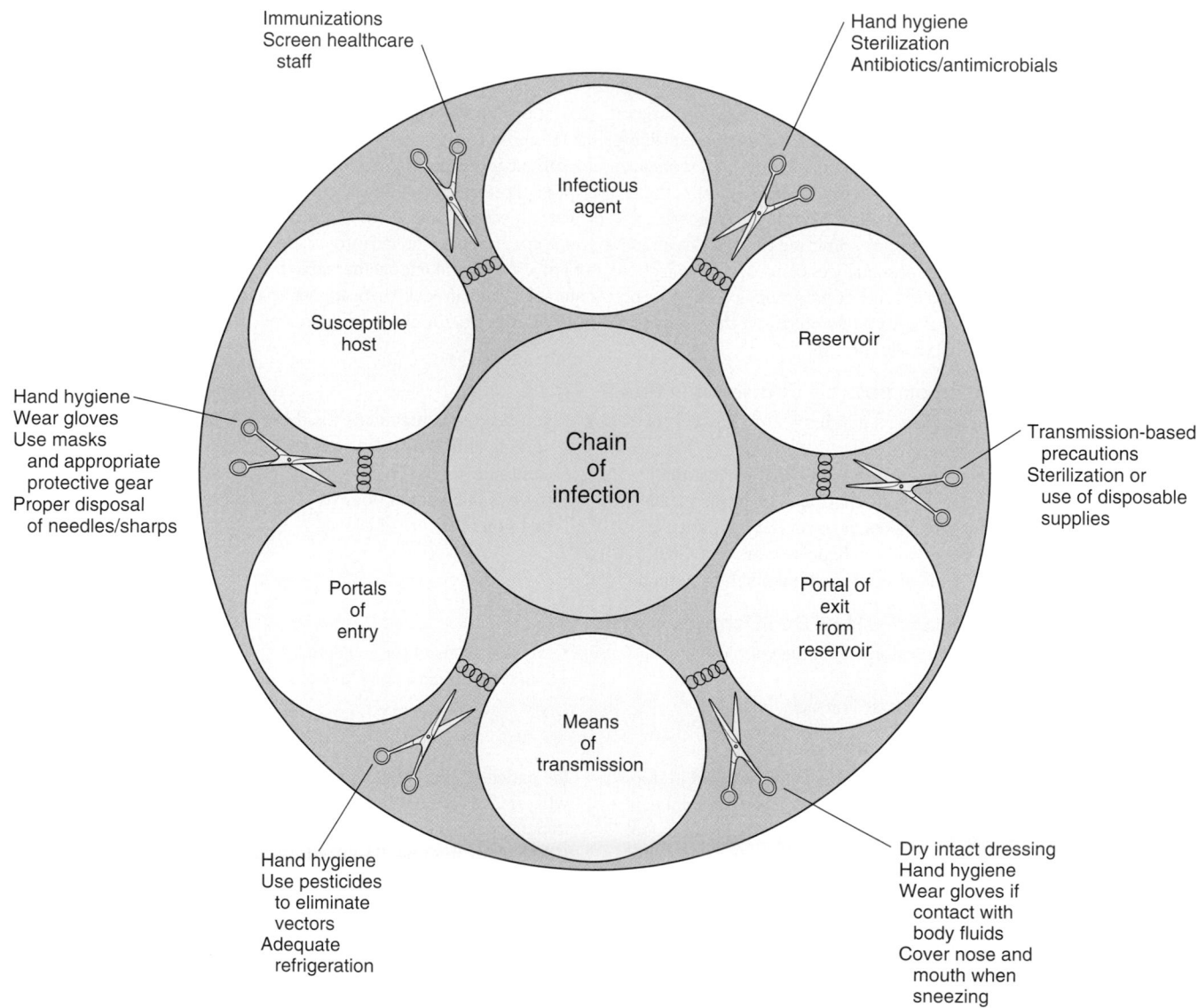

FIGURE 27-1 The infection cycle is demonstrated as a chain. The goal is to break the links of the chain to end the cycle. (Adapted from Murphy, D. [1998]. Infectious microbes and disease: General principles. *Nursing Spectrum, 7*(2), 12–14.)

tive against only gram-positive organisms or as broad spectrum and effective against several groups of microorganisms.

Another distinguishing characteristic of bacteria is their need for oxygen. Most bacteria require oxygen to live and grow and are therefore referred to as **aerobic**. Those that can live without oxygen are **anaerobic** bacteria.

A **virus** is the smallest of all microorganisms, visible only with an electron microscope. Many infections are caused by viruses, including the common cold and the deadly disease, acquired immunodeficiency syndrome (AIDS). Antibiotics have no effect on viruses. Antiviral medications that seem to be effective with some viral infections are available. When given in the prodromal stage of certain viruses, these medications can shorten the full stage of the illness.

Fungi, plantlike organisms (molds and yeasts) that also can cause infection, are present in the air, soil, and water. Some examples of infections caused by fungi include athlete's foot, ring worm, and yeast infections. These infections are treated with antifungal medications. However, many infections due to fungi are resistant to treatment.

Not all organisms to which a person is exposed cause disease. An organism's potential to produce disease in a person depends on a variety of factors, including:

- Number of organisms
- **Virulence** of the organism, or its ability to cause disease
- Competence of the person's immune system
- Length and intimacy of the contact between the person and the microorganism

Identifying the type of infection and infectious agent is not always an easy process. Sometimes new diseases appear, with healthcare workers racing to identify them so that treatment can begin. This is the process that occurred with AIDS or, more recently, with severe acute respiratory syndrome (SARS). Other times, a disease appears in different geographical locations, such as with monkeypox and West Nile virus. In cases like these, countries draw information from one another to learn about treatment options.

Under normal conditions, some organisms may not produce disease. Microorganisms that commonly inhabit various body sites and are part of the body's natural defense system are referred to as normal flora. Other factors may intervene, causing this usually harmless organism to generate an infection. Bacteria that normally cause no problem but, with certain factors, may potentially be harmful, are referred to as opportunists. For example, one type of *Escherichia coli* normally resides in the intestinal tract and causes no harm. However, if it migrates to the urinary tract, it can lead to urinary tract infection.

Reservoir

The **reservoir** for growth and multiplication of microorganisms is the natural habitat of the organism. Possible reservoirs that support organisms pathogenic to humans include other humans, animals, soil, food, water, milk, and inanimate objects.

Other Humans

Some humans act as reservoirs for the infectious agent and demonstrate signs and symptoms of the disease. However, other humans act as reservoirs for the infectious agent but do not exhibit any manifestations of the disease. These individuals are considered carriers. Carriers, although asymptomatic, can transmit the disease. For example, a person who has tested positive for the human immunodeficiency virus (HIV) antibody is probably infected with HIV. However, this person may not exhibit any signs and symptoms of the disease at the time of testing. Moreover, the signs and symptoms of AIDS may not occur for years. However, the person may transmit the virus to others; for example, by intimate sexual contact or by sharing a contaminated needle and syringe. An infected pregnant woman may transmit the virus to her child during pregnancy, birth, or breastfeeding. Nurses can also serve as reservoirs and inadvertently transfer pathogenic organisms to patients.

Animals

The rabies virus is an example of a pathogen whose reservoir is various animals, notably dogs, squirrels, and raccoons. The West Nile virus is another example of a pathogen whose reservoir is an animal, most frequently birds, but also horses (Schweon, 2003).

Soil

The soil also can act as a reservoir. For example, the organisms that cause gas gangrene and tetanus are examples of pathogens whose reservoir is soil.

Other Reservoirs

Many other reservoirs exist, being encountered on a daily basis. Water can harbor *Giardia*, *E. coli* 0157-H7, and *Shigella*. Drinking or swimming in contaminated water can begin the infectious cycle in a person. Ground beef and apple products can contain *E. coli* 0157-H7. The Centers for Disease Control and Prevention (CDC) recommends that all ground beef be cooked until well done and that apple products such as apple juice or apple sauce be pasteurized to prevent the spread of infection. Milk can contain listeria unless pasteurized. Influenza may be spread via inanimate objects if a person touches a contaminated article and then touches his or her nose or eyes.

Portal of Exit

The portal of exit is the point of escape for the organism from the reservoir. The organism cannot extend its influence unless it moves away from its original reservoir. Usually, each type of microorganism has a primary exit route. In humans, common portals of exit or escape routes include the respiratory, gastrointestinal, and genitourinary tracts, as well as breaks in the skin. Blood and tissue can also be portals of exit for pathogens.

Means of Transmission

An organism may be transmitted from its reservoir by various means or routes. Some organisms can be transmitted by more than one route. Organisms can enter the body by way of the contact route, either directly or indirectly. Direct contact involves proximity between the susceptible host and an infected person or a carrier, such as touching, kissing, or sexual intercourse. The indirect contact route involves personal contact with an inanimate object, such as touching a contaminated instrument.

> *Recall Esther Bailey, the woman being catheterized in the Reflective Practice box. In this situation, the catheter becomes contaminated. Indirect contact occurs if this catheter is inserted, predisposing her to an infection.*

Contaminated blood, food, water, or inanimate objects (fomites) are vehicles of transmission. **Vectors,** such as mosquitoes, ticks, and lice, are nonhuman carriers that transmit organisms from one host to another.

Microorganisms can also be spread through the airborne route when an infected host coughs, sneezes, or talks, or when the organism becomes attached to dust particles. Another means of transmission is through droplets. Droplet transmission is similar to airborne transmission. However, airborne particles are less than 5 μm and droplet particles are greater than 5μm. Table 27-1 summarizes the means of transmission for several organisms, their reservoirs, and examples of diseases they transmit.

Portal of Entry

The portal of entry is the point at which organisms enter a new host. The organism must find a portal of entry to a host or it may die. The entry route into the new host often is the same as the exit route from the prior reservoir. The urinary, respiratory, and gastrointestinal tracts and the skin are common portals of entry.

Susceptible Host

Microorganisms can continue to exist only in a source that is acceptable (a **host**) and only if they overcome any resistance mounted by the host's defenses. Susceptibility is the degree of resistance the potential host has to the pathogen. Hospital patients are often in a weakened state of health because of illness and have less resistance. Thus they are more susceptible for infection. Many factors influence a host's susceptibility; these are discussed later in the chapter.

> *Remember Giselle Turheis, the woman with leukemia and a compromised immune status. Her susceptibility to infection is increased because of the lack of an adequate functioning immune system.*

Stages of Infection

An understanding of the stages in the development of an infection is necessary to intervene and disrupt the infection cycle. An infection progresses through the following phases:
- Incubation period
- Prodromal stage
- Full stage of illness
- Convalescent period

The course and severity of the infection, as well as the patient's response, influence the type and extent of nursing care provided.

Incubation Period

The incubation period is the interval between the pathogen's invasion of the body and the appearance of symptoms of infection. During this stage, the organisms are growing and multiplying. The length of incubation may vary. For example, the common cold has an incubation period of 1 to 2 days, whereas tetanus has an incubation period ranging from 2 to 21 days.

TABLE 27-1 Organisms Capable of Causing Disease

Organism	Reservoir	Means of Transmission	Disease Transmitted
Staphylococcus aureus	Skin surface	Contact (direct)	Wound infection
	Mouth		Abscess
	Nose		Carbuncle
	Throat		Boil
Hepatitis B virus	Blood	Contact (indirect)	Hepatitis B
	Feces		
	Body fluids and excretions		
Human immunodeficiency virus	Blood	Contact (direct)	Acquired immunodeficiency syndrome
	Semen		
	Vaginal secretions		
	Breast milk	Contact (ingestion)	
Mycobacterium tuberculosis	Sputum (respiratory tract)	Airborne	Tuberculosis
Borrelia burgdorferi	Ticks (sheep, cattle, deer, mice)	Vectors	Lyme disease
Escherichia coli	Feces	Contact (direct)	*E. coli* infection
	Undercooked meat (beef)	Contact (ingestion)	
	Unpasteurized apple juice		

Prodromal Stage

A person is most infectious during the prodromal stage. Early signs and symptoms of disease are present but these are often vague and nonspecific, ranging from fatigue and malaise to a low-grade fever. This period lasts from several hours to several days. During this phase, the patient often does not realize that he or she is contagious. As a result, the infection spreads.

Full Stage of Illness

The presence of specific signs and symptoms indicates the full stage of illness. The type of infection determines the length of the illness and the severity of the manifestations. Symptoms that are limited or occur in only one body area are referred to as localized symptoms, whereas symptoms manifested throughout the entire body are referred to as systemic symptoms.

Convalescent Period

The convalescent period is the recovery period from the infection. Convalescence may vary according to the severity of the infection and the patient's general condition. The signs and symptoms disappear, and the person returns to a healthy state. However, depending on the type of infection, the person may have a temporary or permanent change to his or her previous health state even after the convalescent period.

A person may continually pass through the four phases with the same infectious process, such as with herpes simplex. Although there may have only been one infectious exposure, the infection may continue to cycle through the phases.

The Body's Defense Against Infection

One of the first lines of defense against infection is the body's normal flora. Flora helps to keep potentially harmful bacteria from invading the body. In addition to the normal flora that inhabit various body sites, other defense systems help a person combat infection. These include the inflammatory response and immune response.

The inflammatory response is a protective mechanism that eliminates the invading pathogen and allows for tissue repair to occur. Inflammation helps the body to neutralize, control, or eliminate the offending agent and to prepare the site for repair (Smeltzer & Bare, 2004).

Another defense system is the immune response. The immune response involves specific reactions in the body as it responds to an invading foreign protein, such as bacteria, or in some cases, to the body's own proteins. The complex mechanisms that constitute the immune response occur as the body attempts to protect and defend itself. The foreign material is called an **antigen,** and the body commonly responds to the antigen by producing an **antibody.** This antigen–antibody reaction, also known as humoral immunity, is one component of the overall immune response. The cell-mediated defense, or cellular immunity, involves an increase in the number of lymphocytes (white blood cells) that destroy or react with cells the body recognizes as harmful. Although these complicated chemical and mechanical responses are not completely understood, it is known that they help to defend the body specifically against bacterial, viral, and fungal infections as well as malignant cells.

Factors Affecting the Risk for Infection

The susceptibility of the host depends on various factors:
- Intact skin and mucous membranes protect the body against microbial invasion.

> Think back to Esther Bailey, the woman being catheterized who also has developed a postoperative wound infection. Undergoing abdominal surgery disrupts the integrity of the skin and mucous membranes, thereby increasing her risk for a wound infection.

- The normal pH levels of the gastrointestinal and genitourinary tracts, as well as the skin, help to ward off microbial invasion.
- The body's white blood cells provide resistance to certain pathogens.
- Age, sex, race, and hereditary factors influence susceptibility. Neonates and older adults appear to be more vulnerable to infection. (See the accompanying box, Focus on the Older Adult.)
- Immunization, natural or acquired, acts to resist infection.
- Fatigue, climate, nutritional and general health status, the presence of preexisting illnesses, previous or current treatments, and certain medications may play a part in the susceptibility of a potential host.
- Stress may adversely affect the body's normal defense mechanisms.
- The increasing use of invasive or indwelling medical devices provides exposure to and entry for more potential sources of disease-producing organisms, particularly in a patient whose defenses are already weakened by disease.

Health habits that promote wellness can decrease the susceptibility of a host. Sensible nutrition, adequate rest and exercise, stress-reduction techniques, and good personal hygiene habits can help maintain optimum bodily function and immune response. Unsafe sex practices and sharing intravenous (IV) needles are potentially dangerous and provide an opportunity for pathogens to enter a host and cause an infection.

THE NURSING PROCESS FOR INFECTION CONTROL AND PREVENTION

Assessing

The nurse plays a critical role in controlling infection. This role begins with early detection and surveillance techniques. The extent of nursing interventions depends on the suscepti-

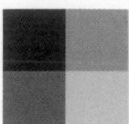

Focus on the Older Adult
Age-Related Changes Predisposing to Infection

Age-Related Changes	Nursing Strategies
Pulmonary Infections	
• Decreased cough reflex	• Place patient in sitting position to eat and drink.
• Decreased elastic recoil of the lungs	• Encourage patient to drink plenty of fluids unless contraindicated.
• Decreased activity of the cilia	• Encourage patient to cough and deep breathe or use incentive spirometer as ordered.
• Abnormal swallowing reflexes	
Urinary Tract Infections	
• Incomplete emptying of the bladder	• Discuss with patient need to void at regular intervals.
• Decreased sphincter control	• Encourage patient to drink plenty of fluids, unless contraindicated.
• Bladder-outlet obstruction due to an enlarged prostate gland	• Administer medications for enlarged prostate (benign prostate hypertrophy) and estrogen depletion as ordered.
• Pelvic floor relaxation due to estrogen depletion	• If patient wears absorbent product, such as an incontinence pad, instruct patient to change pad frequently and perform good "pericare."
• Reduced renal blood flow	• Assess for UTIs (may be atypical in elderly patient*).
	• Discuss need for patient to void immediately after sexual intercourse.
Skin Infections	
• Loss of elasticity	• Encourage patient to drink plenty of fluids, unless contraindicated.
• Increased dryness	• Help patient to perform good hygiene practices daily.
• Thinning of epidermis	• Apply lotion to skin as needed.
• Slowing of cell replacement	• Assess frequently for any breaks in skin integrity, rashes, or changes in skin.
• Decreased vascular supply	

*Atypical clinical manifestations of infection in an older adult include confusion, disorientation, lethargy, anorexia, delayed fever response, falls, incontinence, and failure to thrive.

bility of the host, the virulence of the organism, and the patient's signs and symptoms.

Inquire about the patient's immunization status and previous or recurring infections, observe nonverbal cues, and gather information about the history of the current disease. Nursing assessments include observing for signs and symptoms of a local or systemic infection. A localized infection can result in redness, swelling, warmth in the involved area, pain or tenderness, and loss of function of the affected part. Manifestations of a systemic infection include fever, often accompanied by an increase in pulse and respiratory rate, lethargy, anorexia, and tenderness and enlargement of lymph nodes that drain the area when an infection is present. Laboratory data can provide fur-

ther insight into the presence of an infectious process. Any of the laboratory test results outlined in Box 27-1 may indicate the presence of an infection.

Compilation of this assessment data constitutes a unique nursing database that suggests nursing interventions for patients at risk for infection or those in whom an infection is already present.

Diagnosing

The potential for infection or the presence of an infection in a patient suggests possible nursing diagnoses. The focus of nursing care depends on a nursing diagnosis that accurately

---

BOX 27-1 Laboratory Data Indicating an Infection

- Elevated white blood cell (leukocyte) count—normal value is 5,000 to 10,000/mm³
- Increase in specific types of white blood cells (differential count or percentage of each cell type)

Neutrophils	Normal = 60%–70%	Increased in acute infections that produce pus; increased risk for acute bacterial infection if decreased; may also be increased in response to stress.
Lymphocytes	Normal = 20%–40%	Increased in chronic bacterial and viral infections
Monocytes	Normal = 2%–8%	Increased in severe infections and function as a scavenger or phagocyte
Eosinophil	Normal = 1%–4%	May be increased in allergic reaction and parasitic infection
Basophil	Normal = 0.5%–1%	Usually unaffected by infections

- Elevated erythrocyte sedimentation rate—red blood cells settle more rapidly to the bottom of a tube of whole blood when an inflammation is present
- Presence of pathogen in urine, blood, sputum, or other draining cultures

reflects the patient's condition. The following are examples of nursing diagnoses related to an infectious process:

Risk for Infection related to presence of chronic disease; altered immune response; effects of medication; altered skin integrity; malnutrition; presence of invasive or indwelling medical device; lack of proper immunization

Social Isolation related to presence of communicable disease (AIDS)

Impaired Oral Mucous Membrane related to ineffective dental hygiene; trauma; side effect of medication; presence of invasive medical device

Deficient Diversional Activity related to lack of visitors; restrictions imposed by airborne isolation precautions

Risk for Imbalanced Body Temperature related to infectious process, dehydration

Anxiety related to high risk for infection; social isolation

Risk for Latex Allergy Response related to occupational exposure; history of multiple surgical procedures

Activity Intolerance related to effects of infectious process, generalized weakness.

Outcome Identification and Planning

The nurse develops appropriate patient outcomes after reviewing the assessment data, considering the cycle of events resulting in an infection, and incorporating the principles of infection control. Planning outcomes that prevent infection or interfere with the infection cycle is an exciting challenge, providing an opportunity to see the positive results from one's efforts, that is, effective nursing interventions aimed at controlling or preventing infection. The following examples of expected patient outcomes are appropriate for preventing infection and using infection-control techniques. The patient will:

• Demonstrate effective hand hygiene and good personal hygiene practices
• Identify the signs of an infection
• Maintain adequate nutritional intake
• Demonstrate proper disposal of soiled articles
• Use appropriate cleansing and disinfecting techniques
• Demonstrate an awareness of the necessity of proper immunizations
• Demonstrate stress-reduction techniques
• Verbalize an understanding of health risks associated with a latex allergy

Implementing

The nurse uses aseptic techniques to halt the spread of microorganisms and minimize the threat of infection. To control the number of organisms, medical and surgical asepsis are vital. The practice of **asepsis** includes all activities to prevent infection or break the chain of infection. There are two asepsis categories: medical asepsis and surgical asepsis. Medical asepsis, or clean technique, involves procedures and practices that reduce the number and transfer of pathogens. Medical asepsis procedures, for example, include performing hand hy-

giene and wearing gloves. Surgical asepsis, or sterile technique, includes practices used to render and keep objects and areas free from microorganisms. Surgical asepsis procedures could include inserting an indwelling urinary catheter or inserting an IV catheter.

Using Medical Asepsis

Medical asepsis techniques are used continuously both within and outside health agencies, based on the assumption that pathogens are likely to be present. For example, public drinking cups are considered unsanitary because a person harboring pathogens may transfer them to the cup when used. In a healthcare facility, if a specific pathogen is known to be present, special methods of medical asepsis are used to prevent further spread of the organism. Nearly every nursing activity includes practices of medical asepsis. Therefore the nurse assumes a major responsibility for breaking the cycle of infection by providing safe patient care and protecting the patient as well as one's self from microorganisms that may cause disease. Box 27-2 highlights the basic practices of medical asepsis for nurses to use when giving care to patients.

Hand Hygiene

Hand hygiene is the most effective way to help prevent the spread of organisms. According to recent CDC guidelines, the term hand hygiene is now preferred and applies to either handwashing with plain soap and water, use of antiseptic handrubs including alcohol-based products, or surgical hand antisepsis (CDC, 2002). Although opinions differ as to the proper cleaning agents, the minimum length of time for washing, and the ideal frequency of adequate hand hygiene measures, all agree that hand hygiene is the most important procedure for preventing infections. Nurses need to focus on this simple procedure that can interrupt the cycle of infection.

Bacterial Flora on Hands

Two types of bacterial flora are normally found on the hands: transient bacteria and resident bacteria. Transient bacteria, normally picked up by the hands in the usual activities of daily living, are relatively few (in number and type) on clean and exposed areas of the skin. They are attached loosely on the skin, usually in grease, fats, and dirt, and are found in greater numbers under the fingernails. Transient bacteria, pathogenic as well as nonpathogenic, can be removed with relative ease by washing the hands thoroughly and frequently.

Resident bacteria, normally found in creases in the skin, are relatively stable in number and type. They cling tenaciously to the skin by adhesion and adsorption, requiring considerable friction with a brush for removal. They are less susceptible to antiseptics than transient bacteria. It is not possible to clean the skin completely of all bacteria.

Transient bacteria may adjust to the environment of the skin when they are present in large numbers over a long period. They then become resident bacteria. If pathogenic organisms become resident bacteria on the skin, the hands then become carriers of the particular organism. Therefore, to help prevent transient bacteria from becoming resident bacteria, it is impor-

BOX 27-2 **Practicing Basic Principles of Medical Asepsis in Patient Care**

- Practice good hand hygiene (see Box 27-3).
- Keep soiled items and equipment from touching the clothing. Carry soiled linens or other used articles so that they do not touch your clothing.
- Do not place soiled bed linen or any other items on the floor, which is grossly contaminated. It increases contamination of both surfaces.
- Avoid having patient cough, sneeze, or breathe directly on others. Provide them with disposable tissues, and instruct them, as indicated, to cover their mouth and nose to prevent spread by airborne droplets.
- Move equipment away from you when brushing, dusting, or scrubbing articles. This helps prevent contaminated particles from settling on the hair, face, and clothing.
- Avoid raising dust. Use a specially treated cloth or a dampened cloth. Do not shake linens. Dust and lint particles constitute a vehicle by which organisms may be transported from one area to another.
- Clean the least soiled areas first and then the more soiled ones. This helps prevent having the cleaner areas soiled by the dirtier areas.
- Dispose of soiled or used items directly into appropriate containers. Wrap items that are moist from body discharge or drainage in waterproof containers, such as plastic bags, before discarding into the refuse holder so that handlers will not come in contact with them.
- Pour liquids that are to be discarded, such as bath water, mouth rinse, and the like, directly into the drain to avoid splattering in the sink and onto you.
- Sterilize items that are suspected of containing pathogens. After sterilization, they can be managed as clean items, if appropriate.
- Use practices of personal grooming that help prevent spreading microorganisms. Examples include shampooing the hair regularly, keeping it short or pinned up to limit the possibility of carrying microorganisms on hair shafts, keeping the fingernails short and free of broken cuticles and ragged nail edges, and avoiding wearing rings with grooves and stones that may harbor microorganisms.
- Follow guidelines conscientiously for standard and transmission-based precautions as prescribed by agency.

tant to clean the hands promptly when they are visibly soiled, after each contact with contaminated materials, and after removing gloves.

Cleansing Agents

Various hand hygiene products are available. Soaps and detergents, also referred to as nonantimicrobial agents, are considered adequate for routine mechanical cleansing of the hands and removal of most transient microorganisms. They help remove soil because they lower surface tension and act as emulsifying agents. Bar, liquid, leaflet, and powdered soap are all effective. Use of a particular type in a healthcare agency often depends on personnel or agency preference.

Using handwashing products that contain an **antimicrobial** or antibacterial ingredient is recommended in any setting where the risk for infection is high. When present in certain concentrations, these agents can kill bacteria or suppress their growth. Numerous studies have documented that alcohol-based handrubs more effectively reduce bacterial counts on the hands of healthcare personnel than antimicrobial soap, thus reducing nosocomial spread of disease. Alcohol-based handrubs have an alcohol concentration between 60% and 90% and are available as foam, gel, or lotions. In addition to their ability to reduce overall infection rates, alcohol-based handrubs save time, do not require a sink, and can be made easily available in patient care areas (see the accompanying Research in Nursing box). Studies have indicated that the additional cost of these antimicrobial agents is more than offset by a reduction in the number of hospital-acquired infections (CDC, 2002).

By their nature and when used frequently, alcohol-based products can cause skin irritation and dryness. This defeats the purpose of the product in decreasing the number of surface organisms because damaged skin harbors organisms and is more difficult to clean adequately. Therefore, alcohol-based handrubs containing emollients address these concerns and are more acceptable. Lotions, best applied after patient care is completed, may also be used to soothe damaged skin. Small, nonrefillable containers that are less likely to become contaminated from bacteria are recommended for personal use. Be aware of the possibility that oil-based lotions may adversely affect the integrity of latex gloves (Jones et al., 2000). Check with infection-control personnel to determine whether a particular lotion interferes with the action of soaps or antimicrobial agents used in the agency.

Recommended Techniques

The CDC, the government agency responsible for investigating, preventing, and controlling disease has recently released new recommendations, with the intent of improving hand hygiene practices in healthcare workers (Box 27-3). If a healthcare worker's hands are visibly soiled or contaminated with blood or body fluids, washing the hands with soap and water is required. If the hands are not visibly soiled, an alcohol-based hand rub can be used. See Guidelines for Nursing Care 27-1 for directions on how to use an alcohol-based hand rub.

Effective handwashing requires at least a 15-second scrub with plain soap or disinfectant and warm water. Hands that are visibly soiled need a longer scrub. Many studies have established the merits of handwashing, and several agencies have published directions and recommendations. The Association for Professionals in Infection Control and Epidemiology (APIC) has published guidelines for handwashing in various settings and reviewed the variety of products available for handwashing.

Research in Nursing Making a Difference

Hand Hygiene: Use of Alcohol Hand Sanitizer as an Infection-Control Strategy in an Acute-Care Facility

Hand hygiene is the most important way to prevent the spread of infection. However, due to short staffing, dermatitis from frequent handwashing, poor access to sinks, and deficient knowledge of the healthcare provider, handwashing compliance has been documented to be less than 50%. Hospital-acquired infections account for $4.5 billion annually. To reduce this amount, different ways have been researched to ensure good hand hygiene habits in healthcare providers.

Related Research

Hilburn, J., Hammond, B., Fendler, E., & Groziak, P. (2003). Use of alcohol hand sanitizer as an infection control strategy in an acute care facility. *American Journal of Infection Control, 31*(2), 109–116.

> The study took place in a 498-bed acute-care facility, with 1,700 employees. The study was performed on the orthopedic surgical unit. For 6 months prior to the study, information was gathered regarding handwashing compliance. After this data

was collected, an alcohol-gel hand sanitizer was made available for healthcare providers, patients, and visitors for the next 10 months. The hand sanitizer was placed in patient rooms, on medication carts, and at the nurses' station. Patients were also given information on the importance of hand hygiene and a small bottle of the alcohol gel to keep at their bedside. The most frequent types of infections noted on this floor were urinary tract and surgical site.

Relevance to Nursing Practice

Interventions that increase compliance with hand hygiene can lead to a decrease in the amount of nosocomial infections. During the 10-month period that the alcohol gel was used, there was a 36.1% decrease in infection rates. The average amount saved by the institution during this period was estimated to be $91,257.57, with a range of $13,797 to $316,135. This significant savings should definitely offset the cost of the alcohol hand gel.

BOX 27-3 Recommendation for Hand Hygiene

If hands are visibly soiled or contaminated with blood or other body fluid:

- Wash hands with either a nonantimicrobial soap and water or an antimicrobial soap and water.
- Wash hands before eating and after using the restroom.
- Use warm, not hot, water to prevent further irritation to skin. (See Skill 27-1 for correct handwashing technique.)

If hands are not visibly soiled, use an alcohol-based handrub to decontaminate hands:

- Decontaminate hands before having direct contact with patients, after having direct contact with a patient, before donning sterile gloves for a procedure, and after removing gloves. (See Guidelines for Nursing Care 27-1 for correct technique.)
- Decontaminate hands also after contact with inanimate objects surrounding the patient, and if moving hands from a contaminated site to a clean site on a patient's body during patient care.
- Perform decontamination also after contact with body fluids or excretions, mucous membranes, nonintact skin, and wound dressings.
- Alternatively, wash hands with an antimicrobial soap and water.

Adapted from Centers for Disease Control and Prevention. (2002). Guideline for hand hygiene in health-care settings. *Morbidity and Mortality Weekly Report 2002, 51*(RR16), 1–45.

Most guidelines recommend removing all jewelry except wedding bands, where bacteria tend to accumulate. Rings also increase the likelihood that gloves may tear when donned over the jewelry. Nails are to be kept short, with close attention to the area beneath the fingernails, because most organisms are found under and around the nails. Nail polish does not appear to increase the number of microorganisms as long as the polish is not chipped. A clear polish is preferable to color because the area under the nails is more visible. Artificial nails are not recommended because they harbor more bacteria than natural nails, place the wearer at risk for developing a fungal infection in the nail bed, and are associated with less vigorous scrubbing in the nail area. A recent study suggests that two nurses' long or artificial nails may have been a factor in exposing neonates in a neonatal intensive care unit to an infection caused by *Pseudomonas aeruginosa* (Moolenar et al., 2000). Recommended handwashing techniques for medical asepsis are listed in Skill 27-1.

Guidelines for Nursing Care 27-1
Hand Hygiene: Using an Alcohol-Based Handrub

- Apply product to the palm of one hand, using the amount of product recommended on the package (it will vary according to the manufacturer).
- Rub hands together, making sure to cover all surfaces of the hands, fingers, and in between the fingers.
- Continue rubbing until the hands are dry.

SKILL 27-1   Handwashing

EQUIPMENT

Non-antimicrobial or antimicrobial soap   Paper towels   Oil-free lotion (optional)

ACTION	RATIONALE
1. Stand in front of the sink. Do not allow your clothing to touch the sink during the washing procedure.	The sink is considered contaminated. Clothing may carry organisms from place to place.
2. Remove jewelry, if possible, and secure in a safe place or allow plain wedding band to remain in place.	Removal of jewelry facilitates proper cleansing. Microorganisms may accumulate in settings of jewelry. If jewelry was worn during care, it should be left on during handwashing.
3. Turn on water and adjust force. Regulate the temperature until the water is warm.	Water splashed from the contaminated sink will contaminate your clothing. Warm water is more comfortable and has less tendency to open pores and remove oils from the skin. Organisms can lodge in roughened and broken areas of chapped skin.
4. Wet the hands and wrist area. Keep hands lower than elbows to allow water to flow toward fingertips.	Water should flow from the cleaner toward the more contaminated area. Hands are more contaminated than forearms.
5. Use about 1 teaspoon liquid soap from dispenser or rinse bar of soap and lather thoroughly. Cover all areas of hands with the soap product. Rinse soap bar again and return to soap dish.	Rinsing the soap before and after use removes the lather that may contain microorganisms.
6. With firm rubbing and circular motions, wash the palms and backs of the hands, each finger, the areas between the fingers, the knuckles, wrists, and forearms. Wash at least 1 inch above area of contamination. If hands are not visibly soiled, wash to 1 inch above the wrists.	Friction caused by firm rubbing and circular motions helps to loosen dirt and organisms that can lodge between the fingers, in skin crevices of knuckles, on palms and backs of the hands, and on the wrists and forearms. Cleaning less contaminated areas (forearms and wrists) after hands are clean prevents spreading organisms from the hands to the forearms and wrists.

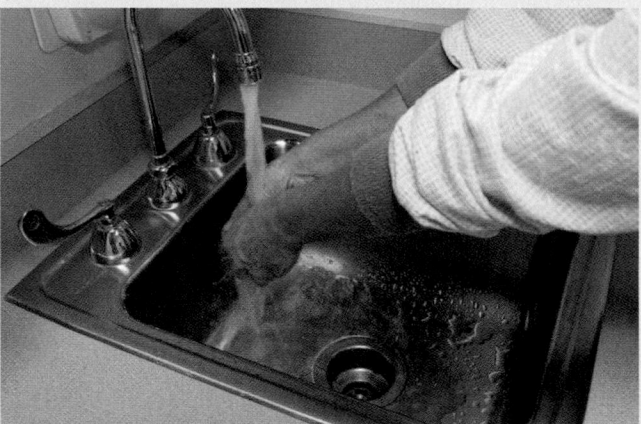

Action 4: Wetting hands and wrists.   (Photo by Rick Brady.)

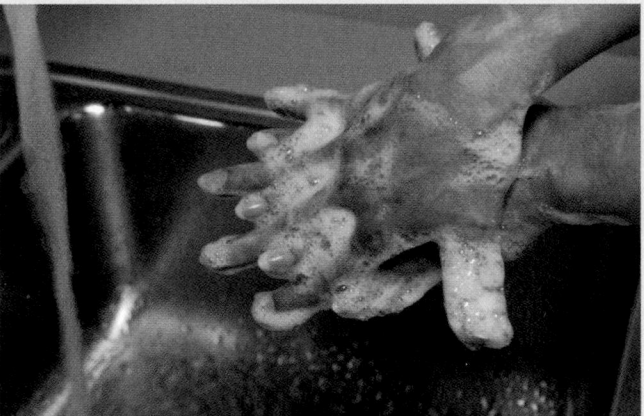

Action 6: Washing hands and forearms with firm rubbing and circular motions. (Photo by Rick Brady.)

7. Continue this friction motion for at least 15 seconds.	Length of handwashing is determined by degree of contamination.
8. Use fingernails of the other hand or a clean orangewood stick to clean under fingernails.	Area under nails has a high microorganism count, and organisms may remain under the nails where they can grow and be spread to others.
9. Rinse thoroughly.	Running water rinses organisms and dirt into the sink.
10. Dry hands, beginning with the fingers and moving upward toward forearms, with a paper towel and discard it immediately. Use another clean towel to turn off the faucet. Discard towel immediately without touching other clean hand.	Drying the skin well prevents chapping. Dry hands first because they are the cleanest and least contaminated area. Turning the faucet off with a clean paper towel protects the clean hands from contact with a soiled surface.

(continued)

Handwashing (continued)

ACTION	RATIONALE
11. Use lotion on hands if desired.	Oil-free lotion helps to keep the skin soft and prevents chapping. It is best applied after patient care is complete and from small, personal containers. Oil-based lotions should be avoided because they can cause deterioration of gloves.

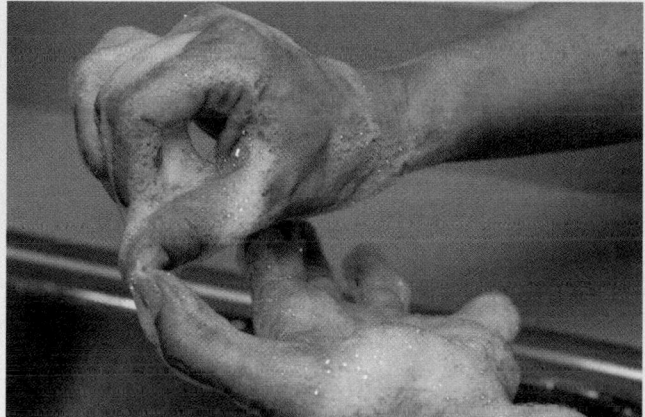

Action 8: Cleaning under fingernails.   (Photo by Rick Brady.)

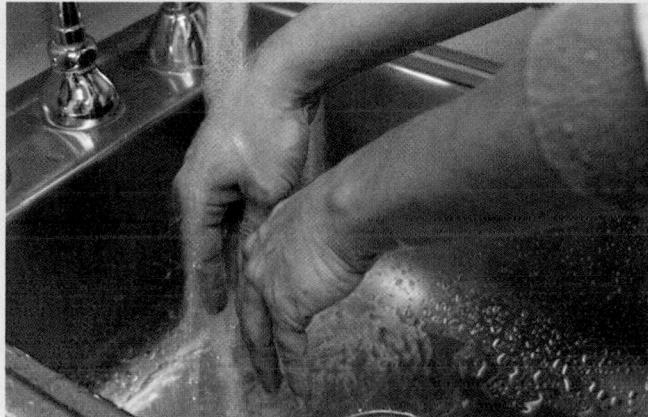

Action 9: Rinsing thoroughly.   (Photo by Rick Brady.)

Child Consideration	Instruct children at early age in proper handwashing techniques.
Special Consideration	An antimicrobial soap product is recommended before an invasive procedure and after exposure to blood or body fluids. The length of the scrub will vary based on need.
	Sinks with various faucet controls are available. In addition to the more common hand faucets, knee- and foot-operated controls may be used. Sinks with elbow controls are generally used in a surgical setting.
	Liquid, bar, granules, or leaflets are all acceptable forms of nonantimicrobial soap.

Even though healthcare personnel know the importance of good hand hygiene, most studies report that compliance with this simple preventive measure is difficult to achieve. Despite intensive educational efforts, hand hygiene is practiced infrequently. Wearing gloves does not eliminate the need for proper hand hygiene. In reality, the warmth and moisture inside gloves create an ideal environment for bacteria to multiply, making it even more important to perform good hand hygiene before and after using gloves. Research also indicates that gloving does not guarantee complete protection from infectious organisms. Gloves provide a barrier but are not impenetrable. It has been shown that many times glove-barrier failure goes undetected by the healthcare worker. Double gloving (putting on two gloves) is recommended if the healthcare worker is going to be exposed to blood or body fluids.

Hand antisepsis before assisting with a surgical procedure involves a more lengthy scrub, reducing resident and transient flora from the forearms and hands. This procedure, known as surgical hand scrub, incorporates surgical asepsis and is described in texts that deal with operating and delivery room procedures. The CDC guideline recommends using an antimicrobial soap or alcohol-based hand rub with persistent activity for surgical hand antisepsis. Scrub time is also reduced significantly when these agents are used.

Control via Sterilization and Disinfection

Cleansing, disinfection, and sterilization help to break the cycle of infection and prevent disease. Most health agencies provide patient-care items that are sterile when purchased and disposed of after use. Some items, such as pitchers, water glasses, and plastic basins, may be used repeatedly but by one patient only; they are then discarded or sent home with the patient on discharge.

Health agencies usually maintain a central supply unit where most reusable equipment is cleaned, kept in good working order, and sterilized as indicated. In the home and in some small health agencies, the nurse sometimes must make decisions about how to prepare equipment and supplies that are safe for patient use. Although nurses may not be directly involved in the actual process, they must be aware of the critical role that nurses play in preventing infection.

Several processes are used to destroy microorganisms. **Disinfection** destroys all pathogenic organisms except spores; **sterilization** is the process by which all microorganisms, including spores, are destroyed. Disinfection can be used when prepping the skin for a procedure or cleaning a piece of equipment that does not enter a sterile body part. Sterilization is usually performed on equipment that is entering a sterile portion of the body. Disinfection and sterilization of contaminated or infected objects and good hand hygiene diminish and often eliminate microorganisms as potential sources of infection.

Factors for Method Selection

Various factors influence the choice of sterilization and disinfection methods, including the following:

Nature of organisms present: The CDC recommends that all supplies, linens, and equipment in a healthcare setting should be treated as if the patient were infectious. Some organisms are easily destroyed, whereas others can withstand certain common sterilization and disinfection methods.

Number of organisms present: The more organisms present on an item, the longer it takes to destroy them.

Type of equipment: Equipment with small lumens, crevices, or joints requires special care. Certain articles that may be damaged by various sterilization and disinfection methods require special handling.

Intended use of equipment: The need for medical or surgical asepsis influences the preparation and cleaning of equip-ment. In the home, it may be safe to use equipment and supplies that are clean, but most health agencies prefer to use sterilized articles for patient care.

Available means for sterilization and disinfection: The choice of chemical or physical means of sterilization and disinfection depends on the nature and number of organisms, the type and intended use of the equipment, and the availability and practicality of the means. (Table 27-2 lists the types of methods for sterilization and disinfection.)

Time: Time is a key factor when sterilizing or disinfecting articles. Failure to follow the recommended time periods is grossly negligent.

Cleaning of Supplies and Equipment

Proper cleaning of items used in healthcare before they are sterilized or disinfected is essential to reduce the number of organisms and to dislodge them from crevices and from under layers of contaminating substances. The following techniques are recommended for cleaning equipment:

• Wear waterproof gloves at all times.
• Rinse the articles first with cold running water to remove organic material. Heat coagulates certain organic material, which makes removal more difficult.
• Wash the articles, after rinsing them, in warm water that contains detergent or soap. The combination of warm water and soap facilitates emulsification and removal of dirt and debris.

TABLE 27-2 Methods of Sterilization and Disinfection

Method	Discussion	Caution
Physical		
Steam	Higher temperature caused by higher pressure destroys organisms (eg, autoclaving)	Most plastic and rubber devices are damaged by autoclaving.
Boiling water	Frequently used in the home—simple and inexpensive; boil item for at least 10 minutes	Spores and some viruses are not destroyed by boiling.
Dry heat	Alternative sterilization method for home. Used for metal items. Heat oven to 350°F for 2 or more hours.	Insufficient to destroy all microorganisms. Not used in healthcare agencies.
Radiation	Used for pharmaceuticals, foods, plastics, and other heat-sensitive items	Object must be directly exposed to ultraviolet radiation on all surfaces. Poses risk to personnel.
Chemical		
Ethylene oxide gas	Destroys microorganisms and spores by interfering with metabolic processes in cells. Gas is released while items (oxygen and suction gauges, blood-pressure equipment) are contained in autoclave.	Precautions necessary because gas is toxic to humans.
Chemical solutions	Generally used for instrument and equipment disinfection and for housekeeping disinfection. Chlorines are useful for disinfecting water and for housekeeping purposes. A solution of sodium hypochlorite (household bleach) in a 1:100 dilution effectively inactivates human immunodeficiency virus. Betadine and alcohol are also used as disinfectants.	Method does not destroy all spores and may cause corrosion on metal surfaces.

- Use a brush with stiff bristles, as indicated, to clean the articles thoroughly. Friction aids in the removal of organisms and debris from difficult-to-reach areas.
- Rinse and dry the article thoroughly.
- Prepare the cleaned equipment for sterilization or disinfection.
- Consider the brush, gloves, and the sink or basin in which the articles were cleaned as highly contaminated, and treat or discard them accordingly.

Home Care Considerations

The increasing number of individuals who are ill or immunocompromised, coupled with increasingly virulent organisms, poses sterilization and disinfection concerns for home environments. After thorough cleaning, some contaminated items may be disinfected by placing them in boiling water or using common household disinfectants such as bleach, isopropyl alcohol (70%), or acetic acid (white vinegar).

Transmission-Based Precautions and Barrier Techniques for Infection Prevention and Control

The transfer of pathogens from person to person can be decreased by limiting the dissemination of pathogens. The most practical way to accomplish this is through the use of barriers that prevent common vehicles from transmitting the pathogens. Figure 27-2 shows how barriers break the infection cycle. Barriers are ways to decrease the spread of pathogens and include personal protective equipment, hand hygiene, and barrier techniques.

Personal Protective Equipment and Supplies

According to the 1992 Occupational Safety and Health Administration (OSHA) ruling, healthcare agencies must provide employees with the equipment and supplies necessary to minimize or prevent exposure to infectious material. This personal protective equipment includes gloves, gowns, masks, and protective eye gear. Skill 27-2 illustrates the proper use of this equipment.

Gloves

Gloves, not a substitute for good hand hygiene, are worn only once and discarded appropriately according to agency policy. Then hands are thoroughly decontaminated with meticulous hand hygiene. Each patient interaction requires a clean pair of gloves, and some care activities for an individual patient may necessitate changing gloves more than once. Gloves are not necessary when care activities do not involve the possibility of soilage of hands with body fluids. Activities such as turning a patient, feeding a patient, taking vital signs, and changing IV fluid bags do not require the use of gloves as long as the potential contact with body fluids is not present. While wearing gloves, never do the following: leave the patient's room (unless transporting a contaminated item or a patient requiring transmission-based precautions), write in the patient's chart, or use the computer keyboard or telephone in the nurses' station. Recent studies have also indicated that healthcare workers should not touch their pagers without performing good hand hygiene first (Beyea, 2002).

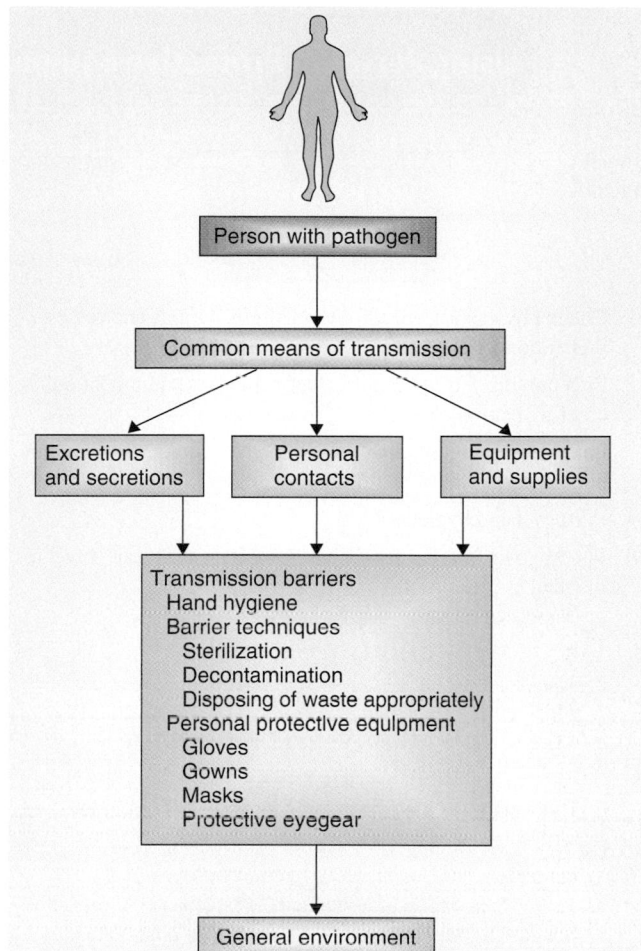

FIGURE 27-2 Transmission barriers help prevent the transporting of pathogens from the infected person to the general environment.

As mentioned earlier, gloves are not always an impenetrable barrier. In high-risk settings such as the operating room, glove failure is common. Reports indicate that during surgery, particularly operative procedures longer than 3 hours, gloves fail more than 50% of the time (Graves & Twomey, 2002). Being exposed to body fluids and blood and handling many surgical instruments are both factors contributing to glove failure. For example, tiny tears or cuts that occur in the gloves often are not observed until the gloves are removed after surgery and blood is visible on the hands. In an effort to provide a safer working environment, electronic glove-monitoring devices combined with ongoing education about safe gloving technique and injury prevention are being used. In addition, double gloving with a colored glove under a translucent outer glove is an alternative solution to detect a breach in glove integrity. (Graves & Twomey, 2002).

Latex Allergy. Approximately 700,000 healthcare workers have reported a latex sensitivity, with reactions ranging from local skin reactions to urticaria (hives) to systemic anaphylaxis, an exaggerated allergic reaction that can result in death. The initial CDC recommendation for universal precautions contributed to an increased use of latex gloves for patient-care activities. In 1980, latex glove use was around 785 million; by

Using Personal Protective Equipment

EQUIPMENT
Gloves
Gown
Mask (surgical or particulate respirator)
Protective eyewear

ACTION	RATIONALE
1. Check physician's order for type of precautions and review precautions in Infection-Control Manual.	Mode of transmission or organism determines type and degree of precautions.
2. Plan nursing activities and gather necessary equipment before entering patient's room.	Organization facilitates performance of task and adherence to precautions.
3. Provide instruction about precautions to patient, family members, and visitors.	An explanation encourages cooperation of patient and family and reduces apprehension about precaution procedures.
4. Perform hand hygiene.	Hand hygiene deters the spread of microorganisms.
5. Put on gown, gloves, mask, and protective eyewear, if recommended as precaution:	Equipment interrupts chain of infection. Protects patient and nurse.
a. Tie gown securely at neck and waist.	Gown should protect all clothing. Obtain waterproof gown if soiling is likely.
b. Use clean disposable gloves. If worn with gown, draw glove cuffs over gown sleeves.	Gloves protect hands and wrists from microorganisms.
c. Mask must be securely tied and fitted to face.	Masks protect nurse or patient from droplet nuclei and large-particle aerosols.
d. Eyewear must have protection on side of face or side shields.	Eyewear protects mucous membranes in the eye from splashes.
6. When patient care is completed, remove gloves first.	Gloves have been involved in patient care and are most soiled.
a. Untie waist strings of gown first. Grasp outside of one glove and turn inside out to remove. Continue to hold on to glove.	Ungloved hand is clean and should not touch contaminated areas. Waist strings of gown are considered contaminated.
b. Insert fingers of ungloved hand inside the cuff of the remaining glove. Grasp glove on inside and remove by turning inside out. Drop in appropriate container.	

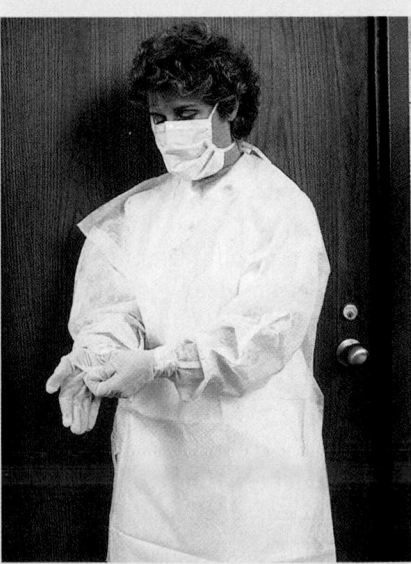

Action 6a: Grasping outside of first glove and pulling it off inside out.

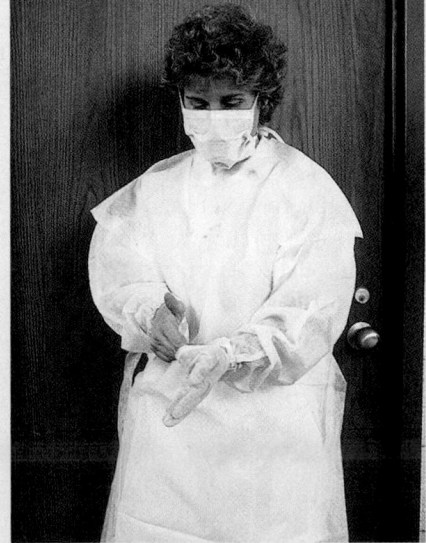

Action 6b: Placing fingers of ungloved hand inside cuff of the remaining glove.

7. After gloves are removed, remove mask: *Surgical mask*	
a. Untie mask and drop by strings into waste container.	Center of mask is contaminated. Strings are considered clean.

(continued)

ACTION	RATIONALE
Particulate respirator a. Use hand to hold respirator in place. b. Pull bottom strap up and over head. c. Pull top strap over head. d. Remove respirator from face and save for future use or discard according to manufacturer's directions.	This method prevents respirator from falling off face onto floor.
8. Remove gown: a. Gown that is not visibly soiled requires no particular technique for removal	
For gown that is visibly soiled: a. Untie neck strings of gown. Remove gown without touching outside of gown by keeping one hand up and under the gown cuff and using this protected hand to pull the opposite sleeve down and off. b. Use ungowned arm and hand to grasp the gown from the inside and remove from the remaining arm. Remove gown and turn inside out and drop in appropriate container.	Neck strings are considered clean. Outside of gown is contaminated.

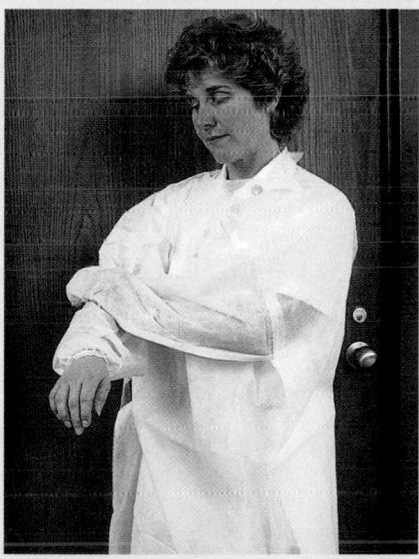

Action 8b: Using protected hand to pull the opposite sleeve down and off.

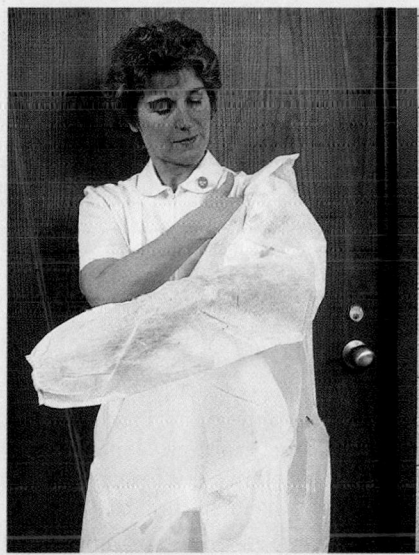

Action 8c: Using ungowned hand to grasp gown from the inside.

ACTION	RATIONALE
9. Remove eyewear last and clean according to agency policy.	Eyewear is reusable.
10. Perform hand hygiene.	Hand hygiene prevents spread of microorganisms.

1995, latex glove use had elevated to 9.5 billion (Gehring & Ring, 2000). Changes in the manufacturing process to meet supply demands may also have been a factor. The cornstarch powder or talc used to make gloves easier to put on is a major causative factor in any latex allergy. The powder binds with the latex protein and becomes airborne, where it can remain for 5 to 12 hours after healthcare workers don or remove gloves. People can be exposed to latex in many different ways. The powder particles may be inhaled, be absorbed into skin or mucous membranes, or enter the bloodstream. Re-

peated exposures have been shown to lead to a latex sensitivity. If the person continues to be exposed to latex after a sensitivity has developed, the person may demonstrate signs of a latex allergy.

Recommendations for Latex Allergy. The National Institute for Occupational Safety and Health (NIOSH) recommends that nonlatex gloves or powder-free, low-allergen latex gloves (if latex gloves are used) be available for employees. Nitrile gloves, gloves made of a synthetic material that resembles latex but has no latex proteins, are now also available. Nitrile has demonstrated adequate barrier qualities, but tears easily (Graves & Twomey, 2002). For patients with a latex allergy, a "latex-safe" healthcare environment is essential. A 1998 FDA ruling required all products or packaging containing natural rubber latex to carry a warning that these products may cause allergic responses in sensitive individuals. All healthcare facilities are required to have a written policy that identifies how to deal with latex-sensitive employees and patients. Before admission, the room for a patient with known or suspected latex allergy must be cleaned to remove any trace of residual glove powders. A latex-safe environment involves removal or covering of any natural latex rubber items, such as wall-mounted blood pressure cuffs, sharps containers, injection port caps on IV tubing, and urinary catheters. Awareness of an allergy to latex is also important for safe home care. Nurses need to ask whether patients have experienced any unusual signs or symptoms when blowing up balloons, using latex condoms, or wearing rubber gloves for dishwashing or cleaning. Box 27-4 summarizes information on latex allergy for healthcare personnel and patients.

Gowns

Gowns are usually worn to prevent soiling of the healthcare worker's clothing by the patient's blood and body fluids. They provide barrier protection and are donned immediately before entering the patient's room. Individual gown technique is recommended; this means that a gown is worn only once and is then discarded appropriately according to agency policy. A waterproof gown is used if there is an increased likelihood of contact with the patient's blood or body fluids. If a gown becomes heavily soiled or moistened with blood or body fluids when caring for a patient, remove it, perform thorough hand hygiene and put on a clean gown. There is no one special technique for applying a gown used as a barrier, but recommended practices for removing a soiled gown are described previously in Skill 27-2.

Masks

Masks help prevent the wearer from inhaling large-particle aerosols, which usually travel short distances (about 3 feet), and small-particle droplet nuclei, which can remain sus-

---

BOX 27-4 Latex Allergy Summary

Risk Factors:

Healthcare workers who wear latex gloves

People with allergic tendencies

People with food allergies, specifically banana, papaya, avocado, potatoes, kiwi fruit, chestnuts, and pineapples

Latex-industry workers

People with asthma, spina bifida, or a history of multiple surgical procedures or exposures to latex

Types of Reactions:

Irritant contact dermatitis: nonallergic dermatitis, restricted to area that has made contact with the latex. Gloves may cause erythematous and pruritic hands.

Delayed hypersensitivity: allergic contact dermatitis, displayed as dry, crusty bumps, erythema, pruritis, scaling vesicles, papular lesions at site of contact, including the palms; not a life-threatening reaction, however, person should be aware of latex contact.

Immediate hypersensitivity: systemic reactions, displayed as rhinitis, conjunctivitis, angioedema, bronchospasm, shock, and/or systemic anaphylactic reactions; this is a life-threatening sensitivity.

Diagnosis:

RAST: blood test for IgE antibodies to latex

Skin prick: small amount of serum derived from latex placed on small prick in skin

Patch test: small piece of latex taped to patient for 48–96 hours with periodic checking for any sign of latex reactions listed above

Glove challenge: patient wearing a latex glove for period of time, with periodic checking for any signs of latex reactions listed above

CAUTION: Any time a person with suspected latex allergies is exposed to latex, emergency equipment should be available.

Dipstick test: drop of blood placed on test strip; can be done without other equipment (not available yet)

Treatment:

Avoidance of latex-containing products

Localized reaction treated with oral diphenhydramine, cool compresses, and hydrocortisone 1% cream

Systemic reaction possibly treated with epinephrine (see below) subcutaneously, systemic steroids, antihistamines, with transport to the emergency department

Protocols for Patients With Latex Allergies:

• Place allergy sticker on chart, Caution sign on door, and allergy wrist band.

• Remove all latex-containing articles from room.

• Place three-way stopcocks in IV lines for medication administration. Place tape over any injection ports on IV tubing.

• Remove rubber stoppers from vials before drawing up medications.

• If available, place a cart containing all latex-free supplies in or outside of patient's room.

• Use glass syringes if no latex-free alternative is available.

• Cover latex portion of blood-pressure cuff or stethoscope before using on patient.

Frequently Used Products That Contain Latex:

Blood-pressure cuffs	Stethoscopes
Electrode pads	Tourniquets
IV tubing	Syringes
Foley catheters	Surgical masks
Baby bottle nipples	Pacifiers

Adapted from Gehring, L., & Ring, P. (2000). Latex allergy: Creating a safe environment. *Dermatology Nursing, 12*(3), 197–201.

pended in the air and travel longer distances. Masks also discourage the wearer from touching the eyes, nose, and mouth, thus limiting contact of organisms with mucous membranes.

Various mask practices are used. In some instances, all personnel and all the patient's visitors wear masks; in other situations, a patient requiring specific precautions wears the mask when transported outside his or her room to protect healthcare personnel and other patients from any exposure to pathogens.

A mask is worn only once and never lowered around the neck and then brought back over the mouth and nose for reuse. How long one can wear one mask while caring for one patient is the subject of debate. It should certainly be changed before it becomes damp from the wearer's exhalations. (See Skill 27-2 for the recommended practice for applying and removing a mask.)

The serious increase in the number of multidrug-resistant tuberculosis cases prompted new guidelines to prevent the transmission of this disease. According to CDC guidelines, either a high-efficiency particulate air (HEPA) filter respirator or N95 respirator certified by NIOSH must be worn when entering the room of a patient with known or suspected tuberculosis.

Think back to Jackson Ray Ivers, the son coming to visit his mother who is hospitalized with tuberculosis. The nurse would incorporate knowledge of tuberculosis transmission and appropriate barriers to explain to Mr. Ivers about the need for wearing a mask, or, in this case, a respirator.

These respirators filter inspired air, whereas surgical masks filter only expired air. Caregivers have expressed difficulty wearing the HEPA-style respirator for extended periods of time, but the N95 respirator, which is designed to filter out particles as small as 1 μm with 95% efficiency, fits more comfortably against the face (Fig. 27-3). The N95 mask also costs considerably less than the HEPA filter respirators. The elastic straps on these respirators provide more protection and a better fit than the ties on regular surgical masks.

Protective Eyewear

Protective eyewear, such as goggles or a face shield, must be available whenever there is a risk of contaminating the mucous membranes of the eyes. For example, suctioning a tracheostomy or assisting with an invasive procedure that may result in splattering of blood or other body fluids requires protection for the caregiver. Plain glasses are unacceptable because side shields are required.

Other Supplies and Procedures

Used equipment may be disposed of after use or, if reusable, bagged according to agency policy, sent to a central cleaning area, and sterilized or disinfected. Double bagging may be required if the single bag is not secure or is soiled on the outside. A contaminated item must never be used for another patient.

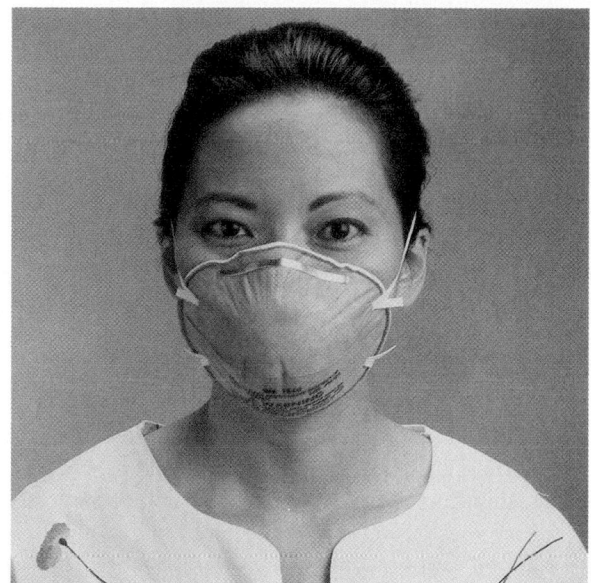

FIGURE 27-3 The Type N95 healthcare particulate respirator is NIOSH approved. It meets CDC guidelines for tuberculosis exposure control and is designed specifically for use in a healthcare setting. (Courtesy of 3M Health Care.)

Double bagging of trash and linen is usually needed only if the outside of the bag is visibly soiled. Some linen bags are water soluble and dissolve in hot water, making it unnecessary for workers to handle the contaminated linen. The use of paper trays and plastic eating utensils does not prevent transmission of organisms and is no longer recommended. The combined hot water and detergent used in commercial dishwashers sufficiently decontaminates dishes, glasses, and utensils. All spills of body fluids or substances must be immediately cleaned with the appropriate chemical germicide or disinfectant.

When collecting a specimen, take care to prevent the outside of the container from becoming contaminated with any secretions or body fluids. Place all laboratory specimens in plastic bags and seal the bags to prevent leakage during transportation. A bag marked "BIOHAZARDS" is used to dispose of trash that contains liquid or semi-liquid blood or other potentially infective material (OPIM), trash contaminated with blood or OPIM that would release these substances if compressed, and trash that is caked with dried blood or OPIM and is capable of releasing these materials during handling.

Specialized Infection-Control Precautions

In addition to barriers, specific precautions have been established to prevent the transmission of infection. Historically, the term **isolation,** a protective procedure that limits the spread of infectious diseases among hospitalized patients, hospital personnel, and visitors has been used. Currently the CDC has developed specific guidelines for transmission-based precautions (see discussion later in this chapter).

Historical Perspective

Early practices involved isolating or quarantining infected patients together in a separate facility where few, if any, aseptic techniques were employed. At the beginning of the 20th century, efforts at isolation moved toward placing infected individuals together in one hospital (infectious disease hospitals) or a hospital ward where caregivers used gowns and antiseptic solutions for handwashing as barriers to disease transmission. Eventually, infectious disease hospitals closed, including those set aside for people with tuberculosis. Patients who were considered infectious were routinely placed on general hospital units in separate rooms or in multiple-patient rooms with other patients who had the same infection.

Early CDC Guidelines

By 1970, the CDC was actively involved in developing and recommending infection-control practices and procedures for hospitals. Initial guidelines from the CDC included procedures for category-specific isolation, in which all infectious diseases that required similar infection-control techniques were grouped together in categories. The CDC recommended that hospitals use the specific isolation techniques to prevent transmission of all the diseases in each category.

In 1983, rather than group similar infectious diseases together, the CDC initiated disease-specific isolation, which listed each infectious disease separately, along with the individual interventions and barriers necessary to prevent transmission of that specific pathogenic organism. This system eliminated unnecessary isolation practices because caregivers responded to specific directions for that disease and thus individualized care for each patient based on the specific pathogenic organism. Because of the many diseases and modes of transmission, this isolation method required knowledgeable practitioners and accurate medical diagnoses and laboratory reports so that the correct isolation category was chosen.

Universal Precautions

Concern about the transmission of bloodborne diseases (eg, AIDS, hepatitis B virus [HBV]) and the increasing incidence of hospital-acquired infections caused a shift in the focus of infection-control programs. In 1987, in an effort to protect healthcare workers, the CDC issued recommendations for universal precautions. The CDC recommended that healthcare workers use gloves, gowns, masks, and protective eyewear when exposure to blood or body fluids was likely and that all patients should be considered potentially infected. Blood, semen, vaginal secretions, breast milk, cerebrospinal, synovial, pleural, peritoneal, pericardial, and amniotic fluids were included in universal precautions. However, the precautions did not extend to possible exposure involving feces, nasal secretions, sputum, sweat, tears, urine, and vomitus, unless they contained visible blood. The risk of HIV or HBV being transmitted through these materials was thought to be very low or nonexistent.

Universal precautions also recommended the use of puncture-resistant containers for disposing of all needles and sharps. Needles were not to be recapped because most needlestick injuries occur during recapping. The use of universal precaution strategies was not meant to replace other isolation system safeguards. The CDC recommended using universal precautions along with category-specific or disease-specific isolation systems.

OSHA Regulations

OSHA, a government agency that administers the Occupational Safety and Health Act of 1970, establishes minimum health and safety standards for workers. In 1991, OSHA issued regulations for use of universal precautions in all situations and settings in which occupational exposures to blood and other potentially infectious materials were possible. This ruling reinforced CDC guidelines for universal precautions and made violations punishable with severe fines. Recognizing that HBV poses the greatest bloodborne risk to healthcare workers, OSHA also required that employers offer HBV vaccine free of charge to employees to prevent its transmission. The American Nurses Association is urging OSHA to extend this directive to provide immunization and mandate protection against bloodborne diseases for nursing students who practice in these healthcare facilities.

OSHA has also fined hospitals that fail to use equipment or devices that reduce the risk for needlestick injuries for employees.

Body Substance Precautions

Body substance precautions (or body substance isolation) are an extension of universal precautions. First implemented at Harborview Medical Center in Seattle in 1985, they were designed to reduce the risk for cross-transmission of organisms between patients and to minimize the risk for infection in healthcare personnel. Body substance isolation precautions consider all body substances potentially infectious regardless of a person's diagnosis, advocating the consistent use of barriers whenever healthcare personnel have contact with moist body substances, mucous membranes, and nonintact skin. The more inclusive term "body substance" includes not only blood and blood-tinged fluids but also feces, urine, wound drainage, oral secretions, vomitus, and any other body substance. Advocates of body substance isolation consider it a simple, straightforward approach to infection control.

Using body substance isolation precautions eliminates the need for category-specific or disease-specific systems except for certain airborne diseases that require special precautions. Varicella (chickenpox), influenza, and pulmonary tuberculosis are examples of airborne diseases that require a private room with the door closed and a "Stop Sign Alert" on the door that requests visitors to check with the nurse before entering the room. Mask use depends on the organism and the visitor's immune status. By its design, body substance isolation reduces risks for patients and personnel by treating all people in a similar manner, thus minimizing potential infection from unknown, undiagnosed diseases.

In this system, disposable gloves and needle disposal containers are placed in every room. Each patient interaction requires good hand hygiene technique before and after care. Clean gloves are required for each patient, and high-stress care situations often require that gloves be changed several times while caring for one patient. When gloves are removed, this system recommends hand hygiene only if hands are visibly soiled. Some healthcare experts have cited this lack of emphasis on handwashing after glove removal as a disadvantage of this system.

Body substance isolation precautions also provide a consistent approach to soiled linen, trash disposal, and laboratory specimens. Laundry bags are secured and transported in the usual manner. Visible soiling on the outside requires double bagging. Laundry workers wear heavy gloves when handling soiled linen and must follow good handwashing technique. Trash is disposed of in securely tied plastic bags according to hospital policy or local and state requirements.

Some hospitals still use body substance precautions but have replaced the "Stop Sign Alert" for certain airborne disease with one indicating airborne-based transmission precautions. The Joint Commission on Accreditation of Healthcare Organizations (JCAHO) has recommended that only the means of transmission, rather than the patient's particular disease, be listed on any posting outside the patient's room to ensure patient confidentiality. The CDC encourages healthcare facilities to review their current recommendations and modify them according to the needs of their agency.

Current CDC Guidelines

The latest CDC guidelines replace all previous recommendations. In conjunction with the Hospital Infection Control Practices Advisory Committee (HICPAC), the CDC revised isolation precautions for use in healthcare facilities. The latest guidelines include the major features of universal and body substance precautions but use new terminology so as not to be confused with the previous systems. This guideline recognizes the importance of body fluids, secretions, and excretions in the transmission of hospital-acquired pathogens. Nurses must understand the various precautions or barrier techniques if they are to use them correctly and minimize infection risks to patients as well as to themselves (see Promoting Health 27-1: Infection-Control Precautions and Barrier Techniques).

The revised guideline designates two tiers of precautions:

Standard precautions: precautions used in the care of all hospitalized individuals regardless of their diagnosis or possible infection status. These precautions apply to blood, all body fluids, secretions, and excretions except sweat (whether or not blood is present or visible), nonintact skin, and mucous membranes.

Transmission-based precautions: precautions used in addition to standard precautions for patients in hospitals with suspected infection with pathogens that can be transmitted by airborne, droplet, or contact routes. These precautions encompass all the diseases or conditions previously listed in the disease-specific or category-specific classifications. These categories recognize that a disease may have multiple routes of transmission.

Recall Jackson Ray Ivers, the son of a patient with tuberculosis. Based on the nurse's knowledge of disease transmission, the nurse institutes airborne precautions for the patient and instructs Mr. Ivers in the need for proper hand hygiene and the use of a mask.

Promoting Health 27-1 *Infection Control Precautions and Barrier Techniques*

Use the assessment checklist to determine how well you are observing infection control or barrier precautions as you care for patients in a healthcare facility or in a community setting. Then develop a prescription for self-care by choosing appropriate behaviors from the list of suggestions.

ASSESSMENT CHECKLIST

almost always / sometimes / almost never

1. Perform hand hygiene before and after contact with a patient.
2. I wear gloves if contact with blood or body fluids is a possibility.
3. I use additional protective equipment (gowns, masks, goggles) when necessary.
4. I avoid recapping any needles.
5. I place needles or other sharp objects in a puncture-proof disposable container.
6. I dispose of used or contaminated objects and equipment in a leak-resistant plastic trash bag.

SELF-CARE BEHAVIORS

1. Read infection control standards published by OSHA and CDC.
2. Attend programs that provide updates on current CDC/OSHA policies.
3. Maintain strict personal hygiene habits.
4. Obtain immunizations when available.
5. Assess for any signs and symptoms of an infection.
6. Perform hand hygiene frequently.
7. Perform hand hygiene immediately after removing gloves.
8. Protect myself with the barriers necessary to prevent exposure to blood, body fluids, or secretions.
9. Follow agency policy if any exposure to blood or body substance occurs.
10. Never eat, drink, smoke, apply cosmetics or lip moistener, or handle contact lenses in an area where occupational exposure is possible.

The three types of transmission-based precautions (airborne, droplet, or contact) may be used alone or in combination, but always in addition to standard precautions. Box 27-5 summarizes the CDC guidelines along with specific recommendations for both tiers of precautions. Hospitals are encouraged to modify these recommendations as needed for implementation of their infection-control strategy.

The CDC continues to recommend the use of puncture-resistant containers for disposal of all needles and sharps. Since most needlestick injuries occur during recapping, **never** recap needles. The most serious risk associated with needlestick injury is the possible exposure to bloodborne pathogens such as HBV, hepatitis C virus (HCV), and HIV. The greatest risk of seroconversion (development of antibodies in response to an infection) after a needlestick injury occurs with hepatitis B (10%–30%); hepatitis C has a smaller rate of seroconversion (4%–10%); HIV has the smallest possible rate of seroconversion after a needlestick injury (0.1%–0.3%) (Shiao, Guo, & McLaws, 2002). Most hospitals now purchase needleless or protected or recessed IV systems. Although more expensive, studies have determined that higher costs for the newer equipment may be almost totally offset by lower costs of treatment and follow-up of needlestick injuries to employees. Although alternative equipment is available, nurses must still be accountable for their own safe work practices. In certain situations, as when access to a needle-disposal unit is not immediately possible, it may be necessary to recap a needle. Figure 27-4 illustrates an example of how to recap a needle to prevent needlestick injuries.

BOX 27-5 Summary of CDC Recommended Practices for Standard and Transmission-Based Precautions

Standard Precautions (Tier 1)
- Follow hand hygiene techniques (see Box 27-3).
- *Wear clean nonsterile gloves* when touching blood, body fluids, excretions of secretions, contaminated items, mucous membranes, and nonintact skin. Change gloves between tasks on the same patient as necessary and remove gloves promptly after use.
- *Wear personal protective equipment* such as mask, eye protection, face shield, or fluid-repellent gown during procedures and care activities that are likely to generate splashes or sprays of blood or body fluids. Use gown to protect skin and prevent soiling of clothing.
- *Avoid recapping used needles.* If you must recap, never use two hands. Use a needle-recapping device or the one-handed scoop technique (see Fig. 27-4). Place needles, sharps, and scalpels in appropriate puncture-resistant containers after use.
- *Handle used patient care equipment that is soiled with blood or identified body fluids, secretions, and excretions carefully* to prevent transfer of microorganisms. Clean and reprocess items appropriately if used for another patient.
- *Use adequate environmental controls* to ensure that routine care, cleaning, and disinfection procedures are followed.
- *Review room assignments carefully.* Place patients who may contaminate the environment in private rooms (such as an incontinent patient).

Transmission-Based Precautions (Tier 2)
The following precautions are recommended in addition to standard precautions:

Airborne Precautions
- Use these for patients who have infections that spread through the air, such as tuberculosis, varicella (chicken pox), and rubeola (measles).
- Place patient in private room that has monitored negative air pressure in relation to surrounding areas, 6 to 12 air changes per hour, and appropriate discharge of air outside or monitored filtration if air is recirculated. Keep door closed and patient in room.
- Use respiratory protection when entering room of patient with known or suspected tuberculosis. If patient has known or suspected rubeola (measles) or varicella (chicken pox), respiratory protection should be worn unless person entering room is immune to these diseases.
- Transport patient out of room only when necessary and place a surgical mask on the patient if possible.
- Consult CDC Guidelines for additional prevention strategies for tuberculosis.

Droplet Precautions
- Use these for patients with an infection that is spread by large-particle droplets, such as rubella, mumps, diphtheria, and the adenovirus infection in infants and young children.
- Use a private room, if available. Door may remain open.
- Wear a mask when working within 3 feet of patient.
- Transport patient out of room only when necessary and place a surgical mask on the patient if possible.
- Keep visitors 3 feet from the infected person.

Contact Precautions
- Use these for patients who are infected or colonized by a microorganism that spreads by direct or indirect contact, such as MRSA, VRE, or VISA.
- Place the patient in a private room if available.
- Wear gloves whenever you enter the room. Change gloves after having contact with infective material. Remove gloves before leaving the patient environment, and wash hands with an antimicrobial or waterless antiseptic agent.
- Wear a gown if contact with infectious agent is likely or patient has diarrhea, an ileostomy, colostomy, or wound drainage not contained by a dressing.
- Limit movement of the patient out of the room.
- Avoid sharing patient-care equipment.

Adapted from http://www.phppo.cdc.gov/cdcrecommends/showarticle.asp?a_artid=p0000419.

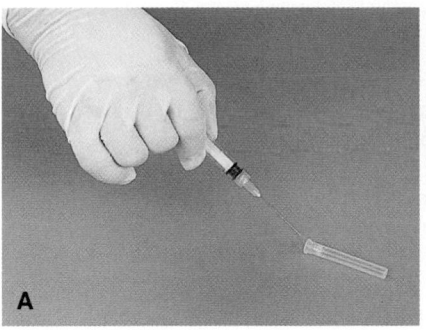 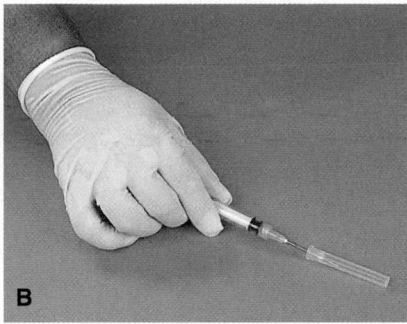 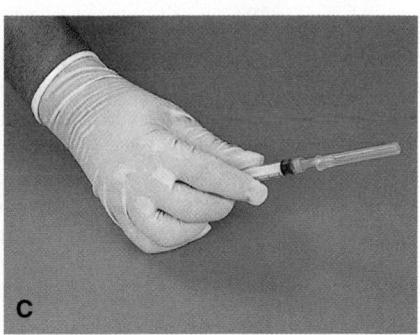

FIGURE 27-4 If it is necessary to a recap a needle, use a one-handed scoop technique: (**A**) Preparing to slide needle into cap. (**B**) Lifting cap onto needle. (**C**) Covering needle with cap. Alternatively, a needle-recapping device may be used.

Special Situations

When caring for a patient with methicillin resistant staphylococcus aureus (MRSA) or vancomycin resistant enterococcus (VRE), the nurse plays a major role in helping to contain the infection. When either of these two situations are identified, the CDC guideline for standard precautions applies to all patients, and the second level of transmission-based precautions, particularly contact precautions (see Box 27-5), are implemented. To help prevent the spread of these organisms, the following additional measures are effective (adapted from Gewanter, Klein, & Jones, 2002):

- Wear nonsterile gloves when entering the room of a patient who may have an antibiotic-resistant bacteria.
- After care, remove gloves and perform good hand hygiene before contact with other patients.
- Avoid wearing rings, bracelets, or watches.
- Do not use the same blood pressure cuff, stethoscope, thermometer, or other patient-care items on other patients.
- Change gloves after each task to avoid contaminating other areas of patient's body.
- Enforce transmission-based contact precautions (as discussed in Box 27-5).

Occasionally, nurses need to use neutropenic precautions for a patient whose immune system is compromised (eg, one recovering from transplantation surgery or receiving chemotherapy). Those who are immunosuppressed more often than not become infected by organisms harbored in their own bodies rather than by pathogens present in the environment or transmitted from other people. As with all patients, standard precautions are required, but some additional measures are helpful when a patient's ability to withstand any bacterial invasion is compromised. Recommendations in this situation include the following:

- Provide a healthy caregiver.
- Restrict visits from friends and family members who have colds or contagious illnesses.
- Avoid standing collection of water in the room (eg, with flowers or in humidifiers) to prevent bacteria typically found in this water.

Using Surgical Asepsis

Surgical asepsis techniques, used regularly in the operating room, labor and delivery areas, and certain diagnostic testing areas, are also used by the nurse at the patient's bedside. Procedures that involve the insertion of a urinary catheter, sterile dressing changes, or preparing an injectable medication are examples of surgical asepsis techniques. An object is considered sterile when all microorganisms, including pathogens and spores, have been destroyed. For example, the needle for an injection must be handled so that it is sterile when inserted into a patient. Sterile forceps or gloves are used to handle sterile dressings to protect against contamination. The basic principles of surgical asepsis are listed in Box 27-6.

When observing medical asepsis, areas are considered contaminated if they bear or are suspected of bearing pathogens. When following surgical asepsis, areas are considered contaminated if they are touched by any object that is not also sterile. One of the most important aspects of surgical and medical asepsis is that the effectiveness of both depends on faithful and conscientious practice by those carrying them out. It is far better to err on the side of safety when using surgical asepsis than to take the slightest chance of possible contamination. Being a patient advocate requires vigilant aseptic technique and a willingness to speak up if the patient's safety has been compromised by improper procedures.

> Think back to Esther Bailey, the woman described in the Reflective Practice display. The nurse acted appropriately by speaking up about the possible contamination of the catheter. Had this catheter been used, the patient's safety would have been compromised.

Explaining the surgical asepsis procedure to patients facilitates their cooperation. Inform the patient about which objects and areas may not be touched, and direct the patient to avoid sudden movements that might contaminate the equipment. This helps the patient assist in maintaining the sterility of the procedure.

Opening a Sterile Package and Preparing a Sterile Field

Commercially prepared sterile items may be sealed in paper or packaged in plastic containers. Sterile packages may be opened on a flat surface or while held in the hands. Skill 27-3 illustrates how to open a sterile package and prepare a sterile field.

BOX 27-6 Practicing Basic Principles of Surgical Asepsis

- Allow only a sterile object to touch another sterile object. Unsterile touching sterile means contamination has occurred.
- Open sterile packages so that the first edge of the wrapper is directed away from the worker to avoid the possibility of a sterile surface touching unsterile clothing. The outside of the sterile package is considered contaminated. Opening a sterile package is shown and described in Skill 27-3.
- Avoid spilling any solution on a cloth or paper used as a field for a sterile setup. The moisture penetrates through the sterile cloth or paper and carries organisms by capillary action to contaminate the field. A wet field is considered contaminated if the surface immediately below it is not sterile.
- Hold sterile objects above the level of the waist. This will ensure keeping the object within sight and preventing accidental contamination.
- Avoid talking, coughing, sneezing, or reaching over a sterile field or object. This helps to prevent contamination by

droplets from the nose and the mouth or by particles dropping from the worker's arm.
- Never walk away from or turn your back on a sterile field. This prevents possible contamination while the field is out of the worker's view.
- Keep all items sterile that are brought into contact with broken skin, or used to penetrate the skin to inject substances into the body, or to enter normally sterile body cavities. These items include dressings used to cover wounds and incisions, needles for injection, and tubes (catheters) used to drain urine from the bladder.
- Use dry, sterile forceps when necessary. Forceps soaked in disinfectant are not considered sterile.
- Consider the edge (outer 1 inch) of a sterile field to be contaminated.
- Consider an object contaminated if you have any doubt as to its sterility.

A sterile item should be covered if it is not used immediately. Reapply the cover by touching only the outside of the wrapper and reversing the opening order.

Pouring Sterile Solutions

Care is necessary when pouring sterile liquids onto a sterile dressing or into a sterile basin. The outer surfaces of the bottle and cap are considered unsterile, whereas the inside areas and the solution are considered sterile. After a solution has been opened, the outer bottle should be labeled and dated if it is to be reused. Most solutions are considered sterile for 24 hours after they are opened. When pouring from a bottle, grasp the bottle so that the label is in the palm of your hand. This action prevents any of the liquid from running over the label and making it illegible. If you are pouring from a bottle that has been previously used, "lip" it by pouring a small amount out into a waste receptacle to "clean" the rim of the bottle (see Skill 27-3).

Adding Sterile Supplies to a Sterile Field

After establishing a sterile field, it may be necessary to add items such as instruments or additional supplies to the sterile field. Actions 8 through 10 in Skill 27-3 demonstrate this technique. Once a sterile field is established, objects on a field may only be handled by using sterile forceps or with hands wearing sterile gloves.

Putting on Sterile Gloves

Sterile gloves are donned in a way that allows only the inside of the gloves to come in contact with the hands. Skill 27-4 describes the proper technique for putting on sterile gloves. After the gloves are on, only sterile items may be handled with the sterile-gloved hands. Careful removal of the gloves reduces any hand contact with contaminated materials. Good hand hygiene technique before and after putting on sterile gloves is imperative.

Positioning a Sterile Drape

The sterile drape, which ideally is waterproof, may be used to extend the sterile working area. Using sterile gloves allows the nurse to handle the entire drape surface. For protection when positioning, fold the upper edges of the drape over the sterile-gloved hands (Fig. 27-5). When sterile gloves are not worn, the nurse can touch only the outer 1 inch (2.5 cm) of the drape. Use caution when shaking the drape open so as not to touch one's clothing or an unsterile object. Holding the drape by the 1-inch upper edge, position the drape over the desired area. Do not reach over the drape because this would contaminate a sterile area.

Preventing Nosocomial Infections

For various reasons and sometimes despite best efforts, certain patients in health agencies develop infections that were not noted to be present on admission. The term **nosocomial** infection is used to describe a hospital-acquired infection. In its broad meaning, nosocomial means that the infection results while the patient is receiving healthcare, and the source may be either exogenous or endogenous. An infection is referred to as **exogenous** when the causative organism is acquired from other people. An **endogenous** infection occurs when the causative organism comes from microbial life harbored in the person. An infection is referred to as **iatrogenic** when it results from a treatment or diagnostic procedure. Not all nosocomial infections are iatrogenic.

Prevention of nosocomial infections is a major challenge for healthcare providers. In the United States, nosocomial infections affect approximately two million people annually (CDC, 2000). Nosocomial infections are the fifth leading cause of death in acute care settings, killing 90,000 people annually (Stone, Larson, & Kawar, 2002). The cost of the additional hospital care days necessary to treat a nosocomial infection is staggering, particularly in light of the efforts to control spiraling healthcare expenses. Based on analysis of

(*text continues on page 678*)

Preparing a Sterile Field

EQUIPMENT

Sterile wrapped drape or commercially
prepared sterile package

Additional sterile supplies as needed
(dressings, container, solution)

ACTION	RATIONALE

Initially Preparing the Field

1. Explain procedure to patient.

   An explanation encourages patient cooperation and reduces apprehension.

2. Gather equipment.

   Preparation provides for an organized approach to task.

3. Perform hand hygiene.

   Hand hygiene deters the spread of microorganisms.

4. Check that sterile wrapped drape or package is dry and unopened. Also note expiration date.

   Moisture contaminates a sterile package. Expiration date indicates period that package remains sterile.

5. Select a work area that is waist level or higher.

   Work area is within sight. Bacteria tend to settle, so there is less contamination above waist level.

6. Open sterile wrapped drape or commercially prepared sterile package.
   a. For *sterile wrapped drape*, open outer covering. Remove sterile drape, lifting it carefully by its corners. Shake open, hold away from your body, and lay drape on selected work area.

   Outer 1 inch (2.5 cm) of drape is considered contaminated. Any item touching this area is also considered contaminated.

   b. Place *commercially prepared package* in center of work area. Touching outer surface only, carefully reach around item and fold topmost flap of wrapper away from you. Open right and left flap before grasping the nearest flap and opening toward you.

   Proper placement prevents contamination by reaching across sterile field. Touching outer side of wrapper maintains sterile field.

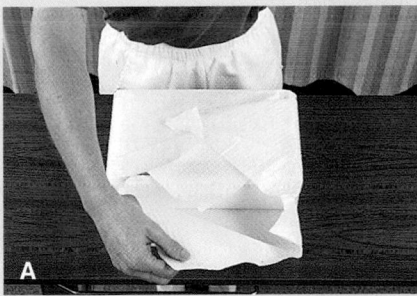 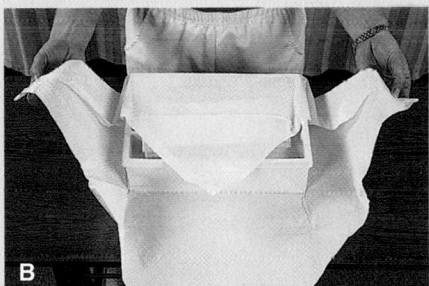 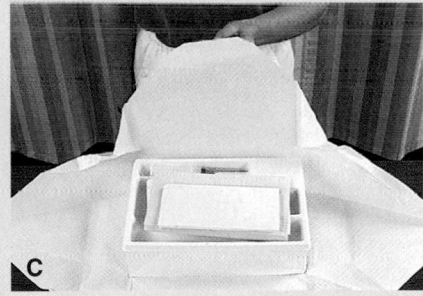

Action 6b: Opening a commercially prepared sterile package: (**A**) The nurse folds the topmost part of the covering wrapper away from her body. (**B**) She then opens the next layer of the wrapper to the sides. (**C**) The nurse opens the last layer of the wrapper toward her to prevent any reaching over the sterile field.   (Photos by Rick Brady.)

7. Place additional sterile items on field as needed.

   Sterile field is maintained.

Adding a Sterile Item to a Sterile Field

8. Open agency-prepared item or commercially packaged item:
   a. Hold *agency-wrapped item* in one hand, with top flap opening away from you. With other hand, unfold top flap and both sides. Keeping a secure hold on item, grasp the corners of the wrapper and pull back toward wrist, covering hand and wrist.

   Only sterile surface and item are exposed before dropping onto sterile field.

   b. If *commercially packaged item* has an unsealed corner, hold package in one hand and pull back on top cover with the other hand. If edge is partially sealed, use both hands to carefully peel apart.

   Contents remain uncontaminated by hands.

(continued)

ACTION

RATIONALE

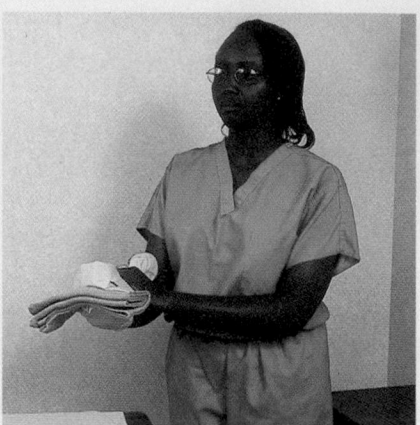

Action 8a: Preparing to drop sterile towel onto sterile field.

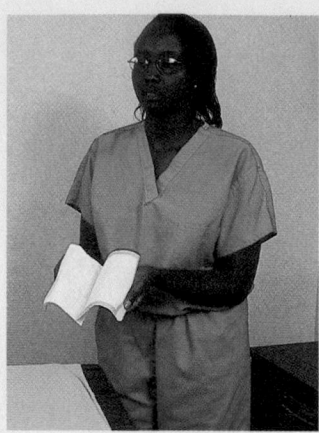

Action 8b: Using both hands to peel apart edges of a commercially packaged item.

9. Drop sterile item onto sterile field from a 6-inch (15 cm) height or add item to field from the side. Be careful to avoid 1-inch border.

Wrapper does not contaminate sterile field. Any items landing on 1-inch border are considered contaminated.

10. Discard wrapper.

A neat work area promotes proper technique.

Pouring a Sterile Solution

11. Obtain appropriate solution and check expiration date.

Once opened, a bottle should be labeled with date and time. Solution remains sterile for 24 hours.

12. Open solution container according to directions and place cap on table with edges up.

Sterility of inside cap is maintained.

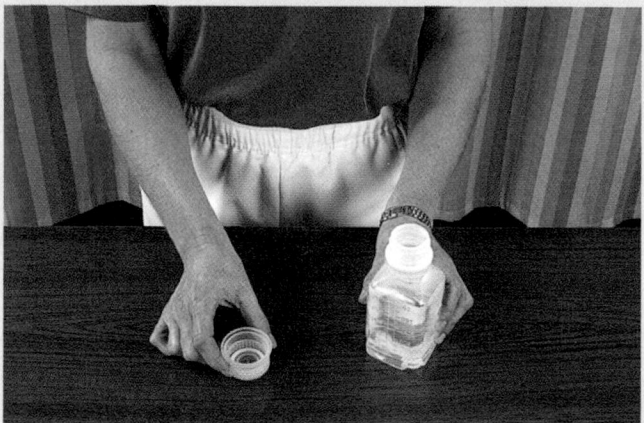

Action 12: Opening solution container.   (Photo © B. Proud.)

13. If bottle has previously been opened, "lip" it by pouring a small amount of solution into waste container.

This cleanses the lip of the bottle.

14. Hold bottle outside the edge of the sterile field with the label side facing the palm of your hand and prepare to pour from a height of 4 to 6 inches (10–15 cm). The tip of the bottle should never touch a sterile container or dressing.

Label remains dry, and solution may be poured while reaching across sterile field. Minimal splashing occurs from that height. Accidentally touching the tip of the bottle to a container or dressing contaminates both items.

15. Pour required amount of solution steadily into sterile container positioned at side of sterile field. Avoid splashing any liquid.

Moisture contaminates sterile field.

(continued)

Preparing a Sterile Field (continued)

ACTION	RATIONALE

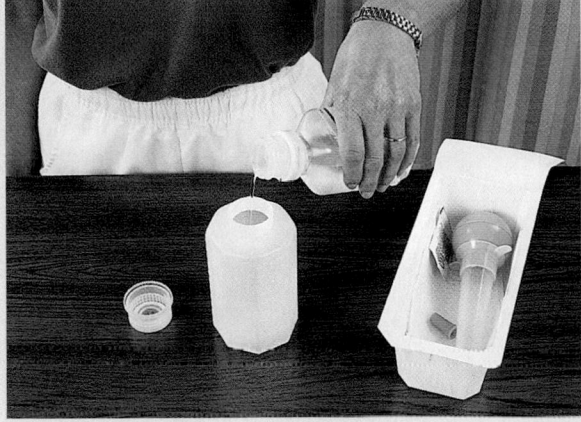

Action 15: Pouring solution into sterile container.   (Photo © B. Proud.)

16. Touch only the outside of the lid when recapping.	Solution remains uncontaminated.

Donning and Removing Sterile Gloves

EQUIPMENT

Sterile gloves (size of gloves is indicated on outer wrapping; select appropriate size)

ACTION	RATIONALE

To Apply Gloves

1. Perform hand hygiene.	Hand hygiene deters the spread of microorganisms. Gloves are easier to don when hands are dry.
2. Place sterile glove package on clean, dry surface above your waist.	Moisture could contaminate the sterile gloves. Any sterile object held below the waist is considered contaminated.
3. Open the outside wrapper by carefully peeling the top layer back. Remove inner package, handling only the outside of it.	This maintains sterility of gloves in inner packet.

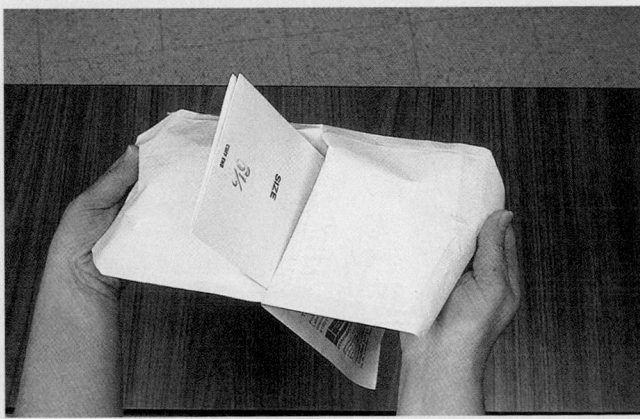

Action 3: Peeling back top layer of outer package.

(continued)

ACTION	RATIONALE
4. Carefully open the inner package and expose the sterile gloves with the cuff end closest to you.	The inner surface of the package is considered sterile.

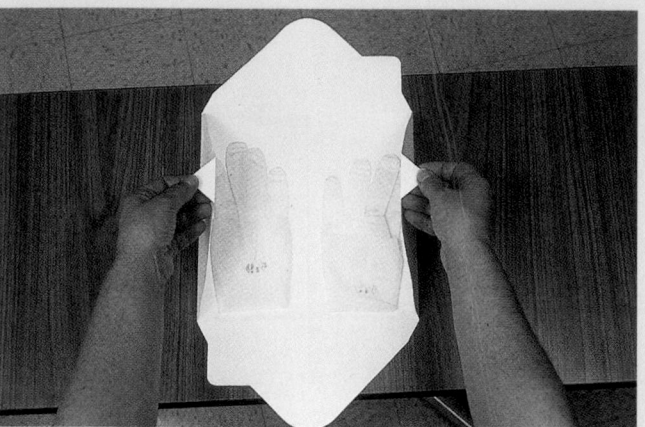

Action 4: Opening inner package.

ACTION	RATIONALE
5. With the thumb and forefinger of nondominant hand, grasp the folded cuff of the sterile glove for dominant hand.	Unsterile hand only touches inside of glove. Outside remains sterile.

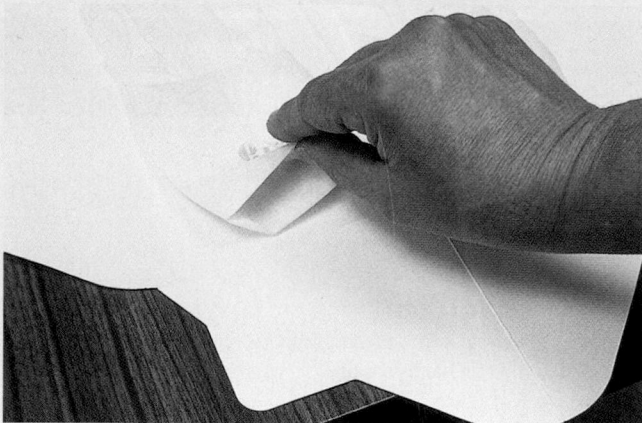

Action 5: Grasping edge of folded cuff.

ACTION	RATIONALE
6. Lift and hold glove with fingers down. Be careful it does not touch any unsterile object.	Glove is contaminated if it touches unsterile objects.

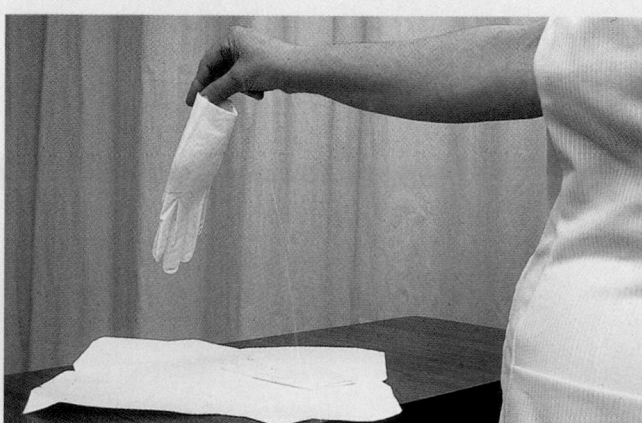

Action 6: Lifting and holding glove with fingers down.

(*continued*)

SKILL 27-4 Donning and Removing Sterile Gloves (continued)

ACTION	RATIONALE
7. Carefully insert the dominant hand into glove and pull glove on. Leave cuff folded down until other hand is gloved.	Attempts to turn upward with unsterile hand may result in contamination of sterile glove.

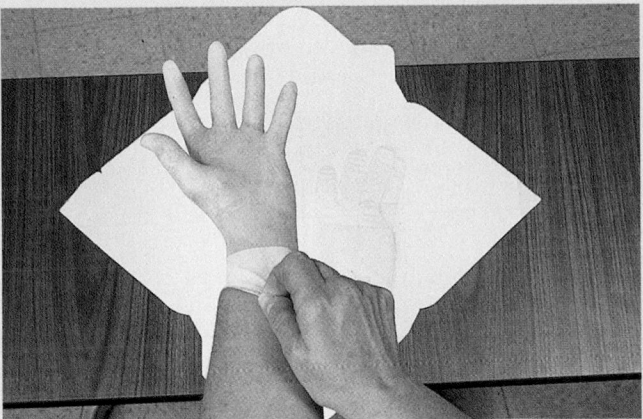

Action 7: Pulling first glove on with cuff folded.

| 8. Holding thumb outward, slide fingers of gloved hand under cuff of remaining glove and lift glove upward. | Thumb is less likely to become contaminated if held outward. If thumb touches the inside of the opposite glove, it is considered contaminated because of the powder on the inside of the glove. |

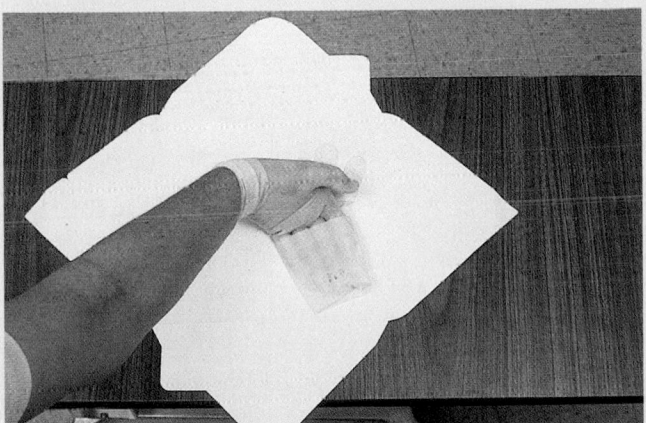

Action 8: Sliding fingers of gloved hand under cuff of second glove.

| 9. Carefully insert nondominant hand into glove. Adjust gloves on both hands touching only sterile areas. | Sterile surface touching sterile surface prevents contamination. |

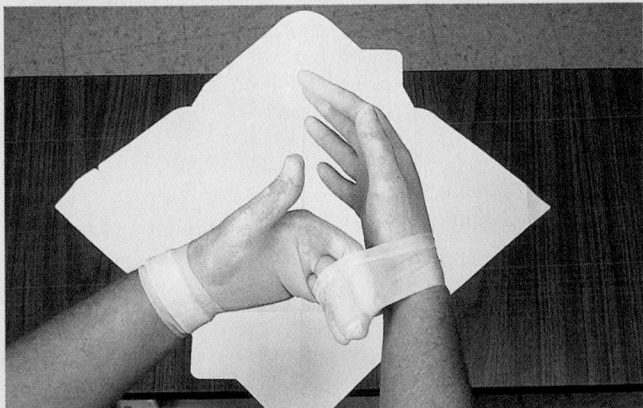

Action 9: Inserting hand with cuff folded.

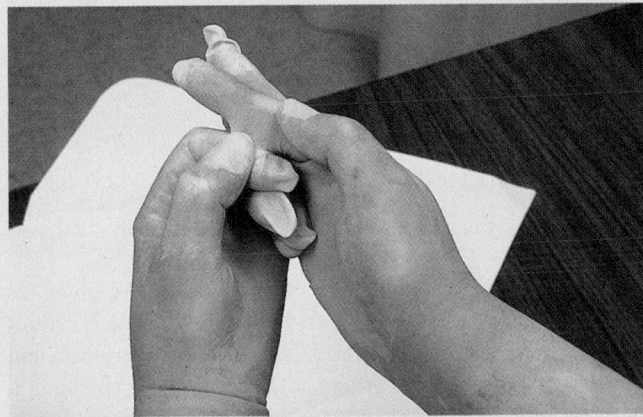

Action 9: Adjusting glove on both hands.

(continued)

SKILL
27-4 **Donning and Removing Sterile Gloves** (continued)

ACTION

RATIONALE

To Remove Gloves

1. Using dominant gloved hand, grasp other glove near cuff end and remove by inverting it, keeping the contaminated area on the inside. Continue to hold on to glove.

Contaminated area does not come in contact with hand or wrist.

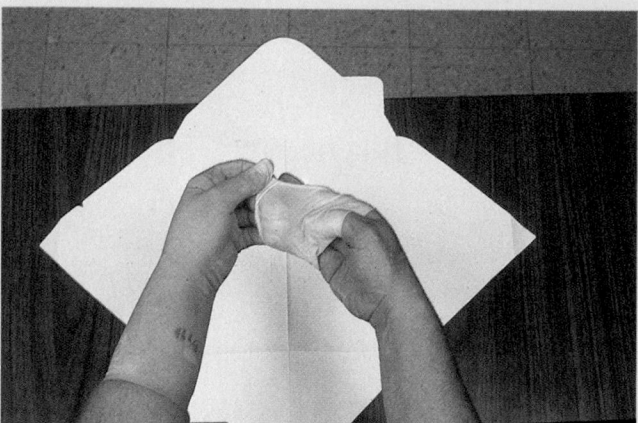

Action 1: Inverting glove as it is removed.

2. Slide fingers of ungloved hand inside the remaining glove. Grasp glove on inside and remove by turning inside out over hand *and other* glove.

Contaminated area does not come in contact with hand or wrist.

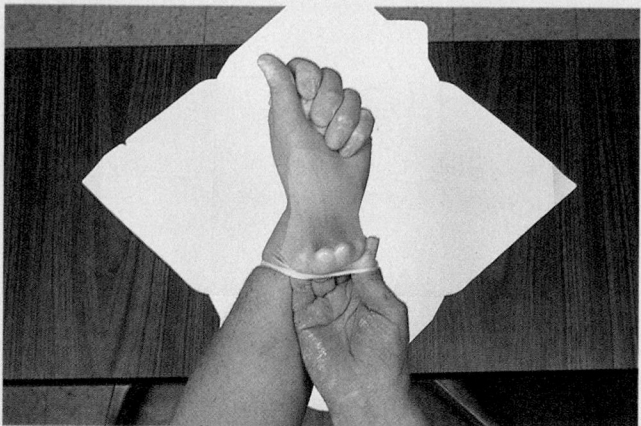

Action 2: Sliding ungloved fingers inside second glove.

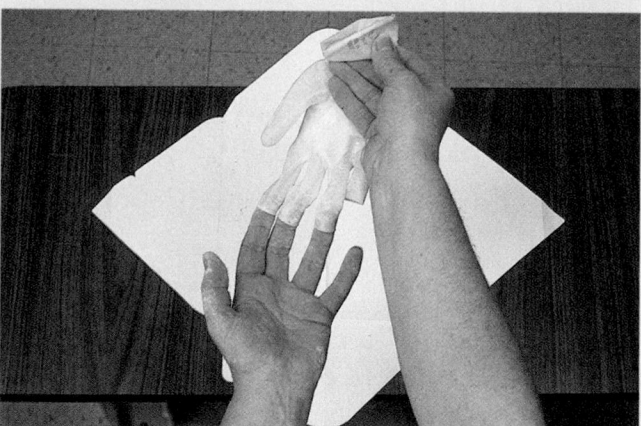

Action 2: Removing second glove inside out

3. Discard gloves in appropriate container and perform hand hygiene.

Hand hygiene reduces the spread of microorganisms.

---

past research, the cost of nosocomial infections in 2001 was estimated at $5.7 billion dollars (Stone et al., 2002).

Recently, staffing issues have been associated with an increase in nosocomial infections. Staffing takes into account registered nurse-to-patient ratio, level of RN experience, and the use of temporary workers. Many times, nurses have a heavy patient load and do not feel that they have time to thoroughly wash their hands. If the nurse is new, he or she may

feel overwhelmed with the patient assignment and forget to perform proper hand hygiene.

Invasive Medical Devices

Most hospital-acquired infections are caused by bacteria, such as *E. coli, Staphylococcus aureus, Streptococcus faecalis, Pseudomonas aeruginosa,* and *Klebsiella* species. Urinary tract infections, pneumonia, and bloodstream infections are

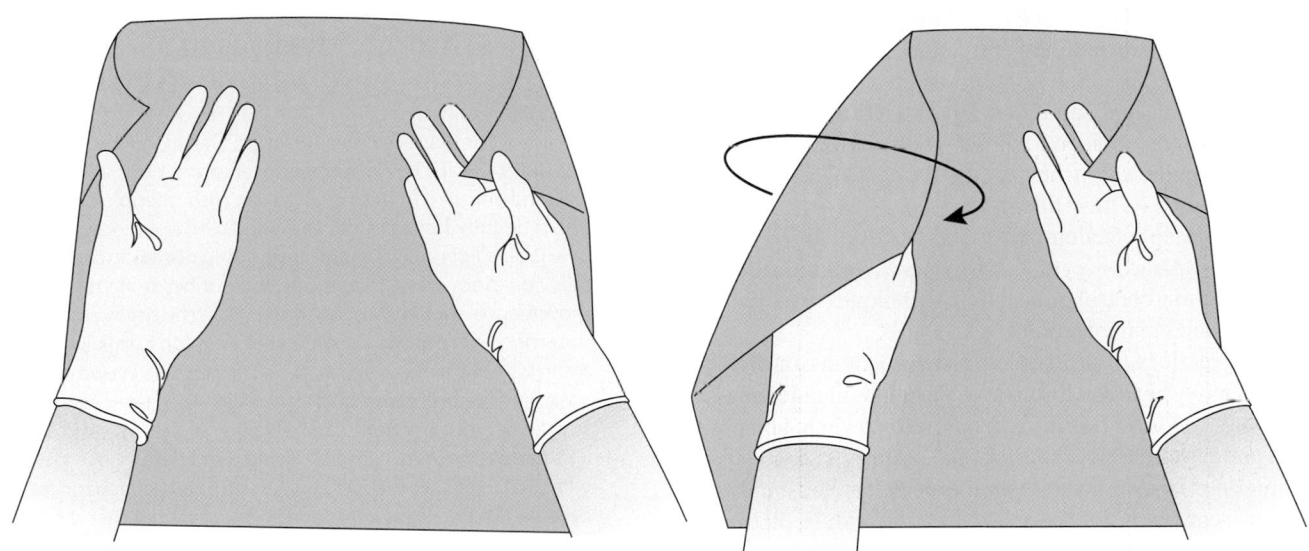

FIGURE 27-5 Techniques of cuffing a sterile drape over gloved hands.

the three most common sources for nosocomial infections, most of which can be traced to an invasive device such as a urinary catheter or venous access catheter. Surgical wounds are also a common site for infections to develop.

> Consider Esther Bailey, the 72-year-old woman who has had abdominal surgery and developed a wound infection. The patient already has one infection. However, insertion of the catheter increases her risk for an additional infection, directly related to the use of the catheter.

The increasing use of biomedical equipment is often cited as a causative factor. In addition to indwelling urinary catheters and venous access catheters, other devices associated with causing infection include hemodynamic monitoring lines, hemodialysis equipment, and respiratory equipment. Patients receiving mechanical ventilation are especially at risk for nosocomial pneumonia. Often, the hands of the healthcare worker using the instruments or equipment are the most significant means for the transmission of the pathogens.

Antibiotic-Resistant Organisms

A significant and disturbing trend continues to be the development of hospital-acquired pathogens resistant to antibiotics. The indiscriminate use of broad-spectrum antibiotics has allowed once-susceptible bacteria to develop defenses against antibiotics. As a result, resistant organisms, such as methicillin-resistant *S. aureus* (MRSA) have emerged. When *S. aureus,* a common cause of nosocomial wound and skin infections postoperatively, developed resistance to methicillin, vancomycin became the drug of choice. However, vancomycin intermediate-resistant *S. aureus* (VISA) has emerged, with eight reported cases in the United States as of June 2002 (Goldrick, 2002). Also, as epidemiologists had expected, in June 2002, the United States had its first diagnosed case of a *S. aureus* fully resistant to vancomycin (Bauer, 2002). This has

presented a formidable challenge because other antibiotics that are able to treat this organism are limited.

Vancomycin resistant enterococcus (VRE) is another serious pathogen in hospitals. Enterococci, a species of streptococcus often found in normal intestinal and female genital tracts, can cause nosocomial infections with a high mortality rate if the organism is vancomycin resistant. Originally treated with penicillin, ampicillin, and then gentamycin, the enterococci became resistant to each drug. Subsequently, physicians again prescribed vancomycin as the drug of choice. However, resistance has developed. Several new drugs are being investigated that may become alternatives for treating drug-resistant bacteria. The U.S. Food and Drug Administration (FDA) recently approved a new antibiotic, linezolid (Zyvox), that is effective against the deadliest enterococcal pathogens and provides an alternative if vancomycin resistance develops (Wooten & Salkind, 2003). Linezolid, administered IV or orally, is more expensive than vancomycin, and should not be used if other antibiotics are effective against a particular organism. A culture of a wound, blood, or other body fluids can identify the specific organism present; a sensitivity test determines which antibiotic is most effective against the organism.

Strategies to Protect the Patient

Nurses are in a unique position to prevent the transmission of nosocomial infections. MRSA and VRE most often are transmitted by the hands of healthcare providers. Both MRSA and VRE can also be spread through patient contact with a contaminated surface, such as side rails or an overbed table. However, VRE lives much longer in the environment and therefore is more likely to be spread in this manner than is MRSA. Careful assessment and evaluation of high-risk patients and situations, coupled with strict observance of medical and surgical asepsis techniques, including the use of barriers, help to minimize infection and reduce the unnecessary suffering imposed on patients. Using nursing diagnoses to generate appropriate nursing interventions makes a significant difference.

Healthcare agencies have found the following measures to be successful in reducing the incidence of nosocomial infections:

- Instituting constant surveillance by infection-control committees and nurse epidemiologists. Their work can reduce infections significantly when aggressive control measures are initiated based on their findings.
- Having written infection-prevention practices for all agency personnel. Adherence to hand-hygiene recommendations and infection-control precaution techniques can prevent many nosocomial infections.
- Using practices to promote and keep patients in the best possible physical condition. Measures include meeting the patient's needs for nutrition, fluids, rest, oxygen, and physical and psychological comfort and security.

Outbreaks of nosocomial infection in acute care hospitals and long-term care facilities are costly, frequently difficult to control, and debilitating for patients. Infection-control measures save lives and reduce the risk for transmission of pathogens to patients as well as personnel.

With their increased focus on patient safety, the Joint Commission on Accreditation of Healthcare Organizations (JCAHO) has recently mandated that death or serious injury caused by a nosocomial infection must be reported to JCAHO as a sentinel event (JCAHO, 2003).

Meeting Needs of Patients Requiring Infection-Control Precautions

The psychological implications of infection-control precautions are usually great, whether the patient is strictly separated from others or needs only to observe relatively simple precautions (see the accompanying box, Through the Eyes of a Student).

The current standard precautions of the CDC treat all people in a similar manner and greatly minimize the psychological trauma of feeling unclean and undesirable that often occurred with earlier measures. Sensory deprivation and loss of self-esteem may occur, however, with transmission-based precautions. Friends and relatives, as well as healthcare personnel, may be inclined to spend less time with the patient because they are afraid that they will contract the disease or because of the inconvenience of coping with specific transmission precaution procedures. Nursing measures to help prevent sensory deprivation and loss of self-esteem are discussed in Chapters 31 and 34.

Health teaching about transmission-based precautions can ease the fears of patients and family members. Both must understand the pertinent epidemiologic facts and how to carry out the specific precautions. It is helpful to emphasize the following:

- Precautions are temporary.
- The precautions and protective equipment worn by the staff protect the patient, the caregiver, and other patients.
- Proper hand hygiene before and after visiting the patient is the most effective measure to prevent spread of the disease.
- Continued explanations about procedures and continued updates on progress help to minimize anxiety.

Through the Eyes of a Student

She was the cutest little girl I have ever known. She was infected with HIV from birth. Her mother was an IV drug user and engaged in unprotected sex with multiple partners. This little girl, who came into the world with an innocent, fresh, new face full of unconditional love, could not walk, could not talk, could not chew, could not control her urine or bowel movements—but boy could she smile! In the beginning I was so terrified of contracting AIDS that I couldn't walk into her room without a mask, gown, gloves, protective eyewear, and basically a full protective body spacesuit. At the end, I wanted to take her into my home and give her all the love, support, and care she needed. I am not saying that I didn't wear gloves when I changed her diapers or when I flushed her heparin lock because I did . . . I was very careful. But I realized that she is a person, a person full of feelings, a person who needed me, and from whom I could learn. People with AIDS virus are just that—people. We need to learn to treat them as such.

I also learned not to fear the person who is diagnosed with HIV infection or AIDS. I know that I will take the proper safety precautions with this person. The person I need to fear is the cute little old man who would never have AIDS because "he's not the type." If I don't use precautions, it is possible that one day I'll become infected through contact with someone who is "not the type." If that should ever happen, I hope everyone who cares for me will treat me as a real person and not be afraid.

—Karmi N. Soder, Georgetown University
Washington, DC

Nurses must document their health teaching about barrier precautions in the patient's plan of care. A well-informed nurse who understands how to protect both self and patients and a well-informed patient who is cooperating in his or her care represent superior communicable disease precautions.

Raising Ethical Concerns About Infection Risks

Infection-control and precautions minimize infection risks for patients as well as healthcare workers. However, the increasing numbers of people infected with HIV, HBV, and HCV have led to serious ethical concerns and controversy related to the risk for transmitting these diseases. At issue are the rights of the patient versus the rights of the healthcare worker and the healthcare agency. Questions such as the following are being debated:

- Should all hospital patients be routinely tested for HIV infections?
- Should HIV testing be mandatory for all healthcare workers?
- Should healthcare workers infected with HIV be permitted to perform exposure-prone invasive procedures?
- What procedures should be considered exposure prone?
- Will healthcare facilities be liable if they allow HIV-positive staff to care for patients?

- Should pregnant healthcare providers be expected to care for patients with infectious diseases?

The CDC and various medical and nursing groups are seeking consensus on these issues, based on scientific information and valid statistical evidence. Although the CDC has issued guidelines related to these topics, not all states have adopted the guidelines. Additionally, some states have revised them. All agree, however, that healthcare workers who conscientiously adhere to appropriate infection-control precautions seriously reduce the risk for infection for patients and themselves.

Accidental Exposure Reporting

Nurses are accountable for their own safety. Any needlestick injury or accidental exposure to blood or body fluids must be reported immediately so that appropriate interventions can be used. Failure to notify an employer of an exposure may result in personal jeopardy as well as loss of compensation if an infection develops. An agency's plan for this type of exposure typically includes the following:

- Washing the exposed area immediately with warm water and soap
- Reporting the incident to the appropriate person and completing an incident or injury report if required by the agency
- Informing the agency of the source (patient's name) and nature of the exposure
- Consenting to an initial baseline blood test, if agreeable, to determine personal HIV and HBV status, with repeat blood test 6 weeks after exposure and at 3-month, 6-month, and 1-year intervals
- Consenting to postexposure prophylaxis, if recommended, at the appropriate time
- Awaiting blood test results of the involved patient (with his or her consent) to determine HIV and HBV status. State laws may vary concerning this practice. Some institutions may also test for HCV.
- Attending counseling session regarding safe practices to protect self and others

Using the Infection-Control Nurse

In the hospital, the infection-control nurse is responsible for educating patients and staff about effective infection-control techniques and for collecting statistics about infections. Many hospitals rely on this specialized practitioner to survey laboratory reports and review records for patients at risk, as well as suggest approaches to potentially dangerous situations. Intensive investigative strategies create a positive environment that significantly reduces the incidence of hospital-acquired infections in healthcare facilities. The infection-control nurse knows the devastating effects of infection and is intent on promoting health and fostering a systematic approach to infection control.

In the home, the infection-control nurse's duties include surveillance for agency-associated infections, education, consultation, epidemiologic investigation, quality-improvement activities, and policy and procedure development. OSHA regulations state that home care agencies must have an infection-

control program and that OSHA infection-control standards and policies must be available to all staff for reference.

Teaching About Infection Control

Teaching about medical asepsis and infection control is a challenging nursing responsibility. Patients need to be aware of techniques that prevent the spread of infection. Use of the nursing process in infection control protects both the patient and the nurse.

Medical asepsis techniques are appropriate for most procedures in the home, except for self-injection technique and venous catheter care, which require surgical asepsis. The patient frequently must make adjustments and improvise with the resources and supplies available for his or her use. In addition, the nurse emphasizes effective hand hygiene and other hygiene practices that interrupt the infection cycle. To satisfy OSHA requirements, many home care agencies have either a full-time or part-time infection-control practitioner.

Patients should be taught to use basic principles of asepsis at home and in public facilities. These involve the activities of daily living (see Chap. 37 for a discussion of personal hygiene). Following are examples of medical asepsis practices recommended in the home:

- Washing hands before preparing food and before eating
- Preparing foods at temperatures high enough to ensure that they are safe to eat, the most common example being the preparation of fresh meat
- Using care with cutting boards and utensils, and washing hands before and after handling raw meat
- Keeping foods refrigerated, especially those containing mayonnaise
- Washing raw fruits and vegetables before serving them
- Using pasteurized milk and fruit juices
- Washing hands after using the bathroom
- Using individual personal care items, such as washcloths, towels, and toothbrushes, rather than sharing

Think back to Giselle Turheis, the woman with leukemia and a compromised immune system. When teaching the patient about measures to prevent infection, the nurse would stress the use of proper practices in the home to reduce the patient's risk for infection.

Prevent infection in public facilities by following these guidelines:

- Wash hands after using any public bathroom.
- Use paper towels or hot-air dryers in restrooms.
- Use individually wrapped drinking straws.
- Use tongs to lift food from common service trays in cafeterias, food stores, and salad bars.

The community reinforces medical asepsis practices in various ways, including the following:

- Using sterilized combs and brushes in barber and beauty shops
- Performing examination of food handlers for evidence of disease

- Encouraging food handlers to receive the hepatitis A vaccination
- Enforcing frequent handwashing by food handlers

Evaluating

Nurses as primary caregivers can intervene in and positively affect a patient's outcome. By assessing the person at risk, selecting appropriate nursing diagnoses, planning, and intervening to maintain a safe environment, the nurse can reduce a patient's potential for developing an infection. Evaluation of the plan of care determines whether the individual's need for safety is being met effectively. Ongoing systematic evaluation is crucial for nurses who strive to maintain a secure environment for their patients as well as themselves. If patient goals have been met and evaluative criteria have been satisfied, the patient will accomplish the following:

- Correctly use techniques of medical asepsis
- Identify health habits and lifestyle patterns that promote health
- State the signs and symptoms of an infection
- Identify unsafe situations in the home environment

▓ Developing Critical Thinking Skills

1. A nurse cannot help but notice that whenever a particular surgeon makes rounds, he ignores basic principles of asepsis. He will move from one patient to another, touching dressings without washing his hands between patients. He is also inconsistent in his practice of sterile technique. You suspect that there is a higher rate of postoperative infection among his patients. What do you do?
2. A friend who is a nursing student always wears gloves when doing anything for ill patients. You are more selective in your use of gloves. She tells you that you are a fool for "taking chances" because you never know what you may pick up and bring home. Should this be a matter of personal preference? Is one position more consistent with good nursing? Are your instructors consistent in how they would respond to the above question?

▓ Practicing for NCLEX

1. The smallest infectious agents capable of causing an infection are:
   a. Bacteria
   b. Viruses
   c. Molds
   d. Yeasts
2. Your patient has developed a low-grade fever and states that she has felt very tired lately. This phase of an infection is known as the:
   a. Incubation period
   b. Prodromal stage
   c. Full stage of illness
   d. Convalescent period
3. The highest mortality rate is associated with nosocomial infections that involve the:

a. Respiratory tract
b. Integumentary system
c. Urinary tract
d. Intestines

4. A patient develops a urinary tract infection after an indwelling urinary catheter has been inserted. This would most accurately be termed:
   a. A viral infection
   b. A chronic infection
   c. An iatrogenic infection
   d. An opportunistic infection
5. The nurse has opened the sterile supplies and donned two sterile gloves to complete a sterile dressing change. Maintaining surgical asepsis requires the nurse to:
   a. Keep splashes on the sterile field to a minimum
   b. Cover the nose and mouth with gloved hands if a sneeze is imminent
   c. Use the dominant hand to cleanse the incision with a moist saline sponge and then apply the dry dressing
   d. Consider the outer 1 inch of the sterile field as contaminated
6. The CDC standard precaution recommendations apply to:
   a. Only patients with diagnosed infections
   b. Only blood and body fluids with visible blood
   c. All body fluids including sweat
   d. All patients receiving care in hospitals
7. In addition to standard precautions, the nurse caring for a patient with rubella would plan to implement:
   a. Droplet precautions
   b. Airborne precautions
   c. Contact precautions
   d. Universal precautions
8. When caring for a patient with latex allergy, the nurse creates a latex-safe environment by:
   a. Carefully cleaning the wall-mounted blood pressure device before using it
   b. Donning latex gloves outside the room to limit powder dispersal
   c. Using a latex-free pharmacy protocol
   d. Placing the patient in a semiprivate room
9. The guidelines for minimum protection standards for infection prevention and control were initially developed by:
   a. OSHA
   b. Individual healthcare facilities
   c. The state governing body
   d. The CDC
10. The recommended sequence for removing soiled personal protective equipment when the nurse prepares to leave the patient's room is to remove:
    a. Gown, goggles, mask, gloves, and exit the room
    b. Gloves, wash hands, remove gown, mask, and goggles
    c. Gloves, mask, gown, goggles, and wash hands
    d. Goggles, mask, gloves, gown, and wash hands

11. For a nurse under normal conditions with unsoiled hands, effective hand hygiene between patients requires:
    a. At least a 15-second scrub with plain soap and water
    b. At least a 23-minute scrub with an antimicrobial soap
    c. Use of an alcohol-based antiseptic hand rub
    d. That a mask be worn when scrubbing
12. Which hospitalized patient is most at risk for developing a nosocomial infection?
    a. Mr. Y, a 60-year-old patient who smokes two packs of cigarettes daily
    b. Mrs. J, a 40-year-old patient who has a white blood cell count of 6000/mm³
    c. Mr. L, a 65-year-old patient who has an indwelling urinary catheter in place
    d. Mrs. M, a 60-year-old patient who is a vegetarian and slightly underweight
13. A patient develops food poisoning from contaminated potato salad. The means of transmission for the infecting organism is:
    a. Direct contact
    b. Vector
    c. Vehicle
    d. Airborne
14. A nurse is caring for an obese 62-year-old patient with arthritis who has developed an open reddened area over his sacrum. A priority nursing diagnosis is:
    a. Imbalanced Nutrition: More Than Body Requirements related to immobility
    b. Impaired Physical Mobility related to pain and discomfort
    c. Chronic Pain related to immobility
    d. Risk for Infection related to altered skin integrity
15. The nurse teaches a patient at home to use clean technique when changing a wound dressing. This is:
    a. The nurse's preference
    b. Safe for the home setting
    c. Unethical behavior
    d. Grossly negligent

▪ Answers With Rationale

1. The correct response is *b*. A virus is the smallest of all microorganisms and can only be seen with a special microscope. Molds and yeasts (fungi) and bacteria are larger infectious agents.
2. The correct response is *b*. During the prodromal stage, the person has vague signs and symptoms, such as fatigue and a low-grade fever. There are no obvious symptoms of infection during the incubation period, and they are more specific during the full stage of illness, before disappearing by the convalescent period.
3. The correct response is *a*. Urinary tract infections and surgical wounds are common sites for nosocomial infections to develop, but the highest mortality rate is associated with those infections that involve the respiratory tract. The intestine is not particularly prone to nosocomial infections.

4. The correct response is *c*. An infection that develops as a result of the insertion of an indwelling catheter is termed iatrogenic. Because this infection just developed, it is not chronic, nor did it occur because of any altered physiology that may give an opportunistic organism a chance to cause infection. Urinary infections are bacterial, not viral.
5. The correct response is *d*. Considering the outer inch of a sterile field as contaminated is a principle of surgical asepsis. Moisture contaminates the sterile field, and sneezing would contaminate the sterile gloves. The sterile hand that cleaned a wound should not be used or should be regloved before applying a sterile dressing.
6. The correct response is *d*. Standard precautions apply to all patients receiving care in hospitals regardless of their diagnosis or possible infection status. These recommendations include blood, all body fluids, secretions, and excretions except sweat, nonintact skin, and mucous membranes.
7. The correct response is *a*. Rubella is an illness transmitted by large-particle droplets and requires droplet precautions in addition to standard precautions. Airborne precautions are used for patients who have infections spread through the air with small particles, for example, tuberculosis, varicella, and rubeola. Universal precautions and body-substance isolation are incorporated into the new CDC standard precautions recommendations.
8. The correct response is *c*. A latex-free pharmacy protocol is a vital component when creating a safe environment for this patient. Wall-mounted blood pressure devices have latex tubing and should not be touched or used on the patient. Latex gloves could cause a serious allergic response; only synthetic gloves are allowed in a latex-free environment. A private room is best to minimize the possibility of latex exposure from something used for the other patient.
9. The correct response is *d*. The CDC established the initial minimum requirements for infection prevention and control. OSHA has issued and monitors regulations for use of universal precautions in situations and settings in which exposure to blood and other infectious materials is possible.
10. The correct response is *c*. Gloves are always removed first because they are most likely to be contaminated, and hands should be washed thoroughly after the equipment has been removed and before leaving the room.
11. The correct response is *c*. Hands that are not visibly soiled can be effectively cleaned with an alcohol-based hand rub. Neither a mask nor an antimicrobial soap is required in this situation or setting. Hands that are visibly soiled require a wash with either a nonantimicrobial soap and water or an antimicrobial soap and water.
12. The correct response is *c*. Indwelling urinary catheters have been implicated in most nosocomial

infections. Cigarette smoking, a normal white blood cell count, and a vegetarian diet have not been implicated as risk factors for nosocomial infections.

13. The correct response is *c*. Contaminated food is a vehicle for transmitting an infection. Direct contact requires proximity between the susceptible host and an infected person. A vector is a nonhuman carrier, such as an insect, and the airborne means of transmission carries the organism in droplet nuclei or with dust.

14. The correct response is *d*. The priority diagnosis in this situation is the possibility of an infection developing in the open skin area. The others may be potential or probable diagnoses for this patient and may also require nursing interventions after the first diagnosis is addressed.

15. The correct response is *b*. In the home setting, where the patient's environment is more controlled, medical asepsis is usually recommended, with the exception of self-injection. This is the appropriate procedure for the home and is neither unethical nor grossly negligent.

Bibliography

Afif, W., Huor, P., Brassard, P., & Loo, V. (2002). Compliance with methicillin-resistant *staphylococcus aureus* precautions in a teaching hospital. *American Journal of Infection Control, 30*(7), 430–433.

Bauer, J. (Ed.). (2002). Clinical highlights. *RN, 65*(10), 18.

Beyea, S. (2002). Hospital pagers and bacteria. *AORN Journal, 76*(3), 520–522.

Brooke, P. (2001). Legally speaking: The legal realities of HIV exposure. *RN, 64*(12), 71–73, 76–77.

Centers for Disease Control and Prevention. (2000). Monitoring hospital-acquired infections to promote patient safety— US, 1990—1999. *Morbidity and Mortality Weekly Report 2000, 49*(08), 149–153.

Centers for Disease Control and Prevention. (2002). Guideline for hand hygiene in health-care settings. *Morbidity and Mortality Weekly Report 2002, 51*, (RR16), 1–45.

Duffy, J. (2002). Nosocomial infections: Important acute care nursing-sensitive outcomes indicators. *AACN Clinical Issues, 13*(3), 358–366.

Gehring, L., & Ring, P. (2000). Latex allergy: Creating a safe environment. *Dermatology Nursing, 12*(3), 197–201.

Gewanter, B., Klein, R., & Jones, S. (2002). Antibiotic-resistant bacteria on the rise: Patients face greater risks than healthy workers do. *American Journal of Nursing, 102*(3), 116.

Girard, N. (2003). OR masks—safe practice or habit? *AORN Journal, 77*(1), 12–15.

Goldrick, B. (2002). First reported case of VRSA in the United States: An alarming development in microbial resistance. *American Journal of Nursing, 102*(11), 17.

Graves, P., & Twomey, C. (2002). The changing face of hand protection. *AORN Journal, 76*(2), 248–264.

Hedrick, E. (2000). Where's the science? *American Journal of Infection Control, 28*(1), 66–67.

Hilburn, J., Hammond, B., Fendler, E., & Groziak, P. (2003). Use of alcohol hand sanitizer as an infection control strategy in an acute care facility. *American Journal of Infection Control, 31*(2), 109–116.

Jackson, M., Chiarello, L., & Gaynes, R. (2002). Nurse staffing and health care-associated infections: Proceedings from a working group meeting. *American Journal of Infection Control, 30*(4), 199–206.

Joint Commission on Accreditation of Healthcare Organizations. (2003). 2004 National Patient Safety Goals. Available at http://www.jcaho.org/accredited+organizations/patients+safety/04+npsg/04_npsg/04_npsg.htm.

Jones, R., Jampani, H., Mulberry, G., et al. (2000). Moisturizing alcohol hand gels for surgical hand preparation. *AORN Journal, 71*(3), 584–599.

Lenehan, G. (2002). Latex allergy: Separating fact from fiction. *Nursing, 32*(3), 58–63.

Moolenar, R., Crutcher, M., SanJoaquin, V., Sewell, L., Hutwagner, L., Carson, L., Robinson, D., Smithee, L., & Jarvis, W. (2000). A prolonged outbreak of *Pseudomonas aeruginosa* in a neonatal intensive care unit: Did staff fingernails play a role in disease transmission? *Infection Control and Hospital Epidemiology, 21*(2), 80–85.

Murray, B. (2000). Drug therapy. Vancomycin-resistant enterococcal infections. *New England Journal of Medicine, 342*(10), 710–721.

Rees, J., Davies, H., Birchall, C., & Price, J. (2000). Psychological effects of source isolation nursing: Patient satisfaction. *Nursing Standard, 14*(29), 32–36.

Saiman, L., Lerner, A., Saal, L., Todd, E., Fracaro, M., Schneider, N., Connell, J., Castellanos, A., Scully B., & Drusin, L. (2002). Banning artificial nails from health care settings. *American Journal of Infection Control, 30*(4), 252–254.

Schweon, S. (2003). West Nile virus: Get ready for its return. *RN, 66*(4), 56–60.

Shiao, J., Guo, L., & McLaws, M. (2002). Estimation of the risk of blood borne pathogens to health care workers after a needlestick injury in Taiwan. *American Journal of Infection Control, 30*(1), 15–20.

Smeltzer, S., & Bare, B. (2004). *Brunner & Suddarth's Textbook of medical-surgical nursing* (10th ed.), Philadelphia: Lippincott Williams & Wilkins.

Stone, P., Larson, E., & Kawar, L. (2002). A systematic audit of economic evidence linking nosocomial infections and infection control interventions: 1990–2000. *American Journal of Infection Control, 30*(3), 145–152.

Winslow, E., & Jacobson, A. (2000). Can a fashion statement harm the patient? *American Journal of Infection Control, 100*(9), 63, 65.

Wooten, J., & Salkind, A. (2003). Superbugs: Unmasking the threat. *RN, 66*(3), 37–43.

Worthington, K. (2001). Latex allergy: What's the facility's responsibility, and what's yours? *American Journal of Infection Control, 101*(7), 88.

Worthington, K. (2002). Are your medical gloves really protecting you? Take an active role in purchasing the right glove for the job. *American Journal of Infection Control, 102*(10), 108.

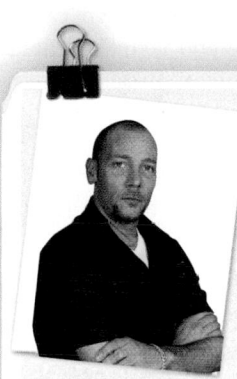

Brian Legett, a 30-year-old man with a long history of back problems due to a work injury, comes to the clinic for evaluation. He states, "I've had so many kinds of treatment, and nothing seems to work. Maybe I should see a chiropractor?"

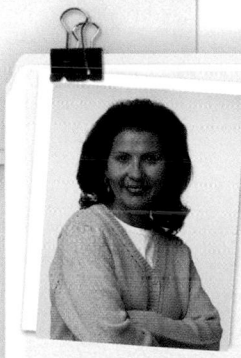

Sylvia Puentes, a middle-aged woman, is scheduled for abdominal surgery next week. She comes to the outpatient clinic for preoperative evaluation and laboratory testing and says, "I'm really anxious about the surgery, but I don't want to take any medicines. Is there anything I can do to help me relax?"

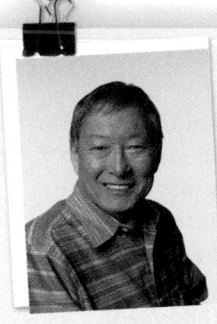

Lee Chen, a 65-year-old man dying of lung cancer, was brought to the United States from China by his two daughters, who believed that U.S. medicine would cure him. Mr. Chen did not respond to any of the therapies that were attempted, and the team wants to transition to palliative care. The daughters are unwilling to authorize removal of ventilatory support or sign a do-not-resuscitate order. They request an acupuncturist, but the physician refuses their request.

Focusing on Blended Skills

The types of blended skills you'll need to respond to the case scenarios include:

Cognitive Skills

- Knowledge of available and appropriate complementary and alternative modalities
- Ability to obtain information about complementary and alternative modalities
- Knowledge of the underlying mechanisms of action for complementary and alternative modalities such as chiropractic science, mind–body modalities, and acupuncture
- Ability to safely incorporate knowledge of complementary and alternative modalities into a patient's plan of care
- Knowledge of the use of complementary and alternative modalities by various cultures

Technical Skills

- Strong assessment skills to identify the patient's belief in, request for, and use of complementary and alternative modalities
- Ability to integrate complementary and alternative modalities with technical nursing assistance necessary to meet the needs of a patient with a chronic back injury, an anxious woman scheduled for surgery, and a terminally ill patient
- Ability to ask for assistance as necessary when dealing with complementary and alternative modalities as a component of a patient's plan of care
- Ability to demonstrate competent teaching skills related to different complementary and alternative modalities, such as chiropractic science, mind–body modalities, and acupuncture

Interpersonal Skills

- Ability to establish a trusting nurse–patient relationship with patients interested in complementary and alternative modalities
- Ability to work collaboratively with other members of the healthcare team to promote culturally competent care that includes the use of complementary and alternative modalities
- Ability to use therapeutic communication skills to meet the needs of patients at various stages of health and illness, such as a patient with chronic back problems, an anxious woman scheduled for surgery, and a terminally ill patient
- Demonstration of respect for a patient's human dignity when implementing the plan of care

Ethical and Legal Skills

- Commitment to implementing the patient's plan of care successfully, within the scope of nursing practice
- Ability to participate as a trusted and effective patient advocate, such as for a terminally ill patient, with a commitment to securing the best possible care for patients and families
- Value for the importance of incorporating culture when assessing and planning care for patients and their families
- Demonstration of a strong sense of accountability for the health and well-being of patients that translates into a commitment to getting patients the information and help they need
- Demonstration of accountability for all actions performed, including the ability to practice nursing in an ethically and legally defensible manner
- Ability to incorporate knowledge of the nurse's ethical and legal responsibilities when providing care that involves the use of complementary and alternative modalities

Learning Outcomes

After completing the chapter, the learner should be able to accomplish the following:

1. Explain how neuropeptides contribute to mind–body healing.
2. Use energy concepts to explain energy healing modalities.
3. Explain the physiologic processes involved in modalities focusing on stress reduction.
4. Discuss ways in which nurses can use knowledge of complementary and alternative modalities in providing patient care.
5. Discuss ways in which nurses can use selected complementary and alternative modalities for self-care and health promotion.

Key Terms

acupuncture
allopathy
aromatherapy
aura
Ayurveda
chakra
chiropractic
dosha
Healing Touch (HT)
holism
holistic nursing
homeopathy
imagery
integrative care
intercessory prayer
meridian
naturopathic medicine
relaxation response
shamanism
Therapeutic Touch (TT)
traditional Chinese medicine (TCM)
qi
qi gong
yin/yang

Many people in the United States are using complementary and alternative modalities (CAM) to promote health and assist with healing from illness. The widely used term "complementary and alternative medicine" refers to interventions that are complementary (they can be used with traditional interventions and thus complement them) as well as alternative (not included in the scope of traditional medical care). However, the reality is that people without medical degrees practice many of these modalities. Therefore, many nurses are using the term "complementary and alternative *modalities*," since it is more inclusive. This chapter takes that approach.

Nurses should be knowledgeable about CAM primarily for three reasons. First, patients, families, physicians, and institutions are increasingly expecting practicing nurses to be knowledgeable about CAM. Many institutions are providing selected CAM to inpatients as part of total patient care or as an option for patients to purchase. It is estimated that at least 15% of hospitals are offering CAM to their patients either as part of the patient care package or on a private-pay basis.

Second, many nurses are expanding their clinical practice by incorporating CAM. Almost half of state Boards of Nursing recognize selected alternative/complementary modalities as part of nursing practice and include provisions for the safe practice of these modalities by registered nurses (Sparber, 2001).

Finally, although CAM may seem totally safe, there are some potentially harmful situations. For example, certain herbs may interact with each other or with pharmaceutical agents, causing negative effects. A basic, working knowledge of CAM contributes to the nurse's effectiveness (see the Reflective Practice box for an example).

INTRODUCTION TO COMPLEMENTARY AND ALTERNATIVE MODALITIES

Prevalence of CAM in the United States

Studies report that about 50% of adults in the United States use CAM as part of their healthcare. CAM is particularly effective for chronic illness, the incidence of which is rapidly rising in the United States. Eisenberg et al. (1993), in a groundbreaking study, found that "alternative therapies were used most frequently for chronic conditions, including back problems, anxiety, depression, and headaches" (p. 1569).

Many people also use CAM for stress management/ reduction. Techniques such as relaxation with focused breathing, meditation, imagery, biofeedback, and massage are used in all stages of health and illness to promote healing and/or manage symptoms. Since stress can contribute to illness, CAM can sometimes be effective in reducing symptoms and enhancing quality of life.

Recall Sylvia Puentes, the anxious patient scheduled for surgery. The nurse's knowledge of CAM would be important in helping this patient to reduce her preoperative anxiety. The nurse could discuss various methods available, allowing the patient to select the one that seems best for her. Such actions help develop a trusting nurse–patient relationship and foster a sense of self-esteem in the patient by allowing her to participate in the plan of care and decision making.

Growth of CAM Industry

Eisenberg et al. (1998) "conservatively" estimated that consumers spent $27 billion on CAM in 1997. Eighty-five percent of schools of nursing responding to a survey reported that CAM was included in their curricula (Fenton & Morris, 2003). Approximately two thirds of medical schools in the United States offer courses in CAM, either as elective or required courses. Some insurers pay for selected CAM for particular identified conditions. Scores of private organizations provide classes and workshops for consumers as well as education and practical experience for healthcare providers.

Many private and governmental organizations have been developed to deal with CAM. For example, the Foundation for Alternative Medicine (NFAM) is engaged in international research to determine "best practices" for cancer treatment. The National Center for Complementary and Alternative Medicine (NCCAM) in the National Institutes of Health in the federal government funds research on CAM. The special White House Commission on Complementary and Alternative Medicine Policy (WHCCAMP) issued an extensive report in March 2002, addressing policy issues specific to CAM. The U.S. Food & Drug Administration (FDA) is seeking to increase regulations for dietary supplements.

PRINCIPLES OF AND APPROACHES TO CAM

Allopathy (or biomedicine), the term generally used to describe "traditional" medical care, has been dominant for about 100 years and has spearheaded remarkable advances in biotechnology, surgical interventions, pharmaceutical approaches, and diagnostic tools. Allopathic care is particularly effective when aggressive treatment is needed in emergency or acute situations.

However, allopathic care has not been very effective in dealing with chronic illness, the current primary health problem. "The medical model has met impressive challenges, but the rise of progressive chronic and stress-related diseases has added a burden to the Western quality of life not mitigated by biomedicine" (Bright, 2002, p. 3). CAM increasingly is being used as an "answer" to the problem of chronic illness. The CAM and allopathic systems differ fundamentally in several ways (Table 28-1). Many CAM modalities are based on a theory and philosophy of holism upon which holistic nursing also is based. Many practitioners and consumers of healthcare choose to combine allopathic modalities and CAM in an integrative approach. These concepts are discussed below.

Reflective Practice
Challenge to Cognitive Skills

This spring, while working on an oncology floor, I was caring for Lee Chen, a 65-year-old man dying of lung cancer. His two daughters, who were living in the United States, had brought him from China to the United States, believing that U.S. medicine would cure him. Unfortunately, Mr. Chen had not responded to any of the therapies that were attempted, and all of his professional caregivers believed that the goal of treatment should now be preparation for a comfortable and dignified death using compassionate palliative care. His daughters, however, were unwilling to accept this goal and would not authorize removing him from ventilatory support or issuing a do-not-resuscitate order. Mr. Chen could no longer speak on his own behalf. One afternoon, one of his daughters informed Mr. Chen's physician that she was going to bring an acupuncturist in to work on her father. The physician told her in no uncertain terms that he would not allow "voodoo medicine" on his unit. I wasn't sure what to do, because both daughters were growing more and more upset, and this answer seemed like the "last straw."

Thinking Outside the Box: Possible Courses of Action

- Accept the status quo and try to comfort the daughters.
- Support the physician's judgment and try to get the daughters to see things his way.
- Learn more about acupuncture and related benefits and harms (I have never seen it done and know very little about what to expect).

- Find out if the physician really had the authority to forbid acupuncture on this patient.
- Advocate for the patient and his family if there is a possibility that acupuncture will benefit him.

Evaluating a Good Outcome: How Do I Define Success?

- Patient receives culturally appropriate care consistent with the goals of compassionate palliative care.
- The patient is not harmed.
- Mr. Chen's daughters feel supported as they struggle with decisions and anticipatory grieving.
- All healthcare team members (including Mr. Chen's physician) learn about acupuncture and other complementary and

alternative therapies as well as about the hospital's policies regarding their use.
- The physician is confronted in a professional manner about the behavior as increasing the stress on the family caregivers.
- I grow in my knowledge of how to incorporate CAM into my care.

Personal Learning: Here's to the Future!

I was so upset by the daughters' distress that I decided to learn more about acupuncture. After searching the Internet and talking with a nurse who was receiving acupuncture treatments, I decided that acupuncture treatments were unlikely to harm the patient; in fact, the treatments just might help to increase his comfort level. At the very least, Mr. Chen's daughters would believe that we respected and supported their efforts to help their father. I was also hopeful that the professional caregiving team would learn more about culturally competent care. When I spoke with the head nurse, she was understanding about my goals and actually confronted Mr. Chen's

doctor and secured his approval for having the acupuncturist visit. I learned that the acupuncturist had to be credentialed by our hospital. While Mr. Chen's cancer did not respond to the acupuncture treatment, he did seem more comfortable, and his daughters couldn't thank me enough. I talked with them about how impressive their devotion to their father was and also mentioned that they may need to give him one last gift, the gift of "letting go." Unfortunately, I never saw this family again because this was my last week on this unit.

Reflection

How do you think you would respond in a similar situation? Why? What does this tell you about yourself and about the adequacy of your skills for professional practice? Can you think of other ways to respond? What factors do you think may have played a role in the physician's answer? How did the nursing student promote culturally competent care? Imagine if the nursing student (rather than the head nurse) had approached the physician to allow the acupuncturist to visit. Do you think that the physician's answer would have

been the same as it was when the head nurse confronted him? Please explain why or why not. What other skills (cognitive, interpersonal, technical, ethical/legal) would you need to respond well in this situation? Do you agree with the criteria to evaluate a successful outcome? Did the nursing student meet the criteria? Please explain.

Melinda Ventura, Georgetown University

Holism

Holism is a theory and philosophy that focuses on connections and interactions between parts of the whole. In contrast, the prevailing scientific approach has focused on reductionism, the goal of which is to reduce all phenomena to the smallest possible atom, particle, or interaction. Using a holistic perspective, all living organisms, including humans, are continuously connecting and interacting with their environment. Further, parts of the organism, whether they are systems, subsystems, or cells, are also continuously interacting and changing. This continual interaction and change means that the body is not the sum of its parts (as in reductionism), but that it is a unified, dynamic whole.

TABLE 28-1 Beliefs Underlying Complementary and Alternative Modalities and the Allopathic Systems

Complementary and Alternative Modalities	Allopathic Medicine
Mind, body, and spirit are integrated and contribute to health and illness.	Illness occurs in either the mind or the body, which are separate entities.
Health is a state characterized by a dynamic balance of mind, body, and spirit.	Health is the absence of disease.
Illness is a manifestation of imbalance or disharmony and is a process.	Illness is an event caused by an external agent (eg, bacteria) or a mechanical problem.
Healing is done by the patient.	Curing is accomplished by external agents.
Healing is a natural, slow process that involves the body, mind, and spirit.	Curing occurs more quickly and seeks to destroy the invading organism or repair the affected part.

Adapted from Ferguson, M. (1987). *Aquarian conspiracy: Personal and social transformation in our time.* New York: J. P. Tarcher.

Although one might view holism as a recently developed belief system, holism in fact was the predominant belief throughout history until sometime before René Descartes, a French philosopher who lived in the early part of the 17th century. He and other influential thinkers asserted that the mind and body were separate from each other. That belief lasted until the early 20th century, when researchers began to prove there was a connection between the mind and the body.

One of the 20th-century researchers, Hans Selye, developed the term "general adaptation syndrome" (GAS) to describe the general holistic pattern that emerges when people experience stress/illness. The GAS reflects a general immune response that occurs in various parts of the body. This theory holds that when a person is sick, he or she is "sick all over," not just where symptoms manifest. Selye also demonstrated that adrenal exhaustion can be caused by emotional tension, such as suppressed rage or frustration. (For more on the GAS, see Chap. 32.)

A holistic philosophy underlies much of CAM. People have a mind, body, and spirit that are connected and function as a unified whole. A change in any part of the organism will be reflected in other parts. When someone feels the emotion of sadness, he or she may have a physical response of crying. And when a person feels stressed and overwhelmed, the face and body language frequently reflect this condition.

Holistic Nursing

Holistic nursing is nursing practice built on a holistic philosophy. Since holism is a philosophy and not a specific nursing role, holistic nurses can be found in all varieties of healthcare settings as well as in independent practice settings. In addition, holistic nurses frequently add CAM to their practice. Most holistic nurses use CAM for self-care, an essential component of holistic practice. Registered nurses can become certified in holistic nursing through the American Holistic Nurses' Association Credentialing Corporation.

Integrative Care

A person who uses **integrative care** uses some combination of allopathic medicine and CAM (Table 28-2). There are several types of integrative care models used throughout the United States, and they can be housed in virtually all healthcare delivery structures. Optimally, these models include healthcare providers who "share the responsibility in coordinating the best possible treatment plan for a client, including the client's choices for care and the providers' expertise in understanding and managing the complexities of conventional/complementary treatment interactions" (Bright, 2002, p. 11).

However, in the Eisenberg et al. study (1998), almost 40% of respondents were using some form of CAM without notifying their physician. For example, a patient who is undergoing surgery may take a homeopathic remedy before and after surgery, may be visited periodically by an energy worker, and may take vitamins to promote healing throughout the surgical experience. An emerging nursing practice opportunity is that of a care coordinator who integrates the modalities that patients receive.

TYPES OF CAM

CAM consists of a large variety of modalities that are based on a set of beliefs different from those of allopathic medicine. Some of these modalities have developed fairly recently (such as imagery), while others have been used for thousands of years as components of ancient healing systems (such as Ayurveda or traditional Chinese medicine). Some modalities can be used effectively without assistance (nutritional approaches), while others (naturopathy) are more effective when used with guidance from practitioners who have particular knowledge and expertise. Many patients use these types of care as outpatients. An understanding of these modalities is important for the nurse because when outpatients use the allopathic system, they may become inpatients.

TABLE 28-2 Integrative Care of the Common Cold

In this example, adding herbs and/or acupuncture to a typical allopathic approach would represent integrative care.

Complementary and Alternative Modalities	Allopathic Approaches
Acupuncture to appropriate areas to reduce sinus congestion	Decongestant over-the-counter medications
Rest and fluids	Rest and fluids
Herbs, vitamin C to stimulate immune system	Vitamin C to stimulate immune system

Many of these modalities are not covered by insurance plans or HMOs, which means that consumers must pay out of their own pockets. In addition, government and professional groups do not regulate the majority of these modalities. Because of this, there can be inconsistencies among the preparation and care provided by practitioners.

CAM Systems

A CAM system consists of a philosophy and set of beliefs about health and illness and specific types of treatment. Ayurveda and traditional Chinese medicine are by far the oldest systems; homeopathy, naturopathy, and chiropractic are newer systems.

Ayurveda

Ayurveda originated in the Vedic civilization of India about 4,000 years ago. "It is a science of life that delineates the diet, medicines, and behaviors that are beneficial or harmful for life. Ayurveda considers that balance among people, the environment, and the larger cosmos is integral to human health" (Bright, 2002, p. 273).

Description

Central to Ayurvedic medicine is understanding the patient's basic constitution, or **dosha** (Table 28-3). People can display one dosha predominately or can be a combination of two or three doshas. A person whose doshas are balanced experiences health and well-being in mind, body, and spirit. Since each dosha has particular characteristics, when a dosha is out of balance, an individual typically displays signs and symptoms (including disease) characteristic of the imbalance. Imbalance in

TABLE 28-3 The Three Doshas in Ayurvedic Medicine

Dosha	Characteristic
Vata	Changeable
Pitta	Intense
Kapha	Relaxed

Adapted from Bright, M. A. (2002). *Holistic health and healing*. Philadelphia: F. A. Davis.

the doshas can be caused by a number of factors, including stress, lifestyle, and improper diet.

Diagnosis is made by information obtained in a detailed holistic history, review of symptoms, and selected physical observations. Many treatment modalities are specific for each dosha and may include nutrition, exercise, herbs, breathing, meditation, massage, aromatherapy, and purification. The quality of care received from an Ayurvedic practitioner can vary considerably based on the practitioner's educational preparation. An individual can be certified as an Ayurvedic practitioner after attending a qualified 2-year program, and there are prerequisites for background preparation.

Nursing Considerations

Special considerations may be necessary for patients who want to want to continue their Ayurvedic program. For example, some may have special dietary (eg, vegetarian) needs, some may need time set aside for self-care such as meditation, and some may desire to continue taking an herbal/supplement regimen.

Yoga

"Yoga has been practiced for thousands of years in India, where it is a way of life that includes ethical models for behavior and mental and physical exercises aimed at producing spiritual enlightenment" (Fontaine, 2000, p. 245). In the United States, yoga is paired frequently with other health-promoting activities that assist people to achieve unity and wholeness.

Description

Generally, yoga consists of various physical postures that are practiced to promote strength and flexibility, increase endurance, promote relaxation, and reduce one's response to stress. Breathing exercises, posture awareness, spiritual practices, and body-mind centering can be added to the basic postures. Basic yoga postures are illustrated in Figure 28-1. There are several branches and schools of yoga that focus on different goals and methods of attaining these goals. Some branches practice more vigorously, while others are gentler.

Nursing Considerations

Yoga can be used throughout the life span. Encourage patients to find a type of yoga that is compatible with their phys-

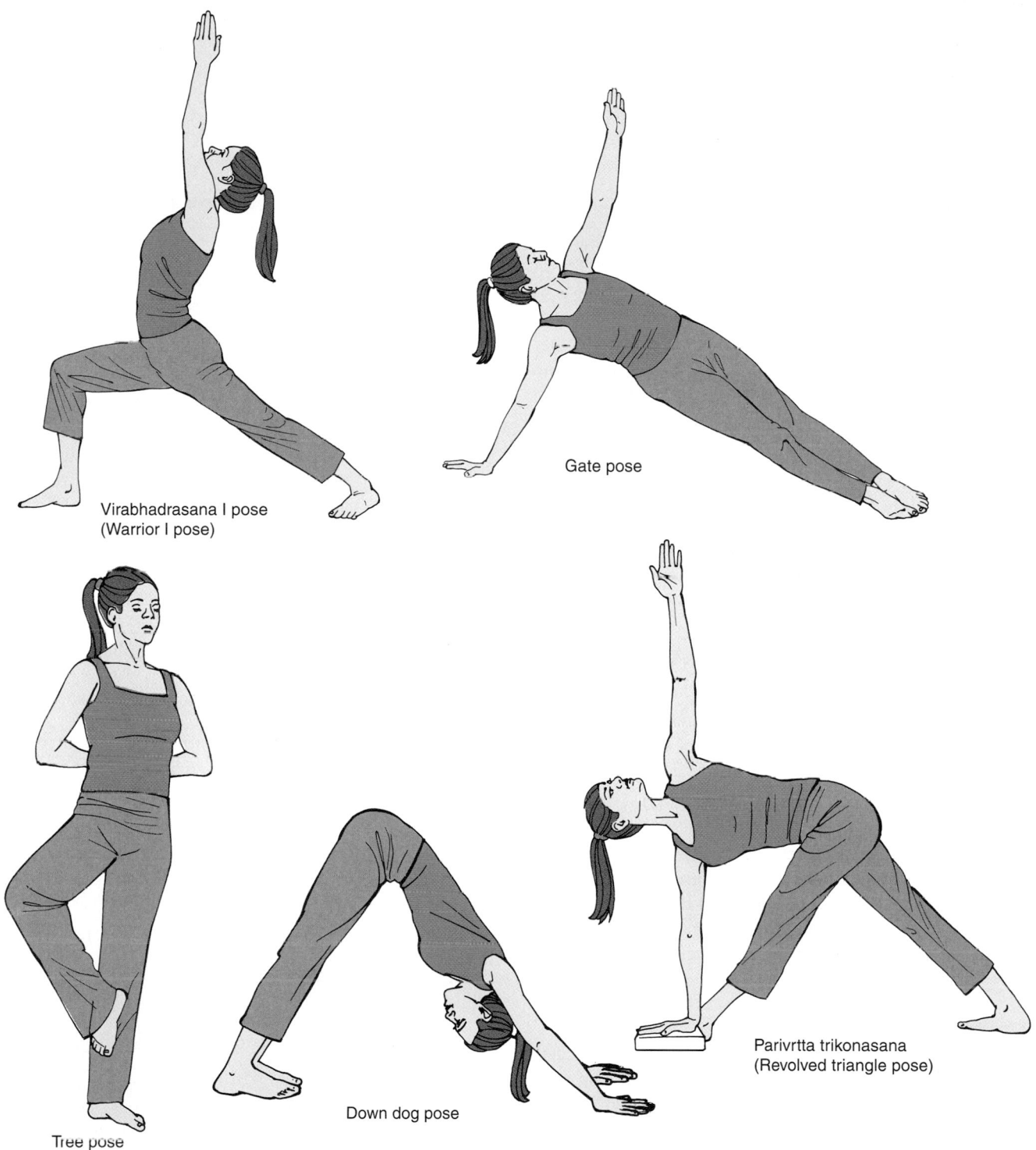

Virabhadrasana I pose
(Warrior I pose)

Gate pose

Tree pose

Down dog pose

Parivrtta trikonasana
(Revolved triangle pose)

FIGURE 28-1 Sample yoga poses.

ical condition and goals. Some postures are contraindicated during menstruation, after surgery, and in the presence of disease. Consumers can buy yoga tapes or DVDs or attend yoga classes. Yoga instructors come from a variety of backgrounds and usually are happy to discuss their preparation and knowledge with potential students.

Traditional Chinese Medicine

Traditional Chinese medicine (TCM) is similar to Ayurveda in at least two ways. First, TCM as a healing system is thousands of years old. Second, TCM believes that the interaction of people with their environment is most significant in creating health.

"The concept most central to TCM is **qi** or chi (pronounced *chee*), which is translated as energy. Qi represents an invisible flow of energy that circulates through plants, animals, and people as well as the earth and sky" (Fontaine, 2002, p. 46–47).

Qi is further viewed as either yin or yang energy. **Yin** and **yang** are opposites and complementary, and health is present when they are in balance in a person and his or her total environment. Conversely, an imbalance of yin and yang is considered to be the cause of illness (Table 28-4).

The goal of the TCM diagnostic process is to arrive at the pattern of disharmony that is manifesting in the person. TCM practitioners obtain a holistic history, observe particular parts of the body such as the tongue, and palpate pulses. Treatment may consist of acupuncture, with or without moxibustion (burning an herb above the acupuncture needle), dietary prescriptions, herbs, massage, and energy exercises such as qi gong. Accredited schools that provide TCM education require extensive college-level coursework followed by an educational program of about 4 years.

> *Remember Lee Chen, the terminally ill patient whose daughters asked for an acupuncturist. When developing the plan of care, the nurse would need to investigate Mr. Chen's culture and examine the beliefs associated with acupuncture. Based on an understanding of this information, the nurse would be better prepared to advocate for the patient and daughters.*

Acupuncture

Although records document the existence of traditional acupuncture treatments in China dating back 5,000 years, **acupuncture** has been prevalent in the United States only since the 1970s (Gerber, 2000). Acupuncture gained national media attention in 1971 when James Reston, a correspondent for the *New York Times,* had an appendectomy in Beijing using acupuncture instead of general anesthesia and postoperative analgesia. Reston's reports of his experience stimulated significant interest in acupuncture and TCM.

Description

Qi is believed to flow vertically in the body through an intricate structure of 72 **meridians,** energy circuits that nourish and support all cells and organs of the body (Bright, 2002) (Fig.

TABLE 28-4 **Characteristics of Yin and Yang**	
Yin	**Yang**
Cool	Hot
Moist	Dry
Dark	Light

Adapted from Bright, M. A. (2002). *Holistic health and healing.* Philadelphia: F. A. Davis.

28-2). Acupuncture consists of placing very thin, short, sterile needles at particular acupoints, believed to be centers of nerve and vascular tissue, along a meridian (Gerber, 2000) (Fig. 28-3). Acupuncture either increases or decreases the flow of chi along the meridian, restoring the balance of yin and yang. This change in the flow of energy contributes to healing.

> *Consider Mr. Chen, the terminally ill patient whose daughters requested that he receive acupuncture. Applying the theory underlying acupuncture's mechanism of action, the nurse would understand that the daughters' request is based on their belief and desire for their father's condition to improve. The nurse would incorporate this understanding in discussions with the daughters about their father's condition. In addition, the nurse would also begin assisting the daughters to "let go" and begin the grieving process should the patient's condition remain unchanged even after the acupuncture.*

Acupuncture is used for a variety of reasons, including reducing pain, promoting adherence to substance abuse programs, and minimizing nausea and vomiting due to chemotherapy and pregnancy. Licensed acupuncturists have graduated from an accredited acupuncture school after significant college-level coursework and passed a licensure examination.

Nursing Considerations

Acupuncture is generally provided in clinics or private offices, although it is possible for acupuncturists to provide acupuncture on inpatients. In this situation, patients may need up to

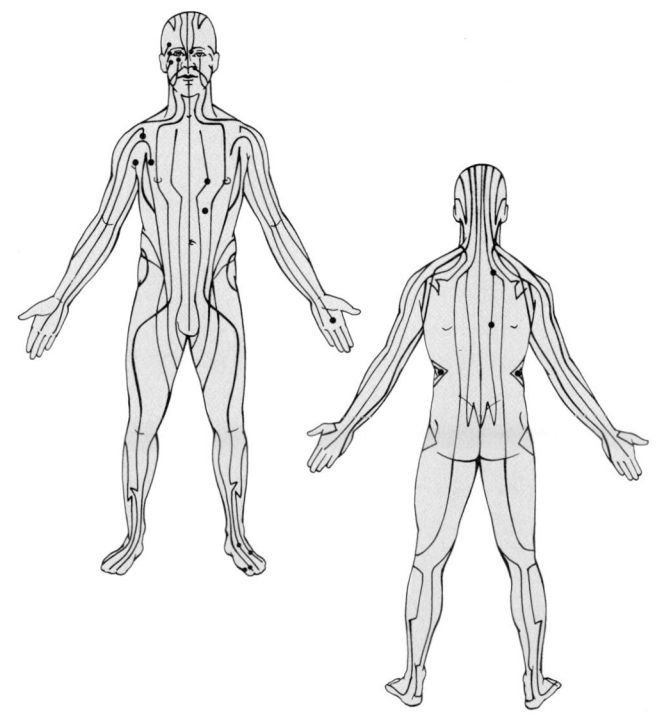

FIGURE 28-2 Acupuncture meridians.

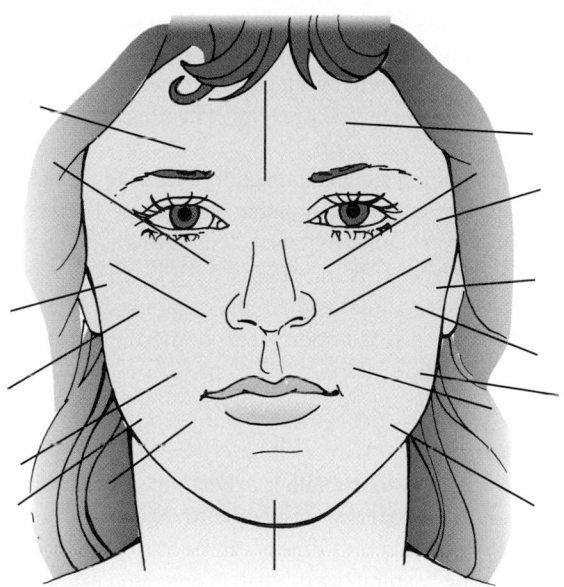

FIGURE 28-3 Placement of acupuncture needles.

1 hour of uninterrupted time in bed while the needles are in place.

Qi Gong

Qi gong is a system of postures, exercises (both gentle and dynamic), breathing techniques, and visualization that regulates the qi.

Description

"The majority of qi gong exercises or meditations enhance systemic health. They are designed to restore the healing system, the body's innate intelligence, so it knows how to correct and heal itself" (Horrigan, 2003, p. 86). For techniques specific to particular diseases, a patient can consult a qi gong teacher. Qi gong postures are illustrated in Figure 28-4. Tai chi, which many say developed from qi gong, has been used successfully in patients in long-term care facilities to promote balance and coordination.

Nursing Considerations

As with yoga, qi gong can be learned through the use of videos/DVDs or in a class. Encourage those interested to ask potential instructors about their background and knowledge.

Homeopathy

Samuel Hahnemann, a German physician, developed **homeopathy** approximately 200 years ago.

Description

The allopathic approach to dealing with illness is frequently to suppress symptoms; for example, acetaminophen can be given to reduce a fever. In contrast, homeopaths believe that when symptoms are suppressed in this manner, the condition "goes deeper" into the body, making it ultimately more difficult to cure. Homeopathy is based on the belief of supporting the body while the symptoms are allowed to "run their course." Homeopaths believe that this process stimulates and strengthens the immune system and promotes healing (Bright, 2002).

Homeopathic practice is based on two fundamental laws. The Law of Similars states that a natural substance that produces a given symptom in a healthy person will cure it in a sick person. The Law of Infinitesimals states that the smallest dose possible will have the desired effect. Although these concepts may seem unusual, they are the same concepts that underlie contemporary immunization practice (Bright, 2002).

Classical homeopathy looks for individual patterns. "Homeopaths believe people get sick in individual ways, showing distinctive patterns of symptoms. . . . Homeopaths do not believe in the existence of 'disease entities' . . . Rather, they concern themselves only with identifying the particular pattern of symptoms of an individual patient" (Weil, 1988, p. 8–9). Health is viewed as a condition of well-being and vitality.

Diagnosis is based on a thorough, holistic history and a determination of the pattern of the individual. Treatment (applying the Law of Similars) consists of matching the pattern the patient is exhibiting with a remedy that would create the same symptom pattern in a healthy person. Remedies in the proper dosages are prepared by clinicians.

Hahnemann himself took many of the remedies to establish what symptoms the remedies produced (Bright, 2002). Homeopathic remedies were effective against the epidemics of cholera, typhus, and scarlet fever in the 19th century in the United States and other countries. Despite this demonstrated effectiveness and the popularity of the modality, homeopathic medical schools closed in the early 1900s when the American Medical Association used its power and influence to close most non-

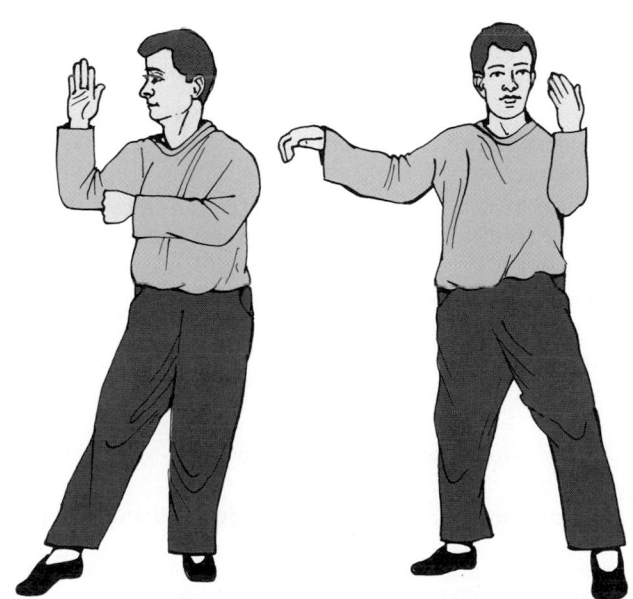

FIGURE 28-4 Qi gong postures.

allopathic schools of medicine. Today, homeopathy is practiced widely and is a part of the healthcare system in countries such as France, Great Britain, and Brazil. It is becoming more available in the United States (Bright, 2002).

There are several levels of homeopathic practitioners. A basic practitioner has completed a 2-year certification program after completing prerequisites after high school. Advanced practitioners complete additional work in homeopathy and can use additional titles.

Nursing Considerations

Remedies can be counteracted by things such as strong chemicals, herbs, and pharmaceuticals. If a patient is using homeopathy for postoperative recovery, the remedy may be repeated several times because of all the potential antidotes in the environment. Because homeopathic practitioners want the illness to "run its course," it is not uncommon for symptoms to get worse before they get better.

Clinical homeopathy is a newer branch of homeopathy that treats particular constellations of symptoms. These remedies are available over the counter in health-food stores and some drugstores. Teaching to Promote Health at Home 28-1: Using Herbs and Supplements also applies to over-the-counter homeopathic preparations.

Naturopathy

Naturopathy is a relatively new system of medicine that began in the early 1900s in the United States. "**Naturopathic medicine** is not only a system of medicine but also a way of life, with emphasis on client responsibility, client education, health maintenance, and disease prevention. It may be the model health system of the future with the movement toward healthy lifestyles, healthy diets, and preventive health care" (Fontaine, 2000, p. 134).

Naturopathic physicians engage in a rigorous educational program similar to that of allopathic physicians. They practice as primary care providers and use a scientific method for diagnosis and treatment. Naturopaths believe in the "vitalist doctrine," which maintains that "the organism's vitality and susceptibility are just as important as, or more important than, the causes of disease" (Bright, 2002, p. 187).

Description

Naturopaths believe that health is a dynamic state of being that provides abundant energy for people to deal with life in our complex society. Much of illness can be attributed, at least in part, to ignoring "natural laws," such as engaging in a sedentary lifestyle without adequate time for exercise; exposing oneself to environmental toxins; eating processed, overcooked foods; engaging in negativity or harboring negative thoughts; and not getting adequate rest or relaxation.

Therapies strive to support the self-healing mechanism of the body. Naturopaths employ an eclectic group of modalities including acupuncture, clinical nutrition, herbal medicine, hydrotherapy (therapeutic use of water), osteopathy (massage and manipulation), and TCM. Licensed naturopathic physicians (ND) complete a 4-year graduate-level medical school after 3 years of standard premedical courses.

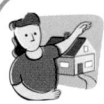

Teaching to Promote Health at Home 28-1
Using Herbs and Supplements

Teaching Tip	Why Is This Important?
Get information from knowledgeable and reliable sources.	Advertising media and many sources on the Internet frequently seek primarily to sell the product, not educate the consumer.
Buy name-brand products that are produced by reputable companies to increase your chances of getting a high-quality product.	Since this industry is not regulated, contamination and inconsistency in the amount of product sometimes occur.
The word "standardized" on an herbal product means that it consistently contains the percentage of the herb stated on the label.	A standardized product means that it contains a certain amount of active ingredient.
Whenever possible, buy single products.	If the product contains several ingredients and you have a reaction or positive response, you won't know which ingredient was the causative agent.
Take the proper dose and monitor side effects.	Herbal remedies are natural medicines and can be toxic in higher-than-recommended doses.
Give the product adequate time to work.	Herbs frequently take longer to produce a therapeutic effect than allopathic preparations.
Become knowledgeable about the product and your reason for using it.	Consumers who initiate any type of self-care tend to make better decisions if they are well informed.

Modified from Fontaine, K. L. (2000). *Healing practices.* Upper Saddle River, NJ: Prentice-Hall, pp. 126–127.

Nursing Considerations

Naturopathic physicians may have responsibility for their patients while they receive inpatient care. Patients who are being treated by a naturopathic physician will probably have a different plan of care than those being treated by allopathic physician.

Chiropractic

Chiropractic science investigates the relationship between the structure (the spine) and function (mainly the nervous system) of the human body to restore and preserve health. The underlying principle is that the functions of the body are controlled by the nervous system, mainly 31 pairs of spinal nerves that feed all organs of the body after branching off the spinal column. Since these nerves are surrounded by vertebrae and other musculoskeletal components, any distortion of the structure of the musculoskeletal system affects the nervous system (Bright, 2002).

The nervous system problem is sometimes caused by a subluxation, which occurs when a joint such as a vertebral bone is out of alignment. By adjusting the spine the joint is brought into proper alignment and the pressure on the nerve is released.

> *Recall Brian Legett, the patient with chronic back problems who has experienced little relief and is asking about seeing a chiropractor. When responding to Mr. Legett, the nurse would need to explain the underlying principles of chiropractic science. In addition, the nurse, in conjunction with other healthcare team members involved in the patient's plan of care, would need to review the patient's history thoroughly to identify (if possible) the underlying cause of his back problems and the various treatments attempted. This review would be important in determining if a referral to a chiropractor would be appropriate.*

Diagnosis can be made by health history, physical examination, and x-rays if needed. Treatments consist of manipulation and other modalities to decrease discomfort and aid the healing process, including ice, heat, ultrasound, electrical muscle stimulation, massage, herbs, and nutritional supplements (Bright, 2002). Doctors of chiropractic (DC) are licensed and attend 4 years of chiropractic school after prerequisite coursework. At this time, most chiropractic treatment is conducted on outpatients.

Mind–Body Modalities

Most people acknowledge that there is a mind–body connection. Situations such as insomnia related to anxiety the night before a major examination, or a migraine headache triggered by a fight with a spouse or good friend indicate that some connection does indeed exist. Recent research has expanded our knowledge of how the mind and body communicate with each other.

Knowing how this communication occurs assists in the understanding of the mind–body modalities of relaxation, meditation, and imagery. These three therapies can be useful for patients as well as self-care for nurses.

> *Think back to Sylvia Puentes, the anxious preoperative patient. The nurse would need to incorporate an understanding of the mind–body connection when discussing possible suggestions for anxiety relief.*

The scientific field of psychoneuroimmunology (PNI) studies neurochemicals such as neuropeptides that are now believed to be the messenger molecules that connect the body and mind. Neuropeptides have properties that allow them to affect neurologic and physiologic tissue receptors. Many neuropeptide receptor sites lie along the gastrointestinal tract; this explains why people can experience a large variety of gastrointestinal symptoms in response to emotional situations. Neuropeptides are produced as needed and travel through all spaces of the body in blood as well as other body fluids. Because they frequently travel and act quickly and are produced only as needed, there is as yet no way to measure them in the body (Pert, 1999).

Benson (1975) studied the **relaxation response** extensively. Dossey et al. (2000) described this response as "an alert, hypometabolic state of decreased sympathetic nervous system arousal" (p. 498). The response can also be viewed as the opposite of Selye's GAS response. Relaxation, which included meditation, was the most popular CAM therapy reported in the Eisenberg studies (Eisenberg et al., 1993, 1998).

Relaxation

Relaxation techniques promote parasympathetic activity, helping to reduce sympathetic activity and restore the balance of the two systems.

Description

Sympathetic system dominance, characterized by increased epinephrine levels in the body, can contribute to symptoms such as hypertension, cool hands and feet, tight muscles, increased heart rate, and increased respiration rate (Dossey et al., 2000). The ultimate goal is to increase the parasympathetic system influence in the body–mind and thus reduce the effect of stress and stress-related illness on the body.

Relaxation can be useful whether a patient is experiencing a single stressful event such as surgery or if the stress is more chronic. For examples of the usefulness of relaxation, refer to Box 28-1: Benefits of Relaxation for Patients and Nurses.

Dossey et al. (2000) discussed several relaxation modalities, including autogenic training, biofeedback, body scanning, hypnosis, meditation, and progressive muscle relaxation. Since these modalities are quite different, the type of relaxation modality chosen needs to be individually suited to the patient.

> *Recall Mr. Chen, the terminally ill patient described in the Reflective Practice display. When developing the plan of care, the nurse needs*

to include the patient's daughters. Therefore, when interacting with the patient's daughters, the nurse would also assess their stress level as they cope with their father's deteriorating condition. This assessment could provide valuable information about the cultural beliefs and values of each daughter, leading the nurse to suggest possible culturally appropriate methods for relaxation.

Nursing Considerations

Nurses can assist patients to begin to achieve a relaxation response by focusing on their breath. Patients can breathe into a stressful or painful area, lengthen their breathing, or focus on abdominal or diaphragmatic breathing. Benson (1975) found it helpful to use a mental device such as a repetitive phrase to remind the body to relax. Many types of relaxation tapes are available for purchase.

Meditation

Meditation has been part of many spiritual and healing traditions for hundreds of years.

Description

Meditation seeks to change one's physiology to a more relaxed state and alter one's perception to an increased acceptance of reality (Wright, 2001). Dossey et al. (2000) listed several types of meditation, including mindfulness meditation, Transcendental Meditation, and relaxation response meditation. Kabat-Zinn (1990) developed mindfulness-based stress reduction (MBSR) and established the first program in 1979 at the University of Massachusetts Medical Center. More than 200 MBSR programs modeled on the original program have been offered at healthcare settings in the United States (Roth & Stanley, 2002). Although mindfulness meditation comes from the Buddhist tradition, it can be practiced in any context. According to Kabat-Zinn (1990), "Mindfulness is basically just a particular way of

paying attention" (p. 12). Participants learn sitting and walking meditation, techniques such as body scanning and breathing techniques, and methods of handling physical and emotional pain (see Box 28-2: Outcomes of Mindfulness-Based Stress Reduction Programs).

Nursing Considerations

Patients seeking inpatient care might have a meditation practice they want to continue. Nurses can provide the time necessary for this. Nurses too could benefit from a meditation practice and could experience a brief meditation during breaks from patient care activities.

Imagery

Imagery has been used for years to prepare for particular events. For example, athletes have used a "rehearsal" form of imagery to improve performance (Shames, 1996). Guided imagery was first used in the 1970s by children with leukemia as an adjunct to chemotherapy. These children imagined their white blood cells "gobbling up" the cancer cells.

Description

Imagery involves using all five senses to imagine an event or body process unfolding according to a plan. When all senses are involved in the experience, the imaginary situation is more fully encoded in the body and more likely to take place. A relaxation technique is frequently used to prepare the mind and body before beginning an imagery session.

According to Rossman (2000), "The ultimate mechanisms of imagery are still a mystery" (p. 18). He believes differences in left and right brain processing help to explain imagery. The left brain processes information in a linear fashion, while the right brain processes information simultaneously. "The imagery it [right brain] produces often lets you see the big picture and experience the way an illness is related to events and feelings you might not have considered important" (p. 19).

Research studies have demonstrated that imagery assists patients with AIDS and cancer to extend their lives as well as enhance their quality of life. People experiencing migraine headaches and fibromyalgia have received symptomatic relief (Bright, 2002).

Nursing Considerations

Nurses can assist clients with imagery in several ways:

- Many kinds of imagery tapes with scripts are available that patients can use independently. If some of these are available on the nursing unit, patients can determine what types of tapes they would like to use or purchase. Patients can also be assisted to write a script and record it for their own use.
- Nurses can work with patients using "outcome imagery," which might consist of using a picture or photograph to visualize the desired outcome in a body part or in a situation. Patients can add to the visual cue and develop a total image.
- During a painful or stressful event, such as an intravenous line being started, the patient can "go to a favorite place" and imagine being there with all the pleasant experiences related to that space.

Think back to Sylvia Puentes, the anxious patient scheduled for surgery. Any of these types of imagery techniques would be appropriate suggestions for the patient. However, the nurse needs to assess the patient's preferences, beliefs, and ability to participate in these techniques to determine the best recommendation.

The Nurses Certificate Program in Imagery is endorsed by the American Holistic Nurses' Association (AHNA). See the website at the end of the chapter for information.

Energy Healing Approaches

Without realizing it, you may have heard a person talk about energy. The terms "resonance" ("I really resonate with you") and "wavelength" ("We are on the same wavelength") were used in Einstein's theory of physics. Today, Einstein's theory of physics, or energy theory, has been added to the sciences of biology and chemistry to express ideas about health and illness as well as to explain the human organism (Gerber, 2001).

All organisms are dependent on a subtle vital force that creates order in the system (Gerber, 2001). This vital force has been known to healing systems and people in various cultures for centuries and has been called a variety of names throughout history, such as vital life force (general usage), *pneuma* (ancient Greece), *qi* or *chi* (China and Japan), and *pran* (India) (Hover-Kramer, 2002). Many traditions consider this subtle energy to reflect the spiritual nature of people and to refer to individuals as mind, body, and spirit.

This life force feeds and nourishes the organism and is carried via two energetic structures that interact with each other: chakras and the etheric body. **Chakras** are concentrated areas of energy aligned vertically in the body that relate to each other as well as to specific areas of the body, mind, and spirit

(Fig. 28-5). The etheric body (**aura**) consists of at least seven layers of energy that surround the body and relate to the chakras (Fig. 28-6). There is scientific evidence that following conception, energetic structures are the first to develop and, in some cases, serve as templates for cellular and organ development (Gerber, 2000). This finding supports the expression, "We are energy first." Energy therapies used for healing are based on the belief that they can affect this primary life force and thus contribute to physiologic healing.

The North American Nursing Diagnosis Association (NANDA) recognizes disturbed energy field as a nursing diagnosis. Defining characteristics of the disturbed field relate to movement, sounds, temperature change, visual changes, and disruption. There are many forms of energy work that seek to reduce disturbance in the energy field. Two types of this energy work have been developed by nurses: Therapeutic Touch and Healing Touch.

Therapeutic Touch

Therapeutic Touch, founded by Delores Krieger in the 1970s, is described as "the use of the hands on or near the body with the intent to help or heal" (Horrigan, 1996, p. 69). The TT process consists of centering, assessing the energy field, and rebalancing the field using modulation, "unruffling," and other techniques (Krieger, 1993).

TT uses four primary scientific premises:

1. All the life sciences agree that, physically, a human being is an open energy system.
2. Anatomically, a human being is bilaterally symmetrical.
3. Illness is an imbalance in an individual's energy field.
4. Human beings have natural abilities to transform and transcend their conditions of living. (Krieger, 1993, p. 12–13).

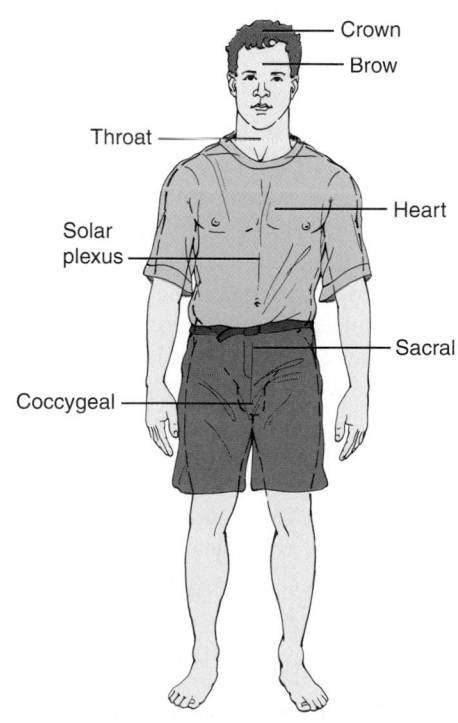

FIGURE 28-5 Location of the seven major chakras.

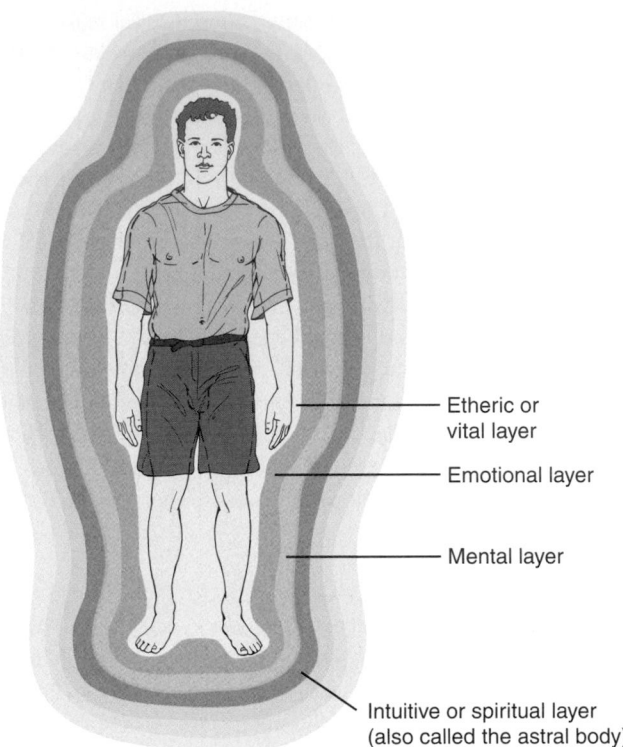

Etheric or
vital layer

Emotional layer

Mental layer

Intuitive or spiritual layer
(also called the astral body)

FIGURE 28-6 First four layers of the human aura.

Healing Touch

Healing Touch (HT), founded by Janet Mengten in the 1980s, uses a collection of energy techniques to assess and treat the human energy system, thus affecting physical, emotional, mental, and spiritual health and healing. The current HT textbook contains about 20 specific energy techniques to be used in particular patient situations. The goal of HT is to restore wholeness through harmony and balance (Hover-Kramer, 2002).

Nursing Considerations for Energy Modalities

Workshops and other learning opportunities are available for nurses to learn energy healing techniques. Energy work can assist patients in virtually all settings and all age groups, although advanced knowledge is necessary to work with babies and other vulnerable populations.

Registered nurses can become credentialed in TT. Details are available on the website.

Box 28-3 describes when HT can be used. Certification in HT for people from various backgrounds is available through Healing Touch International after completion of a series of classes and experiences. The program is endorsed by AHNA, and class information is available on the website.

Botanicals and Nutritional Supplements

Botanical agents (herbs) and nutritional supplements are chemical compounds that are ingested with the hope of achieving a therapeutic goal. They are becoming increasingly popular with consumers, who can buy many of these preparations over the counter or from company distributors. Currently there is no FDA regulation of dietary supplements (which include herbs and nutritional supplements) as long as FDA labeling requirements are followed. Some product sample analyses have revealed inconsistencies in the amount of active ingredients. Because of these inconsistencies as well as for other reasons, the FDA has taken the initiative to pass legislation giving the federal agency more control over herbs and supplements.

Botanicals

Some consumers and practitioners are attracted to herbs because they are "natural" plant products, which are perceived as more compatible with the body than manufactured pharmaceutical agents. In fact, some pharmaceutical agents (eg, Digitalis) were first produced as natural products derived from plants and now are produced chemically.

In many countries, herbal products are regulated and available through the primary healthcare system. In Germany, for example, their "Commission E" reviews scientific data and establishes prescriptive standards for pharmaceuticals, including conventional drugs and plant products used for healing.

Nutritional Supplements

Nutritional supplements are chemical compounds that contain ingredients (vitamins, minerals, enzymes, amino acids, and essential fatty acids) believed to promote health. These products have a wide range of safety and effectiveness.

Nursing Considerations for Botanicals and Nutritional Supplements

Extensive specialized education is required before a nurse can be competent to advise patients on the use of herbs and supplements. However, nurses are finding that information about certain herbs adds an aspect of safety to their practice. For example, some herbs and/or supplements may interact with prescribed medications patients are taking. Ginkgo biloba, the most widely sold herb in Europe and used by many to improve memory, affects platelet function and thus should not be used concurrently with warfarin or aspirin (Sierpina, 2001). Some nursing pharmacology courses include information on commonly used herbs. For information to use in teaching patients about this subject, refer to Teaching to Promote Health at Home 28-1.

Spiritual Approaches

Many cultures throughout the ages have believed that illness involves the human spirit. Shamanism, Native American beliefs, and contemporary prayer studies provide examples of ways in which this belief extends to practice.

Shamanism

Shamanism, according to Achterberg (1985), has been the most widely practiced type of medicine on our planet. In shamanism, illness is thought to originate in the spirit world and usually involves a loss of power. Treatment consists first of restoring the individual's power and then treating symptoms. Since some cultures in the United States practice forms of shamanism, the nurse should have some knowledge of shamanistic practice. Shamanism as a part of cultural traditions is discussed in Chapter 3.

Native American Traditions

Traditional North American healing practices are being increasingly used by both Native Americans and others. Many of these healing practices can be used alone or to complement other treatments. Native American healing practices are grounded in their cultural views. Some cultural concepts identified in a research study (Mehl-Madrona, 1999) include:

- Healing takes time, and time contributes to healing.
- The distractions of modern life interfere with potential healing agents.
- Modern culture encourages us to maintain a low level of emotional awareness.
- Ceremony is important to receive guidance and assistance from the spiritual dimension.

General healing techniques involve native plants and herbs, animals, ritual, ceremony, and purification techniques.

Intercessory Prayer

Intercessory prayer involves praying for the benefit of another person to the Judeo-Christian God. Dossey (1993) thoroughly explored this subject, exploring areas such as beliefs about prayer, the process of praying, and whether a physician's beliefs are important in the healing relationship. This area can be controversial and needs to be explored with patients using sensitivity and cultural competence. Although the effectiveness of prayer is considered difficult to measure, a classic study on intercessory prayer done in 1988 has withstood many critiques and is accepted as a valid study (see the Research in Nursing display).

Other Healing Modalities

The following represent an eclectic group of miscellaneous therapies. Used by practitioners and healthcare consumers and seen in a variety of patient settings, they include nutritional therapy, aromatherapy, music therapy, structural modalities, and humor therapy.

Nutritional Therapy

The eating habits of people in the United States are being scrutinized because of the alarming increase in obesity, particularly in children, and chronic illnesses in all age groups. The so-called typical diet consisting of prepared and processed foods and large amounts of meat, dairy products, and sugar is highly suspect. Many popular eating plans that purport to address these health problems have been endorsed by people with a variety of credentials. The diversity of these approaches is understandably very confusing to the consumer. Although an examination of these popular diets is beyond the scope of this book, it does appear that people have individual needs and preferences with respect to foods. In fact, this belief has been a cornerstone of

 **Research in Nursing** Making a Difference

Positive Therapeutic Effects of Intercessory Prayer in a Coronary Care Unit Population

Byrd, R. (1988). Positive therapeutic effects of intercessory prayer in a coronary care unit population. *Southern Medical Journal, 81*(7), 826–829.

Relevance to Nursing Practice

This double-blind, quantitative clinical study conducted at San Francisco General Hospital involved 393 patients in the coronary care unit. Subjects were randomly assigned to "prayed for" and "not prayed for" groups (prayer group, N = 192; control group, N = 201). Intercessors (people who participated in the experiment by praying) practiced an active prayer life and came from Protestant and Roman Catholic traditions. Intercessors were provided with the patient's first name, diagnosis, and general condition along with pertinent updates in the patient's condition. Intercessors prayed outside the hospital and prayed daily for a rapid recovery and for prevention of complications and death, in addition to other areas of prayer they believed to be beneficial to the patient.

Each patient's hospital course was graded as good, intermediate, or bad based on the development of new diagnoses, problems, or necessary therapies; levels of morbidity; risk of death; and actual death. Eighty-five percent of the patients in the prayer group were graded as good, 73% of the control group; 1% of the patients in the prayer group were graded as intermediate, 5% of the control group; and 14% of the patients in the prayer group were graded as bad, 22% of the control group. Results were significant at $p < 0.01$.

holistic nutritional approaches for centuries in the TCM and Ayurvedic systems. (See also Chap. 42, Nutrition.) For patient teaching guidelines on this subject, see Teaching to Promote Health at Home 28-2. It is common to find many of these approaches endorsed by naturopathic practitioners.

Aromatherapy

Aromatherapy using essential oils was practiced in ancient Egypt and India more than 6,000 years ago. Oils were used in religious ceremonies, for medicinal purposes, and in perfumes and cosmetics. Today one cannot go to a shopping mall without seeing scented candles and various other "aromatherapy" products.

Medicinally, aromatherapy is the "use of essential oils of plants to treat symptoms and as such has no theory of health and illness nor a system of diagnosis" (Fontaine, 2000, p. 153). The fragrance of these oils is believed to ultimately affect the very sensitive amygdala of the limbic system in the brain, where emotional memories are stored and released. "Thus, the sense of smell can evoke powerful memories in a split second

and change people's perceptions and behaviors" (Fontaine, 2000, p. 157).

Commonly used essential oils in a healthcare setting are ginger or peppermint for nausea and lavender or chamomile for insomnia (Fontaine, 2000). Essential oils vary in quality and potency depending upon the manufacturing processes. If specific essential oils are approved for use in an inpatient setting, education on these oils should be provided and one manufacturer should be chosen. In addition, some people are highly sensitive to strong fragrances, particularly concentrated essential oils. This might preclude their use in some patient settings.

Certification in Aromatherapy for Health Professionals is available. This course is endorsed by AHNA, and information is available on the web site listed at the end of the chapter.

Music in Healing

Music is another modality that has been viewed as therapeutic for thousands of years. Today music has demonstrated effectiveness in reducing pain, decreasing anxiety, promoting re-

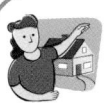

Teaching to Promote Health at Home 28-2
Holistic Approaches to Food Choices

Teaching Tip	Why Is This Important?
Reduce amounts of processed foods.	Processing frequently reduces the nutrients available for absorption. For example, canned foods frequently have lower nutritional values than frozen foods.
Reduce/eliminate soft drinks (colas).	They are "fake food" and have no nutritional value.
Avoid eating foods with preservatives.	Preservatives are artificial substances that the body ultimately needs to excrete, usually through the urine or feces. This excretion process uses energy the body could use for other processes.
Reduce intake of refined and natural sugars.	The "average" individual in the United States consumes an unhealthy amount of glucose. Among other things, excess glucose places an increased demand on the pancreas, kills the natural bacterial flora found in the gastrointestinal tract that is necessary for absorption, and interferes with cellular absorption of nutrients.
Reduce intake of artificial sweeteners, including aspartame.	Since aspartame is not a food, it needs to be excreted, and there is some evidence that it is toxic to humans. In some countries (Japan), aspartame is extensively regulated. Replace aspartame with stevia, a natural sweetener available in liquid or granulated form.
Eat organically grown foods.	If grown according to rigorous organic regulations, these foods contain no pesticides or chemical byproducts, which are toxins in the body.
Reduce intake of dairy products.	Many dairy cows are regularly given antibiotics and, in some cases, hormones. Breakdown products from these substances may be found in milk.
Consider adopting a vegetarian diet.	Animals are increasingly fed antibiotics and potentially contaminated foods. Increasingly, fish are being contaminated with mercury and other pollutants.
Eat foods in season.	Foods produced "out of season" are treated with chemicals to ripen them since they are picked before ripening.
Be aware of genetically engineered, radiated food.	Become informed about these processes before you make a decision as to whether you want to eat these foods.

laxation, and in distracting persons from unpleasant sensations so they are empowered to heal (McCaffrey & Locsin, 2002).

Music consists of sound waves that vibrate at particular frequencies. When these frequencies are harmonious with our bodies, we experience the music as pleasant. Mozart's music has been found to be particularly healing because of its musical qualities (Campbell, 1997). Some music (eg, "grunge rock") could be perceived to be detrimental to healing since it was found to increase hostility, sadness, tension, and fatigue and decrease relaxation and mental clarity (McCraty et al., 1998).

Music can be used to promote healing in several ways. Patients can be provided with their selected CDs to listen to prior to surgery or other stressful events, during imagery, and while relaxing.

> *Remember Sylvia Puentes, the anxious preoperative patient described at the beginning of the chapter. Based an assessment of the patient's likes and dislikes, the nurse might suggest music therapy as a means to reduce the patient's preoperative anxiety.*

Music is frequently played in operating rooms and harp or piano music is played in patient lounges and lobbies.

Structural Modalities

Structural modalities include a variety of "bodywork" techniques such as Rolfing, shiatsu, Feldenkrais, Alexander, myofascial release, and others. These techniques can be painful while they work to oxygenate tissues, break up lymphatic congestion, release muscle tightness, and promote circulation. The goal is to promote communication between body–mind structures and thus improve body functioning. These techniques require specialized preparation and are typically useful in rehabilitation or health-promotion types of settings.

Humor Therapy

Norman Cousins was a well-known editor of the *Saturday Review* when he contracted ankylosing spondylitis in 1964. He wrote about using humor in his therapy program to treat his acute and debilitating illness. He found that after watching 10 minutes of Marx Brothers (comedians) tapes and "belly-laughing," his sedimentation rate (a measure of inflammation in the body) decreased by at least five points permanently (Cousins, 1979). More recent research (Bennett et al., 2003) found that improved immune response was correlated with experiences of "mirthful laughter."

NURSING AND CAM

The development of CAM continues to be a market-driven and, in some respects, a patient-driven phenomenon. Patients/consumers seem to be increasingly unsatisfied with allopathic treatments and are turning to CAM for relief of symptoms and healing. Since healthcare currently operates on a business model, it is probable that more CAM will become available to deal with real or perceived market needs. Currently there is minimal coordination of the development of new CAM. FDA oversight is minimal, and regulation of practitioners is in its infancy. There is a great opportunity here for nurses to expand their practice to meet existing patient needs as well as to promote health. See the Focused Assessment Guide 28-1: Holistic Care for an identification of areas in which a holistic nurse can improve patient care. As new modalities demonstrate their effectiveness, they can be added to the assessment.

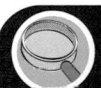

Focused Assessment Guide 28-1

Holistic Care

Factors to Assess	Questions and Approaches
Stress	What measures does the patient use to reduce stress? If the patient wants to continue a meditation, relaxation, or imagery practice while receiving care, explore ways in which that can be accomplished.
Music/sound preferences	What preferences does the patient have for music or environmental sounds (eg, ocean waves, birds) either while meditating or relaxing? The patient could provide his or her own music if preferred music is not available.
Diet	What dietary preferences does the patient have (eg, vegetarian, no processed foods)? Communicate these preferences to nutritional services.
Environmental sensitivity	Is the patient sensitive to environmental odors or fragrances? If so, can an air purifier be brought to the room?
Use of herbs and supplements	Is the patient is taking any herbs or supplements as directed by a CAM practitioner or purchased over the counter? If so, obtain the names of the herbs/supplements, dosages, and reasons for their use. If the patient has these substances in his or her possession, follow applicable institutional policies.
Use of CAM healthcare provider	Is the patient planning to use a primary CAM provider while receiving allopathic care? If so, convey appropriate information to the primary allopathic provider.

Nursing is expanding its knowledge base to include information that explains selected CAM. For example, pharmacology courses in schools of nursing frequently include information on herbs. Certification in holistic nursing for nurses with a baccalaureate degree is available through the American Holistic Nurses' Credentialing Corporation (AHNCC). Graduate-level specialization in holistic nursing is available at some universities. Further, the AHNCC plans to develop an advanced practice certification in holistic nursing for nurses with master's degrees. It is expected that CAM will become a larger part of the practice of some nurses.

Developing Critical Thinking Skills

1. You are caring for a culturally diverse population. How would you appropriately assess for and implement CAM into your care while maintaining cultural sensitivity?
2. The text mentioned digitalis as a pharmaceutical agent first produced by natural products derived from plants that is now produced chemically. Can you think of other examples? The text also mentioned some interactions you must be aware of, such as ginkgo biloba affecting platelet function and being contraindicated with warfarin or aspirin use. Can you think of other examples?

Preparing for NCLEX

1. Which CAM uses meridian energy circuits to nourish and support all cells and organs of the body?
   a. Energy healing approaches
   b. Acupuncture
   c. Chiropractic science
   d. Therapeutic Touch
2. Complementary and alternative modalities are:
   a. Safe interventions to supplement traditional care
   b. Used by a minority of inpatients
   c. Recognized by half of the state Boards of Nursing
   d. Relatively new
3. A combination of traditional medical care and CAM is called:
   a. Integrative care
   b. Holism
   c. Allopathy
   d. Traditional Chinese medicine
4. This CAM uses the Law of Similars and the Law of Infinitesimals:
   a. Energy healing approaches
   b. Ayurveda
   c. Allopathy
   d. Homeopathy
5. Which CAM is most similar to the current health promotion/disease prevention models?
   a. Naturopathic medicine
   b. Chiropractic science
   c. Nutritional supplements
   d. Acupuncture
6. Neuropeptides are messenger molecules for which type of CAM?
   a. Holism
   b. Mind–body modalities
   c. Energy healing approaches
   d. Botanical supplements
7. A CAM that involves active participation by the patient and is often used in pre- and postoperative pain control is:
   a. Acupuncture
   b. Therapeutic Touch
   c. Botanical supplements
   d. Guided imagery
8. The relaxation response is opposite of which person's ideas?
   a. Einstein
   b. Selye
   c. Descartes
   d. Kabot-Zinn
9. Energy healing approaches:
   a. Have a North American Nursing Diagnosis Association (NANDA)-recognized nursing diagnosis
   b. Have an American Holistic Nursing Association certification in energy imagery
   c. Result from Einstein's theory of relativity
   d. Have an underlying principle that the functions of the body are controlled by the nervous system

Answers With Rationale

1. The correct answer is *b*. Acupuncture consists of placing very thin, short, sterile needles at particular acupoints, believed to be centers of nerve and vascular tissue, along a meridian. Energy healing uses the chakras. Chiropractic science uses the spine and nervous system. Therapeutic Touch uses energy fields.
2. The correct answer is *c*. These modalities are not always safe. You may not be aware of who uses CAM, so assessment is imperative. Some of these modalities are thousands of years old.
3. The correct answer is *a*. Holism is interaction between parts of a whole. Allopathy is traditional medical care. Traditional Chinese medicine involves an interaction of people and their environment.
4. The correct answer is *d*. The Law of Similars states that a natural substance that produces a given symptom in a healthy person will cure it in a sick person. The Law of Infinitesimals states that the smallest dose possible will have the desired effect. Although these concepts may seem unusual, they are the concepts that underlie contemporary immunization practice.

5. The correct answer is *a*. Naturopathic medicine is not only a system of medicine but also a way of life, with emphasis on client responsibility, client education, health maintenance, and disease prevention. It may be the model health system of the future with the movement toward healthy lifestyles, healthy diets, and preventive health-care. The other modalities have received recent re-acceptance.

6. The correct answer is *b*. The scientific field of psychoneuroimmunology (PNI) studies neurochemicals, including neuropeptides, which are now believed to be the messenger molecules that connect the body and mind. Neuropeptides have properties that allow them to affect neurologic and physiologic tissue receptors.

7. The correct answer is *d*. Imagery involves using all five senses to imagine an event or body process unfolding according to a plan. A patient can be encouraged to "go to a favorite place." With the other modalities, the patient is more passive.

8. The correct answer is *b*. Hans Selye developed the term "general adaptation syndrome" (GAS) to describe the general holistic pattern that emerges when people experience stress or illness. The relaxation answer is an alert, hypometabolic state of decreased sympathetic nervous system arousal. Einstein developed the theory of energy. Descartes "separated" mind and body. Kabot-Zinn developed the mindfulness-based stress reduction concept.

9. The correct answer is *a*. Disturbed energy field is an accepted nursing diagnosis. AHNA has certificate programs in Healing Touch, a type of energy modality. Einstein's related theory was the "theory of energy." Answer *d* is a definition of chiropractic science.

Bibliography

Achterberg, J. (1985). *Imagery in healing: Shamanism and modern medicine.* Boston: Shambhala.

Bennett, M. P., Zeller, J. M., Rosenberg, L., et al. (2003). The effect of mirthful laughter on stress and natural killer cell activity. *Alternative Therapies, 9*(2), 38–43.

Benson, H. (1975). *The relaxation response.* New York: William Morrow & Co.

Benson, H. (1984). *Beyond the relaxation response.* New York: Times Books.

Bright, M. A. (2002). *Holistic health and healing.* Philadelphia: F. A. Davis.

Bulbrook, M. J., & Mentgen, J. (2002). *Healing Touch level 1 notebook* (4th ed.). Carrboro, NC: North Carolina Center for Healing Touch.

Byrd, R. (1988). Positive therapeutic effects of intercessory prayer in a coronary care unit population. *Southern Medical Journal, 81*(7), 826–829.

Campbell, D. (1997). *The Mozart effect.* New York: Avon Books.

Chopra, D. (2000). *Perfect health.* New York: Three Rivers Press.

Cousins, N. (1979). *Anatomy of an illness.* New York: Bantam Books.

Dossey, B. M., Keegan, L., & Guzzetta, C. E. (2000). *Holistic nursing. A handbook for practice* (3rd ed.). Gaithersburg, MD: Aspen.

Dossey, L. (1993). *Healing words.* New York: HarperCollins.

Eisenberg, D. M., Kessler, R. C., Foster, C., et al. (1993). Unconventional medicine in the United States. *New England Journal of Medicine, 275*(4), 246–252.

Eisenberg, D. M., Davis, R. B., Ettner, S. L., et al. (1998). Trends in alternative medicine use in the United States, 1990–1997. *New England Journal of Medicine, 280*(18), 1569–1575.

Fenton, M. V., & Morris, D. L. (2003). The integration of holistic nursing practices and complementary and alternative modalities into curricula of schools of nursing. *Alternative Therapies in Health and Medicine, 9*(4), 62–67.

Ferguson, M. (1987). *Aquarian conspiracy: Personal and social transformation in our time.* New York: J. P. Tarcher.

Fontaine, K. L. (2000). *Healing practices.* Upper Saddle River, NJ: Prentice Hall.

Gerber, R. (2000). *Vibrational medicine for the 21st century.* New York: HarperCollins.

Gerber, R. (2001). *Vibrational medicine* (3rd ed.). Rochester, VT: Bear & Company.

Horrigan, B. (1996). Janet Quinn, RN, PhD: Therapeutic Touch and a healing way. *Alternative Therapies in Health and Medicine, 2*(4), 69–75.

Horrigan, B. (1999). Michael Murray, ND: A natural approach to health. *Alternative Therapies in Health and Medicine, 5*(2), 77–84.

Horrigan, B. (2003). Ken Cohen, MA, MSTH: Healing through ancient traditions: Qigong and Native American medicine. *Alternative Therapies in Health and Medicine, 9*(3), 83–91.

Hover-Kramer, D. (2002). *Healing Touch. A guidebook for practitioners.* Albany, NY: Delmar.

Kabat-Zinn, J. (1990). *Full catastrophe living.* New York: Delacorte Press.

Krieger, D. (1993). *Accepting your power to heal.* Santa Fe, NM: Bear & Company.

McCaffrey, R., & Locsin, R. C. (2002). Music listening as a nursing intervention: A symphony of practice. *Holistic Nursing Practice, 16*(3), 70–77.

McCraty, R., Barrios-Choplin, B., Atkinson, M., et al. (1998). The effects of different types of music on mood, tension, and mental clarity. *Alternative Therapies, 4*(1), 75–84.

Mehl-Madrona, L. E. (1999). Native American medicine in the treatment of chronic illness: Developing an integrated program and evaluating its effectiveness. *Alternative Therapies, 5*(1), 36–44.

Pert, C. (1999). *Molecules of emotion: The science behind mind-body medicine.* New York: Simon & Schuster.

Rossman, M. L. (2000). *Guided imagery for self-healing.* Tiburon, CA: H. J. Kramer.

Roth, B., & Stanley, T-W. (2002). Mindfulness-based stress reduction and healthcare utilization in the inner city: preliminary findings. *Alternative Therapies, 8*(1), 60–66.

Shames, K. H. (1996). *Creative imagery in nursing.* Albany, NY: Delmar.

Sierpina, V. S. (2001). *Integrative healthcare.* Philadelphia: F. A. Davis.

Sparber, A. (2001). State boards of nursing and scope of practice of registered nurses performing complementary therapies. *Online Journal of Issues in Nursing, 6*(2), 6–7.

Weil, A. (1988). *Health and healing.* Boston: Houghton Mifflin.

Wright, L. D. (2001). Meditation: Myths and misconceptions. *Alternative Therapies, 7*(2), 96–97.

Websites

Aromatherapy for Health Professionals: http://www.rjbuckle.com.

Healing Touch International: http://www.healingtouch.net.

Nurses Certificate Program in Imagery: http://www.IMAGERYRN.com.

Nurse Healers-Professional Associates International (Therapeutic Touch): http://www.therapeutic-touch.org.

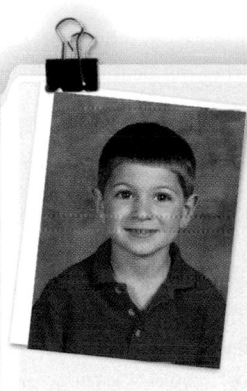

Jacob Shoolin, a 5-year-old boy, is admitted to the hospital diagnosed with pneumonia and an exacerbation of his asthma. He is receiving antibiotic therapy intravenously and bronchodilators orally and via nebulization.

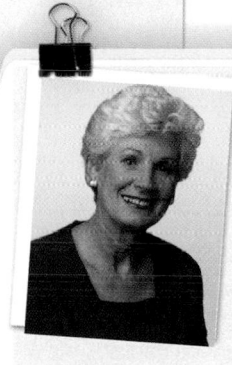

Mildred Campbell, a 65-year-old woman with a history of arthritis, comes to the clinic for evaluation of her painful joints. She states, "I just saw this new medicine advertised on television that is supposed to be really helpful in relieving joint pain. What do you think? Is it something I should try?"

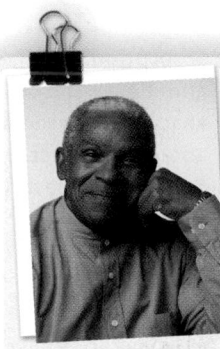

François Baptiste is an elderly man with a wound infection requiring intravenous antibiotic therapy. He is scheduled to receive his next dose at 10 a.m. The medication delivered by the pharmacy is labeled with the correct drug and dose, but with another patient's name.

Focusing on Blended Skills

The types of blended skills you'll need to respond to the case scenarios include:

Cognitive Skills

- Basic knowledge of pharmacology (pharmacodynamics and pharmacokinetics); drug names, types of preparations, types of orders; drug classifications and actions; adverse effects; drug dose calculations
- Knowledge of proper and safe preparation and administration of medications by various routes
- Knowledge of how to develop teaching plans to meet patient needs specific to medication administration
- Knowledge of resources to contact when encountering questions about medications, including dosage parameters, preparation, and administration techniques
- Ability to incorporate knowledge of developmental considerations when administering medications to patients across the life span

Technical Skills

- Ability to use equipment correctly and implement techniques for safe and effective preparation and administration of medications
- Strong assessment skills related to areas that may affect drug action and administration, including previous and current drug use, medication schedule, response to medications, attitude toward drugs and their use, compliance with regimen, and storage
- Ability to calculate drug doses correctly
- Ability to demonstrate competence in administering medications via various routes
- Ability to adapt techniques and skills appropriately when dealing with patients of different ages requiring medications

Interpersonal Skills

- Strong people skills; ability to communicate and interact effectively with individuals and groups
- Ability to establish trusting relationships with patients, families, and colleagues as a basis for teaching and counseling with respect to medication regimens
- Ability to use therapeutic communication effectively to meet the needs of patients requiring medication therapy
- Ability to mobilize necessary support and guidance to administer medications safely and effectively

Ethical and Legal Skills

- Commitment to safety and quality; strong sense of responsibility, accountability; strong advocacy abilities
- Ability to integrate ethical and legal principles into all aspects of medication administration, including documentation
- Commitment to reporting medication errors and to following agency policy for working to prevent their recurrence
- Demonstration of adherence to the five rights of medication administration
- Commitment to administering medications safely within the scope of legal practice
- Knowledge of pertinent drug legislation and policy

Learning Outcomes

After completing the chapter, the learner should be able to accomplish the following:

1. Discuss drug legislation in the United States.
2. Describe drug names, types of preparations, and types of drug orders.
3. Identify drug classifications and actions.
4. Discuss adverse effects of drugs, including allergy, tolerance, cumulative effect, idiosyncratic effect, and interactions.
5. Calculate drug dosages, using the various systems of equivalents.
6. Obtain patient information necessary to establish a medication history.
7. Describe principles used to prepare and administer medications safely by the oral, parenteral, topical, and inhalation routes.
8. Develop teaching plans to meet patient needs specific to medication administration.

Key Terms

absorption	peak level
ampule	pharmacology
anaphylactic reaction	placebo
antagonist effect	p.r.n. order
cumulative effect	stat order
enteral	subcutaneous
excretion	injection
generic name	synergistic effect
half-life	teratogenic
idiosyncratic effect	therapeutic
inhalation	range
intradermal injection	topical
intramuscular injection	application
intravenous route	trade name
metabolism	trough level
official name	vial
parenteral	Z-track

Medication administration is a basic nursing function that involves skillful technique and consideration of the patient's development and safety. The nurse administering medications needs a knowledge base about drugs, including drug names, preparations, classifications, adverse effects, and physiologic factors that affect drug action (see the accompanying box, Through the Eyes of a Student).

Through the Eyes of a Student

I entered my patient's room, knowing that she had had surgery less than 12 hours before my arrival, and introduced myself. I asked how she was feeling, to which she immediately responded, "I need pain medication—now!" I told her that I would check the medication orders and be back as soon as possible. I walked quickly to the medication Kardex, and there it was glaring at me in neatly printed black and white: "Demerol, 100 mg IM q 3–4 hr p.r.n." My mind raced as I thought, "I have never given an IM injection. There has to be something else ordered for pain." I knew there wasn't. I found my clinical instructor and announced, "My patient needs an IM injection." Given the anxiety I was feeling, everything went surprisingly well as we prepared the medication. I went over the procedure one last time before entering the patient's room.

We approached the patient just in time for her to look at us in sheer terror and cry, "I hope that shot isn't for me; I hate them," which did nothing for my already shaking hands. I explained that she couldn't take a pill because she could not have anything by mouth because of the nature of her surgery. My instructor and I positioned the patient on her side—a feat in itself—so that I could give her the shot in the dorsogluteal area. I marked the landmarks at least half a dozen times, wiped the area with alcohol, and asked her if she was ready for the injection. *Big mistake!* She swiftly replied, "No, but get it over with."

A little voice in my head repeated the words my *technologies* professor had said a million times, "Darting action is the key to a successful injection." So I aimed at the bull's-eye that appeared in front of my eyes. My hand, which seemed to be moving in slow motion, propelled downward at a 90-degree angle. Secretly I prayed that I would not hit my own hand. I must have closed my eyes because the next thing I remember was the loudest scream I had ever heard! I looked down and it was a bull's-eye, thank God, but the needle had not penetrated the muscle! The patient successfully tensed her muscle tight enough to intercept the needle midflight. At that moment she relaxed, probably because she thought the worst was over, and I pushed the needle into place. I slowly drew back the plunger to make sure no blood appeared in the syringe. I began injecting the Demerol slowly, watching my hands shake. Then I withdrew the needle and gently applied pressure over the site. It was over and I wanted to scream, "I did it!" but I kept my composure to feign the experience I lacked. Giving my first IM injection was not as bad as I thought it would be!

—*Alison L. Moriarty, Georgetown University, Washington, DC*

The nursing process can be applied to the fundamental nursing skill of medication administration. Assessment includes a comprehensive medication history as well as ongoing assessments of the patient's response during and after drug therapy. Nursing diagnoses are developed from the assessment data. Patient-centered outcomes are evaluated after implementation of the plan of care, tailored to the patient's needs.

A drug or medication is any substance that modifies body functions when taken into the body. The study that deals with chemicals that affect the body's functioning is called **pharmacology.** A pharmacist is a person licensed to prepare and dispense drugs. The physician is legally responsible for prescribing medications, although in some states nurse practitioners have this privilege also. The physician or nurse practitioner conveys the medication plans to others by an order called a prescription. After the pharmacist prepares the medication, the nurse administers the medication to the patient. This chain provides a check-and-balance system for medication administration. If an error is made when the order is written, the pharmacist or nurse administering the medication should note the discrepancy. If the pharmacy provides the wrong medication, the administering nurse should note this discrepancy. (See the accompanying Reflective Practice box for an example.)

Some medications are given frequently, and the nurse becomes familiar with the facts about these drugs. With other medications not given often, the nurse needs information before administering the drugs. Information about specific drugs is available in pharmacology texts. Many hospitals now have computer programs with medication information available at nursing stations. Nurses can use numerous drug references to increase their knowledge of medications.

DRUG LEGISLATION

In 1906, the Pure Food and Drug Act designated the United States Pharmacopeia and the National Formulary as official standards of drugs and empowered the federal government to enforce these standards. This legislation was updated in 1938 by the Federal Food, Drug and Cosmetic Act. The Food and Drug Administration (FDA) enforces this law. Extensive testing of new drugs is required before they may be marketed for use. An amendment to the Federal Food, Drug and Cosmetic Act in 1952 distinguished prescription drugs from nonprescription (over-the-counter) drugs and provided directions for dispensing prescription drugs.

The Comprehensive Drug Abuse Prevention and Control Act, also known as the Controlled Substances Act, was passed in 1970. This law regulates the distribution of narcotics and other drugs of abuse. Such drugs have been categorized according to their therapeutic usefulness and potential for abuse. Government programs for the prevention and treatment of drug abuse were established.

Reflective Practice
Challenge to Ethical and Legal Skills

During my clinical rotation for Complex Care a few weeks ago, I met François Baptiste, an elderly man with a wound infection requiring intravenous antibiotic therapy. He was due for a certain IV antibiotic to be hung at 10 a.m. When I checked his drawer at 8 a.m. and 09 a.m., the antibiotic was not there. However, the nurse I was working with told me not to call pharmacy about it yet since the pharmacy staff often comes and replaces the drawers in the medication carts before 10 a.m. anyway. So I didn't call pharmacy. Sure enough, a pharmacy representative came up that hour and changed the medication drawers. At 10 a.m., I went to look in my patient's drawer. What I found confused me a great deal! Yes, the bag of medication was in there. Yes, it was the right drug and the right dose. However, it was the wrong patient! The label on the bag in my patient's drawer had another patient's name on it. I looked that other patient up, and it turned out he was also a patient on the unit. This patient was also receiving the same drug at the same dose but at a different time. Should I hang this bag for my patient since he is due for it now, I wondered, even though it had someone else's name and medical record number on the label? It was, after all, the same drug and the same dose.

Thinking Outside the Box: Possible Courses of Action

- Change the patient's name on the label and hang the bag.
- Call pharmacy to ask about the mix-up. If the bag did, indeed, contain the same medication at the same dose, then change the patient's name on the label and hang it for my patient.
- Check the other patient's medication administration record (MAR) to confirm that he is, indeed, receiving the same drug at the same dose as my patient, and if so, use this bag for my patient (since it was in my patient's drawer and my patient is due for it now).

- Ask my nurse and/or preceptor what to do. Is it okay, safe, and legal to use this bag if someone else's name is on the label? If they say yes, check with the nurse caring for the patient whose name is on the label to make sure she does not need the medication right now.
- Send the bag back to pharmacy, requesting they send up a new one with an accurate label.
- Call pharmacy, ask them to send up a new bag with an accurate label, and tell them I am giving the other bag to the other patient's nurse.

Evaluating a Good Outcome: How Do I Define Success?

- The right patient receives the right drug, at the right dose, at the right time, via the right route, with the right documentation.
- I do not give my patient someone else's medication unless it has been triple-confirmed by other experts to be the same medication that is ordered for my patient.
- The patient feels comfortable and safe with the drug being administered to him.
- The needs of my patient and those of the patient whose name was on the bag are assessed and met. Both patients have the

medication available to them when they need it and are due for it.
- My education and my license, along with that of my nurse and preceptor, are not put at risk by an avoidable medication error.
- My legal skills are sharpened by thinking through and working through the situation.

Personal Learning: Here's to the Future!

Ultimately, I addressed the situation step by step to make sure all the bases were covered. First, I checked the other patient's drawer to see if he had a bag of this IV antibiotic. He did not, which led me to believe that either his bag was placed in my drawer by accident, or his bag had not been made yet (that the bag in my patient's drawer was intended for my patient but had the wrong label on it). Then I checked my patient's MAR and that of the other patient. Indeed, both were ordered to receive the same drug at the same dose via the same route. However, my patient was due for it at 10 a.m.; the other patient was due for it at 2 p.m. Next, I brought the medication bag, the MARs, and my other paperwork to my clinical preceptor and to the nurses caring for my patient and the other patient. They all agreed that the bag that was in my drawer was the right drug at the right dose, even though it had the wrong name on the label. They told me to change the name on the label and hang the bag. The other patient's nurse assured me she did not need the medication for her patient right now and that I should feel free to use it for my patient. After checking everything over myself again, I felt sure it was safe and legal to administer this medication to my patient. So I changed the name on the label and hung the bag. Everything was fine. My patient did not have an adverse reaction, the other patient got his medication when it was due, and no mistakes were made by any of the nurses. The

only mistake that was made was by pharmacy, then, who put the wrong label on the bag and then put the bag in the drawer.

I learned that checking and double-checking medication labels is extremely important. After a while, we all have a tendency to get into the habit of glancing at things when we are in a hurry, especially when it involves labels we look at all the time, feeling confident that we would recognize a problem. This is not the first time I could have missed a change on the label—there have been several times when I did not think to check every single thing on a label. That's because after giving it so many times, I felt it had become routine. But every time I am tempted not to double-check a label, I am reminded of this situation. As a result, I triple-check things, because those are the times when I am not paying as close attention as I need to be.

I do not think my professional legal skills are quite as adequate as they need to be. Because I do not have my license yet, I am not quite as driven to protect it by knowing all the laws pertinent to nurses as I should or will be. However, as a student nurse, I am careful to avoid any mistakes that could place me in jeopardy, legally, for areas of which I *am* aware. In addition, I am always careful to protect my education and my future as a nurse by not doing things about which I am uncertain. I always ask my preceptor or my

(continued)

Personal Learning: Here's to the Future!

nurse for help or advice when I need it. Moreover, I have carried professional liability malpractice insurance since the day I started nursing school, fearing for the financial viability of my life and my future. Therefore, while my legal skills probably need some work, they are certainly not terrible, and my skills and I are moving in the right direction.

Reflection

How do you think you would respond in a similar situation? Why? What does this tell you about yourself and about the adequacy of your skills for professional practice? Would it have been appropriate for the nursing student to contact the pharmacy? Why or why not? Can you think of other ways to respond? What legal principles did the nursing student adhere to with the described actions? Suppose the nursing student had given the medication without double-checking all of the information. What legal principles might have been violated? What other skills (cognitive, interpersonal, technical, ethical/legal) would you need to respond well in this situation? Do you agree with the criteria to evaluate a successful outcome? Did the nursing student meet the criteria? Please explain.

Tracey Sara Miller, Georgetown University

INTRODUCTION TO PHARMACOLOGY

This introduction to pharmacology will cover drug nomenclature, types of drug preparations, how drugs are classified, mechanisms of drug action, adverse drug effects, and factors affecting drug action.

Drug Nomenclature

Drugs have several names. The chemical name is a precise description of the drug's chemical composition; it identifies the drug's atomic and molecular structure. This name is of significance to the pharmacist. The **generic name** is the name assigned by the manufacturer that first develops the drug. Often, the generic name is derived from the chemical name. The **official name** is the name by which the drug is identified in the official publication, United States Pharmacopeia and National Formulary (USP and NF). The **trade name,** also referred to as the brand name or proprietary name, is selected by the drug company that sells the drug and is copyrighted. A drug can have several trade names when produced by different manufacturers.

Nurses should be familiar with a drug's generic and trade names. For example, acetaminophen (generic name) has trade names such as Tylenol, Tempra, and Liquiprin.

Types of Drug Preparations

Drugs are available in many forms, or preparations. The form in which the drug is prepared may determine the route of administration. Some drugs may be prepared in only one form to be administered by a certain route. Others may be supplied in several preparations, allowing them to be given through various routes. One type of preparation may be desirable in a given situation. For example, a liquid preparation of a medication would be indicated for a young child who cannot swallow solid preparations, such as tablets. Drug preparations are available for oral, topical, and injectable administration. Table 29-1 describes drug preparations commonly used by nurses.

> *Recall Jacob Shoolin, the 5-year-old boy receiving intravenous antibiotics and oral and nebulized bronchodilators for his pneumonia and exacerbation of asthma. The nurse would incorporate knowledge of various drug preparations when planning to administer the prescribed bronchodilators.*

Drug Classifications

How do nurses organize the vast amount of information about medications? Where do nurses begin their study of medications? They should begin with a focus on drug classifications.

Drugs are classified from different perspectives. For example, drugs may be classified by body systems (eg, drugs that affect the respiratory system, drugs that affect the cardiovascular system), by the symptom relieved by the drug, or by the clinical indication for the drug (eg, analgesic, antibiotic).

Mechanisms of Drug Action
Pharmacodynamics

Drugs act at the cellular level to achieve the desired effects. The process by which drugs alter cell physiology and cause effects on the body is called pharmacodynamics (Kee & Hayes, 2003). One mechanism of drug action is a drug–receptor interaction in which the drug interacts with one or more cellular structures to alter cell function. These specialized structures are called receptor sites. The drug fits the receptor as a key fits a lock. Drugs may also combine with enzymes to achieve the desired effect, which is referred to as a drug–enzyme interaction. Some drugs act on the cell membrane or alter the cellular environment.

TABLE 29-1 Common Types of Drug Preparations

Preparation	Description
Capsule	Powder or gel form of an active drug enclosed in a gelatinous container, may also be called liquigel
Elixir	Medication in a clear liquid containing water, alcohol, sweeteners, and flavor
Enteric coated	A tablet or pill coated to prevent stomach irritation
Extended release	Preparation of a medication that allows for slow and continuous release over a predetermined period; may also be referred to as CR or CRT (controlled release), SR (sustained or slow release), SA (sustained action), LA (long acting), or TR (timed release)
Liniment	Medication mixed with alcohol, oil, or soap, which is rubbed on the skin
Lotion	Drug particles in a solution for topical use
Lozenge	Small oval, round, or oblong preparation containing a drug in a flavored or sweetened base, which dissolves in the mouth and releases the medication; also called *troche*
Ointment	Semisolid preparation containing a drug to be applied externally; also called an *unction*
Pill	Mixture of a powdered drug with a cohesive material; may be round or oval
Powder	Single or mixture of finely ground drugs
Solution	A drug dissolved in another substance (eg, in an aqueous solution)
Suppository	An easily melted medication preparation in a firm base such as gelatin that is inserted into the body (rectum, vagina, urethra)
Suspension	Finely divided, undissolved particles in a liquid medium; should be shaken before use
Syrup	Medication combined in a water and sugar solution
Tablet	Small, solid dose of medication, compressed or molded; may be any color, size, or shape; *enteric-coated tablets* are coated with a substance that is insoluble in gastric acids to reduce gastric irritation by the drug
Transdermal patch	Unit dose of medication applied directly to skin for diffusion through skin and absorption into the bloodstream

Pharmacokinetics

Pharmacokinetics is the study of the movement of drug molecules in the body in relation to the drug's absorption, distribution, metabolism, and excretion.

Absorption

Absorption is the process by which a drug is transferred from its site of entry into the body to the bloodstream. Absorption of a drug is influenced by several factors, which are discussed below.

Route of Administration. Injected medications are usually absorbed more rapidly than oral medications.

Drug Solubility. Liquid medications are absorbed more rapidly than solid preparations. Liquid preparations do not have to be dissolved in the gastrointestinal fluids. Most drugs are weak acids and bases. When in solution, drugs are a mixture of ionized and nonionized forms. The nonionized form is lipid soluble and absorbed more readily, whereas the ionized form is not easily absorbed and is lipid insoluble. This factor is important because cell membranes have a fatty acid layer, and a drug that is more lipid soluble can be absorbed more readily and pass through the cell membrane.

pH. The form in which the drug is found depends on the pH of the environment. Acidic drugs are well absorbed in the stomach. Drugs that are basic remain ionized or insoluble in an acid environment. These drugs are not absorbed before reaching the small intestine. The concept of acid–base balance is further discussed in Chapter 46, Fluid, Electrolyte, Acid–Base Balance.

Local Conditions at the Site of Administration. The more extensive the absorbing surface, the greater the absorption of the drug and the more rapid the effect. A patient with burns would have poor absorption from an intramuscular injection, for example. Food in the stomach can delay the absorption of some medications or enhance the rate of absorption of other drugs. Drug absorption can be manipulated with sustained-release preparations or enteric-coated preparations. Enteric-coated preparations are resistant to the digestive action of the stomach.

Drug Dosage. A loading dose, or a larger than normal dose, is usually given when a patient is in acute distress and the maximum therapeutic effect is desired as quickly as possible. If drug toxicity occurs, it can be detected quickly and treated in the controlled hospital environment. A maintenance dose is a lower dosage that becomes the usual or daily dosage. Patients who receive digoxin or phenobarbital may receive loading doses when therapy is initiated.

Serum Drug Levels. After a drug has been absorbed, its serum level can be monitored by drawing a blood specimen and measuring the drug's peak and trough levels. This is recommended for certain medications (eg, aminoglycoside antibiotics, digoxin, and warfarin) to ensure that a therapeutic range is maintained. A drug's **therapeutic range** is that concentration of drug in the blood serum that produces the desired effect without causing toxicity. The **peak level,** or highest plasma concentration, of the drug should be measured when absorption is complete. The peak level may be affected by factors that affect drug absorption as well as the route of administration. The **trough level** is the point when the drug is at its lowest concentration, and this specimen is usually drawn in the 30-minute interval before the next dose. The dosage schedule, as well as the half-life of the drug, can modify the trough level. Simply stated, a drug's **half-life** is the amount of time it takes for half a dose of a drug to be eliminated from the body. Monitoring these levels ensures that therapeutic ranges are obtained without reaching toxic levels.

Distribution

After a drug has been absorbed into the bloodstream, it is distributed throughout the body. The drug accumulates in specific tissues for its action. Distribution depends on the rate of perfusion and capillary permeability to the drug. Certain other factors may also influence distribution. The drug may bind to plasma proteins, which causes unequal distribution and may prevent the drug from reaching its intended site of action. The blood–brain barrier is poorly permeable to water-soluble drugs. Some drugs fail to penetrate the tissues of the central nervous system as readily as others. The placenta, on the other hand, is not a selective barrier to the distribution of drugs. Drugs move across the placenta readily, and many produce harmful effects in the fetus.

Metabolism

Metabolism, or biotransformation, is the breakdown of the drug to an inactive form. The liver is the primary site for drug metabolism. Various processes and enzymes are involved in metabolism. Physiologic changes associated with aging or the presence of liver disease may complicate the process. Pharmacology texts provide more detailed explanations of metabolism.

Excretion

After the drug is broken down to an inactive form, **excretion** of the drug from the body occurs. The kidneys excrete most drugs. The lungs are the primary route for the excretion of gaseous substances, such as inhalation anesthetics. Many drugs are excreted through the intestines. The sweat, salivary, and mammary glands are also routes of drug excretion.

Some medications may be contraindicated, or dosages may need to be adjusted downward if renal excretion is affected by age or disease. Manufacturers are required by law to include specific information regarding implications for geriatric patients on the package inserts of certain drugs. Of particular concern are details concerning the excretion of these drugs in older adults whose renal function has declined. This law affects psychotropic drugs, nonsteroidal anti-inflammatory agents, oral hypoglycemic agents, anticoagulants, certain broad-spectrum antibiotics, and cardiac drugs.

Adverse Drug Effects

Although therapeutic effect is the desired outcome in medication administration, sometimes adverse effects or side effects occur. Secondary drug effects that often are predictable and can usually be tolerated are referred to as side effects. Not all side effects are necessarily adverse. On the other hand, adverse effects are more severe and may require discontinuation of the drug, depending on whether the benefit of the drug outweighs the harm from the adverse effect.

One study reported that nearly 20% of medication orders resulted in an error, and of those 7% had the potential to cause adverse drug events (ADEs; Barker et al., 2002). Most often heparin, insulin, morphine, warfarin, and potassium chloride are involved.

Serious adverse drug reactions must be documented according to agency policy and reported to the FDA MEDWATCH program. According to FDA criteria, a serious adverse drug event is defined as an action that is life threatening, requires intervention to prevent death or permanent impairment, and leads to death, hospitalization, disability, or congenital anomaly. Nurses and healthcare professionals are encouraged to complete a form that provides information on a medication or medical product that they suspect either has caused harm or has the potential to cause harm and submit the form to the MEDWATCH program. This provides a national tracking of all serious adverse drug reactions.

There are various categories of ADEs. One example is the development of an iatrogenic disease caused unintentionally by drug therapy. Neutropenia caused by chemotherapy is an example of this. Other categories of adverse effects discussed below include allergic effects, toxic effects, idiosyncratic effects, and drug interactions.

Allergic Effect

A drug allergy occurs in a person who has been previously exposed to the drug and has developed antibodies. Drug allergies can be manifested in a variety of symptoms ranging from minor to serious. The reaction can occur immediately after the patient receives the medication or be delayed for hours to days. Some of the signs and symptoms of a drug allergy are rash, urticaria, fever, diarrhea, nausea, and vomiting. A life-threatening immediate reaction is called an **anaphylactic reaction** and results in respiratory distress, sudden severe bronchospasm, and cardiovascular collapse. This reaction is treated with epinephrine, bronchodilators, and antihistamines.

Cumulative Effect

Drug tolerance occurs when the body becomes accustomed to a particular drug over a period of time. Larger doses of the drug must be taken to produce the same effects. A **cumulative effect** occurs when the body cannot metabolize one dose of a drug before another dose is administered. The drug is taken in more frequently than it is excreted, and each new dose increases the total quantity in the body. If allowed to reach toxic levels, some drugs may cause permanent damage to the body's organs, such as the kidneys or liver.

Idiosyncratic Effect

An **idiosyncratic effect** is any abnormal or peculiar response to a drug that may manifest itself by overresponse, underresponse, or response different from the expected outcome.

Older patients often have unpredictable or erratic responses to medications. Idiosyncratic effects are thought to be the result of genetic enzyme deficiencies that lead to an abnormal mechanism of drug breakdown.

Drug Interactions

In a drug interaction, the combined effect of two or more drugs acting simultaneously produces an effect either less than that of each drug alone (**antagonist effect**) or greater than that of each drug alone (**synergistic effect**). Alcohol and barbiturates, for example, when taken together create a synergistic effect. Nurses must be knowledgeable and alert for drug interactions and the effects of drug therapy.

Drug interactions become a serious risk with the elderly population. Many times elderly patients see more than one physician and do not always remember to bring the medications that they are taking. This leads to polypharmacy (the taking of more than two medications at a time), which can result in serious drug interactions.

Think back to Mildred Campbell, the 65-year-old woman with arthritis asking about a recently advertised medication for joint pain relief. The nurse would need to assess the patient's medication history to determine her current medication regimen. This information would be crucial to obtain so that the nurse could evaluate for possible polypharmacy and potential risks for drug interactions, even before discussing whether the advertised medication would be appropriate.

Another problem with drug interactions is herbal remedies. Many patients do not consider herbal remedies a medication, since they can purchase them at a nutrition store, but some herbal remedies will interact with medications. When asking patients if they are taking any medications, nurses should specifically ask if they are taking any herbal supplements.

Factors Affecting Drug Action

Certain variables influence the action or effect of a medication.

Developmental Considerations

During pregnancy, most drugs are contraindicated because of their possible adverse effects on the fetus, and certain drugs, referred to as **teratogenic,** are known to have the potential to cause developmental defects in the embryo or fetus. Examples of teratogenic drugs include cocaine, alcohol, phenytoin (Dilantin, an anticonvulsant), and isotretinoin (Accutane, a medication used to treat severe acne). Breastfed infants are also at risk for adverse effects from drugs in the mother's circulation. A child's dose for medication is smaller than an adult's dose. Infants are especially responsive to medications because of the immaturity of their organs. Older people are responsive to medications because their bodies have experienced physiologic changes associated with the aging process, including

decreased gastric motility, muscle mass, acid production, and blood flow, which affect drug absorption. Small body size, reduced weight, and reduced body water also alter distribution, as do decreases in cardiac output and organ perfusion. Decreased plasma binding increases the possibility of drug toxicity. Liver function declines with advancing age and changes occur in the hepatic enzymes involved in drug metabolism. Blood flow to the liver decreases secondary to a decrease in cardiac output. Drugs are excreted more slowly from the body as a result of changes in kidney function. Receptor sensitivity is altered in older people, and their sensitivity to certain drugs increases. The physiologic changes in older people that increase drug susceptibility are summarized in the accompanying display, Focus on the Older Adult.

Recall Mr. Baptiste, the elderly patient receiving intravenous antibiotics for a wound infection. The nurse would need to consider age-related changes that might interfere with the drug action, being especially alert for signs and symptoms of drug toxicity.

Weight

Expected responses to drugs are based largely on those reactions that occur when the drugs are given to healthy adults (18 to 65 years of age, 150 lb [68 kg]). Nurses should know the usual dose for a medication before administering it. Drug doses for children are calculated by weight or body surface area (BSA).

Remember Jacob Shoolin, the boy described at the beginning of the chapter. The nurse would need to verify that the dosage prescribed for this 5-year-old is within the appropriate range for the child's weight or BSA.

Sex

The difference in the distribution of body fat and fluids in men and women is a minor factor affecting the action of some drugs. To date, most research on drugs and their actions and effects has been conducted on men. Future clinical drug trials are expected to include more women to document the effects of hormonal fluctuations.

Genetic and Cultural Factors

Differences in the responses of patients receiving the same medication may result from genetic and cultural differences. Pharmacoanthropology is the science that studies the differences in drug response in various ethnic or racial groups. Enzyme deficiencies or metabolic disturbances can alter the way the body handles medication or metabolizes a drug. For example, Asian patients may require smaller doses of a drug because they metabolize it at a slower rate. A drug dose that is normal for a white patient may cause unexpected side effects in an Asian; differences in body heights and weights do not appear to be a factor in this response. African Americans appear to require larger doses of some medications that are used to lower

Focus on the Older Adult
Altered Drug Response in Older People

Age-Related Changes	Nursing Interventions
Stomach irritation and ulceration • Decreased gastric emptying time and increased pH of gastric juices	Assess for symptoms of stomach discomfort. Test stools for blood.
Increased possibility of drug toxicity • Increased adipose tissue and decreased total body fluid in proportion to the total body mass • Decreased number of protein-binding sites • Decline in liver function and enzyme production needed for drug metabolism • Decreased kidney function, resulting in diminished filtration and excretion	Assess for early signs of drug interactions or toxicity. Monitor blood levels of drugs. Monitor laboratory values such as blood urea nitrogen (BUN) and creatinine.
More pronounced hypotensive effects from medications (particularly antihypertensives and diuretics) • Altered peripheral venous tone	Monitor vital signs. Caution patient to change position slowly.
Increased risk for dizziness and confusion, particularly with beta blockers • Changes in blood–brain barrier allowing for easier penetration of fat-soluble drugs	Assess for dizziness and lightheadedness. Be aware of safety precautions.

blood pressure. Culturally related health beliefs can also affect compliance and response to a medication regimen. Herbal treatments that are popular in some cultures may interfere with or counteract the action of prescribed medication. Nurses who are aware of the specific needs and beliefs of culturally diverse patients are better able to communicate effectively with them. Box 29-1 gives guidelines for effective communication about medication with culturally diverse patients.

Psychological Factors

The patient's expectations of the medication affect the response to the medication, as, for instance, in studies of drug effects in which some patients receive a placebo. A **placebo** is a pharmacologically inactive substance. In clinical drug trials, one group of patients receives the active drug, whereas another group receives a placebo to study the drug's effects. Some patients appear to have the same response with the placebo as with the active drug.

Pathology

The presence of disease can affect drug action. The liver is the primary organ for drug breakdown, so pathologic conditions that involve the liver may slow metabolism and alter the dosage of the drug needed to reach a therapeutic level.

Environment

The patient's environment may influence his or her response to medications. Sensory deprivation and overload may affect drug responses. The relative oxygen deprivation at high alti-

BOX 29-1 Communicating Effectively About Medication With Culturally Diverse Patients

- Acquire basic information about health beliefs and practices of various cultural groups in your healthcare setting.
- Be alert to atypical drug responses or unexpected side effects that may occur in certain ethnic groups.
- Ask specifically about the use of folk or home remedies prescribed by a nontraditional healer.
- Utilize printed or audiovisual information that is in the language spoken by your patients.
- Encourage cultural sensitivity in healthcare workers in your particular setting.
- Recognize that diversity exists within cultural groups. For example, the Hispanic population includes Mexicans, Cubans, Puerto Ricans, and other Latino groups.
- Emphasize threads or messages in health teaching that are common to all cultures (eg, concern about family, faith, and home).
- Include culturally sensitive information in all basic health teaching.
- Help culturally diverse patients to value and understand the importance of communicating concerns and asking questions about prescribed medications.

Adapted from Eisenhauer, L., Nichols, L., Spencer, R. & Bergan, F. (1998). *Clinical pharmacology and nursing management* (5th ed.). Philadelphia: Lippincott Williams & Wilkins.

tudes may increase sensitivity to some drugs. The patient who receives pain medication or a sedative in an active, noisy environment may not be able to benefit fully from the medication's effects, while those receiving pain medication in a quiet environment and using an additional relaxation method, such as guided imagery, may have a longer benefit from the pain medication. Nutritional state can also affect the body's reaction to certain drugs.

Timing of Administration

The presence of food in the stomach delays the absorption of orally administered medications. Some medications should be given with food to prevent gastric irritation, and the nurse should consider this when establishing a patient's medication schedule. Other medications may have enhanced absorption if taken with certain foods. Circadian rhythms and cycles may also influence drug action.

PRINCIPLES OF MEDICATION ADMINISTRATION

Medication Orders

No medication may be given to a patient without a medication order from a physician or, in some states, a nurse practitioner. Each health agency has a policy specifying the manner in which a physician writes an order. In most instances, orders are written on a form designed specifically for a physician's order. This becomes part of a patient's permanent record. Many healthcare facilities use a computer-generated pharmacy order system and can receive a medication order by fax from the physician. Some hospitals are beginning to use a computer entry system where the physician enters the drug order into a computer. The computer sends the order directly to the pharmacy and enters the order into the patient's permanent record. This prevents any guessing when handwriting is illegible or drug names are similar. This system also provides physicians with recommended doses of medications, indicates laboratory tests that monitor the action of the drug, and lists potential interactions that may occur with other medications or food (Carroll, 2003). A computerized order entry system can reduce ADEs.

Safe practice dictates that a nurse follows only a written order, because a written order by a physician is least likely to result in error or misunderstanding. Under certain circumstances, such as in an emergency, a verbal order from the physician may be given to a registered nurse or a pharmacist. In most settings, a student nurse is not permitted to accept a verbal order from a physician. The legal implications for dispensing and administering an agent without a written order vary, and nurses must be familiar with the exact agency policy whenever called on to administer therapeutic agents. The legal implications of verbal orders are discussed in Chapter 7, Legal Implications.

Usual hospital policy dictates that when a patient is admitted, unless specific orders to the contrary are written, all drugs

that the physician may have ordered while the patient was at home are discontinued. This can be a problem when a patient brings medications from home to the hospital. To avoid the possibility of having the patient continue to take the home medications while receiving the same ones or others under new orders, all medications should be sent home with the family or removed from the patient's unit and placed in safekeeping. This requires an explanation to the patient and the family of how the patient's drug plan is to be implemented.

In some inpatient facilities, patients keep their medications at their bedside and learn or continue to administer them as they would at home. It is believed that this approach helps to promote patients' independence. The nurse should be aware when patients are allowed to take their own medications while hospitalized and should know each agent's purpose and possible adverse effects. Also, a notation should be made on the patient's plan of care so that everyone knows the patient has medications at the bedside.

When a patient has had surgery or is transferred to another clinical service or another health agency, it is general practice that all orders related to drugs are discontinued and that new orders are written. Nurses must then carefully check that all medications that are appropriate are reordered. To keep physicians aware of the orders in effect, some hospitals specify a day of the week when orders are to be rewritten, or they are discontinued automatically.

Types of Orders

There are several types of orders that a physician may write. A standing order is carried out as specified until it is canceled by another order. Many physicians whose practices are limited to a particular clinical area have a specified set of written orders for all their hospitalized patients. These are also referred to as standing orders. Occasionally, a physician writes a standing order and its cancellation simultaneously; that is, the physician specifies that a certain order is to be carried out for a stated number of days or times. After the stated period has passed, the order is canceled automatically.

The physician may write a **p.r.n. order** ("as needed") for medication. The patient receives medication when it is requested or needed. A p.r.n. order commonly is written for postoperative pain medication.

Another type of order is called a single order; that is, the directive is carried out only once, at a time specified by the physician. Medication to be administered immediately before surgery is an example of a single order. A **stat order** also is a single order, but it is carried out immediately. A stat order for epinephrine or an antihistamine would be carried out immediately for a patient who is experiencing an anaphylactic drug reaction.

Parts of the Medication Order
The medication order consists of seven parts:
1. Patient's name
2. Date and time the order is written
3. Name of drug to be administered
4. Dosage of the drug

5. Route by which the drug is to be administered
6. Frequency of administration of the drug
7. Signature of person writing the order

Patient's Name

The patient's full name is used. The middle name or initial should be included to avoid confusion with other patients. In most agencies, the patient's full name and identification number and the physician's name are imprinted mechanically on all sheets on the patient's chart, including the physician's order sheet. Be extremely careful when administering medications when there is more than one patient on the unit with the same last name. Not only can the nurse give the wrong patient the wrong medication, but also a physician may write an order in the wrong patient's chart.

Date and Time the Order Is Written

The date the order is written is given, sometimes including the time as well. Because the nursing staff in inpatient agencies changes several times during each 24-hour period, the date and time help to prevent errors of oversight as different nurses take charge of a unit. When an order is to be followed for a specified number of days, the date and time are important so that the discontinuation date and time can be determined accurately. State law determines the length of time an order for a narcotic remains valid. Therefore, the date and time the order is written are essential for determining when the order for a narcotic becomes invalid.

Name of Drug to Be Administered

The name of the drug is stated in the order, either by the brand name or by the generic name. Certain brand names are well known, but the practice of using the generic name is considered safest and is required by some healthcare agencies.

A nurse unfamiliar with a drug can use several sources to obtain information. The USP and NF are the official sources in the United States. Most other countries have similar references that describe official therapeutic agents. Many agencies also provide their own book listing the official drugs commonly used by the agency. Agencies are also beginning to provide access to online medication information sites. The *Physicians' Desk Reference* (PDR) is another source of information that is supplied by pharmaceutical companies. In addition, the nurse may obtain information about drugs from the hospital pharmacist, the physician, and any of several texts written specifically for the nursing role in the management of drug therapy.

Dosage of the Drug

The dosage of a drug can be stated in either the apothecary or the metric system. The metric system has been adopted internationally. These systems are described in a following section.

Apothecary measurements are used less frequently. A medication error may occur if nurses are unfamiliar with the apothecary system, if the physician's handwriting is illegible, or if administration equipment, such as syringes, cups, or reference sources, uses only metric measurement. Self-administered drugs are commonly labeled in household measurements to fa-

cilitate administration. Most agencies post a table of common equivalent dosages for people who have learned to use one system and find that the agency for which they work uses the other system. Although these tables are convenient and useful, the nurse should be prepared to convert from one system to the other because such tables are not available in every situation. The nurse should also be familiar with common equivalent measurements when using household equipment, such as teaspoons and tablespoons, because the home is usually not equipped with special measuring devices; however, patients should be instructed to use measuring spoons and not silverware if administration equipment is not available due to the variability of the amount silverware can hold. The most common equivalents can be found in Appendix A.

Certain standard abbreviations are used to indicate drug amounts, and the nurse should know the common abbreviations before administering drugs. See Tables 17-1 and 17-2 in Chapter 17, Documenting, Reporting, and Conferring, for common abbreviations used in drug orders.

Route by Which the Drug Is to Be Administered

The route to be used when administering a medication is stated clearly because some drugs can be given in more than one way and others may be used safely through only one route. Table 29-2 describes common routes by which medications are administered. See "The Nursing Process for Administering Medications" for guidelines on administering drugs by these routes.

Frequency of Administration of the Drug

The time and frequency with which a drug is to be administered are usually stated in standard abbreviations in the medication order. Common abbreviations used in writing prescriptions, including time and frequency, are listed in Chapter 17, Table 17-1.

The nursing service department of inpatient facilities usually determines the hours at which routine drugs are given. For example, if certain drugs are to be given every 4 hours, the nursing service policy indicates the times. Every-4-hour administration may be at the times of noon, 4 p.m., 8 p.m., midnight, 4 a.m., and 8 a.m. Another agency may use the hours 1 p.m., 5 p.m., 9 p.m., 1 a.m., 5 a.m., and 9 a.m. To lessen the risk for error, some healthcare facilities use the 24-hour clock (or military time), which designates midnight as 0000 hours and runs until 2400 hours. If an administration order states that the drug it is to be given before or after meals, the time of administration depends on the hours at which meals are served. It is a nursing responsibility to check that times for medication administration correspond to safe practice for that drug.

If a drug is to be given only once or twice a day, the decision about which hours to use depends on the nature of the drug and the patient's plan of care. Whenever possible, the patient's choice of time should be considered.

Drugs should be administered punctually as ordered. A nurse administering drugs to several patients, however, cannot give all of the drugs exactly on the hour indicated. Agency policies vary, but a common one is that drugs should be administered within a half-hour before or after the indicated hour.

TABLE 29-2 Routes for Administering Drugs

Terms Used to Describe Route	How Drug Is Administered
Oral route	Having patient swallow drug
Enteral route	Administering drug through an enteral tube
Sublingual administration	Placing drug under tongue
Buccal administration	Placing drug between cheek and gum
Parenteral route	Injecting drug into
Subcutaneous injection	Subcutaneous tissue
Intramuscular injection	Muscle tissue
Intradermal injection	Corium (under epidermis)
Intravenous injection	Vein
Intraarterial injection	Artery
Intracardial injection	Heart tissue
Intraperitoneal injection	Peritoneal cavity
Intraspinal injection	Spinal canal
Intraosseous injection	Bone
Topical route	Inserting drug into
Vaginal administration	Vagina
Rectal administration	Rectum
Inunction	Rubbing drug into skin
Instillation	Placing drug into direct contact with mucous membrane
Irrigation	Flushing mucous membrane with drug in solution
Skin application	Applying transdermal patch
Pulmonary route	Having patient inhale drug

Thus, a drug to be administered at 9 a.m. can be administered any time between 8:30 a.m. and 9:30 a.m. using this policy. However, this policy does not apply to all drugs. A preoperative medication ordered to be given at 7:30 a.m. should be administered at that hour because the time was planned in relation to the time surgery is to begin. Preoperative medications may also be given when the nursing unit receives a call from the operating room to premedicate the surgical patient. This also holds true when patients are given drugs before certain diagnostic procedures and with stat orders.

Signature of Person Writing the Order
The signature, with title, of the person writing the order follows the order. The signature, with title, is important for legal reasons because the authority to prescribe drugs is defined by state laws. Also, if there is a question about the order, the signature indicates who should be contacted.

Checking the Medication Order
Agency policy specifies the manner in which the medication order is checked. Various systems are used, and nurses should be familiar with the system used in the agency where they work and should implement it correctly to minimize errors.

In many institutions, the order is copied onto the patient's medication record, often called a Kardex or MAR (medication administration record). Increasing numbers of healthcare facilities are computerizing patient records, including medication records (CMAR [computerized medication administration record]). The nurse is responsible for checking that the medication order was transcribed correctly by comparing it with the original order. The nurse is also responsible for double-checking the dosage of the medication.

Questioning the Medication Order
Nurses are legally responsible for the drugs they administer. Any drug order suspected to be in error should be questioned. The suspected error may be in any part of the order. The legal implications are serious in a situation in which there is an error in a drug order and the nurse could be expected, based on knowledge and experience, to have noted and reported the error.

On occasion, the nurse may not think that there is an error in the order but may not understand why the medication has been prescribed. In such instances, the nurse should ask how the order relates to the patient's plan of care. This may prevent a medication error if the wrong medication has been ordered.

Confusion over the placement of a decimal point can lead to a medication error. A zero should always precede a decimal point (eg, 0.1 mg) for clarity, but there is no need to use a zero after a decimal point (eg, 1.0 mg) because this can cause confusion if the decimal point is unclear or missed completely.

A drug to which the patient is allergic may be prescribed inadvertently. The patient may describe past adverse reactions with the drug. It is general practice to indicate any drug allergies clearly on the patient's chart. The drug should not be given and the order should be questioned when, in the nurse's judgment, the patient is allergic to a drug. In many healthcare facilities, the patient may also wear a wristband that indicates specific allergies. An allergic reaction can be life threatening to the patient.

A drug may be ordered that would potentially interact with another medication that the patient is taking. All medications that a nurse is unfamiliar with should be verified before administration to avoid possible drug interactions. If a nurse has difficulty reading an order, guessing is gross carelessness; checking with the person who wrote the order is the only safe procedure.

Nurses have the right to refuse to administer any medication that, based on their knowledge and experience, may be harmful to the patient. Although this situation seldom occurs, the nurse needs to understand that the patient's safety is a primary objective in the administration of medications. The nurse must also notify the physician of the refusal to administer the medication.

Medication Supply Systems

Medications are supplied in a number of ways. With a stock supply system, large quantities of medications are kept on the nursing unit. The stock supply has advantages and disadvantages. The medications are immediately available to the nurse, but this eliminates the double-check system by the pharmacy. With an individual supply system, each patient is supplied with the medication needed for a period of time. The nurse is responsible for accurately measuring the dosage from the medication containers. In the unit dose system, the pharmacist simplifies medication preparation by packaging and labeling each dosage for a 24-hour period.

Some nursing units use a medication cart for the administration of medications. The standard cart contains individual drawers into which the medications for each patient are placed. The drawer is labeled with the patient's name. The nurse moves the cart from room to room when dispensing medications. A computerized medication system usually remains in a central area, has drawers stocked with approved medications, and provides access to the medications ordered for each patient. A computerized medication dispensing system is shown in Figure 29-1. Another medication cart uses bar codes to help eliminate medication errors. With this system, the patient's wrist identification band has a bar code. When this bar code is scanned, a computer screen displays all of the patient's current medications. Each medication also has a bar code, and if any of the five rights (right medication, right dosage, right route, right time, and right patient) are incorrect for the medication, an alert message will appear on the screen notifying the nurse of the discrepancy (Carroll, 2003).

Dosage Calculations

Systems of Measurement

Nurses need to be proficient in the use of weights and measures as well as systems of measurement to calculate drug dosages and prepare medications for administration. Three systems of measurement are used for administering medications: the metric system, the apothecary system, and the household system. All three systems of measurement are in use in the United States. The nurse may be called on to convert dosages from one system to another. It is then extremely important that the nurse

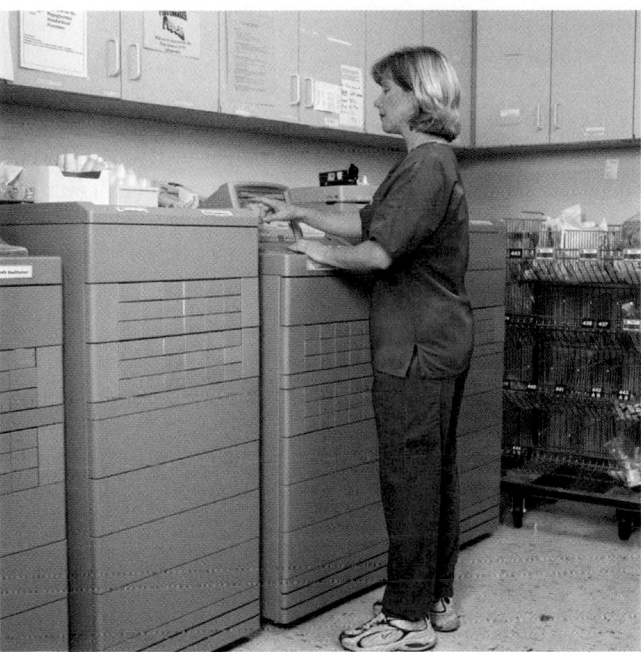

FIGURE 29-1 Computerized medication dispensing system.

is able to calculate commonly used equivalents, as listed in Appendix A. Practice the Medication Calculation Problems at the end of this chapter to develop your dose calculation skills.

Metric System

The metric system is the most widely accepted and convenient system. The basic units of measurement are the meter (linear), the liter (volume), and the gram (weight). The metric system is a decimal system, in which each unit can be divided into multiples of 10 (10, 100, 1000). Calculations in the metric system often involve moving the decimal point to the right or left. In the preparation of medications, the nurse usually uses the following metric units:

- Weight
  - 1 kilogram = 1,000 grams
  - 1 gram = 1,000 milligrams
  - 1 milligram = 1,000 micrograms
- Volume
  - 1 liter = 1,000 milliliters or cubic centimeters

It may be necessary to convert drug dosages to a different unit in the metric system. To convert a larger unit into a smaller unit, move the decimal point to the right (the new number is larger than the original). To convert a smaller unit into a larger unit, move the decimal point to the left (the new number is smaller than the original). *Example 1:* 0.5 g equals how many milligrams? Move the decimal point three places to right; the answer is 500 mg. *Example 2:* 900 mg equals how many grams? Move the decimal point three places to the left; the answer is 0.9 g.

Apothecary System

The apothecary system is less convenient and precise than the metric system and is infrequently used. The basic unit of weight is the grain. The minim, dram, ounce, pint, and quart are used for volume. In the apothecary system, Roman numerals are used to express numbers (grains X) and quantities less than 1 are written in fraction form (grains 1/4).

Household System

The household system is the least accurate system of measurement and is not used widely except in home settings. Teaspoon, tablespoon, teacup, and glass are commonly used household measures. As discussed previously, teaspoon and tablespoon refer to measuring spoons, not silverware.

Formulas for Computing Drug Dosages

Drugs are sometimes prepared and supplied in the amount ordered by the physician, and the nurse can see when checking the medication label that no calculation is necessary. At other times, drugs are not prepared and supplied in the exact quantities called for in the medication order, and the nurse must do a dosage calculation to determine what quantity of medication the patient is to receive.

Several formulas can be used to calculate drug dosages. One such formula consists of ratios to set up a proportion and can be used to calculate dosages for both solid and liquid preparations. A ratio shows the relation between numbers. A proportion contains two ratios. The nurse is usually seeking the quantity of on-hand medication that is equal to the desired dosage (the dosage ordered). The formula is as follows:

$$\frac{\text{dose on hand}}{\text{quantity on hand}} = \frac{\text{dose desired}}{X \text{ (quantity desired)}}$$

The dosage must be in the same unit of measurement. This applies to the quantity as well. Dosages are on the top line of the proportion, quantities on the bottom line. After the numbers are placed in the proportion, the nurse cross-multiplies to find the desired quantity.

Example: Amoxicillin, 625 mg PO, is ordered. It is supplied as a liquid preparation containing 250 mg in 5 mL. How much does the nurse administer?

$$\frac{250 \text{ mg}}{5 \text{ mL}} = \frac{625 \text{ mg}}{X \text{ mL}}$$

Cross-multiply:

$$3125 = 250X$$
$$X = 12.5 \text{ mL}$$

Example: Phenobarbital, gr i PO, is ordered. It is available in 30-mg tablets. How many tablets does the nurse administer?

There are two systems of measurement in this problem. The nurse checks the list of equivalents to learn that 60 mg is equivalent to grains i.

$$\frac{30 \text{ mg}}{1 \text{ tablet}} = \frac{60 \text{ mg}}{X \text{ tablets}}$$
$$60 = 30X$$
$$X = 2 \text{ tablets}$$

Another formula that can be used to calculate drug dosages is as follows:

$$\frac{\text{dose desired}}{\text{dose on hand}} \times \text{quantity on hand} = \frac{\text{desired}}{\text{quantity}}$$

This formula can be used for both liquid dosages and fractions of tablets.

A newer way that is used to solve medication dosages is dimensional analysis (Curren & Munday, 2001). When using dimensional analysis, the first numerator must be what you are solving for. For instance, in the amoxicillin example, you would set up the equation like this:

$$\text{mL} = (5 \text{ mL}/250 \text{ mg}) \times 625 \text{ mg} = 12.5 \text{ mL}$$

Dimensional analysis can also encompass conversion factors all in the same formula. For instance, the nurse is to administer 50 mcg fentanyl. The pharmacy supplies the nurse with an ampule of fentanyl 0.1 mg/2 mL. How much should the nurse administer? To solve the problem, the mg needs to be converted to mcg. This can all be done in the same calculation.

$$\text{mL} = (2 \text{ mL}/0.1 \text{ mg}) \times (1 \text{ mg}/1{,}000 \text{ mcg}) \times 50 \text{ mcg} = 1 \text{ mL}$$

Pediatric Calculations

Pediatric dosages are calculated according to the child's body weight or body surface area (BSA). The most frequently used and most convenient method involves calculating a child's dose according to weight. Most drug reference books publish the pediatric dosages per weight. This is due to the large size difference from infants to toddlers to school-aged children. When calculating pediatric drug dosages, the nurse must check whether the formula is per dose or per 24-hour period; a medication overdose can occur if the nurse does not note that the calculation is per 24 hours and gives the total amount of medication in one dose.

> *Remember Jacob Shoolin, the 5-year-old boy with pneumonia and asthma. The nurse would need to obtain the child's weight accurately and then verify that the dosages of medications ordered are within the appropriate range.*

The BSA formula provides the most accuracy in calculating pediatric dosages because it considers weight and height. This formula is used in specific medications such as acyclovir. To find a child's BSA, the West nomogram is used (Fig. 29-2). The child's height is located at a point in the left column and the weight is located at a point in the right column. The two points are connected with a straight line. The point at which the line crosses the surface area column is the child's BSA. The formula for calculating the child's dosage is as follows:

$$\frac{\text{BSA (child)}}{\text{BSA (adult)}} \times \text{adult dose} = \text{child's dose}$$

The average adult BSA is 1.7 square meters.

A less commonly used formula is Clark's rule for children aged 2 years or younger. This formula assumes that the average adult weighs 150 lb (68 kg) and is calculated as follows:

$$\frac{\text{usual adult}}{\text{dose}} \times \frac{\text{weight of child in pounds}}{150} = \frac{\text{child's}}{\text{dose}}$$

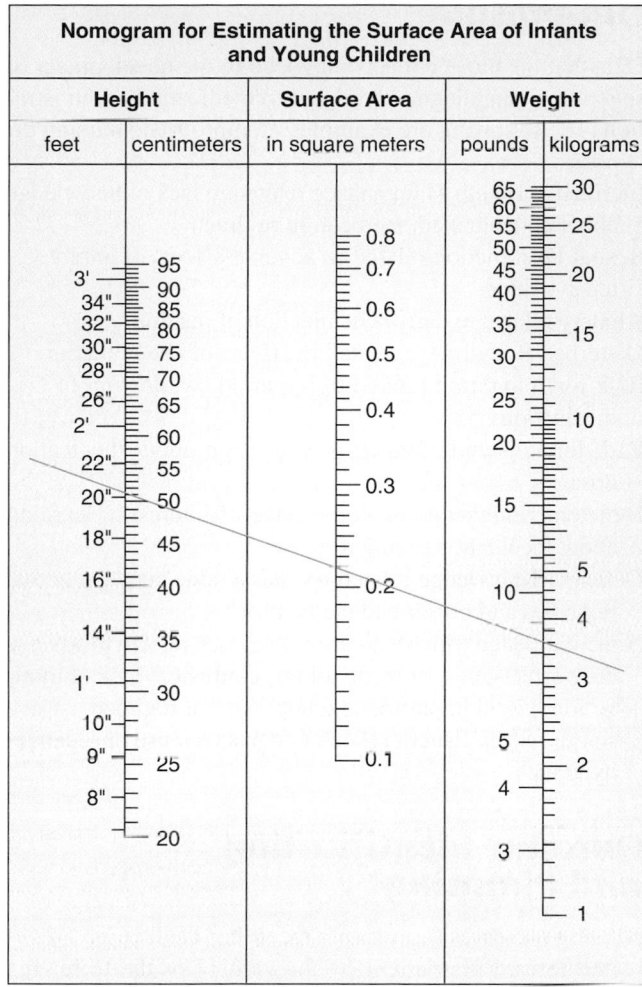

Nomogram for Estimating the Surface Area of Infants and Young Children				
Height		**Surface Area**	**Weight**	
feet	centimeters	in square meters	pounds	kilograms

FIGURE 29-2 Body surface area nomogram. To determine the surface area of the child, draw a straight line between the point representing his or her height on the left vertical scale and the point representing weight on the right vertical scale. The point at which this line intersects the middle vertical scale represents the child's surface area in square meters.   (Courtesy of Abbott Laboratories.)

Using Safety Measures While Preparing Drugs

Three Checks and Five Rights

Medication errors have been said to cause 150 deaths per day and 1.3 million injuries per year (Phillips et al., 2001). Safety is of the utmost importance in preparing and implementing drug administration. The nurse observes the three checks and the five rights when administering medications.

The label on the medication container should be checked three times during medication preparation. The label should be read (1) when the nurse reaches for the container or unit dose package, (2) immediately before pouring or opening the medication, and (3) when replacing the container to the drawer or shelf or before giving the unit dose medication to the patient.

The five rights help to ensure accuracy when administering medications. The nurse gives the (1) right medication to the (2) right patient in the (3) right dosage through the (4) right route at the (5) right time.

The importance of the three checks and the five rights cannot be overemphasized. The safe nurse does not allow automatic habits of preparing medications to replace constant thinking, purposeful action, and repeated checking for accuracy.

Think back to Mr. Baptiste, the patient described in the Reflective Practice display. By adhering to the five rights, the nurse would be able to determine that the medication delivered by the pharmacy was labeled incorrectly.

Maintaining a Safe Environment

An environment that promotes safety and good working habits contributes to accuracy in the preparation of drugs for administration. Good lighting must be present when preparing drugs. Also, the nurse who is preparing drugs should work alone. This practice helps to avoid distractions and interruptions, which may lead to errors.

After the nurse begins to prepare drugs for administration, they should not be left unattended. If it is imperative to leave for a short time, the drugs that have been prepared should be placed in a locked area, such as in the medication cart. The nurse who prepares the medication also administers the drug and records the drug administration. When the nurse is not working at the medication cart, it should be locked. The locking of the medication cart is a requirement of the certifying bodies of hospitals.

Caring for Controlled Substances Safely

Controlled substances are kept in a locked drawer or container as a safety measure. Narcotics or controlled substances may be ordered only by physicians, and in some states nurse practitioners, who are registered with the Department of Justice, Bureau of Narcotics and Dangerous Drugs. According to federal law, a record must be kept for each narcotic that is administered. Healthcare agencies provide forms for keeping such records, and these forms are kept with the narcotics. Although the forms differ, the following information usually is required:

- Name of the patient receiving the narcotic
- Amount of the narcotic used
- Hour the narcotic was given
- Name of the physician who prescribed the narcotic
- Name of the nurse who administered the narcotic

It is common practice to check narcotics daily at specified intervals. In hospitals, checking is usually performed at each shift change. The amount of narcotics on hand is counted, and each used narcotic must be accounted for on the narcotic record. Some agencies use a computerized system for dispensing narcotics. The nurse has a secure identification code that provides access into the system, identifies the patient by name or identification number, and verifies the count for each drug as it is removed. Since this secure identification code is equivalent to the nurse's signature, it should never be given out to other staff members. Unless the narcotic count is incorrect, this eliminates the need to check the narcotic count at specific intervals each day. A narcotic count that does not check properly must be reported immediately. The law requires these special precautions to aid in the control of drug abuse.

The nurse administering narcotics has an important responsibility to see that the federal law is observed. If for any reason a narcotic prepared for administration has to be discarded, a second nurse should act as a witness, and that person should also sign the narcotic sheet. Nurses should also document with a witness any time a full dosage is not given and some of the narcotic needs to be disposed of. For instance, if 3 mg of a narcotic has been ordered and the nurse uses a 4-mg syringe, the remaining 1 mg should be disposed of while a witness is watching, and both nurses should sign the document.

Identifying the Patient

The nurse prepares medications, considering safety at all times, as discussed in the previous sections. Positive identification of the patient is essential to safe drug administration. Before administering the drug, check carefully to see that the right drug is being given to the right patient. Patients in inpatient healthcare agencies usually wear identification bracelets. Identify the patient by checking the identification bracelet, as shown in Figure 26-7 in Chapter 26, Safety. Also, ask the patient to state his or her name if possible. It is considered unsafe to call the patient by name because the patient may respond even if the nurse uses the wrong name. In some long-term care facilities a current photograph of the resident, displayed above the resident's bed, can also be used as a form of identification. The 2004 National Patient Safety Goals established by JCAHO state that whenever administering patient medications, two methods to identify that patient should be used.

THE NURSING PROCESS FOR ADMINISTERING MEDICATIONS

Assessing

Assessment of the patient receiving medications begins during a nursing history. One component of this is the medication history. During the interview, the nurse can adapt questions to meet the patient's needs and level of understanding. The nurse should avoid using medical jargon that the patient may not understand but instead should use familiar terms. For instance, the patient may refer to a diuretic as the "water pill" or to an anticoagulant as a "blood thinner." Areas to be included in the medication history are listed in the accompanying Focused Assessment Guide.

The nurse caring for Mildred Campbell would need to incorporate this information when assessing the patient. This information is extremely important to prevent possible drug interactions should the patient decide to use the medication advertised on television.

The nurse not only assesses the patient with regard to medications during the nursing history but also continues the assessment during and after medication administration. The accompanying box describes medication self-care behaviors for healthcare workers.

Diagnosing

Data that the nurse collects may lead to the development of several nursing diagnoses related to medication administration. The following are examples of appropriate nursing diagnoses:

Ineffective Health Maintenance related to lack of knowledge about anticoagulant medication regimen

Sexual Dysfunction related to adverse effects of antihypertensive drug

Anxiety related to daily self-injection of insulin

Disturbed Body Image related to effects of chemotherapy

Risk for Aspiration related to impaired swallowing of oral medications

Risk for Poisoning related to confusion about medication dosages

Deficient Knowledge related to lack of interest in learning about medication regimen

Deficient Knowledge related to interactions between herbal remedies and prescribed medications

Noncompliance with Medication Regimen related to adverse drug effects, cost of medications, confusion, lack of motivation, visual impairment, complexity of regimen

Disturbed Sleep Pattern related to consistent use of sedative-hypnotics

Outcome Identification and Planning

Nursing measures for patients receiving medication are directed toward the patient's achievement of the following goals:

- Clinical observations will improve. For example, the patient's pain will be relieved, or vital signs will return to baseline.
- The patient will receive a dosage that reaches the therapeutic level.
- The patient will demonstrate education regarding his or her medication.

Implementing: Administering a Medication

Remain with the patient and see that the medication is taken. If the patient receives several drugs, offer them separately so that if one is refused or dropped, positive identification can be made and the drug can be recorded or replaced. Never leave medications at the bedside for the patient to take later. This is an unsafe practice because the patient may forget to take the medication, or someone else may take the medication. Record medication administration as soon as possible after the patient takes the medication. Some agencies allow patients to self-administer certain drugs to promote the patient's independence. Be familiar with agency policy on this matter.

Nursing responsibilities for administering drugs by any route are listed in Box 29-2.

Focused Assessment Guide 29-1

Medications

Factors to Assess	Questions and Approaches
Previous and current drug use	What medications are you taking that the doctor prescribed for you?
	What over-the-counter medications or herbal supplements are you taking on a regular basis?
	Do you use nonmedicinal drugs (eg, alcohol, caffeine, home remedies)?
	How often do you use them?
	What is the reason for taking the medication?
	What medications have you taken during the past year and for what reasons?
	Is there anything else you have tried to alleviate your symptoms?
Medication schedule	At what times do you take your medications?
	Is there any special way your medication has to be prepared (eg, crushing and mixing with applesauce)?
	Do you have any special method for remembering to take your medications?
Response to medications	Have the medications had the expected effects?
	Have you ever experienced any adverse or unexpected reactions to the medications?
	Is there a family history of this type of reaction to medication?
	Do you have any allergies to medications?
	What happens when you take this medication?
Attitude toward drugs and use of drugs	How do you feel about taking medications?
	Why do you take the medications?
Compliance with regimen	Can you tell me your understanding of the reason for taking the medications?
	Can you describe how you follow the medication schedule?
	Are there any problems that prevent you from following the medication regimen?
Storage	Where are your medications stored at home?
	How long do you keep medications in the home?
	Can you show me any medications you have on hand?

Promoting Health 29-1 *Medications*

Use the following assessment checklist to determine how well you are meeting your own need for safe medication practices. Then develop a prescription for self-care by choosing appropriate behaviors from the list of suggestions.

ASSESSMENT CHECKLIST

almost always / sometimes / almost never

1. I store medications in a safe place (eg, a cool, dry place, away from direct sunlight, out of the reach of children).
2. I discard medications that have passed their expiration date.
3. I wear a Medic Alert tag or carry information that identifies a drug allergy or required medication.
4. I am cautious about combining prescribed medication with OTC drugs, herbal supplements, alcohol, or foods that can interact with the drug.

SELF-CARE BEHAVIORS

1. Finish all prescriptions as ordered by physician or nurse practitioner.
2. Avoid foods, alcohol, or over-the-counter drugs and herbal supplements that may interact with a prescribed drug.
3. Use available resources (textbooks, pharmacist, physician) to verify the potential for drug interactions or possible side effects of a medication.
4. Use a reminder system to maintain medication schedule.
5. Avoid sharing medications or taking someone else's prescribed pills.
6. Complete any laboratory tests necessary for maintenance or adjustment of a medication regimen.
7. Practice safe behaviors when storing medications.
8. Purchase drugs from the same pharmacy as an additional safeguard with multiple medication regimens.

Administering Oral Medications

Drugs given orally are intended for absorption in the stomach and small intestine. The oral route is the most commonly used route of administration. It is usually the most convenient and comfortable and is the safest for the patient. Occasionally, a patient may unintentionally or intentionally hide a medication in the mouth, or "cheek" it. Check that the medication was actually swallowed before recording that it has been taken. After oral administration, drug action has a slower onset and a more prolonged but less potent effect. There are certain situations in which oral medications would not be administered, such as when the patient has difficulty swallowing, is unconscious, is to receive nothing by mouth, or is vomiting.

Oral medications are available in solid and liquid form. Solid preparations include tablets, capsules, and pills. Some tablets are scored for easy breaking if a partial quantity is needed. Enteric-coated tablets are covered with a hard surface that impedes absorption until the tablet has left the stomach. Absorption takes place in the small intestine because the active ingredient of the drug is irritating to the stomach mucosa. Enteric-coated tablets should not be chewed or crushed. Other forms of oral medications that should not chewed or crushed without checking include any of the extended-release forms, such as SR (sustained release), XL (extended release), CR or CRT (controlled release), SA (sustained action), LA (long acting). Certain narcotics that were previously administered parenterally can now also be administered in a lollipop or oral-transmucosal form.

Liquid preparations include elixirs, spirits, suspensions, and syrups. Some are water-based solutions and others are alcohol-based solutions. If the patient has had a previous drug or alcohol addiction, medications containing alcohol should be avoided. Disposable, calibrated cups are available for the administration of liquid medications. For patients who find it difficult to take liquids from a cup, the medication can be placed in the mouth directly using a plastic syringe without a needle. The syringe should be placed between the gum and cheek and the liquid given to the patient slowly. This technique, in addition to having the patient in an upright or side-lying position, helps prevent the patient from choking and aspirating the medication. When administering a drug with a syringe, do not place the safety cap back over the syringe after drawing up the medication. This could pose an aspiration risk if the safety cap was not removed before administering the dose and the cap was accidentally injected into a patient's mouth.

If a label becomes difficult to read or accidentally comes off the container, the container should be returned to the pharmacy. A medication should never be given from a bottle without a label or with a label that cannot be read with accuracy. Because of the danger of error, unused medications should not be returned to their bottles. Care should be exercised in pouring to prevent unnecessary loss. Medications should not be transferred from one pharmacy container to another. Many medication bottles now have an identification code number on them. If similar medications were mixed and a patient had a reaction, it would be difficult to identify which drug was responsible. A medication with an unexpected precipitate should not be used, nor should one that has changed color. Skill 29-1 describes the techniques for preparing and administering oral medications.

Special Techniques

Certain drugs that are given orally can discolor the teeth or damage the enamel. Such a medication should be mixed well with water or some other liquid; the patient takes it through a drinking straw, and water is taken after administration. This practice reduces the strength of the drug that comes in contact with the teeth.

Some patients object to the taste of certain medications. The following techniques help disguise or mask an objectionable taste:

- Crush the medication and add it to food or a drink so that the patient can swallow it. Many times the food or drink will mask the flavor of the medication. However, as previously discussed, some drugs cannot be crushed (eg, enteric-coated and sustained-release capsules). Check with the pharmacist or a pharmacology reference if you are uncertain about crushing a medication.
- Allow the patient to suck on a small piece of ice for a few minutes before taking the medication. The ice numbs the taste buds, and the objectionable taste is less discernible.
- Store oily medications in the refrigerator. Cold oil is less aromatic than oil at room temperature.
- Place the medication in a syringe, and place the syringe well back on the tongue, being careful not to trigger the patient's gag reflex. This places the medication on the part of the tongue with few taste buds.
- Offer oral hygiene immediately after giving the medication.
- Give the medication with generous amounts of water or other liquids, if permitted, to dilute the taste.

(text continues on page 726)

Administering Oral Medications

EQUIPMENT

Medication in disposable cup or oral syringe
Liquid with straw if not contraindicated

Medication Kardex or computer-generated MAR

Medication cart or tray

ACTION	RATIONALE
1. Gather equipment. Check each medication order against the original physician's order according to agency policy. Clarify any inconsistencies. Check the patient's chart for allergies.	This comparison helps to identify errors that may have occurred when orders were transcribed. The physician's order is the legal record of medication orders for each agency.
2. Know the actions, special nursing considerations, safe dose ranges, purpose of administration, and adverse effects of medications to be administered.	This knowledge aids the nurse in evaluating the therapeutic effect of the medication in relation to the patient's disorder and can also be used to educate patients about their medications.
3. Perform proper hand hygiene	Hand hygiene prevents the spread of microorganisms.
4. Move the medication cart to the outside of the patient's room or prepare for administration in the medication area.	Organization facilitates error-free administration and saves time.
5. Unlock the medication cart or drawer.	Keeping the cart or drawer locked safeguards each patient's medication supply. Hospital accrediting bodies require medication carts to be locked when not in use.
6. Prepare medications for one patient at a time.	This prevents errors in medication administration.
7. Select the proper medication from the drawer or stock and compare with the Kardex or order. Check expiration dates and perform calculations if necessary.	Comparison of medication to the physician's order reduces errors in medication administration. Verify calculations with another nurse if necessary. This is the first safety check.
a. Place unit dose-packaged medications in a disposable cup. Do not open wrapper until at the bedside. Keep narcotics and medications that require special nursing assessments in a separate container.	a. The label is needed for an additional safety check. Prerequisites to giving certain medications may include monitoring of certain vital signs.
b. When removing tablets or capsules from a bottle, pour the necessary number into the bottle cap and then place the tablets in a medication cup. Break only scored tablets, if necessary, to obtain the proper dose.	b. Pouring medication into the cap allows for easy return of excess medication to the bottle. Pouring tablets or capsules into the nurse's hand is unsanitary.
c. Hold liquid medication bottles with the label against the palm. Use the appropriate measuring device when pouring liquids, and read the amount of medication at the bottom of the meniscus at eye level. Wipe the lip of the bottle with a paper towel.	c. Accuracy is possible when the appropriate measuring device is used and then read accurately. Liquid that may drip onto the label makes the label difficult to read.

Action 7: Comparing medication with Kardex or order.   (Photo by Rick Brady.)

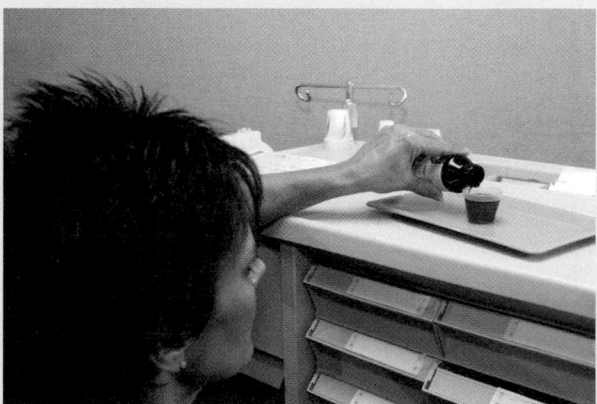

Action 7c: Measuring at eye level.   (Photo by Rick Brady.)

(continued)

SKILL 29-1 Administering Oral Medications (continued)

ACTION	RATIONALE
8. Recheck each medication package or preparation with the order as it is poured.	This is a second check to guard against a medication error.
9. When all medications for one patient have been prepared, recheck once again with the medication order before taking them to the patient.	This is a third check to ensure accuracy and to prevent errors.
10. Transport medications to the patient's bedside carefully, and keep the medications in sight at all times.	Careful handling and close observation prevent accidental or deliberate disarrangement of medications.
11. See that the patient receives the medications at the correct time.	Check agency policy, which may allow for administration within a period of 30 minutes before or 30 minutes after the designated time.
12. Identify the patient carefully. There are three correct ways to do this: a. Check the name on the patient's identification band. b. Ask the patient his or her name. c. Verify the patient's identification with a staff member who knows the patient.	Identifying the patient is the nurse's responsibility to guard against error. a. This is the most reliable method. Replace the identification band if it is missing or inaccurate in any way. b. This requires an answer from the patient, but illness and strange surroundings often cause patients to be confused. c. This is another way to double-check identity. Do not use the name on the door or over the bed because these may be inaccurate.

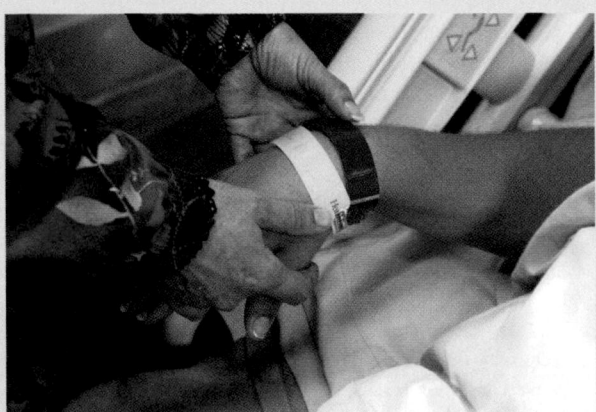

Action 12a: Checking patient identity.   (Photo by Rick Brady.)

ACTION	RATIONALE
13. Complete necessary assessments before administration of medications. Check allergy bracelet or ask the patient about allergies. Explain the purpose and action of each medication to the patient.	Assessment is a prerequisite to administration of medications.
14. Assist the patient to an upright or lateral position.	Swallowing is facilitated by proper positioning. An upright or side-lying position protects the patient from aspiration.
15. Administer medications: a. Offer water or other permitted fluids with pills, capsules, tablets, and some liquid medications. b. Ask the patient's preference regarding medications to be taken by hand or in a cup and one at a time or all at once. c. If the capsule or tablet falls to the floor, it must be discarded and a new one administered. d. Record any fluid intake if intake and output measurement is ordered.	a. Liquids facilitate swallowing of solid drugs. Some liquid drugs are intended to adhere to the pharyngeal area, in which case liquid is not offered with the medication. b. This encourages the patient's participation in taking the medications. c. This prevents contamination. d. This provides for accurate documentation.

(continued)

SKILL 29-1 Administering Oral Medications (continued)

ACTION	RATIONALE
16. Remain with the patient until each medication is swallowed. Unless the nurse has seen the patient swallow the drug, it cannot be recorded that the drug was administered.	The patient's chart is a legal record. Only with a physician's order can medications be left at the bedside.
17. Perform hand hygiene	Hand hygiene prevents the spread of microorganisms.
18. Record each medication given on the medication chart or record using the required format.	Prompt recording avoids the possibility of accidentally repeating the administration of the drug.
a. If the drug was refused or omitted, record this in the appropriate area on the medication record and notify the physician.	a. This verifies the reason the medication was omitted and ensures that the physician is aware of the patient's condition.
b. Recording of administration of a narcotic may require additional documentation on a narcotic record stating drug count and other specific information.	b. Controlled substance laws necessitate careful recording of narcotic use. If using a computerized medication station, the machine may document needed information upon withdrawal of the medication.

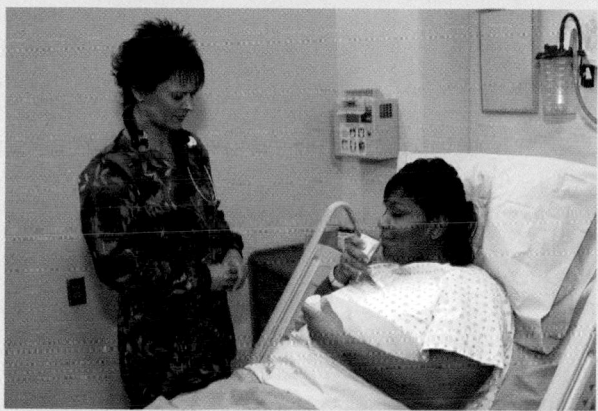

Action 16: Observing patient swallowing medication.
(Photo by Rick Brady.)

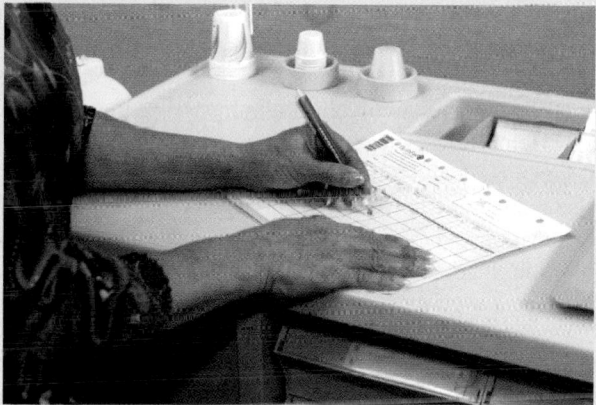

Action 18: Documenting administration of medication.
(Photo by Rick Brady.)

19. Check on the patient within 30 minutes to verify his or her response to medication.	This provides an opportunity for further documentation and additional assessment of the effectiveness of pain relief and adverse effects of medications.

Infant and Child Considerations

• Special devices, such as oral syringes and calibrated nipples, are available in a pharmacy to ensure accurate dose administration for young children and infants.

• Some creative ways to administer medications to children include the following: have a "tea party" with medicine cups; place a syringe (without needle) or dropper in the space between the cheek and gum and slowly administer the medication; save a special treat for after the medication administration (e.g., movie, playroom time, or a special food if allowed).

• The FDA has received reports of infants choking on the plastic caps that fit on the end of syringes when used to administer oral medications. They recommend the following: remove and dispose of caps before giving syringes to patients or families, caution family caregivers to dispose of caps on syringes they buy over the counter, and report any problems with syringe caps to the FDA. Companies have begun to manufacture syringes labeled "oral use" without the caps on them.

Older Adult Considerations

Elderly patients with arthritis may have difficulty opening child-proof caps. On request, the pharmacist can substitute a cap that is easier to open. A rubber band twisted around the cap may provide a more secure grip for older patients.

Home Care Considerations

• Encourage the patient to discard outdated prescription medications.

• Discuss safe storage of medications when there are children and pets in the environment.

• Discuss with parents the difference in over-the-counter medications made for infants and medications made for children. Many times parents do not realize that there are different strengths to the actual medications, leading to under- or overdosing.

• Encourage patients to carry a card listing all medications, dosage, and frequency in case of an emergency.

(continued)

ACTION	RATIONALE

Special Considerations

- If the patient questions a medication order or states the medication is different from the usual dose, always recheck and clarify with the original order and/or physician before giving the medication.
- If the patient's level of consciousness is altered or his or her swallowing is impaired, check with the physician to clarify the

route of administration or alternative forms of medication. This may also be a solution for a child or a confused patient who is refusing to take a medication.

- Patients with poor vision can request medication labels printed in larger type. A magnifying lens also may prove helpful.

Children. It can be challenging and frustrating to administer medications to infants and children. Children younger than 5 years have difficulty swallowing tablets and capsules. Most medications are available in liquid form. Nursing responsibility also includes teaching and preparing family members to administer medications to a child at home. In addition to understanding the medication order and the reason for the medication, the caregiver should be able to demonstrate any special techniques involved in administering the prescribed drugs. Helpful strategies for administering oral medications to children include the following:

- Use a dropper to give infants or very young children liquid medications while holding them in a sitting or semisitting position. Place the medication between the gum and cheek to prevent aspiration.
- Crush uncoated tablets or empty a soft capsule and mix the medication with soft foods, such as potatoes, pudding, or cooked or hot cereal, for patients who are likely to aspirate liquids. Proper absorption may not occur if coated tablets or hard capsules are added to food.
- If a medication has an objectionable taste, warn the child, if he or she is old enough to understand. Failing to warn the child is likely to decrease the child's trust in the nurse.
- Take care when selecting the food to be mixed with the medication. The item should not be an essential part of the child's diet, such as formula or the child's favorite food. The child may refuse to eat a food associated with medications.
- Offer the child a flavored ice pop or frozen fruit bar immediately before taking the medication. It numbs the tongue, making the taste of the medication less evident.
- Praise the child for a job well done after he or she swallows the medication.

> *Consider Jacob Shoolin, the school-aged boy described at the beginning of the chapter who is to receive oral bronchodilator therapy. The nurse would incorporate knowledge of these strategies in conjunction with his developmental level when preparing to administer the oral medication to Jacob.*

Older Adults. Techniques for administering medications to older people include the following:

- Allow extra time to administer medications to older patients, because their reflexes may be slowed and their understanding of the treatment decreased.
- Older patients may have difficulty swallowing medications and may find it easier to take their medications when crushed or given in liquid form. Initiate swallowing by massaging the laryngeal prominence or the area just below the chin prominence. The pressure from the gentle massage creates the desire to swallow. A speech therapist may offer additional suggestions for patients who have difficulty swallowing.
- Reevaluation of the drug dosage is necessary with the older patient. Weight and age should be used as criteria for determining the dosage.
- Assist the older patient to set up a schedule as a reminder to take medications as scheduled at home.
- Monitor the patient carefully for adverse effects that may result from the drug regimen. These may be magnified in older individuals.
- Teach patients the names of drugs rather than distinguishing them by color. Manufacturers may vary the colors of generic drugs, and the visual changes associated with aging may make it more difficult to identify medications by their color.

In older adults, compliance is influenced heavily by the education about medications provided by nursing staff. Winland-Brown and Valiante (2000) found that compliance with medications in the elderly population was affected by "confusion over doses and schedules, forgetfulness, toxic interactions, and excessive financial expense" (see the Research in Nursing box). Adequate patient teaching can prevent many of these issues.

Administering Medications Through an Enteral Feeding Tube

Patients with a gastrointestinal tube (nasogastric, nasointestinal, percutaneous endoscopic gastrostomy [PEG], or J tube) often receive medication through the tube. The insertion of the tube and care of the patient with an enteral feeding tube are described in Chapter 42, Nutrition. The following are suggestions for giving medications through the tube:

- Use liquid medications or medications that can be crushed and combined with liquid.

Research in Nursing Making a Difference
Enhancing Medication Compliance in Elderly People Living in the Community

Noncompliance with a medical regimen places an individual at risk for complications from disease, leading to an increase in physician visits and hospitalizations. Many previous studies have documented that elderly individuals living at home who require medication for chronic diseases are particularly at risk for noncompliance with their medication schedules. Managed care and the accompanying cuts in home care reimbursement limit the nurse's ability to improve compliance, yet simple measures that serve as reminders for this population can have a positive effect on management of symptoms and overall well-being.

Related Research
Winland-Brown, J., & Valiante, J. (2000). Effectiveness of different medication management approaches on elders' medication adherence. *Outcomes Management for Nursing Practice, 4*(4), 172–176.

Participants, ranging in age from 70 to 100 years old, who lived in an independent living facility and had a chronic illness were recruited to participate in the study. All participants were cognitively intact and had a previous hospitalization due to a medication noncompliance issue or medication management concern. The participants were randomly placed in three groups. The con-

trol group performed self-administration of medications. The second group used the pillbox method as the approach to medication management, and the third group had a voice-activated medication dispenser. During the study, the number of doses of medications taken by the patient was recorded, as well as the effect of medication compliance on the medical diagnosis. The voice-activated medication dispenser showed the highest rate of medication compliance, with the pillbox method coming in second. The lowest rate of medication compliance was with the self-administration of medications. This study demonstrated the need for individualized medication administration methods for elderly persons living in the community.

Relevance to Nursing Practice
Interventions that enable the nurse to increase medication compliance in a group such as the elderly can lead to a direct decrease in the number of hospitalizations and physician visits as well as a higher quality of life for the patient. The interventions studied here not only increased compliance but also allowed the subjects to continue to feel independent. The nurse can play an essential role in helping elderly people to remain compliant with their medications while keeping their independence.

- Bring the liquid medication to room temperature. Cold liquids may cause patient discomfort.
- Remove the clamp from the tube and use the recommended procedure for checking tube placement in the stomach or intestine before administering the drug.
- Flush the tube with 15 to 30 mL water (5 to 10 mL for children) before giving the medication and immediately after giving the medication. Flushing before may warn you if the tube is clogged and helps to maintain tube patency.
- Give medications separately and flush with water between each drug. Some medications may interact with each other or become less effective if mixed with other drugs.
- If the tube is connected to suction, keep it disconnected from the suction and clamped for 20 to 30 minutes after administration of the medication to allow absorption.
- Disconnect a continuous tube feeding before giving medications, and leave the tube clamped for a short period of time after the medication has been given, according to agency protocol.
- Document the water intake and liquid medication by tube on the intake and output record. Adjust the amount of water used if the patient's fluid intake is restricted.

Administering Sublingual and Buccal Medications
Certain drugs, such as nitroglycerin, are administered sublingually; that is, a tablet is placed under the patient's tongue. Another method is to administer the medication between the cheek and gum (buccal administration). These areas are rich in superficial blood vessels, which allows the drug to be ab-

sorbed relatively rapidly into the bloodstream for quick systemic effects. Sublingual and buccal medications should not be swallowed but rather held in place so that complete absorption can occur. Before administering a sublingual or buccal drug, the nurse may offer the patient a drink of water (if the patient is permitted to have fluids) or oral care (if the patient is NPO). This ensures that the tablet will dissolve appropriately.

Administering Parenteral Medications
Enteral means within the intestines; **parenteral** means outside the intestines or alimentary canal. Therefore, one way of administering a medication by the parenteral route involves injecting the medication into those body tissues outside of the intestines or alimentary canal. Table 29-2 defines terms used to describe various types of injections. Advanced injection techniques consist of injecting medications into an artery, the peritoneum, heart tissues, the spinal canal, and bones. Techniques for injecting medications into these areas are discussed in clinical texts. In most instances, physicians are responsible for these procedures, and nurses assist.

Absorption occurs more rapidly with an injection than when other routes are used. Intravenous injections are absorbed more rapidly than intramuscular ones, but the effects of intramuscular injections usually last longer due to the increased absorption time. Absorption is also more nearly complete; therefore, the results are more predictable, and the desired dosage can be determined with greater accuracy. Giving drugs by injection is necessary if the drug is available in no other form. Injections are particularly desirable for patients who are unconscious, who have gastrointestinal disturbances, or who are uncooperative. The injection of drugs also is used in emergencies because absorption and desired results occur rapidly.

Needles and Syringes

Needles are available in various lengths and gauges, with different sizes of bevels. Figure 29-3 shows the parts of a needle. The most commonly used needle lengths vary from 5/16″ to 2″ (0.8 to 5.1 cm). The needle length used depends on the route of administration. The gauge is determined by the diameter of the needle. Needle gauges are numbered 18 through 30. As the diameter of the needle increases, the gauge number decreases: for instance, an 18-gauge needle is larger than a 30-gauge needle. The bevel of the needle is its sloped edge, designed to make a narrow, slitlike opening that closes quickly.

Syringes are supplied in various sizes. Most syringes are plastic and disposable. Some syringes are supplied with the needle attached; others are not, in which case you should select an appropriate needle.

Choose the equipment needed for an injection based on the following criteria:

- Route of administration: A longer needle is required for an intramuscular injection than for an intradermal or a subcutaneous injection.
- Viscosity of the solution: Some medications are more viscous than others and require a large-lumen needle to inject the drug.

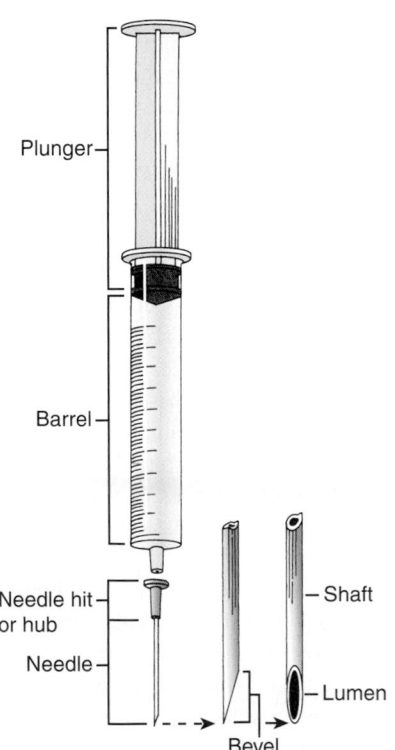

FIGURE 29-3 Parts of a needle and syringe.

Plunger

Barrel

Needle hit
or hub

Needle

Shaft

Lumen

Bevel

- Quantity to be administered: The larger the amount of medication to be injected, the greater the capacity of the syringe.
- Body size: An obese person requires a longer needle to reach muscle tissue than a thin person.
- Type of medication: There are special syringes for certain uses. An example is the insulin syringe used to inject insulin. Some medications, such as iron dextran injection (Imferon), are irritating to subcutaneous tissue, so a longer needle should be used to ensure proper placement of the medication in the muscle tissue.

After use, needles and syringes are placed in puncture-resistant containers without being recapped; most needlestick injuries occur during recapping. The one-handed technique is used when a needle must be recapped. This technique and additional measures to protect healthcare workers from accidental transmission of infectious diseases are discussed in Chapter 27, Asepsis. Many manufacturers have now placed retractable needle sheath covers on prefilled syringes. With these syringes, once the needle is contaminated, the top slides forward and over the needle to prevent a needlestick injury.

For parenteral injections, techniques of surgical asepsis must be followed strictly to avoid introducing organisms into the body. The parts of the syringe and needle that must be kept sterile during the procedure of preparing and administering an injection are the inside of the barrel, the part of the plunger that enters the barrel, the tip of the barrel, and the needle, except for the needle hub. Surgical asepsis also applies to cleaning the skin for an injection. The skin is cleaned with alcohol or povidone-iodine (Betadine) in a circular motion, working from the center of the designated site outward.

Needleless Systems

The risk for accidental needle sticks and exposure to bloodborne pathogens is reduced significantly with the use of needleless devices or protected needles. Chapter 27 describes the rationale for these systems of protection for healthcare workers. These devices prevent needlestick injuries in a variety of ways. Examples include needles that can be sheathed in a plastic guard after the needle is withdrawn from the skin and syringes that have a retractable needle that locks and seals inside the syringe barrel. Needleless systems are also available for intravenous use, including recessed and shielded intravenous needle connectors as well as blunt cannulas that are inserted into special receptor sites on tubing or lock setups. A new needleless device (Injex) is available for insulin delivery. This system uses pressure to inject the insulin through the skin and into the subcutaneous tissue. It is virtually pain-free, but its use is contraindicated in very thin patients and those taking anticoagulants (Clarke, 2002). All needleless devices or blunt cannulas are discarded in special containers that are puncture-proof, leak-proof, and clearly labeled; these containers are available at various locations on each healthcare unit. Figure 29-4 shows an example of a needleless device.

Preparing Medications for Administration by Injection

Drugs that are administered by injection are packaged in several ways. Those that deteriorate in solution are usually dis-

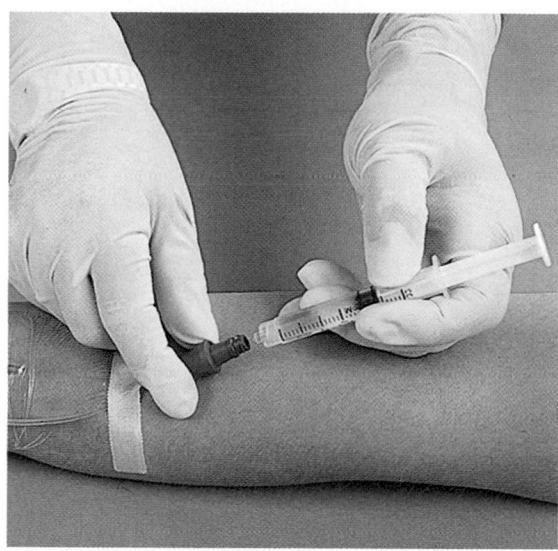

FIGURE 29-4 Syringe prepared to inject into needleless port.

pensed as powders and are reconstituted immediately before injection. Drugs that remain stable in solution are usually dispensed in ampules, bottles, or vials in an aqueous or oily solution or suspension. Drugs may be dispensed in single-dose glass ampules, single-dose rubber-capped vials, multidose rubber-capped vials, and prefilled cartridges. Figure 29-5 shows several types of ampules and vials as well as prefilled cartridges.

Ampules. An **ampule** is a glass flask that contains a single dose of medication for parenteral administration. There is no way to prevent airborne contamination of any unused portion of medication after the ampule is opened, so if not all the medication is used, the remainder must be discarded. Medication is removed from an ampule after its thin neck is broken. Take special care when breaking the ampule so as not to cut yourself. If you cut yourself on the ampule, discard the ampule and medication. Because of the risk of small glass shards falling into the ampule, use a filter needle to remove the medication from the vial and then discard

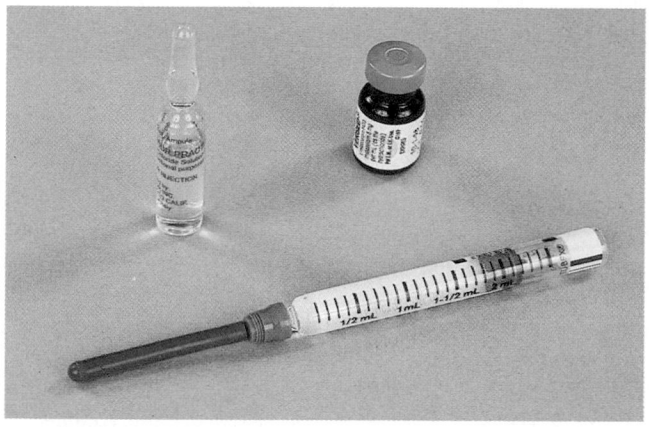

FIGURE 29-5 Ampule, vial, and prefilled cartridge. (Photo © B. Proud).

it appropriately before administering the medication to the patient. The ampule can be inverted or placed on a flat surface to draw the solution into the syringe. Care must be taken not to contaminate the needle by touching the rim of the ampule. Skill 29-2 shows how to remove medication from an ampule.

Vials. As Figure 29-5 shows, a **vial** is a glass bottle with a self-sealing stopper through which the medication is removed. For safety in transporting and storing, the single-dose rubber-capped vial is usually covered with a soft metal cap that can be removed easily. The rubber stopper that is then exposed is the means of entrance into the vial.

Some drugs are dispensed in vials that contain several doses. This means that the nurse can remove several doses from the same container. To prevent microbial growth in the vial, each multidose vial is usually good for only 24 hours. Label the vial with the time and date when first used. After the initial use of the multidose vial, wipe the rubber stopper with alcohol each time the medication is removed from the vial. To facilitate removal of medication, inject air into the vial. The amount of air injected into the vial is the same amount as the desired quantity of solution. Skill 29-3 details how to remove medication from a vial.

Prefilled Cartridges. Prefilled cartridges provide a single dose of medication. Insert the cartridge into a reusable holder. Before giving the injection, check the dosage in the cartridge and clear the cartridge of excess air. Most prefilled cartridges are overfilled; therefore, eject any excess medication to give an exact dose and avoid a medication error. Tubex and Carpuject are two types of prefilled cartridges. Examples of prefilled cartridges are shown in Figure 29-5.

Similar to prefilled cartridges are prefilled syringes. These are syringes that are already filled with a medication and usually have their own needle attached. Like prefilled cartridges, these syringes also come with excess air. In some cases, this air is accounted for and does not need to be expelled before administering the medication. Lovenox is an example of a syringe where the air should not be expelled before administering.

Mixing Medications in One Syringe

Preparation of medications in one syringe depends on how the medication is supplied. When using a single-dose vial and a multidose vial, air is injected into both vials and the medication in the multidose vial is drawn into the syringe first. This prevents the contents of the multidose vial from being contaminated with the medication in the single-dose vial. First, it is important to ensure that the two drugs are compatible. The steps to follow when preparing medications from two multidose vials in one syringe are illustrated in Figure 29-6.

When preparing medications from an ampule and a vial, the medication in the vial is prepared first. The medication in the ampule is drawn up after the medication in the vial. Nurses must be aware of drug incompatibilities when preparing medications in one syringe. Certain medications, such as

SKILL 29-2 Removing Medication From an Ampule

EQUIPMENT

Sterile syringe and filter needle
Alcohol swab or gauze pad
Ampule of medication

Medication Kardex or computer-generated
MAR

Needle (optional; for medications that are
to be given IM, size depends on medication being administered and patient)

ACTION	RATIONALE
1. Gather equipment. Check the medication order against the original physician's order according to agency policy.	This comparison helps to identify errors that may have occurred when orders were transcribed.
2. Perform hand hygiene.	Hand hygiene deters the spread of microorganisms.
3. Tap the stem of the ampule or twist your wrist quickly while holding the ampule vertically.	This facilitates movement of medication in the stem to the body of the ampule.
4. Wrap a small gauze pad or dry alcohol swab around the neck of the ampule.	This protects the nurse's fingers from the glass as the ampule is broken.
5. Use a snapping motion to break off the top of the ampule along the prescored line at its neck. Always break away from your body.	This protects the nurse's face and fingers from any shattered glass fragments.

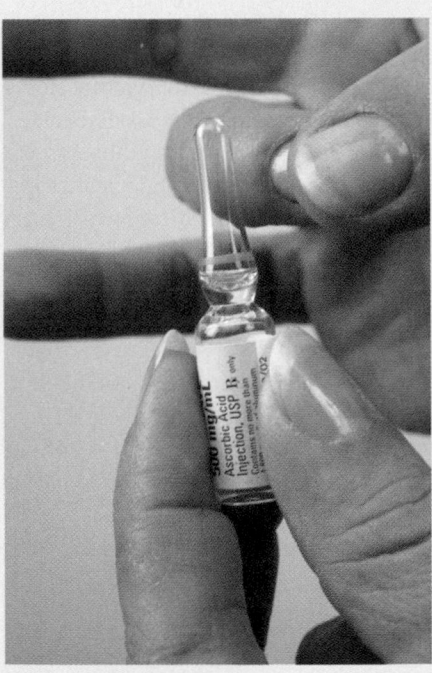
Action 3: Tapping stem of ampule.
(Photo by Rick Brady.)

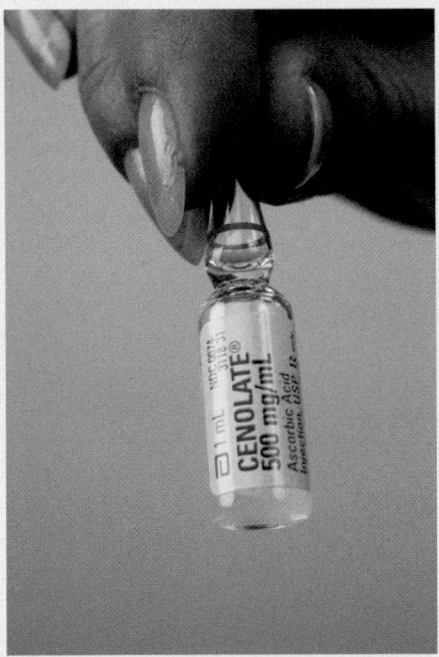
Action 3: Twisting motion of wrist while holding ampule.   (Photo by Rick Brady.)

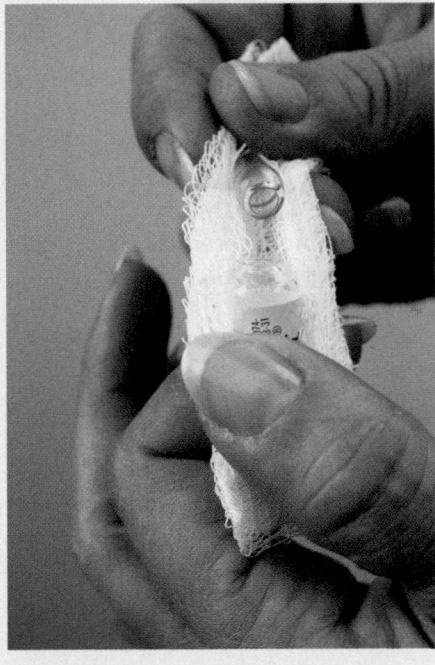
Action 5: Snapping off top of ampule.
(Photo by Rick Brady.)

6. Remove the cap from the filter needle by pulling it straight off. Insert the filter needle into the ampule, being careful not to touch the rim.	The rim of the ampule is considered contaminated. Use of a filter needle prevents the accidental withdrawing of small glass particles with the medication.
7. Withdraw medication in the amount ordered plus a small amount more (~30%). Do not inject air into solutions. Use either of the following methods:	By withdrawing a small amount more of medication, any air bubbles in the syringe can be displaced once the syringe is removed, while still having ample medication in the syringe.
a. Insert the tip of the needle into the ampule, which is up-right on a flat surface, and withdraw fluid into the syringe. Touch the plunger at the knob only.	a. The contents of the ampule are not under pressure; therefore, air is unnecessary and will cause the contents to overflow. Handling the plunger at the knob only will keep the shaft of the plunger sterile.

(continued)

ACTION	RATIONALE

b. Insert the tip of the needle into the ampule and invert the ampule. Keep the needle centered and not touching the sides of the ampule. Withdraw the fluid into the syringe. Touch the plunger at the knob only.

b. Surface tension holds the fluids in the ampule when inverted. If the needle touches the sides or is removed and then reinserted into the ampule, the surface tension is broken and fluid runs out. Handling the plunger at the knob only keeps the shaft of the plunger sterile.

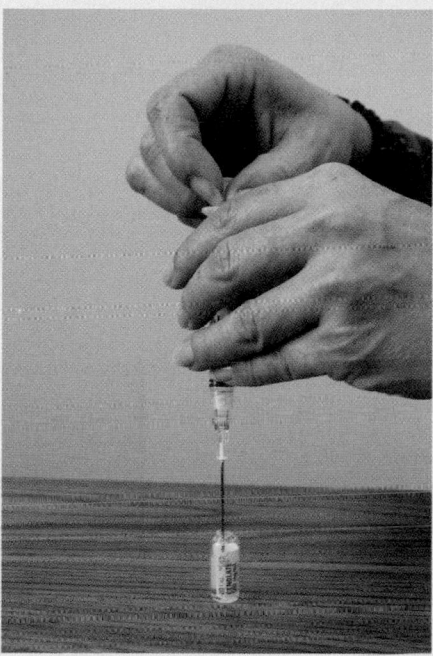

Action 7a: Withdrawing medication from upright ampule.   (Photo by Rick Brady.)

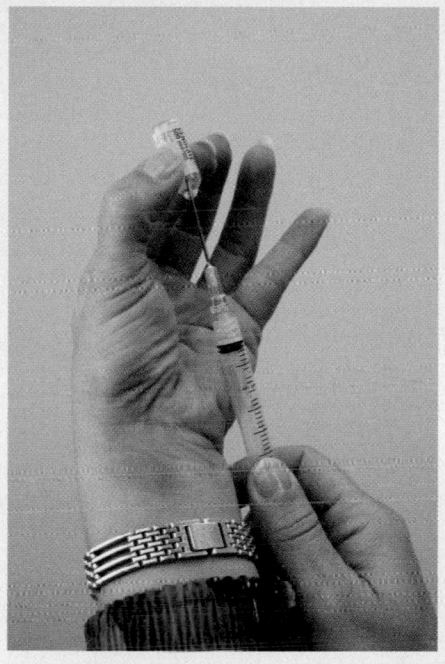

Action 7b: Withdrawing medication from inverted ampule.   (Photo by Rick Brady.)

8. Do not expel any air bubbles that may form in the solution. Wait until the needle has been withdrawn to tap the syringe and expel the air carefully. Check the amount of medication in the syringe and discard any surplus.

Ejecting air into the solution increases pressure in the ampule and can force the medication to spill out over the ampule. Ampules may have overfill. Careful measurement ensures that the correct dose is withdrawn.

9. Discard the ampule in a suitable container after comparing with the medication Kardex.

If not all of the medication has been removed from the ampule, it must be discarded because there is no way to maintain the sterility of the contents in an unopened ampule.

10. Discard the filter needle in a suitable container. If the medication is to be given IM or if agency policy requires the use of a needle to administer medication, attach the selected needle to the syringe.

The filter needle used to draw up the medication should not be used to administer the medication to prevent any glass shards from entering the patient. If your agency has a needleless IV system, the medication is ready to be given.

11. Perform hand hygiene.

Hand hygiene deters the spread of microorganisms.

---

diazepam (Valium), are incompatible with other drugs in the same syringe. Other drugs have limited compatibility and should be administered within 15 minutes of preparation. Incompatible drugs may become cloudy or form a precipitate in the syringe. Such medications are discarded and re-prepared in separate syringes. Mixing more than two drugs in one syringe is not recommended. If it must be done, the pharmacist should be contacted to determine the compatibility of the three drugs as well as the compatibility of their pH values and the preservatives that may be present in each drug. A

drug compatibility table should be available to nurses who are preparing medications.

Mixing Insulins in One Syringe

Insulin, a naturally occurring hormone produced by the islets of Langerhans in the pancreas, enables cells to use carbohydrates. Patients with diabetes mellitus produce no insulin or produce insulin in insufficient amounts. Several types of insulin are available for use by patients with diabetes mellitus. Insulins vary in their onset and duration of action and are

Removing Medication From a Vial

EQUIPMENT

Sterile syringe and needle (size depends
  on medication being administered and
  patient)

Vial of medication
Medication Kardex or computer-generated
  MAR

Alcohol swab
Filter needle (optional)
Second needle (optional)

ACTION	RATIONALE
1. Gather equipment. Check medication order against the original physician's order according to agency policy.	This comparison helps to identify errors that may have occurred when orders were transcribed.
2. Perform hand hygiene.	Hand hygiene deters the spread of microorganisms.
3. Remove the metal or plastic cap on the vial that protects the rubber stopper.	The metal or plastic cap prevents contamination of the rubber top.
4. Swab the rubber top with the alcohol swab.	Alcohol removes surface bacteria contamination. This should be done the first time the rubber stopper is entered, and with any subsequent re-entries into the vial.
5. Remove the cap from the needle by pulling it straight off. (Some agencies recommend use of a filter needle when withdrawing premixed medication from multidose vials.) Draw back an amount of air into the syringe that is equal to the specific dose of medication to be withdrawn.	Before fluid is removed, injection of an equal amount of air is required to prevent the formation of a partial vacuum because a vial is a sealed container. If not enough air is injected, the negative pressure makes it difficult to withdraw the medication. (Use of a filter needle prevents any solid material from being withdrawn through the needle.)
6. Pierce the rubber stopper in the center with the needle tip and inject the measured air into the space above the solution. (Do not inject air into the solution.) The vial may be positioned upright on a flat surface or inverted.	Air bubbled through the solution could result in withdrawal of an inaccurate amount of medication.
7. Invert the vial and withdraw the needle tip slightly so that it is below the fluid level.	This prevents air from being aspirated into the syringe.
8. Draw up the prescribed amount of medication while holding the syringe at eye level and vertically. Be careful to touch the plunger at the knob only.	Holding the syringe at eye level facilitates accurate reading, and the vertical position makes removal of air bubbles from the syringe easy. Handling the plunger at the knob only will keep the shaft of the plunger sterile.
9. If any air bubbles accumulate in the syringe, tap the barrel of the syringe sharply and move the needle past the fluid into the air space to reinject the air bubble into the vial. Return the needle tip to the solution and continue withdrawing the medication.	Removal of air bubbles is necessary to ensure that the dose of medication is accurate.
10. After the correct dose is withdrawn, remove the needle from the vial and carefully replace the cap over the needle. If a filter needle has been used to draw up the medication and the medication needs to be administered through a needle, remove the filter needle and replace it with a new needle. (Some agencies recommend changing needles, if needed to administer the medication, before administering the medication.)	This prevents contamination of the needle and protects the nurse against accidental needle sticks. A one-handed recapping method may be used as long as care is taken not to contaminate the needle during the process. A filter needle used to draw up medication should not be used to administer the medication to prevent any solid material from entering the patient.

(continued)

Removing Medication From a Vial (continued)

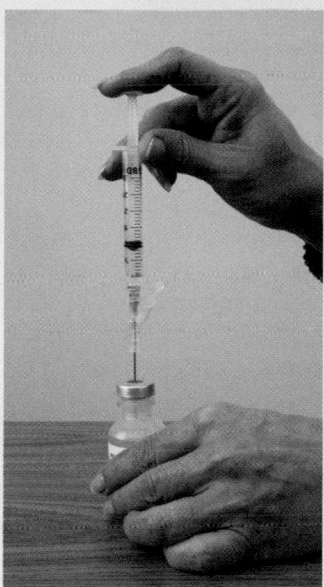

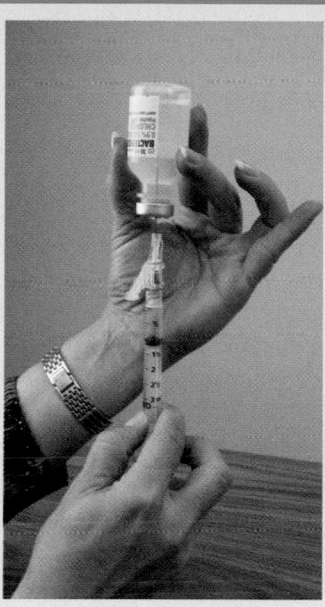

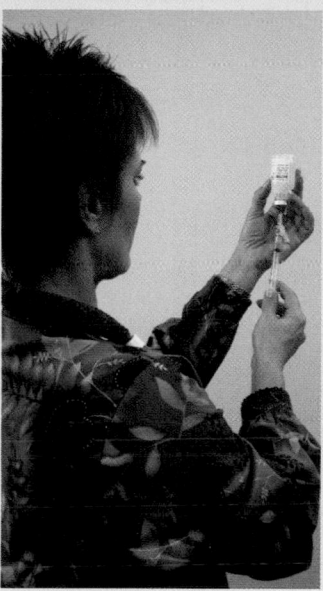

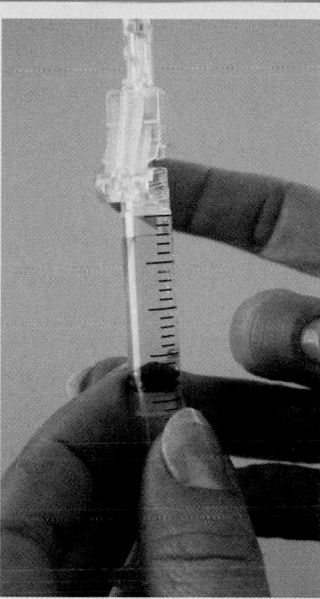

Action 6: Injecting air with vial upright. (Photo by Rick Brady.)

Action 7: Positioning needle tip in solution. (Photo by Rick Brady.)

Action 8: Withdrawing medication from inverted vial. (Photo by Rick Brady.)

Action 9: Tapping to remove air bubbles. (Photo by Rick Brady.)

ACTION	RATIONALE
11. If a multidose vial is being used, label the vial with the date and time opened, and store the vial containing the remaining medication according to agency policy.	Because the vial is sealed, the medication inside remains sterile and can be used for future injections. Labeling the opened vials with a date and time limits its use after a specific time period.
12. Perform hand hygiene.	Hand hygiene deters the spread of microorganisms

classified as short acting, intermediate acting, and long acting. Some insulins have a modifying protein that slows absorption. The modifying proteins are globin and protamine (NPH, globin zinc, protamine zinc). Before administering any insulin, the nurse should be aware of the onset time and ensure that proper food is available.

Insulin dosages are calculated in units. The scale commonly used is U100, which is based on 100 units of insulin contained in 1 mL of solution. Due to the small amounts of insulin to be administered in children, the physician may order a special concentration made by the pharmacist, such as U25 (25 units of insulin in 1 mL of solution). An insulin syringe is calibrated in units also. Before drawing up the insulin, make sure that the syringe is calibrated for the correct insulin; for example, if you have U100 insulin, the syringe should say U100. Before administering insulin, check the dosage with the physician's orders. Many cases of diabetes mellitus are regulated with a combination of two insulins (eg, regular and NPH insulins). Typically, preparations of regular insulin are clear, while intermediate- or long-acting insulins are cloudy. It is no longer safe, however, to use the terms "clear" and "cloudy" to designate types of insulin preparation. Insulin glargine (Lantus) is a clear but long-acting insulin (24-hour du-

ration). Skill 29-4 gives the steps for mixing two types of insulins in the same syringe.

The importance of rotating injection sites for insulin administration cannot be overemphasized. Injection sites are discussed in the later section, Administering Medications Subcutaneously. A 10-mL vial of unrefrigerated insulin may be used safely for 1 month if stored in a cool place. If stored in the refrigerator, it may be kept for 3 months (Kee & Hayes, 2003).

Reconstituting Powdered Medications

Occasionally, a drug is supplied as a powder in a vial. A liquid, or diluent, must be added to the powder before it is administered as a solution. The technique of adding a diluent to a powdered drug is called reconstitution. Information needed for reconstitution, such as what solution to use for the diluent and dosage calculation, is usually found on the vial label. Additional sources of information about reconstitution of medications are package inserts and the pharmacist.

Another form that powdered medications may come in is called an Actovial. Actovials have the diluent and powder in the same vial but separated by a rubber stopper. When the nurse is ready to administer the medication, the rubber

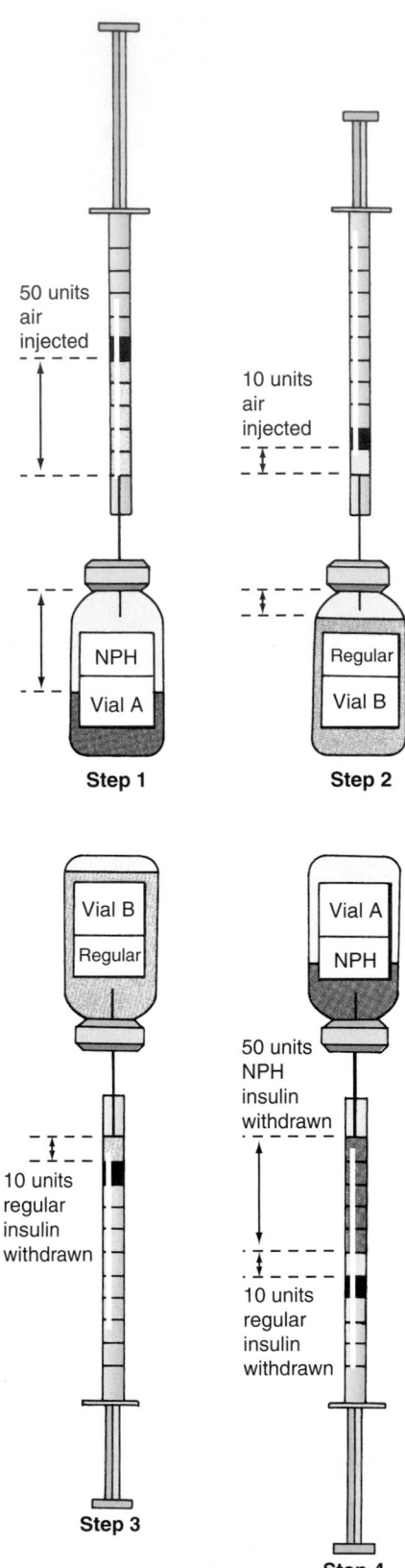

50 units
air
injected

10 units
air
injected

NPH

Vial A

Regular

Vial B

Step 1

Step 2

Vial B

Regular

Vial A

NPH

10 units
regular
insulin
withdrawn

50 units
NPH
insulin
withdrawn

10 units
regular
insulin
withdrawn

Step 3

Step 4

FIGURE 29-6 Mixing medications in one syringe.

stopper is deployed and the actovial is gently agitated to mix the diluent and powder.

Administering Medications Intradermally

The intradermal route has the longest absorption time of all parenteral routes. For this reason, intradermal injections are used for diagnostic purposes, such as the tuberculin test and tests to determine sensitivity to various substances. The advantage of the intradermal route for these tests is that the body's reaction to substances is easily visible, and degrees of reaction are discernible by comparative study.

Intradermal injections are placed just below the epidermis. Sites commonly used are the inner surface of the forearm, the dorsal aspect of the upper arm, and the upper back. Equipment used for an intradermal injection includes a tuberculin syringe calibrated in tenths and hundredths of a milliliter. A ¼″ to ½″ (0.6 to 1.3 cm), 26- or 27-gauge needle is used. The dosage given intradermally is small, usually less than 0.5 mL. Skill 29-5 shows how to administer an intradermal injection.

Administering Medications Subcutaneously

Subcutaneous tissue lies between the epidermis and the muscle. Because there is subcutaneous tissue all over the body, various sites are used for **subcutaneous injections.** These sites are the outer aspect of the upper arm, the abdomen (from below the costal margin to the iliac crests), the anterior aspects of the thigh, the upper back, and the upper ventral or dorsogluteal area. Figure 29-7 shows the sites on the body where subcutaneous injections can be given. This route is used to administer insulin, heparin, and certain immunizations.

Equipment used for a subcutaneous injection depends on the medication to be given. For instance, insulin is prepared with an insulin syringe. Heparin is prepared with a tuberculin syringe or supplied in a prefilled cartridge. A 5/16″ to 1″, 25- to 30-gauge needle is used for this route. Ordinarily, no more than 1 mL of solution is given subcutaneously. Giving larger amounts adds to the patient's discomfort and may predispose to poor absorption.

The skin is cleaned for a subcutaneous injection in the same manner as for an intradermal injection. Research has questioned the need to clean the skin with an alcohol prep before an insulin injection. The combination of a small-gauge needle that limits the number of bacteria that can pass through it and bacteriostatic additives in insulin preparations makes skin preparation before an insulin injection unnecessary, but this cleansing is still commonly performed.

Choose the angle of needle insertion based on the amount of subcutaneous tissue present and the length of the needle. In most cases, a 5/8″ needle is inserted at a 45-degree angle and a ½″ needle is inserted at a 90-degree angle. The patient's size may also determine the angle of needle insertion. For a thin patient, it is best to bunch the skin to create a skin fold and insert the needle at a 45-degree angle. The risk for injecting a

Mixing Insulins in One Syringe

EQUIPMENT

Two vials of insulin
Sterile insulin syringe with 25 to 31-gauge
   needle

Medication Kardex or computer-
   generated MAR

Alcohol swabs

ACTION	RATIONALE
1. Gather equipment. Check medication order against the original physician's order according to agency policy.	This comparison helps to identify errors that may have occurred when orders were transcribed. The nurse must verify the type of insulin that has been prescribed. "Clear" and "cloudy" cannot safely be used to designate types of insulin.
2. Perform hand hygiene.	Hand hygiene deters the spread of microorganisms.
3. If necessary, remove the metal cap that protects the rubber stopper on each vial.	The metal cap prevents contamination of the rubber top.
4. If insulin is a suspension (NPH, Lente), roll and agitate the vial to mix it well.	There is some controversy regarding how to mix NPH insulin properly. Some say to roll the vial; others say to shake the vial. Regardless of the method used, the suspension must be mixed well to avoid administering an inconsistent dose. Regular insulin or clear insulin does not need to be mixed before withdrawal.
5. Cleanse the rubber tops with alcohol swabs.	It is questionable whether cleaning with alcohol actually disinfects or, instead, transfers resident bacteria from the hands to another surface. Because it is difficult in a healthcare facility to keep an insulin vial in its original box as recommended, cleansing with alcohol will most likely continue.
6. Remove the cap from the needle. Inject air into the modified insulin preparation (eg, NPH insulin). Touch the plunger at the knob only. Use an amount of air equal to the amount of medication to be withdrawn. Do not allow the needle to touch the medication in the vial. Remove the needle.	Regular, or short-acting, insulin should never be contaminated with NPH or any insulin modified with added protein. Placing air in the NPH insulin first without allowing the needle to contact the insulin ensures that regular insulin is not contaminated with the additional protein in the NPH. Handling the plunger by the knob only ensures the sterility of the plunger shaft.
7. Inject air into the regular insulin without additional protein. Use an amount of air equal to the amount of medication to be withdrawn.	An equal amount of air must be injected into the vacuum to allow easy withdrawal of medication.
8. Invert the vial of regular insulin and aspirate the amount prescribed. Remove the needle from the vial.	Regular insulin that contains no additional protein is not contaminated by insulin that contains globulin or protamine.
9. Cleanse the rubber top of the modified insulin vial. Insert the needle into this vial, invert it, and withdraw the medication. Carefully replace the cap over the needle.	Previous addition of air eliminates the need to create positive pressure. Capping the needle prevents contamination and protects the nurse against accidental needle sticks. A one-handed recap method may be used as long as care is taken to ensure that the needle remains sterile.
10. Store the vials according to agency recommendations.	Insulin need not be refrigerated but must be protected from temperature extremes.
11. Perform hand hygiene.	Hand hygiene deters the spread of microorganisms.

(continued)

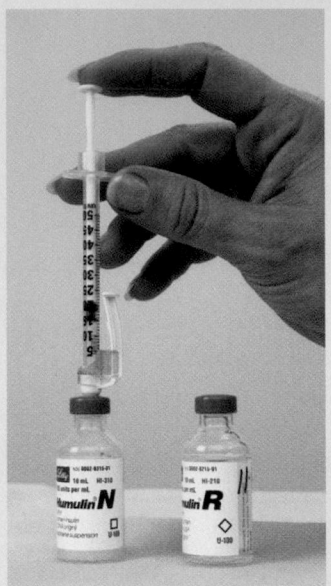

Action 6: Injecting air into modified insulin preparation.   (Photo by Rick Brady.)

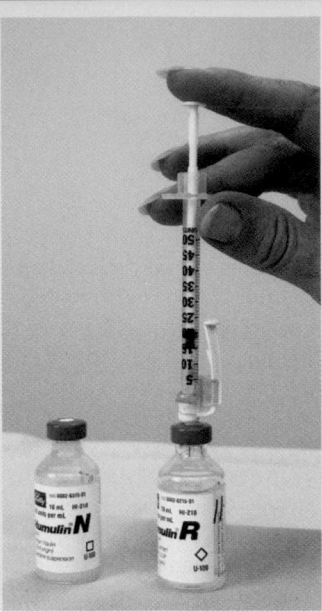

Action 7: Injecting air into clear insulin. (Photo by Rick Brady.)

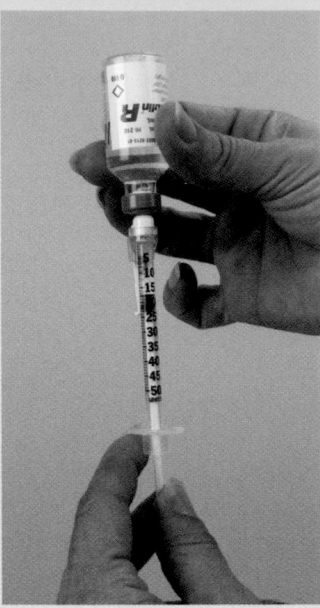

Action 8: Withdrawing clear insulin. (Photo by Rick Brady.)

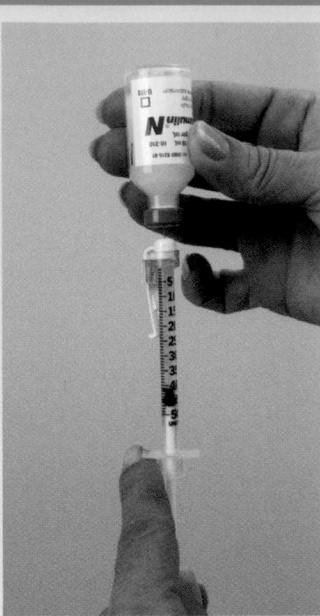

Action 9: Withdrawing modified insulin.   (Photo by Rick Brady.)

Special Considerations

• An insulin-dependent diabetic patient who is visually impaired may find it helpful to use a magnifying apparatus that fits around the syringe.

• An insulin-cartridge pen (the Novalin Pen) is available that allows the patient to dial the correct dose of insulin and press a button to release the dose quickly through a short, fine, 27-gauge needle.

• Before attempting to explain or demonstrate devices to help low-vision diabetic patients to prepare their medication, the nurse should attempt to use the device under similar circumstances. Practice using the aid with eyes closed or in a poorly lit room to detect any difficulties the patient may experience.

medication intramuscularly is lower for a heavier person, and a 90-degree angle may be used. Because the needle used for insulin injections is thinner (30 gauge) and shorter (5/16″), the angle of needle insertion is less important. It is unlikely, even in a thin person, that this smaller needle will reach muscle tissue.

Heparin is also administered subcutaneously; the abdomen is the most commonly used site. The area 2″ around the umbilicus and the belt line must be avoided. The manufacturer's directions for subcutaneous administration of low-molecular-weight heparin preparations (eg, Lovenox) include specific instructions to pinch the tissue gently and insert the needle at a 90-degree angle into a fat pad on either side of the abdomen. Aspiration or pulling back on the plunger is not recommended with administration of heparin because this action can result in hematoma formation. Aspiration after an insulin

injection is also unnecessary and has not proved to be a reliable indicator of needle placement. For a subcutaneous injection, the site is gently massaged after the medication has been given, except in the case of heparin and insulin, because massaging the site can increase the rate of absorption of these agents.

It is necessary to rotate sites or areas for injection if the patient is to receive frequent injections. This helps to prevent buildup of fibrous tissue and permits complete absorption of the medication. Insulin is absorbed most quickly in the abdomen, followed by the arms, thighs, and buttocks. It is recommended that patients administering their own insulin use the same area of the body at the same time every day to ensure more consistent absorption (Fleming, 1999). For instance, every morning the patient may use the abdomen for insulin injection and every evening before dinner the patient may inject

Administering an Intradermal Injection

EQUIPMENT

Medication
Alcohol swab
Disposable gloves
Medication Kardex or computer-
  generated MAR

Sterile syringe and needle (25- to
  27-gauge, ¼″ to ⅝″ long)

Acetone and 2″ × 2″ sterile gauze square
  (optional)

ACTION	RATIONALE
1. Assemble equipment and check the physician's order.	This ensures that the patient receives the right medication at the right time by the proper route. Many intradermal drugs are potent allergens and may cause a significant reaction if given in an incorrect dose.
2. Explain the procedure to the patient.	Explanation encourages cooperation and reduces apprehension.
3. Perform hand hygiene. Don disposable gloves.	Hand hygiene deters the spread of microorganisms. Gloves act as a barrier and protect the nurse's hands from accidental exposure to blood during the injection procedure.
4. If necessary, withdraw medication from an ampule or vial as described in Skills 29-2 and 29-3.	
5. Select an area on the inner aspect of the forearm that is not heavily pigmented or covered with hair. The upper chest and upper back beneath the scapulae also are sites for intradermal injections.	The forearm is a convenient and easy location for introducing an agent intradermally. Hair or lesions at the injection site may interfere with assessments of skin changes at the site.
6. Cleanse the area with an alcohol swab while wiping with a firm, circular motion and moving outward from the injection site. Allow the skin to dry. If the skin is oily, clean the area with a pledget moistened with acetone.	Pathogens on the skin can be forced into the tissues by the needle. Introducing alcohol into tissues irritates the tissues and is uncomfortable for the patient. Acetone is effective for removing oily substances from the skin.
7. Remove the needle cap with the nondominant hand by pulling it straight off.	The cap protects the needle from contact with microorganisms. This technique lessens the risk of an accidental needlestick.
8. Use the nondominant hand to spread the skin taut over the injection site.	Taut skin provides for an easy entrance into intradermal tissue.
9. Place the needle almost flat against the patient's skin, bevel side up, and insert the needle into the skin so that the point of the needle can be seen through the skin. Insert the needle only about ⅛″.	Intradermal tissue is entered when the needle is held as nearly parallel to the skin as possible and is inserted about ⅛″.

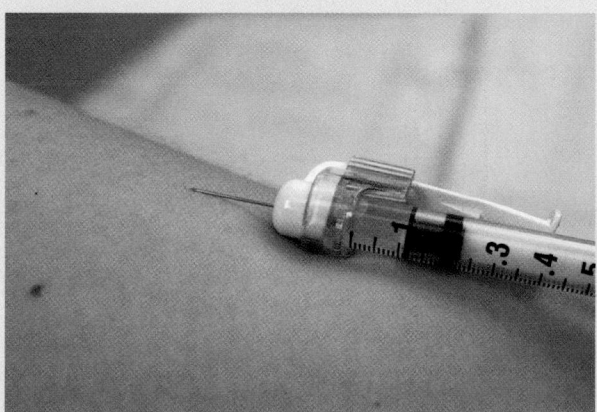

Action 9: Inserting the needle almost level with the skin.
(Photo by Rick Brady.)

| 10. Slowly inject the agent while watching for a small wheal or blister to appear. If none appears, withdraw the needle slightly. | If a small wheal or blister appears, the agent is in the intradermal tissue. |

(continued)

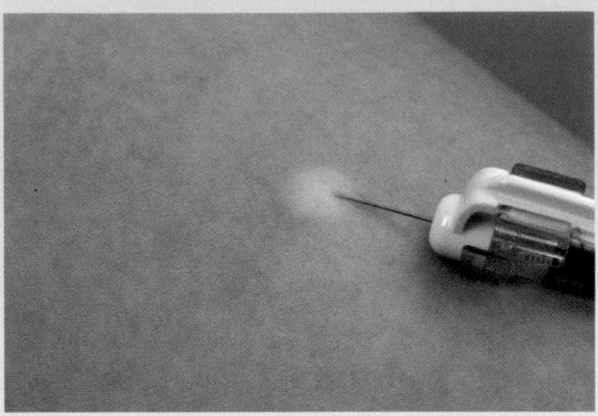

Action 10: Observing for wheal while injecting medication.
(Photo by Rick Brady.)

ACTION	RATIONALE
11. Withdraw the needle quickly at the same angle that it was inserted.	Withdrawing the needle quickly and at the angle at which it entered the skin minimizes tissue damage and discomfort for the patient.
12. Do not massage the area after removing the needle.	Massaging area may interfere with test results by spreading medication to underlying subcutaneous tissue.
13. Do not recap the used needle. Discard the needle and syringe in the appropriate receptacle.	Proper needle disposal protects nurse from accidental injection. Most accidental puncture wounds occur when recapping needles.
14. Assist the patient to a position of comfort.	This provides for the well-being of the patient.
15. Remove gloves and dispose of them properly. Perform hand hygiene.	Hand hygiene deters the spread of microorganisms.
16. Chart the administration of the medication as well as the site of administration. Charting may be documented on the CMAR, including location. Some agencies recommend circling the injection site with ink.	Accurate documentation is necessary to prevent medication error. Circling the injection site allows for easy identification of the injection site and permits careful observation of the exact area.

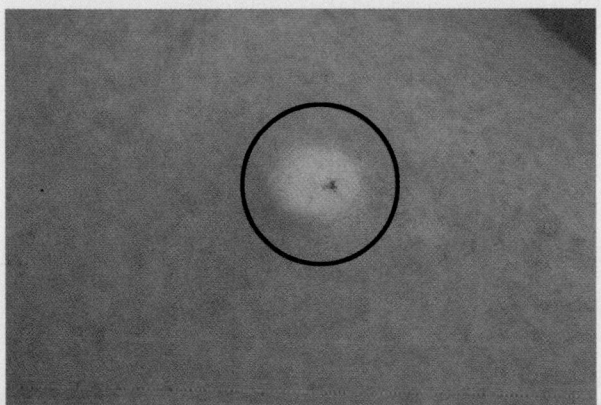

Action 16: Drawing a circle around wheal on skin.   (Photo by Rick Brady.)

| 17. Observe area for a reaction at ordered intervals, usually at 24- to 72-hour periods. Inform the patient of inspection. | With many intradermal injections, the nurse will need to look for a localized reaction (after a period of time) in area of injection. |

Special Considerations

- Since the needle is entering only the dermal portion of tissue, where there are no large blood vessels, aspiration (pulling back on the plunger) is not recommended for an intradermal injection.

- Some agencies recommend administering intradermal injections with the bevel down versus the bevel up.

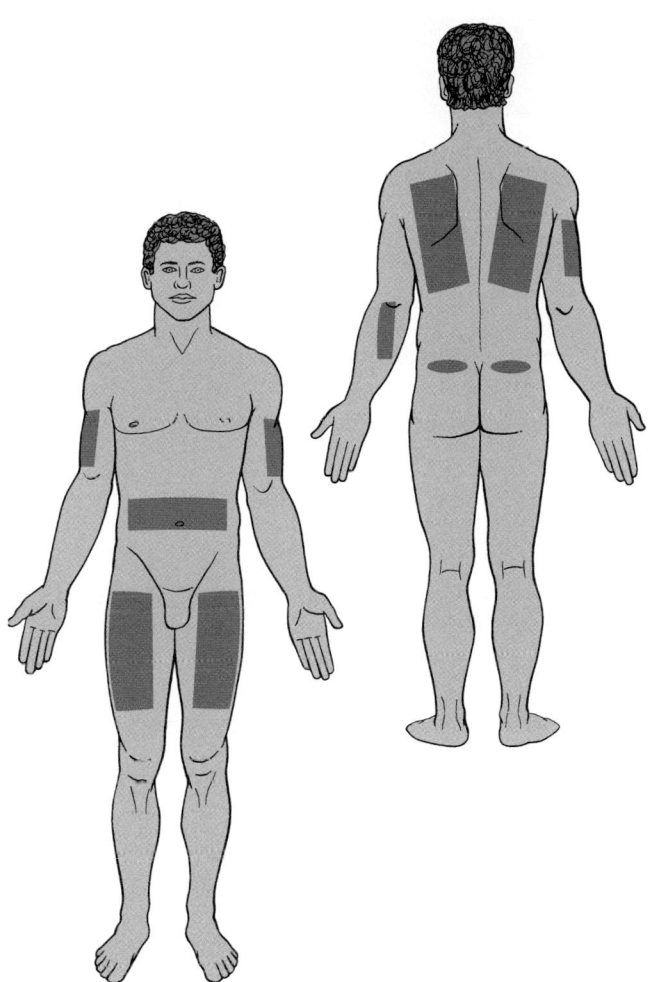

FIGURE 29-7 Sites on the body where subcutaneous injections can be given.

the insulin into the arms or thighs. In each case, the injections should be given an inch away from the previous injection site so that the same area will not be used again in the same month. A small spot bandage or piece of tape can be used to mark the first injection site, with subsequent injections rotated in a circle around that site. After this area has been used, an adjacent site, an inch away, can be selected, using the same rotation format. A marked diagram incorporated into the patient's plan of care is also helpful for noting alternative sites. Do not rely on memory: not even the patient can always recall the site of the previous injection, so the site of administration is recorded in the patient's record.

Skill 29-6 shows the procedure for administering medications subcutaneously. Techniques for reducing discomfort in subcutaneous administrations are listed after the section on Administering Medications Intramuscularly.

Some medications, such as insulin and terbutaline, may be administered continuously via the subcutaneous route. Figure 29-8 shows a patient wearing an insulin pump. A subcutaneous infusion of terbutaline can be used to stop preterm labor. Advantages include the longer rate of absorption via the subcutaneous route and convenience for the patient.

Administering Medications Intramuscularly

The intramuscular route is often used to administer drugs that are irritating, because there are few nerve endings in deep muscle tissue. If a sore or inflamed muscle is entered, however, the muscle may act as a trigger area, and severe referred pain often results. It is best to palpate a muscle before injection. Select a site that does not feel tender to the patient and where the tissue does not contract and become firm and tense.

Absorption occurs as in subcutaneous administration but more rapidly because of the greater vascularity of muscle tissue. Five milliliters is considered the maximum to be given in one site for an adult with well-developed muscles, although the patient's size and the site used (eg, deltoid muscle) may require a smaller amount (Nicoll & Hesby, 2002).

Intramuscular Injection Sites

An important part of administering an **intramuscular injection** is the selection of a safe site away from large nerves, bones, and blood vessels (Fig. 29-9). If care is not taken, common complications include abscesses, necrosis and skin slough, nerve injuries, lingering pain, and periostitis (inflammation of the membrane covering a bone).

The sites for injecting intramuscular medications should be rotated when therapy requires repeated injections. The sites described in this chapter may all be used on a rotating basis. Whatever pattern of rotating sites is used, a description of it should appear in the patient's plan of nursing care.

Ventrogluteal Site. The ventrogluteal site (see Fig. 29-9A) involves the gluteus medius and gluteus minimus muscles in the hip area. The ventrogluteal site is recommended for both adults and children older than 7 months of age as a safe site for most intramuscular injections: there are no large nerves or blood vessels in the injection area, the site is removed from bone tissue, the area is clean (fecal contamination is rare at this site), and the patient can be on the back, abdomen, or side for the injection. To relax the gluteal muscle, the patient may flex the knees while lying on the back, point the toes inward while lying in the prone position, and flex the upper leg in front of the lower leg in the side-lying position. Although any of the three positions just described may be used when injecting the ventrogluteal site, nurses increasingly prefer the side-lying position.

To locate the ventrogluteal site, place the palm of your hand over the greater trochanter, with your fingers facing the patient's head. The right hand is used for the patient's left hip, or the left hand for the right hip, to identify landmarks. The index finger is placed on the anterosuperior iliac spine and the middle finger extends dorsally, palpating the crest of the ilium. A triangle is formed, and the injection is given in the center of the triangle.

Vastus Lateralis Site. The vastus lateralis muscle is recommended frequently for the injection of medications if the ventrogluteal site cannot be used (see Fig. 29-9B). It is a thick muscle, and there is little or no danger of serious injury. There are no large nerves or vessels in its proximity, and it does not cover a joint. The muscle covers the anterolateral aspect of the thigh. It is bounded by the midanterior thigh on the front of the

(text continues on page 742)

Administering a Subcutaneous Injection

EQUIPMENT

Medication
Alcohol swabs
Disposable gloves

Medication Kardex or computer-generated
MAR

Sterile syringe and needle (size depends on
medication being administered and patient)

ACTION	RATIONALE
1. Assemble equipment and check the physician's order.	This ensures that the patient receives the right medication at the right time by the proper route.
2. Explain the procedure to the patient.	An explanation encourages patient cooperation and reduces apprehension.
3. Perform hand hygiene.	Hand hygiene deters the spread of microorganisms.
4. If necessary, withdraw medication from an ampule or vial as described in Skills 29-2 and 29-3.	
5. Identify the patient carefully. Check the identification band on the patient's wrist and ask the patient his or her name. Close the curtain to provide privacy. Don disposable gloves.	It is the nurse's responsibility to guard against error. Gloves act as a barrier and protect the nurse's hands from accidental exposure to blood during the injection procedure.

6. Have the patient assume a position appropriate for the most commonly used sites.
  a. Outer aspect of upper arm: The patient's arm should be relaxed and at the side of the body.
  b. Anterior thighs: The patient may sit or lie with the leg relaxed.
  c. Abdomen: The patient may lie in a semirecumbent position.
	Injection into a tense extremity causes discomfort.

7. Locate the site of choice according to the directions given in this chapter. Ensure that the area is not tender and is free of lumps or nodules.	Good visualization is necessary to establish the correct location of the site and avoid damage to tissues. Nodules or lumps may indicate a previous injection site where absorption was inadequate.
8. Clean the area around the injection site with an alcohol swab. Use a firm, circular motion while moving outward from the injection site. Allow the antiseptic to dry. Leave the alcohol swab in a clean area for reuse when withdrawing the needle.	Friction helps to clean the skin. A clean area is contaminated when a soiled object is rubbed over its surface.

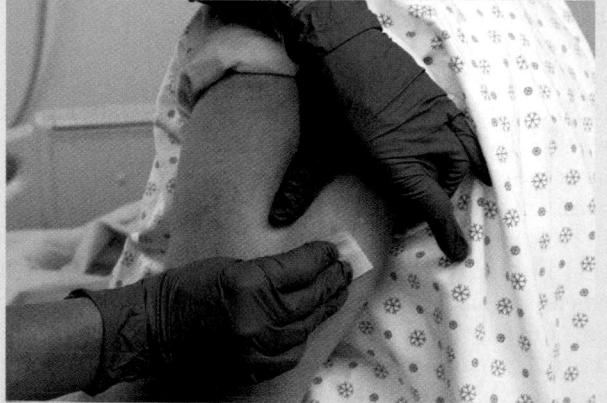

Action 8: Cleaning injection site.   (Photo by Rick Brady.)

ACTION	RATIONALE
9. Remove the needle cap with the nondominant hand, pulling it straight off.	The cap protects the needle from contact with microorganisms. This technique lessens the risk of an accidental needlestick.
10. Grasp and bunch the area surrounding the injection site or spread the skin at the site.	This provides for easy, less painful entry into the subcutaneous tissue. The decision to pinch or spread tissue at the injection site depends on the size of the patient. If the patient is thin, skin needs to be bunched to create a skin fold.

(continued)

SKILL
29-6   **Administering a Subcutaneous Injection** (continued)

ACTION	RATIONALE

11. Hold the syringe in the dominant hand between the thumb and forefinger. Inject the needle quickly at an angle at 45 to 90 degrees, depending on the amount and turgor of the tissue and the length of the needle.

Inserting the needle quickly causes less pain. Subcutaneous tissue is abundant in well-nourished, well-hydrated people and spare in emaciated, dehydrated, or very thin persons. For a thin person, it is best to insert the needle at a 45-degree angle.

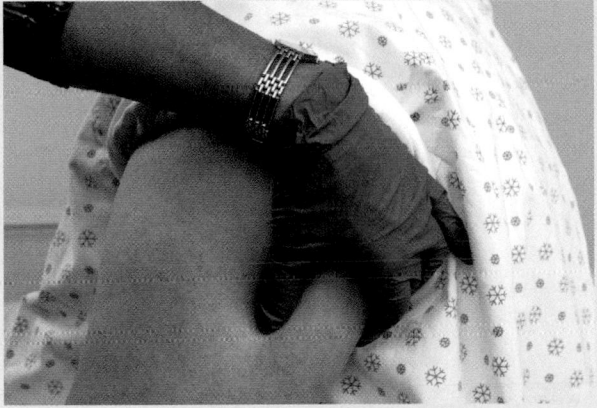

Action 10: Bunching tissue around injection site.   (Photo by Rick Brady.)

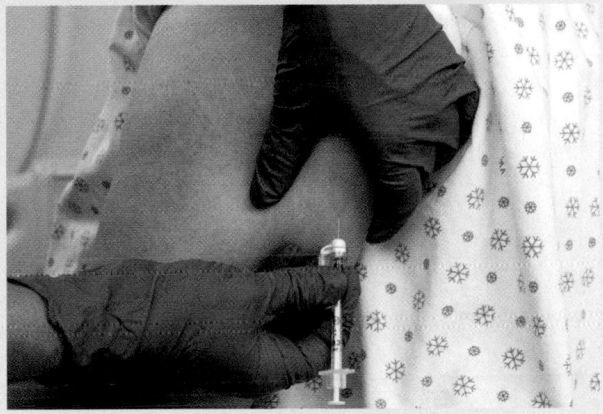

Action 11: Inserting needle.   (Photo by Rick Brady.)

12. After the needle is in place, release the tissue. If you have a large skin fold pinched up, ensure that the needle stays in place as the skin is released. Immediately move your nondominant hand to steady the lower end of the syringe. Slide your dominant hand to the tip of the barrel.

Injecting the solution into compressed tissues results in pressure against nerve fibers and creates discomfort. If there is a large skin fold, the skin may retract away from the needle. The nondominant hand secures the syringe and allows for smooth aspiration.

13. Aspirate, if recommended, by pulling back gently on the plunger of the syringe to determine whether the needle is in a blood vessel. If blood appears, the needle should be withdrawn, the medication syringe and needle discarded, and a new syringe with new medication prepared. Do not aspirate when giving insulin or any form of heparin.

Discomfort and possibly a serious reaction may occur if a drug intended for subcutaneous use is injected into a vein. Heparin is an anticoagulant, and bruising may be produced if the nurse aspirates during injection. Because the insulin needle is so small, aspiration after insulin has proved unreliable in predicting needle placement.

14. If no blood appears, inject the solution slowly.

Rapid injection of the solution creates pressure in the tissues, resulting in discomfort.

15. Withdraw the needle quickly at the same angle at which it was inserted.

Slow withdrawal of the needle pulls the tissues and causes discomfort. Applying countertraction around the injection site helps to prevent pulling on the tissue as the needle is withdrawn. Removing the needle at the same angle at which it was inserted minimizes tissue damage and discomfort.

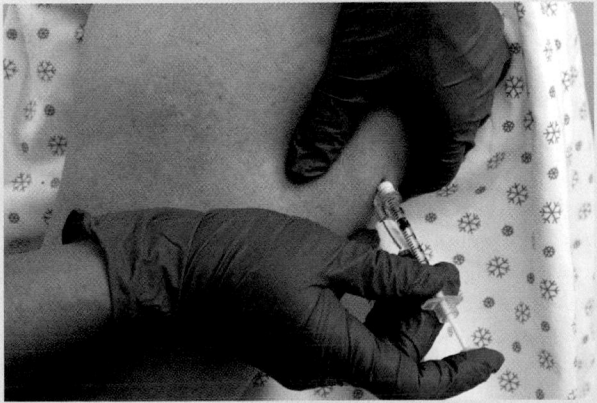

Action 14: Injecting medication.   (Photo by Rick Brady.)

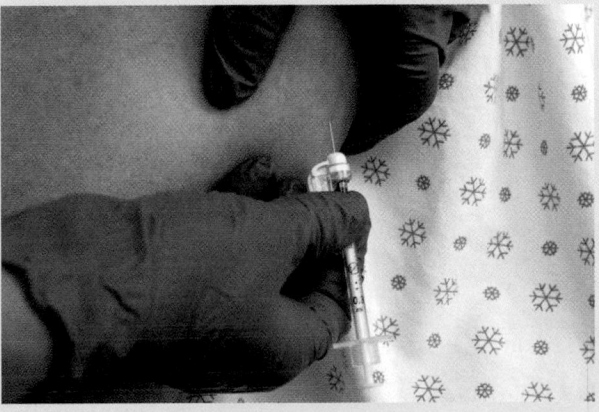

Action 15: Withdrawing needle.   (Photo by Rick Brady.)

(continued)

SKILL 29-6 Administering a Subcutaneous Injection (continued)

ACTION	RATIONALE
16. Massage the area gently with the alcohol swab. Do not massage a subcutaneous heparin or insulin injection site. Apply a small bandage if needed.	Massaging helps to distribute the solution and hastens its absorption Massaging the site of a heparin injection causes additional bruising. Massaging after an insulin injection may contribute to unpredictable absorption of the medication.
17. Do not recap the used needle. Discard the needle and syringe in the appropriate receptacle.	Proper disposal of the needle protects the nurse from accidental injection. Most accidental needle sticks occur when recapping needles.
18. Assist the patient to a position of comfort.	This provides for the well-being of the patient.
19. Remove gloves and dispose of them properly. Perform hand hygiene.	Hand hygiene deters the spread of microorganisms.
20. Chart the administration of the medication, including the site of administration. This charting can be done on the CMAR.	Accurate documentation is necessary to prevent medication error.
21. Evaluate the patient's response to the medication within an appropriate time frame.	Reaction to medication given by the parenteral route may occur within 15 to 30 minutes after injection.

Infant and Child Considerations

Do not tell a child that an injection will not hurt. You can describe the feel of the injection as a pinch. Assure the child that it will hurt for only a short time. A child who believes you have been dishonest with him or her is less likely to cooperate with future procedures.

Older Adult Considerations

Many elderly patients have less adipose tissue, so adjust the angle of the needle accordingly; you do not want to inadvertently give a subcutaneous medication intramuscularly.

Home Care Considerations

According to the American Diabetes Association, reuse of insulin syringes in the home setting appears safe. Once the needle is dull, it should be discarded (usually after 2 to 10 uses).

---

leg and the midlateral thigh on the side. The thigh is divided into thirds horizontally and vertically, and the injection is given in the outer middle third. This space provides a large number of injection sites. The vastus lateralis site is particularly desirable for infants and children, whose gluteal muscles are poorly developed. The vastus lateralis can be accessed easily while restraining an infant by placing the child's knees at the end of

the examination table or bed and leaning against the infant's lower leg (Fig. 29-10).

Deltoid Muscle Site. The deltoid muscle is located in the lateral aspect of the upper arm (see Fig. 29-9C). It is not often used because it is a small muscle and is not capable of absorbing large amounts of solution. Damage to the radial nerve and artery is a risk of the deltoid site. Intramuscular injections into the deltoid muscle should be limited to 1 mL of solution and given only for adults. The deltoid muscle is not developed enough in infants and children to absorb medication adequately.

The deltoid muscle can be located by palpating the lower edge of the acromion process. A triangle is formed at the midpoint in line with the axilla on the lateral aspect of the upper arm. Hepatitis B virus vaccine is one medication that should be given in the deltoid muscle in adults to induce adequate levels of the antibody.

Dorsogluteal Site. The dorsogluteal site (see Fig. 29-9D), located in the buttock, has been a common site for administering intramuscular injections. However, because of the potential for injury to the sciatic nerve and the presence of major blood vessels and bone mass near the site, the dorsogluteal muscle is not recommended. Therefore, refer to your institutional policy when considering the dorsogluteal site. The posterosuperior

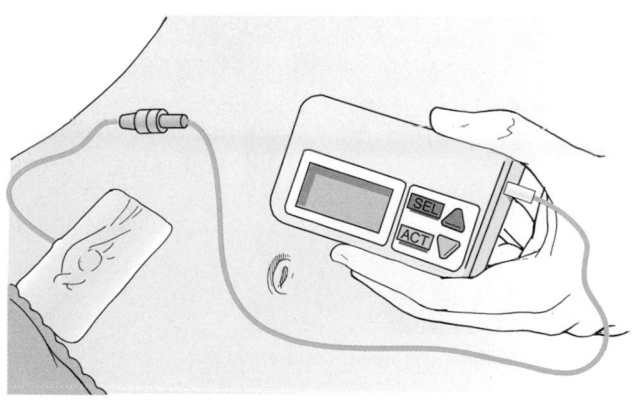

FIGURE 29-8 Patient wearing insulin pump.

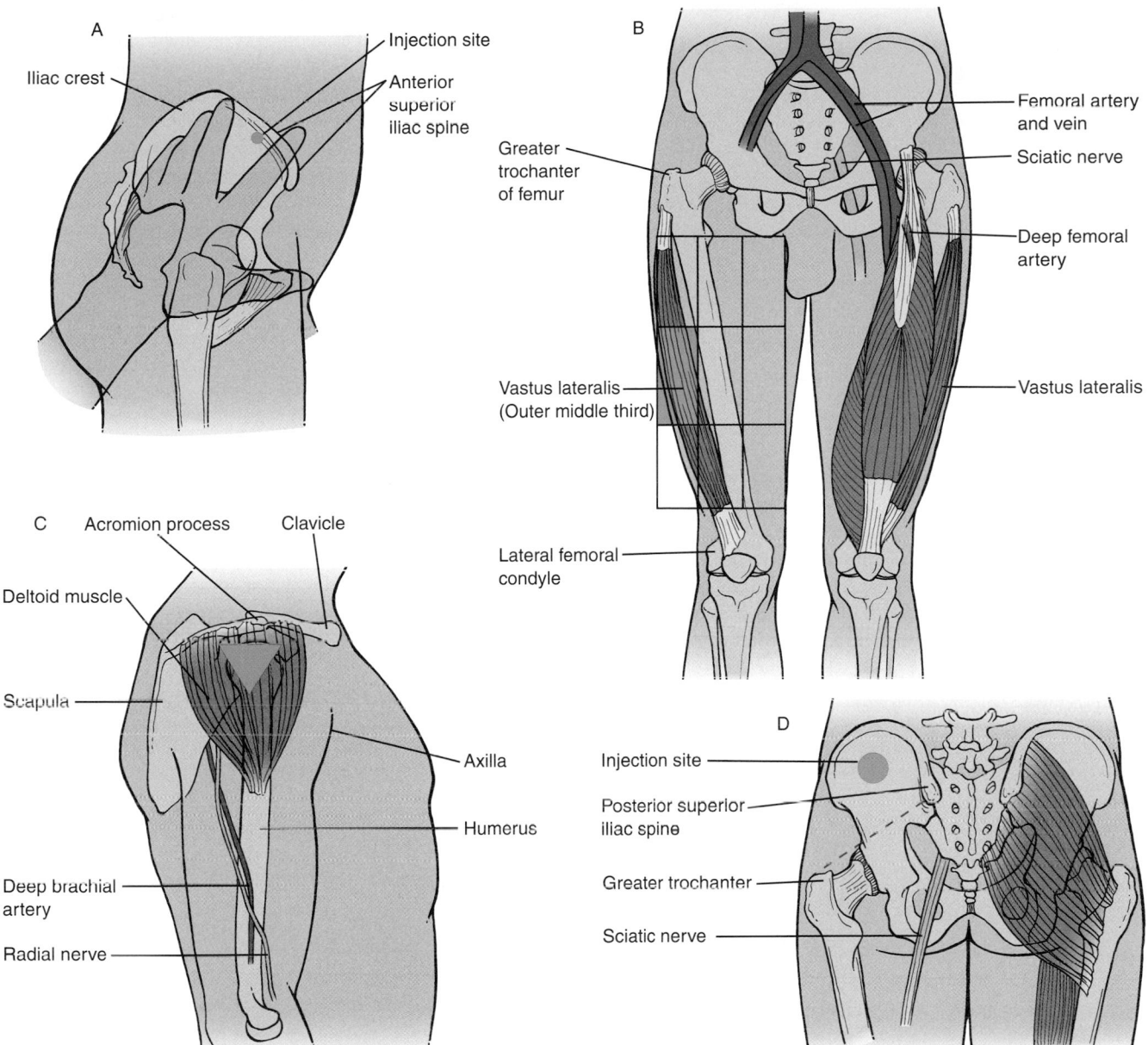

FIGURE 29-9 Sites for intramuscular injections. Descriptions for locating the sites are given in the text. (**A**) The ventrogluteal site is located by placing the palm on the greater trochanter and the index finger toward the anterosuperior iliac spine. (**B**) The vastus lateralis site is identified by dividing the thigh into thirds, horizontally and vertically. (**C**) The deltoid muscle site is located by palpating the lower edge of the acromion process. (**D**) The dorsogluteal site is lateral and slightly superior to the midpoint of a line drawn from the trochanter to the posterior superior iliac spine.

iliac spine and the greater trochanter represent the anatomic landmarks. An imaginary line is drawn between the posterosuperior iliac spine and the greater trochanter. The injection site is lateral and slightly superior to the midpoint of the line. Walking develops the gluteal muscles; therefore, the dorsogluteal site should not be used for children younger than 3 years of age because their gluteal muscles are too small.

Good visualization of the entire area and careful mapping are necessary to locate the proper site. This necessitates adequate exposure by lowering the undergarments; merely raising one side of the underclothing permits only a partial vi-sualization of the area. The patient should be in a prone position with the toes pointed inward, or in the side-lying position with the upper knee flexed and the upper leg in front of the lower leg. These positions promote maximum muscle relaxation and, therefore, minimum discomfort. This site should not be used with the patient in a standing position because the gluteus muscle is tense.

Intramuscular Injection Procedure

No more than 5 mL should be injected into a single site for an adult with well-developed muscles. The less-developed mus-

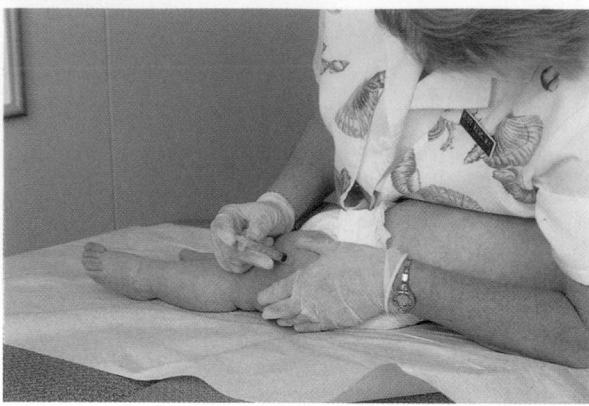

FIGURE 29-10 Nurse restraining infant for intramuscular injection into the vastus lateralis.

cles of children and elderly people limit the intramuscular injection to 1 to 2 mL. The needle should enter the skin between 72 and 90 degrees (Katsma & Katsma, 2000). Equipment commonly used for an intramuscular injection includes a 1.5″ (3.8 cm), 21- to 23-gauge needle. The needle length should be selected with care. Prepackaged, loaded syringes usually have a needle that is 1″ long. If there is any question about whether the belly of the target muscle can be reached, the medication should be transferred to another syringe with the appropriate needle size. A short needle does not minimize discomfort, and a longer one does not increase discomfort. The patient's anatomy should dictate the needle length chosen. The most important consideration is to use a needle with a tip that will reach deep into the muscle.

The addition of an air bubble to the syringe is unnecessary and potentially dangerous because it could result in an overdose of medication. Disposable syringes are calibrated to deliver a correct dose without the use of an air bubble, with the exception of Lovenox. The technique for administering an intramuscular injection is outlined in Skill 29-7. Figure 29-11 compares the angles for needle insertion for different forms of injections.

Z-Track Technique

Any intramuscular injection may be given using the **Z-track** technique. This method prevents seepage of the medication into the needle track and reduces pain and discomfort, particularly for patients receiving injections over an extended period. The Z-track method is also suggested for elderly patients who have decreased muscle mass. Some agents, such as iron,

(*text continues on page 747*)

SKILL 29-7   **Administering an Intramuscular Injection**

EQUIPMENT

Medication
Alcohol swab
Dry sponge
Disposable gloves

Medication Kardex or computer-generated MAR

Sterile syringe and needle (size depends on medication being administered and patient)

ACTION	RATIONALE
1. Assemble equipment and check the physician's order.	This ensures that the patient receives the right medication at the right time by the proper route.
2. Explain procedure to patient.	Explanation encourages cooperation and alleviates apprehension.
3. Perform hand hygiene.	Hand hygiene deters the spread of microorganisms.
4. If necessary, withdraw medication from an ampule or vial as described in Skills 29-2 and 29-3.	
5. Do not add air to the syringe.	Adding air to the syringe is potentially dangerous and may result in an overdose of medication.
6. Identify the patient carefully. There are three correct ways to do this: a. Check the name on the patient's identification bracelet. b. Ask the patient his or her name. c. Verify the patient's identification with a staff member who knows the patient.	Identifying the patient is the nurse's responsibility to guard against error. a. This is the most reliable method. Replace the identification band if it is missing or inaccurate in any way. b. This requires an answer from the patient, but illness and strange surroundings often cause patients to be confused. c. This is another way to double-check identity. Do not rely on the name on the door or over the bed, because these may be inaccurate.
7. Provide for privacy. Have the patient assume a position appropriate for the site selected.	Injection into a tense muscle causes discomfort.

(*continued*)

SKILL 29-7 Administering an Intramuscular Injection (continued)

ACTION	RATIONALE

a. Ventrogluteal: The patient may lie on the back or side with the hip and knee flexed.

b. Vastus lateralis: The patient may lie on the back or may assume a sitting position.

c. Deltoid: The patient may sit or lie with arm relaxed.

d. Dorsogluteal: The patient may lie prone with toes pointing inward or on the side with the upper leg flexed and placed in front of the lower leg.

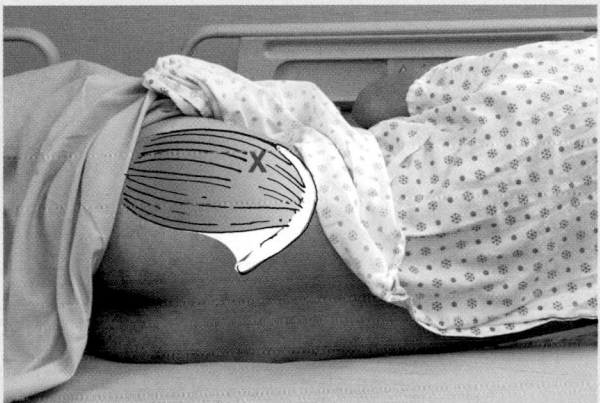

Action 7a: Positioning for ventrogluteal site injection.
(Photo by Rick Brady.)

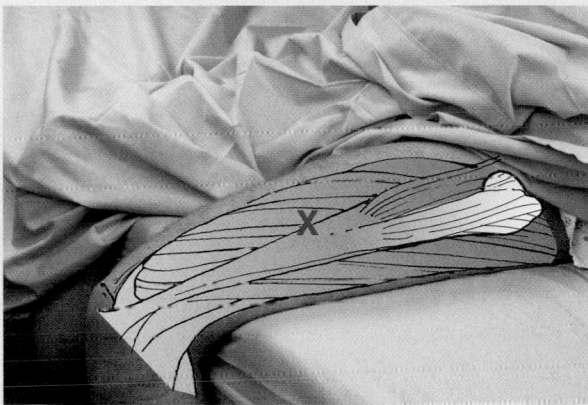

Action 7b: Positioning for vastus lateralis site injection.
(Photo by Rick Brady.)

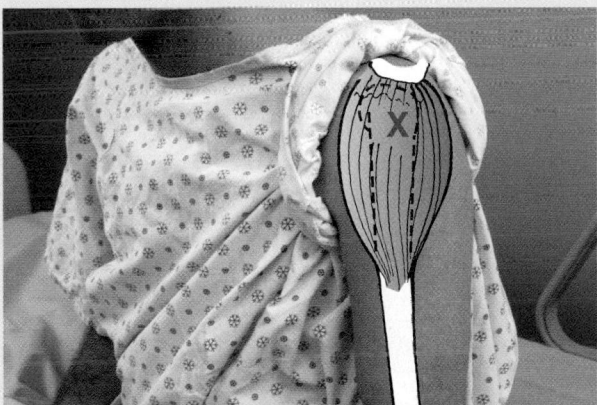

Action 7c: Positioning for deltoid muscle site injection.
(Photo by Rick Brady.)

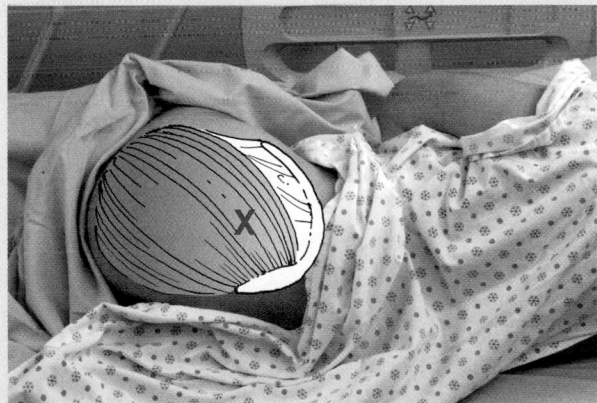

Action 7d: Positioning for dorsogluteal site injection.
(Photo by Rick Brady.)

8. Locate the site of choice according to the directions given in this chapter. Ensure that the area is not tender and is free of lumps or nodules. Don disposable gloves (see Fig. 29-9).

Good visualization is necessary to establish the correct location of the site and avoid damage to tissues. Nodules or lumps may indicate a previous injection site where absorption was inadequate. Gloves act as a barrier and protect the nurse's hands from accidental exposure to blood during the injection procedure.

9. Clean the area thoroughly with an alcohol swab, using friction. Allow alcohol to dry.

Pathogens present on the skin and alcohol can be forced into the tissues by the needle.

10. Remove the needle cap by pulling it straight off.

The cap protects the needle from contact with microorganisms. This technique lessens the risk of an accidental needlestick and also prevents inadvertently unscrewing the needle from the barrel of the syringe.

(continued)

ACTION	RATIONALE
11. Displace the skin in a Z-track manner (see Fig. 29-12) or spread the skin at the site using your nondominant hand.	This makes the tissue taut and minimizes discomfort. Using the Z-track technique prevents the medication from seeping into the needle track and is less painful.

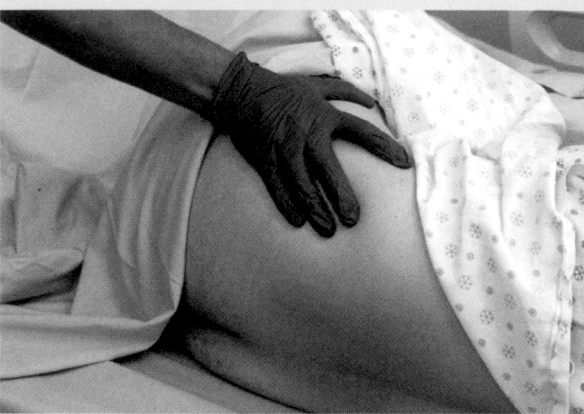

Action 11: Spreading the skin at vastus lateralis site.   (Photo by Rick Brady.)

ACTION	RATIONALE
12. Hold the syringe in your dominant hand between the thumb and forefinger. Quickly dart the needle into the tissue at a 72- to 90-degree angle.	A quick injection is less painful. Inserting the needle at a 72- to 90-degree angle facilitates entry into muscle tissue.
13. As soon as the needle is in place, use your nondominant hand to hold the lower end of the syringe. Slide your dominant hand to the tip of the barrel.	This acts to steady the syringe and allows for smooth aspiration.
14. Aspirate by slowly (for at least 5 seconds) pulling back on the plunger to determine whether the needle is in a blood vessel. If blood is aspirated, discard the needle, syringe, and medication, prepare a new sterile setup, and inject at another site.	Discomfort and possibly a serious reaction may occur if a drug intended for intramuscular use is injected into a vein. Aspirating slowly facilitates backflow of blood even if the needle is in a small, low-flow blood vessel.
15. If no blood is aspirated, inject the solution slowly (10 seconds per mL of medication).	Injecting slowly reduces discomfort by allowing time for the solution to disperse in the tissues.

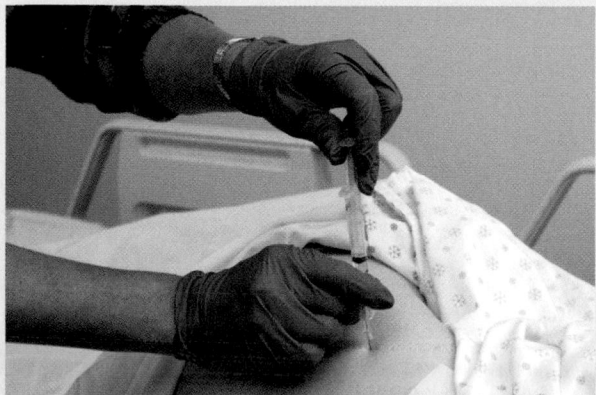

Action 14: Aspirating.   (Photo by Rick Brady.)

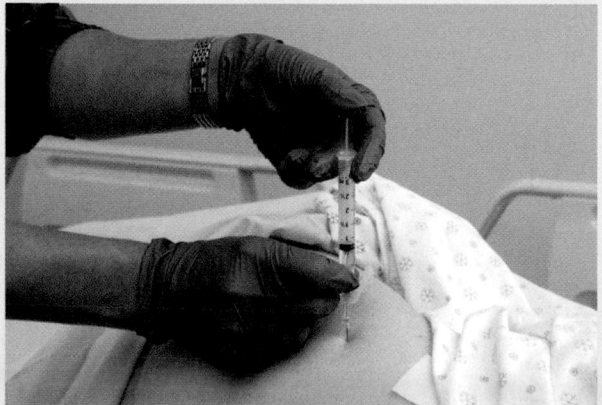

Action 15: Injecting.   (Photo by Rick Brady.)

ACTION	RATIONALE
16. Remove the needle slowly and steadily. Release the displaced tissue if the Z-track technique was used.	Slow withdrawal allows the medication to begin to diffuse through the muscle.
17. Apply gentle pressure at the site with a small, dry sponge.	Light pressure causes less trauma and irritation to the tissues. Massaging can force medication into the subcutaneous tissues.

(continued)

Administering an Intramuscular Injection (continued)

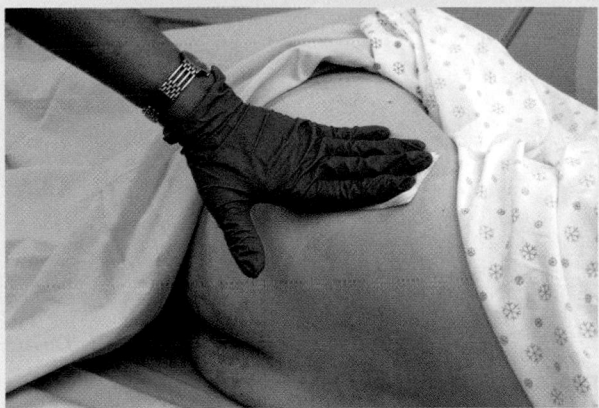

Action 17: Applying pressure at the site.   (Photo by Rick Brady.)

ACTION	RATIONALE
18. Do not recap the used needle. Discard the needle and syringe in the appropriate receptacle.	Proper disposal of the needle protects the nurse from accidental needlestick. Most accidental needle sticks occur when recapping needles.
19. Assist the patient to a position of comfort. Encourage the patient to exercise the extremity used for the injection, if possible.	Exercise promotes absorption of the medication.
20. Remove gloves and dispose of them properly. Perform hand hygiene.	Hand hygiene deters the spread of microorganisms.
21. Chart the administration of the medication, including the site of administration. This may be documented on the CMAR.	Accurate documentation is necessary to prevent medication error.
22. Evaluate the patient's response to the medication within an appropriate time frame. Assess the site, if possible, within 2 to 4 hours after administration.	Reaction to medication given by the parenteral route is a possibility. Assessment of the site detects any untoward effects.

Infant and Child Considerations

Safe injection into an infant's vastus lateralis muscle may require use of a 1″ needle rather than the commonly used ⅝″ needle. A 1″

needle consistently allows penetration into the muscle and safe administration of the medication.

are best given via the Z-track method due to the irritation and discoloration associated with this agent.

In the Z-track technique, a clean needle is attached to the syringe after the syringe is filled with the medication; this prevents the injection of any residual medication on the needle into superficial tissues. The needle should be at least 1.5″ (3.8 cm) long. The ventrogluteal, vastus lateralis, or dorsogluteal site can be used for this procedure. The skin is pulled down or to one side about 1″ (2.5 cm) and held in this position with the left hand (for a right-handed person). The needle is inserted and the nurse aspirates carefully to detect the presence of blood. The medication is injected slowly, the needle is steadily withdrawn, and the displaced tissue is released and allowed to return to its normal position. Massage of the site is not recommended because it may cause

irritation by forcing the medication to leak back into the needle track, but gentle pressure may be applied with a dry sponge.

The procedure for administering a Z-track injection is outlined in Figure 29-12.

Reducing Discomfort in Subcutaneous and Intramuscular Administrations

The following are recommended techniques to reduce discomfort when injecting medications subcutaneously or intramuscularly:

- Select a needle of the smallest gauge that is appropriate for the site and solution to be injected, and select the correct needle length.

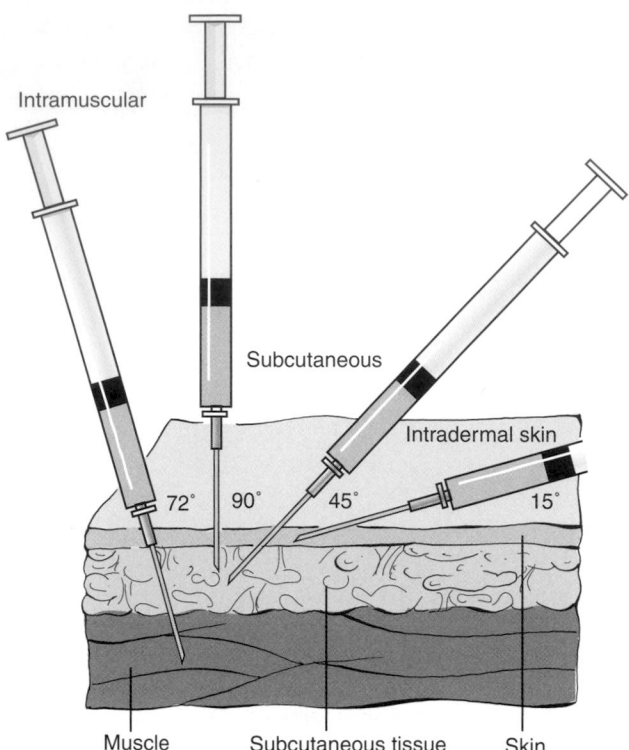

FIGURE 29-11 Comparison of the angles of insertion for intramuscular, subcutaneous, and intradermal injections.

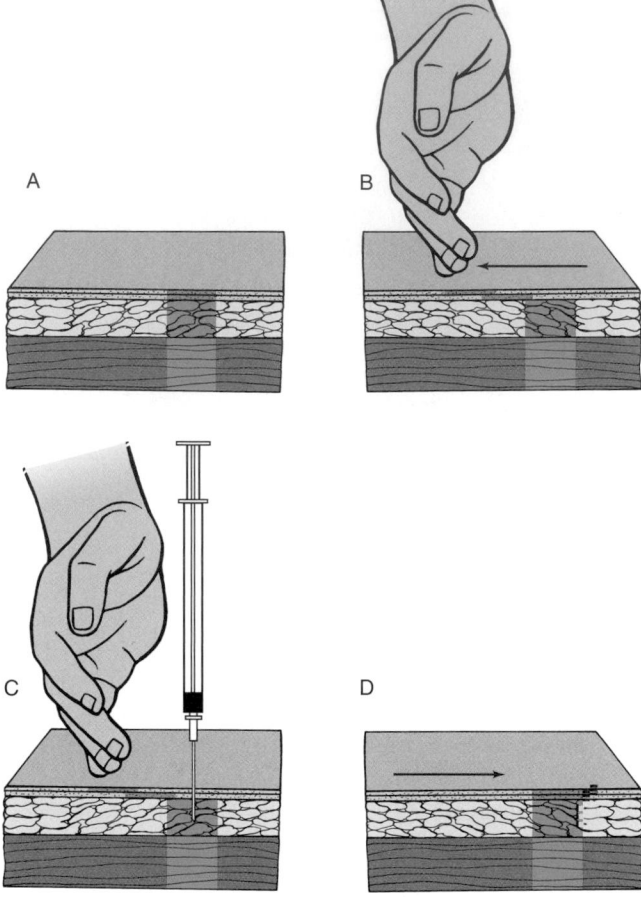

FIGURE 29-12 The Z-track or zigzag technique is recommended for intramuscular injections. (**A**) Normal skin and tissues. (**B**) Moving the skin to one side. (**C**) Needle is inserted at a 90-degree angle, and the nurse aspirates for blood. (**D**) Once the needle is withdrawn, displaced tissue is allowed to return to its normal position, preventing the solution from escaping from the muscle tissue.

- Be sure the needle is free of medication that may irritate superficial tissues as the needle is inserted. Recommended procedure is to use two needles—one to remove the medication from the vial or ampule and a second one to inject the medication. If medication is in a prefilled syringe with a nonremovable needle and has dripped back on the needle during preparation, gently tap the barrel to remove the excess solution.
- Use the Z-track technique for intramuscular injections to prevent leakage of medication into the needle track, thus minimizing discomfort.
- Inject the medication into relaxed muscles. There is more pressure and discomfort when the medication is injected into a contracted muscle.
- Do not inject areas that feel hard on palpation or tender to the patient.
- Insert the needle with a dartlike motion without hesitation, and remove it quickly at the same angle at which it was inserted. These techniques reduce discomfort and tissue irritation.
- Do not administer more solution in one injection than is recommended for the site. Injecting more solution creates excess pressure in the area and increases discomfort.
- Inject the solution slowly so that it may be dispersed more easily into the surrounding tissue (10 seconds per 1 mL).
- Apply gentle pressure after injection, unless this technique is contraindicated.

- Allow the patient who is fearful of injections to talk about his or her fears. Answer the patient's questions truthfully, and explain the nature and purpose of the injection. Taking the time to offer support often allays fears and decreases discomfort.
- Rotate sites when the patient is to receive repeated injections. Injections in the same site may cause undue discomfort, irritation, or abscesses in tissues.
- Determine whether the patient is a candidate for the needless insulin delivery device. This method is pain-free but is more costly than traditional methods.

Administering Medications Intravenously

Medications administered intravenously have an immediate effect. The **intravenous route** is the most dangerous route of administration: because the drug is placed directly into the bloodstream, it cannot be recalled, nor can its actions be slowed. Intravenous administration is the route used in most emergency situations when immediate absorption is required. There also are many nonemergency clinical situations in which drugs are administered intravenously. Patient-controlled analgesia (PCA) allows the patient to control administration of an intravenous analgesic for pain management (see Chap. 41). Skill 46-1 in Chapter 46 describes the basic technique for administering an intravenous infusion. There are several ways to administer medications intravenously.

Medications via Intravenous Solution. Medications may be added to the patient's infusion solution. The recommended procedure is for the pharmacist to add the prescribed drug to a large volume of intravenous solution, but sometimes the drug is added in the nursing unit, in which case sterile technique must be maintained. Steps for adding medications to intravenous solutions are given in Skill 29-8.

SKILL 29-8 Adding Medications to an Intravenous Solution Container

EQUIPMENT
Medication prepared in a syringe with a 19- to 21-gauge needle, blunt needle or needleless device (follow agency policy)

Alcohol swab
Intravenous fluid container (bag or bottle)
Label to be attached to the intravenous container

Medication Kardex or computer-generated MAR

ACTION	RATIONALE
1. Gather all equipment. Check the medication order with the physician's order. Take equipment to patient's bedside.	Checking the orders ensures that the patient receives the correct medication at the correct time and in the right manner. Having equipment available saves time and facilitates performance of the task.
2. Perform hand hygiene.	Hand hygiene deters the spread of microorganisms.
3. Identify the patient by checking the identification band on the patient's wrist and asking the patient his or her name. Check for any allergies that patient may have.	This ensures that the medication is given to the right person.
4. Explain the procedure to the patient.	Explanation allays the patient's anxiety.
5. Add the medications to the intravenous solution that is infusing:	
a. Check that the volume in the bag or bottle is adequate.	a. The volume should be sufficient to dilute the drug.
b. Close the intravenous clamp.	b. This prevents backflow directly to the patient of improperly diluted medication.
c. Clean the medication port with an alcohol swab.	c. This deters entry of microorganisms when the needle punctures the port.
d. Steady the container and uncap the needle or needleless device and insert it into the port. Inject the medication.	d. This ensures that the needle or needleless device enters the container and medication can be dispersed into the solution.
e. Remove the container from the intravenous pole and gently rotate the solutions.	e. This mixes the medication with the solution.
f. Rehang the container, open the clamp, and readjust the flow rate.	f. This ensures the infusion of the intravenous solution with the medication at the prescribed rate.
g. Attach the label to the container so that the dose of medication that has been added is apparent.	g. This confirms that the prescribed dose of medication has been added to the intravenous solution.

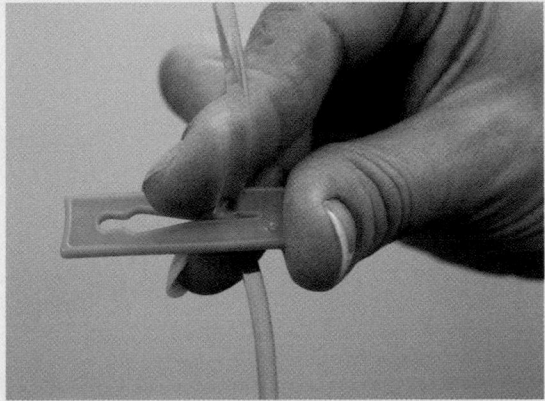

Action 5b: Closing the IV clamp.   (Photo by Rick Brady.)

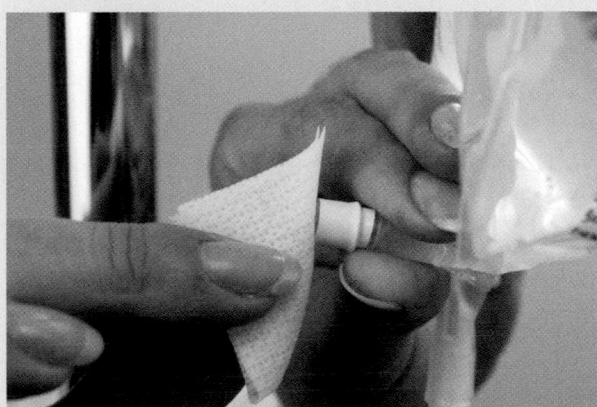

Action 5c: Cleaning the medication port.   (Photo by Rick Brady.)

(continued)

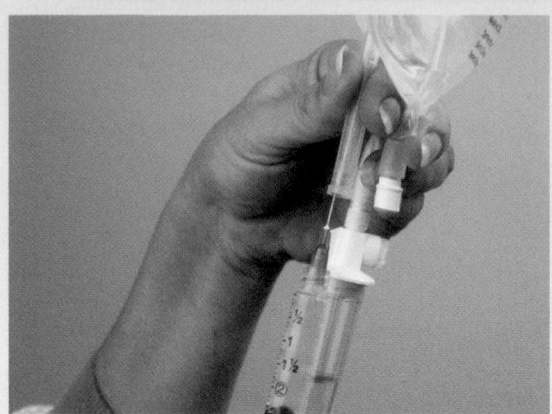

Action 5d: Steadying bag and uncapping needle.
(Photo by Rick Brady.)

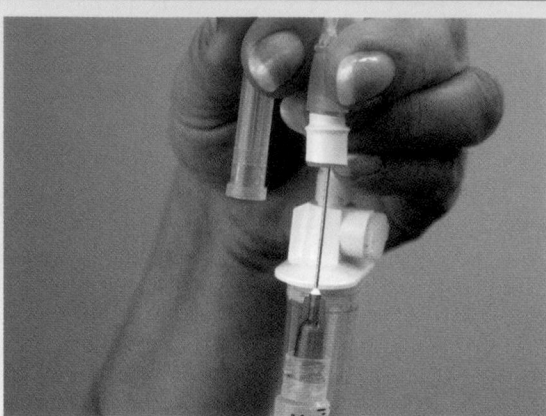

Action 5d: Inserting the needle or needleless device into the port.
(Photo by Rick Brady.)

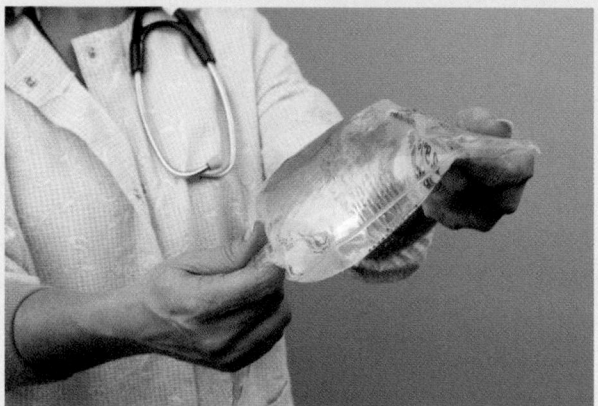

Action 5e: Rotating solution to distribute medication.   (Photo by Rick Brady.)

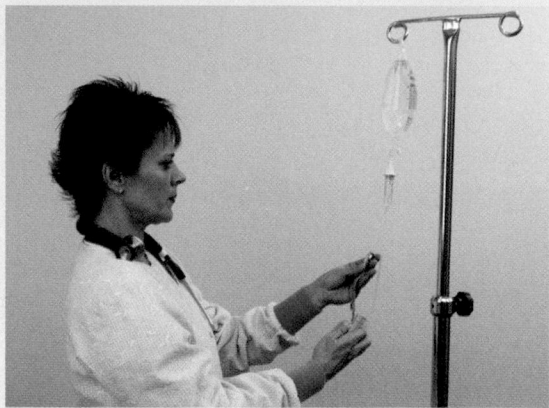

Action 5f: Readjusting flow rate.   (Photo by Rick Brady.)

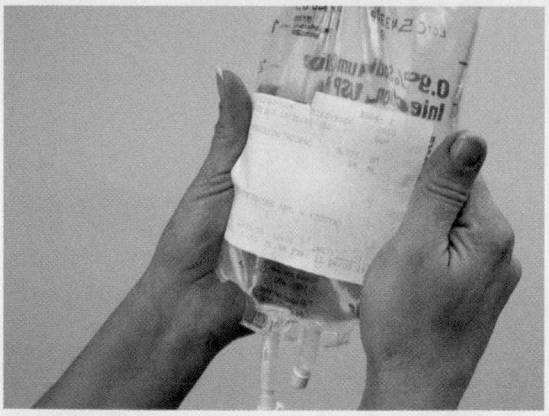

Action 5g: Labeling container to show medication.
(Photo by Rick Brady.)

ACTION	RATIONALE
6. Add the medication to the intravenous solution before the infusion:	
a. Carefully remove any protective cover and locate the injection port. Clean with an alcohol swab.	a. This deters entry of microorganisms when the needle punctures the port.
b. Uncap the needle or needleless device and insert into the port. Inject the medication.	b. This ensures that the needle enters the container and that medication can be dispersed into the solution.

(continued)

Adding Medications to an Intravenous Solution Container (continued)

ACTION	RATIONALE
c. Withdraw and insert the spike into the proper entry site on the bag or bottle.	c. This punctures the seal in the intravenous bag or bottle.
d. With tubing clamped, gently rotate the intravenous solution in the bag or bottle. Hang the intravenous bag or bottle.	d. This mixes the medication with the solution.
e. Attach the label to the container so that the dose of medication that has been added is apparent.	e. This confirms that the prescribed dose of medication has been added to the intravenous solution.
7. Dispose of equipment according to agency policy.	This prevents inadvertent injury from the equipment.
8. Perform hand hygiene.	Hand hygiene deters the spread of microorganisms.
9. Chart the addition of medication to the intravenous solution. This may be done on the CMAR.	Accurate documentation is necessary to prevent medication errors.
10. Evaluate the patient's response to the medication within the appropriate time frame.	Careful observation is needed because medications given by the intravenous route may have a rapid effect.

When medication is administered by continuous infusion, the patient receives it slowly and over a long period. Although this can be an advantage when it is desirable to give the medication slowly, it is a disadvantage when the patient needs to receive the drug more quickly. Also, if for some reason not all of the solution can be infused, the patient will not receive the prescribed amount of the medication. The patient receiving medication by a continuous intravenous infusion should be checked for possible adverse effects at least every hour.
Medications via an Intravenous Bolus or Push. A medication can be administered as an intravenous bolus or push.

This involves a single injection of a concentrated solution directly into an intravenous line (Skill 29-9).
Medications via Intermittent Intravenous Infusion. Medications can be administered by intermittent intravenous infusion. The drug is mixed with a small amount of the intravenous solution, such as 50 to 100 mL, and administered over a short period at the prescribed interval (eg, every 4 hours). As mentioned earlier, needleless devices are recommended by the Centers for Disease Control and Prevention and the Occupational Safety and Health Administration; they prevent needle sticks and provide access to the primary venous line. Either

Adding a Bolus Intravenous Medication to an Existing Intravenous Infusion

EQUIPMENT

Alcohol swab	Medication prepared in a syringe with needless device or 23- to 25-gauge, 1″ needle (if needleless system in use, a needle is not needed)	Medication Kardex or computer-generated MAR
Watch with second hand, or stopwatch		
Disposable gloves		

ACTION	RATIONALE
1. Bring equipment to the patient's bedside. Check the medication order with the physician's order. Check a drug resource to clarify if medication needs to be diluted before administration.	Having equipment available saves time and facilitates performance of the task. Checking the orders ensures that the patient receives the correct medication at the correct time and in the right manner.
2. Explain the procedure to the patient.	Explanation allays the patient's anxiety.
3. Perform hand hygiene. Don clean gloves.	Hand hygiene deters the spread of microorganisms. Gloves protect the nurse from exposure to bloodborne pathogens.
4. Identify the person by checking the identification band on the patient's wrist and asking the patient his or her name.	This ensures that the medication is given to the right person.
5. Assess the intravenous site for inflammation or infiltration.	Intravenous medication must be given directly into a vein for safe administration.

(continued)

ACTION	RATIONALE
6. Select the injection port on the tubing that is closest to the venipuncture site. Clean the port with an alcohol swab.	Using the port closest to the needle insertion site minimizes dilution of the medication. Cleaning with alcohol deters entry of micro-organisms when the needle punctures the port.

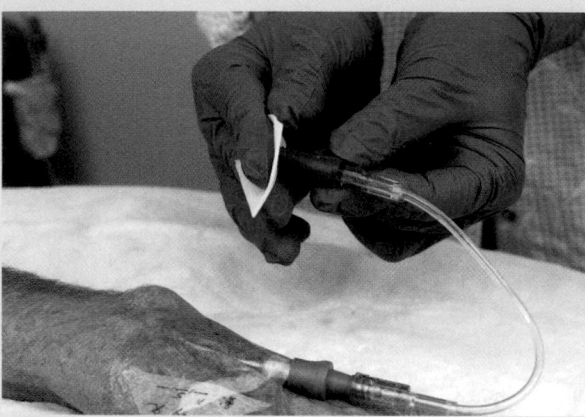

Action 6: Cleaning injection port.   (Photo by Rick Brady.)

ACTION	RATIONALE
7. Uncap the syringe. Steady the port with your nondominant hand while inserting the needleless device or needle into the center of the port.	This supports the injection port and lessens the risk for accidentally dislodging the intravenous line or entering the port incorrectly.
8. Move your nondominant hand to the section of intravenous tubing just beyond the injection port. Fold the tubing between your fingers to temporarily stop the flow of the intravenous solution.	This minimizes the dilution of the intravenous medication with the intravenous solution.
9. Pull back slightly on the plunger just until blood appears in the tubing. If no blood appears, medication may still be administered while assessing the intravenous insertion site for signs of infiltration.	This ensures that the medication is injected into a vein.
10. Inject the medication at the recommended rate (see Special Considerations below).	This delivers the correct amount of medication at the proper interval according to the manufacturer's directions.

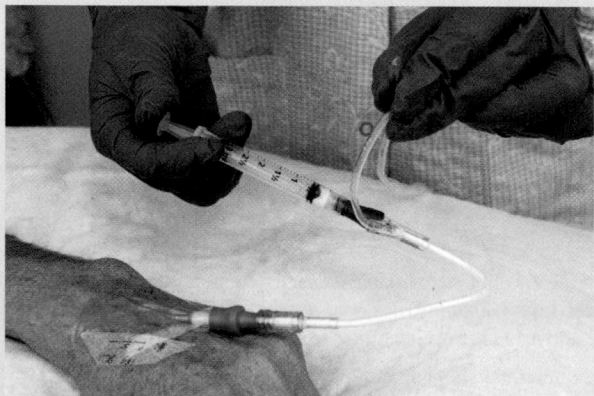

Action 10: Injecting medication while interrupting IV flow.
(Photo by Rick Brady.)

ACTION	RATIONALE
11. Remove the needle. Do not cap it. Release the tubing and allow the intravenous fluid to flow at the proper rate.	This prevents accidental needlestick.

(continued)

Adding a Bolus Intravenous Medication to an Existing Intravenous Infusion (continued)

ACTION	RATIONALE
12. Dispose of the syringe in the proper receptacle.	Proper disposal prevents accidental injury and spread of microorganisms.
13. Remove gloves and perform hand hygiene.	Hand hygiene deters the spread of microorganisms.
14. Chart the administration of the medication. This may be done on the CMAR.	Accurate documentation is necessary to prevent medication errors.
15. Evaluate the patient's response to the medication within the appropriate time frame.	The patient requires careful observation because medications given by an intravenous bolus injection may have a rapid effect.

Special Considerations

- Agency policy may recommend the following variations when injecting a bolus intravenous medication: (1) Release the folded tubing after a portion of the drug has been administered at the prescribed rate to facilitate delivery of the medication. (2) Use a syringe with 1 mL of normal saline to flush the tubing after an intravenous bolus is delivered to ensure that residual medication in the tubing is not delivered too rapidly. (3) Consider how fast the intravenous fluid is flowing to determine whether a flush of

normal saline is in order after administering medication. If the fluid is flowing at less than 50 cc/hour, it may take the medication up to 30 minutes to reach the patient. This depends on the type of tubing that is used in the agency.
- If the intravenous line is a small gauge (22 to 24 gauge) placed in a small vein, the patient may complain of stinging and pain at the site while medication is being administered due to irritation of the vein. A warm pack placed over the vein may ease discomfort.

---

blunt-ended cannulas or recessed connection ports may be used. A patient with an intravenous line in place can receive the solution containing the medication by way of a piggyback setup, a volume-control administration set (eg, Pediatrol or Volutrol), or a mini-infusion pump. The intravenous piggyback delivery system requires the intermittent or additive solution to be placed higher than the primary solution container. An extension hook provided by the manufacturer provides for easy lowering of the main intravenous container. The port on the primary intravenous line has a back-check valve that automatically stops the flow of the primary solution, allowing the secondary or piggyback solution to flow when connected. A tandem delivery setup is similar except that both solutions remain at the same height and there is no back-check valve at the secondary port on the primary line. This type of setup is used infrequently because the solution from the primary intravenous line will back up into the tandem line if this intermittent infusion is not clamped immediately after it is infused. Because manufacturers' designs vary, the nurse should check the directions carefully for the systems used in the agency. The nurse is responsible for calculating and manually adjusting the flow rate of the intravenous intermittent infusion or regulating the infusion with an infusion pump or controller. Intravenous administration of medications using additive sets is explained in Skill 29-10.

For Jacob Shoolin, the 5-year-old boy receiving intravenous antibiotic therapy, and Mr. Baptiste, the elderly patient receiving antibiotic therapy for a wound infection, the nurse would select

the most appropriate type of additive set to use when administering the prescribed antibiotic (unless the physician ordered a specific type).

Medications can also be placed in a controlled-volume administration set for intermittent intravenous infusion. The medication is diluted with a small amount of solution and administered through the patient's intravenous line (see Skill 29-10). This type of equipment is also used for infusing solutions into children and older patients when the volume of fluid infused must be monitored carefully.

The minisyringe pump for intermittent infusion is battery operated and allows medication mixed in a syringe to be connected to the primary line and delivered by mechanical pressure applied to the syringe plunger (see Skill 29-10).

A heparin or saline lock, or intermittent venous access device, is used for patients who require intermittent intravenous medication but not a continuous intravenous infusion. This device consists of a needle or catheter connected to a short length of tubing capped with a sealed injection port. An intravenous lock is shown in Skill 29-11. After the catheter is in place in the patient's vein, the catheter and tubing are anchored to the patient's arm so that the catheter remains in place until the patient no longer requires the repeated medication intravenously.

An intravenous lock allows the patient more freedom than a continuous intravenous infusion. The patient is connected to the intravenous line when it is time to receive the medication and disconnected when the medication is completed. A saline flush rather than a heparin flush is used in

(text continues on page 757)

Administering Intravenous Medications by Piggyback, Volume Control Administration Set, or Mini-Infusion Pump

EQUIPMENT

For piggyback or mini-infusion pump:
Gloves (optional)
Medication prepared in labeled piggyback set or syringe (5 to 100 mL)
Secondary infusion tubing (microdrip or macrodrip)
Needleless device, stopcock, or sterile needle (21 to 23 gauge)

Alcohol swab
Tape
Metal or plastic hook
Mini-infusion pump
Date label for tubing
For volume control set:
Gloves (optional)

Volume control set (eg, Volutrol, Buretrol, Burette)
Medication (in vial or ampule)
Syringe with needleless device attached or a 20- or 21-gauge needle
Alcohol swab
Medication label

ACTION	RATIONALE
1. Gather equipment and bring to the patient's bedside. Check the medication order against the original physician's order according to agency policy.	Having equipment available saves time and facilitates performance of the task. Checking the orders ensures that the patient receives the correct medication at the correct time and in the right manner.
2. Identify the patient by checking the identification band on the patient's wrist and asking the patient his or her name.	This ensures that the medication is given to the right person.
3. Explain the procedure to the patient.	Explanation allays the patient's anxiety.
4. Perform hand hygiene and don gloves.	Hand hygiene deters the spread of microorganisms. Gloves protect the nurse when connecting setup to an existing intravenous line.
5. Assess the intravenous site for inflammation or infiltration.	The medication must be administered directly into a vein that is not inflamed to avoid injuring surrounding tissue.

FOR PIGGYBACK INFUSIONS

6. Attach the infusion tubing to the piggyback set containing diluted medication. Place the label on the tubing with the appropriate date, and attach the needle or needleless device to the end of the tubing according to the manufacturer's directions. Open the clamp and prime the tubing (see action 4, Procedure 46-1). Close the clamp.	This removes air from the tubing and preserves the sterility of the setup. Tubing for piggyback setup may be used for 48 to 72 hours, depending on agency policy.
7. Hang the piggyback container on the intravenous pole, positioning it higher than the primary intravenous container according to the manufacturer's recommendations. Use a metal or plastic hook to lower the primary intravenous container.	The position of the container influences the flow of the intravenous fluid into the primary setup.
8. Use an alcohol swab to clean the appropriate port.	This deters entry of microorganisms when the piggyback setup is connected to the port.
9. Connect the piggyback setup to:	
a. Needleless port	a, b. Needleless systems and stopcock setup eliminate the need
b. Stopcock: turn stopcock to open position	for a needle and are recommended by the Centers for Disease Control and Prevention.
c. Primary intravenous line: uncap the needle and insert it into the secondary intravenous port closest to the top of the primary tubing. Use a strip of tape to secure the secondary set tubing to the primary infusion tubing. The primary line is left unclamped if the port has a backflow valve.	c. The tape stabilizes the needle in the infusion port and prevents it from slipping out. The backflow valve in the primary line secondary port stops the flow of the primary infusion while the piggyback solution is infusing. Once completed, the backflow valves opens and the flow of the primary solution resumes.
10. Open the clamp on the piggyback set and regulate the flow at the prescribed delivery rate, or set the flow rate for the secondary infusion on the infusion pump. Monitor the medication infusion at periodic intervals.	Delivery over a 30- to 60-minute interval is usually a safe method of administering an intravenous medication. It is important to verify the safe administration rate for each drug to prevent adverse effects.

(continued)

SKILL
29-10

Administering Intravenous Medications by Piggyback, Volume Control Administration Set, or Mini-Infusion Pump (continued)

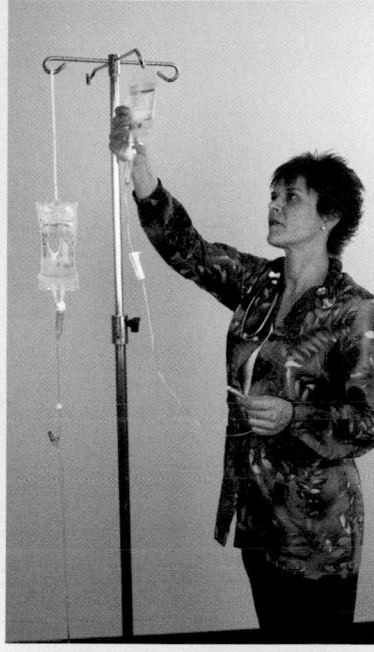

Action 7: Positioning the piggyback container on the IV pole.   (Photo by Rick Brady.)

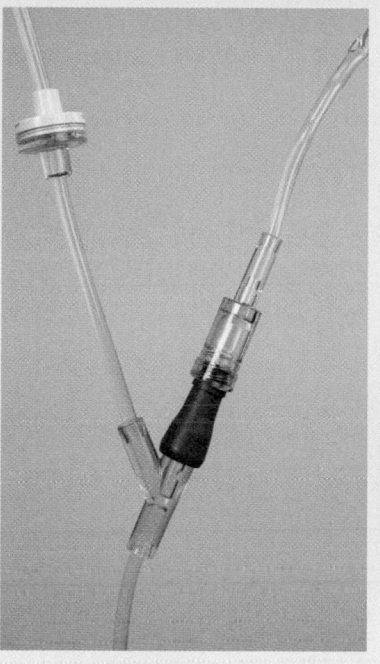

Action 9a: Piggyback setup connected to a needleless port.   (Photo by Rick Brady.)

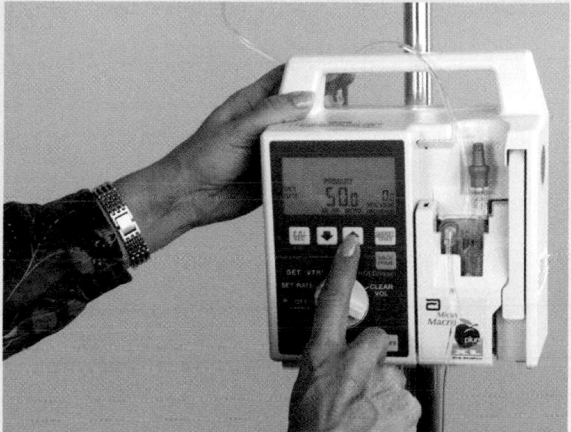

Action 10: Adjusting pump rate.   (Photo by Rick Brady.)

ACTION	RATIONALE
11. Clamp the tubing on the piggyback set when the solution is infused. Follow agency policy regarding disposal of equipment.	This reduces the risk for contaminating the primary intravenous setup.
12. Readjust the flow rate of the primary intravenous solution.	Piggyback medication administration may interrupt the normal flow rate of the primary intravenous fluid. Readjustment of the rate may be necessary.

USING A MINI-INFUSION PUMP

ACTION	RATIONALE
13. Connect the prepared syringe to the mini-infusion tubing.	Special tubing is used to connect the prepared medication to the primary intravenous line.
14. Fill the tubing with the medication by applying gentle pressure to the syringe plunger.	This removes air from the tubing.
15. Insert the syringe into the mini-infusion pump according to the manufacturer's directions.	The syringe must fit securely in the pump apparatus for proper operation.
16. Use an alcohol swab to cleanse the appropriate connector. Connect the mini-infusion tubing to the appropriate connector as in action 9.	This deters entry of microorganisms when the piggyback setup is connected to the port. Proper connection allows the intravenous medication to flow into the primary line.
17. Program the pump to begin the infusion. Set the alarm if recommended by the manufacturer.	The pump delivers the medication at a controlled rate. An alarm is recommended for use with an intravenous lock apparatus.
18. Recheck the flow rate of the primary intravenous fluid once the pump has completed delivery of the medication.	The normal flow rate of the primary intravenous fluid may have been altered by the mini-infusion pump.

(continued)

Administering Intravenous Medications by Piggyback, Volume Control Administration Set, or Mini-Infusion Pump (continued)

ACTION	RATIONALE

USING A VOLUME-CONTROL ADMINISTRATION SET

19. Withdraw the medication from the vial or ampule into the prepared syringe. See Skill 29-2 or 29-3.	The correct dose is prepared for dilution in the intravenous solution.
20. Open the clamp between the intravenous solution and the volume-control administration set or secondary setup. Follow the manufacturer's instructions and fill with the desired amount of intravenous solution. Close the clamp.	This dilutes the medication in the minimal amount of solution. Reclamping prevents the continued addition of fluid to the volume to be mixed with medication.
21. Use an alcohol swab to clean the injection port on the secondary setup.	This deters entry of microorganisms when the needle punctures the port.
22. Remove the cap and insert the needle or blunt needleless device into the port while holding the syringe steady. Inject the medication. Mix gently with intravenous solution.	This ensures that the medication is evenly mixed with the solution.

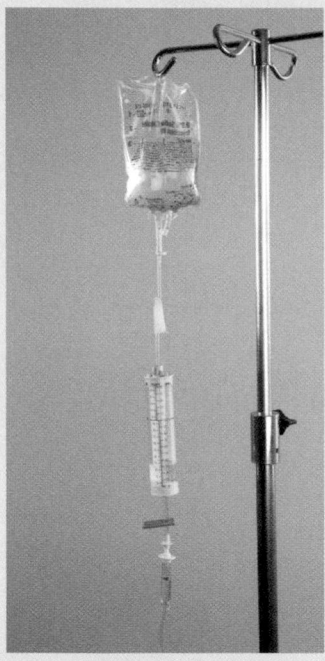

Action 20: Bag with burette and tubing.   (Photo by Rick Brady.)

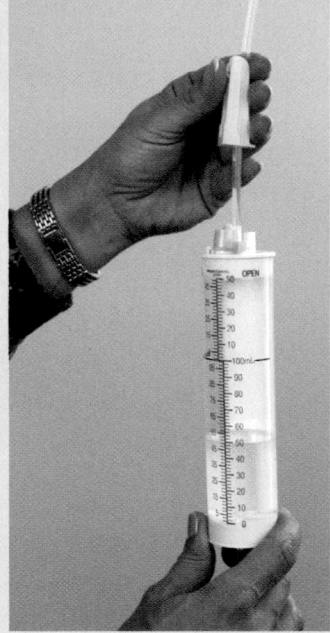

Action 20: Adjusting clamp between bag and burette.   (Photo by Rick Brady.)

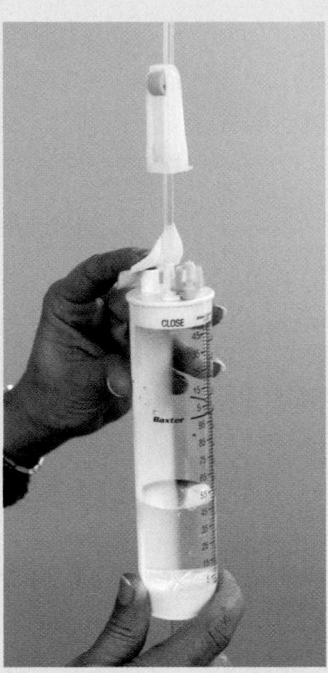

Action 21: Cleaning injection port. (Photo by Rick Brady.)

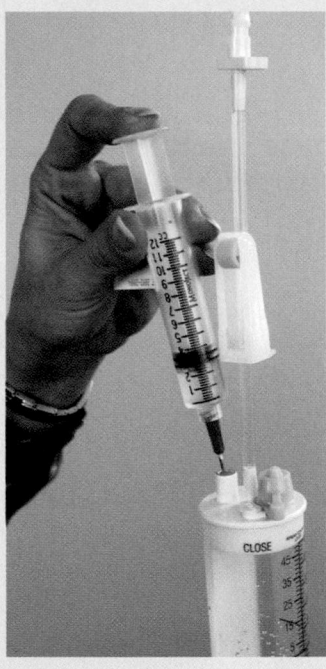

Action 22: Injecting medication into port.   (Photo by Rick Brady.)

23. Open the clamp below the secondary setup and regulate at the prescribed delivery rate. Monitor the medication infusion at periodic intervals.	Delivery over a 30- to 60-minute interval is a safe method of administering intravenous medication.
24. Attach the label to the volume-control device.	This prevents medication error.
25. Place the syringe with the uncapped needle in the designated container.	Proper disposal of the needle protects the nurse from accidental needlestick. Most accidental needle sticks occur when recapping needles.
26. Perform hand hygiene.	Hand hygiene deters the spread of microorganisms.

(continued)

SKILL 29-10

Administering Intravenous Medications by Piggyback, Volume Control Administration Set, or Mini-Infusion Pump (continued)

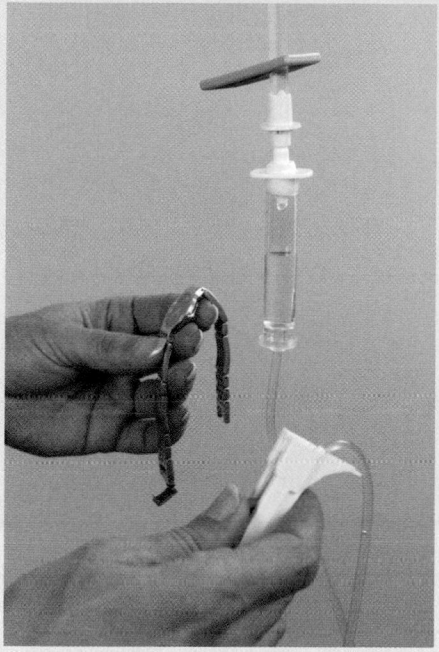

Action 23: Adjusting flow rate of primary fluid.
(Photo by Rick Brady.)

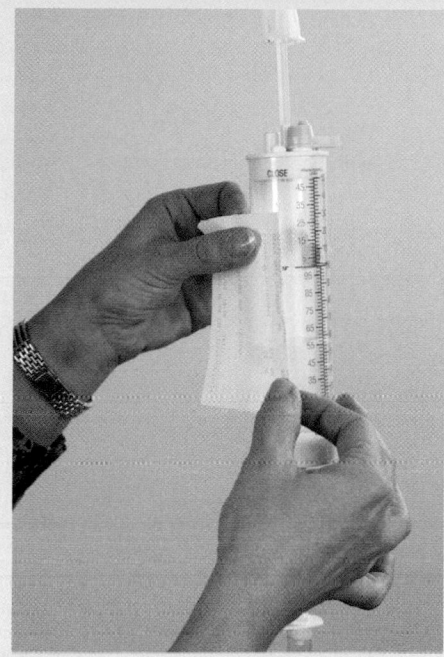

Action 24: Applying medication label to burette.
(Photo by Rick Brady.)

ACTION	RATIONALE
27. Chart the administration of medication after it has been infused. This can be done on the CMAR.	Accurate documentation is necessary to prevent medication errors.
28. Evaluate the patient's response to the medication within the appropriate time frame.	The patient requires careful observation because medications given by the parenteral route may have a rapid effect.

Infant and Child Considerations

Small infants and children with fluid restriction requirements may not tolerate the added intravenous fluid needed to administer with piggyback or volume-control systems. For these children, the nurse should consider using the mini-infusion pump.

many agencies to maintain the patency of the lock. Using saline eliminates any possible systemic effects on coagulation, development of a heparin allergy, and drug incompatibility, which may occur when a heparin solution is used. The intermittent infusion is not started until the nurse confirms intravenous placement. The saline lock is flushed after the infusion is completed to clear the vein of any medication and to prevent clot formation in the needle. The procedure for flushing an intravenous lock with saline is discussed in Skill 29-11. The intravenous site is assessed for complications (see Chap. 46). If infiltration or phlebitis occurs, the lock is removed and replaced in a new site.

In addition to a peripheral intravenous line, intermittent intravenous medication may be administered through a centrally placed line into the subclavian or internal jugular veins or through a peripherally inserted central catheter (PICC). These venous access devices are discussed in more detail in Chapter 46. Medications are prepared under laminar flow in a sterile environment if they are to be administered through a central intravenous line, such as a Hickman catheter. Laminar flow is a technique that helps regulate airflow to prevent bacterial contamination and collection of hazardous chemical fumes. Aseptic technique is observed when the nurse administers medications through a central intravenous line. All connections are cleaned with povidone-iodine or an antiseptic agent.

Administering Topical Medications

When a drug is applied directly to a body site, it is called a **topical** application. Topical applications are usually intended for

(text continues on page 760)

Introducing Drugs Through a Heparin or Intravenous Lock Using the Saline Flush

EQUIPMENT

Medication
Medication Kardex or computer-generated
 MAR
Saline vial
Sterile syringe (2) with needleless device
 or 25-gauge needle

Alcohol swabs
Watch with second hand or stopwatch
Gloves (optional)
For bolus injection:
 Sterile syringe (2) with needleless
  device or 25-gauge needle

For intermittent intravenous delivery:
 Intravenous setup with needleless device
  attached to tubing or a 25-gauge needle
Adhesive tape (optional)

ACTION	RATIONALE
1. Assemble the equipment and check the physician's order.	This ensures that the patient receives the right medication at the right time by the proper route.
2. Identify the patient by checking the identification band on the patient's wrist and asking the patient his or her name. Explain the procedure to the patient.	This ensures that the right patient is receiving the medication. Explanation alleviates the patient's apprehension about intravenous drug administration.
3. Perform hand hygiene.	Hand hygiene deters the spread of microorganisms.
4. Withdraw 1 to 2 mL of sterile saline from the vial into the syringe as described in Skill 29-3.	Using saline eliminates the concerns about drug incompatibilities and the effect on the systemic circulation that exists with heparin.
5. Don clean gloves.	Gloves protect the nurse's hands from contact with the patient's blood.
6. Administer the medication. For bolus intravenous injection: a. Check the drug package for the correct injection rate for the intravenous push route. b. Clean the port of the lock with an alcohol swab. c. Stabilize the port with your nondominant hand and insert the needleless device or needle of the syringe of normal saline into the port. d. Aspirate gently and check for blood return (blood return does not always occur even though the lock is patent). e. Gently flush with 1 mL of normal saline. Remove the syringe. f. Insert the needleless device or needle of the syringe with medication into the port and gently inject the medication, using a watch to verify the correct injection rate. Do not force the injection if resistance is felt. If the lock is clogged, it must be changed. Remove the medication syringe and needle when administration is completed. g. Remove the syringe with medication from the port. Stabilize the port with your nondominant hand and insert the needleless device or needle of the syringe of normal saline into the port. Slowly flush the reservoir with 1 to 2 mL of sterile saline using positive pressure. To gain positive pressure, you can either clamp the intravenous tubing as you are still flushing the last of the saline into the intravenous line or remove the syringe as you are still flushing the remainder of the saline into the intravenous line. Remove the syringe and discard uncapped needles and syringes in the appropriate receptacle. Remove gloves and discard appropriately.	a. Using the correct injection rate prevents speed shock from occurring. b. Cleaning removes surface bacteria at the lock entry site. c. This allows for careful insertion into the center circle of the lock. d. Blood return usually indicates that the catheter is in the vein. e. Saline flush ensures that the intravenous line is patent. A patient's complaint of pain or resistance to the flush detected by the nurse may indicate that the line is not patent. f. Easy installation of medication usually indicates that the lock is still patent and in the vein. If force is used against resistance, a clot may break away and cause a blockage somewhere else in the body. g. Positive pressure prevents blood from backing into the intravenous catheter and causing the intravenous line to clot off.

(continued)

**Introducing Drugs Through a Heparin or Intravenous Lock
Using the Saline Flush** (continued)

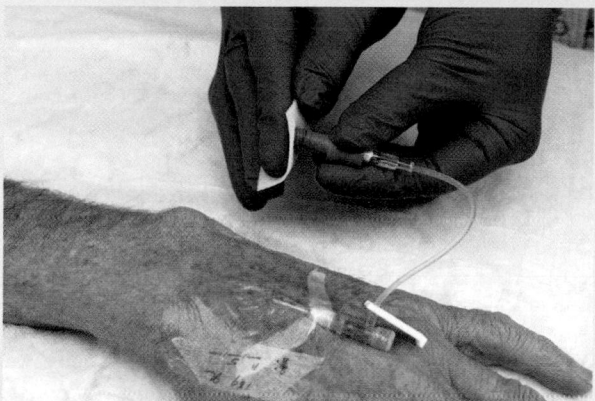

Action 6b: Cleansing the port with an alcohol swab.   (Photo by Rick Brady.)

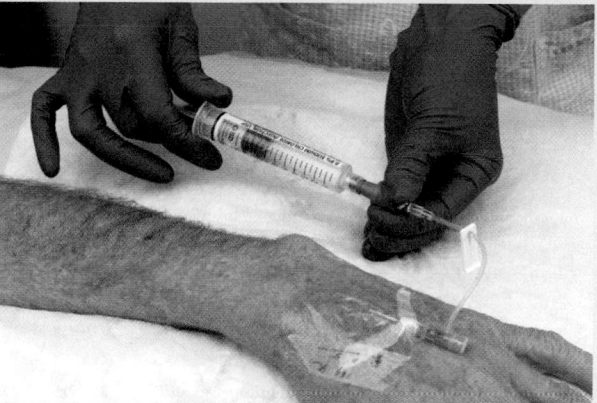

Action 6c: Inserting syringe with blunt needle into port.
(Photo by Rick Brady.)

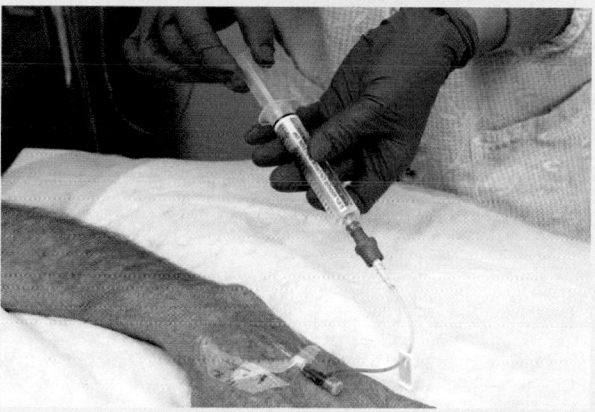

Action 6d: Aspirating for a blood return.   (Photo by Rick Brady.)

ACTION	RATIONALE

For administration of a drug by way of an intermittent delivery system:

a. Use a drug resource book to check for the correct flow rate of the medication (the usual is 30 to 60 minutes).

b. Connect the infusion tubing to the medication setup according to the manufacturer's directions. Hang the intravenous setup on a pole. Open the clamp and allow the solution to clear the intravenous tubing of air. Reclamp the tubing.

c. Attach a needleless connector or a sterile 25-gauge needle to the end of the infusion tubing.

d. Clean the port of the lock with an alcohol swab.

e. Stabilize the port with your nondominant hand and insert the needleless device or needle of the syringe of normal saline into the port.

f. Aspirate gently and check for blood return (blood return does not always occur even though the lock is patent).

g. Gently flush with 1 mL of normal saline. Remove the syringe.

h. Insert the blunt needleless device or needle attached to the tubing into the port. If necessary, secure with tape.

a. Using the correct injection rate prevents speed shock from occurring.

b. This removes air from the tubing and preserves the sterility of the setup.

c. A small-gauge needle prevents damage to the lock.

d. Cleaning removes surface bacteria at the lock entry site.

e. This allows for careful insertion into the port.

f. Blood return usually indicates that the catheter is in the vein.

g. Saline flush ensures that the intravenous line is patent.

h. Tape secures the needle in the lock port.

(continued)

SKILL
29-11
Introducing Drugs Through a Heparin or Intravenous Lock
Using the Saline Flush (continued)

ACTION	RATIONALE
i. Open the clamp and regulate the flow rate or attach to an intravenous pump or controller according to the manufacturer's directions. Close the clamp when the infusion is complete.	i. This ensures that the patient receives the medication at the correct rate.
j. Remove the needleless connector or needle from the lock. Carefully replace the uncapped, used needle or needleless device with a new sterile one. Allow the medication setup to hang on the pole for future use according to agency policy.	j. This prevents possible needlestick with a contaminated needle. Agency policy specifies the length of time for safe use of intravenous infusion tubing.
k. Stabilize the port with your nondominant hand and insert the needleless device or needle of the syringe of normal saline into the port. Slowly flush the reservoir with 1 to 2 mL of sterile saline using positive pressure. To gain positive pressure, you can either clamp the intravenous tubing as you are still flushing the last of the saline into the intravenous line or remove the syringe as you are still flushing the remainder of the saline into the intravenous line. Remove the syringe and discard uncapped needles and syringes in the appropriate receptacle. Remove gloves and discard appropriately.	k. Saline clears the line of medication with fewer of the systemic effects of the heparin flush. Positive pressure prevents blood from backing into the intravenous catheter and causing the intravenous line to clot off.
7. Perform hand hygiene.	Hand hygiene deters the spread of microorganisms.
8. Check the injection site and intravenous lock at least every 8 hours and administer a small amount of saline (2 to 3 mL) if medication is not given at least every 8 to 12 hours.	This ensures the patency of the system for continuing injections.
9. Change the heparin lock at least every 72 to 96 hours or according to agency policy. A lock that is not patent should be changed immediately.	Changing a heparin lock regularly and having it free of clotted blood reduces the risks for infection and emboli in the circulating blood.
10. Chart the administration of the medication or saline flush.	Accurate documentation is necessary to prevent medication error.

Infant and Child Considerations

If the volume of medication being administered is small (<1.0 ml), always include the amount of flush solution as part of the total amount to be injected and take this into account when determining how fast to push a medication. For example, if the medication is to be injected at a rate of 1.0 mL per minute and the total amount of solution to be injected is 2.25 mL (0.25 mL medication volume plus

2.0 mL saline flush solution volume equals 2.25 mL), then the medication would be injected over a period of 2 minutes and 15 seconds.

Special Considerations

Some agencies recommend the use of single-dose saline vials without preservative in the solution. Preservatives may be linked to an increased incidence of phlebitis with heparin locks.

direct action at a particular site, although some systemic effect may also occur. The action depends on the type of tissue and the nature of the agent.

If the site of application is readily accessible, such as the skin, an agent can easily be placed on it. If it is a cavity, such as the nose, or is enclosed, such as the eye, a mechanical applicator is needed to introduce the drug.

Skin Applications

The skin is a mechanical and chemical barrier that protects the underlying tissues. It is a sense organ, with receptors that respond to touch, pain, pressure, and temperature. The skin helps in excretion, in regulating body temperature, and in storing essentials to the body, such as water, salts, and glucose.

When a drug is incorporated in an agent such as an ointment and rubbed into the skin for absorption, the procedure is referred to as an inunction. On normal skin, drugs are absorbed into the lining of the sebaceous glands. Absorption is hindered because of the protective outer layer of the skin, which makes penetration difficult, and because of the fatty substances that protect the lining of the glands. Cleaning the skin thoroughly with soap or detergent and water before administration and then rubbing the medicated preparation into the skin can enhance absorption. Absorption can also be improved by using a drug mixed in an ointment or added to a liniment that will mix with the fat in the gland lining. When indicated, local heat applied to the application area can improve blood circulation and promote absorption. To prevent any absorption by the nurse's skin, gloves should be worn whenever applying topical medications. The following are typical preparations applied to skin areas:

- Powders are used to promote drying of the skin and prevent friction on the skin. Use caution when applying to prevent inhalation of the powder.
- Ointments provide prolonged contact of a medication with the skin and soften the skin. They are usually thoroughly massaged into intact skin.
- Creams and oils lubricate and soften the skin and prevent drying of the skin. If a large part of the body is to be covered, the preparation should be warmed in the hands or fingers to prevent chilling.
- Lotions protect and soothe the skin. Shake lotions thoroughly before using, and apply with cotton balls or gauze.

The transdermal route is being used more frequently to deliver medication. This involves applying to the skin a disk or patch that contains medication intended for daily use or for longer intervals. Transdermal patches are commonly used to deliver hormones, narcotic analgesics, and nicotine. Medication errors have occurred when patients applied multiple patches at once or failed to remove the overlay on the patch that exposes the skin to the medication. Narcotic analgesic patches are associated with the most adverse drug effects. Clear patches have a cosmetic advantage but can be difficult to find on the patient's skin when they need to be removed or replaced. Despite a slow onset of action, transdermal drug patches maintain consistent serum drug levels (see the accompanying Guidelines for Nursing Care: Applying Transdermal Patches).

Eye Instillations and Irrigations

The receptors for the sense of sight are located in the eye. The outer layer of the eyeball is called the sclera. The cornea is the transparent part of the sclera in front of the eyeball. The sclera is fibrous and tough, but the cornea is easily injured by trauma. For this reason, applications to the eye seldom are placed directly onto the eyeball.

Because direct application cannot be made onto the sensitive cornea, applications intended to act on the eye or the lids are placed onto, or instilled or irrigated into, the lower conjunctival sac.

The eye is a delicate organ, highly susceptible to infection and injury. Although the eye is never free of microorganisms, the secretions of the conjunctiva have a protective action against many pathogens. For maximum safety for the patient, the equipment, solutions, and ointments introduced into the conjunctival sac should be sterile. If this is not possible, the most careful guidelines for medical asepsis should be followed.

Eyedrops. Eyedrops are instilled for their local effects, such as for pupil dilation or constriction when examining the eye, for treating an infection, or for controlling intraocular pressure in patients with glaucoma. The type and amount of solution depend on the purpose of the instillation. See the accompanying box, Guidelines for Nursing Care: Instilling Eyedrops.

Guidelines for Nursing Care 29-1
Applying Transdermal Patches

- Wear gloves when applying or removing patches. Hand hygiene is also a necessity.
- Remove the old patch before applying the new one.
- Gently wash the area where the old patch was with soap and water.
- Dispose of old patches carefully. Keep out of the reach of children and away from pets.
- Rotate application sites.
- Follow directions and use the patch as prescribed. Remove the patch from its protective covering and then remove the clear plastic covering without touching the adhesive. Apply the patch and use the palm to press firmly for about 10 seconds.
- Apply the patch at the same time of the day and write your initials, the date, and time on the patch.
- Document site of application on the CMAR.
- Monitor the patient's response carefully. Be alert for adverse effects specific to the medication applied.
- Check for dislodgement of the patch if the patient is active. Read information about the patch or consult with the pharmacist to determine reapplication schedule and procedure.
- Assess for any skin irritation. If necessary, remove the patch, wash the area carefully with soap and water, and allow skin to air dry.
- Aluminum backing on a patch necessitates precautions if defibrillation is required. Burns and smoke may result.

Ointments. Various types of medication in ointment form may be prescribed for the eye. These ointments are usually used for a local infection or irritation. Eye ointments are dispensed in a tube. A small amount of ointment is distributed along the exposed lower conjunctival sac after the eyelids and eyelashes have been cleansed. About ½″ of ointment is squeezed from the tube along the exposed sac. After the application, the eyes should be closed. The warmth helps to liquefy the ointment. Instruct the patient to move the eye, because this helps to spread the ointment under the lids and over the surface of the eyeball. Explain that the ointment may temporarily blur vision; encourage the patient not to rub the eye.

Eye Irrigation. An eye irrigation is performed to remove secretions or foreign bodies or to cleanse and soothe the eye. In an emergency, eye irrigation can be used to remove chemicals that may burn the eye. Copious amounts of tap water should be used to remove chemicals such as acid. The irrigation should continue for at least 15 minutes, and then professional help should be sought. Many emergency rooms have eye flush stations to help with eye irrigations. Care should be taken so that the overflowing irrigation fluid does not contaminate the other eye. The techniques for administering an eye irrigation are described in Skill 29-12.

Guidelines for Nursing Care 29-2
Instilling Eyedrops

- Perform hand hygiene before putting on gloves.
- Offer the patient paper tissues to remove solution and tears that may spill from the eye during the procedure.
- Clean the eyelids and eyelashes of any drainage with cotton balls or gauze pledgets moistened with normal saline solution, because debris can be carried into the eye when the conjunctival sac is exposed. Use each cotton ball for only one stroke, moving from the inner toward the outer canthus to prevent carrying debris to the lacrimal ducts.
- Tilt the patient's head back slightly if sitting, or place the patient's head over a pillow if lying down. The head may be turned slightly to the affected side to prevent solution or tears from flowing toward the opposite eye.
- Remove the cap from the medication bottle, being careful not to touch the inner side of the cap.
- Invert the monodrip plastic container that is commonly used to instill eyedrops.
- Have the patient look up while focusing on something on the ceiling.
- Place the thumb or two fingers near the margin of the lower eyelid immediately below the eyelashes, and exert pressure downward over the bony prominence of the cheek. The lower conjunctival sac is exposed as the lower lid is pulled down.
- Hold the dropper close to the eye but avoid touching the eyelids or lashes, which may startle the patient and cause blinking. Also, avoid touching the eyeball with the dropper, because this could easily injure the eye.
- Squeeze the container and allow the prescribed number of drops to fall in the lower conjunctival sac. Do not allow drops to fall onto the cornea because of the dan-

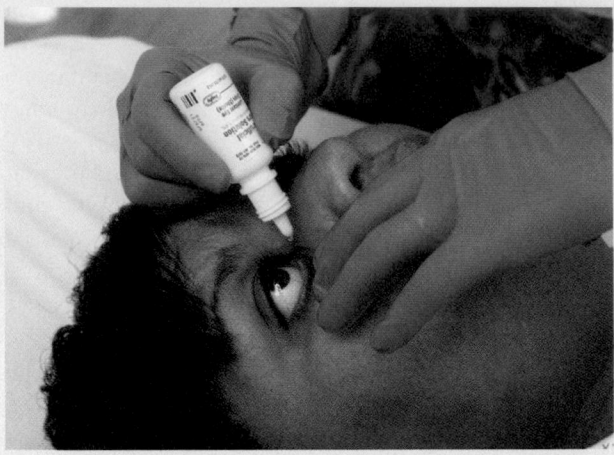

With the lower lid pulled down, the nurse prepares to administer the eyedrops on the lower conjunctival sac.

ger of injuring it and the unpleasant sensation it causes the patient.
- Release the lower lid after the eyedrops are instilled. Ask the patient to close the eyes gently.
- Apply gentle pressure over the inner canthus to prevent the eyedrops from flowing into the tear duct. This minimizes the risk of systemic effects from the medication.
- Instruct the patient not to rub the affected eye.
- Remove gloves and perform hand hygiene.
- Chart the administration of medication after the drops have been administered. This may be done on the CMAR.
- Evaluate the patient's response to the medication within the appropriate time frame.

Eye Medication Disks. An eye medication disk is flexible and resembles a contact lens; it contains medication that is gradually released into the conjunctival sac. It can remain in place for up to a week before being removed and discarded. When properly placed, the disk is completely covered by the lower eyelid, allowing the patient to wear contact lenses, swim, and sleep with the disk in place. The nurse should wear gloves when applying and removing the disk. Additional nursing guidelines for inserting and removing an intraocular disk include the following:

- Position the disk with the convex side adhering to your fingertip.
- Ask the patient to look up, and use the other hand to pull the patient's lower eyelid down gently.
- Place the disk in the conjunctival sac and lift the lower eyelid up and over the disk. If properly positioned, the disk should not be visible at this time.
- For removal, expose the disk by pulling down on the patient's lower eyelid.

- Use the forefinger and thumb of the other hand to gently pinch the disk and lift it out of the patient's eye.

Eye medication disks are usually applied at bedtime because they initially cause blurring of vision.

Ear Instillations and Irrigations

The ear contains the receptors for hearing and equilibrium. It consists of the external ear, the middle ear, and the inner ear. The external ear consists of the auricle or pinna and the exterior auditory canal. The auditory canal serves as a passageway for sound waves. Drugs or irrigations are instilled into the auditory canal for their local effect. They are used to soften wax, relieve pain, apply local anesthesia, destroy organisms, or destroy an insect lodged in the canal, which can cause almost intolerable discomfort. If the ear canal has swollen to the point that medication cannot pass, a long piece of cotton material called a wick is inserted so that one end is near the middle ear and the other end is external. This cotton then acts as a wick to help medication get to the inner ear.

SKILL
29-12   **Administering an Eye Irrigation**

EQUIPMENT

Sterile irrigating solution (warmed to 37°C
  [98.6°F])
Sterile irrigation set (sterile container and
  irrigating or bulb syringe)

Emesis basin or irrigation basin
Cotton balls
Waterproof pad

Towel
Disposable gloves

ACTION	RATIONALE
1. Explain the procedure to the patient.	Explanation facilitates cooperation and reassures the patient.
2. Assemble the equipment at the patient's bedside.	This provides for an organized approach to the task.
3. Perform hand hygiene.	Hand hygiene deters the spread of microorganisms.
4. Have the patient sit or lie with the head tilted toward the side of the affected eye. Protect the patient and the bed with a waterproof pad.	Gravity aids the flow of solution away from the unaffected eye and from the inner canthus of the affected eye toward the outer canthus.
5. Don disposable gloves. Clean the lids and the lashes with a cotton ball or washcloth moistened with normal saline or the solution ordered for the irrigation. Wipe from the inner canthus to the outer canthus. Discard the cotton ball or use a different corner of the washcloth with each wipe.	Materials lodged on the lids or in the lashes may be washed into the eye. This cleaning motion protects the nasolacrimal duct and the other eye.

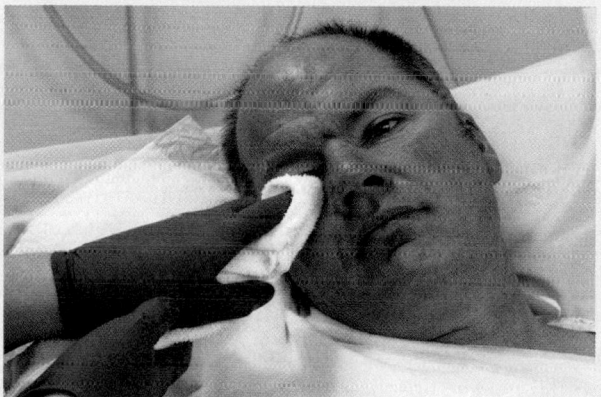

Action 5: Cleaning lids and lashes from inside of eye to outside.
(Photo by Rick Brady.)

ACTION	RATIONALE
6. Place the curved basin at the cheek on the side of the affected eye to receive the irrigating solution. If the patient is sitting up, ask him or her to support the basin.	Gravity aids the flow of solution.
7. Expose the lower conjunctival sac and hold the upper lid open with your nondominant hand.	The solution is directed onto the lower conjunctival sac because the cornea is sensitive and easily injured. This also prevents reflex blinking.
8. Hold the irrigator about 2.5 cm (1″) from the eye. Direct the flow of the solution from the inner to the outer canthus along the conjunctival sac.	This minimizes the risk for injury to the cornea. Solution directed toward the outer canthus helps to prevent the spread of contamination from the eye to the lacrimal sac, lacrimal duct, and nose.
9. Irrigate until the solution is clear or all of the solution has been used. Use only enough force to remove secretions gently from the conjunctiva. Avoid touching any part of the eye with the irrigating tip.	Directing solutions with force may cause injury to the tissues of the eye as well as to the conjunctiva. Touching the eye is uncomfortable for the patient and may cause damage to the cornea.
10. Have the patient close the eye periodically during the procedure.	Movement of the eye when the lids are closed helps to move secretions from the upper to the lower conjunctival sac.

(continued)

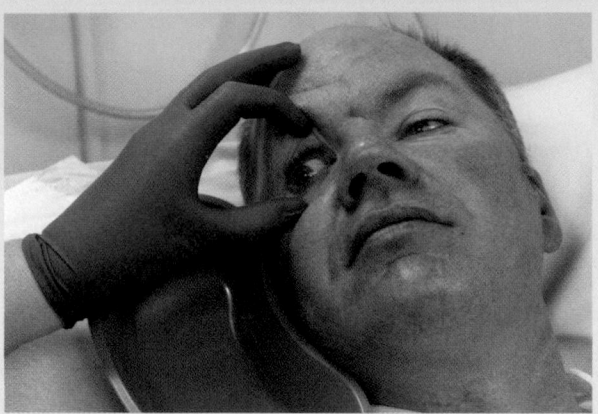

Action 7: Holding eye in position.   (Photo by Rick Brady.)

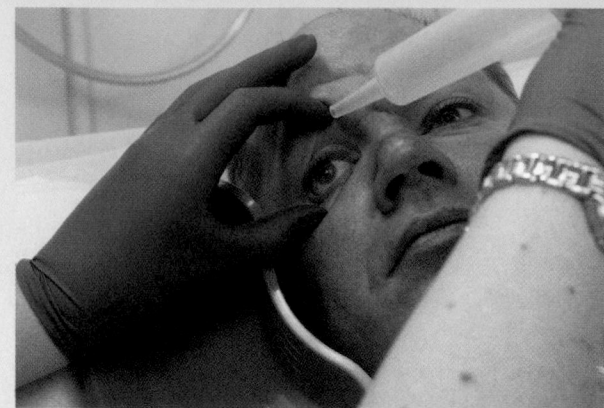

Action 8: Preparing to irrigate the eye.   (Photo by Rick Brady.)

ACTION	RATIONALE
11. Dry the area after the irrigation with cotton balls or a gauze sponge. Offer a towel to the patient if the face and neck are wet.	Leaving the skin moist after an irrigation is uncomfortable for the patient.
12. Remove gloves and perform hand hygiene.	Hand hygiene deters the spread of microorganisms.
13. Chart the irrigation, appearance of the eye, drainage, and the patient's response.	This provides accurate documentation.

The tympanic membrane separates the external ear from the middle ear. Normally, it is intact and closes the entrance to the middle ear completely. If it is ruptured or has been opened by surgical intervention, the middle ear and the inner ear have a direct passage to the external ear. When this occurs, instillations and irrigations should be performed with the greatest of care to prevent forcing materials from the outer ear into the middle ear and the inner ear. Sterile technique is used to prevent infection.

Ear Drops. Follow the techniques listed in the accompanying box, Guidelines for Nursing Care: Instilling Ear Drops, when placing drops in the external auditory canal.

Ear Irrigations. Irrigations of the external auditory canal are ordinarily done for cleaning purposes or for applying heat to the area. Typically, normal saline solution is used, although an antiseptic solution may be indicated for local action. To prevent pain, the irrigation solution should be at least at room temperature. An irrigation syringe is used in most instances. An irrigating container with tubing and an ear tip may also be used, especially if the purpose of the irrigation is to apply heat to the area. The techniques for administering an irrigation of the external auditory canal are described in Skill 29-13.

Nasal Instillations

Besides serving as the olfactory organ, the nose functions as an airway to the lower respiratory tract and protects the tract by cleaning and warming the air taken in by inspiration. Cilia project on most of the surfaces of the nasal mucous membrane and help remove particles of dirt and dust from the inspired air. The nose also serves as a resonator when speaking and singing.

Nasal instillations are used to treat allergies, sinus infections, and nasal congestion. Medications with a systemic effect, such as vasopressin, may also be prepared as a nasal instillation. The nose is normally not a sterile cavity, but because of its connection with the sinuses, medical asepsis should be observed carefully when using nasal instillations. See the accompanying box, Guidelines for Nursing Care: Instilling Nose Drops.

Solutions instilled by drops may also be applied to the nasal mucous membrane in a spray. A small atomizer is used. The end of the nose is held up, and the tip of the nozzle is placed just inside the naris and directed backward. Only enough force is used to bring the spray into contact with the membrane; too much force may drive the solution and contamination into the sinuses and eustachian tubes.

Vaginal Applications

A healthy vagina contains few pathogens but many nonpathogenic organisms. The nonpathogens are important because they protect the vagina from the invasion of pathogens. The normal secretions in the vagina are acidic and further serve to protect the vagina from microbial invasion. Therefore, the normal mucous membrane is its own best protection.

Creams, foams, and tablets can be applied intravaginally using a narrow, tubular applicator with an attached plunger. Suppositories that melt when exposed to body heat are also

Guidelines for Nursing Care 29-3
Instilling Ear Drops

- Warm the solution to be instilled to body temperature to minimize discomfort for the patient.
- Perform hand hygiene and don gloves (gloves are to be worn if drainage is present).
- Offer a tissue to the patient.
- Clean the external ear of drainage with cotton balls moistened with normal saline solution, as necessary.
- Place the patient on the unaffected side in bed, or if ambulatory, have the patient sit with the head well tilted to the side so that the affected ear is uppermost. This positioning prevents the drops from escaping from the ear.
- Draw up the amount of solution needed in the dropper. Excess medication should not be returned to a stock bottle. A monodrip plastic container may also be used.
- Straighten the auditory canal by pulling the cartilaginous portion of the pinna up and back in an adult, straight back for a school-age child, and down and back in an infant or a child under age 3 years. Pulling on the pinna as described helps to straighten the canal properly for ear instillation.

- Hold the dropper in the ear with its tip above the auditory canal. For an infant or an irrational or restless patient, protect the dropper with a piece of soft tubing to help prevent injury to the ear.
- Allow the drops to fall on the side of the canal. It is uncomfortable for the patient if drops fall directly onto the tympanic membrane.
- Release the pinna after instilling the drops, and have the patient maintain the position to prevent the medication from escaping.
- Gently press on the tragus a few times to help move the medication from the canal toward the tympanic membrane.
- If ordered, loosely insert a cotton ball to prevent medication from leaking out.
- Wait 5 minutes before instilling drops in the second ear, if ordered.
- Remove gloves and perform hand hygiene.
- Document the medication administration and any drainage from ear noted.

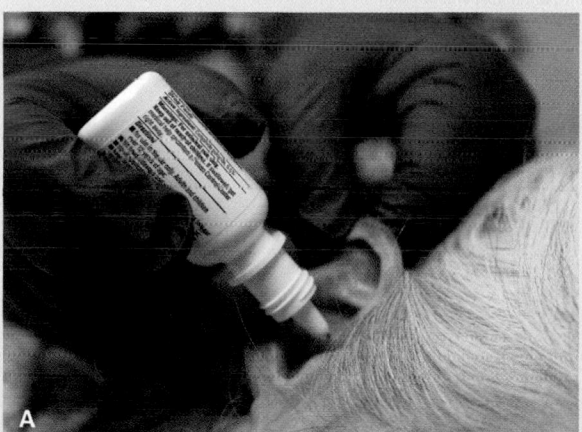

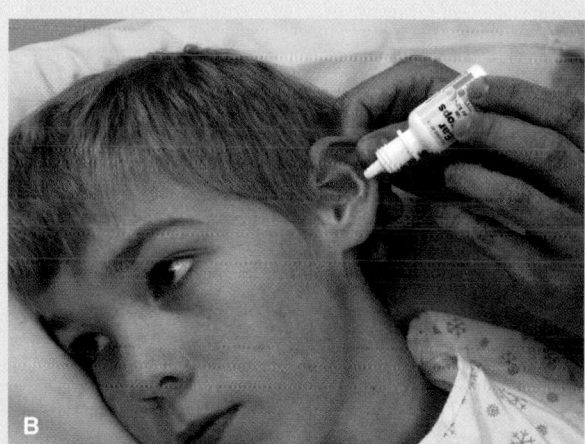

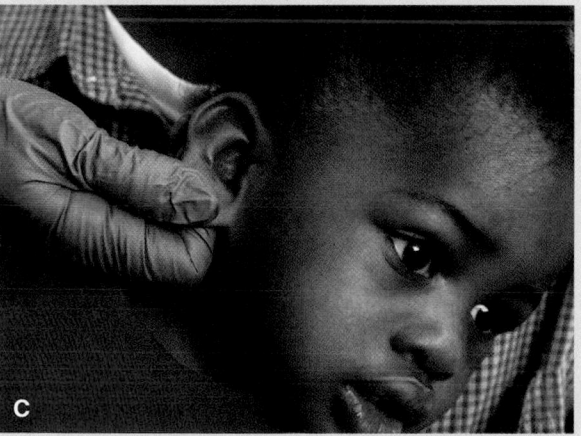

(A) Adult patient positioned for eardrop instillation; nurse straightens the auditory canal by pulling the cartilaginous portion of the pinna up and back. (B) School-age child positioned for eardrop instillation; nurse straightens the auditory canal by pulling the cartilaginous portion of the pinna straight back. (C) Child under 3 years of age ready for eardrop instillation; nurse straightens the auditory canal by pulling the cartilaginous portion of the pinna down and back. Child can be held by parent.

SKILL
29-13   **Administering an Ear Irrigation**

EQUIPMENT

Prescribed irrigating solution (warmed to 37°C [98.6°F])
Irrigation set (container and irrigating or bulb syringe)

Waterproof pad
Emesis basin
Cotton-tipped applicators

Disposable gloves (optional)
Cotton balls

ACTION	RATIONALE
1. Explain the procedure to the patient.	Explanation facilitates cooperation and provides reassurance.
2. Bring the equipment to the patient's bedside. Check the physician's order. Protect the patient and bed linens with a moisture-proof pad.	This provides for an organized approach to the task.
3. Perform hand hygiene.	Hand hygiene deters the spread of microorganisms.
4. Have the patient sit up or lie with the head tilted toward the side of the affected ear. Have the patient support the basin under the ear to receive the irrigating solution.	Gravity causes the irrigating solution to flow from the ear to the basin.
5. Clean the pinna and the meatus at the auditory canal as necessary with moistened cotton-tipped applicators dipped in warm tap water or the irrigating solution.	Materials lodged on the pinna and at the meatus may be washed into the ear.
6. Fill the bulb syringe with the warm solution. If an irrigating container is used, allow air to escape from the tubing.	Air forced into the ear canal is noisy and therefore unpleasant for the patient.
7. Straighten the auditory canal by pulling the pinna up and back for an adult, straight and back for a child over 3 years of age, and down and back for an infant or child up to 3 years of age (see Guidelines for Nursing Care 29-3).	Straightening the ear canal helps allow the solution to reach all areas of the canal easily.
8. Direct a steady, slow stream of solution against the roof of the auditory canal, using only enough force to remove secretions. Do not occlude the auditory canal with the irrigating nozzle. Allow the solution to flow out unimpeded.	Directing solution at the roof of the canal helps prevent injury to the tympanic membrane. Continuous in-and-out flow of the irrigating solution helps prevent pressure in the canal.

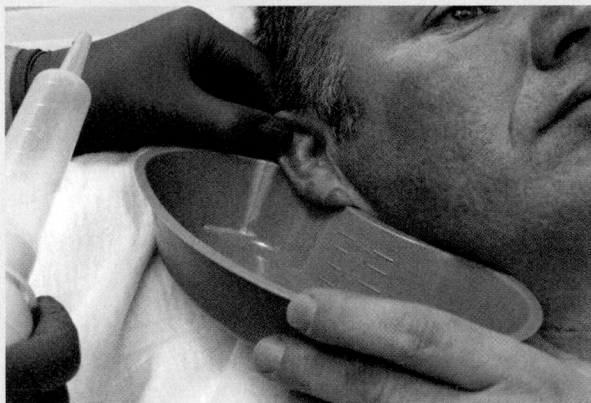

Action 7: Straightening the auditory canal.   (Photo by Rick Brady.)

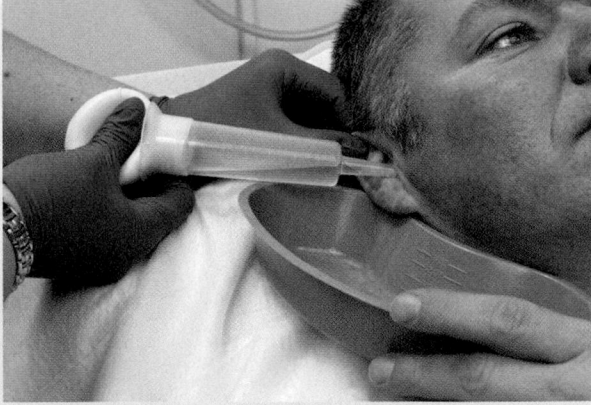

Action 8: Instilling irrigation fluid.   (Photo by Rick Brady.)

9. When the irrigation is completed, place a cotton ball loosely in the auditory meatus and have the patient lie on the side of the affected ear on a towel or absorbent pad.	The cotton ball absorbs excess fluid, and gravity allows the remaining solution in the canal to escape from the ear.
10. Perform hand hygiene.	Hand hygiene deters the spread of microorganisms.
11. Chart the irrigation, the appearance of the drainage, and the patient's response.	This provides accurate documentation.
12. Return in 10 to 15 minutes and remove the cotton ball and assess drainage.	Drainage or pain may indicate injury to the tympanic membrane.

Guidelines for Nursing Care 29-4
Instilling Nose Drops

- Perform hand hygiene and don gloves (gloves are to be worn if drainage is present).
- Provide the patient with paper tissues and ask that the patient blow his or her nose before instilling the nose drops.
- Have the patient sit up with head tilted well back; if the patient is lying down, tilt the head back over a pillow. These positions allow the solution to flow well back into the naris.
- Draw sufficient solution into the dropper for both nares. Excess solution should not be returned to a stock bottle.
- Hold up the tip of the nose and place the dropper just inside the naris about one third of an inch. Instill the prescribed number of drops in one naris and then into the other. Protect the dropper with a piece of soft tubing if the patient is an infant or young child. Avoid touching the nares with the dropper because it may cause the patient to sneeze.
- Have the patient remain in position with the head tilted back for a few minutes to prevent the solution from escaping.
- Remove gloves and perform hand hygiene.
- Document the medication administration and any drainage from the nose noted. The medication documentation may be done on the CMAR.

administered by vaginal insertion. Suppositories should be refrigerated for storage.

Ask the patient to void before inserting the medication. Position the patient so that she is lying on her back with the knees flexed. Maintain privacy with draping. Adequate light should be available to visualize the vaginal opening. See the accompanying box, Guidelines for Nursing Care: Inserting Vaginal Suppository or Cream.

Rectal Instillations

Rectal suppositories are used primarily for their local action, such as laxatives and fecal softeners. Systemic effects are also achieved with rectal suppositories. Acetaminophen suppositories are used for an antipyretic effect, and many antiemetics are available in suppository form to relieve nausea and vomiting.

Use clean disposable gloves to prevent contamination with feces and microorganisms. See the Nursing Guidelines for Inserting a Rectal Suppository in Chapter 44, Bowel Elimination. After the suppository is inserted, the patient should remain in that position for 5 minutes. If the suppository is for laxative purposes, it must remain in position for 35 to 45 minutes, or until the patient feels the urge to defecate.

Administering Medications by Inhalation

The lungs are supplied richly with blood and have a large surface area. These characteristics allow drugs to be absorbed easily from the lower respiratory tract. The smaller the particles of inhaled medication, the lower in the respiratory tract the medication tends to travel. A disadvantage of using this route is that the drug dosage is difficult to establish.

Drugs classified as bronchodilators and decongestants commonly are administered by **inhalation.** They act to decrease resistance to airflow by enlarging air passageways. Decongestants are local vasoconstrictors. Bronchodilators promote relaxation of musculature in the tracheobronchial tree. The relaxed passages produce less resistance to airflow and provide an opened respiratory passageway. Bronchodilators are further discussed in Chapter 45, Oxygenation.

Drugs for inhalation may be administered by a hand atomizer or a nebulizer. These devices break up the medication into a mist for more efficient inhalation. The hand-held, metered-dose inhaler (MDI) is often used incorrectly and the correct dose of medication is not delivered. For better medication delivery, a spacer should be used whenever using an MDI in a child. (See nursing guidelines for using an inhaler in Chapter 45.)

Nebulization may also result from the force of an oxygen stream or compressed air passed through the fluid in a nebulizer or an atomizer. This method is valuable for patients who require inhalation of a drug several times a day when the hand atomizer is fatiguing. Infants and toddler can also benefit from nebulized medications. With the use of an oxygen mask, a child can receive medications with minimal interruption of his or her activities. The oxygen stream is also useful in the production of vapors when high humidity is needed continuously for long periods.

> *Recall Jacob Shoolin, the school-age boy receiving bronchodilator therapy via nebulization. Using an oxygen mask for delivery might be frightening for Jacob, so the nurse should prepare him carefully for this treatment.*

One of the most common means of administering a nebulized drug using air pressure is the intermittent positive-pressure breathing machine (see Chap. 45).

Documenting Medication Administration

The medication record is a legal document. Recording each dose of medication as soon as possible after it is given provides a documented record that can be consulted if there are any questions about whether the patient received the medication. Do not record medications before they are given; if the medication were then not given, the medication record would show falsely that the patient received the medication. Different forms are used for recording medications; an example is given in Figure 29-13. The name of the medication, dosage, route of administration, time given, and nurse's initials are noted on the form. The site used for an injection should be

Guidelines for Nursing Care 29-5
Inserting Vaginal Suppository or Cream

- Perform hand hygiene and wear disposable gloves.
- Fill a vaginal applicator with the prescribed amount of cream, or have a suppository ready.
- Lubricate the applicator with water, as necessary. A suppository may be lubricated with a water-soluble gel. Ordinarily, lubrication is unnecessary but it may be used to reduce friction while inserting the applicator or suppository.
- Use clean aseptic technique to administer the medication.
- Spread the labia well with the fingers, and clean the area at the vaginal orifice with a washcloth and warm water to remove discharge, as necessary. Use a different corner of the washcloth with each stroke, moving from above the orifice downward toward the sacrum. These techniques prevent contamination of the vaginal orifice with debris surrounding the anus.
- Introduce the applicator gently in a rolling manner while directing it downward and backward to follow the normal contour of the vagina for its full length. Push the plunger to its full length, and then gently remove the applicator with the plunger depressed. After the applicator is properly positioned, the labia may be allowed to fall in place to free the nurse's hand for manipulating the plunger. Insert a suppository with gloved fingers well into the vagina.
- Ask the patient to remain in the supine position for 5 to 10 minutes after insertion.
- Offer the patient a perineal pad to collect excess drainage.
- Remove gloves and perform hand hygiene.
- Document the medication administration, any drainage from the vagina noted, and the condition of skin in the

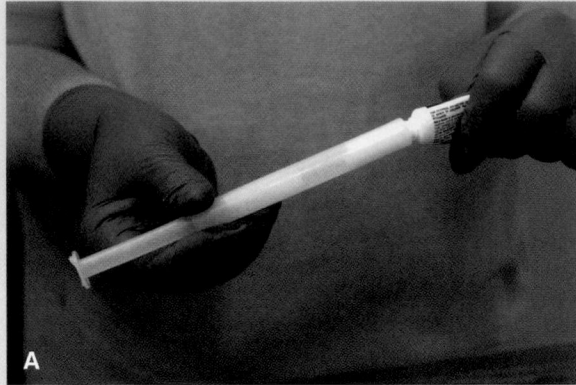

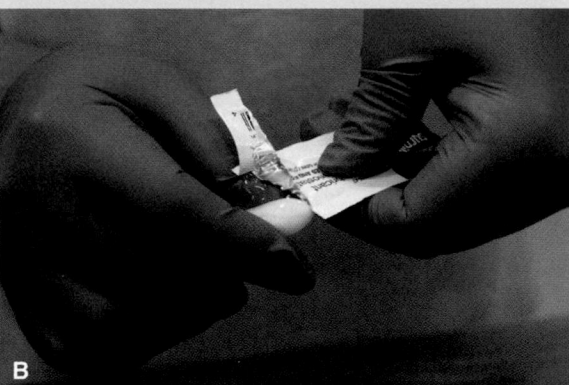

(A) Filling vaginal applicator with cream. **(B)** Lubricating vaginal suppository.

perineal area. Medication documentation may be performed on the CMAR.
- Teach proper techniques to the patient who wants to administer vaginal suppositories and creams herself.

---

recorded. The nurse's full signature and title must appear on the form for initial identification. Other specific patient information may be required. For instance, the pulse rate may be recorded when administering some cardiac drugs, or a description of the effects on the patient's pain when administering analgesics may be recorded.

Omitted Drugs

Drugs may be omitted intentionally or inadvertently. The omission and the reason for it are documented on the patient's record. Drugs may be omitted intentionally for the following reasons:

- The patient is to have a diagnostic test and is to fast before the test. Oral drugs are usually omitted, or their administration is delayed, depending on the physician's orders.
- The problem for which the medication is intended no longer exists. For example, a laxative has been ordered for a patient. The patient has had a bowel movement and no longer needs the laxative. The laxative is then omitted.

- The patient is suspected of having an allergy to the medication. Any suspected allergy should be reported to the physician.

To reduce the incidence of medication errors, many healthcare facilities are using computerized medication administration record systems. These automated records give the pharmacy the ability to track statistical information, maintain inventory control of drugs, and integrate this information with the central billing system (see Focused Critical Thinking Guide 29-1).

Refused Drugs

If the patient refuses to take a drug that is considered essential to the therapeutic regimen, report this promptly. The nurse can often determine the reason for the refusal and can help the patient accept needed drugs. If the patient is not persuaded by reasonable efforts and adamantly refuses to take a medication, it is unwise to continue urging the patient. Patients have the right to refuse therapy; recognize

CROZER-CHESTER MEDICAL CENTER
MEDICATION ADMINISTRATION + PARENTERAL THERAPY RECORD

FORM NS-MAR-1

Allergies: Operative Date:
                               Procedure:

Penicillin

Legend for Injection Sites
RA- Right Arm   RT- Right Thigh
LA- Left Arm   LT- Left Thigh
RB- Right Buttock R.Abd.- Right Abdomen
LB- Left Buttock   L.Abd.- Left Abdomen

STANDING ORDERS (MEDICATION ORDERED PER ROUTINE SCHEDULE OR WITH SPECIFIC NUMBER OF DOSES)

ORDER DATE & RN INIT.	EXP. DATE & TIME	MEDICATION, DOSAGE, FREQUENCY, ROUTE	HOURS	11/29 INJ. SITE	11/29 INIT.	11/30 INJ. SITE	11/30 INIT.	12/1 INJ. SITE	12/1 INIT.	12/2		12/3		12/4		12/5		12/6		12/7		12/8	
11/29/05 SM		Digoxin 0.25 mg po QD	10A		AC		AC		CL														
					AR =88		AR =92		AR =86														
11/29/05 SM		Lasix 20 mg QD po	10A		AC		AC		CL														
11/29/05 SM		Trental 400 mg TID Po	10A		AC		AC		CL														
			2P		AC		AC		CL														
			6P		PR		PR		PR														
11/29/05 SM		Slow K++ po QD	10A		AC		AC		(CL)														
11/29/05 SM		Serax 15 mg Po q. 8°	6A		SP		SP		MS														
			2P		AC		AC		CL														
			10P		PR		PR		PR														
11/29/05 SM		Procardia 20 mg po TID	10A		AC		AC		CL														
			2P		AC		AC		CL.														
			6P		PR		PR		PR														

SINGLE ORDERS (STAT, PRE-OP, ONE TIME DOSE, ON CALL, DIAGNOSTIC PREP)

ORDER DATE & RN INIT.	MEDICATION, DOSAGE, ROUTE	TO BE GIVEN DATE	TO BE GIVEN TIME	INJ. SITE	RN INIT.	ORDER DATE & RN INIT.	MEDICATION, DOSAGE, ROUTE	TO BE GIVEN DATE	TO BE GIVEN TIME	INJ. SITE	RN INIT.
11/29 PR	Dalmane 15 mg po now	11/29	11P	—	PR						
11/30	Dulcolax Tab. iii po at 6 pm	11/30	6P		PR						

FIGURE 29-13 Example of a medication record.

PRN MEDICATIONS (ENTER DATE, TIME GIVEN, INJECTION SITE AND RN INITIALS)															
ORDER DATE & RN INIT.	EXP. DATE & TIME	MEDICATION, DOSES, FREQUENCY, ROUTE		DOSES GIVEN											
11/29/05 sm		Tylox tab ii po q 3° prn	DATE	11/29	11/30										
			TIME	1q	3A										
			INJ. SITE												
			RN INIT.	AC	SP										
11/29/05 sm		Maalox 30cc po q 6° prn	DATE												
			TIME												
			INJ. SITE												
			RN INIT.												
			DATE												
			TIME												
			INJ. SITE												
			RN INIT.												

PARENTERAL THERAPY			DOCUMENTATION FOR MEDICATION WITHHELD			
ORDER DATE & RN INIT.	I.V. SOLUTIONS	SCHEDULE	DATE	TIME	MEDICATION	REASON FOR WITHHOLDING
11/29/05 sm	1000 cc D5W	q. 8°	12/1	10A	Slow K tab ii	patient refused

RN IDENTIFICATION								
INIT.	SIGNATURE	INIT.	SIGNATURE	INIT.	SIGNATURE			
AC	a. Christopher RN							
PR	P Rogers RN							
SP	S. Pointer RN							
CL	C. Lewis RN							

FIGURE 29-13 *Continued*

and respect that right. The refusal to take prescribed drugs and the manner in which the situation was managed should be described on the patient's record and reported according to agency policy.

Medication Errors

Nurses should take every precaution to avoid errors when administering therapeutic agents. Common types of medication errors include the following:

- Inappropriate prescribing of the drug (eg, incorrect dose, quantity, or route, or inadequate instruction)
- Extra, omitted, or wrong doses
- Administration of a medication to a patient that was not ordered for him or her
- Administration of a drug by an incorrect route or at in incorrect rate
- Failure to give a medication within the prescribed time interval
- Incorrect preparation of a drug before administration
- Improper technique when administering a drug
- Giving a drug that has deteriorated

Prompt acknowledgment of errors may minimize their possible detrimental effect. The immediate priority is the safety of the patient. The following steps are recommended when a medication error occurs:

1. Check the patient's condition immediately when the error is noted. Observe for the development of adverse effects related to the error.
2. Notify the nurse manager and the physician to discuss possible courses of action, depending on the patient's condition.
3. Write a description of the error on the patient's medical record, including remedial steps that are taken.
4. Complete the form used for reporting errors, as dictated by agency policy. These forms, called accident, incident, or unusual occurrence reports, require an objective, complete account of the medication error. Include the steps taken after the error was recognized. For legal reasons, the error must be described fully and accurately. Medication errors are a common allegation in nursing liability cases. The fact that an incident report was filed should not be documented in the patient's record.

Although incident reports have a negative connotation for many nurses, they can provide vital information that can be used to prevent the error from being repeated in the future. These tools can provide tracking of errors throughout the institution, providing information that may prevent future medication errors. The emphasis should be on the collaborative efforts necessary to provide safe patient care and decrease the

Focused Critical Thinking Guide 29-1

Medications

You are caring for two residents in a long-term care facility. One of your residents is scheduled to receive a B$_{12}$ injection, and because it will be your first intramuscular injection, it has you more than a little apprehensive. You are eagerly awaiting the moment when your instructor will be free to supervise your injection. Meanwhile, she has cleared you to administer the 10 a.m. meds, and you bring a multivitamin, a diuretic, and an anti-inflammatory agent to one of your assigned residents. When you go to record the medications you administered, you suddenly realize to your horror that you brought them to the wrong resident. When you grab your buddy and confide your error, she says, "Whatever you do, don't tell Miss McMullen [the clinical instructor]. She gets spastic about med errors and has a reputation for gleefully failing students!" You remember that the resident who received the wrong medications has no known drug allergies and think that she probably wouldn't suffer any adverse effects from the meds she received. What should you do?

1. Identify Goal of Thinking
Determine how you ought to respond to the realization that you administered medications to the wrong resident.

2. Assess Adequacy of Knowledge
Pertinent circumstances: A resident has received three medications that were not ordered for her. *You are a nursing student in your first clinical rotation* and fear your clinical instructor's response should you inform her about your error. You are unsure of the harm that might result from the resident receiving the wrong medication.

Prerequisite knowledge: To decide how you should respond in this situation you need to understand your professional obligations, which include your moral and legal accountability for having committed a medication error. You will need knowledge of the pharmacologic action of each of the medications you administered and their potential adverse effects on the resident who received them (possible interactions with other medications she is receiving, contraindications with related adverse effects, etc.). You recognize that there is no way for you to get the knowledge you need to make a morally and legally defensible response unless you admit your error to a responsible party.

Room for error/Time constraints: Because you do not know the effects of these medications, you are not in a position to judge how much room there is for error, nor are you able to make a prudent decision about how much time you have to act. The only defensible response is to seek help to clarify your position immediately because a resident's well-being is potentially at stake. No imagined personal costs would justify a delay in your admission of your error.

3. Address Potential Problems
The most serious obstacle to critical thinking in this situation would be an inability to think rationally about your obligation to report the error because of your fear of being censured by your clinical instructor. You will want to examine critically your friend's claim that your instructor will respond harshly because this may, in fact, not be the case. You will also want to test your friend's unstated assumption that your primary obligation in this sort of situation is to take care of yourself—even if this course of action results in harm to a patient. It would be helpful to think through the consequences of every healthcare professional behaving in this manner.

4. Consult Helpful Resources
Given that you are new to medication administration and are unable to assess the potential harm caused to the resident who received the wrong medications, you will find that your most helpful resource is your instructor and you will need to enlist her assistance immediately. She will probably want to contact the resident's physician to determine whether there are any contraindications to this resident's receiving the medications you administered or possible interactions with other medications. A pharmacist may also need to be consulted. You will want to be familiar with the institution's policy on medication errors and will need to know how to complete an incident report. If the nursing home has a risk manager, you may want to consult him or her.

5. Critique Judgment/Decision
You have two options here: admit your error and initiate appropriate follow-up, or attempt to cover up your error and "hope for the best." Your decision will basically be made on the strength of your moral conviction that your primary obligation is to safeguard patient well-being, even should this involve some self-sacrifice. Once you recognize the potentially disastrous consequences of patients not being able to trust healthcare professionals to act in their best interests, you decide that there really is only one professionally acceptable response in this situation, and you inform your instructor. It turns out that the resident who received the wrong medications suffered no adverse reactions. You, on the other hand, spend an awful morning following up on your error and even have to delegate your B$_{12}$ injection to another student while you are admitting your error to the resident, her attending, and the charge nurse and completing the incident report. At the end of the day, your instructor compliments you for your honesty and sense of responsibility and cautions you not to repeat the mistake. You are grateful that your worst fears (*failing*) weren't confirmed and leave the unit having learned a powerful lesson about the costs of being accountable.

incidence of errors. Peer review committees have proved effective in some healthcare settings.

Another effort to prevent medication errors involves the assignment of pharmacists to patient care areas in the hospital. The pharmacists spend time on the units and interact directly with the nurses and physicians to ensure safe medication delivery. They review patient profiles, discuss side effects of drugs and potential drug interactions, and ensure that medications are administered at appropriate times across nursing shifts. This team approach has the potential to significantly reduce medication errors.

Teaching About Medications and Abuse

Teaching about medications is an ongoing process and should begin as soon as the patient is admitted to the healthcare facility. In many cases, patients continue a prescribed medication regimen at home after discharge from the hospital. A factor that affects the patient's compliance with the medication regimen at home is education about the prescribed medications. Teaching should be tailored to the patient's level of understanding. Written instructions can be used as a reference for the patient (see Teaching to Promote Health at Home).

Explain the techniques of medication administration to the patient and family. Before being discharged from a healthcare facility, the patient should practice the necessary techniques under the supervision of a nurse to acquire sufficient skill for safe administration. Many patients have learned to give themselves injections, as well as many other medications, when the teaching was planned well and the patient was able and willing to learn.

Emphasize the importance of taking medications as prescribed and for as long as prescribed. A common error made by patients is simply omitting a drug, either through carelessness or because they believe that missing a dose is not important. Various aids are available to remind the patient to take his or her medication on schedule. Medication containers that beep when a dose is due to be taken, scratch-off dots on a medication label, and an electronic cap that signals dosage time and records each time the cap is removed are available. Advise patients to keep their medications with them when they travel. If luggage is lost or misplaced, refilling the prescription may be difficult.

Instruct the patient not to alter the dosage without consulting the physician. Medications should not be discontinued when symptoms disappear. Drugs used to maintain health, such as those used to control high blood pressure,

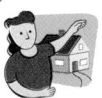

Teaching to Promote Health at Home 29-1
Medications

Health Topic	Teaching Tip	Why Is This Important?
General information	• Medication name and dosage • Intended effects of medication • Expected side effects of medication	Patients should know the names and reasons for medications in case of medical emergencies. Patients should also know expected side effects of the medication so they do not stop taking the medication.
Taking the medication	• Medications should be taken at the same time every day. • Teach whether food, beverages, or other medications have any effect on the medication. • Teach what patient should do if a dose is missed. • Teach patient to take medications as prescribed for as long as prescribed. • Teach not to alter drug dosage without consulting healthcare provider.	If patients make taking medications a part of their daily routine, they are less likely to miss a dose. Some medications require food to prevent stomach irritation; absorption of other medications is impeded by food in the stomach. Patients are likely to miss a dose of medication and need to know what to do if this happens. Some medications have severe consequences if stopped abruptly; others need to be taken for a set period of time and at a recommended dosage to be effective.
Special instructions	• Teach what to do when adverse effects occur. • Keep medications with them when traveling. • Do not share medications with other people. • Proper storage	Patients need to know whom to contact if any adverse effects occur. Luggage can be lost or misplaced. Teach patients that just because someone else has similar symptoms does not mean that the same medication should be taken. Medication should be kept out of the reach of children and pets. For labeling purposes, medications should be kept in the container in which they were dispensed. Some medications are sensitive to humidity and light; keep medications in a cool, dry place.

need to be continued as ordered to avoid recurrence of symptoms.

Caution the patient not to share prescribed medications with other family members or with friends and neighbors. Inappropriate use of another person's drugs can have serious consequences.

Nurses have a responsibility to teach about drug abuse. Teaching may take place on an individual basis or on a family or community level. Drug abuse is a major public health concern worldwide, especially among teenagers and young adults. Continued public and individual education is indicated, and nurses are also expected to set high standards for their own behavior and the use of drugs. Because drug abuse is increasingly common in healthcare providers, nurses who suspect that a colleague is abusing drugs must observe, document, and intervene for the patient's safety.

Evaluating

The effectiveness of drugs can be assessed in several ways. Clinical observation is the first method. Subjective data from the patient (eg, "My pain has disappeared") can be collected. Objective data (eg, the patient's vital signs) help the nurse evaluate medication effectiveness. Nurses also assess the patient for adverse drug effects.

Measurement of drug levels in body fluids provides data about the patient's response to a particular medication. For many drugs, including digoxin, warfarin, anticonvulsants, and aminoglycoside antibiotics, monitoring blood levels is an important component of therapy. The patient is tested to determine whether the drug level in the blood is within the therapeutic range. Drug dosages may be adjusted based on the serum drug level.

Monitoring systems can also assist the nurse in evaluating drug effectiveness. For the patient with an arrhythmia, for example, a cardiac monitor can show a change in heart rhythm.

The patient should be educated about the medication. The patient should be able to verbalize the following:
- How and when to administer the medication
- When to notify the healthcare provider
- Expected side effects and adverse effects

■ Developing Critical Thinking Skills

1. You are scheduled to give an intramuscular injection in the ventrogluteal site and remember learning that it should be administered using the Z-track technique. When you mention this to the nurse in the hospital who has been taking care of your patient, she tells you to be sure to remember the air lock. You remember your instructor telling you *not* to use an air lock. What do you do?

2. You are caring for two patients and have just completed giving medications to the first when you realize that you gave her the medications ordered for your other patient. What should you do?

■ Preparing for NCLEX

1. The name selected by the pharmaceutical company selling the drug and copyrighted by it is the drug's:
   a. Chemical name
   b. Generic name
   c. Official name
   d. Trade name

2. The process by which a drug is transferred from its site of entry into the body to the bloodstream is known as:
   a. Absorption
   b. Distribution
   c. Metabolism
   d. Excretion

3. A patient has an abnormal, unexpected response to a drug. This is defined as:
   a. Drug tolerance
   b. A cumulative effect
   c. An idiosyncratic effect
   d. An anaphylactic reaction

4. A medication order reads: "Digoxin, 0.125 mg PO qod." The nurse correctly gives this drug
   a. Daily before bedtime
   b. By mouth every other day
   c. Twice a day by the oral route
   d. Once a week after recording an apical rate

5. You are to administer a medication to Mr. Brown. In addition to checking his identification bracelet, you can correctly verify his identity by:
   a. Asking the patient his name
   b. Reading the patient's name on the sign over the bed
   c. Asking the patient's roommate to verify his name
   d. Asking, "Are you Mr. Brown?"

6. You are to administer a medication using a nasogastric tube. Before giving the medication, you should:
   a. Crush the enteric-coated pill for mixing in a liquid
   b. Flush open the tube with 60 mL of very warm water
   c. Check for proper placement of the nasogastric tube
   d. Take the patient's vital signs

7. The medication order reads: "Meperidine, 50 mg IM stat." The prefilled cartridge is available with a label reading 50 mg/1 mL. The cartridge contains 1.2 mL of meperidine. You should:
   a. Give all the medication in the cartridge because it expanded when it was mixed
   b. Call the pharmacy and request the proper dose
   c. Refuse to give the medication
   d. Dispose of 0.2 mL correctly before administering the drug

8. A patient requires 40 units of NPH insulin and 10 units of regular insulin daily subcutaneously. The correct sequence when mixing insulins is:
   a. Inject air into the regular insulin vial and withdraw 10 units; then, using the same syringe, inject air into the NPH vial and withdraw 40 units of NPH insulin.

b. Inject air into the NPH insulin vial, being careful not to allow the solution to touch the needle; next, inject air into the regular insulin vial and withdraw 10 units; then, withdraw 40 units of NLH insulin.

c. Inject air into the regular insulin vial, being careful not to allow the solution to touch the needle; next, inject air into the NPH insulin vial and withdraw 40 units; then, withdraw 10 units of regular insulin.

d. Inject air into the NPH insulin vial and withdraw 40 units; then, using the same syringe, inject air into the regular insulin vial and withdraw 10 units of regular insulin.

9. Ms. Hall has an order for meperidine, 100 mg q 4 h p.r.n. The nurse notes that according to Ms. Hall's chart, she is allergic to Demerol. The order for medication was signed by Dr. Long. Which of the following would be the correct procedure in this situation?

a. Administer the medication; the doctor knows best.

b. Call Dr. Long and ask that she change the medication.

c. Ask the supervisor to administer the medication.

d. Ask the pharmacist to provide a medication to take the place of Demerol.

10. The nurse manager on your unit prepared medications for Mr. Giles. She is called to the phone and asks you to give the patient his medications. Which is the best response to this request?

a. Give Mr. Giles the medication and record it in his chart.

b. Tell the nurse manager that you do not have time and ask her to get someone else.

c. Tell the nurse manager that because you did not pour the medication, you cannot administer it.

d. Give the medication to Mr. Giles but have the nurse manager chart it.

11. Why is the intravenous method of medication administration is called the "most dangerous route of administration"?

a. The vein can take only a small amount of fluid at a time.

b. The vein may harden and become nonfunctional.

c. Blood clots may become a serious problem.

d. The drug is placed directly into the bloodstream, and its action is immediate.

12. Mr. King is receiving heparin subcutaneously. Which of the following demonstrates correct technique for this procedure?

a. Aspirate before giving and gently massage after the injection.

b. Do not aspirate; massage the site for 1 minute.

c. Do not aspirate before or massage after the injection.

d. Massage the site of the injection; aspiration is not necessary but will do no harm.

13. A patient refuses to take her noon medication, saying that she does not need it. Which of the following would be the best response?

a. Tell her that she must take the medication because the doctor ordered it.

b. Tell her that you went through a lot of preparation to get her medications ready, and it's the least she can do.

c. Tell her that you don't care whether she takes the medications or not.

d. Tell her that you will return the medications to the cart but would like to discuss her reasons for refusing to take the medications.

14. A nurse discovers that she has made a medication error. Which of the following should be her first response?

a. Record the error on the medication sheet.

b. Notify the physician regarding course of action.

c. Check the patient's condition to note any possible effect of the error.

d. Complete an incident report, explaining how the mistake was made.

15. The nurse takes an 8 a.m. medication to the patient and properly identifies her. The patient asks the nurse to leave the medication on the bedside table and states that she will take it with breakfast when it comes. What is the best response to this request?

a. Leave the medication and return later to make sure that it was taken.

b. Tell her that it is against the rules, and take the medication with you.

c. Tell her that you cannot leave the medication but will return with it when breakfast arrives.

d. Take the drug from the room and record it as refused.

▪ Answers With Rationale

1. The correct answer is *d*. The chemical name identifies the drug's chemical composition and molecular structure. The generic name is assigned by the manufacturer who develops the drug. The official name is the name that identifies the drug in the official publication.

2. The correct answer is *a*. Distribution, metabolism, and excretion occur after the drug has been absorbed.

3. The correct answer is *c*. Drug tolerance results when the body becomes accustomed to the drug over time. A cumulative effect occurs when the body cannot metabolize one dose of a drug before another one is given. An anaphylactic reaction is a life-threatening, immediate response to a drug.

4. The correct answer is *b*. The abbreviation "qod" refers to every-other-day administration.

5. The correct answer is *a*. A sign over the patient's bed may not always be current. The roommate is an

unsafe source of information. The patient may not hear his name but may reply in the affirmative anyway (eg, a person with a hearing deficit).

6. The correct answer is *c.* Tube placement should always be checked before administering any medication to prevent the possibility of aspiration if the tube is not in the stomach. Enteric-coated pills should never be crushed, and very warm water may injure stomach mucosa. Taking vital signs is not necessary unless a particular medication requires it before administration.

7. The correct answer is *d.* Many cartridges are over-filled, and some of the medication needs to be discarded. Giving the excess medication in the cartridge may result in adverse effects for the patient. For this dose, it is not necessary to call the pharmacy or refuse to give the medication, provided the order is written correctly.

8. The correct answer is *b.* Regular or short-acting insulin should never be contaminated with NPH or any insulin modified with added protein. Placing air in the NPH vial first without allowing the needle to contact the solution ensures that the regular insulin will not be contaminated.

9. The correct answer is *b.* The nurse is responsible for any medications he or she gives and must contact the doctor to inform her of the patient's allergy to the drug. The nurse should not give the medication and might speak with the supervisor only if he or she is uncomfortable with the physician's answer once she is notified. The nurse is legally unable to order a replacement medication, as is the pharmacist.

10. The correct answer is *c.* Nurses should never give medications prepared by someone else because they are responsible for what they administer.

11. The correct answer is *d.* The intravenous route is a direct access to the bloodstream, and medications act quickly when given intravenously. The condition of the veins is not as important as the rapid effect of the medication administered intravenously.

12. The correct answer is *c.* When giving heparin subcutaneously, do not aspirate or massage, so as not to cause trauma or bleeding in the tissues.

13. The correct answer is *d.* The patient has the right to refuse medications, but the nurse should assess the patient's reasons for refusal, document them, and report them to the physician.

14. The correct answer is *c.* The nurse's first responsibility is the patient, and careful observation is necessary to assess for any effect of the medication error. The other nursing actions are pertinent, but only after checking the patient's welfare.

15. The correct answer is *c.* Safe nursing practice requires that a medication never be left at the patient's bedside. It is not correct to say that the patient has refused medication in this situation.

Medication Calculation Problems

1. Metoprolol (Lopressor), 25 mg PO, is ordered. Metoprolol is available as 50-mg tablets. How many tablets would the nurse administer?

2. Phenytoin (Dilantin), 100 mg PO, is ordered to be given through a nasogastric tube. Phenytoin is available as 30 mg/5 mL. How much would the nurse administer?

3. Captopril (Capoten), 12.5 mg PO, is ordered. Captopril is available as 25-mg tablets. How many tablets would the nurse administer?

4. Potassium chloride (K-Dur), 20 mEq, is ordered. Potassium chloride is available as 10 mEq per tablet. How many tablets would the nurse administer?

5. Digoxin (Lanoxin), 0.0625 mg PO, is ordered. Digoxin is available as 0.125-mg tablets. How many tablets would the nurse administer?

6. Propantheline bromide (Pro-Banthine), 15 mg, is ordered. Propantheline bromide is available as 7.5-mg tablets. How many tablets would the nurse administer?

7. Ciprofloxacin (Cipro), 500 mg PO, is ordered. Ciprofloxacin is available as 250-mg tablets. How many tablets would the nurse administer?

8. Furosemide (Lasix), 20 mg PO, is ordered. Furosemide is available as 40-mg tablets. How many tablets would the nurse administer?

9. Theophylline elixir, 100 mg PO, is ordered by way of a percutaneous endoscopic gastrostomy tube. Theophylline elixir is available as 8 mg/15 mL. How much would the nurse administer?

10. Clonidine (Catapres), 0.1 mg PO, is ordered. Clonidine is available as 0.2-mg tablets. How many tablets would the nurse administer?

11. Vitamin K, 10 mg given IM, is ordered. Vitamin K is available as 5 mg/mL. How much would the nurse administer?

12. Meperidine (Demerol), 35 mg IM, is ordered. Meperidine is available as 50 mg/mL. How much would the nurse administer?

13. Midazolam (Versed), 3 mg IM, is ordered. Midazolam is available as 5 mg/mL. How much would the nurse administer?

14. Hydroxyzine (Vistaril), 50 mg IM, is ordered. Hydroxyzine is available as 25 mg/mL. How much would the nurse administer?

15. Epoetin alfa (Epogen), 2,000 units SC, is ordered. Epoetin alfa is available as 4,000 units/mL. How much would the nurse administer?

16. Nalbuphine (Nubain), 1.5 mg IM, is ordered. Nalbuphine is available as 1 mg/mL. How much would the nurse administer?

17. Octreotide acetate (Sandostatin), 50 µg SC, is ordered. Octreotide is available as 100 µg/mL. How much would the nurse administer?

18. Morphine sulfate, 4 mg SC, is ordered. Morphine sulfate is available as 8 mg/mL. How much would the nurse administer?
19. Prochlorperazine (Compazine), 7.5 mg IM, is ordered. Prochlorperazine is available as 5 mg/mL. How much would the nurse administer?
20. Glycopyrrolate (Robinul), 0.4 mg IM, is ordered. Glycopyrrolate is available as 0.2 mg/mL. How much would the nurse administer?

Answers to Medication Calculation Problems

1. $\dfrac{\text{dose on hand}}{\text{quantity on hand}} = \dfrac{\text{dose required}}{X \text{ (quantity desired)}}$

   $\dfrac{50 \text{ mg}}{1 \text{ tablet}} = \dfrac{25 \text{ mg}}{X}$

   cross-multiply:

   $50X = 25$

   $X = 0.5 \text{ or } \frac{1}{2} \text{ tablet}$

2. $\dfrac{\text{dose on hand}}{\text{quantity on hand}} = \dfrac{\text{dose desired}}{X \text{ (quantity desired)}}$

   $\dfrac{30 \text{ mg}}{5 \text{ ml}} = \dfrac{100 \text{ mg}}{X}$

   cross-multiply:

   $30X = 500$

   $X = 16.66 \text{ or } 17 \text{ ml}$

3. $\dfrac{\text{dose on hand}}{\text{quantity on hand}} = \dfrac{\text{dose desired}}{X \text{ (quantity desired)}}$

   $\dfrac{25 \text{ mg}}{1 \text{ tablet}} = \dfrac{12.5 \text{ mg}}{X}$

   cross-multiply:

   $25X = 12.5$

   $X = 0.5 \text{ or } \frac{1}{2} \text{ tablet}$

4. $\dfrac{\text{dose on hand}}{\text{quantity on hand}} = \dfrac{\text{dose desired}}{X \text{ (quantity desired)}}$

   $\dfrac{10 \text{ mEq}}{1 \text{ tablet}} = \dfrac{20 \text{ mEq}}{X}$

   cross-multiply:

   $10X = 20$

   $X = 2 \text{ tablets}$

5. $\dfrac{\text{dose on hand}}{\text{quantity on hand}} = \dfrac{\text{dose desired}}{X \text{ (quantity desired)}}$

   $\dfrac{0.125 \text{ mg}}{1 \text{ tablet}} = \dfrac{0.0625 \text{ mg}}{X}$

cross-multiply:

$0.125X = 0.0625$

$X = 0.5 \text{ or } \frac{1}{2} \text{ tablet}$

6. $\dfrac{\text{dose desired}}{\text{dose on hand}} \times \dfrac{\text{quantity}}{\text{on hand}} = X \text{ (desired quantity)}$

   $\dfrac{15 \text{ mg}}{7.5 \text{ mg}} \times 1 \text{ tablet} = X$

   $2 \times 1 = 2 \text{ tablets}$

7. $\dfrac{\text{dose desired}}{\text{dose on hand}} \times \dfrac{\text{quantity}}{\text{on hand}} = X \text{ (desired quantity)}$

   $\dfrac{500 \text{ mg}}{250 \text{ mg}} \times 1 \text{ tablet} = X$

   $2 \times 1 = 2 \text{ tablets}$

8. $\dfrac{\text{dose desired}}{\text{dose on hand}} \times \dfrac{\text{quantity}}{\text{on hand}} = X \text{ (desired quantity)}$

   $\dfrac{20 \text{ mg}}{40 \text{ mg}} \times 1 \text{ tablet} = X$

   $\frac{1}{2} \times 1 = X$

   $X = \frac{1}{2} \text{ tablet}$

9. $\dfrac{\text{dose desired}}{\text{dose on hand}} \times \dfrac{\text{quantity}}{\text{on hand}} = X \text{ (desired quantity)}$

   $\dfrac{100 \text{ mg}}{80 \text{ mg}} \times 15 \text{ ml} = X$

   $\dfrac{1500}{80} = X$

   $X = 18.75 = 19 \text{ ml}$

10. $\dfrac{\text{dose desired}}{\text{dose on hand}} \times \dfrac{\text{quantity}}{\text{on hand}} = X \text{ (desired quantity)}$

    $\dfrac{0.1 \text{ mg}}{0.2 \text{ mg}} \times 1 \text{ tablet} = X$

    $\frac{1}{2} \times 1 = X$

    $X = \frac{1}{2} \text{ tablet}$

11. $\dfrac{\text{dose on hand}}{\text{quantity on hand}} = \dfrac{\text{dose desired}}{X \text{ (quantity desired)}}$

    $\dfrac{5 \text{ mg}}{1 \text{ mL}} = \dfrac{10 \text{ mg}}{X}$

    cross-multiply:

    $5X = 10$

    $X = 2 \text{ mL}$

12. $\dfrac{\text{dose on hand}}{\text{quantity on hand}} = \dfrac{\text{dose desired}}{X \text{ (quantity desired)}}$

    $\dfrac{50 \text{ mg}}{1 \text{ mL}} = \dfrac{35 \text{ mg}}{X}$

cross-multiply:

$$50X = 35$$

$$X = 0.7 \text{ mL}$$

13. $\dfrac{\text{dose on hand}}{\text{quantity on hand}} = \dfrac{\text{dose desired}}{X \text{ (quantity desired)}}$

$$\frac{5 \text{ mg}}{1 \text{ mL}} = \frac{3 \text{ mg}}{X}$$

cross-multiply:

$$5X = 3$$

$$X = 0.6 \text{ mL}$$

14. $\dfrac{\text{dose on hand}}{\text{quantity on hand}} = \dfrac{\text{dose desired}}{X \text{ (quantity desired)}}$

$$\frac{25 \text{ mg}}{1 \text{ mL}} = \frac{50 \text{ mg}}{X}$$

cross-multiply:

$$25X = 50$$

$$X = 2 \text{ mL}$$

15. $\dfrac{\text{dose on hand}}{\text{quantity on hand}} = \dfrac{\text{dose desired}}{X \text{ (quantity desired)}}$

$$\frac{4000 \text{ U}}{1 \text{ mL}} = \frac{2000 \text{ U}}{X}$$

cross-multiply:

$$4000X = 2000$$

$$X = \tfrac{1}{2} \text{ mL}$$

16. $\dfrac{\text{dose desired}}{\text{dose on hand}} \times \dfrac{\text{quantity}}{\text{on hand}} = X \text{ (desired quantity)}$

$$\frac{1.5 \text{ mg}}{1 \text{ mg}} \times 1 \text{ mL} = X$$

$$1.5 \times 1 = X$$

$$X = 1.5 \text{ mL}$$

17. $\dfrac{\text{dose desired}}{\text{dose on hand}} \times \dfrac{\text{quantity}}{\text{on hand}} = X \text{ (desired quantity)}$

$$\frac{50 \text{ μg}}{100 \text{ μg}} \times 1 \text{ mL} = X$$

$$\tfrac{1}{2} \times 1 = X$$

$$X = \tfrac{1}{2} \text{ mL}$$

18. $\dfrac{\text{dose desired}}{\text{dose on hand}} \times \dfrac{\text{quantity}}{\text{on hand}} = X \text{ (desired quantity)}$

$$\frac{4 \text{ mg}}{8 \text{ mg}} \times 1 \text{ mL} = X$$

$$\tfrac{1}{2} \times 1 = X$$

$$X = \tfrac{1}{2} \text{ mL}$$

19. $\dfrac{\text{dose desired}}{\text{dose on hand}} \times \dfrac{\text{quantity}}{\text{on hand}} = X \text{ (desired quantity)}$

$$\frac{7.5 \text{ mg}}{5 \text{ mg}} \times 1 \text{ mL} = X$$

$$1.5 \times 1 = X$$

$$X = 1.5 \text{ mL}$$

20. $\dfrac{\text{dose desired}}{\text{dose on hand}} \times \dfrac{\text{quantity}}{\text{on hand}} = X \text{ (desired quantity)}$

$$\frac{0.4 \text{ mg}}{0.2 \text{ mg}} \times 1 \text{ mL} = X$$

$$2 \times 1 = X$$

$$X = 2 \text{ mL}$$

Bibliography

Abrams, A. (2001). *Clinical drug therapy* (6th ed.). Philadelphia: Lippincott Williams & Wilkins.

Ahmed, D., & Fecik, S. (2000). MAOIs: Still here, still dangerous. *American Journal of Nursing, 100*(2), 29–30.

Barker, K., Flynn, E., Pepper, G., et al. (2002). Medication errors observed in 36 health care facilities. *Archives of Internal Medicine, 162*(16), 1897–1903.

Carroll, P. (2003). Medication errors: The bigger picture. *RN, 66*(1), 52–58.

Clarke, K. (2002). No needles needed. *Nursing, 32*(5), 49–51.

Curren, A., & Munday, L. (2001). *Dimensional analysis for meds* (2nd ed.). Clifton Park: Delmar Learning.

Eisenhauer, L., Nichols, L., Spencer, R., & Bergan, F. (1998). *Clinical pharmacology and nursing management* (5th ed.). Philadelphia: Lippincott Williams & Wilkins.

Fleming, D. (1999). Challenging traditional insulin injection practices. *American Journal of Nursing, 99*(2), 72–74.

Haddad, A. (2001). Ethics in action. *RN, 64*(9), 25–28.

Jech, A. (2001). The next step in preventing med errors. *RN, 64*(4), 46–49.

Johanson, L. (2001). Complacency can kill. *RN, 64*(8), 49–50.

Karch, A., & Karch, F. (2001). Let the user beware. *American Journal of Nursing, 101*(2), 25.

Karch, A., & Karch, F. (2001). Take part in the solution: How to report medication errors. *American Journal of Nursing, 101*(10), 25.

Katsma, D., & Katsma, R. (2000) The myth of the 90-degree-angle intramuscular injection. *Nurse Educator, 25*(1), 34–37.

Kee, J., & Hayes. E. (2003). *Pharmacology: A nursing process approach* (4th ed.). Philadelphia: Saunders.

Koschel, M. (2001). Question of practice: Filter needles. *American Journal of Nursing, 101*(1), 75.

Kuhn, M. (1998). *Pharmacotherapeutics: A nursing process approach* (4th ed.). Philadelphia: F. A. Davis.

McKenry, L., & Salerno, E. (2002). *Pharmacology in nursing* (21st ed.). St. Louis: C. V. Mosby.

Morris, M. (2002). When a phone order differs from the written one. *RN, 65*(1), 71.

Nicoll, L., & Hesby, A. (2002). Intramuscular injection: An integrative research review and guideline for evidence-based practice. *Applied Nursing Research, 16*(2), 149–162.

North American Nursing Diagnosis Association. (2002). *Nursing diagnoses: Definitions and classification 2002–2003.* Philadelphia: Author.

Phillips, J., Beam, S., Brinker, A., et al. (2001). Retrospective analysis of mortalities associated with medication errors. *American Journal of Health Systems & Pharmacy, 58*(19), 1835–1841.

Trooskin, S. (2002). Low-technology, cost-efficient strategies for reducing medication errors. *American Journal of Infection Control, 30*(6), 351–354.

Wentz, J., Karch, A., & Karch, F. (2000). You've caught the error—Now how do you fix it? *American Journal of Nursing, 100*(9), 24.

Winland-Brown, J., & Valiante, J. (2000) Effectiveness of different medication management approaches on elders' medication adherence. *Outcomes Management for Nursing Practice, 4*(4), 172–176.

Wolf, Z., Serembus, J., & Beitz, J. (2001). Clinical inference of nursing students concerning harmful outcomes after medication errors. *Nurse Educator, 26*(6), 268–270.

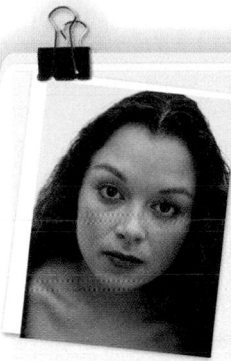

Molly Greenbaum, a 38-year-old woman who is scheduled for a vaginal hysterectomy later in the day, arrives at the hospital at 6:30 a.m. With tears in her eyes and wringing her hands, she states, "I really didn't sleep very much last night. I kept thinking about the surgery."

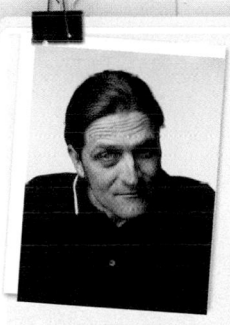

Ron Johnson, a middle-aged man with an extensive medical history, including gunshot wounds, bilateral leg amputations, paraplegia, and several surgeries, has been hospitalized in the past for long periods of time. Yesterday he underwent creation of a urinary diversion and is NPO. He asks, "Why won't anybody give me anything to eat? My doctor said that I would be able to eat the day after surgery. I want some food and I want it now!"

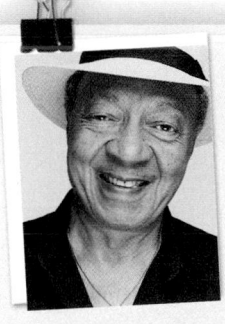

Marcus Benjamin, a 73-year-old man, has just had a total hip replacement under general anesthesia and is transferred to the postanesthesia care unit (PACU). His vital signs are stable. He has an intravenous catheter in his right antecubital space, infusing at 125 cc/hr, and an indwelling urinary catheter in place, draining clear yellow urine. The dressing over the surgical site is clean and dry, without any drainage.

Focusing on Blended Skills

The types of blended skills that you'll need to respond to the case scenarios include:

Cognitive Skills

- Basic knowledge of the surgical experience, including perioperative phases, categories of surgery, types of anesthesia, informed consent, and related nursing care
- Ability to integrate the nursing process to develop an individualized plan of care for patients undergoing surgery during each phase of the surgical experience
- Knowledge of the impact of physiologic age-related changes on a patient's risk during the perioperative period
- Knowledge of wound care
- Knowledge of intravenous therapy techniques and rationales for use
- Ability to identify the common psychological patient responses before and after surgery
- Ability to incorporate knowledge of the topics related to the surgical experience into a patient teaching plan
- Knowledge of physical and psychological preparation necessary for the patient who is to undergo surgery
- Ability to integrate knowledge of potential postoperative complications when developing a patient's postoperative plan of care, including appropriate preventive interventions
- Knowledge of resources to contact when encountering questions about the surgical experience or care with which you are unfamiliar

Technical Skills

- Strong assessment skills to identify risk factors and potential problems that may affect a patient's perioperative experience
- Ability to use equipment correctly and competently when providing perioperative care
- Ability to ask for assistance as necessary when performing new or technologically complex procedures or working with unfamiliar equipment
- Ability to implement techniques for safe and effective nursing care of patients in each perioperative phase

- Incorporation of principles of asepsis and intravenous therapy when providing care to a patient throughout each perioperative phase
- Ability to complete preoperative checklist accurately

Interpersonal Skills

- Ability to communicate to the patient concern about the patient and his or her well-being
- Ability to demonstrate respect for the patient's human dignity when implementing the perioperative plan of care
- Ability to work collaboratively with interdepartmental members of the healthcare team, using clear, accurate, and professional communication skills
- Ability to establish trusting relationships with patients, families, and colleagues as a basis for quality perioperative care
- Ability to identify and respond to the needs of the patient and family during the perioperative period, a naturally stressful situation

Ethical and Legal Skills

- Commitment to implementing the perioperative plan of care safely within the scope of nursing practice
- Ability to participate as a trusted and effective patient advocate, including advocating for the patient who is fearful or demonstrates demanding behavior
- Consistent use of appropriate legal safeguards when implementing the perioperative plan of care
- Demonstration of knowledge of informed consent
- Knowledge of pertinent agency policy for perioperative nursing responsibilities
- Knowledge of the ethical and legal principles that guide decision making about perioperative care measures for any patient, regardless of the type of surgery being performed

Learning Outcomes

After completing the chapter, the learner should be able to accomplish the following:

1. Describe the surgical experience, including perioperative phases, classification of surgery, types of anesthesia, informed consent and advance directives, and ambulatory surgery.
2. Conduct a preoperative nursing history and physical assessment to identify patient strengths as well as factors that increase the risks for surgical and postoperative complications.
3. Prepare a patient physically and psychologically for surgery.
4. Identify assessments and interventions specific to the prevention of complications in the immediate and early postoperative phases.
5. Use the nursing process to develop an individualized plan of care for the surgical patient during each phase of the perioperative period.

Key Terms

anesthesia
atelectasis
conscious sedation/analgesia
elective surgery
embolus
emergency surgery
hemorrhage
hypovolemic shock
perioperative nursing
perioperative period
pneumonia
thrombophlebitis

The treatment of a wide variety of illnesses and injuries includes some type of surgical intervention. Surgery may be planned or unplanned, major or minor, invasive or non-invasive and may involve any body part or system. A surgical procedure of any extent is a stressor that requires physical and psychosocial adaptations for both the patient and the family. The patient's recovery from a surgical procedure requires skill-

ful and knowledgeable nursing care whether the surgery is done on an outpatient basis or in the hospital. (See the accompanying Reflective Practice box for an example of nursing care for a patient who has had surgery.)

Nursing care provided for the patient before, during, and after surgery is called **perioperative nursing.** All phases of the nursing process are used to make assessments and provide in-

Reflective Practice
Challenge to Intellectual Skills

During a recent clinical experience on a level II ICU, I worked with a Ron Johnson, a middle-aged male patient who had an extensive medical history that included gunshot wounds, bilateral leg amputations, paraplegia, and several surgeries. Because of this, he had lengthy hospital stays and was known by the staff as being a difficult and manipulative patient. During my encounter with him, he was first day postop from a urinary diversion surgery. The patient was ordered to be NPO for the first 2 to 3 days following the surgery. However, this patient claimed that his surgeon had told him that he would be able to eat the day after the surgery, and he was demanding that I give him food and fluids. "I want some food and I want it now!" I told the patient that I had to follow the orders in his chart and that it was unlikely that he would be able to have anything by mouth during my shift. He asked me to explain the reasons for being NPO after surgery and I did my best under the time constraints by telling him that the bowel is affected by anesthesia and it is not ready to handle the intake of food and fluids. In all honesty, I did not know the major consequences of eating or drinking after surgery; however, I did not admit this to him. He was obviously not satisfied with my explanation because when I returned from my lunch break, he was sitting in front of a lunch tray with a large glass of fluids. He had talked some of the nursing assistants into getting him the items. He made the decision to act against my instructions and the instructions of his surgeon because I was not able to give him a clear, articulate explanation of his NPO status.

Thinking Outside the Box: Possible Courses of Action

- Tell the patient that I was unable to give him the best explanation of his NPO status, informing him that I would return in 5 to 10 minutes after consulting with a nurse and deciding the best way to articulate to him the consequences of ignoring the order.
- Avoid giving him any explanation at all, assuming that because of his extensive surgical history he knew the reasons why he must not eat or drink.

- Ask another nurse or even the dietitian to explain the NPO order.
- Alert the surgeon that this patient was at risk for being non-compliant and ask him to come to see the patient as soon as possible.

Evaluating a Good Outcome: How do I Define Success?

- The patient verbalizes an understanding of my explanation and the consequences of his actions.
- The patient complies with the physician's orders and with my instructions.

- The patient remains free of injuries/complications.
- I feel competent in my explanations and actions.
- I am able to take responsibility for the patient's actions.

Personal Learning: Here's to the Future!

This patient taught me a great deal. He taught me that sometimes, rather than giving an inadequate explanation, it would be better to admit that you do not know or that your knowledge is not up to par in a particular area. I should have been honest with Mr. Johnson, admitting that I was unsure about why he wasn't allowed to eat or drink. It would have been more advantageous to consult with someone else before giving him a more thorough explanation. I also should have recognized that Mr. Johnson was exhibiting extreme frustration and depression, placing him at

high risk for noncompliance. All he needed was someone to take the extra time with him, offering compassion and support. Unfortunately, the patient did not comply with the order and thus was at risk for developing serious complications such as a bowel obstruction. I alerted the surgeon of the patient's actions, and luckily the surgeon was understanding. In the future, I will make a major effort to gather the appropriate information to give patients a thorough, understandable explanation when they ask for specific information.

Reflection

How would you respond in a similar situation? Why? What does this tell you about yourself and about the adequacy of your skills for professional practice? What cognitive skills did the nursing student use? What cognitive skills were lacking or would have been helpful? How might the patient's past history have influenced the nursing student's actions? Explain. If you were this nursing student, would you have been influenced by his past history? Why

or why not? Can you think of other ways to respond? What other skills (cognitive, interpersonal, technical, ethical/legal) would you need to respond well in this situation? Do you agree with the criteria to evaluate a successful outcome? Did this nursing student meet the criteria? Why or why not?

Colleen Kilcullen, Georgetown University

terventions to promote the recovery of health, prevent further injury or illness, and facilitate coping with alterations in physical structure and function.

A conceptual model for perioperative nursing care is shown in Figure 30-1. In this model, the patient is at the center of all care activities. The three critical domains for patient care are safety, physiologic responses, and the patient and family behavioral responses. For each of these domains, there are desired outcomes. These, rather than the usual progression of the nursing process, which begins with assessment, are identified first in the model because perioperative nursing is preventive in nature. Therefore, perioperative nurses base their plans of care on already known and recognized desired outcomes. The patient is assessed for the relevance of the outcome, nursing diagnoses are then identified, and interventions are planned. The domain in the model that relates to the health system is intended to represent the structure elements and other system activities that must be present to support safe, effective, high-quality patient care.

The type of surgery scheduled influences the desired outcomes, nursing diagnoses, assessments, and interventions carried out by the nurse. For example, the nurse's role when caring for the patient having ambulatory surgery may involve providing patient care from admission through discharge. The nurse's role for hospital-based surgery is usually specific to one phase.

This chapter discusses preparing the patient for surgery, supporting the patient during surgery, and assisting with recovery after surgery. Selected nursing diagnoses and expected outcomes are included for each phase of care of the surgical patient.

THE SURGICAL EXPERIENCE

Regardless of the surgical intervention required or the setting in which the surgery is performed, all patients progress through specific perioperative phases, require some type of anesthesia, and give their consent for surgery. The following sections describe those components of the surgical experience.

Phases of the Perioperative Period

The patient who is having surgery progresses through several distinct phases, called the **perioperative period.** The three

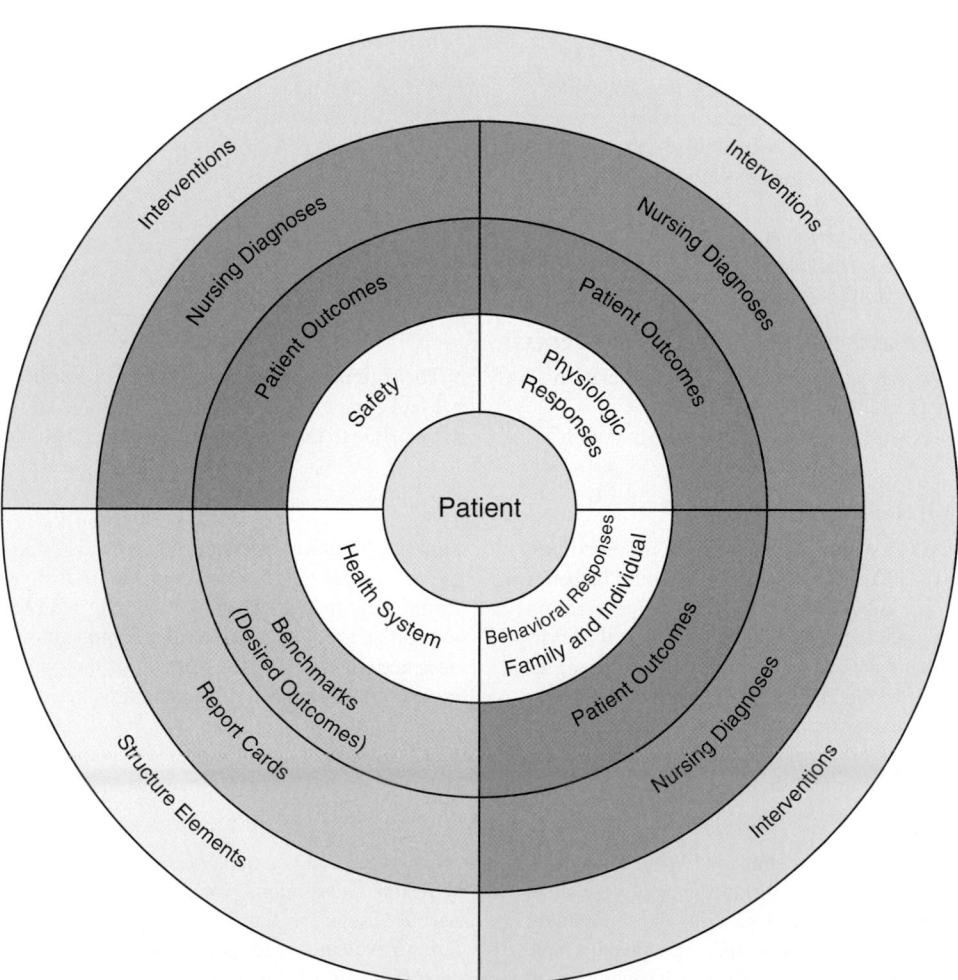

FIGURE 30-1 Association of periOperative Registered Nurses Perioperative Patient-Focused Model. (Reproduced with permission, *AORN Perioperative Patient Focused Model.* Copyright © AORN, Inc., 2170 S. Parker Road, Suite 300, Denver, CO 80231.)

phases of perioperative patient care are the preoperative phase, beginning with the decision that surgical intervention is necessary and lasting until the patient is transferred to the operating room bed; the intraoperative phase, extending from admission to the surgical department (or operating room) to transfer to the recovery area; and the postoperative phase, lasting from admission to the recovery area to complete recovery from surgery.

The postoperative phase can further be broken down into phase I (providing patient care from a totally anesthetized state to one requiring less acute nursing interventions), phase II (preparing the patient for self or family care or for care in a phase III extended care environment), and phase III (providing ongoing care for patients requiring extended observation or intervention after transfer or discharge from phase I or II) (American Society of PeriAnesthesia Nurses [ASPAN], 1998).

With an increasing trend toward short-stay or same-day surgical treatment, the nursing interventions in each phase of perioperative or postanesthesia nursing care may vary somewhat, but they remain basically the same. The nursing process is used during each phase to meet physical and psychosocial needs and to facilitate the patient's return to health. Each of these phases, with related patient needs and nursing activities, is described in detail in this chapter.

Surgical Procedure Classification

Surgical procedures usually are classified according to urgency, risk, and purpose. Table 30-1 lists each classification,

TABLE 30-1 Classification of Surgical Procedures

Classification	Purpose	Examples
Based on Urgency		
Elective: Delay of surgery has no ill effects; can be scheduled in advance based on patient's choice	• To remove or repair a body part • To restore function • To improve health • To improve self-concept	Tonsillectomy, hernia repair, cataract extraction and lens implantation, hemorrhoidectomy, hip prosthesis, scar revision, facelift, mammoplasty
Urgent: Usually done within 24–48 hours	• To remove or repair a body part • To preserve or restore health • To restore function • To prevent further tissue damage	Removal of gallbladder, coronary artery bypass, surgical removal of a malignant tumor, colon resection, amputation
Emergency: Done immediately	• To preserve life (plus purposes listed above)	Control of hemorrhage; repair of trauma, perforated ulcer, intestinal obstruction; tracheostomy
Based on Degree of Risk		
Major: may be elective, urgent, or emergency	• To preserve life • To remove or repair a body part • To restore function • To improve or maintain health	Carotid endarterectomy, cholecystectomy, nephrectomy, colostomy, hysterectomy, radical mastectomy, amputation, trauma repair
Minor: Primarily elective	• To restore function • To remove skin lesions • To correct deformities	Teeth extraction, removal of warts, skin biopsy, dilation and curettage, laparoscopy, cataract extraction, arthroscopy
Based on Purpose		
Diagnostic	• To make or confirm a diagnosis	Breast biopsy, laparoscopy, bronchoscopy, exploratory laparotomy
Ablative	• To remove a diseased body part	Appendectomy, subtotal thyroidectomy, partial gastrectomy, colon resection, amputation
Palliative	• To relieve or reduce intensity of an illness; is not curative	Colostomy, nerve root resection, débridement of necrotic tissue, balloon angioplasties, arthroscopy
Reconstructive	• To restore function to traumatized or malfunctioning tissue • To improve self-concept	Scar revision, plastic surgery, skin graft, internal fixation of a fracture, breast reconstruction
Transplantation	• To replace organs or structures that are diseased or malfunctioning	Kidney, liver, cornea, heart, joints
Constructive	• To restore function in congenital anomalies	Cleft palate repair, closure of atrial–septal defect

with purposes and examples for each. No matter what the defined degree of risk, any surgical procedure imposes physical and psychological stress and is seldom considered minor by the patient.

> *Recall Molly Greenbaum, the 38-year-old woman who is to undergo a vaginal hysterectomy. The nurse would incorporate knowledge about the various classifications of surgery to plan appropriate care before and after surgery.*

Surgery Based on Urgency

Surgery may be classified as **elective surgery** (the procedure is preplanned and based on the patient's choice); urgent surgery (the surgery is necessary for the patient's health but not an emergency); and **emergency surgery** (the procedure must be done immediately to preserve the patient's life, body part, or body function).

Surgery Based on Degree of Risk

Surgery is classified as minor or major based on the degree of risk for the patient. Minor surgery is almost always performed in settings such as a physician's office, an outpatient clinic, or a same-day, ambulatory surgery setting. This classification means that the surgical procedure is usually brief, carries a low risk, and results in few complications. In contrast, major surgery may require hospitalization, is usually prolonged, has a higher degree of risk, involves major body organs or life-threatening situations, and has a greater risk for postoperative complications. Advances in the use of laser techniques and minimally invasive approaches involving very small incisions have made major surgery less traumatic, requiring shortened hospital stays. New surgical approaches using minimally invasive techniques continue to evolve. Many surgical procedures, even though they are classified as major, may now be performed on an ambulatory basis or as a 23-hour hospital stay.

Surgery Based on Purpose

Some terms used to classify surgical procedures based on purpose include diagnostic, ablative, palliative, reconstructive, transplantation, and constructive (see Table 30-1).

Anesthesia

Anesthesia, depending on its classification as general or regional, produces such states as loss of consciousness, analgesia, relaxation, and loss of reflexes. General anesthesia produces all of these responses, whereas regional anesthesia does not cause narcosis but results in analgesia and reflex loss. Anesthesiologists (medical doctors) or certified registered nurse anesthetists (CRNAs) administer anesthetic agents. Nurse anesthesia is an advanced nursing specialty, with CRNAs administering about 65% of the 26 million anesthetics given to patients in the United States each year (American Association of Nurse Anesthetists, 2003). Both physicians and nurses who administer anesthesia perform preoperative physical assessments, conduct preoperative teaching, administer anesthesia during the surgical procedure, and oversee the patient's postoperative recovery from the anesthetic.

General Anesthesia

General anesthesia involves the administration of drugs by the inhalation, intravenous (IV), rectal, or oral route to produce central nervous system depression. The desired actions of general anesthesia are loss of consciousness, analgesia, relaxed skeletal muscles, and depressed reflexes. Choices of route and type of anesthesia are made primarily by the anesthesia provider after discussion with the patient. Many factors influence these choices, including the type and length of surgery and the physical and psychological status of the patient. Inhalation anesthesia is often used because it has the advantage of rapid excretion and reversal of effects.

The three phases of general anesthesia are induction, maintenance, and emergence. Induction begins with administration of the anesthetic agent and continues until the patient is ready for the incision. Maintenance continues from this point until near the completion of the procedure. Emergence starts as the patient begins to emerge from the anesthesia and usually ends when the patient is ready to leave the operating room; the length of time depends on the depth and length of anesthesia (Rothrock, Smith, & McEwen, 2003). New anesthetic agents enable patients to emerge from anesthesia and "wake up" in a fraction of the time required in the past. As these agents become more commonly used, patients will frequently bypass the postanesthesia care unit (PACU). This will enable more surgical procedures to be safely done in doctors' offices.

The advantages of general anesthesia are that it can be used for patients of any age and for any surgical procedure, with the patient unaware of the physical trauma of the surgery. There are, however, major associated risks for circulatory and respiratory depression, postoperative nausea and vomiting, and alterations in thermoregulation.

> *Remember Marcus Benjamin, the 73-year-old man who had a total hip replacement. The nurse would need to incorporate knowledge about the risks associated with general anesthesia along with knowledge of the physiologic changes associated with aging when developing an appropriate plan of care for this patient. Key to this plan of care would be measures that prevent or minimize the patient's risk for complications.*

Regional Anesthesia

Regional anesthesia occurs when an anesthetic agent is injected near a nerve or nerve pathway in or around the operative site, inhibiting the transmission of sensory stimuli to central nervous system receptors. The patient receiving regional anesthesia remains awake but loses sensation in a specific area or region of the body. In some instances, reflexes may also be lost. Regional anesthesia may be accomplished through major nerve blocks or through spinal (subarachnoid block), caudal, or epidural blocks.

Nerve Blocks

Nerve blocks are accomplished by injecting a local anesthetic around a nerve trunk supplying the area of surgery, such as the jaw, face, and extremities. Onset and duration of the block depend on the anesthetic drug, its concentration, the amount injected, and the addition of epinephrine, which prolongs the block.

Spinal Anesthesia

Spinal anesthesia is achieved by injecting a local anesthetic into the subarachnoid space through a lumbar puncture, causing sensory, motor, and autonomic blockage. This type of anesthesia is used for surgery of the lower abdomen, perineum, and legs. Adverse effects of spinal anesthesia may include hypotension, headache, and urine retention.

Caudal and Epidural Anesthesia

Caudal anesthesia is the injection of the local anesthetic into the epidural space through the caudal canal in the sacrum; it may be used for procedures on the lower extremities or perineum.

Epidural anesthesia involves the injection of the anesthetic through the intervertebral spaces, usually in the lumbar region (although it may also be used in the thoracic or cervical regions).

Although regional anesthesia may be selected for numerous types of surgery and patients, research indicates that it is especially useful in reducing postsurgical pain, bowel dysfunction, and length of hospital stay for older adult patients (Goodwin, 1999).

Topical and Local Anesthesia

Topical anesthesia is used on mucous membranes, open skin surfaces, wounds, and burns. Cocaine in a 4% to 10% solution is the most commonly used agent; others are lidocaine (Xylocaine) and benzocaine.

Local anesthesia is the injection of an anesthetic agent such as lidocaine, bupivacaine, or tetracaine to a specific area of the body. It is administered by the surgeon in minor, short-term surgical or diagnostic procedures such as tissue biopsy.

Conscious Sedation/Analgesia

Conscious sedation/analgesia is used for short-term procedures. The patient maintains cardiorespiratory function and can respond to verbal commands while the IV administration of sedatives and analgesics raises the pain threshold and produces an altered mood and some degree of amnesia. This type of anesthesia is often administered by a perioperative nurse with specialized training and competence in administering the medications and monitoring the patient's cardiac rate and rhythm, respiratory rate, oxygen saturation, level of consciousness, blood pressure, and skin condition.

Informed Consent and Advance Directives

Informed consent is the patient's voluntary agreement to undergo a particular procedure or treatment (such as surgery)

after having received the following information, which should be provided in understandable words (layman's terms) by the physician:

- Description of the procedure or treatment along with potential alternative therapies
- The underlying disease process and its natural course
- Name and qualifications of the person performing the procedure or treatment
- Explanation of the risks involved, including risk for damage, disfigurement, or death, and how often they occur
- Explanation that the patient has the right to refuse treatment and that consent can be withdrawn

Informed consent protects the patient, the physician, and the healthcare institution. The signed form is a legal document as well as an ethical imperative. The responsibility for securing informed consent from the patient lies with the person who will perform the procedure; this is usually the physician. The nurse may sign as a witness, signifying that the patient signed the consent form without coercion and was alert and aware of the act. The patient always has the right to refuse treatment.

Consent forms are not legal if the patient is confused, unconscious, sedated, mentally incompetent, or a minor (as determined by state laws). Consent may be given in those instances by a parent, spouse, next of kin, or legal guardian. Most states have a list prioritizing authorized next of kin in signing operative consents. It is important to know who is authorized to contact the proper person in case a question arises. In emergency situations, the physician may obtain consent over the telephone or by court order. More detailed information about informed consent is included in Chapter 7.

Advance directives, another type of legal document, allow the patient to specify instructions for his or her healthcare treatment should he or she be unable to communicate these wishes postoperatively. This allows the patient to discuss his or her wishes with family members in advance of the surgery. Two common forms of advance directive include living wills and durable power of attorney for healthcare. If the patient should experience a serious, life-threatening complication, such as intraoperative cardiac arrest, the family has previous knowledge of the patient's wishes regarding cessation of treatment, resuscitative efforts, or end-of-life decisions. It is important to discuss and document the exact do-not-resuscitate (DNR) wishes of the patient and family members before surgery.

Ambulatory Surgery

Surgical procedures performed in ambulatory (also referred to as outpatient or same-day) surgical settings have become common as the healthcare system has reduced the length of hospital stay to lower healthcare costs. These surgical settings may be found as freestanding units, in hospitals, and in physicians' offices. Some freestanding ambulatory surgery centers specialize in selected types of surgery, such as orthopedics or hernia repair. Others perform a wide variety of surgical interventions, including major surgical procedures that formerly required a 3-week stay in a hospital (Pessagno, 1999).

By allowing the patient to spend the night before surgery at home and to return to his or her own home to convalesce, much of the stress associated with surgery is eliminated.

> *Think back to Molly Greenbaum, the 38-year-old woman described at the beginning of the chapter. She arrived at the hospital on the morning of her surgery. Although she is fearful about the surgery, consider what her fear might have been had she spent the night before her surgery in the hospital.*

Patients who are older or chronically ill or who do not have support systems or access to resources to provide the care needed after surgery may require additional teaching and referral for home care services.

PREOPERATIVE NURSING CARE

Patients who require surgical intervention and nursing care enter the healthcare setting in a wide variety of situations, ranging from essentially healthy people who have planned elective procedures to emergency admissions for treatment of trauma. Surgical patients may be any age and at any point on the health–illness continuum. It is the nurse's responsibility to identify factors that affect the risk of a surgical procedure. This includes assessing the physical and psychosocial needs of the patient and family and establishing a plan of care, based on appropriate nursing diagnoses. Also included are interventions to meet the patient's needs and facilitate his or her recovery as the patient progresses through the perioperative period.

> *Consider Ron Johnson, the middle-aged man who has a history of previous surgeries and had urinary diversion surgery 1 day ago. The nurse would need to obtain a thorough history of the patient's previous surgeries and postoperative course to identify the patient's risk for problems with the current surgical procedure. Key to this assessment would be information about the patient's psychosocial needs, especially related to difficult and manipulative behavior.*

Some of the desired outcomes of the plan of care for the surgical patient, outlined by the Association of periOperative Registered Nurses (Association of periOperative Registered Nurses [AORN], 2002), are that the patient will meet the following goals:

- Be free from injury and adverse effects related to positioning, retained foreign objects, or chemical, physical, or electrical hazards
- Be free from infection
- Maintain fluid and electrolyte balance and skin integrity
- Demonstrate an understanding of the physiologic and psychological responses to the planned surgery
- Participate in a rehabilitation process following surgery

THE NURSING PROCESS FOR PREOPERATIVE CARE

Assessing

The importance of preoperative assessment cannot be overemphasized. Surgery is a major trauma to the body, and preoperative assessments identify factors that may place the patient at greater risk for complications during and after surgery (see Examples of NIC). Assessment of the surgical patient includes a health history and physical assessment to establish baseline data, identify risk factors, and determine the teaching and psychosocial needs of the patient and family. The assessment is often conducted several days before surgery as part of preoperative laboratory screening and teaching; this is referred to as preadmission testing. It may be conducted in the hospital, a surgical clinic, an office, or even in the patient's home.

Preoperative nursing assessments and teaching are key processes of care for ambulatory surgical patients (Fig. 30-2). Preoperative teaching can often be combined with preoperative screening tests, which are usually done 2 to 5 days before the scheduled surgery. Preoperative teaching for ambulatory surgery includes instructions to the patient and family (Box 30-1).

Health History

The health history identifies risk factors and strengths in the patient's physical and psychosocial status and helps the nurse to individualize the preoperative assessment. Health history information significant to the surgical experience includes the patient's developmental level; medical history; medications; previous surgeries; perceptions and knowledge of the surgery to be done; nutrition; use of alcohol, illicit drugs, or nicotine; activities of daily living and occupation; coping patterns and support systems; and sociocultural needs.

Examples of Nursing Interventions Classification (NIC)
Risk Identification

- Review past medical history and documents for evidence of existing or previous medical and nursing diagnoses.
- Identify patients with continuing care needs.
- Determine community support systems.
- Determine financial resources.
- Determine educational status.
- Identify patient's usual coping strategies.
- Determine past and current level of functioning.
- Initiate referrals to healthcare personnel and/or agencies, as appropriate.

McCloskey, J. C., & Bulechek, G. M. (Eds.) (2000). *Nursing interventions classification (NIC)* (3rd ed., pp. 565). St. Louis: Mosby. A full listing of nursing activities for each nursing intervention can be found in this book.

PREADMISSION TEACHING/TESTING PERIOPERATIVE ASSESSMENT

Planned Surgery And Date: _Arthroscopy, debridement_
foreign body ① knee   8/7/06

Date Of Visit: _7/14/06_

Surgical History: _① Knee arthroscopy x3_
(1997 = most recent with little improvement.) ® inguinal hernia repair 10
years ago.

Anesthesia History: _No problems_

Systems Review: _____   Allergy: _NKA_
                                Dental: _N/A – no bridges or crowns_

Contact Lens/IOL: _N/A_
Hearing Aid: _N/A_

Cardiovascular
Angina: —	Stroke: —
Rheumatic Fever: —	Murmur: —
Hypertension: —	Infarction: —
Date Last EKG: _1997_	Pacemaker: —

Respiratory
Pneumonia: —	Smoke: —
Asthma: —	Recent URI: —
Date Last CXR: _1997_	

Hematology
Bleeding Tendency: _On ASA – to D/C 8 days pre-op._

GI
Recent Vomiting: —	Diarrhea: —
Jaundice: —	Hepatitis: —

GYN
L.M.P.: _N/A_	Para: _____
	Gravida: _____

GU
UTI/Problems: —

Neuropsych
Syncope: —	Epilepsy: —

Musculoskeletal
	Neck Or
Arthritis: _① Knee_	Back Inj.: —
R.O.M.: _Limit = ① Knee only_	Prothesis: —
Skin Integrity: _No problems noted_	

Metabolic
Diabetes: —	
Thyroid: —	

Medications (including over-the-counter, herbal):
ASA daily
Lipitor 40 mg (each evening)

B/P _130/82_   T. _98²_   P. _86_   R. _20_   Wt. _185_
                                          Ht. _6'1"_

Advance Directive: _Done_
Escort Name/Phone: _Wife (207) 143-4444_

Lab Ordered:
H & H – results WNL

Abnormal Lab work called to

Dr. _____ on _____ Initials _____

X-ray _Chest xray – Normal_
AP/Lat ① knee – Medial joint line spurs, lateral compartment well preserved

Abnormal X-ray called to

Dr. _____ on _____ Initials _____

EKG
NSR – WNL

Abnormal EKG work called to

Dr. _____ on _____ Initials _____

Pre-op Teaching Guidelines

✓ Pre-Op Medications	✓ Skin Prep
✓ Transported to Holding Room	✓ Awake in Postanesthesia Care Unit
✓ Visitors to Waiting Room	✓ Oxygen Delivery
✓ I.V. Fluids	✓ Deep Breaths and Cough
__ Sequential Compressive Device (Appr. Surg.) Leggings (Cysto or GYN)	✓ Frequent Check BP & P
✓ Taken to O.R.	✓ Fluid and Food Restrictions
✓ Safety Belt	✓ Cannot Drive Self Home
✓ BP Cuff, Monitor Pads, Pulse Oximeter	✓ Jewelry, Make-up Left Home
✓ Electrosurgical Pad	✓ Wear Loose Clothing
✓ Use of Pain Scale	__ Video _____
	✓ Hand-out Packet _____

Notes: _____
Scheduled for knee classes

Postanesthesia Care Unit Follow Up: _Has voided. Using ice bag_
on ① knee. Pain 2 on scale 1 → 10. Has post-op appt made. Reviewed signs
and symptoms that should be called to MD.

Post-Op Follow Up: _____
Will do knee rehab unless contradicted by physician

Phone: _(207) 143-4444_

FIGURE 30-2 Example of an ambulatory surgery assessment record.

Preoperative Information for Ambulatory Surgery

Provide verbal and written instructions for patients having ambulatory surgery as follows:

- List medications routinely taken, and ask the physician which should be taken or omitted the morning of surgery.
- Notify the surgeon's office if a cold or infection develops before surgery.
- List allergies, and be sure the operating staff is aware of these.
- Remove nail polish and do not wear makeup for the procedure.
- Leave all jewelry and valuables at home.
- Wear clothing that buttons in front; short-sleeved garments are better for surgery on the hands.
- Have someone available for transportation home after recovery from anesthesia.

Inform patient of:

- Limitations on eating or drinking before surgery, with a specific time to begin the limitations
- When and where to arrive for the procedure, as well as the estimated time when the procedure will be performed

Remember Ron Johnson, the patient described in the Reflective Practice display. Because the patient has undergone previous surgeries, the nurse might assume that the patient understands the meaning of and rationale for maintaining NPO status. However, the nurse needs to investigate the patient's understanding about this area to ensure compliance with it.

Developmental Considerations

Infants and older adults are at a greater risk from surgery than are children and young or middle-aged adults.

The infant has a lower total blood volume, making even a small loss of blood a serious consideration because of the risk for dehydration and the inability to respond to the need for increased oxygen during surgery. The infant also has difficulty maintaining stable body temperature during surgery because the shivering reflex is not well developed, making hypothermia or hyperthermia more likely. The renal system has a lower glomerular filtration rate and creatinine clearance, leading to a slower metabolism of drugs that require renal biotransformation. Because the liver is immature until after the first year of life, the effects of muscle relaxants and narcotics may be prolonged.

Physiologic changes associated with aging (described in Chap. 20) increase the surgical risk for older patients. These changes, summarized in Focus on the Older Adult, decrease older adults' ability to respond to the stress of surgery, alter the response to preoperative and postoperative medications and anesthesia, and prolong or alter wound healing processes. With an increasing older adult population, assessing physiologic changes is crucial to providing knowledgeable, safe, holistic

nursing care to older surgical patients. Chronic illnesses, more common in the older population, also increase surgical risk and may require usual perioperative procedures to be altered. For example, a patient with congestive heart failure may be more easily fatigued and thus unable to be up and about as rapidly after surgery.

Consider Marcus Benjamin, the 73-year-old man who had a total hip replacement. Due to his age, the nurse would need to be alert to potential complications specifically associated with age-related changes and use of general anesthesia, IV therapy, urinary catheterization, and reduced mobility.

Medical History

The medical history provides information about past and current illnesses. Pathologic changes associated with past and current illnesses increase surgical risk as well as the risk for postoperative complications. Preoperative assessments and documentation are necessary to provide a database for individualized assessments and interventions in the intraoperative and postoperative phases of care. The following sections highlight selected examples and associated risks.

Cardiovascular Diseases. Cardiovascular diseases, such as thrombocytopenia, hemophilia, recent myocardial infarction or cardiac surgery, congestive heart failure, and dysrhythmias, increase the risk for hemorrhage and hypovolemic shock, hypotension, venous stasis, thrombophlebitis, and overhydration with IV fluids.

Respiratory Diseases. Respiratory disorders, such as pneumonia, bronchitis, asthma, emphysema, and chronic obstructive pulmonary diseases, increase the risk for respiratory depression from anesthesia as well as postoperative pneumonia, atelectasis, and alterations in acid–base balance.

Kidney and Liver Diseases. Kidney and liver diseases influence the patient's response to anesthesia, affect fluid and electrolyte as well as acid–base balance, alter the metabolism and excretion of drugs, and impair wound healing.

Endocrine Diseases. Endocrine diseases, especially diabetes mellitus, increase the risk for hypoglycemia or acidosis and slow wound healing and present an increased risk for postoperative cardiovascular complications.

Medications

The use of prescribed, over-the-counter, or herbal drugs can affect the patient's reaction to and increase the risk from the stress of surgery and the effects of the anesthetic agent. Many medications are canceled before the surgery, but the nurse should know the purposes and actions of the patient's drugs as well as the physician's orders. Specific medications may be given even when the patient is going to surgery (eg, patients with heart or cardiovascular problems or diabetes mellitus). Surgical risk is increased by drugs in the following categories:

- Anticoagulants (may precipitate hemorrhage)
- Diuretics (may cause electrolyte imbalances, with resulting respiratory depression from anesthesia)

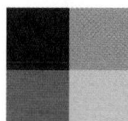

Focus on the Older Adult
Nursing Interventions to Address Age-Related Increased Surgical Risk

Age-Related Changes	Nursing Interventions
Cardiovascular	
Decreased cardiac output, stroke volume and cardiac reserve Decreased peripheral circulation Increased vascular rigidity	• Obtain and record baseline vital signs. • Assess peripheral pulses. • Teach leg exercises, turning, and ambulating. • Document normal activity levels and tolerance of fatigue. • Monitor fluid administration rate. • Allow sufficient time for effects of medications to occur.
Respiratory	
Reduced vital capacity Diminished cough reflex Decreased oxygenation of blood Decreased chest expansion and strength of intercostal muscles and diaphragm	• Obtain and record baseline respiratory depth and rate. • Teach coughing and deep-breathing exercises. • Teach use of incentive spirometer. • Assess color of skin. • Explain use of pulse oximeter for monitoring postoperative oxygenation.
Central Nervous System	
Decreased reaction time and coordination Reduced short-term memory Sensory deficits Decreased thermoregulation ability	• Orient to surroundings. • Institute safety measures, such as keeping environment clear of clutter and using a night-light. • Allow additional time for teaching. • Use appropriate measures to conserve body heat.
Renal	
Decreased renal blood flow Reduced bladder capacity	• Monitor amount and times of voiding. • Monitor fluid and electrolyte status. • Maintain and record intake and output.
Gastrointestinal	
Increased gastric pH Prolonged gastric-emptying time Decreased hepatic blood flow, liver mass, and enzyme function	• Obtain baseline weight. • Monitor nutritional status (weight, laboratory data). • Observe for prolonged effects of medications.
Integumentary	
Decreased vascularity Decreased skin moisture and elasticity Decreased subcutaneous fat	• Assess skin status. • Monitor fluid status. • Pad and protect bony prominences. • Monitor skin for pressure areas. • Use minimal amounts of tape on dressings and intravenous sites.

- Tranquilizers (may increase the hypotensive effect of anesthetic agents)
- Adrenal steroids (abrupt withdrawal may cause cardiovascular collapse in long-term users)
- Antibiotics in the mycin group (when combined with certain muscle relaxants used during surgery, may cause respiratory paralysis)

Previous Surgery

Data about previous surgeries are important for meeting the patient's physical and psychological needs throughout the perioperative period. Physical implications of previous surgeries are important to the intraoperative and postoperative phases (eg, previous heart or lung surgery may necessitate adaptations in anesthesia and in positioning during surgery). Complications during or after prior surgery, such as malignant hyperthermia, latex sensitivity, pneumonia, thrombophlebitis, or surgical site infection, may necessitate careful postoperative monitoring or alter intraoperative care.

The patient's past experiences with surgery also affect the plan of care established in the preoperative phase, especially if a past experience was negative. When the interview elicits negative feelings about the surgical experience, pain management, or nursing interventions carried out to prevent complications during previous surgeries, teaching and mutual goal setting are even more important.

In addition to experiences with past surgery, the patient's perceptions and knowledge of the surgical procedure to be performed should be assessed. The patient's questions or statements are important for meeting psychological and family needs when preparing the patient for surgery and planning for patient and family teaching and preparation for discharge.

Nutrition

Both malnutrition and obesity increase surgical risk. Surgery increases the body's need for nutrients that are necessary for normal tissue healing and resistance to infection. A patient who is malnourished is at higher risk for alterations in fluid and electrolyte balance, delay in wound healing, and wound infection. Obese patients are at increased risk for respiratory, cardiovascular, and gastrointestinal problems. Fatty tissue has a poor blood supply and therefore has less resistance to infection; postoperative complications of delayed wound healing, wound infection, and disruption in the integrity of the wound are more common.

Use of Alcohol, Illicit Drugs, or Nicotine

Patients with a large habitual intake of alcohol require larger doses of anesthetic agents and postoperative analgesics, increasing the risk for drug-related complications. Patients who use illicit drugs are at risk for interactions with anesthetic agents. These are specific to the illicit drug used and should be noted on the medical record for safe anesthetic management.

Patients who smoke are at higher risk for respiratory complications after surgery. All patients retain pulmonary secretions during anesthesia, but smokers, who already have increased mucous secretions and decreased ciliary action in the tracheobronchial tree, have more difficulty clearing the respiratory passages after surgery. In addition, the tracheobronchial mucosa is irritated chronically in people who smoke; anesthesia increases this irritation.

Activities of Daily Living and Occupation

Exercise, rest, and sleep habits are important for preventing postoperative complications and facilitating recovery. A patient with a well-established exercise program has improved cardiovascular, respiratory, metabolic, and musculoskeletal function, thereby lowering the risks of surgery. Rest and sleep are essential to physical and emotional adaptation and recovery from the stress of surgery. Information from the health history allows the nurse to individualize interventions to promote rest and sleep.

Many surgical procedures require a delay in returning to a career or occupation or may affect how the patient earns a living. Knowledge of a patient's usual work and concerns about returning to work help the nurse plan necessary teaching and referrals.

Coping Patterns and Support Systems

Assessment of the patient's psychological, sociocultural, and spiritual dimensions is as important as the physical history and examination. Surgery is a major psychological stressor and affects coping patterns, support systems, and individual human needs.

A surgical procedure, whether it is planned or unexpected, major or minor, causes anxiety and fear. While obtaining the health history, the nurse can use cues from the patient's and family's verbal and nonverbal communication to identify fears and concerns and to plan nursing interventions to provide the information and emotional support necessary to successful recovery from surgery.

Surgery is an unfamiliar experience over which a person has no control; the resulting anxiety may be expressed in many ways, such as anger, withdrawal, apathy, confrontation, or questioning. Therapeutic communication skills are essential for establishing the trusting nurse–patient relationship that is necessary to identify and resolve fear. Patients often fear the unknown, pain or death, and changes in body image and self-concept. The patient has fears about the surgery itself, the anesthesia, the diagnosis, the future, financial and family responsibilities, response to pain, or possible disfigurement or disability. Common fears are that the anesthesia will not "put me to sleep"; that death will occur during surgery; or that the patient will not be able to handle postoperative pain. Surgical procedures often leave the patient with permanent changes in body structure, function, or appearance. Patients commonly fear alterations in physical attractiveness, social relationships, lifestyle, and sexuality.

> *Recall Molly Greenbaum, the 38-year-old woman who is fearful of surgery. The patient's statements about the inability to sleep, in conjunction with the tears in the patient's eyes and wringing of hands, would be clues to the nurse that the patient is experiencing stress. Exploring the patient's fears, past coping mechanisms, and support systems would be valuable in developing the patient's plan of care, both before and after surgery. Doing so would help to promote a positive perioperative experience for the patient. In addition, the nurse would need to investigate what fears the patient may be experiencing related to a vaginal hysterectomy, such as changes in physical attractiveness, marital relationship, and sexuality.*

Encourage the patient to identify and verbalize fears; often simply talking about fears helps to diminish their magnitude. At the same time, incorrect knowledge can be identified and corrected, strengths can be identified, and teaching can be done. The reduction of fear is of major importance in preoperative preparation; emotional stress added to the physical stress of surgery increases the surgical risk. The nursing history should elicit the ways in which a patient provides self-support to reduce stress. These are discussed in Chapter 32 and range from listening to music to practicing active relaxation techniques.

Coping with stress can be facilitated through the support systems identified in the assessment phase of preoperative nursing care. As much as possible, family members or significant others should be part of the initial interview and should be included in discussions of fears and concerns. Encourage family members to provide support before and after surgery.

By identifying the patient's spiritual beliefs in the nursing history, the nurse can support the patient's spiritual needs through acceptance, participation in prayer or other rituals, or referral to a spiritual leader. Faith in a higher being provides support and helps to reduce fears in many people.

The need for other support systems can also be identified in the initial interview. For example, a patient having a colostomy, heart transplant, or mastectomy may have many questions answered and anxieties reduced by a preoperative visit from a person who has had the same operation and adapted successfully.

Sociocultural Needs

A person's perceptions of and reactions to the surgical experience are influenced by individual factors, including family health beliefs and practices, economic factors, and cultural/ethnic background. As discussed in Chapter 2, each person is influenced by family health beliefs and practices. A patient who requires surgery but has grown up in a family that believes that surgical intervention is the last possible option for treating illness may be hesitant about the surgery or may be convinced that death will result. The resulting anxiety may make this patient even more susceptible to surgical risk. Reactions to teaching, physical care, and pain are also influenced by family values and cultural/ethnic identity. For example, a male patient reared with the belief that it is unmanly to acknowledge pain may demonstrate a stoic acceptance of pain and refuse needed medications postoperatively.

Cultural and ethnic influences also affect the patient's responses to and perceptions of the surgical experience. The patient's cultural background may require that nursing interventions be individualized to meet needs in such areas as language, food preferences, family interactions and participation, personal space, and health beliefs and practices. For example, a patient from a culture that believes that bed rest is the most important treatment for illness or injury may have difficulty accepting the need for postoperative exercises and early ambulation.

Physical Assessment

Assessing the patient's current physical status provides data for interventions to decrease surgical risk and potential postoperative complications. Depending on the situation, the physical assessment is conducted as described in Chapter 25. See the Focused Assessment Guide 30-1.

Presurgical Screening Tests

Various presurgical screening tests provide objective data of normal body function. In cases of abnormalities, such tests provide data for medical interventions to improve the patient's physical status and thus decrease the risks for surgical complications. The nurse's role is to ensure that the tests are explained to the patient, the results are recorded in the

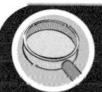

Focused Assessment Guide 30-1

Preoperative Physical Assessment

Factors to Assess	Questions and Approaches
General survey	• Note general state of health. • Note body posture and stature. • Take and record vital signs.
Skin	• Inspect skin for color, characteristics, and location and appearance of lesions. • Assess skin over bony prominences. • Palpate skin turgor.
Chest and lungs	• Observe chest excursion and diameter and shape of thorax. • Auscultate breath sounds. • Palpate for any pain or tenderness.
Cardiovascular system	• Inspect for jugular vein distention. • Auscultate apical rate, rhythm, and character. • Auscultate heart sounds. • Assess for peripheral edema. • Palpate character of peripheral pulses.
Abdomen	• Ask time of last bowel movement. • Inspect abdominal contour. • Auscultate bowel sounds.
Neurologic system	• Note orientation, level of consciousness, awareness, and speech. • Assess reflexes. • Assess motor and sensory ability. • Assess visual and hearing ability.
Musculoskeletal system	• Inspect and note joint range of motion. • Palpate muscle strength. • Assess ability to ambulate.

patient's record before surgery, and abnormal findings are reported. Additionally, abnormal results are data for determining additional nursing diagnoses and collaborative problems.

Usual presurgical screening tests include chest x-ray, electrocardiography, complete blood count, electrolyte levels, and urinalysis. Normal findings for laboratory tests are found in Appendix B. Significant abnormal findings include an elevated white blood cell count (presence of infection), decreased hematocrit and hemoglobin level (presence of bleeding, anemia), hyperkalemia or hypokalemia (increased risk for cardiac problems), elevated blood urea nitrogen or creatinine levels (possible renal failure), and abnormal urine constituents (indicating infection or fluid imbalances).

Diagnosing

Nursing diagnoses for patients in the preoperative phase may be identified for various problems that exist or for which a patient is at risk. These are derived from the analysis of subjective and objective data obtained from the health history and physical examination as well as information from other health team members and screening tests. Many diagnoses reflect assessment of risk and are made to guide interventions for patient needs in the intraoperative and postoperative phases. Nursing care throughout the perioperative period must be consistent and documented; the preoperative nursing diagnoses provide the basis for consistent, holistic care from admission through recovery. See Examples of NANDA Nursing Diagnoses appropriate to the preoperative period.

Outcome Identification and Planning

Preoperative nursing care is affected by the length of the preoperative phase. For patients who enter the hospital through the emergency department needing immediate surgery and those who have ambulatory surgery, there may not be enough time for comprehensive assessments and teaching. There has been a tremendous increase in the number of ambulatory and short-stay surgeries, in which patients are admitted early on the morning of surgery. In such cases, the nurse must use standardized preoperative plans and individualize the plans for the particular patient and family. Outcome criteria are standard for all patients having surgery, but nursing interventions are designed to meet the priority needs of individual patients and situations.

Planning for the entire perioperative period is done in the preoperative phase and includes expected outcomes that are discussed and mutually agreed on by the nurse, the patient, and the family. Specific appropriate outcomes are as follows:

- Is physically and emotionally prepared for surgery
- Demonstrates turning, coughing, and deep-breathing exercises
- Verbalizes understanding of postoperative pain management
- Maintains fluid intake and nutritional balance to meet needs

Implementing

Preoperative nursing interventions provide the patient with the necessary psychological and physical preparation for surgery and the postoperative phase. This section discusses implementing the plan of care to meet established patient

---

Examples of NANDA Nursing Diagnoses | The Preoperative Patient

Nursing Diagnoses	Related Factors	Sample Defining Characteristics
Anticipatory Grieving	Any condition that is perceived as a potential loss, such as physical ability and appearance following surgery	• Verbalizations of distress at the potential loss • Denial of the potential loss • Altered eating habits, sleep patterns, activity level, and/or libido
Anxiety	Any condition that is perceived as a threat or danger, such as effects of surgery on ability to carry out family roles and responsibilities Any condition that is perceived as a danger, such as the possibility of dying while under anesthesia	• Restlessness, poor eye contact, fidgeting, quivering voice, hand tremor • Increased pulse and respirations • Abdominal pain, sweating, dry mouth, fatigue, nausea, urinary frequency • Preoccupation, forgetfulness, decreased attention span • Verbalizations of distress, worry, being afraid
Risk for Infection	Any condition that interferes with normal inflammatory healing process	*Risk Factors* • Obesity • Aging • Immunosuppression • Malnutrition

goals. Skill 30-1, Preoperative Patient Care: Hospitalized Patient, outlines the actions and rationale for preoperative patient care.

Preparing the Patient Psychologically Through Communicating

Surgery is almost always viewed as a life crisis and evokes anxiety and fear. Anxiety can be reduced and recovery facilitated by nursing actions that focus on therapeutic communications and patient and family teaching.

The nurse uses therapeutic communication skills and techniques, as described in Chapter 21, to establish a supportive and trusting nurse–patient relationship and to facilitate psychological safety and security. Nursing interventions to meet the psychological needs of the surgical patient through communication are outlined in Box 30-2.

Each patient is a unique individual and responds to the surgical experience in a unique way. One note of caution: avoid false reassurance. In an attempt to allay anxiety and fear, the nurse may be tempted to reassure the patient that he or she will

---

SKILL 30-1   Preoperative Patient Care: Hospitalized Patient

ACTION	RATIONALE
General	

1. Identify patients for whom surgery is a greater risk:
  a. Very young and elderly patients
  b. Obese or malnourished patients
  c. Patients with fluid and electrolyte imbalances
  d. Patients in poor general health from chronic diseases and infectious processes
  e. Patients taking certain medications (ie, anticoagulants, antibiotics, diuretics, depressants, steroids)
  f. Patients who are extremely anxious
	This allows for recognition of patients who may be prone to complications after surgery.

2. Review nursing database, history, and physical examination. Check that baseline data are recorded; report those that are abnormal.	Review identifies patients who are surgical risks.
3. Check that diagnostic testing has been completed and results are available; identify and report abnormal results.	This check may influence type of surgery and anesthetic as well as timing of surgery or need for additional consultation.
4. Promote optimal nutrition and hydration status.	This promotes wound healing.

5. Identify learning needs of patient and family. Conduct preoperative teaching regarding the following:
  a. Coughing and deep-breathing exercises; respiratory therapy regimens
  b. Management of pain after surgery
  c. Leg exercises and early ambulation
  d. Postoperative equipment and monitoring devices
  e. Home care requirements
	This enhances surgical recovery and allays anxiety by preparing patients for postoperative convalescence, discharge plans, and self-care.

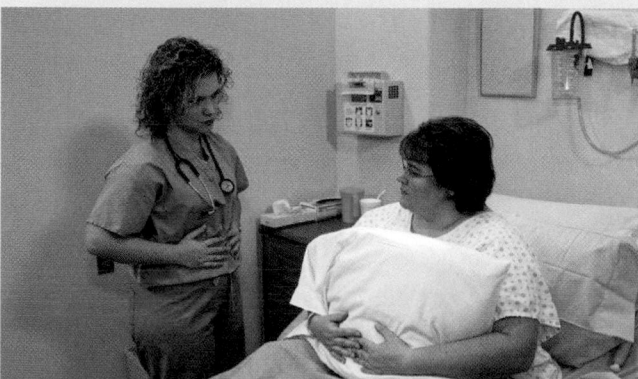

Action 5a: Teaching patient to splint incision before coughing.

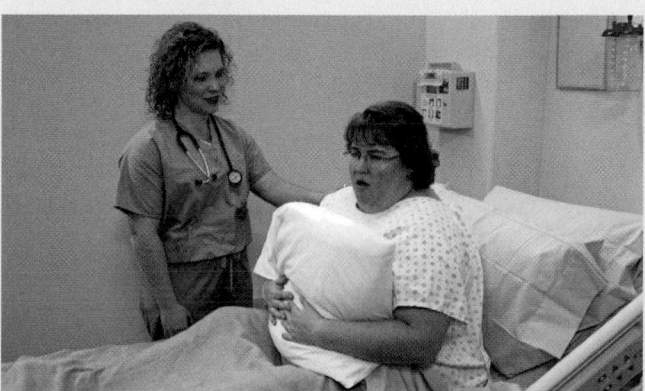

Action 5a: Teaching patient to cough.

(continued)

ACTION	RATIONALE
Day Before Surgery	
6. Provide emotional support. Answer questions realistically. Provide spiritual assistance if requested. Include family when possible.	This allays family and patient misconceptions and fears.
7. Follow preoperative fluid and food restrictions.	This reduces risk for vomiting and aspiration during surgery. Anesthetic agents temporarily depress gastrointestinal function and processes.
8. Prepare for elimination needs during and after surgery.	Anesthetic agents and abdominal surgery interfere with normal elimination function. A urinary catheter inserted preoperatively minimizes risk for inadvertent trauma to bladder during surgery.
9. Attend to patient's special hygiene needs (ie, use of antiseptic cleaning agents to prepare surgical site).	This decreases risk for infection.
10. Provide for adequate rest.	Rest minimizes stress before surgery.
Day of Surgery	
11. Check that proper identification band is on patient.	Double-checking ensures identity of patient.
12. Check that preoperative consent forms are signed, witnessed, and correct, that advance directives are in medical record (as applicable), and that medical record is in order.	This fulfills legal requirement related to informed consent and educates patients regarding advance directives.
13. Check vital signs. Notify physician of any pertinent changes (ie, rise or drop in blood pressure, elevated temperature, cough, symptoms of infection).	This provides baseline data for comparison.
14. Provide hygiene and oral care. Remind patient of food and fluid restrictions and time when NPO for surgery.	This promotes comfort and prevents intraoperative complications during anesthesia induction.
15. Continue nutritional and hydration preparation.	This prepares patient for operative procedure.
16. Remove cosmetics and prostheses (eg, contact lenses, false eyelashes, dentures, and so forth). Assess for loose teeth.	These interfere with assessment during surgery.
17. Have patient empty bladder and bowel before surgery.	An empty bladder and bowel minimize risk for injury or complications during and after surgery.
18. Place valuables in appropriate area. Hospital safe is most appropriate place for valuables. They should not be placed in narcotics drawer.	This ensures safety of valuables and personal possessions.
19. Attend to any special preoperative orders.	This prepares patient for operative procedure.
20. Complete preoperative checklist and record of patient's preoperative preparation.	This ensures accurate documentation and communication with perioperative nurse caring for patient.
21. Administer preoperative medication as prescribed by physician/anesthesia provider.	Medication reduces anxiety, provides sedation, and diminishes salivary and bronchial secretions.

bc fine. Such a response denies the patient's emotional needs, shuts off therapeutic communications and trust, and may not be true.

Preparing the Patient Psychologically Through Teaching

Teaching about postoperative activities is implemented in the preoperative phase and is the nurse's responsibility. Patients and families need to know about surgical events and sensations, how to manage pain, and how to perform the physical ac-

tivities necessary to decrease the risk for postoperative complications and facilitate recovery. The teaching–learning process (see Chap. 22) is individualized to meet common and individual patient needs.

The timing of teaching is a significant consideration: teaching too far in advance of surgery or when the patient is anxious is less effective. In today's healthcare system, patients often enter the hospital the day before or the day of surgery, and teaching must be adapted to this schedule. Many institutions provide teaching sessions before admission to prepare the pa-

BOX 30-2 **Nursing Interventions to Meet Psychological Needs of Patients Having Surgery**

- Establish and maintain a therapeutic relationship, allowing the patient to verbalize fears and concerns.
- Use active listening skills to identify and validate verbal and nonverbal messages revealing anxiety and fear.
- Use touch, as appropriate, to demonstrate genuine empathy and caring.
- Be prepared to respond to common patient questions about surgery:
  Will I lose control of body functions while I'm having surgery?
  How long will I be in the operating room and PACU?
  Where will my family be?
  Will I have pain when I wake up?
  Will the anesthetic make me sick?
  Will I need a blood transfusion?
  How long will it be before I can eat?
  What kind of scar will I have?
  When will I be able to be sexually active?
  When can I go back to work?

tient for surgery. Whether done before or after admission, a preoperative teaching checklist gives nurses organized and comprehensive guidelines for instruction. Box 30-3 provides a sample of preoperative teaching with associated surgical events.

Nursing research has indicated that the success of preoperative teaching varies with the timing of the teaching, the individual patient and his or her support systems, the type of surgery, and group versus individual sessions. Preoperative teaching has proved beneficial in decreasing postoperative complications and length of stay as well as positively influencing recovery.

Teaching about Surgical Events and Sensations

Patients and their families need to know when surgery is scheduled; about how long the surgery and postanesthesia care will last; and what will be done before, during, and after surgery (eg, procedures, medications, equipment). If the surgery is elective, a tour of the operating suite may be helpful in reducing anxiety and fear of the unknown; although especially helpful for children, this is also useful in preparing adult patients. An explanation of surgical events includes a description of the various members of the healthcare team.

Patients also need to know what sensations they will experience during the perioperative period. Although the sensa-

BOX 30-3 **Sample Preoperative Teaching: Activities and Events for In-Hospital Surgery**

Preoperative Phase
- ☐ Exercises and physical activities
  - ☐ Deep-breathing exercises
  - ☐ Coughing
  - ☐ Incentive spirometry
  - ☐ Coughing
  - ☐ Turning
  - ☐ Leg exercises
- ☐ Pain management
  - ☐ Meaning of PRN orders for medications
  - ☐ Timing for best effect of medications
  - ☐ Splinting incision
  - ☐ Nonpharmacologic pain management options
- ☐ Visit by anesthesiologist
- ☐ Physical preparation
  - ☐ NPO
  - ☐ Sleeping medication the night before
  - ☐ Preoperative checklist (review items)
- ☐ Visitors and waiting room
- ☐ Transported to operating room by stretcher

Intraoperative Phase
- ☐ Holding area
  - ☐ Skin preparation
  - ☐ Intravenous lines and fluids
  - ☐ Medications

- ☐ Operating room
  - ☐ Operating room bed
  - ☐ Lights and common equipment (eg, cardiac monitor, pulse oximeter, warming device, etc.)
  - ☐ Safety belt
  - ☐ Sensations
  - ☐ Staff

Postoperative Phase
- ☐ Postanesthesia care unit
  - ☐ Frequent vital signs, assessments (eg, orientation, movement of extremities, strength of grasp)
  - ☐ Dressings/drains/tubes/catheters
  - ☐ Intravenous lines
  - ☐ Pain medications/comfort measures
  - ☐ Family notification
  - ☐ Sensations
  - ☐ Airway/oxygen therapy/pulse oximetry
  - ☐ Staff
- ☐ Transfer to unit (on stretcher)
  - ☐ Frequent vital signs
  - ☐ Sensations
  - ☐ Pain medications/nonpharmacologic strategies
  - ☐ NPO, diet progression
  - ☐ Exercises
  - ☐ Early ambulation
  - ☐ Family visits

tions differ depending on the type of surgery, teaching should include information about dry mouth and drowsiness from preoperative medications, a sore throat from an endotracheal tube, a gradual return of feeling and movement after spinal anesthesia, and pain from the surgical incision.

Teaching about Pain Management

Pain is a normal part of the surgical experience and a major concern for the patient and family. Guidelines for the management of acute surgical pain have been established by the Agency for Health Care Policy and Research (1992). The guidelines are based on these principles: (1) the pain reported by the patient is the determining factor of pain control; (2) pain must be assessed as often as every 2 hours after major surgery; and (3) the older patient is at risk for both undertreatment and overtreatment of pain.

Teach the patient and family that medications to relieve pain will be ordered by the physician and administered by the nurse. The physician may order pain medications to be given on a regular basis or on an as-needed (p.r.n.) basis. If medication is ordered p.r.n., there is a time restriction between doses (eg, every 2–4 hours). The patient needs to ask for the medication and should do so before the pain becomes severe. If the medication does not control the pain, a different one can be ordered. There is little danger of addiction to pain medications used in the postoperative management of pain. In addition, the use of relaxation techniques (eg, deep breathing, music, and guided imagery) enhances the effects of pain medications.

Alternative methods of pain control, including transcutaneous electrical nerve stimulation (TENS) and patient-controlled analgesia (PCA), may be used after surgery. A discussion of TENS and information about nursing interventions when using PCA are in Chapter 41. Before surgery, teach the patient how to use these methods of pain control. After surgery, assess the effectiveness of the pain relief using these methods. Pain management is further discussed in Chapter 41.

Teaching Physical Activities

The most common causes of postoperative complications are cardiovascular and respiratory alterations, including atelectasis, pneumonia, thrombophlebitis, and emboli. Physical activities to reduce the risk for these complications are deep breathing, coughing, incentive spirometry, leg exercises, and turning in bed. These activities are taught in the preoperative period. The patient should be able to state the purpose and demonstrate the activities before going to surgery. (This section gives the rationale for the activities; postoperative complications are discussed later in the chapter.)

Deep Breathing. During surgery, the cough reflex is suppressed, mucus accumulates in the tracheobronchial passageways, and the lungs do not ventilate fully. After surgery, respirations often are less effective as a result of the anesthesia, pain medications, and pain from the incision. Patients who have thoracic or high abdominal incisions are especially prone to shallow breathing because of incisional pain with deeper

respirations. As a result, alveoli do not inflate and may collapse, and secretions are retained, increasing the risk for atelectasis and respiratory infection. Deep-breathing exercises hyperventilate the alveoli and prevent them from collapsing again, improve lung expansion and volume, help to expel anesthetic gases and mucus, and facilitate oxygenation of tissues. See the Guidelines for Nursing Care 30-1 for teaching the patient deep-breathing techniques.

Coughing. Coughing helps remove retained mucus from the respiratory tract and is usually is taught in conjunction with deep breathing. Coughing is especially important in patients with an increased risk for respiratory complications. Because coughing is often painful, the patient should be taught how to splint the incision (ie, support the incision with a pillow or folded bath blanket, as shown in Skill 30-1) and to use the period after pain medication has been administered to best advantage. See the Guidelines for Nursing Care 30-2 for teaching the patient how to cough effectively.

Incentive Spirometry. An incentive spirometer is often ordered for patients having surgery, and the proper technique for using it should be practiced preoperatively. This device helps to increase lung volume and inflation of alveoli and facilitates venous return. A gauge on the incentive spirometry device allows the patient to measure his or her progress and provides immediate positive reinforcement for the breathing efforts. See Guidelines for Nursing Care 30-3 for teaching the patient how to use the incentive spirometer.

Leg Exercises. During surgery, venous blood return from the legs slows; some surgical positions also decrease venous return. With circulatory stasis of the legs, thrombophlebitis and resultant emboli are potential complications. Leg exercises increase venous return through flexion and contraction of the quadriceps and gastrocnemius muscles. Leg exercises must be individualized to patient needs, physical condition, physician

---

Guidelines for Nursing Care 30-1
Deep Breathing

- Place the patient in semi-Fowler's position, with the neck and shoulders supported.
- Ask the patient to place the hands over the rib cage, so he or she can feel the chest rise as the lungs expand.
- Ask the patient to:
  - Exhale gently and completely.
  - Inhale through the nose gently and completely.
  - Hold his or her breath for 3 to 5 seconds and mentally count "one, one thousand, two, one thousand," and so forth.
  - Exhale as completely as possible through the mouth with lips pursed (as if whistling).
  - Repeat three times.
- This exercise should be done every 1 to 2 hours while the patient is awake for the first 24 to 48 hours after surgery and as necessary thereafter, depending on risk factors and pulmonary status.

Guidelines for Nursing Care 30-2
Effective Coughing

- Place the patient in a semi-Fowler's position, leaning forward.
- Provide a pillow or folded bath blanket to use in splinting the incision.
- Ask the patient to:
  - Inhale and exhale deeply and slowly through the nose three times.
  - Take a deep breath and hold it for 3 seconds.
  - "Hack" out for three short breaths.
  - With mouth open, take a quick breath.
  - Cough deeply once or twice.
  - Take another deep breath.
- Repeat the exercise every 2 hours while awake.

preference, and agency protocol. Guidelines for teaching the patient leg exercises are given in Figure 30-3.

Turning in Bed. Turning in bed improves venous return, respiratory function, and gastrointestinal peristalsis and prevents the unrelieved pressure that would occur if the patient were to remain in one position only. Although turning in bed sounds like a simple procedure, incisional pain makes it difficult, and it should be practiced before surgery. To turn in bed, the patient should raise one knee, reach across to grasp the side rail on the side toward which he or she is turning, and roll over while pushing with the bent leg and pulling on the side rail. A small pillow is useful for splinting the incision while turning. The patient should turn and change positions in bed every 2 hours.

Preparing the Patient Physically

The physical preparation of the patient for surgery varies, depending on the patient's physical status and special needs, type of surgery, and physician's orders. Certain nursing interventions are appropriate for all surgical patients in the areas of hygiene and skin preparation, elimination, nutrition and fluids, and rest and sleep. The nurse is also responsible for the preparation and safety of the patient on the day of surgery.

Hygiene and Skin Preparation

Intact skin is the body's first line of defense against microorganisms, and an alteration in skin integrity (eg, the surgical incision) provides a potential source of infection. Therefore, the skin is prepared to minimize skin contamination and decrease the risk for postoperative surgical site infection.

The skin is cleaned at the operative site with an anti bacterial soap or solution to remove bacteria. The patient can do this while taking a bath or shower. Ideally, a shower is taken the evening before or the morning of surgery. Shampooing the hair and cleaning the fingernails also help to reduce the number of organisms present.

The incisional area may require removal of hair before surgery. The need for hair removal depends on the amount of hair, the location of the incision, and the type of surgical procedure being performed. This may be done on the unit or in the surgical suite immediately before the operation, usually in the surgical holding area. If hair must be removed, depilatory creams or hair clippers are recommended by the Centers for Disease Control and Prevention rather than shaving the surgical site, as was done in the past. If the surgeon requires a shave prep, it should be done as close to the time of surgery as possi-

Guidelines for Nursing Care 30-3
Teaching Patients to Use an Inceptive Spirometer

- Assist patient to upright position if possible.
- Remove dentures if they fit poorly.
- Medicate with ordered pain medication if needed.
- Demonstrate how to steady device with one hand and hold mouthpiece with other hand.
- Instruct the patient to exhale normally and then place lips securely around mouthpiece.
- Instruct patient not to breathe through his or her nose. Use a nose clip if necessary.
- Instruct the patient to inhale slowly and as deeply as possible through the mouthpiece.
- Tell patient to hold breath and count to three. Check position of gauge to determine progress and level attained.
- Instruct patient to remove lips from mouthpiece and exhale normally.
- Tell patient to complete breathing exercises about 10 times every hour if possible. Rest in between breaths as necessary.

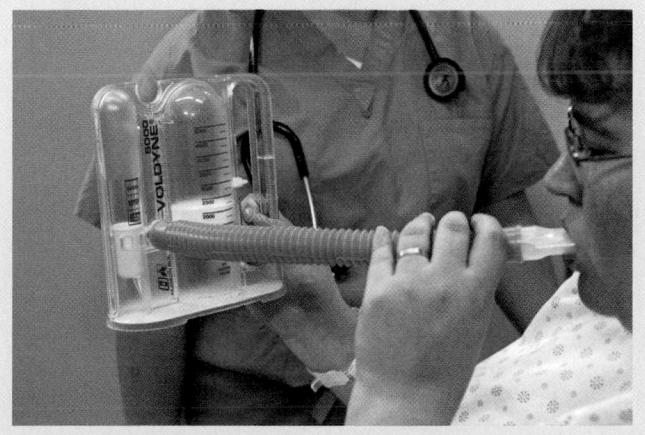

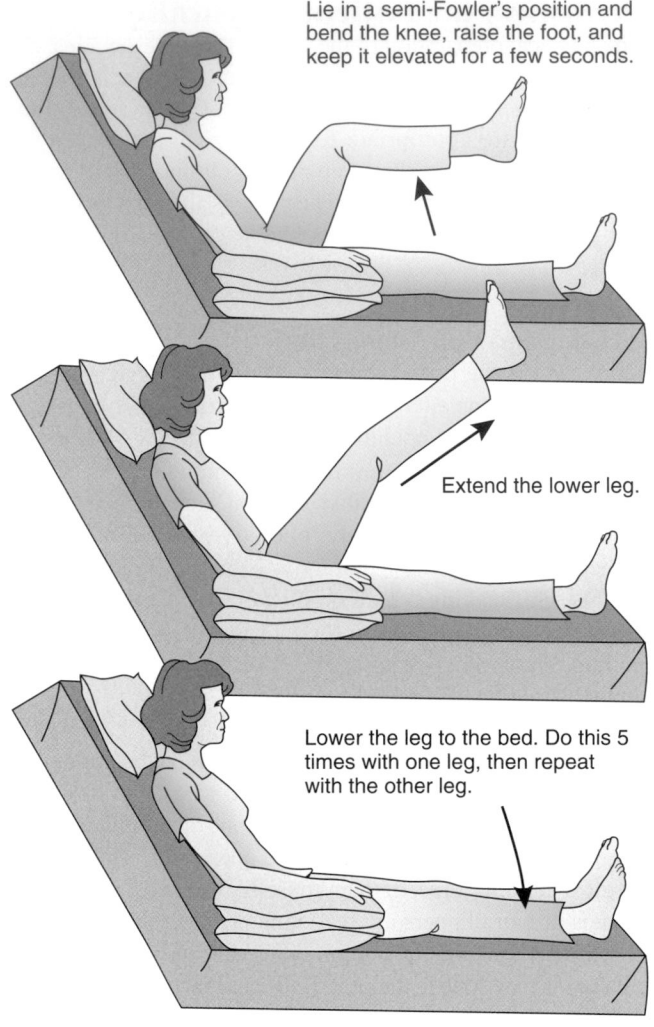

Lie in a semi-Fowler's position and bend the knee, raise the foot, and keep it elevated for a few seconds.

Extend the lower leg.

Lower the leg to the bed. Do this 5 times with one leg, then repeat with the other leg.

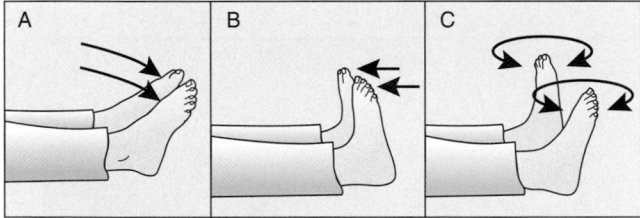

A. Point the toes of both feet toward the foot of the bed. Relax both feet.
B. Pull toes toward the chin. Relax both feet.
C. Make circles with both ankles. First circle to the right, then to the left. Repeat 3 times. Relax feet.

FIGURE 30-3 Leg exercises to increase venous return.

ble. Agency protocol should be followed for the timing, people responsible, and documentation of the condition of the skin and method of preparation.

Elimination

Emptying the bowel of feces is no longer a routine procedure before surgery, but the nurse should use preoperative assessments to determine the need for an order for bowel elimination. If the patient has not had a bowel movement for

several days or has had preoperative barium diagnostic tests, an enema helps to prevent postoperative constipation.

If the patient is scheduled for surgery of the gastrointestinal tract, a cleansing enema is usually ordered. Peristalsis does not return for 24 to 48 hours after the bowel is handled, so preoperative cleansing helps to decrease postoperative constipation. An empty bowel also prevents contamination of the surgical area during surgery.

Insertion of an indwelling urinary catheter may be ordered before surgery, especially in patients having pelvic surgery, to prevent bladder distention or accidental injury. If an indwelling catheter is not in place, the patient should void immediately before receiving preoperative medications to ensure an empty bladder during surgery.

Nutrition and Fluids

The diet order for a patient having surgery depends on the type of surgery and type of anesthesia to be used. In the past, most surgical patients could not eat or drink anything for 8 to 12 hours before the surgery. More current practice is to allow patients to drink clear liquids up to 2 hours before surgery with the permission of the physician. Clear liquids, which must be carefully defined for the patient, include water, fruit juices without pulp, carbonated beverages, clear tea, and black coffee.

According to the American Society of Anesthesiologists, patients, especially children, may be less anxious, better hydrated, and have fewer headaches and nausea after surgery with these revised practice guidelines for preoperative fasting (Crenshaw & Winslow, 2002). See the accompanying Research in Nursing box. The nurse explains the reason for being NPO to the patient and, at the appropriate time, removes all food and fluids from the bedside and places a sign over the bed so that all health team members and visitors know about the restriction. If the patient eats or drinks, the physician should be notified at once.

Review the patient scenario involving Ron Johnson, described in the Reflective Practice display. Because the patient had undergone previous surgeries, the nurses may have assumed that the patient understood the restrictions associated with being NPO and the reasons why. Knowledge of the patient's history is important. However, it would be just as important to assess the patient's knowledge about food and fluid restrictions to ensure that the patient does have a good understanding of these restrictions.

Patients need to be well nourished and hydrated before surgery to counterbalance fluid, blood, and electrolyte loss during surgery and to facilitate tissue healing after surgery. Preoperative assessments provide a base for physical preparation for surgery, including the need for supplemental nutrition, fluids, or electrolytes. A patient who is undernourished may require parenteral nutrition (see Chap. 42) and IV electrolyte

Research in Nursing Making a Difference

Preoperative Fasting

Although having a patient remain NPO after midnight prior to the day of surgery has been a traditional practice, this is now being challenged. The American Society of Anesthesiology (ASA) revised its practice guidelines in 1999 for healthy patients undergoing elective surgery. These recommendations, based on research findings that pulmonary aspiration is rare following surgery with modern anesthesia, allow clear liquids up to 2 hours before elective surgery, a light breakfast (such as tea and toast) 6 hours before surgery, and a heavier meal 8 hours before surgery.

Related Research

Crenshaw, J., & Winslow, E. (2002). Preoperative fasting: Old habits die hard. *American Journal of Nursing, 102*(5), 36–45.

The purpose of this study was to determine if publication of these guidelines had changed preoperative fasting guidelines. The authors interviewed 155 patients in a large hospital about their preoperative fasting, comparing instructed, actual, and rec-

ommended fasting times for both solid food and liquids. They found that most of the patients continued to be instructed to have nothing to eat or drink after midnight, regardless if they were scheduled for early or late surgery.

Based on these findings, the conclusion was that in actual practice little has changed in preoperative fasting in answer to the revised ASA guidelines.

Relevance to Nursing Practice

It is important that nurses be knowledgeable about current practice guidelines and related research. Nurses are the healthcare providers who most often provide preoperative teaching. It is important that nurses and physicians collaborate to ensure that agency policy and procedures are congruent with the ASA guidelines and are understandable to patients. In addition, as thirst is a common problem with any length of NPO, nurses should teach patients how to decrease this discomfort by interventions such as brushing teeth, chewing gum, or sucking on hard candy.

---

replacements. If the patient's screening tests show a hemoglobin level of less than 10 g/dL and a hematocrit of less than 33%, blood or blood component therapy may be given preoperatively to maintain volume and increase the oxygenation of tissue during surgery.

Rest and Sleep

Rest and sleep are important in reducing the stress before surgery and for healing and recovery after surgery. The nurse can facilitate rest and sleep in the immediate preoperative period by meeting psychological needs, carrying out teaching, providing a quiet environment, encouraging relaxation or comfort measures that are personally effective for the individual patient, or administering the prescribed bedtime sedative medication for hospitalized surgical patients.

Preparing the Patient on the Day of Surgery

The preoperative checklist outlines the nurse's responsibilities on the day of surgery; these activities must be completed before the patient is transported to surgery. An example of a preoperative checklist is provided in Figure 30-4. Some of these activities have already been described (eg, NPO, preoperative teaching, informed consent, skin preparation, screening tests, bladder elimination).

Preoperative medications that might be prescribed are as follows:

- Sedatives, such as diazepam (Valium), midazolam (Versed), or lorazepam (Ativan) to alleviate anxiety and decrease recall of events related to surgery
- Anticholinergics, such as atropine and glycopyrrolate (Robinul), to decrease pulmonary and oral secretions and to prevent laryngospasm

- Narcotic analgesics, such as morphine and meperidine hydrochloride (Demerol), to facilitate patient sedation and relaxation and to decrease the amount of anesthetic agent needed
- Neuroleptanalgesic agents, such as fentanyl citrate-droperidol (Innovar), to cause a general state of calmness and sleepiness
- Histamine receptor antihistaminics, such as cimetidine (Tagamet) and ranitidine (Zantac), to decrease gastric acidity and volume

See Guidelines for Nursing Care 30-4 for further preoperative interventions the day of surgery.

Evaluating

Evaluating the plan of care for the preoperative phase is based on the expected outcomes. The plan is effective if the patient is physically and emotionally prepared for surgery, can verbalize expected events and sensations of the perioperative period, and can demonstrate postoperative exercises and activities.

INTRAOPERATIVE NURSING CARE

The intraoperative phase of surgery begins with admission of the patient to the surgical area and lasts until the patient is transferred to the PACU. Although the surgeon has a dominant role during this phase, the perioperative nurse has critical responsibilities and roles in collaboratively meeting patient needs. The nursing process uses the preoperative data and plan as a basis for the intraoperative plan of care.

Preoperative Checklist

	YES	NO	N/A	INITIALS
Identification band in place	✓			*PL*
NPO	✓			*PL*
Pre-op bath or shower completed	✓			*PL*
Enema/douche given			✓	*PL*
Hospital gown	✓			*PL*
Underwear removed	✓			*PL*
Voided on call/Foley in place *voided*	✓			*PL*
Height & weight recorded _68 in_ Height _151 lbs._ Weight				*AK*
Nail polish removed			✓	*AK*
Make-up removed			✓	*AK*
Hair ornaments removed			✓	*AK*
Jewelry removed (earrings, necklaces, bracelets, rings)	✓			*AK*
Valuables given to family or placed in safe	✓			*AK*
Dentures removed, placed/given to _____			✓	*AK*
Prosthesis removed, placed/given to _____			✓	*AK*
Contact lenses/(glasses) placed/given to _family_	✓			*AK*
Operative permit signed	✓			*PL*
Anesthesia permit signed	✓			*PL*
Hemeprofile, UA (report in chart)	✓			*PL*
EKG (report on chart)	✓			*PL*
Chest X-ray (report on chart)	✓			*PL*
Computer cards, addressograph plate with chart	✓			*PL*
Medication record in chart and discontinued	✓			*PL*
Pre-op teaching completed by _P. LeMone, RN_ (see plan)				*PL*
Side rails up	✓			*AK*
Allergy sticker on chart front/allergy bracelet on	✓			*AK*
Correct operative site marked with an X	✓			*PL*
If no, was the surgeon notified?				
Oxygen _____ liters per nasal cannula _____% per face mask			✓	*PL*
History and physical updated with last 7 days	✓			*PL*
Type and cross match done. Number of units of blood set up _2_	✓			*PL*

Preoperative vital signs: ___98.4 - 68 - 16 - 126/78___

Allergies: ___none___

Preoperative medications given (time and route) _to be given in preop holding_

Comments: ___family will be in surgery waiting room___

Transported to OR per: _cart_   Accompanied by _wife_

Date: _10/02/04_   Time: _1300_   Signed ___P. LeMone, RN___
                                      (RN or LPN)

                               Signed ___A. Koeplin___
                                        (transport personnel)

FIGURE 30-4 Example of a preoperative checklist.

> ## Guidelines for Nursing Care 30-4
> ### Patient Preparation the Day of Surgery
>
> - Obtain and record vital signs and assess for and report any abnormal findings (eg, an elevated temperature).
> - Have the patient remove all personal clothing and put on an operating room gown.
> - Remove all hairpins or hairpieces, makeup, and fingernail polish.
> - Remove all prostheses, such as dentures or partial plates, eyeglasses, contact lenses, and artificial limbs.
> - Remove jewelry, including body-piercing jewelry. If the patient prefers not to remove a wedding band, it can be securely taped to the finger (in some types of surgery, leaving jewelry on is not allowed). When jewelry is removed, it should be given to a family member or locked in a safe place and its disposition noted.
> - Leave on a hearing aid, and be certain that perioperative and PACU nurses know the patient has one.
> - Be sure that the patient's identification bracelet is in place.
> - Note allergies according to institutional policy (eg, on the front of the patient's record or on an allergy bracelet).
> - Carry out any special procedures ordered, such as inserting a nasogastric tube, starting an intravenous line, or applying antiembolic stockings or compression devices.
> - Give the prescribed preoperative medications at either the scheduled time or "on call" (the operating room per-
>
> sonnel call to tell the nurse to give the medication). With ambulatory surgery and rapid recovery tracks, much less premedication is prescribed.
> - Elevate the side rails, lower the bed (if possible), apply a safety restraint, and instruct the patient to stay in bed or on the stretcher.
> - Tell the family of the hospitalized surgical patient where the patient will be taken after surgery (if a different location, such as the intensive care unit). Describe the waiting area and take the family there after the patient leaves for the operating room. Ambulatory surgery patients usually wait in the waiting area with family members until it is time for surgery. Tell the family that the surgeon will come to the waiting area to tell them what happened in surgery.
> - Document, through checklists and narrative charting, the nursing interventions carried out.
> - Assist in moving the patient from the bed to the operating room stretcher when it is time to transport the patient to surgery, ensuring accurate identification.
> - Prepare the hospitalized patient's bed (make a surgical bed) and room for postoperative care.
> - Have necessary equipment and supplies in the room for postoperative care.

THE NURSING PROCESS FOR INTRAOPERATIVE CARE

Assessing

The first room the patient enters when transferred to the surgical area is usually the holding area. Nurses in surgical scrub attire identify the surgical patient, assess the patient's emotional and physical status, and verify the information on the preoperative checklist. They may also carry out required immediate preoperative care, including performing skin preparation, starting IV fluids, and giving preoperative medications. The patient's response to the procedures is assessed, and the events of surgery are explained. When the operating room is prepared, a perioperative nurse helps transport the patient to the operating room.

In the operating room, the patient is positioned on the operating bed, anesthetized, and draped. The perioperative nurse assesses the patient and reviews preoperative data, paying particular attention to factors that increase surgical risk. The nurse also assesses the patient during positioning and monitors supplies used to maintain safety for the patient.

Diagnosing

Patient problems in the intraoperative period may occur in relation to the position of the patient during the procedure, the ef-

fects of the anesthesia, equipment used and potential hazards, disruption of tissues during surgery, and the incision. See Examples of NANDA Nursing Diagnoses during the intraoperative period.

Outcome Identification and Planning

The planning phase of the nursing process focuses on identifying actions most effective for preventing complications, resolving patient problems, and ensuring patient safety. Some expected outcomes are that the patient will:

- Remain free of neuromuscular injury
- Maintain intact skin surfaces
- Have symmetric breathing patterns
- Be free of injury from burns, retained foreign objects (inaccurate count of supplies), and wound contamination

Implementing

During surgery, nurses function as scrub nurses and circulating nurses, in an expanded role as registered nurse first assistants (RNFAs), or in an advanced practice role as acute care nurse practitioners (APNs). The scrub nurse is a member of the sterile team who maintains surgical asepsis while draping and handling instruments and supplies. The circulating nurse assesses the patient on admission to the operating room, collaborates in safely positioning the patient on the operating bed, assists with monitoring the patient during surgery, provides additional supplies, maintains environmental safety, and, throughout the surgical procedure, counts the number of instruments, needles, and sponges used during the surgery to prevent the accidental loss of an item in the wound. The RNFA actively assists the surgeon by providing exposure, hemostasis, and wound closure. The APN coordinates care activities, collaborates with physicians and nurses in all phases of perioperative and postanesthesia care, and integrates case management, critical paths, and research into care of the surgical patient. Additional educational preparation is required for the roles of the RNFA and the APN.

Positioning

The patient is placed in a specific operative position after anesthesia has produced loss of consciousness and reflexes. Ensure patient safety and comfort in positioning to prevent alterations in integumentary, respiratory, vascular, and neuromuscular function (Rothrock, Smith, & McEwen, 2003). The risk for skin injury is avoided by lifting, rather than rolling or pulling, the patient into the surgical position. Rolling or pulling can cause a shearing force, in which two or more tissue layers slide on each other, stretching subcutaneous blood vessels, obstructing blood flow, and contributing to pressure ulcers.

Although all of the operative positions are not described here, perioperative nurses need to know the position to be used and significant nursing considerations for that position. Two examples are the Trendelenburg position and the lithotomy position. The Trendelenburg position requires lowering the upper torso and raising the feet. It is commonly used in minimally invasive surgery of the lower abdomen or pelvis. The displacement of the abdominal viscera toward the head decreases diaphragm movement and respiratory exchange; blood pools in the upper torso, and blood pressure increases; hypotension can result with return to the supine position. Shearing with resultant tissue damage is also a significant risk in this position. The lithotomy position is used for gynecologic, rectal, and uro-

logic procedures. The placement of legs in stirrups causes pooling of blood in the legs, increasing the risk of thrombophlebitis. Pressure can also damage the peroneal nerve, with resultant footdrop.

Draping

Drapes are used to create and maintain a sterile field around the operative site, preventing the passage of microorganisms, particulate matter, and fluids between sterile and nonsterile areas. The only area left exposed is the incision site. Plastic adhesive drapes may be used to form a complete seal over the skin; with these drapes, skin color is visible, and the incision is made through the impermeable adhesive drape.

Documenting

Throughout surgery, the perioperative nurse documents ongoing patient assessment, item counts (sponges, sharps, instruments), monitoring data (eg, vital signs, urine output, blood loss, pulse oximetry results), positioning, medications, dressings and drains, and so forth on the intraoperative record. This documentation includes planning and implementation of perioperative nursing activities and evaluation of the achievement of patient outcomes.

Transferring to the Postanesthesia Care Unit

After the surgery, the patient is moved carefully from the operating bed to a stretcher. This is a critical time: sudden or rough handling can cause severe hypotension or potentially lethal cardiac or respiratory arrest. The patient is then transported to the PACU, and the nurse verbally communicates relevant preoperative and intraoperative assessments and interventions to the PACU nurses to ensure continuity of care.

Evaluating

Evaluation of the effectiveness of the plan of care for the intraoperative phase is based on the expected outcomes. If met, the plan was effective.

POSTOPERATIVE NURSING CARE

The postoperative phase can be divided into two stages—immediate care (usually provided in the PACU in both in-hospital and ambulatory surgery centers) and ongoing postoperative care (lasting from return to the unit through convalescence). Nursing assessments and interventions are consistent with those in the preoperative and intraoperative phases and are carried out to maintain function, promote recovery, and facilitate coping with alterations in structure or function. See the accompanying Through the Eyes of a Student account. Assessments and nursing interventions are combined in discussing immediate postoperative care; the phases of the nursing process are used to describe ongoing postoperative care.

Immediate Postoperative Care

Care in the PACU involves assessing the postoperative patient, with emphasis on preventing complications from anesthesia or the surgery. Assessments are continuous and ongoing, using preoperative and intraoperative data as bases for comparison. The assessments made in the PACU include respiratory status, cardiovascular status, central nervous system status, fluid status, wound status, and general condition. These assessments

Through the Eyes of a Student

The first time I took care of a patient with "multiple tubes," I was horrified at the thought of actually touching the patient. I hadn't really been exposed to that many critically ill patients until my last semester as a student nurse. I remember being assigned a patient in the cardiothoracic intensive care unit in the hospital where I trained. The patient was a "fresh heart"—a cardiopulmonary bypass graft patient who had just been operated on that morning.

I remember walking into the room and thinking, "What do I do with all of these tubes?" and then with horror thinking, "What if one of them falls out?" Needless to say, I was overwhelmed and frightened but at the same time excited at the challenge that faced me. I asked my preceptor what each tube was for and where it was hooked up and whether it would fall out if I touched it. She answered all my questions with patience and understanding and asked me if I wanted to handle the lines. I looked at her as if she were insane, but went ahead and did it. Would you believe that nothing fell out! I must admit that the experience taught me a lot, but it also got me over the fear of tubes.

I now chuckle every time I see a nursing student's face with that same look of horror as I had, and I try to answer every question with the same degree of patience and understanding that my preceptor had for me.

—Lynda L. Ullmer, RN
Gaithersburg, MD

initially are made every 10 to 15 minutes. The average PACU stay is about 2 hours, but it will vary depending on the type of surgery, length of anesthesia, and patient response.

Mr. Benjamin, the older adult who has had a total hip replacement, will require frequent assessments during his stay in the PACU, specifically vital signs, cardiovascular status, respiratory status, IV therapy, wound status, and urinary elimination.

Respiratory Status

Respiratory function is assessed by monitoring respiratory rate, rhythm, and depth; by auscultating breath sounds; and by noting the oxygen saturation level. During a surgical procedure with general anesthesia, an endotracheal tube may be inserted to administer the anesthetic gases and maintain patent air passages. The airway is not removed until the laryngeal and pharyngeal reflexes return, allowing the patient to control the tongue, cough, and swallow. The airway is assessed for patency, humidified oxygen is administered, and pulse oximetry is initiated. Cardiovascular and mental status assessments provide additional data about oxygenation. Ineffective respiratory function is indicated by restlessness and anxiety; unequal chest expansion with use of accessory muscles; shallow, noisy respirations; cyanosis; and tachycardia.

Respiratory obstruction is the most common PACU emergency. It may occur as a result of secretion accumulation, obstruction by the tongue, laryngospasm (a sudden, violent contraction of the vocal cords), or laryngeal edema. Respiratory obstruction is indicated by assessments of ineffective respiratory function plus observing for wheezing or crowing sounds with respiratory effort. Positioning, administering humidified oxygen, encouraging the patient to take deep breaths, and suctioning may be used to maintain a patent airway and tissue oxygenation.

Cardiovascular Status

Cardiovascular function is assessed by taking vital signs, monitoring electrocardiogram rate and rhythm, and observing skin color and condition. Blood pressure findings are compared with baseline data from the preoperative period; hypotension may be the result of varied factors, including anesthetic agents, preoperative medications, position changes, blood loss, respiratory alterations, and peripheral blood pooling. Transient hypertension can also occur as a result of anesthetic effects, respiratory insufficiency, the surgical procedure, or the excitement phase of recovery from anesthesia. Oxygen administration, deep breathing, leg exercises, verbal stimulation (to help expel anesthetic gases and facilitate increasing level of consciousness), and maintaining accurate IV flow rates can increase low blood pressure.

Patients are at risk for altered body temperature related to the surgical procedure, its length, anesthetic agents, a cool surgical environment, age, and use of cool irrigating or infusion fluids. Inadvertent hypothermia (temperature below 35.5°C [96°F]) can lead to complications of poor wound healing, hemodynamic stress, cardiac disturbances, coagulopathy, delayed emergence from anesthesia, and shivering and its associated discomfort. Measure the patient's body temperature, usually by the oral or tympanic route, and initiate interventions if the patient complains of being cold or is hypothermic. Warmed blankets placed on the patient's body and head and forced warm-air devices are used for rewarming.

Assess all pulses for bilateral equality, rhythm, rate, and character. Of special significance are assessments of abnormal function—an irregular rhythm, absence of pulses, or tachycardia. Tachycardia, an early symptom of shock, must be carefully evaluated. Other related assessments are cyanosis, edema, a cool skin temperature, and a decrease in urine output.

Central Nervous System Status

The return of central nervous system function is assessed through response to stimuli and orientation. Consciousness returns in reverse order, with the usual pattern being: (1) unconsciousness; (2) response to touch and sounds; (3) drowsiness; (4) awake but not oriented; and (5) awake and oriented. Nurses in the PACU verbally reorient the patient by touching and calling him or her by name.

Fluid Status

Fluid imbalance may result from factors such as preoperative fluid restriction, fluid loss during surgery, wound drainage, or the surgical stress response (with retention of sodium and water). Imbalanced fluid volume (deficit or excess) is a risk for all surgical patients but is an especially important one in children and older adults. Assessing fluid status includes skin turgor, vital signs, urine output, wound drainage, and IV fluid intake. IV fluid administration assessments include the type of fluid infused, the rate, location of lines, condition of the IV insertion site, and the security and patency of the tubing.

Wound Status

The nurse in the PACU assesses the wound dressing for amount, consistency, and color of drainage as well as for any tubes or drains and the amount and type of drainage by that route. See the accompanying Through the Eyes of a Student account.

Large amounts of bright-red drainage, combined with other abnormal physical status assessments (restlessness, pallor, cold moist skin, decreasing blood pressure, increasing pulse and respiratory rates), may indicate hemorrhage and hypovolemic shock. Report these symptoms immediately.

Pain Management

Pain is both a subjective and an objective experience. Clinical practice guidelines developed by the Agency for Health Care Policy and Research recommend the assessment of pain using a rating scale. The scale may be verbal (ranging from no pain to worst possible pain), numeric (with 10 on a scale of 0 to 10 being the worst possible pain), or a "faces" rating scale, ranging from a smiley face indicating no pain to a face that has frowns and tears for worst possible pain. (see Chap. 41). Early administration of analgesia, using nonsteroidal anti-inflammatory drugs and opiates, occurs in the PACU. Opiates may be delivered by PCA, allowing the patient to control the analgesic administration. Nonpharmacologic methods to decrease pain and improve comfort include positioning, verbal reassurance, touch, applications of heat or cold, massage, music therapy, humor therapy, meditation, and guided imagery. Preoperative assessments, noting methods that are personally effective for the patient, assist in effective implementation in the PACU. These should supplement, not substitute for, pharmacologic pain relief.

General Condition

Other assessments and interventions are made to ensure physical and emotional comfort and safety. Constant reorientation and reassurance that the surgery is completed provide psychological comfort. Careful assessments, proper positioning, and use of side rails and restraints maintain physical safety.

The patient is discharged from the PACU when his or her physical status and level of consciousness are considered stable. The family is notified that the patient is being transferred back to his or her room, and the PACU nurse gives a verbal report to the unit nurse about the assessments and interventions during the intraoperative and immediate postoperative phases.

Ongoing Postoperative Care

Ongoing postoperative care is planned to facilitate recovery from surgery and coping with alterations. The plan of care includes promoting physical and psychological health, preventing complications, and teaching self-care when the patient returns home. Skill 30-2, Postoperative Care When Patient Returns to Room, outlines ongoing postoperative patient care.

THE NURSING PROCESS FOR ONGOING POSTOPERATIVE CARE

Assessing

The nurse on the unit assists PACU personnel in transferring the patient to the bed in the unit room and makes an initial assessment using data from the preoperative and intraoperative phases. A postoperative checklist or flow sheet (Fig. 30-5) may be used. The initial assessment is often combined with the implementation of postoperative physician's orders. See Table 30-2 for focused assessments and interventions.

After assessment, document the time of arrival and all assessment data. Follow agency protocol for assessment routines: common time frames are every 15 minutes until stable, changing to every 1 to 2 hours for the first 24 hours, and every

SKILL 30-2   Postoperative Care When Patient Returns to Room

ACTION	RATIONALE
Immediate	
1. Place patient in safe position (high Fowler's or side-lying). Note level of consciousness.	A sitting position facilitates deep breathing; side-lying with neck slightly extended prevents aspiration and airway obstruction.
2. Monitor and record vital signs frequently. Assessment order may vary, but usual frequency includes taking vital signs every 15 minutes the first hour, every 30 minutes the next 2 hours, every hour for 4 hours, and finally, every 4 hours.	Comparison with baseline preoperative vital signs may indicate impending shock or hemorrhage.
3. Provide for warmth. Assess skin color and condition.	Hypothermia is uncomfortable and may lead to cardiac dysrhythmias and impaired wound healing.
4. Check dressings for color, odor, and amount of drainage, and feel under patient for bleeding.	Hemorrhage and shock are life-threatening complications of surgery.

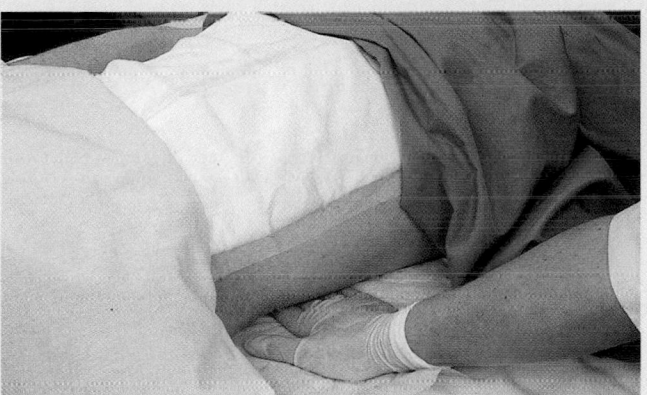

ACTION	RATIONALE
5. Verify that all tubes and drains are patent and equipment is operative; note amount of drainage in collection device.	This ensures maintenance of vital functions.
6. Maintain intravenous infusion at correct rate.	This prevents dehydration and electrolyte imbalances.
7. Provide for a safe environment. Keep bed in low position with side rails up. Have call bell within patient's reach.	This prevents accidental injury.
8. Relieve pain by administering medications ordered by physician. Check record to verify if analgesic medication was administered in the postanesthesia care unit.	Analgesics are used for relief of postoperative pain.
9. Record assessments and interventions on chart.	This provides for accurate documentation.
General	
10. Promote optimal respiratory function: a. Coughing and deep breathing b. Incentive spirometry c. Monitor oxygen saturation. d. Frequent position change/early ambulation e. Administration of oxygen as ordered	Anesthetic agents may depress respiratory function: patients who have existing respiratory or cardiovascular disease or abdominal or chest incisions or who are obese or elderly or in a poor state of nutrition are at greater risk for respiratory complications.
11. Maintain adequate circulation: a. Frequent position changes b. Early ambulation c. Application of antiembolic stockings or pneumatic compression devices, if ordered by physician d. Leg and range-of-motion exercises if not contraindicated	Preventive measures can improve venous return and circulatory status.
12. Assess urinary elimination status: a. Promote voiding by offering bedpan at regular intervals b. Monitor catheter drainage if present c. Measure intake and output	Anesthetic agents may temporarily depress bladder tone and response.

(continued)

ACTION	RATIONALE

13. Promote optimal nutrition status and return of gastrointestinal function:
   a. Assess for return of peristalsis
   b. Assist with diet progression
   c. Encourage fluid intake
   d. Monitor intake
   e. Medicate for nausea and vomiting as ordered by physician
	Anesthetic agents and narcotics depress peristalsis and normal functioning of gastrointestinal tract.

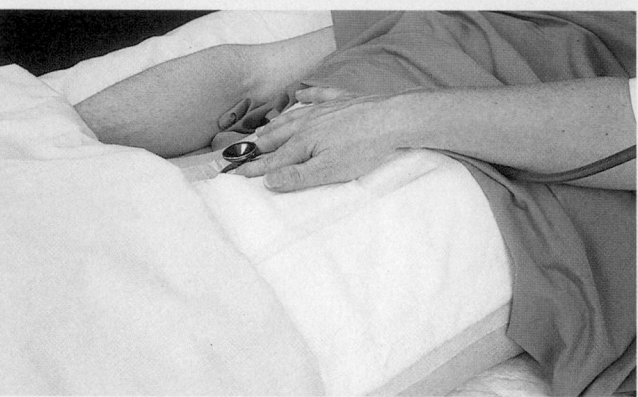

ACTION	RATIONALE

14. Promote wound healing:
   a. Use surgical asepsis
   b. Assess condition of wound
   c. Assess any drainage
	Alterations in nutrition, circulatory, and metabolic status may predispose patients to infection and delayed healing.

15. Provide for rest and comfort.	This shortens recovery period and facilitates return to normal function.
16. Provide emotional and spiritual support.	This facilitates individualized care and patient's return to normal health.

4 hours thereafter. Although agency protocols are used for guidelines in the immediate postoperative period, the nurse is responsible for adjusting the frequency and priorities of assessment to the specific needs of each patient.

Diagnosing

Nursing diagnoses in the postoperative phase may represent actual problems or those for which the patient is at risk. When making nursing diagnoses, the nurse uses assessment data and plans of care established before and during surgery and includes the family. See Examples of NANDA Nursing Diagnoses appropriate to the preoperative period.

Outcome Identification and Planning

The plan of care in the postoperative phase begins in the preoperative phase, when nursing activities to reduce stress and teach postoperative activities are carried out. From admission,

the patient and family are prepared for uneventful recovery and self-care after discharge. Specific expected outcomes are individualized based on risk factors, the surgical procedure, and the patient's unique needs. Examples of desired postoperative outcomes for a patient after major surgery are as follows: The patient will

- Carry out leg exercises every 2 to 4 hours
- Deep breathe and cough effectively every 2 hours
- Verbalize decreasing levels of pain
- Have a balanced intake and output
- Regain normal bowel and bladder elimination
- Have a well-healed surgical incision
- Remain free of infection
- Verbalize any concerns about appearance of wound
- Verbalize and demonstrate wound self-care

Implementing

Many nursing interventions in the postoperative phase have already been discussed in this chapter or are fully discussed in

Name Dale Courtney

M.R. # 302-59910

**POSTOP
PROGRESS FLOW RECORD**

Date	8/7/00									
Time	10	10¹⁵	10³⁰	11	11¹⁵	11³⁰	12	12³⁰		
BP	120/80	126/82	128/80	130/80	130/82	130/80	130/82	128/80		
Pulse	90	88	88	90	88	86	86	86		
Respirations	22	24	22	20	20	22	20	20		
Temperature	98⁸	98⁸	98⁸	98⁸	98⁸	98⁸	98⁸	98⁸		
I.V.	D₁d							→	Discharged to home with wife	
Wound	DD&I						→			
Drain(s)	N/A									
LOC	AAA x3							→	Reviewed D/C instructions	
Pain	SPA				→	+4 (Iced)	+3	+3	+2	Immobilizer on for D/C
Nausea	No							→		
Foley/Other Cath or Voiding	No						Voided 45cc		Voided	
Turn, Cough Deep Breathe	C & DB							→	Ambulated	
Moves All Extremities	+4							→	Returned to baseline	
Initials	JCR	JCR	JCR	JCR	JCR	JCR	JCR			

Key _____ _____

_____ _____

FIGURE 30-5 Example of a postoperative progress record.

other chapters; therefore, this section focuses on nursing interventions to meet the expected outcomes of the plan of care. Nursing care to prevent complications, promote a return to health, and facilitate coping with alterations is discussed.

Preventing Postoperative Complications

A wide variety of factors increase the risk of postoperative complications. These have been described in the preoperative and intraoperative sections of this chapter and include age, health habits, physical condition, medical history, psychological status, and surgical intervention (eg, anesthesia, positioning, wound). Ongoing postoperative assessments and interventions are implemented to decrease the risk for postoperative complications. If postoperative complications occur, the nurse provides physical assessments and care, provides emotional support to the patient and family, and carries out prescribed treatments.

TABLE 30-2 Postoperative Assessments and Interventions on Return to the Unit

Factors to Assess	Assessments and Interventions
Vital signs	• Temperature, blood pressure, pulse and respiratory rates • Note, report, and document deviations from preoperative and PACU data as well as symptoms of complications.
Color and temperature of skin	• Skin color (pallor, cyanosis), skin temperature, and diaphoresis
Level of consciousness	• Orientation to time, place, and person • Reaction to stimuli and ability to move extremities
Intravenous fluids	• Type and amount of solution, flow rate, security and patency of tubing • Infusion site
Surgical site	• Dressing and dependent areas for drainage (color, amount, and consistency) • Drains and tubes; be sure they are intact, patent, and properly connected to drainage systems.
Other tubes	• Assess indwelling urinary catheter, gastrointestinal suction, and others for drainage, patency, and amount of output. • Be sure dependent drainage bags are hanging properly and suction drainage is attached and functioning. • If oxygen is ordered, ensure placement of ordered application and flow rate.
Comfort	• Assess pain (location, duration, and intensity), and determine whether analgesics were given in the PACU. • Assess for nausea and vomiting. • Cover the patient with a blanket. • Reorient to the room as necessary. • Allow family members to remain with the patient after the initial assessment is completed.
Position and safety	• Place the patient in an ordered position, or • If the patient is not fully conscious, place in the side-lying position. • Elevate the side rails and place the bed in low position.

Preventing Cardiovascular Complications

Nursing interventions to prevent or monitor for cardiovascular complications are listed in Box 30-4. Specific cardiovascular complications include hemorrhage, shock, thrombophlebitis, and pulmonary embolus.

Hemorrhage. Hemorrhage is an excessive internal or external blood loss. Hemorrhage may lead to hypovolemic shock. It may occur from a slipped suture, a dislodged clot in the wound, or stress on the surgical site; it may also be the result of pathophysiologic conditions or certain medications. Common indications of hemorrhage are restlessness, anxiety, and frank bleeding as well as hypotension; cold, clammy skin; a weak, thready, and rapid pulse; cool, mottled extremities; deep, rapid respirations; decreased urine output; thirst; and apprehension. The primary purposes of care for the patient having a hemorrhage include stopping the bleeding and replacing blood volume. If bleeding occurs, apply a pressure dressing to the bleeding site and be prepared to have the patient return to the operating room if bleeding cannot be stopped or is massive.

Shock. Shock is the body's reaction to acute peripheral circulatory failure as the result of an alteration in circulatory control or a loss of circulating fluid. The type of shock most commonly seen in postoperative patients is **hypovolemic shock,** which occurs from a decrease in blood volume.

Common indications of shock are the same as those for hemorrhage.

The primary purpose of care for a patient in shock is to improve and maintain tissue perfusion by eliminating the cause of the shock. Nursing interventions include establishing and maintaining the airway; placing the patient in a flat position with the legs elevated 30 to 45 degrees; administering oxygen therapy; monitoring vital signs, hematocrit, blood gas results, and general condition; maintaining body warmth with covers; and administering medications. The nurse must also be prepared to assist with the insertion of IV lines and to administer fluids as well as whole blood or its components.

Thrombophlebitis. Thrombophlebitis is an inflammation of a vein associated with thrombus (blood clot) formation. Thrombophlebitis from venous stasis is most commonly seen in the legs of postoperative patients (Porth, 2002). Indications of thrombophlebitis are pain and cramping in the calf or thigh of the involved extremity, redness and swelling in the affected area, elevated temperature, and an increase in the diameter of the involved extremity.

Care for the patient with thrombophlebitis includes preventing a clot from breaking loose and becoming an embolus that travels to the lungs, heart, or brain and preventing further clot formation. Nursing interventions include administering medications (eg, anti-inflammatory agents, anticoagulants,

Examples of NANDA Nursing Diagnoses | The Postoperative Patient

Nursing Diagnoses	Related Factors	Sample Defining Characteristics
Risk for Infection	Any condition that interferes with normal inflammatory healing process or provides an entry for infectious agents	*Risk Factors* • Obesity • Aging • Immunosuppression • Malnutrition • Presence of incision • Decreased ability to cough, deep breathe, use incentive spirometer • Presence of drains, tubes, and catheters • Insertion site for intravenous therapy
Disturbed Body Image	Any condition that causes confusion in the mental image of oneself, including surgical incision, removal of body part, and inability to use body as one did before surgery	• Verbalization of altered view of one's body in appearance, structure, or function • Refusal to look at incision or area of surgical treatment • Actual change in one's body from surgery or trauma • Actual missing body part • Verbalizations of negative feelings about body
Acute Pain	Any condition that causes actual tissue damage, such as the surgical incision	• Rating pain as severe on a scale of 1 to 10 (ie, as a 9) • Positioning or guarding self to avoid pain • Inability to sleep • Loss of appetite • Diaphoresis, changes in vital signs, dilated pupils • Moaning, crying, sighing
Urinary Retention	Any condition that causes incomplete emptying of the bladder, such as neurologic effects of anesthesia	• Urine not eliminated for more than 8 hours • Distended, palpable bladder • Small, frequent voiding • Residual urine

---

BOX 30-4 Nursing Interventions to Prevent or Monitor Postoperative Cardiovascular Complications

- Assess and document vital signs as ordered and as the patient's status dictates, using preoperative assessments as a baseline.
- Provide covers, forced warm air, or other warming device or techniques as necessary to prevent shivering and hypothermia.
- Maintain fluid balance.
- Maintain accurate intake and output.
- Monitor rate, type, and access site of intravenous fluids.
- Assess skin turgor and hydration of mucous membranes.
- Monitor amount, color, and consistency of wound drainage (dressings and drains or tubes).

- Implement leg exercises and turning in bed every 2 hours.
- Assist with ambulation. Ambulation usually begins the evening of surgery and increases as tolerated; blood pressure and pulse and respiratory rates are used to monitor tolerance.
- Apply and follow protocols for antiembolic stockings or compression devices, if ordered.
- Administer anticoagulant medications, if prescribed.
- Measure bilateral calf and thigh circumference daily.
- Avoid positioning that impedes venous return (eg, do not mechanically raise the knee portion of the bed or place pillows under the knees).

analgesics), maintaining the patient on bed rest, applying external heat, applying high antiembolic stockings or sequential pneumatic compression devices (Box 30-5), and measuring bilateral calf or thigh circumference every shift. Teach the patient not to massage the legs.

Pulmonary Embolus. An **embolus** is a blood clot or foreign substance that is dislodged and travels through the bloodstream until it lodges in a smaller vessel. In postoperative patients, the embolus is often part of a thrombus that breaks free from a vein wall. If the embolus lodges in the pulmonary vessels, it is called a pulmonary embolus. Indications of a pulmonary embolus include dyspnea, chest pain, cough, cyanosis, rapid respirations, tachycardia, and anxiety. This is a life-threatening condition, and immediate treatment is necessary. The primary goals of care are to stabilize cardiovascular and respiratory function and to prevent further emboli. Nursing interventions include notifying the physician immediately if symptoms occur, maintaining the patient on bed rest in the semi-Fowler's position, assessing vital signs frequently, administering oxygen therapy, administering medications (eg, anticoagulants, analgesics), and instructing the patient to avoid Valsalva's maneuver (forced exhalation against a closed glottis, such as straining to have a bowel movement) to prevent increased intrathoracic pressure and, possibly, increased emboli.

Preventing Respiratory Complications

Nursing interventions to prevent or monitor for respiratory complications include monitoring vital signs, implementing deep breathing, coughing, incentive spirometry, and turning in bed every 2 hours; ambulating; maintaining hydration; avoiding positioning that decreases ventilation; and monitoring responses to narcotic analgesics. Specific respiratory complications include pneumonia and atelectasis.

Pneumonia. Pneumonia is an inflammation of the alveoli as the result of an infectious process or the presence of foreign material. Pneumonia may occur postoperatively as a result of aspiration, infection, depressed cough reflex, increased secretions from anesthesia, dehydration, and immobilization. Indications of pneumonia are an elevated temperature, chills, a cough that produces rusty or purulent sputum, crackles and wheezes, dyspnea, and chest pain. The goals of care are to treat the underlying infection, maintain respiratory status, and prevent the spread of microorganisms. Nursing interventions include those used to prevent or monitor for respiratory complications and promoting full aeration of the lungs by positioning the patient in semi-Fowler's or Fowler's position, administering oxygen therapy, administering medications (eg, antibiotics, expectorants, analgesics), providing frequent oral hygiene, and ensuring rest and comfort.

Atelectasis. Atelectasis is the incomplete expansion or collapse of alveoli with retained mucus, involving a portion of lung and resulting in poor gas exchange. Indications of atelectasis include decreased lung sounds over the affected area, dyspnea, cyanosis, crackles, restlessness, and apprehension. The primary goals of care are to ensure oxygenation of tissues, prevent further atelectasis, and expand involved lung tissues. Nursing interventions include those used to prevent or monitor for respiratory complications, and positioning the patient in semi-Fowler's position, administering oxygen therapy, and administering analgesics for pain.

BOX 30-5 **Pneumatic Compression Devices**

Pneumatic compression devices are composed of an air pump, connecting tubes, and an extremity sleeve. The sleeve may cover the entire leg or may extend from the foot to the knee. A variety of types are available; the accompanying figure provides one example. The devices apply brief pressure to the legs to enhance blood flow and venous return, thereby decreasing the risk for thrombophlebitis after surgery. The devices may apply either intermittent or sequential pressure. Intermittent pneumatic compression devices fit over the entire leg, with inflation and deflation of the sleeve covering the leg alternating from one leg to the other by a preset timer. Sequential pneumatic compression devices are designed so that pressure moves up the leg in increments. They may inflate and deflate by alternating from one leg to the other, or they may do so for both legs at once.

Nursing Care
- Explain the purpose of the device to the patient.
- Apply the device so that two fingers fit between the leg and the sleeve.
- Position the tubing so the patient can move about without interrupting the air flow.

- Remove the sleeves at least once a day for skin care and assessment.
- Assess the extremities for peripheral pulses, edema, changes in sensation, and movement on a regular schedule.
- Ensure that all chambers are inflating in proper sequence once per shift.

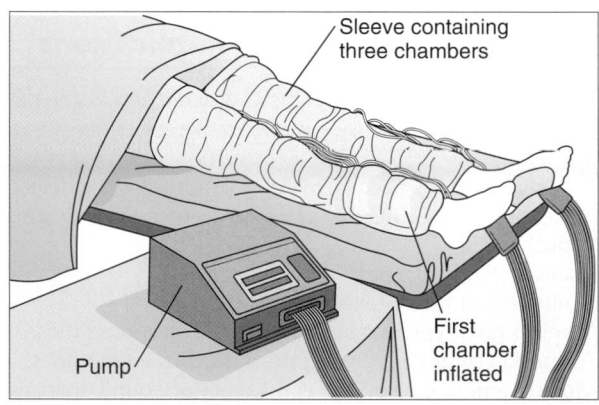

Preventing Surgical Site Complications

The nurse assesses and cares for the surgical site to promote healing and prevent complications. Wound care is discussed in Chapter 38. Nursing interventions to prevent and monitor for complications at the surgical site are monitoring vital signs, especially temperature elevation; maintaining hydration; maintaining nutritional status; encouraging a diet high in proteins, carbohydrates, calories, and vitamins; using proper hand hygiene; and following aseptic technique when changing dressings at the surgical site and exit sites for tubes and drains. Soiled gloves and dressings should be disposed of following standard precautions.

Promoting a Return to Health

Nurses provide interventions during postoperative recovery to promote physical and psychological functioning at as near a normal state as possible. The plan of care to achieve this goal includes activities to meet elimination, fluid and electrolyte, nutrition, and rest and comfort needs.

Meeting Elimination Needs

Both urinary and bowel elimination can be altered by anesthesia, manipulation of organs during surgery, inactivity, and altered fluid and food intake during the perioperative period. Assessments and nursing interventions to promote the return of normal bowel and urinary elimination are outlined in Box 30-6.

Meeting Fluid and Nutrition Needs

Nursing assessments and interventions to meet fluid needs are met by monitoring patterns of intake and output, maintaining prescribed IV fluid infusion rates, and assessing skin turgor and mucous membranes for dehydration. Nutrition needs are met by monitoring weight, providing oral hygiene before meals and as needed, monitoring postoperative dietary progression (often from clear to full liquids, then from soft to regular diet), maintaining an environment conducive to appetite (clean, neat, and free of odors), encouraging the patient to sit up in bed or a chair for meals, and encouraging family participation in meals.

Meeting Comfort and Rest Needs

Comfort needs are a priority after surgery. Factors that interfere with comfort include nausea, vomiting, thirst, hiccups, and pain at the surgical site. Nursing interventions that promote rest and comfort by providing relief for these problems are listed in Guidelines for Nursing Care 30-5. Comfort and rest are also promoted by providing personal hygiene, keeping bed linens clean, providing quiet rest periods, and allowing family members to remain with the patient.

Helping the Patient Cope

Surgery may alter the patient's physical appearance as well as his or her physiologic function, leading to the risk for or actual alterations in self-concept and body image. Changes in a person's self-perception can influence all of the human dimensions and areas of human functioning, including self-

---

BOX 30-6 Nursing Assessments and Interventions to Meet Postoperative Elimination Needs

Bowel Elimination

- Assess for the return of peristalsis by auscultating bowel sounds every 4 hours when the patient is awake.
- Assess abdominal distention, especially if bowel sounds are not audible or are high-pitched (indicative of possible paralytic ileus, which is an absence of intestinal peristalsis).
- Assess ability to pass flatus and stool.
- Assist with movement in bed and ambulation to relieve gas pains, a common postoperative discomfort.
- Encourage food and fluid intake when ordered, especially fruit juices and high-fiber foods.
- Maintain privacy when patient is using the bedpan, urinal, commode, or bathroom.
- Administer suppositories, enemas, or medications, such as stool softeners, as prescribed.

Urinary Elimination

- Monitor patterns of intake and output.
- Assist in assuming normal position to void by using an upright position when on a bedpan and using a bedside commode or bathroom when able, or by assisting the male patient to stand upright to void with a urinal.
- Assess for bladder distention by palpating above the symphysis pubis if the patient has not voided within 8 hours after surgery or if the patient has been voiding frequently in amounts of less than 50 mL; notify the physician of abnormal assessment results.
- Maintain prescribed intravenous fluid infusion rates.
- Encourage oral fluid intake when prescribed.
- Provide privacy when the patient is using bedpan, bedside commode, urinal, or bathroom.
- Initiate urinary catheterization if prescribed.

---

esteem, relationships with others, sexual identity, spiritual beliefs, sociocultural values, and independent and fulfilling engagement in activities of daily living.

Many surgical patients have the same reaction to loss of a body part as to a death (see Chap. 33). The response and adaptation to it are influenced by multiple factors, including age, cultural values and beliefs, sociocultural background, significance of the body part, visibility of the body part, time to prepare for the change, and support people available. A surgical patient's grief is a normal, appropriate response. It is unique to the person experiencing it, and although there are stages and phases of grief, there is no timetable for it. The nurse must be aware of the patient's needs and provide interventions to meet those needs in coping with change.

Remember Mr. Johnson, who had a urinary diversion. The patient already has experienced changes in body image related to his bilateral amputations and paraplegia. Now the patient

Guidelines for Nursing Care 30-5
Promoting Postoperative Rest and Comfort

Nausea and Vomiting
- Avoid giving the patient a large amount of fluids or food at one time, especially after being NPO.
- Administer prescribed medications.
- Provide oral hygiene as needed.
- Maintain clean environment.
- Avoid use of a straw.
- Avoid strong-smelling food.
- Assess for possible allergy to medications, such as antibiotics or analgesics.
- Maintain bowel elimination.

Thirst
- Offer sips of water or ice chips when NPO (if permitted).
- Maintain oral hygiene.

Hiccups
- Have the patient do the following:
  - Take several swallows of water while holding the breath (if not NPO).
  - Rebreathe into a paper bag.
  - Eat a teaspoon of granulated sugar.

Surgical Pain
- Assess pain frequently; administer prescribed analgesics every 2 to 4 hours on a regular schedule during the first 24 to 36 hours after surgery.
- Reinforce preoperative teaching for pain management.
- Offer nonpharmacologic measures to supplement medications: massage, position changes, relaxation, guided imagery, meditation, music.

BOX 30-7 Nursing Interventions to Facilitate Postoperative Coping and Adaptation

- Accept each patient as a unique individual.
- Identify through verbal and nonverbal cues patients who are at risk for alteration in self-concept. The risk is increased if the patient has little support from others, a visible alteration, or an alteration that will seriously affect functional ability.
- Allow time for patients and families to verbalize their feelings about the alteration, and do not assume that all patients will have problems.
- Identify and support strengths and effective coping mechanisms.
- Encourage the patient and family to be part of goal setting and decision making throughout the surgical experience.
- Provide teaching and honest information to the patient and family about all aspects of care.
- Work collaboratively with other members of the health team to provide referrals and resources as necessary to meet physical, psychological, and spiritual needs.

Evaluating

The achievement of desired outcomes for postoperative recovery and rehabilitation may be evaluated in a number of ways. Because the final resolution of some desired outcomes may not be apparent or measurable at the time of discharge, many institutions use follow-up telephone calls or surveys that are mailed to patients. It may also be possible to work with the physician's office to have a patient complete a survey on the first postoperative visit. Whatever mechanism is selected, important outcomes, such as the absence of surgical site infection, the patient's satisfaction with pain management measures, return to former levels of mobility and activity, and the absence of postoperative complications for which the patient was at risk, should be included as part of evaluative criteria.

must learn to adapt to another alteration, a urinary diversion. The nurse needs to investigate the patient's previous beliefs, values, and coping mechanisms to assist the patient in adapting to this most recent alteration.

The nursing process is used to implement interventions, beginning with the patient's decision to have surgery and continuing through convalescence. Nursing interventions to facilitate coping and adaptation are outlined in Box 30-7.

Providing Ambulatory Surgery Postoperative Care

Evaluating the patient's postoperative status after ambulatory surgery focuses on ensuring that the patient can be safely cared for at home. After surgery and recovery from the anesthetic, the patient is asked to sit up and drink liquids. A patient who is no longer drowsy or dizzy, has stable vital signs, and has voided is allowed to go home accompanied by a responsible adult. The patient is not allowed to drive a car to go home. The usual length of time from completion of surgery to discharge is 1 to 3 hours, provided that established criteria have been met. Written and verbal instructions for home care are given to the patient and family.

◼ Developing Critical Thinking Skills

1. You are providing the immediate preoperative care for a woman scheduled for surgery to remove a brain tumor. She tells you she does not want the surgery because she knows she is dying and just wants to go home to be with her husband and children. She also knows that her husband cannot accept the fact that she is dying and wants her to have the surgery. What do you do?

2. You are assigned to discharge a woman from your same-day surgery unit to her home. You strongly believe that she is not ready to go home, and there is no caretaker in her home. When you voice your concern to the surgeon, you are told that this is not your problem and that there is nothing anyone can do about the situation because her insurer will not approve hospitalization. How do you respond?

Practicing for NCLEX

1. Mrs. Ogg requires surgery for treatment of a ruptured spleen as the result of an automobile accident. This type of surgery belongs in which of the following categories?
   a. Minor, diagnostic
   b. Minor, elective
   c. Major, emergency
   d. Major, palliative

2. A general anesthetic is given for specific purposes during a surgical procedure. Which one of the following purposes is not included?
   a. Loss of consciousness
   b. Relaxation of skeletal muscles
   c. Reduction of reflex action
   d. Localized loss of sensation

3. You have been asked to witness a patient signature on an informed consent form for surgery. You recognize that the document is valid for which one of these patients?
   a. A 92-year-old patient who is severely confused
   b. A 45-year-old patient who is oriented and alert
   c. A 10-year-old patient who is oriented and alert
   d. A 36-year-old patient who has had a narcotic premedication

4. Although surgical patients may be taking any number of medications before surgery, which of the following categories of drugs would be most likely to increase surgical risk?
   a. Anticoagulants
   b. Antacids
   c. Laxatives
   d. Sedatives

5. An obese patient who has surgery is at risk for which of the following postoperative complications?
   a. Hunger
   b. Impaired wound healing
   c. Hemorrhage
   d. Gas pains

6. Which of these teaching methods would be most effective in preoperative teaching for ambulatory surgery?
   a. Lecture with video
   b. Discussion
   c. Audiovisuals
   d. Written instructions

7. Mr. Ying is scheduled for surgery. He says to you, "I am so frightened—what if I don't wake up?" What would be your best response?
   a. "You have a wonderful doctor."
   b. "Let's talk about how you are feeling."
   c. "Everyone wakes up from surgery!"
   d. "Don't worry, you will be just fine."

8. A PCA pump allows postoperative patients to:
   a. Be totally pain free
   b. Take unlimited amounts of medication
   c. Choose the type of pain medication
   d. Administer their own analgesic

9. Mr. Moreno has had a surgical procedure that necessitated a thoracic incision. You anticipate that he will have a higher risk for postoperative complications involving which body system?
   a. Respiratory system
   b. Circulatory system
   c. Digestive system
   d. Nervous system

10. While assessing a patient in the PACU, the perianesthesia nurse notes increased wound drainage, restlessness, a decreasing blood pressure, and an increase in the pulse rate. The most probable cause for these findings is:
    a. Thrombophlebitis
    b. Atelectasis
    c. Infection
    d. Hemorrhage

11. Your patient tells you she is having pain in her right lower leg. You assess the presence of thrombophlebitis by:
    a. Palpating the skin over the tibia and fibula
    b. Measuring and documenting calf circumference daily
    c. Taking and recording vital signs four times a day
    d. Noting difficulty with ambulation

12. Gas pains are a common postoperative discomfort. Which of the following nursing actions implemented in the plan of care would be most likely to relieve gas pains?
    a. Cough and deep breathe every 2 hours.
    b. Maintain NPO status for 48 hours.
    c. Encourage frequent ambulation.
    d. Take vital signs every 4 hours.

13. Which of the following surgical patients is at a greater risk for alterations in body image?
    a. Female, aged 19 years, large facial laceration
    b. Female, aged 42 years, gallbladder surgery
    c. Male, aged 14 years, fractured clavicle
    d. Male, aged 52 years, hernia repair

14. Older adults often have reduced vital capacity as a normal physiologic change. Which nursing action would be most important for the postoperative care of an older surgical patient specific to this change?
    a. Take and record vital signs every shift.
    b. Turn, cough, and deep breathe every 4 hours.
    c. Encourage increased intake of oral fluids.
    d. Assess bowel sounds daily.

15. The rationale for the use of leg exercises after surgery is that leg exercises:
    a. Promote respiratory function
    b. Maintain functional abilities
    c. Provide diversional activities
    d. Increase venous return

Answers With Rationale

1. The correct answer is *c*. This surgery would involve a major body organ, has the potential for postoperative complications, requires hospitalization, and must be done immediately to save the patient's life.
2. The correct answer is *d*. Whereas *a, b,* and *c* are all purposes of a general anesthetic, a localized loss of sensation occurs with a regional anesthetic.
3. The correct answer is *b*. A consent form is not legal if the patient signing the form is confused, sedated, or a minor.
4. The correct answer is *a*. Anticoagulant drug therapy would increase the risk for hemorrhage during surgery. The other categories of drugs normally would not increase surgical risk.
5. The correct answer is *b*. Fatty tissue is less vascular and therefore less resistant to infection and more prone to delayed wound healing.
6. The correct answer is *d*. Although all of the answers might be useful in teaching patients and families before ambulatory surgery, written instructions are most effective in providing information.
7. The correct answer is *b*. This answer allows the patient to talk about his feelings and fears and is therapeutic. The other answers give false reassurance.
8. The correct answer is *d*. A PCA pump allows the patient to administer his or her own analgesic. Use of this device does not allow the patient to take unlimited amounts of medication, choose the type of pain medication, or be totally pain free.
9. The correct answer is *a*. A thoracic incision makes it more painful for the patient to take deep breaths or cough. Shallow respirations and ineffective coughing increase the risk for respiratory complications.
10. The correct answer is *d*. Increased wound drainage, restlessness, decreasing blood pressure, and increasing pulse rate are assessment findings that indicate hemorrhage.
11. The correct answer is *b*. Inflammation from thrombophlebitis increases the size of the affected extremity and can be assessed by measuring circumference on a regular basis.
12. The correct answer is *c*. Frequent ambulation stimulates peristalsis and relieves gas pains. The other answers are incorrect in this situation.
13. The correct answer is *a*. The reaction of the patient to an accidental or intentional incision is influenced by age, time to prepare for the change, and visibility of the trauma. Large facial wounds increase the risk for an alteration in body image.
14. The correct answer is *b*. Reduced vital capacity in older adults increases the risk for respiratory complications, including pneumonia and atelectasis. Having the patient turn, cough, and deep breathe every 4 hours maintains respiratory function and helps to prevent complications.
15. The correct answer is *d*. Leg exercises in the postoperative period do increase venous return. As a result, the patient has a decreased risk for thrombophlebitis and emboli.

Bibliography

Adams, A. (2001). Preventing surgical site infection: Guidelines at a glance. *Nursing Management, 32*(8) OR Edition, 46.

Agency for Health Care Policy and Research. (1992) *Acute pain management: Operative or medical procedures and trauma.* Clinical practice guidelines. DHHS Pub. No. (AHCPR) 920032. Silver Spring, MD: Author.

Allen, G. (2002). Malnutrition and its effect on wound healing. *AORN Journal, 76*(5), 893.

American Association of Nurse Anesthetists. (2003). *CRNA.* Available at http://www.aana.com/crna/careerqna.asp.

American Society of PeriAnesthesia Nurses. (1998). *Standards of perianesthesia nursing practice.* Thorofare, NJ: Author.

Arnstein, P. (2002). Optimizing perioperative pain management. *AORN Journal, 76*(5), 812–818.

Association of periOperative Registered Nurses. (1997). *AORN's age-specific competency series.* Denver, CO: Author.

Association of periOperative Registered Nurses. (2002). *AORN standards, recommended practices and guidelines.* Denver, CO: Author.

Borchardt, M. (1999). Review of the clinical pharmacology and use of the benzodiazepines. *Journal of Perianesthesia Nursing, 14*(2), 65–72.

Christie, F. (1998). Pulmonary embolism. *American Journal of Nursing, 98*(11), 36–37.

Collins, N. (2003). Obesity and wound healing. *Advances in Skin & Wound Care: The Journal for Prevention and Healing, 16*(1), 45–47.

Crenshaw, J., & Winslow, E. (2002). Original research: Preoperative fasting. Old habits die hard. *American Journal of Nursing, 102*(5), 36–45.

Goodwin, S. A. (1999). Notes from the American Society of Anesthesiologists meeting. *Journal of Perianesthesia Nursing, 14*(2), 102–105.

Kost, M. (1999). Conscious sedation: Guarding your patient against complications. *Nursing, 29*(4), 34–39.

Noble, K. (1999). PACU: Ensuring a safe experience. *Advance for Nurses, 1*(5), 11–13.

Patton, C. M. (1999). Preoperative nursing assessment of the adult patient. *Seminars in Perioperative Nursing, 8*(1), 42–47.

Pessagno, J. J. (1999). Ambulatory care: Adjusting to the evolution of a changing health care system. *Advance for Nurses, 1*(8), 20–21.

Pessagno, J. J. (2002). Recommended practices for managing the patient receiving local anesthesia. *AORN Journal, 75*(4), 849–852.

Porth, C. M. (2002). *Pathophysiology: Concepts of altered health states* (5th ed.). Philadelphia: Lippincott.

Rothrock, J., Smith, D., & McEwen, D. (Eds.). (2003). *Alexander's care of the patient in surgery* (12th ed.). St. Louis: Mosby.

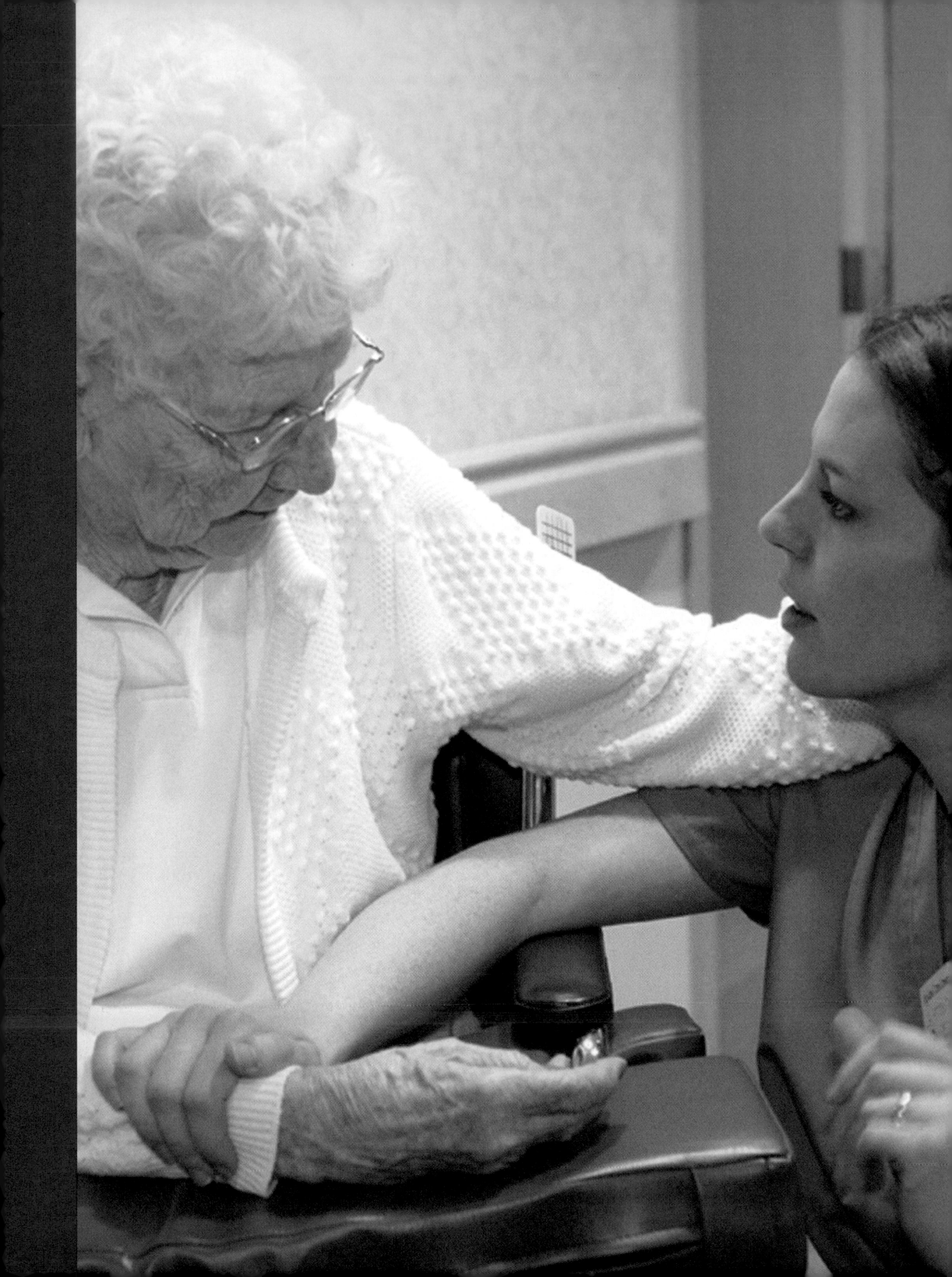

Promoting Healthy Psychosocial Responses

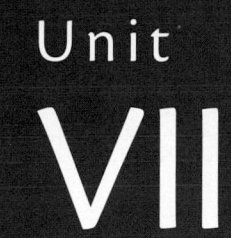

The unique function of the nurse is to assist the individual . . . in the performance of those activities contributing to health or its recovery (or to peaceful death) that he would perform unaided if he had the necessary strength, will or knowledge . . . in such a way as to help him gain independence as rapidly as possible.

Virginia Henderson (1897–1996)
the "first lady of nursing," whose career spanned almost 70 years as both author and researcher; her works on nursing principles are research based and have been translated into 25 languages

Every person is a composite of interrelated physiologic, psychosocial, and spiritual dimensions; alterations in one dimension affect the others. Unit VII discusses psychosocial considerations in holistic patient care, focusing on sense of self; stress and adaptation; loss, grief, and dying; sensory stimulation; sexuality; and spirituality.

Each individual's sense of self is critical to that person's attitudes toward health and may affect self-care abilities positively or negatively. Additionally, the relative presence or absence of developmental or experiential stressors can motivate or thwart psychosocial growth and self-actualization. Nursing interventions to promote healthy psychosocial responses, including maintaining, strengthening, or changing self-concept are basic to all aspects of patient care. Because sense of self constitutes the foundation upon which a person's ability to respond to healthcare interventions is built, nurses are aware of the importance of this vital area of human experience and include assessment and intervention to promote a positive sense of self.

Loss, grief, and dying are universal human experiences that most nurses encounter in some form on a daily basis. Effective nurses are competent and willing to assist people struggling with loss, grief, and dying.

Intact and functioning senses are necessary for life, normal growth and development, communication, and pleasurable experiences. Alterations in any of the senses require caring, knowledgeable, and individualized nursing interventions to meet needs, enhance individual independence, and prevent further overload or deprivation.

Sexuality and spirituality are important components of human functioning. These dimensions are an integral part of each person's identity and are critical elements in holistic patient care. Nurses recognize the importance of these areas for optimal health and use their knowledge and skills to assist patients to enhance wellness in these areas.

To facilitate wellness in each of these psychosocial spheres, nurses must develop self-awareness, including knowledge of their own personal characteristics, attitudes, and perceptions, as well as understanding how others' attitudes, perceptions, values and practices differ from their own. Nurses understand that their own personal biases, including the ability to accept others who have cultural, spiritual, racial, ethnic, or sexual identity characteristics that differ from their own, affect their ability to plan and to provide optimal care. Nursing interventions and therapeutic interpersonal skills are used to elicit concerns, identify needs, implement teaching, make referrals, and demonstrate empathic caring and acceptance.

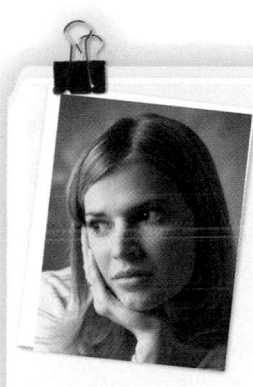

Lourie Ackerman, a 16-year-old single teenager, confides to the school nurse that she is pregnant and is going to keep the baby. She states "My life is over. My mother told me I'd never amount to anything."

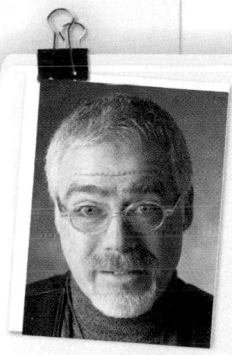

Anthony Santorini is a middle-aged man with a history of diabetes. He recently underwent a below-the-knee amputation due to complications resulting from poor glucose control. One morning, he states "I feel like damaged goods. I'm not a whole man anymore."

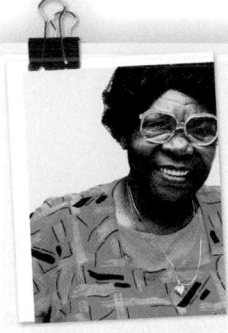

Delores Sparks is a 72-year-old African American widow, diagnosed with advanced lung cancer 14 months ago. She was living alone in a small apartment until 9 months ago, when she had to move in with her daughter after a lengthy hospital stay because she was no longer capable of living alone, and had a probable prognosis of, at most, 3 months to live. A recent home visit revealed that the patient was increasingly depressed and feeling like a burden to her daughter. She stated "I'm just an old dish rag, not good for anything anymore."

The types of blended skills you'll need to respond to the case scenarios include:

Cognitive Skills

- Knowledge of various theoretical principles related to self-concept, including the three dimensions of self-knowledge, self-expectation, and self-evaluation
- Knowledge of the variables that influence the development and maintenance of self-concept, and the relationship between self-concept and health and health behaviors
- Knowledge of growth and development and effect on self-concept for an adolescent, a middle-aged man, and an older woman
- Knowledge of measures to modify a negative self-concept for a pregnant adolescent, a middle-aged man with an amputation, and an older woman feeling like a burden
- Ability to incorporate knowledge of the nursing process to identify, diagnose, and resolve self-concept disturbances
- Knowledge of how to teach others to use self therapeutically to meet the healthcare needs of individuals at different developmental stages and different health conditions

Technical Skills

- Ability to provide technical nursing assistance necessary to assess and meet the needs of a pregnant adolescent, a middle-aged man with an amputation, and an older woman feeling like a burden
- Ability to adapt techniques to address changes in self-concept for patients at different developmental stages
- Ability to seek out help as necessary when providing technical nursing assistance while caring for patients with negative self-concept.

Interpersonal Skills

- Capacity to develop skills of self-reflection, enabling the nurse to identify his or her own biases that may negatively affect provision of optimal care, including self-awareness of own self-concept when dealing with patients experiencing issues involving self-concept
- Strong interpersonal skills to establish trusting relationships with a pregnant adolescent, a middle-aged man with an amputation, and a woman with terminal cancer feeling like a burden to her daughter

- Ability to use self therapeutically to enhance the self-concept of patients, family caregivers, and colleagues
- Ability to help patients find the motivation to develop new health and coping behaviors
- Ability to communicate and interact effectively with patients at different developmental stages and issues involving self-concept and their families
- Ability to demonstrate respect, empathy, and caring regardless of whether the patient's exhibits a positive or negative self-concept
- Ability to interact effectively and work collaboratively with other members of the healthcare team to meet the needs of patients with issues involving self-concept
- Demonstration of respect for the patient's human dignity and autonomy, regardless of whether the patient is a pregnant adolescent, a middle-aged male with an amputation, or an older woman who feels as if she is a burden to her family

Ethical and Legal Skills

- Demonstration of a strong sense of accountability for the health and well-being of patients at different developmental stages with issues involving self-concept
- A commitment to patient advocacy, including getting them the help they need to achieve their health goals—within the scope of one's nursing responsibilities and available resources
- Ability to integrate knowledge of ethical and legal principles concerning issues involving self-concept when providing care, including the need to document nursing assessment, diagnosis, outcome identification and planning, implementation, and evaluation
- A willingness to hold one's self accountable for safe, high-quality care for patients at different developmental stages with problems involving self-concept
- Ability to practice in an ethically and legally defensible manner, including familiarity with facility policy and role responsibilities related to managing the care of patients with issues involving self-concept

Learning Outcomes

After completing the chapter, the learner should be able to accomplish the following:

1. Identify three dimensions of self-concept: self-knowledge, self-expectation, and self-evaluation (self-esteem).
2. Describe major steps in the development of self-concept.
3. Differentiate positive and negative self-concept and high and low self-esteem.
4. Identify six variables that influence self-concept.
5. Use appropriate interview questions and observations to assess a patient's self-concept.
6. Develop nursing diagnoses to identify disturbances in self-concept (body image, self-esteem, role performance, personal identity).
7. Describe nursing strategies that are effective in resolving self-concept problems.
8. Plan, implement, and evaluate nursing care related to select nursing diagnoses for disturbances in self-concept.

Key Terms

body image
false self
global self
ideal self
personal identity
role performance
self-actualization
self-concept
self-esteem

An individual's self-concept is crucial to his or her health and well-being throughout life. One's self-image or **self-concept** has the power to either encourage or thwart personal growth. People with deficient self-concept might lack the motivation to learn self-care behaviors in response to illness, injury, and trauma. Nursing efforts aimed at teaching new health behaviors might fail until the patient values himself or herself enough to want to invest energy in self-care. Some patients observing aspects of their negative self-concept that affect their health behaviors might desperately want to make modifications but have no idea how to do so. The experience of illness, diagnostic testing, and treatment can severely threaten the self-concept of a patient. Nurses sensitive to patients' expressions of self-concept can use each nurse–patient interaction to enhance a patient's sense of self and to assist the patient in resolving self-concept disturbances. (See the accompanying Reflective Practice box for an example.)

As people move through the hierarchy of human needs to higher levels, needs for self-esteem and self-actualization arise, as discussed in Chapter 2. Both of these variables are components of self-concept. The need for **self-esteem** is the need to feel good about oneself and to believe that others hold one in high regard. The need for **self-actualization** is the need to reach one's potential through full development of one's unique capability.

Study of this chapter provides knowledge of the dimensions of self-concept, formation of self-concept, and key factors affecting self-concept. Practical interview guides are offered for assessing self-concept (personal identity, body image, self-esteem, role performance). Strategies for enhancing the self-esteem of the nurse are provided. Numerous examples of nursing diagnoses are given, and specific nursing strategies for assisting patients to meet self-concept outcomes are described. These guides and the concluding Nursing Plan of Care for Mrs. Motsky illustrate how the nurse's knowledge of self-concept may be combined with skilled nursing interventions and caring to successfully resolve disturbances in self-concept.

Reflective Practice
Challenge to Interpersonal Skills

Mrs. Delores Sparks is a 72-year-old widowed African American woman. Before her diagnosis of advanced lung cancer 14 months ago, she lived alone in a small apartment. Nine months ago, following a lengthy hospital stay, she moved in with her daughter, where it was determined that she was no longer capable of living alone and probably had, at most, 3 months to live. I was visiting her during my home health nursing experience and growing more and more concerned with her depression. Mrs. Sparks verbalized that she felt like a burden to her daughter, who has three children herself and was currently taking care of a granddaughter born to her eldest, unmarried daughter. Mrs. Sparks was being treated for her depression, but I was concerned about the effects all this was having on her self-concept. She told me she was like "an old dish rag" that wasn't good for anything anymore.

Thinking Outside the Box: Possible Courses of Action

- Try to cheer her up at each visit.
- Ignore her deteriorating self-concept, since focusing on it may only make her feel worse; it is certainly true that she has enough bad stuff going on in her life to make her feel bad.
- Explore sources of positive affirmations of her worth; try to use my professional relationship with her to communicate "you are a person of worth and I care about you!"

Evaluating a Good Outcome: How Do I Define Success?

- Mrs. Sparks' self-concept improves.
- I learn how to communicate a sense of worth to vulnerable patients.
- I learn how to address problems with self-concept.

Personal Learning: Here's to the Future!

Unfortunately, this situation got worse before it got better. Mrs. Sparks did not always take her meds for depression, and her daughter voiced increasing frustration with her mother's mood. "Mom talks all the time now about how even God doesn't want her. She says that she may have to take her own life since God doesn't seem to be doing it!" The daughter also said that Mrs. Sparks apologized to her constantly for being such a bother. Things didn't start to change until I learned that Mrs. Sparks used to be a very important member of her Baptist church community. She stopped attending services when she got too weak to go out. This was clearly a major loss for her. When I successfully got her minister to visit, he literally turned her life around, providing her with lots of positive reinforcement for how she could use her illness to do God's work. She seemed much more peaceful now. I've also encouraged her to tell me stories about the church work she did in the past and these reminiscences seem to be helpful.

Reflection

How do you think you would respond in a similar situation? Why? What does this tell you about yourself and about the adequacy of your skills for professional practice? Can you think of other ways to respond? What factors may have contributed to the patient's feelings of being a burden to her daughter? Describe the patient's self-concept using the dimensions of self-knowledge, self-expectations, and self-evaluation. What other skills (cognitive, interpersonal, technical, ethical/legal) would you need to respond well in this situation? Do you agree with the criteria to evaluate a successful outcome? Did the nursing student meet the criteria? Please explain your answer.

OVERVIEW OF SELF-CONCEPT

Dimensions of Self-Concept

Self-concept is the mental image or picture of self. All the feelings, beliefs, and values associated with "I" or "me" compose self-concept. Specific components of self-concept include personal identity, body image, self-esteem, and role performance. Crucial to each component are the dimensions of self-concept, which include self-knowledge, self-expectations, and self-evaluation.

People with a positive self-concept usually have greater and more diversified self-knowledge, more realistic perceptions and expectations, and higher self-esteem, whereas those with negative self-concept tend to exhibit poorer self-knowledge, less realistic perceptions and expectations, and lower self-esteem.

Consider Anthony Santorini the patient with a below-the-knee amputation. Analysis of the patient's comments would indicate that the patient is experiencing a negative self-concept. The nurse would need to assess Mr. Santorini more closely to determine his self-knowledge, self-expectations, and self-evaluation for each component of self-concept. This would help the nurse identify possible factors contributing to his status and gain a fuller picture of the patient's current condition.

Self-Knowledge: "Who Am I?"

Global self is the term used to describe the composite of all the basic facts, qualities, traits, images, and feelings one holds about oneself. These strongly influence a person's ability to manage life events and ensure emotional stability. A person's self-knowledge includes:

- Basic facts (sex, age, race, occupation, cultural background, sexual orientation)
- Person's position within social groups
- Qualities or traits that describe typical behaviors, feelings, moods, and other characteristics (generous, hot-headed, ambitious, intelligent, sexy)

Although some labels cannot be changed (eg, age and race), most are subjective and sensitive to change. Some conditions associated with alterations in self-concept or global self-worth include developmental changes, life crisis, illness, and loss.

Think back to Dolores Sparks, the older woman with advanced lung cancer who feels like a burden. When assessing the patient's global self-worth, the nurse would need to identify any developmental changes that Mrs. Sparks is experiencing that may be contributing to her current status, such as changes related to her increasing age. In addition, information about role changes, including the inability to care for herself and the need to be dependent due to her illness, in conjunction with the knowledge of her terminal condition and anticipatory griev-

ing related to her death, would be essential for determining her feelings of global self-worth.

Self-Expectations: "Who or What Do I Want to Be?"

Expectations for the self flow from various sources. The **ideal self** constitutes the self one wants to be. These self-expectations develop unconsciously early in childhood and are based on the image of role models such as parents, other caretaking figures, and public figures. These personal expectations might be healthy or unhealthy. Contrast the significance of a child's identifying a rock star or drug dealer as his hero rather than parents, government leaders, or other professional people. A **false self** might develop in individuals who have the emotional need to respond to the needs and ambitions significant people, such as parents, have for them.

Consider Lourie Ackerman, the pregnant adolescent. Her revelation of her mother's comment about not amounting to anything indicates the patient's false self. The nurse would need to gather additional data about Lourie's desire to keep the baby. This information would be valuable in determining if Lourie is unconsciously trying to convince herself that she will be a failure to maintain her mother's approval or if this is something that she truly wants.

Self-Evaluation: "How Well Do I Like Myself?"

Self-esteem is the evaluative and affective component of the self-concept, sometimes termed self-respect, self-approval, or self-worth. According to Maslow (1954, p. 90), all people "have a need or desire for a stable, firmly based, usually high evaluation of themselves, for self-respect or self-esteem, and for the esteem of others." Accordingly, he identified two subsets of esteem needs: (1) self-esteem needs (strength, achievement, mastery and competence, confidence in the face of the world, independence, and freedom), and (2) respect needs or the need for esteem from others (status, dominance, recognition, attention, importance, and appreciation). For Maslow, self-esteem comes from two major sources: how competent children think they are in various aspects of life and how much social support they receive from other people. One's self-esteem, like the various self-images that make up one's self-concept, varies considerably depending on a specific relationship or situation.

Coopersmith (1967) identified the four bases of self-esteem as (1) significance—the way a person feels he or she is loved and approved of by the people important to that person; (2) competence—the way tasks that are considered important are performed; (3) virtue—the attainment of moral–ethical standards; and (4) power—the extent to which a person influences his or her own and others' lives. According to Coopersmith, people with high, medium, and low self-esteem differ in their expectations of the future, in their affective reactions, and in their basic styles of adapting to environmental demands. People with high self-esteem are accustomed to being well received and successful. They are able to approach people, tasks, and new situations freely, with confidence in their ability to interact and to get along with people and to respond successfully to life's challenges.

Harter (1986) emphasized that an individual's judgment about his or her competency in areas of greatest importance to that person are most likely to affect the level of self-worth a person experiences. Harter (1999) described three major self-evaluation feelings or affects in children: (1) pride, based on a positive self-evaluation; (2) guilt, based on behaviors incongruent with ideal self; and (3) shame, associated with low global self-worth. These affects are learned in early childhood within relationships with significant others and maintained through practice.

Sullivan (1953) proposed the self-representations of "good-me" and "bad-me" based on reflected appraisals of the self learned in the context of a child's early relationship with significant others, especially parents. The child's feelings of self-esteem and self-worth develop out of his or her perceptions of the parenting figure's feelings, or affects, expressed in caring for the child. Sullivan posited that children perceived their parents' relative anxiety through a process he termed "empathy." Children exposed to higher levels of parental anxiety are at risk for developing lower self-esteem and a greater self-representation of "bad-me." As the child developed further, he or she would begin to behave in ways that confirmed the earlier self-appraisals.

> *Recall Lourie Ackerman, the pregnant adolescent? Her statement about not amounting to anything reflects the description of "bad-me." Applying Sullivan's concepts, Lourie is behaving in a way that confirms her perception of her mother's feelings.*

Sullivan and his most important interpreter within nursing, Hildegarde Peplau (1997; 1952), emphasized the fluidity of self-appraisals throughout the lifespan. They taught that positive interaction at any point in a person's life with new significant others (such as nurses) who are less anxious and more accepting and nurturing than prior figures can have a positive, growth-promoting effect on that person's self-esteem and self-concept.

Bowlby (1969) developed attachment theory, which describes modes by which a young child develops and maintains feelings about the self as well as values and beliefs about the world. Attachment is a process by which the child maintains felt security via an interpersonal bond with close caretakers, most notably parents. Through a learning process based on the child's perception of the caretaker's thoughts and reactions toward him or her, the child forms a sense of self as secure or insecure, calm or anxious, likable or not. Through this process, children also develop beliefs and feelings about others as well as individual perceptions of situations and events. Depending on how healthy the child's attachment experience is with the early caretaker, the growing child's self-esteem might vary greatly. The child's thoughts and feelings about events might closely match reality or might be distorted and out of touch with reality. Such patterns tend to remain relatively fixed into adulthood.

Formation of Self-Concept

Although self-concept is largely considered to be a social creation that develops as a result of interactions with others (Fig. 31-1), contemporary nursing researchers and others recognize that certain inborn tendencies, such as temperament when interacting with social and interpersonal experiences, are crucial in the formation of self-concept (McClowry, 2003). Psychoanalysts have also emphasized the importance of inborn traits, such as innate aggression, because they affect a child's interpersonal experiences and shape self-concept (Freud, 1927). According to the theoretical formulations stated above, the formation of self-concept includes the following:

1. An infant learns that the physical self is different from the environment. If basic needs are met, warmth and affection are experienced, and the caretakers' anxiety is minimized, then the child begins life with positive feelings about self.
2. The child next internalizes (incorporates into self) other people's attitudes toward self, including attitudes directed toward the child's innate tendencies such as temperament and aggression. This internalization forms the foundation of self-concept. Parents or other direct caretakers play the most influential role; peers play the second most influential role. Later, the child continues to behave in ways that confirm this early self-concept.
3. The child or adult internalizes the standards of society.

Stages in the development of the self include self-awareness (infancy), self-recognition (18 months), self-definition (3 years), and self-concept (6–7 years).

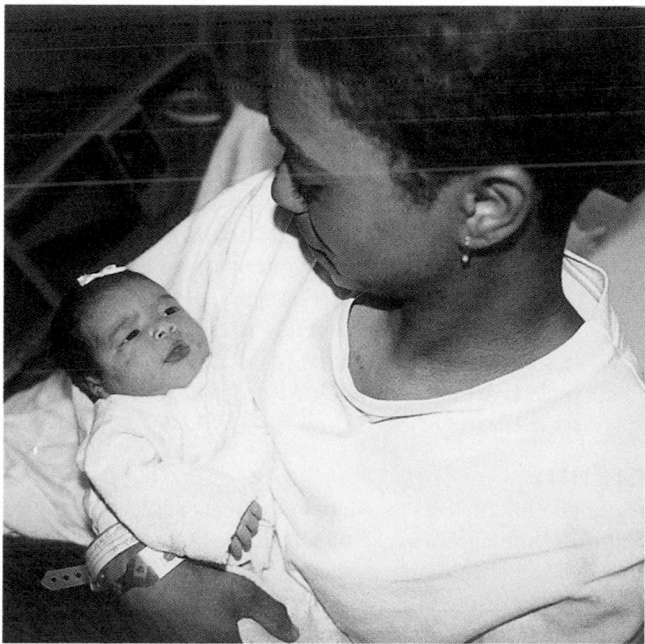

FIGURE 31-1 Interaction between caregivers and the infant are important to the child's development. Feeding, holding, cuddling, and cooing are forms of interaction.

Coleman, Morris, and Glaros (1990) identified the following psychological conditions that foster healthy development of the self in children:
- Emotional warmth and acceptance
- Effective structure and discipline
- Clearly defined standards and limits, so that children understand what goals, procedures, and conduct are approved
- Adequately defined roles for both older and younger members of the family
- Established methods of handling children that produce the desired behavior, discourage misbehavior, and deal with infractions when they occur
- Encouragement of competence and self-confidence
- Helping children meet challenges
- Appropriate role models
- A stimulating and responsive environment

Formation of self-concept is further described in developmental theories, especially in Erikson's stages of development, Piaget's cognitive developmental stages, and Havighurst's developmental tasks (see Chaps. 18 and 19).

Factors Affecting Self-Concept

Almost any life experience can influence a person's self-concept. Key factors include developmental considerations, culture, internal and external resources, history of success and failure, stressors, and illness or trauma.

Developmental Considerations

As a person matures, the criteria that mark the experiences necessary for a positive self-concept change. Although the infant needs a supportive environment in which all human needs are met, the growing child needs the freedom to explore and develop the ability to meet increasing personal needs. Table 31-1 highlights developmental changes affecting self-concept, related implications for nursing, and potential causes of self-concept disturbances.

> *Think back to Anthony Santorini, the middle-aged patient with an amputation. For the adult, society emphasizes an intact body, fitness, style and beauty as important to fulfill role expectations. However, for Mr. Santorini, the amputation is an irreversible body change that affects these areas, ultimately altering his view of how he can function. As a result, he feels that he can no longer function in his role as a man.*

Culture

As a child internalizes the values of parents and peers, culture begins to influence a sense of self. If the culture is relatively stable, little tension might be experienced between what culture expects of the child and what the child expects of self. When parents, peers, and the adult world confront the child with different cultural expectations, the sense of self might be confused. For example, an adolescent might realize his or her parents live by the work ethic and believe it is necessary to rise

early every day and put in a full day's work. The adolescent's peer group has few demands placed on it and encourages the adolescent to hang out with the group. The adolescent's vocational aptitudes, meanwhile, are leading him or her to consider a music career in a rock group, which will keep the adolescent out late many nights doing something the parents do not classify as work.

Children of immigrants whose values and practices of their culture of origin vary from the culture of adoption face cultural dissonance. Parents might expect children to behave according to their own cultural norms; peers and society, as well as the adolescent's desire to "belong," create the desire to abandon old cultural beliefs, attitudes, and practices among many of these children. Conflict between parents and children, as well as cultural confusion, might occur.

Internal and External Resources

The personal strengths an individual recognizes, develops, and uses are powerful but subjective determinants of self-concept. For example, one person might use humor as both an effective coping mechanism and a successful interpersonal tool. Another person might use humor to avoid facing conflict and might feel badly about being known as a joker or clown. The degree to which an individual integrates healthy, useful internal resources or personal strengths is associated with how well a person has been able to establish a positive self-concept in the context of nurturing experiences. Self-concept is also associated with the ability to identify and use external resources such as a network of support people (see accompanying Research in Nursing box), adequate finances, and organizational supports. People who feel more positively about themselves tend to feel connected to others and to society; they can identify and use more external resources. On the other hand, people who feel disconnected and alone tend to perceive and use fewer environmental resources.

> *Remember Delores Sparks, the older adult woman who feels like a burden? The nurse would need to assess the situation more closely to determine what external resources and supports are available for Mrs. Sparks. In the Reflective Practice display, the patient's minister helped to provide one means of support. Subsequently, Mrs. Sparks began to feel better about herself.*

History of Success and Failure

People with a history of repeated failure (in school, friendships, work, or marriage) might perceive themselves as failures and actually perpetuate this image by unconsciously encouraging others to treat them this way. They might come to fear success and actually find it easier to fail even though they do not like themselves that way. Thus, failure influences an individual's self-concept negatively (eg, Sullivan's "bad-me" self-representation), and his or her self-concept instructs the person to continue to fail. On the other hand, a series of successful experiences, especially when experienced in the context of an accepting, nurturing, caring relationship, might condition a person to strive for the next success, and a posi-

TABLE 31-1 Developmental Changes Affecting Self-Concept

Developmental Period	Changes Affecting Self-Concept	Implications for Nursing	Potential Causes of Disturbances in Self-Concept
Infancy	• No self-concept at birth • Beginning differentiation of self and nonself	• Teach parents the critical importance of providing consistent and affectionate parenting • Assess if the parents have reasonable expectations of the infant: sleeping, eating, other awake behaviors	• Unmet basic human needs • Lack of adequate body and sensory stimulation • Parents' lack of acceptance of the infant's appearance or behavior • Poor match between parent's and child's temperament or needs
Childhood	• An intact body is important to the young child, who fears bodily mutilation • During middle childhood, a sense of being trusted and loved, of being competent and trustworthy develops • Differences between self and others are strong	• If invasive procedures are indicated, explain simply to the child what is being done and offer the child support • Assess the parents' ability to provide the type of developmental environment in which the child's self-concepts can evolve positively	• Dysfunctional family • Too much or too little structure • Sensory perceptual impairments
Adolescence	• Development of secondary sex characteristics; rapid body changes • Sense of self is consolidated • Emphasis on sexual identity • Parental influences on self concept are often rejected; peers become more important; movement is toward development of own identity	• Assess adolescent's self-knowledge and understanding of body changes • Counsel adolescent regarding mature and healthy use of independence he or she craves • Provide anticipatory guidelines regarding hazards to life, health, human functioning	• Inability to accept body • Inability to resolve competing pulls to be both a child and an adult • Unhealthy peer pressure • Identify confusion
Adulthood	• Society places emphasis on intactness of body, fitness, energy, sexuality, style, sophistication, beauty • Important to meet role expectations well	• Assess how realistic the adult's expectations are and the incentive they provide for growth and development • Assist patient to deal constructively with negative influences in self-image • Preretirement counseling	• Inability to fulfill conflicting role expectations • Failure to accept role responsibility (eg, parenting responsibilities) • Unreasonable expectations • Irreversible body change related to trauma, illness • Unsatisfying job • Failure to develop new goals to give meaning and purpose to life • Multiple stressors
Later years	• Declining physical and possibly mental abilities • Multiple losses • Increasing dependency • Impending death • Diminished choices/options	• Assess how the older person is adjusting to effects of aging • Counsel regarding meaningful use of time • Explore resources • Assess depression; substance abuse • Recognize and value elders' life experience	• Loss of significant work (retirement); feelings of uselessness • Death of spouse, significant others • Diminished physical attractiveness, strength, overall health • Multiple stressors • Fear of dependency • Change may be more difficult

tive self-concept might be forged that expects success and makes it happen.

Crisis or Life Stressors

Life stressors or crises (eg, marriage, divorce, acute or chronic illness, an exam, a new job or job loss, a gray hair, a fire) might call forth a personal response and mobilize an individual's talents, resulting in good feelings about oneself, or it might result in emotional paralysis with diminished self-concept. People vary greatly in their perception of what constitutes a crisis or stressor, as well as the degree to which such experiences might disrupt or diminish self-concept. However, major stressors

Research in Nursing Making a Difference

Promoting Enhanced Self-Concept Through Social Support, Satisfaction With Healthcare, and Role Function

Social support, positive role function, and satisfaction with health-care have been demonstrated to have a positive influence on the experience of dealing with illness.

These three conditions have been evaluated as predictors of adjustment and perceived overall health factors in women who have breast cancer.

Related Research

Hoskins, C. N. (2001). Promoting adjustment among women with breast cancer and their partners. *Journal of the New York State Nurses Association, 32*(2), 19–23.

This ongoing program of nursing research focuses on evaluating predictors of adjustment outcomes in women diagnosed with breast cancer and their partners. Questionnaires were administered during various phases of the breast cancer experience to gather data about the study factors. The researchers developed and are evaluating a videotaped health-education intervention and a telephone-counseling program for these individuals. To date, the study data support the conclusion that greater social support from partners, the patient's ability to perform life roles, and greater satisfaction with healthcare are strongly predictive of patients' perception of better overall health status and greater psychological well-being.

Relevance for Practice

Nurses need to take factors related to self-concept into consideration in planning care, as these factors have been shown to have a direct relationship to how people adjust to health problems. Nurses can also provide effective care via media programs such as videotapes or long-distance via telephone.

place anyone at relative risk for maladaptive responses, such as withdrawal, isolation, depression, extreme anxiety, substance abuse, or exacerbation of physical illness. How the person perceives the stressor (threat, challenge, defeat) and his or her ability to mobilize personal strengths and other resources are determined largely by that person's self-concept, which, in turn, is influenced by the response the person chooses.

Aguilera (1994) described three factors that determine a person's response to crisis: (1) the person's perception of the event or situation; (2) the person's situational supports (external resources); and (3) the coping mechanisms the person possesses (internal resources.) All of these factors are related to self-concept. The degree of strength an individual has in each area is related to his or her precrisis self-concept. Similarly, each of these conditions can alter self-concept either positively or negatively during or after crisis. Intervention to strengthen any of these three areas can help people better cope with crisis and emerge with enhanced self-concept.

Recall Anthony Santorini, the patient who had an amputation? To promote an enhanced self-concept, the nurse would need to assess his perception of the situation and his coping mechanisms to gain further insight into Mr. Santorini's self-concept. In addition, the nurse would need to investigate any support systems available to Mr. Santorini, such as family, friends, and community resources that might be helpful in fostering a more positive self-concept.

Aging, Illness, or Trauma

Many people take a healthy body for granted. Society encourages a kind of denial of the eventuality of aging, chronic illness, and the necessity to integrate crisis and change throughout each person's lifetime. Society emphasizes and rewards youth, health, and narrow norms for physical attractiveness while devaluing seniors, those with chronic illness, and those whose appearance does not correspond to movie-star standards. Thus, even the suggestion of disease, the sudden impact of illness, trauma, or bodily disfigurement, or signs of the aging process might pose serious threats to the self (Fig. 31-2). People vary greatly in their response to aging, illness, and trauma. This is due to the threats to self-concept and internal beliefs about the self that these conditions may pose.

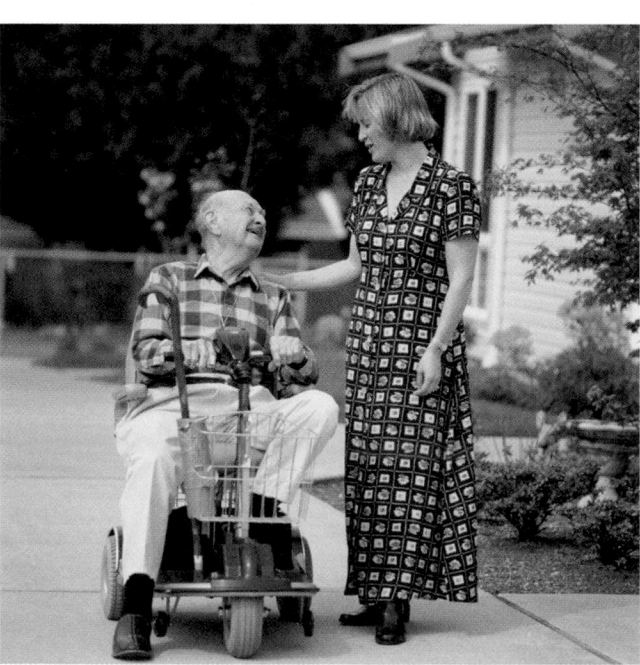

FIGURE 31-2 An illness or alteration in function may present a crisis situation, which affects the patient's self-concept.

Consider Delores Sparks, the woman described in the Reflective Practice display. Aging, by itself, can influence one's self-concept. However, the patient also is faced with the loss of independence and personal space, reliance on others for daily care, knowledge that she has a terminal illness, and the prospect of death in the near future. All of these factors are contributing to Mrs. Sparks' current status.

THE NURSING PROCESS

Before nurses can successfully identify and resolve self-concept disturbances in patients, they must be comfortable with themselves and possess an adequate self-concept. See Box 31-1.

Assessing

The nurse assessing self-concept focuses on the patient's personal identity, body image, self-esteem, and role performance. A general assessment of self-concept should be included in every comprehensive nursing assessment. It is as important to identify and label a patient's positive self-concept as it is to note problems.

Remember Lourie Ackerman, the pregnant adolescent described at the beginning of the chap-

ter? Although she states that her "life is over," the nurse would need to assess her for any indications of a positive self-concept. For example, the nurse would need to question Lourie further about her feelings of parenting and previous experiences with parenting, such as with younger siblings. In addition, the nurse would investigate Lourie's future goals and plans and availability of supports The nurse would then use this information, building on positive aspects to foster a positive self-concept as Lourie prepares for motherhood.

Patients experiencing illness or trauma resulting in body disfigurement, altered functioning, or life crises that arrest development and thwart the achievement of life goals are at high risk for problems related to self-concept and should be assessed more carefully. If potential problems surface during the interview, a more thorough assessment should be carried out.

Think back to Anthony Santorini, the patient who had an amputation. The patient's statement about being "damaged goods" would lead the nurse to suspect an alteration in self-concept. However, the nurse needs to investigate the patient's comments more closely to determine the underlying reason. Although the loss

---

BOX 31-1 Enhancing Self-Concept for Nursing Professionals

Important goals for enhancing self-concept include the following:

- Identify basic unmet human needs, exploring positive means to meet these needs.
- Schedule time every day to meet personal needs.
- Assess the effect of feedback from significant others on self-esteem.
- Describe personal strengths accurately.
- Develop a realistic plan to achieve goals for personal growth and development.

Specific strategies for enhancing self-concept in relation to one's professional practice follow:

Dispel the myth that it is necessary to know all there is to know about nursing to be a good nurse. At no one point in time does any nurse ever have it all together. Acceptance of the need to learn new theories or new procedures frees you from having to practice defensively (ie, pretend to be on top of every new development) and is a great stimulus for professional growth and development.

Realistically evaluate strengths and weaknesses. Build a periodic review into your practice and be fair in your self-evaluation. "I think I'm giving better care than ever before and I know my patients are appreciative, but I'm sensing a lot of tension between myself and a couple of the other nurses. . . ."

Accentuate the positive. Many of us have a knack for forgetting the 99 things we did well and focusing on our one error.

Errors need to be taken seriously and evaluated but not to the exclusion of overlooking positive accomplishments.

Develop a conscious plan for changing weaknesses into strengths. Professional growth and development depend on strong motivation to become better at what you do. "Realizing that I never know what to say when a patient receives bad news, I can try to avoid these patients or consciously plan to develop better interpersonal skills." Nurses are tremendous resources for each other. Tapping into each other's strengths is a great way to build self-esteem mutually. "You always seem to know the right thing to say or do with patients. Do you mind if I observe for a while and then 'try on' some of your behaviors?"

Work to develop team self-esteem. A basic interpersonal principle that seems to work well in practice is to offer to others what you want yourself. Because our sense of self is strongly influenced by the feedback we receive from others, positive reinforcement of our strengths and sincere offers to help correct deficiencies are needed by everyone.

Actively demonstrate your commitment to nursing and concern about nursing's public image. To feel good about yourself, you need to be able to experience pride in your profession. Active participation in professional organizations can offer many personal rewards—not the least of which is enthusiasm and pride in being a nurse. Monitoring the media's portrayal of nursing and providing appropriate feedback contributes to individual and corporate nursing self-esteem.

of his leg may be paramount, the patient's statements may be related to feelings of guilt for not having complied better with his diabetic regimen to reduce his risk of complications. Mr. Santorini may be blaming himself for his current state. Or possibly the patient fears how others will react to him. Once the information is obtained, the nurse can individualize Mr. Santorini's care. If this information is overlooked, the patient may be at higher risk for problems later on in the future. Thus, a thorough assessment is key.

The accompanying Focused Assessment Guide highlights elements common to any self-concept assessment and high-risk factors.

It is important for the nurse conducting this assessment to realize the limitations of self-reporting. A patient might give what he or she believes are the desired or socially acceptable responses to interview questions. "Why, of course I like myself. I'm a pretty good person. Yes, I have friends." For this reason, the nurse must evaluate the patient's responses in relation to observations made about the patient and what is known about the patient from other sources. (See the accompanying Promoting Health 31-1) When the nursing assessment reveals a clustering of these behaviors, it is important to discuss this finding with the patient. This is especially true when there is a discrepancy between the patient's words and behavior. "You've told me that you feel in control of your situation right now and are committed to the treatment plan, but I notice you're not taking your medications regularly and you did mention that you are drinking more heavily. . . ."

Personal Identity

When assessing self-concept, the information needed first is the patient's description of self. **Personal identity** describes an individual's conscious sense of who he or she is. "How would you describe yourself to others?" The nurse pays special attention to the labels used by the patient and the order in which they appear. A simple exercise consists of asking patients to "Make a list of 10 labels that you believe identifies yourself

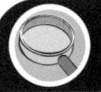

Focused Assessment Guide 31-1

Self-Concept

Factors to Assess	High-Risk Factors	Questions and Approaches
Personal identity	• Developmental changes • Trauma • Gender dissonance • Cultural dissonance	How would you describe yourself to others? 　• Personal characteristics and traits 　• Strengths 　• Fears
Body image	• Loss of body part or function • Disfigurement • Developmental changes	Describe your body to me. What do you like most/least about your body? Is there anything about your body that you would like to change?
Self-esteem	• Unhealthy interpersonal relationships • Failure to achieve developmental milestones • Failure to achieve life goals • Failure to live up to personal moral code • Sense of powerlessness	Tell me something about your sense of satisfaction with yourself. Tell me about your relationship with others. Who would you like to be? Who or what has influenced your self-expectations? Are these expectations realistic? 　• *Significance:* What is your response when you feel unloved or unappreciated by those who are important to you? 　• *Competence:* How do you feel about your ability to do the things in life that are important to you? 　• *Virtue:* To what degree are you satisfied with the way you are able to live up to your moral standards? 　• *Power:* To what extent do you feel able to control what happens to you in life? How does this make you feel?
Role performance	• Loss of valued role • Ambiguous role expectations • Conflicting role expectations • Inability to meet role expectations	How do you feel about your ability to do all the things your roles demand of you? Are these roles satisfying for you?

Promoting Health 31-1 *Self-Concept*

Use the assessment checklist to determine how well you are meeting your need for positive self-concept. Then develop a prescription for self-care by choosing appropriate behaviors from the list of suggestions.

ASSESSMENT CHECKLIST

almost always	sometimes	almost never	
☐	☐	☐	1. I have established appropriate expectations and goals for myself.
☐	☐	☐	2. I have effective and satisfying relationships with others.
☐	☐	☐	3. I cope effectively with change and loss.
☐	☐	☐	4. I accept and feel good about myself.

SELF-CARE BEHAVIORS

1. Accept normal variations in physical appearance and capabilities.
2. Use problem-solving and decision-making strategies to define expectations and set goals.
3. Set priorities and accept that no one person can be all things to all people.
4. Forget past mistakes; carrying around "excess baggage" is unhealthy.
5. Emphasize strengths and abilities in self.
6. Take an active part in group activities in school, work, church, or the community.
7. Volunteer time, talents, or services.
8. Avoid excessive alcohol and drugs.
9. Live life one day at a time.
10. Get help for self-concept disturbances that interfere with healthy social and professional activities.

(eg, gay man, student, Italian American, opera fan, premed major). Put the most important label first, and then list the others in order of decreasing importance. (What if the order were reversed?) To what extent do you think your way of organizing information about yourself affects your behavior?"

It is important to discover whether individuals are comfortable with their perceived identity. Developmental changes, trauma, and cultural and gender dissonance might all place a patient at risk for personal identity disturbances.

Personal Strengths

Many patients focus naturally on their deficiencies; asking pointed questions about personal strengths can help a patient identify positive factors:

"What are some of your personal strengths . . . qualities you are proud of . . . things you do well?"

"What special talents or abilities do you have?"

"What has helped you cope in the past when things were tough?"

> Consider Delores Sparks, the woman described in the Reflective Practice display. Obtaining information about Mrs. Sparks' personal strengths would be key to planning appropriate interventions to foster a positive self-concept. Assessment revealed that one of the areas important to her was her participation in her church community. The nurse used this information, contacting her minister, to provide support.

Body Image

Body image is the subjective view a person has about his or her physical appearance. Body image disturbances are expectable with any alteration in bodily appearance, structure, or function.

When a disturbed body image is suspected, the nurse carefully interviews and observes the patient to identify the nature of the threat to the person's body image (functional significance of the part involved, importance of physical appearance, and visibility of the part involved): the meaning the patient attaches to the threat; the adequacy of the patient's coping abilities; response of family members and significant others; and help available to the patient and his or her family.

The patient's response to the deformity or limitation is assessed, including changes in independence–dependence patterns and in socialization and communication.

> Recall Anthony Santorini, the middle-aged male who had an amputation? The patient voiced concerns that he was not "whole" anymore. The nurse would need to assess the underlying factors associated with this feeling. Is the feeling related to the actual loss of a body part, fear of further disfiguration due to continued complications, inability to function independently, or fear of how others will react to the loss? Additional inquiry is needed to determine the value Mr. Santorini places on physical appearance and the meaning he attaches to his extremities, such as ability to walk, work, or just get around the house or his environment. The nurse could then work with the patient and assist with adapting to the loss of his leg. Incorporating information about the use of a prosthesis may be helpful as he begins to adapt to his body change.

Response to Deformity or Limitation

Adaptive and maladaptive responses to deformity or limitation follow:

- *Adaptive responses:* Patient exhibits signs of grief and mourning (shock, disbelief, denial, anger, guilt, acceptance).
- *Maladaptive responses:* Patient continues to deny and to avoid dealing with the deformity or limitation, engages in self-destructive behavior, talks about feelings of worthlessness or insecurity, equates deformity or limitation with whole person, shows a change in ability to estimate relationship of body to environment.

Independence–Dependence Patterns

Adaptive and maladaptive responses to changes in independence–dependence patterns follow:

- *Adaptive responses:* Patient assumes responsibility for care (makes decisions); develops new self-care behaviors; uses available resources; interacts in a mutually supportive way with family.
- *Maladaptive responses:* Patient assigns responsibility for his or her care to others; becomes increasingly dependent or stubbornly refuses necessary help.

Self-Esteem

When a patient has shared perceptions of self, the nurse questions if the patient likes himself or herself, if the patient is pleased with his or her expectations, and the progress the patient is making to realize these expectations. For example, the nurse might state:

"Tell me what you like about yourself."

"What would you change about yourself if you could?"

Using a graphic description of self-esteem as the discrepancy between the "real self" (what we think we really are) and the "ideal self" (what we think we would like to be), the nurse can obtain a quick indication of a patient's self-esteem by having the patient plot two points on a line—real self and ideal self (Fig. 31-3). The greater the discrepancy, the lower the

High self-esteem

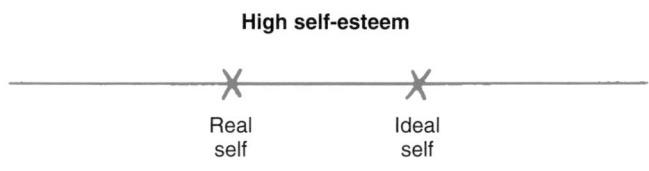

Low self-esteem

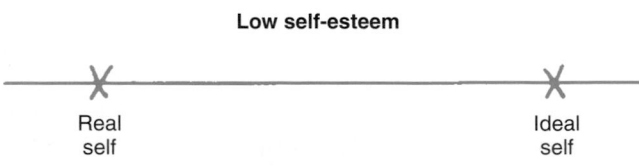

FIGURE 31-3 The patient who perceives his or her real self as relatively close to the ideal self has high self-esteem. The patient who perceives his or her real self as far from his ideal self has low self-esteem.

self-esteem; the smaller the discrepancy, the higher the self-esteem.

A person's ideal self may differ dramatically from the current sense of self and positively or negatively influence behavior and personal development. If indicated, the nurse questions the patient about self-expectations:

"You've told me something about who you are and how you view yourself now. Tell me who you would like to be in the future."

"What life goals are important to you?"

"Where do you see yourself 5 years from now? In 10 years?"

"Are these expectations realistic?"

"Are your expectations stemming from who you would like to be or from who you think you should be?"

"Who or what has influenced your self-expectations?"

> Remember Lourie Ackerman, the pregnant adolescent who feels her life is over? The nurse could use these questions to determine Lourie's ideal self and compare it with her current sense of self. This information would be important in planning Lourie's care and preparing her for her role as a mother.

The nurse is assessing whether the patient possesses life goals that are positively motivating personal development. Unrealistic expectations need to be identified, and their source needs to be explored with the patient. For example:

"You seem to feel that it is necessary to be all things to all people—no matter what this costs you. How might this belief have developed? Is it helpful to you?"

"What I'm hearing is that your performance must always be perfect, that although you allow others to make mistakes, you cannot allow yourself this luxury. Tell me more about this."

"Then, unless you graduate at the top of your class, you will not be satisfied? Why is this so important? Is this type of achievement realistic with your abilities? What will this success both benefit and cost you?"

"You state you have no goals for the future. When you wake up each morning, what gets you out of bed? What keeps you moving?"

If the need for a more detailed assessment is indicated, the nurse next explores the concepts of socialization and communication, significance, competence, virtue, and power.

Socialization and Communication

- *Adaptive responses:* Maintains usual social patterns, communicates needs and accepts offers of help, serves as support for others
- *Maladaptive responses:* Isolates himself or herself, exhibits superficial self-confidence, is unable to express needs (becomes hostile, ashamed, frustrated, depressed)

To assess the quantity and quality of the patient's interpersonal relationships, as information in this area identifies the level of social support and relatedness the person has, the nurse might ask:

"Tell me about the people in your life."

"Who do you feel is important to you?"

"Is there anyone you feel you can depend on for help if you need it?"

"How do you feel about your relationships?"

"Tell me about changes you've noticed in your ways of meeting and interacting with others."

"Many people have 'people' problems. Are your relationships causing you any problems right now?"

Significance

To assess the patient's feelings of significance, the nurse might ask:

"Are there people in your life with whom you share a close relationship?"

"To what extent do you feel loved and approved of by the key people in your life?"

"Does it bother you when you feel unloved or when others fail to appreciate you?"

"In what ways do you let family members and friends know that you like them or are proud of their accomplishments?"

Competence

To assess the patient's feelings of competence, the nurse might ask:

"What are the things you need to do to feel important?"

"Is anything interfering with your ability to execute these tasks?" ("How does this make you feel?")

"How important to you is it to feel that others value your work?"

Virtue

To assess the patient's sense of virtue, the nurse might ask:

"Tell me something about the moral–ethical principles that govern your life."

"How must you live to describe yourself as a 'good' person?"

"How do you feel about your ability to live this way?"

"Describe any difficulties you experience in living up to your moral principles that you would like to discuss."

"In what ways can the nurses help you to live better according to your moral standards?"

Power

To assess the patient's sense of virtue, the nurse might ask:

"How important is it to you to 'be in control' of your life (health)?"

"To what extent did you feel 'in control' of your life (health) before this illness (trauma, crisis, and so forth)?"

"To what extent do you feel 'in control' of your life (health) currently?"

"What is it that makes you feel not in control?"

"How might you change this? How can nurses help you to develop and gain more control?"

Role Performance

We all play many roles. Life roles such as our occupation or profession can constitute a major portion of our identity. Our ability to successfully execute societal as well as our own ex-

pectations regarding role-specific behaviors, or our **role performance**, is easily compromised by illness and injury. Often, illness or developmental processes such as aging make it necessary to alter or relinquish previous roles. Generally, people experience such alterations as major losses. Thus, all people whose roles are altered or compromised are at risk for disturbances in self-concept. With any patient who has experienced compromised role performance, the following questions are indicated:

"What major roles describe you—son, daughter, spouse, parent, employer or employee, student, club member, and so on?"

"How important is it to you to be good in each of these roles?"

"Tell me how successful you think you are in each of these roles."

"What roles or expectations would you change if you could?"

"How do you feel about the need for changes in your current role?"

"What new skills or behaviors might be necessary to help you resume or modify current roles?"

"What is it like for you to lose a role that's been important to you?"

"How is life going to be different now? What other role options do you have?"

"How can I help you identify other role options or direction?"

Think back to Dolores Spurks, the woman with advanced lung cancer now living with her daughter. The change in living situation and dependence on her daughter for everyday activities has definitely affected the patient's role performance. Once living alone and fairly self-sufficient, Mrs. Sparks now relies on her daughter. The above questions would be extremely important to ask Mrs. Sparks to determine the actual impact her illness and change in living situation has had on her self-concept.

Diagnosing

Disturbances in Self-Concept as the Problem

Specific disturbances in self-concept that can be treated by independent nursing interventions receive one of four nursing diagnostic labels:

- *Disturbed Body Image:* The state in which an individual experiences or is at risk for experiencing a disruption in the way one perceives one's body image
- *Chronic Low Self-Esteem* or *Situational Low Self-Esteem:* The state in which an individual experiences or is at risk for experiencing negative self-evaluation about self or capabilities
- *Ineffective Role Performance:* The state in which an individual experiences or is at risk for experiencing a

disruption in the way he or she perceives his or her role performance
- *Disturbed Personal Identity:* The state in which an individual experiences or is at risk for experiencing an inability to distinguish between self and nonself (Carpenito, 2004)

Common etiologies and defining characteristics for these diagnoses are found in the accompanying box, Examples of NANDA Nursing Diagnoses: Disturbances in Self-Concept.

Disturbance in Self-Concept as the Etiology

Because disturbances in self-concept have the potential to affect so many other areas of human functioning, they may serve as etiologies for numerous problem statements. Examples of these follow:

- Impaired Adjustment related to change in health status (increasing dependency, need for ongoing medical evaluation and treatment, and so forth)
- Anxiety related to irreversible change in body image (eg, amputation, mastectomy, burn); delayed development of secondary sex characteristics (body image); discrepancy between real and ideal self (self-esteem); perceived incompetence in important roles; loss of key roles (child or spouse dies, separation, retirement, graduation)
- Ineffective Coping related to inability to identify personal strengths, low self-esteem, "I know I can't manage this"; role conflict
- Anticipatory or Dysfunctional Grieving related to change in body image, loss of key roles
- Ineffective Health Maintenance related to low self-esteem—"Why bother?"

Examples of NANDA Nursing Diagnoses | Disturbances in Self-Concept

Nursing Diagnoses	Related Factors	Sample Defining Characteristics
Disturbed Body Image	Irreversible changes in body image such as amputation, mastectomy, hysterectomy, colostomy, scars, burns, disfiguring skin disorder	"Look at me. Nothing can ever be the same again. I feel less whole. When I look in the mirror, all I see is my (stump, missing breast, scar). I know when others look at me they feel repulsed or at the very least pity me."
	Effects of treatment (eg, braces, casts)	Thirteen-year-old adolescent girl with scoliosis wearing a Milwaukee brace (covers pelvic area and has rods in the front and back that extend up to the chin): "I feel dumb in this thing . . . it's bad enough that my back is crooked but this makes me look like a freak. Besides, it's hot. Must I wear it to school?"
	Difficulty accepting development of secondary sex characteristics or delayed development of same	Fifteen-year-old adolescent boy, sophomore in high school, height 5'1", weight 88 lb: "When am I going to grow up and start looking like the other guys in my class?" No pubic hair; penis, testes, and scrotum are the same size and proportion as in childhood
	Extreme thinness or obesity	Twenty-year-old woman, height 5'7"; weight 200 lb: "I hate my body . . . I've been fat all my life and I'm always on a diet. Why can't I be like everyone else?"
Low Self-Esteem	Feeling unloved or unapproved of by significant others	Twelve-year-old son of parents in the process of getting a divorce: "No matter what I do to make my dad like me he acts like I don't exist. When he's home, he fights with mom, but mostly he's away. I wouldn't even care if he yelled at me so long as he noticed me. I wonder why he doesn't like me?"
	Feelings of incompetence	Forty-two-year-old car salesperson, with company for 18 years: "What's wrong with me? I do my job, I'm also never absent, I have a good sales record, but I keep getting passed over for promotions. I think I'm too old to move to a different company, but I don't want to just sell cars for someone else for the rest of my life!"
	Failure to live according to personal moral ethical code	Thirty-three-year-old single computer programmer: "I should have known I'd get pregnant—I deserve it. I knew I was wrong to go to bed with this guy. Basically I've tried to live the way I think I should all my life up until now. What if something's wrong with the baby because of my sin?"

(continued)

Examples of
NANDA
Nursing Diagnoses
Disturbances in Self-Concept (Continued)

Nursing Diagnoses	Related Factors	Sample Defining Characteristics
	Powerlessness	Sixty-seven-year-old alert widow with degenerative joint disease: "It may be hard for me to move around now, but darn it—there's nothing wrong with my mind. The kids think they are helping me by making all my decisions, but they aren't. I'm not a doddering old lady in a nursing home."
Ineffective Role Performance	Rejection of role	Twenty-two-year-old mother 2 days after birth of her second son (first son is 15 months old): "I don't know who my husband got to watch our son. I never wanted to be a mother anyway. My husband and I have never had any time for ourselves—and things aren't going to get any better."
	Role conflict Role fatigue Multiple life stressors	Twenty-one-year-old, full-time junior nursing student who failed a major exam; is married and the mother of an 18-month-old daughter; works every other weekend in a hospital as an ECG technician: "I'm trying so hard to get my grades up, but I don't know what else I can do. My husband seems to be losing patience with me more and more and I sometimes feel awful about neglecting my daughter. I'd stop working but we need the money. I want nursing so bad but I'm getting awfully tired."
	Changing personal resources (physical health, mental abilities, motivation)	Fifty-year-old college chemistry teacher begins exhibiting signs of early Alzheimer's disease; forgets where she is and what she is doing; began rambling in class and saying things that made no sense—much to the class's amusement. Later cried and called herself "stupid."
Disturbed Personal Identity	Unresolved crisis	Eighty-eight-year-old man who lost his wife 6 months ago; wife took care of all his needs; sits alone in the house all day: "We always did everything together. I wish I had died first. What shall I do?"
	Declining physical, mental, or sensory abilities	Same 88-year-old man 3 months after admission to long-term care institution, medical diagnosis "rule out depression/dementia"; has become increasingly withdrawn, never initiates conversation; responses to questions are sometimes inappropriate: "What do you mean, what's my name? Who cares? I want to go home to my wife."
	Rejection of membership in minority group	Fifteen-year-old Cambodian girl recently emigrated to the United States with family; in constant conflict with parents as she rejects her family's culture in hopes of fitting in with peer group: "Sometimes I feel like I no longer know who I am or how I should act. I feel lonely inside and afraid."

- Hopelessness related to low self-esteem, overwhelming role demands, belief that nothing will change (destiny is controlled externally)
- Deficient Knowledge: How to help children develop High Self-Esteem related to lack of experience with parenting
- Noncompliance (specify) related to low self-esteem
- Altered Parenting related to disturbance in role performance (rejection of parent role)
- Posttrauma syndrome related to disturbance in personal identity
- Self-Care Deficit related to learned helplessness, low self-esteem—"I can't"
- Disturbed Sensory Perception related to disturbance in personal identity (ability to distinguish between self and nonself)
- Ineffective Sexuality Patterns related to changed body image, disturbance in self-concept
- Impaired Social Interaction or Social Isolation related to low self-esteem, disturbance in personal identity
- Disturbed Thought Processes related to disturbance in personal identity
- Risk for Self-Directed Violence related to disturbance in self-concept, overwhelmed by failure to live according to moral–ethical standards

Important Distinctions

When assessment data point to an alteration in self-concept, the nurse's first task is to determine whether the altered self-concept is the problem, the cause of the problem (etiology), or merely a sign that a problem exists (defining characteristics). Self-concept data seem to fit well in all three categories. It is important that an accurate determination be made because this directs the outcomes developed for the patient and related nursing interventions. Table 31-2 presents three different diagnoses that might be written for the same patient.

Consider Delores Sparks and the following nursing diagnoses:

Situational Low Self-Esteem related to perceived failure in role of mother and grandmother manifested by feelings of being a bother and not good for anything anymore. Assessment data point to a disturbance in self-esteem as the priority problem. Nursing energies will be directed to helping the patient evaluate herself positively despite the stress of the illness and loss of independence.

Ineffective Health Maintenance related to decreased self-esteem as manifested by feelings of depression. Here, low self-esteem is contributing to the patient's problem of failing to maintain her health as much as possible by following through with actions, and by voicing thoughts of ending her own life. Nursing energies will be best directed to improving the patient's use of health resources; one of the means used will be to help her to value herself enough to choose healthy behaviors.

Ineffective Coping related to difficulty accepting changes in health status and role resulting from terminal illness as manifested by low self-esteem statements ("I feel like an old dish rag, not good for anything anymore") and thoughts about ending her life ("since God isn't doing it.") Here, low self-esteem statements are the cues that led to the identification of the problem statement. One of the criteria used to evaluate nursing intervention to increase the patient's coping skills will be a reduction in or elimination of low self-esteem statements.

Outcome Identification and Planning

Whenever nurses care for patients, nursing interventions need to be supportive of the following patient outcomes. The patient will achieve the following:

- Describe self realistically, identifying both strengths and deficiencies
- Verbalize realistic expectations for self based on who he or she would like to be
- Verbalize that self is liked, or at least "OK"
- Communicate his or her feelings and needs in a way that is comfortable and effective in meeting needs
- Nurture relationships in which needs for love and worth are mutually met (significance)
- Assume role-related responsibilities with confidence (competence)
- Express satisfaction with ability to live according to one's moral–ethical standards (virtue)

TABLE 31-2 Type of Nursing Diagnosis: Effect on Nursing Care

Type of Nursing Diagnosis	Nursing Diagnosis	Nursing Care
Problem	Situational Low Self-Esteem related to perceived failure in role of wife (recent divorce) as manifested by neglect of personal appearance and inability to accept positive reinforcement	Assessment data point to a disturbance in self-esteem as the priority problem. Nursing energies will be directed to helping the patient evaluate herself positively despite the stress of the divorce.
Etiology	Ineffective Health Maintenance related to decreased self-esteem as manifested by failure to follow through on referrals (support group, stress-management class, etc.); "Why bother? Nothing ever works for me anyway."	Low self-esteem is contributing to the patient's problem of failing to follow through with health-seeking behaviors. Nursing energies will be best directed to improving the patient's use of health resources; one of the means used will be to help her to value herself enough to choose healthy behaviors.
Defining characteristic	Ineffective Coping related to inability to accept recent divorce as manifested by low self-esteem statements: "I never should have gotten married—my mother said I'd be a rotten wife." "I know I can't make it on my own." "Why did he do this to me?"	Low self-esteem statements are the cues that led to the identification of the problem statement. One of the criteria used to evaluate nursing intervention to increase the patient's coping skills will be a reduction in or elimination of low self-esteem statements.

- Demonstrate confidence in ability to accomplish what is desired (power)

    Sample outcomes for patients with specific disturbances in self-concept follow:

- Describe the relation between self-concept and behavior
- Identify faulty thinking that reinforces a negative self-concept (distortions and denials, faulty categorizing, inappropriate standards)
- Integrate positive self-knowledge into self-concept
- Report feeling better about himself or herself

Implementing

Nursing interventions to assist patients to develop and maintain a positive self-concept might vary tremendously from one patient to another. Nurses must be comfortable with their own self-concept before they can address problems in patients. Specific nursing strategies addressed in this section include helping patients identify and use personal strengths, helping at-risk patients maintain a sense of self, enhancing or modifying the self-concept, developing a positive body image, and working with parents and educators to develop self-esteem in children, adolescents, and older adults. These and other nursing interventions are summarized in the accompanying box, Example of Nursing Interventions Classification (NIC): Selected Self-Awareness Enhancement Activities.

Helping Patients Identify and Use Personal Strengths

When confronted with a major stressor, many people forget that they have histories of successful coping and numerous personal strengths. Patients at high risk for giving up are those with low self-esteem or multiple stressors perceived as being overwhelming.

Although attributing strength to a patient sounds like something nurses would do naturally, nurses frequently fall into the trap of "doing" for patients (ie, solving their problems rather than helping them to identify and tap their personal power and strengths). Moreover, patients continually instruct nurses about how they should be perceived, and some patients successfully communicate a manipulative helplessness that encourages the nurse to take charge. An appropriate nursing response in this case is "I wonder why you want me to speak with your physician about treatment alternatives. I'm sure you would feel much better hearing this information firsthand. If you'd like, I will stay here while you talk with the physician."

Patients experiencing powerlessness might need help to recognize their strengths (Fig. 31-4). Examples of personal strengths that might better equip a person to respond to life's challenges include:

healthy functioning body	meaningful work
ability to adjust to/function with chronic bodily malfunction	hobbies and other interests
	education
cognitive abilities	life experience and a past
positive self-concept	history of effective
interpersonal skills	coping
sense of meaning and purpose in life	good sense of humor
	spirituality
belief system	healthy nutritional state
social support network	ability to make decisions

Recall Delores Sparks? Her feelings of depression and feelings of being a bother may be related to feelings of loss of control over her life. Her minister provided support for Mrs. Sparks and helped to reinforce her worth as a person through her religion, providing positive reinforcement of her life and strengths.

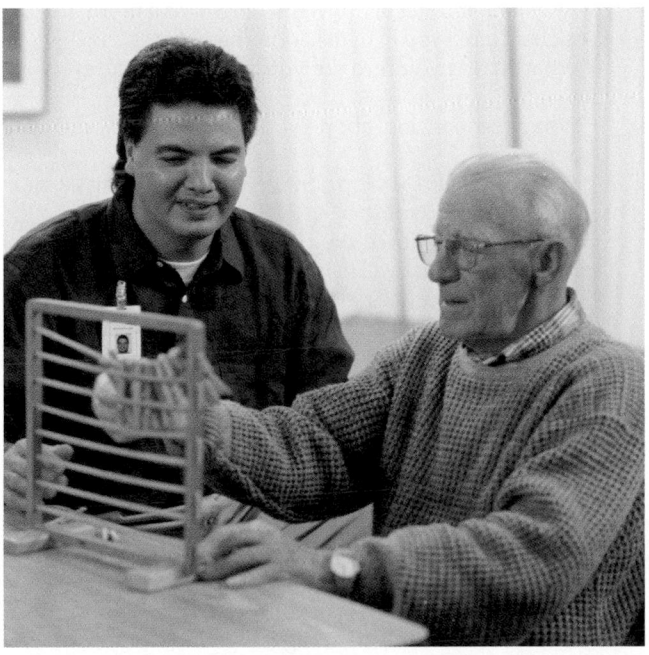

FIGURE 31-4 The nurse helps the patient recognize his self-worth and strengths.

Examples of Nursing Interventions Classification (NIC) Selected Self-Awareness Enhancement Activities

- Encourage patient to recognize and discuss thoughts and feelings.
- Assist patient to realize that everyone is unique.
- Assist patient to realize the impact of illness on self-concept.
- Assist patient to change view of self as victim by defining own rights, as appropriate.
- Assist patient to be aware of negative self-statements.
- Assist patient to identify guilty feelings.
- Explore with patient the need to control.
- Assist patient to identify positive attributes of self.

From McClosky, J., & Bulechek, G. (2000). *Nursing interventions classification (NIC)* (3rd ed.) (p. 574). St. Louis: C. V. Mosby. A full listing of nursing activities for each nursing intervention can be found in this book.

Specific strategies nurses can use to help patients identify and use personal strengths include the following:

- Encourage patients to identify their strengths.
- Replace self-negation with positive thinking (see Box 31-2).
- Notice and reinforce patient strengths.
- Encourage patients to will for themselves the strengths they desire and to try them on.
- Help patients cope with necessary dependency resulting from aging or illness.

Helping At-Risk Patients Maintain a Sense of Self

People who are acutely ill are often separated not only from their strengths but also from any real sense of self. This is largely because, as patients in healthcare facilities, they are removed from their personal roles, environments, and belongings, and stripped of their individuality by staff caring for them. One patient, a college president who was recovering from serious complications after surgery for ovarian cancer, shared the following:

When I first got sick, it didn't matter how people treated me because I knew who I was. As I've grown sicker and weaker, I become whomever people make me. If a nurse walks in here and moves me like meat, I become a slab of meat. My sense of self seems more and more dependent on how people respond to me.

Nurses can help patients maintain a sense of self and worth by doing the following:

- Use looks, speech, and judicious touch to communicate worth.
- Acknowledge the patient's status, roles, individuality.
- Speak to the patient respectfully and in a nonpatronizing manner.
- Converse with the patient about his or her life experience.
- Address the patient by preferred name whenever entering the patient's room.
- Offer the patient a simple explanation before initiating any procedure.
- Move the patient's body respectfully if the patient is unable to do this.
- Respect the patient's privacy and sensibilities.
- Acknowledge and allow expression of negative feelings.
- Help the patient to recognize strengths and explore alternatives.

It is important for nurses to keep in mind that patients are people first and foremost. A person's illness does not define who that person is. Too often there is a tendency for all healthcare professionals to focus primarily on a patient's illness, and the whole person is forgotten or ignored, with potential negative consequences for that patient's sense of self, such as lack of motivation to learn or execute important healthcare behaviors. The way nurses care for patients can directly impact self-concept; self-concept, in turn, directly impacts health. This type of caring does not require additional nursing time or energy. It does require from the nurse continual reaffirmation that nursing is a person-centered profession and that nothing is more important at any moment of a nurse's workday than the person being served.

Modifying a Negative Self-Concept

The time is ripe for change when a patient realizes that a negative self-concept is hindering personal development related to healthcare. Nurses might use a cognitive–behavioral approach to assist the patient in modifying self-concept. The general principle involved here is to help the patient alter his or her perspective of a situation from a more negative view to a more positive view, a process known as "reframing." Once a person can view his or her situation more positively, a wider variety of behavioral options, coping mechanisms, or internal or external supports can be identified and activated. While any person's self-concept is usually firmly entrenched and naturally resists change, the nurse should remain optimistic that change is possible, if even in small increments. Helpful nursing interventions include the following:

- Help the patient identify and describe in detail how he or she thinks and feels about situations related to self-concept (identify the patient's faulty thinking patterns).
- Explore with the patient alternative ways of viewing the same situation (reframe the patient's thinking about the situation).

BOX 31-2 Exploring and Developing the Positive

Example: Twenty-year-old mother who perceives herself as "a failure in everything I try"; states husband feels child-rearing is the woman's responsibility and she is terrified.

Immediate goal: Assist mother to better understand her feelings of failure by exploring them with her. This paves the way for her to recognize her strengths as a mother.

- Ask her to tell you in detail about her failures.
  "What makes you feel like you are a failure at everything?"
  "What terrifies you about your responsibilities as a mother?"
  Long-term goal: Develop confidence in parenting skills, see herself as good mother.

- Explore and reinforce the patient's personal qualities and strengths that will help her to reach her goal.
  "You look like a natural mother when you hold your baby; some women are afraid at the beginning to even hold their infants."
  "That's good that you are talking with your baby. Babies quickly sense how a parent feels about them."

- Teach the patient how to substitute positive self-talk for negative self-talk.
  Negative self-talk (mother during feeding): "She's awfully fussy tonight, I mustn't be doing this right. . . . It was probably dumb luck that she took to breast so well this morning. . . ."
  New positive self-talk: ". . . but she fed so well this morning and the nurse said her weight is good. I wonder what else might be making her fussy . . . maybe she's wet. . . ."

- Teach the patient to "red flag" faulty thinking behavior as soon as he or she is aware of it. The goal is to replace the negative thinking and self-talk with thinking and self-talk that will develop a more positive self-image.
- Help the patient explore the positive dimensions of himself or herself that he or she wishes to develop, and incorporate this new knowledge into the self-concept.

> *The nurse would incorporate actions to maintain a sense of self and worth when planning and implementing the care for Anthony Santorini. The nurse would focus on Mr. Santorini as a person, rather than an amputee. Doing so would help to treat the patient as an individual, demonstrating respect for his unique situation. In addition, the nurse would employ reframing techniques to help the patient view himself in a more positive manner, helping to change his view of himself as "damaged goods" to one of being a whole person.*

Developing a Positive Body Image

Interventions for body image disturbances vary according to the nature of the disturbance. Interventions may include any combination of the following:

- Express interest in and acceptance of the patient through verbal and nonverbal expression. Allow the patient to share his or her feelings openly. Sitting quietly by the patient for a few minutes, with a few words such as "How are things?" or "Tell me what's going on with you" communicates to the patient your willingness and readiness to share his or her experience.
- Explore with the patient his or her feelings about altered body image and his or her perceptions about the meaning and consequences of such alteration.
- Support the patient through the various stages of loss, grief, and mourning (shock, disbelief, denial, anger, guilt, acceptance), remembering that there is no one right way to proceed through these stages. Rather, patients may move fluidly in and out of various stages, sometimes returning to earlier stages. Some patients may need to learn that it is okay to cry, to be angry, or to feel depressed.
- Use play therapy with children so that they can describe their feelings and work through their grief using the nonthreatening medium of dolls or animals.
- Use self-reflection to gain awareness of your attitudes and feelings toward the patient. Be careful that facial expressions, words, or body positioning do not communicate to the patient disgust, fear, or rejection.
- While communicating support to the patient who is slow to develop and use appropriate self-care behaviors, firmly insist that the patient participate in his or her care to the extent that the patient is able. Whenever possible, provide the patient with honest answers to his or her questions or put the patient in touch with the appropriate person to give the answers.
- Strengthen the decision-making ability of the patient by honestly exploring alternatives; help the patient to imagine living with the consequences of different courses of action.
- Reinforce the patient's personal strengths and help the patient and family to identify all possible resources.
- Assess the response of the patient's significant others and intervene if they negatively influence the patient.

Developing Self-Esteem in Children and Adolescents

Nurses who work in practice settings where they have access to groups of parents, adult caregivers, or teachers can offer specific guidelines for creating developmental environments that build high self-esteem. Box 31-3 offers five strategies for building self-esteem in children. Because some parents and educators may not have experienced these aids to personal growth themselves, it is beneficial for the nurse to role-model these behaviors when interacting with children.

Important learning tasks for children include understanding and accepting oneself, feelings, and others; independence; goals and purposeful behavior; mastery, competence, and resourcefulness; emotional maturity; and choices and consequences.

Enhancing Self-Esteem in Older Adults

The many losses associated with aging (eg, diminished strength and physical health, interpersonal losses, retirement, and shrinking income) make older adults especially vulnerable to disturbances in self-concept, particularly chronic low self-esteem. Society's generally negative view of aging compounds the problem. Nurses interacting with older adults should employ the following interventions to enhance and maintain self-esteem in this population:

- Identify one's own attitudes and feelings about aging and elders.
- Address seniors respectfully, communicating that you take their concerns seriously.
- Respect and affirm seniors' intellect, individuality, personal strengths, culture, and spirituality.
- Adjust communication style to accommodate any sensory or cognitive deficits.
- Encourage sharing of life experiences.
- Assist individuals to identify strengths and coping mechanisms to deal with present problems.
- Provide a safe environment for elders to communicate such concerns as interpersonal or physical loss, feelings about illness and death, sexuality, or financial issues.
- Advocate for seniors needing help in attaining services necessary to meet their healthcare needs.
- Explore the personal meaning of dependency for the person, and help seniors adapt both physically and emotionally to any necessary dependency.

The Focus on Older Adults box describes nursing interventions to promote self-esteem in older adults.

Evaluating

Nurses who are sensitive to the relationship between self-concept and general well-being consistently evaluate the

BOX 31-3 Building Self-Esteem in Children

Strategy One: Looking at the Positive and the Negative

Instruct parents to write an honest description of their child for a stranger. Next have the parents underline the child's positive and negative qualities.

To reinforce the positive qualities, (1) notice examples of ability in many different circumstances and point this out to the child; (2) find occasion to frequently and honestly praise the child; and (3) give the child an opportunity to show ability frequently.

To address the negative qualities constructively, ask: (1) What need is being expressed by this behavior? (2) Can I see a positive quality being expressed by this behavior? and (3) How can I help my child express this quality and meet her needs in a more positive way?

Reexamine the list of negative qualities and ignore those that are a matter of taste, preference, or personal style.

Strategy Two: Listening

The following guidelines can help parents to use listening to communicate to a child, "You are important. What you say matters to me. You matter to me."

1. Make sure that you are ready to listen.
2. Give your child your full attention.
3. Minimize distractions.
4. Be an active listener.
5. Invite your child to talk.

Listen for the point of a child's story ("What is she trying to tell me? Why is this important to him?"). Don't feel that you have to fix things. Listen for and respond to the feelings.

Strategy Three: Using the Language of Self-Esteem

Feedback that enhances self-esteem has three components: (1) a description of the behavior (describe the behavior without judging it); (2) your reaction to the behavior (language that shares something about your self); and (3) acknowledgement of the child's feelings. For example, "Thanks for playing with your brother tonight [description]. I was wondering how

I was going to pay attention to our guests if he got fussy and was really grateful when I noticed that you kept him occupied and happy [reaction]. I know that there were other things you might have enjoyed doing more [acknowledgment]."

To give correction using the language of self-esteem, (1) describe the problematic behavior, (2) state a reason for the behavior change, (3) acknowledge the child's feelings, and (4) offer a clear statement of what is expected.

Attacking communications: "Don't let me ever hear you talk that way to your mother again."

Language of self-esteem: "I overheard you telling your mom that she should 'Get a life and get off your case.' [description]. When you talk like that it just makes people angry or sad, which isn't very helpful [reason for behavior change]. You probably feel like you are being picked on, and we may have some expectations that are different from those of your friends' parents. I hope you know that this is because we love you and want the best for you [acknowledgment]. In the future try to talk to others with the same respect you'd like others to show you [statement of expectation]."

Avoid using the following destructive language styles, which tear down self-esteem: overgeneralizations ("You *never* come home on time!"), the silent treatment, and vague or violent threats.

Strategy Four: Helping Children Meet Expectations

To help children meet expectations, (1) be sure that your expectations are reasonable and appropriate for your child's age; (2) plan ahead; (3) be clear about your expectations; (4) focus on the positive; (5) provide choices when possible; and (6) provide rewards.

Strategy Five: Promoting a Feeling of Success

To help children have the courage to try new types of experiences, which results from successfully meeting challenges: (1) let a child know what to expect; (2) let your child practice the necessary skills; (3) be patient; and (4) make it safe to fail.

(Material adapted from McKay, M., & Fanning, P. [1992]. *Self-esteem* [2nd ed.]. Oakland, CA: New Harbinger Publications.)

---

effect the nursing plan of care has on the patient's self-concept.

> *For example, while educating Anthony Santorini, the patient with a history of diabetes who had an amputation due to complications of the disorder, about reducing the risk of further complications, the nurse may detect that the patient is feeling extremely guilty about his lack of compliance in the past. "Why should I even try to change any of these things now? I made myself sick, so I may as well live with the punishment." If the plan of care is to be effective, the nurse must first help this patient value himself sufficiently to want to make the necessary changes.*

When the plan of care includes specific interventions to assist patients with disturbances in body image, self-esteem, role performance, and personal identity, the nurse listens carefully to the patient's self-report and observes patient behaviors to see if the disturbances are being resolved. Basically, the patient should be able to meet the following outcomes:

- Is comfortable with body image and able to use it effectively to meet human needs
- Is able to describe self positively
- Is able to meet realistic role expectations without undue anxiety and fatigue
- Is capable of interacting appropriately with environment while recognizing self to be a separate and distinct entity

See the accompanying Nursing Plan of Care 31-1 for Mrs. Motsky.

Focus on the Older Adult
Promoting Self-Esteem in Older Adults

Area of Concern	Nursing Strategies
Personal identity	• When an older person's sense of self is threatened, assist him or her to find meaning in the experience, to regain mastery to the extent that this is possible, and to evaluate realistically the adequacy of his coping strategy. • Teach older people to identify and develop a game plan for confronting anxiety-producing situations. • Help to identify and secure intervention for treatable depressions. • Treat causes of self-identity disturbances, such as pain, abusive living arrangements, and substance abuse.
Body image	• Notice and affirm positive physiologic characteristics of older adults. • Teach preventive self-care measures that reduce discomforting signs of aging (eg, exercise, which maintains muscle mass and joint flexibility; proper nutrition; and basic hygiene and skin care measures). • Explore new activities (including hobbies) that are within the changing physical capabilities of the older person.
Self-Esteem	• Assist older adults to identify and use personal strengths. • Communicate that you value older people simply for who they are (unconditional affirmation); know and use the name they prefer, ask them questions about their life, interests, or values. • When appropriate, use the expertise of older adults and ask their advice; let them know you value their life experiences. • Engage older people in activities in which they can be successful. • Allow older people to make tough decisions and confront challenging situations when appropriate; teach protective family members the value of older adults confronting situations that invite continued growth. • Empower older people to meet their own needs; provide necessary knowledge, teach new behaviors, instill the belief that they "can manage."
Role performance	• Explore with older people the many roles they have fulfilled throughout their lifetime; invite reminiscences. • Facilitate grieving over valued roles that are no longer able to be performed. • Remedy, whenever possible, factors that prevent older from engaging in valued roles. • Explore new roles.

NURSING PLAN OF CARE 31-1   *for Melissa Motsky*

PATIENT CARE STUDY

Melissa Motsky is a 31-year-old married woman, mother of three children (aged 12, 10, and 8 years) and junior-level nursing student. She works every other weekend as a nurse's aide. She has just received a letter from the nursing division head informing her that she is in academic jeopardy and will fail out of the program unless her grades improve. She presents this to her adviser.

After talking with Ms. Motsky, who calls herself a failure and who cries as she describes her situation at home, her faculty adviser suspects a serious self-esteem problem and helps her to list factors contributing to her current sense of failure and low self-esteem. The following list is generated:

SIGNIFICANCE

- Receives little understanding, affection, approval from husband. "I stay with him because of the kids. I started back to school because I had to get out of the house and want to make something of myself. He doesn't understand this."
+ "The children are very supportive but get impatient when I have to study and can't spend time with them."
- Feels a failure in all the roles that are important to her—wife, mother, and, now, student. "I jeopardized everything to go back to school—if I fail, it's all over for me. There just isn't enough time or energy to do anything well."
+ "They do love me at work, though, which makes me feel like nursing is what I should be doing."

VIRTUE

- "I've always believed that hard work pays off and that if you were faithful to your duty you'd be rewarded by the good life—I'm beginning to doubt that. Maybe I'm a fool for trying so hard."
+ "I do still try to live according to my beliefs and feel okay about this. I treat others as I'd like to be treated."

POWER

- "I always believed I could do anything I put my heart and soul into. But I can't seem to change my marriage, and if I fail out of school, that will be the end of all my dreams."

Key indicators of low self-esteem that also surfaced in the interview included overeating (10-lb weight gain during the past year); difficulty sleeping; fatigue; new sensitivity to criticism; and expressions of feeling unloved, alone, and no longer able to manage. Personal strengths included history of "can do" mentality, high motivation to succeed, and past history of success as mother and nurse's aide.

(continued)

NURSING PLAN OF CARE 31-1 — *for Melissa Motsky* (continued)

NURSING DIAGNOSIS	Situational Low Self-Esteem related to decreased sense of significance, competence, virtue, and power as manifested by expressions of being a failure, powerlessness, fatigue, tears, weight gain, low academic performance (test grades 68, 74)
EXPECTED OUTCOME	By this time next month, 11/2/06, the client will demonstrate increased self-esteem by: • Expressing positive statements about herself

Nursing Interventions

Assist patient to rediscover and "own" personal strengths: identify personal qualities and strengths that have pleased her in the past and explore why this has changed; recommend that she make at least one positive statement about herself each morning and evening.

Consistently interact with the patient as if she had the power to weather the crisis successfully (ie, "will" strength to her). Role-model positive self-concept behaviors.

Rationale

Patients can lose touch with their strengths, especially when multiple stressors seem to create impossible demands.

Once the patient senses that an authority believes in her power and expects her to use it, she may internalize this knowledge and act on it.

Evaluative Statement

11/3/06   Outcome partially met. Patient's statements are of the "This is good, *but . . .*" variety. "I think I'm doing better in school but I don't know if it will continue."

Recommendation: Continue to identify and reinforce personal strengths.

C. Taylor, RN

EXPECTED OUTCOME	By this time next month, 11/2/06, the patient will demonstrate increased self-esteem by: • Reporting ability to receive negative feedback without falling apart

Nursing Interventions

Explore with patient to what degree she allows the opinions of others to influence her self-concept.

Teach how the self-concept filters life experiences; thus, if I feel that I am a failure, I may interpret the words and behaviors of others as confirming this, even though that was not their intention.

Explore with the patient ways she can enhance her self-concept independently of others (eg, take time each day for herself). Encourage patient to draw on personal strengths.

Teach the patient how to analyze feedback constructively and respond appropriately; *cancel negative thinking*. For example, patient receives care plan back with many corrections and the notation, "sloppy work."

Maladaptive response: "She hates me. See, this proves I'll never be a good nurse. I wasted my time even doing this."

Adaptive response: "I spent as much time as I had on this . . . now let me see what I did wrong. Maybe I should make an appointment with my instructor so she can show me how to improve."

Rationale

Significance—sense of being loved and approved of by significant others—is a critical component of self-esteem.

Principle of self-consistency: once I am down, I may reinforce this by distorting what I feel, hear, and experience.

This facilitates internal locus of control versus external. Spending time on self communicates that self is valuable.

It is important to break the cycle of negative thinking, which reinforces negative self-concept.

Evaluative Statement

11/3/06   Outcome partially met. Patient reports being able to handle everything except putdowns from her husband.

Recommendation: Explore origin of power she has given to her husband to influence her sense of self and what she wants to do about this.

C. Taylor, RN

(continued)

NURSING PLAN OF CARE 31-1   *for Melissa Motsky* (continued)

EXPECTED OUTCOME   By this time next month, 11/2/06, the patient will demonstrate increased self-esteem by
• Getting a passing grade on her next quarterly examination

Nursing Interventions	Rationale	Evaluative Statement
Explore study skills with patient; recommend study group.	Poor study skills may also be contributing to her low academic performance. A study group will meet both her social and academic needs.	11/3/06 Outcome met. Grade: 82 *C. Taylor, RN*
Discuss importance of how she *perceives* present situation. If present failures are equated with *defeat*, she may be unable to mobilize her resources to succeed; if present failures represent *challenge*, it may call forth her best efforts and result in success.	The meaning given to present stressor can dramatically affect the patient's response to it and condition her for success or failure.	
Discuss importance of breaking cycle of failure leading to another failure.	If this short-term goal is met, it will set the stage for future successes and contribute to the patient's positive self-concept.	

EXPECTED OUTCOME   By this time next month, 11/2/06, the patient will demonstrate increased self-esteem by:
• Verbalizing that the way she is living her life is okay

Nursing Interventions	Rationale	Evaluative Statement
Assist patient to examiner her moral–ethical standards; explore sources of these standards and whether the patient feels comfortable with them.	Moral–ethical standards may be uncritically internalized and place the patient in conflict.	11/3/06 Outcome met. Patient stated: "I guess I'm living the best way I know how right now. If things are meant to be different someone is going to have to show me how."
Identify unrealistic standards; patient may need "permission" to be human.	Unrealistic standards (perfectionism, conventionality) may constantly undermine the patient's self-esteem.	*Recommendations:* Reinforce self-acceptance.
Refer if appropriate for counseling.	Support groups on campus (counseling centers, ministries) may be able to meet patient's needs.	*C. Taylor, RN*

EXPECTED OUTCOME   By this time next month, 11/2/06, the patient will demonstrate increased self-esteem by:
• Reporting two recent instances when personal power was effective in accomplishing desired goals

Nursing Interventions	Rationale	Evaluative Statement
Identify and affirm patient's use of personal power to accomplish goals.	A negative self-concept may deny or distort personal successes; outside intervention may be necessary to bring these to consciousness.	11/3/06 Outcome met . . . with difficulty. Needed considerable prompting to identify successful use of her personal power. Was ready to attribute passing grade to luck rather than her own efforts. *Recommendations:* Have patient make daily record of her use of personal power and results. *C. Taylor, RN*

(continued)

NURSING PLAN OF CARE 31-1   *for Melissa Motsky* (continued)

SAMPLE DOCUMENTATION

10/2/06   Nursing

Melissa Motsky presented today after receiving academic jeopardy letter. She is strongly motivated to complete nursing program successfully and seems to have the ability to do this. Current multiple life stressors—lack of support from husband; need to mother three children (12, 10, 8); part-time nurse's aide job (necessary for financial reasons); and current academic jeopardy (test grades 68, 74) are all contributing to her low self-esteem and overwhelming sense of being a failure. We together developed a care plan that it is hoped will help her to do better academically as well as begin to feel better about herself. See attached. She will return 11/2/06 at 10 AM for follow-up.

C. Taylor, RN

SOAP Format

10/2/06, 12:30 PM, nursing

Academic jeopardy—Melissa Motsky

S: "I jeopardized everything to go back to school—if I fail, it's all over for me." Reports lack of support from husband; grief that she does not have enough time for children; failure of personal work ethic ("hard work pays off"); and sense of powerlessness.
O: Nursing II quarterly exam grades: 68, 74; weight gain of 10 lb during past year; facial and body expressions of fatigue, profuse tears
A: Low Self-Esteem related to decreased sense of significance, competence, virtue, and power
P: See attached plan of care.

C. Taylor, RN

■ Developing Critical Thinking Skills

1. The personal strengths an individual recognizes, develops, and uses are powerful but subjective determinants of self-concept. Identify the strengths that have been major determinants of your self-concept (eg, power, intelligence, physical attractiveness, goodness, humor, "can-do" attitude) and explore how this is helping you to succeed in nursing. Discuss with another student ways that nurses can assist patients to recognize, develop, and use personal strengths to cope better with the stress of injury and illness.

2. Role play with another student your responses to the following patients, and then reverse roles. Reflect on the effects different types of nursing presence and response have on a patient's self-concept. Discuss the nursing responses that would be most helpful to patients at risk for self-concept disturbances.
   - A male patient who was recently passed over for a promotion states "I can't believe I've got to deal with this ulcer. It's just one more thing holding me back from succeeding in this business."
   - An anorexic teenager tells you that she can't possibly eat the dinner you brought her, and states "I can't do my usual workout in here, and look how fat I'm getting."
   - "I need to talk with someone about how it feels to be a woman trapped in a man's body."

   - A woman, after mastectomy, refuses to look at the incision site and notes "If I can't bring myself to look at this, how can I ever expect my husband to want me again?"
   - A resident in a nursing home says "Don't trouble yourself about me. I'm sure you have lots of people to take care of who are more deserving of your time and attention."

■ Practicing for NCLEX

1. Robert, aged 19 years, has Down syndrome and is mildly developmentally disabled with an intelligence quotient of 82. He told his nurse "I'm a good helper. You see I can carry these trays because I'm so strong. But I'm not very smart, so I have just learned to help with the things I know how to do." Robert most likely has
   a. Negative self-concept and low self-esteem
   b. Negative self-concept and high self-esteem
   c. Positive self-concept and fairly high self-esteem
   d. Positive self-concept and low self-esteem
2. Joe was asked to make a list of 20 words that describe him. After 15 minutes, Joe listed the following: 25 years old, male, named Joe; then declared he couldn't think of anything else. Joe has demonstrated
   a. Lack of self-esteem
   b. Deficient self-knowledge

c. Unrealistic self-expectation

d. Inability to evaluate himself

3. Joe was able to list only three facts, traits, or qualities to describe himself. The nurse then asked him to list facts, traits, or qualities that he would like to be descriptive of himself or that he thinks he should have. Joe quickly listed 25, all of which were characteristic of a successful man. When asked if he knew anyone like this, he replied "My father." This discrepancy between Joe's description of himself as he is and as he would like to be indicates

a. Negative self-concept

b. Joe's modesty (lack of conceit)

c. Body image disturbance

d. Joe's affection for his father

4. David and his wife decided that she will get a job so that David can go to pharmacy school, as he has wanted to do for some time. Their three teenagers, who were involved in the decision, are also getting jobs to buy their own clothes. David plans to work 12 to 16 hours weekly. He states "I was always an A student, but I may have to settle for Bs now because I don't want to neglect my family, and I need to work a few hours so that my wife won't have to work overtime." David's self-expectations are

a. Realistic and positively motivating his development

b. Unrealistic and negatively motivating his development

c. Unrealistic but positively motivating his development

d. Realistic but negatively motivating his development

5. Which of the following statements made by the parent of a child you are seeing in clinic needs to be followed up with teaching about how to foster healthy development of the self in children?

a. "I love my child so much I 'hug him to death' every day."

b. "I think children need challenges, don't you?"

c. "My husband and I both grew up in very restrictive families. We want our children to be free to do whatever they want."

d. "My husband and I have different ideas about discipline, but we're talking this out because we know it's important for Johnny that we be consistent."

6. Which intervention would you take first to assist a woman who states that she feels incompetent as the mother of a teenage daughter?

a. Recommend that she discipline her daughter more strictly and consistently

b. Make a list of things her husband can do to help her improve

c. Assist the mother to identify both what she believes is preventing her success and what she can do to improve

d. Explore with the mother what the daughter can do to improve her behavior

7. Which of the following patients is least likely to develop problems related to self-concept?

a. 55-year-old woman television news reporter undergoing a hysterectomy (removal of uterus)

b. Young clergyperson whose vocal cords are paralyzed after a motorbike accident

c. 32-year-old accountant who survives a massive heart attack

d. 23-year-old model who just learned that she has breast cancer

For questions 8 to 11, read the patient data below and use the following letters to indicate the diagnosis that data suggest (each response may be used only once):

a. Personal Identity Disturbance

b. Body Image Disturbance

c. Self-Esteem Disturbance

d. Altered Role Performance

8. Juanita Sanchez has only been in the United States 3 months and has recently suffered the loss of her husband and job. She states that nothing feels familiar . . . "I don't know who I am supposed to be here" and she misses home (Nicaragua) terribly.

9. Jim Boa, a sophomore in high school, has missed a lot of school this year because of leukemia. He said he feels like he is falling behind in everything and misses "hanging out at the mall" with his friends most of all.

10. "Why did I have to be born into a family of big bottoms and short fat legs! No one will ever ask me out for a date. Oh why can't I have long thin legs like everyone else in my class? What a frump I am."

11. Marissa Yule, a 33-year-old businessperson, is now in counseling attempting to deal with a long-repressed history of sexual abuse by her father. "I guess I should feel satisfied with what I've achieved in life, but I'm never content, and nothing I achieve makes me feel good about myself . . . I hate my father for making me feel like I'm no good. This is an awful way to live."

12. Nancy, 36 years old, who was divorced 5 years earlier, entered the emergency department with severe burns and cuts on her face after an auto accident in a car driven by her fiancé of 3 months. Three weeks later, her fiancé has not yet contacted her. Nancy states that he is so busy and she is too tired to have visitors anyway. Nancy frequently lies with her eyes closed and head turned away. These data suggest that

a. There is no disturbance in self-concept.

b. This patient has ego strength and high self-esteem but may have a disturbance of body image.

c. The area of self-esteem has very low priority at this time and should be ignored until much later.

d. It is probable that there are disturbances in self-esteem and body image.

13. Which of the nursing interventions below is least likely to assist a severely ill patient with cancer to maintain a positive sense of self?
    a. Making it a point to address the patient by name each time you enter the room
    b. Fatiguing the patient as little as possible by performing all procedures in silence
    c. Continuing to respect the patient's privacy and sensibilities
    d. Offering the patient a simple explanation before moving her in any way

14. Doris, 16 years old, has a nursing diagnosis of Body Image Disturbance related to severe acne. In planning nursing care, an appropriate goal for this nursing diagnosis is "The patient will
    a. Make above-B grades in all tests at school."
    b. Demonstrate by diet control and skin care increased interest in control of acne."
    c. Report that she feels more self-confidence in her music and art, which she enjoys."
    d. Express that she is very smart in school."

15. A 4½-year-old boy required stitches for a laceration on the eyebrow. After the doctor held him, visited with him, and explained what was going to be done and that his eye would get better and look just like it did before, the boy placed his hands under his hips as instructed and quietly permitted the procedure. He then expressed pride in himself. Evaluation of the effect of this healthcare experience is best expressed in which of the following?
    a. The doctor did an excellent job.
    b. The child's self-esteem was enhanced and fear of bodily mutilation decreased, and the parents were given an excellent role model.
    c. The child was made the center of attention and the situation exaggerated, thus encouraging the child to become self-centered.
    d. These interventions consumed too much physician time to be evaluated positively.

■ Answers With Rationale

1. The correct response is c. The data point to Robert's having a positive self-concept ("I'm a good helper") and fairly high self-esteem (realizes his strengths and limitations). The statement "But I'm not very smart" is accurate and is not an indication of a negative self-concept (a and b).

2. The correct response is b. Jerry's inability to list more than three items about himself indicates deficient self-knowledge. There are not enough data provided to determine whether he lacks self-esteem (a), has unrealistic self-expectations (c), or is unable to evaluate himself (d).

3. The correct response is d. Low self-esteem is characterized by great discrepancy between the ideal and real selves. There are no data in this item to suggest that Jerry has either a negative self-concept (a) or a body image disturbance (c). The data do indicate something more serious than modesty (b).

4. The correct response is a. David's self-expectations are realistic, given his multiple commitments, and seem to be positively motivating his development.

5. The correct response is c. Each option with the exception of c correctly addresses some aspect of fostering healthy development in children. Because children need effective structure and development, giving them total freedom to do as they please may actually hinder their development.

6. The correct response is c. The first intervention priority with a mother who feels incompetent to parent a teenage daughter is to assist the mother to identify what is preventing her from being an effective parent and then to explore solutions aimed at improving her parenting skills. The other interventions may prove helpful, but they do not directly address the mother's problem with her feelings of incompetence.

7. The correct response is a. Based simply on the facts given, the 55-year-old news reporter would be least likely to experience body image or role performance disturbance because she is beyond her childbearing years, and the hysterectomy should not impair her ability to report the news. The young clergyperson's inability to preach (b), the 32-year-old's massive myocardial infarction (c), and the model's breast resection (d) have much greater potential to result in self-concept problems.

8. The correct response is a. An unfamiliar culture, coupled with traumatic life events and loss of husband and job, had resulted in this patient's total loss of her sense of self: "I don't know who I am supposed to be here." Her very sense of identity is at stake, not merely her body image, self-esteem, or role performance.

9. The correct response is d. Important roles for Jim are being a student and a friend. His illness is preventing him from doing either of these well. This self-concept disturbance is basically one that concerns role performance.

10. The correct response is b. Clearly, this patient's concern is with his or her body image.

11. The correct response is c. Marissa's self-concept disturbance is mainly one of devaluing herself and thinking that she is no good. This is a self-esteem disturbance.

12. The correct response is d. The traumatic nature of Nancy's injuries, her fiancé's failure to contact her, and Nancy's response, that is, her withdrawal, all point to potential problems with both body image and self-esteem. It is not true that self-esteem needs are of low priority.

13. The correct response is b. Each option with the exception of b should assist the patient to maintain a

positive sense of self. Working in silence with the patient may be preferable to idle chatter, but the ideal is to address the patient by name, give simple explanations of procedures, and communicate by simple words of caring that he or she is a person of worth.

14. The correct response is *b*. All of these patient goals may be appropriate for Doris, but the only goal that directly addressed her body image disturbance is *b*.

15. The correct response is *b*. The physician enhanced the child's self-esteem by teaching him how to participate effectively, decreased his fear of bodily mutilation by telling him that his eyebrow would heal and look normal, and gave the parents an excellent role model.

Bibliography

Aguilera, D. C. (1994). *Crisis intervention: Theory and methodology* (7th ed.). St. Louis: Mosby.

Atwater, W. E. (1996). *Adolescence* (4th ed.). Upper Saddle River, NJ: Prentice-Hall.

Bello, L. K., & McIntire, S. N. (1995). Body image disturbances in young adults with cancer. *Cancer Nursing, 18*(2), 138–143.

Bensink, G. W., Godbey, K. L., Marshall, M. J., & Yarandi, H. N. (1992). Institutionalized elderly: Relaxation, locus of control, self-esteem. *Journal of Gerontological Nursing, 18*(4), 30–36.

Bowlby, J. (1969). *Attachment and loss: Vol I: Attachment.* NY: Basic Books.

Carpenito, L. J. (2004). *Nursing diagnosis: Application to clinical practice* (10th ed.). Philadelphia: Lippincott Williams & Wilkins.

Coleman, J. C., Morris, C. G., & Glaros, A. G. (1990). *Contemporary psychology and effective behavior* (7th ed.). Glenview, IL: Scott, Foresman.

Coopersmith, S. (1967). *The antecedents of self-esteem.* San Francisco: Freeman.

Freud, S. (1927). The ego and the id. In J. Strachey (Ed.) (1961), *The standard edition of the complete psychological works of Sigmund Freud* (Vol. XIX, 3–63.). London: The Hogarth Press.

Harter, S. (1986). Processes underlying the construction, maintenance and enhancement of the self-concept in children. In J. Suls & A. G. Greenwald (Eds.), *Psychological perspectives on the self* (Vol. 3, 137–181). Hillsdale, NJ: Erlbaum.

Harter, S. (1999). *The construction of the self.* New York: Guilford.

Hoskins, C. N. (2001). Promoting adjustment among women with breast cancer and their partners: A program of research. *Journal of the New York State Nurses Association, 32*(2), 19–23.

LeMone, P. (1991). Analysis of a human phenomenon: Self concept. *Nursing Diagnosis, 2*(3), 126–130.

Maslow, A. (1954.) *Motivation and personality.* New York: Harper and Row.

McCloskey, J., & Bulechek, G. (2000). *Nursing interventions classification (NIC)* (3rd ed.). St. Louis: C. V. Mosby.

McClowry, S. G. (2003). *Your child's unique temperament: Insights and strategies for responsive parenting.* Champaign, Il: Research Press.

McKay, M., & Fanning, P. (1992). *Self-esteem* (2nd ed.). Oakland, CA: New Harbinger Publications.

Peplau, H. E. (1952). *Interpersonal relations in nursing.* New York: G.P. Putnam & Sons.

Peplau, H. E. (1997). Peplau's theory of interpersonal relations. *Nursing Science Quarterly, 10*(4), 162–167.

Stein, K. F. (1995). Schema model of the self-concept. *Image— The Journal of Nursing Scholarship, 27*(3), 187–193.

Sullivan, H. S. (1953). *The interpersonal theory of psychiatry.* New York: W. W. Norton & Co.

Taylor, C. (1982). The need for self esteem. In H. Yura & M. B. Walsh (Eds.), *Human needs and the nursing process.* Norwalk, CT: Appleton-Century-Crofts.

Stress and Adaptation

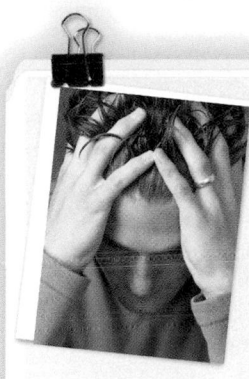

Peter Bainbridge is the husband of a pregnant woman who is brought into the emergency department with multiple injuries after a motor vehicle crash. He is screaming, "Save my wife! Save my baby!"

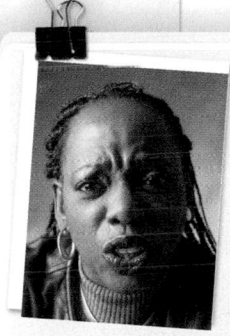

Joan Rogerrio, a middle-aged woman with a history of inflammatory bowel disease, comes to the outpatient clinic with complaints of increasing episodes of diarrhea. She says, "I think my bowel disease is flaring up again." Further assessment reveals she started a new job a month ago after being out of the workforce for the past 15 years. "Since the children are in school most of the day, my husband and I decided it was time for me to go back to work to help out financially," she says.

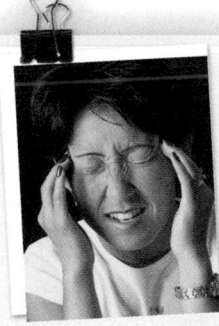

Sarah Keller, a nursing student, comes to the student health center complaining that she feels sick. She says, "I'm supposed to start my critical care rotation tomorrow and I'm terrified not only of the tubes and machines, but of my instructor. I had her for my health assessment rotation and it was really a disaster. I feel a migraine coming on."

Focusing on Blended Skills

The types of blended skills you'll need to respond to the case scenarios include:

Cognitive Skills

- Knowledge about the relationship between stressors, stress, and adaptation
- Knowledge about the physiologic and psychological responses to stress
- Ability to integrate knowledge about healthy lifestyles, support systems, stress management techniques, and crisis intervention into nursing care
- Ability to recognize the warning signs when stressors are exceeding coping mechanisms—in yourself and others
- Knowledge of stress management resources available for the individual and in the community

Technical Skills

- Strong assessment skills to identify physiologic and psychological responses to stress and use of defense mechanisms
- Ability to use correctly the equipment necessary to provide care to patients experiencing different stressors and responses and to diagnose and treat problems related to inadequate coping
- Ability to provide technical nursing interventions necessary to assess and meet the needs of the husband of a injured pregnant woman, a middle-aged woman experiencing an exacerbation of her bowel disease since returning to work, and a nursing student complaining of feeling ill secondary to stress
- Ability to adapt techniques to address patients at different developmental stages experiencing various degrees of stress

Interpersonal Skills

- Demonstration of self-reflection to identify your own responses to stress
- Strong interpersonal skills to establish trusting relationships with the husband of an injured pregnant patient, a woman returning to the workforce, and a nursing student complaining of feeling ill due to the stress of school
- Ability to assist patients to develop positive coping mechanisms to deal with stress
- Ability to communicate and interact effectively with patients and their caregivers even in times of extreme stress or crisis
- Demonstration of respect for the patient's human dignity and autonomy

Ethical and Legal Skills

- Demonstration of a strong sense of accountability for the health and well-being of patients experiencing various degrees of stress
- A commitment to patient advocacy, including getting patients the help they need to cope with stress
- Familiarity with agency policy and role responsibilities related to stress management
- Ability to integrate knowledge of ethical and legal principles concerning issues of crisis, coping, and stress management in the plan of care for the husband of an injured pregnant woman, a middle-aged woman with an exacerbation of her bowel disease, and a nursing student complaining of being ill when faced with the stress of a new clinical rotation
- Ability to practice in an ethically and legally defensible manner when providing care to patients experiencing various degrees of stress and crisis

Learning Outcomes

After completing the chapter, the learner should be able to accomplish the following:

1. Describe the mechanisms involved in maintaining physiologic and psychological homeostasis.
2. Explain the interdependent nature of stressors, stress, and adaptation.
3. Describe the physical and emotional responses to stress, including local adaptation syndrome, general adaptation syndrome, mind–body interaction, anxiety, and coping and defense mechanisms.
4. Discuss the effects of short-term and long-term stress on basic human needs, health and illness, and the family.
5. Compare and contrast developmental and situational stress, incorporating the concepts of physiologic and psychosocial stressors.
6. Recognize and cope effectively with stress unique to the nursing profession.
7. Integrate knowledge of healthy lifestyle, support systems, stress management techniques, and crisis intervention into hospital-based and community-based care.

Key Terms

adaptation
anxiety
burnout
caregiver burden
coping mechanisms
crisis
crisis intervention
defense mechanisms
fear
fight-or-flight response
general adaptation syndrome (GAS)
homeostasis
inflammatory response
local adaptation syndrome (LAS)
psychosomatic disorder
reflex pain response
stress
stressor

Stress is a part of life: everyone feels stress at one time or another. Books and magazines are full of articles about stress, discussing everything from the negative stressful effects of performing one's job to the positive stress of holidays. Television advertisements for over-the-counter remedies promise fast relief from stress headaches and upset stomachs. Stress is blamed for excessive weight gain, drinking, and smoking as well as for divorce and child abuse. Feeling "stressed out" is common, and taking "stress breaks" to do physical exercise is recommended in many work settings. With stress such a part of everyday life, it is easy to see that any additional problem, such as an illness or injury, can increase the effects of stress on the person experiencing the problem.

The experience of stress and the ways one responds to it are unique to each individual. The process of responding to stress is constant and dynamic and is essential to the person's physical, emotional, and social well-being. Stress and adaptation are major components in health and illness. Nurses need to understand the concepts and levels of stress when providing nursing care to patients in all settings. Nurses themselves are subject to stress from the demands of their career, and they need to know healthy ways of responding (see the accompanying Reflective Practice display for an example).

This chapter discusses stress from a holistic perspective, including both physical and psychological stress. Elements discussed include homeostasis, stress and adaptation, and nursing actions to promote stress reduction. The concluding nursing plan of care illustrates how the nurse promotes coping and adaptation by providing interventions specific to individualized stress and coping.

BASIC CONCEPTS OF STRESS AND ADAPTATION

The basic concepts of stress and adaptation are stress, stressors, adaptation, and homeostasis.

Reflective Practice
Challenge to Technical Competency

I went to the student health center this afternoon because I was feeling sick. Tomorrow I am supposed to begin my critical care rotation. My instructor is the same one that I had for health assessment and that rotation was really a disaster. She has the reputation for the being the hardest instructor in the school. She terrifies me. But I'm just as terrified of the tubes and machines that I'm going to be faced with in the critical care unit. Skilled with my hands I am definitely not! I'm not even in the unit and already I am quaking. I tried to switch rotations but no luck. Now I have to decide what to do tomorrow. I already feel a migraine coming on!

Thinking Outside the Box: Possible Courses of Action

- Call in sick! Obviously this can't be a long-term strategy.
- Grin and bear it! Just try to do my job and for the most part fade into the woodwork.

- Try to find a preceptor in critical care to whom I can explain my fears and have her/him help me develop the skills (and comfort!) I definitely need.
- Be honest with my instructor about my fears and the stress I am experiencing and ask for HELP!

Evaluating a Good Outcome: How Do I Define Success?

- I develop the skills (and comfort) I need to effectively provide care in a high-tech environment.
- No patient is harmed because of my lack of skill.

- I learn to manage my stress and use it to my advantage.
- I pass this rotation with flying colors!

Personal Learning: Here's to the Future!

After some hard reflection (and the wise counsel of my mother), I decided I was giving my fear of this rotation (and instructor!) way too much power over me! I realized that nursing would continue to put me in new and frightening situations. But escape just couldn't be my "modus operandi." So urging myself to "bite the bullet," I got to the clinical area. Immediately after pre-conference, I literally grabbed my instructor and told her I had to talk

to her before I began giving care. While she'll never be called "warm and fuzzy," she surprised me by being understanding. Then she spent some extra time orienting me to the unit and helping me develop comfort with a lot of equipment I'd be using that day. I learned an important lesson in confronting fear and not letting it get the best of me. Hopefully I can remember this the next time "flight" seems more attractive than "fight!"

Reflection

How do you think you would respond in a similar situation? Why? What does this tell you about yourself and about the adequacy of your skills for professional practice? Can you think of other ways to respond? Explain the autonomic nervous system responses the nursing student was experiencing. Describe the defense mechanisms the nursing student was used. What other skills (cognitive, interpersonal, technical, ethical/legal) would you need to respond well in this situation? How did the nursing student use task-oriented reactions and attack behavior? What personal factors may have influenced the nursing student's reaction. Propose some strategies that would be appropriate for the nursing student to use to cope with stress. Do you agree with the criteria to evaluate a successful outcome? Did the nursing student meet the criteria. Please explain your response.

Sarah Keller, Georgetown University

Stress

Stress is a condition in which the human system responds to changes in its normal balanced state. Stress results from a change in the environment that is perceived as a challenge, a threat, or a danger, and can have both positive and negative effects. The major sources of stress in our society arise from interpersonal relationships and performance demands rather than from actual physical threat (Pender, 2002). Not only is stress a part of everyday experience, but a person's responses to stress are also necessary to life. Stress affects the whole person in all the human dimensions (physical, emotional, intellectual, social, and spiritual).

> *Think back to Sarah Keller, the nursing student complaining of feeling ill. By her own reports, she was feeling overwhelmed and extremely anxious about her upcoming critical care clinical rotation. The stresses included lack of confidence with the equipment and machines of the unit and the demands that might be placed on her by the instructor. As a result, she exhibited physiologic responses to these stresses. These stresses could also affect her ability to function intellectually and socially.*

The perception of stress and the responses to it are highly individualized, not only from person to person but also from one time to another in the same person. Because stress is individual and holistic, there is no commonly accepted definition or measurement.

Stressors

A **stressor** is anything that is perceived as challenging, threatening, or demanding. Stressors may be either internal (eg, an illness, a hormonal change, or fear) or external (eg, loud noise or cold temperature). As with stress, the perception and effects of the stressor are highly individual. Stressors themselves are neither positive nor negative, but they can have positive or negative effects as the person responds to change.

> *Consider Joan Rogerrio, the middle-aged woman who was returning to the workforce and experiencing an exacerbation of her inflammatory bowel disease. The decision to return to work was fostered by the family's financial need, which could be considered a stressor. This stressor had a positive effect in that it prompted Joan to return to work. However, the stressor of returning to work after a 15-year absence exerted a negative effect, resulting in frequent episodes of diarrhea.*

Adaptation

When a person is in a threatening situation, immediate responses occur. Those responses, which are often involuntary, are called coping responses. The change that takes place as a result of the response to a stressor is **adaptation.** Adaptation is, to some degree, an ongoing process as a person strives to maintain balance in his or her internal and external environments (Fig. 32-1). Adaptation also occurs in families and groups. Adaptation is necessary for normal growth and development, the ability to tolerate changing situations, and the ability to respond to physical and emotional stressors.

Homeostasis

Our bodies are always interacting with a constantly changing environment. The environment includes the external environment, which surrounds our bodies, and the internal environment, which includes the mechanisms that regulate body functions and the fluids that surround body cells. To maintain health, the body's internal environment must remain in a balanced state. Various physiologic mechanisms within the body respond to internal changes to maintain relative constancy in the internal environment, which is called **homeostasis.**

W. B. Cannon introduced the concept of homeostasis in 1939, although throughout history people have believed that health is the result of a balanced state. Some of the most important people in medical history, including Hippocrates (the father of medicine) and Claude Bernard (the father of physiol-

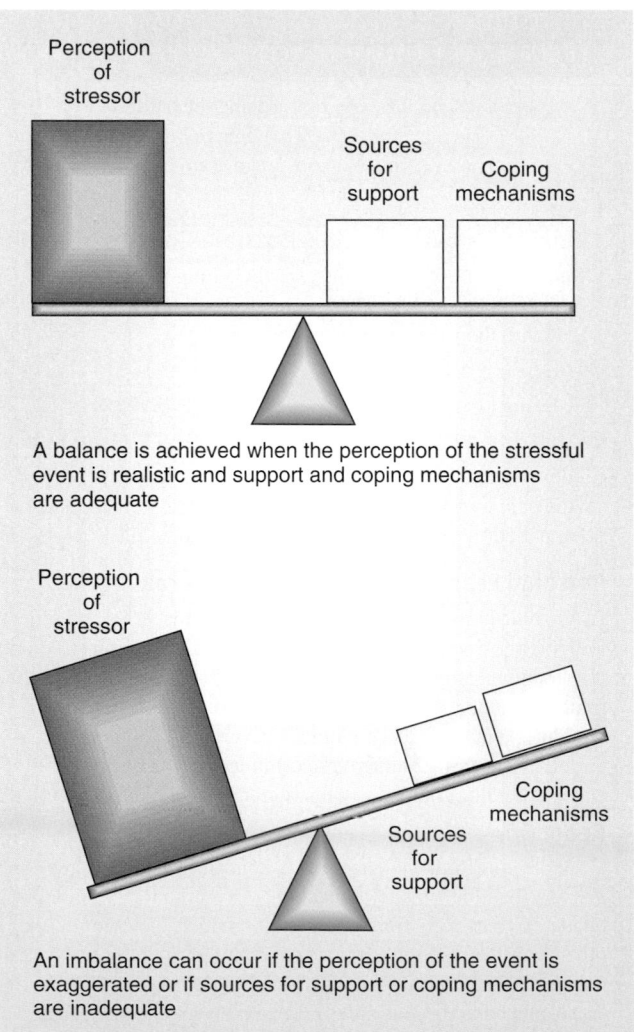

A balance is achieved when the perception of the stressful event is realistic and support and coping mechanisms are adequate

An imbalance can occur if the perception of the event is exaggerated or if sources for support or coping mechanisms are inadequate

FIGURE 32-1 A realistic perception of a stressful event, sources for emotional support, and appropriate coping mechanisms are components of a system of balances during stress.

ogy), believed in and wrote about this balanced state. Originally the focus was on life processes that occur within the body, such as heart rate, blood pressure, and water balance. The concept of homeostasis has been expanded, however, to include both physiologic and psychological balance.

MAINTAINING PHYSIOLOGIC AND PSYCHOLOGICAL HOMEOSTASIS

The effects of physiologic and psychological stress are interrelated, as are the mechanisms that are consciously or unconsciously used to maintain homeostasis in response to stress. For example, the mechanisms described below, including the general adaptation syndrome (GAS) and mind–body interaction, are physiologic responses to either physical or emotional stressors.

Physiologic Homeostasis

Long before you entered nursing, you knew that sweating when you were hot and shivering when you were cold occur to help maintain a stable body temperature. These are examples of homeostatic mechanisms that regulate the body's internal environment.

The autonomic nervous system and the endocrine system primarily control homeostatic mechanisms. Involved to a lesser degree are the respiratory, cardiovascular, gastrointestinal, and renal systems. These mechanisms are self-regulating, occur without conscious thought, and usually function to correct abnormal conditions. On a simple level, they are like a thermostat regulating a furnace. When the temperature in a house falls below the preset temperature on the thermostat, the thermostat turns on the furnace, which heats the house to the desired temperature and then shuts off.

The regulatory mechanisms of the body are reacting constantly to changes to maintain homeostasis and health. The homeostatic mechanisms of the body systems are summarized in Table 32-1. They are important in understanding the consequences of both short-term and long-term stress, which can threaten physiologic homeostasis and result in illness. Box 32-1 provides examples of illnesses known to be associated with stress.

Local Adaptation Syndrome

The **local adaptation syndrome (LAS)** is a localized response of the body to stress. It involves only a specific body part (tissue, organ) instead of the whole body. The stress precipitating the LAS may be traumatic or pathologic. LAS is a primarily homeostatic short-term adaptive response. Although the body has many localized stress responses, the two most common responses that influence nursing care are the reflex pain response and the inflammatory response.

Reflex Pain Response

The **reflex pain response** is a response of the central nervous system to pain. It is rapid and automatic, serving as a protective mechanism to prevent injury. The reflex depends on an intact, functioning neurologic reflex arc and involves both sensory and motor neurons. For example, if you step into a bathtub of dangerously hot water, your skin senses the heat and immediately sends a message to the spinal cord. A message is then sent to a motor nerve, which activates the muscles in your leg to pull back your foot. All of this happens before you consciously realize that the water is too hot to be safe.

Inflammatory Response

The **inflammatory response** is a local response to injury or infection. It serves to localize and prevent the spread of infection and promote wound healing. When you cut your finger, for example, you often develop the symptoms of the inflammatory response—pain, swelling, heat, redness, and changes in function. The three phases in the inflammatory response are outlined here and discussed more fully in Chapter 38, Skin Integrity.

In the first phase, bleeding is controlled initially by vasoconstriction (narrowing) of the blood vessels at the injury site. After the bleeding has been controlled, histamines are released and capillary permeability increases, allowing increased flow of blood and white blood cells to the area. The blood flow then returns to normal, but the white blood cells remain to help resist infection.

During the second phase, exudate (made up of fluid, cells, and inflammatory byproducts) is released from the wound. The amount of exudate depends on the size, location, and severity of the wound. During the third and final phase, damaged cells are repaired by either regeneration (replacement with identical cells) or formation of scar tissue. Some body tissues (skin, bone) are easily reproduced and regain their former function; others (nervous system, intestines) do not regenerate but form nonfunctional scar tissue.

General Adaptation Syndrome (GAS)

The **general adaptation syndrome (GAS)** is a biochemical model of stress developed by Hans Selye (1976). The GAS describes the body's general response to stress, a concept essential in all areas of nursing care. The three stages in the GAS (Fig. 32-2) are the alarm reaction, resistance, and exhaustion. Although the alarm stage is short term (minutes to hours), the length of the resistance and exhaustion stages varies greatly, depending on such variables as the severity and duration of the stressor, the previous health of the person, and the immediacy and effectiveness of healthcare interventions.

> Recall Peter Bainbridge, the husband whose wife was injured in a motor vehicle crash. His initial statements about saving his wife and his baby indicate that he is in the alarm reaction stage identified by the GAS.

The Alarm Reaction

The alarm reaction is initiated when a person perceives a specific stressor, and various defense mechanisms are activated. The perception of threat may be conscious or unconscious. The autonomic nervous system initiates the **fight-or-flight response,** preparing the body to either fight off the stressor or to run away from it; however, this is most often not in a literal sense. Hormone levels rise to prepare the body to react. This phase of the alarm reaction, called the shock phase, is charac-

TABLE 32-1 **Homeostatic Regulators of the Body**

System	Action	Effect
Autonomic Nervous		
Parasympathetic—Functions under normal conditions and at rest (Cranial and sacral nerves)		
	· Regulates heart rate	· Slows rate
	· Stimulates secretion of digestive juices and digestive tract smooth muscle	· Improves digestion, increases peristalsis
	· Stimulates insulin secretion	· Increases uptake of glucose by cells
Sympathetic—Functions under stress conditions to bring about the fight-or-flight response		
	· Stimulates heart rate and force	· Increases rate, strengthens contractions, increases cardiac output
	· Dilates skeletal muscle blood vessels	· Increases muscle strength
	· Dilates blood vessels to the brain	· Increases mental alertness
	· Stimulates release of glycogen stores	· Increases blood glucose levels
Endocrine		

Pituitary	· Secretes hormones:
	    Adrenocorticotropic hormone (ACTH)
	    Thyroid-stimulating hormone (TSH)
		· Stimulates the adrenal cortex
		· Stimulates the thyroid

Adrenals	· Medulla produces epinephrine and norepinephrine	· Prepares the person for emergencies; supports the sympathetic system
	· Cortex secretes mineralocorticoids, glucocorticoids, and androgens	· Mineralocorticoid aldosterone regulates fluid and electrolytes · Glucocorticoids raise glucose levels (for energy) and increase resistance to physical stress
Thyroid	· Secretes thyroid hormone and calcitonin	· Regulates metabolic rate and growth
Other		
Cardiovascular	· Serves as transport system and pump	· Provides oxygen and nutrients and removes carbon dioxide and wastes from cells
Renal	· Filters, excretes, and reabsorbs metabolic products and water	· Maintains fluid, electrolyte, and acid–base balance
Respiratory	· Intake and output of oxygen and carbon dioxide	· Necessary for metabolism; helps maintain acid–base balance
Gastrointestinal	· Takes in food and fluids · Eliminates waste products	· Energy sources; maintains fluids and electrolytes

---

BOX 32-1 **Examples of Physical Illnesses Associated With Stress**

Autoimmune disorders
  Graves' disease (hyperthyroidism)
  Rheumatoid arthritis
  Ulcerative colitis
  Psoriasis
  Myasthenia gravis
Cardiovascular disorders
  Hypertension
  Coronary artery disease
Respiratory disorders
  Asthma
Gastrointestinal disorders
  Esophageal reflux
  Constipation
  Diarrhea
  Ulcerative colitis

---

terized by an increase in energy levels, oxygen intake, cardiac output, blood pressure, and mental alertness. (If you recall the last time you almost had a car accident, you can easily identify these body reactions!) During the second phase of the alarm reaction, countershock, there is a reversal of body changes.

Resistance

Having perceived the threat and mobilized its resources, the body now attempts to adapt to the stressor. Vital signs, hormone levels, and energy production return to normal. If the stress can be managed or confined to a small area (LAS), the body regains homeostasis. If the damage to the body is too great (eg, with severe injury and bleeding or a major illness such as cancer or a heart attack), the adaptive mechanisms fail.

Exhaustion

Exhaustion results when the adaptive mechanisms are exhausted. Without defense against the stressor, the body may either rest and mobilize its defenses to return to normal or reach total exhaustion and die.

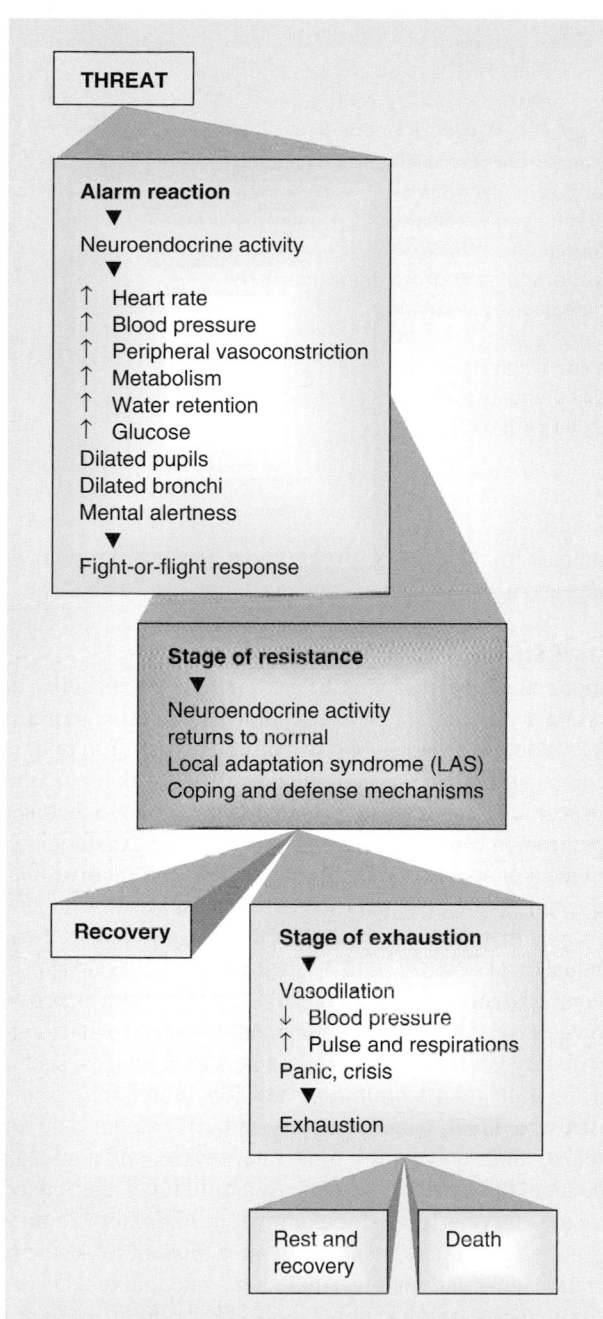

FIGURE 32-2 The general adaptation syndrome (general response to stress).

The GAS is a physiologic response to stress, but it is important to remember that the response results from either physical or emotional stressors. The stages occur with either physical or psychological damage to the person. Obvious examples are seen in patients with severe injury or an illness, but GAS is also a factor in mental illness, social isolation, and loss (or lack) of human relations.

Psychological Homeostasis

To maintain mental well-being, humans also must maintain psychological homeostasis. As discussed in Chapter 2, Health

of the Individual, Family, and Community, each person needs to feel loved and a sense of belonging, to feel safe and secure, and to have self-esteem. When these needs are not met or a threat to need fulfillment occurs, homeostatic measures in the form of coping or defense mechanisms help return the person to emotional balance.

Everyone frequently encounters physical, psychological, and social changes in their internal and external environments. A person's perception of these changes may be conscious or unconscious. If the person has the necessary resources, adaptation takes place and balance is maintained. If the resources cannot reestablish balance, a state of stress results. The person's responses and the degree of stress depend in part on the nature, intensity, timing, number, and duration of stressors. Adaptation to stress also depends on a person's age, developmental level, past experiences, support systems, and coping mechanisms (see the display Focus on the Older Adult). Adaptive responses include the mind–body interaction, anxiety, and coping/defense mechanisms.

Mind–Body Interaction

Consider the following examples of mind–body interaction:
- Tomorrow you are scheduled to take a final examination, and you must make a passing score to pass the course and remain in the nursing program. After being awake most of the night, you cannot swallow any food at breakfast, you have a rapid heartbeat, you are filled with feelings of apprehension, and you have diarrhea.
- Since his wife was killed in a car crash, Tom Green has been the sole support of his 4-year-old son, who is developmentally delayed and hyperactive. Tom has been coming to the neighborhood health clinic with increasing frequency over the past 5 months, complaining of weight loss, headaches, and stomach pain.

Remember Sarah Keller, the nursing student who said she felt a migraine coming on due to her upcoming clinical rotation in the critical care unit and anticipation of having a strict instructor. As a result of her anticipated fears and lack of confidence, she physiologically responded to the stressors by feeling that she was developing a migraine. However, by communicating her concerns to the instructor and receiving additional guidance, her ability to cope with the situation improved, and no migraine developed.

These examples illustrate the relationship between psychological stressors and the physiologic stress response. In the first example, as you begin the test and discover that you know most of the answers, your symptoms disappear rapidly. Tom's stress, however, is always present and is long term, increasing his risk for developing an illness.

What causes this link between psychological stressors and the physiologic stress response? Although the exact cause is not well understood, it is thought that humans react to threats of danger as if they were physiologic threats. A person per-

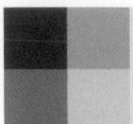

Focus on the Older Adult
Sources of Stress with Aging

Stress, with resultant anxiety, is a risk in the older population. Although the prevalence of anxiety is lower in older adults compared to younger age groups, it tends to be more clinically significant (Moorhead & Brighton, 2001). As the number of older adults increases in the population, anxiety is now, and increasingly will be, a significant problem. Not all older patients will experience stress to the point of anxiety, but the following possible causes should always be considered when providing nursing care:

- Invasive or health-related tests or examinations
- Surgical procedures

- Diagnosis of chronic illnesses, including diabetes, cancer, and cardiovascular diseases
- Declining physical and/or mental capabilities
- Retirement
- Loss of spouse and/or significant others
- Increased social isolation
- Chronic pain
- Alcohol abuse
- Loss of independence in living arrangements, driving, and activities of daily living

---

ceives the threat on an emotional level, and the body prepares itself either to resist the danger or to run away from it (the fight-or-flight response).

> *Recall Sarah Keller, the nursing student described in the Reflective Practice display. Her description of her behavior and subsequent actions demonstrate her ability to "fight" the danger, rather than flee ("flight").*

Each person reacts in her or his own way. With prolonged stress, some may develop chronic diarrhea; others may develop headaches. Such illnesses are real and are called **psychosomatic disorders** because the physiologic alterations are thought to be at least partially caused by psychological influences. Box 32-2 lists physiologic indicators of stress.

Another component of mind–body interaction is the effect of life changes on a person. Researchers have found that the number of changes a person has in his or her life (both positive and negative) is correlated with illness. A life change is defined as an event in a person's life that requires energy for adaptation. When energy is expended to adapt to the event, the person's resistance to illness is lowered. For example, although a holiday celebration with family and friends is considered a positive event in one's life, stressful factors include the time necessary

to prepare for the party, worrying about how everyone will get along, and trying to decide how much money to spend.

Anxiety

Various emotional responses to stress may occur, including depression and anger. The most common human response is **anxiety.** Anxiety is a vague, uneasy feeling of discomfort or dread accompanied by an autonomic response; the source is often nonspecific or unknown to the individual. It is also a feeling of apprehension caused by anticipating a danger. Anxiety is experienced at some time by all people and can involve one's body, self-perceptions, and social relationships. It is an altering signal that warns of impending danger and enables the individual to take measures to deal with threat (NANDA, 2003). In contrast, **fear** (a feeling of dread) is a cognitive response to a known threat. Anxiety is the emotional response to that threat.

Anxiety is often present before new experiences, such as starting college or beginning a new job, which may be perceived as a threat to one's identity and self-esteem. The four levels of anxiety are mild, moderate, severe, and panic, and each level has different effects. At a mild level, anxiety can have a positive effect—for example, mild anxiety about an upcoming examination can motivate a student to do the required reading and review. Anxiety beyond that level is generally negative and has unpleasant effects. In an attempt to neutralize, deny, or counteract the anxiety, the person develops individual patterns of coping.

Mild Anxiety

Mild anxiety is present in day-to-day living. It increases alertness and perceptual fields (eg, vision and hearing) and motivates learning and growth. Although mild anxiety may interfere with sleep, it also facilitates problem solving. Mild anxiety is often manifested by restlessness and increased questioning.

Moderate Anxiety

Moderate anxiety narrows a person's perceptual fields so that the focus is on immediate concerns, with inattention to other communications and details. Moderate anxiety is manifested by a quavering voice, tremors, increased muscle tension, a complaint of "butterflies in the stomach," and slight increases in respirations and pulse.

BOX 32-2 Physiologic Indicators of Stress

Backache
Constipation or diarrhea
Dilated pupils
Dry mouth
Headache
Increased urination
Increased pulse, blood pressure, and respirations
Loss of appetite
Nausea
Sleep disturbances
Stiff neck
Sweaty palms

Severe Anxiety

Severe anxiety creates a very narrow focus on specific detail, causing all behavior to be geared toward getting relief. The person has impaired learning ability and is easily distracted. Severe anxiety is manifested by difficulty verbally communicating, increased motor activity, a fearful facial expression, headache, nausea, dizziness, tachycardia, and hyperventilation.

Panic

Panic causes the person to lose control and experience dread and terror. The resulting disorganized state is characterized by increased physical activity, distorted perception of events, and loss of rational thought. The person is unable to learn, concentrates only on the present situation, and often experiences feelings of impending doom. This level of anxiety can lead to exhaustion and death. Panic is manifested by difficulty communicating verbally, agitation, trembling, poor motor control, sensory changes, sweating, tachycardia, hyperventilation, dyspnea, palpitations, a choking sensation, and sensations of chest pain or pressure.

Consider Peter Bainbridge, the man whose wife was admitted to the emergency department. Although he did not experience some of the manifestations listed previously, such as choking sensations or chest pain or pressure, his level of anxiety was most likely quite high, possibly even to the panic stage, as evidenced by his screaming to save his wife and baby. One could assume that he was probably hyperventilating, trembling, and possibly shaking.

Coping Mechanisms

Anxiety often is managed without conscious thought by **coping mechanisms,** which are behaviors used to decrease stress and anxiety. Many coping behaviors are learned, based on one's family, past experiences, and sociocultural influences and expectations. Typical behaviors include the following:
- Crying, laughing, sleeping, cursing
- Physical activity, exercise
- Smoking, drinking
- Lack of eye contact, withdrawal
- Limiting relationships to those with similar values and interests

Moderate, severe, and panic levels of anxiety are greater threats and involve more complex coping mechanisms as the person strives to reduce the stress and anxiety. Coping mechanisms often used at higher levels of anxiety are categorized as task-oriented reactions. Task-oriented reactions involve consciously thinking about the stress situation and then acting to solve problems, resolve conflicts, or satisfy needs. These reactions include attack behavior, withdrawal behavior, and compromise behavior.

Attack behavior occurs when a person attempts to overcome obstacles to satisfy a need; it may be constructive, with assertive problem solving, or destructive, with feelings and actions of aggressive anger and hostility. Withdrawal behavior involves physical withdrawal from the threat, or emo-

tional reactions such as admitting defeat, becoming apathetic, or feeling guilty and isolated. Compromise behavior is usually constructive, often involving the substitution of goals or negotiation to partially fulfill one's needs.

Defense Mechanisms

Other unconscious reactions to stressors, called **defense mechanisms,** often occur. These mechanisms protect one's self-esteem and are useful in mild to moderate anxiety. When extreme, however, they distort reality and create problems with relationships. At that point, the mechanisms become maladaptive instead of adaptive. Common defense mechanisms are summarized in Table 32-2. You will learn more about them in your study of mental health nursing.

EFFECTS OF STRESS

Physiologic and psychological stress affects all of the human dimensions. It strongly influences how one attains basic human needs; it is a factor in health and illness; and it becomes a component in family reactions to illness. Both long-term stress and crisis situations may seriously affect a person's physical and emotional health.

Stress and Basic Human Needs

Basic human needs, described in Chapter 2, are common to all people. Stress, too, is common to all people. Both the attainment of these needs and the adaptation to stress require energy and motivate behaviors. As a person strives to meet basic human needs at each level, stress can be either a stimulus or a barrier.

How a person meets basic human needs and responds to stress is unique to the individual, depending on his or her sociocultural background, priorities, and past experiences (Box 32-3). In all people, the failure to meet needs results in an imbalance in homeostatic mechanisms and, eventually, illness.

Stress in Health and Illness

The health–illness continuum (described in Chap. 4, Health and Illness) is also affected by stress. Health and homeostatic balance are at one extreme of the continuum; exhaustion and death are at the other extreme.

Stress in a healthy person may promote health and prevent illness. For example, the fear of developing lung cancer may motivate a person to stop smoking, or anxiety about baby care may prompt prospective parents to attend prenatal classes and read childcare books. Stressors in health also facilitate normal growth and development, provide the stimulus for learning constructive adaptive behaviors, stimulate problem-solving abilities, encourage social relationships, and help develop spiritual strength.

The effects of stress on a sick or injured person are, in contrast, usually negative. Stress can cause illness, and illness causes stress; see one example in the Research in Nursing box. The presence of an illness or a disability demands new coping skills at a time when homeostasis is challenged.

TABLE 32-2 Commonly Occurring Defense Mechanisms

Defense Mechanism	Causes	Example
Compensation	A person attempts to overcome a perceived weakness by emphasizing a more desirable trait or overachieving in a more comfortable area.	A student who has difficulty with academics may excel in sports.
Denial	A person refuses to acknowledge the presence of a condition that is disturbing.	Despite finding a lump in her breast, a woman does not seek medical treatment.
Displacement	A person transfers (displaces) an emotional reaction from one object or person to another object or person.	An employee who is angry with a coworker kicks a chair.
Introjection	A person incorporates qualities or values of another person into his or her own ego structure. This mechanism is important in the formation of conscience during childhood.	An older sibling tells his preschool sister not to talk to strangers, expressing his parents' values to his younger sister.
Projection	A person's thoughts or impulses are attributed to someone else.	A person who denies any sexual feelings for a coworker accuses him of sexual harassment.
Rationalization	A person tries to give a logical or socially acceptable explanation for questionable behavior ("behavior justification").	A patient who forgot to keep a healthcare appointment says, "If patients didn't have to wait 3 months to get an appointment, they wouldn't forget them."
Reaction formation	A person develops conscious attitudes and behavior patterns that are opposite to what he or she would really like to do.	A married woman is attracted to her husband's best friend but is constantly rude to him.
Regression	A person returns to an earlier method of behaving.	Children often regress to soiling diapers or demanding a bottle when they are ill.
Repression	A person voluntarily excludes an anxiety-producing event from conscious awareness.	A father may not remember shaking his crying baby.
Sublimation	A person substitutes a socially acceptable goal for one whose normal channel of expression is blocked.	An individual who is aggressive toward others may become a star football player.
Undoing	An act or communication used to negate a previous act or communication	A husband who was physically abusive to his wife may bring her an expensive present the next day.

Remember Joan Rogerrio, the woman experiencing an exacerbation of her bowel disease. The negative effects of stress exacerbated her illness. As a result, Joan needs to develop new coping skills to deal with the demands of working to minimize the effects of this stressor on her illness.

People who enter healthcare settings are also subjected to situational stressors.

Adaptation to acute and chronic illness involves two sets of adaptive tasks:

1. General tasks (as in the case of any situational stress) involve maintaining self-esteem and personal relationships and preparing for an uncertain future.
2. Illness-related tasks include such stressors as losing independence and control, handling pain and disability, and carrying out the prescribed medical regimen.

Every situation is different, and each person perceives and reacts to stressors in an individual manner. There is no one "best" way to cope with a given situation. Nursing considerations include the person's major concern, specific illness, sociocultural background, and available resources. For example, an older woman may be anxious about the cost of treatment for her hip fracture, whereas her roommate, with the same injury, is seriously concerned about the care of her cats while she is in the hospital. As another example, Mary and Jane have both entered the hospital with the medical diagnosis of breast cancer. Mary is worried about possible disfigurement and death, but she believes that with the help of surgery and chemotherapy, she can overcome the cancer. Jane, on the other hand, comes from a community that has strong fundamental religious beliefs. She believes that the cancer is a punishment from God and refuses treatment, even though she fears death.

Prolonged Stress

Prolonged or long-term stress is a serious threat to physical and emotional health. As the duration, intensity, or number of stressors increases, a person's ability to adapt is lessened. The failure of adaptive mechanisms is also influenced by a person's state of health and past experiences with stress.

Long-term stress affects physical status, increasing the risk for disease or injury. Recovery and return to normal function are also compromised by prolonged stress. High levels of stress are associated with cardiovascular disease, gastro-intestinal disorders, and cancer. It is believed that these diseases are the result of various factors, including the effects of the fight-or-flight response, eating patterns, lifestyle, and coping mechanisms. A person who reacts to stress by overeating, smoking, using alcohol or illegal drugs, or becoming hyperactive puts additional strain on the body. Homeostasis cannot be maintained, and illness results.

Family Stress

The stress that affects an ill person also affects the person's family members or significant others. When the family is viewed as a system, the behavior of the individual is influenced by the family, and any alterations in the individual's behavior in turn affect the family. Stressors for the family include changes in family structure and roles, anger and feelings of helplessness and guilt, loss of control over normal routines, and concern for future financial stability. The family thus is an integral part in the assessment, planning, nursing interventions, and evaluation of actions to promote adaptation to stress.

> *Consider Joan Rogerrio, the woman with an exacerbation of her bowel disease. Her family is already experiencing changes related to her return to work. These changes could be possible stressors for the family. These family stressors are increased by Joan's illness, which may ultimately affect her role performance. Thus, the nurse would need to assess the family situation closely for the impact of these stressors on the family.*

The family, both as individuals and as a unit, uses many of the same coping and defense mechanisms described previously. Family members may be overly protective, deny the seriousness of the illness, or blame healthcare providers for the

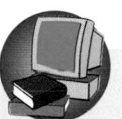

Research in Nursing Making a Difference

Effects of Worry and Stress on Blood Pressure

High blood pressure (hypertension) is a major health problem in the United States and is more prevalent in the African-American population. It has been suggested that stress is a major risk factor in hypertension and in the management of hypertension. Little research has been conducted to explore the concept of "worry" and how that personal experience affects one's response to stress. This is especially true in the African-American population.

Related Research

Boutain, D. (2001). Discourses of worry, stress, and high blood pressure in rural South Louisiana. *Journal of Nursing Scholarship, 33*(3), 225–230.

The purpose of this study was to explore how a sample of African-American residents in rural Louisiana related worry and stress to their high blood pressure. Fifteen men and 15 women with diagnosed hypertension were interviewed twice, and a seven-stage data analysis of all passages containing words related to worry and stress was conducted. The main themes identified were "making a way out of no way," "keep going on: uplift of self and health," and "envisioning a future in the present: uplift of children, kin and community." Findings of stress as a primary factor in hypertension supported the findings of other studies. Racial prejudice was viewed as a stress among participants, related primarily to economic status and gender. Worry about self, children, kin, and community health caused stress, making hypertension more difficult to manage or control.

Relevance to Nursing Practice

Nurses are often the healthcare providers who consistently interact with people with hypertension, and they provide holistic care by assessing and identifying factors in each patient's life that may make medical management more difficult. Patients may be reluctant to discuss environmental and day-to-day living factors affecting their health, so both initial and ongoing assessments should include questions about these factors. It is also important to use culturally competent language when exploring the social processes identified as affecting patients' abilities to manage hypertension. Research supports that a patient- and community-based approach to healthcare enables individuals with hypertension to seek healthcare, to have their blood pressure managed, and to view themselves as partners in hypertension control.

patient's condition or behaviors. On the other hand, the family can provide the social support necessary to help the patient manage and adapt to stress. Emotional support from family members allows open expression of feelings and helps meet love and belonging needs. The inclusion of family members in problem solving, teaching and learning activities, and physical care helps both the patient and the family to maintain their self-esteem and feeling of worth.

Caring for a family member at home for long periods can also cause prolonged stress. Called **caregiver burden,** this stress response includes chronic fatigue, sleep problems, and an increased incidence of stress-related illnesses, such as high blood pressure and heart disease.

Prolonged stress can seriously threaten mental health. As coping or defense mechanisms become ineffective, a person may try less effective coping patterns or maladaptive defense mechanisms. As anxiety increases despite these measures, the person may experience difficulties on the job, with personal relationships, and with self-esteem. These problems in turn act as additional stressors, and mental illness may result.

Crisis

A **crisis** is a disturbance caused by a precipitating event, such as a perceived loss, a threat of loss, or a challenge, that is perceived as a threat to self (Stuart & Laraia, 2001).

Crises may be maturational, situational, or adventitious. Maturational crises occur during developmental events that require role change, such as when a teenager moves into adulthood. Situational crises occur when a life event disrupts a person's psychological equilibrium, such as loss of a job or death of a loved family member. Adventitious crises are accidental and unexpected events, resulting in multiple losses and major environmental changes, such as fires, earthquakes, and floods that involve not only individuals but also entire communities.

In a crisis, the person's usual methods of coping are ineffective, resulting in increasingly greater levels of anxiety. This failure produces high levels of anxiety, disorganized behavior, and an inability to function adequately. After the precipitating event, the person's anxiety increases, and phases of the crisis emerge. First, the anxiety activates the person's usual methods of coping. If these are not effective, the person experiences more anxiety because the coping mechanisms are not working. As the crisis continues, the person tries new methods of coping or redefines the threat. This may lead to resolution of the crisis or, if not effective, may result in severe or panic levels of anxiety. The crisis is more likely to be successfully resolved if the person realistically views the event, if effective coping mechanisms are present, and if situational support systems are available.

> Think back to Peter Bainbridge, the husband who is screaming in the emergency department. Peter is experiencing a crisis due to the injuries to his pregnant wife. When dealing with Peter, the nurse needs to assist him in viewing the situation realistically if possible and enlisting the aid of support persons such as family and friends.

FACTORS AFFECTING STRESS AND ADAPTATION

Stress and adaptation are affected by the sources of stress, the types of stressors experienced, and personal factors.

Sources of Stress

Although there are an almost infinite number of sources of stress, they can be categorized into two broad areas—developmental stress and situational stress. Both create major demands for adaptive responses.

Developmental Stress

Developmental stress, or a developmental crisis, occurs as a person progresses through the normal stages of growth and development from birth to old age (these are described in Chaps. 19, Conception Through Young Adults, and 20, The Aging Adult). Within each stage, certain tasks must be achieved to resolve the crisis and reduce the stress. Examples of developmental stress include the following:

- The infant learning to trust others
- The toddler learning to control elimination
- The school-aged child socializing with peers
- The adolescent striving for independence
- The middle-aged adult accepting physical signs of aging

Situational Stress

Situational stress is different from developmental stress. It does not occur in predictable patterns as one progresses through life. Rather, situational stress can occur at any time, although the person's ability to adapt may be strongly influenced by his or her developmental level. Examples of situational stress, which may be either positive or negative, include the following:

- Illness or accident
- Marriage or divorce
- Loss (belongings, relationships, family member)
- New job
- Role change

> Recall the three individuals described at the beginning of the chapter. All three are experiencing situational stress, but each is responding differently: Peter is screaming, Joan is experiencing an exacerbation of her bowel disease, and Sarah is developing physiologic complaints.

Consider pregnancy as an example. A young married couple may be overjoyed at the prospect of becoming parents, whereas an unmarried adolescent may be panic-stricken when she discovers she is pregnant. The situations and the developmental levels of the young couple and the adolescent will have a major effect on the adaptations they will make. A person's physical and psychosocial capacities to cope with the situation depend not only on his or her stage of maturation but also on the support systems available.

Types of Stressors

Stressors may be physiologic and psychosocial. A physiologic stressor may in turn cause psychosocial stress, and vice versa.

Physiologic Stressors

Physiologic stressors have both a specific effect and a general effect. The specific effect is an alteration of normal body structure and function. The general effect is the stress response. Primary physiologic stressors include chemical agents (drugs, poisons), physical agents (heat, cold, trauma), infectious agents (viruses, bacteria), nutritional imbalances, hypoxia, and genetic or immune disorders.

Psychosocial Stressors

There are an almost infinite variety of psychosocial stressors, which become so much a part of our daily lives that we often overlook them. To illustrate the many types of psychosocial stressors, consider those listed in Box 32-4. Psychosocial stressors include both real and perceived threats. The person's responses are continuous and include individualized coping mechanisms for responding to anxiety, guilt, fear, frustration, and loss. The mechanisms serve to maintain psychological homeostasis.

Personal Factors

A person's adaptation to stress, whether positive or negative, is influenced by a number of personal factors. One's physiologic reserve and genetic inheritance are important in maintaining homeostasis and adapting to stressors. The ability to

adapt is decreased in the very young, the very old, and those with altered physical or mental health, who do not have the necessary physiologic reserve to cope with physical changes such as dehydration or fluid excess. Adequate nutrition and sleep are necessary for enzyme function, immune responses, wound healing, and energy production and restoration. Malnutrition, dietary deficits or excess, and sleep deprivation all impair one's ability to adapt to stress. Social factors and life events are also implicated in adaptation to stress, with people who have strong support systems and relationships better able to adapt to stress and remain healthy (Porth, 2002).

STRESS AND ADAPTATION IN THE NURSING PROFESSION

Nursing involves activities and interpersonal relationships that are often stressful (Fig. 32-3). Activities identified as highly stressful include the following:

- Assuming responsibilities for which one is not prepared
- Working with unqualified personnel
- Working in an environment in which supervisors and administrators are not supportive
- Caring for a patient during a cardiac arrest or for a patient who is dying
- Experiencing conflict with peers

The stress is even greater for two groups of nurses—new graduates, who must adjust to an environment different from

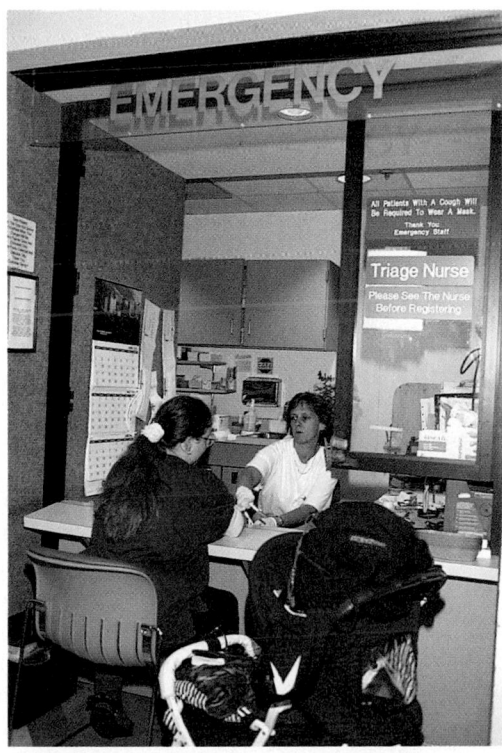

FIGURE 32-3 Some nursing specialties can be more stressful than others. To prevent burnout and alleviate personal stress, a nurse may need to work in another area of nursing temporarily or permanently. (Photo © Kathy Sloane.)

BOX 32-4 Examples of Psychosocial Stressors

- Accidents: cause stress for the victim, the person who caused the accident, and the families of both
- Stressful or traumatic experiences of family members and friends
- Horrors of history, such as Nazi concentration camps, the dropping of the atomic bomb on Hiroshima, and the Sept. 11, 2001, terrorist attacks
- Fear of aggression or mutilation, such as muggings, rape, murder, and terrorism
- Events of history that are brought into our homes through television, such as wars, earthquakes, and violence in schools
- Rapid changes in our world and the way we live, including changes in economic and political structures and rapid advances in technology

what they experienced as students, and nurses who work in settings such as intensive care and emergency care. In the present healthcare reform climate, many healthcare institutions are downsizing and increasing nurses' patient care assignments, also creating stress for nurses. Nurses may worry not only about the future of their positions but also about the safety of their patients. The anxiety is complicated by the expectations of nurses. Even though they may have strong negative feelings and reactions, their role does not include behaviors and verbal expressions that are less than positive and supportive.

Student nurses also experience stress and may have difficulty adapting to the requirements and responsibilities of caring for others. Factors causing stress in student nurses include the following:

- Fear of failing the classroom or clinical laboratory components of each course
- Fear of failing the licensure examination after graduation
- The demands of the nursing program
- Fear of injuring patients
- The need to balance work and study
- The need to meet financial and family responsibilities

> Recall Sarah Keller, the nursing student described in the Reflective Practice display. She was feeling overwhelmed with the responsibilities of caring for patients in a high-tech environment. This feeling was compounded by her concerns about the assigned instructor. In addition, she probably was affected by the factors identified above. Subsequently, Sarah began to feel ill. She needs to learn how to adapt to these stressors.

Most nurses and student nurses thoroughly enjoy their education and work and cope with physical and emotional demands effectively. Some, however, become overwhelmed and develop symptoms of anxiety and stress. The complex of behaviors is called **burnout.** Burnout can be compared with the exhaustion stage of anxiety and is characterized by a wide range of behaviors. Some nurses try to become "supernurses," expecting perfection in themselves and others. Some withdraw and do only minimal work; still others resort to drugs or alcohol. Many nurses who cannot handle the stress leave the profession.

What can graduate and student nurses do to help reduce stress and prevent burnout? The first step in preventing a stress level high enough to cause burnout is to identify and accept the stress. The same stress reduction techniques that are used for patients have positive benefits for nurses as well (see "Encouraging Use of Stress Management Techniques" in the Nursing Process section). Nurses must accept that they have the same needs and are as individual as their patients. By recognizing the early signs of stress and taking steps to reduce it, nurses can continue to be effective and productive as well as satisfied in the profession. (See the Focused Critical Thinking Guide 32-1.)

THE NURSING PROCESS FOR THE PATIENT WITH STRESS AND ANXIETY

Before reading further, use the accompanying Promoting Health 32-1 to see how well you are meeting your own needs for adaptation and role-modeling healthy behaviors when you are stressed. This tool can also be used with others to develop assessment and teaching skills for healthy responses to stress.

> Remember Joan Rogerrio, the woman returning to work after an absence of 15 years. The nurse could use the tool in Promoting Health 32-1 as part of the patient's assessment. Then the nurse could use those items identified as "sometimes" and "almost never" as a basis for teaching Joan measures to adapt and cope with her stressors.

Assessing

Stress and anxiety are problems that nurses encounter in patients of all ages and in all settings. Stress is assessed through a health assessment, including a nursing history and physical assessment. Risk factors for, or indicators of, stress may be identified through standardized tests or open-ended questions to elicit information. The patient's willingness to share information is affected by the level of stress experienced as well as the coping or defense mechanisms in use.

Nursing History
The nursing history assists the nurse in identifying stressors and how the person perceives and copes with stress. Manifestations of anxiety, as well as questions and leading statements to identify stress and anxiety, are listed in the Focused Assessment Guide 32-1.

Physical Assessment
There are no specific guidelines for the physical assessment of stress. Physical indicators of stress, in addition to those listed in the Focused Assessment Guide, may include cardiac dysrhythmias, chest pain, headache, hyperventilation, diarrhea, tense muscles, and skin lesions such as eczema. These manifestations are the result of the mind–body interaction described earlier.

Diagnosing

Assessment data may reveal stress and anxiety to be the problem or the etiology of a problem.

Anxiety as the Problem
The following nursing diagnoses may be made when anxiety is the cause of the problem:

Focused Critical Thinking Guide 32-1

Stress and Anxiety

You are a senior nursing student in your community health course. You have been assigned to visit and provide ongoing assessments for Charles Obedide, a 28-year-old man who was involved in a serious motorcycle accident a year ago and is paralyzed from the waist down. Charles initially participated fully in his rehabilitation and has been living independently in an apartment that is wheelchair accessible. However, a month ago, Charles was ill for 2 weeks, lost his job, and broke up with his girlfriend. When you made your last home visit, Charles was restless, had an increased pulse, and did little talking. At this visit, Charles is wearing dirty clothes and has a strong body odor, and there are several empty beer cans on the table in the kitchen. Charles begins to cry, saying, "I am so upset—I can't sleep or eat—I need help." What would you do?

1. Identify Goal of Thinking
Identify the level of anxiety experienced by Charles and begin interventions to help Charles decrease his level of anxiety.

2. Assess Adequacy of Knowledge
Pertinent circumstances: Charles has had numerous losses in the past year, including loss of body function and changes in body image. He has recently lost his job, a major source of economic support and self-concept. He lost his girlfriend, a major source of support. Previously, Charles was clean and well-groomed. There was no previous evidence of drinking. His parents live nearby and are supporting and loving.

Prerequisite knowledge: Before you decide what to do in this situation, you need to assess the level of anxiety experienced by Charles. You need to know the typical behaviors of each level and be able to recognize that Charles has severe anxiety. You must recognize that Charles needs interventions to regain equilibrium.

Room for error: Charles requires and has asked for help. You are unsure of your abilities to help him to deal effec-

tively with his anxiety. You realize that his frustration with the situation could make him angry. You also know that depression and the potential for self-violence are risks unless something is done to reduce his anxiety.

Time constraints: Although you are not certain about how serious his problem is, you understand that Charles needs help in reducing his anxiety soon. There is time for you to ask for guidance from your instructor.

3. Address Potential Problems
There are several potential barriers to critical thinking in this situation. You realize Charles needs help in reducing his level of stress, which in turn causes you anxiety. You are also somewhat frightened about his appearance and behavior. You do not believe your own abilities are developed well enough to help Charles adequately, but at the same time, you do know he needs help.

4. Consult Helpful Resources
Your best source of information is Charles himself. You ask him what you can do to help him. He replies, "Just get someone here to help me." You ask his permission to call his mother, and he agrees. His mother says she will be there in 5 minutes. You call your instructor, and she tells you to call the home health agency for further instructions.

5. Critique Judgment/Decision
When his mother arrives, she says she had no idea he was so distressed. She talks to the home health agency staff, who report that they have called Charles's physician and will continue to follow up on needed care and referrals for professional counseling. You believe you made the right decisions: you identified that Charles needed help, you contacted his mother to provide support, you contacted your instructor, and you contacted the home health agency. You also remained calm during the situation, despite your own anxiety.

- Anxiety related to conflicts about values and goals in life, threat to self-concept, threat of death, threat of or change in health status, threat to or change in environment or role, situational/maturational crisis, or unmet needs.
- Ineffective Coping related to inability to maintain marriage
- Defensive Coping related to loss of job and economic security
- Disturbed Thought Processes related to panic state
- Ineffective Denial related to continued smoking behavior
- Decisional Conflict related to placement of parent in nursing home
- Disabled Family Coping related to lack of knowledge about home care of child on ventilator
  Samples of three of these diagnoses are given in Examples of NANDA Nursing Diagnoses.

Anxiety as the Etiology
Stress and anxiety may affect many other areas of human functioning. In the following nursing diagnoses, stress and anxiety are involved in the etiologies of other problems:
- Imbalanced Nutrition: Less Than Body Requirements related to inadequate caloric intake while striving to excel in gymnastics
- Caregiver Role Strain related to long-term stress of care for parent with Alzheimer's disease
- Social Isolation related to feelings of worthlessness and apprehension following failure in school
- Spiritual Distress related to inability to accept diagnosis of terminal illness
- Hopelessness related to presence of disabling physical injuries
- Disturbed Sleep Pattern related to anxiety about terminally ill spouse

Promoting Health 32-1 *Stress and Adaptation*

Nurses who design care plans for patients to reduce stress must also examine themselves as a factor in the success of that plan of care. The nurse who wishes to encourage healthy adaptation to stress must demonstrate behaviors that support a healthy lifestyle. Use the assessment checklist to determine how well you are adapting to stress. Then develop a prescription for self-care by choosing the appropriate behaviors from the list of suggestions.

ASSESSMENT CHECKLIST

almost always	sometimes	almost never	
☐	☐	☐	1. I have realistic perceptions of new situations, self, and others.
☐	☐	☐	2. I understand my own personal physical and emotional responses to stress.
☐	☐	☐	3. I anticipate and prepare for change.
☐	☐	☐	4. I have the ability to satisfactorily solve problems and make decisions.

Further information may be found on the following web sites:
- Blue Cross Blue Shield. (2003). Coping with stress. http://www.fepblue.org/toyourhealth/tyhhlthwatch/tyhhwcopngstress
- Campusaccess.com. (2003). Academic life—Coping with stress. http://www.campusaccess.com/campus_web/student/s3acad_cope

SELF-CARE BEHAVIORS

1. Accept as positive indicators of growth the changes that come with different parts and stages of life.
2. Maintain an open mind about change—change what you can, and accept what you cannot change.
3. Avoid self-defeating behaviors to cope with stress, such as smoking, alcohol, and drugs.
4. Practice methods of stress management that work best for you: relaxation techniques, exercise, hobbies.
5. Set realistic goals.
6. Develop problem-solving strategies for use in stressful situations.
7. Accept help from others.
8. Take life one day at a time.

- National Mental Health Association. (2003). Stress—Coping with everyday problems. http://www.nmha.org/infoctr/factsheet/41
- University of South Florida. (2003). Coping with stress in college. http://isis2.admin.usf.edu/counsel/self-hlp/stress

Outcome Identification and Planning

The nurse plans and implements care to decrease anxiety and facilitate adaptation in the patient with anxiety. The expected outcomes of the plan must be mutually determined with the patient or family members. The expected outcomes of the plan of care may include that the patient will achieve the following:

- Decrease the level of anxiety by verbalizing feelings and using support systems
- Develop effective coping skills through problem-solving skills and anxiety-reducing techniques
- Describe a reduction in anxiety and an increase in comfort

Implementing

Nurses may use a variety of interventions to help patients decrease stress and to facilitate coping. If the patient's anxiety seems too great or the nurse is uncomfortable with the interventions, a referral should be made. Referrals may be made, for example, to a professional counselor, to individuals who have experienced the same type of surgery or health problem, or to the patient's rabbi, minister, or priest.

The nursing interventions discussed in this section include teaching healthy activities of daily living, encouraging use of support systems, and practicing stress management techniques. See Examples of Nursing Interventions Classification activities to reduce anxiety. Methods should be selected carefully, based on the person's physical and emotional characteristics, family and social structure, and previously used coping mechanisms that were successful. Guidelines for Nursing Care 32-1 lists nursing interventions to reduce anxiety for patients as they enter a healthcare setting.

Teaching Healthy Activities of Daily Living

A person's normal lifestyle greatly influences his or her perceptions of and reactions to stressors. For example, a person who is overweight, sedentary, and chronically tired is at increased risk for developing an illness as a result of stress. These factors are also stressors and further increase the risk. Exercise, rest, and good nutrition are important components of stress reduction.

> *Think about Sarah Keller's lifestyle as a nursing student. The workload involved with school and the factors associated with stress in nursing students described previously place Sarah at risk for stress. In addition, other factors, such as demands from family members or a need to work part-time, decrease her ability to maintain a healthy lifestyle with exercise, rest, and good nutrition.*

Exercise

Regular exercise helps to maintain physical and emotional health. The benefits of exercise include an improved musculo-skeletal system, more effective cardiovascular function, weight

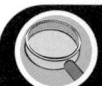 **Focused Assessment Guide 32-1**

Anxiety

Factors to Assess	Questions and Approaches
Subjective data:	• "Have you noticed that you sometimes feel your heart beating or have difficulty breathing?"
Heart palpitations	
Difficulty breathing	• "Tell me about your appetite and sleep."
Problems with appetite or sleep	• "Of the following, which best describes how you are feeling: sad, apprehensive, angry, mistrustful, helpless, hopeless?"
Feelings of sadness, apprehension, anger, mistrust, helplessness, hopelessness	• "Tell me about any changes you have noticed in your sexual desire."
Changes in sexual desire	• "How does your body feel when you are upset?"
Objective data:	• Note body posture and movements.
Dry mouth	• Inspect skin and mucous membranes.
Increased perspiration	• Take and record vital signs.
Tremors	• Note general affect.
Tachycardia	
Increased blood pressure	
Dilated pupils	
Crying	
Restlessness	
Rapid speech	
Pacing around the room	
Lack of facial expression	
Ability to verbalize anxiety	• "You have been very quiet today. Has something happened since our last visit?"
	• "It must be very frightening to be told that you have cancer."
	• "I notice you seem upset. Would you like to talk about it?"
	• "What has caused you to feel stressed in the past?"
	• "What do you do to feel better when you feel anxious?"

control, and relaxation. Exercise improves one's general sense of well-being, relieves tension, and enables one to cope better with day-to-day stressors. General health guidelines recommend that an exercise program consist of 30 to 45 minutes of moderate activity three or four times a week. People who are overweight, chronically ill, or older than 35 years of age should have a thorough physical examination before beginning such a program. The type of exercise depends on what the person enjoys—for example, walking, jogging, bicycling, swimming, or sports such as golf or tennis.

Rest and Sleep

Rest and sleep help the body to maintain homeostasis and restore energy levels. Adequate rest can provide "insulation" against stress, but stress may interfere with one's ability to sleep. Although each person has individual needs, 7 to 8 hours of sleep a day is recommended. Relaxation techniques can be used during both health and illness to facilitate rest and sleep. Hospitalized patients may require additional nursing interventions to relieve pain and promote comfort to get needed rest.

Nutrition

Nutrition plays an active role in maintaining the body's homeostatic mechanisms and in increasing resistance to stress. (Nutrition is discussed in detail in Chap. 42.) Obesity and malnutrition are major stressors and greatly increase the risk

for illness. People of all ages should maintain a normal body weight and should follow these guidelines established by the U.S. Senate Committee on Nutrition and Human Needs:

• Reduce intake of salt, refined sugar, animal fat, and cholesterol.

• Eat more fruit, vegetables, and whole grains.

• Eat less red meat and more fish and poultry.

Consider Joan Rogerrio, the woman who has returned to work and is experiencing an exacerbation of her bowel disease. The demands of her new job may interfere with her ability to eat properly; she may need to work through lunch or grab fast food or takeout for dinner. As a result, her resistance to stress is decreased.

Encouraging Use of Support Systems

Support systems provide emotional support that helps a person identify and verbalize feelings associated with stress. Other valuable contributions include providing information and services, maintaining positive self-concept, and establishing an avenue for new relationships and social roles. In addition, families and support groups provide an accepting environment, allowing the person to explore problem-solving methods and try out new coping skills. There are support groups for almost every situation; examples are listed in Box 32-5.

Examples of NANDA Nursing Diagnoses | Stress and Adaptation

Nursing Diagnoses	Related Factors	Sample Defining Characteristics
Anxiety	Unmet needs, situational/maturational crises, threat to self-concept, stress, threat to or change in role status, health status, interaction patterns, role function, environment, economic status	**Behavioral:** • Restlessness, fidgeting, insomnia • "I am so worried about my son getting married." **Affective:** • Irritable, jittery, focused on self, worried, apprehensive • "I just know I won't be able to do what I have to in this new job." **Physiologic:** • Tremors, increased pulse and respirations, urinary urgency, perspiration, diarrhea, dry mouth, nausea, respiratory difficulties • "I can't eat or sleep, and my heart feels like it's going to jump out of my chest." **Cognitive:** • Preoccupation, confusion, decreased attention and concentration, tendency to blame others • "What did you just tell me? I can't seem to remember, and it's all my husband's fault for leaving me."
Ineffective Coping	Inability to appraise stressors, inadequate choices of practical responses, and/or inability to use available resources	• "I know my bad grades are my fault, but I just can't make myself go to class or study." • "I have been so down lately, so I just go out and drink a lot and feel better for a while." • "When I get upset, I just get in my car and drive down the highway at 90 miles an hour."
Ineffective Denial	A conscious or unconscious attempt to disavow the knowledge or meaning of an event to reduce anxiety, but leading to detriment of health	• "I know I have a lump in my breast, but it's probably just nothing." • "I do have a lot of heartburn, but I just take something I bought at the store and it feels better." • "I have noticed some bright red blood when I have a bowel movement, but I figure it's just my hemorrhoids."

Examples of Nursing Interventions Classification (NIC)
Anxiety Reduction

• Use a calm, reassuring approach.
• Clearly state expectations for the patient's behavior.
• Explain all procedures, including sensations likely to be experienced during the procedure.
• Seek to understand the patient's perspective of a stressful situation.
• Encourage parents to stay with child, as appropriate.
• Listen attentively.
• Encourage verbalization of feelings, perceptions, and fears.
• Help the patient identify situations that precipitate anxiety.
• Support the use of appropriate defense mechanisms.
• Instruct the patient on the use of relaxation techniques.

McCloskey, J. & Bulechek, G. (Eds.) (2000). *Nursing interventions classification (NIC)* (3rd ed., p. 146). St. Louis: Mosby.

Encouraging Use of Stress Management Techniques

Stress creates emotional distress that often produces physical signs and symptoms. One person may have tension headaches; another becomes irritable; another clenches his fists. Many people take legal or illegal drugs, drink or smoke to excess, or eat compulsively. These behaviors can be modified and adaptive mechanisms strengthened through specific techniques aimed at managing stress. Only a few techniques are included here, but the literature describes many stress reduction methods, including exercise, prayer, art therapy, music therapy, massage, and therapeutic touch. Chapter 28, Complementary and Alternative Modalities, provides further information. Students should learn different methods they can use for themselves and in varied clinical situations.

Relaxation

Relaxation techniques are useful in many situations, such as childbirth, pain, anxiety, sleeplessness, illness, and anger, and

Guidelines for Nursing Care 32-1
Reducing Anxiety on Admission to a Healthcare Facility

1. Assess physical status, sensory status, and cognitive status.
2. Assess cultural/ethnic background, including beliefs about healthcare, dietary restrictions, and language spoken.
3. Assess past experiences with the healthcare system, including medical-surgical treatment for illness or injury.
4. Assess concerns and stressors.
5. Assess amount and type of support systems available.
6. Provide information about the environment:
   a. All healthcare providers should introduce themselves by name and title.
   b. Explain policies and routines.
   c. If the hospital is the setting, provide verbal and written guidelines for use of equipment, telephone, television, meals, and visiting hours.
7. Provide and discuss the patient's rights specific to care in the agency or institution.
8. Mutually determine expected outcomes of the plan of care.
9. Provide information about all diagnostic procedures, surgical procedures, activity, and diet.

Guidelines for Nursing Care 32-2
Relaxation Activities

Deep Breathing
1. Sit comfortably and place your hands on your stomach. Inhale slowly and deeply, letting your abdomen expand as much as possible. Hold your breath for a few seconds.
2. Exhale slowly through your mouth, blowing through puckered lips. When your abdomen feels empty, begin again with a deep inhalation.

Progressive Muscle Relaxation
1. Tighten your hand into a fist and notice how it feels. Hold the tension for a few seconds.
2. Loosen your grip, relax the muscles in your hand, and let the tension slip away.
3. Continue to tighten-hold-relax each muscle group: hands, arms, shoulders, face, chest, back, abdomen, legs, feet.

other uses are being discovered. Relaxation promotes a body reaction opposite to that of the fight-or-flight response: respiratory, pulse, and metabolic rates, blood pressure, and energy use are all decreased.

Relaxation can be taught to individuals or groups and is especially helpful because it allows a person to control his or her feelings and behaviors. Various techniques can be used, but most involve rhythmic breathing, reduced muscle tension, and an altered state of consciousness (Stuart & Laraia, 2001). Relaxation is discussed as a comfort measure in Chapter 40, Rest and Sleep. Two relaxation activities, to be practiced three or four times at each session, are deep breathing and progressive muscle relaxation (see Guidelines for Nursing Care 32-2).

BOX 32-5 Examples of Support Groups

Alcoholics Anonymous
Overeaters Anonymous
Weight Watchers
Parents Without Partners
Reach to Recovery (cancer)
Ostomy clubs
Child abuse support groups
Sudden infant death support groups
Stroke clubs
Assertiveness training groups

Meditation
Meditation has four components: quiet surroundings, a passive attitude, a comfortable position, and a word or mental image on which to focus. A person practicing meditation sits comfortably with closed eyes, relaxes the major muscle groups, and repeats the selected word silently with each exhalation. Alternatively, the person may focus on a pleasant scene and mentally place himself or herself in it while breathing slowly in and out. This exercise should be performed for 20 to 30 minutes twice a day.

> Sarah Keller, the nursing student, could learn to perform relaxation exercises or practice meditation. Both techniques would be helpful in reducing stress, and in addition Sarah would be able to do these by herself.

Anticipatory Guidance
Anticipatory guidance focuses on psychologically preparing a person for an unfamiliar or painful event. Nurses use this technique to teach patients about procedures and the surgical experience. When patients know what to expect, their anxiety is reduced and their coping mechanisms are more effective. For example, before changing a dressing, teaching would include all the information about the pain involved—onset, severity, cause, and methods of relief. With this knowledge, the patient feels less threatened and tolerates the procedure more easily.

A related process is anticipatory socialization, in which people prepare themselves for roles to which they aspire but do not yet occupy. This process may be used, for example, to prepare expectant parents for the role of parenting, thereby enhancing the potential of the child to experience normal growth and development.

Guided Imagery
In guided imagery, a person creates a mental image, concentrates on the image, and becomes less responsive to stimuli (in-

cluding pain). The nurse sits by the patient and reads a description of a scene or an experience that the patient has described as happy, pleasant, or peaceful. The patient is then "guided" through the image. For example, using a soothing, soft voice, the nurse might start as follows: "You are floating in your swimming pool. The water is cool and comfortable. Birds are singing in the trees. The roses are perfuming the air." As the patient becomes more and more focused on the scene, the nurse needs only verbally "paint the picture" at intervals.

Biofeedback

Biofeedback is a method of gaining mental control of the autonomic nervous system and thus regulating body responses, such as blood pressure, heart rate, and headaches. A measurement device (eg, skin temperature sensors) is used, and the patient tries to control the readings through relaxation and conscious thought. Over a period of time, the feedback of the change in readings teaches the person to control physiologic functions that normally are considered involuntary responses. The process is still being researched.

Providing Crisis Intervention

As defined earlier, a crisis is a situation that cannot be resolved by usual coping mechanisms. As a result, the person cannot function normally and requires interventions to regain equilibrium. **Crisis intervention** is a five-step problem-solving technique designed to promote a more adaptive outcome, including improved abilities to cope with future crises. The steps are as follows:

1. Identify the problem. This may be more difficult than it appears, as the cause of the crisis is often difficult for the person to identify accurately. Until it is clear, a solution is impossible.
2. List alternatives. All possible solutions to the problem need to be listed. An appropriate solution to a problem is much more likely if many options are considered.
3. Choose from among alternatives. Each option needs to be carefully considered, using a "what would happen if" approach. The alternative chosen will be highly individualized, based on the person's priorities and values.

4. Implement the plan. The alternative chosen is put into action. The nurse may need to provide support and encouragement so that action is taken.
5. Evaluate the outcome. In this final step, the effectiveness of the plan needs to be carefully considered. If it did not work as well as expected, another alternative should be chosen. If it did work, it has the positive benefit of improving self-confidence and future problem-solving efforts.

The major factor in helping patients adapt to high levels of stress is to identify and plan individually for situations causing the stress. Help the person recognize his or her own stress level and specific responses to stress. Encourage the person to adopt a philosophy of accepting what cannot be changed and changing what cannot be accepted. Stress the importance of accepting help from others and giving support to others when needed, as well as being actively involved in problem solving and decision making. Nurses must use therapeutic communication skills in all interactions.

> *Remember Peter Bainbridge, the man whose pregnant wife was injured in a car crash. The nurse would incorporate crisis intervention when developing the plan of care. The key is to assist Peter to identify the underlying problem, using appropriate therapeutic techniques.*

Evaluating

The evaluation of the plan of care is based on the mutually established expected outcomes. It is important to observe both verbal and nonverbal cues when evaluating the usefulness of the plan. In general, the plan is considered to be successful if the patient and family achieve the following:

- Verbalize causes and effects of stress and anxiety
- Identify and use sources of support
- Use problem solving to find solutions to stressors
- Practice healthy lifestyle habits and anxiety-reducing techniques
- Verbalize a decrease in anxiety and an increase in comfort
  See the Nursing Plan of Care 32-1.

NURSING PLAN OF CARE 32-1   *for Mei Fu*

Mei Fu is a 24-year-old graduate student. She is married and has two small children; her husband is also a graduate student. Although she lived in China until 3 years ago, she speaks English well. After several months of headaches and diarrhea, Mrs. Fu made an appointment at the student health clinic.

The nurse practitioner at the clinic conducted a health history and physical assessment of Mrs. Fu and noted the following data:

- Patient is a thin woman who appears her stated age. She is currently in school and expects herself to make the highest grades. She also cares for her two children and her husband. Although her husband encourages her to go to school, he believes it is the wife's responsibility to provide all child and house care. She has had no previous serious illnesses or surgery.

- Patient reports having frequent headaches, rating the pain as a 3 on a scale of 0 (no pain) to 10 (worst possible pain). She also reports having 4 to 6 bowel movements each day, sometimes with abdominal cramping. The diarrhea does not seem to be related to any type of foods eaten. Both the headaches and the diarrhea have been present for the past 2 months. During the interview, the patient appeared restless and talked rapidly. Questions often had to be repeated.

- Physical assessment reveals slight tachycardia, a fine hand tremor, and visible perspiration. Large muscle groups are tense and fists clenched. No tenderness is noted on abdominal palpation. Pupils are equal in size and react to light and accommodation. Nasal mucosa is normal.

(continued)

NURSING PLAN OF CARE 32-1   *for Mei Fu* (continued)

NURSING DIAGNOSIS   Anxiety related to stress of achievement in school and care of family as manifested by rapid speech, tachycardia, tremor, tense muscles, headache, and diarrhea.

EXPECTED OUTCOME   By her return appointment in 2 weeks, 10/20/06, Mrs. Fu will:
• Identify sources of and responses to stress

Nursing Interventions	Rationale	Evaluative Statement
Ask Mrs. Fu to keep a diary of hours spent in school-related activities and family care, number and times of headaches, and circumstances that occurred before diarrhea.	Identifying sources of stress and the physical responses to stress is the first step in planning coping strategies to reduce stress.	10/20/06 Outcome met. Mrs. Fu kept a diary as requested. She identified that she does not have any time for herself. Her headaches are worse during the week. She often has diarrhea when papers are due or when her husband and children are demanding of her time. *S. Aird, RN, FNP*

EXPECTED OUTCOME   By her return appointment, 10/20/06, Mrs. Fu will:
• Identify sources of personal strength and support

Nursing Interventions	Rationale	Evaluative Statement
Ask Mrs. Fu to make a list of the people who are important to her and provide her comfort. Ask her to discuss how these people can help her cope with her situation. Ask Mrs. Fu to describe her strengths as a woman, a mother, a wife, and a student.	Identifying support people and areas of personal strength provides the patient with the means to manage stress and enhances self-concept.	10/20/06 Outcome met. Mrs. Fu stated that her family is her greatest source of support, but they are in China and she misses them very much. She does have a very good friend who is also a good listener. She identified her strengths as being a person who cares for others and a good student. She said she is also a good artist, but has not had time for art for months. *S. Aird, RN, FNP*

EXPECTED OUTCOME   By her return appointment, 10/20/06, Mrs. Fu will:
• Describe lifestyle changes that include eating a well-balanced diet with three meals a day, walking for 20 to 30 minutes four times a week, and sleeping restfully 7 hours a night

Nursing Interventions	Rationale	Evaluative Statement
Discuss with Mrs. Fu the food pyramid and the importance of eating foods from each group. Also discuss why she should eat three meals a day.	Adequate nutrition helps maintain the homeostatic mechanisms of the body and increases resistance to stress.	10/20/06 Outcome met. Mrs. Fu was given a copy of the food pyramid, and food preparations were discussed. Although the Fu's have a healthy diet, Mrs. Fu often was too busy to eat more than a few bites. She said that she is making a big effort to eat three times a day.

(continued)

NURSING PLAN OF CARE 32-1   *for Mei Fu* (continued)

Discuss with Mrs. Fu the benefits of regular exercise in reducing stress.	Exercise improves well-being, relieves tension, and facilitates coping with daily stressors.	She is walking to school and enjoys the time by herself. She arranged this time by asking her husband to take the children to school.
Discuss with Mrs. Fu the importance of sleep in reducing stress.	Adequate rest and sleep restore energy and facilitate coping with stressors.	She is sleeping better, and averages 7 hours most nights.

S. Aird, RN, FNP

EXPECTED OUTCOME

By her return appointment, 10/20/06, Mrs. Fu will:
• Practice relaxation for 20 minutes each day

Nursing Interventions	Rationale	Evaluative Statement
Teach and have Mrs. Fu practice progressive muscle relaxation. Suggest that she buy a tape to facilitate the technique (tapes for relaxation are widely available). Recommend that she plan a time when she can be alone and use 20 minutes to complete the technique.	Relaxation promotes a response opposite to the stress response; decreases heart rate, respiratory rate, blood pressure, and metabolic processes.	10/20/06 Outcome met. Mrs. Fu said that at first she had difficulty in finding time to be alone, but she feels so much better after she relaxes that she insists on the time. She did buy a tape and says it helps her very much.

S. Aird, RN, FNP

EXPECTED OUTCOME

By her return appointment, 10/20/06, Mrs. Fu will:
• Report a decrease in headaches and diarrhea and an increase in her ability to provide self-care to manage stress

Nursing Interventions	Rationale	Evaluative Statement
Assess frequency and severity of headaches and bowel movements. Assess patient's self-report of coping with stressors.	Decreasing stress in daily life often is effective in decreasing physical responses. Self-care of stress is critical in effective management.	10/20/06 Outcome met. Mrs. Fu reports she has noticed fewer headaches in the past week, and the diarrhea is almost gone. Mrs. Fu verbalized the importance of continuing to practice a healthy lifestyle and relaxation. She said she has spent time with her friend and has gotten out her sketch pad. She stated that she believes she can manage her life much better now.

S. Aird, RN, FNP

SAMPLE DOCUMENTATION

10/06/06, 10 am, nursing

Initial visit to student health center by Mrs. Fu to discuss physical problems of headache and diarrhea. History and physical assessment findings indicated large number of personal stressors, manifested by physical signs and symptoms. Assessment data supported nursing diagnosis: Anxiety related to stress of achievement in school and care of family. Discussion centered on identifying sources of stress, physical responses to stress, sources of support, and personal strength. Teaching strategies included diet, exercise, sleep, and progressive muscle relaxation. Patient's progress will be monitored at next visit on 10/20/06.

S. Aird, RN, FNP

Developing Critical Thinking Skills

1. Identify the nursing activities and relationships that cause you the most stress. What are your personal warning signs that a situation is becoming stressful? What do you do to decrease your level of stress? Who is most important in helping you do this?

2. List nursing interventions you would use to reduce stress in the following situations:
   - A newly married young woman who found a lump in her breast and is undergoing a breast biopsy
   - The parents of a 2-year-old who are sitting in the surgical waiting room as their child undergoes brain surgery
   - The daughter (and caretaker) of a woman with severe Alzheimer's disease

Practicing for NCLEX

1. Stress is a condition in which the human system:
   a. Becomes increasingly disorganized
   b. Responds to changes in its normal balanced state
   c. Responds to negative changes in its internal environment
   d. Is less likely to respond appropriately to stimuli

2. Which of the following is an external stressor?
   a. High environmental temperature
   b. Changes in hormone levels
   c. Fear of the dark
   d. Having an infection of the intestine

3. The body maintains the internal environment at a constant state through:
   a. Internalization
   b. Adaptation
   c. Cellular integrity
   d. Homeostasis

4. Which of the following is developmental stress?
   a. An infant learns to turn over.
   b. A school-aged child learns how to add and subtract.
   c. An adolescent gets a job.
   d. A young adult has a variety of friends.

5. The reflex pain response and the inflammatory response are examples of:
   a. Localized responses of the body to stress
   b. Negative responses of the body to stress
   c. Generalized responses of the body to stress
   d. Ways in which the body controls stress

6. What response is expected during the shock phase of the general adaptation syndrome?
   a. Decreasing pulse
   b. Increasing sleepiness
   c. Increasing energy levels
   d. Slow respirations

7. A vague feeling of discomfort or dread with an unknown source is:
   a. Fear
   b. Concern
   c. Panic
   d. Anxiety

8. Toward the end of the semester, as final examinations near, you find yourself sleeping more than usual. This behavior is probably your form of a:
   a. Coping mechanism
   b. Defense mechanism
   c. Offense mechanism
   d. Adapting mechanism

9. Your patient has just been diagnosed with cancer but responds as though this is impossible. Which of the defense mechanisms is being demonstrated here?
   a. Projection
   b. Denial
   c. Displacement
   d. Repression

10. Home care of patients by family members for long periods of time can cause long-term stress and increased risk for illness. The name for this stress response is:
    a. Home care chronicity
    b. Patient burnout
    c. Residual stress
    d. Caregiver burden

11. All but one of the following responses are typical of relaxation techniques. Which is not typical?
    a. Rhythmic breathing
    b. An increased pulse rate
    c. Reduced muscle tension
    d. An altered state of consciousness

12. Which type of stress reduction activity would probably be most useful for a patient before an unfamiliar or painful event?
    a. Progressive muscle relaxation
    b. Meditation
    c. Anticipatory guidance
    d. Biofeedback

13. What is the first step in crisis intervention through problem solving?
    a. Identify the problem.
    b. List alternatives.
    c. Implement a plan.
    d. Evaluate the outcome.

14. Biofeedback is a method of gaining mental control of what part of the body?
    a. Skin
    b. Senses
    c. Autonomic nervous system
    d. Central nervous system

15. What setting is considered most stressful for nurses?
    a. Cancer treatment center
    b. Nursing home
    c. Operating room
    d. Intensive care unit

■ Answers With Rationale

1. The correct answer is *b*. Individuals perceive and respond to stress in highly individualized ways. Stress evokes both positive and negative responses to changes in the internal and external environment.

2. The correct answer is *a*. The other answers are internal stressors.

3. The correct answer is *d*. To maintain health, the internal environment must remain in balance; this balance is maintained through various physiologic mechanisms as they respond to internal changes.

4. The correct answer is *c*. Although the other choices are milestones for a certain developmental age, the adolescent who gets a job is seeking independence, a major task for that level of growth and development.

5. The correct answer is *a*. The local adaptation syndrome is a localized response of the body to stress. These responses are homeostatic and short-term; the most common are the reflex pain response and the inflammatory response.

6. The correct answer is *c*. The body perceives a threat and prepares to respond by increasing the activity of the autonomic nervous and endocrine systems. The initial or shock phase is characterized by increased energy levels, oxygen intake, cardiac output, blood pressure, and mental alertness.

7. The correct answer is *d*. Panic is an experience of terror. A concern is a worry. Fear has a known cause. Only anxiety is a psychological response to an unknown threat.

8. The correct answer is *a*. Mild anxiety is often handled without conscious thought through the use of coping mechanisms, which are behaviors used to decrease stress and anxiety. Sleeping is a coping mechanism.

9. The correct answer is *b*. Denial occurs when a person refuses to acknowledge the presence of a condition that is disturbing.

10. The correct answer is *d*. Reactions to home care of family members for long periods of time, called caregiver burden, include chronic fatigue, sleep disorders, and an increased incidence of stress-related illnesses, such as hypertension and heart disease.

11. The correct answer is *b*. No matter what the technique, relaxation involves rhythmic breathing, reduced muscle tension, and an altered state of consciousness.

12. The correct answer is *c*. Anticipatory guidance focuses on psychological preparation of the patient for an unfamiliar or painful event. When patients know what to expect, their anxiety is reduced and their coping mechanisms are more effective.

13. The correct answer is *a*. Although identifying the problem may be difficult, a solution to a crisis situation is impossible until the problem is identified.

14. The correct answer is *c*. Biofeedback is a method of gaining control of the autonomic nervous system and regulating body responses to stress such as increased blood pressure, increased heart rate, and headaches.

15. The correct answer is *d*. Patients in intensive care units have complex needs and are at greater risk for death; their care is often stressful.

Bibliography

Boutain, D. (2001). Discourses of worry, stress, and high blood pressure in rural South Louisiana. *Journal of Nursing Scholarship, 33*(3), 225–230.

Carpenito, L. J. (2002). *Nursing diagnosis: Application to clinical practice* (9th ed.). Philadelphia: Lippincott.

Cherry, G., Thiele, J., & Schodde, G. (2003). You tell us: How do you take care of yourself so that you can take care of your patients? *ONS News, 18*(2), 6.

Frasca-Beaulier, K. (1999). Interior design for ambulatory care facilities: How to reduce stress and anxiety in patients and families. *Journal of Ambulatory Care Management, 22*(1), 67–73.

Kwong, E., & Kwan, A. (2003). How older people manage stress. *Nursing Older People, 15*(3), 18–21.

McCloskey, J., & Bulechek, G. (Eds.). (2000). *Nursing interventions classification (NIC)*. (3rd ed.). St. Louis: Mosby.

Moorhead, S., & Brighton, V. (2001). Anxiety and fear. In M. Maas, K. Buckwalter, M. Hardy, et al. *Nursing care of older adults: Diagnoses, outcomes, & interventions* (pp. 571–592). St. Louis: Mosby.

North American Nursing Diagnosis Association. (2003). *Nursing diagnoses: Definitions & classification 2003–2004*. Philadelphia: Author.

Pender, N. (2002). *Health promotion in nursing practice* (4th ed.). Upper Saddle River, NJ: Prentice Hall.

Porth, C. M. (2002). *Pathophysiology: Concepts of altered health states* (6th ed.). Philadelphia: Lippincott.

Selye, H. (1976). *The stress of life*. New York: McGraw-Hill.

Spence, L., & Kaiser, L. (2002). Companion animals and adaptation in chronically ill children. *Western Journal of Nursing Research, 24*(6), 639–656.

Stuart, G., & Laraia, M. (2001). *Principles and practice of psychiatric nursing* (7th ed.). St. Louis: Mosby.

Tsai, P. (2003). A middle-range theory of caregiver stress. *Nursing Science Quarterly, 16*(2), 137–145.

Ward, K. (2002). Managing stress: An essential of leadership. *SCI Nursing, 19*(2), 80–81.

Weckman, H. (2001). Moving from distress to de-stress: Some suggestions for managing the stress in your life. *SCI Nursing, 18*(3), 148–149.

Loss, Grief, and Dying

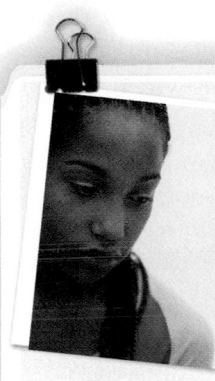

Yvonne Malic, a 20-year-old, single woman, has just given birth to a baby, 11 weeks premature. The neonate weighs 2 pounds 2 ounces (1,021 g) and is immediately admitted to the neonatal intensive care unit because of severe respiratory distress. Up until this point, Yvonne had a normal pregnancy and was expecting a healthy baby girl. "I was so happy to be pregnant and I wanted to be a mother so much. But my baby is so tiny! And now the doctors are telling me that she has less than a 50% chance of surviving the next 24 hours."

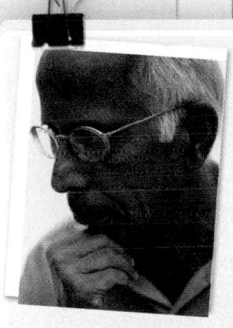

Manuel Perez is a 68-year-old man who 2 months ago moved to a retirement community with his 69-year-old wife. "We were looking forward to traveling and playing lots of golf. But she had this stroke, and now she has permanent brain damage." Mr. Perez can be seen sitting at his wife's bedside, holding her hand, and crying. "The doctors are asking me if I want to continue all these treatments that are keeping her alive. And they mentioned something about donating her organs. I don't know what to do. We never talked about what either of us would want."

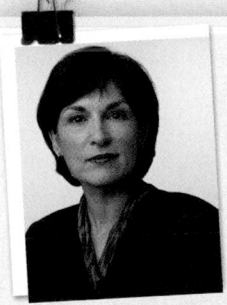

Anna Maria Giordano, a 49-year-old female attorney, has recently suffered a major cerebral hemorrhage. Her prognosis is considered extremely poor by one physician, but possibly hopeful by another. Her advance directives found on the chart very clearly state that if she was in a comatose condition with no hope for recovery, she did not want life-sustaining treatment. Her family is called to make a decision about continuing life-sustaining treatment.

Focusing on Blended Skills

The types of blended skills you'll need to respond to the case scenarios include:

Cognitive Skills
- Basic knowledge about loss and grieving and the factors that affect loss, grief, and dying
- Ability to incorporate knowledge about the stages of grief into the treatment of patients experiencing loss, grief, or death
- Ability to identify the impact that loss, grief, and death and dying have on the patient and his or her family members
- Knowledge about quality end-of-life outcomes and the competencies necessary for nurses to provide high-quality care to patients and families during the transition at the end of life
- Ability to use the nursing process to care for patients with problems related to loss, grief, and dying

Technical Skills
- Ability to use correctly the equipment and protocols necessary to identify and treat problems related to loss, grief, and dying
- Ability to use and adapt technical nursing assistance appropriately in situations involving individuals in different age groups and developmental stages

Interpersonal Skills
- Ability to communicate and interact effectively with patients and their family caregivers

- Ability to establish trusting relationships, even in times of great crisis related to loss (anticipatory and actual loss)
- Ability to clarify information and misconceptions for family members who are overwhelmed
- Ability to affirm dignity and worth in times of stress and grieving; ability to communicate caring
- Ability to facilitate decision making, especially when the decisions to withhold or withdraw life-sustaining treatment may result in the death of a loved member of the family

Ethical and Legal Skills
- Commitment to safety and quality; strong sense of responsibility and accountability; strong advocacy skills
- Familiarity with the ethical and legal guidelines concerning the authorization for and the withholding or withdrawing of life-sustaining medical interventions
- Familiarity with federal and state legislation related to end-of-life care and organ donation
- Ability to apply knowledge of agency policy and role responsibilities for end-of-life care and organ donation
- Knowledge of the state's requirements for advance directives
- Ability to incorporate knowledge about the rights of dying patients into a patient's plan of care
- Ability to advocate for the patient who has an advance directive

Learning Outcomes

After completing the chapter, the learner should be able to accomplish the following:

1. Differentiate the types of loss.
2. Describe the grief process and the stages of grief.
3. Describe Kübler-Ross's stages of dying.
4. Compare and contrast three definitions of death.
5. Identify ethical and legal issues concerning end-of-life care.
6. Identify six factors that affect loss, grief, and dying.
7. Describe physiologic, psychological, and spiritual care of a dying patient and family.
8. Use the nursing process to plan and implement care for dying patients and their families.
9. Articulate and defend a personal response to a patient's plea, "Please help me die."
10. List the clinical signs of approaching death.
11. Outline nursing responsibilities after death.
12. Discuss the role of the nurse in caring for a dying patient's family.

Key Terms

active euthanasia
actual loss
advance directive
anticipatory loss
assisted suicide
bereavement
comfort-measures-only order
death
do-not-hospitalize order
do-not-resuscitate order
dysfunctional grief
grief
loss
maturational loss
mourning
palliative care
perceived loss
physical loss
psychological loss
situational loss
terminal illness
terminal weaning

At any stage of one's life there is the potential for loss, grief, and death. This is especially true for persons experiencing altered health and for members of their family. A wide variety of losses may occur, including loss of a body part or function; loss of one's ability to care for oneself or to perform valued family or work roles; and death, which may be the most difficult loss of all. Death may be as difficult for healthcare professionals as it is for surviving family members. The goals of nursing focus on health maintenance and health restoration, with an emphasis on facilitating maximum potential in wellness. Other aims of nursing, however, are to promote "good dying" through compassionate palliative care and to facilitate coping with disability and death. The nurse is often the key person in providing support and care when loss or death occurs. To provide effective care, the nurse must have accepted his or her own feelings about death and understand the stages of grieving and dying. (For an example, see Reflective Practice: Challenge to Ethical and Legal Skills.)

LOSS AND GRIEVING

Loss

Loss occurs when a valued person, object, or situation is changed or made inaccessible so that its value is diminished or removed. There are several types of loss, all of which everyone may experience at some time. **Actual loss** can be recognized by others as well as by the person sustaining the loss; loss of a limb, of a spouse, of a valued object such as money, and of a job are all examples of actual loss. **Perceived loss** is felt by the person but is intangible to others; loss of youth, of financial independence, and of a valued environment are examples of perceived loss. Directly related to actual and perceived loss are physical and psychological loss. A person who loses an arm in an automobile accident suffers from both the **physical loss** of the arm and the **psychological loss** that may be caused by an altered self-image and the inability to return to his or her occupation. These losses are simultaneously physical, psychological, and actual. A person who is scarred but does not lose a limb may suffer a perceived and psychological loss of self-image.

> *Recall Mr. Perez, whose wife has brain damage from a recent stroke. The nurse could use knowledge of the types of losses to help Mr. Perez deal with all the recent changes in his life, including the loss of his wife's ability to be his partner.*

There is also maturational and situational loss. **Maturational loss** is experienced as a result of natural developmental processes. The first child may experience a loss of status when her sibling is born. Similarly, the stay-at-home parent of a single child may experience a sense of loss when the child begins school. **Situational loss,** on the other hand, is experienced as a result of an unpredictable event, including traumatic injury, disease, death, or national disaster.

Another type of loss is **anticipatory loss,** in which a person displays loss and grief behaviors for a loss that has yet to take place. Anticipatory loss is often seen in the families of patients with serious and life-threatening illnesses and serves to lessen the impact of the actual loss of a family member.

> *Think back to Yvonne Malic, the 20-year-old single mother of the premature neonate described in the beginning of the chapter. The nurse could use knowledge of anticipatory loss to assist Yvonne in coping with the seriousness of her neonate's condition.*

Grieving

Grief is the emotional reaction to loss. It occurs with loss caused by separation as well as with loss caused by death. Many people who divorce experience grief; loss of a body part, a job, a house, or a pet may cause grief. **Bereavement** is the state of grieving during which a person goes through a grief reaction. **Mourning** is the period of acceptance of loss and grief during which the person learns to deal with the loss. Bereavement, which is experienced by both the patient and the family, may have profound health consequences that require additional care. Bereaved people often neglect their health to an extreme, whereas mourning is characterized by a return to more normal living habits.

Grief Reactions

Reactions to grief and dying are similar. The stages of these reactions overlap and vary among individuals (see Factors That Affect Grief and Death, later in this chapter). One person may skip a reaction stage, whereas another may repeat an earlier stage. Each person is different, and patients and family members may be at different reaction stages.

Engel (1964) was among the first to define stages of grief. Engel's six stages are:
1. Shock and disbelief
2. Developing awareness
3. Restitution
4. Resolving the loss
5. Idealization
6. Outcome

Shock and disbelief are usually defined as refusal to accept the fact of loss, followed by a stunned or numb response: "No, not me." Developing awareness is characterized by physical and emotional responses such as anger, feeling empty, and crying: "Why me?" Restitution involves the rituals surrounding loss; with death, it includes religious, cultural, or social expressions of mourning, such as funeral services. Resolving the loss involves dealing with the void left by the loss. Idealization is the exaggeration of the good qualities that the person or object had, followed by acceptance of the loss and a lessened need to focus on it. Outcome, the final resolution of the grief process, includes dealing with loss as a common life occurrence.

> *Remember Yvonne, the single mother of the premature neonate. The nurse could use knowledge of the stages of grief when assessing Yvonne to establish the most appropriate interventions for her plan of care.*

Reflective Practice
Challenge to Ethical and Legal Skills

Anna Maria Giordano was a 49-year-old female attorney who had recently suffered a major cerebral hemorrhage. I came in contact with Ms. Giordano on one of my off-site clinical rotations when I accompanied a social worker for a day at a large medical center. According to most of the nurses and physicians, and the documentation in her chart, her prognosis looked very poor. Due to the fact that she was a lawyer, her advance directives were very clear, appearing to say exactly what she wanted. In essence, her advance directive stated that if she was in a comatose condition and that it appeared as if there was no hope for recovery, she did not want life-sustaining treatment. Although testing did not reveal brain death, almost all the physicians agreed that her condition had little to no hope for improvement. However, one neurosurgeon felt that her condition was improving, with hopes for her recovery; therefore, he had no intention of stopping the life-sustaining treatment. Her family members from Boston had come earlier in the week to discuss treatment options and were given two points of view by two different physicians. Upon hearing the determination of a poor prognosis along with seeing no improvement in the patient's condition over the past few weeks, it was clear from her advance directives that this is not what she wanted.

Thinking Outside the Box: Possible Courses of Action

- Ignore the entire situation: it didn't entirely concern me, since I was only observing as a nursing student for 1 day.
- Talk to the social worker about what I thought was stated in the advance directives, and ask why it wasn't being followed.
- Challenge the doctor as to why he was telling the family that the patient was improving when her assessments for the past 3 weeks had shown no improvement.

Evaluating a Good Outcome: How Do I Define Success?

- The patient is properly diagnosed and her wishes from her advance directives are followed as clearly as they are stated.
- Since the patient is unable to speak, her power of attorney is able to convey what the patient would want.
- The family and the patient's power of attorney are fully informed about the patient's condition so that they can make an educated decision based on what the patient would want.
- My personal and professional integrity are affirmed.

Personal Learning: Here's to the Future!

I chose to talk to the social worker about the patient's advance directives. The social worker was very aware of the situation, explaining that in the past, this neurosurgeon had given other patients' families more optimistic views of the situation, refusing to stop life-sustaining treatment. The social worker explained that she was in the process of bringing this issue to an ethics committee to discuss the situation and hoped that something would be resolved. She also explained that advance directives are often difficult to follow precisely. If the patient is unable to communicate, then the power of attorney takes over, trying his or her best to do what the patient would want. At these times, it can become very subjective. Therefore, follow-

ing the advance directives is not as simple as one would think it would be.

Although my actions were not extraordinary in this situation, I felt that I learned a quite a bit about advance directives, especially trying to honor the patient's and family's wishes. I had learned about advance directives in the past in my previous classes. However, this was the first time I had ever had to deal with them in actual practice. I was able to see how difficult it can be when making such an important decision. I was impressed by the way that the social worker was handling the case; I only hope that I would act in a similar fashion if I were ever faced with a situation like this in the future.

Reflection

How do you think you would respond in a similar situation? Why? Are there any factors that might affect your response? If so, explain what these factors are and their possible effect. What do you think might be influencing the neurosurgeon's refusal to end the life-sustaining treatment? How would you respond to this neurosurgeon? In what stage of grief do you think that the neurosurgeon is? The nursing student? The social worker? What does this tell you about yourself and about the adequacy of your skills for professional practice? Can you think of other ways to respond? What

other skills (cognitive, interpersonal, technical, ethical/legal) would you need to respond well in this situation? Have you ever been involved in a situation involving an advance directive? If so, were the patient's wishes followed? If not, why not? Do you agree with the criteria used to evaluate a successful outcome? Was professional integrity affirmed? Explain.

Kathryn Southerton, Georgetown University

Kübler-Ross (1969), considered a pioneer in the study of grief and death reactions, defined five stages of reaction similar to Engel's. These stages—(1) denial and isolation, (2) anger, (3) bargaining, (4) depression, and (5) acceptance—are discussed in detail in Responses to Dying and Death. Other theorists describe similar stages. More important than the actual

stages of any given grief reaction, however, is the idea that grief is a process that varies from person to person.

Normal Versus Dysfunctional Grief

Both normal and dysfunctional grief may be delayed, and normal grief may be either abbreviated or anticipatory. Abbreviated grief is of short duration but is genuine; anticipatory grief occurs before the actual loss, as in the extended terminal illness of a family member. Assessment priorities, expected outcomes, and interventions for patients and families experiencing anticipatory grieving are illustrated in Examples of NANDA Nursing Diagnoses.

Dysfunctional grief is abnormal or distorted; it may be either unresolved or inhibited. In unresolved grief, a person may have trouble expressing feelings of loss or may deny them; unresolved grief also describes a state of bereavement that extends over a lengthy period. In inhibited grief, a person suppresses feelings of grief and may instead manifest somatic symptoms.

DYING AND DEATH

Dying may occur suddenly as a result of an accident, injury, or pathologic crisis, such as a heart attack; or it may occur after a prolonged experience of debilitating disease, such as cancer, acquired immunodeficiency syndrome (AIDS), or multiple sclerosis. Whereas some welcome death and even hasten death, choosing the time and manner of their dying, others fear death and will try anything to delay it. Given the choice, some choose to die at home surrounded by loved ones. Others die alone or in intensive care units surrounded by healthcare professionals and technological equipment. A patient's wishes should, if possible, be followed. See the Research in Nursing box, Promoting Quality End-of-Life Care. Rights of dying people are listed in Box 33-1.

> *Think back to Anna Maria Giordano, the 49-year-old woman described in the beginning of this chapter. Knowledge about the rights of dying people would provide the nurse with a basis for ensuring that the patient's advance directive wishes are followed.*

Signs of Impending Death

The clinical signs of impending or approaching death include:
- Inability to swallow
- Pitting edema
- Decreased gastrointestinal and urinary tract activity
- Bowel and bladder incontinence
- Loss of motion, sensation, and reflexes
- Elevated temperature, but cold or clammy skin; cyanosis
- Lowered blood pressure
- Noisy or irregular respiration
- Cheyne-Stokes respirations

The patient may or may not lose consciousness. It is often helpful to prepare family members and significant others for the transformations that signal impending death. Nuland's popular books *How We Die* (1994) and *The Wisdom of the Body* (1997) are useful resources.

Definitions of Death

In 1981, the President's Commission for the Study of Ethical Problems in Medicine and Biomedical and Behavioral Research defined **death** as present when an individual has sustained either (1) irreversible cessation of circulatory and respiratory functions, or (2) irreversible cessation of all functions of the entire brain, including the brain stem.

A Harvard University committee stated that the following characteristics must be present for at least 24 hours before death can be declared:
- Lack of receptivity and responsiveness
- Lack of movement or breathing
- Lack of reflexes
- Flat encephalogram

In the United States, there are currently three definitions of death in the literature—the traditional heart–lung definition, the whole-brain definition, and the higher-brain definition.

Heart–lung death is the irreversible cessation of spontaneous respiration and circulation; the accepted criterion for death until the 1960s emerged as a definition of death from the historical idea that the flow of body fluids was essential for life.

Whole-brain death is the irreversible cessation of all functions of the entire brain, including the brain stem; this definition emerged in the 1960s from the belief that neocortical functioning is the key to the definition of a human being. Most protocols require two separate clinical examinations, including induction of painful stimuli, pupillary responses to light, oculovestibular testing, and apnea testing. To enhance accuracy, standard practice is not to perform brain death testing while a patient is hypothermic, hypotensive, or under the influence of neuromuscular blocking agents or barbiturates.

Higher-brain death is the irreversible loss of all "higher" brain functions, of cognitive function; this definition was suggested in the 1970s and emerged from the belief that the brain is more important than the spinal cord and that the critical functions are the individual's personality, conscious life, uniqueness, and capacity for remembering, judging, reasoning, acting, enjoying, and worrying (Ott, 1995).

Good Dying

Since the 1995 publication of the Study to Understand Prognoses and Preferences for Outcomes and Risks of Treatments (SUPPORT), there has been a concentrated focus in the United States on improving the care given to dying persons and their families (SUPPORT Principal Investigators, 1995). An example is the Last Acts project funded by the Robert Wood Johnson Foundation. At the end of 2002, Last Acts published the report *Means to a Better End: A Report on Dying in America Today*. The 50 states and the District of Columbia were rated on eight "key elements" of end-of-life care (state advance directive policies, location of death, hospice use, hospital end-of-life services, care in intensive care units at the end of life, pain among nursing home residents, state pain policies, and palliative care–certified physicians and nurses). Referred to as a "state-by-state report card," America was seen as doing "a mediocre job of caring for its most seriously ill and dying patients (Robert Wood Johnson Foundation, 2002). Additionally, Last Acts reported that almost 60% of 1,000 persons interviewed rated the health care system's care

Grieving may be defined as the state in which an individual or family experiences a natural human response involving psychosocial and physiologic reactions to an actual or perceived loss (person, object, function, status, relationship). NANDA nursing diagnoses include the following:

Anticipatory Grieving: Intellectual and emotional responses and behaviors by which individuals work through the process of modifying self-concept based on the perception of potential loss (NANDA, 1994)

Dysfunctional Grieving: Extended, unsuccessful use of intellectual and emotional responses by which individuals attempt to work through the process of modifying self-concept based upon the perception of loss (NANDA, 1994)

Because nurses encounter patients dealing with anticipatory grieving more frequently than patients dysfunctionally grieving, assessment priorities, expected outcomes, and interventions will be given for anticipatory grieving.

Assessment Priorities
- Determine the exact nature of the anticipated or potential loss.
- Explore factors that are contributing to the importance or significance of the anticipated loss.
- Assess concerns, fears, feelings, and hopes related to the anticipated loss.
- Assess adequacy of knowledge and coping mechanisms.
- Recognize personal strengths and available resources, including present support system.

Expected Outcomes
The patient will:
- Express grief openly and progress through stages of grief with appropriate grief work
- Share concerns with significant others and seek needed help
- Make decisions about the future that advance best interests
- Demonstrate eventual resolution of grief by self-report, appearance, and resumption of usual activities of daily living

Interventions
Interventions for anticipatory grieving are determined by the type of loss (eg, body part; death of self, a significant other, or child), the extent of the loss to the individual and family, and what other support the individual or family has. Examples of interventions are the following:
- Use interpersonal skills to demonstrate empathy for patient's situation and commitment to patient's well-being.
- Encourage the patient to share concerns, feelings, fears, and hopes openly.
- Respond to inquiries honestly, compassionately, and in a manner that does not deprive the patients of realistic hope.
- Promote grief work through each stage of grieving (see box below). Support the patient and "nudge" the patient to begin the next stage of grieving as appropriate.
- Make appropriate referrals (see earlier listing of bereavement resources).
- Alert the patient who is moving through the grief work slowly of the signs of dysfunctional grieving and instruct about how to obtain help should this happen; referral for counseling may be indicated.

Stages of Grief and Related Grief Work
Denial
- Initially support and then strive to increase the development of awareness (when individual indicates readiness for awareness).
Isolation
- Listen and spend designated time consistently with person and family.
- Offer the person and family opportunity to explore their emotions.
- Reflect on past losses and acknowledge loss behavior (past and present).
Depression
- Begin with simple problem solving and move toward acceptance.
- Enhance self-worth through positive reinforcement.
- Identify the level of depression and indications of suicidal behavior or ideas.
- Be consistent and establish times daily to speak with the person and family.

Anger
- Allow for crying to release this energy.
- Listen to and communicate concern.
- Encourage concerned support from significant others as well as professional support.
Guilt
- Listen and communicate concern.
- Allow for crying.
- Promote more direct expression of feelings.
- Explore methods to resolve grief.
Fear
- Help the person and family recognize the feeling.
- Explain that this will help cope with life.
- Explore the person's and family's attitudes about loss, death, etc.
Rejection
- Allow for verbal expression of this feeling state to diminish the emotional strain.
- Recognize that expression of anger may create a rejection of self to significant others.

(From Carpenito-Moyet, L. J. [2004]. *Nursing diagnosis: Application to clinical practice* [10th ed., 349–350]. Philadelphia: Lippincott Williams & Wilkins. Used with permission.)

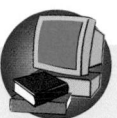

Research in Nursing Making a Difference
Promoting Quality End-of-Life Care

National studies continue to report poor patient and family satisfaction with end-of-life care in all settings.

Related Research
Kirchoff, K. T., Spuhler, V., Walker, L., Hutton, A., Cole, V., & Clemmer, T. (2000). Intensive care nurses' experiences with end-of-life care. *American Journal of Critical Care, 9*(1), 36–42.

The purpose of this project was to address end-of-life care by intensive care unit (ICU) nurses through focus groups with nurses and to listen to the stories of the people who are major witnesses and providers of that care. The research questions addressed in the study were: (1) What do ICU nurses consider "good" end-of-life care? (2) How do nurses describe their experiences of shifting from curative nursing interventions to end-of-life care? (3) What are ICU nurses' perceptions of care

dilemmas and barriers to providing quality end-of-life care? "Good" end-of-life care in the ICU was described as ensuring that the patient is as pain free as possible and that the patient's comfort and dignity are maintained. Involvement of the patient's family is crucial. A clear, accurate prognosis and continuity of care are important. Switching from curative care to comfort care is awkward.

Relevance to Nursing Practice
These researchers noted that disagreement among patients' family members or among caregivers, uncertainty about prognosis, and communication problems further complicate end-of-life care in ICUs. Changes in the physical environment, education about end-of-life care, staff support, and better communication would improve care of dying patients and their families.

of dying patients as fair or lower, while only 10% ranked the system as very good or excellent.

Participants in a recent study identified six major components of a good death: (1) pain and symptom management, (2) clear decision making, (3) preparation for death, (4) completion, (5) contributing to others, and (6) affirmation of the whole person. The six themes are process-oriented attributes of good death, and each has biomedical, psychological, social, and spiritual components. Physicians' discussion of a good death differed greatly from those of other groups. Physicians offered the most biomedical perspective, and patients, families, and other healthcare professionals defined a broad range of attributes integral to the quality of dying (Steinhauser et al., 2000).

The accompanying Focus on the Older Adult displays quality indicators for end-of-life care. While the American Geriatric Society developed these indicators, they apply to persons of all

ages. Nurses play a critical role in focusing the team's attention on meeting the needs of dying persons and their families.

Responses to Dying and Death

Although each person reacts to the knowledge of impending death or to loss in his or her own way, there are similarities in the psychosocial responses to the situation. Kübler-Ross has studied the emotional responses to death and dying in depth, and nursing and other helping professions have used her findings extensively.

The stages of dying, much like the stages of grief, may overlap, and the duration of any stage may range from as little as a few hours to as long as months. The process varies from person to person. Some people may be in one stage for such a short time that it seems as if they skipped that stage. Sometimes a

---

BOX 33-1 The Dying Person's Bill of Rights

I have the right to be treated as a living human being until I die.

I have the right to maintain a sense of hopefulness, however changing its focus may be.

I have the right to be cared for by those who can maintain a sense of hopefulness, however changing this might be.

I have the right to express my feelings and emotions about my approaching death in my own way.

I have the right to participate in decisions concerning my care.

I have the right to expect continuing medical and nursing attention even though "cure" goals must be changed to "comfort" goals.

I have the right not to die alone.

I have the right to be free from pain.

I have the right to have my questions answered honestly.

I have the right not to be deceived.

I have the right to have help from and for my family in accepting my death.

I have the right to die in peace and dignity.

I have a right to retain my individuality and not be judged for my decisions, which may be contrary to beliefs of others.

I have the right to discuss and enlarge my religious and/or spiritual experiences, whatever these may mean to others.

I have the right to expect that the sanctity of the human body will be respected after death.

I have the right to be cared for by caring, sensitive, knowledgeable people who will attempt to understand my needs and will be able to gain some satisfaction in helping me face my death.

Reprinted with permission from Barbus, A. J. (1975). The dying person's bill of rights. *American Journal of Nursing, 75*(1), 99.

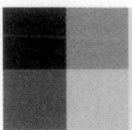

Focus on the Older Adult
Measuring Quality of Care at the End of Life

The American Geriatric Society developed the following statement of principles about quality care at the end of life, but these indicators would seem to work well for persons of all ages:

1. *Physical and emotional symptoms.* Pain, shortness of breath, fatigue, depression, fear, anxiety, nausea, skin breakdown, and other physical and emotional problems often destroy the quality of life at its end. Symptom management is regularly deficient. Care systems should focus on these needs and ensure that people can count on a comfortable and meaningful end of their lives.
2. *Support of function and autonomy.* Even with an inevitable and progressive decline with fatal illness, much can be done to maintain personal dignity and self-respect. Achieving better functional outcomes and greater autonomy should be valued.
3. *Advance care planning.* Often, the experience of patient and family can be improved just by planning ahead for likely problems, so that decisions can reflect the patient's preferences and circumstances rather than responding to crises.
4. *Aggressive care near death—site of death, CPR, and hospitalization.* Although aggressive care is often justified, most patients would prefer to have avoided it when short-term outcome is death. High rates of medical interventions near death should prompt further examination of provider judgment and care system design.
5. *Patient and family satisfaction.* The dying patient's peace of mind and the family's perception of the patient's care and comfort are extremely important. In the long run, we can hope that the time at the end of life will be especially precious, not merely tolerable. We must measure both patient and family satisfaction with these elements: the decision-making process, the care given, the outcomes achieved, and the extent to which opportunities were provided to complete life in a meaningful way.

6. *Global quality of life.* Often a patient's assessment of overall well-being illuminates successes and shortcomings in care which are not apparent in more specific measures. Quality of life can be good despite declining physical health, and care systems that achieve this should be valued.
7. *Family burden.* How health care is provided affects whether families have serious financial and emotional effects from the costs of care and the challenges of direct caregiving. Current and future pressures on funding health care are likely to displace more responsibility for services and payment onto families.
8. *Survival time.* With pressures upon health care resources likely to increase, there is new reason to worry that death will be accepted too readily. Purchasers and patients need to know survival times vary across plans and provider systems. In conjunction with information about symptoms, satisfaction, and the other domains listed here, such measures will allow insights into the priorities and tradeoffs within each care system.
9. *Provider continuity and skill.* Only with enduring relationships with professional caregivers can patient and family develop trust, communicate effectively, and develop reliable plans. The providers also must have the relevant skills, including rehabilitation, symptom control, and psychological support. Care systems must demonstrate competent performance on continuity and provider skill.
10. *Bereavement.* Often health care stops with the patient's death, but the suffering of the family goes on. Survivors may benefit with relatively modest interventions.

Used with permission, The American Geriatric Society.

---

person returns to a previous stage. According to Kübler-Ross, the five stages of dying are:

1. Denial and isolation
2. Anger
3. Bargaining
4. Depression
5. Acceptance

In the denial and isolation stage, the patient denies that he or she will die, may repress what is discussed, and may isolate himself or herself from reality. The patient may think, "They made a mistake in the diagnosis. Maybe they mixed up my records with someone else's."

In the anger stage, the patient expresses rage and hostility and adopts a "why me?" attitude: "Why me? I quit smoking and I watched what I ate. Why did this happen to me?"

In the bargaining stage, the patient tries to barter for more time: "If I can just make it to my son's graduation I'll be satisfied. Just let me live until then." Many patients put their personal affairs in order, make wills, and fulfill last wishes, such as trips, visiting relatives, and so forth. It is important to meet

these wishes, if possible, because bargaining helps patients move into later stages of dying.

In the depression stage, the patient goes through a period of grief before death. The grief is characterized by crying and not speaking much: "I waited all these years to see my daughter get married. And now I may not be here to see her walk down the aisle. I can't bear the thought of not being there for the wedding—and of not seeing my grandchildren."

When the stage of acceptance is reached, the patient feels tranquil. She or he has accepted death and is prepared to die. The patient may think, "I've tied up all the loose ends: made the will, made arrangements for my daughter to live with her grandparents. Now I can go in peace knowing everyone will be fine."

Terminal Illness

In the case of a **terminal illness,** an illness in which death is expected within a limited space of time, the physician is usually responsible for deciding what, when, and how the patient should be told. The nurse, along with members of the clergy and other healthcare professionals, may be involved with these decisions and in discussing the patient's condition with him or her. Most patients want to know their diagnosis and prognosis as soon as possible so that they can begin appropriate planning and take care of business and personal affairs. It is critical for terminally ill patients and their families to have some sense of how the disease is most likely to progress and what this will mean for the patient. All who are involved with the patient's care should know exactly what the patient and the family have been told; members of the patient's healthcare team need to communicate among themselves. Cultural influences may dictate how much information is desired and which family members are to be informed.

An expert in "breaking bad news" suggests six basic rules to facilitate better patient outcomes (Buckman, 1992):

1. Sit face-to-face in a private place and have the discussion at a time when the patient is not distracted or in great pain.
2. Ask the patient how much he or she already knows about the condition, so you can align your discussion at the proper level of detail.
3. Ask the patient how much he or she wants to know.
4. Give the information in "small chunks" and stop occasionally to check that the information is being understood.
5. Acknowledge any emotional reaction from the patient and respond to that reaction with sincerity and empathy.
6. Summarize, ask for questions, and have a clear idea of when you will meet again.

Impact on Patient

Many patients realize without being told that they are suffering from a terminal illness; they often pick up this knowledge from nonverbal communication by their families and by healthcare professionals. Patients must be allowed to go through the stages of the grieving process and to make decisions about their care; they must be supported in their decision making. Competent patients have the right to consent to and refuse any and all indicated medical treatment—even life-sustaining treatment—and should be made aware of this right. In the past, patients and family members complained about receiving care they did not want and of not being allowed to die. In today's climate of cost-conscious decision making, some patients and family members are complaining that they are being denied costly life-sustaining treatment because of inadequate personal funds or insurance or because they are deemed a poor "investment" of scarce resources.

Impact on Family

The family and significant others of terminally ill patients should be encouraged to participate in planning the patient's care. Healthcare personnel should be available to discuss the patient's condition with family members and should offer support and care as the family begins the grieving process. The family may want to make arrangements with the patient for funeral or memorial services, depending on which stage of grief both the patient and the family members are in.

Palliative Care

Palliative care means taking care of the whole person—body, mind, and spirit, heart and soul. It looks at dying as something natural and personal. The goal of palliative care is to give patients with life-threatening illnesses the best quality of life they can have by the aggressive management of symptoms. Palliative care is sometimes called hospice care. Box 33-2 illustrates the five principles of palliative care.

Ethical and Legal Dimensions

The ethical and legal implications of nursing are discussed in general in Chapters 6 and 7. A brief discussion of nursing's ethical and legal responsibilities in end-of-life care follows. Multiple treatment options and sophisticated life-support technologies may make it difficult to draw the line between promoting life and needlessly prolonging the dying process. In these cases, healthcare decision making is complicated for patients and healthcare professionals alike. Patients have a legally and morally protected right to consent to and refuse any and all indicated medical therapies. Legal foundations for the patient's freedom to choose include the common law right of self-determination and the constitutionally supported right of privacy. Calls to legalize physician-assisted suicide and physician-administered lethal injections ("aid in dying") pose new ethical challenges. As patients and families struggle with end-of-life treatment decisions, they are increasingly looking to nurses for information, advice, and support. Nursing care priorities are highlighted in the accompanying Examples of Nursing Diagnoses box. See Box 33-3 for related Internet re-

---

BOX 33-2 Five Principles of Palliative Care

1. Palliative care respects the goals, likes, and choices of the dying person and his or her loved ones . . . helping them to understand the illness and what can be expected from it, and to figure out what is most important during this time.
2. Palliative care looks after the medical, emotional, social, and spiritual needs of the dying person . . . with a focus on making sure he or she is comfortable, not left alone, and able to look back on his or her life and find peace.
3. Palliative care supports the needs of family members . . . helping them with the responsibilities of caregiving and even supporting them as they grieve.
4. Palliative care helps to gain access to needed healthcare providers and appropriate care settings . . . involving various kinds of trained providers in different settings, tailored to the needs of the patient and his or her family.
5. Palliative care builds ways to provide excellent care at the end of life . . . through education of care providers, appropriate health policies, and adequate funding from insurers and the government.

Used with permission. The Robert Wood Johnson Foundation, Last Acts Palliative Care Task Force, "Five Principles of Palliative Care," 1999. Special supplement to *Advances, 2, 3*

Examples of NANDA Nursing Diagnoses | Decisional Conflict

Patients and the surrogate decision makers for incompetent patients frequently feel overwhelmed when they need to make life-and-death decisions about end-of-life care. The NANDA diagnosis for this response follows:

Decisional Conflict: The state of uncertainty about course of action to be taken when choice among competing actions involves risk, loss, or challenge to personal life values (NANDA, 1994)

Assessment Priorities

The objective of assessment is to identify individuals and families who are at high risk for decisional conflict and to provide the support they need to make appropriate end-of-life care decisions that advance the patient's interests before problems develop. Potential problems when this need is overlooked include postponement of decision making, which interferes with the patient receiving optimal care; vacillation in decision making, which disturbs continuity of care for the patient; and escalation of conflict concerning decision making, which may result in a standoff between participating parties—the patient, individual family members, and healthcare professionals.

- Detect difficulties with making decisions: fear; insufficient or erroneous information; inadequate support; conflict between religious convictions, personal moral beliefs, and choice one wants to make; reluctance to assume responsibility for making life-and-death decision.
- Identify what is causing the decision making to be hard for the patient or family and what type of information or support could reverse this.
- Identify potential conflicts between what the patient wants and what his or her family or caregivers believe should be done.
- Observe the patient or his or her surrogate decision makers for physical signs of distress that reflect feeling overwhelmed by the decision that needs to be made: signs of fatigue and general exhaustion; signs of agitation and distress; signs of growing anger and alienation.
- Read the chart carefully to identify decisions that are pending and note the lack of movement toward a decision or toward resolution of existing conflict.

Expected Outcomes

The morally and legally valid decision-maker will achieve the following:

- Describe care options (including the option of nontreatment), listing the advantages and disadvantages of each
- Seek clarification of options, if necessary, and whatever support is needed
- Express fears, concerns, and hopes
- Make an informed and voluntary choice
- Make end-of-life decisions that reflect the patient's values and goals, advancing his or her interests
- Make end-of-life decisions that are consistent with the aims of medicine and nursing

Interventions

Nursing measures revolve around identifying and supporting the morally and legally valid decision maker. The following should be considered:

- Competent patients—those who can (1) understand the information needed to make the decision, (2) reason in accord with a relatively consistent set of values, and (3) communicate a preference—have the right to consent to and to refuse any and all indicated medical treatment.
- Surrogates of previously competent patients are to be guided by what is known about the patient's values and preferences. These surrogates may be designated in an advance directive, or there may be state or province law designating a hierarchy of surrogates, such as spouse, parent, adult child, sibling; the morally valid surrogate is the one who best knows the patient and the patient's preferences.
- Surrogates deciding for a never-competent patient (child or profoundly retarded adult) must be guided by a determination of what is in the patient's best interests by referring to more objective and socially shared values.

The nurse clarifies the goal of treatment (cure, stabilization of functioning, preparation for a comfortable and dignified death) and makes sure that treatment decisions are consistent with this goal. Nursing intervention may be helpful in making sure that everyone is clear about the goal of care and changes in the goal of care as the patient's condition changes. Because some physicians are reluctant to accept preparation for a comfortable, dignified death as an appropriate goal of medicine, some patients have received unwanted care that needlessly prolonged their dying. Conversely, decisions are being made today for financial and other reasons that deprive patients of wanted end-of-life care.

The nurse serves as an advocate for the patient and the family unless what the patient or family wants violates the profession of nursing and nursing's code of ethics or one's own conscience. Interventions include the following:

- Providing whatever information and support the patient or family needs to make an informed and voluntary decision
- Referring the patient or family to sources that can clarify problematic aspects of the decision, such as religious authority, ethicist, legal counsel
- Identifying and addressing coercive influences on decision making, being sensitive to cultural norms; for example, whereas a controlling husband may be violating his wife's freedom to make autonomous choices in one culture, in another, it is customary for the husband (or male elder in the family) to make choices for a woman.

Documentation of end-of-life care preferences of competent, or previously competent, patients is important. This includes a written record of communication, a living will, durable power of attorney for healthcare, and a medical advance directive. These preferences must be communicated to those who are ordering care.

- Mediating sources of conflict
- Referring patient or family to ethics consult team or ethics committee if conflict cannot be resolved

---

BOX 33-3 Internet Resources for End-of-Life Care

Aging With Dignity

http://www.agingwithdignity.org

A not-for-profit organization founded to affirm and safeguard human dignity and to promote better care of the dying. Makes available the "Five Wishes" living will.

Choice in Dying

http://www.choices.org

A national, not-for-profit organization devoted to right-to-die issues and end-of-life decision making. The site features a wide range of educational materials as well as state-specific advance directives that can be downloaded from the site at no charge.

End of Life Physician Education Resource Center (EPERC)

http://www.eperc.mcw.edu

A central repository for educational materials and information about end-of-life issues.

Last Acts

http://www.lastacts.org

A call-to-action campaign to improve care at the end of life. Its goals are to bring death-related issues out in the open and help individuals and organizations pursue better ways to care for the dying. Among this organizations many resources is the video *Asking About Advance Directives: Scenarios for Healthcare Providers*.

Tool Kit for Nurturing Excellence at End-of-Life Transitions (TNEEL)

http://www.son.washington.edu/departments/bnhs/pain/tneel.asp

Available on CD-ROM, this tool kit addresses six areas: ethical concerns, goals of comfort (includes pain management), communication and relationships, grief, the impact of dying (epidemiology, economics, service and delivery systems of care, resource utilization), and well-being (includes quality of life, spirituality, complementary therapies).

Supportive Care of the Dying: A Coalition for Compassionate Care

http://www.careofdying.org

Thirteen Catholic healthcare organizations and the Catholic Health Association have joined together to promote culture change that will bring supportive care, compassionate relief of suffering, and pain and symptom management to persons with life-threatening illness and their caregivers. The overall goal of the coalition is to develop and test innovative projects and to provide support to member organizations as they initiate systemic change in the care of persons affected by life-threatening illness.

---

sources for patients and families experiencing conflict about decision making.

Advance Directives

Decisions about healthcare are becoming increasingly complex. Patients, family members, and healthcare professionals alike are voicing frustration as they grapple with complex decisions about prolonging life. Some of the most difficult cases involve patients who are no longer able (competent) to indicate their treatment preferences. Two kinds of written **advance directives** can minimize difficulties by allowing individuals to state in advance what their choices would be for healthcare should certain circumstances develop. Living wills provide specific instructions about the kinds of healthcare that should be provided or foregone in particular situations. A durable power of attorney for healthcare appoints an agent the person trusts to make decisions in the event of subsequent incapacity. A combination directive is illustrated in Figure 33-1. One popular directive in the United States entitled *Five Wishes* allows individuals to specify:

1. The person I want to make care decisions for me when I can't
2. The kind of medical treatment I want or don't want
3. How comfortable I want to be
4. How I want people to treat me
5. What I want my loved ones to know.

Many means have been suggested to ensure that adult patients have an opportunity to learn about and use advance directives to indicate their wishes about life-prolonging treat-

ment and to appoint surrogate decision makers should they lose decision-making capacity. Nurses have an important role to play in facilitating this dialog. In the United States, the Patient Self-Determination Act of 1990 requires all hospitals to inform their patients about advance directives. Because the status of advance directives varies from state to state, it is important for nurses to be familiar with federal and state laws concerning these directives. Nurses can also be instrumental in developing institutional policies that ensure that patients on admission are encouraged to talk with family, significant others, and healthcare professionals about their treatment preferences.

> *Recall Anna Maria Giordano, the 49-year-old attorney described in the beginning of the chapter. The nurse would use knowledge of this patient's advance directives to assist with developing an appropriate plan of care that conforms to the legal and ethical guidelines of the state in which the patient is located.*

Do-Not-Resuscitate or No-Code Orders

To prevent the improper use of cardiopulmonary resuscitation, which is designed to prevent unexpected death, some physicians will write do not resuscitate (DNR), or no code, on the chart of a patient if the patient or surrogate has expressed a wish that there be no attempts to resuscitate the patient. A **do-not-resuscitate order** means simply that: that no attempts are to be made to resuscitate a patient who stops breathing or whose

(text continues on page 884)

D.C., Maryland and Virginia

ADVANCE DIRECTIVE

My Durable Power of Attorney for Health Care, Living Will and Other Wishes

I, _____ , write this document as a directive regarding my medical care.

Put the initials of your name by the choices you want.

PART 1. MY DURABLE POWER OF ATTORNEY FOR HEALTH CARE.

_____   I appoint this person to make decisions about my medical care if there ever comes a time when I
                              cannot make those decisions myself:

NAME _____ PHONE HOME _____ WORK _____

ADDRESS _____

_____

           If the person above cannot or will not make decisions for me, I appoint this person:

NAME _____ PHONE HOME _____ WORK _____

ADDRESS _____

_____

_____   I have not appointed anyone to make health care decisions for me in this or any other document.

***I want the person I have appointed, my doctors, my family, and others to be guided by the decisions I
have made below:***

PART 2. MY LIVING WILL.

These are my wishes for my future medical care if there ever comes a time when I can't make these decisions
for myself.

A. **These are my wishes if I have a *terminal condition:***
     Life-Sustaining Treatments

_____   I do not want life-sustaining treatments (including CPR) started. If life-sustaining treatments are
                                          started, I want them stopped.
_____   I want life-sustaining treatments that my doctors think are best for me.

_____   Other wishes: _____

Artificial Nutrition and Hydration

_____   I do not want artificial nutrition and hydration started if it would be the main treatment keeping me
                                          alive. If artificial nutrition and hydration
                                          is started, I want it stopped.
_____   I want artificial nutrition and hydration even if it is the main treatment keeping me alive.

_____   Other wishes: _____

Comfort Care

_____   I want to be kept as comfortable and free of pain as possible, even if such care prolongs my dying
                                          or shortens my life.

_____   Other wishes: _____

B. **These are my wishes if I am ever in a *persistent vegetative state:***

Life-Sustaining Treatments

_____   I do not want life-sustaining treatments (including CPR) started. If life-sustaining treatments are
                                          started, I want them stopped.
_____   I want life-sustaining treatments that my doctors think are best for me.

_____   Other wishes: _____

FIGURE 33-1 Example of an advance directive. (Used with permission of District of Columbia Hospital
Association, Washington, DC.)

Artificial Nutrition and Hydration

_____   I do not want artificial nutrition and hydration started if it would be the main treatment keeping me alive.
If artificial nutrition and hydration is started, I want it stopped.
_____   I want artificial nutrition and hydration even if it is the main treatment keeping me alive.
_____   Other wishes: _____

Comfort Care

_____   I want to be kept as comfortable as possible, even if such care prolongs my dying or shortens my life
_____   Other wishes: _____

C. **Other Direction**

You have the right to be involved in all decisions about your medical care, even those parts not dealing with terminal conditions or persistent vegetative states. If you have wishes not covered in other parts of this document, please indicate them here.

_____

_____

PART 3. OTHER WISHES.

A. **Organ Donation**
_____   I do not wish to donate any of my organs or tissues.
_____   I want to donate all of my organs and tissues.
_____   I only want to donate these organs and tissues: _____
_____   Other wishes: _____

Autopsy
_____   I do not want an autopsy.
_____   I agree to an autopsy if my doctors wish it.
_____   Other wishes: _____

If you wish to say more about any of the above choices, or If you have any other statements to make about your medical care, you may do so on a separate sheet of paper. If you do so, put here the number of pages you are adding: _____

PART 4. SIGNATURES.

You and two witnesses must sign this document for it to be legal.

A. **Your Signature**

By my signature below I show that I understand the purpose and the effect of this document.

SIGNATURE _____ DATE _____

ADDRESS _____

B. **Your Witnesses' Signatures**
I believe the person who has signed this advance directive to be of sound mind, that he/she signed or acknowledged this advance directive in my presence, and that he/she appears not to be acting under pressure, duress, fraud or undue influence. I am not related to the person making this advance directive by blood, marriage or adoption, nor, to the best of my knowledge, am I named in his/her will. I am not the person appointed in this advance directive. I am not a health care provider or an employee of health care provider who is now, or has been in the past, responsible for the care of the person making this advance directive.

Witness #1

SIGNATURE _____ DATE _____

ADDRESS _____

Witness #2

SIGNATURE _____ DATE _____

ADDRESS _____

FIGURE 33-1 _Continued_

heart stops beating. However, many physicians are reluctant to write these orders, especially when this issue is a source of conflict between the patient and family or between individual family members.

In some cases, a physician who believes the patient will not benefit from resuscitative measures may indicate verbally to the nurse that only a slow-code (or "show-code") should be called; that is, in the case of cardiopulmonary or respiratory arrest, calling a code and resuscitating the patient are to be delayed until these measures will be ineffectual. Slow-codes are never good practice, and many healthcare institutions now have policies forbidding their use. It is likely that a nurse could be charged with negligence in the event of a slow-code and resultant patient death.

The standard of care still obligates healthcare professionals to attempt resuscitation if a patient stops breathing or his or her heart stops (cardiopulmonary arrest) and there is no DNR order to the contrary. For this reason, it is important for nurses to clarify a patient's code status if the probable benefits of resuscitation are negligible or if the nurse has reason to believe a patient would not want to be resuscitated. Many states now allow patients living at home to craft special orders that allow emergency medical technicians called to the home in the event of cardiopulmonary arrest to respect the patient's wishes not to be resuscitated.

Comfort Measures Only and Other Special Orders

When a discussion is taking place about resuscitation, it is appropriate to question the use of other life-sustaining interventions, such as the use of dialysis, ventilatory support, artificial nutrition and hydration, blood transfusions, antibiotics and other medications, and surgery. Patients may request a **comfort-measures-only order,** which indicates that the goal of treatment is a comfortable, dignified death and that further life-sustaining measures are no longer indicated. A **do-not-hospitalize order** is being used by patients in nursing homes and other residential settings who have elected not to be hospitalized for further aggressive treatment.

Whereas some patients may want aggressive life-sustaining treatment and such treatment is medically beneficial, other patients may be at a point in their illness at which they choose to terminate all life-sustaining measures and allow the disease to progress naturally to death. This is termed passive euthanasia. There is no moral obligation to initiate or continue the use of life-sustaining treatment that is minimally effective or disproportionately burdensome. Laws may place constraints on those who may decide to withhold or withdraw life-sustaining treatment for incompetent patients. Nurses should be familiar with pertinent federal and state laws and the policies in their institution or agency concerning the withholding or withdrawing of life-sustaining treatment. Nurses should also be familiar with the forms used to indicate patient preferences about end-of-life care.

Terminal Weaning

Terminal weaning is the gradual withdrawal of mechanical ventilation from a patient with a terminal illness or an irre-

versible condition with a poor prognosis. In some cases, competent patients decide that they wish their ventilatory support ended; more often, the surrogate decision makers for an incompetent patient determine that continued ventilatory support is futile. Although it may be expected that a patient will not be able to survive the weaning, death is never a certain outcome, and it is not unusual for a patient to initiate spontaneous respirations once ventilatory support is withdrawn and live for several hours to several days. Competent patients and family members should be prepared for all possibilities. A nurse's role in terminal weaning is to participate in the decision-making process by offering helpful information about the benefits and burdens of continued ventilation and a description of what to expect if terminal weaning is initiated. Supporting the patient's family and managing sedation and analgesia are critical nursing responsibilities; unfortunately, many agencies and institutions do not have policies. Nurses involved in terminal weaning should consult the literature (Campbell, 1994; Rushton & Terry, 1995).

Assisted Suicide and Active Euthanasia

Euthanasia literally means "good dying." Until recently, most societies maintained that the distinction between killing and allowing to die was morally relevant. This meant that passive euthanasia, the withholding or withdrawing of medically ineffective or disproportionately burdensome therapies, was morally and legally justified even when this hastened or directly caused a patient's death. On the other hand, making a lethal combination of drugs available to a patient wishing to die (**assisted suicide**) or administering a lethal injection or carbon monoxide, even when performed with compassionate intent at the request of a patient (**active euthanasia**), was deemed both immoral and illegal. Some are questioning the validity of this distinction today, and there are efforts to legalize assisted suicide and active euthanasia in numerous countries. In the United States, physician-assisted suicide is legal in Oregon. It is important for nurses to understand the arguments for and against assisted suicide and active euthanasia and to clarify what they believe. See Box 33-4: Ethical Challenges.

Arguments in Favor of Assisted Suicide and Active Euthanasia

People who are in favor of assisted suicide and active euthanasia argue that it is a beneficent and compassionate act; that it respects autonomy by preserving the patient's control of the manner, method, and timing of death; and that it takes the matter outside the reach of "medical power" and scrupulosity. They would also argue that it prevents the injustice that allows some patients to choose death by refusal of life-support measures, while denying others the right to do so by active euthanasia. Proponents of assisted suicide and active euthanasia would say that in a pluralistic society, euthanasia must be accepted, whatever its intrinsic morality, because states have no moral justification for intruding into such private decisions.

Proponents of involuntary euthanasia (euthanasia for an individual who cannot consent) argue that, in addition, it is irrational to afford rights of personhood to anencephalics or

BOX 33-4 Ethical Challenges: Thinking Critically About Assisted Suicide and Active Euthanasia

Nurses are often the first to hear a patient's plea, "Please help me die." It is critical for nurses to reflect carefully on what they believe about assisted suicide and active euthanasia and how this influences the responses they make to patients. Assisted suicide is illegal in all states in the United States except Oregon.

- Should the principle of respect for autonomy be expansive enough to embrace respect for, and acquiescence to, a competent patient's request for assistance in dying?
- Does the right to privacy entail a right, in effect, to decide the time and manner of one's death and to gain assistance in implementing that decision?
- Is there such a thing as *rational* suicide?
- If assisted suicide and active euthanasia were to become accepted practices, would this simply represent a logical, defensible extension of the well-established moral basis for refusal of treatment and withholding/withdrawing treatment?
- Are assisted suicide and active euthanasia acts of mercy, morally grounded in the principles of benefiting and not harming patients and expressive of the virtues of compassion and beneficence?
- Is it possible to conceive of situations in which a nurse or a physician has a duty to help a patient die (specifically via active euthanasia/assisted suicide)?
- Is refusal to accede to a patient's request for assisted suicide or active euthanasia a form of abandonment, *or* are there limits to the duty to respect autonomy, right to privacy, and self-determination?
- Are calls for assisted suicide and active euthanasia emblematic of failure to provide adequate palliative care and to address the suffering of the dying?
- If medicine and nursing possess an "internal" morality, are assisted suicide and active euthanasia consistent with that morality?

patients in a permanent vegetative state and unjust to deny them the right to die to which they are entitled. They argue that beneficence to patient, family, and healthcare professionals, as well as conservation of society's resources, makes involuntary euthanasia a positive moral duty of physicians.

Arguments Against Assisted Suicide and Active Euthanasia

People who oppose assisted suicide and active euthanasia argue that it undermines the value of, and respect for, all human life. Guidelines cannot avoid "sliding down the slippery slope" to involuntary euthanasia and selective devaluation of the lives of the most vulnerable among us. Another argument is that euthanasia should be unnecessary because the major reasons for requesting it—intolerable pain and fear of overtreatment—can

now be handled by better palliative care, analgesia, and advance directives. Furthermore, a focus on euthanasia will divert attention from other valuable palliative techniques.

Opponents of assisted suicide and active euthanasia claim that if euthanasia is legal, patients will feel a subtle pressure to conform so as to relieve the economic and emotional burdens they impose on family and friends. They also feel that euthanasia is socially destructive; it undermines trust in physicians and healthcare professionals, desensitizes society to killing, and imperils the grounds already gained in legitimizing passive euthanasia. Many Americans hold the religious belief that human life is the gift of the Creator and that humans are its stewards but not its absolute masters (Pellegrino, 1991).

American Nurses Association Position

In 1994, the American Nurses Association issued position statements stating that assisting in suicide and participating in active euthanasia are in violation of the Code for Nurses, the ethical traditions and goals of the profession, and its covenant with society. Nurses can expect to be confronted by patients who seek their assistance in ending their life. Unless nurses think through this issue carefully, they will be unprepared to respond to the request, "Nurse, please help me die" (see Box 33-4).

Death Certificate

US law requires that a death certificate be prepared for each person who dies. The law specifies what information needs to be supplied. Death certificates are sent to local health departments, which compile many statistics from the information. The mortician assumes responsibility for handling and filing the death certificate with proper authorities. A physician's signature is required on the certificate, as well as that of the pathologist, the coroner, and others in special cases. The nurse's responsibility is to ensure that the physician has signed a death certificate.

Organ Donation

Patients who express a wish to donate functional organs, such as heart, corneas, liver, lungs, and kidneys, can fill out an organ donor consent card (Fig. 33-2). The family of a deceased patient also may decide to donate the patient's functional organs. The nurse should be able to review options and provide consent forms to interested patients and their families. Until recently, most organs were retrieved from totally brain-dead patients. New protocols for retrieving organs from non–heart-beating cadavers are raising multiple practice concerns. Comprehensive attention to optimal patient and family care at the time of withdrawal of life-sustaining therapy needs to remain the nurse's priority. The scarcity of organs has resulted in legislation mandating hospitals and other healthcare agencies to notify transplantation programs of potential donors.

Think back to Mr. Perez, who was asking about advance directives and organ donation after his wife had a stroke. The nurse could incorporate knowledge of organ donation to develop

Signed by the donor and the following two witnesses in the presence of each other:

_____   _____
Signature of Donor   Date of Birth of Donor

_____   _____
Date Signed   City and State

_____   _____
Witness   Witness

This is a legal document under the Uniform Anatomical Gift Act or similar laws in all 50 states

                                    For further information call
Delaware Valley   **800 KIDNEY-1**
TRANSPLANT   2401 Walnut St., Suite 404
PROGRAM   Philadelphia, PA 19103

UNIFORM DONOR CARD

_____
Print or type name of donor
In the hope that I may help others, I hereby make this anatomical gift, if medically acceptable, to take effect upon my death. The words and marks below indicate my desires.
I give: a) _____ any needed organs or parts
       b) _____ only the following organs or parts

_____
Specify the organ(s) or parts(s)
for the purpose of transplantation, therapy, medical research or education:
       c) _____ my body for anatomical study if needed

_____
Limitations or special wishes, if any

FIGURE 33-2 Example of an organ donor card.

an appropriate teaching plan for Mr. Perez so that he can make the most informed decision possible.

Autopsy

An autopsy is an examination of the organs and tissues of a human body after death. Obtaining consent for autopsy is a legal requirement. The closest surviving family member or members usually have the authority to determine whether an autopsy is performed. Some religious groups prohibit autopsies except for legal purposes.

It is commonly the physician's responsibility to obtain permission for an autopsy. Sometimes the patient may grant this permission before death. The nurse can assist by explaining the reasons for an autopsy. Many relatives find comfort when they are told that the knowledge gained from an autopsy may contribute to advances in medical science as well as establish the exact cause of death.

If death is caused by accident, suicide, homicide, or illegal therapeutic practice, the coroner must be notified, according to law. The coroner may decide that an autopsy is advisable and can order that one be performed, even though the patient's family has refused consent. In some cases, a death that occurs within 24 hours of admission to the hospital must be reported to the coroner.

FACTORS THAT AFFECT GRIEF AND DYING

Many factors, including age, family relationships, socioeconomic position, and cultural and religious influences, affect a person's reaction to and expression of grief, and like the stages of grief reaction, they vary from person to person.

Developmental Considerations

Children do not understand death on the same level as adults do, but their sense of loss is just as great. Both terminally ill children and their siblings are likely to talk and ask questions about death in an attempt to understand it. Terminally ill children require parental love and support as well as social interaction with other children. Death of a parent or another significant person can retard a child's development or may cause the child to regress developmentally. Children need to go through the same grief reactions as adults to accept such a loss and maintain emotional well-being.

The loss of a parent by a middle-aged adult helps to prepare the adult for the loss of a spouse or significant other and to accept his or her own eventual death. Older people may lose a spouse or friends and relatives their own age. As this happens, they reminisce about life, put their lives and the purpose of living in perspective, and prepare themselves for their own inevitable death.

Family

Family roles have an important impact on a person's reactions to and expressions of grief. For example, the eldest sibling may feel a need to "be strong" and therefore may not grieve openly; a person who loses a spouse may display the same type of behavior to "protect the children."

The death of a child is usually a devastating experience for the family. The family needs time to accept the reality of the situation, opportunities to talk and to be listened to, and the experience of expressing themselves behaviorally in a nonjudgmental environment. The family of a terminally ill child may express feelings of guilt by wondering if they were responsible for the impending death. A sibling may suppress a guilt feeling for having wished the ill child (or a parent) dead.

Socioeconomic Factors

A bereaved family may suffer more acutely if there is no health or life insurance or pension after the death of the family provider. Such families face not only the loss of a loved one but also an economic loss that may further disrupt family life. Older people especially may be placed in a difficult position because the death of a spouse may result in the decrease or even elimination of a source of retirement income for the surviving spouse. This reduction in income may lead to loss of home, community, and support systems.

Cultural Influences

Both the physical and emotional manifestations of grief may be culturally influenced. Clinical symptoms of grief include repeated somatic distress, tightness in the chest, choking or shortness of breath, sighing, empty feeling in the abdomen, loss of muscle power, and intense subjective distress. Other symptoms include vomiting, dizziness, fainting, fatigue, weight loss, headaches, and chest pains.

Culture also influences a person's expression of grief. In many families in the Western culture, grief is a private matter shared only with the family. As such, many people internalize their feelings of grief and may not express their feelings of loss to others. On the other hand, cultural background may necessitate that the patient's and family's public display be emotional and distressed, with loud weeping and moaning.

Although sex roles have become less differentiated in the past few decades, male and female reactions to death may differ. The widow who has a job may not be as emotionally distraught as the woman who needed her husband for support. Likewise, the widower who has not taken care of the children or the house may view the future more bleakly than the man who has cooked meals and changed diapers. Some ethnic traditions may be ingrained in certain people, and the woman may be expected to be weak and need support, whereas the man may be expected to be emotionally supportive. This varies from culture to culture and from person to person.

Religious Influences

Faith and religious practices play an important role in the expression of grief and provide comfort and solace to the person experiencing loss. Many people who have put spiritual matters in the background of their lives have found death to be an impetus for a return to earlier practices of religion. At the same time, others may blame God for the death of their loved one and turn away from God (see Chap. 36).

Cause of Death

The grief response often depends on the cause of death. Many deaths are sudden and involve shock as well as normal grieving in the survivors. Death from disease may generate several types of response, including the belief that the death is a punishment (eg, when AIDS was first diagnosed in homosexuals and drug users), terror and panic (eg, when people are reminded of the devastation caused by plagues of earlier centuries), and guilt (eg, when family and friends believe that they could have prevented the death).

Accidental death is often associated with feelings of bad luck. The guilt response can be enormous, especially when children die as the result of an accident. Death while defending a country usually is viewed by most of society as honorable and necessary. Violent deaths occur daily, especially in larger cities. Suicide accounts for a great number of violent deaths; in fact, among teenagers, it has become a major concern. It is also believed that many accidental deaths are actually suicides.

THE NURSE AS ROLE MODEL

Holistic care of the terminally ill patient and family almost always involves some personal emotional investment. It is unrealistic and unfair to expect nurses to handle circumstances surrounding death without feelings. The best policy seems to be taking the time to explore one's own feelings and express them; see Promoting Health 33-1.

The nurse who neglects to deal with personal feelings about life, dying, and death is in a questionable position for analyzing and considering the needs of patients facing death. A nurse's own feelings play a major role in determining how he or she cares for a patient with a terminal illness. The following are some questions the nurse should use to help clarify his or her thinking and feelings about dying and death:

- If I could control the events that result in my own death, where would I want to be? What cause of death would I choose? Whom would I want to have present during my terminal illness?
- What fears do I have about death?
- How would I answer these same questions for a patient for whom I have been caring?
- How could I improve the quality of care for a terminally ill patient for whom I am caring?
- If I were a member of the patient's family, what things would I want a nurse to do for me?

The nurse who cares for a patient for an extended period will undergo a grief reaction when the patient dies. Grief after the death of a patient is natural, and the nurse should allow himself or herself to go through the grieving process rather than shut off the grief. The nurse should also address personal health needs.

THE NURSING PROCESS FOR GRIEVING OR DYING PATIENTS AND FAMILIES

The nursing process is a helpful tool when caring for patients who are grieving or dying and their families and significant others. Box 33-5 presents the competencies necessary for nurses to provide high-quality care to patients and families during the transition at the end of life.

Assessing

Focused assessment for those experiencing loss, grief, and dying is directed toward determining the adequacy of the patient's and family's knowledge, perceptions, coping strategies (see Chap. 32), and resources. Pertinent interview questions are in Focused Assessment Guide 33-1. Physical assessment of both the dying patient and of concerned family, friends, and family caregivers is essential to diagnosing some problems.

(*text continues on page 890*)

Promoting Health 33-1 *Grieving*

If a past or current loss is influencing your everyday functioning, use the assessment checklist to see how well you are responding to the losses in your life. Then develop a prescription for self-care by choosing appropriate behaviors from the list of suggestions.

ASSESSMENT CHECKLIST

almost always / sometimes / almost never

1. I can name the personal losses that are currently influencing my state of well-being.
2. I have a plan for coping with these losses that is in place and helping me to cope.
3. I understand the importance of grieving, and I actually set time aside for this self-care measure.
4. I am comfortable with my feelings and am able to give them expression.
5. There is someone who knows and accepts me well enough to allow me to share openly and honestly.
6. I value being a supportive presence for people with life-threatening illnesses.
7. I respond genuinely to the concerns and feelings of dying patients and their families; I am not afraid to cry with patients and to allow my feelings to show.

SELF-CARE BEHAVIORS

1. Make a list of the losses that are interfering with your present state of well-being. These may include the loss of health, valued role, image/reputation, relationship, material object, job, person.
2. Determine whether or not you are addressing these losses in a conscious fashion, and identify coping strategies that may be of help.
3. Try implementing a "tried and true" or new coping strategy.
4. Talk about one of these losses with a friend, religious leader, or counselor/therapist. Assess your comfort level in sharing your feelings openly. Ask the person you are sharing with how he or she thinks you are responding.
5. Be honest about any maladaptive coping strategies you may be using to cope, such as addictions, apathy ("Who cares?"), withdrawal and passivity, depression, acting out. Get any help you need to replace these maladaptive coping measures.
6. Reflect upon what your level of comfort in being with people who are dying reveals about your own acceptance of the fact that we will all die.

BOX 33-5 Competencies Necessary for Nurses to Provide High-Quality Care to Patients and Families During the Transition at the End of Life

1. Recognize dynamic changes in population demographics, healthcare economics and service delivery that necessitate improved professional preparation for end-of-life care.
2. Promote the provision of comfort care to the dying as an active, desirable, and important skill and an integral component of nursing care.
3. Communicate effectively and compassionately with the patient, family and healthcare team members about end-of-life issues.
4. Recognize one's own attitudes, feelings, values, and expectations about death and the individual, cultural, and spiritual diversity existing in these beliefs and customs.
5. Demonstrate respect for the patient's views and wishes during end-of-life care.
6. Collaborate with interdisciplinary team members while implementing the nursing role in end-of-life care.
7. Use scientifically based standardized tools to assess symptoms (eg, pain, dyspnea [breathlessness], constipation, anxiety, fatigue, nausea/vomiting, and altered cognition) experienced by patients at the end of life.
8. Use data from symptom assessment to plan and intervene in symptom management using state-of-the-art traditional and complementary approaches.
9. Evaluate the impact of traditional, complementary, and technological therapies on patient-centered outcomes.
10. Assess and treat multiple dimensions, including physical, psychological, social, and spiritual needs, to improve quality at the end of life.
11. Assist the patient, family, colleagues, and self to cope with suffering, grief, loss, and bereavement in end-of-life care.
12. Apply legal and ethical principles in the analysis of complex issues in end-of-life care, recognizing the influence of personal values, professional codes, and patient preferences.
13. Identify barriers and facilitators to patients' and caregivers' effective use of resources.
14. Demonstrate skill at implementing a plan for improved end-of-life care within a dynamic and complex healthcare delivery system.
15. Apply knowledge gained from palliative care research to end-of-life education and care.

(Used with permission. American Association of Colleges of Nursing [1999]. Competencies necessary for nurses to provide high-quality care to patients and families during transition at the end of life. Washington, DC: Author.)

Focused Assessment Guide 33-1

The Experience of Loss, Grief, Dying, and Death

Assessment Priorities

Patient and family's understanding of medical condition, prognosis, and dying process

Patient and family's attitude toward death and dying and knowledge of the dying process

Patient's preferences for end-of-life treatment and care: desire to be at home or in a hospital or hospice setting; decisions concerning aggressiveness of treatment, resuscitation, advanced life support, organ donation, etc.

Documented evidence of advance care planning

Existence of advance directive **[It is critical that the authorized decision maker be known to all members of the healthcare team]**

Religious beliefs

Cultural influences

Stage of grief and death reaction (denial and isolation, anger, bargaining, depression, acceptance)

Adequacy of coping behaviors

Adequacy of resources

Physiologic needs of the patient: personal hygiene, pain control, nutritional and fluid needs, movement, elimination and respiratory care needs

Psychological needs of the patient and family: fear of the unknown, pain, separation, leaving loved ones, dependence; loss of dignity; unfinished business; powerlessness

Spiritual needs of the patient and family: need for meaning and purpose, for love and relatedness, for forgiveness, for hope

Factors to Assess	Questions and Approaches
Adequacy of knowledge base	What have you been told about your condition? What do you know about this condition? Please describe what you have been told about your treatment options. Is there anything you don't understand about what your doctor is recommending? What else would you like to know about your present condition and treatment options? Do you know how to contact your doctor and to get the information you need/desire? *Objective is to identify whether or not the knowledge the patient and family possess will allow them to make informed decisions that will serve their best interests.*
Realism of expectations/perceptions	Have you had any previous experiences with this condition or with the death of someone you love? What are your expectations in this case? How do you see the next few weeks (days) playing out? What are your fears, hopes, concerns, worries? What good do you think might be happening in the midst of all this? *Objective is to discover whether the patient and family have unrealistic expectations or misperceptions about the diagnosis, prognosis, and care options that will interfere with their decision making and coping.*
Adequacy of coping strategies	Dealing with our own dying is a once-in-a-lifetime experience, and sometimes we begin the process feeling totally unprepared. Tell me something about how you think you are coping with all this. How well do you think those around you are coping? How can I help you develop or tap the resources that will help you to cope better? *Objective is to identify whether the patient and the patient's family are using effective coping strategies. If you detect problems, try to identify coping strategies they have used effectively in the past. Also identify and address destructive habits that have not served them well in the past such as addictions, destructive relationships, passivity, acting out. Creatively problem-solve about new strategies they might try.*
Adequacy of resources	What is helping you to get through this? Do you think the resources available to you are adequate? If the sky was the limit, what help would you wish for? What is interfering with your getting the help you need? What are some of the community resources that might be of help to you? Are you using these? *Objective is to assess the adequacy of the human, financial, spiritual, and psychological resources available to the patient. Questions should be directed to determining what, if anything, is interfering with the patient using whatever resources are available to facilitate coping.*
Physical response	A physical assessment of the patient and the patient's family and caregivers should be performed to detect problems with coping that result in fatigue, decreased energy, decreased self-care (deficient grooming, unplanned weight loss), and other maladaptive responses.

Diagnosing

The data the nurse collects about how a patient or the patient's caregivers are responding to loss, actual or anticipated, or impending death may lead to several different nursing diagnoses. Samples of these diagnoses are given in the accompanying Examples of NANDA Nursing Diagnoses.

Response to Loss as the Problem

Nursing diagnoses that specifically address human responses to loss and impending death in the problem statement include Impaired Adjustment, Caregiver Role Strain, Decisional Conflict, Ineffective Denial, Ineffective Coping, Anticipatory or Dysfunctional Grieving, Hopelessness, Ineffective Therapeutic Regimen Management, and Powerlessness. Sample

---

Examples of NANDA Nursing Diagnoses | Loss and Impending Death

Nursing Diagnoses	Related Factors	Sample Defining Characteristics
Impaired Adjustment	Newly diagnosed terminal illness	"This can't be happening to me. . . . I know I'm going to die. . . . Why should I try and fight this? Mother fought this same diagnosis and died, why should I hope to be any different?"
Caregiver Role Strain	Hospital discharged dying patient because of inadequate insurance	Spouse has dark circles under eyes, reports unable to sleep through night, decreased appetite, and general lack of energy. "I want to do everything I can for Tony, but I feel so overwhelmed. . . . I don't think anyone prepared me for everything I now find myself needing to do for him. . . . I'm always afraid that I'll hurt him or do something wrong." "I don't want to complain, but I miss being able to go out with my friends. Last week I didn't even get to church because Tony wasn't feeling well Sunday morning and asked me not to leave. . . . Sometimes I think I'll just go crazy."
Decisional Conflict	Repeat hospitalizations for aspiration pneumonia and new inability to swallow	Family has requested ethics consult because they are split about pending decisions for initiation of artificial nutrition and hydration and advisability of future hospitalizations and continued aggressive treatment; patient has Alzheimer's disease and has been in a nursing home for last 5 years.
Ineffective Coping	Inability to accept death of 42-year-old son who died of a heart attack 2 years ago; failure of coping mechanisms that worked in the past	70-year-old widow who lived alone with son until his death 2 years ago has become a recluse and eats just enough to keep herself alive, seems to exist on gin, cigarettes, and chocolate. "Mothers aren't supposed to outlive their children . . . why didn't God take me first? I just want to die and be with Bernie. . . ."
Ineffective Denial	Inability to believe that she has AIDS and that husband was bisexual	Patient who is just "getting her life back in order" (left abusive husband 1 year ago and is newly happily remarried) learns that she has AIDS. "This can't be happening to me . . . after all I've been through . . . I hear what you are saying but I don't believe you . . . there must be some mistake. . . ." Breaks next appointment and refuses to respond to repeated urgings to seek treatment.
Anticipatory Grieving	Knowledge that fetus is anencephalic	"I don't know how this can be happening to us. . . . We've tried to do everything right. . . . We've waited for this baby for so long. . . . It's hard to believe that our baby won't be normal and that if what the doctors say is true she will only live for a few hours or days at most. . . ."
Dysfunctional Grieving	Inability to accept death of anencephalic infant; no grief resolution	Two years after birth of anencephalic infant who died 3 days after delivery, couple has failed to come to peace with child's death; divorce pending; wife has lost 15 pounds, and her husband complains that she "really let herself go, she quit her job, mopes around the house all day, and isn't interested in anything anymore."

(continued)

Examples of NANDA Nursing Diagnoses
Loss and Impending Death (Continued)

Nursing Diagnoses	Related Factors	Sample Defining Characteristics
Hopelessness	Inability to accept son's diagnosis of leukemia and favorable prognosis linked to knowledge of death of neighbor's son who had similar diagnosis	"Don't be leading us on. . . . We know what leukemia means, we have neighbors who lost a son to leukemia. . . . It's not true that you can treat this. . . ." Parents refuse to believe favorable prognosis; after hearing diagnosis, they become apathetic and withdrawn. "Marge and Joe tried to do everything to save their son and failed, why should we even try? Nothing else in our lives has worked out."
Ineffective Therapeutic Regimen Management (also, Powerlessness)	Suddenness of injury and inability to prepare sufficiently to provide needed in-home care	"One minute our life was perfect and then, WHAM, all of a sudden everything went wrong. If only my husband hadn't gone out that night and if only he could get his leg back. I should be doing more to help him but I just want to sit and cry. This isn't what I bargained for when we got married. I don't think I can spend the rest of my life with a cripple." Home health nurse notes that neither the patient nor his wife is following through with recommended exercises, and he has broken several appointments at the rehabilitation center. Both the patient and his wife seem to have given up and express no interest in therapeutic regimen.

---

defining characteristics for these diagnoses appear later in the box in the Implementing section.

Response to Loss as the Etiology

Difficulty responding to loss or impending death may also affect other areas of human functioning and result in different diagnoses. Examples of nursing diagnoses for which the experience of loss as the etiology are:

- Anxiety related to inability to predict how the last stage of illness will play itself out
- Nausea related to complications of chemotherapy for end-stage breast cancer
- Interrupted Family Processes related to stress of caring for dying mother
- Fatigue related to constant demands of caring for dying family member
- Fear related to perceived loss of control and increasing need to be dependent in final stages of illness
- Deficient Knowledge related to lack of experience in caring for dying family member at home
- Noncompliance related to denial of gravity of illness and impending death
- Situational Low Self-Esteem related to inability to accept need for assistance as disease progresses
- Spiritual Distress related to inability to reconcile diagnosis and pain with belief in a loving God
- Self-Care Deficits related to waning strength as terminal illness progresses

Outcome Identification and Planning

Nursing care should be directed toward the achievement of the following goals or outcomes for grieving and dying patients and their families. The patient or family will achieve the following:

- Demonstrate freedom to express feelings, needs, fears, and concerns
- Identify and use effective coping strategies
- Accept need for help as appropriate and use available resources
- Make healthcare decisions reflecting personal values and goals; ultimately feel peaceful about role in decision making
- Declare preferences regarding treatment options
- Report sufficient relief of pain to interact meaningfully with family and to attend to everyday concerns
- Experience a dignified and comfortable death
- Family or significant others: resolve grief after a suitable period of mourning and resume meaningful roles and daily activities

The patient and the family should take an active role in planning for care. Such planning takes the patient's preferences into consideration, facilitates the acceptance of death by the patient and the family, and provides interventions to meet holistic needs.

Implementing

The nurse's aims in caring for dying patients and their families include facilitating coping of the dying person and family and promoting health and preventing illness of the family. The accompanying box Examples of Nursing Interventions Classification (NIC) suggests standardized nursing interventions for specific NIC dying care activities.

Developing a Trusting Nurse–Patient Relationship

Communication is a lifelong need up to the moment of death and should be maintained at all times with the patient and family. To develop meaningful communication, the nurse must develop a trusting relationship with the patient. This relationship is explored throughout this text. The nurse needs to develop listening skills and the ability to recognize both verbal and nonverbal cues given by the patient and family. These skills are discussed in Chapter 21.

The nurse should be willing to discuss the patient's fears and doubts openly and to serve as a nonjudgmental listener. A caring nurse feels at ease in crying with the grieving person and sharing experiences with fears, loneliness, and death. This allows the griever the freedom to express his or her deepest concerns. Nonverbal communication is equally important. A smile, a touching hand or stroke, and eye-to-eye contact are all meaningful. The warmth behind the gesture and the honest concern of the nurse are what count.

The sense of hearing is believed to be the last sense to leave the body; many patients retain a sense of hearing almost to the moment of death. It is kind and thoughtful of the nurse to speak to the comatose patient and to encourage family members to do likewise. The nurse should explain to the patient the nursing care being given and the noises in the unit.

Explaining the Patient's Condition and Treatment

All involved healthcare personnel should know exactly what the patient and family have been told. Telling them different things puts the nurse and other team members at cross-purposes and sets up distrust on the part of the family. Because patients and families often direct questions about the patient's prognosis to the nurse, it is up to the nurse to take the initiative in determining a means to be consistent in terminology, prognosis, and description of progress.

The patient's condition and treatment should be explained to both the patient and the family. Patience is required during explanations. They may be so grieved by the diagnosis that they do not hear all the information that is shared with them. The nurse can question them to learn how much they have retained; then the information they missed can be repeated. Care options, as well as the expected outcomes of each option, should be fully explained.

Teaching Self-Care and Promoting Self-Esteem

The patient should be encouraged to retain independence and make decisions as long as possible. Personal hygiene practices and self-feeding should also be managed by the patient as long as possible. After the patient is confined to bed, the creative nurse and family caregivers should attempt to find self-care activities the patient can perform. When physical abilities fail, determining when to take medication, for example, may be all the control the patient can retain.

Having familiar objects in view can help make the patient feel more comfortable and secure. Whether the patient is at home or in a healthcare agency, it is desirable to have the environment reflect personal preferences. This gives the patient some degree of control when health and other activities of daily living have slipped out of the patient's reach, and it supports self-esteem.

In the transition from independence to interdependence and ultimately to dependence, the patient may experience depression and express frustration and grief about "being a burden." It is crucial for professional and nonprofessional caregivers to respond to the dying patient as a person of worth whose life has meaning and value. Chapter 11 discusses practical ways in which nurses can use looks, touch, words, and actions to communicate respect and caring.

Teaching Family Members to Assist in Care

Preparing family members to assist in nursing care competently and confidently yields benefits to both the patient and family members. Having loved ones near comforts the patient, and family members are comforted by knowing that they helped comfort the patient. The nurse must supervise family members providing nursing care to the patient. Family members may not want to provide care themselves but may want to know what to expect and how they can psychologically aid the patient. The nurse can help by explaining the patient's condition, what treatment the patient is undergoing, and what result the family can expect from the treatment. Knowing the facts may help family members to cope better with impending loss.

Meeting the Needs of Dying Patients
Physiologic Needs

Physiologic care of the patient involves meeting physical needs such as personal hygiene, pain control, nutritional and fluid needs, movement, elimination, and respiratory care. Personal hygiene includes cleanliness of the skin, hair, mouth, nose, and eyes. Frequent baths and linen changes may be necessary. The mouth and nose should be kept free of mucus, and secretions should be wiped from the eyes. The physician will determine the medication and dosage needed for pain control, but the patient's wishes should be considered. (See Chap. 41 for a further discussion of pain control.) Some patients prefer and are able to control their own medication. Many dying patients suffer from malnutrition and dehydration, and nutritional and fluid needs must be addressed. The patient may require nutritional support but should be encouraged to take sips of water if still able to swallow. The dying patient may also elect to forego artificial nutrition and hydration because the burdens of feeding and hydrating artificially may outweigh the benefits. See the classic article by Zerwekh (1983) for a discussion of these benefits and burdens. Periodic movement should also be allowed; regular changes of position help prevent pressure ulcers. Problems with elimination include the development of incontinence, constipation, and urinary retention. Absorbent pads or a nearby bedpan may be used for incontinent patients, laxatives or enemas may be used for relieving constipation, and catheterization may be required for urinary retention. Bed linens should be changed often. Repositioning the conscious patient in semi-Fowler's position can provide respiratory care; the unconscious patient should be positioned in a semi-prone position that allows drainage of saliva and mucus. Oxygen therapy may be necessary for some patients.

Psychological Needs

When people speak of their fears of death, responses typically include fear of the unknown, pain, separation, leaving loved ones, loss of dignity, loss of control, and unfinished business. Kübler-Ross believes that there is still another, more overwhelming and more significant fear that often is repressed and unconscious: that of the catastrophic, destructive force that has befallen a person and that the person cannot change. Kübler-Ross points out that terminally ill people communicate this fear of a destructive force but do so largely through symbolic language. A person may use nonverbal language, such as a facial expression, a particular kind of handclasp, or, in the case of children, drawings and manner of play with toys. Verbal communication may also be used symbolically. Two nurses have provided an excellent study of the special awareness, needs, and communications of the dying (Callanan & Kelley, 1992).

A fear of isolation, of having to face death alone, is a primary concern of the dying patient. The nurse supports the patient by indicating his or her presence, giving full attention, and showing that he or she cares. The presence of family members in the room should be encouraged. Reminiscences should be shared.

Sexual Needs

Dying patients and their sexual partners may feel uncomfortable discussing their sexual needs. Frequently, partners may wish to be physically intimate with the dying person but are afraid of "hurting" him or her and also afraid that an open expression of sexuality is somehow "inappropriate" when someone is dying. Nurses who are sensitive can help by encouraging discussion and by suggesting ways to be physically intimate that will meet the needs of both partners. A loving foot massage or tender, cradling body embrace may be exactly what a dying person needs in his or her last moments.

Spiritual Needs

Many terminally ill patients find great comfort in the support they receive from their religious faith. The nurse should aid in obtaining the services of clergy as each situation indicates.

Although not all patients follow specific spiritual or religious beliefs, most require some form of spiritual care. Most patients need to feel that their lives have meaning; many feel a need for hope in the face of death. See Box 33-6 for examples of specific interventions to enable hope in the terminally ill. The nurse should not impose his or her beliefs on the patient but should let the patient know that his or her beliefs are important. The nurse should arrange for visits from a spiritual adviser if desired. Spiritual needs are discussed more fully in Chapter 36.

Meeting Family Needs

The nurse can provide care for the family facing loss by listening to their concerns. Family members need to verbalize their worries and fears, and nurses and other healthcare personnel can provide support by being nonjudgmental listeners. Likewise, nursing care of the grieving family involves communication and listening. Application of the communication skills discussed in Chapter 21 and earlier in this section aids the nurse in being a nonjudgmental listener. Feedback to the family can be provided by summarizing or paraphrasing, without questioning the validity of the family's emotions. All family members, including children, should be part of the grieving process. Family members may need to be reminded to get rest and to eat. Too many visitors may tire the patient; when explanations are offered, most relatives readily understand this. When they want to remain at the hospital, they should be directed to a quiet place where they may relax.

The reality of death can be made less painful by preparing the family ahead of time. When the process has been explained to the family, they are better prepared to understand the needs of the dying person and how to support him or her.

The steps of the grieving process should be explained to all family members ahead of time so that they will recognize the specific stages as they experience them and understand that the process is normal. They will be able to recognize that other members of the family are going through the same stages, perhaps at different times. This preparation allows for better understanding and communication within the family.

Death creates a change in family roles. As one person (the dying person) leaves a role, adjustments must be made within the family to compensate. Each member plays a part in that compensation, and the nurse can help with these adjustments.

BOX 33-6 Enabling Hope in the Terminally Ill

These guidelines are the product of an interdisciplinary team of those providing care for the terminally ill. They are presented to encourage anyone providing care for the terminally ill to consider the crucial place of hope in their caring and also their own potential to enable such hope.

Hope

Hope is the ingredient in life that enables an individual both to consider a future and to actively bring that future into being. Hope originates in imagination but must become a valued and realistic possibility for that individual in order to energize action. Hope has the capacity to embrace the reality of individual's suffering without escaping from it (false hope) or being suffocated by it (despair, helplessness, hopelessness).

Hope is unique to each person. During terminal illness, the future being considered will become more focused, yet hope is essential for an individual to transcend despair and complete crucial life tasks.

Enabling Hope
Acknowledging Individual Uniqueness

To enable such hope, the care provider must acknowledge *the uniqueness of the individual* and take seriously the dreams of the terminally ill person within the changing nature of the illness. Steps that can be taken to translate hope into accomplishment must be considered. For this to happen, care providers need to do the following:

- Consider all language used, and appreciate how easily hopes can be disabled by such terms as "hopeless situation" or "nothing more can be done."
- Encounter the individual's feelings at his or her own level; be willing to stay at that individual's level and allow him or her to lead.
- Be willing to take the necessary time to establish rapport with the individual in order that his or her hopes can be shared in a supportive atmosphere. Where appropriate, use physical contact to build trust.
- Realize the changing nature both of the disease and the accompanying hopes. At one point, a hope for cure may be the necessary activating force for an individual to undergo treatment; at another, a hope to consider one's dying may give the energy to complete crucial life tasks or endure the many losses of terminal illness.

Granting Control

A factor crucial to the nourishing of hope within an individual is that of *control*. An individual must be willing to take the necessary action to achieve what is hoped for. Terminal illness places many restrictions upon an individual and often robs that person of a feeling of being able to control the situation, thus leading to increasing helplessness and hopelessness. To counter this, efforts must be made not only to support an individual in hoping, but also to grant the person control in bringing realistic hopes into being.

To help support an individual's sense of control in order to enable active hoping, care providers need to do the following:

- Provide honest and accessible information regarding the progress of the illness.
- Allow an individual to express and work through many hopes in order to develop those hopes appropriate to him or her in the present context.
- Allow for freedom of choice regarding treatment options to the degree possible within the setting.
- Maximize the present possibilities for achieving hopes while allowing for the changing realities of terminal illness.

Being Aware of One's Own Feelings

Hope is strengthened by those who care for and support a terminally ill individual. Within the context of illness and suffering, hope may be fragile and must be nurtured in relationships with professional caregivers, family, and friends. To enable hope, care providers must be aware of their own hope for that individual.

Care providers need to do the following:

- Recognize their own assumptions regarding that particular individual and how those assumptions may inhibit the enabling of hope for that person.
- Be aware of how their own hope for that individual may differ from the hope being expressed by that person.
- Resist judging expressed hope and be willing to explore such hope further.
- Accept the individual's present suffering. Avoid giving "false hope" that minimizes the reality of the situation ("It can't be that bad," or "Don't worry, everything will be fine") or encouraging despair by focusing only upon the illness ("God can't possibly heal you now. That cancer's all through you!").

Supporting Spirituality

A component of hope is *spirituality*. Supported by faith in God, hope is the capacity to transcend present suffering, to lift one's perspective to future possibilities, and so to enable that individual to accomplish important life tasks. This capacity to transcend is facilitated by one's belief in the presence of God within the changing context of terminal illness.

To enable this spiritual aspect of hope, care providers need to do the following:

- Accept the individual's own spiritual journey and present level of faith (or lack of).
- Be open to expressed hopes that link with religious belief (eg, "God will cure me" or "I pray that God will take me home soon").
- Allow for spiritual struggle and its resultant emotions (eg, anger when "the cancer is back and God has failed to cure me!"). Recognize that the level of spiritual struggle during terminal illness may increase to enable the accomplishment of crucial hope for life tasks such as reconciliation and forgiveness.
- Be prepared to accept the reality of death as an aspect of hope. Accept an individual who has shifted hope to how he or she wishes to die, to life after death, to a meeting with deceased loved ones, etc.
- Enable an individual to have access to whatever means and rites of religion that will encourage his or her hope.

Courtesy of Ted Creen, D.Min., Palliative Care Pastoral Consultant, 865 2nd Ave. West, Owen Sound, Ontario, Canada; 519-376-7886

Providing Postmortem Care

When a patient dies, the nurse's responsibilities include caring for the patient's body, caring for the family, and discharging specific legal responsibilities. The latter involve ensuring that a death certificate is issued and signed, labeling the body, and reviewing organ donation arrangements, if any.

Care of the Body

After the patient has been pronounced dead, the nurse is responsible for preparing the body for discharge. The body is placed in normal anatomic position to avoid pooling of blood, soiled dressings are replaced, and tubes are removed. In most cases, it is unnecessary to wash the body; the mortician normally attends to this. Some religions strictly forbid washing of the body, whereas in others a special person must perform it. In cultures in which the family's washing of the deceased's body is considered the last service a family can give a loved one, the family should be given the necessary supplies and left alone in the room with the body. If an autopsy is to be performed, any tubes that were in place should not be removed. In such cases, the nurse should follow the hospital's policy.

The nurse is legally responsible for placing identification tags on either the shroud or garment the body is clothed in and the ankle to ensure that the body can be identified even if it is separated from its shroud. The nurse should also place an identification tag on the patient's dentures or other prostheses to ensure that the mortician receives these. The patient's body may have to be placed in the hospital's morgue refrigerator if mortuary arrangements were not made before the patient's death. The importance of proper and complete identification cannot be overemphasized.

If the patient died of a communicable disease, the body may require special handling to prevent the spread of disease. Requirements for such handling are usually specified by local laws and are contingent on the disease-causing organism, mode of transmission, and other characteristics.

Care of the Family

After a patient has died, the nurse provides support and care to the patient's family (see Through the Eyes of a Student). In most cases, this involves listening to the family's expressions of grief, loss, and helplessness. Because comforting words are often difficult to find, the nurse should offer solace and support by being an attentive listener. Family members may need to see the patient's body to accept the death fully; in such cases, the nurse should arrange for family members to view the body before it is discharged to the mortician.

Sudden death creates unique problems for the family. In the case of sudden injury or illness, the physical needs of the patient are paramount to the healthcare team. This means that family members are not provided as much emotional support or information as they would be if the patient's illness were prolonged, nor are they permitted to exercise as many options regarding the patient's care. The family that loses a member unexpectedly has not had an opportunity to begin the grieving process or to share in grieving with the deceased person. Family members should be allowed to express grief and

Through the Eyes of a Student

We had had several day-shift clinical rotations, but this was our first evening clinical experience. We were unsure as to what the evening would be like. We knew the evening would provide us with a new outlook on nursing, but we were not prepared for what unfolded.

I had been taking care of a patient when another nursing student asked if I would check in on her patient while she had her dinner break. This patient was known to each of the students because we all had the pleasure of caring for him. I was told he was lying in bed watching television and that he had changed his code status to "DNR" (do not resuscitate) just that day. When I went to check on him, I found him lying in bed but not watching television. His eyes were closed as if he were sleeping peacefully. I spoke his name several times without a response. At the same time, I was also checking for a radial pulse. When I couldn't find his pulse, I swiftly walked to find the instructor. Together we went back to him and assessed his condition. There were no radial or carotid pulses. His chest was not rising and the instructor listened to his heart with a stethoscope. There wasn't a heartbeat. I stood there feeling helpless and low-spirited. This was a man to whom we had all grown close. His family came to see him and to say a few final words. Tears were shed not only by his family but by those of us who had cared for him.

Our first evening clinical was an extremely emotional night. We were all quiet as we walked down the hallway to go home. The student who was caring for him that night was stopped by his daughter and two young granddaughters. One granddaughter was wearing his hat and the other was carrying his belt. This man's daughter was broken-hearted by his death, yet needed to know that he wasn't alone when he died. The student told her that I had been the one with him. The daughter seemed relieved to know that he was not by himself when he died.

As I look back on that evening, I'm sad that this man is no longer with us. I did not know him for very long, but he touched me in a way that helped me understand the true meaning of nursing: not only to care for the sick, disabled, or enfeebled, but also to be human and offer support for grieving families.

—Joyce A. Shearman, Delaware County
Community College, Media, Pennsylvania

should be given emotional support. Most often, the family is in the emergency department waiting room when death is confirmed. They are stunned, bewildered, and numb. They should not be rushed from the waiting room, but rather provided a private place to begin their grieving. The nurse should acknowledge their shock and listen to their grief. The family needs guidance in making plans and help in making decisions.

It is proper for the nurse who was caregiver or who took care of the patient for a prolonged period to attend the funeral. It also is appropriate for the nurse to make a follow-up call to the patient's family after the funeral or memorial service to offer both concern and care for the family's well-being. Follow-up visits are important to give support to the family. If the nurse assesses that the family is not coping well (dysfunctional grief), appropriate referral should be made.

Care of Other Patients

Because it is not unusual for nurses in institutional settings to provide care to more than one patient at a time, after the death of one patient, the nurse must continue to provide care to the other patients. Other patients are often aware of a death and may need to be consoled; this is particularly true of a patient who has shared a room with the deceased patient. Other patients may have grief reactions and should be supported through the grief process by the nurse. Death of a patient may cause depression in other patients and may make them more aware of their own future deaths.

Evaluating

The plan of nursing care for dying patients is effective if patients meet the outcome of a comfortable, dignified death and family members resolve their grief after a suitable time of mourning and resume meaningful life roles and activities. See the Nursing Plan of Care 33-1.

NURSING PLAN OF CARE 33-1   *for Mrs. Esposita and Her Family*

The Espositas have been married for 19 years and have two children, Jorge, who is 16, and Marita, who is 13. It has been 2 years since Mrs. Esposita was diagnosed with ovarian cancer, and this period has been difficult for the entire family. She has had several hospitalizations because of bowel obstructions and returned home more debilitated each time. At present, she is extremely cachexic and in the end stage of her illness. She initially tried aggressive treatment, and several chemotherapy regimens failed. During her last hospitalization 2 months ago, a decision was made not to continue aggressive therapy, and Mrs. Esposita insisted on returning home to die.

The nurse who has been visiting Mrs. Esposita at home asked for assistance from her colleagues in devising a plan of care for Mr. Esposita. Until now, Mrs. Esposita wanted nothing to do with the local hospice because of a reported "bad experience" a neighbor had. Her insurance will not provide for all the home nursing care she needs, and her husband and children have been trying to meet her needs for nursing as well as run the house and meet their own needs. A demanding woman, Mrs. Esposita never seems satisfied with anything anyone does, and the family is looking utterly frustrated, angry, and fatigued. Jorge is coping by "opting out"; he frequently spends the night with friends and doesn't even call home to report on his whereabouts. Marita's grades have fallen, and she has dropped out of cheerleading and other school activities so that she can take care of her mother. Mr. Esposita, who has been silent until now, recently confided that he doesn't know how much longer he can go on this way, and seemed horrified to hear himself say, "I just wish she would die already and get this all over with!" He is very concerned about the changes in his children and feels powerless to change what is happening. For her part, Mrs. Esposita seems oblivious to her family's needs and, even in her weakened state, multiplies pleas for assistance. She seems to be afraid of dying and never wants to be left alone.

NURSING DIAGNOSIS	Caregiver Role Strain related to multiple losses and burdens associated with caregiving responsibilities as manifested by self-report, breakdown in family relationships, fatigue, and anger.
EXPECTED OUTCOME	• Mr. Esposita will talk openly about his feelings and share his frustrations about his present situation.

Nursing Interventions	**Rationale**	**Evaluative Statement**
Plan visits for when there is time for private conversation with Mr. Esposita; initiate conversations by telling him that it is not unusual for family caregivers to feel fatigued, powerless, frustrated, angry, and emotionally distant. Encourage him to talk about what he is feeling: "You seemed surprised at yourself when you said that you wished your wife would 'just die.' This isn't an unusual wish for someone in your situation. . . . Tell me more about what you are feeling now. . . ."	This will normalize what Mr. Esposita is experiencing and communicate that someone cares about him and about what he is experiencing. Simply giving voice to what he is feeling and sharing this with a healthcare professional may help him to accept and address what he takes to be negative and possibly shameful feelings.	10/15/06 Outcome partially met. Mr. Esposita states that he feels better now that he is sharing some of what he's been holding in for such a long time, but he still believes that if he was really a good husband he wouldn't feel this way. Also states that it is hard for him to find words to express everything that he is feeling. *Revision:* Continue to encourage Mr. Esposita to talk about what he is experiencing and provide a private opportunity for this to happen. *E. McLoughlin, RN*

(continued)

NURSING PLAN OF CARE 33-1

for Mrs. Esposita and Her Family (continued)

EXPECTED OUTCOME
- By 10/17/06 Mr. Esposita will develop a realistic caregiving plan that matches his ability to care with his wife's need for care and that identifies other resources for his wife's unmet needs.

Nursing Interventions	Rationale	Evaluative Statement
Assist Mr. Esposita to identify what his wife's actual needs for care are; how much of this care it is reasonable to expect the family to provide; and other potential caregiving sources.

Explain to Mrs. Esposita that her family may not be able to meet all her needs for care but that every effort will be made to ensure these needs are met by other caregivers.

Assist Mr. Esposita to identify and use new resources: identify at least one new support person who can sit with Mrs. Esposita and relieve the family of some of this burden; explore the family's reluctance to use hospice and evaluate other community resources. Use appropriate referrals. | Mr. Esposita may need "permission" to not meet his wife's unrealistic needs. The nurse's authority may be useful in helping him to believe that he can be a good and faithful husband and still fail to meet her expectations. Identifying other caregiving resources will ensure that Mrs. Esposita's needs will be met.

Even if the nurse's sympathies are with the family, it is critical to communicate to the patient that you are committed to her and intent on doing all in your power to ensure that her needs are met. If the patient's needs are met, it will improve her relationships with her family.

The family may be feeling unnecessarily overwhelmed because they have failed to explore the availability of other resources. A gentle push may be needed to make this happen. If a "sitter" can be obtained for several hours in the evening, this would give Mr. Esposita time after work to do something with his children or for himself. | 10/17/06   Outcome not met. To date, Mr. Esposita has been unable to identify any additional caregivers for Mrs. Esposita and continues to feel the need to assume all responsibility for her care when he is home.

Revision: Bring list of community resources to Mr. Esposita, including church group, and plan with him to contact these sources. Reinforce that it is OK to ask for help.

E. McLoughlin, RN |

EXPECTED OUTCOME
- By 10/20/06 Mr. Esposita will report feeling more in control and less depressed and angry.

Nursing Interventions	Rationale	Evaluative Statement
Lead Mr. Esposita in a discussion that aims to identify everything that is making him feel powerless; then list those factors over which he has no control and those he can influence or change.

Provide opportunities for Mr. Esposita to control decision making over those aspects of his life and his wife's care for which he can exert control. Affirm constructive decision making and ask him how it feels to be "back in control" of at least some aspects of his life. Discuss with Mr. Esposita those factors he can change, and assist him in making decisions. | This will break the cycle of his thinking that there is nothing at present over which he can exert control. Simply making the list is a first step toward taking action.

This is an example of "guided discovery"; you are allowing Mr. Esposita to experience himself as once again in charge and to allow this experience to define his self-image. Reinforcement of his success affirms his self-image of one who is in charge. Types of support that can be given to caregivers include emotional (concern, trust), appraisal (affirms self-worth), informational (useful advice), and instrumental assistance or tangible goods. | 10/20/06   Outcome met. Mr. Esposita reports that even though most of his situation remains unchanged, he no longer feels powerless and is less depressed and angry. He expressed gratitude for this intervention and says it has given him new energy.

E. McLoughlin, RN |

(continued)

NURSING PLAN OF CARE 33-1   *for Mrs. Esposita and Her Family* (continued)

SAMPLE DOCUMENTATION

10/17/06, 12 PM, Nursing

Met with Mr. Esposita this morning and talked about the plan to identify other caregivers who might be able to "sit" with his wife on some evenings in order to give him time to do things for his children and himself. He reported no progress in identifying anyone but also stated that he hadn't really made any efforts to locate someone: "Who would want to help us? Besides, I wouldn't want to inflict my wife and her moods on anyone right now." I explained that there are many individuals and groups who provide exactly this type of assistance and that his wife's moods were not uncommon for someone in her situation. We then made a list of possible caregiver resources, including some family members who had earlier expressed an interest in helping out, the parish nurse service from his church, and finally the local hospice. If the first two sources do not work out, will explore family reluctance to use hospice resources more carefully because this may be their best hope. Will evaluate progress made on 10/21/06.

E. McLoughlin, RN

Developing Critical Thinking Skills

1. Recall personal losses (death of a family member or friend; loss of a significant relationship, job, or opportunity) and recollect what you were experiencing at the time. Try to remember what your expectations were from those you looked to for support, and how your ability to cope was influenced by whether those expectations were met. Remembering that no two people respond to loss in exactly the same way, develop a list of nursing measures to help patients dealing with loss. Compare your list with those of other students and incorporate their ideas.

2. Compare and contrast the care a patient dying of cancer would receive in a critical care unit and at home with hospice care. Identify the advantages and disadvantages of each. Talk with family members and friends about their preferences. Use your analysis to help describe these options to prospective patients. Role-play a situation with a peer in which you counsel a woman with cancer who is told that cure is no longer an option and that she has less than 6 months to live. Reflect on how your experiences, beliefs, and values might affect what you say to patients and how you say it.

Practicing for NCLEX

1. A woman who is firmly committed to natural childbirth and who has attended each natural childbirth class in preparation for labor and delivery undergoes a cesarean delivery when her fetus displays signs of distress. Inconsolable, she cries and calls herself a failure as a mother. Her loss may best be described as:
   a. Actual
   b. Perceived
   c. Psychological
   d. Combination of the above

2. The period of acceptance of loss and grief during which the person learns to deal with experienced loss is best termed:
   a. Anticipatory grieving
   b. Bereavement
   c. Mourning
   d. Stages of death and dying

3. When you interview an 82-year-old resident of a nursing home, she tells you that she has never gotten over the death of her son 20 years ago. She reports that her life fell apart after that and she never again felt like herself or was able to enjoy life. This type of grief is best described as:
   a. Abbreviated
   b. Anticipatory
   c. Dysfunctional
   d. Inhibited

4. A patient with AIDS whom you have been visiting at home tells you, "I'm no longer afraid of dying. I think I've made my peace with everyone, and I'm actually ready to move on." This reflects his progress to which stage of death and dying?
   a. Acceptance
   b. Anger
   c. Bargaining
   d. Denial

5. When you next visit this dying patient with AIDS, he breaks down and cries and tells you that it is unfair that he should have to die now when he's finally made peace with his family and wants to live. You are shocked by this change in his mood. Your best reply would be:

a. "You can't be feeling this way. You have to proceed through the stages of dying in an orderly progression, and you've just moved backward."

b. "It does seem unfair. Tell me more about how you are feeling."

c. "You'll be all right; who knows how much time any of us has to enjoy relationships with those we love? You're lucky to have had the opportunity to make your peace."

d. "Tell me about your pain. Did it keep you awake last night?"

6. Which definition of death is gaining in popularity, as more people believe that critical human functions are personality, conscious life, and the capacity for remembering, judging, reasoning, acting, enjoying, and worrying?

a. Heart–lung death

b. Higher-brain death

c. Personhood death

d. Whole-brain death

7. If your patient tells you that he has no one he trusts to make healthcare decisions for him should he become incapacitated, you should help him to prepare:

a. Combination advance medical directive

b. Durable power of attorney for healthcare

c. Living will

8. Which of the following nurse responses would be endorsed by the American Nurses Association?

a. A nurse promises a dying patient that he will do everything possible to keep her comfortable but that he cannot administer an injection or overdose to cause her death.

b. A nurse tells a dying patient who is on a ventilator that under no condition can he be removed from the ventilator because this is active euthanasia and is expressly forbidden by the Code for Nurses.

c. After exhausting every intervention in her bag of tricks to keep a dying patient comfortable, the nurse says, "I think you are now at a point where I'm prepared to do what you've been asking me. Let's talk about when and how you want to die."

d. In response to a patient who asks for assistance in committing suicide, a nurse replies, "I'm personally opposed to assisted suicide, but I'll find you a colleague who can help you."

9. You are caring for a comatose patient whose primary diagnosis is breast cancer but who has suffered multiple complications and who is now in the end stages of her illness. She has been in the medical intensive care unit for 3 weeks. Her husband tells you that he and his wife often talked about the end of her life and that she was very clear about not wanting aggressive treatment that would merely prolong her dying. You both agree that this seems to be all that therapy is now doing for her. Which of the following orders

would you recommend the husband speak to her physician about?

a. Comfort-measures-only

b. Do-not-hospitalize

c. Do-not-resuscitate

d. Slow-code-only

10. If you are involved in the terminal weaning of a patient, you will want to do all of the following except:

a. Participate in the decision-making process by offering the family information about the advantages and disadvantages of continued ventilatory support

b. Explain to the family what will happen at each phase of the weaning and offer support

c. Check the orders for sedation and analgesia and make sure that the anticipated death is comfortable and dignified

d. Tell the family that death will occur almost immediately after the patient is removed from the ventilator

11. All of the following diagnoses may apply to a young couple who gave birth to a premature infant with serious respiratory problems who has been in the neonatal intensive care unit for the last 3 months. The couple has a 22-month-old son at home. Which diagnosis best fits the following set of assessment data: report of chronic fatigue and decreased energy, guilt about neglecting son at home, shortness of temper with one another, apprehension about continued ability to go on this way?

a. Anticipatory Grieving

b. Ineffective Coping

c. Caregiver Role Strain

d. Powerlessness

12. Which of the nursing actions described below would you correct if you saw a nursing assistant doing this?

a. Talking to a comatose patient

b. Sitting on the bed of a dying patient holding her hand and crying

c. Agreeing with the daughter of a dying resident with Alzheimer's disease that the burdens associated with artificially feeding her father may outweigh the benefits

d. Telling a dying patient to sit back and relax and that she will wash him because it's easier that way

13. Which of the following nursing actions violates the standards of caring for the body after a patient has been pronounced dead?

a. Keeping the patient in a comfortable sitting position until the family has arrived and said their good-byes

b. Placing identification tags on both the shroud and the ankle

c. Removing soiled dressings and tubes

d. Preparing to transfer the body to the morgue

14. The family of a patient who has just died asks to be alone with the body and asks for supplies to wash the body. You know that the mortician usually washes the body. Your best response is:
   a. Inform the family that there is no need for them to wash the body since the mortician does this
   b. Explain that hospital policy forbids their being alone with the deceased patient and that hospital supplies are to be used only by hospital personnel
   c. Give the supplies but watch the family so that nothing unusual happens
   d. Provide the requested supplies and ask if this request is linked to their religious or cultural customs and if there is anything else you can do to be of assistance

15. A 70-year-old woman who has had a number of strokes refuses further life-sustaining interventions, including artificial nutrition and hydration. She is competent, understands the consequences of her actions, is not depressed, and persists in refusing treatment. Her doctor is adamant that she cannot be allowed to die this way, and her daughter agrees. An ethics consult has been placed. Who is the appropriate decision maker?
   a. Patient
   b. Daughter
   c. Doctor
   d. Ethics consult team

■ Answers With Rationale

1. The correct answer is *d*. Each of the above is only partially correct because there are elements of the loss of the type of delivery she values, which are actual, perceived, and psychological.

2. The correct answer is *c*. Mourning is defined as the period of acceptance of loss and grief during which the person learns to deal with experienced loss. The text offers other definitions for anticipatory grieving, bereavement, and the stages of death and dying.

3. The correct answer is *c*. Abbreviated grief and anticipatory grief are both types of normal grief, and given the length of time this resident's grief has lasted and its effects on her life, it is not normal. Because she is able to give expression to her grief, inhibited grief is not the correct answer. By a process of elimination, the correct answer is dysfunctional grief.

4. The correct answer is *a*. The patient's statement does not reflect anger, bargaining, or denial; hence, by a process of elimination, acceptance is the correct choice.

5. The correct answer is *b;* you want to validate that you have heard what the patient is saying and invite him to share more of his feelings, concerns,

and fears. You do not want to offer false reassurance (*c*) or use diversion (*d*): both of these strategies would communicate your lack of interest in what he is really feeling. It is simply not true that people have to move through these stages in an orderly fashion (*a*).

6. The correct answer is *b* because the functions described are controlled by the cortex, or higher brain. There is no such thing as personhood death.

7. The correct answer is *c*. The living will is a document whose precise purpose is to allow individuals to record specific instructions about the type of healthcare they would like to receive in particular end-of-life situations. Both the combination directive and the durable power of attorney involve appointing someone to make decisions, which is something this patient is reluctant to do.

8. The correct answer is *a*. The American Nurses Association states that nurse-assisted suicide and participation in active euthanasia violate the Code for Nurses and the ethical traditions of the profession. This makes *c* and *d* incorrect because it does not matter if a nurse's personal morality allows him or her to accept assisted suicide. Removing ventilatory support is not necessarily active euthanasia and is not expressly forbidden by the Code for Nurses.

9. The correct answer is *a*, comfort-measures-only order, because she would want all aggressive treatment to be stopped at this point and all care to be directed to a comfortable, dignified death. Because she is already in the hospital, there is no need for *b* at this point, and a do-not-resuscitate order is not sufficiently comprehensive. One should never recommend performing a slow-code-only order because it violates good practice.

10. The correct answer is *d; a, b,* and *c* are all nursing interventions that should be carried out by the nurse involved in terminal weaning. Because there are no guarantees how any patient will respond once removed from a ventilator, and because it is possible for the patient to breathe on his or her own and live for hours, days, and, rarely, even weeks, the family should definitely not be told that death will occur immediately.

11. The correct answer is *c;* although it is true that each of the diagnoses listed might apply to the couple described, the defining characteristics for the NANDA diagnosis Caregiver Role Strain fit the set of assessment data provided.

12. The correct answer is *d*. Answers *a* and *b* are acceptable and desirable nursing interventions, and if the nursing assistant is experienced, he or she may very well be in a position to do *c*. Because it is good to encourage dying patients to be as active as possible for as long as possible, it is generally not good practice to perform basic self-care measures the patient

can perform simply because it is "easier" to do it this way.

13. The correct answer is *a*. The other answers are all indicated nursing interventions and consistent with standards of care. Because the body should be placed in normal anatomic position to avoid pooling of blood, leaving the body in a sitting position is contraindicated.

14. The correct answer is *d*. Answer *a* ignores the needs of the family and reflects an ignorance of or insensitivity to cultural and religious practices; *b* is simply not true; and *c* presumes that the family is up to no good purpose and, unless you have reason to suspect something out of the ordinary, is simply uncalled-for.

15. The correct answer is *a*. Because this patient is competent, she has the right to refuse therapy that she finds to be disproportionately burdensome, even if this hastens her death. Neither her daughter nor her doctor has the authority to assume her decision-making responsibilities unless she asks them to do this. The ethics consult team is not a decision-making body; it can make recommendations but has no authority to order anything.

Bibliography

American Association of Colleges of Nursing. (1999). *Competencies necessary for nurses to provide high-quality care to patients and families during the transition at the end of life*. Washington, DC: Author.

American Geriatrics Society Ethics Committee. (1995). The care of dying patients: a position statement from the American Geriatrics Society. *Journal of the American Geriatrics Society, 43*, 577–578.

American Nurses Association. (1991). *Position statement on promotion of comfort and relief of pain in dying patients*. Washington, DC: Author.

American Nurses Association. (1995). *Position statement on assisted suicide*. Washington, DC: Author.

Buckman, R. (1992). *How to break bad news*. Baltimore: John Hopkins University Press.

Caplan, A. L., Snyder, L., & Faber-Langendoen, K. (2000). The role of guidelines in the practice of physician-assisted suicide. *Annals of Internal Medicine, 132*(6), 476–481.

Callanan, M., & Kelley, P. (1992). *Final gifts*. New York: Poseidon Press.

Campbell, M. L. (1994). Terminal weaning. *Nursing, 24*(9), 34–39.

Carpenito, L. J. (1995). *Nursing diagnosis: Application to clinical practice* (6th ed.). Philadelphia: J. B. Lippincott.

Edwards, B. S. (1994). When the family can't let go. *American Journal of Nursing, 94*(1), 52–56.

Ehrle, R. N., Shafer, T. J., & Nelson, K. R. (1999). Determination and referral of potential organ donors and consent for organ donation: Best practices—a blueprint for success. *Critical Care Nurse, 19*(2), 21–33.

Engel, G. L. (1964). Grief and grieving. *American Journal of Nursing, 64*(9), 93–98.

The Hastings Center. (1987). *Guidelines on the termination of life-sustaining treatment and the care of the dying*. Bloomington, IN: Indiana University Press.

Holmquist, M., Chabalewski, F., Blount, T., Edwards, V. M., & Pietroski, R. (1999). A critical pathway: Guiding care for organ donors. *Critical Care Nurse, 19*(2), 84–98.

Irish, D. P., Lundquist, K. F., & Nelsen, V. J. (Eds.). (1993). *Ethnic variations in dying, death, and grief*. Washington, DC: Taylor & Francis.

Jansen, L. A., & Sulmasy, D. P. (2002). Sedation, alimentation, hydration, and equivocation: Careful conversation about care at the end of life. *Annals of Internal Medicine, 136*(11), 845–849.

Kirchoff, K. T., Spuhler, V., Walker, L., Hutton, A., Cole, V., & Clemmer, T. (2000). Intensive care nurses' experiences with end-of-life care. *American Journal of Critical Care, 9*(1), 36–42.

Kübler-Ross, E. (1969). *On death and dying*. New York: Macmillan.

Last Acts. (2002). *Means to a better end: A report on dying in America today*. http://www.lastacts.org.

Lauterbach, S. S. (Ed.). (1995). The experience of loss. *Holistic Nursing Practice, 9*(3).

Lynn, J., & Goldstein, N. E. (2003). Advance care planning for fatal chronic illness: Avoiding commonplace errors and unwarranted suffering. *Annals of Internal Medicine, 138*(10), 812–818.

McCue, J. D. (1995). The naturalness of dying. *Journal of the American Medical Association, 273*(13), 1039–1043.

North American Nursing Diagnosis Association. (1994). *NANDA nursing diagnoses: Definitions and classifications 1995–1996*. Philadelphia: Author.

Nuland, S. B. (1994). *How we die*. New York: Alfred A. Knopf.

Nuland, S. B. (1997). *The wisdom of the body*. New York: Alfred A. Knopf.

Ott, B. B. (1995). Defining and redefining death. *American Journal of Critical Care, 4*(6), 476–480.

Ott, B. (1999). Advance directives: The emerging body of research. *American Journal of Critical Care, 8*(1), 514–519.

Pellegrino, E. D. (1991). Ethics. *Journal of the American Medical Association, 265*(23), 3118–3119.

Pellegrino, E. D. (2000). Decisions to withdraw life-sustaining treatment. *Journal of the American Medical Association, 283*(8), 1065–1067.

President's Commission for the Study of Ethical Problems in Medicine and Biomedical and Behavioral Research. (1981). *Defining death*. [Pub. No. 81-600150]. Washington, DC: U.S. Government Printing Office.

Quill, T. E., & Byock, I. R. (2000). Responding to intractable terminal suffering: The role of terminal sedation and voluntary refusal of food and fluids. *Annals of Internal Medicine, 132*(5), 408–414.

Quill, T. E., Lee, B. C., & Nunn, S. (2000). Palliative treatments of last resort: choosing the least harmful alternative. *Annals of Internal Medicine, 132*(6), 488–493.

Robert Wood Johnson Foundation. (2002). *First state-by-state report of dying in American today.* http://www.rwjf.org/news/releaseDetail.jsp?id=1037586523372.

Rushton, C., & Terry, D. B. (1995). Neuromuscular blockade and ventilator withdrawal: Ethical controversies. *American Journal of Critical Care, 4*(2), 112–115.

Saver, C. L. (1994). Decoding the ACLS algorithms. *American Journal of Nursing, 94*(1), 27–36.

Scanlon, C. (May 23, 1996). Euthanasia and nursing practice: Right question, wrong answer. *New England Journal of Medicine, 334*(21), 1401–1402.

Scanlon, C., & Rushton, C. (1996). Assisted suicide: Clinical realities and ethical challenges. *American Journal of Critical Care, 5*(6), 397–405.

Scanlon, D. (2003). Ethical concerns in end-of-life care. *American Journal of Nursing, 103*(1), 48–56.

Schroeder, S. A. (1999). The legacy of support [editorial]. *Annals of Internal Medicine, 131*(10), 780–781.

Schwarz, J. K. (1999). Assisted dying and nursing practice. *Image: The Journal of Nursing Scholarship, 31*(4), 367–373.

Schwartz, J. K. (2003). Understanding and responding to patients' requests for assistance in dying. *Journal of Nursing Scholarship, 35*(4), 377–384.

Seguin, M., & Smith, C. K. (1994). *A gentle death.* Toronto: Key Porter Books.

Sittser, G. L. (1995). *A grace disguised.* Grand Rapids, MI: Zondervan Publishing House.

Steinhauser, K. E., Clipp, E. C., McNeilly, M., et al. (2000). In search of a good death: Observations of patients, families, and providers. *Annals of Internal Medicine, 132*(10), 825–832.

Sullivan, J., Seem, D. L., & Chabalewski, F. (1999). Determining brain death. *Critical Care Nurse, 19*(2), 37–46.

SUPPORT Principal Investigators. (1995). A controlled trial to improve care for seriously ill hospitalized patients: The study to understand prognoses and preferences for outcomes and risks of treatment (SUPPORT). *Journal of the American Medical Association, 274,* 1591–1598.

Zerwekh, J. V. (1983). "The dehydration question?" *Nursing, 13*(1), 47–51.

Sensory Stimulation

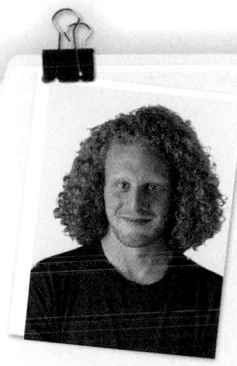

Ori Soltes, a 28-year-old man, is in the intensive care unit after a motor vehicle crash that resulted in multiple internal injuries as well as fractures. He is being monitored continuously and receiving mechanical ventilation. On the 5th day after the crash, he began to exhibit transient episodes of acute confusion.

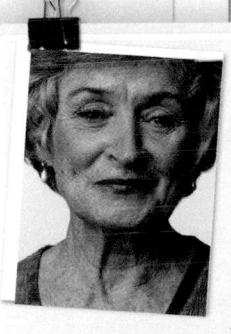

Dolores Pirolla, a 74-year old woman, comes to the older adult clinic with her 77-year-old husband who was diagnosed with macular degeneration and progressive vision loss. She states "Now I've noticed he's also having difficulty hearing me. I'm worried because he doesn't want to leave the house and we hardly see any of our friends anymore. We used to go out to the movies or dinner at least once a week. Lately, if we get out once a month, that's a lot!"

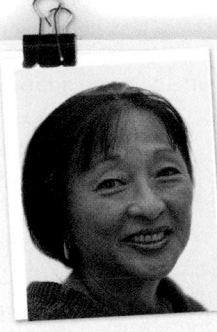

Muriel Hao is a 56-year-old woman who had surgery 2 days ago. She denies any complaints of pain or discomfort. She is receiving intravenous therapy via an infusion pump. She states "Please stop that beeping. It's driving me nuts and I can't rest."

Focusing on Blended Skills

The types of blended skills you'll need to respond to the case scenarios include:

Cognitive Skills

- Knowledge of the sensory experience, including the major components and conditions necessary to experience the world
- Knowledge of the arousal mechanism and how the body responds, including sensoristasis and adaptation
- Ability to integrate knowledge of sensory alterations, including factors contributing to disturbed sensory perceptions
- Knowledge of the manifestations of sensory overload, sensory deprivation, and sensory deficits
- Ability to incorporate knowledge of appropriate interventions when developing the plan of care for patients experiencing disturbed sensory perception, such as the patient in the intensive care unit, the wife of a patient with vision and hearing deficits, and a patient with sensory overload
- Knowledge of how to meet the safety and emotional needs of individuals with disturbed sensory perception, such as the wife of a patient with vision and hearing deficits

Technical Skills

- Strong assessment skills related to sensory overload, sensory deprivation, and sensory deficits
- Competence in using technical nursing assistance when providing care to patients with different disturbed sensory perceptions
- Ability to seek out assistance as necessary when performing technical nursing assistance

Interpersonal Skills

- Demonstration of the ability to empathize with and to communicate and interact effectively with patients and their caregivers, such as the patient in the intensive care unit, the wife whose husband has hearing and vision deficits, and the woman who is upset about the beeping of her equipment

- Ability to establish trusting nurse–patient relationships—even when confronted by patients with sensory problems
- Demonstration of teaching and counseling skills to assist patients and their caregivers with the measures to cope with disturbed sensory perception
- Ability to demonstrate respect for a patient's human dignity and autonomy throughout the patient's care
- Special interpersonal competence to interact with other healthcare team members, seeking out appropriate assistance when needed
- Ability to coordinate and facilitate the efforts of the healthcare team and community resources to meet the needs of patients experiencing disturbed sensory perception and their family caregivers

Ethical and Legal Skills

- Strong sense of accountability for the health and well-being of patients, which translates into a commitment for getting them the help they need within the scope of nursing responsibilities and available resources
- A willingness to hold one's self accountable for safe, high-quality care regardless of the patient's sensory problem
- Ability to practice in an ethically and legally defensible manner, including familiarity with facility policy and role responsibilities related to managing the care of patients with disturbed sensory perception
- Ability to integrate knowledge of ethical and legal principles related to sensory experiences in the intensive care unit, safety and emotional needs associated with sensory deficits, and use of technological equipment

Learning Outcomes

After completing the chapter, the learner should be able to accomplish the following:

1. Describe the four conditions that must be met in each sensory experience.
2. Explain the role of the reticular activating system in sensory experience.
3. Identify etiologies and perceptual, cognitive, and emotional responses to sensory deprivation and sensory overload.
4. Perform a comprehensive assessment of sensory functioning using appropriate interview questions and physical assessment skills.
5. Develop nursing diagnoses that correctly identify sensory/perceptual alterations that may be treated by independent nursing intervention.
6. Describe specific nursing interventions to prevent sensory alterations, to stimulate the senses, and to assist patients with sensory difficulties.
7. Develop, implement, and evaluate a plan of nursing care to help patients meet individualized sensory/perceptual outcomes.

Key Terms

adaptation
arousal
culturally competent care
disturbed sensory perception
kinesthesia
reticular activating system (RAS)
sensoristasis
sensory deficit
sensory deprivation
sensory overload
sensory perception
sensory reception
stereognosis
stimulus
visceral

A person's senses are vital to survival, growth and development, and the experience of bodily pleasure. For example, awareness of the intensities and sources of sound, ways to control noise, and the assessment of patients' perceptions of and responses to sound can provide nurses with a basis for therapeutic manipulation of the environment.

Nurses encounter many patients who have impaired sensory functioning that places them at risk for injury, disturbed growth and development, and decreased well-being. Moreover, the stress of illness or trauma and the need for diagnosis and treatment may quickly result in sensory deprivation or overload, with serious disturbances in visual, perceptual, cognitive, or emotional functioning (see the accompanying Reflective Practice box for an example).

This chapter provides knowledge of the process of sensation, the role of the arousal mechanism, sensory alterations, and factors affecting sensory stimulation. Practical suggestions are given for performing an assessment of sensory functioning. Examples of nursing diagnoses are provided, identifying specific disturbances in sensory perception as the etiology and many diagnoses describing the effects of disturbed sensory perception in other areas of human functioning. Patient outcomes for preventing and managing sensory alterations are described. Specialized nursing interventions for patients with

Reflective Practice
Challenge to Technical Skills

All throughout nursing school we are taught theory, and from that theory we are to use critical thinking to determine how to care for a particular patient, focusing on the patient, not the machines surrounding them. "You'll learn that later" they say.

I was assigned to care for Muriel Hao, a 56-year-old woman who had surgery 2 days ago. As I walk into her room, I check to see if she is comfortable and whether she needs anything at that particular point in time. She asks me one favor. "Please stop that beeping. It's driving me nuts and I can't rest." So I look at the machine, dumbfounded, and worried that the patient is going to think I am incompetent because I cannot even work a simple machine. No theory from a classroom is going to teach me how to make the machine stop beeping. To make things worse, every facility has different machines. As nursing students, we go from one facility to another, trying to get accustomed to the equipment and technologies of each one. I assume that things will get easier once I have steady employment in a facility. If that particular facility changes its technologies, I would hope that there would be an in-service on the new technology. But what do I do now, as a nursing student?

Thinking Outside the Box: Possible Courses of Action

- Press the buttons on the machine, and hope that the beeping goes away.
- Seek out someone who does know how to work the machine and have them fix it so I don't do more damage.
- Find someone who knows how to work the machine, have them fix it, and then have them explain to me how to fix it so I can do it next time.

Evaluating a Good Outcome: How Do I Define Success?

- Personal integrity is maintained (if I can't fix it, I feel stupid, and that's an insult to my integrity).
- Professional integrity remains intact (if I can't fix it, I will feel incompetent as a nurse—if I can't even fix a machine, how am I supposed to help a person?).
- The patient expresses relief that the beeping has stopped and she is now able to rest.

Personal Learning: Here's to the Future!

Although this does not seem like a huge or very troublesome problem, every nursing student can probably attest to feeling this way at least once. The first few times it happened to me, I just asked someone to fix it for me, thinking it was a one-time problem. Then I realized that this is something that I was facing over and over again. So I asked someone to show me how to fix the problem if it should occur again. I understood what to do and knew how to do it. Then we switched hospitals and I was confused once again. In today's environment of ever-changing technology, I realized that it is not just the students who feel this way. Nurses, too, have these same feelings. We all learn new things every day, whether it's from a patient, another nurse, a doctor, or a technical specialist. We just need to know that it's okay to ask questions. Moreover, not knowing how to work with a piece of equipment does not mean that you are incompetent with people. Learning in the healthcare field is an ongoing process.

Reflection

How do you think you would respond in a similar situation? Why? What does this tell you about yourself and about the adequacy of your skills for professional practice? Are there any other possible courses of actions that the nursing student should have identified? If so, please explain. What patient needs was the nursing student addressing? What personal needs? Describe the patient's sensory experience, addressing the major components and four conditions necessary to experience the world. Can you think of other ways to respond? What other skills (cognitive, interpersonal, technical, ethical/legal) would you need to respond well in this situation? What measures might have been appropriate for the nursing student to do in preparation for this patient assignment? Do you agree with the criteria to evaluate a successful outcome? Did the nursing student meet the criteria? Please explain why or why not?

Michele Jordan, Georgetown University

vision or hearing impairment, confusion, and altered consciousness also are presented.

THE SENSORY EXPERIENCE

Components and Conditions

The sensory experience consists of two components: reception and perception. **Sensory reception** is the process of receiving data about the internal or external environment through the senses. The senses by which individuals maintain contact with the external environment are vision (visual), hearing (auditory) smell (olfactory), taste (gustatory), and touch (tactile). **Stereognosis** is the sense that perceives the solidity of objects and their size, shape, and texture. In addition, individuals orient themselves internally by the kinesthetic and visceral senses. (**Kinesthesia** refers to awareness of positioning of body parts and body movement; **visceral** pertains to inner organs.) The kinesthetic and visceral senses arise internally from muscles and hollow organs, respectively, and are the body's basic orienting systems.

Sensory perception is the conscious process of selecting, organizing, and interpreting data from the senses into meaningful information. Perception is influenced by the intensity, size, change, or representation of stimuli, as well as by past experiences, knowledge, and attitudes.

For a person to receive the necessary data to experience the world, four conditions must be met:
- A **stimulus**—an agent, act, or other influence capable of initiating a response by the nervous system—must be present.
- A receptor or sense organ must receive the stimulus and convert it to a nerve impulse.
- The nerve impulse must be conducted along a nervous pathway from the receptor or sense organ to the brain.
- A particular area in the brain must receive and translate the impulse into a sensation.

Think back to Muriel Hao, the 56-year-old woman unable to rest because of the machine's beeping. The nurse would incorporate knowledge of sensory reception and perception to determine that the patient is experiencing a continuous and large amount of auditory stimuli from the beeping of the machine. In addition, the nurse would need to keep in mind other sources of stimuli, such as possible visual stimuli from the lighted numbers on the machine, tactile stimuli from being touched to determine the possible problem associated with machine, and internal stimuli associated with pain and discomfort from surgery.

Arousal Mechanism

To receive stimuli and respond appropriately, the brain must be alert or aroused. The **reticular activating system** (RAS), a poorly defined network that extends from the hypothalamus to the medulla, mediates arousal. The optimal arousal state of the RAS is a general drive state called **sensoristasis**. Nerve impulses from all the sensory tracts reach the RAS, which then selectively allows certain impulses to reach the cerebral cortex and be perceived. The mesencephalic portion of the RAS appears to be the center of the system. Stimulation of this area produces the most pronounced and long-lasting effects on the cerebral cortex (Fig. 34-1). With its many ascending and descending connections to other areas of the brain, the RAS serves to monitor and to regulate incoming sensory stimuli, thus maintaining, enhancing, or inhibiting cortical **arousal.** States of arousal or awareness are described in Box 34-1.

The body quickly adapts to constant stimuli. In addition, the repeated stimulus of a continuing noise, such as city traffic, or a noxious odor eventually goes unnoticed. Therefore, a stimulus must be variable or irregular to evoke a response. This phenomenon is termed **adaptation**. Impulses that are not acted on when received may be used at a later date in response to the same or similar stimuli The memory process involves the storage of that material. For example, thought and memory are used when a new sensory experience occurs and the organism uses a response based on previous knowledge and experience.

DISTURBED SENSORY PERCEPTION

When a patient is admitted to a health agency, he or she is confronted with stimuli that are different in quality and quantity than that to which he or she is accustomed. For example, a patient confined to bed rest may receive many fewer stimuli,

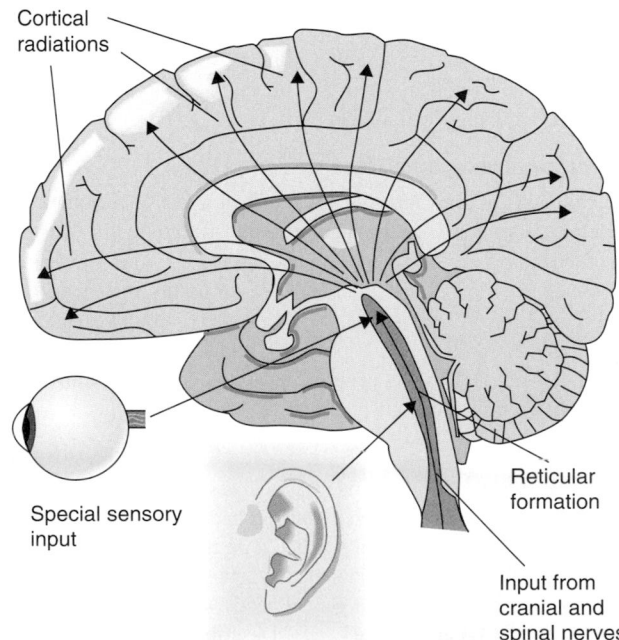

Cortical radiations

Special sensory input

Reticular formation

Input from cranial and spinal nerves

FIGURE 34-1 Nerve impulses from all the sensory tracts reach the reticular activating system (RAS), which then selectively allows certain impulses to reach the cerebral cortex and to be perceived.

BOX 34-1 States of Awareness

Conscious States

Delirium	Disorientation, restlessness, confusion, hallucinations, agitation, alternating with other conscious states
Dementia	Difficulties with spatial orientation, memory, language, changes in personality
Confusion	Reduced awareness, easily distracted, easily startled by sensory stimuli, alternates between drowsiness and excitability; resembles minor form of delirium state
Normal consciousness	Aware of self and external environment, well-oriented, responsive
Somnolence	Extreme drowsiness, but will respond normally to stimuli
Chronic vegetative state	Conscious but unresponsive, no evidence of cortical function

Unconscious States

Asleep	Can be aroused by normal stimuli (light touch, sound, etc.)
Stupor	Can be aroused by extreme and/or repeated stimuli
Coma	Cannot be aroused and does not respond to stimuli (coma states can be further subdivided according to the effect on reflex responses to stimuli) (see Glasgow Coma Scale, Chapter 25)

---

whereas one undergoing multiple diagnostic tests may receive a greater-than-normal level of sensory input. These and other typical experiences are likely to result in disturbed sensory perceptions experienced by the patient. The nurse's sensitivity to how color, sound, and touch are stimulating the patient combined with attention to the patient's need for privacy and for social interaction can significantly reduce disturbances in sensory perception.

Severe sensory alterations can occur, especially in certain areas, such as the critical care or intensive care units (termed intensive care unit [ICU] psychosis). Factors contributing to severe sensory alteration include sensory overload, sensory deprivation, sleep deprivation, and cultural care deprivation.

Consider Ori Soltes, the young man in the ICU. The nurse would need to assess Mr. Soltes closely for underlying reasons for his confusion. Although the possible causes are numerous and most likely multiple in nature, the nurse would need to address the possibility of sensory deprivation and overload as contributing to the patient's confusion.

Table 34-1 provides an overview of sensory deprivation and sensory overload with related nursing interventions. The accompanying Research in Nursing box addresses the experiences of patients in ICUs.

Sensory Deprivation

Sensory deprivation results when a person experiences decreased sensory input or input that is monotonous, unpatterned, or meaningless. With decreased sensory input, the RAS is no longer able to project a normal level of activation to the brain. As a result, the individual may hallucinate simply to maintain an optimal level of arousal. Factors placing a patient at high risk for sensory deprivation include the following:

- An environment with decreased or monotonous stimuli (such as institutionalized patients or those confined to a small living area at home, on bed rest, or in isolation)
- Impaired ability to receive environmental stimuli (patients with impaired vision or hearing; with bandages or casts that interfere with vision, hearing, or tactile stimulation; or with affective disorders who "close out" the environment)

Remember Dolores Pirolla, the wife of the older man with vision deficits who was developing hearing deficits? The nurse would incorporate knowledge of risk factors for sensory deprivation when developing the patient's plan of care. In this case, Mr. Pirolla's sensory deficits involving vision and now hearing are impacting his ability to receive environmental stimuli. Thus, the nurse would develop a plan of care that addresses measures to ensure that the patient and his wife receive adequate stimulation from the environment.

- Inability to process environmental stimuli (patients with spinal cord injuries or brain damage, those who are confused or disoriented, or are taking prescribed or recreational drugs affecting the central nervous system)

Sensory deprivation can lead to various effects. These effects include perceptual, cognitive, and emotional disturbances *Perceptual responses* involve the inaccurate perception of sights, sounds, tastes, smells, and body position, coordination, and equilibrium. These responses can range from mild distortions such as daydreams, to gross distortions such as hallucinations. *Cognitive responses* involve the patient's inability to control the direction of thought content. Typically, attention span and ability to concentrate are decreased. The patient may demonstrate difficulty with memory, problem solving, and task performance. *Emotional responses* typically are manifested by

TABLE 34-1 Overview of Sensory Deprivation and Sensory Overload

Sensory Deprivation   Insufficient quantity or quality of stimuli; may result from decreased sensory input or monotonous, unpatterned, and unmeaningful input

Defining Characteristics	Contributing Factors	Patients at Risk
Physical behaviors: drowsiness, excessive yawning *Escape behaviors:* eating, exercising, sleeping, running away to escape the deprived environment *Changes in perception:* unusual body sensations; preoccupation with somatic complaints (dry mouth, palpitations, difficulty breathing, nausea); change in body image; illusions and hallucinations *Changes in cognitive behavior:* decreased attention span, inability to concentrate, decreased problem solving and task performance *Changes in affective behavior:* crying, increased irritability and annoyance over small matters, confusion, panic, depression	*Decreased environmental stimuli:* institutionalized environment; separation from significant others and usual sources of stimuli; treatments that decrease access to stimuli, such as bed rest or isolation *Impaired ability to receive environmental stimuli:* impaired vision, hearing, taste, smell, touch resulting from treatments such as bandages or body casts that interfere with reception of stimuli, or as a result of depression and other affective disorders *Inability to process environmental stimuli:* spinal cord injuries, brain damage, confusion, dementia, medications that depress the central nervous system	Institutionalized patients, especially those in long-term care settings Patients with communicable disease (eg, AIDS) Patients confined to bed Patients with sensory alterations (eg, impaired vision or hearing, or patients with eye patches or body casts) Patients who are depressed Patients from a different culture Patients with a disturbance of the nervous system

Nursing Interventions

Maintain sufficient level of arousal by increasing sensory stimuli from all sensory modalities:
- Instruct the patient in self-stimulation methods: counting, singing, reading, reciting poetry.
- Structure meaningful tangible stimuli into patient's external environment; include a variety of people, ideas, sensations; a pet may provide excellent stimulation.
  - Visual stimulation

    Colorful sheets, pajamas, robes   Clocks, calendars, wrist watches
    Colorful uniform tops for the nurse   Pictures, flowers, greeting card
    Face-to-face human contact
  - Auditory stimulation

    Call person by name   Reading to the patient
    Conversation that communicates caring   Television, radio
        as well as orients patient
  - Gustatory and olfactory stimulation

    Attention to oral hygiene and properly fitting dentures
    Food of different textures, colors, temperatures served attractively
    Smelling food before eating it and recalling pleasurable aromas from the past
    Seasoning foods or having favorite foods brought from home
  - Tactile stimulation

    Backrubs and foot soaks   Hair brushing, combing, washing
    Turning and repositioning   Hugs
    Passive range-of-motion exercises   Touching of arms or shoulders
  - Cognitive input

    Orient patient to environment
    Encourage patient participation in self-care
    Discuss current events or patient's occupation, hobbies, or interests
    Reinforce reality without arguing with a patient who is hallucinating. "No, I don't see a man standing there but the linen hamper may be confusing you."
  - Emotional input

    Encourage patient to share fears, concerns, and perceptions; reassure patient that illusions and misperceptions do occur with sensory deprivation
- Incorporate culturally assistive, supportive, facilitative acts into nursing care.
- *Caution:* Because it can be difficult to distinguish the behavioral manifestations of sensory deprivation from sensory overload, introduce more stimulation cautiously. If the added stimulation only increases the patient's maladaptive behaviors, consider reducing sensory input because the patient may be experiencing sensory overload.

(continued)

TABLE 34-1 (Continued)

Sensory Overload Excessive stimuli over which an individual feels little control; brain is unable meaningfully to respond to or ignore stimuli

Defining Characteristics	Contributing Factors	Patients at Risk
Similar to those observed in sensory deprivation Elderly patients and patients who have suffered a stroke are more likely to experience a confusion or agitation. Young patients are more likely to seek the comfort of their parents' embrace to block out sensory overload.	*Increased internal stimuli:* pain, pressure and discomfort of intrusive tubes (eg, intravenous lines [IVs], catheters; endotracheal tubes, nasogastric tubes), worry about state of health or need to make treatment decisions *Increased external stimuli:* unfamiliar healthcare environment, such as lights, noises, sounds, odors, movement, and constant presence of strangers, many of whom touch the body; intrusive procedures such as diagnostic tests and treatments; scratchy linens *Inability perceptually to disregard or selectively ignore some stimuli:* nervous system disturbances, medications such as caffeine that stimulate the central nervous system arousal mechanism	Acutely or chronically ill patients Patients in pain Patient with intrusive monitoring or treatment equipment Hospitalized patients, especially those in critical care settings Patients with disturbances of the nervous system

Nursing Interventions

- Provide a consistent, predictable pattern of stimulation to help the patient develop a sense of control over the environment.
- Offer simple explanations before procedures, tests, and examinations.
- Establish a schedule with the patient for routine care such as eating, bathing, turning, positioning, coughing, and exercising.
- Speak calmly with the patient and move slowly; communicate confidence.
- Explore with the patient what stimuli are most distressing and develop a plan to reduce or eliminate these (eg, incoming phone calls, visitors); ear plugs or pain medication may be indicated.
- Be careful not to cause sensory deprivation
- Identify and, wherever possible, eliminate culturally inappropriate stimuli.

(Adapted from Lee, K. A. [1991]. Sensory overload, sensory deprivation, and sleep deprivation. In M. L. Patrick, S. I. Woods, R. F. Craven, J. S. Rokosky, & P. M. Bruno [Eds.], *Medical-surgical nursing* [2nd ed.]. Philadelphia: J. B. Lippincott.)

Research in Nursing Making a Difference
Promoting Improved Intensive Care Experiences

Critical care staff may have difficulty comprehending how patients experience a stay in an intensive care unit. Barriers to the usual means of achieving shared understanding, such as patients' inability to speak because of intubation or fluctuating levels of consciousness, led these authors to search the literature for systematic research into patients' perceptions of critical care.

Related Research

Stein-Parbury, J., & McKinley, S. (2000). Patients' experiences of being in an intensive care unit: A select literature review. *American Journal of Critical Care, 9*(1), 20–27.

The authors reviewed a total of 26 research studies on patients' experiences of being in an intensive care unit. Patients recalled not only experiences that were negative but also ones that were neutral or positive. Positive experiences included a sense of safety and security promoted especially by the nurses. Negative experiences included impaired cognitive functioning and discomforts, such as problems with sleeping, pain, and anxiety. The review indicates steps that critical care staff can take to develop better ways to understand patients' experiences.

Relevance to Nursing Practice

This is an excellent example of using research findings to improve practice: to improve the quality of patients' experiences and to reduce anxiety and offset potential adverse effects of being a patient in an intensive care unit.

apathy, anxiety, fear, anger, belligerence, panic, or depression. Rapid mood changes also may occur (see Table 34-1 for additional information). Wahl and Heyl (2003), in a discussion of the relationships among visual impairment, loss of hearing, and cognitive function in older adults, found that cognitive capacity and nonimpaired sensory function were closely related to higher cortical functions.

Sensory Overload

Sensory overload is the condition that results when a person experiences so much sensory stimuli that the brain is unable to either respond meaningfully or ignore the stimuli. The person feels out of control and may exhibit all of the manifestations observed in sensory deprivation. The amount and quality of stimuli necessary to produce overload may differ greatly from one individual to another and are influenced by factors such as age, culture, personality, and lifestyle.

In some patients, especially those coming from a quiet environment with unvarying stimuli, the experience of being hospitalized quickly results in sensory overload. In such patients, the brain is assaulted by the constant presence of strangers who not only demand to be spoken to but also touch and poke at the body; by the strange sights, odors, sounds, and feels of the unfamiliar environment; by the constant presence of pain or discomfort from dressings, intravenous (IV) lines, drainage tubes, or endotracheal tubes; and by the ever-present worries about the meaning and course of the illness.

Recall Muriel Hao, the woman upset about the beeping of her machine? Assessment of Ms. Hao would most likely reveal that she is experiencing sensory overload.

Nursing care focuses on reducing distressing stimuli and helping the patient to gain control over the environment (see Table 34-1).

Now consider Ori Soltes, the young man in the ICU. When assessing Mr. Soltes and his confusion, the nurse would need to be alert for factors that would contribute to sensory overload, such as bright lights, noises from the various monitoring devices, and frequent examinations. In addition, the nurse would need to assess for possible factors contributing to sensory deprivation. For example, the patient is receiving mechanical ventilation. As a result, healthcare team members may limit verbal communication with the patient, thus reducing some auditory stimuli that he would receive. Additionally, the patient is in bed with multiple injuries, also restricting his ability to interact with the environment.

Sensory Deficits

Impaired or absent functioning in one or more senses is termed **sensory deficit.** Examples of sensory deficits include impaired sight and hearing, altered taste, numbness and paralysis that result in altered tactile perception, and impaired kinesthetic sense. These deficits may be reversible or permanent, may occur gradually or all at once, and may be present at birth or evolve later. Awareness of a patient's sensory deficits is necessary to determine whether the patient is able to compensate for the deficit. Illness and hospitalization may threaten a patient's usual adaptive patterns and require new self-care abilities. Patients with evolving deficits will require assistance in coping and in learning to compensate skillfully.

Remember Dolores Pirolla, the wife of the man with vision and hearing deficits? The nurse would need to assess both the patient and his wife to determine how each is coping. From the description at the beginning of the chapter, Mr. Pirolla appears to be experiencing problems coping with the vision changes. As a result, both Mr. and Mrs. Pirolla are beginning to experience social isolation. The nurse would incorporate this information when developing a plan of care for the patient and his wife.

FACTORS AFFECTING SENSORY STIMULATION

The amount of stimuli different individuals consider optimal appears to vary considerably. Factors influencing the amount and quality of stimuli needed to maintain cortical arousal include developmental considerations, culture, personality and lifestyle, stress, and illness and medication.

Developmental Considerations

Different types of sensory stimulation are needed for growth as sensory receptors and organs and the nervous system mature. Although the newborn is capable of rudimentary perceptual discrimination at birth, many neural pathways are immature and must be stimulated to develop, become refined, and function adequately. Appropriate stimulation includes soothing, holding, rocking and changes of position (tactile and kinesthetic sensations), singing and being talked to (auditory sensations), and changing patterns of light and shade, such as through the use of mobiles and bright objects (visual sensations).

Taquino and Lockridge (1999) identified strategies to promote and improve developmental outcomes when caring for critically ill infants. They found that the neonatal ICU is a source of inappropriate sensory stimulation. To facilitate developmentally supportive care, it is recommended that medically fragile infants have limited light and visual and vestibular stimulation to simulate being in the womb.

For children, engaging in developmentally appropriate play will develop muscles and coordination, provide an outlet for surplus physical energy, develop communication skills, provide sources of learning, act as a stimulant to creativity, develop social skills, teach sex roles, provide an outlet for the release of emotional energy, and develop self-insights.

Sensory functioning tends to decline progressively through-out adulthood as the result of aging or chronic illness. The adult may experience the need to compensate for the loss of one type of stimulation by increasing other sources of sensory stimuli. See the accompanying box, Focus on the Older Adult: Sensory Stimulation.

Culture

An individual's culture may dictate the amount of sensory stimulation considered normal. For example, the amount of touching a child experiences in a Puerto Rican family may be different from that experienced by a child in a German family. Similarly, male and female roles may be culturally defined; for example, although the man is expected to respond to the chal-lenge of out-of-the-home sensory stimuli, the woman who at-tempts to do so may be scorned if her place is considered to be in the home. Ethnic norms, religious norms, income group norms, and the norms of subgroups within a culture all influ-ence the amount of sensory stimulation sought by an individual and perceived as meaningful.

Moreover, sensory deprivation, sensory overload, and sleep deprivation are all related to or affected by an individual's cul-tural practices, values, and beliefs. The nurse who is sensitive to the patient's culture attempts to determine what constitutes acceptable levels of stimuli from the patient's viewpoint. For example, in certain cultures, touching is viewed as a natural and welcome custom, whereas other cultures may view it as in-sulting or offensive. Similarly, patients may find comfort in cultural and religious symbols of care and healing that are absent in a hospital environment. Thus, nurses must be aware of the aspects of the patient's culture to deliver **culturally com-petent care.**

Personality and Lifestyle

Apart from a person's culture, different personality types de-mand different levels of stimulation. One person may thrive on a steady stream of fast-paced changes and excitement, whereas another may feel best when daily routines are rigidly structured and life sends no challenges necessitating changes. Lifestyle choices can dramatically influence the quantity and quality of stimuli received by an individual. The nurse who elects to work in the emergency room of a large city hospital is exposed to vastly different stimuli than the nurse making home visits in a rural setting.

Stress

Increased sensory stimulation may be sought during periods of low stress simply to maintain cortical arousal. During high-stress periods, multiple stressors may already be overloading the sensory system, and decreased sensory stimulation is de-sired. Illness, a time of stress, can affect the reception of sen-

Focus on the Older Adult
Sensory Stimulation

Age-Related Changes	Nursing Strategies
Decrease in vision	• Ensure the patient is using corrective lenses such as contacts, glasses, and/or magnifiers. • Administer medications that enhance vision, such as medications that lower intraocular pressure in older adult patients with glaucoma. • Provide adequate lighting and clear pathways of clutter to prevent injury. • Provide enlarged print. • Encourage the patient to visit the ophthalmologist annually.
Decrease in hearing	• Ensure the patient is using hearing assistive devices. • When communicating with the patient, use a lower tone. • Speak to the patient so that he/she can visualize mouth movements.
Decreased sense of touch	• Protect the patient's skin from temperature extremes. • Assess the extremities for breaks in the skin, blisters, drainage, or open wounds. • Ensure the patient is ambulating with assistive devices.
Sensory deprivation	• Discourage the use of sedatives. • Assess the effect of medications on the patient's central nervous system. • Provide interaction with children and pets. • Encourage the patient to participate in exercise classes and provide activity therapy. • Ensure that institutionalized elderly adults share meals with four individuals per table. • Ensure homebound elderly adults have frequent visits from family and community resources such as Meals on Wheels or church volunteers.
Sensory overload	• Orient the patient to person, place, and time. • Decrease environmental noise. • Encourage patient to participate in nursing care.

sory stimuli and their transmission and perception. Therefore, the stress of physical illness, pain, hospitalization, testing, surgery, or treatment may provide more stimulation than an individual can process and respond to without assistance.

> *Think back to Muriel Hao, the woman who had surgery 2 days ago. Most likely, Ms. Hao is experiencing sensory overload from all of the events of the past several days. In addition, the constant beeping of the equipment is adding to this overload.*

Medication

Medications that alert or depress the central nervous system may interfere with the perception of sensory stimuli. Certain medications may also contribute to the impairment of sensory functioning by decreasing reception (eg, captopril, an antihypertensive agent, can cause taste alteration).

THE NURSING PROCESS FOR SENSORY STIMULATION

Assessing

When assessing a patient for disturbed sensory perceptions, interview the patient and examine him or her for sensory deficits and manifestations of sensory deprivation or overload. Be sure to include an assessment of the patient's environment to determine whether it is providing adequate sensory stimulation for healthy development.

Assessment of the Sensory Experience

When assessing the patient's sensory experience, structure it based on the components of the sensory experience—stimulation, reception, and transmission–perception–reaction. See the Focused Assessment Guide 34-1. Because patients may adapt

 Focused Assessment Guide 34-1

Sensory Stimulation

Factors to Assess	Questions and Approaches
Stimulation	"Does your current environment overly, insufficiently, or appropriately stimulate you?" "Are you bored? Why?" "Are you able to read? Watch television? Knit? Why not?" "Are there other people in your home during the day? Do you spend much time together? How do you spend the time?" "Who visits you while you are in the hospital?" Note reduction in the patterns or meaningfulness of stimulation in each sensory modality; changes in stimulation other than decreases (eg, new or unusual stimulation); or developmental appropriateness of stimulation.
Reception	"Does anything interfere with the functioning of your senses?" "Describe any corrective devices you use for sensory impairments."
Assess for visual disturbances.	"Please read my name tag (or this page of print)." Note if the patient can correctly identify objects directly in front of the eyes as well as those requiring peripheral vision. Note eye rubbing; squinting; movements indicating faulty vision (bumping into furniture, overreaching or underreaching for objects); changes in the appearance of the eye (cataracts, swelling); and complaints of eye pain, spots, halos, or other visual disturbances.
Assess for auditory disturbances.	"Repeat the words that I will speak softly close to each ear." Note if the patient is able to hear equally well from both ears, distinguish voices, locate the direction of a sound, if the patient needs to face the person speaking and relies on lip reading, if the patient's responses to questions include blank looks, many nods, smiling, or inappropriate responses indicating faulty hearing. Note complaints of ringing or buzzing in ears.
Assess for gustatory (taste) disturbances.	"Close your eyes, stick out your tongue, and tell me if what I place on your tongue is sweet, sour, bitter, or salty." "Have you been experiencing any strange tastes (bitter, metallic) or aftertastes lately?" Note if the patient is able to differentiate sweet, sour, bitter, or salty tastes or reports unusual, persistent taste sensations. Note deficient oral hygiene, ill-fitting dentures, braces, or anything else that might contribute to gustatory disturbances.

(continued)

Focused Assessment Guide 34-1

Sensory Stimulation (Continued)

Factors to Assess	Questions and Approaches
Assess for olfactory (smell) disturbances.	"Close your eyes and tell me what you smell." "Have you smelled odors lately that others cannot smell, or have you been especially sensitive to odors?" Note if the patient can correctly identify common odors (coffee, vanilla) or has noticed increased sensitivity to odors.
Assess for tactile (touch) disturbances.	"Close your eyes and tell me when you feel something (brush skin with cotton ball), if what you feel is dull or sharp (use both ends of safety pin), hot or cold (use items from food tray). Now, keep your eyes closed and tell me what I am placing in your hand (coin, cotton ball, paper clip)." Note if the patient can correctly sense touch and distinguish sharp and dull, hot and cold, and different shapes. Note if the patient reports decreased sensation in any part of the body; numbness, pins and needles, tingling; or abnormal sensitivity to pain or touch.
Assess for kinesthetic and visceral disturbances.	Note if the patient withdraws from being touched. "Have you noticed any changes in the way you perceive your body?" "Do you feel any unusual pressure or pain inside your body?" Note if the patient seems unsure of his or her body parts or body position and if he or she experiences new internal sensations (fullness, pressure, pain).
Transmission–perception–reaction	"Are you aware of any problems with your nervous system?" "Have you found it difficult to communicate verbally?" Note consciousness, orientation, appropriateness of responses, ability to perform usual self-care activities, ability to follow simple commands, decision-making abilities, pathology affecting central nervous system, or prescribed or recreational drug use that affects the central nervous system.
Behavioral manifestations of sensory deprivation or overload	
Perceptual responses	Mild to gross sensory distortions (illusions, hallucinations)
Cognitive responses	Thought disorganization, slowness of thought, decreased attention/concentration, difficulty with problem solving and task performance
Emotional responses	Rapid mood changes, anxiety, panic

to sensory impairments, it may be helpful to include someone the patient knows well (eg, spouse or parent) in the assessment to see if that person has noticed behavioral characteristics in the patient that suggest a sensory disturbance (eg, "I've noticed he turns the television volume much louder than ever before.").

Stimulation

Assess whether there have been any recent changes in sensory stimulation, for example, reduction of stimulation from one or more sensory modalities ("Since my husband died, no one touches me anymore. It sounds crazy, but I'm hungry to be touched!") or new or unusual stimulation ("Ever since my granddaughter moved in with me, my house is always noisy. I can't stand the constant noise and her smoking."). Assess whether the type of stimulation present is developmentally appropriate. High-risk patients for problems related to stimulation include children in nonstimulating environments, older people, terminally ill patients, patients on bed rest, patients in

isolation, and patients requiring intensive nursing in a critical care setting.

Reception

Assess for anything that may interfere with sensory reception and describe any corrective devices the patient uses for sensory impairments (eyeglasses, contact lenses, hearing aids). The Reception section of the Focused Assessment Guide 34-1 highlights assessment strategies for each sense. Patients at high risk for reception problems include people with visual, auditory, or other sensory impairments.

Consider Dolores Pirolla and her husband who has visual and hearing deficits. The nurse would need to assess the amount and type of stimulation Mr. Pirolla is receiving. In addition, the nurse would need to investigate what measures the couple uses to adapt to the progressive visual changes. Doing so would pro-

vide a sound basis on which to build the plan
of care.

Transmission–Perception–Reaction

Be alert for patients at high risk for transmission–perception–reaction problems, such as the patient who is confused or has a nervous system impairment. Use everyday interactions as multiple opportunities to assess patients' abilities to transmit, perceive, and react to stimuli.

Defining Characteristics of Sensory Deprivation and Overload

Complete the assessment of the patient's sensory functioning by assessing for specific indicators of sensory deprivation or overload (see Table 34-1 earlier in the chapter). Observe for boredom, inactivity, slowness of thought, daydreaming, increased sleeping, thought disorganization, anxiety, panic, illusions, and hallucinations. Be knowledgeable of the patient's usual state to enhance ability to identify changes stemming from sensory deprivation or overload.

> Think back to Muriel Hao, the woman who had surgery 2 days ago. The patient's complaints of inability to rest due to the machine's beeping should alert the nurse to the possibility of sensory overload. Additionally, to confirm the suspicions, the nurse would need to review the patient's medical record to gather more data about the patient's usual state and behavior.

Physical Assessment

Physical examination skills related to the senses are discussed in Chapter 25. Ear and eye tests, whether performed by a physician or nurse, should be considered when planning care. Problems with the neurologic system indicate the necessity of further assessment of the sensory experience.

Diagnosing

Disturbed Sensory Perception as the Problem

When assessment data point to sensory disturbances that can be treated independently by nursing interventions, nursing diagnoses are developed and labeled. The North American Nursing Diagnosis Association (2003) recognizes the following diagnostic labels for sensory/perceptual problems:

- *Disturbed Sensory Perception:* A state in which the individual or group experiences or is at risk for a change in the amount, pattern, or interpretation of incoming stimuli. These alterations may be further specified as visual, auditory, gustatory, olfactory, tactile, or kinesthetic. Sensory deprivation, sensory overload, and uncompensated sensory loss may also be used to further specify the disturbed sensory perception and in some cases may be the etiology.
- *Acute Confusion:* The abrupt onset of a cluster of global, transient changes and disturbances in attention, cognition,

psychomotor activity level of consciousness, or sleep–wake cycle
- *Chronic Confusion:* An irreversible, long-standing, or progressive deterioration of intellect and personality characterized by decreased ability to interpret environmental stimuli or decreased capacity for intellectual thought processes and manifested by disturbances of memory, orientation, and behavior
- *Impaired Memory:* The state in which an individual experiences the inability to remember or recall bits of information or behavior skills. Impaired memory may be attributed to pathophysiologic or situational causes that are either temporary or permanent.

Common etiologies for disturbed sensory perception include the following:
- Altered environmental stimuli: excessive or insufficient
- Altered sensory reception, transmission, or integration
- Chemical alterations: endogenous (eg, electrolytes) or exogenous (eg, drugs)
- Psychological stress

Sample nursing diagnoses in which the disturbed sensory perception is the problem are listed in the accompanying box.

Disturbed Sensory Perception as the Etiology

Because disturbed sensory perceptions affect many other areas of human functioning, they serve as etiologies for multiple problem statements. Examples may include the following:

Activity Intolerance related to impaired balance and coordination (kinesthetic alteration)

Anxiety related to paranoia stemming from hearing impairment, sensory deprivation (specify setting), sensory overload

Impaired Verbal Communication related to difficulty receiving, transmitting, and perceiving sensory stimuli

Ineffective Coping related to sensory overload (multiple stressors)

Deficient Diversional Activity related to impaired vision or hearing

Delayed Growth and Development related to nonstimulating home environment

Risk for Injury related to decreased or impaired sensation (specify visual, auditory, tactile, kinesthetic)

Deficient Knowledge about means to Compensate for Sensory Impairment (blindness, deafness, and so forth) related to lack of previous experience with this problem, unavailability of resources

Deficient Knowledge of providing a Developmentally Stimulating Environment related to lack of experience with children's growth and development

Impaired Physical Mobility related to impaired balance and coordination (kinesthetic alteration)

Impaired Parenting associated with failure to Provide Stimuli for Growth related to lack of knowledge, decreased motivation to provide for child's growth and development

Powerlessness related to inability to interact meaningfully with environment

Examples of NANDA Nursing Diagnoses | Disturbed Sensory Perception

Nursing Diagnoses	Related Factors	Sample Defining Characteristics
Disturbed Sensory Perception: Sensory Deficit or Excess Visual	Eye patches after surgery	"I never realized before how sight-dependent I am. I don't know what time of day it is now unless I have the radio on or smell food coming in." "It's frightening not to know who is in my room and what they are doing." Patient observed sitting in room with blank facial expression; frequently comments on how bored he or she is and how slowly time is passing; hesitant to move about room without assistance although he or she has been oriented repeatedly
Auditory	Effects of aging	"You're right. I don't always hear what people are saying anymore so I try not to get involved in conversations. If people insist on talking, I just nod and hope I'm giving the right response." Able to hear moderately spoken word close to right ear; cannot hear same from left ear; often startled when someone approaches from left side Sits close to television and radio; loud volume, no history of hearing testing
Gustatory or olfactory	Chemotherapy	"I always seem to have a bitter taste in my mouth now and can't stomach certain foods at all that I used to enjoy, like beef, tomatoes, coffee. . . . I also can't take sweets, and I used to be a real sweets junkie." "Sometimes the very smell of certain foods or even the thought of eating nauseates me." Patient has been receiving vincristine (cancer chemotherapeutic agent) for past 3 months; some nausea and vomiting; history of poor oral hygiene
Tactile	Psychological stress	"I don't know why I feel this way, but I'm hypersensitive to touch. If anyone even brushes against me I feel burning pain. Even the weight of my clothes against my skin bothers me. I'm trying to move my body as little as possible and keep it protected—but that's obviously impossible when even a breeze assaults me." Patient observed holding the body stiffly looking like he or she does not know what to do with the arms and legs; dressed only in a loose-fitting outfit; reports that he or she sits at home all day afraid to go out
Kinesthetic	Clinitron bed therapy	"I've been in this bed for 2 weeks now and I've lost all sense of my body . . . it's a curious weightless feeling that I have . . . sort of like floating in Jell-O. I'm no longer sure where my body begins and ends, and when I try to lift an arm or leg I feel like I'm in slow motion. I hope I'll be able to walk when I get out of here."
Disturbed Sensory Perception : Sensory Deprivation	Isolation	"One of the worst things that has happened to me since I found out I had AIDS is that everyone is afraid of me—and no one touches me. I'm so lonely. I've always needed a lot of people around." "Here in the hospital I think I'm going crazy. I can't leave this room. Everyone who comes in looks the same dressed in those yellow gowns. Lately I've seen some bizarre things that I know can't be real. I look at the clock and it turns into a swirling sun with a sad face that keeps coming closer and closer to me and I'm terrified I'll burn up if it gets too close. That's crazy, isn't it? I'm really losing it now." Disturbed sleep for past 2 weeks; during the day yawns excessively and cat-naps; limited attention span; states he or she is unable to concentrate on anything.
Disturbed Sensory Perception: Sensory Overload	Trauma of rape and aftercare	"When is everyone going to stop touching me? First he wouldn't stop. Now everyone here is poking at me, looking at me, asking me hundreds of questions. . . . Why did I have to report this and come to the hospital? Oh please leave me alone. Get out of here everyone."

Self-Care Deficit: (specify) related to visual impairment, auditory impairment, tactile impairment

Disturbed Body Image related to kinesthetic impairment (distorted sense of body parts), sensory deprivation

Low Self-Esteem related to effects of disturbed sensory perception (specify visual, auditory, and so forth)

Ineffective Role Performance related to sensory/perceptual alteration (blindness, deafness, and so forth)

Disturbed Personal Identity related to sensory deprivation or overload

Sexual Dysfunction related to decreased sensation

Impaired Skin Integrity related to absent tactile sensation (injury)

Disturbed Sleep Pattern related to sensory deprivation or overload

Impaired Social Interaction related to inability to receive and process interactional stimuli

Social Isolation related to visual or auditory impairment

Disturbed Thought Processes (specify: illusions, hallucinations, decreased attention or concentration, and so forth) related to sensory deprivation or overload

Outcome Identification and Planning

In whatever setting nurses encounter and care for patients, optimal sensory stimulation is a priority. Nursing care focuses on the patient outcomes that follow. The patient will:

- Live in a developmentally stimulating and safe environment
- Exhibit a level of arousal that enables the brain to receive and meaningfully organize patterns of stimulation
- Demonstrate intact functioning of the senses: vision, hearing, taste, smell, touch, kinesthetic and visceral awareness
- Maintain orientation to time, place, and person
- Respond appropriately (verbally and nonverbally) to sensory stimuli while executing self-care activities

   Patients with impaired sensory functioning require individualized outcomes similar to the following. The patient will:

- Report feeling safe and in control of the environment
- Describe different types of meaningful stimuli present in the environment
- Demonstrate (describe) appropriate self-care behaviors for visual impairment, hearing impairment, or other sensory impairment
- Verbalize acceptance of the sensory deficit

Implementing

The nurse can assist patients to improve sensory functioning by teaching patients and significant others methods for stimulating the senses, teaching patients with intact and impaired senses appropriate self-care behaviors, and interacting therapeutically with patients experiencing sensory impairments. Safety is always a special concern for patients with sensory alterations. Ensure that the patient's environment is as free of danger as possible and assist the patient to develop new self-care behaviors to compensate for sensory impairments. Safety considerations are discussed in Chapter 26 in more detail. The nursing interventions described here relate to preventing sensory alteration, stimulating the senses, meeting the needs of vision- and hearing-impaired people, communicating with a confused person, and communicating with an unconscious person. Communication guidelines for patients with sensory deficits are also highlighted in Chapter 21.

Preventing Disturbed Sensory Perception and Stimulating the Senses

The most effective means by which sensory alteration can be managed is prevention. The key to prevention is, with the patient's help, to create a functional and meaningful environment while keeping limitations in mind. The creation of such an environment requires careful observation, analysis, and creative planning.

   Although numerous nursing measures can be considered in planning care, determining their appropriateness depends on the circumstances. Promote the patient's well-being by offering care that provides rest and comfort (see Chaps. 40 and 41). Attempt to control patient discomfort whenever possible.

> *Recall Muriel Hao, the woman who had surgery 2 days ago? The patient verbalizes an inability to rest due to the "beeping of the machine." The initial priority would be to stop the machine from beeping. The nurse would need to investigate the underlying problem related to the machine's beeping, such as a low battery or an occlusion. Once the cause is determined, the nurse can then focus on comfort measures.*

Be aware of the need for sensory aids and prostheses, such as eyeglasses, contact lenses, hearing aids, dentures, canes, and artificial limbs, making them available as needed. Social activities, as shown in Figure 34-2, help to stimulate the senses and mind. Enlist the aid of family members to participate in or encourage these activities. Also encourage physical activity and exercise, which help maintain normal sensory perceptions

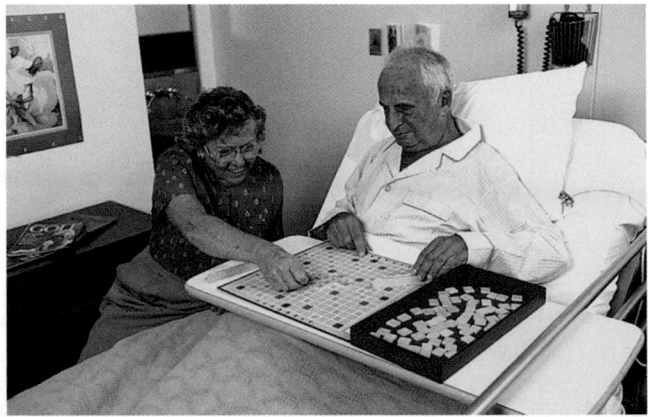

FIGURE 34-2 The nurse helps the patient find methods for stimulating his or her senses. Family members may participate in sensory activities.

and decrease the likelihood of sensory alteration (exercises are discussed in Chap. 39).

Provide stimulation for as many senses as possible. Varied sights, sounds, smells, body positions, and textures can be helpful in providing a variety of sensations. For example, music therapy has been found to benefit selected physiologic variables such as pulse rate, respiratory rate, and mood state in patients receiving mechanically ventilation. Listening to music can ameliorate the stress response and promote nonpharmacologically induced relaxation for the study subjects. All nurses, but especially critical care nurses, can be confident in implementing this nonpharmacologic, independent intervention to promote relaxation without worry of untoward side effects, which are sometimes caused by pharmacologic sedation. Consider cultural factors when stimulating senses and when offering nursing care. This is especially important when caring for patients from cultures different from the nurse's.

Teaching About Sensory Experiences

Teaching is a significant nursing responsibility. Help prepare patients for sensory experiences. An informed patient is better able to handle fears, frustration, and confusion. Therefore, explain procedures before performing them or having the patient experience them. Explanations also help prevent the patient from feeling that his or her space and body are being invaded.

Allow individuals experiencing perceptual and thought distortions the opportunity to acknowledge that fact. Discussing such experiences and being reassured that these experiences are normal and usually temporary generally eases anxiety.

Remember Ori Soltes, the young man in the ICU who becomes confused? The nurse needs to acknowledge the patient's confusion, reorienting him frequently. In addition, the patient's ability to communicate is limited as a result of the ventilator. Therefore, the nurse should provide the patient with alternative means to communicate, such as paper and pencil or a blackboard to write on so that the patient can make his needs known. The nurse also would need to reinforce explanations about all the equipment and technologies to which the patient is being exposed. Doing so may help to alleviate some of his anxiety.

Patients and family members can be guided in sensory self-stimulation, and parents can be aided in stimulation of newborns, infants, and children. Teaching to Promote Health at Home 34-1 gives helpful suggestions for teaching

---

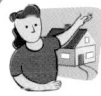

Teaching to Promote Health at Home 34-1
Sensory Stimulation

Health Topic	Teaching Tip	Importance
Hearing	• Avoid loud noise that is concentrated at the ear canal, such as with ear phones. • Decrease background or loud noises. • Use ear plugs when using loud machinery, including lawn mowers, grass trimmers, or industrial equipment. • Have regular hearing assessments. Children should be assessed in school yearly. • Do not insert objects such as cotton-tipped applicators into the ear. • Avoid cleaning of the ear. • Have ear pain evaluated by a physician or nurse practitioner. • Instruct the patient on the signs and symptoms of hearing loss.	Hearing loss occurring as an individual ages is called **presbycusis**. Presbycusis is the deterioration of nerves and structures within the inner ear. Many occupations result in hearing loss due to increased noise. Thus, the use of ear-protective devices can decrease the development of hearing loss. Instructing the patient on signs and symptoms of hearing loss and interventions to be implemented can help to slow the development of hearing loss.
Vision	• Protect the eye from damage due to ultraviolet rays with sunglasses and tinted windows. • Provide adequate light for working or reading. • Stimulate vision with colors and shapes. • Use large print to assist in readability. • Have an annual eye examination. • Avoid rubbing the eyes. • Use cleaning products or aerosol products safely in a well-ventilated area. • Use eye shields when in contact with harmful or toxic products, such as blood or body fluids or cleaning products. • Avoid nonprescription eye drops.	The education of the patient to maintain adequate eye function enhances the patient's quality of life. The avoidance of strain on the eye stimulates vision, thus enhancing sensory perception.

(continued)

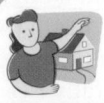

Teaching to Promote Health at Home 34-1
Sensory Stimulation (Continued)

Health Topic	Teaching Tip	Importance
Taste (gustatory)	• Practice oral care three times per day to prevent infection and decay. • Visit the dentist biannually for dental cleaning and examination. • Notify the dentist about pain or sensitivity to hot or cold. • Provide nutritional foods that are high in fiber, low in fat and sugar. • Enhance taste with use of spices.	Prevention of mouth disease enhances the taste and enjoyment of foods.
Smell	• Use aromatherapy to reduce stress. • Protect the nose from noxious fumes. • Eliminate disturbing odors with adequate ventilation. • Visit the physician or nurse practitioner when experiencing nasal congestion or diminished sense of smell. • Avoid wearing heavy colognes or perfumes. • Enhance the sense of smell by remembering pleasant odors.	The sense of smell is important in assisting the individual to relax, particularly during times of stress. It is important to evaluate any difficulty with the sense of smell and nasal congestion, since the nose lies in close proximity to the ear and the brain. Thus the prevention of infection is a primary aspect of care.
Touch	• Protect the skin from extremes in temperature. • Provide various textures in the environment. • Provide touch such as during the bath or massage therapy. • Instruct on all aspects of invasive procedures.	Protecting the skin from temperature changes decreases damage to the skin and underlying tissues. The use of a variety of textures stimulates nerve fibers and tactile sense.
Sensory Overload	• Reduce the number and type of stimuli. • Provide periods of rest. • Provide explanation of sounds and activities within the environment. • Use relaxation techniques to enhance rest.	Sensory overload can be prevented by using these measures. As a result, the patient is able to organize stimuli to decrease anxiety and stress.
Sensory deprivation	• Provide reading material, audiovisual stimulation, and interactive activities. • Provide stimulation through the visitors, phone conversations, and e-mail. • Use therapeutic touch. • Encourage the use of assistive devices such as hearing aids and glasses. • Provide a radio and television. • Orient to time, place, and person.	Increasing sensory perception enhances the patient's responses, helping to create a meaningful environment.

patients about sensory stimulation and includes suggestions that the nurse can use in a variety of situations.

Meeting the Needs of Patients With Reduced Vision

Always check with the physician to discover if a visual problem is temporary, permanent, partial, or complete, and the degree to which the problem is likely to affect the patient's everyday functioning. This information is vital to developing a realistic teaching plan or plan of care.

The first priority is to teach patients self-care behaviors for maintaining vision and preventing blindness. Lindberg and Kruszewski (1983) offered the following suggestions:

• Avoid rubbing eyes.
• Avoid eyestrain.
• Avoid damage from ultraviolet rays.
• Protect eyes from foreign bodies.
• Keep eyeglasses clean, protected, adjusted.
• Avoid nonprescription eyedrops and seek attention for symptoms.
• Avoid cleaning eyes or contact lenses with soiled articles.
• Use caution with aerosol sprays.
• Use caution with ammonia, lye, and so on.
• Visit your physician frequently if you are prone to eye problems.

- Know the danger signals that indicate serious eye problems: persistent eye redness; pain or discomfort, especially after injury; visual disturbances; crossing eyes; growth on or near the eyes; discharge or increased tearing; and pupil irregularities.

When communicating with patients with reduced vision, follow these guidelines:
- Acknowledge your presence in the patient's room. Identify yourself by name.
- Speak in a normal tone of voice. Remember that the blind person is unable to pick up most nonverbal cues during communication.
- Explain the reason for touching the person before doing so.
- Keep the call light or bell within easy reach of the person and place the bed in the lowest position.
- Orient the person to sounds in the environment.
- Orient the person to the arrangement of the room and its furnishings. Clear pathways for the person and do not rearrange furnishings. Clarify this fact with housekeeping personnel also.
- Assist with ambulation by walking slightly ahead of the person, allowing the person to grasp your arm.
- Stay in the person's field of vision if he or she has partial or reduced peripheral vision.
- Provide diversions using other senses.
- Indicate to the person when the conversation has ended and when you are leaving the room.

Meeting the Needs of Patients With Reduced Hearing

Temporary hearing losses are most often conductive in nature, that is, they are due to a problem with the external or middle ear (wax buildup, foreign-body obstruction, infection). However, sensorineural hearing losses caused by inner ear or central nervous system problems may not be totally correctable. Health teaching to prevent hearing problems includes the following recommendations for patients (Lindberg & Kruszewski, 1983, pp. 307, 312):
- Avoid excessive noise.
- Avoid inserting sharp objects into ears.
- Avoid excessive cleaning of ears.
- Avoid practices that can cause infection; treat infection early.
- Know the symptoms of hearing loss: asking frequently that statements be repeated, inability to hear at a distance, need to see the person who is talking, leaning forward or turning an ear toward the speaker, answering inappropriately, talking too loudly, inability to carry on a phone conversation, strained facial expression.

When communicating with patients who have hearing deficits or impairments, follow these guidelines:
- Orient the person to your presence before initiating conversation. This may be done by moving so you can be seen or by gently touching the person.

- Decrease background noises (television, radio) if possible before you speak.
- Make sure that hearing aids (if applicable) are working optimally.
- Position yourself so that the light is on your face and the person can see your lips and expressions.
- Talk directly to the person while facing him or her or angle the chair so that your voice reaches the ear that hears best. If the person is able to lip-read, use simple sentences and speak in a quiet, natural manner and pace. Be aware of nonverbal communication.
- Do not chew gum, cover your mouth, or turn away when talking with the person.
- Demonstrate or pantomime ideas you wish to express, as appropriate.
- Use sign language or finger spelling, as appropriate.
- Write any ideas that you cannot convey to the person in another manner.

Aids for individuals with reduced hearing include TDD (telecommunication devices), infrared systems, computers, voice amplifiers, amplified telephones, low-frequency door bells and telephone ringers, closed-caption TV decoders, flashing alarm clocks, and flashing smoke detectors.

Consider Dolores Pirolla, the wife of the patient who has a visual deficit and is now demonstrating signs of a hearing deficit. The nurse would incorporate knowledge of the guidelines (for communicating both with persons with reduced vision and hearing) when developing a teaching plan to assist Mrs. Pirolla in dealing with her husband's condition. In addition, the nurse could enlist the aid of social services to help Mrs. Pirolla in obtaining supportive services for her husband's visual impairment and for obtaining assistive devices for her husband to minimize the effects of the hearing deficit.

Communicating With a Patient Who is Confused

The patient who lacks the mental ability to process environmental stimuli may be aware of this inability and find it frustrating. This patient needs the nurse's support to make adjustments to this limitation.

Most likely, Ori Soltes, the patient in the ICU who becomes confused is experiencing a high level of frustration. Due to his accident, the patient suddenly is thrust into an environment filled with unfamiliar sights, sounds, and activities, leading to feelings of being overwhelmed physically and emotionally. His level of frustration may be further increased by his inability to speak, secondary to receiving mechanical ventilation.

Other patients may be oblivious of the deficiency. In both instances, always protect the safety of the patient while providing optimal sensory stimulation. Nursing interventions include the following:

- Using frequent face-to-face contact to communicate the social process (use touch when appropriate, walk arm in arm, hug, give a back rub)
- Speaking calmly, simply, and directly to the patient and allowing sufficient time for the patient to think before responding
- Orienting and reorienting the patient to the environment and filling the patient's personal space with as many personal objects as possible
- Using conversation, watches, clocks, calendar, newspaper, television, radio, and other such devices to orient the patient to time, place, and person
- Clearly communicating that the patient is expected to perform all self-care activities of which the patient is capable
- Keeping the emphasis on patient strengths rather than on deficiencies and verbally reinforcing strengths
- Offering the patient simple explanations for care, new activities, and so on
- Varying environmental stimuli gradually while keeping the environment structured enough that the patient feels comfortable and at home

- Using objects from the patient's past (baseball, picture of a train, photograph) to spark reminiscences and discussions
- Reinforcing reality if the patient is delusional

Refer to Box 34-2 for specific suggestions when caring for older adults with confusion. A list of selected cognitive stimulation activities may be found in Chapter 21.

Communicating With a Patient Who is Unconscious

The following are recommended guidelines for communicating with a patient who is unconscious:

- Be careful of what is said in the person's presence. Hearing is believed to be the last sense lost; therefore the person is often likely to hear what is being said, even though there does not appear to be a response.
- Assume the person can hear you. Talk with the person in a normal tone of voice about things you would ordinarily discuss.
- Speak to the person before touching. Remember that touch can be an effective means of communicating with the unconscious person.
- Keep environmental noises at as low a level as possible. This helps the person focus on the communication.

BOX 34-2 Stimulating the Senses

	Teaching Patients	Nursing Interventions
Vision	Surround yourself with different colors and with an environment that changes (walk through a mall, sit by a window where you see people come and go). Develop a sensitivity to changes in nature (weather patterns, dawn-to-night cycle, changing seasons, changes in a plant or animal). Use visual devices to keep oriented (watches, calendars, newspaper, television). Use crossword puzzles and games to stimulate mental activities. Create favorite scenes in your mind, paying attention to tiny details.	Wear visually stimulating and comforting colors. Keep meaningful visual stimuli such as photos, greeting cards, toys, or flowers near patient. Position patients with impaired mobility where they can see out a window or watch local traffic on the unit.
Hearing	Decrease or eliminate distressing auditory stimuli (change bedroom, talk with family members about noise of stereos and other such equipment, use earplugs, use headphones to listen to soft music). Develop sensitivity to different sounds (music, chirping birds, night sounds, different voices). Use the telephone to maintain contact with family and friends. Use television, radio, cassettes to keep current and to stimulate mental activities. Recall favorite sounds of the past with the situations in which they were heard.	Speak in a warm and pleasant tone and communicate caring to the patient. Use your voice to orient patient to environment and current situation (eg, procedure, treatment). Avoid speaking about the patient to others within the patient's hearing. Remember that patients overhearing snatches of conversation outside their room often presume it is about *them!* Decrease extraneous noise (intercom, movement of carts, loud conversations of staff); use carpets and sound-absorbing material whenever possible.

(continued)

BOX 34-2 (Continued)

	Teaching Patients	Nursing Interventions
Taste	Experiment with foods of different tastes (seasonings), colors, temperature, and textures; realize that as taste buds age, things will no longer taste the same.	Consult with the dietitian about preparing meals with varied taste sensations; serve meals attractively.
	Practice thorough oral hygiene and have regular dental examinations.	Perform routine oral hygiene for patients who are unable to do this for themselves.
	Recall foods that tasted especially good in the past and the events surrounding these tastes (eg, grandparent baking cookies or homemade bread).	
Smell	Consciously savor smells that are pleasant; decrease or eliminate noxious odors.	Keep the patient's room well ventilated, using opportunities when the patient is out of the room to air it out.
	Recall pleasant aromas or smells from the past and the events surrounding them (eg, smell of the ocean as the vacation house was neared, smell of fresh pine in the house at Christmas, the body scent of a loved person or animal).	Remove dressings, drainage, and any equipment with odors from the patient's room as quickly as possible.
		Encourage patients to focus on pleasant or familiar smells, such as coffee, newspaper, or flowers.
		Avoid wearing heavy perfumes.
Touch	Consciously surround yourself with different textures and let yourself feel and enjoy them (scratchy afghan; a puppy's moist, wet tongue; soft petal of a flower; smooth silk scarf; mug of hot chocolate).	Include different textures in the patient's environment (silky pillow sham from home, soft sheepskin, wooly blanket).
	Allow these textures to evoke memories of past tactile experiences (grandchild's hug may bring back memories of hugs from own children, scrap of fabric may recall a prom dress or wedding gown or baby blanket).	Respect the patient's need and desire to be touched or not touched (touch the patient's forearm or shoulder, hug the patient).
	Recognize need to be touched and tell someone, "I need a hug today!"	Use physical care (bath time, foot soaks, hair care, back massages, turning and positioning, passive range of motion) to provide tactile stimulation.
	Receive tactile stimulation from a pet.	Limit intrusive procedures and times when the patient needs to be uncomfortably manipulated.

General Nursing Strategies in the Hospital or Other Residential Care Setting	Encourage the patient to participate in activities that require exploration of the environment (exercise, feeling, tasting, touching, moving, listening).
	Use conversation to explore areas of interest to the patient.
	Encourage the patient to share feelings.
	Familiarize the environment by encouraging the patient to wear own clothes and keep personal items nearby.
	Suggest the use of self-stimulation techniques—humming, singing, whistling, reciting, memory review, and problem solving.

Evaluating

While implementing a plan of nursing care designed to decrease excessive sensory stimuli or increase meaningful stimuli, evaluate the plan's effectiveness by observing for a decrease in the behavioral manifestations of sensory deprivation or overload. It may be concluded that the plan of care is working if a patient who had begun to withdraw and spend most of the day lying in bed with a blank facial expression appears more alert and begins to initiate conversations and to take an interest in personal care. Also evaluate the patient's ability to interact appropriately with the environment while practicing necessary self-care behaviors, and the patient's need for nursing care versus his or her ability to manage the plan of care independently.

Ideally, the patient and family learn to manipulate the environment to promote optimal sensory stimulation for growth and development. Patients with specific sensory impairments are evaluated for their knowledge of the impairment, acceptance and management of the treatment regimen, and their ability to perform necessary self-care activities. See Nursing Plan of Care 34-1 for Mrs. Philomela Palikias.

NURSING PLAN OF CARE 34-1   *for Philomela Palikias*

Two days ago, Mrs. Philomela Palikias delivered by cesarean birth a 32-week-old, small-for-gestational-age infant girl weighing 3 lb, 8 oz. Because of her size and respiratory distress, the infant was placed in the neonatal intensive care unit (NICU). Postpartal assessments indicate that Mrs. Palikias's physical progress is satisfactory. However, the nurses are concerned about her mental status. Mrs. Palikias arrived in the United States 3 months ago with her husband. Both speak only Greek and neither has family in the United States.

Recorded in the patient's progress notes the evening of her 2nd postpartal day is the following nursing assessment:

12/4/06, 9 PM, nursing

Patient refused to get out of bed again this evening—demonstrates no interest in seeing baby; to date has not ambulated to NICU. Refusing to learn and participate in self-care activities—expressing breast milk or performing perineal care. Nurses throughout the day reported sudden mood changes—apathy, frustration, panic, and hostility. Unable to find someone who speaks Greek to serve as translator. Husband does not speak English but appears concerned about his wife.—*N. Gable, RN*

NURSING DIAGNOSIS

Disturbed Sensory Perception: Mixed Sensory Deprivation and Overload related to unfamiliar hospital environment (different culture) and stress of cesarean birth and infant's prematurity as manifested by patient not demonstrating interest in baby or self-care activities; limited ability to concentrate on new tasks (pericare, expressing breast milk); sudden mood changes—apathy, frustration, panic, hostility

EXPECTED OUTCOME

Before discharge, the patient will:
• Demonstrate increased comfort in the hospital environment (decreased or absent mood swings—apathy, frustration, panic, hostility)

Nursing Interventions	Rationale	Evaluative Statement
Secure assistance of an interpreter and work with the interpreter to do the following:		12/6/06 Outcome met. Patient is quiet but no longer apathetic, fearful, or hostile. Moving about in hospital with more confidence.
• Orient the patient to her surroundings (explaining reasons for equipment, procedures, treatment).	Sensory deprivation results from *meaningless*, unpatterned stimuli; once the patient understands her environment, she can respond to it appropriately.	*N. Gable, RN*
• Reassure the patient that what she is experiencing is normal given her recent stresses (moving to new country, cesarean birth of first child, infant's prematurity).	Patients experiencing strange perceptual, cognitive, and affective responses to sensory deprivation and overload often fear they are going crazy and hesitate to share their feelings.	
• Determine the patient's needs.	The patient herself is best able to voice her needs.	
Have the interpreter teach the nurse several Greek words and make recommendations about how the patient can personalize her environment, such as having her husband provide her with usual food, music, and other familiar items.	Contributing to sensory deprivation is the absence of familiar sounds (native languages, sights, tastes, or scents). Having access to familiar food and the like may reduce sensory deprivation.	
See if the interpreter can explain usual customs regarding childbirth and aftercare in Greece.	Including culturally familiar childbirth and aftercare customs in the plan of care enhances patient well-being and cooperation in the plan of care.	
Limit the number of nurses and other persons interacting with the patient; attempt to have the same nurse caring for her each shift.	A trusting nurse–patient relationship can develop.	
Schedule care to allow for uninterrupted periods of sleep and rest.	Sleep deprivation contributes to other sensory alterations.	

(*continued*)

NURSING PLAN OF CARE 34-1

for Philomela Palikias (continued)

EXPECTED OUTCOME

Before discharge, the patient will:
• Resume independent self-care activities

Nursing Interventions	Rationale	Evaluative Statement
Use services of interpreter to teach patient importance of ambulating and becoming independent again in self-care measures.	Regaining independence enhances patient's sense of well-being.	12/6/06 Outcome partially met. Patient is ambulating, but she resists pericare and is fearful when expressing breast milk.
Have interpreter write simple directions for follow-up care, times when baby may be visited after patient is discharged, and so on. Share these instructions with the patient's husband.	Cognitive responses to sensory deprivation and overload include decreased attention span and concentration and problem-solving ability. Written instructions and husband's knowledge reinforce the patient's learning.	*Recommendation:* Continue teaching with assistance of interpreter. *N. Gable, RN*
See if husband has bilingual friends or work acquaintances who might be willing to help the patient when she gets home until she has established a comfortable routine of care for the baby and is knowledgeable about community resources.	Careful discharge planning is necessary to ensure that the patient can manage new parenting responsibilities in an unfamiliar country.	

EXPECTED OUTCOME

Before discharge, the patient will:
• Demonstrate interest in her baby by visiting the NICU, holding the baby, expressing her milk, and other such activities.

Nursing Interventions	Rationale	Evaluative Statement
Learn and respect cultural norms for new mothering behaviors.	Nursing care that is not culturally sensitive is deficient.	12/6/06 Outcome met. Patient is now visiting baby in the unit on her own.
Assist the patient to ambulate to unit to see the baby; if interpreter is available, have the person explain equipment surrounding the baby and answer the patient's questions about the baby.	The patient may be refusing to visit the unit to protect herself from barrage of frightening stimuli (sensory overload); the goal is for her to become familiar with the unit so she is able to focus on bonding with her daughter.	*N. Gable, RN*

SAMPLE DOCUMENTATION

Traditional Note Format

12/5/06, 10 AM, nursing

First session with interpreter and patient at 9 AM. Patient's face brightened as soon as she heard someone speak to her in Greek. Basically, patient shared she did not care too much about what was happening to her but she was terrified about the baby and afraid of what everyone was doing to the baby. Directed interpreter to orient patient to her environment, daily routine, and NICU. Patient appeared anxious when she first saw baby but looked content when able to hold her. Schedule teaching session for tomorrow AM when interpreter will come for 1 hour. Patient currently resting comfortably.

N. Gable, RN

SOAP Format

12/5/06, 9 PM, nursing

Sensory/Perceptual Alterations: Mixed Sensory Deprivation and Overload related to unfamiliar hospital environment stress of cesarean birth and infant's prematurity

(continued)

NURSING PLAN OF CARE 34-1   for Philomela Palikias (continued)

SAMPLE DOCUMENTATION

S: —

O: Cried after husband left this evening; refused postpartal check; turned away from nurses

A: Still feels overwhelmed by newness of all that is happening to her and tries to shut out what she cannot handle

P: Continue to intervene with help of interpreter; focus on helping patient develop more control over her situation; proceed at slow pace; referral to social services for follow-up care.

N. Gable, RN

■ Developing Critical Thinking Skills

1. Describe the practical measures you would take to stimulate the senses of the following sensory-impaired patients. Think carefully about the special sensory needs that accompany different conditions.
   - A deaf child
   - A confused older adult
   - An adult man who has just lost his sight
   - A premature infant whose skin is extremely fragile

2. Visit a critical care unit with other students and list all the factors that contribute to sensory overload or deprivation. Try to identify how the critical care culture evolved in ways that are actually harmful to patients. Discuss which of these factors are unavoidable and which could be modified to better meet patient needs. Identify individualized nursing strategies to minimize sensory overload and deprivation.

■ Practicing for NCLEX

1. When assessing a patient's sensory experience, which of the following would the nurse identify as the major components?
   a. The kinesthetic and visceral senses
   b. Reception and perception
   c. The intensity, size, change, or representation of stimuli
   d. Vision, hearing, smell, taste, and touch

2. When evaluating a patient's sensory experience, which four conditions would be essential for a person to receive data and experience the world?
   a. A stimulus, a receptor, an intact nerve pathway, and a functioning brain
   b. The visual, auditory, olfactory–gustatory, and tactile senses
   c. The basic orienting systems arising from muscles, joints, hollow organs, and movement
   d. The reticular activating system, variable stimuli, memory, and motivation

3. When planning the care for a patient related to disturbed sensory perception, the nurse would integrate knowledge of which system as responsible for monitoring and regulating incoming sensory stimuli to maintain, enhance, or inhibit cortical arousal?
   a. General adaptation system
   b. Kinesthetic/visceral system
   c. Reticular activating system
   d. Sensory/perceptual system

4. You notice that Mr. Wong, who has cataracts, is sitting closer to the television than usual. The nurse would interpret the etiologic basis of his sensory problem is an alteration in which of the following?
   a. Environmental stimuli
   b. Sensory reception
   c. Nerve impulse conduction
   d. Impulse translation

5. Which of the following would be most important to include in the plan of care for a patient who is 85 years old and has presbycusis?
   a. Obtaining large-print written material
   b. Speaking distinctly using lower frequencies
   c. Decreasing tactile stimulation
   d. Initiating a safety program to prevent falls

6. Peter Almone is in the late stages of AIDS, which is now affecting his brain as well other major organ systems. He confides to you that he feels terribly alone because most of his friends are afraid to visit. The nurse determines that which of the following would be the least likely underlying etiology for his sensory problems?
   a. Stimulation
   b. Reception
   c. Transmission–perception–reaction
   d. Emotional responses

7. Which factor is least likely to place a patient at high risk for sensory deprivation?
   a. An environment with decreased or monotonous stimuli
   b. Impaired ability to receive environmental stimuli
   c. Impaired ability to process environmental stimuli
   d. Impaired ability to respond to environmental stimuli

8. Which patient would the nurse assess as being at greatest risk for sensory deprivation?

a. An elderly man confined to bed at home after a stroke

b. An adolescent in an oncology unit working on homework supplied by friends

c. A woman in labor

d. A toddler in a play room awaiting same-day surgery

9. A patient in an intensive care burn unit for 1 week is in pain much of the time and has his face and both arms heavily bandaged. His wife visits every evening for 15 minutes at 6, 7, and 8 PM. A heart monitor beeps for a patient on one side, and another patient moans frequently. Assessment would suggest that that the patient probably is experiencing which of the following?

a. Sufficient sensory stimulation

b. Deficient sensory stimulation

c. Excessive sensory stimulation

d. Both sensory deprivation and overload

10. Richard's spinal cord was severed, and he is paralyzed from the waist down. When obtaining data about this patient, which component of the sensory experience would be most important to assess?

a. Transmission of tactile stimuli

b. Adequate stimulation in the environment

c. Reception of visual and auditory stimuli

d. General orientation and ability to follow commands

11. An 11-year-old 6th grader whose grades have dropped has difficulty completing her work on time, frequently rubs her eyes, and squints. Her visual acuity on a Snellen's eye chart was 160/20. Which nursing diagnosis would be most appropriate?

a. Deficient Knowledge related to visual impairment

b. Ineffective Role Performance (Student) related to visual impairment

c. Disturbed Body Image related to visual impairment

d. Delayed Growth and Development related to visual impairment

12. Of the four items listed below, which nursing intervention would be best to prevent sensory alterations for a man with a severe hearing deficit who reads lips well?

a. Turn the radio or television volume up very loud and close the door to his room.

b. Prevent embarrassment and emotional discomfort as much as possible.

c. Provide daily opportunity for him to participate in a social hour with six or eight people.

d. Encourage daily participation in exercise and physical activity.

13. In a boarding home where most patients have slight to moderate visual or hearing impairment and some are periodically confused, which of the following would be the nurse's first priority in caring for sensory concerns?

a. Maintaining safety and prevent sensory deterioration

b. Insisting that every patient participate in as many self-care activities as possible

c. Emphasizing and reinforcing individual patient strengths

d. Encouraging reminiscence and life review in groups

14. The nursing diagnosis for 8-month-old Sally was Disturbed Sensory Perception: Sensory Deprivation related to inadequate parenting. Since that time, both parents have attended parenting classes. However, both parents work while Sally stays with her 86-year-old grandmother, who has reduced vision. The parents provide appropriate stimulation in the evening. At an evaluation conference at age 11 months, Sally lays on the floor sucking her thumb and rocking her body. Her facial expression is dull, and she vocalizes only in a low monotone ("uh-h-h"). Which statement accurately reflects evaluation about the child's sensory deprivation?

a. Her parents lack motivation to provide necessary stimulation.

b. Her grandmother is unable to improve Sally's care.

c. Sally's sensory deprivation is still severe.

d. This is normal behavior for a child of Sally's age.

15. Which nursing interventions would be least appropriate for an elderly woman in a nursing home with a nursing diagnosis of Disturbed Sensory Perception: Chronic Sensory Deprivation related to the effects of aging? She had walked out the door unobserved and was hit by a car.

a. Ignore when the patient is confused or go along to prevent embarrassment.

b. Encourage self-care and independent decisions.

c. Take walks around the grounds and to the garden daily.

d. Provide daily contact with children, community people, and pets.

■ Answers With Rationale

1. The correct response is *b*. Reception and perception are the major components of any sensory experience. All other choices are merely part of the sensory experience.

2. The correct response is *a*. A stimulus, a receptor, an intact nerve pathway, and a functioning brain are the four conditions necessary for a person to receive data and experience the world.

3. The correct response is *c*. The reticular activating system maintains, enhances, or inhibits cortical arousal by monitoring and regulating incoming sensory stimuli. The general adaptation system (*a*) is the system responsible for responding to stress. Kinesthetic and

visceral (*b*) are senses that arise internally from muscles and hollow organs and are the body's basic orienting systems. Sensory and perceptual systems (*d*) are the two components of the sensory experience.

4. The correct response is *b*. Cataracts are interfering with the patient's ability to receive visual stimuli— altered sensory reception. The nature of incoming stimuli (*a*), the conduction of nerve impulses (*c*), and the translation of incoming impulses (*d*) in the brain are not a problem here.

5. The correct response is *b*. Presbycusis is a normal loss of hearing as a result of the aging process. Speaking distinctly in lower frequencies is indicated. The other choices refer to interventions for other sensory problems.

6. The correct response is *d*. Emotional responses are an effect of sensory deprivation and although may be occurring with this patient, they are not the underlying etiology for his condition. This patient is receiving decreased environmental stimuli (*a*) (eg, from his friends); is more than likely experiencing problems with reception because of major organ involvement (*b*); and his impaired brain function will impair impulse transmission–perception–reaction (*c*).

7. The correct response is *d*. An impaired ability to respond to environmental stimuli places a patient at risk for problems other than sensory deprivation. The other options all pertain to components of the sensory experience that, if impaired, may place a patient at high risk for sensory deprivation.

8. The correct response is *a*. The patient confined to bed rest at home is at risk for greatly reduced environmental stimuli. All of the other patients are in environments where environmental stimuli are at least adequate.

9. The correct response is *d*. This patient's bandages may result in deficient sensory stimulation (sensory deprivation), and the monitors and other sounds in the intensive care burn unit may cause a sensory overload. All other options are incomplete responses.

10. The correct response is *a*. Below-the-waist paralysis makes the transmission of tactile stimuli a problem. Although the other options may be assessed, they are indirectly related to his paralysis and of lesser importance at this time.

11. The correct response is *b*. An important role for an 11-year-old is that of student. Her impaired vision is clearly disturbing her role performance as a student, as evidenced by her lower grades. Although the other options may also represent accurate diagnoses for this patient, they do not flow from the data that were presented.

12. The correct answer is *c*. Although all the options listed are appropriate, providing daily opportunities for this patient to participate in a social hour builds on his strength of being able to lip-read and provides sufficient sensory stimulation to prevent sensory

deprivation resulting from his hearing loss, thereby meeting his needs.

13. The correct answer is *a*. Safety is a basic physiologic need that must be met before higher-level needs, such as love and belonging, self-esteem, and self-actualization, can be met.

14. The correct response is *c*. Although the data show that the parents have been motivated to improve their parenting skills, it is clear from the data presented that Sally's sensory deprivation is still severe. The data suggest that the grandmother is not improving Sally's care, but there is nothing to suggest that she is unable to do so (*b*) if shown how.

15. The correct response is *a*. Even if well motivated, ignoring a patient's confusion to prevent embarrassment may be dangerous, as it was in this case in which the appropriate safety precautions were never implemented. The other options are all appropriate for this patient.

Bibliography

Broussard, A. B. (1990). Incorporating infant stimulation concepts into prenatal classes. *Journal of Obstetric, Gynecologic, and Neonatal Nursing, 19*(5), 381–387.

Fine, J. I., & Rouse-Bane, S. (1995). Using validation techniques to improve communication with cognitively impaired older adults. *Journal of Gerontological Nursing, 21*(6), 39–45.

Glynn, N. J. (1992). The music therapy assessment tool in Alzheimer's patients. *Journal of Gerontological Nursing, 18*(1), 3–9.

Hall, G. R., & Wakefield, B. (1996). Confusion in the elderly. *Nursing 96, 26*(7), 32–37.

Hancock, C. K., Munjas, B., Berty, K., & Jones, J. (1994). Altered thought processes and sensory perceptual alterations: A critique. *Nursing Diagnoses, 5*(1), 26–30.

Harrison, L. L., & Woods, S. (1991). Early parental touch and preterm infants. *Journal of Obstetric, Gynecologic, and Neonatal Nursing, 20*(4), 299–306.

Luckmann, J. (1999). *Transcultural communication in nursing*. Albany, NY: Delmar Publishing.

Kloosterman, N. D. (1991). Cultural care: The missing link in severe sensory alteration. *Nursing Science Quarterly, 4*(3), 119–122.

Larsen, P. D., Hazen, S. E., & Hoot Martin, J. L. (1997). Assessment and management of sensory loss in elderly patients. *AORN Journal, 65*(2), 432–437.

Lindberg, J. B., & Kruszewski A. Z. (1983). Special senses and the environment. In J. Lindberg, M. Hunter, & A. Kruszewski (Eds.). *Introduction to person-centered nursing* (pp. 297–315). Philadelphia: J. B. Lippincott.

Lindblade, D. D., & McDonald, M. (1995). Removing communication barriers for the hearing-impaired elderly. *MEDSURG Nursing, 4*(5), 379–385.

McConnell, E. A. (1996). Caring for a patient who has a vision impairment. *Nursing 96, 26*(5), 28.

Moore, J. R., & Gilbert, D. A. (1995). Elderly residents: Perceptions of nurses' comforting touch. *Journal of Gerontological Nursing, 21*(1), 6–13.

North American Nursing Diagnosis Association. (2003). *NANDA nursing diagnoses: Definitions and classifications 2003–2004.* Philadelphia: Author.

Oehler, J. M. (1991). Beyond technology: Meeting developmental needs of infants in NICUs. *Maternal–Child Nursing, 16*(3), 148–151.

Palumbo, M. V. (1990). Hearing access 2000: Increasing awareness of hearing impaired. *Journal of Gerontological Nursing, 16*(9), 26–31, 37–38.

Pope, D. S. (1995). Music, noise, and the human voice in the nurse–patient environment. *Image—The Journal of Nursing Scholarship, 27*(4), 291–296.

Poroch, D. (1995). The effect of preparatory patient education on the anxiety and satisfaction of cancer patients receiving radiation therapy. *Cancer Nursing, 18*(3), 206–214.

Seyfrit, M. (1995). Going blind. *American Journal of Hospice and Palliative Care, 12*(3), 31–40.

Snyder, M., Egan, E. C., & Burns, K. R. (1995). Interventions for decreasing agitation behaviors in persons with dementia. *Journal of Gerontological Nursing, 21*(7), 34–40.

Standley, J. M., & Moore, R. S. (1995). Therapeutic effects of music and mother's voice on premature infants. *Pediatric Nursing, 21*(6), 509–512.

Stein-Parbury, J., & McKinley, S. (2000). Patients' experiences of being in an intensive care unit: A select literature review. *American Journal of Critical Care, 9*(1), 20–27.

Suedfeld, P. (1985). Stressful levels of environmental stimulation. *Issues in Mental Health Nursing, 7*(1/4), 83–104.

Taquino, L. T., & Lockridge, T. (1999). Caring for critically ill infants: Strategies to promote physiological stability and improve development outcomes. *Critical Care Nurse, 19*(6), 64–79.

Wahl, H., & Heyl, V. (2003). Connections between vision, hearing, and cognitive function in old age. *Generations, 27*(6), 39–44.

Wang, J. F. (1995). Caregiver–child interaction in Japan, Taiwan, and the United States. *Journal of Obstetric, Gynecologic, and Neonatal Nursing, 24*(4), 353–361.

Zahr, L. K., & Balian, S. (1995). Responses of premature infants to routine nursing interventions and noise in the NICU. *Nursing Research, 44*(3), 179–185.

Sexuality

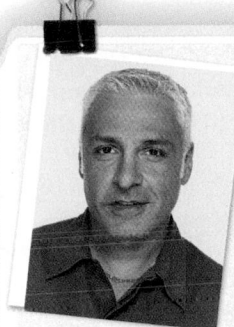

Jefferson Smith, a middle-aged man, has a history of diabetes and hypertension and is receiving numerous medications as treatment. During a routine visit to his primary care physician, Mr. Smith confides that he has been having problems "in the bedroom." He reports difficulty attaining and maintaining an erection.

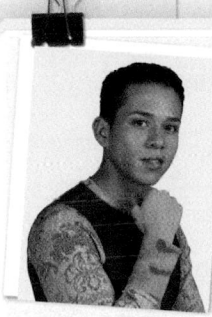

Paul Rojas is a young adult homosexual diagnosed with AIDS. He comes to the clinic today for infusion therapy, which usually takes several hours. Mr. Rojas comments to the nurse "You don't feel comfortable with me, do you?"

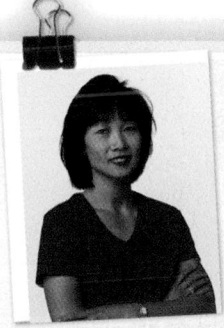

Amy Liu is a middle-aged woman who had a hysterectomy about 1 year ago for excessive uterine bleeding due to multiple uterine fibroids. She comes to the clinic for a checkup and begins to cry during the assessment. She says, "I don't feel like a woman anymore. My husband and I used to have a wonderful sexual relationship, but now I rarely want to have sexual intercourse and when I do, it hurts. My husband is being so patient, but I don't know how much longer he'll put up with me! What's wrong with me?"

The types of blended skills you'll need to respond to the case scenarios include:

Cognitive Skills

- Strong knowledge base about human sexuality, including anatomy and physiology, growth and development, sexual myths, and current issues
- Knowledge of terminology associated with sexual health, including gender identity, gender role behavior, and sexual orientation
- Knowledge of methods of sexual expression and factors affecting sexuality, such as diabetes and hypertension treatment, changes in body image and self-concept resulting from surgery, and homosexuality and AIDS
- Ability to integrate knowledge about sexual health into nursing care, including the ability to identify areas of sexual dysfunction for the patient with a history of diabetes and hypertension experiencing impotence, the middle-aged woman experiencing pain on intercourse and changes in sexual desire, and a homosexual patient with AIDS
- Ability to identify patients with problems related to sexuality and to develop and implement appropriate plans to address these problems

Technical Skills

- Strong assessment skills for interviewing a patient with concerns about sexuality or with a sexual preference different from your own
- Ability to use correctly the products and equipment necessary to meet the sexual needs of patients
- Ability to provide technical nursing assistance to assess and meet the needs of a patient experiencing impotence, a woman experiencing a decrease in sexual desire after surgery, and a homosexual patient with AIDS
- Ability to adapt techniques for patients with problems affecting sexual health
- Ability to seek help when necessary when caring for patients with problems affecting sexual health

Interpersonal Skills

- Strong interpersonal skills to establish trusting relationships and build rapport with a patient experiencing impotence, a woman experiencing problems with sexual desire and pain on intercourse after a hysterectomy, and a homosexual patient diagnosed with AIDS
- Demonstration of a nonjudgmental attitude to avoid bias, which would impede trusting nurse–patient and nurse–colleague relationships
- Counseling skills to reduce patient anxiety involving problems related to sexual health
- Sense of your own sexuality and comfort with sexual issues
- Ability to help patients find motivation to develop new health and coping behaviors related to sexual health issues and problems
- Ability to demonstrate respect, empathy, and caring regardless of the patient's sexual preference or orientation
- Ability to interact effectively and work collaboratively with other members of the healthcare team to meet the needs of patients with issues involving sexual health
- Demonstration of respect for the patient's human dignity and autonomy, regardless of the patient's sexual preference, orientation, or sexual health issue

Ethical and Legal Skills

- Commitment to safety and quality when providing care to patients with varying sexual health problems
- Strong sense of accountability for the health and well-being of patients with wide-ranging problems involving sexual health
- A commitment to patient advocacy, including getting patients the help they need to achieve sexual health goals, within the scope of nursing responsibilities and available resources
- Familiarity with agency policy and role responsibilities related to meeting the sexual health needs of patients
- Ability to practice in an ethically and legally defensible manner when providing care to patients with different issues involving sexual health

Learning Outcomes

After completing the chapter, the learner should be able to accomplish the following:

1. Describe male and female reproductive anatomy and physiology.
2. Describe the sexual response cycle, differentiating male and female responses.
3. Identify factors that affect an individual's sexuality.
4. Perform a sexual assessment, using suggested interview questions and appropriate physical assessment skills.
5. Describe types of sexual dysfunctions and the assessment priorities for each.
6. Develop nursing diagnoses identifying a problem with sexuality that may be remedied by independent nursing actions.
7. Describe five areas in which the nurse can educate the patient about sexuality.
8. Plan, implement, and evaluate nursing care related to selected nursing diagnoses involving problems of sexuality.

Key Terms

biologic sex
bisexual
contraception
erogenous zones
gender identity
gender role behavior
heterosexual
homosexual
impotence
masturbation
menarche
menopause
menstruation
orgasm
premenstrual (tension) syndrome
sexual dysfunction
sexual harassment
sexual health
sexual orientation
sexuality
transsexual
transvestite

Sexuality is a concern in professional nursing care because it permeates an individual's life, both in illness and in health. **Sexuality** is the degree to which a person exhibits and experiences maleness or femaleness physically, emotionally, and mentally. Sexuality is defined not only by a person's genitalia but also by attitudes and feelings. It can also be defined as learned behaviors in how a person reacts to his or her own sexuality and by how one behaves in relationships with others. Culture profoundly influences learned behaviors about sexuality. Sexuality is an integral part of a person's identity and is present in one's demeanor through actions, communications, and physical appearance. See the accompanying Reflective Practice box for an example.

This chapter discusses sexual health, reproductive anatomy and physiology, the sexual response cycle, and factors that affect sexuality. Obtaining a sexual history as part of a comprehensive patient history is presented, as well as interview questions that specifically address a patient with a sexual dysfunction. Nursing priorities with regard to assessment of the reproductive system are presented. Analysis of assessment data is discussed, with examples of corresponding nursing diagnoses. The patient case scenarios and nursing plan of care provide the nurse with examples of how the information presented in the chapter can be used in a clinical setting to nurture and promote aspects of sexuality in patients.

SEXUAL HEALTH

The World Health Organization defines **sexual health** as "the integration of the somatic, emotional, intellectual and social aspects of sexual being, in ways that are positively enriching and that enhance personality, communication, and love" (1975, p. 6). Because our sexuality is so basic to our sense of self, nurses need to value sexuality as a critical element of health and well-being in general and must be skilled in identifying and meeting problems related to sexual self-concept, body image, and sexual identity.

Reflective Practice
Challenge to Interpersonal Skills

During my clinical experience in the HIV/infectious disease clinic, I met Paul Rojas, a single young adult homosexual who was diagnosed with AIDS. One day he came to the clinic for infusion therapy, which usually takes several hours.

I was a 20-year-old, single white female with no personal experience with gay or lesbian friends or with individuals who are bisexual, transsexual, or transvestites. I was confused and uncertain about how to respond to him. How should I approach him? What would we talk about during these several hours at the clinic? I was sure my instructor thought this would be a "great learning experience," but what was I supposed to learn? Usually quite self-confident, I was confused, uncomfortable, and uncertain as to how to act.

Thinking Outside the Box: Possible Courses of Action

- Hide my discomfort and simply provide the technical nursing care Paul needs; spend as little time as possible in his room.
- Refuse this assignment because I am unsure I can provide the care Paul needs.
- Talk with my instructor or another experienced nurse whom I respect about my questions and concerns.
- Share with Paul that this is my first experience working with a homosexual patient and ask him what I should know; spend extra time getting to know him and his experiences with other healthcare professionals.

Evaluating a Good Outcome: How Do I Define Success?

- Provide the nursing care he needs in an manner that is respectful.
- Learn from this experience how to be respectful of all patients and to interact in a way that affirms their human dignity.
- Gain knowledge about gender identity and expression through this experience.

Personal Learning: Here's to the Future!

I didn't know how to raise my questions, so I met Paul totally at a loss and did exactly what I didn't want to do: I completed the technical nursing care such as vital signs and intravenous care and then got out of the room as quickly as possible. It wasn't until almost the end of his treatment that he asked me, "You don't feel comfortable with me, do you?" When I answered truthfully that I didn't, all of a sudden wonderful sharing began. When I look back now and think that I almost allowed my fear to prevent me from getting to know Paul and his world, I could kick myself. I hope I always remember to let patients teach me about their world.

Reflection

How do you think you would respond in a similar situation? Why? What does this tell you about yourself and about the adequacy of your skills for professional practice? Can you think of other ways to respond? Propose possible factors that may have influenced the nursing student's response to the patient. What other skills (cognitive, interpersonal, technical, ethical/legal) would you need to respond well in this situation? With what issues was the nursing student dealing? The patient? Explain how the nursing student's truthful response to the patient's question affected the therapeutic relationship. Do you agree with the criteria to evaluate a successful outcome? Did the nursing student meet the criteria? Please explain your answer.

Think back to Amy Liu, the woman who reported changes in sexual desire and pain on intercourse. As a result of these changes, she reported not feeling like a woman anymore. The nurse would interpret her statements as reflecting a change in her self-concept and body image secondary to the sexual health issues.

Sexual identity encompasses a person's self-identity, biologic sex, gender identity, gender role behavior or orientation, and sexual orientation or preference. **Biologic sex** is the term used to denote chromosomal sexual development: male (XY) or female (XX), external and internal genitalia, secondary sex characteristics, and hormonal states. **Gender identity** is the inner sense a person has of being male or female, which may be the same as or different from his or her biologic gender. **Gender role behavior** is the behavior a person conveys about being male or female, which, again, may or may not be the same as biologic gender or gender identity (Pillitteri, 2003).

Consider Paul Rojas, the homosexual patient with AIDS. The nurse would need to assess his gender identity and gender role behaviors to gain a fuller understanding of his sexual identity and to provide appropriate care.

People experience sexual gratification in many ways, and what is considered normal differs from one individual to another and among cultures. **Sexual orientation** refers to the preferred gender of the partner of an individual. The origins of sexual orientation are unknown, but there are studies claiming a genetic basis. Certainly, some sexual preferences are culturally determined and may be dictated by opportunity.

Common sexual orientations are as follows:

- A **heterosexual** is one who experiences sexual fulfillment with a person of the opposite gender.
- A **homosexual** is one who experiences sexual fulfillment with a person of the same gender. Homosexual males often use the term "gay"; homosexual females use the term "lesbian." Heterosexuality and homosexuality can be placed at opposite ends of a continuum, with many variations in between.
- A **bisexual** is a person who finds pleasure with both opposite-sex and same-sex partners. Homosexual or heterosexual people may have bisexual relationships at times.
- A **transsexual** is a person of a certain biologic gender who has the feelings of the opposite sex. The person feels trapped within the body of the wrong sex. The reason behind this is unknown, although many factors are believed to be involved. For many transsexuals, the solution is to change their bodies, through surgery and hormone therapy, to match their inner feelings.
- A **transvestite** is an individual who desires to take on the role or wear the clothes of the opposite sex. Most transvestites are heterosexual, and many keep their lifestyle hidden.

PHYSIOLOGY

Female

The female genitalia are represented by both internal and external structures. The appearance of the external genitalia (see Fig. 25-46 in Chap. 25) varies slightly among individuals.

External Genitalia
Mons Pubis
The mons pubis is a pad of fatty tissue that lies over the part of the bony pelvis called the symphysis pubis. In the physically mature female, the mons pubis is covered with coarse pubic hair. It contains many nerve endings that make the mons pubis sensitive to touch and pressure.

Labia Majora and Labia Minora
The labia majora consist of two rounded folds of fatty tissue. The outer lips separate downward from the mons pubis and meet again below the vaginal introitus. The labia majora contain a multitude of sebaceous and sweat glands. They respond to touch during sexual activity. The labia minora are the smaller lips located within the labia majora. They are thin and sensitive structures and are pale pink. When stimulated by touch, the labia minora may turn a darker pink or even red owing to the presence of many blood vessels. The labia minora have no hair and are smooth.

Clitoris
The clitoris is found above the urinary meatus at the joining of the labia minora, called the clitoral hood. The clitoris is a small, button-like structure similar to the penis in its reaction to stimuli. The clitoris contains erectile tissue, blood vessels, and nerves. It is extremely sensitive. The opening of the vagina lies between the urinary meatus and the anus. It may contain a structure called the hymen, which is a thick membrane with no apparent function. At one time, the hymen was thought to represent virginity (not having experienced sexual intercourse), but this is erroneous. Remnants, or "tags," of the hymen may be noted at the vaginal introitus in both sexually active and inactive women.

Internal Genitalia
The internal genitalia—the ovaries, fallopian tubes, uterus, and vagina—are located deep within the pelvis of the female.

Ovaries
The female body normally contains two ovaries, one on each side. The ovaries closely resemble an almond in size and shape. When a girl is born, each of her ovaries contains some 200,000 to 400,000 follicles. This number steadily decreases until puberty, when 100,000 to 200,000 follicles remain, and the number continues to decline over the reproductive years. The process of ovulation is discussed later in this chapter. The ovaries also secrete the hormones estrogen and progesterone.

Fallopian Tubes

The fallopian tubes are slender structures that extend from either side of the uterus and end in a fringed fashion near each ovary. Their function is to transport a mature ovum (female reproductive cell) from an ovary to the uterus. Fertilization of the ovum by a sperm usually occurs in the tube. The fertilized ovum then travels the rest of the way to the uterus, where it implants. An unfertilized ovum travels the same path but does not implant and is eventually expelled from the body during menses. Because the lumen of each tube is so narrow, it can easily be damaged by the effects of infection and surgery.

Uterus

The uterus is a pear-shaped organ about 3″ long located between the urinary bladder and the rectum. Its primary purpose is to house and nurture a pregnancy (the condition of carrying a developing embryo in the uterus). The uterus comprises three layers:

1. The outermost layer, the perimetrium, consists of elastic tissue.
2. The middle layer, the myometrium, is muscular.
3. The innermost layer, the endometrium, comprises tissue that thickens and sloughs off with menses.

The cervix is the structure at the lower portion of the uterus that connects the uterus and the vagina. The cervix is usually closed, but during the birth process, it dilates and thins out extensively to permit the birth of a baby. The cervix is a smooth pink structure that possesses few nerve endings. When touched, the sensation resembles that of touching the end of one's nose.

Vagina

The vagina is a tubular, hollow organ that lies between the urethra and the rectum. Its size and shape vary among women. The walls of the vagina are composed of rugae, or ribbed tissue. The vagina serves three purposes: it is (1) a receptacle for the penis during sexual intercourse, (2) a birth canal for the passage of a baby, and (3) an exit for menstrual flow from the uterus. During sexual activity, the walls of the vagina secrete, or "sweat," a thin watery material, sometimes in copious amounts. This lubrication is necessary for the comfortable placement and movement of the penis in the vagina.

> *Recall Amy Liu, the middle-aged woman complaining of pain with intercourse. The nurse would need to determine if she is experiencing a change in vaginal secretions, possibly due to her surgery or other changes, such as the onset of menopause.*

Breasts

Although the breasts are not considered part of the internal or external genitalia, they are an important aspect of female physical sexuality. The breasts consist of fatty and glandular tissues and the nipples. Their size and shape vary widely among women. The nipples are pale to deep pink. Caressing of the breasts can be pleasurable during sexual activity, and many women can be brought to orgasm by this action alone.

Menstruation

Menstruation is a cycle during which the body prepares for the presence of a fertilized ovum. Cycles are about 28 days long but may vary from 21 to 40 days. The first menstrual period, called **menarche,** is experienced at about 12 years of age, but the age of menarche is individual and may occur anywhere between 8 and 17 years of age. **Menopause,** the cessation of a woman's menstrual activity, occurs between the ages of 45 and 55 years. The woman may experience irregular menses over time before menstruation ends.

The Menstrual Cycle

The menstrual cycle is controlled by a series of reactions that rely on feedback from the ovaries to the pituitary gland. Actually, two cycles occur simultaneously: one in the ovaries and one in the uterus (Fig. 35-1).

In the ovaries, in a typical 28-day cycle, the phase from day 4 to 14 is called the follicular phase. During this phase, a number of follicles mature, but only one produces a mature ovum. At the same time, in the uterus, the endometrium is becoming thick and velvety in preparation for receiving a fertilized egg. This phase in the uterus is called the proliferation phase. Ovulation generally occurs on day 14. The mature ovum ruptures from the follicle and the surface of the ovary and is swept into the fallopian tube. If sperm are present, the ovum is fertilized at this time. Some women can detect ovulation by the presence of a sharp, cramping pain over the ovulating ovary; this pain is called mittelschmerz, or middle pain, because it occurs in the middle of the cycle.

From day 15 to day 28, the phase in the ovaries is called the luteal phase. The leftover empty follicle fills up with a yellow pigment and is then called the corpus luteum, or yellow body. The purpose of the corpus luteum is to produce hormones that encourage a fertilized egg to grow. If fertilization does not occur, the corpus luteum begins to disintegrate. During the luteal phase in the ovaries, the uterus also undergoes changes. This phase is called the secretory phase. The endometrial lining thickens. However, in the absence of a fertilized egg, the corpus luteum dies and the endometrial lining disintegrates.

At day 28, menses, or the menstrual flow, begins as a result of the uterus shedding the useless portion of its endometrium. Menses lasts for 3 to 7 days, the average length of flow being 5 days. The menstrual discharge is a bloody fluid that also contains endometrial debris, mucus, and enzymes. It is odorless until exposed to the air, when the woman may notice a light, fleshy, pungent odor. Deodorized pads and tampons do little to minimize odor and can cause chemical irritation to the vulva and vagina. Good hygiene and regular bathing are much more effective during menses to prevent odor. Normal blood loss averages 30 to 80 mL. Pads and tampons should be changed frequently to prevent odor and irritation from wetness. Women using tampons should read and follow the manufacturer's suggestions to reduce the risk for toxic shock syndrome. Usually, the flow is the heaviest and is bright red on the first day or two of menses, gradually tapering off to light-

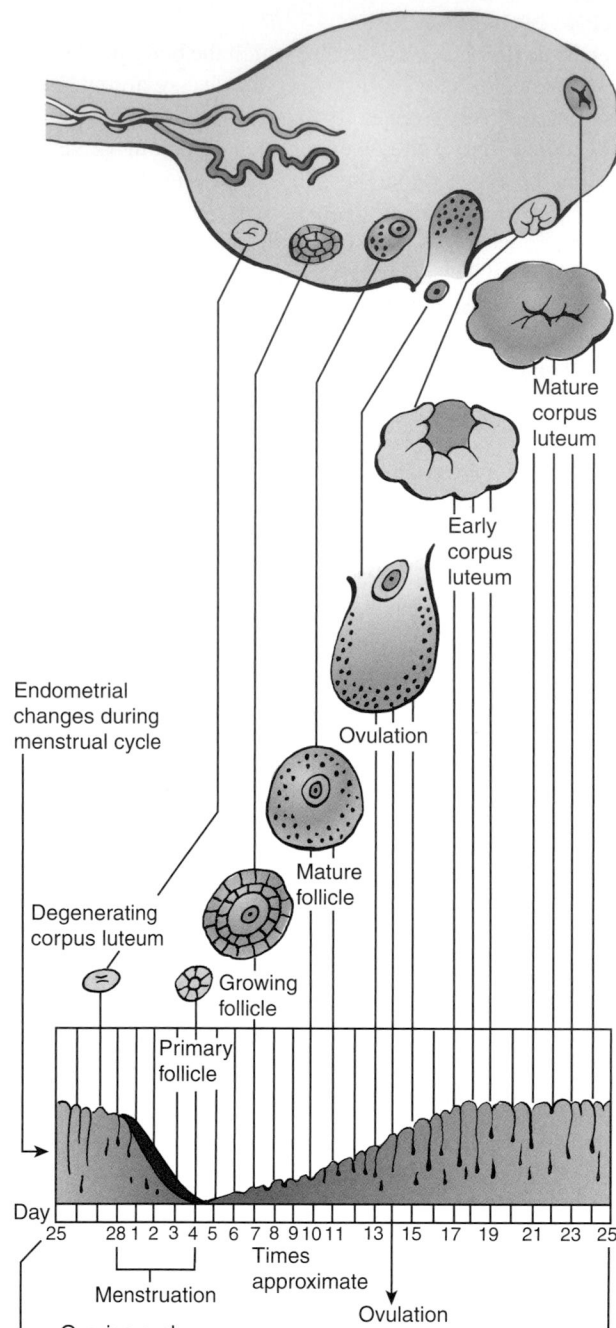

FIGURE 35-1 Schematic representation of one ovarian cycle and the corresponding changes in the endometrium.

brown staining. Many women experience some degree of discomfort either premenstrually or during menses.

There is no scientific rationale supporting abstinence from sexual activity during menses. Many women enjoy sex during menses owing to the increase in vascularity in the pelvic region, which heightens enjoyment. Men may also enjoy the warm wetness the menstrual flow provides to the vagina. If flow is heavy, a diaphragm can be used to hold it back during sexual activity, or a towel can be used to protect the bedding. Some women who experience abdominal cramping during

menses, or dysmenorrhea, find that sexual activity and orgasm relieve their discomfort.

Premenstrual (Tension) Syndrome

Menstrual cycle–related distress, commonly called **premenstrual (tension) syndrome** (PMS), reportedly occurs in 50% to 90% of the female population. PMS is characterized by the appearance of one or more of the following several days before the onset of menstruation: irritability, emotional tension, anxiety, mood changes, headache, breast tenderness, and water retention. Although it is often used to explain unusual behavior (and has been used as a legal defense), its etiology is still uncertain (both physiologic and psychogenic theories have been postulated), as are its effects on women's roles and relationships. Most of the current PMS literature perpetuates a twofold myth: (1) biology and physiology are destiny (many females do and should experience premenstrual distress) and (2) female biology and physiology result in psychiatric disorder, destruction, and violence (Winter, Ashton & Moore, 1991). Nurses have a great role to play in researching PMS and ensuring that women and the public correctly understand its effects.

Male

External Genitalia

Unlike the female genitalia, the male genitalia (illustrated in Fig. 25-47 in Chap. 25) are found primarily outside the body.

Testes

The testes, which are about the size of walnuts, feel smooth and are freely movable within the scrotum. Normally, two testes are present. The testes produce sperm and the hormones necessary for the maintenance of male sex characteristics. The primary hormone secreted by the testes is testosterone, which is responsible for a man's deep voice, beard growth, and body hair.

Scrotum

The scrotum is the loose, baglike structure that houses the testes. The scrotum hangs between a man's upper thighs. The area around the base of the penis and the scrotum is covered with pubic hair. The looseness of the scrotum is intentional to provide expansion and contraction. When exposed to cool temperatures, the scrotum contracts and draws the testes closer to the body for warmth. In warm temperatures, the scrotum become loose and allows the testes to hang farther away from the heat of the body. The testes are sensitive organs and can suffer discomfort, sometimes extreme, if handled roughly or jostled. It is important for men and boys to wear a properly fitted athletic supporter, or jockstrap, when engaged in strenuous physical activity. However, the continuous use of such a support can cause the temperature within the scrotum to rise and the delicate sperm to die because of constant exposure to high temperatures. Snug-fitting garments such as tight jeans can have the same effect on a man's fertility. The scrotum can be a source of sexual pleasure when lightly stroked, fondled, or caressed during sexual activity.

Penis

The penis is a tubular structure located above the scrotum. It functions to eliminate urine from the bladder, to ejaculate semen and impregnate a woman, and as a sex organ for sexual pleasure. It consists of the shaft and the glans (head of the penis). In the uncircumcised male, the glans is covered by loose skin (foreskin) that can be retracted. In the circumcised male, the foreskin has been surgically removed, and the glans is exposed. Penis size and shape vary among individuals. Normally, the penis is soft and flaccid and 2.5″ to 4″ long. The dimensions of the penis in no way dictate the man's ability to perform effectively during sexual activity. When an erection occurs, the blood vessels in the shaft of the penis become congested, and the penis becomes hard and erect. The size of the penis during an erection may increase to 5.5″ to 7″ in total length. The penis, particularly the glans, is extremely sensitive to stimulation. Stroking and handling of the shaft of the penis are also pleasurable during sexual activity.

The stimulation that prompts an erection varies. A full bladder on awakening in the morning can cause an erection. Fantasy, memories of a past sexual encounter, and accidental brushing by an attractive stranger can all lead to an erection. An erection in the male does not always signify desire for sexual activity. Exposure of the male patient by the nurse during a bed bath may cause an erection. An erection is a normal physiologic response and not something the man can voluntarily control. The erection ceases if no further stimulation is added.

Internal Genitalia

Tubules from the testes drain into the epididymis, which in turn drains into the vas deferens and ejaculatory ducts. These ducts then drain directly into the urethra. It is believed that the vas deferens acts as a reservoir for sperm between ejaculations.

The seminal vesicles, prostate gland, and Cowper's glands produce a liquid called seminal plasma. The seminal plasma and the sperm collectively make up the semen. The plasma aids in the transport of sperm and also provides energizing nutrients for the sperm. It contains a form of sugar (fructose), mucus, salts, water, base buffers, and coagulators to aid the sperm in their journey. Semen is a thick, creamy white fluid with the consistency of mucus or egg whites.

Breasts

Male breasts contain little real breast tissue, but they still may be stimulated during sexual activity. Although the area of sensitivity is usually limited to the nipple and areola, its stimulation can be as pleasurable an experience for the male as it is for a female.

Ejaculation

Ejaculation is the expulsion of semen by the rhythmic contractions of the penis. The penis engages in short, jerky movements that produce a spurt of semen with each motion. The period of ejaculation is short, and the penis becomes flaccid after ejaculation. The normal amount of semen per ejaculate is 2 to 6 mL. A fertile man dispels 120 to 160 million sperm per ejaculate. Cowper's glands produce small droplets of fluid during sexual activity that neutralize the acidity of the male urethra and aid in the transport of sperm. This fluid may contain sperm. Therefore, contraceptive measures, if used, must be taken before this fluid can be introduced into the vagina.

Many males, particularly adolescent boys, may experience a phenomenon known as a nocturnal emission, or "wet dream." These ejaculatory episodes occur during sleep without physical stimulation. They are perfectly normal and do not represent any sort of deviation.

SEXUAL RESPONSE CYCLE

The physiologic responses to sexual activity of females and males are more similar than different (Fig. 35-2). Also, body response is essentially the same regardless of the source of stimulation; that is, fantasy, masturbation, and sexual intercourse can all bring about the same body reactions. The sexual response cycle is not limited to the genital organs but is a total-body response that causes many physiologic changes throughout the body. The cycle has four phases: (1) excitement, (2) plateau, (3) orgasm, and (4) resolution; there is a smooth progression from one phase to the next. Although only physiologic responses are discussed here, the emotional and mental involvement of sexual response contributes a great deal to the pleasure and satisfaction of sexual activity.

The human body contains many **erogenous zones,** areas that when stimulated cause sexual arousal and desire. The genitals are an obvious source of sexual pleasure for both men and women, but other areas of the body are also considered erogenous zones. The skin is the largest erogenous zone. Other areas include the ears, lips, thighs, and breasts. Some people can reach orgasm simply by stimulation of erogenous zones other than the genitals. The most important body organ for sexual arousal and stimulation is the brain. It allows individuals freedom to enjoy a sexual experience but also may prevent satisfaction by inhibitions, doubts, and guilt.

> *Think back to Amy Liu, the woman experiencing a decrease in sexual desire and pain on intercourse. The nurse would incorporate knowledge of erogenous zones when discussing sexual arousal with Mrs. Liu. Mrs. Liu and her husband may find some of this information helpful to increase her sexual desire and arousal.*

Excitement

The excitement phase is initiated by erotic stimulation and arousal. Some of the physiologic changes common in both men and women include an increase in heart rate and blood pressure and the appearance of a pink flush to the skin. This sex flush, which is more evident in women than in men, spreads over the face, neck, back, and upper torso. Congestion of the genitals with increased blood flow begins in the excitement phase and causes even more arousal. The length of the excitement phase varies greatly among individuals and even from

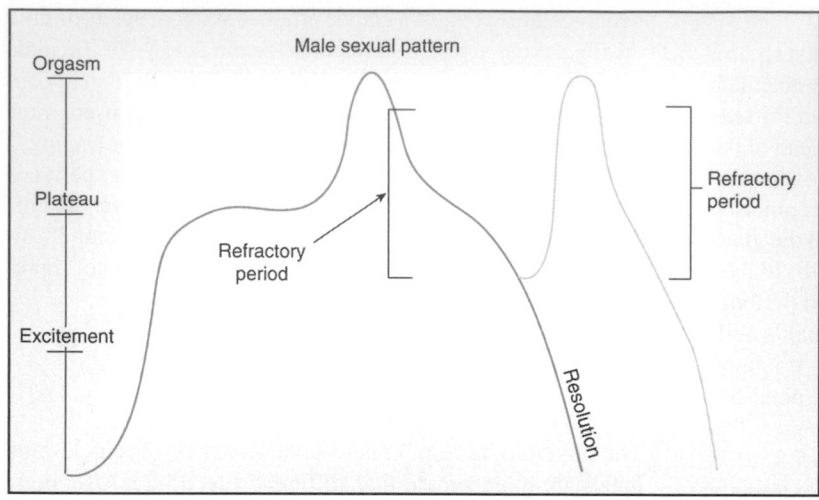

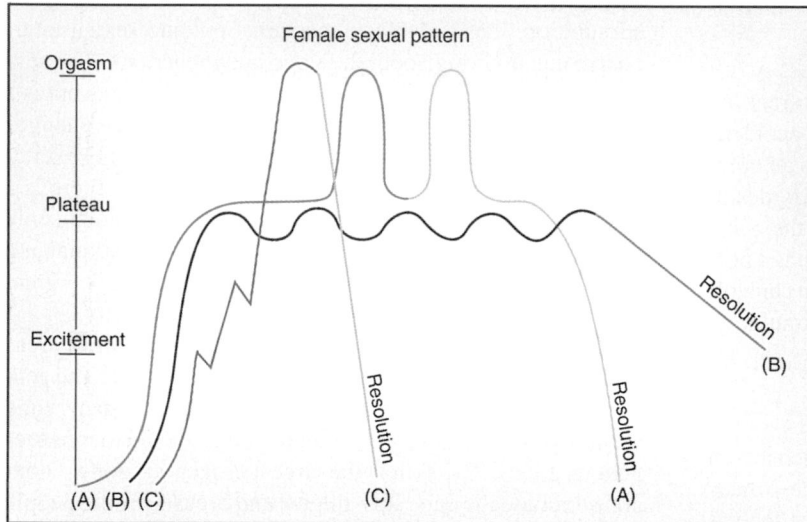

FIGURE 35-2 Male and female sexual response patterns. There are three female patterns shown. (**A**) Steady progression to plateau stage is followed by intense orgasm; subsequent orgasms may occur; resolution is slower. (**B**) Slower progression to plateau stage is followed by minor surges toward orgasm, causing prolonged pleasurable feelings without definitive orgasm; resolution is slowest. (**C**) Rapid progression to plateau stage with some peaks and dips; one intense orgasm follows with rapid resolution. This most closely resembles the male pattern.

one experience to another. Women usually enjoy a more prolonged period of stimulation than do men.

During the excitement phase, the woman's breasts swell and the nipples become erect and hard to the touch. Lubrication of the vagina seeps to the outside of the body along the vulvar creases and makes stimulation of the genitals more pleasurable by decreasing friction. The upper two thirds or so of the vagina enlarge and expand. The clitoris enlarges and emerges slightly from the clitoral hood. The labia also enlarge and separate and turn a deep rosy red with arousal.

The first obvious sign of arousal in the man is an erection of the penis caused by increased pelvic congestion of blood. The scrotum noticeably elevates, thickens, and enlarges. The skin of the penis and scrotum turns a deep reddish-purple in response to congestion and arousal. Male nipples may also harden and become erect.

Plateau

The intensity of the plateau phase is greater than that of excitement but not enough to begin orgasm. Desire and arousal continue to build and intensify. This phase varies from a few

minutes to 15 to 20 minutes. In the female, the clitoris retracts and disappears under the clitoral hood. It is thought that the clitoris performs in this mysterious way as the body's protection against overstimulation. In the male, secretions from Cowper's glands may appear at the glans of the penis during the plateau phase.

Orgasm

The term **orgasm** defines the climax and sexual explosion of the tension that has been building over the preceding phases. Orgasm lasts only seconds, but it is an extremely intense reaction. Characteristics of the orgasm phase are the involuntary spasmodic contractions of the genital organs. The number of contractions felt by the individual depends on the intensity of the orgasm.

The orgasm phase in the female begins with a heightened feeling of physical pleasure, followed by overwhelming release and involuntary contractions of the genitals. Loss of muscular control can also be seen in spastic contractions and twitching of the arms and legs. The number of contractions can be as few as 4 or as many as 20. Areas of the body that contract spasmodically are the uterus, anal sphincter, rectum, and urethral sphincter. It is believed that women achieve orgasm in a variety of ways. Although some women can achieve orgasm by penile thrusting in the vagina alone, most women need clitoral stimulation to reach orgasm.

During orgasm in the male, involuntary spasmodic contractions occur in the penis, epididymis, vas deferens, and rectum. The male orgasm is most often accompanied by ejaculation of semen from the urinary meatus of the penis. It is not necessary for ejaculation and orgasm to occur simultaneously; rather, it is a coincidence that the two events usually happen at the same time.

Resolution

The resolution phase is characterized by a return to normal body functioning present before the excitement phase. Feelings of relaxation, fatigue, and fulfillment are common. Some people have a need to be held, fondled, and caressed. Physical demonstrations of affection may initiate the sexual response cycle once again. The woman is physiologically capable of immediate response to sexual stimulation. Because of this, many women can achieve multiple orgasms. The man experiences a period during which he is incapable of sexual response, called the refractory period. The length of the refractory period is individual; it might be a few minutes or even days before the man's body responds readily to continued sexual stimulation.

SEXUAL EXPRESSION

The methods by which people gain satisfaction through sexual stimulation are varied. Touch, smell, sight, sounds, feelings, thoughts, and fantasy can all contribute to sexual fulfillment in any form of expression chosen by individuals. Feelings of love for another person are closely associated with desire.

Forms of sexual stimulation include kissing, hugging, stroking, squeezing, breast stimulation, manual stimulation of the genitals, oral–genital stimulation, and anal stimulation. Sexual stimulation may be physical or psychological. Erotic stimulation through the use of films, magazines, and photographs is common. Fetishism, usually practiced by a male, is sexual arousal with the aid of an inanimate object not generally associated with sexual activity. Items such as shoes, leather, rubber, and women's undergarments might be used.

Masturbation

Masturbation is a technique of sexual expression in which an individual practices self-stimulation. Many myths and misinformation surround masturbation. It is a way for a person to learn what he or she prefers during stimulation and what feels good. Men masturbate by holding and stroking the shaft of the penis. Women find manual stimulation of the clitoris enjoyable, although variations of technique are numerous. People masturbate regardless of sex, age, or marital status. People might not masturbate because they feel guilty about it or believe self-stimulation is wrong. Masturbation is not "dirty" and will not lead to blindness or insanity.

Sexual Intercourse
Vaginal Intercourse
Heterosexual genital intercourse is the most common image that comes to mind when sexuality is mentioned. The act of intercourse (coitus or copulation) usually begins by stimulation of the senses in some way, followed by a period of activity known as foreplay. "Petting" is part of foreplay; it can involve simple stroking of the breasts, arms, back, and neck without genital involvement or may lead to mutual masturbation and orgasm.

The act of placing the penis in the vagina, penile–vaginal intercourse, can be accomplished in various positions. The most common position in Western cultures is the missionary position, in which the woman lies horizontally underneath the man. (This position was named by the Polynesians because it was the preferred position for intercourse used by religious missionaries.) Couples may find other positions to be more stimulating and comfortable. Clitoral stimulation is difficult to achieve in the missionary position. Lying side by side, female on top, and rear entry are some examples of coital positions that enable clitoral stimulation. Sexually inhibited people may believe they need "permission" to engage in alternative sexual positions.

When the penis is pushed into the vagina, the man begins rhythmic thrusting movements of his hips to move the penis back and forth along the vaginal walls. The woman might match her partner's hip movements with movements of her own body. These movements continue until orgasm is attained by one person or both.

Simultaneous orgasms, or both people attaining orgasm at the same moment, are difficult to achieve, and a preoccupation with attaining simultaneous orgasms might disrupt the ultimate intimacy and satisfaction possible during coitus.

The period after coitus is just as significant as the events leading up to it. Caressing, hugging, and kissing deepen the couple's intimacy and should be nurtured, not rushed.

Anal Intercourse
Anal intercourse, the act of inserting the penis into the anus and rectum of a partner, is another form of intercourse. Commonly practiced by gay men, it is also used by heterosexual couples. Once the penis (or any object) is placed in the rectum, it should not be introduced into the vagina without thorough cleansing because many microorganisms present in the rectum can cause vaginal infections. Care should be used to avoid injury to the delicate rectal mucosa, and lubrication is essential for comfort. Condoms are now recommended for both types of intercourse to prevent sexually transmitted infections (STIs).

Oral–Genital Stimulation

Stimulation of the genitals by the mouth and tongue might be used during foreplay or as a way to reach orgasm. Cunnilingus is stimulation of the female genitals by licking and sucking the clitoris and surrounding structures. Fellatio is stimulation of the male genitals by licking and sucking the penis and surrounding structures. These techniques may be used by one partner or both simultaneously (*soixante-neuf*).

Celibacy

Celibacy is abstinence from genital sexual activity. Celibacy might be practiced for many reasons. Dissatisfaction with the harmful consequences of the "sexual revolution" of the 1960s is leading an increasing number of adolescents and adults to choose celibate lifestyles. Many members of religious orders live celibate lives.

Alternative Forms of Sexual Expression

Alternate forms of sexual expression include voyeurism, sadism, masochism, sadomasochism, and pedophilia.
- Voyeurism is the achievement of sexual arousal by looking at the body of another. Some voyeurs develop complex means to spy on others that involve violations of privacy.
- Sadism refers to the practice of gaining sexual pleasure while inflicting abuse on another person.
- Masochism refers to gaining sexual pleasure from the humiliation of being abused.
- Sadomasochism is the act of practicing sadism and masochism together. It might involve being tied up, biting, hitting, spanking, whipping, pinching, and other activities.

- Pedophilia is a term used to describe the practice of adults gaining sexual fulfillment by performing sexual acts with children.

FACTORS AFFECTING SEXUALITY

Many factors influence a person's sexuality and produce personal feelings regarding sexuality. The brain, rather than the genitals, plays the most significant role in how people perceive themselves as sexual beings.

Developmental Considerations

The process of human development affects the psychosocial, emotional, and biologic aspects of life, and these in turn affect an individual's sexuality. Sexuality is the only distinguishing trait present at conception. From birth onward, gender, or sex, influences behavior throughout life. Table 35-1 summarizes sexuality throughout the life span and the nursing implications for each stage.

Culture

The manner in which sexuality is perceived by a society in turn influences the individual. Every culture has its own norms regarding sexual identity and behavior. To some degree, culture dictates the duration of sexual intercourse, methods of

TABLE 35-1 Developmental Aspects of Sexuality Through the Life Span

Stage	Characteristics	Nursing Implications and Teaching Guidelines
Infancy: Birth to 18 mo	• Needs affection and tactile stimulation • Boys have penile erections, and girls have orgasmic potential • Gradually can differentiate self from others • Obtain pleasure from touching genitals • Dressed according to gender • Toys are gender related	• Avoid early weaning to prevent oral deprivation. • Encourage parents to provide ample physical touch, deprivation of which may cause physical and mental underdevelopment. • Self-manipulation of genitals is normal behavior; avoid denoting this as "bad." • Avoid confusion of sex by consistent use of male or female role reinforcement.
Toddler: Age 1–3 yr	• Establishes control over bowels and bladder • Both sexes enjoy fondling genitals • Able to identify own gender • Develops vocabulary related to anatomy	• Allow toddler to designate his or her readiness to toilet-training. Strict measures may lead to compulsive behaviors later. • Punishment of genital fondling may lead to guilt and shame regarding sexual behavior later in life. • Use proper terms for body parts.
Preschooler: Age 4–6 yr	• By age 6, sexuality has been internalized and preference for sexual partners determined • Methods of play and dress are in accordance with gender • Enjoys exploring body parts of self and playmates • Engages in masturbation	• Parents may cause anxiety in the child by intolerance of inconsistency of sex-role behavior. • Negative overreaction by parents of child's masturbating behavior can lead to a belief that the genitals and sex are bad and dirty. *(continued)*

TABLE 35-1 (Continued)

Stage	Characteristics	Nursing Implications and Teaching Guidelines
School-age: Age 6–10 yr	• There is attachment to the parent of the opposite sex • Tendency toward having same-sex friends • Curiosity about sex and sharing of fears • Increasing self-awareness	• Same-sex preference for relationships is not related to heterosexual or homosexual tendencies. • Give child the information desired in a clear, factual form. May look to peers for information that may be incorrect.
Preadolescence: Age 10–13 yr	• Puberty begins for most boys and girls with development of secondary sex characteristics • Menarche takes place • May test behavioral limits	• Information is necessary regarding body changes to alleviate fears. This information should be given to the young person before pubertal changes begin. • Parents need to find a satisfactory middle ground for role setting. Rules that are either too rigid or too lenient can interfere with the development of self-confidence and internal value system. • Treat body image changes with a positive attitude to prevent poor self-image.
Adolescence: Age 13–19 yr	• Begins to develop opposite-sex relationships • Sexual fantasies are common • Masturbation is common • May begin to partake in sexual activity ranging from light to heavy petting to full genital intercourse • Girls concerned with reputations and self-image • Boys preoccupied with competitiveness of sexual activity • Incidence of adolescent pregnancies is increasing	• Parents share their beliefs and moral value systems with their children. • Teenagers may share their feelings with parents. Not taking them seriously may lead to lack of trust and communication gap. • Teens need information regarding contraceptive measures and the potential for contracting sexually transmitted infections.
Young adulthood: Age 20–35 yr	• Premarital sex is common • Although many young adults choose cohabitation instead of marriage, most marry and begin families before age 30 yr • Knowledge regarding sexual response and activity increases pleasure of relationship • May experiment with various sexual expressions • Develops own value system and respects values of other people • Many couples share financial responsibilities as well as household tasks	• Encourage communication between partners regarding sexual needs and differences. • Teach use of abstinence and contraceptive measures to prevent unwanted pregnancies. • Counsel against promiscuous behavior to guard against sexually transmitted diseases and loss of trust of partner. • Daily communication is necessary to vent stresses and work out difficulties.
Adulthood: Age 35–55 yr	• Bodily changes as a result of menopause • Couples focus on quality rather than quantity of sexual experiences • Divorce is common • Grown children begin their own lives and sexual experiences • Sexual satisfaction may actually increase because of loss of fear of pregnancy	• Both men and women need positive reinforcement of what is good about themselves and their relationships. • Teach parents that *empty nest syndrome* (feelings of loss caused by children leaving) is common. Accentuate positive aspects of this situation. • Encourage couple to use this period as one of renewal for themselves.
Late adulthood and elderly: Age 55 yr and older	• Orgasms may become shorter and less intense in both men and women • Vaginal secretions decrease, and period of resolution in men lengthens • May feel need to conform to stereotypes regarding the aging process and cease sexual activity • Fear of loss of sexual abilities	• Sexual activity need not be hindered by age. • Teach couples that adaptation to bodily changes is possible with use of comfortable positions for intercourse and increased time for stimulation. • Teach alternatives to coitus, such as caressing, hugging, and stroking, when coitus is impossible because of illness or disability. • Couples who have been consistently sexually active throughout their lives may continue their intimate relationship for as long as they desire.

sexual stimulation, and sexual positions. In some cultures, women might be expected merely to tolerate sex; in others, the woman's participation is encouraged.

> *Remember Amy Liu, the woman who was described at the beginning of the chapter. It would be important for the nurse to assess the patient's culture to determine if this is playing a role in her feelings. For example, the nurse would investigate how her culture views women who have had a hysterectomy and thus can no longer reproduce. This view may be affecting Mrs. Liu's feeling that she is not a woman anymore. This in turn affects her self-concept and her sexual health.*

Religion

Some people view organized religion as having a generally negative effect on the expression of sexuality. Many forms of sexual expression other than male–female coitus are considered unnatural by some religions. Also, over time, the concept of virginity came to be synonymous with purity, and sex became synonymous with sin. Double standards and rigid regulations have inflicted a considerable amount of guilt and anxiety on many individuals. A number of sexual dysfunctions can be related to an individual's anguish over the negative connotation of sex as dictated by some religious groups. Most major religions are reexamining their teachings on sexuality in response to challenges posed by their members. Many have recognized the importance of solid sex education within the realm of the church. There is also a new interest in the spirituality of marriage, and churches are examining their role in supporting the intimate/sexual relationship of married couples.

Ethics

Healthy sexuality depends on freedom from guilt and anxiety. What one person believes is wrong might be perfectly natural and correct to another. Some individuals might feel that certain forms of sexual expression are bizarre and the people who participate in them are perverted. If the sexual expression is performed by consenting adults, is not harmful to them, and is practiced in privacy, it is not considered a deviant behavior. Individuals should personally decide with which aspects of sexual expression they are comfortable. Frequently, all an individual needs to alleviate guilt and consequently enhance sexual satisfaction is permission from a healthcare professional to engage in a different form of expression.

Lifestyle

Modern lifestyles greatly affect sexuality and its expression. Both men and women are exposed to stress, and many are under considerable strain to perform and function in the workplace as well as at home. Stressors might be external, such as job and financial demands, or internal, such as a competitive

nature. These varied responsibilities place a time restraint on communication between a couple as well as on the energy level and motivation for sexual satisfaction. Although some couples view sexual activity as a release from the stressors of everyday life, most place sex far from the top of the list of things to do. It is crucial to a relationship's survival that a couple set aside priority time—if not for lovemaking, then for intimate, quiet contact.

Childbearing Considerations

All sorts of questions surround childbearing, and the ability (or lack of ability) to procreate can put great pressure on a sexual relationship: Are we ready to be parents? What does it mean to be a responsible parent—especially in this age when an increasing number of prenatal interventions are available to maximize fetal outcomes (quality control)? Should life partners be chosen only if genetic testing reveals a good match for reproduction? If we choose to be sexually active and not have children, what are the best means to prevent unwanted pregnancies? If we become pregnant and choose not to continue the pregnancy, what are our options? If we desperately want a child and discover one or both parties to be infertile, what are our options? The age of biotechnology promises "designer babies" and raises hard questions for individuals and society. Individuals frequently look to nurses for help in sorting through how they ought to respond to these challenges. Experienced nurses are good at detecting when a fear of pregnancy or inability to conceive is interfering with a couple's normal sexual expression or when a changing developmental stage (eg, menopause) is interfering with normal sexual expression.

Sexually Transmitted Infections

The term "sexually transmitted infections" is used to describe infections that are almost always transmitted through direct sexual contact. While the fear of getting (or transmitting) an STI may impair sexual functioning for some, it is also true that many people engage in risky sexual behaviors without giving sufficient thought to their health. Table 35-2 lists common types of STIs and their signs and symptoms. The number of cases and varieties of STIs has increased over the years, and many are at epidemic proportions. STIs are hard to control because the partner or partners also need treatment; this is usually difficult if the partner is promiscuous or a one-time contact.

Sexuality educators caution patients that having sexual contact with someone means also having sexual contact with everyone else that person has had contact with in the past. The only sure way to avoid exposure to an STI is for a virgin to have sexual contact with another virgin. Condoms are not foolproof in preventing STIs: the disease can be spread if the condom slips or tears during intercourse.

Some STIs can be treated easily and effectively, whereas others have long-term implications. For instance, women may suffer severe consequences from an STI by developing pelvic inflammatory disease (PID); the resulting adhesions damage delicate reproductive structures and may lead to infertility.

TABLE 35-2 Sexually Transmitted Infections

Disease	Characteristics
Acquired immunodeficiency syndrome (AIDS)	• Human immunodeficiency virus (HIV) • Positive ELISA and Western Blot tests • Incidence high in IV drug users and homosexual and bisexual men; increased heterosexual transmission • Fatigue, diarrhea, weight loss, enlarged lymph nodes, fever, anorexia, and night sweats
Cervical intraepithelial neoplasia (CIN) Cervical cancer	• Abnormal Pap smears • Women with multiple sex partners, women who began sexual activity before age 18, and women whose partners have multiple female partners • Asymptomatic • Possible vaginal bleeding or spotting
Chlamydia trachomatis Nongonococcal urethritis (NGU) Chlamydia	• The most prevalent STD to date • Intracellular bacteria • Vaginal discharge, burning on urination, urinary frequency, dysuria, and urethral soreness • Many women do not have symptoms.
Cytomegalovirus (CMV)	• A virus in the same family as herpes and Epstein-Barr • May be asymptomatic or may be confused with another disease such as pneumonia, mononucleosis, or hepatitis • Not exclusively sexually transmitted.
Nonspecific vaginitis *Gardnerella vaginalis*	• Mixed anaerobic bacteria • Foul-smelling, thin, grayish white vaginal discharge • Male partners do not have symptoms.
Neisseria gonorrhoeae "The clap" or "the drip" Gonorrhea	• Gram-negative bacteria • Both men and women may not have symptoms. • Symptoms in men: purulent penile discharge, dysuria, frequency of urination • Symptoms in women: dysuria, abnormal menses, vaginal discharge, pelvic inflammatory disease • Symptoms of pharyngitis if oral sex practiced • May be accompanied by chlamydial infection • Detected by gonorrhea culture of cervix or penile discharge from men • Newborns exposed at birth are at risk for blindness and pneumonia. • Untreated gonorrhea can result in infertility, skin rash with lesions, and acute arthritis.
Herpes simples virus type 1 and 2 "Cold sores" Herpes	• A DNA virus • Lesions develop mostly in oral and genital areas. • Appear as single or multiple painful vesicles, which rupture and form ulcer-like lesions; these form scabs as they heal. • First infections last about 10 to 14 days, whereas subsequent infections are shorter in duration. • Recurrences are usually preceded by prodromal symptoms of tingling and fullness.
Human papilloma virus (HPV) Condylomata acuminata Genital warts Venereal warts	• A DNA virus • Pale, soft, papillary lesions found around the internal and external genitalia and perianal and rectal areas of the body; vary in size • Profuse watery vaginal discharge, dyspareunia, intense pruritus, and vulvar irritation • Women with HPV are at risk for cervical cancer. • Male partner may or may not have lesions.
Treponema pallidum Syphilis	• A spirochete detected through serologic blood test (VDRL, RPR, STS) • Three stages to disease if left untreated *Primary:* Single painless genital lesion 10 days to 3 months after exposure *Secondary:* Generalized skin rash, enlarged lymph nodes, fever that may appear 2 to 4 weeks after appearance of primary lesion; may last for several years *Latent:* Usually no clinical symptoms present for as long as 20 years; may continue to involve and damage neurologic and cardiovascular organs; dementia, confusion, paralysis, and paresis may occur
Trichomoniasis "Trich" Trichomonas vaginalis	• Protozoan with flagella • Identified on wet-mount microscopic examination of vaginal discharge • May be identified on Pap smear • Usually asymptomatic in male patients • Foul-smelling vaginal discharge, thin, foamy, and green in color, causes itching of vulva and vagina, burning on urination and dyspareunia; "strawberry" cervix may be seen on speculum examination

(Data from Center for Disease Control/National Center for HIV, STD and TB Prevention [2002]. Sexually transmitted disease guidelines 2002 [Electronic Versions]. *Morbidity and Mortality Weekly Report*, 51; Garbach, S., Bartlett, J. & Blacklaw, N. [1998]. *Infectious disease* [2nd ed]. Philadelphia: Saunders; Mandell, G., Bennett, J. & Dolin, R. [2000]. *Principles and practice of infectious diseases* [5th ed] Philadelphia: Churchill Livingstone. Baldwin, K., & Goodwin, K. [1985]. The Papanicolaou smear. *Journal of Nurse–Midwifery* 30[6]: 327–331; Bourcier, K., & Seidler, A. [1987]. Chlamydia and condylomata acuminata; An update for the nurse practitioner. *Journal of Obstetric, Gynecologic, and Neonatal Nursing* 16[1], 17–21; Fromer, M. [1983]. *Ethical issues in sexuality and reproduction*. St. Louis: C. V. Mosby; Hatcher, R., et al. [1986]. *Contraceptive technology*. New York: Irvington.)

Having an STI might affect one's self-concept and keep an individual from becoming intimate for fear of spreading the infection. Some STIs, such as acquired immunodeficiency syndrome (AIDS), are deadly because there is no cure.

> *Recall Paul Rojas, the homosexual patient with AIDS. The nurse would need to assess the patient's sexual practices and instruct him about sex practices to prevent the transmission of AIDS. In addition, the nurse would need to investigate the effect that this STI has had on his sexuality.*

Sexual Dysfunction

Sexual dysfunction is a problem that prevents an individual or couple from engaging in or enjoying sexual intercourse and orgasm. Dysfunctions might occur as a result of physiologic malfunctions, conflicts with cultural norms, interpersonal problems, or any combination of these. Anxieties and fears concerning the sexual act are almost always present. Patients with severe sexual dysfunctions require intensive professional therapy from a qualified sex therapist.

Male Primary Sexual Dysfunctions
Erectile Failure

Erectile failure, also called **impotence,** is the inability of a man to attain or maintain an erection to such an extent that he cannot have satisfactory intercourse. Common causes of impotence (which may be physiologic or psychological) include various illnesses, treatments for these illnesses, and personal anxieties. New medications have revolutionized treatment for erectile dysfunction.

> *Remember Jefferson Smith, the patient with diabetes and hypertension who is having problems with erections. The nurse would review the pathophysiologic effects of diabetes and hypertension on sexual response and would evaluate his current status, including a review of all medications that he is taking, to determine possible contributory factors.*

Premature Ejaculation

Premature ejaculation is a condition in which a man consistently reaches ejaculation or orgasm before or soon after entering the vagina. The result is that his partner usually does not have time to reach sexual satisfaction. Causes of the problem are rarely physical.

Retarded Ejaculation

Retarded ejaculation, also called ejaculatory incompetence, refers to a man's inability to ejaculate into the vagina, or delayed intravaginal ejaculation. The causes of this problem are similar to those of impotence. When it occurs after the man has experienced normal ejaculations, the cause is most probably due to interpersonal problems.

Female Primary Sexual Dysfunctions
Inhibited Sexual Desire

Inhibited sexual desire consists of an inhibition in sexual arousal so that congestion and vaginal lubrication are absent or minimal. Causative factors may be anxiety, negative emotions, fear, interpersonal problems, or physical factors. Orgasmic dysfunction is defined as the inability of a woman to reach orgasm. The causes are similar to those of inhibited sexual desire.

Dyspareunia

Dyspareunia is painful intercourse. Although it is most often described by women, some men may also suffer from this disorder. The cause is usually physical, although psychological problems such as fear and anxiety can cause pain in some women.

> *Consider Amy Liu, the woman who had a hysterectomy and is experiencing pain on intercourse. The nurse would review the patient's history to determine if the problem is physiologic secondary to changes in the reproductive tract from surgery, or psychological, secondary to the changes in self-concept and feelings of not being a woman.*

Vaginismus

Vaginismus is a rare condition in which the vaginal opening closes tightly and prevents penile penetration. Vaginismus is due to involuntary spastic contractions of the muscles at and around the vaginal opening and the levator ani muscles. The cause of vaginismus may be physical, psychological, or both.

Vulvodynia

Vulvodynia, a chronic vulvar discomfort or pain characterized by burning, stinging, irritation, or rawness of the female genitalia that interferes with sexual activity, is particularly problematic because little is known about its cause or treatment.

Other Health Conditions

A healthy body, mind, and emotions are necessary for sexual wellness. A primary sexual dysfunction can affect a person's sexual expression. Similarly, any trauma or stress that interferes with an individual's ability to perform daily functions will also affect the expression of sexuality. Illness is no exception.

> *Think back to Paul Rojas, the homosexual patient with AIDS. In addition to the issues he faces about sexual orientation, he must also face the effect of AIDS on his daily functioning as well as his sexual health.*

Diabetes Mellitus

Diabetes mellitus is a hormonal disease in which an inadequate amount of insulin is secreted by the pancreas. Although almost all hormonal disorders affect sexuality in some way, diabetes is the most prevalent and well known. Erectile dysfunction, or impotence, is a great concern among diabetic men. Treatment to date depends largely on the degree of erectile ability lost. Some men might be candidates for a penile prosthesis, which was developed in 1973. The prosthesis is surgically implanted below the base of the penis, and inflation of the device produces an erection when sexual activity is desired. Pharmacologic management (eg, sildenafil citrate [Viagra]) might also be indicated.

> *Think back to Jefferson Smith, the patient with diabetes and hypertension. The nurse would explore with Mr. Smith his feelings about the effect of his disorder on his sexual function and sexuality. Additional consultation with other members of the healthcare team would be necessary to determine the most appropriate plan for treatment of Mr. Smith's impotence.*

It is not uncommon for diabetic women to experience loss of capacity for orgasm (orgasmic dysfunction). Difficulty experiencing arousal and loss of vaginal lubrication have also been reported. Frequent *Monilia* infections of the vagina are also common and can cause discomfort during coitus.

Cardiovascular Disease

Cardiovascular disease is prevalent in North America, and the sexual response cycle can greatly increase the demands on the heart and other structures. A person with a cardiovascular disease might experience much anxiety over the effect the illness will have on sexuality and sexual functioning.

Hypertension

The most significant difficulty a hypertensive person faces regarding sexuality is that the medication used to control the disease frequently causes a change in sexual functioning. These sexual dysfunctions may be relieved by modifying the dose of the medication or switching to a different medication.

> *Consider Jefferson Smith, the patient with a history of diabetes and hypertension. The nurse would obtain a complete medication history from the patient to determine if his pharmacologic therapy is the underlying cause of his impotence or if the medication is contributing to a preexisting problem associated with his diabetes. This investigation would provide information about whether an adjustment in medication dosage might minimize or alleviate Mr. Smith's impotence.*

Myocardial Infarction (Heart Attack)

The primary goal after a myocardial infarction (MI) is to allow the heart ample time to heal. Activities of daily living, including sexual activity, should be resumed gradually, and stressors such as overexertion, alcohol consumption, and emotional upheavals should be avoided. In an uncomplicated MI, sexual activity may begin at about the third week of recovery, beginning with masturbation to partial erection in the male. Generally, this activity is gradually increased until 3 months after the MI, when sexual intercourse may be resumed. A comfortable position that places the least stress on the affected partner should be used.

Diseases of the Joints and Mobility

Joint diseases and disorders affect young and old people. Pain, fatigue, stiffness, and loss of range of motion can accompany any of the dozens of known diseases of the joints. The disease itself does not affect sexual functioning, although the manifestation of it can cause discomfort and anxiety.

Surgery and Body Image

Surgery is performed to remove diseased tissue and repair body organs, and it usually requires an incision with resulting scars. The most devastating kinds of surgery are those used to remove cancerous tissue and surrounding structures. Patients are almost always distressed about a diagnosis of cancer and possible death. After surgery, patients need to adjust to major alterations in their bodies. Changes in body image also affect a person's self-perception as a sexual being.

> *Remember Amy Liu, the woman who had had a hysterectomy. The uterus, because it is a female reproductive organ, is often associated with childbearing and is a major component of a woman's "femaleness." The nurse would interpret the significance of the uterus to the patient's self-concept and how the surgery to remove it has affected her overall feelings of "femininity" and "femaleness." Using this information, the nurse would then correct any misconceptions that Mrs. Liu may have about this reproductive organ and develop an appropriate teaching plan.*

Mastectomy is a surgical procedure to remove a breast and surrounding tissue. After such surgery, a woman's return to sexual functioning depends on many factors, such as support of her partner, the value placed on the breast by the man or woman, and fear of discomfort during sexual activity.

An ostomy is a surgical opening placed on the outside of the body to allow for the passage of secretions and elimination into a closed drainage bag. Grieving over the loss of the natural means to eliminate waste, such as urine or feces, accompanies learning to live with an obvious artificial device. Many people are anxious as to how this apparatus will affect their sex lives and how accepting their partners will be of it.

Spinal Cord Injuries

Thousands of people are victims of spinal cord injuries each year as a result of various types of accidents. This type of injury almost always results in some degree of permanent disability. Such people face multiple adaptations in their lifestyles, including those related to mobility, bowel and bladder control, sexual functioning, and role expectations. The extent of sexual response that remains after a spinal cord injury depends primarily on the level and extent of the injury. Ejaculation and orgasm are most likely to remain with low spinal injuries. Women are more likely to experience orgasm than men, but they complain more about the lack of physical sensations during the excitement phase than do men. Many people find that other erogenous zones become more easily stimulated after the injury.

Chronic Pain

Many chronic illnesses are accompanied by constant pain, and an individual with persistent pain might not desire any sexual contact. However, the desire for human warmth and contact does not cease because of pain. Altered or modified positions for coitus are sometimes necessary; these are discussed in more detail later in this section.

Mental Illness

Various psychological and physical disorders can cause mental illness. The mind plays a powerful role in sexuality, and any disruption of its functioning will no doubt cause some disturbance in sexual functioning. Even a disorder such as mild depression can affect desire and sexual functioning. Sometimes, it is difficult for the partner of a patient who has developed a mental illness to continue the sexual relationship. People afflicted with Alzheimer's disease can lose the memory of any contact with a partner or spouse. At times, patients with mental illness act out in a sexual manner, such as touching themselves or removing their clothing at inappropriate times and places.

Medications

Some medications have side effects that may affect sexual functioning. Some people use illegal drugs because of their reputed ability to heighten the sexual experience; these drugs can have serious and even deadly side effects. The accompanying display lists some of the categories of medications and their possible effects on sexual functioning.

THE NURSE AS ROLE MODEL

A nurse's attitudes, biases, and prejudices regarding sexuality are readily transmitted to patients through his or her actions, manner of speech, avoidance of certain circumstances, and types of discussion (see Focused Critical Thinking Guide). The level of knowledge a nurse has about sexual issues can inhibit or promote discussions of sexual health. The nurse who does not have a sound knowledge base of reproductive anatomy and physiology, sexual response, sexual expression, and other issues surrounding sexuality will be unable to assess, teach, or counsel the patient with sexual concerns. The nurse must also feel comfortable with himself or herself as a sexual being (see Promoting Health).

Recall Paul Rojas, the patient described in the Reflective Practice box. The nurse caring for

Mr. Rojas needs to be comfortable with his or her own sexuality to ensure that he or she provides nonjudgmental care. In addition, the nurse needs a solid knowledge foundation about sexual orientation and sexual preference to develop an appropriate, unbiased plan of care that meets Mr. Rojas' needs.

Nursing goals to enhance interactions with patients and to promote individual sexual health are as follows: The nurse will be able to:
* Feel comfortable as a sexual being
* Develop self-awareness regarding sexual topics
* Develop communication skills that promote discussion of sexual concerns with patients
* Identify patients with problems related to sexuality and intervene competently and comfortably to meet these needs
* Practice responsible sexual expression

THE NURSING PROCESS FOR THE PATIENT WITH A SEXUAL HEALTH NEED

Assessing

Sexual History

The comprehensive health history should include information regarding a patient's reproductive and sexual health, depending on the circumstances in which the patient is receiving care. As a rule, three general categories of patients should have a sexual history recorded by the nurse:
* Any inpatient or outpatient receiving care for pregnancy, STI, infertility, or contraception
* Any patient experiencing sexual dysfunction
* Any patient whose illness will affect sexual functioning and behavior in any way

Information is best obtained from the patient by beginning with nonthreatening questions and progressing to more sensitive concerns (see the accompanying Focused Assessment Guide). Patients usually have no difficulty answering questions regarding their bodies and general reproductive issues such as, "When did your menstrual periods first begin?"

Nurses should explain to patients that this information might be helpful in assisting them in the plan of care and in identifying any sexual problems or concerns. The assessment provides an excellent opportunity for the nurse to teach by helping the patient confront fears. Four general levels of sexual history are:

Level 1: Sexual history as part of a comprehensive health history—obtained by a nurse

Level 2: Sexual history—obtained by a nurse with education and training in sexuality

Level 3: Sexual problem history—obtained by a sex therapist

Level 4: Psychiatric/psychosocial history—obtained by a psychiatric nurse clinician

Each level acquires more specific information from the patient regarding sexual health and also requires the interviewer

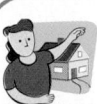

Teaching to Promote Health at Home 35-1
Factors Affecting Sexuality

Health Topic	Teaching Tip	Why is This Important?
Medications and their effects on sexual functioning	**Amyl nitrite:** Peripheral vasodilator used in the past for treating angina; has become popular as sex enhancer among male homosexuals in particular; when inhaled at time of orgasm, the resulting vasodilation is felt to cause an intensified orgasmic release. Loss of erection, hypotension, and faintness may occur.	Health problems may require treatment with a variety of medications. Many medications can contribute to sexual dysfunction. Educating patients about the effects of medications on sexual function is a critical component of nursing and healthcare planning. The nurse should educate the patient about strategies to deal with the sexual side effect of the medications.
	Anticonvulsants: Dilantin (phenytoin) has sedative effects, which may decrease desire and reduce sexual response.	
	Antidepressants:	
	Tricyclic compounds	
	Monoamine oxidase inhibitors	
	Lithium carbonate	
	Similar to antihypertensive drugs. Male impotence is significant.	
	Male impotence and ejaculatory dysfunction in 25% to 30% of men.	
	Decreases serum testosterone levels in men. Some antidepressants have been found to cause prolonged painful erections known as *priapism;* one such drug is trazodone.	
	Antihistamines: May have sedative effect that decreases desire; may also cause decreased vaginal lubrication.	
	Antihypertensives:	
	Methyldopa	
	Clonidine	
	Reserpine	
	May decrease desire in both men and women	
	Erectile failure in 24% of men; no adverse effect on female patients	
	Decreased desire in women; erectile and ejaculation dysfunctions in men	
	Antipsychotics: Cause decreased desire in 10% to 20% of patients; may also cause erection and ejaculatory dysfunctions	
	Small amount of the antipsychotic drug may be found in the semen; the partner may experience a resulting genital rash. Wear condoms while taking therapy.	
	Antispasmodics: These drugs relax smooth muscle; male impotence may occur.	
	Barbiturates: In low initial doses, sexual pleasure may be increased due to loss of inhibitions. However, long-term use commonly causes decreased desire and orgasmic dysfunction. Male impotence is not uncommon.	
	Cocaine: Reported to increase quality of sexual experience, but chronic use results in sexual dysfunction and loss of desire in both men and women.	
	Ethyl alcohol: In moderate amounts, decreases inhibitions and consequently improves sexual functioning. Continued consumption decreases sexual functioning. Chronic alcoholics are impotent and often sterile. Testicular damage and permanent dysfunction are common. Female alcoholics experience decreased desire and orgasmic dysfunction.	
	Marijuana: Release of inhibitions may cause feeling of increased sexual functioning. Marijuana users have an increased incidence of decreased desire and male impotence.	
	Narcotics: Serious impairment of sexual functioning with increased dependence. Erectile and ejaculatory dysfunctions common in men. Testosterone levels and amount of semen decreased. High incidence of decreased desire in both men and women.	

(Data from Crenshaw, T., & Goldberg, J. [1996]. *Sexual pharmacology: drugs that affect sexual functioning.* New York: Norton; Fuentes, R. [1983]. Sexual side effects. What to tell your patients, what not to say. RN, 46[2], 34–41; Woods, N. F. [1984]. *Human sexuality in health and illness.* St. Louis, MO: C. V. Mosby.)

Focused Critical Thinking Guide 35-1

Situation

A 33-year-old Caucasian male with AIDS who is living alone at home asks you, the visiting nurse, about the nurse who was substituting for you during your vacation. "I don't like to complain, but he was overly friendly—if you get what I mean. . . . I wasn't comfortable with the way he was touching me and I'd rather not have help with my bath than have him back here." You have to decide how to respond.

1. Identify Goal of Thinking

Clarify what the patient is saying and make a judgment about the behavior behind his concern so that you can respond appropriately.

2. Assess Adequacy of Knowledge

Pertinent circumstances: You have been visiting the patient for the last 2 months following his discharge from a local hospital because of AIDS-related complications. Apart from his clinical picture, you know very little about the patient, who has always seemed private and reserved during your visits. You "feel sorry" that the patient is as sick as he is at this point in his life, and your instinct is to trust him. You really don't know the colleague who was substituting for you because he is a "new hire."

Prerequisite knowledge: Before you can make a judgment about the patient's concern, you need to know more about what actually happened between him and your colleague. You do not know your colleague well because he is a "new hire" and has only been working in the agency for 3 months. You have heard reports that he is gay. You know that the patient is single but do not know his sexual orientation. You will need to talk with your colleague to get his description of his encounter with the patient. You will also need to know more about what touch means to both the patient and your colleague because culture and individual preference can profoundly influence the meaning different individuals give to touch.

Room for error: Life and death do not hinge on how you respond to this patient. However, the well-being of the patient and your colleague's reputation are at stake, so the matter is grave.

Time constraints: You must make some immediate response to the patient. Because you do not have sufficient information to judge what happened, you should not feel pressured to make a definitive response. The patient's well-being will not be jeopardized if you postpone a complete response until you have investigated the complaint.

3. Address Potential Problems

The most serious obstacles to critical thinking in this situation would be false assumptions you (and the patient) might have about homosexuality in general and male homosexual nurses in particular, and the failure to reason carefully about the situation. Your tendency to "go to bat" for patients and

to believe whatever a patient tells you "no matter what" may result in your unfairly and prematurely judging a colleague.

4. Consult Helpful Resources

Your colleague is the first resource you should consult because you need to hear his side of the event before you can think critically about what happened. When you do meet with him, he thanks you for bringing up the subject because he was similarly disturbed by his encounter with this patient. "I guess I'm a touchy-feely kind of guy and generally find that patients respond well to human touch. In the past, patients have told me how much it means to them to have someone massage their back, stroke a forearm, or greet them with a hug. Touch is certainly a big part of the 'therapeutic package' I give each of my patients. I did sense rather quickly, though, that Jim didn't like to be touched and modified my approach. My sense, from a few comments he made, is that he's probably homophobic [afraid of homosexuals]."

After listening to your colleague, you decide you need to learn more about touch, touch as a therapeutic intervention, and homophobia. You can consult the literature or local experts.

5. Critique Judgment/Decision

Wanting to explore the situation more fully, you responded to the patient initially by saying, "I am sorry that you felt uncomfortable by my colleague's care. I want to talk with him about his sense of what happened and will then discuss this with you when I return on Wednesday." After talking with your colleague you are reasonably assured that he was not intending, inappropriately, to communicate anything of a sexual nature to the patient. On your return visit to the patient you inform him about your research and judgment and say, "Touch can mean different things to different people. My sense is that Dave simply wanted to communicate that he cares. If he is going about this in the wrong way, he wants to know what he should be doing differently. We certainly don't want this to be a problem for you or any other patient. Would you like to talk more about this or to file a report?"

You initially think you have three options: (1) to agree at the outset that your colleague has behaved in a sexually inappropriate and unprofessional manner, (2) to investigate the incident and conclude that your colleague was in the wrong, or (3) to investigate the incident and conclude that your colleague was in the right. You chose the third and are relieved when the patient seems to accept your explanation. Two months later, when you receive a similar complaint from another male patient, you are troubled. You realize now that there was a fourth option, and that this is the one you should have taken. Convinced by your colleague's sincerity and good intent, you might nonetheless have informed Dave that you need to communicate this patient concern to your supervisor so that if future incidents are reported there will be a record of repeat complaints.

Promoting Health 35-1 *Sexuality*

Use the assessment checklist to determine how well you are meeting your sexuality needs. Then develop a prescription for self-care by choosing appropriate behaviors from the list of suggestions.

ASSESSMENT CHECKLIST

(columns: almost always / sometimes / almost never)

- ☐ ☐ ☐ 1. I feel good about my sexual identity.
- ☐ ☐ ☐ 2. I have satisfying relationships with others.
- ☐ ☐ ☐ 3. I accept sexual needs as a normal part of life.
- ☐ ☐ ☐ 4. I am comfortable with physical actions that indicate love and belonging (such as touching and hugging).

SELF-CARE BEHAVIORS

1. Avoid stereotyping typical gender roles.
2. Learn the biologic aspects of sexual functioning.
3. Ask questions about sexual needs and sexual activity when necessary.
4. Enjoy close relationships with others who love you.
5. Give a hug to someone you love.
6. Accept touch from others as a sign of caring and affection.
7. Practice safer sex (eg, use contraceptives or condoms, and choose partner carefully).
8. Recognize how age, illness, or disability influences sexual needs and expression.

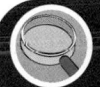

Focused Assessment Guide 35-1

Sexuality

Factors to Assess	Questions and Approaches
Reproductive history	Ask women their date of menarche, date of last menstrual period, duration and length of flow in days, number of pregnancies, living children, miscarriages, abortions, method of birth control. Ask men the number of children they have fathered and method of birth control used. Ask both men and women of childbearing age if they have any concerns about their fertility and determine whether there is any interest in the new reproductive technologies and genetic testing options.
History of sexually transmitted diseases	"Do you or a sexual partner have a history of sexually transmitted infections? Many people today have questions about sexually transmitted infections that they are reluctant to express. Do you have any questions? Have you noticed any signs that might indicate a problem?"
History of sexual dysfunction	"Have you ever experienced a problem such as erectile dysfunction, failure to achieve orgasm, or pain during intercourse?"
Sexual self-care behaviors	"Do you perform the breast self-exam (testicular self-exam) on a monthly basis? When was your last gynecologic (urologic) examination (Pap smear, mammogram)? Is there a family history of breast disease, ovarian cancer, testicular cancer, colon cancer? With all the attention on safer sex today and responsible parenting, many people have questions about their sexual self-care behaviors. Do you have any such concerns?" (It is important for nurses to ascertain whether patients possess the knowledge, attitudes, and skills necessary to promote their own sexual health and that of others.)
Sexual self-concept	
Sexual identity	"How do you feel about yourself as a man or woman? Is anything changing the way you feel about yourself?"
Sexual body image	"Many people have concerns about their sexual body image. Are you comfortable with your physical maleness or femaleness? Have you experienced any physical changes (eg, baldness, weight loss or gain, impotence, menopause, mastectomy, hysterectomy, sterilization) that are troubling to you?"
Sexual self-esteem	"We all have certain expectations of ourselves. Are you comfortable with the way you are currently expressing yourself sexually and meeting your sexual needs?"
Sexual role performance	"Has anything interfered with your ability to be a spouse, sexual partner, parent (any other valued sex-related roles)?"
Sexual functioning	"It's not unusual for people with health concerns (name specific medical problem, if appropriate) to have questions related to sexuality and sexual functioning. Do you have any questions or concerns that I can help you with? Has anything [if appropriate, substitute the name of a specific disease, surgery, or medication] changed your ability to function sexually?" (Asking patients if they have questions about resuming their usual sexual activity is an appropriate part of discharge planning for many patients.)

to have more sophisticated preparation and skills. The professional nurse usually performs a sexual history on level 1.

The nurse sets the tone or atmosphere for the interview. The nurse's attitudes will greatly affect the patient's response to the sexual history, and patients will be more cooperative if they sense the nurse's security and ease during the interview. Privacy is essential for the sexual history; doors should be closed and no interruptions allowed. The nurse sits close to the patient and speaks in a quiet, relaxed, objective tone of voice. Eye contact and open body posture are used. The nurse explains to the patient that no one will have access to this information unless it is significant to the patient's care.

Reproductive health information should be obtained first, followed by the sexual health history. The best approach is to begin with general open-ended questions and progress to more specific ones. The nurse should use the language used by the patient because the patient might be reluctant to admit that he or she does not understand certain terms for fear of appearing ignorant or foolish. For example, the patient might use the term "come" to mean climax or orgasm.

It is useful to begin questions with "many people like" or "many people feel." This gives patients security in knowing they are not alone in how they feel and will encourage them to talk about their problems or concerns. For example: "Many people feel that it's helpful to discuss their concerns about sex with their partner. What do you think about this?"

One helpful structure for obtaining information about sexual problems follows:

- Description of the problem: "How would you describe the problem?"
- Onset and cause of the problem: "What do you think caused the problem, or what was happening when you first noticed it?"
- Past attempts at resolution: "What have you tried in the past to correct the problem?"
- Goals of the patient: "What do you wish to accomplish?"

A narrative form of recording a sexual history is generally used because it allows the interviewer to document the data in many of the patient's own words. If a patient is seeking help for a sexual problem, a more specific format will be used in recording information obtained by a skilled therapist.

A few of the major dysfunctions and assessment priorities are briefly discussed in Table 35-3. See also Focus on the Older Adult.

Physical Assessment

Physical examination of the reproductive or genitourinary system for either male or female patients is necessary under the following circumstances:

- As part of a routine physical examination
- Annual women's healthcare examination, including a Pap smear
- Suspected STI
- Suspected pregnancy
- Workup for infertility

- Unusual lump, discharge, or appearance of the genital organs noticed by the patient
- Request for birth control
- Change in urinary function

The examiner may routinely perform a complete physical examination along with assessment of the reproductive system if the patient has not had contact with the healthcare system within 1 year or if the assessment findings from a complete examination would be useful in diagnosing an ailment or complaint. See Chapter 25 for a detailed description of how to examine the female and male genitalia.

The nurse should initially ask whether the patient has had this type of examination in the past (if this information is not evident by the patient's records). Depending on the patient's knowledge base, the nurse should explain the progressive steps of the examination and what the patient may feel during the examination. This will give the patient some feeling of control and security during the examination. The nurse's responsibilities during an examination of the reproductive system are as follows:

- Provide information about the examination
- Teach the patient
- Provide support to the patient during the examination
- To assist the examiner, if appropriate, with any procedures or laboratory studies

Keeping the patient comfortable and respecting his or her privacy and modesty should be primary nursing considerations. Some female patients might be uncomfortable with male examiners and vice versa for religious, cultural, or other reasons. Sensitivity to these concerns allows the examiner to adapt to these concerns (eg, to ensure that a female nurse is in the room when a female patient is undergoing a pelvic examination by a male physician).

Diagnosing

Nursing diagnoses written to address problems of sexuality belong to one of two categories:

- *Ineffective Sexuality Patterns:* The state in which an individual experiences or is at risk for a change in sexual health. Sexual health is the integration of somatic, emotional, intellectual, and social aspects of sexual being in ways that are enriching and that enhance personality, communication, and love.
- *Sexual Dysfunction:* The state in which an individual experiences or is at risk for change in sexual function that is viewed as unrewarding or inadequate

A related diagnosis is Rape-Trauma Syndrome.

Ineffective Sexuality Patterns or Sexual Dysfunction as the Problem

Before a nursing diagnosis can be made regarding a sexual problem, the nurse must carefully review the assessment data to determine whether the situation can be corrected by independent nursing interventions. Although many problems of

TABLE 35-3 Sexual Dysfunction and Nursing Assessment

Sexual Dysfunction	Assessment Priorities
Male	
Erectile failure (impotence)	• History of diabetes, spinal cord trauma, cardiovascular disease, surgical procedure, alcoholism • Use of certain medications such as antihypertensives, antidepressants, or illicit drugs • Determine degree of mental depression that may be present • Obtain specific information regarding the degree of impotence, length of time of disorder, continuing life factors
Premature ejaculation	• Assess what patient defines as his dysfunction and ability to control ejaculation • Assess any causative relationship factors, such as anxiety, guilt, lack of time, new partner, and so on
Retarded ejaculation	• History of neurologic disorders, Parkinson's disease, or use of certain medications • Same assessment priorities as for premature ejaculation
Female	
Inhibited sexual desire	• Use of oral contraceptives or other hormonal therapy, use of alcohol or certain medications • History of sexual abuse, rape or incest, depression, or other sexual dysfunctions • Assess any other contributing or relationship factors.
Orgasmic dysfunction	• Assess knowledge level regarding sexual response cycle and anatomy • Assess communication pattern between patient and her partner • Assess usual sexual pattern and behavior between patient and her partner • Assess any other contributing factors
Dyspareunia	• History of diabetes, hormonal imbalance, vaginal infection, endometriosis, urethritis, cervicitis, or rectal lesions • Use of antihistamines, alcohol, tranquilizers, or illicit drugs • Assess patient's ability for vaginal lubrication during sexual act • Assess patient's use of coital positions • Assess use of cosmetic or chemical irritants to genitals, such as deodorant tampons, contraceptive creams, or jellies or condoms • Physical assessment of internal and external genitalia • Assess any other contributing factors
Vaginismus	• Assess knowledge regarding anatomy and sexual response • Assess pattern of sexual activity: how often, level of arousal, orgasm • Assess presence of other sexual dysfunctions • History of sexual abuse, trauma, or rape • Assess patient's feelings regarding her partner • Assess any other causative factors, such as fear of pregnancy, anxiety, guilt • Physical assessment of internal and external genitalia

sexuality experienced by a patient in a healthcare situation are amenable to nursing action, some require the expertise of other specialties.

> An impotent diabetic patient, such as Jefferson Smith described at the beginning of the chapter, who would benefit from a penile implant needs medical consultation. A patient with a serious sexual dysfunction or one who practices destructive sexual expression needs intensive therapy by a clinical psychologist, sex therapist, or counselor. Appropriate referrals by the nurse should follow the identification of such problems.

Sexual dysfunction may be specified as erectile failure (impotence), premature ejaculation, retarded ejaculation, inhibited sexual desire, orgasmic dysfunction, vaginismus, or dyspareunia. Common etiologies for sexual dysfunction include effects of medication (specify), effects of alcohol consumption, effects of disease process (specify), history of abuse (specify rape, incest), feelings of depression, guilt, anxiety, fear of rejection, miscommunication with partner, fear of pain, effects of birth control method (specify), lack of knowledge, or effects of surgical procedure (specify).

The nursing diagnosis Ineffective Sexuality Patterns can be further specified by loss of desire (to abstinence), increased desire (to promiscuity), or change in sexual expression. Common etiologies for Ineffective Sexuality Patterns include stress (lifestyle, job, family, finances, marital conflict), isolation from partner, effects of pregnancy (specify), feelings of depression, loss of privacy, loss of communication with partner, relationship change (new partner), effects of disease process (sexual position, frequency, mode of expression), change in body image, change in self-concept, or loss of partner. Some nursing diagnoses concerning sexuality are given in Examples of NANDA Nursing Diagnoses: Sexuality.

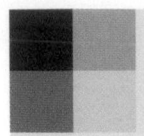

Focus on the Older Adult
Nursing Strategies to Address Age-Related Changes in Sexuality and Sexual Function

Factors that contribute to sexual dysfunction in the older adult are essentially the same as those that affect performance at any age: disease or mutilating surgery of the genitourinary tract, diverse systemic diseases, and emotional disturbances coupled with societal attitudes.

Age-Related Changes	Nursing Strategies
Use of multiple medications	• Educate elderly patients, intimate partners, and family about the sexual side effects of specific medications. Sometimes a change in medication dosage or modification in the treatment regimen can reduce sexual dysfunction.
Dependence on alcohol or marijuana to cope with discomforts of aging, resulting in weakened erection, reduced desire, delayed ejaculation	• Before the patient can decide to stop using alcohol or drugs, he or she must realize the need to change his or her behavior. The nurse can assist in attitude and value clarification about substance use, sexuality, and sexual behavior. Refer the elderly patient to a counselor who can assist with sexual performance problems as well as emotional and dependence problems.
Age-related metabolic disorders such as anemia, diabetes, malnutrition, and fatigue may affect the quality of life and cause impotence.	• Symptoms may be initially discussed with the nurse. The patient may be hesitant to discuss sexual problems openly. Listen carefully. Acknowledge that sexual problems in the elderly are not unusual. Even if the nurse does not know all the answers, active listening on the nurse's part may encourage the patient to visit his or her healthcare provider or a counselor. Encourage elderly patients to have a thorough physical evaluation by a healthcare provider.
Obesity may damage cardiac and vascular integrity and reduce self-esteem, resulting in decreased sexual performance and interest.	• Encourage the patient to seek the advice of his or her healthcare provider and to explore weight reduction and health promotion programs.
Many elderly persons are concerned that sexual activity might increase the risk for illness or even death due to stress on the heart or blood pressure.	• Teach the patient that sexual intercourse and similar forms of sexual expression are not considered dangerous for anyone able to walk around a room and may actually offer physiological benefits.
Radical surgery or dysfunction of the genitourinary tract affects sexual capacity and libido. Extensive surgery due to malignancy may make intercourse difficult or impossible.	• Patients need support and guidance in adjusting to these changes. Provide specific suggestions for how to accommodate to the surgical changes while still maintaining a sexually satisfying relationship. The nurse should acknowledge the need for sexual expression in some form or other and should provide an open, nonjudgmental response when patients display a need for warmth, close contact, and companionship. Touch is particularly important. An atmosphere of trust between the nurse and the elderly patient is essential.
Loss of a spouse	• Explore alternative forms of sexual expression with patients who are widows and widowers. Encourage them to attend a support group and become active socially. The nurse should acknowledge that human sexuality crosses a wide spectrum, and the pattern for each individual is an outcome of his or her development, experiences, and sense of personal identity. The basic pattern is not altered by age or loss of a spouse or loved one. It continues to influence one's capacity for involvement in all life activities.

Murray, R., & Zentner, J. (2000). *Health promotion strategies through the life span.* New Jersey: Prentice Hall.

Ineffective Sexuality Patterns or Sexual Dysfunction as the Etiology

Changes in sexuality can affect other areas of human functioning. In the following nursing diagnoses, problems of sexuality are the etiology of another problem:

• Impaired Adjustment related to loss of sexual partner, loss of sexual body part

• Anxiety related to fear of pregnancy, loss of sexual functioning or desire, effects of disease process on sexual functioning
• Pain related to sexual position, penile penetration, effects of genital surgery, lack of vaginal lubrication
• Ineffective Coping related to effects of body image on sexual expression, change in sexual partner

Examples of NANDA Nursing Diagnoses | Sexuality

Nursing Diagnoses	Related Factors	Sample Defining Characteristics
Sexual Dysfunction: Erectile Failure	Use of antihypertensive medication	• 45-year-old man with 3-year history of hypertension • Maintained normotensive on reserpine, 0.25 mg daily • "I have had trouble keeping an erection. My wife and I haven't made love in months. We don't talk about it anymore. I guess that part of my life is over." • Patient appears resigned and saddened.
Sexual Dysfunction: Dyspareunia	Effects of menopausal process	• 54-year-old woman whose last menses was 1 year ago • "Whenever my husband and I make love, my vagina burns and stings." • States decrease in vaginal lubrication during past several months
Altered Sexuality Patterns: Change in Sexual Expression	Loss of privacy due to hospitalization	• 23-year-old man hospitalized for past 6 weeks with injuries resulting from car crash; has been in traction for fractured right femur • "I can't take this place anymore! Everyone barges in here whenever they want to—nobody cares about my feelings—a guy can't even act like a guy around here. I wish I could be alone with my wife for a while with no interruptions."
Altered Sexuality Patterns: Loss of Desire	Change in body image due to body-altering surgery	• Surgery for bowel cancer with construction of permanent colostomy 1 month ago • "I know the colostomy was necessary to save my life, but it is so disgusting. I'll never be able to have a relationship with my husband again. It's a real turn-off to me—just imagine what he'll think—how can I expect him to want to make love to a freak?"
Alteration in Comfort: Pain	Abduction of hips in sexual positioning	• 60-year-old woman with history of osteoarthritis for 6 years • "The act of intercourse hurts my hips so bad that I'm in pain the whole next day. I don't want to stop having intercourse with my husband, but I'm going to have to if this pain gets worse." • Patient states that the missionary position is the only position used during sex with her husband throughout their 40-year-marriage.

• Fear related to pain during sexual intercourse, history of sexual abuse
• Anticipatory Grieving related to loss of sexual functioning, effects of surgical excision of genital body part
• Delayed Growth and Development related to sexual exploitation or abuse, sexual guilt, effects of hormonal imbalance, lack of information about sexuality
• Deficient Knowledge (specify: contraceptive methods, spread of STIs, sexual response, genital anatomy, modes of sexual expression, self-examination, effects of disease or medications) related to misinformation, sexual myths, lack of interest in learning, cognitive limitation
• Disturbed Body Image (specify: surgical excision of genital body part, loss of or gain in body weight) related to fear of rejection

• Impaired Social Interaction related to effects of marital separation or divorce
• Social Isolation related to fear of contracting STI, fear of sexual encounter

Outcome Identification and Planning

Nurses should value sexuality as an important aspect of who the patient is and how the patient is identified as a unique human. Specific patient outcomes to promote sexual health follow: The patient will:
• Define individual sexuality
• Establish open patterns of communication with significant others

- Develop self-awareness and body awareness
- Describe responsible sexual health self-care practices, identifying appropriate resources
- Practice responsible sexual expression (eg, by 5/1/06, the patient will use rubber condoms during all sexual encounters)

Specific patient outcomes will depend on the nature of the patient's problem or concern. Expected outcomes should be patient-oriented—that is, something the patient desires to do or has the ability to accomplish. For example, it is not enough to advise a method of birth control; rather, the nurse needs to know which method the patient is motivated and able to use.

Implementing

Establishing a Trusting Nurse–Patient Relationship

It is impossible to address a patient's sexuality if trust has not been developed between the nurse and the patient (see Through the Eyes of a Student). The nurse needs to project an objective,

Through the Eyes of a Student

I knew it was going to happen sooner or later. Male nurses are not unheard of in this day and age, but some people just aren't yet ready for us—especially Ethel, a 68-year-old black woman with a deep religious conviction. I concluded this because she called on Jesus for help when I told her that I was her student nurse for the day, and that I would be giving her a bath.

"You're my nurse?" she said. "Help me, Jesus. . . . No, no, you just go on and help somebody else, honey. I've already had my bath," she insisted.

Accordingly, I told her she was mistaken and that I understood her anxiety. Then I proceeded to exaggerate the truth by saying that I had done this before, when really I had given baths before, but not to members of the opposite sex. She thought *she* was having anxiety!

Next I asked my instructor, Lynn, for help. She quickly assessed the situation and tried to comfort Ethel by vouching for my professional character and abilities, but still no go. Then I tried appealing to her logic.

"This is a hospital where male doctors examine you all the time. Why is this any different?" I asked. "Because you are not a doctor" was her logical reply.

I felt inadequate. I could not give this woman the care she needed because of my gender. Luckily, in the next bed, Michele was about to give her patient a bath. She offered to give Ethel her bath if I would help her with her patients.

Consequently, Ethel got her bath, and I learned that a nurse has to be flexible as well as willing to ask for and accept help when the patient's quality of care is at stake. This is something I hope to remember throughout my nursing career.

—*Daniel E. Zirolli,*
Delaware County Community College,
Media, Pennsylvania

nonthreatening, and nonjudgmental attitude and needs to stress that the information the patient gives will be kept confidential. The nurse who is aware of his or her behavior and verbal and nonverbal cues and anticipates the patient's concerns will help the patient trust the nurse with information of an intimate nature. It is important to establish respect for the patient and empathy before discussing sexual issues. The nurse should consider all of the patient's circumstances and life experiences and should view them using a therapeutic, not a pitying, approach. Only when the nurse is accepted as a trusted, caring person will the patient reveal details of his or her private life, including sexual concerns.

Review the Reflective Practice display for this chapter. Note how the nursing student initially avoided interpersonal contact with the patient, performing the technical aspects of care but ignoring the patient as a person. Communication and trust did not occur until the patient asked the nursing student about the level of discomfort and the nursing student responded truthfully.

Teaching About Sexuality and Sexual Health

Most nursing interventions pertaining to a patient's sexuality involve teaching to promote sexual health. Major goals of patient teaching are a change in knowledge, a change in patient attitude, or a change in behavior. In some situations, patients need assistance in defining or redefining their sexuality and its importance to their lives. Offering information, dispelling fears, and providing positive reinforcement are some ways nurses can assist patients to increase their knowledge about their bodies and sexual functioning. Patients might need assistance in modifying behaviors or learning new skills to increase the quality of sexual health and functioning.

Correcting Sexual Myths and Promoting Body Awareness

Many people believe things about sex that they have heard from family or friends or as part of their culture that are not true or are not based on scientific data. The nurse may refute sexual myths and teach factual information during the assessment or while providing care (Table 35-4).

Patients might need assistance in becoming familiar with what they believe and feel about their sexual selves. The nurse can be helpful in a situation in which a patient has difficulty accepting or developing his or her sexuality by promoting self-confidence and a good self-concept in the patient. When patients feel comfortable about themselves and their sensual feelings, they can begin to focus on how they feel about their sexual functioning and specific sexual expressions.

Getting to know one's physical body is important to healthy sexual development. Every man and woman, sexually active or not, needs to be aware of the appearance of his or her genitalia. Some people, because of their background, feel ashamed and repulsed by their bodies; others feel that touching the body

TABLE 35-4 **Sexual Myths and Facts to Refute Them**

Sexual Dysfunction	Assessment Priorities
Each person is born with a certain amount of sexual drive, which if overdrawn in youth leaves little reserve for later years.	Actually, the correlation between sexual activity and length of time it persists throughout life is just the opposite. The more consistently sexually active a person is, the longer the activity continues into the later years of life.
The need for expressing one's sexuality becomes less important in the latter half of one's life.	Physiologically, sexual desire and ability do not decrease markedly after middle age. The expression of one's sexuality, as an integral part of development, follows the overall pattern of health and physical performance.
Sexual abstinence is necessary in training for sports.	Physiologically, the achievement of orgasm is rarely more demanding than most activities encountered in daily life. The desire for sleep that often follows is most commonly due to factors other than physical exhaustion from sexual activities. There is no scientific evidence that sex "weakens" a person.
Excessive sexual activity can lead to mental illness.	The biologic significance of human sexuality has no greater effect on total development than any other necessary biologic function. There is no scientific basis for believing that one will develop a mental or physical illness with excessive or no sexual activity.
Wet dreams are indicators of sexual disorders.	Erotic dreams that culminate in orgasms are normal common physiologic phenomena in at least 85% of men. They can occur at any age after puberty. Some women also report in clinical studies that their sexual dreams culminate in orgasm. In women, this phenomenon is believed to increase with advancing age.
Because of the anatomic nature of the sex organs, women are passive and men are aggressive.	Physiologic studies disprove this myth by showing the woman to be far from passive. Maximum gratification requires each partner to be both passive and aggressive in participating mutually and cooperatively.
It is unnatural for a woman to have as strong a desire for sex as a man—women should not enjoy sex as much as men.	These myths have been reinforced by a society that has traditionally taught women that they are to suppress sexual desires to gain love, security, and society's respect, based on the assumption that it is the basic nature of women to be submissive, dependent, and subordinate. Physiologic studies indicate that, in some respects, the woman's sex drive is not only as strong but may be even stronger than that of the man.
Women who have multiple orgasms or who readily come to climax are nymphomaniacs or promiscuous.	Physiologic studies at this time suggest that we do not know women's sexual potential; these studies indicate that there is a wide range of intensity and duration of orgasmic experience, and the potential for multiple or frequent orgasms within a brief period is not at all uncommon. Therefore, women normally may have greater orgasmic capacity than men with regard to duration and frequency of orgasm.
There is a difference between vaginal orgasm and clitoral orgasm.	Physiologic misunderstanding has produced the myth of separate clitoral and vaginal orgasms rather than their interrelations. Female orgasm is normally initiated by clitoral stimulation, but because it is a total-body response, there are marked variations in intensity and timing. There is no reason to believe that the female response to the sex act is due to a vaginal rather than a clitoral orgasm.
A mature sexual relationship requires the man and woman to achieve simultaneous orgasm.	Although simultaneous orgasm may be desirable, it is unrealistic. Often, it is possible only under the most ideal circumstances and is not a determinant of sexual achievement or of satisfaction (except to someone who accepts this as dogma).
It is dangerous to have intercourse during menstruation.	Because the source of the menstrual flow is from the uterus rather than the vagina, there is no basis for concern about tissue damage to the vagina. Actually, the desire for sex increases during the menses as a result of increased pelvic vasocongestion. There is no physiologic basis for abstinence during the menses.
The larger penis has greater possibilities for producing orgasm in the woman.	Physiologically, there is practically no relation between the size of a man's penis and his ability to satisfy a woman sexually. Furthermore, there is little correlation between penile size and body size and their relation to sexual potency.
The face-to-face coital position is the proper, moral, and healthy one.	Recent knowledge of human sexual practices dispels this myth with the recognition that there is no normal or single most acceptable sexual position. Whatever position offers the most pleasure and is acceptable to both partners is correct for them. Any variation is normal, healthy, and proper if it satisfies both partners.
The ability to achieve orgasm is an indicator of a person's sexual responsiveness.	Achievement of a satisfactory sexual response is the result of numerous physical, psychological, and cultural influences. Too often, the physical fact of orgasm (or lack of orgasm) is taken to be symbolic of sexual responsiveness and seen out of context of the entire relationship between man and woman.

is dirty and might feel guilt and anxiety in stimulating themselves. Patients need assistance in improving body awareness if any of these issues are present. Patients can become accustomed to looking at their bodies by looking at nonthreatening anatomy first and then proceeding to the genitals. This can be done in the shower or with the use of a mirror. Knowing what looks normal can be of great importance so that patients can report the development of an unusual appearance later on.

After patients have developed some degree of comfort in looking at their bodies, they can progress to experiencing touch. Again, patients should progress from nonthreatening parts of the body until the genitals can be touched without stress.

A good exercise for women in developing body awareness is the use of Kegel exercises. These exercises promote good vaginal tone by localizing and strengthening the pubococcygeal muscle. A woman can locate this muscle by stopping a stream of urine midway through urination. Contracting this muscle can be repeated at any time of the day in any circumstance because its performance is undetectable. Women who practice Kegel exercises have found that their sexual satisfaction is greatly improved.

Teaching Self-Examination

It is important for both men and women to learn to examine themselves through inspection and palpation of sexual body parts. Many conditions, some life-threatening, can be detected by self-examination. Early detection of cancer is crucial to its control and cure. Some STIs might also be detected by self-examination.

Breast Self-Examination

According to http://www.breastcancer.org, a nonprofit organization for breast cancer education, a woman in the United States is diagnosed with breast cancer every 3 minutes. Breast cancer is the leading cancer among white and African American women. African American women are more likely to die from this disease. The incidence of breast cancer in women has increased from one in 20 in 1960 to one in eight today.

Breast self-examination (BSE) should be performed monthly; such a routine helps the person become familiar with what is normal. BSE should be performed after each menstrual period, or once a month for a postmenopausal woman. Any contact with a female patient in the healthcare delivery system should include assessment of her knowledge and practice of BSE.

The steps in performing BSE are shown in Figure 35-3 and are as follows:

1. Stand before a mirror with hands on hips to inspect the breasts. Look for indentations, dimpling, or odd position of a nipple. Any discharge from a nipple is abnormal unless the woman is nursing. Report changes in the size or shape of breasts.
2. Lie on the bed with a small pillow under the shoulder on the side of the breast to be examined and the arm over the head. Using the opposite hand, start palpating the outer edge of the breast. Use small circular motions of the flat portions of the fingers. Work inward in a clockwise manner toward the nipple. Gently squeeze the nipple to detect discharge. Repeat this procedure for the

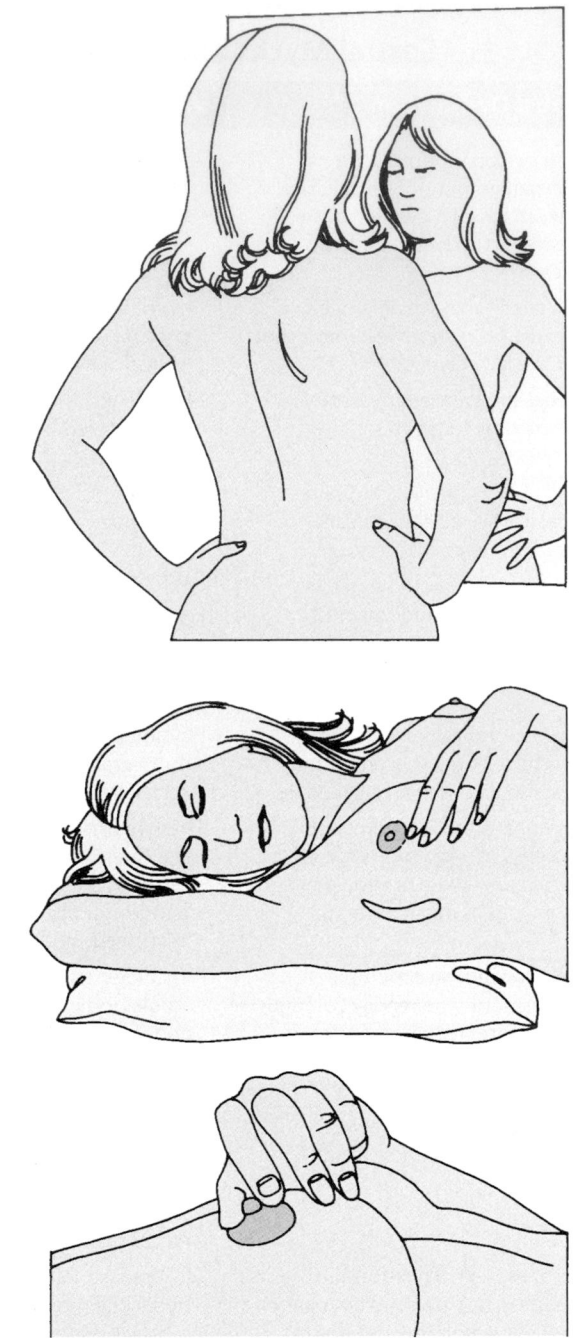

FIGURE 35-3 Breast self-examination is to be performed once a month. It is begun with inspection using a mirror. Attention is given to contours of the breast and to the skin. Pressing down on the hips serves to tense pectoralis major muscles to inspect for any retraction of the skin. Palpatory examination is performed in a supine position with the side to be examined elevated on a pillow or blanket. Self-examination is completed with a squeeze of the nipple to detect abnormal discharge.

opposite breast. Report any unusual lump or tenderness to a healthcare professional.

Testicular Self-Examination

Male patients need to be taught to perform monthly assessment of the testicles. Although testicular cancer is not widespread, it can be easily detected, and the prognosis is good if it is found early. A good time to examine the testes is during a shower, when the scrotum becomes warm and loose. Men should also be taught the importance of examining their breasts.

The steps in testicular self-examination (TSE), shown in Figure 35-4, are as follows:

1. Use the thumb and fingers of each hand to palpate each testicle simultaneously. Systematically palpate the testes, feeling for lumps or differences in texture. The testes should feel smooth.
2. Palpate the epididymis above each testicle. The epididymis feels soft and not as smooth as a testicle.

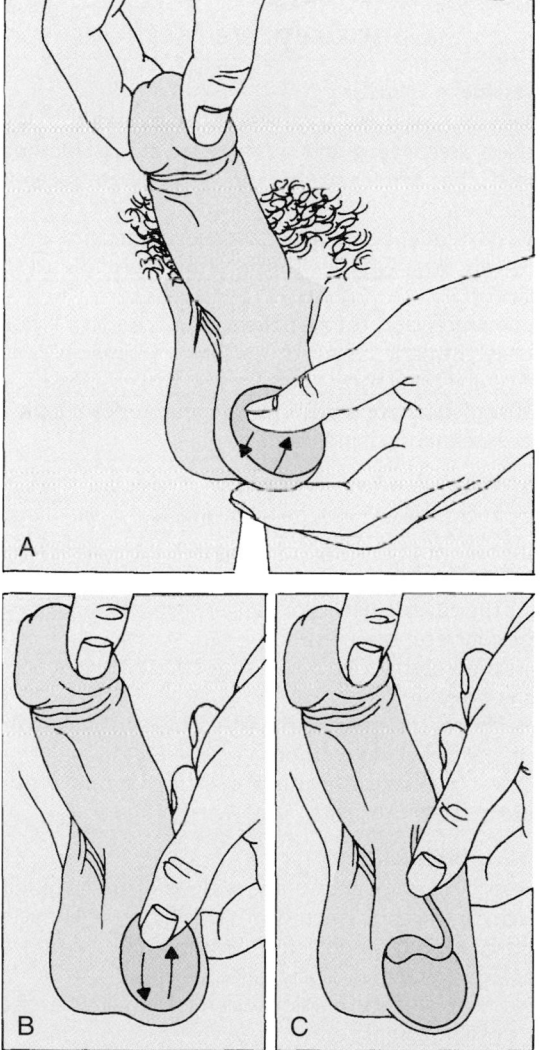

FIGURE 35-4 Testicular self-examination is to be performed once a month. A convenient time is after a warm bath or shower when the scrotum is relaxed. Both hands are used to palpate the testis; the normal testicle is smooth and uniform is consistency. (**A**) With the index and middle finger under the testis and the thumb on top, roll the testis gently in a horizontal plane between the thumb and fingers, feeling for any evidence of a small lump or abnormality. (**B**) Follow the same procedure for palpation in the vertical plane. (**C**) Locate the epididymis (cordlike structure on the top and back of the testicle that stores and transports sperm). Repeat the examination for the other testis; it is normal to find one testis larger than the other. Any evidence of a small, pea-sized lump should be checked by a physician. It may be due to an infection or a tumor growth.

3. The spermatic cord, or vas deferens, extends upward from the scrotum toward the base of the penis. Palpate it for firmness and smoothness in texture.

Promoting Responsible Sexual Expression

Patients need to know how to gain satisfactory sexual experiences while behaving responsibly in their activities. Responsible sexuality encompasses these major areas: the form of sexual expression, the prevention of unwanted pregnancy, the prevention of spread of STIs, and sex education.

Form of Sexual Expression

The form of sexual expression used by patients should not inflict unwanted harm on themselves or others. When sexual expression encroaches on the rights of others, it is neither healthy nor desirable. Sexual acts that violate another's rights are usually considered to be acts of aggression or hostility rather than stemming from sexual need or desire. Rape, in particular, is motivated by the need to dominate and humiliate the victim.

Prevention of Unwanted Pregnancy

Contraception is a process or technique for preventing pregnancy by means of a medication, device, or method that blocks or alters one or more of the processes of reproduction in such a way that sexual union can occur without impregnation. The prevention of unwanted pregnancy must be a conscious decision. Anyone considering the possibility of a sexual encounter who is unprepared for pregnancy should refrain from intercourse or obtain a contraceptive method from a healthcare provider or from the pharmacy; it is too late to think about contraception during sexual intercourse. To practice responsible sexuality, the contraceptive method must be used consistently and according to instructions.

Prevention of STIs

The various STIs are widespread. The only sure way to avoid an STI is to remain a virgin until marriage, to marry a person who is a virgin, and thereafter never to have sex with anyone else. When this is impractical, other practices that can decrease a patient's risk for STIs are the following:

- Limit the number of sexual partners. The risk for an STI rises with the addition of each new partner.
- If a partner has symptoms of an STI, the patient should abstain from any sexual activity.
- If exposure to an STI was possible, the patient should visit a healthcare facility for examination.
- If the patient contracts an STI, he or she should notify all partners and advise them to seek treatment.
- Use condoms for protection against STIs as well as against pregnancy. The patient should keep condoms handy if he or she is in a non-monogamous relationship.

Sex Education

Sex education is critical to healthy sexual development and safe sexual behaviors. See Examples of Nursing Intervention Classifications: Safe Sex Activities. Information received from peers and friends is almost always inadequate and erro-

Examples of Nursing Interventions Classification (NIC)
Safe Sex Activities

- Discuss patient's attitudes about various birth control methods.
- Instruct patient on the use of effective birth control methods, as appropriate.
- Incorporate religious beliefs into discussion of birth control, as appropriate.
- Discuss abstinence as a means of birth control, as appropriate.
- Encourage patient to be selective when choosing sexual partners, as appropriate.
- Stress the importance of knowing the partner's sexual history, as appropriate.
- Instruct patient on low-risk sexual practices, such as those that avoid bodily penetration or the exchange of bodily fluids, as appropriate.
- Instruct patient on the importance of good hygiene, lubrication, and voiding after intercourse, to decrease susceptibility to infections.
- Plan sex education classes for groups of patients as appropriate.

(From McCloskey, J., & Bulechek, G. [2000]. *Nursing interventions classification [NIC]* [3rd ed]. [p. 654]. St. Louis: C. V. Mosby. A full listing of nursing activities for each nursing intervention can be found in this book.)

neous. Parents should be taught to answer children's questions immediately and accurately.

Considering Contraception

Unintended pregnancy remains a significant women's health issue in the United States as well as a critical social issue. In the United States, 50% of all pregnancies are unplanned; in more than half of them (53%), the couple was using some method of contraception. [This and the statistics that follow about contraceptive methods were obtained from Birth Control: Planned Parenthood Federation of America, Inc., http://www.plannedparenthood.com.] Many unintended pregnancies result from the use of less effective methods of contraception, such as condom, spermicide, or barrier methods. The past several years have seen the development of new, easier to use, and more effective methods of contraception. Nurses and nurse practitioners have a responsibility to provide information to women regarding their many contraceptive options.

Patients choose contraception for many reasons and might contact healthcare providers specifically to obtain information about birth control. Some people use contraception for the orderly spacing of pregnancies in a family; others may want to prevent pregnancy from occurring until a family is desired. Some people choose a permanent method to prevent pregnancy from ever occurring. Factors that affect a person's choice of a contraceptive method include age, marital status, desire for future pregnancy, religious beliefs, level of education, cost, and ease of use. Other considerations are the woman's knowledge about available methods, her perceptions of the various

methods, and in many cases her previous experience with contraception.

All contraceptive methods have advantages and disadvantages. The nurse must understand and explain thoroughly the available methods so that the patient can choose the one that will best meet his or her situation and needs (Box 35-1).

When choosing a contraceptive method, the patient should consider the following:
- How well will it fit into my lifestyle?
- How convenient will it be?

BOX 35-1 Knowledge Deficit: Contraceptive Methods

Assessment Priorities
- Determine past use of contraceptive methods.
- Assess effectiveness and satisfaction with past methods.
- Assess the patient's current knowledge of contraceptive methods.
- Assess frequency of the patient's sexual activity.
- Identify any methods that are unacceptable to the patient.
- Assess motivation of the patient to use certain methods.
- Assess the patient's level of comfort with manipulation of genital body parts.
- Obtain complete patient history and perform a physical examination if indicated.

Expected Outcomes
The patient will achieve the following:
- Choose a contraceptive method that the patient is motivated to use.
- List the adverse effects or danger signs associated with the contraceptive method.
- List the steps needed to use the contraceptive method effectively.
- Use the contraceptive with every act of sexual intercourse.
- Choose a back-up method.
- Report back to the healthcare setting for follow-up as directed.

Nursing Interventions
- Describe in terms at the patient's level of understanding each contraceptive method for which the patient needs information (give objective information in matter-of-fact manner to avoid bias by nurse).
- Describe the effectiveness of each method and side effects or possible complications.
- Instruct the patient in the use of a chosen method, giving step-by-step instructions.
- Advise the patient of the importance of having a back-up method on hand.
- Instruct the patient in the use of the back-up method.
- Have the patient obtain a physical examination if indicated by the chosen contraceptive method (eg, the pill).
- Instruct the patient to report back in a specified period for follow-up of use of method if indicated (follow-up visits to a healthcare facility are important, particularly if a patient elects to use the pill).

- How effective will it be?
- How safe will it be?
- How affordable will it be?
- How reversible will it be?
- Will it protect against STIs?

Methods of Contraception

Behavioral

Abstinence is considered a behavioral method of contraception. There are two types of abstinence: continuous and periodic. Choosing abstinence does not mean that a person is sexless. Most people are abstinent at some time in their lives. Abstinence can be a positive way of dealing with sexuality when it represents a well-thought-out decision regarding one's mind, body, spirit, and sexual health.

Continuous abstinence involves not having any sex with a partner at all. It is 100% effective in preventing pregnancy and STIs. However, individuals may find it difficult to abstain for long periods of time. Ending abstinence without being prepared to protect against an unplanned pregnancy or infection might cause additional problems.

Periodic abstinence and fertility awareness methods are two methods of contraception that involve charting a woman's fertility pattern. Periodic abstinence is a method used by some sexually active women to prevent pregnancy. They become familiar with their fertility patterns and abstain from vaginal intercourse on the days they think they could become pregnant. Women who monitor their fertility to prevent pregnancy either abstain from vaginal intercourse for at least one third of each menstrual cycle or use barrier methods during the fertile or "unsafe" period.

Three basic charting methods can be used to predict ovulation in order to plan or prevent pregnancy:

- *Temperature method:* The woman takes her temperature every morning before getting out of bed. Her temperature will rise between 0.4° and 0.8°F on the day of ovulation and will remain at that level until her next period.
- *Cervical mucus method:* The woman observes the changes in her cervical mucus throughout the first part of the menstrual cycle, until after ovulation. Cervical mucus is normally cloudy, but a few days before ovulation it becomes clear and slippery and can be stretched between the fingers. This indicates the most fertile phase of the cycle. The couple must abstain from vaginal intercourse or use a barrier method during this period to avoid pregnancy.
- *Calendar method:* The woman charts her menstrual cycle on a calendar. The couple must refrain from intercourse or use a barrier method during "unsafe" days.

The best approach to monitoring fertility is to use all three methods; the combination of these methods is called the symptothermal method. Of 100 couples who use any of these methods for one year, 20 women will become pregnant with typical use. The failure rate is higher in single women. Using the methods carefully and consistently and avoiding unprotected vaginal intercourse during the fertile phase can give better results.

Coitus interruptus (withdrawal), one of the oldest and most widely used contraceptive methods, is the withdrawal of the penis from the vagina before ejaculation. Pregnancy cannot occur if sperm is kept out of the vagina. Of every 100 women whose partners use withdrawal as a method of contraception, 27 will become pregnant during the first year of typical use. However, pre-ejaculate can contain enough sperm to cause a pregnancy. Pregnancy is also possible if pre-ejaculate or semen is spilled onto the vulva.

Barrier Methods

Barrier methods include the condom, diaphragm, cervical cap, and vaginal sponge used in combination with a spermicidal agent.

Diaphragm. The diaphragm has been used in various forms since ancient times. It is a dome-shaped device made of latex rubber that mechanically prevents semen from coming into contact with the cervix. It is also used to hold a spermicidal jelly in place against the cervix. The diaphragm is placed in the vagina before sexual activity. It fits between the pelvic notch at the front of the vagina to behind the cervix at the back. It should not be detected by either the woman or her partner when correctly situated in the vagina. A diaphragm must be individually fitted during a pelvic examination. The woman needs to be familiar with her body and able to handle her genitals for diaphragm placement and removal. The diaphragm must be worn during each episode of sexual activity and consistently used with a spermicidal agent. Twenty of 100 women who use the diaphragm will become pregnant during the first year of typical use; six will become pregnant with perfect use.

Condom. The traditional condom, or "rubber," is used by men, although it is appropriate for a woman to have a condom available for her partner's use. The condom is rolled over the erect penis and collects the semen after ejaculation occurs. If the condom does not have a nipple receptacle end, a small space should be left at the end of the condom to collect sperm (this prevents breakage). Condoms are available over the counter and have had a surge of popularity with the recent increase in the incidence of AIDS and other STIs.

A female condom is also available. The female condom is a ringed pouch that unrolls in the vagina. Advantages included the fact that the male does not need to have an erection for the pouch to be used, and it offers significant protection from STIs.

Of 100 women whose partners use condoms, about 14 will become pregnant during the first year of typical use; two will become pregnant with perfect use. The latex condom protects against STIs, including HIV. The latex condom offers better protection against STIs than any other birth control method because it blocks the exchange of body fluids that may be infected.

Cervical Cap. The cervical cap is a thimble-shaped rubber device that is placed over the cervix and may be left there for up to 3 days at a time. Its mechanism of action is similar to that of the diaphragm. Not all women can wear a cervical cap because of individual anatomic differences. There is some evidence to suggest that the cervical cap can cause cervical inflammation and increase the risk for pelvic infection.

Spermicides. Spermicides are used with barrier methods but can also be used alone. Spermicides come in creams, jellies, foams, and suppositories. Although readily available, spermicides are not as effective alone as when combined with another method, such as a diaphragm or a condom.

Vaginal Sponge. The vaginal sponge is a barrier method that contains a spermicide. The sponge acts not only as a barrier between the semen and the cervix but also as a reservoir to hold semen. The vaginal sponge carries some risk of toxic shock syndrome (TSS) and is contraindicated for use in women who have a past history of TSS. Women who use the vaginal sponge must follow package directions carefully and remove the sponge within 24 hours. The vaginal sponge is about as effective as the diaphragm.

Hormonal

Hormonal methods are based on the feedback mechanism of hormones of the menstrual cycle. Synthetic estrogens and progestin chemical compounds are used in the form of a pill, shot, or implant to prevent ovulation.

Oral Contraceptives. The oral contraceptive ("the pill") is the most common contraceptive method and the most popular method for women in their 20s. Most of the harmful side effects and dangers associated with taking the pill are related to the estrogen component. However, most pills currently available contain a small dose of estrogen. The pill has many beneficial noncontraceptive effects. It has been shown to protect women against the development of breast, ovarian, and endometrial cancer. Taken consistently and as prescribed, the pill is almost 100% effective in guarding against pregnancy. However, the cost might be prohibitive to some women. The woman must also be motivated to take a pill every day at the same time. A health history and physical examination by a healthcare provider are necessary to obtain a prescription for oral contraceptives. Some women should not take the pill if they have certain physiologic disorders or diseases. Smoking increases the risks associated with oral contraceptives. Women taking the pill should be reminded to take measures to protect themselves from STIs.

Norplant System. The Norplant System is a reversible, 5-year, low-dose progestin-only contraceptive. The system consists of six matchstick-size capsules (made of Silastic tubing) that are placed just under the skin of the woman's upper arm. The average annul pregnancy rate over 5 years is less than 1%. The most common side effect is a change in the menstrual bleeding pattern, including prolonged menstrual bleeding, spotting between menstrual periods, or no bleeding at all.

Implanon. In the Implanon system, a single etonogestrel-containing rod is implanted in the woman through the use of a disposable insertion kit. Removal requires a small incision and takes about 3 minutes. The single-rod system contains 68 mg of etonogestrel in an ethylene vinyl acetate (EVA) copolymer core surrounded by an EVA membrane. The rod releases 67 mcg of etonogestrel daily. This method of contraceptive approaches 100% efficacy. The most common reason for discontinuation is weight gain.

Depo-Provera. Depo-Provera is the brand name of a progestin-only hormonal birth control system. It uses a hormone similar to progesterone, one of the hormones made by a woman's ovaries that regulates the menstrual cycle. It is called depot medroxyprogesterone acetate (DMPA). An injection of DMPA in the buttock or arm can prevent pregnancy for 12 weeks and is 99.7% effective. Protection is immediate if the injection is given on the first day of the woman's period. Irregular bleeding is the most common side effect for women using DMPA. Of every thousand women who use Depo-Provera, only three will become pregnant during the first year of use.

Transdermal Contraceptive Patch. The transdermal contraceptive patch (Evra) supplies continuous daily circulating levels of ethinyl estradiol (20 mcg) and norelgestromin (150 mcg). The patch is applied weekly on the same day of each week for 3 weeks, followed by a patch-free week. It may be applied to any of four sites: lower abdomen, upper outer arm, buttock, or upper torso (excluding the breast). Women who use the contraceptive patch demonstrate more effective use compared with those using oral contraceptive pills. The patch has been found to have an overall annual probability of pregnancy (method failure plus user failure) of 0.8%. This contraceptive method has the same contraindications as oral contraceptives. The most common side effects include breast symptoms, headache, application site reactions, nausea, upper respiratory tract infection, and dysmenorrhea.

Vaginal Ring. The vaginal ring (NuvaRing) is a soft, flexible, transparent ring made of ethylene vinyl acetate copolymer. It releases approximately 120 mcg of etonogestrel and 15 mcg of ethyl estradiol daily. Each ring is inserted into the vagina and used for one cycle, which consists of 3 weeks of continuous use followed by a ring-free week. Women can insert and remove the ring themselves. It does not need to be fitted, nor does it require particular placement within the vagina. The ring works by inhibiting ovulation in much the same way oral contraceptives do. Used appropriately, the vaginal ring is 99.3% effective in protecting against pregnancy. Benefits of the vaginal ring include ease of use, self-insertion, high degree of effectiveness, and low incidence of negative or adverse effects. The most common side effects include headache, vaginal discharge, vaginitis, vaginal discomfort, foreign body sensation, coital problems, and ring expulsion.

Intrauterine Devices

The intrauterine device (IUD) is an object that is placed by a physician or nurse practitioner within the uterus to prevent implantation of a fertilized ovum. IUDs are small devices made of flexible plastic that provide reversible birth control. IUDs usually prevent fertilization of the egg, but the precise mechanism by which it works is unknown. IUDs seem to affect the way the sperm or egg moves. It may be that substances released by the IUD immobilize sperm. Another possibility is that the IUD prompts the egg to move through the fallopian tube too fast to be fertilized. IUDs that contain copper are more effective for two reasons. The copper affects the behavior of enzymes in the lining of the uterus to prevent implantation and also causes the production of increased amounts of prostaglandin. Only 8 of 1,000 women using copper IUDs will become pregnant with perfect use.

Combination hormonal and IUD contraceptive methods include a T-shaped device with a steroid reservoir around the vertical stem (Mirena). It releases 20 mcg of levonorgestrel daily and provides contraception for up to 5 years. Fertilization is prevented because the device causes changes in cervical mucus and endometrial morphology, inhibition of sperm migration, alteration of sperm–egg binding and ovarian function as well as a foreign body reaction by the uterus. Failure of implantation may occur in some women. Estradiol levels are managed within the usual range of women who are not using contraceptives. Normal function of the ovaries and fertility are restored as quickly after discontinuation as with any IUD. Efficacy approaches 100%. An additional benefit of this contraceptive method is that it controls menorrhagia in pre- and perimenopausal women. Adverse side effects peak at 3 months of us and reduce in frequency after that. The most common side effects include bleeding, depression, headache, acne, and weight changes.

Both types of IUDs have a filament string that serves two purposes. It allows for easier removal by a clinician, and it allows the woman or her clinician to check if the IUD is still in the correct position.

Emergency Contraception

Emergency contraception, often called the "morning after" pill, is designed to reduce the risk of pregnancy after unprotected intercourse. Emergency contraception is provided in two ways:

1. Increased doses of specific oral contraceptive pills. Emergency contraceptive pills can reduce the risk of pregnancy when taken up to 120 hours after unprotected intercourse (ideally within 72 hours).
2. Insertion of a copper IUD within 5 to 7 days after unprotected intercourse.

Sterilization

Sterilization methods should be regarded as permanent and irreversible in both men and women. Although sterilization can sometimes be surgically reversed, the results are not always satisfactory. Sexual desire and ability are unaffected by sterilization.

Sterilization in women is accomplished by surgically severing the fallopian tubes. This procedure, known as tubal ligation, prevents the ovum from traveling down the tube. Tubal ligation is usually performed on an outpatient basis, sometimes under local anesthesia. Postoperative care and recovery time are required after a tubal ligation.

Sterilization in men is accomplished by surgically severing the vas deferens, which prevents sperm from entering the semen. The vasectomy is usually performed in a physician's office under local anesthesia. The man and his partner must use an alternative form of contraception until he has produced two semen analyses with zero sperm. It usually takes about 4 to 6 weeks for all stored sperm to be eliminated from the man's ductal system.

Future Trends

Private industry remains a driving force behind contraceptive research and development. More than 100 experimental contra-ceptive methods are being studied around the world. The U.S. government contributes to contraceptive research primarily by funding research conducted at the National Institute of Health.

Almost 40 million women in the United States are at risk for unintended pregnancy. Given that unintended pregnancies are as likely to end in abortion as in birth, there is a clear need to focus on the prevention of unintended pregnancy. Future trends in contraception are likely to be shaped in part by increased awareness of STIs and continuation of the AIDS pandemic. For at-risk women, the emphasis will be on a highly effective primary means of contraception used in conjunction with a barrier method, such as the condom, to prevent STIs.

Female Contraceptives. Most of the contraceptive products that will soon be available for women are refinements of products already available. New barrier methods for women will include enhanced cervical caps and vaginal sponges with microbicides to protect against STIs. New contraceptive pills, patches, and rings for women will use varied combination of hormones. Injectable progestin products might one day protect against pregnancy for up to 90 days. Oral and/or injectable vaccines may one day immunize women against pregnancy. These vaccines might produce antibodies to attack egg or sperm, or the immune system might create antibodies to a crucial type of protein molecule found on the head of sperm. Contraceptive implants designed to remain effective for 2 or 3 years, as well as biodegradable implants with efficacy of up to 18 months, are under development. Computerized fertility monitors that predict ovulation will offer couples who use fertility awareness methods of contraception a much more sophisticated and accurate charting method. Methods for permanent sterilization will expand to include chemical scarring techniques and insertion of fallopian tube chemical plugs and cryosurgery. Temporary sterilization may be effected by the use of silicone plugs.

Unisex Reversible Contraceptives. The concept of unisex reversible contraception is being explored. This method involves a group of drugs called gonadotropin-releasing hormone (GnRH) agonists and can be used to prevent the release of follicle-stimulating hormone (FSH) and luteinizing hormone (LH) from the pituitary gland. The release of FSH and LH triggers ovulation and spermatogenesis. Blocking release of these hormones will temporarily suppress fertility for women or men. In addition, various contraceptive injections, implants, and vaccines for men are being researched.

Male Contraceptives. Methods of contraception for men continue to be explored. The challenge of developing a reversible method of contraception for men is complicated because men are always producing sperm. Because of this continuous fertility, the opportunities for reversible intervention that are permitted by women's fertility cycles are not available in men. Effective contraceptive methods for men that do not permanently impair fertility have proven elusive, but research continues. Most research has focused on a hormonal approach to decrease spermatogenesis. The major problem is that interference with steroidogenesis might also interfere with the other actions of testosterone, such as sexual function, bone and muscle growth, kidney function, and protein anabolism.

Facilitating Coping with Special Sexual Needs

The nurse can help patients cope with sexual concerns generated by diseases and their treatments. The nurse should offer anticipatory guidance and information to patients, stressing the importance of open communication with the patient's partner. The nurse should include the partner in teaching.

Discussion about possible sexual positions that can reduce pain during coitus is useful. The nurse can show the patient drawings of possible sexual positions. The patient will also find that intercourse may be more comfortable if pain medication is taken before beginning sexual activity.

When teaching patients about medications, the nurse should mention any sexual side effects that may occur to prevent anxiety and depression. Patients should alert the physician if these side effects occur because often the drug dosage can be modified or the drug changed. If patients are unaware of this, they may discontinue the medication on their own rather than sacrifice sexual functioning, if this is an important aspect of life for them.

Health Care Needs of Lesbian, Gay Male, Bisexual, and Transgender Individuals

The health of lesbian, gay male, bisexual and transgender (LGBT) individuals requires the nurse to address several issues important to this diverse group. Stigma, as well as a range of other social and cultural factors, affects the health of LGBT people as well as the ability of the healthcare system and providers to care for them. LGBT people come from diverse cultural backgrounds, have varied ethnic or racial identity, and differ in terms of education, age, income, and place of res-

idence. Lesbian, gay, and bisexual people are defined by their sexual orientation, and this definition is complex and variable. Sexual behavior, cultural factors, disclosure of sexual orientation and/or gender identity, prejudice and discrimination, as well as concealed sexual identity each present unique health challenges to this population (Box 35-2).

Other issues that affect healthcare delivery to the LGBT population include the following:

- Public health infrastructure: Efforts to research and address the healthcare needs of LGBT persons are hindered by an inadequate infrastructure to support and fund population-specific initiatives.
- Access to quality health services: Financial, structural, personal, and cultural barriers limit access to screening and prevention services and cause delays in receiving care for acute conditions in the LGBT population.
- Health communication: Negative provider attitudes, lack of provider education regarding unique aspects of lesbian and gay health, and exclusion of same-sex partners in care planning seriously hamper therapeutic communication between members of the LGBT population and those who provide care.
- Educational and community-based programs: Some government agencies, professional organizations, and healthcare organizations address health issues of the LGBT population, but this population still relies heavily on self-created community-based programs to address their special healthcare requirements.

Clearly, significant research is needed regarding the unique experience and healthcare needs of the LGBT population, along with increased education for healthcare providers. Issues of prejudice and inequitable service distribution in the healthcare

---

BOX 35-2 Issues and Related Health Consequences Affecting the Health of the Gay, Lesbian, Bisexual, and Transgender Population

Sexual Behavior
- Hepatitis A and B
- Enteritis
- Human papilloma virus
- Bacterial vaginosis
- Anal cancer
- Other STIs

Cultural Factors
- Body culture: eating disorders
- Socialization through bars: drug, alcohol, and tobacco use
- Nulliparity: breast cancer
- Parenting: insemination questions, mental health concerns
- Gender polarity in dominant culture: conflicts for transgender and intersex persons

Disclosure of Sexual Orientation or Gender Identity
- Psychological adjustment
- Depression

- Anxiety
- Suicide
- Conflicts with family of origin
- Lack of social support
- Physical/economic dislocation

Prejudice and Discrimination
- Provider bias and lack of sensitivity
- Harassment and discrimination in medical encounters, employment, housing, child custody
- Limited access to care or insurance coverage
- "Pathologizing" of gender variant behavior
- Violence against LGBT population

Concealed Sexual Identity
- Reluctance to seek preventive care
- Delayed medical treatment
- Incomplete medical history (eg, concealed risk, sexually related complications, social factors)

Dean, L., Meyer, I. H., Sell, R. I., et al. (2000). Lesbian, gay, bisexual, and transgender health: Findings and concerns. *Journal of the Gay and Lesbian Medical Association, 4*, 101–151.

system will need to be addressed to improve the health of this population.

> *Think back to Paul Rojas, the homosexual patient with AIDS. The nurse needs to be acutely aware of the healthcare delivery system in the community to ensure that Mr. Rojas has access to the most appropriate and needed services. In addition, consultation with social services would be helpful for initiating referrals for appropriate services as Mr. Rojas' condition changes.*

Advocating Sexuality Needs of Patients

A hospital experience or institutionalization puts a strain on a person's individuality and sexual self. Illness may diminish feelings of sexual desire, and the desire for sexual interaction can signal a patient's improving health. The nurse should provide anticipatory guidance because many patients may hesitate to make such a request for fear of being ridiculed. Often, a patient merely desires privacy to hold and caress his or her partner. The intimacy of this act often fulfills the patient's feelings of longing to be needed and loved.

There are many ways the nurse can advocate for a patient's sexual needs. Some may seem obvious and commonplace, whereas others may require the nurse to come to terms with his or her own sexuality (Box 35-3).

Counseling the Patient Regarding Sexuality

Not all patients with sexual concerns need intensive therapy. Some patients benefit greatly from simply having someone listen to their concerns. Voicing their concerns allows patients to put the information into perspective and focus on what the problem is and how to solve it. Nurses counseling patients

should not offer their own advice, because what is right for one person may be wrong for another. Also, offering false reassurances, such as, "It'll be all right," is unproductive. Rather, the nurse should adopt an objective, empathic, and receptive attitude to facilitate open communication between nurse and patient.

Annon (cited in Hatcher et al., 1990) developed the PLISSIT model for counseling to be used by therapists and nontherapists for patients with sexual problems. The four stages to this model, each increasing in intensity with the seriousness of the patient's problem, are listed in Box 35-4.

Abortion Counseling

Abortion remains an issue that deeply divides people. Many believe it is a woman's right to choose whether to continue a pregnancy and then to take safe and legal action if a decision is made to terminate. Others believe that from fertilization onward, a human being exists who commands the full respect and protection we afford adult humans, and thus abortion is always wrong. Some would allow abortion only if it is indicated for a woman's health or in cases of rape. It is important for nurses to know what they believe, why they believe this, and how their beliefs are likely to influence their ability to counsel women and couples.

Counseling in Cases of Abusive Relationships and/or Rape

It is not uncommon for nurses to encounter children, adolescents, women, and sometimes men who experience sexual abuse and rape in their relationships or families. The National Victim Center (http://www.nal.usda.gov/pavnet/cj/cjnatvic.htm) reported the following:

- One out of every eight adult women, or at least 12.1 million American women, have been the victims of forcible rape.

BOX 35-3 Advocating Patients' Sexual Needs

- All patients should be accepted as sexual beings with the right to be treated with dignity and with sensitivity to their feelings.
- All patients have the right to some degree of privacy.
  - Anticipate the patient's desire for privacy by the simple act of drawing a curtain or closing a door.
  - Patients should be given the option of wearing their own sleepwear to promote sexual identity.
- Potentially shaming situations for the patient should be anticipated.
  - Give information regarding what the procedure is and why it needs to be done, and acknowledge that the patient's embarrassment is normal and understandable.
- Healthcare providers should not simply take for granted that patients do not mind intrusive or embarrassing procedures performed on their bodies and private parts.
- Patients have a right to question the physician regarding sexual needs or future sexual functioning.
  - Anticipate these questions for the patient.

- Ask patients if they have any concerns regarding sexuality that can be answered by the nurse.
  - Nurses can interface with the physician to obtain information required by the patient.
- The atmosphere in healthcare settings needs to allow for sexual expression between patients and their partners.
- Confidentiality is a right of every patient.
  - Do not promise confidentiality if that promise cannot be kept.
  - Allow no one access to the patient's personal records who is not directly involved in the patient's care.
  - Allow no information regarding patients to escape into idle conversation.
- All patients should be referred to formally as Mr., Mrs., Miss, Ms., according to the patient's preference.
- Visitors, including a visiting spouse, should be referred to as people with genders, rather than as "the visitor."
- Patients should be allowed to keep some personal possessions, if it is practical to do so.

P—*Permission giving:* The nurse may make a suggestion that the patient can use. Permission giving is not the same as advice. Permission giving implies giving the patient freedom to choose to do something that the authority figure (such as a nurse) deems to be a positive alternative. It may be something the patient wanted to do all along. For example,

> *Patient:* "Aren't some sexual positions perverted?"
> *Nurse:* "Many people enjoy using different positions for sex. Some positions are more pleasurable to some couples than others. You and your partner have the right to use any position for sex that you desire."

LI—*Limited information:* Specific factual information is required by the patient. It often involves some aspect of anatomy and physiology or the specifics of certain sexual expressions.

SS—*Specific suggestions:* Patients need very specific instructions regarding a useful technique. Many patients have a sexual dysfunction for which they are seeking intervention and correction.

IT—*Intensive therapy:* Used primarily by therapists, it involves issues such as marriage, self-concept, and sexual desire, to name a few. If the first three levels of counseling presented were unsuccessful, intensive therapy is indicated.

- Sixty-one percent of all forcible rapes occurred before victims reached the age of 18, 29% occurred when the victim was less than 11 years old, and another 32% occurred between the ages of 11 and 17.
- Rape victims often suffer devastating mental health problems, with 31% developing rape-related posttraumatic stress disorder (PTSD) sometime in their lifetime. Rape-related PTSD dramatically increases the risk for major alcohol and drug abuse problems. They are 13 times more likely to have two or more major alcohol problems and 26 times more likely to have two or more major drug abuse problems.

Clearly, nurses need to be alert to evidence of sexual abuse while taking the history and conducting physical examinations. Abuse crosses all socioeconomic and ethnic groups. Nurses should become familiar with their legal and clinical responsibilities when a victim is identified. The first priority is getting the victim into a safe environment and mobilizing support for the victim and family. Multiple parties may need therapy.

Evaluating

To evaluate the plan of care, the nurse needs to use information from the patient for most outcomes. The nurse cannot evaluate the patient by observing his or her expression of sexuality, but the nurse can evaluate how the patient is progressing toward sexuality-oriented goals by his or her appearance, self-confidence, and manner. For example, a patient who has expressed feelings of anxiety in the past over a sexual concern should be observably more confident and free of anxiety if the patient outcomes are being met. The nurse also needs to ask the patient about progress toward outcomes. Some outcomes need to be "stepping stones," because not all problems are easily resolved with one-time intervention and direction.

When evaluating a patient's progress, it may help to ask: "In what ways have you been able to achieve [orgasm, increased desire, comfortable intercourse, erection]?" "What methods seemed most effective? Which were not?" "What do you think should be the next step?" The nurse should determine from this interaction with the patient whether something more needs to be accomplished. It is not enough to assume that because a set of outcomes has been met, the patient is satisfied with the results. See the Nursing Plan of Care 35-1.

(*text continues on page 966*)

┌───┐
│ **NURSING PLAN**   *for Pete Manheim*   │
│ **OF CARE 35-1**   │
└───┘

Pete Manheim is a 13-year-old adolescent boy attending the area health clinic. He is nervous as he explains to the nurse his need for healthcare. He has noticed "sticky white stuff" around his penis and bedclothes on arising some mornings and fears he may be ill. Pete has also expressed concern about his lack of knowledge regarding sexuality. He has heard a lot of stories from his friends but does not feel he can talk to his parents because the subject has never been broached at home. Also, although Pete is a virgin, he is beginning to feel pressured by his friends, who boast of many sexual experiences.

After spending time in conversation with Pete, the nurse gathered the following data:

- Pete is experiencing nocturnal emissions and has little scientific knowledge about their source.

- Pete is anxious because of the stories regarding sex he has heard from his friends.
- There is no communication or dialogue at home with parents about issues of sexuality.
- Pete is having feelings of insecurity and anxiety about his present virginal status, which he feels he should change.
- Peer pressure from friends is also a concern.

The nurse will work together with Pete to develop a plan of care to correct misinformation and relieve his anxiety. Planning will be directed toward correcting myths and supplying Pete with accurate information. Because Pete has a negligible knowledge base on sexuality, the plan of care will allow for ongoing sessions to augment the initial information. The nurse should outline this plan with Pete to be certain it is acceptable to him.

(continued)

NURSING PLAN OF CARE 35-1   *for Pete Manheim* (continued)

NURSING DIAGNOSIS   Knowledge Deficit: Adolescent Sexuality Concerns related to misinformation and absent family-based sex education as manifested by self-report

EXPECTED OUTCOME   By the end of the teaching session, the patient will:
• Describe the nature of nocturnal emissions

Nursing Interventions	Rationale	Evaluative Statement
Assess patient's present knowledge base on nocturnal emission and the source of his information.	It is necessary to discover what the patient does know and to build on that knowledge.	8/1/06 Outcome met. Patient able to describe the source of nocturnal emissions.
Use terms that the patient has used and language at the level of the patient's understanding.	This facilitates comprehension.	*R. Gordon, RN*
Teach the patient about nocturnal emissions:	Knowledge decreases anxiety.	
• Nocturnal emissions, or "wet dreams," are normal in men of all ages, and they are particularly common in the teenage years. They are not the result of disease.		
• They occur during sleep as the result of erotic dreams. The "white sticky stuff" is the result of ejaculation of semen from the penis.		
• This is an involuntary action over which the male has no control.		

EXPECTED OUTCOME   By the end of the teaching session, the patient will:
• Differentiate sexual myths from sound knowledge

Nursing Interventions	Rationale	Evaluative Statement
Assess what patient has heard from peers regarding sexual information:	The nurse can then specifically address the myths to which the patient has been exposed.	8/1/06 Outcome met. Patient was able to differentiate between truth in sexual issues and what is myth.
Myth 1: "A large penis is better for sex than a small one."	This enables the patient to develop a positive sexual body image based on fact.	*R. Gordon, RN*
Truth: No relation exists between the size of a penis and the man's ability to perform sexually. When a penis becomes erect, it reaches sufficient size to engage in sexual intercourse.		
Myth 2: "Jerking off causes blindness. It is a dirty habit."	The patient is given permission to engage in a sexual activity of a masturbatory nature.	
Truth: Masturbation or self-stimulation is a natural and healthy outlet for sexual urges. Men and women of all ages masturbate. Masturbation can also teach the person what feels good and what does not. Every person has the right to masturbate if he or she wishes to do so.		

(continued)

NURSING PLAN OF CARE 35-1

for Pete Manheim (continued)

Nursing Interventions	Rationale	Evaluative Statement
Myth 3: "It looks bad for a guy to be a virgin—everybody's doing it." Truth: No one, whether male or female, should feel pressured into sexual activity at any age. Engaging in sexual activity carries with it a great deal of responsibility and concerns of pregnancy and spread of sexually transmitted infections (STIs). No one needs to know of another person's status if the person chooses not to discuss it.	The patient is given permission to abstain from sexual activity and not to feel pressured by friends. Almost 39% of teens have had sex by age 16 years.	

EXPECTED OUTCOME By the end of the teaching session, the patient will:
• List the positive aspects of abstinence in a sexual relationship

Nursing Interventions	Rationale	Evaluative Statement
Assess the patient, including previous discussion of sexual myths and knowledge. Instruct the patient on the positive aspects of abstinence, including the following: • Engagement in any sexual activity should be a personal decision and not the result of pressure from friends. • Abstinence will guarantee protection from pregnancy and from most STIs. • People can show affection for each other without sexual involvement. • Every person has the right to say no.	Giving the patient all the information necessary allows him to make an informed decision. Many young people think they are immune to the consequences of their actions. Therefore, it is important to stress that pregnancy and STIs are very probable results of sexual intercourse. It is difficult to understand and undertake all the implications of a sexual relationship during the teenage years. The patient learns that a successful sexual relationship requires intimacy, love, and sharing; it should not be merely an outlet for sexual feelings. The patient has permission to refuse an activity in which he is not sure he wishes to engage.	8/1/06 Outcome partially met. Patient able to list verbally all positive aspects of abstinence but is still undecided. *Revision:* Reinforce to patient that this is a personal decision that he can make for himself with a good knowledge base. Also, he does not have to make a firm decision for or against abstinence immediately. He should take time to think about this information. *R. Gordon, RN*

EXPECTED OUTCOME By the end of the teaching session, the patient will:
• Describe the correct use of rubber condoms

Nursing Interventions	Rationale	Evaluative Statement
Assess what the patient knows about rubber condoms and their use.	Since patient is undecided about whether to initiate a sexual relationship in the future, it is prudent to give him information to protect against pregnancy and STIs.	8/1/06 Outcome met. Patient successfully listed the steps in using a condom. *R. Gordon, RN*

(continued)

NURSING PLAN OF CARE 35-1   *for Pete Manheim* (continued)

Nursing Interventions	Rationale	Evaluative Statement
Inform the patient that rubber condoms are available over the counter in drug stores. Prices vary according to type and style.	Patient should know where to purchase condoms and the variety available.	
Teach patient the steps in using rubber condoms:	Patient should know how to use condoms safely.	
• Roll condom onto the penis as soon as it becomes erect.	Protects against sperm from secretions from Cowper's glands	
• If condom does not have a nipple receptacle end, leave a small space at end of condom to collect semen.	Provides a pocket to collect semen and prevents breakage	
• Immediately after ejaculation, remove penis and condom from vagina by holding onto base of condom.	Prevents spillage of semen into the vagina	
• Discard condom.	Condoms are not meant to be reused. A new condom is used for each act of intercourse.	
Advise the patient to use a condom with every act of intercourse. Spermicides used with condom increase effectiveness.	To be as effective as possible, the condom should be used with every act of intercourse. The rubber condom used with spermicide is effective against pregnancy and the spread of STIs. The woman's use of a spermicide foam in the vagina increases effectiveness.	

EXPECTED OUTCOME

By the end of the teaching session, the patient will:
• Express a decrease in anxiety

Nursing Interventions	Rationale	Evaluative Statement
Assess patient's anxiety level by verbal and nonverbal behavior.	Patient was anxious when he came into clinic. It is important to evaluate level of anxiety before he leaves. If he is still anxious, reassessment should occur because plan of care may have been unsuccessful.	8/1/06 Outcome met. Patient expressed relief that he is normal. Would like to bring a friend to next session. Future teaching sessions to include these topics identified by patient: • STIs, particularly AIDS • Pregnancy—occurrence and prevention • Sexual expression • Further discussion of sexual myths *R. Gordon, RN*

SAMPLE DOCUMENTATION

8/1/06, 11 AM, nursing

Nursing consultation with 13-year-old patient regarding anxiety about cause and source of nocturnal emissions. Patient also expressed concern about sexual myths he has heard from friends. Stated that much peer pressure exists to become sexually active. Patient admits to possessing little knowledge regarding sexual issues. Feels he cannot discuss sexuality with parents because it is not a topic that has been brought up in the past at home. Will conduct initial teaching session with patient to provide information and decrease anxiety about priority concerns. Patient is willing to return to clinic for at least three more teaching sessions to expand knowledge base of sexuality.

R. Gordon, RN

SEXUAL HARASSMENT

Harassment is any annoying or distressing comment or conduct that is known or should be known to be unwelcome. **Sexual harassment** is unwelcome behavior that is sexual or gender-based in nature. This type of harassment usually occurs in the context of an asymmetrical relationship where one person has more formal power than the other (eg, a faculty member over a student) or more informal power (eg, one peer over another). Sexual harassment can be directed toward individuals of any age, either gender, and any sexual orientation. There are two forms of sexual harassment: "quid pro quo" and environmental harassment (also called a "hostile" environment).

"Quid Pro Quo"

"Quid pro quo" means something given or withheld in exchange for something else. "Quid pro quo" harassment occurs when an individual's employment or well-being as an employee is dependent on agreeing to unsolicited and unwelcome sexual demands. This type of harassment is typically initiated by a person in a position of authority who offers either direct or indirect reward or punishment based on the granting of sexual favors. "Quid pro quo" harassment is a clear abuse of power and is legally, morally, and ethically wrong.

Hostile Environment Harassment

Hostile environment harassment occurs when workplace behaviors of a sexual or gender-based nature create a hostile, intimidating environment and when this type of environment hurts an individual's work performance. The negative behaviors in hostile environment harassment are not directly linked to job-related consequences; instead, the employee's willingness to suffer the experience of the demeaning environment becomes a condition of employment. This type of harassment is not necessarily caused by a person with formal power. Hostile environment is sometimes difficult to define, as it is not always easy to determine when offensive speech or behavior actually turns to true harassment. Coworkers and peers can create a hostile work environment for a member of the group through the following:

- Unwelcome sexually oriented and gender-based behaviors
- Sexual bantering
- Sexual jokes
- Offensive pictures and language
- Sexual innuendoes
- Sexual behavior
  See the accompanying Research in Nursing box.

Responding to Patient Advances

Inappropriate sexual behavior by a patient may cause the nurse to respond with either passive avoidance or aggressive retaliation. An assertive response is recommended that supports the nurse in maintaining his or her self-respect and encourages the patient to accept responsibility for his or her behavior:

1. Be self-aware: Do not deny feelings about being harassed.
2. Confront: Provide feedback to the patient in a non-threatening way and clearly state what behavior is or is not acceptable.
3. Set limits: Define clear and reasonable consequences that will be enforced if the behavior continues.
4. Enforce the stated limits: Maintain boundaries.
5. Report: Document the incident and submit to supervisor.

Research in Nursing Making a Difference
Understanding Sexual Harassment

Recognizing and labeling sex-based and sexual harassment is often difficult for people who find themselves in a hostile work environment. Despite much research on the topic during the past two decades, little progress has been made in providing a descriptive language to help individuals convey their experiences in these situations. Registered nurses may struggle to understand and interpret their experiences and often have difficulty helping others understand as well.

Related Research
Madison, J., & Minichiello, V. (2000). Recognizing and labeling sex-based sexual harassment in the health care workplace. *Journal of Nursing Scholarship, 32*(4), 405–410.

   The purpose of this study was to explore how registered nurses recognize and label incidents of sex-based and sexual harassment in the Australian healthcare workplace. A convenience sample of 16 volunteers were interviewed for approximately 1 hour each. The volunteers were registered nurses who were students enrolled in advanced tertiary preparation in nursing, counseling, and healthcare management at an Australian university and who had competed a survey on sexual harassment. The interviews were part of a qualitative study based on the premise that sex-based harassment and sexual harassment are socially constructed symbolic phenomena. The purpose of the interview was to investigate how informants recognized and labeled the harassment experience.

Relevance for Practice
The study findings suggested that education about sexual harassment should be specific and based on structural impediments to a positive workplace as well as on interactive information as reported and interpreted by the harassed persons. Harassment is context-related: behavior overlooked and accepted in the past may now be interpreted by some as harassment. The definitions of sex-based harassment and sexual harassment will continue to change with other changes in the workplace. Two critical conclusions to use in further research are the importance of listening to informants and the suggestion that issues associated with sexual harassment should be purposely raised in the workplace.

Responding to Harassment by Colleagues

The objective of employers should be to create a positive work environment that is characterized by mutually respectful behavior. Many have taken steps to eliminate hostile work environments by educating employees, developing policies against workplace harassment, and outlining guidelines for responding to sexual harassment:

1. If harassed by a coworker, confront the behavior immediately. An assertive statement is sometimes sufficient to stop the behavior.
2. If the harassment continues, document the date and time and describe the behavior.
3. Consult your supervisor.
4. If the harassment still does not stop, file a grievance with administration.
5. Seek legal advice if all previous efforts to stop the behavior have been unsuccessful.

Effects of Harassment

Harassment can cause feelings of helplessness, worthlessness, and guilt in the victim. This can often lead to less career satisfaction and feelings of loss of control. Anger is a common emotion experienced by those who have been harassed and may lead to requests for transfer, resignation, or withdrawal from the workplace. In many cases, job performance is affected due to reduced levels of concentration. Loss of job motivation and skill confidence, along with reduced job satisfaction and organizational commitment, are common.

■ Developing Critical Thinking Skills

1. Role-play with another student the interview you would use to obtain a sexual history from the following individuals. Think about how you modified the interview in each situation and why. Identify what made you feel uncomfortable as either the nurse or the patient. Discuss how you can best address this discomfort:
   - Mother voices concern that her 9-year-old son is frequently playing with his penis.
   - Adult man appears distressed when he notes that he has suddenly become impotent with his partner of many years.
   - A high-school girl says that her mother tells her something is wrong with her because she is attracted only to women.
   - A new resident in a nursing home complains that he misses his privacy and has nowhere to make love.
2. Describe how you would respond to a newly diagnosed HIV-positive woman with multiple partners who tells you that it is none of your business how she acquired the virus or what she plans to do now that she has it. Think carefully about what is at stake in terms of your response.

3. You know a patient is uncomfortable about undergoing a pelvic examination, and you ask the male physician to wait for you to give a med before he begins the examination. He tells you he can't wait and doesn't need your assistance. You know the patient wants another woman in the room. How would you respond, and what is at stake? Does it matter if the reason for the patient's request to have you present is simply preference, is linked to a history of abuse, or is related to her cultural or religious beliefs?

■ Practicing for NCLEX

1. The cessation of a woman's menstrual activity is termed:
   a. Menarche
   b. Premenstrual syndrome
   c. Menopause
   d. Menstrual dysfunction
2. Masturbation is a technique of sexual expression in which an individual practices self-stimulation. Another fact related to masturbation is that:
   a. Only male adolescents masturbate.
   b. There are serious health risks associated with frequent masturbation.
   c. Individuals who masturbate demonstrate sexual dysfunction.
   d. Masturbation is a means of learning what a person prefers sexually.
3. Stimulation of the female genitals by licking and sucking the clitoris and surrounding structures is called:
   a. Fellatio
   b. Soixante-neuf
   c. Cunnilingus
   d. Masturbation
4. The practice of gaining sexual pleasure while inflicting abuse on another person is called:
   a. Pedophilia
   b. Voyeurism
   c. Sadism
   d. Masochism
5. A 52-year-old man asks the nurse if some sexual positions are considered perverted. The nurse responds by saying that many people enjoy different positions for sex and that each couple has the right to use any position for sex that they enjoy. In consideration of the PLISSIT model for counseling patients with sexual problems, this is an example of:
   a. Limited information
   b. Specific suggestion
   c. Permission giving
   d. Intensive therapy
6. A patient tells the nurse that she uses a mechanical barrier for birth control. Which of the following methods fits that category?

   a. Diaphragm
   b. Oral contraceptive pills
   c. Depo-Provera
   d. Evra patch
7. An 18-year-old male patient tells you he uses cocaine regularly to try to boost his sexual performance. Which of the following is true about the effects of cocaine on sexual performance?
   a. Cocaine has no effect on sexuality.
   b. Cocaine can reduce testosterone levels and sperm production.
   c. Even a small amount of cocaine can cause impotence.
   d. Chronic cocaine use results in sexual dysfunction and loss of desire in both men and women.
8. Which of the following statements by a patient indicates a need for teaching about contraception?
   a. "Depo-Provera is not effective against sexually transmitted infections, but contraceptive protection is immediate if I get the injection during the first 5 days of my period."
   b. "The hormonal ring contraceptive, NuvaRing, protects against pregnancy by suppressing ovulation, thickening cervical mucus, and preventing the fertilized egg from implanting in the uterus."
   c. "Abstinence may be an effective method of contraception and may be used as a periodic or continuous strategy."
   d. "Withdrawal is an effective method of birth control as well as an effective method of reducing the spread of sexually transmitted infections."
9. The integration of somatic, emotional, intellectual, and social aspects of sexual being in ways that are positively enriching and that enhance personality is termed:
   a. Gender role behavior
   b. Sexual health
   c. Gender identity
   d. Sexuality
10. Unwelcome behavior that is sexual or gender-based in nature is called:
   a. Intimidation
   b. Sexual harassment
   c. Confrontation
   d. Altercation

Answers With Rationale

1. The correct answer is *c*. Menarche is the first menstrual period. Premenstrual syndrome is characterized by the appearance of one or more of the following characteristics several days before the onset of menstruation: irritability, emotional tension, anxiety, mood changes, headache, breast tenderness, and water retention. Menopause, the cessation of a woman's menstrual cycle, occurs between the ages of 45 and 55 years. The woman may experience irregular menses over time before menstruation ends.

2. The correct answer is *d*. People masturbate regardless of sex, age, or marital status. No known health risks are associated with masturbation. Masturbation is not "wrong" or "dirty." It is a means of learning what a person prefers during stimulation and what feels good.

3. The correct answer is *c*. Fellatio is stimulation of the male genitals by licking and sucking the penis and surrounding structures. Cunnilingus is stimulation of the female genitals by licking and sucking the clitoris and surrounding structures. Masturbation is a practice of self-stimulation. Soixante-neuf occurs when both fellatio and cunnilingus occur at the same time.

4. The correct answer is *c*. Pedophilia is the practice of adults gaining sexual fulfillment by sexual acts with children. Voyeurism refers to sexual arousal achieved by looking at the body of another. Sadism refers to gaining sexual pleasure while inflicting abuse on another person. Masochism refers to gaining sexual pleasure from the humiliation of being abused.

5. The correct answer is *c*. When the nurse encourages and offers support for the patient's choices, the patient accepts this approach as permission to engage in the activity under discussion.

6. The correct answer is *a*. The diaphragm is the only barrier method of contraception listed; all the other methods are hormonal.

7. The correct answer is *d*. When used chronically, cocaine can result in both sexual dysfunction and loss of sexual desire.

8. The correct answer is *d*. Withdrawal offers no protection against sexually transmitted infections.

9. The correct answer is *b*. Gender role behavior is the behavior a person conveys about being male or female, which may or may not be the same as his or her biologic gender or gender identity. Gender identity is the inner sense a person has of being male or female. Sexuality is the degree to which a person exhibits and experiences maleness or femaleness physically, emotionally, and mentally. Sexual health is the term that best fits the definition.

10. The correct answer is *b*. Sexual harassment may be defined as any unwelcome verbal or physical advance or sexually explicit statement—such as leers, pats, grabs, jokes, requests for dates, and even rape—that interferes with a person's ability to do his or her job by making him or her feel humiliated, intimidated, or uncomfortable.

Bibliography

Abrams, S., Skee, D., Natarajan, J., & Wong, F. A. (2002). Pharmacokinetic overview of OrthoEvra/Evra. *Fertility and Sterility, 7*(2), S3–S12.

Alteneder, R. R. (1997). Addressing couples' sexuality concerns during the childbearing period: Use of PLISSIT model. *Journal of Obstetric, Gynecologic, and Neonatal Nursing, 26*(6), 651–658.

American Academy of Pediatrics Committee on Adolescence (1993). Homosexuality and adolescence. *Pediatrics, 92,* 631–633.

Brady, M. (1998). Female genital mutilation. *Nursing, 28*(9), 50–51.

Birth control: Planned Parenthood Federation of America, Inc. http://www.plannedparenthood.rg/bc/index.html.

Bradford, J., Ryan, C., Honnold, J., & Rothblum, E. (2001). Expanding the research infrastructure for lesbian health. *American Journal of Public Health, 91*(7), 1029–1032.

Carter, J., & Verhoef, M. J. (1995). Efficacy of self-help and alternative treatments of premenstrual syndrome. *Women's Health Issues, 4*(3), 130–137.

Centers for Disease Control/National Center for HIV, STD and TB Prevention (2002). Sexually transmitted disease guidelines 2002 (Electronic Version). *Morbidity and Mortality Weekly Report, 51.*

Cholewinski, J. T., & Burge, J. M. (1990). Sexual harassment of nursing students. *Image The Journal of Nursing Scholarship, 22*(2), 106–110.

Clark, M., Landers, S., Linde, R., & Sperber, J. (2001). The GLBT health access project: A state-funded effort to improve access to care. *American Journal of Public Health, 91*(6), 895–896.

Cole, F. L., & Slocumb, E. M. (1995). Factors influencing safer sexual behaviors in heterosexual late adolescent and young adult collegiate males. *Image The Journal of Nursing Scholarship, 27*(3), 217–223.

Dean, L., Meyer, I., Robinson, K., et al. (2000). Lesbian, gay, bisexual, and transgender health: Findings and concerns. *Journal of Gay and Lesbian Medical Association, 4,* 101–151

Doyle, D., Bisson, D., Janes, N., Lynch, H., & Martin, C. (1999). Human sexuality in long-term care. *Canadian Nurse, 95*(1), 26–29.

Fehring, R. J. (1991). New technology in natural family planning. *Journal of Obstetric, Gynecologic, and Neonatal Nursing, 20*(3), 199–205.

Fuentes, R. J., Rosenberg, J. M., & Marks, R. G. (1983). Sexual side effects: What to tell your patients, what not to say. *Registered Nurse, 46*(2), 34–41.

Garbach, S., Bartlett, J., & Blacklaw, N. (1998). *Infectious disease* (2nd ed.). Philadelphia: Saunders.

Harbin, R. E. (1995). Female adolescent contraception. *Pediatric Nursing, 21*(3), 221–226.

Hardingham, L. (1998). Ethics in the workplace. Sexual harassment: being aware of its most common, subtle form. *Alberta RN, 54*(9), 14–15, 23.

Hatcher, R., Guest, S., Stewart, F., Stewart, G. K., Trussell, J., Cerel, S., & Kates, W. (1990). *Contraceptive technology* (15th ed.). New York: Irvington.

Hofland, S. L., & Powers, L. (1996). Sexual dysfunction in the menopausal woman: Hormonal causes and management issues. *Geriatric Nursing, 17*(4), 161–165.

Horsley, J. E. (1990). Don't tolerate sexual harassment at work. *RN, 53*(1), 69, 72, 75.

Hutti, M. (2003). New & emerging contraceptive methods: Nurses can help women make wise choices. *Lifelines, 7*(1), 34–38.

Kaye, J., Donald, C. G., & Merker, S. (1994). Sexual harassment of critical care nurses: A costly workplace issue. *American Journal of Critical Care, 3*(6), 409–415.

MacLaren, A. (1995). Primary care for women: Comprehensive sexual health assessment. *Journal of Nurse-Midwifery, 40*(2), 104–119.

Madison, J., & Minichiello, V. (2000). Recognizing and labeling sex-based sexual harassment in the health care workplace. *Journal of Nursing Scholarship, 32*(4), 405–410.

Mandell, G., Bennett, J., & Dolin, R. (2000). *Principles and practice of infectious diseases* (5th ed.). Philadelphia: Churchill Livingstone.

McGrory, A. (1995). Education for the menarche. *Pediatric Nursing, 21*(5), 439–443.

Pillitteri, A. (2003). *Maternal and child health nursing* (4th ed.). Philadelphia: Lippincott Williams & Wilkins.

Rawlins, S., & Smith, D. (2002). Innovative contraception: New options in hormonal contraception. *American Journal of Nurse Practitioners, 6*(1), 9–28.

Robbins, I., Bender, M., & Finnis, S. (1997). Sexual harassment in nursing. *Journal of Advanced Nursing, 25*(1), 163–169.

Smith, L. L., Taylor, B. B., Keys, A. T., & Gornto, B. A. (1997). Nurse–patient boundaries. Crossing the line: How to recognize signs of professional misconduct and intervene effectively. *American Journal of Nursing, 97*(12), 26–31.

Stockard, S. (1991). Caring for the sexually aggressive patient: You don't have to blush and bear it. *Nursing, 21*(11), 72–73.

Thomas, B., Stamler, L. L., Lafreniere, K., & Dumala, R. (2000). The Internet: An effective tool for nursing research with women. *Computers in Nursing, 18*(1), 13–18.

University of Calgary. (1996). *Annual report, Sexual Harassment Office, July 1, 1993–June 30, 1996.* Calgary: Author.

Varnhagen, C. K. (1991). Sexually transmitted diseases and condoms: High school students' knowledge, attitudes, and behaviors. *Canadian Journal of Public Health, 82*(2), 129–132.

Warner, P. H., & Rowe, T. (1999). Shedding light on the sexual history. *American Journal of Nursing, 99*(6), 34–41.

Williams, A. B. (1992). The epidemiology, clinical manifestations and health maintenance needs of women infected with HIV. *Nurse Practitioner, 17*(5), 27–44.

Winter, E. J. S., Ashton, D. J., & Moore, D. L. (1991). Dispelling myths: A study of PMS and relationship satisfaction. *Nurse Practitioner, 16*(5), 34–45.

Woods, N. F. (1984). *Human sexuality in health and illness.* St. Louis: C. V. Mosby.

World Health Organization. (1975). *Education and treatment in human sexuality: The training of health professionals.* Geneva: Author.

Zook, R. (2000). Sexual harassment in the workplace. *American Journal of Nursing, 100*(12), 24AAAA, 24CCCC.

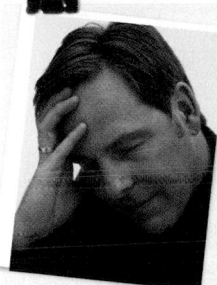

Kevin O'Malley, a 44-year-old devout Irish Catholic parent, asks, "What kind of God allows young people to drink and drive, killing other young people?" His 17-year-old daughter was a victim of a car accident on her prom night about 1 week ago and has been comatose in the critical care unit since then. Her date, one driver, and the driver of the other car, who was intoxicated, were killed in the accident. Physicians give Mr. O'Malley's daughter less than a 50% chance of survival.

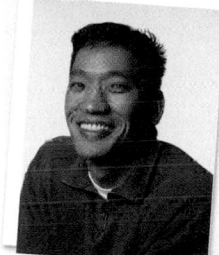

Choi Min Lai, a member of the Hmong culture from Laos, is refusing to allow physicians to perform a series of surgical repairs to correct severe deformities of his 8-year-old son's feet. "In our culture, the deformity is a sign of spiritual favor and good luck. Because of Kou's condition, a warrior ancestor whose feet were wounded in battle will no longer be spiritually trapped. You see, Kou is special."

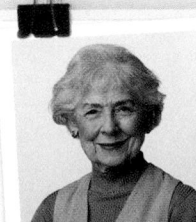

Margot Zeuner, a 75-year-old woman, is taking care of her 80-year-old husband with advanced Alzheimer's disease, who was just discharged from the hospital and requires constant supervision. When visited at home, she says, "I really miss going to church and seeing everyone. They're so supportive. That was the one thing that helped to keep me going."

Focusing on Blended Skills

The types of blended skills you'll need to respond to the case scenarios include:

Cognitive Skills

- Basic knowledge about spirituality, including its influence and that of faith and religion on a person's everyday life and health beliefs
- Ability to demonstrate understanding of factors that influence spiritual development and spiritual health
- Ability to identify spirituality as a source of patient support, strength, or conflict, incorporating this information into the patient's plan of care
- Ability to use the nursing process to meet the spiritual needs of patients at various developmental stages experiencing spiritual distress or conflict

Technical Skills

- Ability to use correctly the equipment and protocols necessary to identify and treat problems and conflicts involving spirituality
- Ability to perform spiritual care interventions confidently and competently, adapting the interventions based on the patient's culture and developmental stage

Interpersonal Skills

- Self-awareness of own spirituality and comfort in dealing with issues involving spirituality
- Ability to communicate and interact effectively with patients and their family caregivers
- Ability to establish trusting relationships, even in times of distress, crisis, and conflict
- Ability to provide supportive presence to meet a patient's spiritual needs
- Ability to demonstrate respect, empathy, and caring
- Ability to be a healing presence

Ethical and Legal Skills

- Commitment to safety and quality; strong sense of responsibility, accountability; strong advocacy skills
- Familiarity with the ethical and legal guidelines of agency policy and role responsibilities related to meeting spiritual needs
- Knowledge of patients' and families' rights related to refusal of care due to cultural religious beliefs

Learning Outcomes

After completing the chapter, the learner should be able to accomplish the following:

1. Identify three spiritual needs believed to be common to all people.
2. Describe the influences of spirituality on everyday living, health, and illness.
3. Differentiate life-affirming influences of religious beliefs from life-denying influences.
4. Distinguish the spiritual beliefs and practices of the major religions practiced in the United States.
5. Identify five factors that influence spirituality.
6. Perform a nursing assessment of spiritual health, using appropriate interview questions and observation skills.
7. Develop nursing diagnoses that correctly identify spiritual problems.
8. Describe nursing strategies to promote spiritual health, and state their rationale.
9. Plan, implement, and evaluate nursing care related to select nursing diagnoses involving spiritual problems.

Key Terms

agnostic
atheist
faith
religion
spiritual beliefs
spiritual distress
spirituality
spiritual needs

Paying attention to the spiritual dimension of health and well-being is integral to holistic care. Patients facing the losses and limits related to injury, disease, and aging begin to evaluate what is important in life and often ask the "eternal questions": Is there a God? Does life have meaning and purpose? Nurses skilled in spiritual care are able to identify and elicit the inner resources that patients and family caregivers have to promote health and healing. Many nurses who describe themselves as professional healers use the terms "vocation" or "calling" to describe the work of nursing. They claim to be "standing on holy ground" when they create that hospitable place where patients can expose their vulnerabilities and ask the hard questions: Will this hurt? Am I dying? Is there anyone I can trust to be with me during this hard time? We learn, with great humility, that sometimes the most important things we do are accomplished simply by being present to those we serve. A Baptist woman with a life-threatening cancer recently wrote to me, "When you made a cross on my forehead with your thumb, it felt very foreign to me. No one has ever done that before. It felt unfamiliar—but perfect. Like a blessing with no conditions—no strings. How liberating. Affirming. Loving. And to think you did it with just your thumb. And your heart. Thank you."

Study of this chapter provides the student with a knowledge base of spirituality, spiritual health, and spiritual care. Practical suggestions for performing a spiritual assessment are given, along with specific interview questions. Sample nursing diagnoses are developed for common problems of **spiritual distress** (spiritual pain, alienation, anxiety, guilt, anger, loss, and despair). Related patient and nursing goals and specific nursing strategies for promoting spiritual health are described. The concluding patient care study illustrates how the nurse's knowledge of spirituality may be combined with skilled nursing interventions and caring to resolve spiritual distress.

SPIRITUAL DIMENSION

The "spirit" dimension of the person was recognized in ancient cultures. "The dual roles of priest and physician were generally held by one individual, and thus the functions and dictates of religion (pertaining to the spirit) and medicine (pertaining to the body) were closely interwoven" (O'Brien, 1982, p. 85). Over the years, however, medicine and religion evolved separately. Not until the holistic health movement took root was the person once again viewed as an integrated whole of body, mind, and spirit. Healthcare practitioners began again to probe the relationships among physical, psychological, social, and spiritual health. Two models are currently being used to illustrate these relationships (Fig. 36-1). In the integrated approach, the bio-psycho-social-spiritual model has four equal dimensions, each of which influences the other. In the unifying approach, the spiritual dimension grounds the biological, psychological, and sociologic dimensions. While it is interesting to interview professional healers about which model is more consistent with their experience, both demand of the nurse greater competence in identifying and meeting spiritual needs than most practicing nurses today display.

Nursing has always had a strongly holistic tradition, and nurses have practiced nursing with sensitivity to the physical, psychosocial, and spiritual needs of people According to Shelly

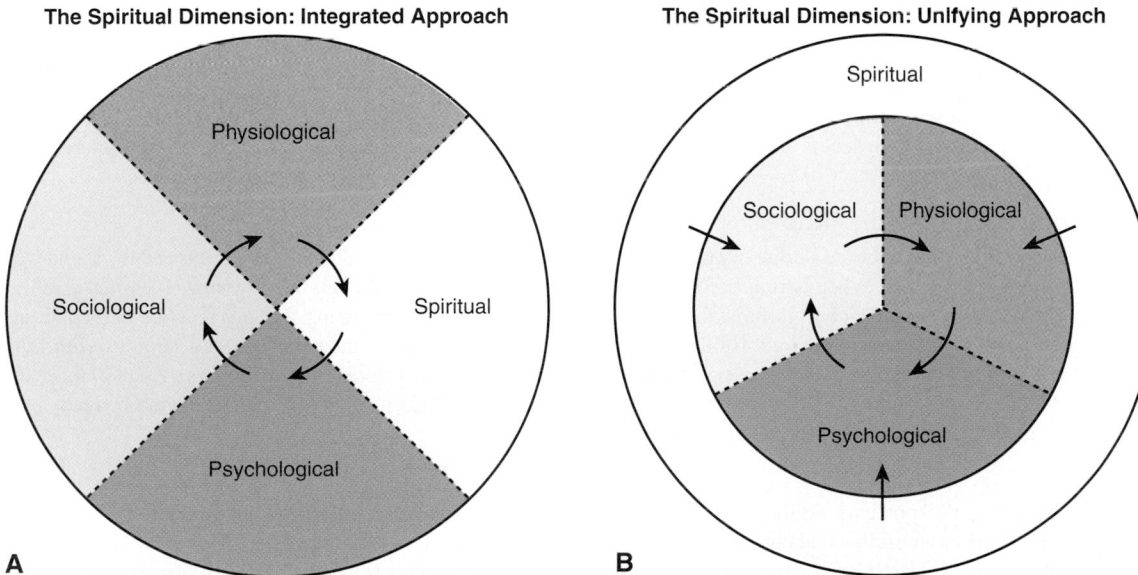

The Spiritual Dimension: Integrated Approach

Physiological

Sociological

Spiritual

Psychological

A

The Spiritual Dimension: Unifying Approach

Spiritual

Sociological

Physiological

Psychological

B

FIGURE 36-1 Spiritual dimensions. No consensus exists about the role of the spiritual dimension in health. (**A**) The *integrated approach* views each of the four dimensions as equal and influencing one another. (**B**) The *unifying model* grounds the biologic, psychological, and social dimensions in the spiritual dimension. (Redrawn from Farran, C. J., Fitchett, G., Quiring-Emblen, C. J., & Burk, J. R. [1989]. Development of a model for spiritual assessment and intervention. *Journal of Religion and Health, 28*[3], 185.)

and Fish (1988), there are three **spiritual needs** underlying all religious traditions and common to all people:

1. Need for meaning and purpose
2. Need for love and relatedness
3. Need for forgiveness

Although nurses may differ in their beliefs about how involved they should become in meeting patients' spiritual needs, it is impossible to nurse individuals well while ignoring the spiritual dimensions of health. Nurses can assist patients to meet spiritual needs by offering a compassionate presence; assisting in the struggle to find meaning and purpose in the face of suffering, illness, and death; fostering relationships (with God/humans) that nurture the spirit; and facilitating the patient's expression of religious or spiritual beliefs and practices. (For an example, see Reflective Practice: Challenge to Intellectual Skills.)

CONCEPTS RELATED TO SPIRITUALITY AND SPIRITUAL HEALTH

Spirituality, faith, and religion, and how these elements influence everyday living and health and illness are important concepts for the nurse to understand when caring for patients. Although some use the words "spirituality," "faith," and "religion" interchangeably, there are distinctions.

Spirituality

Spirituality is anything that pertains to a person's relationship with a nonmaterial life force or higher power. Whereas one person describes spirituality in terms of coming to

---

Reflective Practice
Challenge to Intellectual Skills

During my pediatric rotation I encountered a Hmong family from Laos whose 8-year-old son, Kou, had horribly deformed feet. It seemed as if the entire healthcare team was united to persuade, cajole, and if necessary force Choi Min Lai, Kou's father, and his mother to authorize a series of surgical repairs. But the parents were adamant in their refusal. In their culture, the deformity was a sign of spiritual favor and good luck. They believed that a warrior ancestor whose own feet were wounded in battle would be released from a form of spiritual entrapment because of their son's condition. This made Kou special in their community. I admired their fierce championing of their beliefs, but my heart ached for Kou because of the difficulties he would face in US society if his feet were not repaired. I didn't know anything about the Hmong culture or their beliefs. As a result, I didn't know which side I should support. I also didn't know much about the legal rights of the parents to refuse a procedure, which although not life-saving would clearly benefit their son.

Thinking Outside the Box: Possible Courses of Action

- Remain detached from the conflict and just observe.
- Try to learn more about the family's cultural and religious beliefs to see if this information could be helpful.
- Contact the hospital attorney to find out about the legal rights of the parents to refuse a procedure that while not life-saving would clearly benefit their son.

- Use my relationship with the family to try to persuade them to comply.
- Use my knowledge of Kou and his family to try to persuade the healthcare team to respect their wishes.

Evaluating a Good Outcome: How Do I Define Success?

- The health care team chooses a course of action that is beneficial to Kou and simultaneously respects the family's religious and cultural beliefs.

- We respect the legal rights of this family.
- My knowledge of the Hmong religion and culture is increased.
- I am faithful to my advocacy obligations.

Personal Learning: Here's to the Future!

Unfortunately, this issue was not resolved during my rotation. In fact, the conflict continued to grow. When I completed my rotation, the hospital was appealing to the court to force the parents to accept surgery. I came to believe that the rights of the parents should be respected. Their cultural community was so strong, and they clearly did not see Kou's condition as a correctable "health problem" but rather a blessing to be enjoyed. While a few other

nurses felt the way I did, the physicians and the social worker felt strongly that the parents were wrong. I learned a lot about the Hmong culture, realizing that my practice will continue to surprise me as I encounter patients and families with beliefs and practices very different from mine. As a result of this experience, I hope I will keep an open mind and always be ready to learn.

Reflection

How do you think you would respond in a similar situation? Why? What does this tell you about yourself and about the adequacy of your skills for professional practice? Can you think of other ways to respond? What influence do you imagine the Lais' culture and religion had on their spirituality? How might the spirituality of the physicians influence their actions? The social worker? Other members of the healthcare team? What other skills (cognitive, interpersonal, technical, ethical/legal) would you need to respond well in this situation? Do you agree with the criteria to evaluate a successful outcome? Based on the information provided in Personal Learning, do you think that a successful outcome would be achieved? Why or why not? What would you determine to be a successful outcome?

know, love, and serve God, another speaks of transcending the limits of body and experiencing a universal energy. Spirituality is not something that runs parallel to the rest of human life; rather, it is, in the words of theologian Karl Rahner (1971, p. 229):

> simply the ultimate depth of everything spiritual crea-tures do when they realize themselves—when they laugh or cry, accept responsibility, love, live and die, stand up for truth, break out of preoccupation with themselves to help the neighbor, hope against hope, cheerfully refuse to be embittered by the stupidity of daily life, keep silent, not so that evil festers in their hearts, but so that it dies there—when, in a word, they live as they would like to live in opposition to selfishness and to the despair that always assails us.

Elements of spirituality include:

- Spirituality is experienced as a unifying force, life princi-ple, essence of being.
- Spirituality is expressed and experienced in and through connectedness with nature, the earth, the environment, and the cosmos.
- People express and experience spirituality in and through connectedness with other people.
- Spirituality shapes the self-becoming and is reflected in one's being, knowing, and doing.
- Spirituality permeates life, providing purpose, meaning, strength, and guidance and shaping the journey (Burghardt & Nagai-Jacobson, 1997).

Faith

Faith generally refers to a confident belief in something for which there is no proof or material evidence. It can involve a person, idea, or thing, and it is usually followed by action re-lated to the ideals or values of that belief. For example, if I have faith in my doctor, parish nurse, or healer, I am more likely to adhere to a prescribed regimen/plan of care and to ex-perience benefits. Similarly, patients who believe in a loving and all-powerful God who knows them and cares for them are often better able to cope with the suffering related to injury and illness. The declaration made by the World Conference of the Religions of Peace in Kyoto, Japan, in 1970 is an excellent example of a confident belief in something for which there is no proof or material evidence. Baha'i, Buddhist, Confucian, Christian, Hindu, Jain, Jew, Muslim, Shintoist, Sikh, and others discovered that the things that unite them were more important than those that divided them. They discovered that they shared:

- A conviction of the fundamental unity of the human fam-ily, of the quality and dignity of all human beings
- A sense of the sacredness of the individual person and his conscience
- A sense of the value of the human community
- A belief that love, compassion, unselfishness, and the force of inner truthfulness and of the spirit have ultimately greater power than hate, enmity, and self-interest

- A sense of obligation to stand on the side of the poor and the oppressed as against the rich and the oppressors
- A profound hope that good will finally prevail

Faith is a term that may also be used to describe a cul-tural or institutional religion, such as Judaism, Muslim, or Confucianism.

An **atheist** is a person who denies the existence of a God; an **agnostic** is one who holds that nothing can be known about the existence of a God. The agnostic and the atheist are guided by philosophies of living that do not include a re-ligious faith. They deserve respect for what they choose to believe, just as do those who accept a particular religious creed.

Hope

Hope is the ingredient in life responsible for a positive outlook in even life's bleakest moments. It enables an individual both to consider a future and to actively bring that future into being. Hope originates in imagination but must become a valued and realistic possibility in order to energize action. Hope has the capacity to embrace the reality of the individual's suffering without escaping from it (false hope) or being suffocated by it (despair, helplessness, hopelessness). Hope is unique to each person. Box 33-6 in Chapter 33 contains a set of suggestions for enabling hope in the terminally ill that were developed by an interdisciplinary team of those providing care for the termi-nally ill, but they apply to any situation in which individuals feel hopeless (Creen, 2002).

Love

Above we noted that people express and experience spiritual-ity in and through connectedness with other people. The pop-ular musical "Les Miserables" noted in one of its songs, "To love another person is to see the face of God." Love develops from the basic human need to love and be loved, and we can-not be spiritually whole, spiritually healthy, unless this need is met.

Spiritual Health or Well-Being

Defined most simply, spiritual health or well-being is the condition that exists when the universal spiritual needs for meaning and purpose, love and belonging, and forgiveness are met. Sociologist of religion David Moberg (1979) identi-fied spiritual well-being as relating to the "wellness or health of the totality of the inner resources of people, the ultimate concerns around which all other values are focused, the cen-tral philosophy of life that guides conduct, and the meaning giving center of human life which influences all individual and social behavior" (p. 2). O'Brien's conceptual model of spiritual well-being in illness (Fig. 36-2) identifies three em-pirical referents of spiritual well-being: personal faith, reli-gious practice, and spiritual contentment.

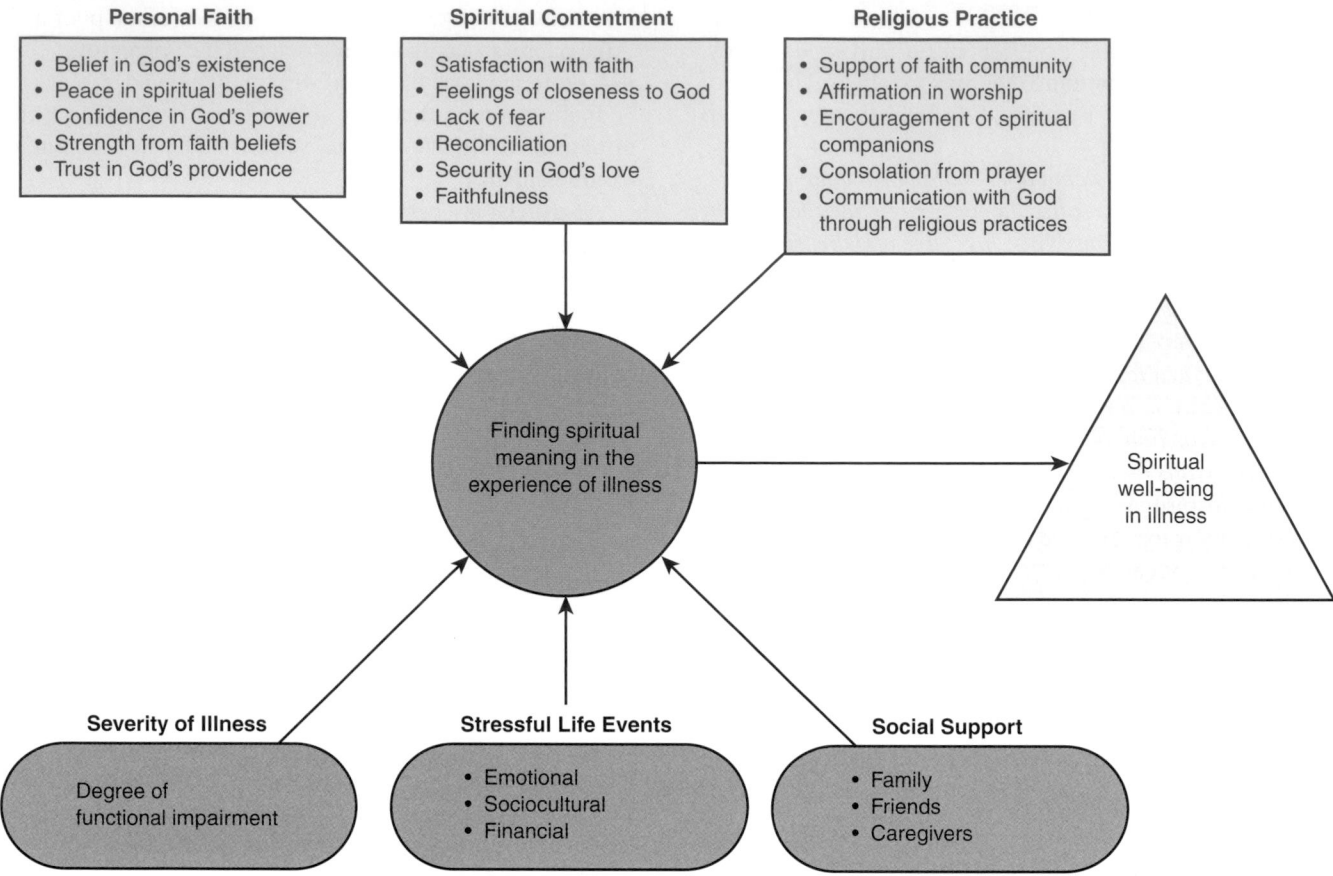

FIGURE 36-2 A conceptual model of spiritual well-being in illness. (Used with permission from O'Brien, M. E. [2003]. *Parish nursing: Healthcare ministry within the church* (p. 109). Boston: Jones and Bartlett.

Religion

Spirituality may include **religion,** which refers to an organized system of beliefs about a higher power. Set forms of worship, spiritual practices, and codes of conduct often characterize religions. Nurses care for people from many different religious traditions. Although it is impossible for nurses to be knowledgeable about all religions, nurses are better able to meet a patient's spiritual needs when they understand his or her religious beliefs and practices. These can directly influence the patient's response to illness and suffering, self-care practices such as diet and hygiene, birth and death rituals, gender roles, spiritual practices, and moral codes. A brief description of the beliefs and health practices of major religious traditions in the United States is provided in Table 36-1. Nurses who are unfamiliar with a patient's religion can gain valuable knowledge by reading (see Carson's [1989] *Spiritual Dimensions of Nursing Practice*) and through discussions with the patient and the patient's family and spiritual adviser.

Recall Choi Min Lai, the father of the 8-year-old boy with foot deformities who is refusing surgical repair based on his cultural and reli-

gious beliefs. Researching information about the patient's beliefs would be essential in planning this family's care and advocating for the patient and his family.

It is important that the nurse never presume to know what a patient's religious beliefs are upon learning that a patient is, for example, Jewish or Muslim because many religious groups and individuals work out their own set of beliefs and practices. Also, the nurse should not interpret the fact that a patient does not belong to an organized religion to mean that the patient has no spiritual needs; a person may be deeply spiritual yet not profess a religion.

Spirituality and Everyday Living

Spiritual beliefs and practices are associated with all aspects of a person's life, including health and illness. According to Quinn (2002), the major wisdom traditions address the invisible Spirit—a creative, mysterious, guiding power—by creating principles and practices that:

• Cultivate love of ourselves, our neighbors, of God, and of nature

TABLE 36-1 Beliefs and Healthcare Practices of Major Religious Traditions in the United States

Religion	Beliefs	Select Healthcare Practices
Adventist	Believe in the individual's choice and God's sovereignty. The body is believed to be the temple of the Holy Spirit.	• The taking of all narcotics and stimulants is prohibited because the body is the temple of the Holy Spirit and should be protected. Many groups prohibit meat. • Many regard Saturday as the Sabbath. • Approach to healthcare is holistic.
American Muslim Mission	Accept the Koran as their sacred scripture (see Islam); most stress the importance of cooperation among blacks in business and education to build self-esteem.	• Members are encouraged to obtain healthcare provided by members of the black community. • Major tenets involve prayer rituals, dietary restrictions (prohibitions against pork and alcohol), hygiene (extreme cleanliness), lifestyle modifications, and marital faithfulness.
Baha'i International Community	Believe in a basic harmony between religion and science	• Seek out competent medical care and pray for health • Obligatory prayers, holy days, and the 19-day fast • Permanent sterilization is prohibited, and abortion is discouraged.
Buddhism	Buddha or "the Great Physician" taught the Four Noble Truths to indicate the range of "suffering," its "origin," its "cessation," and the "way" that leads to its cessation. The real cause of human suffering is ignorant craving. The Noble Eightfold Path, which consists of right views, aspirations, speech, conduct, mode of livelihood, effort, mindfulness, and concentration, leads to the cessation of suffering.	• Buddhist hospitals for sick humans and sick animals antedated anything similar found in the West. • Buddhists do not outwardly proclaim healing through faith. However, spiritual peace and liberation from anxiety attained through the awakening to Buddha's wisdom may be an important factor in expediting healing and the recovery process. • Accepts modern science. The doctrine of avoidance of extremes is applied to the use of drugs, blood, vaccines. • Buddhism does not condone taking lives of any form. • Check with the patient about any special diet restrictions and the observance of holy days.
Christian Scientist	They deny the existence of health crises; sickness and sin are errors of the human mind and can be overcome by altering thoughts, not by using drugs or medicines.	• They will use orthopedic services to set a bone but decline drugs and, in general, other medical or surgical procedures. • They do not allow hypnotism or any form of psychotherapy, which alters the "Divine Mind." • A Christian Science Practitioner may be called to administer spiritual support. • Alcohol and tobacco are not used.
Church of Jesus Christ of Latter Day Saints (Mormons)	Devout adherents believe in divine healing through the "laying on of hands," though many do not prohibit medical therapy. The Church maintains an extensive and well-funded welfare system, including financial support for the sick.	• Disapprove of alcohol, tobacco, and caffeinated beverages • A special undergarment worn by some members should be removed only in an emergency.

(continued)

TABLE 36-1 (Continued)

Religion	Beliefs	Select Healthcare Practices
Confucianism	Inherent in Confucianism is the appreciation of life and the desire to keep the body from untimely or unnecessary death.	• Appreciate life and desire to keep the body from untimely or unnecessary death • Historically emphasized public health solutions to impending health problems
Daoism (Taoism)	Health is a manifestation of the harmony of the universe, obtained through the proper balancing of internal and external forces. Implicit throughout the Daoist tradition is the tendency to understand salvation in the biomedical sense of health and qualitative improvement and prolongation of human life. The universal principle of the Tao is the mysterious biologic and spiritual life rhythm or order of nature.	• There is a "medicinal" concern for maintaining and prolonging human health and life (sheng). Knowing and living a natural life—following the Tao—is the secret of both health and sagehood. • Long tradition of seeking pragmatic medical techniques, along with its religious techniques of meditation and ritual for establishing a harmony of body and spirit, humanity, and nature (holistic approach)
Hinduism	Doctrine of Transmigration. Moral factors, linked with the all-embracing doctrine of "karma," were believed to be significant in promoting health or causing disease.	• Hindu medicine shows a surprising openness to new ideas, at least in respect to practical treatment. • Many Hindu dietary restrictions conform to individual sect doctrine. • The nurse administering medications should avoid touching patient's lips. • Certain prescribed rites are followed after death; disposal of the body is by cremation.
Jehovah's Witnesses	They oppose the "false teachings" of other sects; opposition often extends to modern science, including medicine.	• Blood transfusions violate God's laws and therefore are not allowed. Alternative treatments include use of nonblood plasma expanders, surgical techniques to decrease blood loss, and autotransfusions through use of a heart–lung machine. • The courts have not supported the right of Jehovah Witness parents to refuse life-saving treatment for their children. • Use of alcohol and tobacco are discouraged.
Judaism	Formation closely bound with a divine revelation and with commitment to obedience to God's will. The Hebrew Bible is the authority, guide, and inspiration of the many forms of religion of the Jews (currently Reform, Conservative, and Orthodox).	• For observant Jews: special needs in the areas of diet, birth rituals, male and female contact, and death • Treatment and procedures should not be scheduled on the Sabbath.
Islam	Allah, one God, who is only one, all seeing, all hearing, all speaking, all knowing, all willing, all powerful Must be able to practice the Five Pillars of Islam May have a fatalistic view of health	• Obligatory prayers, holy days, and fasting (Ramadan), and almsgiving • Koranic law and customs that influence birth, diet (eating pork and drinking alcohol are forbidden), care of women, death and prayer rituals • Women are not allowed to make independent decisions, and husbands need to be present when consent is sought.
Native American Religions	Difficult to generalize; notion of cosmic harmony, emphasis on directly experiencing powers and visions and a common view of the cycle of life and death. Death is not the end but the beginning of new life (reincarnation or transcendent hereafter).	• Rituals mark important life changes: birth, puberty, initiation rites, death. • Medicine men and women have specialized spirits from whom they receive the mission to cure. • Common therapeutic measures: sucking, blowing, and drawing out with a feather fan

(continued)

TABLE 36-1 (Continued)

Religion	Beliefs	Select Healthcare Practices
Protestantism	Worship of the one God revealed to the world through Jesus Christ. Love of neighbor is a central tenet. Other beliefs include sin, redemption, salvation, and a final accounting with God. Care of sick encouraged. God the author and giver of life is also the healer. Most accept modern medical science.	• Religious practices vary according to denomination, may include prayer, faith healing, "laying on of hands," and anointing. • Sacraments: baptism, communion, confirmation
Roman Catholicism	Worship of the one God revealed to the world through Jesus Christ. Love of neighbor is a central tenet. Other beliefs include sin, redemption, salvation, and a final accounting with God. Care of sick encouraged. God the author and giver of life is also the healer. Human life is a gift of God. Many take an antiabortion stance, most accept modern medical science.	• Importance of private devotions and Mass attendance on Sunday • Seven sacraments (importance of baptism, eucharist, penance, and the anointing of the sick) • Dietary habits • Sexual ethical norms • Only natural means of birth control; abortion, euthanasia, and sterilization are forbidden
Unification Church	God is the living, eternal person who represents universal love and care. God created the world and humans to reflect his nature. The goal of the Unification Church is to unite Christians everywhere as one family under God.	• Most members are still healthy young adults. There is little information available on their interactions with the healthcare team.
Unitarian Universal Association of Churches and Fellowships	Encourage creativity, reason, and living an ethical life. No member is required to adhere to a given creed or set of religious beliefs. The inherent worth and dignity of every person is affirmed.	• Free to accept what they take to be best for their health

- Cultivate wisdom that helps us find meaning in life, be in relationship with others, be true to ourselves, live in uncertainty and mystery, deal with suffering, sickness, and death, and honor life's transitions (like birth, marriage, and death)
- Cultivate awareness of the sacred dimension of life through practices such as worship, prayer, meditation, and singing
- Respect our connectedness as fellow human beings while acknowledging our differences
- Help us be generous in service to others (pp. 13–14)

Religious influences may be life affirming or life denying. Life-affirming influences enhance life, give meaning and purpose to existence, strengthen one's feelings of self-worth, encourage self-actualization, and are health giving and life sustaining. Life-denying influences restrict or enclose life patterns, limit experiences and associations, place burdens of guilt on individuals, encourage feelings of unworthiness, and are generally health denying and life inhibiting.

Spirituality, Health, and Illness

Spiritual beliefs are of special importance to nurses because of the many ways they can influence a patient's level of health and self-care behaviors.

Guide to Daily Living Habits

Certain practices generally associated with healthcare may have religious significance for a patient. For example, many religions have dietary requirements and restrictions. Acceptable birth-control practices are determined by some religious faiths, as are some types of medical treatments (see Table 36-1; Fig. 36-3).

Source of Support

Many people seek support from their religious faith during times of stress. This support is often vital to the acceptance of an illness, especially if the illness brings with it a prolonged period of convalescence or indicates a questionable outcome. Prayer, devotional reading, and other religious practices often do for the person spiritually what protective exercises do for the body physically.

Think back to Margot Zeuner, the 75-year-old woman caring for her husband with advanced Alzheimer's disease. Assessment reveals that Mrs. Zeuner derived much support from her church group. The nurse, acknowledging the importance of this aspect, could work with Mrs. Zeuner to arrange for assistance at home so that she could attend

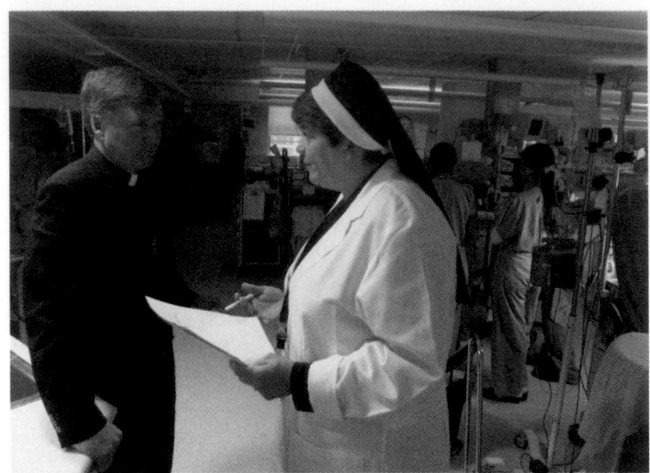

FIGURE 36-3 A nurse ethicist confers with the hospital chaplain before meeting with Catholic parents who have tough decisions to make about how aggressively to treat their newborn.

church activities and continue to receive the support she needs.

Box 36-1 describes how one religion, Buddhism, sees the divine grounding for all human experience, including suffering.

Source of Strength and Healing

The values derived from religious faith cannot be enumerated or evaluated easily. However, the effects attributable to faith are constantly in evidence to healthcare workers. People have been known to endure extreme physical distress because of strong faith. Patients' families have taken on almost unbelievable rehabilitative tasks because they had faith in the eventual positive results of their effort. In "Through the Eyes of a Patient," a woman who was faced with life-threatening events describes what she means by healing, and a caregiver describes a memorable encounter with a burn victim in "Through the Eyes of a Caregiver."

Source of Conflict

Sometimes religious beliefs conflict with prevalent healthcare practices (see Table 36-1). For example, the doctrine of the Jehovah's Witnesses prohibits blood transfusions. In the Islamic religion, humans are regarded as largely helpless in controlling their environment, and illness is accepted as their fate rather than something against which action might be taken. Some Navajos use a lengthy religious ceremony to cure certain diseases, such as tuberculosis. For some people, illness is viewed as punishment for sin and is therefore inevitable.

Such beliefs may require the healthcare worker to modify a treatment plan to accommodate the person's religion. In some instances, acknowledgment of the patient's religious convictions and efforts by health practitioners to accommodate the patient's beliefs can result in quality healthcare without violating the person's religious practices. In other situations, an objective explanation of alternative treatments and the predicted consequences of each may help the patient determine acceptable therapy. Whatever the person's decision about healthcare, the nurse should remember that each person is unique and has a right to pursue his or her own convictions, even though they may differ from those of the healthcare provider.

Health care professionals can reduce conflict by attempting to understand how a particular religious culture influences people's thinking about basic questions of biology and ethics. Some of the major questions that religious beliefs, attitudes, and values can color include:
- What is the meaning of suffering?
- How should we regard the physical body and its functions?
- What is the meaning and role of gender differences, sexuality, and reproduction?
- How are we to understand and respond to birth, aging, and death?
- What constitutes the self, and how is selfhood to be assessed?
- How are sin and moral culpability understood? What makes something sinful, and how is sin relieved or absolved?
- What are the tradition's specific bioethical teachings?

Remember Choi Min Lai, described at the beginning of this chapter. The nurse could use these questions to assess the family's beliefs in greater depth, providing significant data for the healthcare team to incorporate when discussing the possibility of surgery to repair Kou's deformities. Doing so could be helpful in

---

BOX 36-1 The Center Point That Grounds Us . . .

. . . I could scarcely make out the large sitting Buddha near the entrance of the house. But what caught my attention was the metal circle with spokes resembling a wheel, hanging over the figure of the Buddha. . . . I asked our host about the wheel. I was told it represented our eternal journey in this life and continuing into the next. Buddha's teachings say that life is suffering. We cannot avoid suffering as we move around the rim of the wheel, which represents perpetual change and the transitory nature of life. But the wheel also symbolizes wholeness or completion because the wheel revolves around the center axis that does not move. That center point represents the presence of the divine. If we remain aware of this center point, we are strengthened for whatever lies ahead.

. . . It is this center point that grounds us in the midst of the many changes in our lives. It is at the center point where we experience the energy and power that turns the wheel. It is at this center point that we connect with the Everywhere Spirit. When we rest in the center point, we find that we have come home again to the place from which we started. But because of the journey, it is as if we had arrived home for the first time. In our journey around the circles of life, we become new persons over and over again.

(From Susan Gregg-Schroeder, *The Journal of Fellowship in Prayer*, April 1999.)

Through the Eyes of a
Patient

Seven years ago I was faced with three life-threatening events in a period of 3 years. Those life-threatening experiences taught me that it is possible to "heal" and to live fully even when we are in the abyss of suffering. I believe everyone would benefit if we redefined "healing." Here are elements I now include in my definition.

Healing is:
- Becoming whole, a life-long journey of becoming fully human, involving the totality of our being: body, mind, emotion, spirit, social and political context, as well as our relationships with others and with the Divine. Healing does not necessarily mean being happy or getting what we think we want out of life; it means growth, often with pain.
- Becoming our authentic self, releasing old unreal self-images, discovering who we really are, not what we think we should be, knowing why we are here and what we really value, restoring our ability to heed our aspirations.
- Reconnecting lost aspects of ourselves, paying attention to buried feelings and places inside us that are distressed or sick, enabling us to express our self in fullness, both the light and shadow sides.
- Being open to change and new possibilities; responding to problems by changing the picture; being willing to let in more life, to open up to what may have been previously closed or destroyed for us and that which holds promise of giving us new life and fulfillment.
- Facing our fears and refusing to be injured or wounded; changing our belief systems; breaking unnecessary taboos; letting go of what is familiar, and stepping into the unknown.
- Accepting that problems, pain, and suffering are part of life and inseparable from us—not a peripheral relationship, not something isolated and avoidable—enabling us to enter into problems and use suffering, pain, and life-threatening events to enrich our lives.

- Being empowered by the Divine; discovering meaning in our defects, disorders, problems, and disease; experiencing new degrees of creativity and life forces that we might never have imagined before our difficulty; finding that our pains and fears are transformed into relief and confidence.
- Recognizing the value and preciousness of life, knowing that every moment is unique and significant, which usually leads to greater appreciation of the wonder of our minds, bodies, and spirits and of the Divine.
- Having faith and hope—important preconditions for mental and physical health; having a belief in the Divine, the meaning of human life, and the universe; helping us to claim our capacity to create and make something new.
- Finding inner peace, contentment, and tranquility amid the realities of daily life, including its problems, changes, and chaos; experiencing a sense of fullness that makes the burdens of pain or illness lighter.
- Being forgiving of ourselves and others and being forgiven; giving ourselves and others the freedom to let go of rivalry, strife, anger, hatred, fear, and limitations.
- Feeling connected to one another, a sense of interdependence; knowing we are not isolated or autonomous, giving up the illusions of boundaries in life; taking responsibility, acting justly, and accepting that we share our humanity.
- Being loving and loved; loving one's self and wanting to love and serve others, as well as being capable of receiving love; having an ability to trust, a feeling of aliveness, and a sense of greater participation in life.

Used with permission. Carol, J. (2002). What is healing? Sacred Journey, 53(4), 33–35.

---

minimizing the conflict between the family and healthcare team.

FACTORS AFFECTING SPIRITUALITY

Among the many factors that can influence a person's spirituality, the most important are developmental considerations, family, ethnic background, formal religion, and life events.

Developmental Considerations

Because spirituality has to do with the nonmaterial realm of being, a child must have some capacity for abstract thought before he or she can begin to understand the spiritual self. But this is not to say that spirituality is meaningless for children. David Heller (1985) interviewed 40 children between 4 and 12 years

old who were affiliated with one of four major religions (Judaism, Roman Catholicism, Protestantism, or Hinduism) and discovered that the children had definite perceptions of God. Central themes in all the children's descriptions included the following:
- Notion of a God who works through human intimacy and the interconnectedness of lives
- Belief that God is involved in self-change and growth and transformations that make the world fresh, alive, and meaningful
- Attributing to God tremendous and expansive power and then showing considerable anxiety in the face of this power
- Image of light

As the child matures, life experiences usually influence and mature his or her spiritual beliefs. With advancing years, the tendency to think about life after death prompts some individuals to re-examine and reaffirm their spiritual beliefs. Chapter 18 describes the stages of faith development.

Through the Eyes of a Caregiver

What's a nice nurse like me doing in a place like this? I belong in Labor and Delivery, with mothers and babies, not in front of our ER trying to help! It is September 11, 2001. Still can't believe what I hear, what I have seen: the World Trade Center buildings, the Pentagon, Pittsburgh. We are at war—oh no! not us! We are the U.S. We don't do homeland war; we are safe.

Oh God! A motorcycle—the driver screaming, "Wounded! Wounded! Pentagon wounded." A hoax? But wait: this is real. No one here to help but me. "How can I help?"

The Pentagon injured—they're coming! His uniform burned but not past recognition. A soldier of the U.S. Army. A U.S. Army officer on a cardboard stretcher, unloaded from the back of an SUV. Time stands still.

"You rode on the sidewalk to get here? The roads were closed?"

His medals still shine.

"I'm here to help you. I will take care of you. Tell me your name."

"I am Brian, and I know you will take care of me. You and God."

Race. Hurry. Run! Doctors, nurses, technicians. Pull, lift. Monitors, IVs, catheters.

"I'm here to help you. I will take care of you."

"I am Brian, and I know you will take care of me. You and God."

His finger is swelling. His ring, it must come off.

"This will hurt, Brian."

"No problem, Ma'am. Just hurry!"

Pull. Pull again. Try harder. Burned skin comes with it. I put it close to my heart. A pocketed wedding ring of a brave man. I am

going to lose it—but his wife will be here soon. Don't lose it. Another soldier.

"Do you know Brian? Take this ring. It's in your pocket now, officer, find his wife."

ET tubes, EKGs, x-rays. Pain pain pain.

"You must be Brian's wife. I am so sorry."

How to tell the children? Call his mother? He will be spared. Where was he, the E ring? What did he say to you?

"Before he lost consciousness he told me that God and I were caring for him. He told me he would be OK. He told me he loved you very much. His faith was with him every minute."

Burns, creams, bandages. Lungs OK? Head injury? Critical Care.

I am so angry! This is so wrong, unfair, personal now. I am scared! Whop! whop! whop! The helicopter. Unfrozen air space—for Brian. The Washington Hospital Burn Center.

"I am here to help you. They will take care of you. Good-bye, Brian."

The roads have been closed—tough commute—a whole month! They're reopened today. The Pentagon, a first look. I can see it! Oh, my God, help us! The radio, Q107 News.

"Good news tonight. Word from Washington Hospital Center is that Lt. Colonel Brian . . . has been upgraded from critical condition to stable condition."

Brian, we will never forget. Thank you for letting me take care of you, me and God. You are a hero.

Judith Rogers, RN
Clinical Educator, Labor and Delivery
Georgetown University

Family

A child's parents play a key role in the development of the child's spirituality. What is important is not so much what parents teach a child about God and religion but rather what the child learns about God, life, and self from the parents' behavior.

Ethnic Background

Religious traditions differ among ethnic groups. There are clear distinctions between Eastern and Western spiritual traditions as well as among those of individual ethnic groups, such as Native Americans. A person's culture and formal religion have much to do with whether the basic approach to religion is doing something, being someone, or continually striving for harmony.

Formal Religion

Each of the major religious groups discussed earlier in this chapter has several characteristics in common:
- Basis of authority or source of power
- Scripture or sacred word

- An ethical code that defines right and wrong
- A psychology and identity, so that its adherents fit into a group and the world is defined by the religion
- Aspirations or expectations
- Some ideas about what follows death

Life Events

Both positive and negative life experiences can influence spirituality, and they in turn are influenced by the meaning a person's spiritual beliefs attribute to them. For example, if two women who believe in a loving God both lose a child in a car accident, one may bitterly deny God's existence, whereas the other may spend more time in prayer asking God to help her. Similarly, a chain of successful life experiences (marriage, promotion) may cause one person to assume success and experience no need for God, whereas for another it occasions deep gratitude and rejoicing.

Recall Kevin O'Malley, the father of the 17-year-old critically injured in a car accident. As a result of the accident, Mr. O'Malley is questioning his spiritual beliefs. An understanding of the effects of life events on an individual would be important for the nurse when developing a plan of care of Mr. O'Malley.

RELIGION AND LAW, ETHICS, AND MEDICINE

Christian Scientists, Jehovah's Witnesses, and members of faith-healing groups are among those challenging the intricate web of rights and responsibilities among individual, society, church, and state. These religious bodies are asking for protection, under the veil of religious freedom, of their right to exercise individual decisions in accordance with scriptural interpretations, even though those decisions may result in the individual's own death or that of a family member, including a child. The most troubling cases are those in which treatable problems, such as bacterial meningitis, diabetes, and bowel obstruction, resulted in the death of minors whose parents chose religious means of healing over traditional medicine. (See Focused Critical Thinking Guide 36-1.) The American Academy of Pediatrics is urging that all child abuse, neglect, and medical neglect statutes be applied without potential or actual exemption for religious beliefs.

Perhaps even more troubling for nurses are situations in which family members insist on care deemed medically futile (ie, the likelihood of medical benefit is virtually nonexistent) because they believe that God is going to work a miracle. In these cases, simple nursing measures, such as turning or bathing patients, become occasions of pain and torment to both the patient and nurse. Nurses are forced to administer care that they take to be cruel and abusive to patients capable of experiencing pleasure and pain. This nursing care can needlessly prolong a patient's dying. Unfortunately, there are no clear guidelines for drawing the line between promoting life and prolonging the dying process. Although nurses always have the moral right to withdraw from administering care that violates their personal moral code, this does not resolve the problem for the patient. More dialog is needed on the interaction between religion and law, ethics, and medicine. Ideally, the religious freedom of patients and their families is respected, as is the moral autonomy of caregivers and the integrity of the healing professions.

Consider the situation of Choi Min Lai, the father described at the beginning of this chapter. The nurse is required to respect the family's religious freedom and advocate for them while at the same time acting as a professional member of the healthcare team.

PARISH NURSING

Parish nurse programs are a relatively new movement in faith communities from many denominations. They seek to reclaim the church's role in the ministry of healing and focus again on the impact that spirituality, caring relationships, and a responsibly balanced life can have on health and wellness.

According to Nist (2003), parish nurses and health ministry teams work to reintegrate the healing tradition into the life of faith communities by:

- Interpreting the relationship between faith and health
- Promoting personal responsibility for health and wellness
- Serving as health counselors and educators
- Keeping aware of available resources and making appropriate referrals
- Acting as advocates for people who have health needs but only limited resources
- Recruiting and training volunteers
- Visiting church members
- Initiating caring relationships with the elderly, the chronically ill, and the "worried well" (p. 50)

What parish nurses are not are "visiting nurses" or "home health nurses" who provide direct bedside care. The key roles of the parish nurse are health educator, personal health counselor, referral agent, trainer of volunteers, developer of support groups, integrator of faith and health, and health advocate (Holstrom, 1999, p. 69). Nurses who wish to be parish nurses must be registered and compliant with both the state or province practice act and "Scope and Standards of Parish Nursing Practice" (American Nurses Association, 1998).

THE NURSING PROCESS

Before reading further, use the accompanying box, Promoting Health 36-1, to see how well you are meeting your own spiritual needs. This same tool may be used with patients. Many nurses approach professional practice as more than a "job" and use the language of "sacred calling" or "vocation" to describe their career choice. "Through the Eyes of a Caregiver" gives the prayer of one such nurse.

Assessing

Nursing History

Because a person's spirituality and religious beliefs have the potential to influence every aspect of being, an assessment of the patient's spirituality should be included in each comprehensive nursing history. Data are gathered about the patient's spiritual beliefs and practices, the effect of these beliefs on everyday living, spiritual distress, and spiritual needs. O'Brien (1982), Shelly and Fish (1988), and Puchalski and Romer (2000) offer helpful assessment guides. O'Brien's "Spiritual Assessment Guide" (1982, p. 102) divides questions into several categories:

- Spiritual pain: Do you ever feel hurt or pain associated with the spiritual or religious beliefs that you hold? Do you feel pain related to uncertainty or nonbelief?
- Spiritual alienation: Do you frequently feel far away from God? Does it seem that He is remote and far removed from your everyday life?
- Spiritual anxiety: Are you afraid that God might not take care of your needs? That He might not be there when you need Him?

Focused Critical Thinking Guide 36-1

Spirituality

A 16-year-old student approaches you, the school nurse, and confides that she is worried about her brother, who is sick and getting sicker. "My parents are Christian Scientists and have had Christian Science Practitioners in to pray for him, but he seems to be getting worse. I'm afraid he'll die if we don't get him to the hospital." Your first impulse is to visit the student's home to try to see her brother and parents. You immediately remember an article in the paper about the Supreme Court's decision to let stand a Minnesota Court of Appeals ruling upholding an award of $1.5 million to the father of a boy who died in 1989 after his mother, stepfather, and two Christian Scientist Practitioners tried to use prayer to heal his diabetes. Despite their efforts, the boy slipped into a coma and died. What is troubling you is the following comment by Stephen Carter: "By refusing to intervene in *McKown v. Lundman*, the Supreme Court has reinforced a societal message that has grown depressingly common: It is perfectly OK to believe in the power of prayer, so long as one does not believe in it so sincerely that one actually expects it to work—a peculiar fate indeed for our "most inalienable" right" (Carter, S. L. [Jan. 31, 1996]. The power of prayer, denied. *The New York Times*, A17). You do believe in the power of prayer and are not sure how you should respond to the student's plea for help for her brother.

1. Identify Goal of Thinking

Clarify 1) what I believe about prayer's power to heal, and 2) what I believe about a parent's right to substitute prayer for modern medicine when a child is seriously ill. Decide how I should respond. What are my professional obligations?

2. Assess Adequacy of Knowledge

Pertinent circumstances: This is the first time I have encountered a family of Christian Scientists. As a school nurse I am not responsible for my student's brother if he is not in my school and place of employment. That said, I have been asked to help and have the resources to do so.

Prerequisite knowledge: I have no knowledge of what Christian Scientists believe. Moreover, I do not know how the law in our state responds to situations like these. I do not know if any nursing or medical groups have guidelines for situations like these. I immediately get on the Internet to address these deficiencies and also contact my professional nursing organization to see what the law is and if there are any professional organizations that have addressed this issue. I also have to find out how sick the student's brother is and the

probable consequences of his not seeking traditional medical care.

Room for error: The student's brother's very life may depend upon whether or not and how I choose to respond.

Time constraints: Until I learn the exact nature of the boy's medical problems I cannot know how urgent the need to intervene is.

3. Address Potential Problems

In a situation like this, the most obvious impediments to critical thinking would be (1) the unexamined belief that religion trumps all other considerations ("by golly, this country is founded on respect for religious freedom") and (2) the belief that modern medicine is owed to everyone with a life-threatening illness, no matter what other considerations are present.

4. Consult Helpful Resources

I decide to visit the boy's home with the student and call first to seek the parents' permission. After talking with the parents and seeing the boy, I believe that the boy is in a life-threatening situation because the parents were told that their son has diabetes. I am struck by the love and devotion of both parents and I learn via Internet research that they are doing exactly what their religion prescribes. I later consult with a local Christian Scientist group that confirms this. I learn from my professional nursing organization that there is no consensus about how society should respond in situations like these. Many believe that what these parents are doing is neglect and that if the boy dies, they should be held criminally accountable for manslaughter. Others respect their right to practice their religion. Uncertain of how I should respond, I decide to call Child Protective Services and tell them that I am willing to help if they think my relationship with the daughter would be helpful. I explain to my student what I am doing and tell her to keep me informed and to come back for help if she is not getting the assistance she needs.

5. Critique Judgment/Decision

Child Protective Services did intervene immediately, and the boy was hospitalized and treated against the parents' wishes. While I was happy that the boy's condition was stabilized, I did feel uncomfortable about the disrespect shown these obviously intelligent, devout, and loving parents. I decided to learn more about how different states are responding to these challenges and to see if nursing can't get involved in some way.

- Spiritual guilt: Have you ever done things that God would be angry at you for? Are you feeling badly about things that you have done or failed to do in your life?
- Spiritual anger: Are you angry at God for allowing you to be ill? Do you ever feel like blaming God for your illness? Do you think God is unfair to you?

- Spiritual loss: Do you ever feel that you have lost God's love? That you have broken or weakened your relationship with God? Has God turned his back on you?
- Spiritual despair: Do you ever feel that there is no hope of having God's love? Of pleasing him? That God does not love you anymore?

Promoting Health 36-1 *Spirituality*

Use the assessment checklist to determine how well you are meeting spirituality needs. Then develop a prescription for self-care by choosing appropriate behaviors from the list of suggestions.

ASSESSMENT CHECKLIST

almost always | sometimes | almost never

☐ ☐ ☐ 1. I am comfortable with my spiritual beliefs and values.

☐ ☐ ☐ 2. My beliefs meet my needs for love, belonging, forgiveness, meaning, and purpose.

☐ ☐ ☐ 3. I respect the belief systems of others.

☐ ☐ ☐ 4. I derive sufficient strength from my religious beliefs to meet each day's challenges, specially when confronting pain, suffering and death.

SELF-CARE BEHAVIORS

1. Explore personal values and beliefs of self and others.
2. Set aside regular periods to nurture spiritual self.
3. Explore practices that are spiritually supportive.
4. Demonstrate in interaction with others peace, inner strength, warmth, icy, caring, creativity.
5. Respect the belief systems of others.
6. Practice loving relationships with self and others.
7. Seek spiritual assistance to help cope with stress, crisis, or loss.

Additional sample questions are listed in Focused Assessment Guide 36-1.

If the patient reveals a spiritual problem, use interview questions to determine the specific nature of the problem, its probable causes, related signs and symptoms, when it began and how often it occurs, how it affects everyday living, the severity of the problem and whether it can be treated independently by nursing or needs to be referred, and how well the patient is coping with the problem.

Think back to Kevin O'Malley, the father of the 17-year-old girl in the critical care unit. The nurse could use these questions to determine Mr. O'Malley's beliefs, thereby developing a plan of care that addresses his current needs. Additionally, this assessment would provide valuable information about how the father is coping with the current situation.

Through the Eyes of a Caregiver

The Sacred Covenant: A Nurse's Prayer

Gentle God,
   You alone are the source of my strength and the center of my life;
   Bless my nursing that it may always be guided by the sacred covenant of Your loving care.
   Use me as Your instrument in serving the sick;
   Use my eyes to look with compassion on those who are broken in body or in spirit;
   Use my hands to touch with tenderness those who suffer illness or injury;
   Use my lips to speak words of comfort to those who are anxious or afraid.
Dear Lord,
   Let me recognize every sickroom as a tabernacle where You dwell; and
   Let me not forget, as I care for the ill, that
   The ground on which I am standing is holy,
   The vocation to which I am called is holy.
   Help me to be worthy.

*Used with permission. O'Brien, M. E. (2001).
The Nurse's Calling. New York: Paulist Press, p. x.*

Nursing Observation

Because many patients find it difficult to talk about their spiritual beliefs and problems, the nurse also observes the patient's behavior for signs of spiritual distress. A family member or close friend may share significant observations:

- "He's been awfully moody since his heart attack. I can't believe the change in him."
- "I've never seen my father so depressed. He's never in his life been away from the synagogue at Passover. I don't know how to help him."

Significant behavioral observations include sudden changes in spiritual practices (rejection, neglect, fanatical devotion), mood changes (frequent crying, depression, apathy, anger), sudden interest in spiritual matters (reading religious books or watching religious programs on television, visits to clergy), and disturbed sleep. A nurse who observes these behaviors should follow up with appropriate interview questions. Often, problems with spiritual distress do not surface until well after a patient's admission history and examination. Effective questions include the following:

- "You've been lying there so quietly. What are you thinking about?"

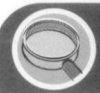

Focused Assessment Guide 36-1

Spirituality

Factors to Assess	Questions and Approaches
Spiritual beliefs	"Are there particular spiritual or religious beliefs that are important to you? Have these beliefs changed recently? Is your illness challenging these beliefs? Do your religious beliefs in any way dictate a course of action that puts you in conflict with what your physicians are recommending?"
Spiritual practices	"Describe your usual spiritual practices and anything interfering with your ability to perform them. Can I help in any way to secure the aids necessary for these practices (prayer shawl, Bible, crystals, beads, icon)?"
Relation between spiritual beliefs and everyday living	"Describe ways your spiritual beliefs affect everyday living (daily schedule, diet, hygiene, sense of self and the world, relationships). Do you find this influence to be healthy (life affirming) or destructive (life denying)?"
Spiritual deficit or distress	"Are your spiritual beliefs currently causing you any distress?"
Spiritual needs	"In what ways can I and the other nurses help you to meet your spiritual needs?" "Would you like me to contact your spiritual adviser or the hospital's pastoral care minister?"
Need for meaning and purpose	"In what ways do your religious beliefs help or hinder you to understand your current situation and face it with peace and courage?"
Need for love and relatedness	"In what ways do your religious beliefs help or hinder you to meet your need to love and be loved?"
Need for forgiveness	"In what ways do your religious beliefs help or hinder you to feel at peace?"
Significant behavioral observations	Be alert to sudden changes in spiritual practices, mood changes, sudden interest in spiritual matters, and sleep disturbances—all of which may point to unresolved spiritual needs.

- "After all you've been through, you must have done a good bit of soul searching. Experiences like these are enough to shake anyone's faith—how is yours holding up?"

Diagnosing

The nurse uses each phase of the nursing process when identifying and treating spiritual problems categorized as nursing diagnoses. The North American Nursing Diagnosis Association (NANDA, 1994) diagnoses related specifically to spirituality are Potential for Enhanced Spiritual Well-Being and Spiritual Distress

Potential for Enhanced Spiritual Well-Being: The process of an individual's developing/unfolding of mystery through harmonious interconnectedness that springs from inner strengths.

Spiritual Distress: Disruption in the life principle that pervades a person's entire being and that integrates and transcends one's biologic and psychosocial nature.

Spiritual distress may be further specified as spiritual pain, alienation, anxiety, guilt, anger, loss, or despair (O'Brien, 1982). Common etiologies for spiritual distress include inability to reconcile current life situation (eg, illness, death of loved person, divorce) with spiritual beliefs ("God is all-powerful, all-loving, all-wise, and He cares about me") or separation from the religious community or supports. Sample nursing diagnoses of spiritual distress are presented in Examples of NANDA Nursing Diagnoses.

Spiritual distress may affect other areas of human functioning. In the following nursing diagnoses, spiritual distress is the etiology of another problem.

- Impaired Adjustment to Illness related to inability to reconcile illness with spiritual beliefs
- Ineffective Individual Coping related to loss of religion as primary support (feels abandoned by God)
- Fear related to feeling unprepared for death and afterlife experience
- Dysfunctional Grieving: Despair related to belief that religion is meaningless
- Hopelessness related to belief that no one cares, including God
- Powerlessness related to feeling victimized by a tyrannical and arbitrary God
- Self-Esteem Disturbance related to failure to live according to dictates of religion
- Sexual Dysfunction related to values conflict
- Sleep Pattern Disturbance related to spiritual distress
- Risk for Self-Directed Violence related to feeling that life is meaningless

Examples of NANDA Nursing Diagnoses | Spiritual Distress*

Nursing Diagnoses	Related Factors	Sample Defining Characteristics
Spiritual Pain	Inability to accept death of son	A 46-year-old woman, agnostic, only son died 6 months ago (lung cancer) "I've often wondered throughout my life if there is a God—thought maybe if I had tried harder I'd have recognized him. Now I don't care if God exists or not because if he allows this I don't want to know him." "My son was my whole life; there's nothing left for me to live for." Lost 10 lb in 6 months since son died; leaves home only when necessary to purchase food, go to bank, and engage in other routine activities.
Spiritual Alienation	Separated from "faith community"	A 72-year-old Orthodox Jewish man, recently admitted to Protestant nursing home following 3-week hospitalization for stroke "I guess Yahweh has written me off; first the stroke that killed half my body and then I'm abandoned here where I can't even observe the Sabbath." "I want to go home."
Spiritual Anxiety	Challenged belief and value system	A 37-year-old previously healthy male executive recovering from massive myocardial infarction "My parents were strict Methodists, but when I left home for college I stopped going to church . . . never gave it much thought . . . there was always something else to do. I started going again but it never meant much." "I haven't exactly done anything awful but I've also not been a saint and I find myself wondering if there is a God, what does he think of me." "Funny, I guess I thought I'd live forever. I sure never thought about dying and what happens after that." Often observed lying quietly in bed awake; asked to see minister.
Spiritual Guilt	Failure to live according to religious rules	A 23-year-old, single, Baptist woman being treated for premenstrual syndrome "I was raised in a strict Baptist home but had to leave . . . I needed more room to be me. I like life here at the university but there's a restlessness in me I can't describe. I've dated several men, one or two I really liked, but I always do something to mess up the relationship. It would kill my mother if she knew I lived with Gary for 3 months." "What it really comes down to is my own sense of betraying myself, my family, and my religion. Who am I anyway?"
Spiritual Anger	Inability to accept illness	A 38-year-old homosexual man recently diagnosed with AIDS "My parents are fundamentalists . . . all I ever heard at home was how much Jesus loves me . . . all the while my mom was beating the daylights out of me. . . . Does He love me? Does He love me so much that He had my parents throw me out when I finally told them I was gay? Does He love me so much that I got AIDS and now no one comes near me?" Facial features are tight; body held rigidly; speech is sharp, appears angry with God, the world, himself.
Spiritual Loss	Terminal illness; anticipatory grieving; inability to find comfort in religion	A 40-year-old mother of three sons who was diagnosed with ovarian cancer 18 months ago; currently in advanced stage of disease

(continued)

Examples of NANDA Nursing Diagnoses — Spiritual Distress* (Continued)

Nursing Diagnoses	Related Factors	Sample Defining Characteristics
		"I've tried hard to do it all right . . . I read my Bible, prayed every day, went to church each Sunday, loved my husband and kids . . . why is this all happening to me? Why must I lose it all? Where is God now that I need him? Some mornings I wish I could shoot myself and end it all—instead another day drags on. Who can help me?" Cries frequently, no longer interested in everyday activities of family, no interest in praying, told family not to have pastor call anymore. *"No one can help now."*
Spiritual Despair	Feeling that no one (not even God) cares	A 92-year-old frail widow who lives alone in a two-room apartment; crippled with arthritis; has two married sons she has not seen for years. Says to community nurse who visits every week, *"No one should have to live like this. If it weren't for the neighbor who comes on Saturday with a few groceries and you I'd be dead. I guess that would be for the best. It's been a long time since I felt like my living or dying would matter to anyone. Because I'm 92 now I guess even God doesn't want me. Couldn't you do something to put me out of my misery?"*

* NANDA-approved nursing diagnosis label.

Outcome Identification and Planning

Enhancing Spiritual Health

Nurses who are sensitive to the role that spiritual beliefs play in influencing both a person's thoughts about self and the world and his or her interactions with the world value spiritual health. Their interactions with any patient who values spirituality are supportive of the following patient outcomes: The patient will

- Identify spiritual beliefs that meet needs for meaning and purpose, love and relatedness, and forgiveness
- Derive from these beliefs strength, hope, and comfort when facing the challenge of illness, injury, or other life crisis
- Develop spiritual practices that nurture communion with inner self, with God, and with the world
- Express satisfaction with the compatibility of spiritual beliefs and everyday living

Addressing Spiritual Distress

Goals and expected outcomes for patients in spiritual distress need to be individualized and may include some of the following. The patient will achieve the following:

- Explore the origin of spiritual beliefs and practices
- Identify factors in life that challenge spiritual beliefs
- Explore alternatives given these challenges: deny, modify, or reaffirm beliefs; develop new beliefs

- Identify spiritual supports (eg, spiritual reading, faith, community)
- Report or demonstrate a decrease in spiritual distress after successful intervention

Implementing Spiritual Care

A variety of interventions are available to the nurse who wishes to help patients meet their spiritual needs. Like other nursing skills, these interventions need to be practiced before the nurse is able to use them confidently, competently, and at the right moment. In this section, the following nursing interventions are presented: offering supportive presence, facilitating the patient's practice of religion, nurturing spirituality, praying with a patient, praying for a patient, counseling the patient spiritually, contacting a spiritual counselor, and resolving conflicts between treatment and spiritual beliefs. These interventions can be used in the home, hospital, or care center in helping patients meet their spiritual needs. See Examples of Nursing Interventions Classification (NIC) for a list of selected spiritual support activities.

Offering Supportive Presence

A nurse's gift of supportive presence must underlie all other types of intervention to meet the patient's spiritual needs. The aim of this intervention is to create a hospitable and sacred space ("holy ground") in which patients can share their vulnerabilities without fear. Supportive presence communicates value and respect (Fig. 36-4). Chapter 21 presents basic communication skills helpful in establishing this type of presence.

The patient who senses that the nurse is sincerely concerned and committed to helping meet human needs is better able to participate in the plan of care. Patients who experience respect and affirmation from other humans find it easier to hold spiritual beliefs that meet their needs for meaning and purpose, love and relatedness, and forgiveness.

Facilitating the Practice of Religion

The following are means the nurse can use to help the patient continue normal spiritual practices in the unfamiliar environment of the hospital or care center:

- Familiarize the patient with the religious services and materials available within the institution.

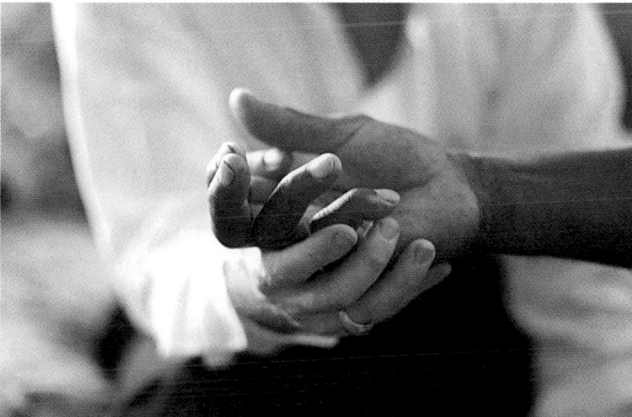

FIGURE 36-4 The nurse offers supportive presence by holding the patient's hand to show that he or she is sincerely concerned, or simply by being present to communicate value and respect.

- Respect the patient's need for privacy or quiet during periods of prayer.
- Assist the patient to obtain devotional objects and protect them from loss or damage.
- Arrange for the patient wishing to receive the sacraments to do so.
- Attempt to meet the patient's religious dietary restrictions.
- Arrange for the patient's minister, priest, or rabbi to visit if the patient so wishes.

If the patient has a conflict between spiritual beliefs and the proposed medical therapy, the nurse can assist the patient in discussing this with the physician. The ill patient in the home may not be able to attend services or meetings to which he or she is accustomed. The nurse can aid the patient in finding ways to express his or her spiritual needs.

Nurturing Spirituality

Some patients who experience a need to get in touch with their spiritual self and to nurture their spiritual development look to the nurse for direction. The person who lives life enmeshed in the action and noises of society may feel strangely uncomfortable when illness forces introspection. The nurse can be helpful in recommending means to develop a relationship with one's inner world and manifest spiritual energy in one's outer world (Hill & Smith, 1990). Box 36-2 lists ways to develop one's inner world and to manifest this energy to the outside world.

Spiritual nurturing for the patient's caregiver also is important. Recent research findings support the importance and value of caregivers' spirituality, yet as a resource it is often overlooked (Kaye & Robinson, 1994). Nurses should consider using interventions that enhance a caregiver's ability to take part in church activities to satisfy his or her spiritual needs and to work with church groups to secure helpful services. Using clergy, prayer, forgiveness, and spiritual reading materials as resources for caregivers may also be helpful.

> *Knowledge of the supportive services provided by the church group of Mrs. Zeuner, the 75-year-old woman taking care of her husband with advanced Alzheimer's disease, would be important to include in the plan of care for Mrs. Zeuner and her husband. Supportive services, such as respite care, parish nursing, and meals, in addition to the emotional support provided by the group, could be extremely helpful for Mrs. Zeuner in her role as caregiver.*

Three ways the nurse can help the patient to nurture his or her own spirituality are by promoting meaning and purpose, promoting love and relatedness, and promoting forgiveness.

Promoting Meaning and Purpose

In the book *Man's Search for Meaning,* psychiatrist Victor Frankl, who survived the horrors of the Nazi concentration camps, writes, "Once an individual's search for meaning is successful, it not only renders him happy, but also gives him the capability to cope with suffering" (1985, p. 163). To help patients searching for meaning, explore with the patient what has given his or her life meaning and purpose up to the present; sources of meaning for other people; and possible meanings for the patient's current experience of illness, pain, suffering, or impending death. If desired by the patient, arrange for referral to a spiritual adviser. Explore with the patient spiritual practices from which strength and hope might be derived (eg, prayer or reading scripture or other spiritual books). Recommend that the patient read spiritual biographies or Harold Kuschner's book *When Bad Things Happen to Good People* (1983) or Kathleen Brehony's book *After the Darkest Hour: How Suffering Begins the Journey to Wisdom* (2000). Referring the patient to appropriate support groups (eg, self-help groups for people with stroke, cancer, and so on) also is helpful.

Promoting Love and Relatedness

First and foremost, treat the patient at all times with respect, empathy, and genuine caring. It is a good idea to encourage the patient to talk about relationships with others and to identify the origin of negative beliefs about people. Box 36-3 may be a good starting point for reflection on loving kindness.

Encourage conversation about God as the patient knows and experiences God (if God is part of the patient's spiritual beliefs). If appropriate, introduce or reinforce the belief that God is a loving and personal God who is concerned about the patient. Whenever possible, encourage and facilitate visits from the patient's family, friends, and spiritual adviser.

Promoting Forgiveness

Offer a supportive presence to the patient that demonstrates your acceptance of the patient. Explore with the patient the

---

> **BOX 36-3 Loving Kindness Meditation**
>
> - May you be at peace.
> - May your heart remain open.
> - May you awaken to the light of your own true nature.
> - May you know the power of your higher self.
> - May peace of mind be your only goal and forgiveness your only task.
> - May you be healed of all pain and hurt.
> - May you be a source of healing for others.
> - May you know the inner beauty of the person you truly are.
> - May you be at peace.
>
> Source unknown.

importance of learning to accept oneself and others, including both strengths and limitations. Explore negative images of God and others that make it difficult for the patient to seek forgiveness and to believe that he or she is forgiven.

Explore the patient's self-expectations and assist the patient to determine how realistic these are. Allow the patient to verbalize shame, guilt, and anger, and counsel about the importance of expressing negative emotions in healthy ways. Refer the patient to a spiritual adviser, if appropriate. Offer the patient examples of how not forgiving others can end up hurting only the one who cannot forgive.

Praying With Patients

Patients accustomed to regular periods of prayer but who feel too ill to pray as they would like or who enjoy praying with others may ask the nurse to pray with them or hope that the nurse will suggest this. Because there are many forms of prayer—quiet reflection, silent communion with God or higher power, reading or recitation of formal prayers, silent or loud calling on God or conversation with God, or reading religious materials—the nurse can take the lead from the patient by asking, "How would you like us to pray?" The religious background of the patient is considered, along with the type of prayers that have been meaningful in the past. It is also helpful to ask the patient if there is a particular prayer request.

The nurse unaccustomed to praying aloud or in public may find it helpful to have a Bible passage or formal prayer readily available. The prayer may also be a simple expression aloud of the patient's needs and hopes. A sample follows:

> *Lord God, our Creator and Healer, I entrust Mrs. Smith and her family to your loving care. Bring peace to her mind and health and strength to her body. Be with her [as her treatment begins today, as she goes for surgery, and so on]. We remember all your blessings to us in the past*

and thank you. We are confident of your help now as we claim your promises.

Prayer should not block communication with the patient. Praying before a patient feels ready to pray may communicate to the patient a lack of interest in the patient's feelings. Because prayer often evokes deep feelings, the nurse should be prepared to spend time with the patient after sharing prayer to respond to these feelings.

Praying for Patients

With research beginning to suggest links between prayer and physical, mental, and spiritual health (Fish, 1995), arguments are being made that healthcare professionals have an obligation to pray for as well as with their patients. At the present time, no one is claiming that healthcare professionals are negligent if they fail to pray for patients. This may, however, be an effective intervention strategy. At the very least, nurses ought to be mediators of the spiritual resources patients and their families need (see the accompanying research box).

Counseling Patients Spiritually

The patient who feels that the nurse is sensitive to spiritual needs and comfortable with his or her own spirituality may choose to share spiritual concerns with the nurse rather than with a religious counselor. The nurse who feels able to counsel the patient may assist the patient to accomplish the following:

- Articulate spiritual beliefs
- Explore the origin of the patient's spiritual beliefs and practices
- Identify life factors that challenge the patient's spiritual beliefs (cause spiritual distress)
- Explore alternatives given these challenges: modify lifestyle; deny, modify, or reaffirm beliefs; develop new beliefs
- Develop spiritual beliefs that meet needs for meaning and purpose, care and relatedness, forgiveness

To be an effective spiritual counselor, the nurse must be open to different spiritual beliefs and forms of spiritual expression and supportive of the patient's efforts to nurture spiritual growth.

Contacting a Spiritual Counselor

Not every nurse feels comfortable in the role of spiritual counselor. The nurse may suggest that the patient talk to a spiritual counselor. When a patient expresses a desire to speak to his or her spiritual counselor, the nurse helps make the appropriate referral. The nurse may offer to contact the patient's own spiritual adviser. Other options are to contact the healthcare facility's pastoral ministry department or use a referral list of clergy in the local community. If a representative of the patient's own religion is unable to visit within the hospital at a particular time, the nurse may suggest a visit from a member of the clergy from another faith. The patient, depending on the situation and the immediacy of the need, may welcome such a suggestion.

The nurse in a care center can assist the spiritual counselor by making the counselor feel welcome, answering questions about the patient, directing the counselor to the patient, and ensuring that the patient is ready to receive the counselor. Preparations of the patient's room for the visit may vary, but the following are generally recommended practices:

- The room should be orderly and free of unnecessary equipment and items.
- There should be a seat for the religious counselor at the bedside or near the patient so that both can be comfortable during the visit.
- The top of the bedside table should be free of items and covered with a clean, white cover if a sacrament is to be administered.
- The bed curtains should be drawn to provide privacy if the patient is in a unit with other patients and is unable to be moved to a more private setting.

Some patients and spiritual advisers may value the nurse's participation in prayers, rituals, or the administration of sacraments. When a nursing diagnosis of Spiritual Distress is made, the nurse and the religious counselor often can collaborate on the plan of care and reinforce each other's efforts to assist the patient to meet goals/outcomes.

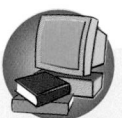

Research in Nursing Making a Difference
Promoting Health

Nurses appreciative of the interrelationship between physical, psychosocial, and spiritual health seek complementary therapeutic interventions.

Related Research
Tacon, A. M., McComb, J., Caldera, Y., & Randolph, P. (2003). Mindfulness meditation, anxiety reduction, and heart disease. A pilot study. *Family and Community Health, 26*(1), 25–33.

The purpose of this small exploratory study was to assess the effectiveness of a mindfulness meditation-based program in reducing anxiety in women with heart disease. The results indicated that women in the intervention group showed improvement in their anxiety scores at the end of the 8-week training.

Relevance to Nursing Practice
Based on preliminary data, the mindfulness meditation-based program holds promise as a complementary therapy to traditional healthcare for individuals with heart disease and may prove similarly effective for other populations.

Resolving Conflicts Between Spiritual Beliefs and Treatments

Both the patient and members of the patient's family may experience conflict between a particular spiritual belief or religious law and a proposed medical treatment or health option. The patient may want the nurse's assistance when conferring with the spiritual adviser about a particular procedure. The nurse's role is to assist the patient in obtaining the information needed to make an informed decision and to support the patient's decision making. Because what the nurse says and the way it is said may powerfully influence the patient's decision, it is important for the nurse to maintain objectivity. Conflicts that resist resolution may be referred to an ethics committee or consult team (see Chap. 6).

Evaluating

The nurse working with a patient and family to achieve specified goals/outcomes to meet spiritual needs can use each patient interaction to evaluate the plan of care. Necessary to the evaluation are sensitivity to what the patient is saying and not saying and observation of the patient when alone as well as when interacting with the family and nurses.

In general, the nurse evaluates the patient's ability to accomplish the following:

- Identify some spiritual belief that gives meaning and purpose to everyday life
- Move toward a healthy acceptance of the current situation: illness, pain, suffering, impending death
- Develop mutually caring relationships
- Reconcile any interpersonal differences causing the patient anguish
- Verbalize satisfaction with relationship with God (if this is important)
- Express peaceful acceptance of limitations and failings
- Express ability to forgive others and to live in the present
- Demonstrate an "interior state of peace and joy; freedom from abnormal anxiety, guilt, or a feeling of sinfulness; and a sense of security and direction in the pursuit of one's life goals and activities" (O'Brien, 1982, p. 98)

The nurse helps the patient to determine whether spiritual beliefs are generally life affirming or life denying and whether there is harmony between these beliefs and the patient's everyday life experiences. See Nursing Plan of Care 36-1.

NURSING PLAN OF CARE 36-1 for Mr. Gargan

Mr. Gargan is a 38-year-old divorced man on a step-down unit after treatment for a myocardial infarction. He owns a small car dealership. His religion is listed as Protestant. Frequently unable to sleep at night, Mr. Gargan often talks with the night nurse and once asked, "Did you ever give much thought to whether or not there is a God?" Sensing much concern behind this question, the nurse asks specific questions to determine whether the patient has spiritual needs that are not being met.

12/26/06, 2 a.m.

Patient again unable to sleep and initiated discussion about God. States was raised in a Lutheran home where everyone went to church on Sunday and tried to live according to God's commandments. Upon leaving home, he stopped going to church (was never a value for his wife) and simply has not given much thought to religion—too busy running his business. Until now has not experienced any need for God. "But when I think how close I was to dying and that I've no idea what to expect after death—I'm actually scared. Do others feel this way?" Wants to explore religious beliefs—feels lack in his life. Said he would like to talk with hospital minister—will arrange for tomorrow.

E. Nolan, RN

NURSING DIAGNOSIS Spiritual Distress: Anxiety related to concerns about relationship with God as manifested by self report

EXPECTED OUTCOME Before discharge, the patient will:
- Identify his religious beliefs

Nursing Interventions	Rationale	Evaluative Statement
Assist the patient to (1) identify the spiritual beliefs he had as a child and the origin of these beliefs; (2) evaluate these beliefs in terms of his life experiences; and (3) reaffirm, modify, or reject these beliefs or develop new spiritual beliefs.	Life experiences may challenge religious beliefs that were uncritically held as a child.	12/30/06 Outcome partially met. Patient states he has a much clearer concept of God and no longer fears that God will reject him for ignoring him for so long . . . but believes he also has a lot to learn. *E. Nolan, RN*

(continued)

NURSING PLAN OF CARE 36-1   *for Mr. Gargan* (continued)

Nursing Interventions	Rationale	Evaluative Statement
Assist the patient to assess whether his newly articulated spiritual beliefs are life affirming or life denying and the degree to which they meet his needs for meaning and purpose, love and relatedness, and forgiveness.	Because spiritual beliefs can exert positive (life-affirming) and negative (life-denying) influences on a person's life, individuals should have some criteria to use when evaluating their beliefs.	(See previous page.)
Refer the patient to the hospital minister for assistance with the above.	Patient may value speaking with a minister.	

EXPECTED OUTCOME

Before discharge, the patient will:
• Reconcile his life up until the present with God

Nursing Interventions	Rationale	Evaluative Statement
Reassure the patient that many people get involved in day-to-day living to the extent that they forget about God, and that in some religions, people believe that God uses illness and other stressors to invite people to rethink their spiritual beliefs. In these traditions, God is often pictured with open arms waiting to welcome a child home.	Images of a stern and unyielding God ready to strike down transgressors may contribute to a patient's spiritual distress.	12/30/06 Outcome met. "This minister has really helped. I wish I had talked to him a long time ago. I've carried so much guilt about my divorce and some other things—thought God would never forgive me. I feel so much more at peace now." *E. Nolan, RN*
Refer the patient to a spiritual advisor for help in experiencing forgiveness if he mentions guilt feelings.	Guilt often inhibits persons from seeking and experiencing the forgiveness they desire.	
Communicate to the patient the importance of people accepting themselves—with all their strengths and weaknesses	Many persons have unrealistic self-expectations	

EXPECTED OUTCOME

Before discharge, the patient will:
• Verbalize that his spiritual beliefs have become a source of strength and peace rather than anxiety

Nursing Interventions	Rationale	Evaluative Statement
Encourage the patient to compare the role of spiritual beliefs in his life before, during, and after hospitalization.	This highlights the positive and negative roles spiritual beliefs can play. It may motivate the patient to continue searching if he values his present experience.	12/30/06 Outcome met. "It's good to be able to feel more peaceful about whatever the future brings. I'm anxious to get out of here because there's a lot I want to do with God's help." *E. Nolan, RN*

EXPECTED OUTCOME

Before discharge, the patient will:
• Increase night sleep to at least 6 undisturbed hours

(continued)

NURSING PLAN OF CARE 36-1   *for Mr. Gargan* (continued)

Nursing Interventions	Rationale	Evaluative Statement
Nurse on the 11 to 7 shift checks on patient at beginning of shift to make sure he is comfortable and ready for sleep.	Nursing supervision of the patient at bedtime rules out other factors that may interfere with sleep.	12/30/06 Outcome met. Patient slept last night from midnight to 6 a.m. Will continue to monitor. *E. Nolan, RN*
Use power of suggestion to enhance sleep: *"I'm sure when I check back you'll be sound asleep."*	Suggestion has been shown to enhance the therapeutic effect of other interventions.	
If sleep remains disturbed, try relaxation exercises or guided imagery (see Chap. 32).	As spiritual anxiety decreases, sleep should improve. If sleep does not improve, other contributing factors and interventions will need to be explored.	

SAMPLE DOCUMENTATION   12/27/06   3 p.m., Nursing

B. Hanks, Protestant minister, here to see patient at 1 p.m. Afterward, patient said he felt "a whole lot better." Reported minister had assured him that many people in the hospital with a serious illness go through exactly what he is experiencing now—and this thought seemed to decrease much of his anxiety. Minister had reinforced nurse's suggestion that he explore his religious beliefs and he has already jotted down some thoughts. "I knew you fixed bodies in hospitals but didn't know you fix souls, too." Patient looking forward to minister's visit tomorrow.

E. Nolan, RN

Developing Critical Thinking Skills

1. Assess your spiritual well-being; that is, to what extent are you able to meet your needs for love and belonging, meaning and purpose, and forgiveness? If confronted with a life-threatening or chronic illness, would you be able to draw on religion or spirituality as a source of strength? Are there any special skills you believe you need to develop to better meet the spiritual needs of your patients? Compare your responses to those of your classmates and explore reasons for the differences you encounter.

2. Poll your classmates and see if they agree strongly, agree, disagree, or disagree strongly with the following statements. Discuss reasons for the differences in your answers and how this is likely to affect your professional practice:
   • Prayer has the power to heal physical, mental, and spiritual illness.
   • Nurses who do not pray for their patients are deficient professional caregivers.
   • Nurses who do not offer to pray with their patients are deficient professional caregivers.

3. How would you respond to a patient who tells you that he isn't very religious but is now wondering if there is a God, and if so, where he stands in relation to God now that his life is in jeopardy? Think about how your personal experience of religion/spirituality colors your response, and determine whether your personal experience of religion/spirituality has prepared you well to respond to these queries.

Practicing for NCLEX

1. Which of the following statements most correctly differentiates between an agnostic and an atheist?
   a. The terms are used interchangeably, both believing there is no God.
   b. An agnostic denies that humans can know anything about God's existence, whereas an atheist denies God's existence.
   c. They both deny the need for a philosophy of living to guide their life.
   d. No aspect of an atheist's life is influenced by spirituality, whereas an agnostic has spiritual values.

2. A nurse who was raised a strict Roman Catholic stated she couldn't assist patients with their spiritual distress because she recognizes only a "field power" in each individual. She said, "My parents and I hardly talk because I've deserted my faith. Sometimes I feel real isolated from them and also God—if there is a God." Analysis of these data reveals which unmet spiritual need?

a. Need for meaning and purpose
b. Need for forgiveness
c. Need for love and relatedness
d. Need for strength for everyday living

3. Which statement is true concerning the influence of spirituality and religion on the various aspects of a person's life?
    a. All aspects of life may be influenced by spirituality.
    b. Activities of daily living (eating, bathing, sleeping, dressing) are rarely influenced by religion.
    c. Work and recreation are not influenced by religion.
    d. Whereas physical illness is seldom influenced by religion, mental illness frequently is.

4. A patient whose last name was Goldstein was served on a paper plate a kosher meal ordered from a restaurant because the hospital made no provision for kosher food or dishes. Mr. Goldstein became angry and accused the nurse of insulting him: "I want to eat what everyone else does—and give me decent dishes." Analysis of these data reveals that:
    a. The nurse should have ordered kosher dishes also
    b. The staff must have behaved condescendingly or critically
    c. Mr. Goldstein is a problem patient and difficult to satisfy
    d. Mr. Goldstein was stereotyped and not consulted about his dietary preferences

5. You are least likely to encounter resistance to emergency life-saving surgery for a patient from which of the following families?
    a. Christian Scientist family
    b. Faith Assembly Healer family
    c. Jehovah's Witness family
    d. Orthodox Jewish family

6. When the family desires baptism for an infant, it is imperative that the nurse provide for baptism to be done because:
    a. Baptism frequently postpones or prevents death or suffering
    b. It is legally required that nurses provide for this care when the family makes this request
    c. It is a nursing function to assure the salvation of the baby
    d. Lack of baptism when desired may increase the family's sorrow and suffering

7. Because the capacity for abstract thought develops as a child grows older, spirituality is understood differently by children of different ages. Which of the following statements is false?
    a. Spirituality and perception of God is meaningless for the 4- to 5-year-old.
    b. Even young children, 4 to 5 years of age, have definite perceptions of God and forms of worship.
    c. Children's perceptions of their "spiritual self" mature as they mature.
    d. Children 5 to 11 years of age may show anxiety concerning the power they believe God has.

8. The most important source of learning about his or her own spirituality for a child is:
    a. His or her church or religious organization
    b. What parents say about God and religion
    c. How parents behave in relationship to one another and their children, to others, and to God
    d. The spiritual adviser for the family

9. Even though a detailed nursing history in which spirituality is assessed is taken on admission, problems with spiritual distress may not surface until days after admission. The probable explanation is that:
    a. Patients usually want to conceal information about spiritual needs
    b. Patients are not concerned about spiritual needs until after their spiritual adviser visits
    c. Family members and close friends often initiate spiritual concerns
    d. Illness increases spiritual concerns, which may be difficult for patients to express in words

10. When a patient needs spiritual counseling, the nurse who is comfortable with his or her own spirituality should:
    a. Always call the patient's own spiritual adviser
    b. Consult with the patient about the spiritual adviser with whom he or she wishes to talk
    c. Attempt to counsel the patient and, if unsuccessful, make a referral
    d. Advise the patient and spiritual adviser concerning health options and the correct decision

11. When assessment data point to a spiritual problem that can be treated by independent nursing intervention, it receives the NANDA-approved diagnostic label:
    a. Spiritual Alienation
    b. Spiritual Despair
    c. Spiritual Distress
    d. Spiritual Pain

12. A patient states she feels so isolated from her family and church and even God "in this huge medical center so far from home." An appropriate goal for the patient to relieve her spiritual distress is as follows. The patient will:
    a. Express satisfaction with the compatibility of her spiritual beliefs and everyday living
    b. Identify spiritual beliefs that meet her need for meaning and purpose
    c. Express peaceful acceptance of limitations and failings
    d. Identify spiritual supports available to her in this medical center

13. A man who is a declared agnostic is extremely depressed after losing his home, his wife, and his children in a fire. His nursing diagnosis is Spiritual Distress: Spiritual Pain related to inability to find meaning and purpose in his current condition. The most important nursing intervention to plan is to:
    a. Ask the patient which spiritual adviser he would like you to call

b. Recommend that the patient read spiritual biographies or religious books
c. Explore with the patient what, in addition to his family, has given his life meaning and purpose in the past
d. Introduce the belief that God is a loving and personal God

14. After having an abortion, the patient told the visiting nurse, "I shouldn't have had that abortion because I'm Catholic, but what else could I do? I'm afraid I'll never get close to my mother or back in the Church again." She then talked with her priest about this feeling of guilt. Which evaluation statement shows a solution to the problem?
    a. Patient states, "I wish I had talked with the priest sooner. I now know God has forgiven me, and even my mother understands."
    b. Patient has slept from 10 p.m. to 6 a.m. for three consecutive nights without medication.
    c. Patient has developed mutually caring relationships with two women and one man.
    d. Patient has identified several spiritual beliefs that give purpose to her life.

15. Mr. Brown's teenage daughter had been involved in shoplifting. He expressed much anger toward her and stated he could not face her, let alone discuss this with her: "I just will not tolerate a thief." Which of the following nursing interventions would you take to assist Mr. Brown with his deficit in forgiveness?
    a. Assure him that many parents feel the same way.
    b. Reassure him that many teenagers go through this kind of rebellion and that it will pass.
    c. Assist the patient to identify how unforgiving feelings toward others only hurt the one who cannot forgive.
    d. Ask him if he is sure he has spent sufficient time with his daughter.

■ Answers With Rationale

1. The correct answer is *b*. An agnostic denies that humans can know anything about God's existence, whereas an atheist denies God's existence. The other options are incorrect.
2. The correct answer is *c*. The data point to an unmet spiritual need to experience love and belonging given her estrangement from her family and God after leaving the church. The other options may represent other needs this patient has, but the data provided do not support them.
3. The correct answer is *a*. Spirituality can influence all aspects of a person's life, including activities of daily living, work and recreation, and all types of illnesses. The other options are incomplete or false.

4. The correct answer is *d*. On the basis of his name alone, the nurse jumped to the premature and false conclusion that this patient would want a kosher diet.
5. The correct answer is *d*. There is no teaching in the Hebrew scriptures that prohibits emergency life-saving surgery; in fact, most Orthodox Jews would be highly motivated to have the surgery because of the high value attached to preserving life. All of the other groups mentioned might have religious grounds for refusing surgery.
6. The correct answer is *d*. Failure to ensure that an infant baptism is performed when parents desire it may greatly increase the family's sorrow and suffering, and this is an appropriate nursing concern. Whether baptism postpones or prevents death and suffering (answer *a*) is a religious belief that is insufficient to bind all nurses. There is no legal requirement regarding baptism, so answer *b* is false. Although some nurses may believe part of their role is to ensure the salvation of the baby (answer *c*), this function would understandably be rejected by many.
7. The correct answer is *a*. It is false that spirituality and perception of God is meaningless for the 4- to 5-year-old. All the other options are correct.
8. The correct answer is *c*. Children learn most about their own spirituality from how their parents behave in relationship to one another, their children, others, and God. Less important sources of learning are each of the other options.
9. The correct answer is *d*. Illness may increase spiritual concerns, which many patients find difficult to express. The other options do not correspond to actual experience.
10. The correct answer is *b*. Even when a nurse feels comfortable discussing spiritual concerns, he or she should always check first with patients to determine the spiritual adviser with whom they wish to talk. Calling the patient's own spiritual adviser (answer *a*) may be premature if it is a matter the nurse can handle. Answers *c* and *d* deny patients the right to speak privately with their spiritual adviser from the outset, if this is what they prefer.
11. The correct answer is *c*. The only NANDA-approved nursing diagnosis among the options is Spiritual Distress. The other options may be further specifications of the broader diagnosis Spiritual Distress.
12. The correct answer is *d*. Each of the four options represents appropriate spiritual goals, but identifying spiritual supports available to her in the medical center demonstrates a decreased sense of isolation.
13. The correct answer is *c*. The nursing intervention of exploring with the patient what, in addition to his family, has given his life meaning and purpose in

the past is more likely to correct the etiology of his problem, Spiritual Pain, than any of the other nursing interventions listed.

14. The correct answer is *a*. Because this patient's nursing diagnosis is Spiritual Distress: Guilt, an evaluative statement that demonstrates diminished guilt is necessary. Only answer *a* directly deals with guilt.

15. The correct answer is *c* because this is the only nursing intervention that directly addresses the patient's unmet spiritual need concerning forgiveness. Answers *a* and *b* may make him feel better initially, but neither addresses his need to forgive. Answer *d* is likely to make him feel guilty.

Bibliography

American Nurses Association. (1998). *Scope and standards of parish nursing practice*. Washington, DC: Author.

Andrews, M. M., & Hanson, P. A. (1995). Religion, culture, and nursing. In M. M. Andrews & J. S. Boyle (Eds.), *Transcultural concepts in nursing care*. Philadelphia: J. B. Lippincott.

Baumann, S. L. (2003). A comparison of three views of spirituality in oncology nursing. *Nursing Science Quarterly, 16*(1), 52–59.

Brehony, K. (2000). *After the darkest hour: How suffering begins the journey to wisdom*. New York: Henry Holt and Company.

Burghardt, M., & Nagai-Jacobson, M. G. (1997). Spirituality and healing. In B. M. Dossey (Ed.), *Core curriculum for holistic nursing*. New York: Aspen Publishers.

Burnhard, P. (1987). Spiritual distress and the nursing response: Theoretical considerations and counseling skills. *Journal of Advanced Nursing, 12*(3), 377–382.

Callahan, D., & Campbell, C. S. (Eds.). (1990). Theology, religious traditions, and bioethics: A special supplement. *Hastings Center Report, 20*(6), 18–19.

Carol, J. (August 2002). What is healing? *Sacred Journey, 53*(4), 12–17.

Carson, V. B. (1989). *Spiritual dimensions of nursing practice*. Philadelphia: W. B. Saunders.

Cohen, C. B., Wheeler, S. E., Scott, D. A., Edwards, B. S., Lusk, P., & the Anglican Working Group in Bioethics. (May–June 2000). Prayer as therapy. *Hastings Center Report, 30*(3), 40–47.

Coles, R. (1990). *The spiritual life of children*. Boston: Houghton Mifflin.

Creen, T. (2002). Enabling hope in the terminally ill. In Anderson, R. C. et al. (Eds.). *Palliative care patient and family counseling manual* (2nd ed., pp. 16–17). New York: Aspen Publishers.

Cutcliffe, J. R. (1995). How do nurses inspire and instill hope in terminally ill HIV patients? *Journal of Advanced Nursing, 22*, 888–895.

Dossey, B. (Ed.). (1989). Spirituality and healing. *Holistic Nursing Practice, 3*(3) [entire issue].

Dossey, B. M., & Dossey, L. (1998). Attending to holistic care. *American Journal of Nursing, 98*(8), 35–38.

Fish, S. (1995). Can research prove that God answers prayer? *Journal of Christian Nursing, 12*(1), 24–27, 46.

Fowler, J. W. (1981). *Stages of faith: The psychology of human development and the quest for meaning*. San Francisco: Harper-Collins.

Frankl, V. (1985). *Man's search for meaning*. New York: Washington Square Press.

Gaskins, S., & Forte, L. (1995). The meaning of hope: Implications for nursing practice and research. *Journal of Gerontological Nursing, 21*(3), 17–24.

Goddard, N. C. (1995). "Spirituality as integrative energy": A philosophical analysis as requisite precursor to holistic nursing practice. *Journal of Advanced Nursing, 22*(4), 808 815.

Gregg-Schroeder, S. (April 1999). A transforming experience: Circles of Life. *Journal of Fellowship in Prayer*, 23–25.

Hauerwas, S. (1990). *Naming the silences: God, medicine, and the problem of suffering*. Grand Rapids: Erdmans.

Heller, D. (1985). The children's God. *Psychology Today, 19*(12), 22–27.

Hill, L., & Smith, N. (1990). *Self-care nursing* (2nd ed.). New York: Appleton & Lange.

Holstrom, S. (1999). Perspectives on a suburban parish nursing practice. In P. A. Solari-Twadell & M. A. McDermott (Eds.), *Parish nursing: Promoting whole person health within faith communities* (pp 67–74). Thousand Oaks, CA: Sage.

Hungelmann, J., et al. (1989). Development of the JAREL spiritual well-being scale. In NANDA (Eds.), *Classification of nursing diagnosis: Proceedings of the eighth conference* (pp. 393–398). Philadelphia: J. B. Lippincott.

Kaye, J., & Robinson, K. M. (1994). Spirituality among caregivers. *Image: The Journal of Nursing Scholarship, 26*(3), 218–221.

Kuschner, H. S. (1983). *When bad things happen to good people*. New York: Avon.

Lo, B., et al. (2002). Discussing religious and spiritual issues at the end of life. *JAMA, 287*(6), 749–754.

Macrae, J. (1995). Nightingale's spiritual philosophy and its significance for modern nursing. *Image: The Journal of Nursing Scholarship, 27*(1), 8–10.

McHolm, F. A. (1992). A nursing diagnosis validation study: Defining characteristics of spiritual distress. In R. M. Carroll-Johnson (Ed.), *Classification of nursing diagnosis: Proceedings of the ninth conference* (pp. 112–119). Philadelphia: J. B. Lippincott.

Moberg, D. O. (1979). The development of social indicators of spiritual well-being and quality of life. In D. O. Moberg (Ed.), *Spiritual well-being: Sociological perspectives* (pp. 1–13). Washington, DC: University Press of America.

Nist, J. A. (2003). Parish nursing programs. *Health Progress, 84*(1), 50–54.

North American Nursing Diagnosis Association. (1994). *NANDA nursing diagnoses: Definitions and classifications 1995–1996.* Philadelphia: Author.

O'Brien, M. E. (1982). The need for spiritual integrity. In H. Yura & M. Walsh (Eds.), *Human needs and the nursing process* (pp. 81–115). Norwalk, CT: Appleton-Century-Crofts.

O'Brien, M. E. (1999). *Spirituality in nursing.* Boston: Jones and Bartlett.

O'Brien, M. E. (2001). *The nurse's calling.* New York: Paulist Press.

O'Brien, M. E. (2003). *Parish nursing: Healthcare ministry within the church.* Boston: Jones and Bartlett.

Parrinder, G. (Ed.). (1983). *World religions.* New York: Facts on File Publications.

Puchalski, C. & Romer, A. L. (2000). Taking a spiritual history allows clinicians to understand patients more fully. *Journal of Palliative Medicine, 3*(1), 129–137.

Quinn, A. (August 2002). Spirituality and the family: What religion should I be? *Sacred Journey, 53*(4), 12–17.

Rahner, K. (1971). How to receive a sacrament and mean it. *Theology Digest, 19,* 229.

Shaffer, J. L. (Ed.). (1989). Spirituality and healing. *Holistic Nursing Practice, 3*(3) [entire issue].

Shelly, J., & Fish, S. (1988). *Spiritual care: The nurse's role* (3rd ed.). Downer's Grove, IL: InterVarsity Press.

Tacon, A. M., McComb, J., Caldera, Y., & Randolph, P. (2003). Mindfulness meditation, anxiety reduction, and heart disease. A pilot study. *Family and Community Health, 26*(1), 25–33.

Widerquist, J., & Davidhizar, R. (1994). The ministry of nursing. *Journal of Advanced Nursing, 19*(4), 647–652.

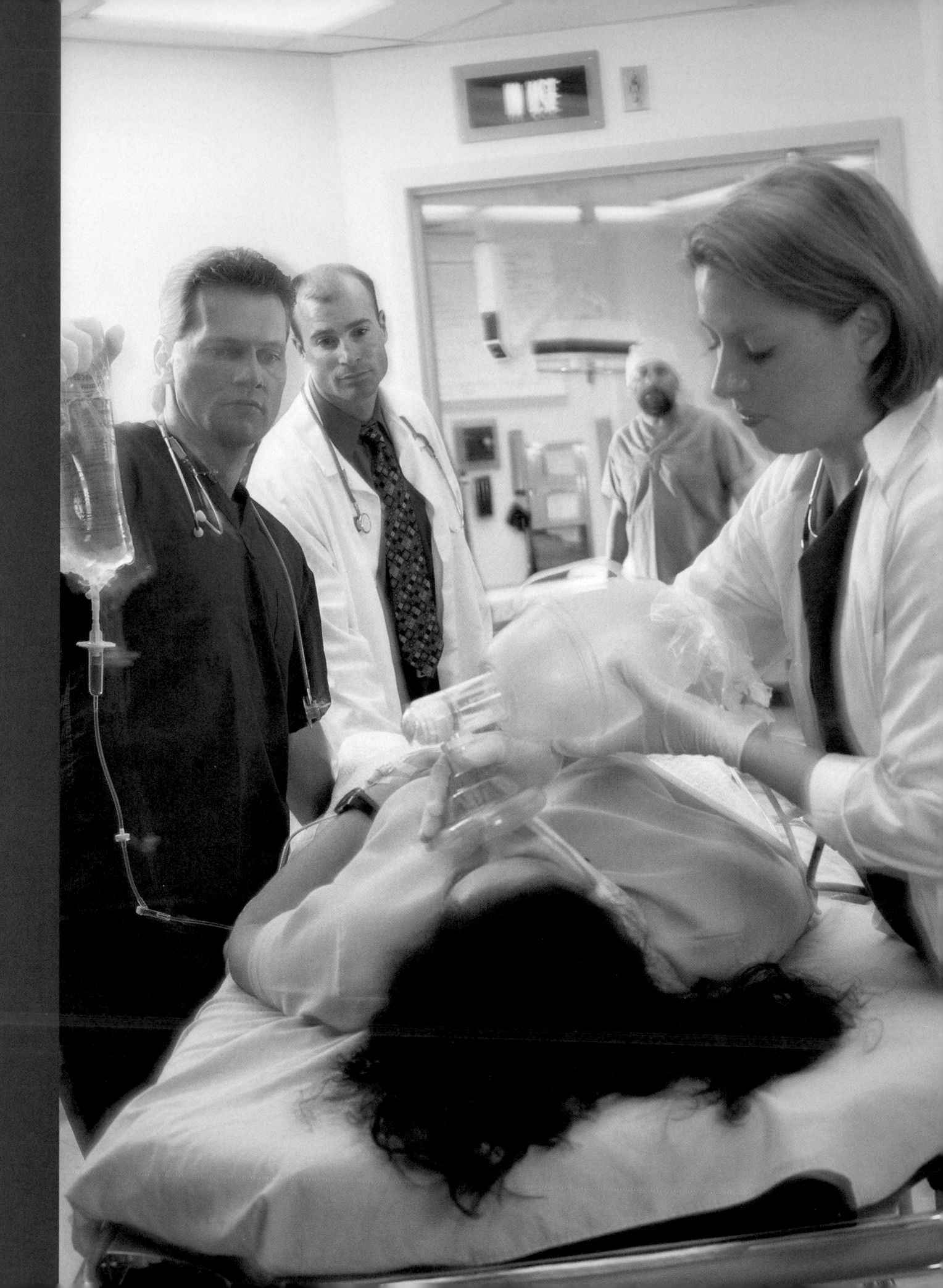

Promoting Healthy Physiologic Responses

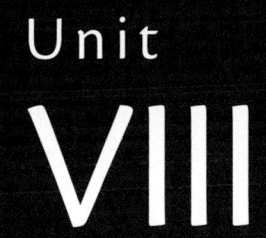

Unit VIII

". . . what nursing has to do is to put the patient in the best condition for nature to act upon him."

Florence Nightingale (1820–1910)
a philosopher, theorist, statistician, humanitarian, and inspirational leader who founded modern nursing through a systematic method of training well-qualified nurses; she also initiated important reforms in military sanitation and hospital construction that greatly improved patient survival

The art and science of caring are blended when nurses implement actions to meet basic human needs and to promote healthy physiologic responses. The chapters in Unit VIII focus on information and guidelines essential to nursing practice in a wide variety of clinical settings and involving both healthy and ill patients of all ages. Included are nursing interventions to promote safety and comfort and to meet basic physiologic needs: hygiene, activity and rest, nutrition, elimination, oxygenation, and fluid–electrolyte balance.

Each basic physiologic need is discussed first with a review of concepts pertinent to the specific area of human function and response, and then with an examination of factors that affect need satisfaction. The steps of the nursing process are used to provide guidelines and information necessary for making accurate assessments, establishing outcomes, and planning, implementing, and evaluating specific nursing interventions to meet needs and promote wellness.

The chapters in Unit VIII enable the beginning nurse to integrate the knowledge and skills necessary to promote healthy physiologic responses in patients in any practice setting. Nursing process skills are further refined to ensure that care is holistic, comprehensive, and individualized.

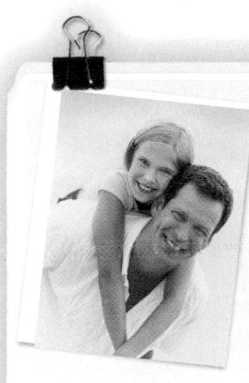

Kylie Simpson is a school-aged child who is brought to the clinic with head lice. Her father says, "I'm so embarrassed and ashamed. We're not dirty people. How could this have happened?"

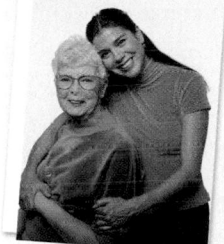

Sonya Delamordo is an older Hispanic woman who has had a stroke (brain attack) resulting in right-sided paralysis. She is being discharged from the hospital and will now live with her daughter, who will be her primary caretaker. Her daughter is eager to learn everything she can about caring for her mother and asks numerous questions, including the best way to keep her mother clean.

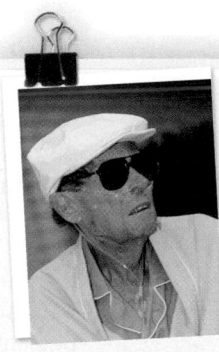

Andrew Craig, age 68, has multiple diagnoses and limited mobility and lives in a long-term care facility. He needs assistance with his morning care. He tells the nurse, "I've already had a complete bath."

Focusing on Blended Skills

The types of blended skills that you'll need to respond to the case scenarios include:

Cognitive Skills

- Basic knowledge about hygiene, hygiene measures, and the products and equipment that facilitate care
- Knowledge about common problems of the skin and mucous membranes and how to treat them
- Knowledge of the effects of various disorders on a patient's ability to perform hygiene measures
- Knowledge of developmental and cultural factors affecting hygiene practices
- Ability to identify patients with self-care deficits related to hygiene and to develop and implement appropriate plans to address these deficits

Technical Skills

- Ability to provide the technical nursing assistance necessary to meet the hygiene needs of patients
- Demonstration of the ability to provide basic hygiene measures
- Ability to use products and equipment correctly to meet the hygiene needs of patients of various ages
- Ability to adapt hygiene care measures to meet the needs of patients at different developmental stages, such as a school-aged child, an older adult with right-sided paralysis, and an older adult with limited mobility and multiple disorders living in a long-term care facility

Interpersonal Skills

- Strong people skills, including the ability to communicate and interact effectively with patients and their caretakers while assisting with hygiene measures
- Ability to interact effectively and work collaboratively with other members of the healthcare team to meet patients' hygiene needs
- Ability to use the time spent assisting patients with hygiene measures to communicate care about the patients and commitment to their health and well-being

- Ability to encourage patients and their caretakers, as appropriate, and colleagues in learning new self-care measures related to hygiene
- Demonstration of knowledge related to personal limitations, with a willingness to seek help when needed
- Ability to demonstrate respect for the patient's human dignity and autonomy, regardless of whether the patient is a school-aged child, an older adult woman with right-sided paralysis being discharged, or a older man living in a long-term care facility

Ethical and Legal Skills

- A strong sense of accountability for the health and well-being of patients (such as a patient with new right-sided paralysis and a patient living in a long-term care facility), which translates into a commitment to getting them the help they need within the scope of nursing responsibilities and available resources
- Ability to integrate knowledge of ethical and legal principles underlying hygiene care, including teaching a patient's daughter about care at home
- Willingness to hold oneself accountable for safe, high-quality care for patients at different developmental stages with different health problems; a willingness to hold colleagues accountable for safe and high-quality practice, such as with an older man living in a long-term care facility
- Commitment to implementing nursing care in different clinical settings within the standards of care and scope of nursing practice
- Ability to document problems with hygiene and nursing's response according to agency policy

Learning Outcomes

After completing the chapter, the learner should be able to accomplish the following:

1. List five functions of the skin, three factors influencing the skin's condition, and four basic principles that guide the practices of skin care.
2. Identify factors affecting skin condition and personal hygiene.
3. Assess the integumentary system and the adequacy of hygiene self-care behaviors using appropriate interview and physical assessment skills.
4. Develop nursing diagnoses related to deficient hygiene measures.
5. Describe the priorities of scheduled hygiene care, early morning care, morning care, afternoon care, and evening care.
6. Identify at least four reasons for including a back massage in daily nursing care.
7. Demonstrate techniques for assisting patients with hygiene measures, including those used when administering various types of baths and those used in cleaning each part of the body.
8. Describe agents commonly used on the skin and scalp, including any precautions necessary for their use.
9. Plan, implement, and evaluate nursing care for common problems of the skin and mucous membranes.

Key Terms

alopecia
caries
cerumen
dermis
epidermis
gingivitis
halitosis
integument
necrosis
pediculosis (lice)
plaque
pyorrhea
sebaceous glands
tartar

Measures for personal cleanliness and grooming, called personal hygiene, promote physical and psychological well-being. Various studies have confirmed that improved personal hygiene practices reduce illness rates (Larson, 2002; Larson & Aiello, 2001). During the 20th century, the large decline in deaths from infectious disease in the United States has been attributed to the development and use of antibiotics, expanded immunization schedules, and the increased focus on personal cleanliness.

Personal hygiene practices vary widely among people. The time of day one bathes and how often one shampoos or changes the bed linens and sleeping garments are relatively unimportant. What is important is that personal care be carried out conveniently and frequently enough to promote personal hygiene.

Ordinarily, well people are responsible for their own hygiene. In some cases, however, the nurse may assist a well person through teaching to develop personal hygiene habits the person may lack.

Illness, hospitalization, and institutionalization generally require modifications in hygiene practices. In these situations, the nurse helps the patient to continue sound hygiene practices and can teach the patient and family members, when necessary, regarding hygiene. Nurses assisting patients with basic hygiene must respect individual patient preferences, providing only the care that patients cannot or should not provide for themselves. (See the accompanying Reflective Practice box for an example.)

This chapter discusses multiple factors that affect personal hygiene and nursing measures that promote personal hygiene. A practical guide for assessing the adequacy of personal hygiene is presented. Because the data the nurse collects when assisting with hygiene may lead to identifying multiple nursing diagnoses and collaborative problems, samples of these are provided. Patient outcomes are presented, as are specific nursing strategies used when performing care of the skin; mouth; eyes, ears, and nose; feet; and perineal and vaginal areas. The concluding nursing plan of care on feminine hygiene illustrates how the nurse uses knowledge of personal hygiene practices and the integumentary system along with specific nursing interventions to resolve nursing diagnoses and to promote the patient's general sense of well-being.

PHYSIOLOGY OF THE SKIN AND ITS APPENDAGES

Integument refers to the skin. The integumentary system is made up of the skin, the subcutaneous layer directly under the skin, and the appendages of the skin (ie, the hair, glands in the skin, and the nails). The skin is one of the body's vital organs and is essential for maintaining life.

The skin has two layers. The superficial portion, the **epidermis,** is composed of layers of stratified epithelial cells. These cells are fused to form a protective, waterproof layer of keratin material. Epithelial cells have no blood vessels of their own and depend on underlying tissues for nourishment and waste removal. When well nourished, epithelium regenerates relatively easily and quickly.

The second layer of skin, the **dermis,** consists of smooth, muscular tissue; nerves; hair follicles; certain glands and their ducts; arteries, veins, and capillaries; and fibrous, elastic tissue. Each hair consists of the shaft, which projects through the dermis beyond the surface of the skin, and the hair follicle, which lies in the dermis. The dermis rests on a subcutaneous fatty tissue layer that anchors the skin layers and serves as a heat insulator for the body. This fatty tissue layer contains blood and lymph vessels, nerves, and fat cells.

The skin covers the entire body and is continuous with mucous membranes at normal body orifices. A cross-section of normal skin is illustrated in Figure 37-1. Glands in the skin include the sebaceous glands, the sweat glands, and the ceruminal glands. The **sebaceous glands** secrete an oily substance called sebum, which lubricates the skin and hair and keeps the skin and scalp pliant. The sweat glands secrete perspiration. The **cerumen** (earwax) in the external ear canals, consisting of a heavy oil and brown pigment, is secreted by the ceruminal glands.

Functions of Skin

The skin serves six major functions: protection, body temperature regulation, sensation, excretion, maintenance of water and electrolyte balance, and vitamin D production and absorption (Table 37-1).

Functions of the Mucous Membranes

Mucous membranes line body cavities that open to the outside of the body. They can also be found in the digestive tract, the respiratory passages, and the urinary and reproductive tracts. Epithelium covers the mucous membrane surfaces and contains cells that secrete mucus. Mucous membranes have receptors that offer the body protection; for example, an irritating substance in the upper respiratory tract causes a person to sneeze, and food caught in the larynx or trachea causes a person to cough. Sneezing and coughing are protective mechanisms that help rid the body of foreign materials. Mucous membranes are insensitive to temperature, except in the mouth and rectum, but are sensitive to pressure. Mucous membranes also function to absorb substances from their surface; for example, digested food is absorbed through the mucous membrane in the small intestine.

FACTORS AFFECTING SKIN CONDITION AND PERSONAL HYGIENE

A firm knowledge base about the functions of the skin and mucous membranes also requires an understanding of the factors that affect skin care and personal hygiene. This information

Reflective Practice
Challenge to Interpersonal Skills

It was our first day of clinical, sophomore year, and we were instructed to do complete a.m. care with our patients. My patient, Andrew Craig, was a 68-year-old man with multiple diagnoses and limited mobility. As I entered the room, he told me he had just had a bed bath a few hours earlier. I wasn't sure what to do, so I asked the tech if my patient had already had a complete bed bath. The tech pulled me into the patient's room and proceeded to scream at the patient, telling him not to lie to me and threatening to make him sit in the chair all day. This patient did not have a hip and had antibiotic beads in the area, so it was very painful for him to sit in a chair because the beads dug into his side. The tech then told me to do the bed bath and left the room. I was left in a very awkward position because the patient was mad at me and I was astounded by how the tech had treated this patient. I was extremely upset as a result of this confrontation.

The day was emotionally very difficult for me, and when I arrived home I became even more upset. The manner in which the tech treated the patient, even though the patient had a tendency to be manipulative, was completely out of line.

Thinking Outside the Box: Possible Courses of Action

- Make the best of a bad situation, but do nothing to change the status quo: "Hey, I'm only a student, right?"
- Confront the tech and tell her about my outrage.
- Report the tech to her supervisor.
- Consult with my instructor about how a professional nurse should respond in a situation like this.
- Be prepared to "go to the top" if initial attempts to reform a bad system don't meet with success.

Evaluating a Good Outcome: How Do I Define Success?

- The patient's basic hygiene needs are met.
- The patient's humanity and integrity are respected.
- Healthcare professionals and technicians are held accountable for incompetent, unethical, and illegal behavior (the tech, nursing leadership, and administration in this nursing home).
- I learn how to be a successful patient advocate.

Personal Learning: Here's to the Future!

I proceeded to talk to my clinical instructor and the coordinator of the class about the incident. The coordinator contacted the nursing home and I had to give a formal statement about the incident. The nurse manager who took my statement was not very receptive and was actually very patronizing.

This entire experience helped me to recognize the type of nurse I want to be. First and foremost, I always want to ensure that I provide a high quality of patient care. At the time of my unfortunate experience, I did not respond immediately to the tech's inappropriate comments. But now that I have gained more experience and become more confident, I would definitely respond immediately if a similar situation ever arose again. I realize that I can't let fear stand in my way when the quality of patient care is suffering. I would encourage any nurse who sees a colleague or anyone treating a patient without the utmost respect and care to speak up and contact appropriate personnel to discuss the situation.

In addition to this one tech's inappropriate behavior, the overall conditions of this nursing home were appalling. I learned a lot this semester about the shortage of nurses (1 RN for 40 patients) and, consequently, how patient care is being jeopardized. During the unfortunate episode to which I was exposed, I was astonished and outraged, but I didn't take any steps to change the conditions except reporting this one incident. At the end of the semester, we reported the conditions to the class coordinator. Now I realize that as an individual, I could have done more to change the conditions in the nursing home. In retrospect, I should have taken a leadership role and notified the outside licensing agency about these conditions (the nursing home ended up losing its accreditation that summer). All nurses are responsible for ensuring the quality of care given to patients, and we must contact whomever necessary to ensure changes are made.

This experience was very difficult for me, but in the end I think it opened my eyes to the importance of nurses acting as leaders.

Reflection

How do you think you would respond in a similar situation? Why? What does this tell you about yourself and about the adequacy of your skills for professional practice? Can you think of other ways to respond? What other skills (cognitive, interpersonal, technical, ethical/legal) would you need to respond well in this situation? What factors may have played a role in the tech's answer to the patient and nursing student? How did the nursing student's actions adhere to ethical and legal principles? Did the nursing student act as a patient advocate? Why or why not? Is it within the nursing student's scope of practice to individually contact a higher authority such as a licensing agency about the situation? Discuss your answer. Do you agree with the criteria to evaluate a successful outcome? Did the nursing student meet the criteria? Please explain your answer.

Catherine Barrell, Georgetown University

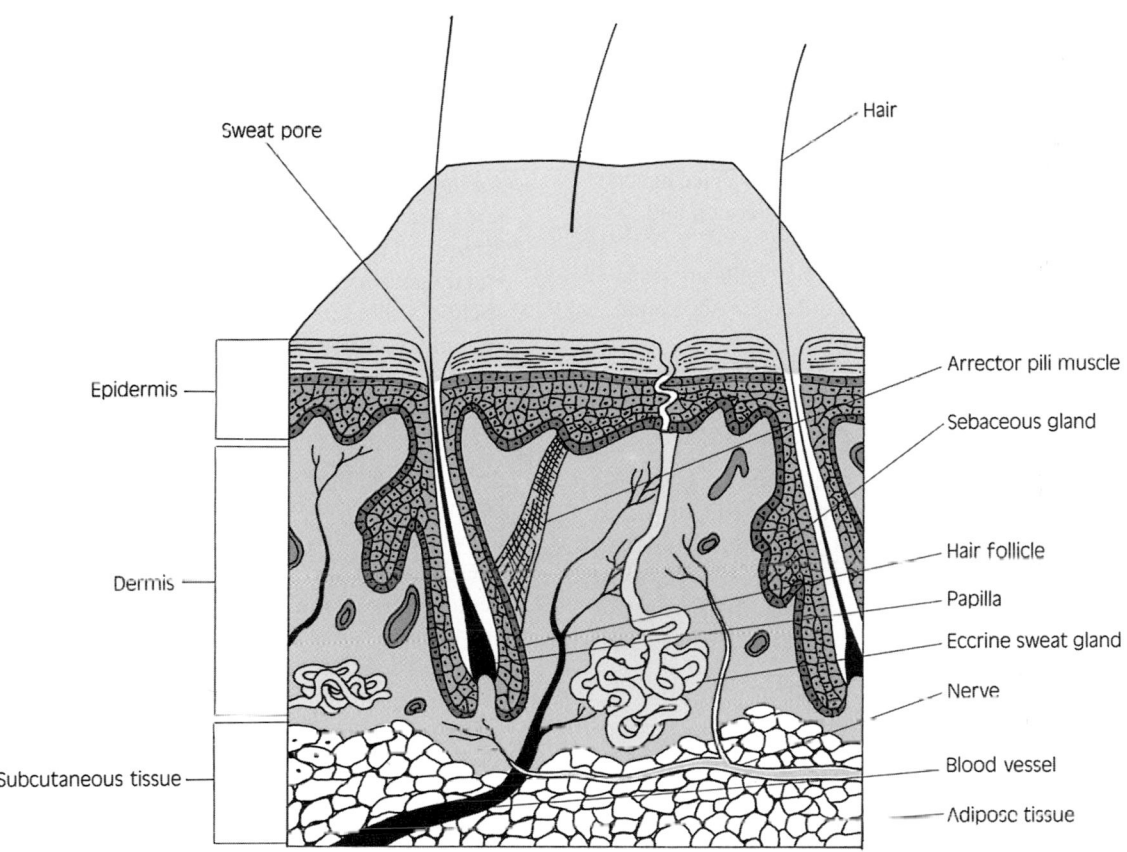

Sweat pore

Epidermis

Dermis

Subcutaneous tissue

Hair

Arrector pili muscle

Sebaceous gland

Hair follicle

Papilla

Eccrine sweat gland

Nerve

Blood vessel

Adipose tissue

FIGURE 37-1 A cross-section of normal skin.

TABLE 37-1 Functions of the Skin

Function	Mechanisms
The skin protects the body	Invasion of the body by bacteria is prevented by intact skin. Injury to underlying tissues and organs is decreased by intact skin.
The skin helps regulate body temperature	The production of perspiration and its loss by evaporation help cool the body. Much heat is lost from the body by radiation and by conduction when the blood supply to the skin is increased by vasodilation. Lack of perspiration and vasoconstriction help the body retain heat. The phenomenon of producing gooseflesh, which is caused by contraction of pilomotor muscles in the skin, helps conserve body heat because the hair standing on end forms a layer of air on the body for insulation.
The skin is a sense organ	There are receptors for pain, touch, pressure, and temperature in the skin that help the body receive stimuli from the environment.
The skin is an excretory organ	Water, salts, and nitrogenous wastes are lost from the skin, although in much smaller quantities than are lost from the kidneys.
The skin helps maintain water and electrolyte balance	The escape of excess water and electrolytes from the body is prevented by the skin.
The skin produces and absorbs vitamin D	A precursor for vitamin D is present in the skin, which, in conjunction with ultraviolet rays from the sun, produces vitamin D.

forms the foundation for certain basic principles related to care of the skin and mucous membranes:

- Unbroken and healthy skin and mucous membranes serve as the first lines of defense against harmful agents.
- Resistance to injury of the skin and mucous membranes varies among people. Factors influencing resistance include the person's age, the amount of underlying tissues, and illness conditions.
- Adequately nourished and hydrated body cells are resistant to injury. The better nourished the cell is, the better able it is to resist injury and disease.
- Adequate circulation is necessary to maintain cell life. When circulation is impaired for any reason, cells receive inadequate nourishment and cannot remove wastes efficiently.

> *Think back to Andrew Craig, the older man described in the Reflective Practice display. His limited mobility, in conjunction with sitting in the chair all day, increases his risk for skin breakdown due to inadequate circulation and pressure. This is essential to keep in mind when planning Mr. Craig's care.*

Skin Condition

Two major factors affecting a person's skin condition are the person's developmental stage and state of health. Each of these factors has various effects on a person's skin.

Developmental Considerations

Specific characteristics of the skin are associated with different developmental stages. Hygiene practices at every age have a direct influence on the status and appearance of the skin.

- An infant's skin and mucous membranes are easily injured and subject to infection. Careful handling of infants is required to prevent injury to and infection of the skin and mucous membranes.
- A child's skin becomes increasingly resistant to injury and infection. However, the skin requires special care and attention to cleanliness following play activities and during toilet training.
- An adolescent's skin ordinarily has enlarged sebaceous glands and increased glandular secretions, caused by hormonal changes in the body. These characteristics predispose adolescents to body odor and acne (discussed later in this chapter).
- Secretions from the skin glands peak during adolescence and continue until about 50 years of age.
- Changes that occur in the skin with aging are discussed in Focus on the Older Adult. These changes are irreversible. Brown spots, called liver spots, often appear. They may begin early as 35 years of age and tend to become more numerous and larger with aging. These spots result from exposure to the wind and sun and are unrelated to the liver.

Focus on the Older Adult
Nursing Strategies to Address Age-Related Skin Alterations

Age-Related Changes	Nursing Strategies
Subcutaneous and dermal tissue become thin: • Skin is more easily injured. • Skin has less capacity to insulate. • Skin wrinkles more easily. • Sensation of pressure and pain is reduced.	• Do not apply tape to skin unless necessary. • Check skin frequently to observe for any signs of a pressure ulcer. • Pad bony prominences if necessary. • Assess pressure tolerance by checking pressure points for redness after 30 minutes.
Activity of the sebaceous and sweat gland decreases: • Skin becomes dryer. • Pruritus (itching) may occur.	• Clean perineal area daily but do not bathe full body on a daily basis. • Apply lotions as needed. • Encourage adequate hydration.
Cell renewal is shorter: • Healing time is delayed.	• Perform careful skin assessments, looking for signs of skin breakdown.
Melanocytes (cells that make the pigment that colors hair and skin) decline in number: • Hair becomes gray-white. • Skin may be unevenly pigmented.	• Assist patient with skin checks, observing for any signs of melanoma or other skin abnormalities.
Nail growth rate diminishes: • Nails become soft and tear easily. • Nails thicken.	• Educate patient to take care of nails. • Advise patient to keep nails short and neat to decrease potential for skin tears and development of an infection.
Collagen fiber is less organized: • Skin loses elasticity.	• Check skin frequently for tears, irritation, or breakdown.

Health State

The state of a person's health has a direct effect on the condition of the skin. For example, some diseases or conditions expose the skin to injury:

- Very thin and very obese people tend to be more susceptible to skin irritation and injury.
- Fluid loss through fever, vomiting, or diarrhea reduces the fluid volume of the body; this is termed dehydration and makes the skin appear loose and flabby.
- Excessive perspiration, often associated with being ill, predisposes the skin to breakdown, especially in skin folds.
- Jaundice, a condition caused by excessive bile pigments in the skin, results in a yellowish skin color. The skin is often itchy and dry, and patients with jaundice are more likely to scratch their skin and cause an open lesion with the potential for infection.
- Diseases of the skin such as eczema and psoriasis often cause lesions that require special care in personal hygiene and therapeutic regimens.

Personal Hygiene

Nurses caring for patients from diverse backgrounds quickly learn that hygiene practices vary widely among individuals. The following factors may influence personal hygiene behaviors.

Culture

Many people in North America place a high value on personal cleanliness and feel unclean unless they shower or bathe at least once daily. Many consider bathing incomplete without the use of products to reduce or mask normal body odors. People from many other cultures often find a weekly bath sufficient and may feel no need to mask normal body odors. Culture may also influence whether bathing is a private or communal activity.

> Consider Sonya Delamordo, the Hispanic woman being discharged to her daughter's home after experiencing a stroke. Although the daughter is very eager to take care of her mother, the nurse would need to investigate the patient's culture to determine how the patient might feel about being cared for by her daughter. Typically, hygiene is a personal matter. The nurse needs to discuss this area with the patient and her daughter to ensure culturally competent care.

Socioeconomic Class

A person's socioeconomic class and financial resources often define the hygiene options available to individuals. For example, a person renting a room in a boarding house may have limited or no access to a tub or shower and may have limited finances to buy soap, shampoo, shaving cream, and deodorant. Homeless people, who often carry all their belongings in a car or shopping cart, may welcome the warm running water and soap available in roadside or public restrooms. Other people

may refrain from using public restrooms because they are perceived as being dirty.

Spiritual Practices

Spiritual practices, including religious beliefs, may dictate ceremonial washings and purifications, sometimes as a prelude to prayer or eating. For example, in the Orthodox Jewish tradition, ritual baths are required for women after childbirth and menstruation. In some religions, contact with a deceased person or a deceased animal may make a person "unclean." Other religions dictate that no modern facilities be installed in homes. This would prohibit some people from having running water and toilets in their homes, which means that they may bathe only once or twice a week.

Developmental Level

Children learn different hygiene practices while growing up. Family practices often dictate practices such as morning or evening baths, the frequency of shampooing and clothing changes, feelings about nudity, and so on. As adolescents become more concerned about their personal appearance, they may adopt new hygiene measures, such as taking more frequent showers and wearing deodorant. As a person ages, bathing frequency commonly decreases, possibly due to limitations in mobility and the natural tendency toward drier skin with age. In addition, older people may avoid the use of deodorant soaps to prevent excessive drying of the skin.

Health State

Disease or injury may reduce a person's ability to perform hygiene measures or motivation to follow usual hygiene habits. Weakness, dizziness, and fear of falling may prevent an individual from entering a tub or shower or from bending to wash the lower extremities. The peripheral vascular complications that often accompany diabetes mellitus require meticulous foot care. Illness may also create a demand for new or modified hygiene measures.

> Remember Kylie Simpson, the school-aged child with lice. The nurse understands that specific measures are necessary to rid the child's hair of lice. As a result, the child and her father need to modify her hygiene practices, specifically hair care, but also other areas as well.

Personal Preferences

People have different preferences with regard to hygiene practices, such as taking a shower versus a tub bath, using bar soap versus liquid soap, and washing to wake oneself or to relax before sleep. A person's self-concept and sexuality also influence personal hygiene practices. For example, in an effort to promote a positive self-image, older adults may use skin care products advertised to prevent wrinkles and diminish signs of aging. Women who are sexually active may use a variety of hygiene products following intercourse that promote cleanliness.

THE NURSING PROCESS FOR SKIN CARE AND PERSONAL HYGIENE

Before attempting to teach patients healthy hygiene practices, nurses need to evaluate their own practices. Promoting Health 37-1 suggests general behaviors to maintain acceptable personal hygiene.

Assessing

Nursing History

As noted above, bathing practices and cleansing habits and rituals vary widely. A clear threat to health must exist before a nurse decides that an individual's hygiene practices are inadequate. The nurse assessing the adequacy of a patient's hygiene practices determines whether the patient has the knowledge, attitude, skills, and resources to care for the skin and mucous membranes; see the Focused Assessment Guide.

Hygiene practices include bathing and care of specific body areas, including the oral cavity, the eyes, ears, and nose, hair, nails, feet, and perineal and vaginal areas. Question the patient about any past or current problems (eg, rashes, lumps, itching, dryness, lesions). When skin problems are present, ask the patient the following:

How long have you had this problem?

Does it bother you?

How does it bother you? Does it itch?

Have you found anything that helps relieve these symptoms?

When documenting the nursing history, be specific, clearly describing the patient's typical hygiene practices and any complaints. The following are two examples of documentation related to hygiene and skin care:

Hygiene: "Showers twice daily, once in the morning and after working out in the evening. Skin tends to be very dry, and moisturizing creams are used daily. Aveeno Oilated baths p.r.n. Allergic to deodorant soaps."

Integument: "History of athlete's foot since high school days with outbreaks every 2 to 3 months. Knowledgeable about appropriate foot care. Uses antifungal agent such as terbinafine hydrochloride (Lamisil DermaGel) or tolnaftate (Tinactin cream), a topical fungicidal agent."

Oral Cavity

The mouth is the first part of the alimentary canal and is also an important part of the respiratory system. The ducts of the salivary glands open into the vestibule of the mouth. The teeth and the tongue, accessory organs in the mouth, play an important role in beginning digestion by breaking up food particles and mixing them with saliva. Saliva is also important as a mechanical cleaner of the mouth.

General good health is as important as cleanliness for maintaining a healthy mouth and teeth. For example, the relationship is well established between good teeth and a diet sufficient in calcium and phosphorus, along with vitamin D, which is necessary for the body to make use of these minerals.

Maintaining good oral hygiene and dental care has several benefits. There is esthetic value in having a clean and healthy mouth. Having one's own teeth contributes to an intact body image. The beginning of the digestive process and gustatory pleasure are enhanced when the mouth and teeth are in good condition.

Assessment of the oral cavity involves obtaining a nursing history related to the oral cavity, including structures such as the teeth, tongue, and salivary glands. When obtaining the nursing history, identify the patient's normal oral hygiene practices and the variables influencing these practices. Note the history of any oral problems and related treatments.

Promoting Health 37-1 *Hygiene*

Use the assessment checklist to determine how well you are meeting your hygiene needs. Then develop a prescription for self-care by choosing appropriate behaviors from the list of suggestions.

ASSESSMENT CHECKLIST

(almost always / sometimes / almost never)

1. I keep my hair clean and neatly styled.
2. My skin is clean.
3. The condition of my mouth indicates satisfactory oral hygiene.
4. My nails are neatly manicured.
5. My body is free of unpleasant odors.

SELF-CARE BEHAVIORS

1. Ensure that diet and exercise are appropriate, since this contributes to clean and intact skin.
2. Brush and floss teeth regularly and visit the dentist at least annually.
3. Keep hair clean, combed, and brushed regularly.
4. Use certain hair care products (eg, hair dyes) cautiously, since they may damage the hair.
5. Clean under nails and maintain nails at an appropriate length. Clip nails straight across and shape or smooth with an emery board or file, if necessary.
6. Bathe and cleanse skin regularly. Apply lotion or cream to dry skin, as necessary. Cleanse the axilla and perineal area thoroughly and apply deodorant or antiperspirant as needed.
7. Appreciate the relationship between hygiene and overall well-being.

Focused Assessment Guide 37-1

Hygiene Practices

Factors to Assess	Questions and Approaches
Daily and weekly bathing habits	Tell me about your daily and weekly bathing habits. Are there special bathing or hygiene products you routinely use or can't use? How can nurses best help you to meet your hygiene needs?
Factors interfering with hygiene practices (sensory, cognitive, endurance, mobility, or motivation)	What recently or in the past has interfered with your hygiene practices? Does anything interfere with your ability to be as clean as you would like?
History of skin or mucous membrane problems (nature, onset of problem and frequency, causes, severity, symptoms, interventions attempted, and results)	Describe any skin problems with rashes, lumps, itching, dryness, lesions, ecchymosis, or masses. What have you used to relieve these symptoms?
Special hygiene practices	
• Mouth	How do you clean your teeth and gums? How often do you have a dental examination? Do you have any dental appliances? Are there any tender areas or lesions in your mouth?
• Eyes, ears, and nose	Do you wear glasses or contact lenses to improve your vision? Do you wear a hearing aid? Have you experienced any discharge or bleeding from or swelling of your eyes, ears, or nose?
• Hair	Have you noticed any unusual dryness of the scalp or changes in hair texture and amount?
• Feet and nails	Is the appearance of the nails normal? How do you normally care for and clean your nails? Is the skin intact on the feet? Have you noticed any swelling of one or both feet? Do you wear any special shoes?
• Perineum	Have you noticed any unusual discharge, swelling, itching, or inflammation? Are you able to complete your own perineal care? Do you follow any special hygiene practices during menstruation? What type of feminine hygiene products (eg, pads, tampons, douches) do you use?

Identify any variables known to cause oral problems, such as deficient self-care abilities, poor nutrition or excessive intake of refined sugars, family history of periodontal disease, or ingestion of chemotherapeutic agents that produce oral lesions. Patients at increased risk for oral problems include those who are seriously ill, comatose, dehydrated, confused, depressed, or paralyzed. Patients who are mouth breathers, who can have no oral intake of nutrition or fluids, who have nasogastric tubes or oral airways in place, and who have had oral surgery are also at increased risk.

Eyes, Ears, and Nose

Begin the nursing history by asking the patient to identify any special eye, ear, or nose care that he or she performs. Also address any specific care measures related to the use and care of visual aids or prostheses (glasses, contact lenses, artificial eye) and hearing aids. Also inquire about any history of eye, ear, and nose problems and related treatments.

Hair

Hair is an accessory structure of the skin. Good general health is essential for attractive hair and skin, and cleanliness is a positive influence. Illness affects the hair, especially when endocrine abnormalities, increased body temperature, poor nutrition, or anxiety and worry are present. Changes in the color or condition of the hair shaft are related to changes in hormonal activity or to changes in the blood supply to hair follicles.

Begin the nursing history by identifying the patient's usual hair and scalp care practices, including styling preferences. Note any history of hair or scalp problems; possible causes of changes in the distribution, texture, or amount of hair; and related treatments. Be alert for any factors that are known to cause hair or scalp problems or that require special care, such as deficient self-care abilities, immobility, malnutrition, and treatments known to result in hair loss (eg, certain chemotherapeutic agents).

Nails and Feet

The nails are an accessory structure of the skin composed of epithelial tissue. The body of the nail is the exposed portion; the root lies in the skin in the nail groove where the nail grows and is nourished. Healthy nailbeds are pink, convex, and evenly curved. With certain pathologic conditions, and to some extent with aging, the nails become ridged and areas become concave.

When obtaining the patient's nursing history, gather information about the patient's normal nail and foot care practices. Include the type of footwear worn and any history of nail or foot problems and their treatments. Foot problems, particularly common in people with diabetes mellitus and peripheral vascular disease, often require hospitalization (Plummer, 2001). A proactive educational approach can prevent many of the serious complications (eg, ulcers, lower extremity amputations) associated with foot problems.

Identify any variables known to cause nail and foot problems, such as deficient self-care abilities, vascular disease, arthritis, diabetes mellitus, history of biting nails or trimming them improperly, frequent or prolonged exposure to chemicals or water, trauma, ill-fitting shoes, or obesity.

Perineal and Vaginal Areas

The perineal area is dark, warm, and often moist, conditions that favor bacterial growth. The patient who cannot clean the perineal area needs the nurse's assistance for this important part of personal hygiene. Neglecting perineal cleaning for the patient who cannot provide self-care often results in physical and psychological discomfort for the patient, skin breakdown, and offensive odors.

When obtaining the nursing history, note any history of perineal or vaginal problems and related treatments. Identify any variables known to cause perineal or vaginal problems or to create a need for special care, such as urinary or fecal incontinence, an indwelling Foley catheter, childbirth, douching, rectal or genital surgery, and diseases such as urinary tract infection, diabetes mellitus, and certain sexually transmitted infections (STIs, eg, herpes).

Physical Assessment

The inspection and palpation skills used to assess the integumentary system are described in detail in Chapter 25, Health Assessment. Assisting patients with basic hygiene measures provides an excellent opportunity for examining a patient's skin. Many individuals are unaware that they have skin lesions, such as precancerous moles, that if untreated could prove fatal. Early detection and treatment of skin problems are important nursing functions.

When examining the skin, pay careful attention to cleanliness, color, texture, temperature, turgor, moisture, sensation, vascularity, and any lesions. If a lesion is detected, document the type, color, size, distribution and grouping, location, and consistency. (Terminology helpful in describing these findings is presented in Chapter 25.) Follow these general guidelines for assessing the skin:

- Proceed systematically in head-to-toe fashion.
- Use a good source of light, preferably daylight.
- Compare bilateral parts for symmetry.
- Use standard terminology to report and record findings.
- Allow data obtained in the nursing history to direct the skin assessment.
- Identify any variables known to cause skin problems, such as deficient self-care abilities, immobility, malnutrition, decreased hydration, decreased sensation, sun exposure, vascular problems (altered tissue perfusion or venous return), or the presence of irritants (body secretions or excretions on the skin, other chemicals, mechanical devices).

Because lifestyle factors, changes in health state, illness, and certain diagnostic and therapeutic measures may adversely affect the skin, be alert for patients who may be at high risk for skin problems, and perform the appropriate skin assessment. Table 37-2 identifies some factors that place a patient at risk for skin alterations. Knowing when to perform the skin assessment and incorporating this into the patient's plan of care is as important as knowing how to do this well.

When documenting the physical assessment of the skin, describe exactly what is observed or palpated, including appearance, texture, size, location or distribution, and any characteristic findings. The following are two examples of documentation of the physical assessment of the skin:

"Skin is pink, warm, dry, and elastic; no petechiae, lesions, or excoriation; multiple moles of small size and regular border and surface."

"Red, macular rash generalized over trunk and thighs; semiconfluent lesions measure 1 to 2 mm; abrupt onset."

Oral Cavity

A physical assessment of the oral cavity involves inspection of the oral cavity and surrounding structures, with particular attention to any unusual odors. When performing the physical assessment of the oral cavity, examine the following:

- Lips: color, moisture, lumps, ulcers, lesions, and edema
- Buccal mucosa: color, moisture, lesions, nodules, and bleeding
- Color of the gums and surface of the gums: lesions, bleeding, edema, and exudate
- Teeth: any loose, missing, or carious (decayed) teeth. Note the presence of dentures or other orthodontic devices.
- Tongue: color, symmetry, movement, texture, and lesions
- Hard and soft palates: intactness, color, patches, lesions, and petechiae
- Oropharynx: movement of the uvula and condition of tonsils, if present

Also, note unusual mouth odors and assess the adequacy of mastication and swallowing. (See Chap. 25 for a further description of the nursing assessment of the oral cavity.)

When inspecting the oral cavity, observe for any oral problems. These problems may be benign or only mildly annoying to patients, but they may also be life-threatening. Identifying

TABLE 37-2 Factors Placing an Individual at Risk for Skin Alterations

Factor	Nursing Implications
Lifestyle Variables	
Homosexuality, history of multiple sexual partners; intravenous drug users; hemophiliacs; bisexual male; partners of the above	• These patients are at high risk for infection with human immunodeficiency virus (HIV) and acquired immunodeficiency syndrome (AIDS). • Assessment needs to include careful examination of the skin for purple blotches that may be indicative of Kaposi's sarcoma.
Occupation that gives a fair, thin-skinned individual prolonged exposure to the sun	• Places individual at high risk for developing skin cancer, which has an excellent prognosis if detected and treated in its early stages but which may be fatal if treatment is delayed. • Assessment needs to include careful examination for a sore that does not heal or a change in size or color of a wart or mole.
Changes in Health State	
Dehydration or malnutrition	• If fluid, protein, and vitamin C intake is deficient, skin loses elasticity and becomes prone to breakdown. • Nursing care is directed toward preventing skin breakdown: frequent changes of patient's position with skin assessment at each change, special mattresses and protection of bony prominences, use of lotions, attention to fluid and nutritional status.
Reduced sensation (paralysis, local nerve damage, circulatory insufficiency)	• Patient's inability to sense temperature extremes, pressure, friction, and other such factors can easily result in injury. • Nursing care incorporates special attention to safety.
Illness	
Diabetes mellitus	• Numerous factors combine to cause skin problems in diabetic patients: cuts and sores that do not heal, lesions on the lower extremities that ulcerate and become necrotic, recurrent bacterial and fungal infections. • The diabetic patient must be taught special hygiene measures to prevent trauma to the skin and learn to assess the skin carefully to detect any alteration.
Diagnostic Measures	
Gastrointestinal (GI) series	• The GI cleansing preparations administered to patients having GI studies done may result in diarrhea, which irritates the sensitive skin in the perianal area—especially if the patient had bouts of diarrhea before the studies; anticipating the problem, noting redness and inflammation, and beginning warm baths and ointments are welcome nursing measures that patients may be too embarrassed to seek.
Therapeutic Measures	
Bed rest	• Bed rest predisposes patients to skin breakdown; the harsh detergents used on hospital laundry compound this problem. • Pressure points need to be examined frequently and protected.
Casts	• Casts easily irritate the skin; careful assessment, covering the rough edges of the cast, and skin care are indicated.
Aquathermia unit	• Wet heat has therapeutic benefit but, if applied to the skin for too long, may macerate the skin; follow protocol in length of application, examine skin carefully between treatments, and allow to dry.
Medications	• Medications may cause allergic skin reactions, such as rashes. • When evaluating the patient's response to a new drug, examine the skin for redness and itching.

the problem and its cause and initiating appropriate treatment are imperative. This may require consultation with a dentist or physician.

Dental Caries

The decay of teeth with the formation of cavities is called **caries.** Caries result from failure to remove **plaque,** an invisible, destructive, bacterial film that builds up on everyone's teeth and eventually leads to the destruction of tooth enamel. A successful plaque-fighting program includes elim-

ination of sweet snacks such as soft drinks, candy, gum, jams, and jellies between meals; thorough cleansing; and regular dental checkups. The use of antiplaque fluoride toothpastes, mouth rinses, and flossing also helps prevent dental caries.

Periodontal Disease

The major cause of tooth loss in adults older than 35 years of age is gum disease. **Gingivitis** is an inflammation of the gingiva, the tissue that surrounds the teeth. **Pyorrhea,** or periodontal disease, is a marked inflammation of the gums that also involves the alveolar tissues. Symptoms include bleeding gums; swollen, red, painful gum tissues; receding gum lines with the formation of pockets between the teeth and gums; pus that appears when gums are pressed; and loose teeth. If unchecked, plaque builds up and, along with dead bacteria, forms hard deposits called **tartar** at the gum lines. The tartar attacks the fibers that fasten teeth to the gums and eventually attacks bone tissue also. The teeth then loosen and fall out. A strong mouth odor (**halitosis**) or a persistent bad taste in the mouth may be the first indication of periodontal disease. Regular treatment by a dentist is imperative.

Other Oral Problems

Other oral problems that may be observed when inspecting the oral cavity include the following:

- Stomatitis, an inflammation of the oral mucosa, has numerous causes, such as bacteria, virus, mechanical trauma, irritants, nutritional deficiencies, and systemic infection. Symptoms may include heat, pain, increased flow of saliva, and halitosis.
- Glossitis, an inflammation of the tongue, can be caused by deficiencies of vitamin B_{12}, folic acid, and iron.
- Cheilosis, an ulceration of the lips (reddened fissures at the angles of the mouth), is most often caused by vitamin B complex deficiencies (especially riboflavin).
- Dry oral mucosa may simply be related to dehydration or may be caused by mouth breathing, an alteration in salivary functioning, or certain medications (eg, anticholinergic drugs).
- Oral malignancies, appearing as lumps or ulcers, must be distinguished from benign mouth problems because early detection may be the difference between cure, radical surgery, or death. Teach patients to see their dentist immediately if they notice white or red patches, persistent sores, swelling, bleeding, numbness, or pain in the mouth.

Eyes, Ears, and Nose

During the eye examination, note the position, alignment, and general appearance of the eye. Check that eyelashes are equally distributed and curl outward. Note the presence of lesions, nodules, redness, swelling, crusting, flaking, excessive tearing, or discharge of eyelids. Check the color of the conjunctivae and test the patient's blink reflex. Assess the patient's gross visual acuity by having the patient read newsprint.

When examining the ear, note its position, alignment, and general appearance. Pay particular attention to a buildup of wax in the canal, dryness, crusting, or the presence of any discharge or foreign body. About one third of older adults have at least one ear obstructed by a wax buildup, and this frequently causes hearing loss that can be reversed (Stone, 1999). Test the patient's gross hearing acuity.

While examining the nose, note its position and general appearance, patency of the nostrils, and presence of tenderness, dryness, edema, bleeding, discharge, or secretions.

Refer to Chapter 25 for additional information related to nursing assessment of the eyes, ears, and nose.

Hair

Assess the condition of the hair. Inspect it for texture, cleanliness, and oiliness. Inspect the scalp for any scaling, lesions, inflammation, or infection. Note any abnormalities such as dandruff, hair loss, or infestations.

Dandruff

Dandruff is a condition characterized by itching and flaking of the scalp and may be complicated by the embarrassment it causes. Persistent, severe cases usually require medical attention, but daily brushing and shampooing with a medicated shampoo may be all that is needed to keep the scalp free of dandruff.

Hair Loss

Hair growth and hair loss are ongoing, daily processes. Hair loss from plaiting, excessive backcombing and teasing, or the use of hair rollers is usually temporary, and hair returns when the tension on the hair shaft is halted. Some people experience hair loss resulting from illness with high fever, certain medications, x-ray therapy of the head, childbirth, or general anesthesia. Some believe that an excessive intake of vitamin A may play a role in hair loss. Some permanent thinning of hair normally accompanies aging.

Absence or loss of hair on the head, also referred to as baldness, is called **alopecia.** It is common in men but rare in women, and it is believed to be hereditary. There is no known cure for baldness, although some medications are currently in use and others are being developed; their long-term efficacy is unknown. For example, minoxidil (Rogaine), a cardiovascular and antihypertensive drug, has reversed balding to some degree when applied to the scalp. Hairpieces, frequently worn by people who are bald, require the same care as normal hair but less frequent washing.

Hair transplantation is a surgical procedure for baldness. Hair is taken from donor sites, usually from the back or sides of the scalp, and transplanted to areas with no hair. The procedure is long and expensive but reportedly has decided benefits for people who find baldness psychologically unpleasant. Complications include serious scalp infections.

Pediculosis

Infestation with lice is called **pediculosis.** There are three common types of lice: *Pediculus humanus capitis,* which infests the hair and scalp; *Pediculus humanus corporis,* which infests the body; and *Phthirus pubis,* which infests the shorter hairs on the body, usually the pubic and axillary hair. Lice lay eggs, called nits, on the hair shafts. Nits are white or light gray and look like dandruff but cannot be brushed or shaken off the hair. Frequent scratching and scratch marks on the body and the scalp suggest the presence of pediculosis. Although anyone may become infested with lice, the continued presence of pediculosis is usually a result of uncleanliness.

Pediculosis can be spread directly by contact with infested areas or indirectly through clothing, bed linen, brushes, and combs. Teaching patients, especially children, not to share personal items is a good way to prevent transmission. The linens and personal care items of a patient with pediculosis require separate and careful handling to prevent spread from person to person.

Several commercial preparations, called pediculicides, are available for the treatment of pediculosis. These drugs destroy the lice and their eggs or nits. However, several treatments are usually necessary before all the nits are destroyed. The procedures and the medications used for the treatment of pediculosis vary among health agencies. The infested hair may be shaved, especially when pubic and axillary hair is infested. In addition, the partners of patients with pubic infestation must be notified.

Recall Kylie Simpson, the school-aged child with lice. The nurse would need to review the methods of transmission with Kylie and her father, reinforcing that anyone can become infested with lice. In addition, the nurse needs to instruct Kylie's father how to handle the items that Kylie has come into contact with since she developed the infestation. Kylie's father also needs education about the use of the prescribed pediculicide to ensure eradication of the infestation. Although the diagnosis of a lice infestation can be quite upsetting, the information and support provided by the nurse can help to minimize the father's anxiety, fears, and feelings of shame and embarrassment.

When educating the patient, stress the importance of finishing the treatment. Many times the patient will shampoo the hair once and not follow through with a second washing. Failure to complete the treatment has produced lice who are now resistant to many of the pediculicides on the market. See Teaching to Promote Health at Home 37-1: Dealing With Head Lice.

Ticks

Ticks are important because they can transmit serious diseases such as Lyme disease, Rocky Mountain spotted fever, and tularemia. Transmission of these diseases can be decreased if the tick is removed within 24 hours of becoming attached. To remove a tick, grasp it with tweezers close to the skin and then steadily pull the tick away (Pauldine, 2003). Once the tick is removed, cleanse the tick bite area with an antiseptic.

Nail and Foot Care

Examine nails for intactness and cleanliness; note capillary refill and the contour of the nailbed; observe the nail base

---

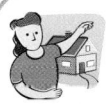

Teaching to Promote Health at Home 37-1
Dealing with Head Lice

Health Topic	Suggested Content	Why is This Important?
Who is at risk for getting head lice?	Preschool and elementary-age children (age 3–10) and their families are most often infested; however, anyone coming in contact with someone who has lice can become infected. African-Americans are less likely to become infected with lice.	Lice can infect any person, regardless of hygiene practices or social status.
How do you become infected with head lice?	By coming in close contact with anyone who has lice; sharing combs, hats, clothing, coats, and scarves with anyone who has lice; lying on a bed, couch, pillow, carpet, or stuffed animal that has recently been in contact with someone who has lice.	One way to prevent the spread of lice is to avoid sharing combs and clothing with people outside of the family.
What are the signs and symptoms of head lice infestation?	Tickling feeling on scalp; itching; sores on the head caused by scratching. The lice may also be seen, especially behind the ears and near the neckline at the back of the neck.	The faster the lice are noticed, the easier they are to eradicate.
How is head lice treated?	Apply a pediculicide according to the manufacturer's directions. Machine wash all washable clothing and bed linens using a hot water cycle. Dry laundry using high heat for at least 20 minutes. Store all clothing, stuffed animals, comforters, and other material things that cannot be washed or dry cleaned in a plastic bag for 2 weeks. Soak all brushes for 1 hour in rubbing alcohol. Vacuum the floor and furniture.	All head lice must be killed or removed or a reinfestation may occur.

Information obtained from http://www.cdc.gov/ncidod/dpd/parasites/headlice/factsht_head_lice.htm

for redness, swelling, bleeding, discharge, and tenderness. Examine the feet for cleanliness and intactness of skin, and note any swelling, inflammation, lesions, tenderness, or orthopedic problems. Examine carefully the skin between the toes. Refer to Chapter 25 for additional information on techniques for assessing the nails and feet.

Perineal and Vaginal Areas

Examine the male genitalia for lesions, swelling, inflammation, excoriation, tenderness, and discharge (amount, color, odor, and source). Examine the female genitalia (pubic area, labia, clitoris, urinary meatus, and perineum) for color, size, lesions, masses, swelling, inflammation, excoriation, tenderness, and discharge (amount, color, odor, and source). Inspect the anal area for cracks, nodules, distended veins, masses, or polyps. Note any perineal odors. Refer to Chapter 25 for additional information about perineal assessment.

Diagnosing

A careful assessment of the skin, mucous membranes, and other body areas may lead to the identification of numerous patient problems that can be classified as nursing diagnoses. Problems concerning deficient hygiene are categorized as self-care deficits. Self-Care Deficit diagnoses address four specific activities necessary to meet daily needs: feeding, bathing and hygiene, dressing and grooming, and toileting. It is important to identify the cause of these problems correctly. If hygiene is deficient because of insufficient knowledge, health education may quickly remedy the problem. If, however, hygiene is viewed as a low priority by the individual or the person lacks the physical ability to perform hygiene measures, these problems must be addressed before health education can be effective. Examples of nursing diagnoses related to hygiene and skin problems are highlighted in the NANDA Nursing Diagnoses box.

In certain situations, a wellness nursing diagnosis may be appropriate as the patient progresses toward an increased level of health awareness and wellness. An example of a wellness diagnosis may be Health-Seeking Behaviors related to oral hygiene practices.

Data collected during the nursing assessment may also lead to the identification of a collaborative problem. For example, a patient receiving intravenous chemotherapy is at risk for developing phlebitis, a complication requiring a collaborative approach. Therefore, when caring for a patient receiving intravenous chemotherapy, checking the infusion site every shift is a priority based on the nurse's knowledge that this complication can occur. In addition, careful preparation and administration of the drug according to the manufacturer's instructions, adherence to nursing protocols for the maintenance of intravenous infusions, and ongoing nursing assessment are key to helping reduce the risk for phlebitis. If redness, warmth, tenderness, or swelling is noted, immediate collaborative intervention is indicated.

Similarly, a nurse may notice a 1.5-cm mole with an irregular border on a patient's back during a bath. Prompt report-ing of this finding to the physician may lead to the detection and early, successful treatment of the medical diagnosis of malignant melanoma.

Outcome Identification and Planning

The plan of nursing care identifies nursing measures to assist the patient to develop or maintain hygiene practices that contribute to a sense of well-being. Appropriate expected outcomes include the following: The patient will:

- Verbalize feeling comfortable and clean
- Participate fully in necessary hygiene measures according to cognitive, sensory, mobility, and endurance abilities
- Maintain intact skin and mucous membranes
- Demonstrate correct skin care measures (when indicated), such as oral care, care of eyes, ears, and nose, nail and foot care, perineal and vaginal care
- Demonstrate signs of healing in existing lesions (oral, scalp, or perineal)
- Exhibit lips, oral mucosa, gums, and tongue that are intact, moist, and free of inflammation and lesions
- Verbalize importance of fluoride use and regular dental examinations
- Demonstrate healthy functioning of eyes, ears, and nose
- Exhibit eyes, ears, and nose that appear clean
- Demonstrate proper use and care of visual or auditory aids
- Exhibit clean hair
- Verbalize satisfaction with appearance
- Participate in hair and scalp care as able
- Exhibit intact, clean, and manicured nails
- Demonstrate intact, clean, and lesion-free foot skin
- Report reduced or absent nail and foot problems (specify: calluses, corns, plantar warts, ingrown nails, athlete's foot)

Implementing

When performing general hygiene measures, the nurse should respect the patient's personal preferences, allow and encourage as much self-care as the patient can perform, meet the patient's need for privacy, and promote physiologic and psychological wellness. The following sections discuss general hygiene measures, including providing scheduled care, helping with bathing, massaging, making the bed, providing environmental care, and teaching patients about skin care.

Providing Scheduled Hygiene Care

When patients require nursing assistance with personal hygiene, it is important to schedule this care at regular intervals. In most hospitals and long-term care settings, the following types of hygiene care are provided. These are individualized according to the patient's personal and cultural preferences.

Remember Andrew Craig, the older man in the long-term care facility who reported that he had already had a complete bath. The nurse would need to investigate this to determine

Examples of NANDA Nursing Diagnoses | Hygiene

Nursing Diagnoses	Related Factors
Bathing/Hygiene Self-Care Deficit	Sensory, cognitive, endurance, mobility, or motivation deficits; low value attached to regular brushing, flossing, and dental examinations
Pain	Skin or mucous membrane alterations
Ineffective Coping	Chronic skin problems
Ineffective Health Maintenance (eg, dental caries, periodontal disease, halitosis)	Deficient oral hygiene practices
Deficient Knowledge	New therapeutic regimen to manage skin or mucous membrane alteration
Impaired Physical Mobility	Painful foot condition (calluses, corns, plantar warts)
Impaired Oral Mucous Membrane	Inadequate oral hygiene, stomatitis, malnutrition, or dehydration
Risk for Infection	Broken skin or traumatized tissue, breaks in oral mucosa and inadequate secondary defenses, traumatized nail base or deficient nail or foot care
Disturbed Body Image	Visible integumentary problems, body odors, loss of teeth, halitosis, dental caries, baldness
Ineffective Sexuality Patterns	Fear of transmitting or acquiring sexually transmitted disease, painful genital lesions
Impaired Skin Integrity	Altered circulation, nutrition and fluid deficit or excess, impaired mobility, irritants (chemical, thermal, mechanical, radiation), scalp laceration (head bandages), pruritus, urinary and fecal incontinence
Risk for Impaired Skin Integrity	Immobility, use of physical restraints, use of an aquathermia device, dehydration, bladder and/or bowel incontinence
Impaired Social Interaction	Negative body image (eg, acne, alopecia), visual or auditory impairment
Impaired Swallowing	Reddened, irritated oropharyngeal cavity
Impaired Tissue Integrity (eg, cornea, mucous membrane, integumentary, or subcutaneous)	Altered circulation, nutrition or fluid deficit or excess, impaired mobility, irritants (chemical, thermal, mechanical, radiation)
Pain	Chemotherapy-induced oral ulceration; corns, calluses, plantar warts, ingrown toenails in foot
Imbalanced Nutrition: Less Than Body Requirements	Painful oral lesions (ill-fitting dentures, gingivitis)
Impaired Oral Mucous Membrane	Dehydration (ineffective oral hygiene, medication)
Disturbed Sensory Perception (Visual, Auditory, or Olfactory)	Psychological stress
Ineffective Health Maintenance	Perceptual impairment (visual or auditory)
Fear	Sudden loss of vision or hearing
Anticipatory Grieving	Increasing visual or auditory impairment
Risk for Injury	Visual impairment

if he had indeed received care. If he had not, then the nurse would need to seek additional information to explain his statement: perhaps the patient was too tired or did not like having to be helped with his care. This information is essential to plan the patient's care effectively.

Early Morning Care

Shortly after the patient awakens, assist him or her with toileting if necessary and then provide comfort measures to refresh the patient and prepare him or her for breakfast (or diagnostic tests). Nursing measures include washing the face and hands and providing mouth care. If needed, supplies necessary for morning care can be ordered at this time.

Morning Care (a.m. Care)

After breakfast, complete morning care. Depending on the patient's self-care abilities, offer assistance with toileting, oral care, bathing, back massage, special skin care measures (eg, pressure ulcer), hair care (includes shaving if indicated), cosmetics, dressing, and positioning for comfort. Cosmetics, if desired, can enhance morale in an ill patient. Agency policies are followed for refreshing or changing bed linens, and the patient's bedside area is tidied. When morning care is completed, the patient should feel refreshed and should be in a comfortable and safe environment.

Morning care is often categorized as self-care, partial care, or complete care. Patients identified as self-care are capable of managing their personal hygiene independently once oriented to the bathroom. However, offer a back massage and spend time assessing the patient's day-to-day needs. Patients identified as partial care most often receive morning hygiene care at the bedside or seated near the sink in the bathroom. They usually require assistance with body areas that are difficult to reach. Patients identified as complete care require nursing assistance with all aspects of personal hygiene. A complete bed bath is done, or the patient is taken to the shower or tub.

Afternoon Care (p.m. Care)

Because hospitalized patients frequently receive visitors in the afternoon or evening or use this time to rest when not scheduled for tests or therapies, ensure the patient's comfort after lunch and offer assistance to nonambulatory patients with toileting, handwashing, and oral care. Straightening bed linens and helping patients with mobility problems to reposition themselves comfortably are other welcome nursing measures.

Hour of Sleep Care (h.s. Care)

Shortly before the patient retires, again offer assistance with toileting, washing of the face and hands, and oral care. Because many patients find that a back massage helps them to relax and fall asleep, offer one routinely. Change any soiled bed linens or clothing and position the patient comfortably. Ensure that the call light and any other objects the patient desires (eg, urinal, radio, water glass) are within easy reach.

As Needed Care (p.r.n. Care)

In addition to scheduled care, offer individual hygiene measures as needed. Some patients require oral care every 2 hours. Patients who are diaphoretic (sweating profusely) may need their clothing and bed linens changed several times a shift. At other times, a nurse may decide to forego hygiene measures because the patient's need for undisturbed rest may be a higher priority.

Helping With Bathing

Bathing serves a variety of purposes, including:
- Cleansing the skin
- Acting as a skin conditioner
- Helping to relax a restless person
- Promoting circulation by stimulating the skin's peripheral nerve endings and underlying tissues
- Serving as a musculoskeletal exercise through activity involved with bathing, thereby improving joint mobility and muscle tonus
- Stimulating the rate and depth of respirations
- Promoting comfort through muscle relaxation and skin stimulation
- Providing sensory input
- Helping to improve self-image
- Providing an excellent opportunity to strengthen the nurse–patient relationship, to thoroughly assess the patient's integumentary system, to observe the patient's physiologic and emotional status closely, to teach the patient as indicated, and to demonstrate care and interest in the patient's general welfare

The simple act of bathing a patient is a vital and caring intervention. In recent years, this basic personal care measure has often been assigned to an unlicensed staff member rather than the professional nurse. It has become a task to be accomplished rather than an opportunity for therapeutic individualized intervention. Although hygiene measures are increasingly being performed by unlicensed assistive personnel, the nurse is responsible for ensuring that hygiene measures were satisfactorily performed. Refer to Chapter 15, Implementing, for a discussion of the nurse's accountability when care is delegated. Nurses whose primary focus is the patient, however, can use the time spent on assisting with bathing to establish a rapport with the patient and to further assess the patient's integumentary system. See Through the Eyes of a Student.

Shower and Tub Baths

A shower or tub bath is the preferred method of bathing for hospitalized patients who are ambulatory. For the most part, even though most patients can do this on their own, the following responsibilities apply:
- Check to see that the bathroom is available, clean, and safe. Showers and tubs should have mats or nonskid strips to prevent patients from slipping and falling.
- Ensure that necessary articles, such as soap, a washcloth, a towel, and a gown, are available for the patient.
- Provide a place for a weak or physically disabled patient to sit in a shower. Most health agencies have a stool or chair that can be used in the shower, and handheld shower heads may facilitate the process. Some nurses have reported that a commode chair with the pan removed serves effectively as a shower chair and offers the patient more support than a stool or chair.
- Assist the patient to the shower or bathroom, as indicated. Patients who are beginning ambulation often need assistance to help prevent falling or fainting.
- Check to see that the water temperature is safe and comfortable—43° to 46°C (110° to 115°F). The lower temperature is recommended for children and elderly patients.
- Help the patient get in and out of the bathtub, as indicated. Have the patient grasp the handrails at the side of

Through the Eyes of a Student

I entered the room with a feeling of dread. How could I possibly bathe the sick, elderly, helpless woman lying in this hospital bed? I had never bathed anyone older than age 2 years, other than myself, of course. How would I be able to move her limp, seemingly lifeless old body? What would an 85-year-old body look like? I could not imagine. I've read all the manuals that describe this procedure, I know what to do, so why am I so nervous? I must be worried that I will hurt her in some way. Maybe she has not been cared for properly before and her hygiene is poor. Well, I might as well get this over with because I'll be doing it the rest of my life. I've got to learn sometime.

I've mustered up enough courage to enter my patient's room. Michelle, her primary nurse, offers to help me because the patient is so difficult to move. Boy, am I relieved! Right before Michelle and I are about to begin, my patient, Mrs. Ash, asks for her teeth. I assume this must mean her dentures and reassure her that I have not seen them but will be happy to look for them as soon as we have completed her bath. Michelle and I each take a side and begin to bathe her. It's truly amazing how those range-of-motion exercises come to mind so easily. I had thought they were long forgotten with the rest of the past semester. Wouldn't my instructors love to hear me now! Suddenly Mrs. Ash yells, "I need the bed pan!" "Oh no!" I thought, as I rushed to the bathroom with soapy gloved hands trying frantically to locate her bed pan before there could be an accident. Michelle, who remained calm during my frenzy, simply stated, "Don't worry, she has an indwelling catheter. She says that every time I bathe her." I knew she had a catheter, how did I forget? Somewhat humbled, I returned to the procedure. I really wanted to put some lotion on her skin because it was so dry. When we were ready to do her back, we prepared to lift her. I pulled her toward me, and Michelle was to continue the bath. We were not prepared for what we saw underneath. Firmly cushioned in Mrs. Ash's lower left buttock were none other than her dentures! On removing them, Michelle and I had to smile at the periodontal grin implanted on Mrs. Ash's bottom. Michelle then asked her how her teeth had gotten to the location where we found them. All she seemed to know was that she needed those teeth back in her mouth STAT! She snatched the dentures from Michelle's hand and attempted to insert them. Michelle and I in unison blurted out, "No, Mrs. Ash, please wait until we clean your teeth before you put them back in your mouth!" Mrs. Ash, somewhat confused, begrudgingly handed over her teeth to be cleaned. Michelle had the honors while I finished the last touches of good hygiene for Mrs. Ash.

What a difference cleanliness can make, not only for the patient but also for me, the student nurse. I felt better knowing that Mrs. Ash was clean and that this procedure was behind me. And to think that I was apprehensive! This was definitely an interesting learning experience.

—Marilyn Johnson,
Holy Family College, Philadelphia

the tub, or place a chair at the side of the tub. The patient sits on the chair and eases to the edge of the tub. After putting both feet into the tub, it is then relatively easy for the patient to reach the opposite side and ease down into the tub. The patient may kneel first in the tub and then sit in it; this process can be reversed when leaving the tub. Use a hydraulic lift, when available, to lower and lift a helpless, heavy patient in and out of a tub.

- Ensure privacy for patients who can safely shower or bathe independently. See that a call device is handy, and make sure the patient knows what the button is for, so that the patient can obtain help if necessary.
- Keep the bathroom door unlocked. Health personnel should be able to enter with ease if the patient needs help. A sign hung on the door ensures privacy. Never leave children alone in the bathroom.
- Help to wash and dry areas of the body that the patient cannot reach, such as the back.
- Make any necessary adaptations. For example, if the patient is confused and becomes agitated by his or her own reflection in the mirror, cover the mirror with a pillowcase before bringing the patient into the tub room (Hilgers, 2003).

Recall Sonya Delamordo, the older Hispanic woman going to her daughter's home after a stroke. Although the responsibilities listed apply to a hospitalized patient, the nurse can incorporate these responsibilities into the teaching plan for Mrs. Delamordo's daughter to ensure the patient's safety with hygiene.

Figure 37-2 illustrates several features that add to the safety of a patient taking a shower or tub bath.

Bed Baths

Some patients must remain in bed as a part of their therapeutic regimen but can still bathe themselves. The following measures help patients to take a bath in bed in several ways:

- Provide the patient with articles for bathing and a basin of water that is a comfortable and safe temperature. Place these items conveniently for the patient on a bedside stand or overbed table.
- Provide privacy for the patient. Make sure the call device is within reach.
- Remove the top linens from the patient's bed and replace them with a bath blanket.
- Place cosmetics in a convenient place for the patient. Provide a mirror, a good light, and hot water for patients who wish to shave with a razor.
- Assist patients who cannot bathe themselves completely. For example, some patients can wash only the upper parts of the body. The remainder of the bath is then completed by nursing personnel.

Bathing procedures for patients who require total nursing assistance vary among health agencies. Skill 37-1 offers one example as a guide. It assumes that the patient can be raised or lowered in bed and that, although the patient may have limited movement, the nurse can manage the patient alone.

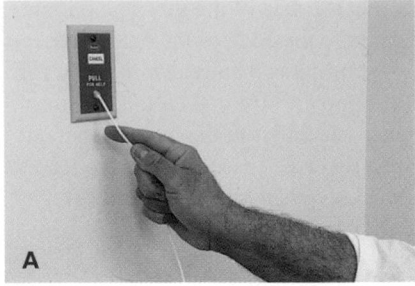 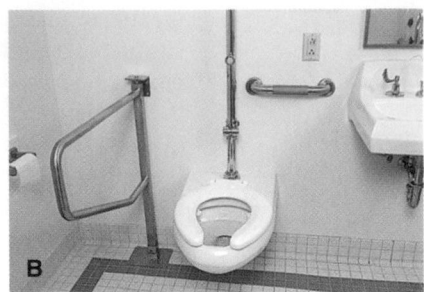 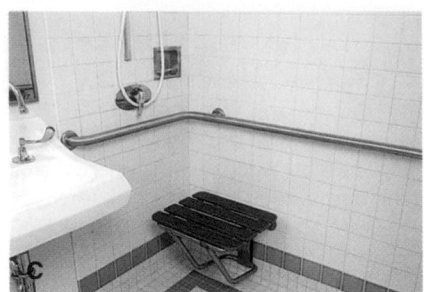

FIGURE 37-2 Examples of features that add to the safety of a patient in bed. (**A**) A call bell equipped with a pull cord. (**B**) Hand rails for use with the commode. (**C**) A shower equipped with a safety seat. (Photo © B. Proud.)

The Bag Bath

Some healthcare agencies recommend use of the "bag bath" as an alternative to the traditional bed bath. This self-contained bathing system consists of a plastic bag containing 8 to 10 pre-moistened washcloths. The bag bath is warmed for a short time (about a minute and a half) in a microwave; experimentation may be needed to find the appropriate time for the washcloths to be warmed to a safe temperature. Each part of the patient's body is cleansed with a fresh cloth. The skin is allowed to air dry (for about 30 seconds) so that the emollient ingredient of the cleaner remains on the skin.

Feedback about this procedure has been overwhelmingly positive. Staff value the time savings when compared with a traditional bed bath and find it effective and easy to perform. Most patients have commented favorably on the bag bath. Patients with mild to moderate skin impairments demonstrated an improved skin condition from consistent use of the bag bath.

(text continues on page 1025)

SKILL 37-1   Giving a Bed Bath

EQUIPMENT

Wash basin
Soap and dish
Washcloths
Bath blanket
Gown or pajamas

Bath thermometer
Bed linen
Towels (2)
Disposable gloves—for anal and perineal care (optional for remainder of bath)

Personal hygiene supplies—deodorant, lotion, and others
Bedpan or urinal
Laundry bag or cart

ACTION	RATIONALE
1. Discuss procedure with the patient and assess the patient's ability to assist in the bathing process as well as personal hygiene preferences. Review the patient's chart for any limitations in physical activity.	This discussion promotes reassurance and provides knowledge about the procedure. Dialogue also encourages patient participation and allows for individualized nursing care.
2. Bring necessary equipment to the bedside stand or overbed table. Remove sequential compression devices and anti-embolism stockings from lower extremities according to agency protocol.	Bringing everything to the bedside conserves time and energy. Arranging items nearby is convenient, saves time, and helps prevent unnecessary stretching and twisting of muscles on the part of the nurse. Most manufacturers and agencies recommend removal of these devices during the bath to allow for assessment.
3. Close the curtains around the bed and close the door to the room if possible.	This ensures the patient's privacy and lessens the possibility of loss of body heat during the bath.
4. Offer the patient the bedpan or urinal.	Voiding or defecating before the bath lessens the likelihood that the bath will be interrupted because warm bath water may stimulate the urge to void.
5. Perform hand hygiene.	Hand hygiene deters the spread of microorganisms.
6. Raise the patient's bed to the high position.	Having the bed in a high position prevents strain on the nurse's back.
7. Lower the side rail nearer to you and assist the patient to the side of the bed where you will work. Have the patient lie on his or her back.	Having the patient positioned near the nurse and lowering the side rail help prevent unnecessary stretching and twisting of muscles on the part of the nurse.

(continued)

SKILL 37-1 Giving a Bed Bath (continued)

ACTION	RATIONALE
8. Loosen top covers and remove all except the top sheet. Place bath blanket over the patient and then remove the top sheet while the patient holds the bath blanket in place. If linen is to be reused, fold it over a chair. Place soiled linen in the laundry bag.	The patient is not exposed unnecessarily, and warmth is maintained. If a bath blanket is unavailable, the top sheet may be used in place of the bath blanket.
9. Assist the patient with oral hygiene, as necessary, and as described in Skill 37-5.	This helps maintain teeth and gums in good condition, alleviates unpleasant odor and taste, and may improve appetite. Some patients may prefer oral care after the bath is completed.
10. Remove the patient's gown and keep the bath blanket in place. If patient has an intravenous line and is not wearing a gown with snap sleeves, remove the gown from the other arm first. Lower the intravenous container and pass the gown over the tubing and the container. Rehang the container and check the drip rate.	This provides uncluttered access during the bath and maintains warmth of the patient. Intravenous fluids must be maintained at the prescribed rate.
11. Raise the side rail. Fill the basin with a sufficient amount of comfortably warm water (between 43° and 46°C [110° to 115°F]). Change as necessary throughout the bath. Lower the side rail closer to you when you return to the bedside to begin the bath.	Side rails maintain patient safety. Warm water is comfortable and relaxing for the patient. It also stimulates circulation and provides for more effective cleansing.
12. Fold the washcloth like a mitt on your hand so that there are no loose ends, as illustrated.	Having loose ends of cloth drag across the patient's skin is uncomfortable. Loose ends cool quickly and feel cold to the patient.

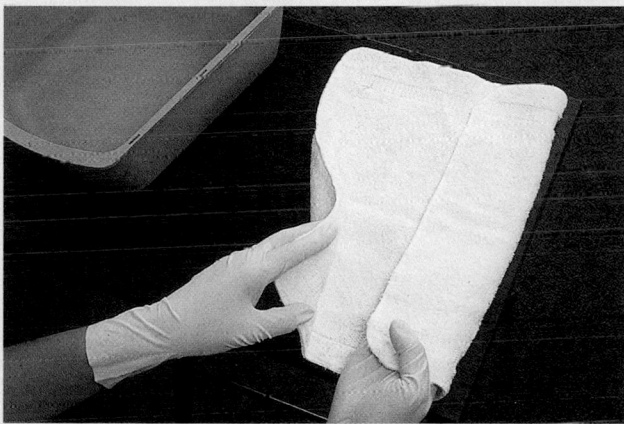

Action 12: Folding washcloth in thirds around hand to make a bath mitt.

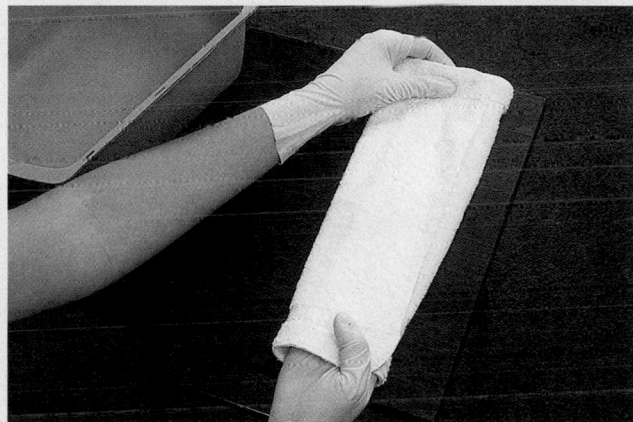

Action 12: Straightening washcloth before folding into mitt.

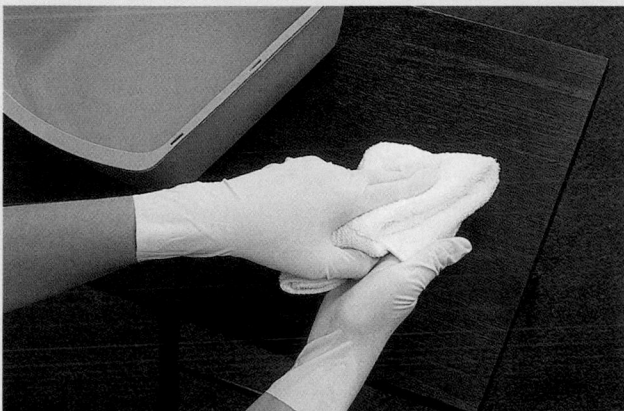

Action 12: Folding ends over and tucking ends under folded washcloth over palm.

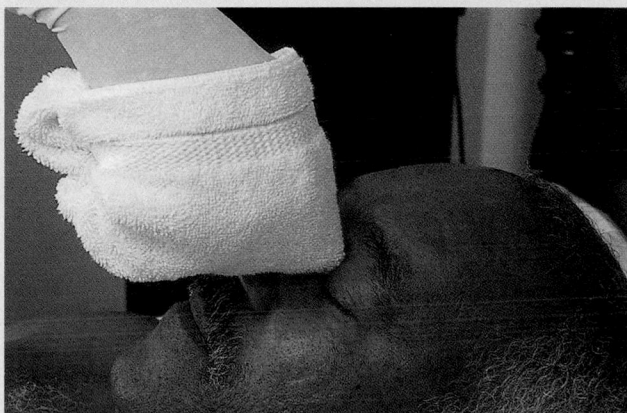

Action 14: Washing from the inner corner of the eye outward.

(continued)

ACTION	RATIONALE
13. Lay a towel across the patient's chest and on top of the bath blanket.	This prevents chilling and keeps the bath blanket dry.
14. With no soap on the washcloth, wipe one eye from the inner part of the eye, near the nose, to the outer part. Rinse or turn the cloth before washing the other eye. (See photo, previous page.)	Soap is irritating to the eyes. Moving from the inner to the outer aspect of the eye prevents carrying debris toward the nasolacrimal duct. Rinsing or turning the washcloth prevents spreading organisms from one eye to the other.
15. Bathe the patient's face, neck, and ears, avoiding soap on the face if the patient prefers.	Soap can be drying and may be avoided as a matter of personal preference.
16. Expose the far arm of the patient and place the towel lengthwise under it. Using firm strokes, wash the arm and axilla, rinse, and dry.	The towel helps to keep the bed dry. Washing the far side first eliminates contaminating a clean area once it is washed. Gentle friction stimulates circulation and muscles and helps remove dirt, oil, and organisms. Long, firm strokes are relaxing and more comfortable than short, uneven strokes.
17. Place a folded towel on the bed next to the patient's hand and put the basin on it. Soak the patient's hand in the basin. Wash, rinse, and dry the hand.	Placing the hands in the basin of water is an additional comfort measure for the patient. It facilitates a thorough washing of the hands and between the fingers and aids removal of debris from under the nails.

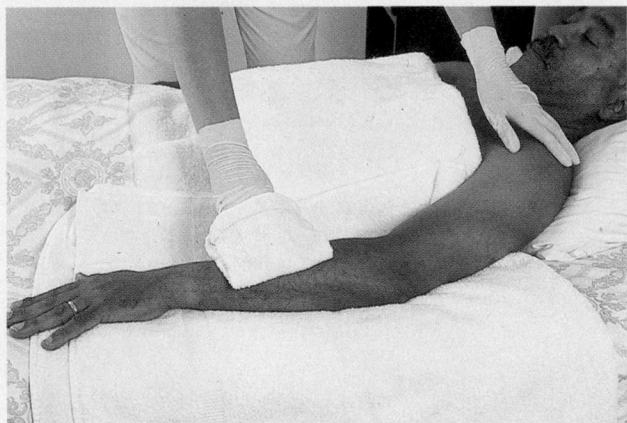

Action 16: Exposing the far arm and washing.

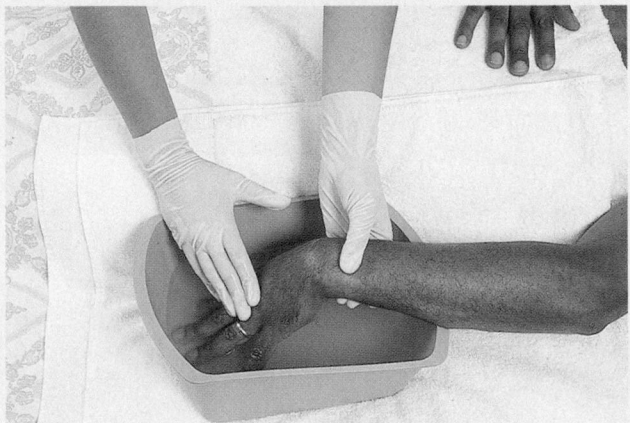

Action 17: Soaking hand in basin.

18. Repeat actions 16 and 17 for the arm nearer to you. (An option for the shorter nurse or one prone to back strain might be to bathe one side of the patient and move to the other side of the bed to complete the bath.)	
19. Spread a towel across the patient's chest. Lower the bath blanket to the patient's umbilical area. Wash, rinse, and dry the patient's chest. Keep the patient's chest covered with the towel between the wash and rinse. Pay special attention to skin folds under the breasts of patients.	Exposing, washing, rinsing, and drying one part of the body at a time avoids unnecessary exposure and chilling. Skin-fold areas may be sources of odor and skin breakdown if not cleansed and dried properly.
20. Lower the bath blanket to the patient's perineal area. Place a towel over the patient's chest.	Keeping the bath blanket and towel in place avoids exposure and chilling.
21. Wash, rinse, and dry the patient's abdomen. Carefully inspect and cleanse the umbilical area and any abdominal folds or creases.	Skin-fold areas may be sources of odor and skin breakdown if not cleansed and dried properly.
22. Return the bath blanket to its original position and expose the far leg of the patient. Place the towel under the far leg. Using firm strokes, wash, rinse, and dry the patient's leg from ankle to knee and knee to groin.	The towel protects linens and prevents the patient from feeling uncomfortable from a damp or wet bed. Washing from ankle to groin with firm strokes promotes venous return.

(continued)

SKILL 37-1 Giving a Bed Bath (continued)

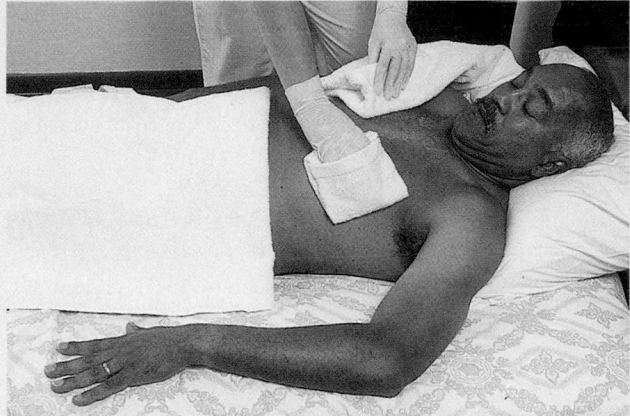

Action 19: Washing the chest area, including the axilla.

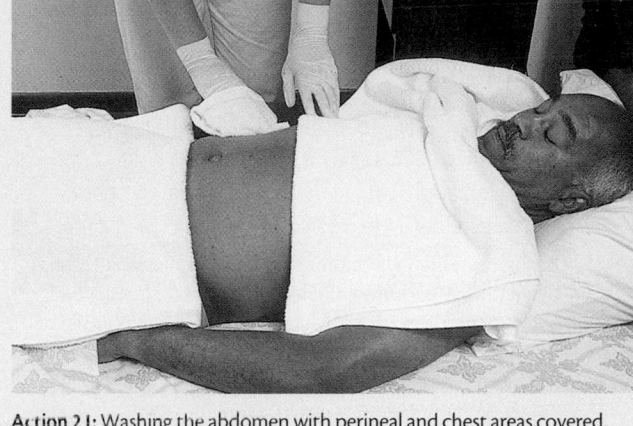

Action 21: Washing the abdomen with perineal and chest areas covered.

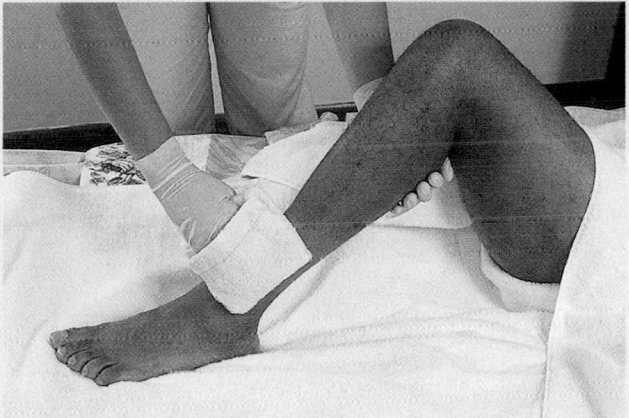

Action 22: Washing and drying far leg, keeping the other leg covered.

ACTION	RATIONALE
23. Fold a towel near the patient's foot area and place the basin on it. Place the patient's foot in the basin while supporting the patient's ankle and heel in your hand and the leg on your arm. Wash, rinse, and dry, paying particular attention to the area between the toes.	Supporting the patient's foot and leg helps reduce strain and discomfort for the patient. Placing the feet in a basin of water is comfortable and relaxing and allows for a thorough cleaning of the feet and the areas between the toes and under the nails.

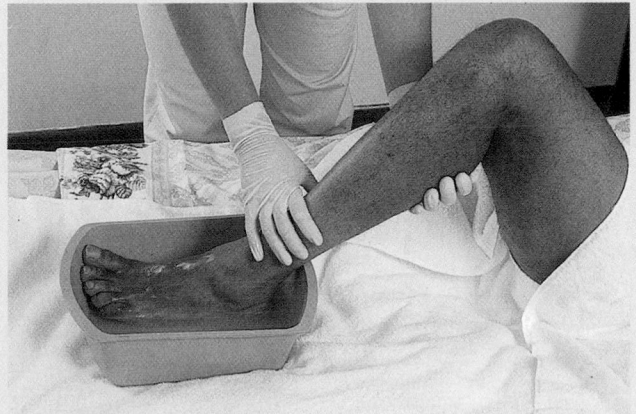

Action 23: Soaking the foot in basin.

(continued)

ACTION	RATIONALE
24. Repeat actions 22 and 23 for the other leg and foot.	
25. Make sure the patient is covered with the bath blanket. Change water or wash cloth at this point or earlier if necessary. Assist the patient onto his or her side.	The bath blanket maintains warmth and privacy. Clean, warm water prevents chilling and maintains the patient's comfort.
26. Assist the patient to a prone or side-lying position. Position the bath blanket and towel to expose only the back and buttocks.	Positioning of the towel and bath blanket protects the patient's privacy and provides warmth.
27. Wash, rinse, and dry the patient's back and buttocks area. Pay particular attention to cleansing between gluteal folds and observe for any indication of redness or skin breakdown in the sacral area.	Fecal material near the anus may be a source of microorganisms. Prolonged pressure on the sacral area or other bony prominences may compromise circulation and lead to development of decubitus ulcer.
28. If not contraindicated, give the patient a backrub, as described in Skill 41-1. Back massage may be given also after perineal care.	A backrub improves circulation to the tissues and is an aid to relaxation. A backrub may be contraindicated in patients with cardiovascular disease or musculoskeletal injuries.

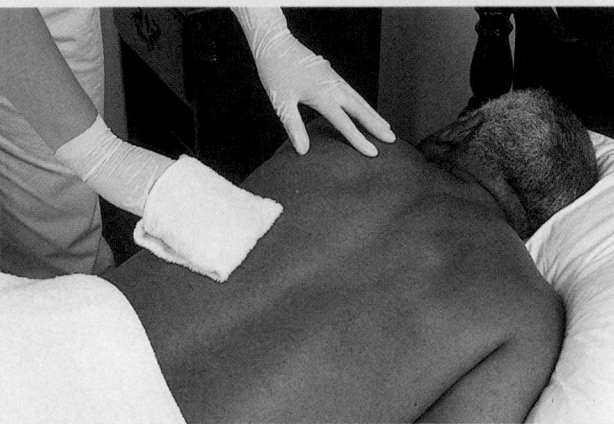

Action 27: Washing the upper back.

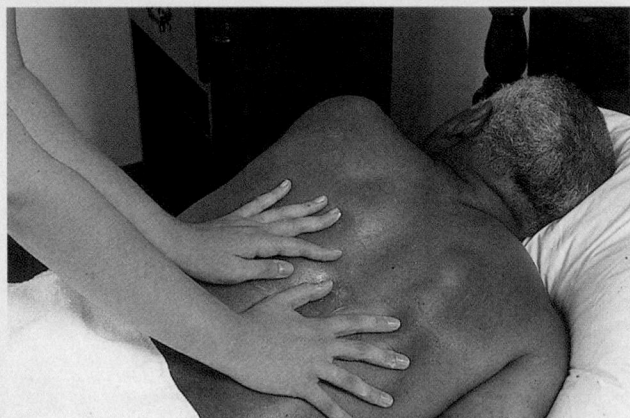

Action 28: Giving a backrub, after washing the lower back.

ACTION	RATIONALE
29. Refill basin with clean water. Discard washcloth and towel.	The washcloth, towel, and water are contaminated after washing the patient's gluteal area. Changing to clean supplies decreases the spread of organisms from the anal area to the genitals.
30. Clean the patient's perineal area or set up the patient so that he or she can complete perineal self-care.	Providing perineal self-care may decrease embarrassment for the patient. Effective perineal care reduces odor and decreases the chance of infection through contamination.
31. Help the patient put on a clean gown and attend to personal hygiene needs.	This provides for the patient's warmth and comfort.
32. Protect the pillow with a towel, and groom the patient's hair, as described in the text.	
33. Change bed linens, as described in Skills 37-5 and 37-6. Remove gloves and perform hand hygiene. Dispose of bed linens according to agency policy.	These actions deter the spread of microorganisms.
34. Record any significant observations and communication on the patient's chart.	A careful record is important for planning and individualizing the patient's care.

(continued)

SKILL 37-1 Giving a Bed Bath (continued)

Special Considerations	Remember that *removal of gown if patient has an intravenous line* necessitates taking the gown off, uninvolved arm first, and then threading the intravenous tubing and bottle or bag through the arm of the gown after the affected arm has been removed from the gown. To replace the gown, place the clean gown on the unaffected arm first and thread intravenous tubing and bottle or bag from inside the arm of the gown on the involved side. *Never* disconnect intravenous tubing to change a gown because this causes a break in a sterile system and introduces the potential for infection.
	Position may have to be modified to accommodate patient's needs. Lying flat in bed during the bed bath may be contraindicated for certain patients.
Infant/Child Considerations	When bathing an infant or young child, have supplies within easy reach and support or hold the child securely at all times to ensure safety. Never leave the child alone.
Older/Adult Considerations	Check temperature of water, particularly before bathing an older patient because sensitivity to temperature may be impaired.
	An older patient who is not incontinent may not require a full bed bath with soap and water every day. If dry skin is a problem, water and skin lotion or bath oil may be used on alternate days.
Home Care Considerations	Evaluate the safety of the bathing area in the home. Tub mats, adhesive strips, grab bars, and shower stools are helpful accessories to prevent falls.

Administering Oral Hygiene

The mouth requires care even during illness, but sometimes care must be modified to meet a patient's needs. If the patient can assist with mouth care while bedridden, provide the necessary materials (Skill 37-2). If the patient is helpless, make certain that the patient's mouth receives care as often as necessary to keep it clean and moist, as often as every 1 or 2 hours if necessary. This is especially important for patients who cannot drink or are not permitted fluids by mouth. Skill 37-3 gives techniques for administering oral hygiene to dependent patients. The nurse should wear disposable gloves, and normal saline solution is recommended. Moisten the mouth with water, if allowed, and lubricate the lips often enough to keep the membranes well moistened.

Following the steps for cleaning the mouth thoroughly is more important than the agent used. This supports the personal experience of many people that no mouthwash, breath freshener, ointment, or paste replaces a thorough mechanical cleaning of the oral cavity.

SKILL 37-2 Assisting the Patient With Oral Care

EQUIPMENT

Toothbrush	Towel	Denture cleaner
Toothpaste	Mouthwash (optional)	$4'' \times 4''$ gauze
Emesis basin	Dental floss (optional)	Washcloth or paper towel
Glass with cool water	Denture-cleansing equipment (if necessary)	Petroleum jelly (optional)
Disposable gloves	Denture cup	

ACTION	RATIONALE
1. Explain the procedure to the patient.	Explanation facilitates cooperation.
2. Perform hand hygiene. Don disposable gloves if assisting with oral care.	Hand hygiene deters the spread of microorganisms. Gloves protect the nurse from exposure to blood and blood-borne infections.
3. Assemble equipment on an overbed table within the patient's reach.	Organization facilitates performance of task.
4. Provide privacy for the patient.	Patient may be embarrassed if cleansing involves removal of dentures.
5. Lower side rail and assist patient to sitting position if permitted, or turn the patient onto the side. Place the towel across the patient's chest. Raise the bed to a comfortable working position.	The sitting or side-lying position prevents aspiration of fluids into the lungs. The towel protects the patient from dampness.

(continued)

SKILL 37-2 Assisting the Patient With Oral Care (continued)

ACTION	RATIONALE

6. Encourage the patient to brush own teeth or assist if necessary:

   a. Moisten the toothbrush and apply toothpaste to bristles.

   Water softens the bristles.

   b. Place brush at a 45-degree angle to gum line and brush from gum line to crown of each tooth. Brush outer and inner surfaces. Brush back and forth across biting surface of each tooth.

   This facilitates removal of plaque and tartar. The 45-degree angle of brushing permits cleansing of all surface areas of the tooth.

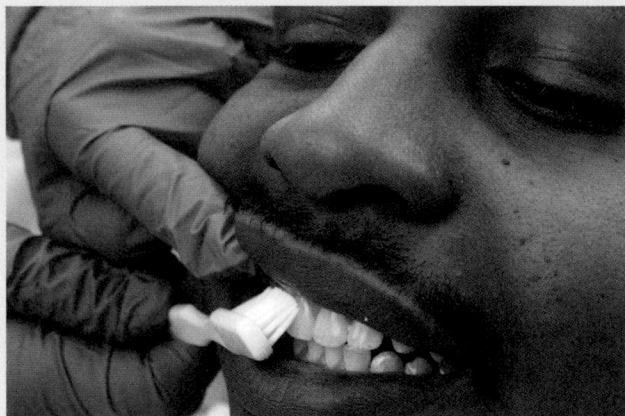

Action 6b: Placing brush at a 45-degree angle to the gum line.

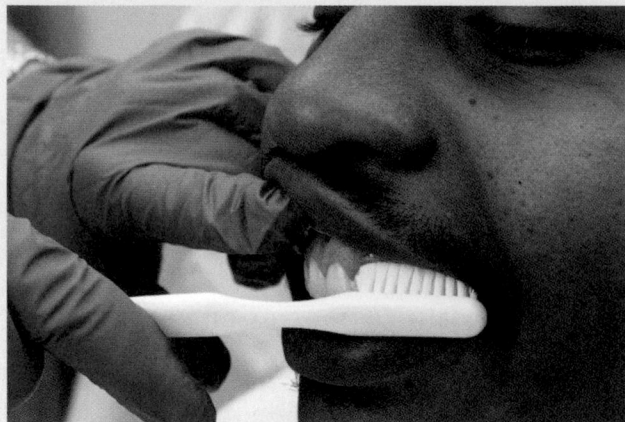

Action 6b: Brushing from the gum line to the crown of each tooth.

   c. Brush tongue gently with toothbrush.

   This removes coating on the tongue. Gentle motion does not stimulate gag reflex.

   d. Have the patient rinse vigorously with water and spit into emesis basin. Repeat until clear. Suction may be used as an alternative for removal of fluid and secretions from mouth.

   The vigorous swishing motion helps to remove debris. Suction is appropriate if swallowing reflex is impaired or absent.

   e. Assist the patient to floss teeth if necessary.

   f. Offer mouthwash if the patient prefers.

   Flossing aids in removal of plaque and promotes healthy gum tissue. Mouthwash leaves a pleasant taste in the mouth.

7. Assist the patient with removal and cleansing of dentures if necessary:

   a. Apply gentle pressure with 4″ × 4″ gauze to grasp upper denture plate and remove. Place it immediately in the denture cup. Lift the lower denture using slight rocking motion, remove, and place in the denture cup.

   Rocking motion breaks suction between the denture and gum. Using 4″ × 4″ gauze prevents slippage and discourages spread of microorganisms.

   b. If the patient prefers, add denture cleanser to the cup with water and follow directions on preparation or brush all areas thoroughly with toothbrush and paste. Place paper towels or washcloth in sink while brushing.

   Dentures collect food and microorganisms and require daily cleansing. Paper towels or washcloth in the sink protects against breakage.

   c. Rinse thoroughly with water and return dentures to the patient.

   Water aids in removal of debris and acts as a cleansing agent.

   d. Offer mouthwash so patient can rinse his or her mouth before replacing dentures.

   Mouthwash leaves a pleasant taste in the mouth and removes food particles, thus permitting proper fit.

   e. Apply petroleum jelly to lips if needed.

   Petroleum jelly prevents cracking and drying of lips.

8. Remove equipment and assist the patient to a position of comfort. Record any unusual bleeding or inflammation. Raise side rail and lower the bed.

   This promotes oral hygiene and provides for oral assessment. Elevated side rails and lowered bed position maintain safety for bedridden patients.

9. Remove disposable gloves from inside out and discard appropriately. Perform hand hygiene.

   This protects the nurse from contact with any microorganism. Hand hygiene deters spread of microorganisms.

SKILL 37-3   Providing Oral Care for the Dependent Patient

EQUIPMENT

Toothbrush
Toothpaste
Emesis basin
Disposable gloves
Cup with cool water
Towel

Mouthwash
Normal saline solution
Denture-cleansing equipment
  (if necessary)
Denture cup
Washcloth or paper towel

Sponge toothette or tongue blades padded
  with 4″ × 4″ gauze sponges
Irrigating syringe with rubber tip (optional)
Petroleum jelly
Suction catheter with suction apparatus
  (optional)

ACTION	RATIONALE
1. Explain the procedure to the patient.	Explanation facilitates cooperation.
2. Perform hand hygiene and don disposable gloves.	Hand hygiene and disposable gloves deter the spread of micro-organisms.
3. Assemble equipment on overbed table within reach.	Organization facilitates performance of task.
4. Provide privacy for the patient. Adjust the height of the bed to a comfortable position. Lower one side rail and position the patient on the side with the head tilted forward. Place the towel across the patient's chest and emesis basin in position under the chin.	The side-lying position with head lowered prevents aspiration of fluid into lungs. Towel and emesis basin protects patient from dampness.
5. Open the patient's mouth and gently insert a padded tongue blade between the back molars if necessary.	Padded tongue blade keeps mouth open for easier cleaning and prevents the patient from biting the nurse's fingers.

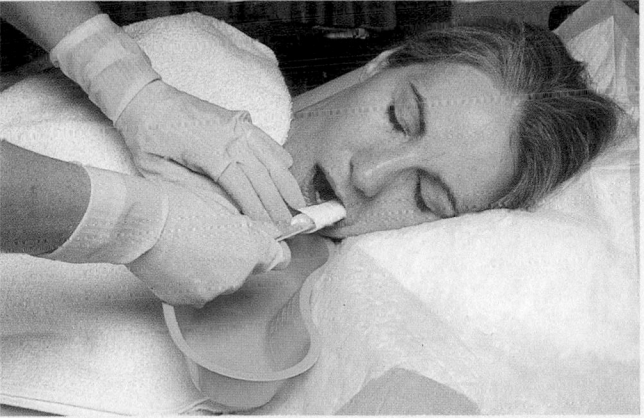

Action 5: Gently inserting padded tongue blade between back molars.

6. If teeth are present, brush carefully with toothbrush and paste. Remove dentures if present and clean before replacing (see action 7 of Skill 37-2). Use toothette or gauze-padded tongue blade moistened with normal saline or dilute mouthwash solution to gently cleanse gums, mucous membranes, and tongue. (See photos on p. 1028.)	Toothbrush or padded tongue blade provides friction necessary to clean areas where plaque and tartar accumulate. Hydrogen peroxide is considered an irritant and no longer recommended. The mechanical action of cleansing is more important than the solution.
7. Use gauze-padded tongue blade dipped in mouthwash solution to rinse the oral cavity. If desired, insert the rubber tip of the irrigating syringe into the patient's mouth and rinse gently with a small amount of water. (See photo on p. 1028.) Position the patient's head to allow for return of water or use suction apparatus to remove the water from oral cavity.	Rinsing helps to cleanse debris from the mouth. Solution that is forcefully irrigated may cause aspiration.
8. Apply petroleum jelly to the patient's lips.	This prevents drying and cracking of lips.
9. Remove equipment and return the patient to a position of comfort. Raise the side rail and lower the bed. Record any unusual bleeding or inflammation.	This promotes oral hygiene and provides for oral assessment. Raised side rail and lowered bed maintain patient safety.
10. Perform hand hygiene.	Hand hygiene deters spread of microorganisms.

(continued)

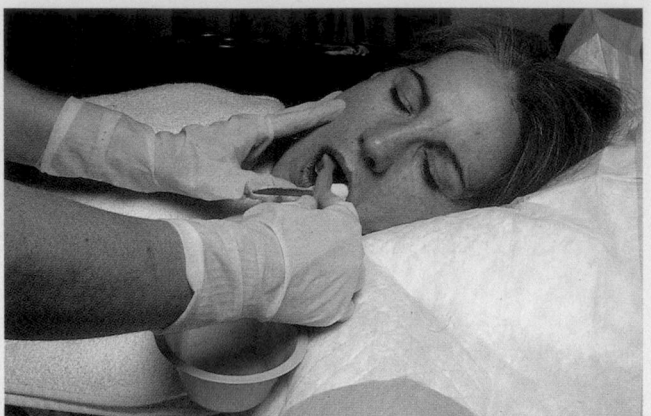

Action 6: Carefully brushing patient's teeth.

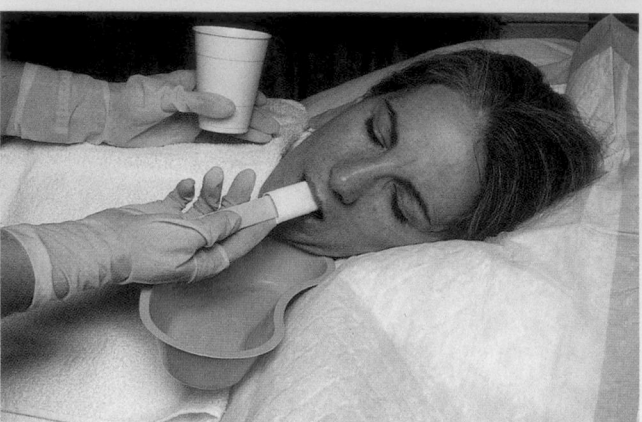

Action 6: Using moistened padded tongue blade to cleanse gums, mucous membranes, and tongue.

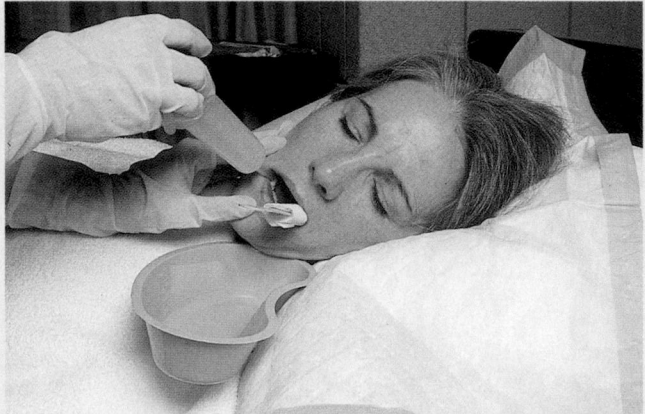

Action 7: Using irrigating syringe and a small amount of water to rinse mouth.

Special Considerations   A patient receiving chemotherapy medication may have bleeding gums and extremely sensitive mucous membranes. Use a soft sponge toothette for cleaning or substitute a salt water rinse (½ teaspoon salt in 1 cup of warm water) for brushing of teeth.

The following is an example of documentation for oral care:

> 10/20/06—Patient generally breathes with mouth open. Sores present on palate, teeth, gums, and oral mucosa. Toothettes dipped in normal saline used for cleansing every 4 hours. Lubricating ointment applied to lips.
>
> —D. Sadowski, RN

Denture Care

Failing to wear dentures for a long period allows the gum line to change, thus affecting the fit of the dentures. If the patient has been instructed to remove dentures while sleeping, a disposable denture cup is convenient and easy to use. Dentures should not be wrapped in toilet tissue or disposable wipes because these are likely to be thrown away. Dentures should be stored in water to prevent drying and warping of plastic materials.

Patients with dentures are more likely to keep them in the mouth if they are kept clean. If the patient cannot care for them, the nurse must ensure that the dentures are clean. Use care when handling a patient's dentures, because they represent a considerable financial investment, and replacement for damage or loss is expensive.

When cleaning dentures, don gloves and hold them over a basin of water or a sink lined with a washcloth or soft towel (Fig. 37-3) so that if they slip from your grasp, they will not fall onto a hard surface and break. If necessary, grasp the dentures with a 4″ × 4″ piece of gauze to help prevent them from slipping out of your gloved hands. Use cool or lukewarm water to cleanse them. Hot water may warp the plastic material of which most dentures are made. Use a brush and a nonabrasive powder or paste. Dentures may be soaked in commercial preparations to help remove stains and hardened

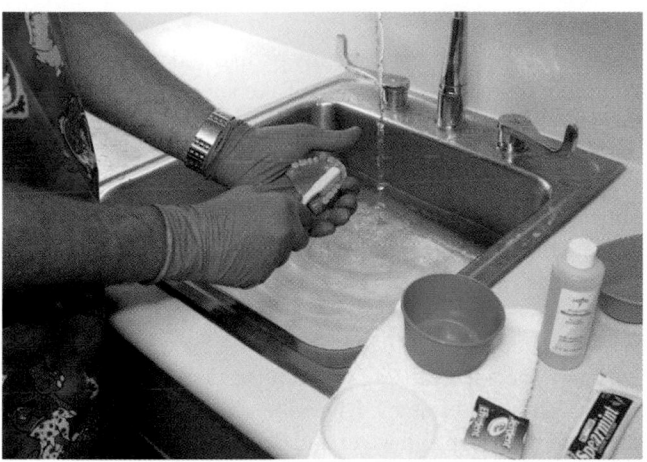

FIGURE 37-3 Proper method of cleaning dentures.

particles and then rinsed well after cleaning. Give the patient the opportunity to brush the gums and tongue and rinse his or her mouth before the dentures are replaced.

Teaching Oral Hygiene
Toothbrushing and Flossing

A toothbrush should be small enough to reach all teeth. The bristles should be sufficiently firm to clean but not so firm that they are likely to injure tooth enamel and gum tissue. Brushes should be cleaned and dried between uses. Most damage is done by bacteria directly after eating, so the teeth should be brushed immediately after eating or drinking. The tongue should also be cleaned with the brush.

Automatic toothbrushes, electric or battery operated, are simple to use and are as good as manual brushes for removing debris and plaque. Pressurized water spray units are available to assist with oral hygiene. However, if too much water pressure is used, particles of debris may be forced into tissue pockets, leading to gum damage. Therefore, their use should be discussed with a dentist.

The toothbrush cannot reach areas between the teeth where food lodges, so flossing once a day is recommended. Flossing removes the debris that the brush cannot and helps to break up colonies of bacteria. Guidelines for Nursing Care 37-1 illustrates a flossing technique.

Toothpastes and powders aid the brushing process and usually have a pleasant taste that encourages brushing, especially by children. Most dentifrices are safe to use, but those containing harsh abrasives may scratch the enamel of the teeth and therefore are not recommended. Salt and sodium bicarbonate are far less expensive than proprietary products on the market and just as effective for short-term use. However, these products lack fluoride and should not be used exclusively. Dentifrices containing stannous fluoride and antitartar

---

Guidelines for Nursing Care 37-1
Flossing

- Wear gloves when flossing a patient's teeth.
- Keep about 1 to 1½ inches of floss held taut between the fingers.
- Do not force the floss between the teeth; insert it gently by moving it back and forth where teeth touch each other.
- Move the floss up and down while using both fingers, first on the side of one tooth and then on the side of the other tooth, until the surfaces are squeaky clean.

- Go to the gum tissue with the floss but not into the gum because this may result in discomfort, soreness, or bleeding.
- Advance the floss from one hand to the other to bring up a fresh section of floss when it has become frayed or soiled.
- Rinse the mouth well with water after flossing to remove food particles and plaque that have been loosened. Also, rinse after eating when flossing or brushing is impossible.

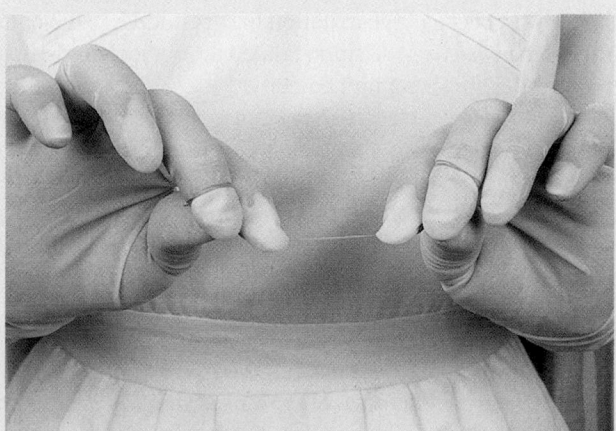

Securing floss around the fingers.

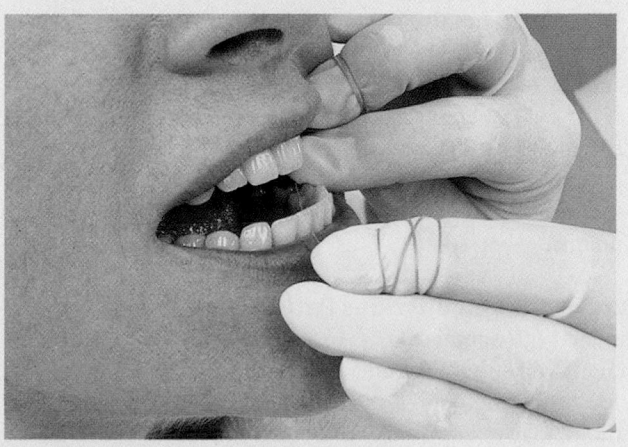

Inserting floss between the teeth.

and antiplaque rinses decrease dental caries and hence are recommended by many dentists.

Mouthwashes

An offensive breath odor (halitosis) is often systemic in nature. For example, the odor of onions and garlic on the breath comes from the lungs, where the oils are being removed from the bloodstream and eliminated with respiration. A mouthwash cannot remove halitosis when odors are being eliminated by respiration.

If the cause of halitosis is poor oral hygiene, cleaning reduces the odor. Commercial mouthwashes may be helpful. If concentrated mouthwashes are used frequently in debilitated patients, however, they may injure oral tissue.

Providing Eye Care

Normally, the eyes are kept clean with lacrimal secretions. Ho during illness, the eyes may produce more secretions than normal and may appear glasslike. Use the following techniques when secretions adhere to the eyelashes and become dry and crusty or when discharge is present:

- Wear gloves during the cleaning procedure.
- Use water or normal saline and cotton balls or a clean washcloth or compress to clean the eyes. Boric acid solution, once popular for cleaning the eyes, is no longer recommended because of its toxicity when absorbed through mucous membranes. Never use soap to clean the eyes, because soap is irritating to eye tissues.
- Position the patient on the same side as the eye to be cleaned so that solution and debris do not run across the bridge of the nose and contaminate the other eye.
- Dampen a cotton ball with the solution of choice and wipe once while moving the cotton ball from the inner canthus to the outer canthus of the eye. This technique minimizes the risk for forcing debris into the area drained by the nasolacrimal duct. Discard the used cotton ball.
- Continue this technique, using one cotton ball for each stroke, until the eye is clean.
- Turn the patient to the opposite side and clean the other eye in the same manner.
- Wipe the lashes dry with a paper tissue or a clean washcloth, exposing a clean area of the tissue or cloth with each stroke.
- If the eyelashes are matted with secretions or debris that cannot be removed by wiping, apply a warm wet compress to the closed eye for 3 to 5 minutes to loosen the secretions so that they may be removed in a painless manner.

Care of the Unconscious Patient's Eyes

Patients with diminished or absent blink (corneal) reflexes and patients whose eyelids remain open require frequent eye care, at least every 4 hours. If the eye is not kept moist, corneal ulceration may result from excessive drying of the eye. Nursing measures include using saline or artificial tears to lubricate the eye and a protective eye shield to keep the eye closed.

Eyeglass Care

Eyeglasses are essential for many people and represent a considerable financial investment. Take special precautions to prevent them from being broken or lost. Encourage patients who need glasses to wear them to avoid eyestrain.

Many eyeglasses have plastic lenses, which are considerably lighter in weight than glass lenses but correct vision just as well. Plastic lenses scratch easily. Whenever setting glasses down, make sure they are placed with the lenses up.

Clean eyeglasses over a terry towel, so that if they slip they will not become scratched or broken. Use warm water and soap or a special cleansing preparation. Hot water may warp plastic lenses and frames. Rinse the glasses well after cleaning them with soap and water and dry with a clean, soft cotton cloth, such as a cotton handkerchief or a special eyeglass cleaning cloth. Paper products that are made of wood pulp increase the risk of scratching the lenses, so do not use a dry paper tissue to clean eyeglasses. Do not use silicone tissues to clean plastic lenses.

Contact Lens Care

A contact lens is a small disc worn directly on the eyeball. It stays in place by surface tension of the eye's tears. Contact lenses are either hard or soft. The older hard lenses are not gas permeable; newer ones are gas permeable and are more comfortable because they allow oxygen to pass directly through the lens to the cornea. Soft lenses are made of a plastic material that absorbs water to become soft and pliable. They are brittle when dehydrated and absorb water when placed in a solution, usually normal saline, or when in contact with tears. Soft lenses may be used for daily wear or extended wear. Disposable soft lenses are also available.

People who wear contact lenses, and the nurses caring for them, need to take special precautions to keep the lenses free of microorganisms that may lead to eye infections and to avoid injuring or scratching the surface of the eye. When providing contact lens care, always perform meticulous hand hygiene and put on gloves before touching eye surfaces and lenses. Caution lens wearers about eye irritation in the presence of noxious vapors or smoke. Also remind lens wearers that lenses should not come into contact with cosmetics, soaps, or hair sprays because eye irritation may result. Urge the patient to report any adverse reaction related to contact lens use to the prescribing physician immediately.

The cornea, which consists of dense connective tissue, does not have its own blood supply. It is nourished primarily by oxygen from the atmosphere and from tears. In a patient who wears contact lenses, the cornea requires more than its normal supply of oxygen because its metabolic rate increases. To allow the cornea to receive a maximal supply of oxygen, hard lenses should not be worn for more than 12 to 16 hours and should be removed before sleeping. Extended-wear soft lenses can be left in place for 1 to 30 days, depending on the manufacturer. Individuals wearing extended-wear lenses should clean them at least once a week. The time that disposable soft lenses should be worn also varies according to the type and the manufacturer. A new type of disposable lens is replaced daily, while other options include lenses that can be worn day and night for 7 days or during waking hours only for 14 days. Excessive tearing, pain, and redness signal the need to remove lenses.

If a patient wears contact lenses but cannot remove them, the nurse is responsible for removing them. This may occur, for example, when the nurse is caring for an unconscious patient. Whenever an unconscious patient is admitted without any family present, always assess the patient to determine whether he or she wears contact lenses. Leaving contact lenses in place for long periods could result in permanent eye damage.

Before removing hard or gas-permeable lenses, use gentle pressure to center the lens on the cornea. A small suction device can also be used in an emergency situation to remove gas-permeable or hard lenses. Figure 37-4 demonstrates removal of hard and soft lenses. Once removed, identify the lenses as being for the right or left eye, because the two lenses are not necessarily identical. If an eye injury is present, do not try to remove lenses because of the danger of causing an additional injury.

Artificial Eye Care

Most patients who wear an artificial eye prefer to care for it themselves. Encourage them to do so when possible. The necessary equipment includes a small basin, soap and water

Removing hard contact lenses

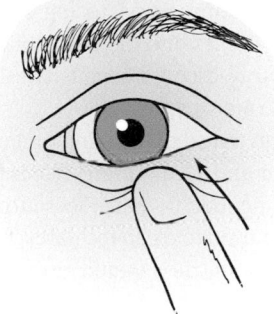

If the lens is not centered over the cornea, apply gentle pressure on the lower eyelid to center the lens.

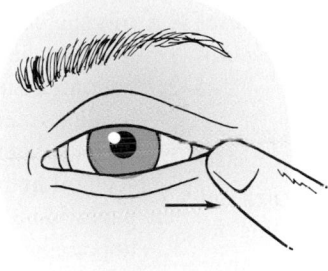

Gently pull the outer corner of the eye toward the ear.

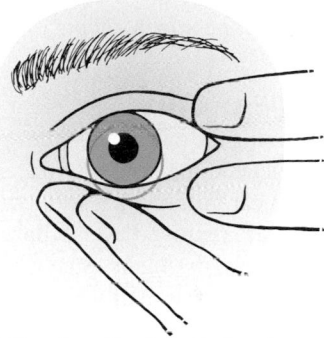

Position the other hand below the lens to receive it and ask the patient to blink.

Or

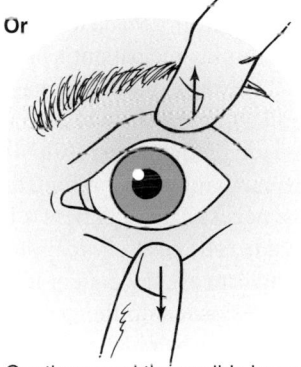

Gently spread the eyelids beyond the top and bottom edges of the lens.

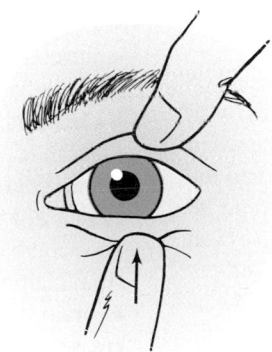

Gently press the lower eyelid up against the bottom of the lens.

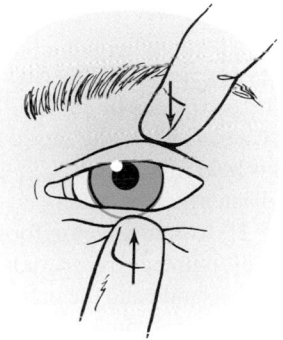

After the lens is tipped slightly, move the eyelids toward one another to cause the lens to slide out between the eyelids.

Removing soft contact lenses

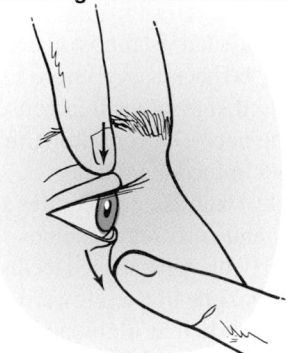

Have the patient look forward. Retract the lower lid with one hand. Using the pad of the index finger of the other hand, move the lens down to the sclera.

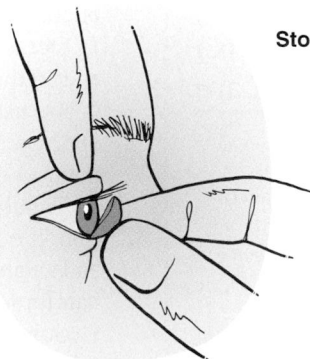

Using the pads of the thumb and index finger, grasp the lens with a gentle pinching motion and remove.

Storing lenses

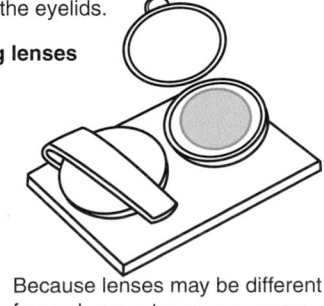

Because lenses may be different for each eye, storage cases are marked L and R, designating left and right lenses. It is important to place the first lens in its designated cup in the storage case before removing the second lens to avoid mixing them up.

FIGURE 37-4 Removing contact lenses.

for washing, and solution for rinsing the prosthesis. Normal saline or tap water can be used for rinsing. Most people have their own method for cleaning the eye socket and the area around it. Ask the patient how he or she does this, and enable the patient to continue with the usual practice. When the nurse is performing the care, the patient should be lying down so that the eye does not accidentally fall to the floor. The socket is ordinarily flushed with normal saline before the eye is replaced.

The following is an example documenting eye care measures:

10/20/06—Patient states, "I can't believe they expect me to take care of this eye. I don't want to touch it!" Has not participated in artificial eye care to date. Patient encouraged to verbalize concerns about artificial eye and assist with care.   —*S. Cohen, RN*

Providing Ear Care

Other than cleaning the outer ears, little intervention is needed for routine hygiene of the ear. After the ears are washed, they should be dried carefully with a soft towel so that water and cerumen (wax) are removed by capillary action. Forcing the towel into the ear for drying or using a cotton-tipped applicator may aid in the formation of wax plugs. Using bobby pins, hairpins, paper clips, or fingernails to remove wax from the ear is extremely dangerous because these may injure or puncture the eardrum. See Examples of Nursing Interventions Classification (NIC).

Hearing Aids

If the patient uses a hearing aid, the batteries must be checked routinely and the ear pieces or ear mold cleaned daily with mild soap and water. A whistling sound that is audible when the hearing aid is held in the hand with the power on and the volume high indicates that the battery is functioning properly. Refer to Chapter 21, Communicator, for strategies nurses can use to promote communication with a hearing-impaired patient. If hearing loss is mild and the patient is not using a hearing aid, the following suggestions may help to improve hearing and should be included in any health teaching:

Examples of Nursing Interventions Classification (NIC)
Ear Care

- Monitor for drainage from ears, as appropriate.
- Avoid placing sharp objects in the ear.
- Determine if cerumen in the ear canal is causing pain or hearing loss.
- Irrigate the ear canal with a Water-Pik (or similar device) on a low setting, using warm water (80° to 90°F), as appropriate.
- Demonstrate proper technique for ear irrigation to caregiver, as appropriate.

From McClosky, J., & Bulechek, G. (2000). *Nursing interventions classification (NIC)* (3rd ed). (p. 265). St. Louis: C. V. Mosby. (This text provides a full listing of nursing activities for each nursing intervention.)

- Avoid noisy places for conversation.
- Choose well-lighted places where it is easier to look at the speaker's face, lips, and hands for cues to the conversation.
- Cup your hand behind your ear.
- Ask people to face you when they are speaking to you.
- Ask people to repeat what they said, if it was not clear to you, and to speak slowly.
- Consider buying amplitude devices so that you can hear your television and radio without turning up the sound.

Figure 37-5 illustrates several types of hearing aids.

Providing Nose Care

The best way to clean the nose is to blow it gently. Both nostrils should be open while doing this. Closing one nostril adds to the danger of forcing debris into the eustachian tubes. Irrigations are usually contraindicated because of the danger of forcing material into the sinuses.

If the external nares are crusted, applying mineral or cottonseed oil helps to soften and remove the crusts. Disposable paper tissues are recommended for nasal secretions. A cotton-tipped applicator may be used to clean the nares, but with great care to avoid injury. The applicator should never be introduced into the nares.

Providing Hair Care

Many cultural overtones are associated with hairstyles, and styles change within a culture from decade to decade. Demonstrate consideration by grooming the patient's hair in the style preferred by the patient. Daily brushing of the hair helps keep it clean and distributes oil along the shaft of each hair. Brushing also stimulates blood circulation in the scalp. Hair that becomes entangled is difficult to comb. Combing tiny sections of hair at a time may be necessary if a patient's hair has not been combed for even 1 day. The best way to protect long hair from matting and tangling is to ask the patient for permission to braid it. Patients usually consent to the procedure if it increases their comfort. Parting the hair in the middle on the back of the head and making two braids, one on either side, prevents the discomfort of lying on one heavy braid on the back of the head. When braiding a patient's hair, ensure that the hair is not pulled too tightly.

Occasionally, a patient's hair is almost hopelessly matted, and cutting the hair may be necessary. Before a patient's hair is cut, usually the patient signs a written consent. Also, as appropriate, discuss the necessity for cutting the hair with a member of the patient's immediate family.

Tightly curled (kinky) hair usually requires special attention. It is normally dry and curly and becomes easily matted and tangled. Use a comb with wide-spaced teeth and work the hair through from the neckline upward toward the forehead.

Some people have their hair straightened, but even after this process, it may be difficult to untangle the hair when the person is confined to bed. Some African Americans style their hair in small braids. The braids are not undone for shampooing and may need to have a lubricant or oil applied daily to prevent hair strands from breaking.

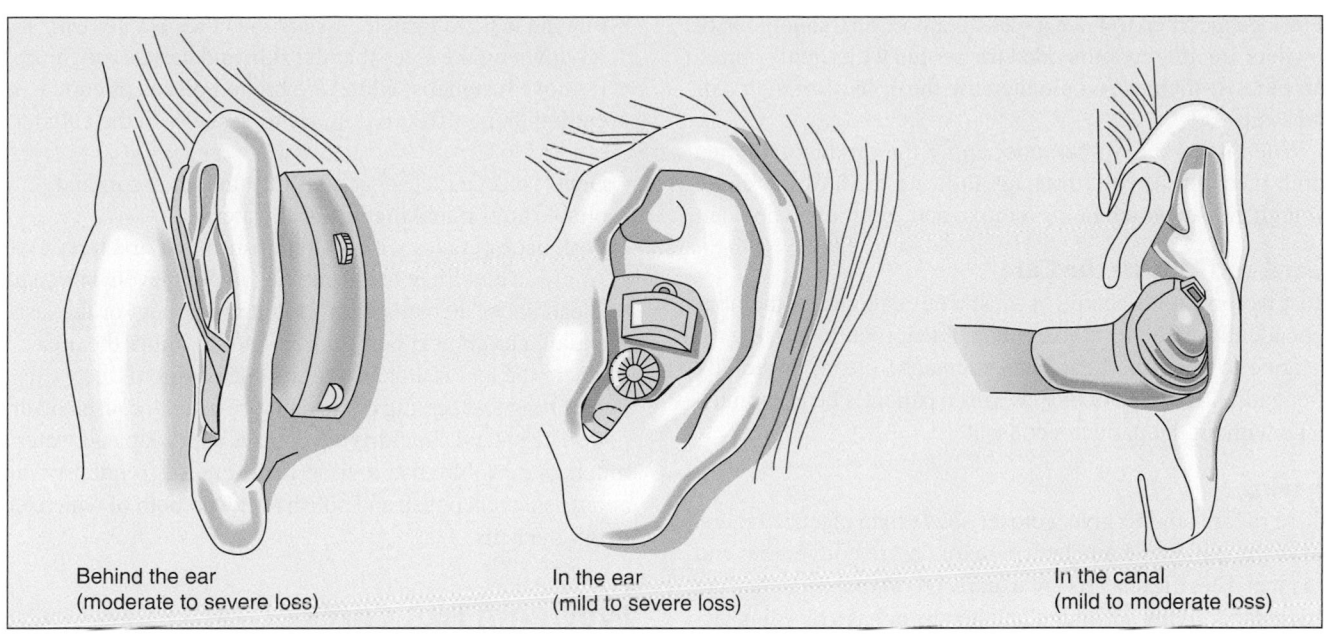

Behind the ear
(moderate to severe loss)

In the ear
(mild to severe loss)

In the canal
(mild to moderate loss)

FIGURE 37-5 Several types of hearing aids.

Shampooing of the Hair

The hair, which is exposed to the same dirt and oil as the skin, requires washing as often as necessary to keep it clean. The comb and brush are washed each time the hair is washed and as frequently as necessary between shampoos. Many health agencies have beauticians and barbers to assist with hair care, including shampooing, but this does not relieve the nurse of the responsibility.

Before shampooing the hair, brush or have the patient brush and comb the hair well to stimulate the scalp and undo tangled hair. The patient may then shampoo the hair while showering, if able. In some hospitals, a physician's order is required for shampooing a patient's hair.

If the patient is on bed rest, whether at home or in the hospital, and unable to shampoo his or her own hair, use the following as a guide:

- Prepare several pitchers of water of a suitably warm temperature for a thorough washing and rinsing, shampoo, one or two towels for drying, and a receptacle to receive wash and rinse water.
- Place a protective pad and a plastic hair-washing tray if one is available (Fig. 37-6) under the head.
- Place the patient in a position over the pad so that water drainage is directed into the receptacle.
- Wet the hair, apply shampoo, and massage the scalp well while washing the hair.
- Rinse the hair and reapply shampoo for a second washing, if indicated.
- Rinse the hair thoroughly.
- Apply conditioner if requested or if the scalp appears dry.
- Dry the hair as quickly as possible to prevent the patient from becoming chilled, and arrange the hair according to the patient's preference.

Think back to Andrew Craig, the older adult in the long-term care facility. Since Mr. Craig has difficulty sitting for long periods of time, it might be necessary to shampoo his hair while he is in bed. The nurse must first discuss this with him to ensure that this meets his needs.

If regular shampooing is inappropriate or is contraindicated by the patient's condition, dry shampoo may be used. Although dry shampoos cannot replace the cleaning benefits of regular shampoos, they are helpful in removing at least some of the dirt, oils, and odors from the hair of patients too

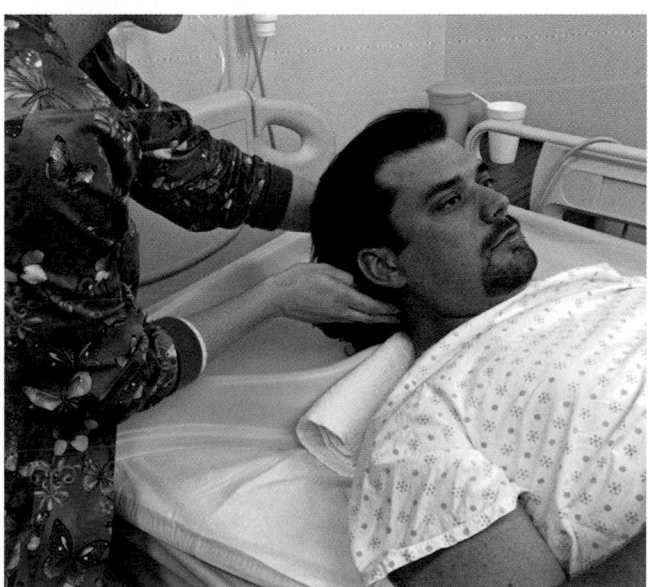

FIGURE 37-6 A nurse uses a protective pad and plastic tray when shampooing a patient's hair.

ill or incapacitated to have a wet shampoo. Dry shampoos or powders are not recommended for people with tightly curled hair because their use would increase the dryness of their hair and scalp.

When using a dry shampoo, apply the product and then comb or brush it from the hair. Pull the teeth of the comb through gauze, which helps remove and capture the powder.

Beard and Moustache Care

Most patients with beards or mustaches can groom them independently. Patients who are dependent require nursing assistance to keep the beard and mustache clean, especially after eating. Never trim or shave off a patient's beard or mustache without the patient's consent.

Shaving

Blade razors tend to give a closer shave than electric razors, but many patients find electric razors more convenient and practical. Electric shavers are usually recommended when the patient is receiving anticoagulant therapy or has a bleeding disorder and are especially convenient for ill and bedridden patients. The technique for shaving patients who cannot shave themselves is described in Guidelines for Nursing Care 37-2.

Providing Fingernail Care

The following are recommended techniques for the care of fingernails:

- File the nails to form an oval at the ends. Do not trim so far down on the sides that the skin and cuticle are injured.
- Remove hangnails, which are broken pieces of cuticle, by cutting them off. Avoid injury to tissue with the cuticle scissors.
- Gently push cuticles back off the nail when soft and pliable after a soaking in warm water.
- Push back cuticles with a blunt instrument or a terry cloth.
- Apply an emollient to the cuticle to help prevent hangnails.
- Clean under the nails with a blunt instrument or the large end of a toothpick, being careful not to injure the area where the nail is attached to the underlying tissue.

Splitting and peeling of the nails are usually caused by dryness. The patient should avoid contact with soap and water as much as possible, use a good hand cream frequently, and avoid using nail polish and polish remover, both of which tend to dry the nails.

Providing Foot Care

Proper foot care is important at any age. It becomes even more so with aging and when conditions such as circulatory disturbances or diabetes mellitus are present. Guidelines for Nursing Care 37-3 highlights the appropriate techniques related to foot care.

The following is an example of documentation of foot care:

10/20/06—Patient states, "I guess I cut that nail too short. It's been hurting for 2 months now." Great toe on right foot is swollen, red, and painful. Skin at base of nail is white. Limps when walking. After bath, patient soaked right foot and dried it carefully. —A. Jones, RN

Providing Perineal Care

It is not always possible for male nurses to attend to male patients and female nurses to attend to female patients. But if perineal cleaning is performed in a matter-of-fact and dignified manner, patients generally do not find care by a person of the opposite gender to be offensive or embarrassing.

> **Remember Sonya Delamordo, who is going home after a stroke to her daughter's home. The patient may be embarrassed to have her daughter help with perineal care. The nurse would encourage the patient to do as much as she can using her left side. By doing so, the patient maintains some control over the situation, thereby promoting her self-esteem and fostering personal hygiene and independence.**

In some cases, a sitz bath may be used to clean and irrigate the perineal and anal areas. The portable type is especially handy in situations where moving a patient to a stationary sitz tub would be cumbersome. The skills associated with administering a sitz bath are discussed in Chapter 38, Skin Integrity.

Perineal care may be carried out while the patient remains in bed. When performing perineal care, follow these guidelines:

Guidelines for Nursing Care 37-2
Shaving

- Wear gloves because contact with blood is possible if any skin nicks occur.
- Apply shaving cream or a warm soap lather to the skin to soften the facial hair and prevent pulling.
- Pull the skin of the face so that it is taut.
- Use short, firm strokes in the direction of hair growth. Patients can often give suggestions on how they shave.
- Wash the patient's face of residual lather and dry.
- Apply aftershave lotion if patient requests it. Aftershave preparations tend to make the patient feel refreshed and have a cosmetic rather than a therapeutic effect.

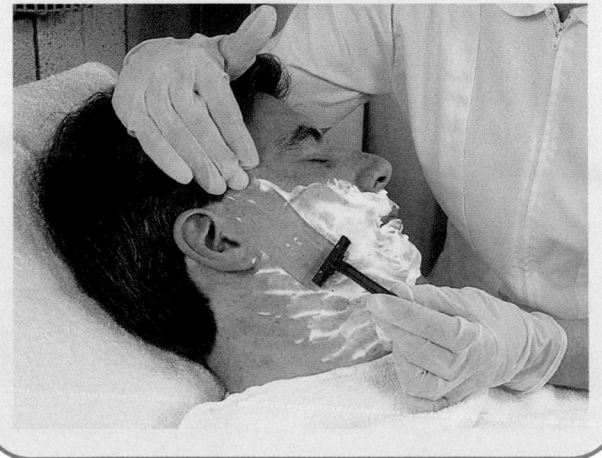

Guidelines for Nursing Care 37-3
Foot Care

- Bathe the feet thoroughly in a mild soap and tepid water solution. Avoid soaking the feet. Be sure to clean the interdigital area.
- Rinse the feet to remove soap residue that can dry and irritate the skin.
- Dry feet thoroughly, including the area between the toes.
- Apply a water-soluble lotion to feet if they are dry. Include the area between the toes.
- Use an antifungal foot powder if necessary to prevent fungal infections, such as athlete's foot.
- For diabetic patients, file the nails; avoid using scissors or nail clippers, which may slip and injure tissues. Non-diabetic patients should avoid digging into or cutting the toenails at the lateral corners when trimming the nails.
- Do not cut off corns or calluses. Commercial removers should be avoided because they may contain ingredients that can lead to development of infection and ulcers. Consult a *podiatrist*, a physician who treats foot disorders, when corns or calluses are present.
- Explain the dangers of going barefoot. Skin on the feet may be injured, or athlete's foot may be acquired in public showers.
- Wear appropriate footwear. Break in new shoes gradually. Improperly fitting shoes can lead to corns, calluses, bunions, and blisters. The soles should be flexible and nonslippery and the heel heights should be safe and offer appropriate support. Shoes with rough ridges, wrinkles, or tears in the linings should be discarded or repaired.
- Wear cotton socks, which provide warmth and absorb perspiration.
- Avoid wearing knee-high stockings, and do not sit with the knees crossed because this can obstruct the circulation to the lower extremities and feet.
- Prop the feet up above the level of the hips a few minutes several times a day if the feet swell.
- Avoid using heating pads and hot-water bottles because of the danger of blistering and burning the feet.
- Report any signs of foot problems to your physician. This is especially important for patients with diabetes.

- Assemble supplies, and provide for privacy.
- Explain the procedure to the patient, and don disposable gloves.
- Wash and rinse the groin area (both male and female patients).
- Always proceed from the least contaminated area to the most contaminated area. For a female patient, spread the labia and move the washcloth from the pubic area toward the anal area to prevent carrying organisms from the anal area back over the genital area. Use a clean portion of the washcloth for each stroke. For a male patient, move the washcloth in a spiral motion from the tip of the penis down its length toward the pubic area (Fig. 37-7).
- In an uncircumcised male patient, retract the foreskin (prepuce) while washing the penis.
- Rinse the washed areas well with plain water.
- Pull the uncircumcised male patient's foreskin back into place over the glans penis to prevent constriction of the penis, which may result in edema and tissue injury.
- Wash and rinse the male patient's scrotum. Handle the scrotum, which houses the testicles, with care because the area is sensitive.
- Dry the cleaned areas and apply an emollient as indicated. Powder the area only if the patient requests it. For the female patient, powder may become a medium for the growth of bacteria.
- Turn the patient on his or her side and continue with cleansing the anal area. Continue in the direction of least contaminated to most contaminated area. In the female, cleanse from the vagina toward the anus. In both female and male patients, change the washcloth with each stroke until the area is clean. Rinse and dry the area.

The following is an example of documentation about teaching perineal care:

10/20/06—Child presented with large amount of smegma under the foreskin and painful urination. Mother and child were instructed in the need and correct technique for cleansing the uncircumcised penis. Child correctly returned the demonstration.   —L. Woo, RN

If the patient has an indwelling catheter and the agency recommends daily care for the catheter, this is usually done after perineal care. Agency policy may recommend use of an antiseptic cleaning agent (eg, povidone–iodine) or plain soap and water on a clean washcloth. Put on clean gloves before cleaning the catheter. Cleanse 6″ to 8″ of the catheter, moving from the meatus downward. Be careful not to pull or tug on the catheter during the cleaning motion. Also inspect the meatus for drainage and note the characteristics of the urine. A physician's order is required if antibiotic ointment is to be applied to the meatus after cleansing. Additional information involving care of an indwelling catheter is discussed in Chapter 43, Urinary Elimination.

When the patient is at home, adaptations related to perineal care and hygiene in general are needed. Guidelines for Nursing Care 37-4 presents general adaptations for hygiene care in the home environment.

Providing Vaginal Care

Vaginal mucous secretions are odor free until they combine with air and perspiration. Thus, for vaginal care, using plain soap and water is the most effective means to control odor. In normal, healthy women, daily douching is believed to be unnecessary and unwise because it tends to remove normal bacterial flora from the vagina, and an acidic solution may irritate or injure normal cells. Douching has also been linked to

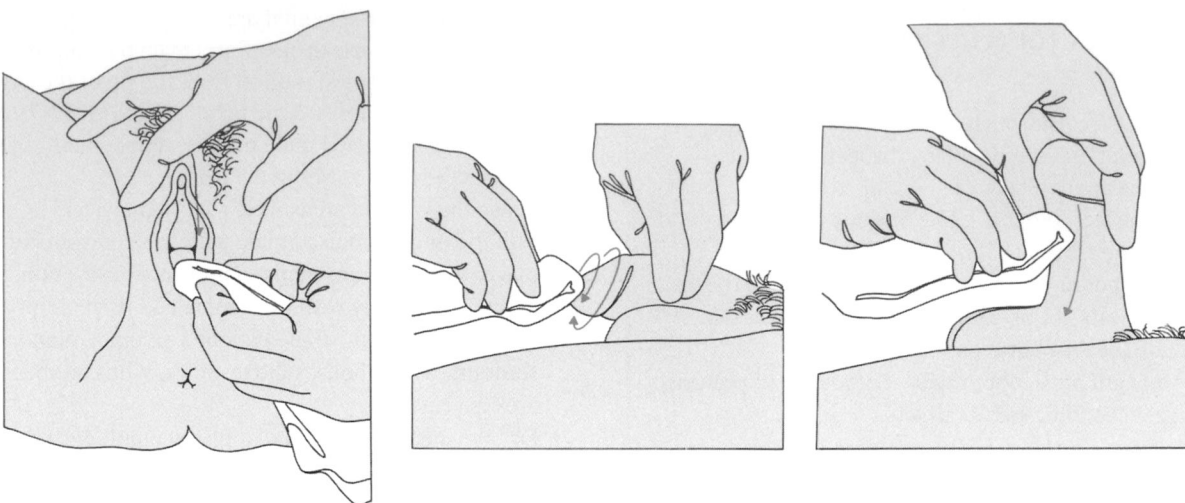

FIGURE 37-7 Performing normal perineal care.

Guidelines for Nursing Care 37-4
Hygiene Needs: General Adaptations for the Home Environment

- Use plastic trash bags or a plastic shower curtain liner to protect the mattress when bathing or shampooing a patient in bed. Disposable washcloths may also be an option to consider. A large plastic container or baby bathtub can effectively serve as a shampoo basin.
- Teach patient and caregiver how to administer oral care and care for dentures. A recent weight loss due to illness can result in dentures that no longer fit properly. Inform the patient that a dentist can reline the dentures for better fit or measure the patient for a new set.
- Review care and cleaning procedures for contact lenses with patient and caregiver. Check that lens case is clearly marked so that each lens is placed in its suitable case (right or left).
- Remind patients or caregivers at home to ask the telephone company about special equipment that can help a hearing-impaired person hear the phone ringing and carry on a phone conversation more easily.
- If linens are soiled with blood or body fluids, instruct family members to wear gloves when handling them. They should be rinsed first in cold water, and then washed separately from other household wash, using hot water, laundry detergent, and bleach.
- Teach family member or caregiver how to perform comfort measures, such as a backrub.
- Instruct caregivers or patients at home with an indwelling catheter to wash the urinary meatus and perineal area twice daily with soap and water. The anal area should also be cleansed after each bowel movement. Careful handwashing is imperative.

bacterial vaginosis, pelvic inflammatory disease, higher rates of HIV transmission, tubal pregnancies, chlamydial infection, and cervical cancer (Cottrell, 2002). Although douching is occasionally ordered to treat a vaginal infection, it is not recommended as a routine hygiene measure.

Deodorants to control odor around the vaginal orifice are unnecessary. Although these deodorants do not contain aluminum salts, which are irritating to the mucous membrane, they are intended for external use only. They should not be placed on sanitary napkins or tampons. Some sprays have been reported as possibly harmful when sprayed into the vagina. Repeated use is not generally recommended because of reported irritation and rashes. In addition, the sprays should not be used on broken skin areas. No therapeutic benefit from their use has been proven to date. Use of these special deodorants is not a substitute for keeping the area clean, and female patients often require teaching on this subject.

Nurses need to be aware of their own feelings related to this area (see Promoting Health 37-2).

If a patient develops a discharge or if irritation and itching around the vaginal orifice persist, notify the physician. See the Nursing Plan of Care 37-1.

Assisting With Antiembolism Stockings

Antiembolism stockings are often used for patients with limited activity to help prevent phlebitis and thrombi formation (described in Chap. 39, Activity). Manufactured by several companies, they are made of elastic material and are available in either knee-high or thigh-high length. Antiembolism stockings help move blood in superficial veins of the legs to deeper veins, prevent stagnation of blood in the veins of the legs, and promote venous return to the heart. A physician's order is required for their use. When assisting with antiembolism stockings, follow these general nursing guidelines:

- Measure the patient's leg to determine the proper size of stocking. The manufacturer whose stockings are being used gives directions for measuring. Some stockings fit either leg; others are designated right or left. An improperly

Promoting Health 37-2 *Feminine Hygiene*

Many women have concerns about feminine hygiene. Personal healthcare practices are influenced by past experiences, cultural knowledge, and societal expectations. It is important for women to feel comfortable with their bodies and to be knowledgeable about self-care practices that promote health and well-being and prevent infection and disease. Use the following assessment checklist to determine how well you are meeting your own need for feminine hygiene, if appropriate. Then develop a prescription for self-care by choosing appropriate behaviors from the list of suggestions.

ASSESSMENT CHECKLIST

almost always / sometimes / almost never

☐ ☐ ☐ 1. I feel comfortable with my body and accept its uniqueness.

☐ ☐ ☐ 2. I am knowledgeable about feminine hygiene practices and products.

☐ ☐ ☐ 3. I value preventive measures that promote health and reduce the likelihood of infection.

☐ ☐ ☐ 4. I understand that changes in vaginal discharge, pain, and bleeding may indicate pathology or disease or may be normal.

☐ ☐ ☐ 5. I am not uncomfortable seeking professional help when symptoms occur.

SELF-CARE BEHAVIORS

1. Wash the perineal area at least once daily. Towels and washcloths should be clean and never shared.
2. Always wipe from front to back after voiding and defecation to avoid introducing bacteria into the vagina or urethra.
3. Avoid sprays, soaps, powders, deodorants, tampons, and pads that are perfumed or irritating in any way.
4. Avoid clothing that is too tight and wear underpants and pantyhose that have a cotton crotch.
5. Avoid douching because it can strip the vagina of its normal flora and introduce bacteria.
6. Change tampons regularly. Use good handwashing technique before and after insertion.
7. Seek professional assistance to distinguish normal symptoms from pathology.
8. Schedule a yearly gynecologic examination with a healthcare professional you trust.

NURSING PLAN OF CARE 37-1 *for Female University Students and Glenda Davis*

Glenda Davis is a nurse practitioner who works in a campus health clinic at a state university. Frequently women ask her questions about feminine hygiene. Realizing that each woman who presents with a question probably represents many other women with similar unvoiced questions, she decides to develop an insert entitled *Self-Care: Feminine Hygiene* for the campus newspaper. The information she plans to include and the population she will address in her checklist are based on the following assessment data:

• Heterogeneous female population is of various ages, cultures, religions, sexual orientation, and family and lifestyle backgrounds.

• Knowledge about feminine hygiene varies widely from almost no knowledge to students who are well read or members of women's health professions.
• Students who present with questions are mostly concerned about the risk of acquiring an STD or the dangers of certain products (eg, tampons and toxic shock syndrome) or have questions related to intercourse and contraception.
• Numerous students report to the clinic with vaginal infections and urinary tract infections.
• Interest is high; ability to comprehend written materials is high.

NURSING DIAGNOSIS   Self-Care Deficit: Feminine Hygiene related to knowledge deficit as manifested by female students presenting to the campus clinic with questions about feminine hygiene; high incidence of vaginal and urinary tract infections; negative attitudes about feminine body frequently expressed.

EXPECTED OUTCOME   Students will:
• Express positive body image, valuing their uniqueness

(continued)

NURSING PLAN OF CARE 37-1

for Female University Students and Glenda Davis (continued)

Nursing Interventions	Rationale	Evaluative Statement
With each student who presents at the clinic for help with a gynecologic concern or problem, take the time to assess her knowledge of the female body and her acceptance of her body and comfort with it.	The women's health movement has encouraged women to feel ownership of their bodies, to appreciate their uniqueness as women, and to increase their awareness of their physical bodies and the feelings associated with them. Many women still feel that the genital area and cyclic phenomena such as the menstrual cycle and the female sexual response cycle are "dirty," and symptoms in this area may evoke fear, guilt, anxiety, and shame.	*Six-month evaluation:* 6/30/06 Outcome partially met: students are beginning to discuss gynecologic concerns more freely, yet great hesitance persists. *Revision:* Continue to help women to know, understand, and accept their bodies and to talk about their bodies. Make this a priority of the nursing staff at the clinic. *G. Davis, RN*
Counsel appropriately.	It is important for nurses to provide women with information about their bodies.	

EXPECTED OUTCOME

Students will:
- Correctly describe feminine hygiene self-care behaviors they are willing to incorporate into their daily lifestyles

Nursing Interventions	Rationale	Evaluative Statement
Assess with each patient her knowledge of feminine hygiene practices (correct any misconceptions) and motivation to use them consistently.	Many women have never been instructed about feminine hygiene, and harmful practices may be "picked up" from the media and other sources (eg, the use of frequent douching and deodorants to eliminate normal body odors).	6/30/06 Outcome met. Following publication of the *Self-Care: Feminine Hygiene* feature and one-on-one counseling using this printed handout, patients are knowledgeable about preventive hygiene measures. *G. Davis, RN*
Address specific concerns related to menstruation, intercourse, other maturational events.	Maturational events, such as menstruation, becoming sexually active, and pregnancy, may result in a need for new or modified hygiene practices.	
Teach the importance of using preventive hygiene measures to reduce the likelihood of acquiring a urinary tract or vaginal infection. Distribute the *Self-Care: Feminine Hygiene* handout and discuss this with the patient.	It is better to prevent a genitourinary infection than to treat it.	

EXPECTED OUTCOME

Campus health clinic records will:
- Demonstrate a reduction in both new and recurrent genitourinary infections

Nursing Interventions	Rationale	Evaluative Statement
Educate women regarding preventive hygiene measures (refer to the *Self-Care* handout).	It is better to prevent a genitourinary infection than to treat it.	6/30/06 Outcome met. Six months after publication and use of the *Self-Care: Feminine Hygiene* handout, the incidence of genitourinary infections is reduced 10%. Will continue to keep education in this regard a priority. *G. Davis, RN*

(continued)

NURSING PLAN OF CARE 37-1

for Female University Students and Glenda Davis (continued)

Nursing Interventions	Rationale	Evaluative Statement
Educate women to distinguish normal from abnormal findings (vaginal discharge, pain, bleeding, problems with urination) and to seek help when appropriate. Nursing measures include teaching preventive measures, instructing in recognition of symptoms, and assisting with self-care activities to prevent and treat infections, including the securing of assistance when indicated.	Early treatment of genitourinary infections reduces the likelihood of residual problems.	
Document new and recurrent genitourinary infections; identify predisposing factors.	Documentation facilitates on-going management of a recurring problem.	

SAMPLE DOCUMENTATION

6/15/06 Nursing

Student visited clinic and expressed need for information about feminine hygiene practices in general as well as those specific hygiene measures for use after intercourse. Also related concern about contracting an STI from partners. Reported that she became sexually active this year and has sexual intercourse once or twice weekly. Stated that "many of my friends use douches" and questioned whether any particular douche products are recommended. We discussed the *Self-Care: Feminine Hygiene* handout and reviewed various healthcare practices. Clarified for student her misconception regarding the advisability of douching. Also counseled her about her right to talk with a sexual partner about STIs and previous contacts with infected individuals. Advised that she refrain from contact or use a condom when she has intercourse. Student reported feeling more "in charge" of body and better able to care for it. Discussed all topics on plan of care and encouraged her to revisit clinic in 6 months for further clarification and evaluation.

G. Davis, RN

---

fitting stocking is uncomfortable and ineffective and possibly even harmful (McConnell, 2002).

- Be prepared to apply the stockings in the morning before the patient is out of bed and while the patient is supine. If the patient is sitting or has been up and about, have the patient lie down with legs and feet elevated for at least 15 minutes before applying the stockings. Otherwise the leg vessels are congested with blood, reducing the effectiveness of the stockings.
- Do not massage the legs. If a clot is present, it may break away from the vessel wall and circulate in the bloodstream.
- Check the legs regularly for redness, blistering, swelling, and pain. Some recommend checking the legs at least once every 8 hours; others recommend twice a day. Remove the stockings completely once a day to bathe the legs and feet.
- Launder the stockings as necessary, but at least every 3 days. Soiled stockings irritate the skin. Dry the stockings on a flat surface to prevent them from stretching. The patient may need two pairs of stockings so that he or she can wear one pair while the second pair is being cleaned.

Always remove antiembolism stockings during morning care and inspect the legs. Then reapply the stockings before the patient is out of bed, as shown in Skill 37-4.

Several manufacturers produce men's and women's hose that apply pressure to the legs from the foot to mid-thigh or higher. Some apply mild pressure; others apply pressure equivalent to that of an elastic bandage. Stockings are available in a variety of colors so that in ambulatory patients other stockings are not needed to cover them. Many people who are on their feet or remain in one position a great deal, such as homemakers, nurses, salespeople, and business people, find them useful. The stockings must be fitted correctly to the person's measurements. Also, instruct patients to apply them immediately on awakening, before getting out of bed and before the legs are in a dependent position.

SKILL
37-4　Applying Antiembolism Stockings

EQUIPMENT

Elastic stockings (in correct size)
For knee-high stockings:
• Measure from heel to popliteal space
• Measure circumference of calf at widest point

Measuring tape
Talcum powder (optional)

For thigh-high stockings:
• Measure from heel to gluteal fold
• Measure circumference of calf and thigh at widest point

ACTION	RATIONALE
1. Explain the rationale for use of elastic stockings to the patient.	Explanation encourages the patient's cooperation.
2. Perform hand hygiene.	Hand hygiene deters the spread of microorganisms.
3. Assist the patient to the supine position. If the patient has been sitting or walking, it is necessary to have him or her lie down with the legs and feet well elevated for at least 15 minutes before applying the stockings.	Dependent position of legs encourages blood to pool in the veins.
4. Provide privacy. Expose legs one at a time, and powder lightly unless patient has dry skin. If the skin is dry, a lotion may be used. Powders and lotions are not recommended by some manufacturers.	Powder and lotion reduce friction and make application of stockings easier.
5. Place hand inside stocking and grasp heel area securely. Turn stocking inside out to the heel area.	Inside-out technique provides for easier application and less compromising of circulation to the extremity from bunched elastic material.

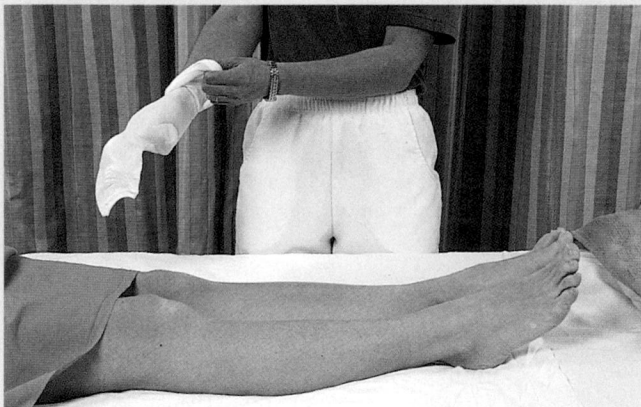

Action 5a: Inserting hand into stocking to grasp heel area.

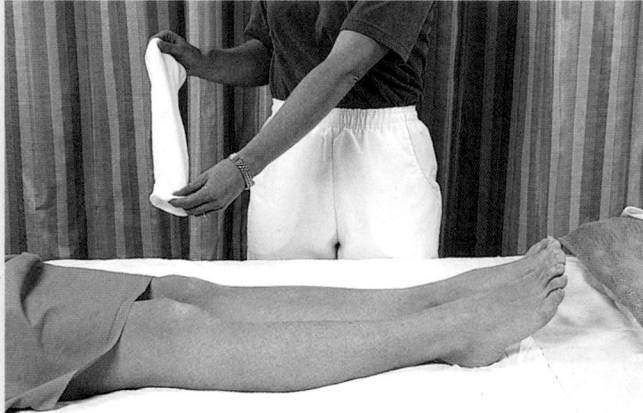

Action 5b: Turning stocking inside out to the heel pocket area.

ACTION	RATIONALE
6. Ease the foot of the stocking over the patient's foot and heel. Check that patient's heel is centered in heel pocket of stocking.	Wrinkles and improper fit interfere with circulation.
7. Using your fingers and thumbs, carefully grasp the edge of the stocking and pull it up smoothly over the ankle and calf until entire stocking is turned right side out. Pull forward slightly on toe section. Repeat for the other leg. Caution the patient not to roll stockings partially down.	Easing the stocking carefully into position ensures proper fit of the stocking to the contour of the leg. Rolling stockings may have a constricting effect on veins. Loosening the toe section provides for comfort in that area.
8. Wash your hands.	Handwashing deters the spread of infection.
9. To remove stocking, grasp the top of the stocking with your thumb and fingers and smoothly pull the stocking off inside out to heel. Support the patient's foot and ease stocking over it.	This preserves elasticity and contour of the stocking.
10. Remove stockings once every shift for 20 to 30 minutes. Wash and air dry as necessary (according to manufacturer's directions).	This allows observation of the patient's circulatory status and condition of the skin on the lower extremity.
11. Record the application of elastic stockings as well as assessment of the patient's circulatory status and skin condition.	This provides accurate documentation of the procedure.

(continued)

Applying Antiembolism Stockings (continued)

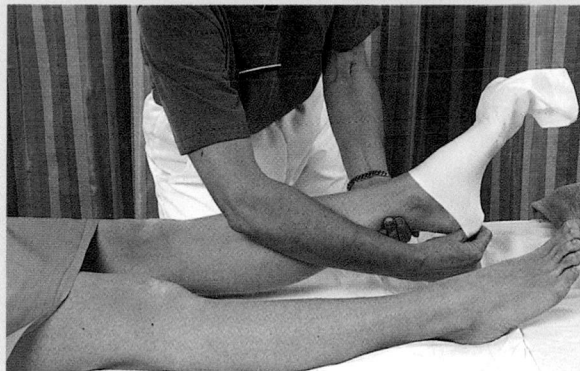

Action 6: Stretching stocking open and easing the foot of the stocking over the patient's foot.

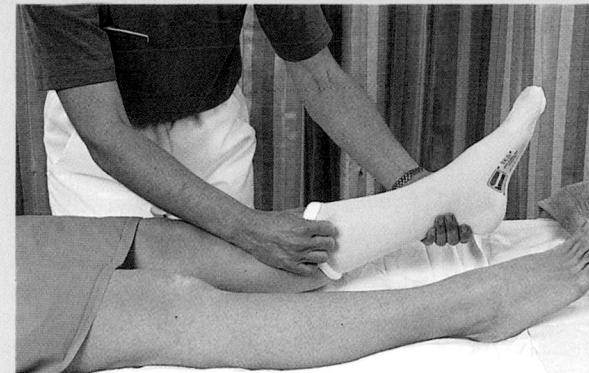

Action 7: Grasping top of stocking to pull up over calf.

Special Considerations	At times, despite the use of elastic stockings, a patient may develop thrombophlebitis. A positive Homans' sign (pain on dorsiflexion of the foot) may be an indication of a deep thrombosis or development of a blood clot in the calf.
Home Care Considerations	Make sure that the patient has an extra pair of stockings ordered during the hospitalization before discharge (for payment and convenience purposes).
	Launder stockings with other "white" clothing. Avoid excessive bleach. Remove from dryer as soon as "low heat" cycle is complete to avoid shrinkage. May also be air dried.

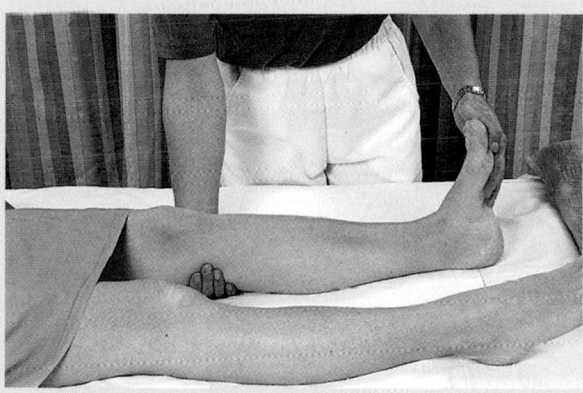

Special consideration: Checking Homans' sign.

Applying Intermittent Pneumatic Compression Stockings

Intermittent pneumatic compression stockings may be used in conjunction with antiembolism stockings. They require a physician's order and are often prescribed for high-risk surgical patients, patients with chronic venous disease, and patients at risk for deep-vein disorders. They consist of a knee-length or thigh-high cuff that is connected to hoses and a pump apparatus. Sequential compression stockings promote venous return by simulating the normal muscle-pumping action in the legs. These stockings are described further in Chapter 30, Perioperative Nursing.

Massaging the Back

A backrub generally follows the patient's bath. A backrub acts as a general body conditioner and can relieve muscle tension and promote relaxation. Some nurses forego giving backrubs to patients due to time pressure. However, giving a backrub allows the nurse to observe the skin for signs of breakdown. A backrub improves circulation; can decrease pain, distress, and anxiety and improve sleep quality; and provides a means of communication with the patient through the use of touch. See the Research in Nursing box.

Because some patients may consider the backrub a luxury and be reluctant to accept it, be sure to communicate its importance and value to the patient. An effective backrub should take 4 to 6 minutes to complete. If a lotion is used, it should be warmed before use.

Be aware of the patient's medical diagnosis when considering giving a backrub. A backrub is contraindicated, for example, if the patient has had back surgery or has fractured ribs. Position the patient on the abdomen or, if this is contra-

Research in Nursing Making a Difference

Evaluating the Power of Therapeutic Massage

After bathing, a backrub has always been a standard of nursing care. With the nursing shortage resulting in understaffing, the backrub has been one of the first cares cut from the to do list of many nurses. Is this best for our patients?

Related Research

Smith, M., Kemp, J., Hemphill, L., & Vojir, P. (2002). Outcomes of therapeutic massage for hospitalized cancer patients. *Journal of Nursing Scholarship, 34*(3), 257–262.

This study evaluated the effects of therapeutic massage on perception of pain, subjective sleep quality, symptom distress, and anxiety in patients being treated for cancer. The sample consisted of 41 participants. Twenty participants received a 15–30 minute light massage three times per week. The massages were at least 24 hours apart and occurred at various times throughout the day. Twenty-one participants received nurse interaction consisting of

20 minutes of deliberate focused communication with the same nurse who had provided massage to the other group.

Prior to the study no differences were found between the groups in relation to pain, symptom distress, subjective sleep quality or anxiety. The groups were monitored using a tool for each variable being researched. The study found that pain, symptom distress, and anxiety decreased in the massage group. Sleep quality remained the same for the massage group. In the nurse interaction group, pain, symptom distress, and subjective sleep quality increased. The mean score for anxiety in the interaction group improved slightly.

Relevance to Nursing Practice

This simple technique has the potential to help patients establish control over their disease process. Sometimes, the simplest nursing action can prove to be an effective caring intervention.

---

indicated, on the side. Recommended techniques for administering a backrub are outlined in Skill 41-1 in Chapter 41, Comfort.

Making a Bed

Usually bed linens are changed after the bath, but some agencies change linens only when soiled. The bed is made for the

ambulatory patient as described in Skill 37-5. If the patient is bedridden, the occupied bed is made as described in Skill 37-6.

Although there are variations in the procedure for making an occupied bed, these minor differences have no real effect on the patient's comfort. In some instances, creativity and flexibility are necessary when changing linens because of

(*text continues on page 1049*)

SKILL
37-5   Making an Unoccupied Bed

EQUIPMENT

Two large sheets (or one large sheet and one fitted sheet)	Bedspread	Protective pad (optional)
Drawsheet (optional)	Pillowcases	Disposable gloves (use if linens are soiled)
Blankets	Linen hamper or bag	
	Bedside chair	

ACTION	RATIONALE
1. Perform hand hygiene	Hand hygiene deters the spread of microorganisms.
2. Assemble equipment and arrange on a bedside chair in the order in which items will be used.	Organization facilitates performance of task.
3. Adjust the patient's bed to the high position, and drop the bed side rails.	Having the bed in the high position and the side rails down reduces strain on the nurse while working.
4. Check bed linens for the patient's personal items and disconnect call bell or any tubes from bed linens.	It is costly and inconvenient when personal belongings are lost. Disconnecting devices prevents damage to the devices and injury to patients.
5. Loosen all linen as you move around the bed from the head of the bed on the far side to the head of the bed on the near side.	Loosening the linen helps prevent tugging and tearing on linen. Loosening the linen and moving around the bed systematically reduce strain caused by reaching across the bed.
6. Fold reusable linens, such as sheets, blankets, or spread, in place on the bed in fourths and hang them over a clean chair.	Folding saves time and energy when reusable linen is replaced on the bed. Folding linens while they are on the bed reduces strain on the nurse's arms. Some agencies change linens only when soiled.

(continued)

ACTION

RATIONALE

7. Snugly roll all of the soiled linen inside of the bottom sheet and place directly into the laundry hamper. Do not place them on the floor or on furniture. Do not hold soiled linens against your uniform.

Rolling soiled linens snugly and placing them directly into the hamper helps prevent the spread of organisms. The floor is heavily contaminated; soiled linen will further contaminate furniture. Soiled linen contaminates the nurse's uniform, and this may spread organisms to another patient.

8. If possible, shift mattress up to the head of the bed.

This allows more foot room for the patient and moves the mattress against the head of the bed.

9. Place the bottom sheet with its center fold in the center of the bed and high enough to have a sufficient amount of the sheet to tuck under the head of the mattress.

Opening linens on the bed reduces strain on the nurse's arms and diminishes the spread of organisms.

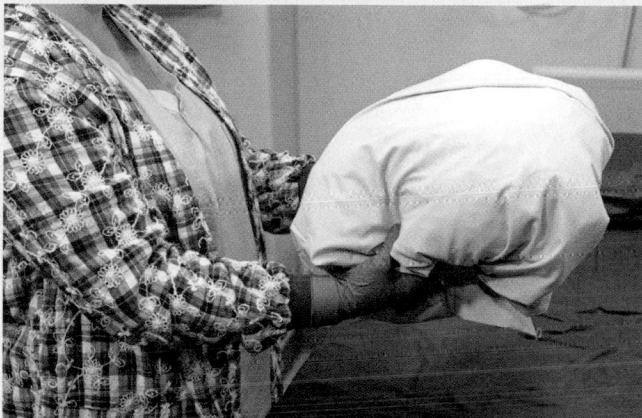

Action 7: Bundling soiled linens in bottom sheet and holding away from body.

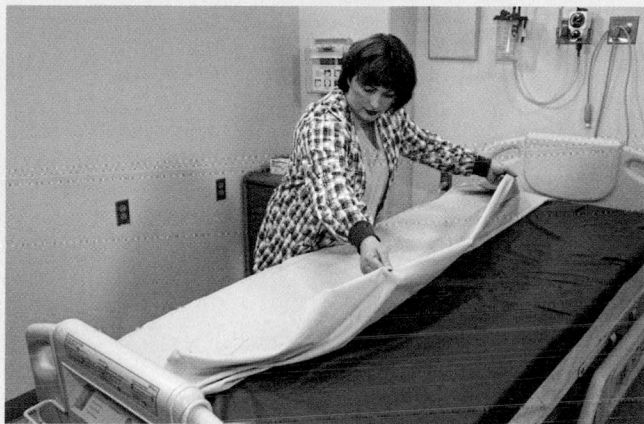

Action 9: Placing clean linens to begin bed making.

10. Place the drawsheet with its center fold in the center of the bed and positioned so it will be located under the patient's midsection. If a protective pad is used, place it over the drawsheet in the proper area. Not all agencies use drawsheets routinely. The nurse may decide to use one.

11. Tuck the bottom sheet securely under the head of the mattress on one side of the bed, making a corner according to agency policy. A mitered corner is shown in the illustrations. Using a fitted bottom sheet eliminates the need to miter corners. Tuck the remaining bottom sheet and drawsheet securely under the mattress. (At this point, before moving to the other side of the bed, top linens may be placed on the bed, unfolded, and secured, allowing the entire side of the bed to be completed at one time as shown in the illustrations.)

When a patient soils the bed, drawsheets can be changed without changing the bottom and top linens on the bed. Having all bottom linens in place before tucking them under the mattress avoids unnecessary moving about the bed. A drawsheet is also an aid when moving the patient in bed.

Making the bed on one side and then completing the bed on the other side saves time. Having bottom linens free of wrinkles reduces discomfort to the bedridden patient.

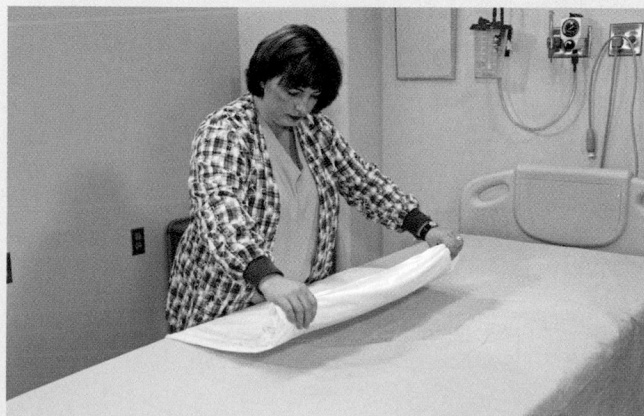

Action 10: Placing the drawsheet on the bed.

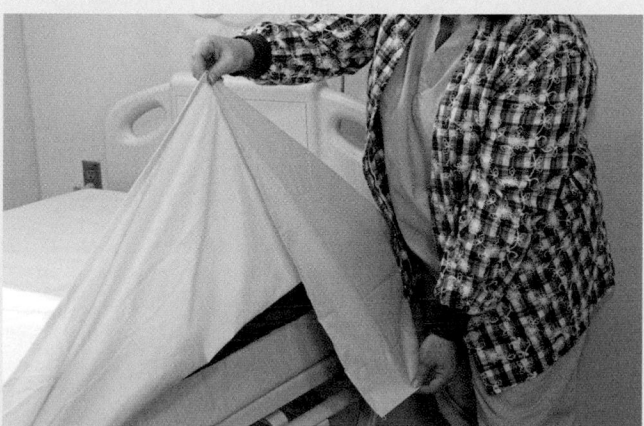

Action 11a: Beginning to make mitered corner by creating a triangular fold.

(continued)

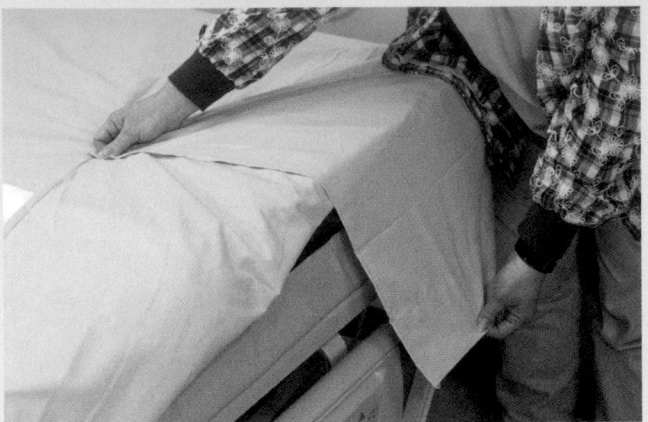

Action 11b: Laying triangular fold on top of bed.

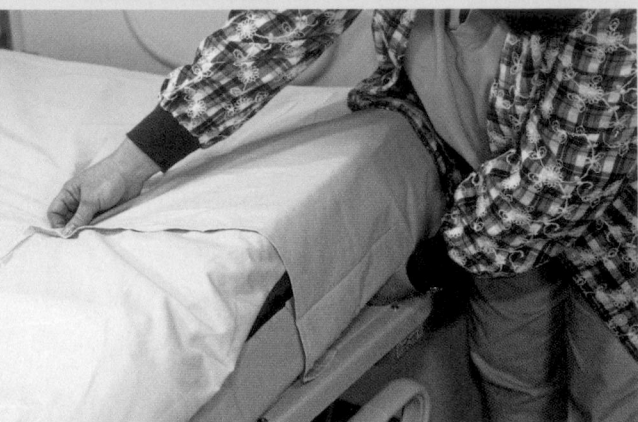

Action 11c: Tucking end of sheet under mattress.

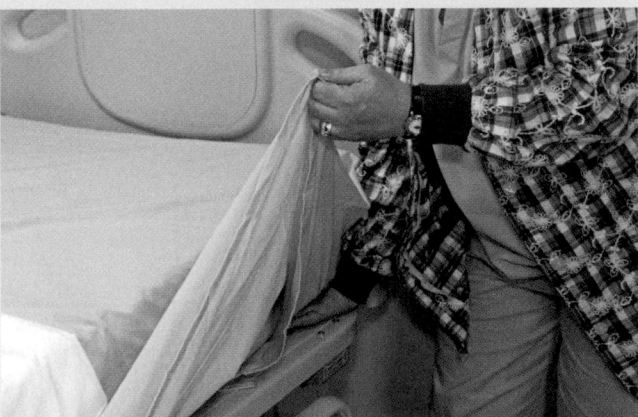

Action 11d: Folding triangular linen fold down over side of mattress.

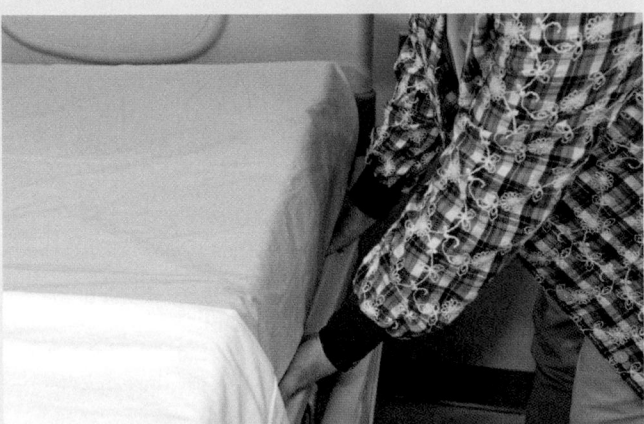

Action 11e: Tucking end of triangular linen fold under mattress to complete mitered corner.

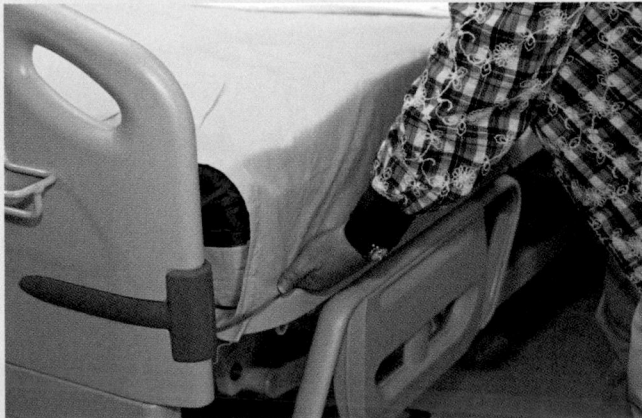

Action 11f: Tucking sheet snugly under foot of mattress.

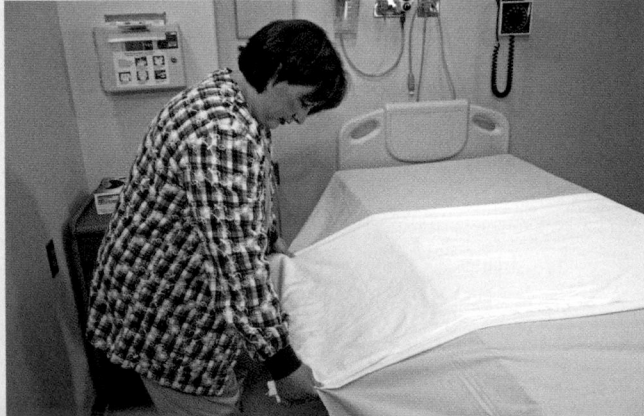

Action 12: Pulling bottom sheet tightly on opposite side of bed.

12. Move to the other side of the bed to secure bottom linens. Secure bottom sheet under the head of the mattress and miter the corner. Pull remainder of sheet tightly and tuck under mattress. Do the same for the drawsheet.

This rids bottom linens of any wrinkles that can cause discomfort for the patient.

(continued)

SKILL
37-5   **Making an Unoccupied Bed** (continued)

ACTION	RATIONALE
13. Place the top sheet on the bed with its center fold in the center of the bed and with the top of the sheet placed so that the hem is even with the head of the mattress. Unfold the top sheet in place, as illustrated. Follow same procedure with top blanket or spread, placing the upper edge about 6 inches below the top of the sheet.	Opening linens by shaking them spreads organisms into the air. Holding linens overhead to open them causes strain on the nurse's arms.
14. Tuck the top sheet and blanket under the foot of the bed on the near side. Miter the corners.	This saves time and energy and keeps the top linen in place.
15. Fold the upper 6 inches of the top sheet down over the spread and make a cuff.	This makes it easier for the patient to get into bed and pull the covers up.

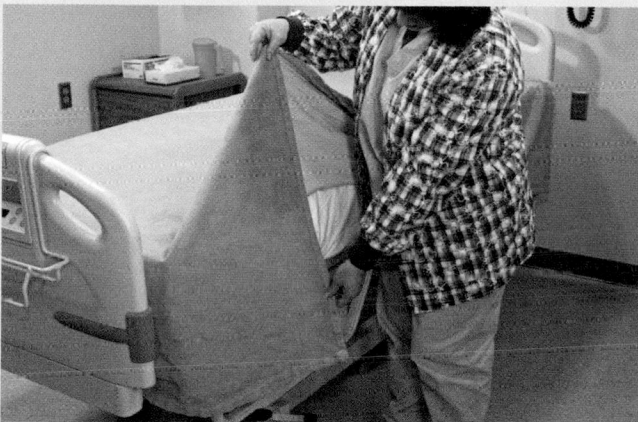

Action 14: Mitering the corner of the top sheet and spread.

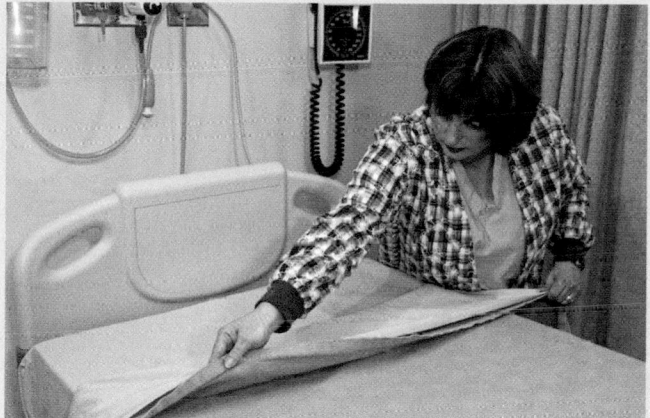

Action 15: Cuffing top linens.

16. Move to the other side of the bed and follow the same procedure for securing top sheets under the foot of the bed and making a cuff.	Working on one side of the bed at a time saves energy and is more efficient.
17. Place the pillows on the bed. Open each pillowcase in the same manner as opening other linens. Gather the pillowcase over one hand toward the closed end. Grasp the pillow with the hand inside the pillowcase. Keeping a firm hold on the top of the pillow, pull the cover onto the pillow.	Opening linens by shaking them causes organisms to be carried around on air currents. Covering the pillow while it rests on the bed reduces strain on the nurse's arms and back.
18. Place the pillow at the head of the bed with the open end facing toward the window.	This provides for a neater appearance.

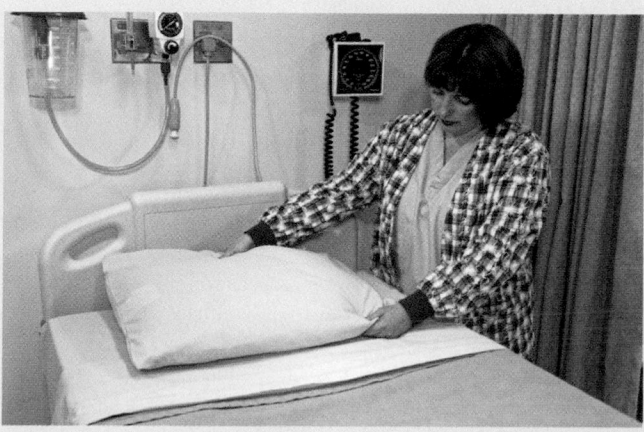

Action 18: Placing pillow on bed.

(continued)

SKILL 37-5 Making an Unoccupied Bed (continued)

ACTION	RATIONALE
19. Fan-fold or pie-fold the top linens.	Having linens opened makes it more convenient for the patient to get into bed.
20. Secure the signal device on the bed according to agency policy.	Having the signal device handy for the patient makes it possible for the patient to call for assistance as necessary.

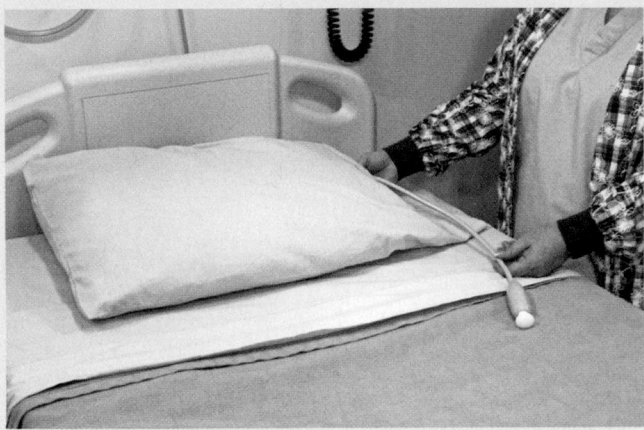

Action 20: Securing signal device to the bed.

ACTION	RATIONALE
21. Adjust the bed to the low position.	Having the bed in the low position makes it easier and safer for the patient to get into bed.
22. Dispose of soiled linen according to agency policy. Perform hand hygiene.	This deters the spread of microorganisms.

SKILL 37-6 Making an Occupied Bed

EQUIPMENT
Two large sheets (or one large sheet and one fitted sheet)
Drawsheet or lift pad
Disposable gloves (use if linens are soiled)

Blanket (optional)
Bedspread
Pillowcases
Linen hamper or bag (optional)

Bedside chair
Protective pad (optional)
Bath blanket (optional)

ACTION	RATIONALE
1. Explain the procedure to the patient. Check the patient's chart for limitations on the patient's physical activity.	This facilitates patient cooperation and determines level of activity.
2. Perform hand hygiene.	Hand hygiene deters the spread of microorganisms.
3. Assemble equipment and arrange on the bedside chair in the order the items will be used.	Organization facilitates performance of task.
4. Close door or curtain.	This provides for privacy.
5. Adjust the patient's bed to the high position. Lower the side rail nearest you, leaving the opposite side rail up. Place the bed in the flat position unless contraindicated.	Having the bed in the high position reduces strain on the nurse while working. Having the mattress flat facilitates making a wrinkle-free bed.
6. Check bed linens for patient's personal items and disconnect the call bell or any tubes from bed linens.	It is costly and inconvenient when personal items are lost. Disconnecting tubes from linens prevents discomfort and accidental dislodging of the tubes.

(continued)

SKILL
37-6 **Making an Occupied Bed** (continued)

ACTION	RATIONALE

7. Place a bath blanket, if available, over the patient. Have the patient hold onto the bath blanket while you reach under it and remove top linens. Leave the top sheet in place if a bath blanket is not used. Fold linen that is to be reused over the back of a chair. Discard soiled linen in a laundry bag or hamper.

This provides warmth and privacy.

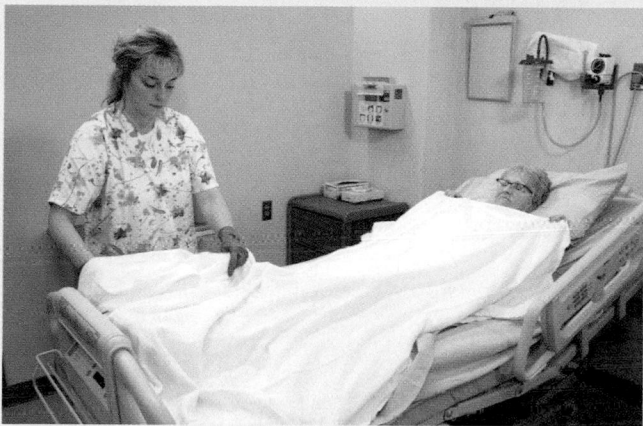

Action 7: Removing top linens from under bath blanket.

8. If possible and another person is available to assist, grasp mattress securely and shift it up to the head of the bed.

This allows more foot room for the patient and positions the mattress against the head of the bed.

9. Assist the patient to turn toward the opposite side of the bed and reposition the pillow under the patient's head.

This allows the bed to be made on the vacant side.

10. Loosen all bottom linens from the head and sides of the bed.

This facilitates removal of linens.

11. Fan-fold soiled linens as close to the patient as possible.

This facilitates removal of linens when the patient turns to the other side.

12. Use clean linen and make near side of bed following actions 9, 10, and 11 of Skill 37-5. Fan-fold the clean linen as close to the patient as possible.

This positions clean linen to make the side of the bed.

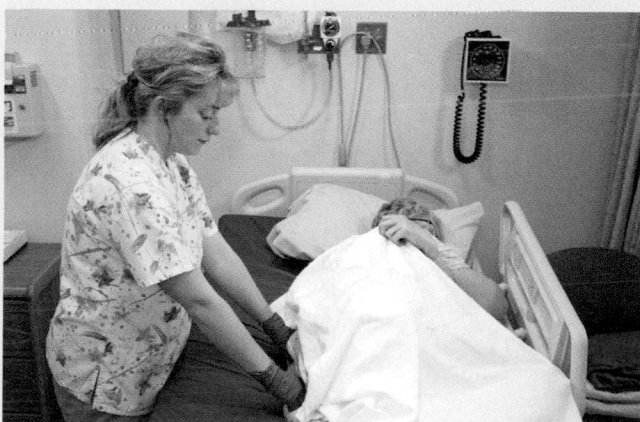

Action 11: Moving soiled linen as close to patient as possible.

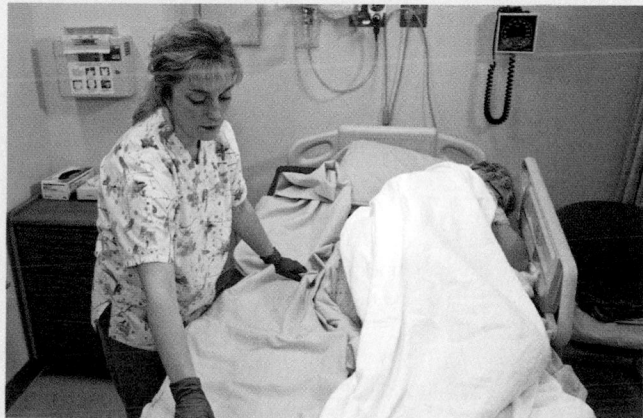

Action 12: Opening and folding clean linens.

13. Raise the side rail. Assist the patient to roll over the folded linen in the middle of the bed toward you. Reposition the pillow and bath blanket or top sheet. Move to the other side of the bed and lower the side rail.

This ensures patient safety. The movement allows the bed to be made on the other side. The bath blanket provides warmth and privacy.

(continued)

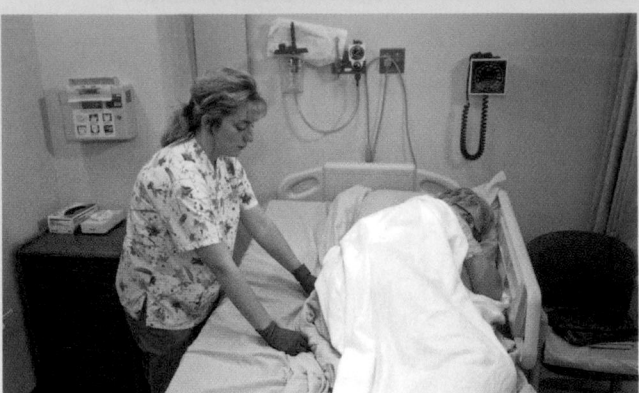

Action 12: Aligning clean bottom sheet on half of bed.

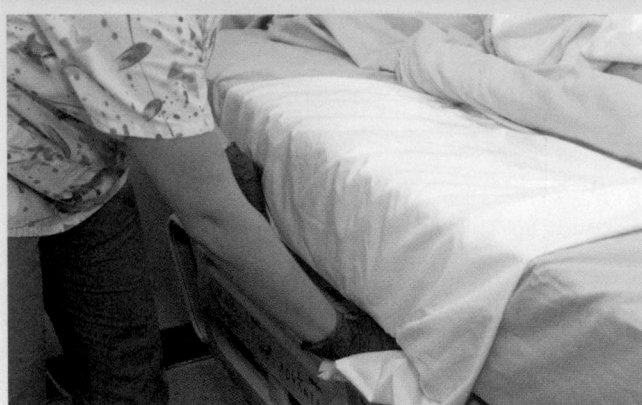

Action 12: Tucking bottom sheet and drawsheet tightly.

ACTION	RATIONALE
14. Loosen and remove all bottom linen. Place these in a linen bag or hamper. Hold soiled linen away from your uniform.	Proper disposal of soiled linen prevents spread of microorganisms.
15. Ease the clean linen from under the patient. Pull taut and secure the bottom sheet under the head of the mattress. Miter corners. Pull the side of the sheet taut and tuck under the side of the mattress. Repeat this with the drawsheet.	This removes wrinkles and creases in the linens, which are uncomfortable to lie on.
16. Assist the patient to return to the center of the bed. Remove the pillow and change the pillowcase before replacing, with open end facing toward the window.	This provides for a neater appearance.
17. Apply top linen so that it is centered and top hems are even with the head of the mattress. Have the patient hold onto the top linen so the bath blanket can be removed.	This allows bottom hems to be tucked securely under the mattress and provides for privacy.

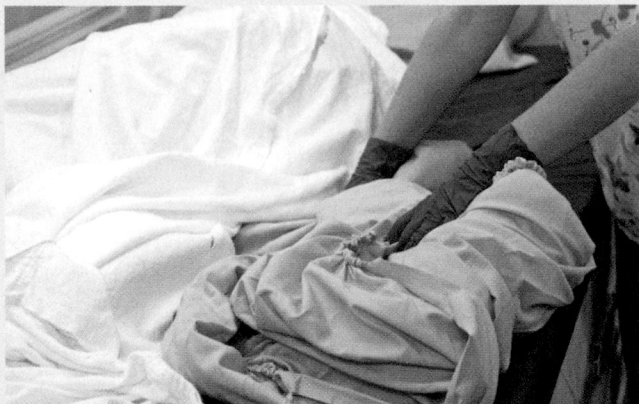

Action 14: Removing soiled bottom linens from other side of bed.

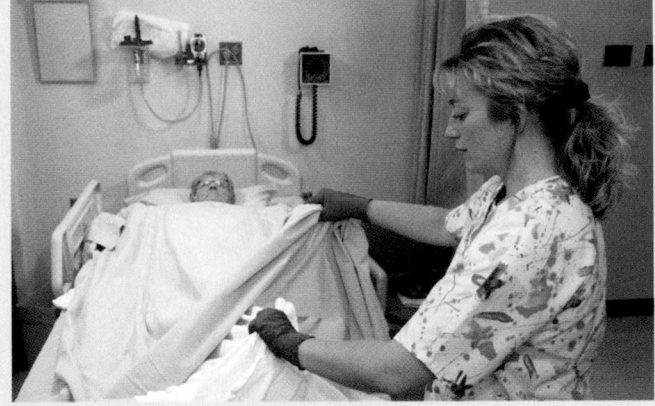

Action 17: Removing the bath blanket from under the top linens.

18. Secure top linens under the foot of the mattress and miter corners. Loosen top linens over the patient's feet by grasping them in the area of the feet and pulling gently toward the foot of the bed.	This provides for a neat appearance. Loosening linens over the patient's feet gives more room for movement.
19. Raise the side rail. Lower bed height and adjust the head of the bed to a comfortable position. Reattach call bell and drainage tubes.	This provides for the patient's safety.
20. Dispose of soiled linens according to agency policy. Perform hand hygiene.	This prevents spread of microorganisms.

Home Care Considerations   Use of a synthetic sheepskin, a soft bath blanket, or flannelette blanket as a bottom sheet may solve the problem of "coldness" for elderly patients with vascular problems or arthritis.

the patient's condition, orthopedic appliances on the bed, or treatments that may be in progress. See Through the Eyes of a Student.

Providing Environmental Care

The environment can improve or detract from the patient's sense of well-being. The patient's environment consists of the bedside unit and the furnishings and equipment in the space around the bed. Ensure that this area is clean, safe, and pleasant.

Bedside Unit

Basic furniture includes the bed, overbed table, bedside stand, and chairs. Standard equipment in the healthcare environment includes the call light, oxygen, suction, and electrical outlets; light fixtures; bath basin; emesis basin; bedpan or urinal; water pitcher and glass; and bed linens. A nursing responsibility is ensuring that necessary equipment and items are in their proper place and functioning properly.

Patients usually store personal items in the bedside stand. Always request permission from alert patients before opening the stand to obtain the bath basin, lotion, or other items. When assisting with hygiene, respecting the patient's right to privacy and ownership of personal goods decreases the patient's sense of powerlessness.

Through the Eyes of a Student

One of my first patients was a man in his late 60s who had suffered a stroke. I was assigned to care for him, and his care included a bed bath and complete linen change—with him in the bed. I was determined to complete this task totally on my own, without asking anyone for help. This was my first mistake.

The patient yelled obscenities at me and had very rough mannerisms. I kept thinking to myself, "I must treat him with gentle care and not show any fear." Inside I was shaking furiously.

I managed to complete his bath and then began to change the sheets. I helped the patient to turn to one side, tucking the dirty linens close to him. I applied the fitted sheets to the upper portion of the bed . . . so far, so good. Immediately going to the foot of the bed, I applied the bottom portion. The top portion popped off—I ran to the top of the bed, reapplied the top portion—the bottom portion popped off—I reapplied it. . . . I must have spent 15 minutes running back and forth trying to get both ends to stay on. By this time sweat was pouring off my face.

When I finally cried "Uncle," I discovered that certain fitted sheets just didn't fit all the mattresses. The usual routine in this case is to walk to the linen closet and get another fitted sheet. That probably takes about 15 seconds!

—Linda A. Keough, Delaware County
Community College, Media Pennsylvania

Before leaving the bedside unit, get into the habit of saying to the patient, "Is there anything else I can do to make you more comfortable?" Checking with the patient communicates genuine caring and can correct for any oversights. Limits regarding what comfort and hygiene measures the nurse can perform may need to be set for patients who are manipulative.

Nurses are responsible for ensuring the safety of the bedside unit. A safe bedside unit includes the following elements:
- Call light functioning and always within reach
- Bed positioned properly, at the appropriate height, and wheels locked
- Side rails safely used when indicated
- Principles of medical asepsis followed
- Electrical equipment safely grounded
- Uncluttered walk space

In addition to safety, another important responsibility is providing a comfortable bedside. This includes attention to ventilation, odors, room temperature, lighting, and noise.

Ventilation and Odors

Because of pathogens and unpleasant odors associated with body secretions and excretions (ie, urine, stool, vomitus, draining wounds, or body odors), good ventilation in patient rooms is imperative. Odors may be decreased by promptly emptying bedpans, urinals, and emesis basins and by being careful not to dispose of soiled dressings or anything with a strong odor in the waste receptacle in the patient's room. Deodorizers may need to be used.

Room Temperature

Patient preferences for room temperature often vary widely. Whenever possible, respect the patient's preference when determining the room temperature. In general, the room temperature should be 20° to 23°C (68° to 74°F).

Lighting and Noise

Because many patients find it difficult to sleep in a healthcare facility and may need to be disturbed frequently for assessment or treatment purposes, be careful to reduce harsh lighting and noises whenever possible, although adequate lighting is necessary for all nursing procedures. Whenever possible, avoid carrying out conversations immediately outside the patient's room. Many patients find this stressful both because the noise disturbs them and because they believe whatever is being said involves them.

Beds

Many people who are ill and hospitalized or are being cared for at home spend a large portion of the day—if not the entire day—in bed, so the bed is an important part of the patient's environment. Nursing responsibilities include ensuring a safe and comfortable bed.

Bed Safety

The typical hospital bed has a motorized metal frame in three sections, which allows the height of the bed to be raised or lowered and the head and foot to be adjusted. Know how to operate the bed and be ready to explain it to the patient. Bed positions are described in Chapter 39.

Hospital beds can also be ordered for use in the home. Because certain positions may be harmful to some patients, instruct the patient and family about advisable bed positions and the use of the bed controls. Hospital beds are generally 66 cm (26″) from the floor. This is higher than most beds at home, thus enabling the nurse or caregiver to reach the patient without undue musculoskeletal strain.

Side rails are used to provide assistance with moving in bed and to prevent the patient from falling (see Chap. 26, Safety, for additional discussion about the use of side rails). Use upper or lower side rails whenever indicated. Also, lock the wheels or casters on the hospital bed whenever the bed is stationary to prevent the bed from moving when the patient is moving from the bed to an upright position or being transferred to a stretcher. The headboard of most hospital beds is removable to allow close patient contact in an emergency situation.

To promote bed safety, ensure the following before leaving the patient's bedside:
- The bed is in its lowest position.
- The bed position is safe for the patient.
- The bed controls are functioning (bed is electrically safe).
- Side rails (upper and lower) are raised if indicated.
- The wheels or casters are locked.

Bed Comfort

The hospital mattress is firm and generally covered with a water-repellent material that can be easily wiped down with a bactericidal solution between patients. A variety of therapeutic beds and mattresses are available to reduce or relieve the effects of pressure on the skin (Fig. 37-8). These are discussed in more detail in Chapter 38.

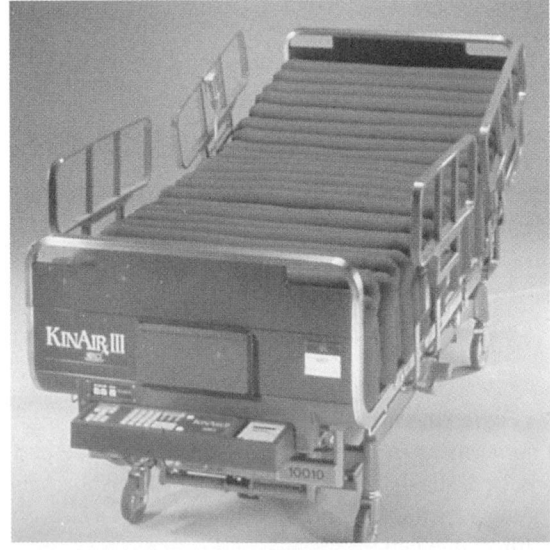

FIGURE 37-8 This special bed is an air-flotation, low-air-loss support surface that provides pressure relief. In this KinAir III there is a microprocessor computer control panel that controls air flow and temperature precisely. A built-in digital scale and heater are included. The bed also has a quick-release level for CPR.   (Photo courtesy of KCI Therapeutic Services, San Antonio, TX.)

Agency policies usually dictate the availability and use of bed linens. Bed linens include mattress covers, sheets, draw-sheets, incontinence pads, pillowcases, blankets, bedspreads, and bath blankets. Towels, washcloths, and patient gowns are often included in linen packs. In some settings, making the bed is not a nurse's responsibility, but ensuring patient comfort is always a priority in nursing, and this often involves creating a comfortable bed environment. To promote bed comfort, ensure the following before leaving a patient:
- Linens are clean and free of crumbs and wrinkles.
- The patient feels comfortably warm.
- Pressure areas are protected from rough sheets, hem edges, and water-repellent material; this is especially important for patients with a nursing diagnosis of Risk for Impaired Skin Integrity.

Teaching Patients About Skin Care

Teaching about skin care can occur at different times. For example, teaching can be done informally during assessment and care procedures. Here the nurse shares information about general skin care measures, including ways to prevent or reduce a patient's risk for skin problems. Occasionally, patients ask for specific information about skin care. In this instance, developing a formal teaching session addressing a specific topic, such as dry skin or acne, would be appropriate. The topics addressed when teaching patients can be wide-ranging. The following section describes common topics related to skin care and skin problems.

Soaps and Detergents

A wide variety of soaps and detergents are available. Soaps are often made from vegetable and animal fats, whereas most detergents are made from petroleum derivatives. Studies have shown that expensive cleansing agents are no more effective than their less expensive counterparts. For most people, the best way to cleanse the skin is with a soap or detergent and water. Review this information with the patient. Also inform patients who are sensitive to soap that often they can use detergents without difficulty.

Deodorants and Antiperspirants

Perspiration is essentially odorless, although it contains some waste products, such as uric acid and ammonia. The odor of perspiration results when bacteria, normally present on everyone's skin, act on the skin's normal secretions.

Inform patients that keeping the body and clothing clean is the best way to prevent body odors. Recommend the use of deodorants and antiperspirants after the skin is clean. Deodorants mask odor, and antiperspirants are intended to reduce the amount of perspiration. They act as astringents and tend to close the exits of the sweat glands. Advise patients to use antiperspirants and deodorants with care and according to directions to prevent skin irritation. Keep in mind that these products are contraindicated in some situations, such as before mammography and during the postoperative period for a patient who has had a mastectomy.

Cosmetics

Cosmetics frequently enhance the appearance of clean and healthy skin. Cosmetics can be used judiciously to help disguise blemishes, improve skin coloring, and make wrinkles appear less obvious. However, certain cultural and religious groups discourage their use.

Periodically, cosmetics containing harmful ingredients have appeared on the market. Be alert to such agents and help consumers avoid their use. The U.S. Department of Health and Human Services, Food and Drug Administration (FDA), enforces federal laws on the purity of foods, drugs, and cosmetics and on the advertising claims of their manufacturers. The FDA is a good source of information.

Remind patients that cosmetics often become contaminated with bacteria and fungi. Advise them to discard cosmetics after they are about 4 months old, especially those applied near the eyes. Encourage patients to keep makeup applicators and puffs immaculately clean and not to share cosmetics.

Common Skin Problems

Assessment frequently reveals dry skin, acne, and skin rashes. Table 37-3 summarizes recommended treatments for these skin problems.

Another skin problem is pressure ulcer formation. Pressure ulcers are areas of cellular **necrosis** caused by the lack

TABLE 37-3 **Skin Care Problems**

Skin Problem	Definition	Treatment
Dry Skin	Is characteristically flaky and is easily susceptible to injury and irritation	• Bathe less frequently. • Rinse off soaps and detergents well. • Use a superfatted soap (eg, Dove) for cleansing. • Avoid wearing wool garments because they tend to irritate the skin. • Use a humidifier to add moisture to the air. • Increase fluid intake when the skin is dry. • Use an emollient to soften, soothe, and protect dry skin after it is cleansed. • Use creams to clean skin that is dry or allergic to soap.
Acne	A condition that is particularly bothersome during adolescence. Hormones cause enlargement of the sebaceous glands and an increase in glandular secretions. Blackheads and pustules appear when secretions become blocked in the sebaceous ducts. Inflammation with infection can also occur.	• Avoid squeezing or picking infected areas because this can spread the infection and cause scarring. • Wash skin and shampoo hair with soap or detergent and hot water to remove oil and debris. • Avoid oily cosmetics, cleansing creams, and emollients. • Use cosmetics sparingly to avoid further blockage of the sebaceous ducts. • Eliminate foods that aggravate the condition. • Be aware that physician may recommend combination therapies that control manifestations of acne but result in *erythema* (redness) and skin peeling. Sun exposure may also be dangerous and should be avoided.
Skin rashes	Eruptions or inflammations of the skin that may be found anywhere on the body. May be precipitated by skin contact with an allergen, overexposure to sun, systemic causes (eg, reaction to a medication). May be described as flat or raised, pruritic or nonpruritic, localized or systemic, or dry or wet.	• Wash area thoroughly with mild cleansing agent and rinse well. • Use a moisturizing lotion on a dry rash to prevent itching and promote healing. • Use a drying agent on a wet rash. • Try tepid baths to help relieve inflammation and itching. • Use antiseptic sprays or lotions to help lessen itching, promote healing, and prevent skin breakdown. • Use over-the-counter products such as Caladryl lotion and hydrocortisone cream, which may prove useful. • Avoid exposure to causative agent if it is known. • See physician if symptoms do not respond to treatment.

of blood circulation to the involved area. At best, they are extremely painful and debilitating to patients; at worst, they may be life-threatening. Preventing pressure ulcers whenever possible and identifying and treating them at the earliest stage possible are critical nursing responsibilities. This topic is explored in detail in Chapter 38.

Evaluating

Performing or assisting with the performance of hygiene measures provides a means of at least daily contact with the patient to determine whether the patient is achieving outcomes related to hygiene and skin care. Indicators that can be used to determine outcome achievement include the following:

- Level of patient's participation in hygiene program
- Elimination of, reduction in, or compensation for factors interfering with the patient's independent execution of hygiene measures (eg, weakness, decreased motivation, lack of knowledge)
- Changes related to specific skin problems—for example, healing of skin lesions, elimination or reduction in causative factors, and independent patient management of the prescribed treatment program

The following are examples of evaluation related to hygiene:
10/26/06—Outcome partially met. Patient's oral mucosa is intact, but thick, dry secretions continue to build up on oral mucosa and gums despite every-4-hour care. Revision: Increase frequency of oral hygiene to every 2 hours. Instruct family. —N. Glynn, RN
10/24/06—Outcome met. Patient demonstrated correct care (cleaning) of artificial eye for the past two mornings. States, "I guess I should be happy to be alive and still able to see." —N. Glynn, RN
10/27/06—Outcome partially met. Patient reports that she is uncomfortable wearing a wig but feels better since its purchase. Revision: Patient still has many questions about effects of chemotherapy; continue teaching and use opportunities to build self-esteem. —A. Jones, RN
10/27/06—Expected outcome met. Patient correctly verbalized rationale for diabetic foot care program and expressed interest in attending the diabetic classes. —A. Diaz, RN
11/20/06—Outcome partially met. Child returned to clinic with clean perineal area and relief of painful urination. Mother reports child spends half the time with her and half with father (parents separated) and that father is not committed to hygiene practices. Revision: Stress again to child importance of retracting foreskin during perineal care. —C. Moser, RN

Developing Critical Thinking Skills

1. Practice the art of back massage with a willing partner until you feel comfortable and confident including this nursing measure in your routine care. Discuss with other students the therapeutic benefits of mas-

sage, and identify nursing situations for which it may be the primary therapy.
2. Interview people of different ages and cultural backgrounds about their hygiene practices. Ask specific questions about the type of nursing assistance they would require if hospitalized and unable to meet their hygiene needs independently. Are there special products or equipment they would need? To what extent are nurses obliged to respect the hygiene preferences of patients?

Practicing for NCLEX

1. When developing a plan of care for an older patient, the nurse pays special attention to the patient's skin based on an understanding of which of the following?
   a. The amount of subcutaneous fat increases.
   b. The sebaceous glands secrete more oil.
   c. The skin becomes increasingly dry.
   d. The skin thickens.
2. Which intervention would be appropriate to include in the plan of care for a patient wearing antiembolism stockings?
   a. Measuring legs before applying stockings to ensure proper fit
   b. Applying stockings while the patient is sitting in a chair
   c. Massaging the legs when the stockings are removed
   d. Leaving stockings in place for 1-week intervals
3. During a bath, the nurse observes that a patient has dry skin. Which action would be best?
   a. Bathe the patient more frequently.
   b. Use an emollient on the dry skin.
   c. Massage the skin with alcohol.
   d. Discourage fluid intake.
4. Which recommendation by the nurse to an adolescent patient with acne would be most appropriate?
   a. Wash the skin frequently using soap.
   b. Use cosmetics liberally to cover blackheads.
   c. Use emollients on the area.
   d. Squeeze blackheads as they appear.
5. The nurse observes a marked inflammation of the gums involving the alveolar tissue and documents this observation using which term?
   a. Glossitis
   b. Caries
   c. Cheilosis
   d. Pyorrhea
6. Which action would be the priority when administering oral care to a dependent patient?
   a. Assisting the patient to the dorsal recumbent position
   b. Wearing disposable gloves
   c. Using a firm toothbrush to cleanse teeth and gums
   d. Irrigating forcefully with hydrogen peroxide

7. Mr. James has an eye infection with a moderate amount of discharge. Which action would be most appropriate for the nurse to use when cleaning his eyes?
   a. Using hydrogen peroxide
   b. Wiping from the outer canthus to the inner canthus
   c. Positioning him on the same side as the eye to be cleansed
   d. Using only one cotton ball per eye

8. Which of the following interventions would the nurse include in the plan of care when providing foot care to an older patient?
   a. Using scissors to correct an ingrown toenail
   b. Trimming toenails as short as possible
   c. Using an alcohol rub if the feet are dry
   d. Bathing the feet at least daily

9. Providing perineal care to a patient requires which of the following?
   a. Using a clean portion of the washcloth for each stroke
   b. Moving from most contaminated to least contaminated area
   c. Using sterile gloves
   d. Leaving the foreskin undisturbed in an uncircumcised male

10. A nurse is caring for an 80-year-old patient who requires total assistance with his personal and oral hygiene. He is thin, has few visitors, and prefers to remain in bed in a semisitting position. Which nursing diagnosis would the nurse identify as the priority?
   a. Risk for Impaired Skin Integrity related to immobility
   b. Bathing/Hygiene Self-Care Deficit related to decreased strength and endurance
   c. Social Isolation related to lack of visitors
   d. Activity Intolerance related to generalized weakness

11. An older patient with an unsteady gait requests a tub bath. Which of the following actions would be most appropriate?
   a. Add Alpha-Keri oil to the water to prevent dry skin.
   b. Allow the patient to lock the door to guarantee privacy.
   c. Assist the patient in and out of the tub to prevent falling.
   d. Keep the water temperature very warm because the patient chills easily.

12. During morning care, the patient asks the nurse to shave him with a disposable razor. Before shaving him, the nurse should:
   a. Have him sign a permission form
   b. Check to see if the patient is taking anticoagulants
   c. Tell him that only a family member may shave a patient
   d. Position him flat in bed

13. To remove gas-permeable contact lenses from an unresponsive patient, the nurse would:
   a. Gently irrigate the eye with an irrigating solution from the inner canthus outward
   b. Grasp the lens with a gentle pinching motion
   c. Don sterile gloves before attempting the removal procedure
   d. Ensure that the lens is centered on the cornea before gently manipulating the lids to release it

14. The nurse is about to bathe a female patient who has an intravenous line in place, and needs to remove her gown. The nurse should:
   a. Temporarily disconnect the IV tubing at a point close to the patient and thread it through the gown
   b. Cut the gown with scissors to allow arm movement
   c. Thread the bag and tubing through the gown sleeve, keeping the line intact
   d. Temporarily disconnect the tubing from intravenous container, threading it through the gown

15. When making an occupied bed, which of the following is most important for the nurse to do?
   a. Keep the bed in the low position
   b. Use a bath blanket or top sheet for warmth and privacy
   c. Constantly keep the side rails raised on both sides
   d. Move back and forth from one side to the other when adjusting the linens

Answers With Rationale

1. The correct answer is *c*. With age, the skin becomes increasingly dry, subcutaneous fat decreases, sebaceous glands secrete less oil, and the skin becomes thinner.

2. The correct answer is *a*. The legs should always be measured according to the manufacturer's directions before ordering antiembolism stockings. Stockings may be uncomfortable if applied while the patient is sitting because leg veins are apt to be congested. Massage is dangerous because it may cause a clot to break away and circulate in the bloodstream. Stockings should be removed once daily.

3. The correct answer is *b*. An emollient soothes dry skin, whereas frequent bathing increases dryness, as does alcohol. Discouraging fluid intake leads to dehydration and, subsequently, dry skin.

4. The correct answer is *a*. Washing the skin frequently with soap removes oil and debris, whereas liberal use of cosmetics and emollients can clog the pores. Squeezing blackheads is always discouraged because it may lead to infection.

5. The correct answer is *d*. Pyorrhea is a marked inflammation of the gums, whereas caries refers to the presence of tooth decay. Cheilosis is ulceration of the lips, and glossitis is an inflammation of the tongue.

6. The correct answer is *b*. Disposable gloves provide a barrier to protect the nurse and patient. The dorsal

recumbent position is unsafe because the patient may easily aspirate any secretions or fluids. A soft toothbrush is recommended to avoid causing irritation and bleeding, and forceful irrigation is never safe. Water would be the choice for any gentle irrigation.

7. The correct answer is *c*. Positioning on the same side as the involved eye discourages contamination of the other eye. Always cleanse from the inner canthus to the outer canthus to avoid forcing debris into the nasolacrimal duct. Water or normal saline should be used for cleansing the eye of any discharge, and one cotton ball should be used for each stroke.

8. The correct answer is *d*. An older patient should have foot care once daily. Correcting an ingrown toenail should be done by a podiatrist, and trimming the toenails may require a physician's order. Cutting the toenails as short as possible exposes tender areas to friction and may lead to the skin being cut during trimming. Alcohol is drying and should not be used when dry skin is usually already a problem.

9. The correct answer is *a*. Using a clean portion of the washcloth for each stroke prevents contamination of other areas. Cleansing should always proceed from the least contaminated to the most contaminated area. Clean gloves, not sterile gloves, are used to provide perineal care. The foreskin in an uncircumcised male should be pulled back to allow cleansing underneath and then gently returned to its former position.

10. The correct answer is *a*. Although Bathing/Hygiene Self-Care Deficit, Social Isolation, and Activity Intolerance may be appropriate nursing diagnoses for this patient, the priority at this time is Risk for Impaired Skin Integrity. A break in his skin, such as from a pressure ulcer, may lead to infection, which at his age could be life-threatening.

11. The correct answer is *c*. Safe nursing practice requires that the nurse assist a patient with an unsteady gait in and out of the tub. Adding Alpha-Keri oil to the bath water is dangerous for this patient because it makes the tub slippery. Although privacy is important, if the patient locks the door, the nurse cannot help if there is an emergency. The water should be comfortably warm at 43° to 46°C. Older patients have an increased susceptibility to burns due to diminished sensitivity.

12. The correct answer is *b*. A patient who is taking anticoagulants should be shaved with an electric razor rather than a blade razor. Shaving a patient does not require permission and can be completed by either the caregiver or a family member. A shave is best completed with the patient in a Fowler's or semi-Fowler's position to prevent soap and water from running behind the patient's head.

13. The correct answer is *d*. The lens must be situated on the cornea, not the sclera, before removal. To remove hard contact lenses, the upper and lower eyelids

are gently maneuvered to help loosen the lens and slide it out of the eye. An attempt to grasp a hard lens might result in a scratch on the cornea. Clean, not sterile, gloves are used if drainage is present.

14. The correct answer is *c*. Threading the bag and tubing through the gown sleeve keeps the system intact. Opening an IV line, even temporarily, causes a break in a sterile system and introduces the potential for infection. Cutting a gown is not an alternative except in an emergency.

15. The correct answer is *b*. Using the bath blanket or top sheet keeps the patient warm and provides privacy. Keeping the bed in the low position and working over raised side rails may strain the nurse's back. Continually moving back and forth to tuck and arrange linen is time-consuming and disorganized.

Bibliography

Aiello, A., & Larson, E. (2002). Causal inference: The case of hygiene and health. *American Journal of Infection Control, 30*(8), 503–510.

Cottrell, B. (2002). Vaginal douching. *Journal of Obstetric, Gynecologic, and Neonatal Nursing, 32*(1), 12–18.

Dougherty, J., & Long, C. (2003). Techniques for bathing without a battle. *Home Healthcare Nurse, 21*(1), 38–39.

Dunn, J., Thiru-Chelvam, B., & Beck, C. (2002). Bathing: Pleasure or pain? *Journal of Gerontological Nursing, 28*(11), 6–13.

Fort, C. (2002). Get pumped to prevent DVT. *Nursing, 32*(9), 50–52.

Hayes, J., Lehman, C., & Castonguay, P. (2002). Graduated compression stockings: Updating practice, improving compliance. *MedSurg Nursing, 11*(4), 163–166, 191.

Hess, C. (2003). Managing a diabetic ulcer. *Nursing, 33*(7), 82–83.

Hilgers, J. (2003). Comforting a confused patient. *Nursing, 33*(1), 48–50.

Larson, E. (2002). The 'hygiene hypothesis': How clean should we be? *American Journal of Nursing, 102*(1), 81–89.

Larson, E., & Aiello, A. (2001). Hygiene and health: An epidemiologic link? *American Journal of Infection Control, 29*(4), 232–238.

Larson, E., Gomez-Duarte, C., Qureshi, K., & Miranda, D. (2001). How clean is the home environment? A tool to assess home hygiene. *Journal of Community Health Nursing, 18*(3), 139–150.

McConnell, E. (2002). Applying antiembolism stockings. *Nursing, 32*(4), 17.

Pauldine, E. (2003). Taking a bite out of Lyme disease. *Nursing, 33*(4), 49–52.

Plummer, S. (2001). Chronic complications. *RN, 64*(5), 34–42.

Stewart, K. (2002). Stopping the itch of scabies and lice. *Nursing, 30*(7), 30–31.

Stone, C. (1999). Preventing cerumen impaction in nursing facility residents. *Journal of Gerontological Nursing, 25*(5), 43–45.

Skin Integrity and Wound Care

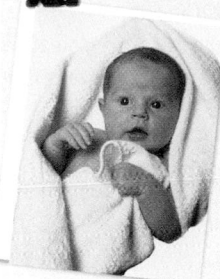

Abigail Karcher, a 5-week-old, small-for-gestational age infant, was born at only 28 weeks' gestation. She is in the neonatal intensive care unit receiving mechanical ventilation. She has chest tubes in place, and several intravenous lines have been inserted for medications and fluids. She also is being monitored with a pulmonary artery catheter.

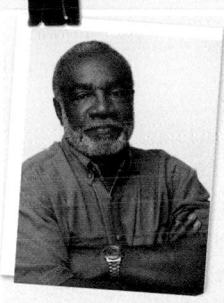

Lucius Everly, who has a history of diabetes and circulatory problems, underwent abdominal surgery several days ago and is in the critical care unit. He is slouched down in bed; his abdominal dressing is moist, and only part of the tape securing the dressing is adhering to the skin. His level of consciousness is decreased, and he responds only to moderate touch and pain. Further assessment reveals the beginning of a pressure ulcer on his heel.

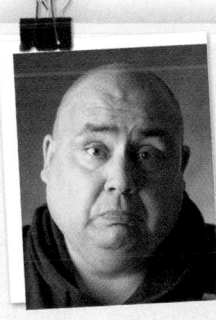

Sam Bentz, a 56-year-old man, has been admitted to the hospital for aggressive treatment of a bone infection that has not responded to usual methods. Mr. Bentz is 5 feet 4 inches tall and weighs more than 300 pounds. He tells you, "Last time I was here, my skin got really irritated and I developed several skin wounds."

Focusing on Blended Skills

The types of blended skills you'll need to respond to the case scenarios include:

Cognitive Skills
- Knowledge of anatomy and physiology related to skin integrity and wound healing
- Ability to identify different types of wounds and their causes
- Knowledge of the phases of wound healing and factors affecting wound healing
- Ability to integrate knowledge of possible complications associated with wound healing for assessment and nursing interventions for prevention
- Knowledge of how to prevent, diagnose, and treat pressure ulcers and other skin alterations
- Familiarity with effective skin, pressure ulcer, and wound care products and equipment
- Knowledge of the principles of asepsis, both medical and surgical

Technical Skills
- Demonstration of strong history and physical assessment techniques to determine a patient's risk for impaired skin integrity, including pressure ulcers
- Demonstration of ability to assess the necessary wound parameters, such as size, depth, and color, for a patient with a wound
- Ability to use correctly the products, protocols, and equipment necessary to prevent and treat pressure ulcers and other skin alterations
- Ability to demonstrate competence in technical nursing assistance to meet the needs of patients who are at risk for or are experiencing a wound or wound complication

- Ability to demonstrate application of the principles of medical and surgical asepsis with wound care measures

Interpersonal Skills
- Ability to establish trusting professional relationships that enlist patients and their caretakers in a plan to prevent or treat pressure ulcers and other skin alterations
- Ability to work collaboratively with the interdisciplinary team to prevent and treat skin alterations
- Strong people skills, with the ability to communicate and interact effectively with patients at various developmental stages
- Ability to demonstrate care and compassion to patients requiring wound care measures

Ethical and Legal Skills
- Commitment to safety and quality; strong sense of responsibility and accountability for skin and wound care
- Ability to advocate for the needs of patients who are unable to communicate these needs
- Ability to document skin and wound care accurately and completely according to agency policy
- Knowledge of special regulations, legislation, and policy detailing nursing responsibilities related to asepsis and wound care

Learning Outcomes

After completing the chapter, the learner should be able to accomplish the following:

1. Discuss the processes involved in wound healing.
2. Describe five factors that affect wound healing.
3. Accurately assess and document the condition of wounds.
4. Implement appropriate dressing changes for different kinds of wounds.
5. Apply heat and cold effectively and safely.
6. Provide information to patients and caregivers for self-care of wounds at home.
7. Identify patients at risk for a pressure ulcer.
8. Describe the four stages of pressure ulcers.
9. Provide nursing interventions to prevent or minimize pressure ulcers in adults.
10. Demonstrate adherence to guidelines for cleaning and dressing a pressure ulcer.

Key Terms

bandage
débridement
dehiscence
dressing
epithelialization
eschar
evisceration
exudate
fistula
granulation tissue
ischemia
necrosis
pressure ulcer
scar
shearing force
wound

The skin is the body's first line of defense protecting the underlying structures from invasion by organisms. Thus, maintaining an intact skin surface is important, because a break or disruption in this integrity is potentially dangerous and possibly life-threatening. The nurse plays a major role in maintaining the patient's skin integrity, in identifying risk factors that predispose a patient to a break in integrity, in intervening to prevent or reduce a patient's risk for impaired skin integrity, and in providing specific wound care when breaks in integrity arise. (See Chap. 37, Hygiene, for additional information about skin and its functions.)

Knowledgeable and skilled wound care is an essential component of nursing care. Using the nursing process, an individualized plan of care is developed to assess the patient and the wound, to identify and prevent complications, to implement and evaluate skills essential to wound care, and to provide physical and emotional support to facilitate healing, adaptation, and self-care. Wound care may be required in any healthcare setting, and increasingly complex wounds are being cared for at home.

This chapter provides information about disruptions in skin and tissue integrity, including wounds and pressure ulcers (see the Reflective Practice box for an example). Because applications of heat and cold are used to treat altered skin integrity, the discussion of those treatment modalities is also included.

WOUNDS

A **wound** is a break or disruption in the normal integrity of the skin and tissues. That disruption may range from a small cut on a finger to a third-degree burn covering almost all of the body. Wounds may result from mechanical forces (such as surgical incisions) or physical injury (such as a burn). Examples of types of wounds and their causes are highlighted in Table 38-1.

Wound Classification

Wounds are classified in many different ways. For example, wounds may classified as intentional or unintentional, open or closed, and acute or chronic. Wounds may also be classified as partial-thickness (all or a portion of the dermis is intact), full-thickness (the entire dermis and sweat glands and hair follicles are severed), or complex (the dermis and underlying subcutaneous fat tissue is also damaged or destroyed).

Intentional Wounds

An intentional wound is the result of planned invasive therapy or treatment. Examples of intentional wounds include those that result from surgery, intravenous therapy, and lumbar puncture. The wound edges are clean, and bleeding is usually controlled. Because the wound was made under sterile conditions with sterile supplies and skin preparation, the risk for infection is decreased, and healing is facilitated.

Think back to Abigail Karcher, the 5-week-old small-for-gestational-age infant in the neonatal intensive care unit. Her numerous intravenous lines would be considered intentional wounds. The nurse would incorporate an understanding of the principles of surgical asepsis when caring for these wound sites to prevent infection.

Unintentional Wounds

Unintentional wounds occur from unexpected trauma, such as from accidents, forcible injury (such as a stabbing or a gunshot), and burns. Because the wounds occur in an unsterile environment, contamination is likely. Wound edges are usually jagged, multiple trauma is common, and bleeding is uncontrolled. These factors create a high risk for infection and a longer healing time.

Open and Closed Wounds

An open wound occurs from intentional or unintentional trauma. The skin surface is broken, providing a portal of entry for microorganisms. Bleeding, tissue damage, and increased risk for infection and delayed healing may accompany open wounds.

A closed wound results from a blow, force, or strain caused by trauma such as a fall, an assault, or a motor vehicle crash. The skin surface is not broken, but soft tissue is damaged, and internal injury and hemorrhage may occur.

Acute and Chronic Wounds

Acute wounds, such as surgical incisions, usually heal within days to weeks. The wound edges are well approximated and the risk of infection is lessened. Chronic wounds, in contrast, do not progress through the normal sequence of repair. The wound edges are often not approximated, the risk of infection is increased, and the normal healing time is delayed. Chronic wounds include deep pressure ulcers and peripheral vascular arterial or venous ulcers.

Wound Healing

Wound healing is a process of tissue response to injury. Injured tissues are repaired by physiologic mechanisms that regenerate functioning cells and replace connective tissue cells with scar tissue. The healing process fills the gap caused by tissue destruction, restoring the structural integrity of the damaged tissue through the orderly release of growth factors and chemical mediators (Porth, 2002). These substances help to increase the blood supply to the damaged area, wall off and remove cellular and foreign debris, and initiate cellular development.

Normally, the healing process occurs without assistance. However, interventions can help to support the process. For example, keeping the injured area free of debris by proper cleaning helps to promote tissue healing, as does positioning the wounded area to promote circulation to that part. These interventions are based on the principles of wound healing, outlined in Box 38-1.

Reflective Practice
Challenge to Ethical and Legal Skills

I had a tough clinical 2 weeks ago while caring for Lucius Everly, a critical care postop patient with a history of diabetes and circulation problems. The nurse I was working with had floated to the unit on this day, but this I didn't know. Mr. Everly appeared to be neglected by other caregivers, and since he was not communicating and had a decreased level of consciousness, he could not express his needs. I saw that he needed bathing, wound care, repositioning in bed, and overall some additional attention. The nurse spoke about Mr. Everly in the room as though he was deaf. In my opinion, the nurse did not respect his inability to communicate. I became frustrated because the nurse I was with did not share this sense of concern for him. I became irritated when I asked what we could do to care for the poor circulation to his feet. My irritation increased when I realized that he was developing a pressure sore on his heel.

Thinking Outside the Box: Possible Courses of Action

- Tell my clinical instructor of my frustrations earlier in the day so my patient's care could have been addressed earlier and my frustrations wouldn't have built up.
- Go to my nurse and tell her that I disagreed with the care she was providing, demanding that more needed to be done for this patient.
- Ask the charge nurse to assess the quality of care that my patient was getting compared to what he needed to be receiving.

Evaluating a Good Outcome: How Do I Define Success?

- Patient receives a higher quality of care.
- The nurse is not insulted by hearing feedback about the care she is providing.
- By addressing the problem earlier in the process, my frustrations do not interfere with the rest of my day.
- The patient is not discriminated against and neglected based on his inability to communicate and his decreased level of consciousness.

Personal Learning: Here's to the Future!

Happy, sad outcome. Although this patient was not verbally communicating, I held his hand, talked to him, and felt that he was able to recognize my caring presence. After our lunch break, I verbalized my frustration about the lack of care to my clinical instructor and I asked if she would come meet him and help me provide the care I saw was due. My clinical instructor agreed that this patient was in need of more care. She, unlike my nurse, did not speak about his condition in front of him as though he could not hear. My instructor also made sure we did everything possible so that this patient was as comfortable as possible. She talked to him as though he was able to hear. In addition, my instructor called in the charge nurse to point out the lack of care this patient had been receiving, wanting to ensure that his future level of care was much improved. My instructor and the charge nurse, in a professional, nondegrading way, expressed to the assigned nurse that this patient needed a higher quality of care due to his critical condition. Having my teacher agree with my concerns for this patient and address the nurse and change nurse made me feel much better about the care my patient would then receive. I later told my teacher that I was frustrated because I felt all the nurse was concerned about was "giving all the medications, and signing off on the right pages"

when in fact talking to this patient, holding his hand, and making him more comfortable was definitely more important. Two days later the patient died. I was sad but so honored to have been able to care for him and hold his hand in his last days.

Although I think I should have gone to my clinical instructor earlier in the day to explain the problem I was having, I think telling her was the right decision. My instructor took my concerns seriously and first helped me care for the patient, then went straight to the charge nurse to ensure proper skin and wound care for the patient. Lastly, she was able to address the nurse without insulting her to make sure we were all on the same page about the care this patient needed but had not been getting. By speaking up, I was able to leave my clinical assignment feeling positive about my actions and advocating for this patient. I still left frustrated with how he had been cared for and realized that all too often as care providers we get too involved in the routine of charting, distributing medications, etc., and can forget how important some simple measures are, such as offering a gentle touch, positioning, providing hygiene and wound care to the best of our ability, and just spending time with them.

Reflection

How do you think you would respond in a similar situation? Why? What does this tell you about yourself and about the adequacy of your skills for professional practice? What factors might have affected the assigned nurse's response to the patient? Would the student have been affected by any of these same factors? Explain. What evidence from the scenario would lead you to suspect that the patient is at risk for impaired skin integrity? What preventive measures might be appropriate? Can you think of other ways to respond? What other skills (cognitive, interpersonal, technical,

ethical/legal) would you need to respond well in this situation? What, if any, ethical and legal principles were demonstrated by the nursing student's actions? Do you agree with the criteria to evaluate a successful outcome? Did the nursing student validate the rationale for the outcome? Would other criteria be appropriate to include? If so, explain.

Carrie Staines, Georgetown University

TABLE 38-1 **Types of Wounds**

Type	Cause
Incision	Cutting or sharp instrument; wound edges in close approximation and aligned
Contusion	Blunt instrument, usually disrupting skin surface; possible resultant bruising
Abrasion	Rubbing or scraping epidermal layers of skin; top layer of skin abraded
Laceration	Tearing of skin and tissue with blunt or irregular instrument; tissue not aligned, often with loose flaps of skin and tissue
Puncture	Pointed instrument puncturing the skin; intentional (such as venipuncture) or accidental
Penetrating	Foreign object entering the skin at high velocity; fragments possibly scattering throughout tissues
Avulsion	Tearing a structure from normal anatomic position; possible damage to blood vessels, nerves, and other structures
Microbial	Secretion of exotoxins or release of endotoxins by living organisms
Chemical	Toxic agents such as drugs, acids, alcohols, metals, and substances released from cellular necrosis
Thermal	High or low temperatures; cellular necrosis as a possible result
Irradiation	Ultraviolet light or radiation exposure

Adapted from: Bullock, B. (1996). *Pathophysiology: Adaptations and alterations in function.* (4th ed.). Philadelphia: Lippincott. Table 15-1, p. 298.

Phases of Wound Healing

Wound healing that ends in the formation of scar tissue involves processes that fill in, cover or seal (**epithelialization**), and shrink the wound (contraction). Wound closure and healing occur by primary intention or secondary intention, depending on the amount of tissue that is lost. Intentional wounds with minimal tissue loss, such as those made by a surgical incision with sutured approximated edges, usually heal by primary intention. Large or open wounds, such as from burns or major trauma, which require more tissue replacement and are often contaminated, commonly heal by secondary intention. If a wound that is healing by first intention becomes infected, it will heal by secondary intention. Wounds that heal by secondary intention take longer to heal and form more scar tissue (Porth, 2002). Connective tissue healing and repair follow the same phases in healing, although differences occur in the length of time required for each phase and in the extent of granulation tissue formed. The phases are:

- inflammatory phase
- proliferative phase
- remodeling phase

Inflammatory Phase

The inflammatory phase begins at the time of injury and prepares the wound for healing. The two major physiologic activities are hemostasis (blood clotting) and the vascular and cellular phase of inflammation.

Immediately after the injury, involved blood vessels constrict and blood clotting begins through platelet activation and clustering. After only a brief period of constriction, these same blood vessels dilate and capillary permeability increases, to allow plasma and blood components to leak out into the area that is injured, forming a liquid called **exudate.** The accumulation of exudate causes swelling and pain. Increased perfusion results in heat and redness. If the wound is small, the clot loses fluid and a hard scab is formed to protect the injury.

The inflammatory cellular phase follows, with movement of white blood cells (leukocytes) to the wound. Neutrophils or polymorphonuclear cells arrive first to ingest bacteria and cellular debris; they are active for 3 or 4 days. About 24 hours after the injury, macrophages (a larger phagocytic cell) enter the wound area and remain for an extended period. Macrophages are essential to the healing process: they not only ingest debris but also release growth factors that are necessary for the growth of epithelial cells and new blood vessels and for attracting fibroblasts that help to fill in the wound, which is necessary for the next stage of healing. During the inflammatory phase, the patient has a generalized body response, including a mildly elevated temperature, leukocytosis, and generalized malaise.

Proliferative Phase

The proliferative phase begins within 2 to 3 days of the injury, possibly lasting up to 2 to 3 weeks in wounds healing by first intention. New tissue is built to fill the wound space, primarily through the action of fibroblasts. Fibroblasts are connective tissue cells that synthesize and secrete collagen and produce specialized growth factors responsible for inducing blood vessel formation as well as increasing the number and movement of endothelial cells. Capillaries grow across the wound, bringing oxygen and nutrients required for continued healing. Fibroblasts form fibrin that stretches through the clot. A thin layer of epithelial cells forms across the wound, and blood flow across the wound is reinstituted. The new tissue, called **granulation tissue,** forms the foundation for scar tissue development. It is highly vascular, red, and bleeds easily. In wounds that heal by first intention, epidermal cells seal the wound within 24 to 48 hours.

Collagen synthesis and accumulation continue, peaking in 5 to 7 days. Depending on the size of the wound, collagen deposit continues for several weeks or even years. By the end of the second week following the injury, the majority of white blood cells have left the wound area, and the wound is lighter in color. The systemic symptoms now typically disappear. During this phase, adequate nutrition and oxygenation, as well as prevention of strain on the suture line, are important patient care considerations.

Remodeling Phase

The final stage of healing begins about 3 weeks after the injury, possibly continuing for as long as 6 months if the wound is

BOX 38-1 Principles of Wound Healing

- Intact skin is the first line of defense against microorganisms. A break in the integrity of the skin increases the risk for infection. Surgical asepsis is used in caring for a wound to minimize the possibility of pathogens entering the site. Careful hand hygiene before caring for a wound is probably the single most effective method for preventing wound infections.
- The body responds systemically to trauma in any of its parts. For example, a surgical incision can cause a variety of systemic reactions, including increased body temperature, increased heart and respiratory rates, anorexia or nausea and vomiting, musculoskeletal tension, and hormonal changes.
- An adequate blood supply is essential for the body's normal response to any injury. The blood transports increased numbers of leukocytes, erythrocytes, and platelets to the site of injury. Antibodies are carried by the plasma. Increased circulation to the injured part removes toxins and debris and provides nutrients and oxygen. Areas of the body with a good blood supply, such as the head and the neck, heal faster than areas in which the blood supply is not as great, such as the distal part of an extremity.
- Normal healing is promoted when the wound is free of foreign material, such as excessive exudate, dead or damaged tissue cells, pathogenic organisms, or embedded fragments of bone, metal, glass, or other substances. In some situations, a collection of pus or foreign body is walled off and healing occurs around it to form an abscess.

- The ability to handle altered skin integrity depends on the extent of the damage and the person's general state of health. The capacity to deal adequately with a wound is limited when a healthy person sustains a massive injury, when the patient has a chronic illness or a depressed immune system, or when the patient is very young or very old.
- The body's response to a wound is more effective if proper nutrition has been maintained.
  - Undernourished patients are at greater risk for developing a wound infection because they have difficulty mounting their cell-mediated defense system associated with T-lymphocyte activity, and some leukocytic functions are diminished in the presence of protein deficiency.
  - Although the role of fatty acids in wound healing is not well understood, certain quantities of glucose are necessary to meet the energy requirements for wound healing.
  - Various vitamins, minerals, and trace elements are also needed for efficient wound healing. Vitamin A is necessary for collagen synthesis and epithelialization. Vitamin B complex serves as a cofactor of enzyme reactions needed for wound healing. Vitamin C is needed for collagen synthesis, capillary formation, and resistance to infection. Vitamin K is needed for the synthesis of prothrombin. Zinc, copper, and iron assist in collagen synthesis. Manganese serves as an enzyme activator.

large. Collagen that was haphazardly deposited in the wound is remodeled, making the healed wound stronger and more like adjacent tissue. New collagen continues to be deposited, which compresses the blood vessels in the healing wound, so that the **scar** (an avascular collagen tissue that does not sweat, grow hair, or tan in sunlight) eventually becomes a flat, thin, white line. Wounds that heal by secondary intention take longer to remodel and form a scar smaller than the original wound; if over a joint or other body structure, the scar may limit movement and cause disability.

> *Recall Sam Bentz, the 56-year-old man admitted for treatment of a bone infection. The nurse would apply the knowledge about the phases of wound healing when reviewing this patient's past history (the wounds he developed on his last admission). In addition, this knowledge would help form the basis for the patient's plan of care should another wound occur during this hospitalization.*

Factors Affecting Wound Healing

Wound healing is affected by a variety of factors. These factors include age, circulation to and oxygenation of tissues, nutritional status, condition of the wound, and the patient's overall health.

Age

Children and healthy adults heal more rapidly than older adults, in whom physiologic changes caused by aging result in diminished fibroblastic activity and circulation. Older adults are more likely to have one or more chronic illnesses, with pathologic changes that impede the healing process. See the accompanying box, Focus on the Older Adult, for other age-related factors affecting wound healing.

Circulation and Oxygenation

Adequate blood flow to deliver nutrients and oxygen and to remove local toxins, bacteria, and other debris is essential for wound healing. Certain physical conditions, because of their effect on circulation and oxygenation, can affect wound healing.

> *Recall Lucius Everly, the patient described in Reflective Practice. The nurse's ability to integrate knowledge of the effects of diabetes on circulation would be important in planning measures to ensure adequate circulation to his extremities as a means to prevent skin breakdown.*

Large amounts of subcutaneous and tissue fat (which has fewer blood vessels) in people who are obese may slow wound healing because fatty tissue is more difficult to suture, is more prone to infection, and takes longer to heal.

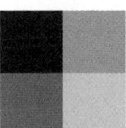

Focus on the Older Adult
Age-Related Factors Affecting Wound Healing

Age-Related Changes	Nursing Interventions
• Skin loses turgor and is more fragile.	• Maintain hydration with intravenous fluids as prescribed. • Maintain record of intake and output. • Use caution when removing tape.
• Decreased secretion of enzymes and absorption of nutrients and minerals may increase risk for delayed wound healing.	• Maintain intake of adequate kilocalories with oral, enteral, or parenteral feedings. • Ensure diet is high in protein, vitamin A, vitamin C, and trace elements (zinc and copper). • Monitor lab results such as serum albumin, total protein.
Risk of infection increases from: • Slower inflammatory response • Reduced antibody production and endocrine system function • Increased incidence of chronic illnesses such as diabetes mellitus and cardiovascular disease that compromise circulation and tissue oxygenation	• Maintain careful hand hygiene and surgical asepsis with dressing changes and care of tubes or drains. • Take and record vital signs, noting and reporting increased temperature. • Monitor wound for manifestations of infection. • Administer medications as prescribed. • Administer supplemental oxygen as prescribed.

Remember Sam Bentz, the middle-aged patient with a bone infection described at the beginning of the chapter. The nurse would incorporate an understanding of this patient's past history and large size to develop an appropriate plan of care to prevent future occurrences of skin breakdown.

Circulation may be impaired in older adults and in people with peripheral vascular disorders, cardiovascular disorders, hypertension, or diabetes mellitus. Oxygenation of tissues is decreased in people with anemia or chronic respiratory disorders and in those who smoke.

Nutritional Status

Wound healing requires adequate proteins, carbohydrates, fats, vitamins, and minerals. Calories and protein are necessary to rebuild cells and tissues. Vitamins A and C are essential for re-epithelialization and collagen synthesis. Zinc plays a role in proliferation of cells. Fluids are necessary for optimal function of cells. All phases of the wound healing process are slowed or inadequate in the patient with poor nutritional status and fluid balance. Nutrition is further discussed in Chapter 42.

Wound Condition

The condition of the wound also affects how quickly and effectively it heals. For example, large, contaminated, infected wounds or wounds that retain foreign bodies heal slowly. Sutures are needed to close surgical wounds. However, sutures also act as foreign bodies, so they are removed as soon as possible.

Health Status

Patients who are taking corticosteroid drugs or require postoperative radiation therapy are at high risk for delayed healing and wound complications. Corticosteroids decrease the inflammatory process, which may delay healing. Radiation depresses bone marrow function, resulting in decreased leukocytes and an increased risk of infection. The presence of a chronic illness (such as cardiovascular disease or diabetes mellitus) or impaired immune function can impair wound healing.

Wound Complications

Wound complications include infection, hemorrhage, dehiscence, and evisceration. These complications increase the risk for generalized illness and death, lengthen the patient's need for healthcare interventions, and add to healthcare costs.

Infection

Bacteria can invade a wound at the time of trauma, during surgery, or at any time after the initial wound occurs. A contaminated wound is more likely to become infected than one that is not contaminated. Additionally, the risk of infection is increased in a surgical wound created during a procedure involving the intestines because the risk for contamination with fecal material is high. Symptoms of wound infection usually become apparent within 2 to 7 days after the injury or surgery; often, the patient is at home. Symptoms of infection include purulent drainage; increased drainage, pain, redness, and swelling in and around the wound; increased body temperature; and increased white blood cell count. Nursing care of infected wounds is discussed later in the chapter.

Hemorrhage

Hemorrhage may occur from a slipped suture, a dislodged clot from stress at the suture line or operative site, infection, or the erosion of a blood vessel by a foreign body (such as a drain). The dressing (and the wound under the dressing if possible) must be checked frequently during the first 48 hours after surgery and no less than every 8 hours thereafter. If excessive bleeding does occur, additional sterile pressure dressings or packing may be necessary, fluid replacement is probably necessary, and surgical intervention may be required. See Chapter 30 for more information about hemorrhage.

Dehiscence and Evisceration

Dehiscence and evisceration (Fig. 38-1) are the most serious postoperative wound complications. **Dehiscence** is the partial or total disruption of wound layers. **Evisceration** is the protrusion of viscera through the incisional area. Patients at greater risk for these complications include those who are obese or malnourished, have infected wounds, or experience excessive coughing, vomiting, or straining. An increase in the flow of serosanguineous fluid from the wound between postoperative days 4 and 5 is a sign of an impending dehiscence. The patient may say that "something has suddenly given way." If dehiscence or evisceration occurs, cover the wound area with sterile towels soaked in sterile 0.9% sodium chloride solution and notify the physician immediately. Both these situations are emergencies that require prompt surgical repair.

Fistula Formation

A **fistula** is an abnormal passage from an internal organ to the skin or from one internal organ to another. Fistulas may be purposefully created (for example, an arteriovenous fistula is created surgically to provide circulatory access for kidney dialysis). However, postoperative fistula formation is most often the result of delayed healing, commonly manifested by drainage from an opening in the skin or surgical site. The pres-

ence of a fistula increases the risk for infection, fluid and electrolyte imbalances, and skin breakdown.

Psychological Effects of Wounds

Because the skin is a sensory organ and plays a major role in communication with others and self-image, wounds require adaptation in the emotional as well as the physical dimension. Although stress and adaptation vary greatly among individuals, actual and potential emotional stressors are common in all patients with wounds. These stressors include pain, anxiety, fear, and changes in body image.

Pain

Pain is part of almost any trauma, from a small cut on the finger to a large incision made during abdominal surgery. Although pain can be considered a physical complication, it also has a large psychological component. Pain from wounds is often increased by activities such as ambulating, coughing, moving in bed, and dressing changes. The actual pain might be worsened by the patient's apprehension about such activities. Nursing interventions to reduce pain can greatly reduce emotional stress. (See Chap. 41 for a more in-depth discussion of pain.)

> Remember Abigail Karcher, the 5-week-old small-for-gestational-age infant described at the beginning of the chapter. Assessment of pain in this patient is crucial because the patient cannot verbalize complaints of pain. The nurse would need to assess the infant closely for behavioral manifestations that would suggest pain.

Anxiety and Fear

Anxiety and fear are common responses to a wound. Patients are apprehensive about the possibility of the wound opening, how much privacy will be lost as the wound is being cared for, and how they and others will react to the appearance and smell of the wound. When caring for patients with wounds, demonstrating acceptance and empathy, encouraging the expression of feelings, answering questions accurately and honestly, and avoiding excessive exposure of body parts when giving wound care are essential.

Changes in Body Image

Body image reflects a person's view of himself or herself as a whole entity. When the skin and tissues are traumatized, that image is changed, requiring the person to adapt and reformulate the concept of self. Wounds and scars that are visible to others, especially on the face, can result in feelings of conspicuousness, ugliness, and diminished self-worth. Large scars, such as from removal of a breast or from creation of a colostomy opening, can seriously affect the person's sexuality, social relationships, and self-concept. (See Focused Critical Thinking Guide 38-1: Wound Care for an example.) Referral to support groups or counselors may be necessary to facilitate coping and acceptance of changes in body structure or function. See Chapter 31 for more information about self-concept.

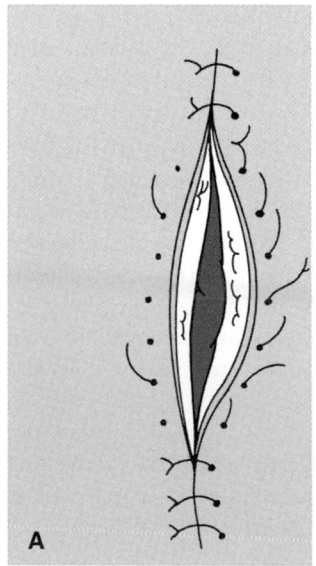
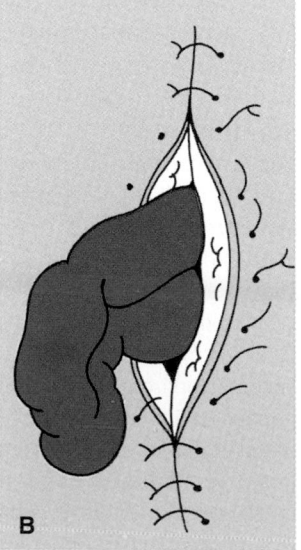

FIGURE 38-1 Wound complications. (**A**) Dehiscence. (**B**) Evisceration.

Focused Critical Thinking Guide 38-1

Wound Care: Promoting Acceptance of Changes in Body Image

During both clinical days in one week you (a female student) have been assigned to care for a middle-aged woman who has had a breast removed because of cancer. The patient, Mrs. Nola, is an attractive woman who is usually cheerful and eager to get better and return home. However, on both days she turned her head away and would not look at the incision when her dressing was changed. She tells you that she "just can't stand to look at herself." Her husband has left the room during the dressing changes after telling you that "it makes me sick to see what happened to my wife." Mrs. Nola is to be discharged to her home the next day and needs to learn how to provide self-care for her wound. What do you do?

1. Identify Goal of Thinking
Determine the most effective way of ensuring wound care and at the same time assisting Mrs. Nola in accepting her altered self-image.

2. Assess Adequacy of Knowledge
Pertinent circumstances: The diagnosis of cancer was made only one day before the surgical removal of the breast. The patient is to be discharged to her home the next day. The wound from her mastectomy has not completely healed and will require dressing changes for another 3 or 4 days. Mrs. Nola has had a disfiguring surgery and is coping with not only a change in body image but also the diagnosis of cancer. She has never before been seriously ill nor had surgery. She has a strong, loving relationship with her husband, but he is unable to deal with the physical disfigurement at this time.

Prerequisite knowledge: Before you decide what to do in this situation, you need to know at what level Mrs. Nola is in coping with the diagnosis of cancer. If she is still in denial about the disease, it is likely that she is also denying the surgical procedure and the changes in her body. You will need to review responses to the diagnosis of cancer as well as the stages of grief and loss. You will have to learn what her sources of support are and how she can best access and use them. You will need to assess how best to help her achieve wound care in the face of her continued refusal even to look at the wound.

Room for error: If she is forced to look at the wound or made to feel inadequate because of her inability to do so,

she will feel threatened and most likely will become angry in response to the perceived threat.

Time constraints: Some decision about wound care must be made before her discharge the next day.

3. Address Potential Problems
There are several potential obstacles to critical thinking in this situation. As a student, you want to exhibit safe, knowledgeable care, and the importance of teaching for home care has been an emphasis in this course. As a woman, you have a sense of what the loss of a breast must mean. Having had a family member die of cancer, you find yourself wanting to do everything for Mrs. Nola. As a novice in nursing, you find it difficult to handle these emotional components of patient care and find yourself wanting to scold both the patient and her husband for being so silly about something as simple as a dressing.

4. Consult Helpful Resources
You must first understand the loss and grief Mrs. Nola is experiencing, and you must then relate that to her response to self-care of the wound. Your best source of information about her coping methods and sources of personal strength is Mrs. Nola herself. You also discuss the most effective way of providing wound care at home with your instructor and the case manager for Mrs. Nola.

5. Critique Judgment/Decision
After talking to Mrs. Nola, your instructor, and the case manager, you mutually agree that Mrs. Nola cannot be hurried into acceptance of her medical diagnosis or her body changes. The case manager consults with Mrs. Nola's physician, who writes an order for a home health nurse to visit for the next 4 days and complete the dressing change. After talking with Mrs. Nola, you identify that she is still very much in denial. You discuss with her the possibility of having a visitor from "Reach to Recovery," a support group for women with breast cancer who have had a mastectomy. Mrs. Nola tells you that she thinks she would like to talk to someone with the same problem, and you call a referral for her. When you tell Mrs. Nola that a home health nurse will be visiting her for the first few days at home to change her dressing, tears come into her eyes. She says "I am so scared, I just don't know what to do." You realize that insisting that Mrs. Nola do her own dressing would have been extremely stressful for her, and that you would have considered the wound as more important than the patient. When you share the situation in postconference, your clinical group supports your decision.

THE NURSING PROCESS FOR WOUNDS

Assessing

Wound assessment involves inspection (sight and smell) and palpation for appearance, drainage, and pain. Included in the

assessment are sutures, any drains or tubes, and manifestations of complications.

Appearance
Wounds are assessed for the approximation of wound edges, color of the wound and surrounding area, drains or tubes, staples or sutures, and signs of dehiscence or evisceration. The

edges of a healthy healing surgical wound appear clean and well approximated, with a crust along the wound edges. Initially, the edges are reddened and slightly swollen. After approximately 1 week, the skin is closer to normal in appearance, with wound edges healing together. The skin surrounding the wound may at first be bruised, but this too returns to normal as blood is reabsorbed.

When infection is present, the wound is swollen and deep red. It feels hot on palpation, and drainage is increased and possibly purulent. A foul odor also may be noted. If dehiscence is impending or present, the wound edges are separated.

Drainage

The inflammatory response results in the formation of exudate, which then drains from the wound. The exudate is composed of fluid and cells that escape from blood vessels and are deposited in or on tissue surfaces. This exudate is called wound drainage and is described as serous, sanguineous, or, if infected, purulent (Box 38-2). Drains may be inserted in or near a wound to promote drainage, thereby reducing the risk of abscess formation and promoting wound healing. Various types of drains are described in Table 38-2.

The amount, color, odor, and consistency of wound drainage are assessed. The amount and color depend on the wound location and size. Typically, larger wounds have more drainage than smaller wounds. Drainage can be assessed on the wound, on the dressings, in drainage bottles or reservoirs, or, depending on the location of the wound and the amount of drainage, under the patient.

Pain

If the patient has increased or constant pain from the wound, further assessments are necessary. Pain, especially when accompanied by an increased or purulent flow of drainage, may indicate delayed healing or an infection. Incisional pain is usually most severe for the first 2 to 3 days and then progressively diminishes.

BOX 38-2 Types of Wound Drainage

- Serous drainage is composed primarily of the clear, serous portion of the blood and from serous membranes. Serous drainage is clear and watery.
- Sanguineous drainage consists of large numbers of red blood cells and looks like blood. Bright-red sanguineous drainage is indicative of fresh bleeding, whereas darker drainage indicates older bleeding. Surgical wounds most commonly have a mixture of serum and red blood cells, called serosanguineous drainage.
- Purulent drainage is made up of white blood cells, liquefied dead tissue debris, and both dead and live bacteria. Purulent drainage is thick, often has a musty or foul odor, and varies in color (such as dark yellow or green), depending on the causative organism.

TABLE 38-2 Common Types of Drains

Type	Purpose	Example
Penrose	Provides sinus tract	After incision and drainage of abscess, in abdominal surgery
T-tube	For bile drainage	After gallbladder surgery
Jackson-Pratt	Decrease dead space by collecting drainage	After breast removal, abdominal surgery
Hemovac	Decrease dead space by collecting drainage	After abdominal, orthopedic surgery
Gauze, iodoform gauze, NuGauze	Allow healing from base of wound	Infected wounds, after removal of hemorrhoids

Sutures and Staples

Skin sutures, which may be black silk, synthetic material, fine wire, or metal skin clips, and metal staples are used to hold tissue and skin together. Retention sutures are used to provide extra support for patients who are obese and for wounds with an increased risk for dehiscence (Fig. 38-2).

Sutures are removed when the wound has developed enough tensile strength to hold the wound edges together during healing. This stage varies from patient to patient, depending on age, nutritional status, and wound location. Silk sutures typically are removed within 6 to 8 days to prevent suture marks, even though collagen formation and remodeling take a total of at least 21 days. This means the scar may still stretch and widen after the silk sutures have been removed. Special subcutaneous techniques have been developed to minimize this problem. In addition, small adhesive wound-closure strips (Steri-Strips) may be applied directly to the wound to help hold it together. Unless otherwise directed, Steri-Strips are not removed during wound care.

Sutures are removed with a suture removal set; staples are removed with a special staple remover. The steps in removing sutures and staples are summarized in the accompanying Guidelines for Nursing Care 38-1. After the removal of skin sutures, Steri-Strips are sometimes applied across the healing wound to give additional support as it continues to heal.

Related Assessments

In addition to assessments of the wound, evaluate the patient's general condition and laboratory test results. Be alert for signs and symptoms of infection, which may cause generalized malaise, increased pain, anorexia, and an elevated body temperature and pulse rate. Laboratory data indicating

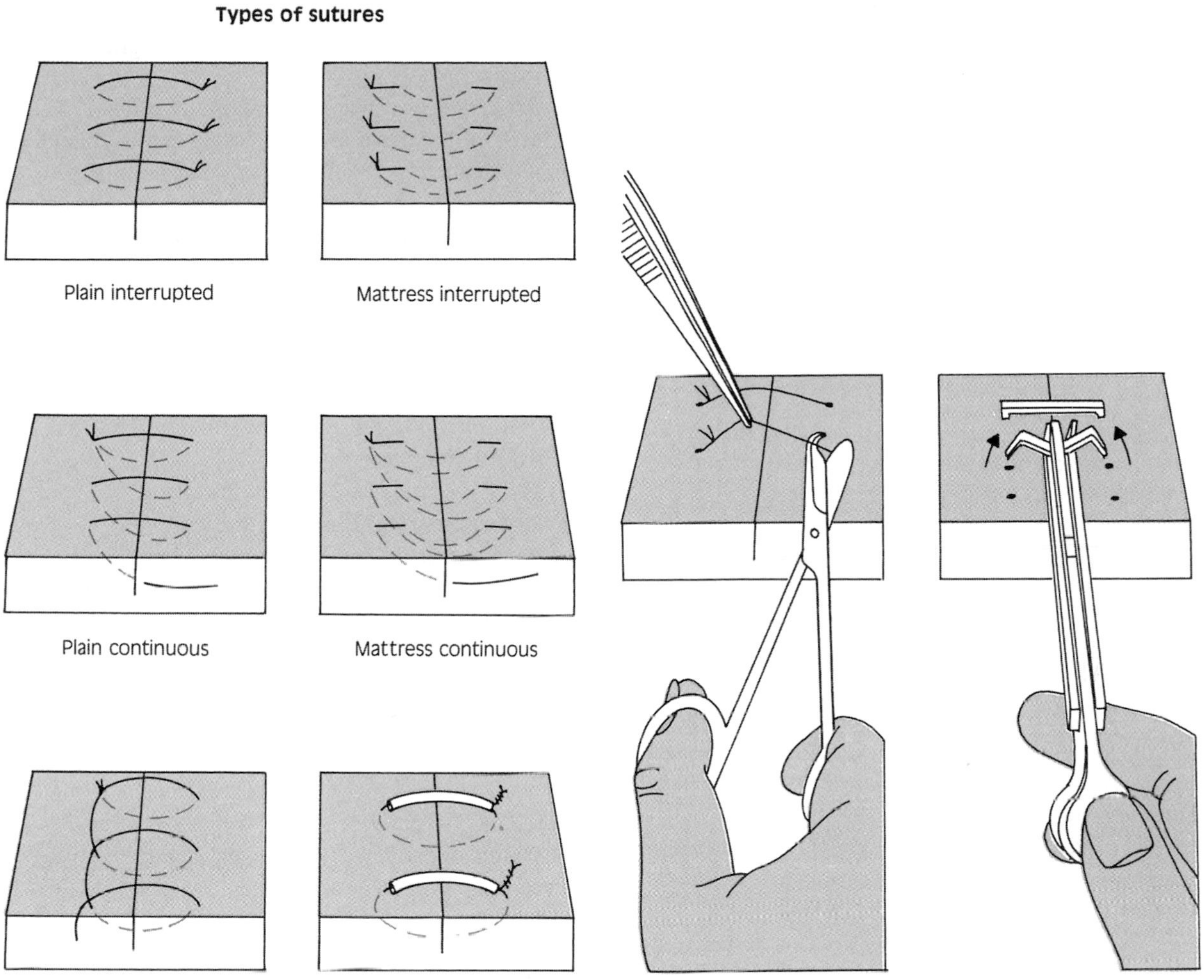

Types of sutures

Plain interrupted   Mattress interrupted

Plain continuous   Mattress continuous

Blanket continuous   Retention   Removing interrupted sutures   Removing staples

FIGURE 38-2 Types of sutures and techniques for removing sutures and staples.

an infection include an elevated white blood cell count and, if a wound culture has been done, a causative organism.

Diagnosing

The patient with a wound is at risk for or has several alterations in health that are supported by assessment. One of the most appropriate nursing diagnoses is Impaired Skin Integrity, defined as a state in which an individual has altered epidermis or dermis (NANDA, 2002). NANDA nursing diagnoses related to wounds are listed in the accompanying Examples of NANDA Nursing Diagnoses: Patient With a Wound.

For patients who request information about wound care at home, the following wellness diagnosis may be appropriate: Readiness for Enhanced Knowledge: Wound Care.

Outcome Identification and Planning

The plan of care is directed toward facilitating the patient's return to health by providing interventions that facilitate

wound healing, reduce the risk for complications, and promote psychosocial adaptation. The following are examples of appropriate outcomes. The patient will:

- Remain free of signs and symptoms of infection
- Verbalize that the pain management regimen relieves pain to an acceptable level
- Be discharged to home within established parameters
- Demonstrate appropriate wound care measures before discharge
- Verbalize understanding of signs and symptoms to report and necessary follow-up care

Implementing

When caring for the patient with a wound, nursing interventions focus on preventing infection and promoting wound healing; preventing further injury or alteration in skin integrity; promoting physical and emotional comfort; and facilitating coping. The accompanying box, Examples of Nursing Interventions Classification, summarizes appropriate interventions for incision site care.

Guidelines for Nursing Care 38-1
Removing Staples and Sutures

The removal of staples or sutures may be done by the physician or by the nurse with a physician's order. Always follow agency protocol; keep in mind these general guidelines:

- Use sterile techniques, following recommended CDC guidelines for care of wounds.
- Perform hand hygiene before and after the procedure.
- Explain the procedure to the patient. Describe the sensation that will be experienced as a pulling or slightly uncomfortable experience.
- Use proper technique to remove and dispose of old dressings.
- Clean the incision from the center of the wound outward, according to agency policy and procedure for type of agent.
- Remove every other suture or staple to be sure wound edges are healed; if they are, remove remaining sutures or staples as ordered.
- Remove or reapply dressing, depending on physician preference and agency policy.
- Remember that some physicians order Steri-Strip application to the healed wound after removal of staples or sutures to give additional support to the wound as it continues to heal. Follow agency protocol and physician preference for placement of these tapes.

Specifics for Suture Removal
1. Use a sterile suture removal kit.
2. Using the sterile forceps, grasp the knot of the first suture and gently lift the knot.
3. Using the sterile scissors, cut one side of the suture below the knot close to the skin.
4. Grasp the knot with the forceps and pull the cut suture through the skin (be sure to pull through the healed wound only the portion of the suture that has been inside the tissue).

Specifics for Staple Removal
1. As directed on the package, gently position the sterile staple remover under the staple to be removed.
2. Firmly close the staple remover to straighten the staple ends (do not lift upward while disengaging staple ends).
3. Carefully lift upward with the closed staple remover to remove the staple from the incision line. It may be necessary to remove one end of the staple and then the other if it does not easily lift out.

Changing Dressings

The goal of wound care is to promote tissue repair and regeneration so that skin integrity is restored. The two methods of caring for wounds are the closed method, in which a **dressing** is used as a protective cover over the wound, and the open method, in which no dressing is used. A moist environment is best for wound healing. When a dressing is placed over a wound, the wound fluid keeps the surface of the wound moist. As a result, epidermal cells migrate more rapidly, maximizing healing.

Most dressings, especially those used for surgical wounds, consist of three layers. The dressing applied directly over the wound, called the contact layer, allows drainage to pass into the middle layer. This contact layer should be able to be removed without causing further tissue damage. The middle layer absorbs the drainage, and the outer layer keeps the two inner layers in place. Many different types of dressings are available, but all essentially have the same purposes:

- Provide physical, psychological, and aesthetic comfort
- Remove necrotic tissue
- Prevent, eliminate, or control infection
- Absorb drainage
- Maintain a moist wound environment
- Protect the wound from further injury
- Protect the skin surrounding the wound

Dressings can rub or stick to the wound, causing further superficial injury. Dressings can also create a warm, damp, and dark environment conducive to the growth of organisms and subsequent potential development of an infection. Most wounds are covered with a dressing, and nurses are responsible for most dressing changes.

Dressing Supplies

The items needed for a dressing change may be gathered individually or may be packaged in a sterile dressing tray, depending on the healthcare setting. Wound care in the home may depend on the supplies provided by the patient or family.

The supplies needed vary with the type, location, and amount of wound drainage; the nursing plan of care identifies the specifics about each patient's dressing procedure and supplies. Materials and supplies include cleaning agents, dressing materials, and materials used to secure the dressing and support the wound.

Cleaning Agents

Although various antiseptic cleaning agents could be used to clean a wound, sterile 0.9% sodium chloride solution is usually the agent of choice. Some authorities question the use of any agent other than 0.9% sodium chloride solution because of their possible caustic effect on skin, tissues, and granulation tissue.

Types of Dressings

The number and types of dressings used depend on the location and size of the wound as well as the amount and type of drainage. The incision line is often covered with sterile petrolatum gauze or a special gauze called Telfa. Telfa's shiny outer surface is applied to the wound and allows drainage to pass through and be absorbed by the center absorbent layer. Both these protective dressings prevent outer dressings from adhering to the wound and causing further injury when removed.

Examples of NANDA Nursing Diagnoses | **Patient with a Wound**

Nursing Diagnoses	Related Factors	Sample Defining Characteristics
Impaired Skin Integrity	Any condition that alters the dermis and/or epidermis, such as a surgical incision or traumatic wound	• Presence of intentional or unintentional wound
Risk for Infection	Any condition that interferes with normal inflammatory healing process or provides an entry for infectious agents	Risk factors: • Disruption in skin integrity • Contaminated wounds • Chronic wounds • Extremes of age • Obesity or malnutrition • Presence of drains, tubes, or catheters • Immunosuppression
Acute Pain	Any condition that causes actual tissue damage, including intentional and unintentional wounds	• Presence of wound • "On a 1-to-10 scale, my pain is 9." • Positioning or guarding self or body part to avoid pain • "I hurt so much that I can't sleep or eat." • Diaphoresis, changes in vital signs, dilated pupils • Moaning, sighing, crying
Disturbed Body Image	Any condition that causes confusion in the mental image of oneself, such as a surgical or traumatic wound	• "I just don't feel like I'm the same person I used to be." • "I'll never be able to do my job if this arm doesn't work." • Refusal to look at incision or area of surgical treatment • Actual change in one's body from surgery or trauma • Actual missing body part

Gauze dressings are commonly used to cover wounds. These dressings come in various sizes (2 × 2 inches, 4 × 4 inches, and 4 × 8 inches) and are commercially packaged as single units or in packs. Special gauze dressings (eg, Sof-Wick) are precut halfway to fit around drains or tubes. Larger dressings (8 × 10 bandages, abdominal pads [ABDs], Surgi-Pads) are placed over the smaller gauze dressings and absorb drainage and protect the wound from contamination or injury.

Transparent dressings (eg, Op-Site) are applied directly over a small wound or tube. These dressings are occlusive, decreasing the possibility of contamination, while allowing visualization of the wound. This type of dressing is often used over intravenous sites, subclavian catheter insertion sites, and noninfected healing wounds.

Think back to Abigail Karcher, the infant described in the beginning of the chapter. The nurse most likely would use a transparent dressing on the infant's intravenous sites, thereby allowing frequent assessment of the site.

Tape
Tape comes in a wide variety of sizes and types, ranging in width from 1 to 4 inches (1-inch-wide tape is the most commonly used). Table 38-3 summarizes the types and purposes of different tapes.

Cleaning a Wound and Applying a Clean Dressing
Prepare the patient for the dressing change before starting the procedure by explaining what will be done. Provide privacy by properly screening the patient. Then help the patient into a position that is comfortable and also convenient for changing the dressing. Expose only the area necessary to perform the wound care while maintaining proper draping.

Using appropriate aseptic techniques when changing the dressing is crucial. Be especially vigilant in performing hand hygiene thoroughly before and after changing dressings and in adhering to standard precautions. Among the most common causes of nosocomial infections is carelessness in practicing asepsis during dressing changes.

The wound is cleaned and the dressing changed as described in Skill 38-1. Dressing changes provide an excellent opportunity for teaching, especially important when the patient will be changing dressings at home. Encourage the patient to help as much as possible.

There is no standard frequency for how often dressings should be changed. It depends on the amount of drainage, the physician's preference, and the nature of the wound. It is customary for the physician to perform the first dressing change, usually within 24 to 48 hours after surgery. Thereafter, nurses change the dressings as needed or daily. The frequency of dressing changes is noted on the patient's plan of care.

Consider the care needed by Lucius Everly, the patient in the critical care unit. Although he has multiple needs, performing incisional wound care cannot be overlooked; otherwise, his risk of infection increases.

Remember, wound contamination occurs through a moist medium. Microorganisms can move from the external surface through the dressing to the wound if a dressing remains in place until it is saturated. Microorganisms can also move from the wound to the outer surface of a saturated dressing. For these reasons, always replace dressings with fresh dressings or reinforce the dressing with additional dressings before drainage causes saturation.

The sight of the wound may disturb a patient. Listen carefully to what the patient is saying and observe nonverbal communication as well. In some instances, the patient may not want to look at the wound, particularly with a wound that in-

TABLE 38-3 Types of Tape

Type	Purpose
Adhesive (can cause occlusion, allergy, skin maceration, shearing)	Used for strength, support, and economy • To secure dressings and splints • To strap joints to prevent athletic injuries • To immobilize or stabilize body parts • To provide pressure • To approximate wound edges
Paper, plastic, acetate	Increased comfort, decreased allergic and skin problems • To close small wounds • To secure dressings
Microfoam	Used for compression or pressure dressings

volves a change in normal body functions or appearance, such as a wound resulting from the removal of a breast, the amputation of an extremity, or the placement of a tube in a draining wound. With patience and emotional support, patients can learn to cope with and adapt to their wound in time.

Wound Drains, Tubes, and Catheters
A variety of drains, catheters, or tubes may be inserted into or near a wound when it is anticipated that a collection of fluid in a closed area would delay healing. After a surgical procedure, the physician places one end of the tube or drain in or near the area to be drained and passes the other end through the skin, either directly through the incision or through a separate opening called a stab wound. Drains and tubes may or may not be sutured in place.

Drains placed directly through the wound (eg, a Penrose drain, an example of an open drainage system consisting of a hollow open-ended tube) usually have a large safety pin attached to the outer portion to prevent the drain from slipping back into the incised area. These types of drains are not sutured in place (Fig. 38-3). Care is necessary to ensure that these drains are not dislodged during dressing changes. Sometimes the physician orders a Penrose drain that is to be shortened each day. To do so, grasp the end of the drain with sterile forceps, pull it out a short distance while using a twisting motion, and cut off the end of the drain with sterile scissors.

Closed drainage systems are used more often than incisional drains like the Penrose drain. Some studies show that the infection rate is cut nearly in half when drains are placed only when necessary and through a separate stab wound rather than in the incision itself. Closed drainage systems consist of a drainage tube that may be connected to an electrical suction device or have a portable built-in reservoir to maintain constant low suction (eg, a Jackson-Pratt drainage tube or a Hemovac; Fig. 38-4). These tubes are usually sutured

Cleaning a Wound and Applying a Sterile Dressing

EQUIPMENT

Sterile gloves
Gauze dressings or squares
Sterile dressing set or suture set
 (contains scissors and forceps)
Cleaning solution
Clean disposable gloves
Sterile basin (optional)

Sterile drape (optional)
Plastic bag for soiled dressings
Waterproof pad
Bath blanket
Tape or ties
Surgi-pads or ABDs

Additional dressing supplies as needed or
 ordered (antiseptic ointments, extra
 dressings)
Acetone or adhesive remover
 (optional)
Sterile normal saline (optional)

ACTION	RATIONALE
1. Explain the procedure to patient.	An explanation encourages patient cooperation and reduces apprehension.
2. Gather equipment.	Preparation provides for organized approach to task.
3. Perform hand hygiene.	Hand hygiene deters spread of microorganisms.
4. Check physician's order for dressing change. Note whether drain is present.	The order clarifies type of dressing.
5. Close door or curtain. Use bath blanket as needed when exposing area to be redressed. Position waterproof pad under patient if desired.	Doing so provides for privacy and warmth.
6. Assist patient to comfortable position that provides easy access to wound area.	Proper positioning provides for comfort.
7. Place opened, cuffed plastic bag near working area.	Soiled dressings may be placed in disposal bag without contaminating outside surfaces of bag.
8. Loosen tape on dressing. Use adhesive remover if necessary. If tape is soiled, don gloves.	It is easier to loosen tape before putting on gloves.
9. Don clean disposable gloves, and remove soiled dressings carefully in a clean to less clean direction. Do not reach over wound. Check position of drains before removing dressing. If dressing is adhering to skin surface, it may be moistened by pouring a small amount of sterile saline onto it. Keep soiled side of dressing away from patient's view.	Using clean gloves protects the nurse when handling contaminated dressings. Cautious removal of dressing is more comfortable for patient and ensures that drain is not removed if one is present. Sterile saline provides for easier removal of dressing.
10. Assess amount, type, and odor of drainage.	Wound healing process or presence of infection should be documented.
11. Discard dressings in plastic disposal bag. Pull off glove inside out and drop it in bag.	Proper disposal of dressings prevents spread of microorganisms by contaminated dressings.
12. Using aseptic technique, open sterile dressings and supplies on work area.	Supplies are within easy reach, and sterility is maintained.
13. Open sterile cleaning solution, and pour over gauze sponges in plastic container or over sponges placed in sterile basin.	Sterility of dressings and solution is maintained.
14. Don sterile gloves.	Using sterile gloves maintains surgical asepsis.
15. Clean wound or surgical incision. Use sterile forceps if desired. a. Clean from top to bottom or from center outward. b. Use one gauze square for each wipe, discarding each square by dropping into plastic bag. Do not touch bag with forceps. c. Clean around drain, if present, moving from center outward in a circular motion. Use one gauze square for each circular motion. d. Dry wound using gauze sponge and same motion. e. Apply antiseptic ointment if ordered.	Cleaning is done from least to most contaminated area. Previously cleaned area is not recontaminated. Movement in this manner ensures cleaning from least to most contaminated area. Moisture provides medium for growth of microorganisms. Growth of microorganisms may be retarded and healing process improved.

(continued)

SKILL
38-1   **Cleaning a Wound and Applying a Sterile Dressing** (continued)

ACTION	RATIONALE
16. Apply a layer of dry, sterile dressings over wound. Use sterile forceps if desired.	Primary dressing serves as a wick for drainage.
17. Use sterile scissors to cut sterile 4 × 4 gauze square to place under and around drain if one is present or use precut sterile gauze.	Drainage is absorbed, and surrounding skin area is protected.
18. Apply second gauze layer to wound site.	Additional layers provide for increased absorption of drainage
19. Place Surgi-pad or ABD dressing over wound as outermost layer.	Wound is protected from microorganisms in environment.
20. Remove gloves from inside out, and discard them in plastic waste bag. Apply tape or tie existing tapes to secure dressings.	Tape is easier to apply after gloves have been removed.

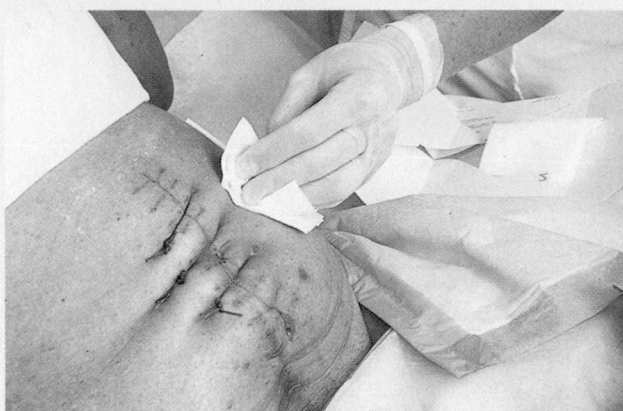

Action 15: Cleaning a surgical incision.

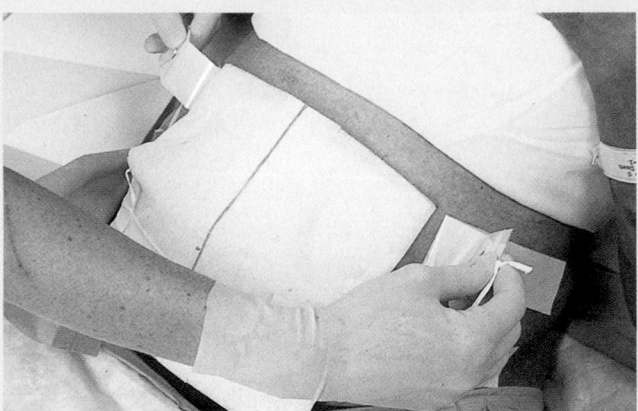

Action 19: Outer layer of dressing in place.

ACTION	RATIONALE
21. Perform hand hygiene. Remove all equipment, and make patient comfortable.	Hand hygiene prevents spread of microorganisms.
22. Check dressing and wound site every shift. Record dressing change and appearance of wound, and describe any drainage in chart.	Accurate documentation of procedure ensures continuity of care and provides information for future assessments.

Infant and Child   To keep a dressing intact or to prevent contamination of wound and supplies on an infant or young child, it may be necessary to restrain the child's hand. An old stocking or piece of stockinette may be used to encircle child's hand and then may be secured to the bed or crib with a tie or safety pin. Care must be taken not to compromise circulation to that extremity.

Home Care Considerations   Reinforce need for thorough handwashing before and after dressing change.

Have plastic bag available for safe disposal of soiled dressings and equipment.

Boil any nondisposable equipment (eg, forceps) for 10 minutes to ensure sterility after washing carefully in warm soapy water.

Inform patient about availability of disposable wound care supplies.

Special Considerations   Instruct patient that any break or interruption in the suture line may require immediate intervention and to notify the surgeon immediately. Instruct patient and family about significant changes that need to be reported to the nurse or physician.

Encourage splinting of wound during activity (coughing, sneezing, sudden movement, or change in position).

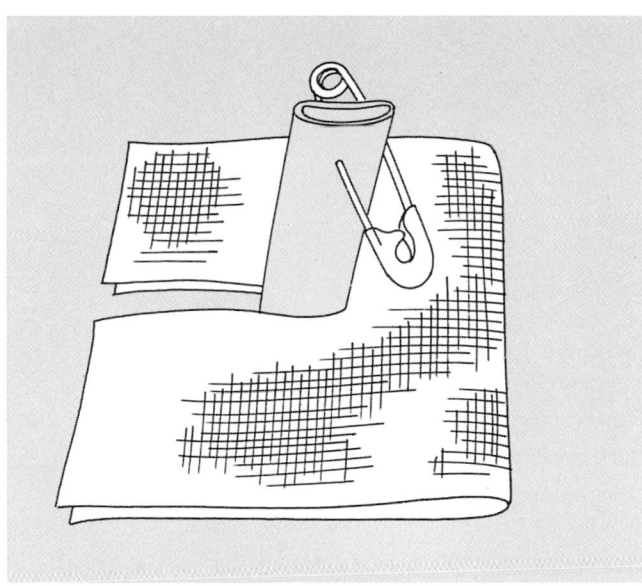

FIGURE 38-3 Penrose drain.

to the skin. The closed drainage system prevents microorganisms from entering the wound from saturated dressings. Closed drainage systems also allow accurate measurement of drainage. Be sure to know which type of drain or tube was inserted during surgery to ensure accurate assessments and interventions.

Portable closed drainage systems have directions for their use printed on the container itself. Do not touch the open port when emptying the drainage system because reflux of drainage from a contaminated port could contaminate the wound.

Collecting a Wound Culture

If assessment of the wound indicates a possible infection, obtain a specimen of the drainage and send it to the laboratory for culture and sensitivity, as outlined in Skill 38-2.

Irrigating and Packing a Wound

An irrigation is a directed flow of solution over tissues. The purposes of an irrigation include cleaning the area of

pathogens and other debris and applying local heat or an antiseptic to the area. Nonsterile solutions are used if the wound is closed. Sterile equipment and solutions are required for irrigating an open wound, even in the presence of an existing infection.

Sterile 0.9% sodium chloride or sterile water, an antiseptic, or an antibiotic solution may be used, depending on the condition of the wound and the physician's order. A sterile, large-volume syringe is used to direct the flow of the solution. Sometimes the physician orders packing to be placed in wounds after irrigation to allow granulation tissue formation and healing by secondary intention to take place. The techniques for irrigating a wound and inserting packing are described in Skill 38-3.

Caring for Draining Wounds

The basic care of a draining wound is similar to that of a wound with little or no drainage. The following interventions are important in caring for a draining wound.

If wound care is uncomfortable, administer a prescribed analgesic 30 to 45 minutes before changing the dressing. Also, plan to change the dressing midway between meals so that the patient's appetite and mealtimes are not disturbed.

Apply a protective ointment or paste if appropriate to cleaned skin surrounding the draining wound. The ointment or paste acts as a protective barrier to prevent skin irritation and excoriation from wound drainage. Protecting the skin is particularly important if the drainage period may be prolonged or the person's skin is especially susceptible to irritation. Remove the protective ointment or paste at least daily, cleaning the skin thoroughly after removal. Use the least amount of rubbing possible to remove the protective material to prevent epithelial cells from being injured by friction.

The first layer of dressing material applied directly to a draining wound is often nonabsorbent but hydrophilic (ie, capable of carrying moisture). This type of material allows drainage from the wound to move into overlying absorbent layers of dressing, helping to prevent maceration and reinfection. Moreover, this type of dressing is less likely to stick

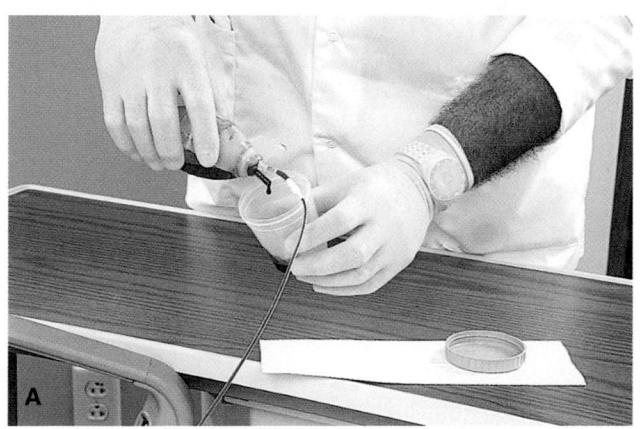
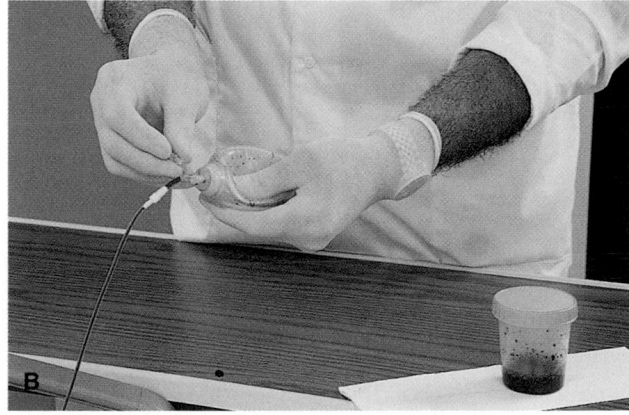

FIGURE 38-4 The Jackson-Pratt drain is a closed drainage system. The nurse empties the drain (**A**) and reapplies suction by compressing the drain reservoir before connecting it to the drain tubing (**B**). (Photo © B. Proud.)

SKILL 38-2   Collecting a Wound Culture

EQUIPMENT

Sterile Culturette tube with enclosed swab
(or culture tube with individual swabs)
Sterile gloves

Clean disposable gloves
Plastic bag for soiled dressing
Label for Culturette tube

Laboratory requisition with rubber band or
plastic bag

ACTION	RATIONALE
1. Explain the procedure to patient.	An explanation encourages patient cooperation and reduces apprehension.
2. Gather equipment.	Proper preparation provides for organized approach to task.
3. Perform hand hygiene.	Hand hygiene deters spread of microorganisms.
4. Don clean disposable gloves. Remove dressing and assess wound and drainage (see Skill 38-1, actions 5 to 11).	Using clean gloves protects nurse from handling contaminated dressings.
5. Using aseptic technique, don sterile gloves and clean wound (see Skill 38-1, Action 15). Remove sterile gloves.	Previous drainage and skin flora are removed.
6. Twist cap to loosen swab in Culturette tube, or open separate swab and remove cap from culture tube, keeping inside un-contaminated.	Supplies are within easy reach, and sterility is maintained.
7. Don clean glove or new sterile glove, if necessary.	Use of Culturette does not require immediate contact with skin or wound. If contact with wound is necessary to collect specimen, wear sterile glove on that hand.
8. Carefully insert swab into wound and roll gently. Use another swab if collecting specimen from another site.	Cotton tip absorbs wound drainage. This prevents cross-contamination of wound.
9. Place swab in Culturette tube, being careful not to touch out-side of container. Twist cap to secure.	Outside of container is protected from contamination with microorganisms.

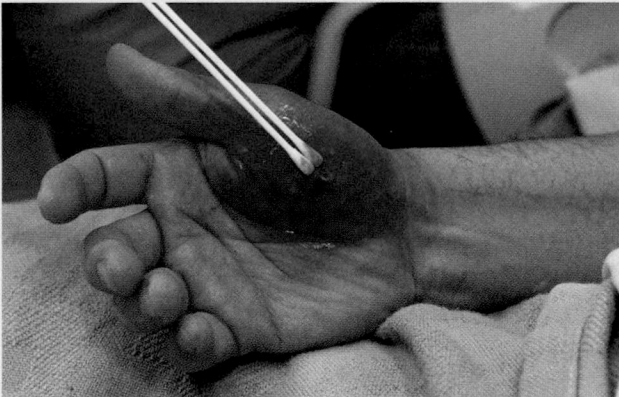

Action 8: Swabbing the wound with the cotton applicator from the Culturette.   (Photo by Rick Brady.)

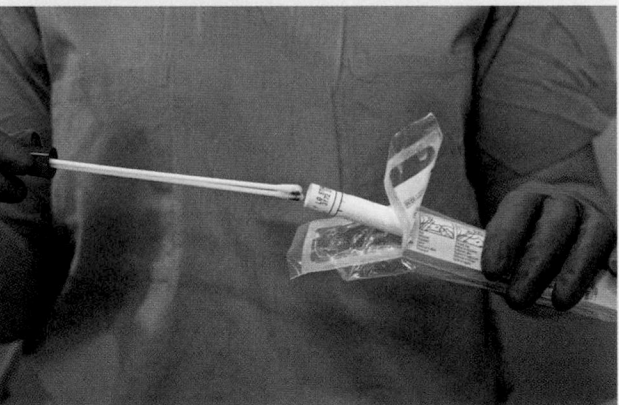

Action 9: Placing the applicator swab back in the Culturette tube. (Photo by Rick Brady.)

10. If using Culturette tube, crush ampule of medium at bottom of tube.	Swab with drainage can be surrounded by culture medium.
11. Remove gloves from inside out, and discard them in plastic waste bag.	Proper disposal prevents spread of microorganisms
12. Perform hand hygiene.	Hand hygiene deters the spread of microorganisms.
13. Apply clean dressing to wound (see Skill 38-1, actions 16 to 20).	Drainage from wound is absorbed.
14. Perform hand hygiene. Remove all equipment and make pa-tient comfortable.	Hand hygiene deters the spread of microorganisms.

(continued)

ACTION	RATIONALE
15. Label specimen container appropriately (patient's name, date, time, nature of specimen). Attach laboratory requisition to tube with rubber band or place tube in plastic bag with requisition attached. Send to laboratory within 20 minutes.	Labeling ensures proper identification of specimen. Overgrowth of other organisms can interfere with test results if specimen remains at room temperature for extended period.
16. Record collection of specimen, appearance of wound, and description of drainage in chart.	Accurate documentation of procedure ensures continuity of care and provides information for comparison of future assessments.

to the wound, making dressing changes more comfortable for the patient.

Material to absorb and collect drainage is then placed over the first layer of nonabsorbent material. This material acts as a wick, pulling drainage out by capillary action. Absorbent cotton has far greater capillarity than untreated cotton. Therefore, cotton-lined gauze sponges soak up more liquid than unlined sponges. The number of gauze sponges used in the dressing depends on the amount of drainage. Loosely packed gauze, the threads of which act as numerous wicks, enhances capillarity and directs drainage upward and away from the wound. Fluffed and loosely packed dressings are more absorbent than tightly packed dressings. The top of the dressing may be further protected by surgical or abdominal pads, which are thick, absorbent pads that help to absorb profuse drainage.

Because a draining wound often requires more frequent dressing changes than a wound without drainage, Montgomery straps are recommended to secure the dressing (Fig. 38-5). These straps do not require changing with each dressing, as tape strips do. Montgomery straps are available commercially or can be made by hand from tape strips. If made of tape, the adhesive end of the strap is placed on the skin well away from the wound. The end of the strap near the wound remains free because the adhesive side is turned back on itself. Gauze or woven strips passed through eyelets or openings are tied over the dressing. When the dressing is changed, the strips are untied and turned back to allow for wound care.

Caring for Infected Wounds

Wounds infected with *Staphylococcus aureus*, beta-hemolytic streptococci, and *Clostridium perfringens* (gas gangrene) often are extensive. Additionally, these wounds usually produce copious amounts of purulent drainage, requiring special techniques. Guidelines for Nursing Care 38-2 summarizes the important points for dressing changes.

Caring for Open Wounds

Caring for open wounds requires an individualized approach. After evaluating each wound, the nurse selects one or more types of dressings. Because cellular migration needed for tissue repair and healing is enhanced by a moist surface, a moist (rather than wet) packing for open wounds is recommended. After soaking packing material in a solution (0.9% sodium chloride solution is the solution of choice), wring out the material so that it is only slightly moist. Next, apply the packing loosely and only to the edges of the wound. Then cover the wound with a secondary dressing to absorb drainage. If the packing dries, soak it with 0.9% sodium chloride solution before removal to prevent it from sticking to the healing tissue and causing injury.

A color classification system termed "R(red) Y(yellow) B(black)" can be used in implementing care for open wounds (Krasner, 1995; Stotts, 1990). This classification, with related interventions, is based on the assessment of wound color. However, many wounds have red, yellow, and black components and are categorized as mixed wounds (Fig. 38-6). When all colors are present, the wound is treated first for the most serious color (black), followed by yellow and finally red.

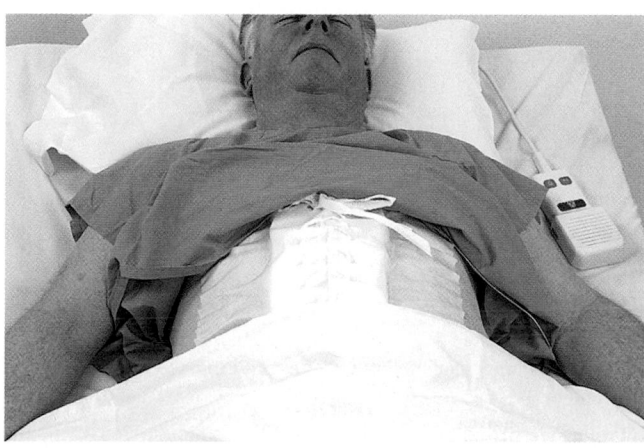

FIGURE 38-5 Montgomery straps make it possible to care for a wound without removing adhesive strips with each dressing change. (Photo © B. Proud.)

SKILL 38-3   Irrigating a Sterile Wound

EQUIPMENT

Sterile irrigation set (basin, container for irrigant, irrigating syringe)
Prescribed irrigating solution (warmed to body temperature or 34°–37°C [93.2°–98.6°F])
Sterile soft catheter (optional)
Plastic bag for soiled dressings

Sterile gloves
Clean disposable gloves
Sterile dressing set or suture set (contains scissors and forceps)
Waterproof pad
Sterile gauze and surgipads or ABDs (for dressing change)

Packing gauze (as specified by physician)
Gown (optional)
Goggles (optional)
Bath blanket
Tape

ACTION	RATIONALE
1. Explain procedure to patient. Check physician's order for irrigation.	Explanation facilitates patient cooperation. The physician's order clarifies procedure and type of supplies required.
2. Gather equipment.	Proper preparation provides for organized approach to task.
3. Perform hand hygiene.	Hand hygiene deters spread of microorganisms.
4. Close door or curtain. Use bath blanket as needed when exposing wound site.	Doing so provides for privacy and warmth.
5. Position patient so that irrigating solution will flow from upper end of wound toward lower end. Place waterproof pad under patient.	Gravity directs flow of liquid from least contaminated to most contaminated area. Waterproof pad protects patient and bed linens.
6. Warm sterile irrigating solution to body temperature.	Warmed solution is more comfortable for patient and promotes vasodilation.
7. Place opened, cuffed plastic bag near working area. Don gown and goggles if recommended.	Soiled dressings and packing may be placed in disposal bag without contaminating outside surfaces of bag. Gown protects uniform from contamination if splashing should occur. Goggles protect mucous membranes of eyes from contact with irrigant fluid.
8. Loosen tape on dressing, and put on clean gloves to remove soiled dressings.	Nurse is protected when handling contaminated dressings.
9. Assess amount, type, and odor of drainage. Observe condition of wound.	Assessment provides information about wound healing process or presence of infection.

Action 9: Assessing wound drainage.

10. Discard dressings in plastic disposal bag. Remove gloves inside out and drop in bag.	Spread of microorganisms by way of contaminated dressings is prevented.
11. Using aseptic technique, open sterile dressings and supplies on work area.	Supplies are within easy reach and sterility is maintained.

(continued)

Irrigating a Sterile Wound (continued)

ACTION	RATIONALE
12. Pour warmed sterile irrigating solution into sterile container. Amount may vary from 200 to 500 mL depending on size of wound.	Doing so facilitates wound irrigation; warming the solution prevents chilling the patient.
13. Put on sterile gloves.	Using sterile gloves maintains surgical asepsis.
14. Position the sterile basin below the wound to collect irrigation fluid with nondominant hand.	Irrigation is facilitated and patient and bed linens are protected from contaminated fluid.
15. Use dominant hand to fill syringe with irrigant. Gently direct a stream of solution into wound, keeping tip of syringe 1 inch (2.5 cm) above upper tip of wound. If using a catheter tip on syringe, insert it gently into wound to point of resistance.	Debris and contaminated solution flow from least contaminated to most contaminated area. Catheter allows introduction of irrigant into wound with small opening or one that is deep.

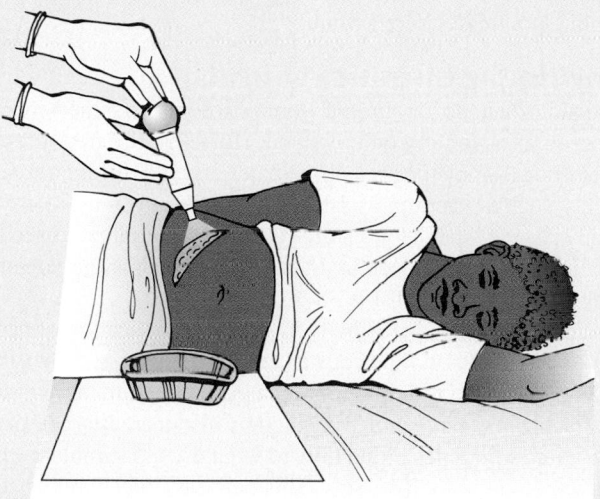

Action 15: Directing stream of solution into the wound.

16. Continue irrigation until solution returns clear. Try to maintain a steady flow of solution.	Irrigation removes exudate and debris.
17. Dry area around wound with a sterile gauze sponge.	Moisture provides medium for growth of microorganisms.
18. Apply layers of sterile dressing.	Drainage is absorbed and surrounding skin area is protected.
19. Remove gloves, and discard them in plastic waste bag. Apply tape to secure dressings.	Tape is easier to apply after gloves have been removed.
20. Perform hand hygiene. Remove all equipment, and make patient comfortable.	Hand hygiene prevents spread of microorganisms.
21. Check dressing and wound site every shift. Record dressing change, appearance of wound, and describe any drainage in chart.	Accurate documentation of procedure ensures continuity of care and provides information for comparison of future assessment.

Special Considerations

If insertion of packing is ordered:
- Use sterile forceps to insert sterile packing into wound gently.
- Be careful not to pack wound excessively because this may impede blood flow and delay healing.
- Cut packing with sterile scissors if necessary.
- Allow a small strip of packing to protrude from small and deep wounds to facilitate removal.

Guidelines for Nursing Care 38-2
Changing Dressings for Infected Wounds

- Perform hand hygiene before donning gloves for wound care.
- Wear a gown while caring for the patient's wound. This gown need not be sterile unless there is a danger of carrying organisms on a clean gown to an already debilitated patient.
- Wear a mask while caring for the wound.
- Be prepared with two pairs of sterile gloves, and change gloves between the removal of the old dressing and the application of the new dressing.
- Use a no-touch technique when handling soiled dressings. Lift soiled dressings with a clamp or forceps. This prevents contamination of the hands.
- Place soiled dressings in a moisture-proof bag, which is then closed securely, double-bagged, and incinerated without being opened.
- Perform thorough hand hygiene again after completing wound care. If organisms accumulate on the hands because proper technique was broken, the organisms not only are likely to be carried to others but eventually may also become resident flora on the nurse's hands.

R = Red = Protect

Red wounds are in the proliferative stage of healing and reflect the color of normal granulation tissue. Wounds in this stage need protection with nursing interventions that include gentle cleansing, use of moist dressings, application of a transparent or hydrocolloid dressing, and changing of the dressing only when necessary.

Y = Yellow = Cleanse

Yellow wounds are characterized by oozing from the tissue covering the wound, often accompanied by purulent drainage. To cleanse these wounds, nursing interventions include irri-

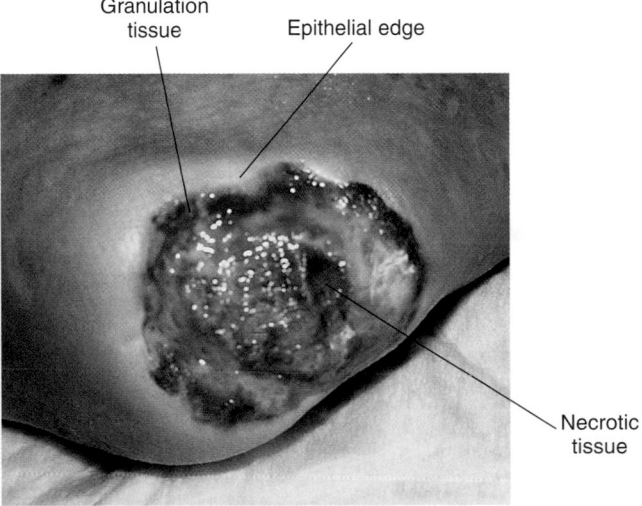

FIGURE 38-6 A wound with various types of wound surface tissue.

Granulation tissue

Epithelial edge

Necrotic tissue

gating the wound; using wet-to-moist dressings; using non-adherent, hydrogel, or other absorptive dressings; and consulting with the physician about using a topical antimicrobial medication to decrease the growth of bacteria.

B = Black = Débride

Black wounds are covered with thick **eschar** (necrotic tissue), which is usually black but may also be brown, gray, or tan. The eschar requires **débridement** (removal) before the wound can heal. These wounds are most often cared for by advanced practice nurses who are educated in the care of more complex wounds. The eschar may be removed by sharp débridement (using a scalpel or scissors to cut away the dead tissue), mechanical débridement (scrubbing the wound or applying a wet-to-moist dressing), chemical débridement (using collagenase enzyme agents), or autolytic débridement (using a dressing that contains wound moisture to help the body produce enzymes to break down the eschar). After débridement, the wound is treated as a yellow wound and then, as healing progresses, a red wound.

Caring for Chronic Wounds

Dressing changes for chronic wounds follow the same general procedures as for any other wound. However, different dressings, such as moisture-retentive materials, and different treatments, such as vacuum-assisted closure therapy, may be used. Many types of special moisture-retentive materials are used to facilitate healing, especially in chronic wounds. Some examples are described in Table 38-4.

Vacuum-assisted closure therapy is the application of negative pressure to pull the cells closer together. This allows the epithelial cells to multiply rapidly and form granulation tissue so that healing can begin. This therapy also increases cell proliferation, stimulates blood flow to wounds, and stimulates the growth of new blood vessels. This painless procedure is used on chronic open wounds, surgical incisions with dehiscence, and stage III and IV pressure ulcers.

Applying Bandages and Binders

Bandages and binders are used to secure dressings, apply pressure, and support the wound. **Bandages** are strips of cloth, gauze (eg, roller gauze, Kerlix, Kling), or elasticized material (eg, Ace bandages) used to wrap a body part. They come packaged in rolls and vary in width from 1 to 6 inches. Binders are designed for a specific body part and include slings, abdominal binders, chest binders, and T-binders. They may be made of cloth (flannel, muslin) or of an elasticized material that fastens together with Velcro. Guidelines for Nursing Care 38-3 highlights important principles for applying bandages and binders.

Roller Bandages

A roller bandage is a continuous strip of material wound on itself to form a cylinder or roll. Plain gauze, elastic webbing, and stretchable roller bandages are made in various widths and lengths. To begin, the free end is held in place with one hand while the other hand passes the roll around the body part. After the bandage is anchored, the roll is passed or rolled around the body part, taking care to exert equal tension in all turns. Keep

TABLE 38-4 Examples of Moisture-Retentive Dressings

Type	Purposes	Use
Transparent films, such as: Acu-derm Bioclusive BlisterFilm Mefilm Polyskin Uniflex Op-Site Tegaderm	• Allow exchange of oxygen between wound and environment • Are self-adhesive • Protect against contamination • Prevent loss of wound fluid • Maintain a moist wound environment • Allow visualization of wound • May remain in place for 24 to 72 hours, resulting in less interference with healing	• Wounds with minimal drainage • Wounds that are small and superficial, such as stage I and II pressure ulcers and superficial burns
Hydrocolloid dressings, such as: DuoDerm Intact Comfeel IntraSite Tegasorb Ultec	• Are occlusive • Absorb drainage • Provide cushioning • Do not allow entry of contaminants • May be left in place for 3 to 5 days, resulting in less interference with healing	• Shallow to moderate-depth skin ulcers • Wounds with drainage • In conjunction with packing for open, deep wounds
Hydrogels, such as: Vigilon IntraSite Gel Aquasorb ClearSite Nu-Gel Hypergel	• Maintain a moist wound environment • Do not adhere to wound • Reduce pain	• Partial- and full-thickness wounds • Necrotic wounds • Burns
Alginates, such as: Sorban AlgiDerm Curasorb Dermacea Melgisorb	• Absorb some exudate • Are compatible with topical medication • Absorb exudate • Maintain moisture	• Infected wounds
Foams, such as: LYOfoam Allevyn	• Maintain moist wound surface • Do not adhere to wound • Insulate wound	• Chronic wounds

Guidelines for Nursing Care 38-3
Applying Bandages and Binders

- Clean the area to be covered and dry it thoroughly before applying a bandage or binder, because prolonged heat and moisture on the skin may cause skin breakdown.
- Bandage the body part in the normal functioning position to prevent deformities and discomfort.
- Apply the bandage or binder with sufficient pressure to provide the amount of immobilization or support desired, to remain in place, and to secure a dressing when present. Do not apply pressure to such a degree that circulation to the body part involved is impeded.
- Maintain equal tension with all bandage turns; avoid unnecessary and uneven overlapping of turns.
- After application, assess circulation and comfort at regular intervals.

tension equal by unwinding the bandage gradually and only with as much of a length as is required. Evenly overlap one-half to two-thirds the width of the bandage with each turn, except for the circular turn (Fig. 38-7).

When removing a roller bandage, cut the bandage with a bandage scissors to prevent excessive manipulation of the part. Cut on the side opposite the injury or the wound, from one end to the other, so that the bandage can be folded open for its entire length. If the bandage is to be reused, it may be unwound by keeping the loose end together and passing it as a ball from one hand to the other while unwinding it.

Circular Turn
A circular turn is used primarily to anchor a bandage. In a circular turn, the bandage is wrapped around the body part with complete overlapping of the previous bandage turn.

Spiral Turn
Once the circular turn anchors the bandage, application continues ascending in a spiral manner using a spiral turn. Each turn overlaps the preceding one by one-half or two-thirds the

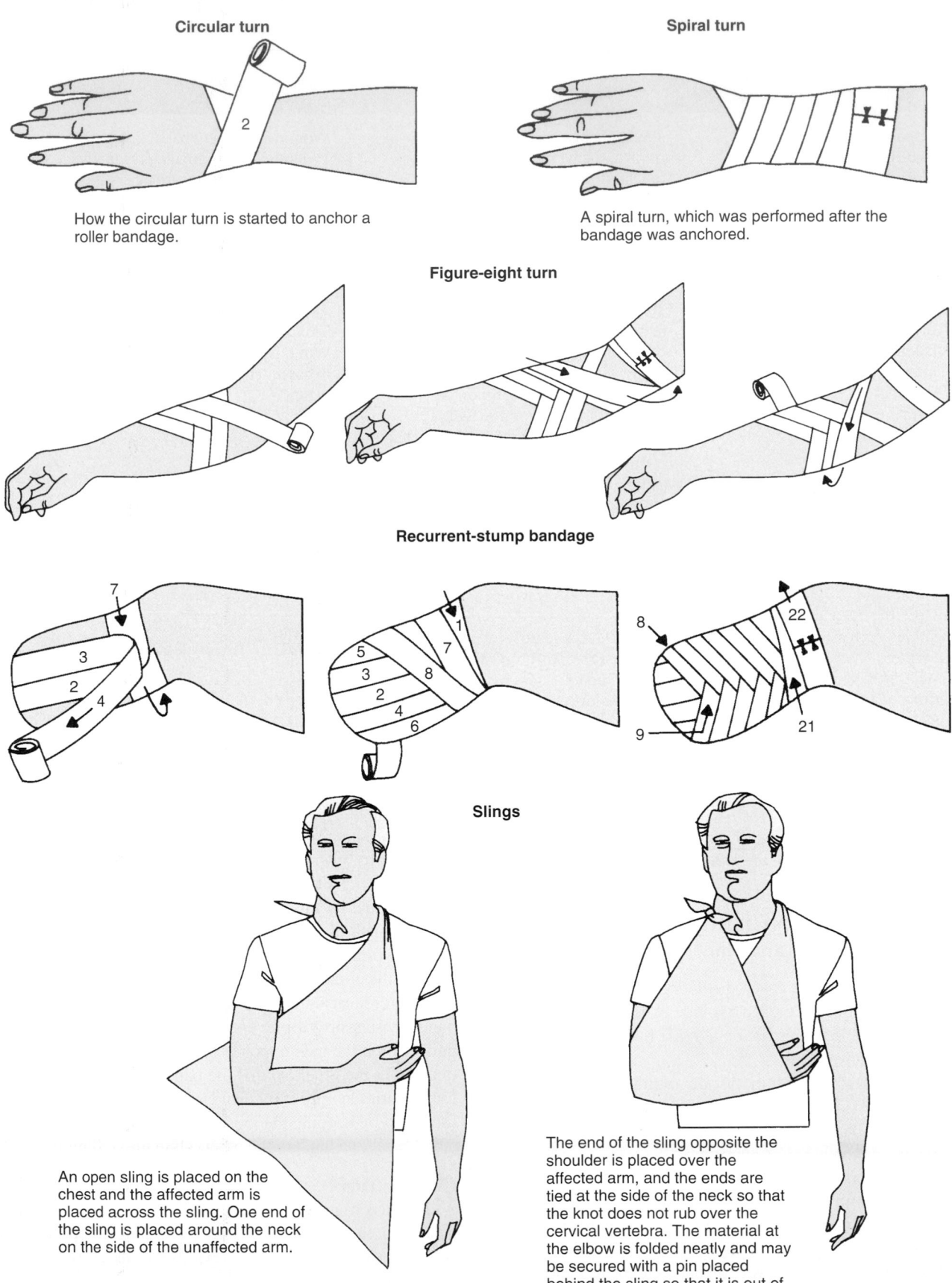

Circular turn

How the circular turn is started to anchor a roller bandage.

Spiral turn

A spiral turn, which was performed after the bandage was anchored.

Figure-eight turn

Recurrent-stump bandage

Slings

An open sling is placed on the chest and the affected arm is placed across the sling. One end of the sling is placed around the neck on the side of the unaffected arm.

The end of the sling opposite the shoulder is placed over the affected arm, and the ends are tied at the side of the neck so that the knot does not rub over the cervical vertebra. The material at the elbow is folded neatly and may be secured with a pin placed behind the sling so that it is out of sight.

FIGURE 38-7 Techniques for applying various bandages.

width of the bandage. The spiral turn is useful for the wrist, fingers, and trunk.

Figure-of-Eight Turn
The figure-of-eight turn consists of making oblique overlapping turns that ascend and descend alternately. It is effective for use around joints, such as the knee, elbow, ankle, and wrist (see Fig. 38-7).

Recurrent Stump Bandage
When applying a recurrent stump bandage, a few circular turns are made to anchor the bandage, and the initial end of the bandage is placed in the center of the body part being bandaged, well back from the tip to be covered. The bandage is passed back and forth over the tip, first on the one side and then on the other side of the center piece of the bandage. Figure 38-7 shows how to apply a recurrent bandage to a stump, using the figure-of-eight turn to finish the bandage. Recurrent bandages are used for fingers, for the head, and for the stump of an amputated limb.

Binders
Of the many different kinds of binders, those used most commonly include straight binders, T-binders, and slings. A straight binder is a straight piece of material, usually about 15 to 20 cm (6 to 8 inches) wide and long enough to more than circle the torso. It is used for the chest and the abdomen. Straight binders may be pinned or, more commonly, fastened with Velcro.

A T-binder might be used to secure dressings on the rectum and perineum and in the groin. The single T-binder is used for female patients, the double T-binder for male patients. The belt is passed around the waist and secured, and the tails are passed between the legs and fastened to the belt.

A sling is used to support an arm. Most healthcare agencies use commercial strap slings or sleeve slings. In the home, a large piece of cloth folded into a triangle can be used as a sling (see Fig. 38-7).

Teaching Wound Care at Home
With the increase in ambulatory surgery and earlier discharge of patients from inpatient settings to home care, teaching patients and their families about wound care is important. Although a nurse may be needed to change dressings and provide wound care in complex situations, family members often are taught how to perform the procedure. To provide the continuity of care that is necessary to prevent infection and promote healing, be sure to include teaching about wound care as part of discharge planning and in interactions with home care patients and families. A summary of teaching content is outlined in Teaching to Promote Health at Home 38-1: Wound Care and Healing.

Evaluating
The plan of care for the patient with a wound is evaluated based on the expected outcomes. Evaluation is ongoing throughout the care of the patient, with the plan being effective if no complications have occurred during wound healing, if the wound is progressing through the healing stages, and if the patient or family has the knowledge and skills necessary for wound care at home.

PRESSURE ULCERS

A **pressure ulcer** is a wound with a localized area of tissue necrosis. Depending on the depth of the ulcer, a pressure ulcer may be an acute wound or a chronic wound. The underlying cause is compression of soft tissue between a bony prominence and an external surface for a prolonged period of time. The terms "pressure ulcer," "decubitus ulcer," and "bedsore" are synonymous. Most people prefer the term "pressure ulcer" because pressure is the most prominent underlying cause.

Pressure ulcers, one of the most common skin and tissue disruptions, are costly in terms of healthcare expenditures. The prevalence of pressure ulcers in the United States has been estimated to be between 1.5 million and 3 million. As many as 60% or more develop in hospitalized patients, 18% develop in nursing homes (with the incidence increased with longer stays), and 7% to 12% of those receiving home health services have pressure ulcers (Mayo Clinic, 2001). Most pressure ulcers occur in older adults as a result of a combination of factors, including aging skin, chronic illnesses, immobility, malnutrition, fecal and urinary incontinence, and altered level of consciousness. Another significant at-risk population includes individuals with spinal cord injuries, traumatic brain injuries, and neuromuscular disorders. When pressure ulcers occur, aggressive intervention and treatment can spare the patient unnecessary pain and discomfort, prevent further tissue deterioration, hasten wound healing, and save millions of healthcare dollars. The accompanying Research in Nursing box highlights the importance of the nurse's role in providing cost-effective pressure ulcer prevention and treatment.

Factors in Pressure Ulcer Development

Pathologic changes at a pressure ulcer site result from blood vessel collapse caused by pressure, usually from body weight. **Necrosis** (death of cells) eventually occurs, leading to the characteristic ulcer. Two mechanisms contribute to pressure ulcer development: (1) external pressure that compresses blood vessels and (2) friction and shearing forces that tear and injure blood vessels.

External Pressure
Pressure ulcers usually occur over bony prominences, where body weight is distributed over a small area without much subcutaneous tissue to cushion damage to the skin. Common sites for pressure ulcers are illustrated in Figure 38-8. Of the susceptible areas, most pressure ulcers occur over the sacrum

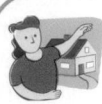

Teaching to Promote Health at Home 38-1
Wound Care and Healing

Health Topic	Suggested Content
Supplies	• Methods for obtaining dressing supplies such as purchasing from pharmacies, drug stores, discount stores, and medical supply stores • Considerations for costs and ease of use • Investigation about reimbursement by insurance company or other source of healthcare financing for supplies
Infection prevention	• Signs and symptoms of infection to be immediately reported to the healthcare provider • Need to watch for increased body temperature, red or separated wound edges, increased pain in the wound, and increased drainage that is thick and has a foul odor • Wearing of disposable gloves when changing the dressing • Hand hygiene before putting on and after removing the gloves • Proper methods for disposal of old dressing, such as wrapping old dressing in several layers of newspaper or putting it in a plastic bag before disposal in a trash container
Wound healing	• Importance of eating well-balanced meals that are high in protein and vitamins • Need to drink 6 to 8 glasses of fluids each day • Rest periods during the day • Modifications in activities of daily living and exercise until healing is complete and approval is given by healthcare provider

and coccyx, followed by the trochanter and the calcaneus (heel). Formation may occur in as little as 1 to 2 hours if the person has not moved for an extended period of time.

The major predisposing factor for a pressure ulcer is external pressure applied over an area, which results in occluded blood capillaries and poor circulation to tissues. Insufficient circulation leads to necrosis and ulcer formation. The skin can tolerate considerable pressure without cell death, but for short periods only. The formation of a pressure ulcer is more affected by the duration of pressure than the amount of pressure.

Research in Nursing Making a Difference
Pressure Ulcer Care in a Long-Term Facility

Much has been written about the importance of preventing and treating pressure ulcers, especially in older adults who require long-term care. For the patient, pressure ulcers are painful and increase the risk of infection and loss of independence in mobility and activities of daily living. For the facility, prevention and treatment are often costly in terms of time and resources. Although the incidence of pressure ulcers in patients varies by facility, longer stays are correlated with an increased probability of developing one or more such wounds.

Related Research
Franz, R., Gardner, S., Specht, J., et al. (2002). Integration of pressure ulcer treatment protocols into practice: Clinical outcomes and care environment attributes. *Outcomes Management for Nursing Practice, 5*(3), 112–120.

The purpose of this study, conducted in a long-term facility, was to determine if a successfully implemented research-based protocol for the treatment of existing pressure ulcers had been sustained over time. Treatment was given by using inexpensive moist wound-healing options. A retroactive chart review was conducted for a 1-year period for all patients who developed pressure ulcers. Data were collected about ulcer characteristics and type, frequency, and duration of treatment; patients were fol-

lowed until the ulcer healed, the patient was discharged or died, or the study ended. Of the 46 ulcers treated during the year, 40 healed, 5 were not healed at the time of death, and 1 was not healed at the end of the study. These findings supported not only the usefulness of the treatment protocol in treating pressure ulcers, but also that pressure ulcers could be completely healed at a relatively low cost to the facility.

In addition, the researchers collected data from nurses working in the facility and identified that management values of maintaining adequate staffing levels and encouraging independent decision making were factors in their success in treating pressure ulcers.

Relevance to Nursing Practice
Nurses must be able to provide care based on knowledge and skill, but they must also be managers of resources and costs of services provided in any setting. This study demonstrates that a relatively simple protocol was successful in all those areas of care. As a further component of the study and of relevance to nursing practice, the values of the facility to maintain staffing levels and to promote staff nurse accountability and decision making were believed to provide the necessary climate to sustain the desired care practices.

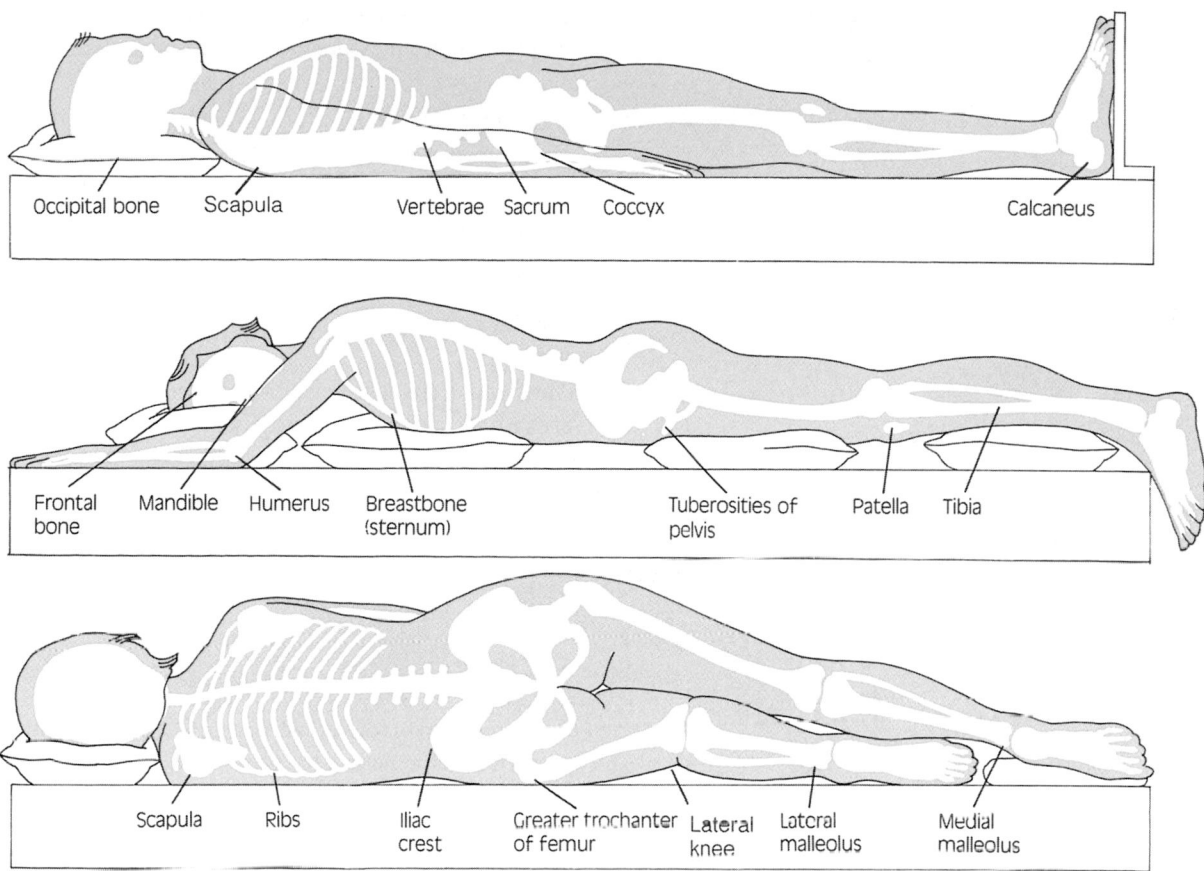

Occipital bone   Scapula   Vertebrae   Sacrum   Coccyx   Calcaneus

Frontal   Mandible   Humerus   Breastbone   Tuberosities of   Patella   Tibia
bone   (sternum)   pelvis

Scapula   Ribs   Iliac   Greater trochanter   Lateral   Lateral   Medial
                   crest   of femur   knee   malleolus   malleolus

FIGURE 38-8 Common sites for development of pressure ulcers.

Consider Mr. Everly, the postoperative patient in the critical care unit described in Reflective Practice. The nurse would integrate knowledge of the patient's condition, including his decreased level of consciousness and confinement in bed, to plan measures such as a turning schedule, proper positioning, and activities to promote movement in bed, thereby preventing body parts from exposure to prolonged pressure.

Friction and Shearing Forces

Friction occurs when two surfaces rub against each other. The injury, which resembles an abrasion, also can damage superficial blood vessels directly under the skin. A patient who lies on wrinkled sheets is likely to sustain tissue damage as a result of friction. The skin over the elbows and heels often is injured due to friction when patients lift and help move themselves up in bed with the use of their arms and feet. Friction burns can also occur on the back when patients are pulled or slid over sheets while being moved up in bed or transferred onto a stretcher.

A **shearing force** results when one layer of tissue slides over another layer. Shearing forces are often responsible for deep pressure ulcers. The small blood vessels and capillaries in the area are stretched and possibly tear, resulting in decreased circulation to the tissue cells under the skin. Figure 38-9 illustrates how shearing forces occur. Patients who are pulled rather than lifted when being moved up in bed or from bed to chair or stretcher are at risk for injury from shearing forces. A patient who is partially sitting up in bed is susceptible to shearing force when the skin sticks to the sheet and underlying tissues move downward with the body toward the foot of the bed. This may also occur in a patient who sits in a chair but slides down.

Risks for Pressure Ulcer Development

Usually, a combination of causes, in addition to pressure, friction, and shearing, contribute to ulcer development. These include immobility, nutrition and hydration, skin moisture, mental status, and age.

Immobility

Someone who sits or lies most of the time is at risk for a pressure ulcer because immobility causes prolonged pressure on body areas. Individuals who are ambulatory do not develop this injury because no part of the body suffers from prolonged pressure. When asleep, healthy people tend to move about in bed freely. Patients who are unconscious and paralyzed are subject to pressure ulcers if they are allowed to remain in any one position. Persons who are emotionally depressed ordinarily do not move around a great deal, placing them at risk for pressure ulcer formation. Additional factors that cause immo-

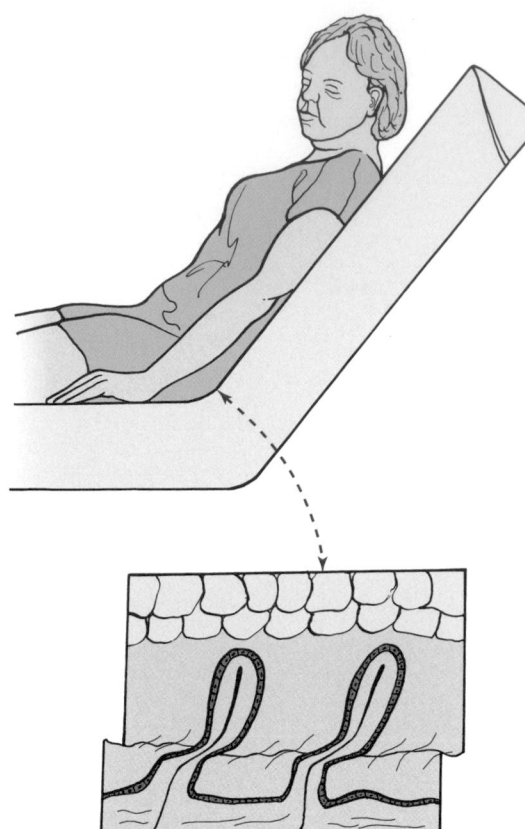

FIGURE 38-9 Shearing forces can occur when a patient is moved carelessly or slides down in bed.

bility and may result in this serious problem are lengthy surgery and the use of tranquilizers or sedatives.

Nutrition and Hydration

Protein-calorie malnutrition predisposes a person to pressure ulcer formation because poorly nourished cells are easily damaged. For example, vitamin C deficiency causes capillaries to become fragile, with resultant poor circulation to the area. Protein deficiency leading to a negative nitrogen balance, electrolyte imbalances, and insufficient caloric intake also predisposes the skin to injury. The condition of the teeth or fit of dentures may also exacerbate the problem of inadequate dietary intake. Dehydration as well as edema can interfere with circulation and subsequent cell nourishment.

Moisture

Prolonged moisture on the skin reduces the skin's resistance to trauma. Warmth increases the cells' demands for oxygen. Therefore, moisture and warmth eventually lead to cell destruction. This is compounded when pressure is present. When skin is damp, less friction is required to blister and abrade skin. Additionally, the moisture associated with urinary incontinence is believed to increase the risk for skin damage more than just due to the chemical irritation from the ammonia in the urine. If personal hygiene is poor, the skin contains many organisms that thrive in the warm, moist environment. Thus, the

increase in organisms increases the risk for the development of an infection in a pressure ulcer that forms.

Mental Status

The more alert an individual is, the more likely he or she is to protect skin integrity by relieving pressure periodically and maintaining adequate skin hygiene. Apathy, confusion, or a comatose state can diminish these self-care abilities and increase the likelihood of skin breakdown.

Age

Older adults are at a greater risk for pressure ulcer formation because the aging skin is more susceptible to injury. Chronic and debilitating diseases, more common in this age group, may adversely affect circulation and oxygenation of dermal structures. Other problems, such as malnutrition and immobility, compound the risk of pressure ulcer development in older adults.

Pressure Ulcer Staging

Appropriate intervention depends on early recognition of the stage of development of the pressure ulcer. Pressure ulcers are commonly classified in four stages. Differentiation of these four stages and a visual representation of the stages are presented in Table 38-5.

The first indication that a pressure ulcer may be developing is blanching (becoming pale and white) of the skin over the area under pressure. Insufficient blood circulation makes the skin appear paler than in areas where circulation is adequate. This local anemia resulting from poor circulation is called **ischemia.** If the pressure continues, circulation is further impaired and a stage I pressure ulcer develops.

When pressure is relieved, ischemia is rapidly followed by hyperemia. The area appears red and feels warm. Reactive hyperemia is a blanchable reddening of the skin that occurs when pressure is removed. The body literally floods the area with blood to nourish and remove wastes from the cells. Reactive hyperemia is not a stage I pressure ulcer. With reactive hyperemia, after a patient who has been lying supine for 2 hours is repositioned onto the side, any reddened area should fade within 60 to 90 minutes. In patients with darkly pigmented skin, hyperemia may best be detected by touch. The skin feels warm, or some change in color is detected.

Recall Mr. Everly, the postoperative patient in the critical care unit who has the beginning of a pressure ulcer on his heel. The nurse would apply knowledge about the stages of pressure ulcer development when assessing his heel.

A stage II pressure ulcer is superficial and may present as a blister or abrasion. Damage to the subcutaneous tissue indicates a stage III lesion, and the extensive destruction associated with full-thickness skin loss is categorized as a stage IV pressure ulcer.

TABLE 38-5 **Comparison of Stages of Pressure Ulcers**

Stage I
An observable pressure-related alteration of intact skin whose indicators, as compared to the adjacent or opposite area on the body, may include changes in one or more of the following: skin temperature (warmth or coolness), tissue consistency (firm or boggy feel), and sensation (pain, itching). The ulcer appears as a defined area of persistent redness in lightly pigmented skin, whereas in darker skin tones, the ulcer may appear with persistent red, blue, or purple hues.

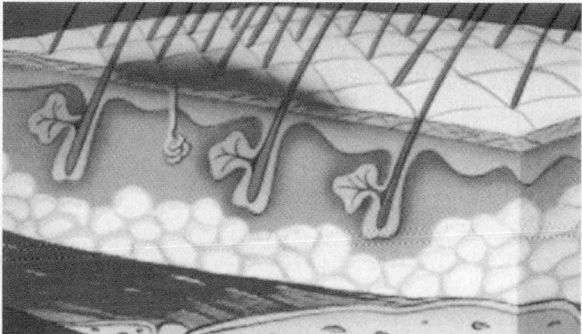

Pressure-relieving measures:
- Frequent turning
- Pressure-relieving devices
- Positioning

Stage II
Partial-thickness skin loss involving epidermis and/or dermis. The ulcer is superficial and presents clinically as an abrasion, blister, or shallow crater.

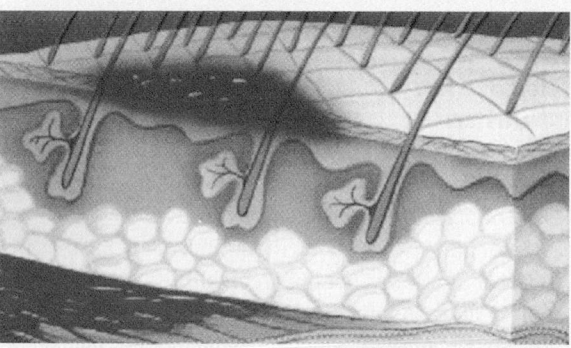

Maintenance of a moist healing environment:
- Saline or
- Occlusive dressing that promotes natural healing but prevents formation of a scar

Stage III
Full-thickness skin loss involving damage or necrosis of subcutaneous tissue that may extend down to, but not through, underlying fascia. The ulcer presents clinically as a deep crater with or without undermining of adjacent tissue.

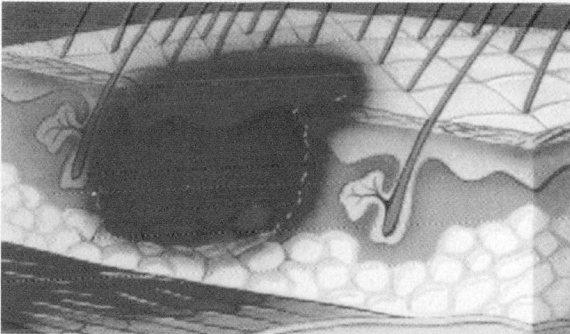

Requires débridement, which can be accomplished by one of the following:
- Wet-to-dry dressings
- Surgical intervention
- Proteolytic enzymes

Stage IV
Full-thickness skin loss with extensive destruction, tissue necrosis, or damage to muscle, bone, or supporting structures (eg, tendon or joint capsule). Sinus tracts may also be associated with stage IV ulcers.

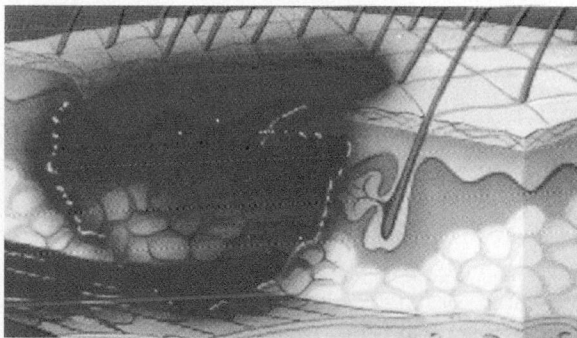

Wounds are treated in the following manner:
- Covered with nonadherent dressing
- Changed every 8–12 hours
- May require skin grafts

From U.S. Department of Health and Human Services. Agency for Health Care Policy and Research. (1992). *Pressure ulcers in adults: Prediction and prevention.* Rockville, MD: DHHS; Porth, C. (1994). *Pathophysiology: Concepts of altered health states.* Philadelphia: JB Lippincott; and National Pressure Ulcer Advisory Panel (NPUAP). http://www.npuap.org.

This staging process has several limitations. If eschar is present, it may be difficult to stage a pressure ulcer. Eschar is a thick, leathery scab or dry crust that is necrotic and must be removed before the stage can be determined accurately. Patients with casts, orthopedic devices, or support stockings require routine assessment of areas where inadequate circulation may be a contributing factor to development of a pressure ulcer.

THE NURSING PROCESS FOR PRESSURE ULCERS

Assessing

Many pressure ulcers can be prevented. It is a nursing priority to perform a comprehensive assessment in all settings and identify patients at risk for pressure ulcers, predisposing factors, or evidence of actual pressure ulcers.

An aggressive approach to prevent a pressure ulcer or manage the care of a patient who already has impaired skin integrity begins with a risk assessment form, which must be simple to use, reliable, and cost-effective. Several different scales are available to assess risk, such as the Norton scale (physical condition, mental condition, activity, mobility, and incontinence) and the Braden scale (mental status, continence, mobility, activity, and nutrition; Fig. 38-10). With these tools, a numeric score is assigned to each assessment area. The degree of risk is based on the patient's total score. For example, a score of 18 or less using the Braden scale indicates risk for pressure ulcer development.

Once a patient's risk has been identified, agencies use different approaches. Many healthcare facilities use a special pressure ulcer assessment form. For patients at risk, a sign placed outside the room or attached to the chart indicates the need for ongoing assessment and special attention to skin integrity.

Documenting assessments is essential to ensure continuity of care, providing the foundation on which to develop the skin plan of care. All caregivers in the home or healthcare agency need to be aware of specific assessments.

Nursing History

When obtaining the nursing history, include questions about the appearance of the skin and patient activities that may contribute to the development of a pressure ulcer. Often a combination of factors places the patient at greatest risk for a pressure ulcer.

Question the patient and family about recent changes in the appearance or condition of the skin and any skin care regimens. Also assess activity status, nutritional state, elimination patterns, cognitive state, and presence of pain associated with altered skin integrity. Nurses have long recognized that patients with pressure ulcers experience pain. Focus assessment on whether dressing changes, positioning in bed or in a chair, or movement elicits any expressions of pain. Even if pain is never verbalized or expressed, always assume that pain is a definite possibility, and focus on comfort needs. The accompanying Focused Assessment Guide 38-1 provides additional suggestions for gathering a nursing history.

Physical Assessment

Physical assessment of the skin is included as part of the initial database collection (skin assessment is described in Chap. 25). Be sure to inspect the skin systematically in a head-to-toe fashion, including bony prominences, on admission and then at regular intervals for all at-risk patients. Reassessment is recommended (Braden & Ayello, 2002), as follows:

- Acute care setting: At least every 48 hours or if the patient's condition changes
- Long-term care setting: Weekly for the first 4 weeks, followed by monthly to quarterly or more frequently if the patient's condition changes
- Home health care: Every visit

According to the Agency for Health Care Policy and Research (AHCPR) Clinical Practice Guideline (USDHHS, 1994), skin assessment for a pressure ulcer specifically includes inspection of the following:

- Location of any lesion or ulcer
- Estimation of the stage
- Dimensions of the ulcer: length, width, depth (Box 38-3)
- Presence of any abnormal pathways in the wound, such as a sinus tract (a cavity or channel underneath the wound that has the potential for infection) or tunneling (a passageway or opening that may be visible at skin level, but with most of the tunnel under the surface of the skin)
- Visible necrotic tissue; necrotic tissue that is in the process of separating from viable portions of the body is referred to as slough.
- Presence of an exudate
- Presence or absence of granulation tissue
- Visible evidence of epithelialization

> With Mr. Everly, the patient described in Reflective Practice, the nurse could use these criteria routinely to ensure consistent assessment of the patient's pressure ulcer.

Mobility

Assessing a patient's mobility status includes evaluating the patient's ability to move, turn, and reposition the body. A patient who is confined to bed or a chair or has limited range of motion is at increased risk for a pressure ulcer. This assessment of activity status is done upon admission to the healthcare facility or during the initial home care interview. The use of any assistive devices to maintain mobility and activity is noted. Additional suggestions for gathering information about mobility are described in Chapter 39.

Nutritional Status

The importance of sound nutrition in the prevention and treatment of a pressure ulcer is well established. Older adults, in particular, need adequate nutrition for optimal health and wound healing. Nutritional assessment is described in Chapter 42. The AHCPR guidelines (USDHHS, 1994) suggest the following laboratory criteria as assessment data indicating that a patient is nutritionally at risk to develop a pressure ulcer:

- Albumin level <3.5 mg/dL (normal, 3.5 to 5 mg/dL)
- Total lymphocyte count <1,800/mm^3 (normal, 1,000 to 4,000/mm^3)
- Body weight decrease of >15%

Moisture and Incontinence

Many studies have documented that moisture makes the skin more susceptible to injury. Whether the moisture is from perspiration, wound drainage, urine, or stool, the skin is compromised. Moisture can create an environment in which microorganisms can multiply and the skin is more likely to blister, suffer abrasions, and become macerated (softening or

Braden Scale for Predicting Pressure Sore Risk

Sensory Perception: Ability to respond meaningfully to pressure-related discomfort
1. **Completely Limited:** Unresponsive (does not moan, flinch, or grasp) to painful stimuli, due to diminished level of consciousness or sedation, OR limited ability to feel pain over most of body surface.
2. **Very Limited:** Responds only to painful stimuli. Cannot communicate discomfort except by moaning or restlessness, OR has a sensory impairment which limits the ability to feel pain or discomfort over half of body.
3. **Slightly Limited:** Responds to verbal commands but cannot always communicate discomfort or need to be turned, OR has some sensory impairment which limits ability to feel pain or discomfort in 1 or 2 extremities.
4. **No Impairment:** Responds to verbal commands. Has no sensory deficit which would limit ability to feel or voice pain or discomfort.

SCORE [ ]

Moisture: Degree to which skin is exposed to moisture
1. **Constantly Moist:** Skin is kept moist almost constantly by perspiration, urine, etc. Dampness is detected every time patient is moved or turned.
2. **Very Moist:** Skin is often but not always moist. Linen must be changed at least once a shift.
3. **Occasionally Moist:** Skin is occasionally moist, requiring an extra linen change approximately once a day.
4. **Rarely Moist:** Skin is usually dry: linen requires changing only at routine intervals.

SCORE [ ]

Activity: Degree of physical activity
1. **Bedfast:** Confined to bed.
2. **Chairfast:** Ability to walk severely limited or non-existent. Cannot bear own weight and/or must be assisted into chair or wheelchair.
3. **Walks Occasionally:** Walks occasionally during the day, but for very short distances, with or without assistance. Spends majority of each shift in bed or chair.
4. **Walks Frequently:** Walks outside the room at least twice and inside room at least once every 2 hours during waking hours.

SCORE [ ]

Mobility: Ability to change and control body position
1. **Completely immobile:** Does not make even slight changes in body or extremity position without assistance.
2. **Very Limited:** Makes occasional slight changes in body or extremity position but unable to make frequent or significant changes independently.
3. **Slightly Limited:** Makes frequent though slight changes in body or extremity position independently.
4. **No Limitation:** Makes major and frequent changes in position without assistance.

SCORE [ ]

Nutrition: Usual food intake pattern
1. **Very Poor:** Never eats a complete meal. Rarely eats more than 1/3 of food offered. Eats 2 servings or less of protein (meat or dairy products) per day. Takes fluids poorly. Does not take a liquid dietary supplement, OR is NPO and/or maintained on clear liquids or IV for more than five days.
2. **Probably Inadequate:** Rarely eats a complete meal and generally eats only about half of any food offered. Protein intake includes only 3 servings of meat or dairy products per day. Occasionally will take a dietary supplement, OR receives less than optimum amount of liquid diet or tube feeding.
3. **Adequate:** Eats over half of most meals. Eats a total of 4 servings of protein (meat, dairy products) each day. Occasionally will refuse a meal, but will usually take a supplement if offered, OR is on a tube feeding or TPN regimen, which probably meets most of nutritional needs.
4. **Excellent:** Eats most of every meal. Never refuses a meal. Usually eats a total of 4 or more servings of meat and dairy products. Occasionally eats between meals. Does not require supplementation.

SCORE [ ]

Friction and Shear
1. **Problem:** Requires moderate to maximum assistance in moving. Complete lifting without sliding against sheets is impossible. Frequently slides down in bed or chair, requiring frequent repositioning with maximum assistance. Spasticity, contractures, or agitation leads to almost constant friction.
2. **Potential Problem:** Moves feebly or requires minimum assistance. During a move skin probably slides to some extent against sheets, chair, restraints, or other devices. Maintains relatively good position in chair or bed most of the time but occasionally slides down.
3. **No Apparent Problem:** Moves in bed and in chair independently and has sufficient muscle strength to lift up completely during move. Maintains good position in bed or chair at all times.

SCORE [ ]

---

3 or 4 = Moderate to Low Impairment	Risk Level	NPO: Nothing by Mouth	
Total Points Possible: 23	19-23 Not at risk	IV: Intravenously	**Total Score:** [ ]
Risk Predicting Score: 16 or Less	15-18 low risk	TPN: Total parenteral nutrition	
	13-14 moderate risk		
	10-12 high risk		
	≤ 9 very high risk		

FIGURE 38-10 Braden Scale for predicting pressure sore risk. (Copyright 1988 by Barbara Braden and Nancy Bergstrom. Reprinted with permission. All rights reserved.)

Focused Assessment Guide 38-1

Skin Integrity and Pressure Ulcer Risk

Factors to Assess	Questions and Approaches
Appearance of skin	• Do you have any skin areas that are discolored? • Do some areas of skin on your body feel warmer or colder than others? • Describe the moisture in your skin: is it damp, dry, oily? • Have you noticed that your skin seems to be thinner? Where? • Have you noticed any swelling in your feet, ankles, or fingers? • Tell me about how you take care of your skin. For example, do you take a tub bath or shower? How often? Do you use oils or lotions?
Recent changes in skin	• Do you have any sores on your body? If so, how many, and where are they? Have they changed in size? Do you have any drainage from them? • Have you noticed that the skin over your hips or backbone gets red if you sit or lie in one position for a long time? Does this disappear in a short time when you are up?
Activity/mobility	• Do you need assistance to walk or move? If so, how much? • Are you confined to your bed or a chair when up? • Can you change your position when you want to?
Nutrition	• Have you gained or lost weight recently? • Describe your usual meals each day. • How many glasses or cups of liquid do you drink each day? • Do you take any food supplements or vitamins? • Do you prepare your own meals? • Do you wear dentures? How do they fit? • Do you have any difficulty swallowing? • Has a doctor ever told you that you are anemic?
Pain	• If you have a sore, is it painful? • Do you take anything for pain? If so, what do you take, and how often? Does it help?
Elimination	• Have you noticed any problems with your bowels or urination? If so, describe. • Have you ever used pads or special pants because you can't control your urine or stools?

disintegration of the skin in response to moisture). Chapter 43 has additional assessment information related to incontinence.

Diagnosing

The stage of the pressure ulcer is a factor in determining the nursing diagnosis. Stage I and II pressure ulcers have superficial skin damage. Thus, Impaired Skin Integrity is the appropriate choice. Stage III and IV pressure ulcers include full-thickness skin loss and damage to underlying tissue; therefore, the diagnosis Impaired Tissue Integrity is more appropriate. For additional information on appropriate nursing diagnoses, see Examples of NANDA Nursing Diagnoses: Pressure Ulcers.

Outcome Identification and Planning

When nurses care for patients who have or are at risk for impaired skin and tissue integrity, nursing interventions are planned and implemented to support the following patient outcomes. The patient will:

• Demonstrate self-care measures to prevent pressure ulcer development and promote wound healing
• Demonstrate progressive healing of the pressure ulcer
• Demonstrate increase in body weight and muscle size
• Remain free of infection at the site of the pressure ulcer
• Develop no new areas of skin breakdown

Implementing

Nursing care is implemented to prevent the formation of pressure ulcers, and to promote healing and prevent complications when a pressure ulcer is present.

Pressure Ulcer Prevention

Many pressure ulcers can be prevented, but some high-risk individuals may develop pressure ulcers that continue to worsen despite aggressive nursing intervention. The AHCPR (USDHHS, 1992) recommends a series of interventions to prevent injury to the skin and promote optimal health. These protocols, displayed in Guidelines for Nursing Care 38-4, also provide the basis for an educational program that promotes on-

BOX 38-3 Measurement of a Pressure Ulcer

In addition to assessing location, stage, drainage, and types of tissue present in the wound, it is imperative that nurses accurately and consistently measure a pressure ulcer. Effective treatment is dependent on precise assessments. The nurse should document the following:

Size of the Wound
- Draw the shape and describe it.
- Measure the length, width, and diameter (if circular).

Depth of the Wound
- Moisten a sterile swab with saline and insert it gently into the wound at a 90-degree angle with the tip down.
- Mark the point on the swab that is even with the surrounding skin surface.
- Remove the swab and measure the depth with a ruler.

Presence of Undermining, Tunneling, or Sinus Tract
- Insert a saline-moistened sterile swab under the wound edge.
- Apply gentle pressure and assess for any abnormal pathways.
- *Never use force when probing with the swab.*
- Measure the location and depth of penetration.

going implementation of preventive measures by caregivers in the home.

Protecting the Skin From External Mechanical Forces

To protect patients at risk from the adverse effects of pressure, implement turning using an every-2-hour schedule in the healthcare setting. Encourage home care patients and caregivers to change body position at least every 2 hours when the patient is seated in a chair or is bedridden (a written schedule or kitchen timer may be helpful). Older adult patients tend to have less tissue tolerance, necessitating more frequent repositioning if redness on bony prominences is noted. The oblique position, an alternative to the side-lying position, results in significantly less pressure on the trochanter area.

Positioning devices such as pillows, foam wedges, or pressure-reducing boots can prove helpful to keep body weight off bony prominences. For example, a standard pillow placed under the calves raises the heels off the bed and alleviates pressure. Never use ring cushions, or "donuts," because they increase venous pressure. Minimize the effects of shearing force by limiting the amount of time the head of the bed is elevated (when possible).

Positioning devices and techniques maintain posture and distribute weight evenly for patients in a chair. Using a trapeze or bed linen to assist in transfers and position changes prevents friction on the skin. Pressure-relieving support surfaces, such as a foam overlay, static flotation mattress, alternating air mattress, low-air-loss bed, and air-fluidized bed, are available. However, there is disagreement about which surfaces are most appropriate. The type of support surface used must be individualized based on the patient's needs. Because none of these devices totally relieves pressure, position changes at regular intervals must still be done.

Pressure Ulcer Care

Despite preventive interventions, pressure ulcers may develop in certain high-risk patients. Aggressive treatment measures by the nurse or caregiver are the key to effective management. Patients, family members and other caregivers, and healthcare

Examples of NANDA Nursing Diagnoses — Pressure Ulcers

Nursing Diagnoses	Related Factors	Sample Defining Characteristics
Impaired Tissue Integrity	Any condition that causes damage to dermal, epidermal, and subcutaneous tissues, such as pressure, friction, shear, or altered circulation	• Presence of stage III or IV pressure ulcer
Ineffective Tissue Perfusion: Peripheral	Any condition that reduces oxygenation of peripheral tissues, such as prolonged pressure	• "I just can't move myself when I sit in the wheelchair." • "I have a sore on my heel." • Presence of ulceration on heel
Chronic Pain	Any condition that causes potential or actual damage to tissues with pain that is constant or recurring without a predictable end and lasts longer than 6 months, such as from a chronic wound or pressure ulcer	• "I've had this bad pain for over a year now." • "I am so tired because this constant pain won't let me sleep." • "I can't do the things I used to do because it just hurts too much." • Presence of pressure ulcer for extended period of time

Guidelines for Nursing Care 38-4
Pressure Ulcer Prevention

- Assess the skin of patients at risk on a daily basis. Pay particular attention to bony prominences.
- Cleanse the skin routinely and whenever any soiling occurs. Use a mild cleansing agent, minimal friction, and avoid hot water.
- Maintain higher humidity in the environment and use skin moisturizers for dry skin.
- Avoid massage over bony prominences.
- Protect the skin from moisture associated with episodes of incontinence or exposure to wound drainage.
- Minimize skin injury from friction and shearing forces by using proper positioning, turning, and transferring techniques. Use lubricants, protective films, dressings, and padding to diminish the effects of friction on the skin.
- Investigate reasons for inadequate dietary intake of protein and calories. Administer nutritional supplements or more aggressive nutritional intervention as needed.
- Continue efforts to improve mobility and activity. If this is unrealistic, attempt to maintain current level of activity, mobility, and range of motion.
- Document measures used to prevent pressure ulcers and the results of these interventions.

providers collaborate to set appropriate treatment goals. The AHCPR guideline on Treatment of Pressure Ulcers specifically outlines measures for caring for a pressure ulcer that reflect knowledge and research (USDHHS, 1994).

Cleaning the Pressure Ulcer

A pressure ulcer that is clean and free of infection should demonstrate some degree of healing within 2 to 4 weeks. Clean the wound with each dressing change, using careful, gentle motions to minimize trauma. Do not use harmful cleaners or antiseptic agents (such as povidone–iodine or hydrogen peroxide) because they damage granulation tissue. Use 0.9% normal saline solution to irrigate and clean the ulcer. Report any drainage or necrotic tissue. Whirlpool treatments may be ordered until the ulcer is considered clean. In addition, surgical excision of necrotic tissue may be necessary.

Dressing the Pressure Ulcer

According to the AHCPR (USDHHS, 1994), the cardinal rule when dressing a pressure ulcer is to keep the ulcer tissue moist and the surrounding skin dry. Therefore, use dressings that continuously keep the wound moist, placing the moist dressing only on the wound surface and keeping the intact, healthy skin surrounding the ulcer dry because it is susceptible to breakdown. Select a dressing that absorbs exudate, if present, but still maintains a moist environment for healing. Use a skin sealant or moisture-barrier ointment on

the surrounding skin and secure the dressing with the least amount of tape that is necessary. Use wet-to-dry dressings only for débridement, when ordered.

Pack wound cavities loosely with dressing material, because overpacking the wound may increase pressure and interfere with tissue healing. If the wound is near the anus, tape all four edges of the dressing, framing it like a picture to keep it intact. As with all wounds, be sure to assess it frequently.

Controlling Infection

Always adhere to standard precautions and use good hand hygiene to prevent infection. AHCPR guidelines (USDHHS, 1994) state that clean gloves and clean dressings may be used to treat pressure ulcers as long as the agency infection-control procedures are followed. Sterile instruments must be used for débridement.

Home Pressure Ulcer Care Teaching

Teaching patients and caregivers how to prevent pressure ulcers requires a comprehensive, organized educational effort. Initially, the healthcare provider presents basic information that explains the terminology, identifies risk factors, explains where and how pressure ulcers develop, and describes various prevention strategies and options. Illustrated instructions written at the level of the learner are a valuable resource. The AHCPR's booklet "Patient Guide for Preventing Pressure Ulcers" outlines specific care measures related to each risk factor and emphasizes the importance of personal involvement in care and treatment decisions; it is available for distribution to consumers. The protocols listed in the Guidelines for Nursing Care boxes also serve as a model for development of a teaching plan that incorporates basic principles and targets individuals at risk. As new information becomes available, education for prevention of pressure ulcers requires updating.

The patient and caregivers must be involved in the plan of care and need a good understanding about causative factors for the pressure ulcer. Instruct them in proper hand hygiene techniques and how to identify the signs and symptoms of infection. Provide the patient and caregivers with simple, easy-to-read instructions. Encourage frequent consultation with the primary healthcare provider about the progress of wound healing and products used. Also ensure that the patient, family, or caregivers understand the need for adequate nutrition to aid in wound healing. Assess the patient's nutritional status and suggest consultation with a dietitian for dietary deficiencies, if necessary.

If dressing changes or wound care is painful, teach the patient to use pain medication as prescribed 30 to 60 minutes before the procedure. Reinforce the importance of hand hygiene before and after the dressing change. When removing a soiled dressing at home, suggest that the caregiver (or patient if he or she is performing wound care) use a small plastic sandwich bag to cover the hand, lifting the dressing off with the covered hand. Then instruct the caregiver to turn the plastic bag inside-out over the hand and soiled dressing before carefully disposing of them.

Other Treatment Options

When other treatment options have failed, surgery may be considered. Surgical procedures may include direct closure of the wound, skin grafting, or various skin flap procedures. The decision is based on the patient's condition and the severity of the ulcer. After surgery, vigilantly protect the surgical site from pressure and contamination.

Several other treatment modalities are being investigated. They include electrical stimulation, hyperbaric oxygen, laser irradiation, ultrasound, and miscellaneous topical agents and systemic drugs.

Evaluating

When evaluating the effectiveness of a plan of care designed to prevent the development of pressure ulcers or treat those already present, the nurse uses each nurse–patient interaction to determine if the patient has met the individualized expected outcomes in the plan of care. Nursing care is considered effective if the patient, family member, or caregiver expresses satisfaction with prevention and treatment measures and is able to accomplish the following:

- Participate effectively in preventive and treatment regimens
- Prevent development of any additional areas of skin breakdown
- Demonstrate progressive healing of pressure ulcer
- Improve overall physical condition (including nutritional state and mobility status)
- Remain free of infection at any pressure ulcer site
- Communicate need for additional support (environmental, physical, psychosocial)

Evaluation is a continuous process that involves ongoing assessment and revised plans and implementations. Color photographs are an excellent method of evaluating the progression of wound healing, allowing visual comparison of the pressure ulcer at the initial assessment and throughout the plan of care through the recovery stages (see Nursing Plan of Care 38-1).

HEAT AND COLD THERAPY

Heat and cold are applied to a specific part or all of a patient's body to bring about a local or systemic change in body temperature for various therapeutic purposes. Physiologic responses to heat and cold are modified by the method and duration of application, the degree of heat and cold applied, the patient's age and physical condition, and the amount of body surface covered by the application. Nurses use heat and cold as nursing interventions in both hospital and community-based settings.

Body temperature is regulated by cells in the hypothalamus in response to signals from thermal (heat and cold) receptors located close to the skin's surface. Stimulation of these receptors sends sensory messages to the anterior hypothalamus to initiate mechanisms to dissipate heat (through vasodilation and sweating) or to preserve warmth through vasoconstriction and piloerection ("goose bumps"). Pain receptors, also located near the skin's surface, are also affected by heat and cold as painful stimuli, with excessive heat perceived as burning and excessive cold experienced as numbness followed by pain.

Effects of Applying Heat

The application of local heat dilates peripheral blood vessels, increases tissue metabolism, reduces blood viscosity and increases capillary permeability, reduces muscle tension, and helps relieve pain. Vasodilation increases local blood flow. In turn, the supply of oxygen and nutrients to the area is increased, and venous congestion is decreased. As local blood flow increases, the viscosity of blood is reduced and increased capillary permeability improves the delivery of leukocytes and nutrients while also facilitating the removal of wastes and prolonging clotting time. These actions, combined with increased tissue metabolism, accelerate the inflammatory response to promote healing.

Heat reduces muscle tension to promote relaxation and helps to relieve muscle spasms and joint stiffness. Heat also helps relieve pain by stimulating specific nerve fibers, closing the gate that allows the transmission of pain stimuli to centers in the brain. Because of these local physiologic effects, heat in various forms is used to treat infections, surgical wounds, inflamed tissue, arthritis, joint and muscle pain, dysmenorrhea, and chronic pain.

The systemic effects of extensive, prolonged heat include increased cardiac output, sweating, increased pulse rate, and decreased blood pressure. This response occurs when heat is applied to a large body area, increasing the blood flow to that area while decreasing it to another part of the body (in effect, causing hypovolemic shock).

Effects of Applying Cold

The local application of cold constricts peripheral blood vessels, reduces muscle spasms, and promotes comfort. Cold reduces blood flow to tissues and decreases the local release of pain-producing substances such as histamine, serotonin, and bradykinin. This action in turn reduces the formation of edema and inflammation. Decreased metabolic needs and capillary permeability, combined with increased coagulation of blood at the wound site, facilitate the control of bleeding and reduce edema formation.

Cold also reduces muscle spasm, alters tissue sensitivity (producing numbness), and promotes comfort by slowing the transmission of pain stimuli. Cold, for these effects, is used after direct trauma, for dental pain, for muscle spasms, after sprains, and to treat some chronic pain syndromes.

Exposure to prolonged or extensive environmental cold produces systemic effects of increased blood pressure, shivering, and goose bumps. Although shivering is a normal body response to cold, prolonged cold may cause tissue injury.

Physiologic Considerations

The rebound phenomenon is important to the therapeutic value of heat and cold and to the safety of patients receiving such therapy. Heat produces maximum vasodilation in 20 to 30 minutes; if heat is continued beyond that time, tissue con-

NURSING PLAN OF CARE 38-1   *for Mary Biesicker*

Mary Biesicker, who is 84 years of age, has been cared for at home by her daughter since being hospitalized last year for a stroke. During the past several months, Mary has been confined to her bed, has had minimal appetite, and has occasionally been confused and disoriented. During the past week, she has had several episodes of bowel and bladder incontinence. Her daughter also reports that Mary has developed a "blister on her lower back at the end of her backbone." She is scheduled for an assessment visit by the nurse from a local home care agency because her daughter is finding it increasingly difficult to care for her mother alone.

The nurse's initial assessment of Mary, relative to skin integrity, revealed the following:

Skin status: Presence of a nickel-sized open area on the sacrum (stage II pressure ulcer), 2 cm in diameter and 1 cm in depth. No abnormal pathways noted. Reddened area (0.5 cm) surrounding lesion. No drainage noted. Reddened area (2.5 cm) also noted on right elbow. Skin dry over all body surfaces.

Nutritional status: Daughter states "usual weight is 115–120 lb, and she has definitely lost some weight." Poor skin turgor.

Elimination status: Wearing "adult diaper," diaper damp with urine and small amount of light brown liquid stool.

Activity status: Lying quietly in bed, moans when area around lesion is palpated.

NURSING DIAGNOSIS

Impaired Skin Integrity related to mechanical factors, inactivity, altered nutritional intake, and incontinence as manifested by stage II pressure ulcer on sacral area and reddened area on right elbow

EXPECTED OUTCOME

6/6/06—at weekly visit, the patient will:
- Experience reduction of pressure on bony prominences (absence of any additional reddened areas)

Nursing Interventions	Rationale	Evaluative Statement
Assess skin for development of any pressure areas (use agency tool).	Pressure results in poor circulation that causes skin breakdown.	6/13/06 Outcome met. Patient has been turned from side to side every 2 hours. Reddened area on right elbow measures 1.25 cm in diameter. No new reddened areas observed.
Avoid sitting or lying on a pressure ulcer.	This facilitates pressure relief in the area and allows blood to reenter capillaries and provide oxygen to the area.	
Reposition from side to side at least every 2 hours.	The duration of pressure is more devastating to skin than the amount of pressure.	*Recommendation:* Arrange for delivery of hospital bed with overbed trapeze setup. Secure a home health aide for limited period of time to assist with repositioning during the night and allow daughter time to rest.
Use pillows to maintain side-lying or oblique position in bed and support right elbow off bed surface.	Pillows relieve pressure on lesion and areas at risk and promote improved circulation to those areas.	*M. Lieb, RN*
Place foam overlay mattress on bed.	Static device provides support and relieves pressure on skin surface.	

EXPECTED OUTCOME

6/6/06—at weekly visit, the patient will:
- Demonstrate a reduction in the size of the stage II pressure ulcer on sacrum

Nursing Interventions	Rationale	Evaluative Statement
Assess condition of pressure ulcer at time of dressing change (refer to previous assessments).	Signs of infection and deterioration can be recognized and treatment plan revised.	6/13/06 Outcome met. Pressure ulcer has decreased slightly in size—1.7 cm in diameter, depth remains the same. No apparent infection noted. Will continue with present treatment regimen.
Irrigate wound with normal saline using a 60-mL piston syringe with a catheter tip.	Normal saline cleanses the wound without harming tissues.	
Dry skin thoroughly surrounding the ulcer.	Moisture makes intact skin more susceptible to injury.	*M. Lieb, RN*

(continued)

NURSING PLAN OF CARE 38-1 *for Mary Biesicker (continued)*

Nursing Interventions	Rationale	Evaluative Statement
Apply moisture-retentive dressing (Tegasorb).	Moisture-retentive dressings create a healing environment by allowing epithelial cells to bridge the wound gap and close it.	
Use clean technique for the dressing change.	In the home, the risk is minimal for cross-contamination of microorganisms.	

EXPECTED OUTCOME

6/6/06—at weekly visit, the patient/caregiver will:
• Demonstrate skills required to promote skin integrity and care for a pressure ulcer

Nursing Interventions	Rationale	Evaluative Statement
Assess caregiver's (daughter) motivation and ability to manage treatment regimen.	Motivation influences readiness to learn and contributes to positive learning outcomes.	6/13/06 Outcome partially met. Daughter able to recognize appearance of pressure areas on skin. Stated she would like to review treatment routine again. Daughter performed assessment and dressing change satisfactorily with nurse in attendance. Clarified and reviewed written instructions again. Daughter states, "I feel much more confident now."
Instruct daughter about causes, skin assessment techniques, and individualized treatment regimen. Provide written instructions and illustrations when possible.	A clear concise teaching guide provides consistent education and is available for reinforcement.	
Provide information about community resources available for assistance with care of mother.	Resources provide opportunity for support and problem solving.	M. Lieb, RN

SAMPLE DOCUMENTATION

6/20/06   Home care visit (nursing)

Mrs. Biesicker was revisited in her home for continued assessment and treatment of pressure ulcer. Nursing diagnosis: Impaired Skin Integrity related to pressure, inactivity, inadequate nutritional intake, and incontinence. According to daughter, patient was turned and repositioned every 2 hours. Foam mattress and pillow supports used for support and pressure reduction. Dressing on pressure ulcer changed. Wound cleansed with normal saline, intact skin surrounding wound, and Tegasorb dressing applied. Granulation tissue noted in wound bed, no evidence of drainage or reddened area around wound. Ulcer has decreased to 1½ cm in size. Reddened area not apparent on right elbow. Reviewed written instructions with daughter for 6/23/04 to discuss healthcare options. Will continue current plan of care and visits every other day.

M. Lieb, RN

gestion and vasoconstriction occur (for unknown reasons). With cold, maximum vasoconstriction occurs when the skin reaches 15°C (60°F); then vasodilation begins.

The ability of the body to adapt to heat and cold is an important consideration when applying heat or cold and when teaching patients and caregivers about heat and cold therapy. Initially, heat and cold skin receptors are strongly stimulated by sudden changes in temperature. For the first few seconds after being stimulated, the response decreases rapidly; it then decreases more slowly for the next 30 minutes, as the receptors adapt to the temperature. A hot application, even if the temperature remains constant, does not feel as warm after adaptation has taken place. Be sure to inform patients that increasing the temperature or lengthening the time of application can seriously damage tissues.

THE NURSING PROCESS FOR HEAT AND COLD THERAPY

Assessing

Before initiating heat or cold therapy, assess the patient's physical and mental status, the condition of the body area to be treated with heat or cold, and the condition of the equipment to be used. Carefully evaluate factors influencing the patient's ability to tolerate heat and cold applications. These factors are the basis for the following considerations with rationale:

- How long will the heat or cold be applied? Prolonged exposure increases tolerance, and rebound effects are undesirable.
- What body part is involved? Some body areas, such as the neck, perineum, and inner aspects of the wrist and forearm, are more sensitive to thermal changes.
- Is the skin intact? Open tissue or abraded skin is more sensitive to thermal changes.
- How large is the area? Applications of heat or cold to large areas of the body cause systemic responses and lower tolerance of temperature change.
- What is the patient's age? Infants, children, and older adults do not tolerate temperature changes as well as adults.
- What is the patient's physical condition? Patients with certain alterations in health, such as those with cardiovascular or peripheral vascular diseases, might have reduced response to or tolerance of thermal changes.

Assessing Physical Status

Assessing the patient's physical status includes obtaining a health history and completing a physical examination. A history of cardiovascular or peripheral vascular impairment, sensory impairment, and alterations in mental status (such as confusion or decreased level of consciousness) indicates the need for caution when using heat or cold because of the danger of tissue damage. Assessments include response to stimuli (sharp and dull), color and appearance of body tissues, circulation (pulses, blanching sign, temperature, and color), level of consciousness, and orientation.

> Consider Mr. Everly, the postoperative patient in the critical care unit, and imagine if the physician had ordered heat or cold applications for this patient. The nurse would need to obtain a thorough assessment of his physical status when planning this care because his history of diabetes and circulation problems, in conjunction with his decreased level of consciousness, would place him at high risk for injury and tissue damage. In addition, the nurse would need to assess him frequently during the application of heat or cold to ensure his safety.

Heat should not be applied to an open wound immediately after the trauma; during hemorrhage; over noninflammatory edema; to an acutely inflamed area, a localized malignant tumor, the testes, or the abdomen of a pregnant woman; or over metallic implants. Conversely, cold should not be used for open wounds or for patients with impaired peripheral circulation or allergy to cold.

Assessing the Area of Application

Baseline assessments are used to ensure safety and to evaluate the outcomes of therapy. The risk for damage to tissues is increased if the area is traumatized or has altered integrity. Assess for open lesions, blisters, wounds, edema, bleeding, or drainage or evidence of altered circulation, such as changes in color, temperature, pulses, and sensation. As with any assessment, compare body parts bilaterally for changes. Tissue with decreased or absent pulses, those that appear pale or cyanotic, and those that feel cold to the touch indicate a decrease in circulation. Subsequently, the risk for injury from heat and cold applications increases.

When the heat or cold is applied, ongoing assessments are made to ensure patient safety and comfort. When heat is applied, assess the patient for undesired responses, including localized redness, blistering, and pain (symptoms of burning), along with possible systemic responses, such as hypotension and changes in consciousness. When cold is applied, assess for localized responses, including pallor, cyanosis, numbness, and pain.

Assessing the Condition of Equipment

The nurse is responsible for checking the equipment used and for maintaining patient safety. Included in this responsibility is checking the condition of cords, plugs, and heating or cooling elements. In addition, inspect the equipment for fluid leaks. Also check to ensure that the equipment distributes and maintains the constant temperature. Do not use faulty equipment; if found, it should be returned for repair.

Diagnosing

The patient's need for and response to the heat or cold suggest possible nursing diagnoses, including the following:
Ineffective Thermoregulation
Ineffective Tissue Perfusion
Acute Pain
Risk for Injury

Outcome Identification and Planning

Heat and cold are used for a variety of therapeutic purposes that are an essential part of planning individualized care and forming the basis for patient outcomes. When applications of heat or cold are part of a plan of care, the following outcomes are appropriate (specific outcomes should be chosen based on the purpose of the application). The patient will:
- Verbalize increased comfort
- Demonstrate evidence of wound healing, decreased muscle spasms, decreased edema, and increased comfort
- Verbalize and demonstrate safe hot or cold application

Implementing

Heat and cold applications may be moist or dry, using many forms and methods. The prescription for the heat and cold application should include the type of application, the body area to be treated, and the frequency and length of time for the applications.

Explain the purpose and steps of the application and the sensations that will be experienced. In the hospital, provide a timer or clock and have the call light within reach. In the home, teach the patient or family member to check the equipment each time to ensure that it is in good working order; to avoid lying or leaning on the equipment; to cover the heating device with a protective cloth; to apply heat only for the prescribed time period; and to report any changes in sensation or discomfort to the healthcare provider.

Applying Heat

Heat is applied by both dry and moist methods. Hot water bottles, electric heating pads, aquathermia pads, or chemical heat packs provide local dry heat by conduction (Skill 38-4). Heat lamps or heat cradles provide dry heat by radiation. Hot compresses or packs, sitz baths, or soaks provide moist heat by conduction.

Dry Heat
Hot Water Bags or Bottles

Hot water bags are a method of dry heat application. Although relatively easy and inexpensive to use, they have

---

SKILL 38-4   Applying an External Heating Device

EQUIPMENT

Hot water bag	40.5° to 43.3°C (105° to 110°F) for	Aquathermia pad
Cover for bag	infants, young children, elderly people,	Electrically controlled unit
Water at the appropriate temperature:	diabetic	Distilled water
46.1° to 51.6°C (115° to 125°F) for older	patients, unconscious	Cover for pad
children and	patients	Gauze bandage or tape
adults	Bath thermometer	(to secure pad)

ACTION	RATIONALE
1. Explain the procedure to the patient.	Explanation facilitates cooperation and provides reassurance for patient.
2. Assess condition of skin where heat is to be applied.	Impaired circulation may affect sensitivity to heat. Elderly people and very young children have the least tolerance to applications of heat.
3. Assemble necessary equipment, and close door or curtain if privacy is desired.	Organization facilitates performance of task.
4. Perform hand hygiene.	Hand hygiene deters the spread of microorganisms.

HOT WATER BAG

5. Check temperature of water with bath thermometer or test on inner wrist. Rinse bag with water, empty, and then fill.	This provides for application of heat within the acceptable range for individual. Rinsing bag with warm water warms the rubber.
6. Fill hot water bag one-half to two-thirds full.	Hot water bottle molds more easily to area and puts less pressure on site.
7. Expel remaining air from bag in one of two ways: Place the bag on a flat surface, permit the water to come to the opening, and then close the bag; or, hold the bag up, twist the unfilled portion to remove the air, and then close the bag. Fasten top securely. Check for leaks.	Air reduces pliability of bag. Securing the top prevents leakage of water and discomfort for patient.
8. Cover bag with towel or other protector, and apply hot water bottle to prescribed area.	Covering the device protects skin from direct contact with rubber. Heat travels by conduction from one object to another.
9. Assess condition of skin and patient's response to heat at frequent intervals. Do not exceed prescribed length of time for application of heat. Remove hot water bag if excessive swelling, redness, or pain occurs, and report to physician.	Maximum therapeutic effects from application of heat occur within 20 to 30 minutes. Extended use of heat (beyond 45 minutes) results in tissue congestion and vasoconstriction. This rebound phenomenon results in increased risk to patient of burns from application of heat.

(continued)

SKILL
38-4   **Applying an External Heating Device** (continued)

HOT WATER BAG

10. After removal, record patient's response and dispose of equipment appropriately.	Accurate documentation of procedure ensures continuity of care.
11. Perform hand hygiene.	Hand hygiene deters the spread of microorganisms.

AQUATHERMIA PAD

12. Check that distilled water is at appropriate level. Use key to adjust temperature at 40.6°C (105°F) if it has not already been preset. Plug in unit, and warm pad before use.	Water temperature is regulated by key. Presetting the temperature eliminates risk of patient adjusting the temperature.
13. Cover pad with pillowcase or other protector, and apply to prescribed area. Do not allow patient to lie on pad if applying to back. Patient should assume prone position and place aquathermia pad on back.	Covering the device protects skin from direct contact with rubber or source of heat. Pressure reduces dissipation of heat.
14. Secure with gauze bandage or tape. Never use safety pins to hold pad in place.	Securing the pad holds it in the proper position on patient. Pins may puncture and damage the pad.
15. Same as actions 9 to 11.	Same as actions 9 to 11.

disadvantages. They may leak, and often the weight of the bag or bottle on the patient's body part can be uncomfortable. Moreover, there is a danger of burns from improper use.

Electric Heating Pads
The electric heating pad can be used to apply dry heat locally. It is easy to apply, is relatively safe to use, and provides constant and even heat. Improper use can, however, result in injury. When applying a heating pad, follow these recommendations:

- Avoid using pins to secure a heating pad. There is a danger of electric shock if a pin touches a wire.
- Place a covering over the pad, preferably one that is moisture-proof. Also prevent wet and moist conditions around the pad. Short-circuiting the heating element may cause an electric shock. Do not cover the heating pad with anything that might be heavy; heat may accumulate and burn the patient when it cannot dissipate normally from the pad.
- Place a heating pad anteriorly or laterally to, not under, the body part. If the heating pad is between the patient and the mattress, heat dissipation may be inadequate, leading to burning of the patient or the bed linens.
- Use a heating pad with a selector switch that cannot be turned up beyond a safe temperature. After heat has been applied and a certain amount of adaptation of heat receptors takes place, the patient often increases the heat when the switch is not permanently preset because the pad does not seem sufficiently warm. Many people have been burned by turning up the heat in an electric pad because they thought the pad was too cool.
- Assess the skin at regular intervals for the effects of excessive exposure to heat, such as increased skin redness, changes in sensation, or discomfort.

- Check agency protocol for the use of heating pads; a release form may need to be signed.

Aquathermia Pads
Aquathermia (Aqua-K) pads are commonly used in healthcare agencies and homes for various health problems, including back pain, muscle spasms, thrombophlebitis, and mild inflammation. These devices are safer to use than a heating pad, but they too must be checked carefully. Guidelines for using aquathermia pads are given in Guidelines for Nursing Care 38-5.

Guidelines for Nursing Care 38-5
Aquathermia Pads

- Keep in mind that the temperature setting is usually set and locked before application.
- If the distilled water in the reservoir runs low, add more at the top of the control unit. Fill two thirds of the control unit. Tighten the cap and then loosen it one-quarter turn to allow heat expansion Do not use tap water.
- Place the unit above the patient so that gravity will help make the water flow.
- Plug in the unit and let it warm for 2 minutes, making sure that the temperature does not exceed 40.6°C (105°F).
- Allow the application to remain in place for only 20 to 30 minutes.
- Assess the patient's skin frequently.

Heat Lamps

Heat lamps provide dry heat to increase circulation to a small area, such as a pressure ulcer. They are available with either infrared or regular 40- to 60-watt bulbs. The lamps (often gooseneck type) are placed 46 to 76 cm (18 to 30 inches) from the area to be treated and applied for 15 to 20 minutes. When using a heat lamp, follow these precautions:

- Clean and dry the area before the treatment to prevent burning.
- Do not cover the lamp or place it under the bedclothes.
- Assess the skin exposed to heat every 5 minutes.

Heat Cradles

A heat cradle is a metal half-circle frame that encloses the body part to be treated with heat. A series of 25-watt bulbs, 16 to 18 inches (41 to 46 cm) from the patient, provides heat over a larger area. The cradle may be covered with a sheet. Treatments usually last for 15 minutes. If the physician orders a heat cradle, follow the recommended precautions to prevent burning as for a heat lamp.

Hot Packs

Commercial hot packs provide a specified amount of dry heat for a specific period. Instructions on the package describe how to activate the pack, either by striking it on a firm surface or by squeezing or kneading it. Follow the same precautions as for other types of dry heat applications.

Moist Heat

Sterile Warm Moist Compresses

Sterile warm moist compresses are used on wounds to promote circulation and wound healing (especially if infected) and to reduce edema. Because moist heat evaporates and cools rapidly, the compresses must be changed frequently and covered with a heating agent (hot water bottle, heating pad, Aqua-K pad) or plastic wrap to maintain heat. Skill 38-5 describes the application of warm sterile compresses to an open wound.

Sitz Baths

Sitz baths are a method of applying tepid or hot water to the pelvic or rectal area by sitting in a tub, special chair, or basin filled with sufficient water to reach the umbilicus. Special basins that fit onto the toilet seat are available. They are designed so that the patient's buttocks fit into a rather deep seat that is filled with water of the desired temperature; the legs and feet remain out of the water. The basins are disposable and economical for home or healthcare agency use. A regular bathtub is not as satisfactory for a sitz bath because the heat causes generalized vasodilation, altering the effect desired. Techniques for administering a sitz bath are given in Guidelines for Nursing Care 38-6.

Warm Soaks

The immersion of a body area into warm water or a medicated solution is called a soak. The purposes of soaks vary: to increase blood supply to a locally infected area; to aid in cleaning large, sloughing wounds, such as burns; to improve circulation; and to apply medication to a locally infected area. A soak has the added advantage of making manipulation of a painful area much easier because the body part is buoyed by the weight of water it displaces. If a warm soak is ordered, follow these general guidelines:

- If a soak is prescribed for a large wound (eg, an entire arm or lower leg or even an area of the torso), expect to adapt sterile technique. For example, the container into which the body area is placed is sterilized before use if possible; if not, the container is cleaned scrupulously. Tap water may be used for soaks because it is accepted as being free from pathogens.
- Unless the temperature of the soak is prescribed otherwise, set the temperature of the water within a range of 40.5° to 43°C (105° to 109°F), which is considered to be physiologically effective and comfortable for the patient.
- Position the container holding the fluid so that the part to be immersed is comfortable and the patient is in good body alignment.
- During the treatment, which usually takes 15 to 20 minutes per soak, maintain the temperature of the soak as constant as possible. This may be done by discarding some of the fluid every 5 minutes and replacing it or by adding solutions at a higher temperature while agitating the water. When replacing or adding fluids, have the patient remove the extremity from the soak.

Applying Cold

Cold is applied by both dry and moist methods. Dry cold is provided with ice bags, cold packs, or a hypothermia blanket (or pad). Cold compresses are a method of applying moist cold.

Dry Cold

Ice Bags

Ice bags, like their counterpart hot water bottles or bags, are relatively easy and inexpensive methods for applying cold to an area. They have essentially the same disadvantages as hot water bags. When using an ice bag, follow these recommendations:

- Fill the bag with small pieces of ice to about two-thirds full. This makes the bag light in weight. Using ice chips, rather than cubes, makes it easier to mold the bag to the body part.
- Remove air from the ice bag in the same manner as removing air from a hot water bag.
- After securing the cap, test the ice bag for leaks and wipe off excess moisture.
- Place a cover on the ice bag to provide comfort and to absorb moisture that may accumulate on the outside of the bag.
- Apply an ice bag for 30 minutes and then remove it for about an hour before reapplying it. This technique prevents the effects of prolonged exposure to cold.
- In the home setting, a bag of frozen vegetables (such as peas) makes a good substitute for an ice bag.

SKILL
38-5   **Applying Warm Sterile Compresses to an Open Wound**

EQUIPMENT

Prescribed solution (warmed to about 40°
  to 43°C [105° to 110°F])
Sterile container for solution
Sterile gauze dressings or compresses
Sterile gloves

Clean disposable gloves
Waterproof pad
Dry bath towel
Bath blanket
Tape or ties

Aquathermia or external heating
  device (optional)
Sterile bath thermometer (if available, to
  check temperature of solution)

ACTION	RATIONALE
1. Assess patient for any circulatory impairment to area where compress is to be applied (numbness, tingling, impairment in temperature sensation, or cyanosis).	Circulatory impairment may interfere with patient's ability to perceive heat and place him or her at risk of injury from the application of heat.
2. Check physician's order for warm compresses. Explain procedure to patient.	An explanation encourages patient cooperation and reduces apprehension.
3. Gather equipment.	This provides for organized approach to task.
4. Perform hand hygiene.	Hand hygiene deters spread of microorganisms.
5. Close door or curtain. Use bath blanket as needed when exposing area for application of warm compresses. Position waterproof pad under patient.	Closing door or curtain provides for privacy and warmth
6. Assist patient to comfortable position that provides easy access to area.	Proper positioning allows comfort and ease of application of compresses.
7. Place opened, cuffed plastic bag near working area.	Soiled dressings may be placed in disposal bag without contaminating outside surfaces of bag.
8. Prepare aquathermia pad or external heating device (optional).	External heating device allows compress to retain heat for longer interval.
9. Using sterile technique, open dressings, and warmed solution. Pour solution into sterile container, and carefully drop gauze for compresses into sterile solution.	Sterile technique is used for warm moist compresses to an open wound.
10. Don clean disposable glove, and remove any dressing carefully. Discard dressing in disposable plastic bag. Pull off soiled glove inside out, and drop it in bag.	Using gloves prevents spread of microorganisms by contaminated dressings.
11. Assess wound healing or presence of infection.	Assessment documents condition of wound before application of compress.
12. Don sterile gloves.	Gloves maintain surgical asepsis.
13. Retrieve sterile compress from warmed solution, and squeeze moisture from it. Apply carefully, and gently mold around wound. Be alert for patient's response to heat.	Excess moisture may contaminate surrounding area and is uncomfortable for patient. Molding compress to skin promotes retention of warmth around wound site.
14. Cover the gauze compresses with dry bath towel, and secure in place if necessary.	Towel provides additional insulation.
15. Apply aquathermia pad or external heating device over towel (optional).	Temperature is controlled, extending therapeutic effect of compress.
16. Monitor condition of skin and patient's response to warm compress at frequent intervals.	Impaired circulation may affect sensitivity to heat
17. After 30 minutes (or time ordered by physician), remove warm compress. Carefully observe condition of skin around wound and patient's response to application of heat.	Maximum therapeutic effects of heat occur within 20 to 30 minutes. Extended use of heat (beyond 45 minutes) results in tissue congestion and vasoconstriction. This rebound phenomenon results in increased risk to patient of burns from application of heat.
18. Apply sterile dressing to wound (see Skill 38-1).	Dressing protects wound from microorganisms in environment.
19. Dispose of equipment appropriately. Perform hand hygiene.	Proper disposal deters spread of microorganisms.
20. Record patient's response and condition of wound and surrounding skin area.	Accurate documentation of procedure ensures continuity of care.

Guidelines for Nursing Care 38-6
Sitz Bath

- Test the water in a sitz bath with a thermometer before the patient enters the water.
- If the purpose of the sitz bath is to apply heat, use water at a temperature of 34° to 37°C (109°–115°F) for 15 minutes to produce relaxation of the parts involved after a short initial period of contraction. Warm water should not be used if considerable congestion is already present.
- If the purpose of the sitz bath is to produce relaxation or to promote healing in a wound by cleansing it of discharge and debris, use water at a temperature of 34° to 37°C (93°–99°F). Check agency protocols for the correct temperature.
- Assist the patient into the tub or onto the sitz bath and position properly. The patient should be able to sit in the basin or tub with the feet flat on the floor without any pressure on the sacrum or thighs.
- Wrap a blanket around the shoulders to protect from chilling and exposure.
- Monitor the patient closely for signs of weakness and fatigue, and discontinue the bath if faintness, pallor, a rapid pulse rate, or nausea is noted.
- Test the water in the tub several times, and keep it at the desired temperature. Additional hot water may be added by pouring it slowly from a pitcher or by opening the hot water faucet slightly. The water should be agitated by stirring it as hot water is added to prevent burning the patient.
- Do not leave the patient alone if there are any questions about safety.
- Help the patient out of the tub when the bath is completed. A sitz bath should take 15 to 30 minutes. Help the patient dry, and cover him or her adequately.

Cold Packs

Commercially prepared ice packs are available in many healthcare agencies and may be purchased commercially. These bags are sealed containers filled with a chemical or a nontoxic substance. Depending on the type, the bags are frozen in the freezer or (if not frozen) are squeezed to activate the chemical that produces the cold. These packs are advantageous because the frozen solution remains pliable and can be easily molded to fit the body part. They are covered with a ribbed cotton sleeve so that the bag can be slipped onto an extremity, or the bag can simply be placed on a body part, such as the head. The skin beneath the pack should be assessed periodically for symptoms of numbness and pain.

Hypothermia Blankets

Body temperature may be lowered by placing the patient on a special hypothermia blanket or pad. This apparatus has coils through which a refrigerated solution circulates. It operates much like an Aqua-K heating unit, except that the liquid is cooled instead of heated. When applying a hypothermia blanket, follow these steps:

- Place the hypothermia blanket on the bed and cover it with a sheet so the patient's skin does not come in direct contact with the cold blanket. Position the patient on the blanket.
- Connect the cooling blanket to the machine and select the cool temperature setting.
- Insert the probe into the patient's anus to monitor body temperature. Monitor the rectal temperature every 15 minutes and all vital signs every 30 minutes.
- Set the temperature control at 98.6°F (37°C) to begin, then decrease it 2° to 3° every 15 minutes until the temperature that is ordered or that is agency policy is reached.
- When the treatment is discontinued, turn off the machine and continue to monitor temperature every 2 hours for 24 hours.

In addition to vital signs, assess the patient for shivering (shivering increases heat production, and is often controlled with medications), fluid status, edema, and altered skin integrity.

Moist Cold

Moist, cold local applications are called cold compresses. They might be used for an injured eye, a headache, a tooth extraction, and sometimes for hemorrhoids. The texture and thickness of the material used depend on the area to which it is applied. For example, eye compresses could be prepared from surgical gauze compresses, which have a small amount of cotton filling. A washcloth makes an excellent compress for the head or face.

Immerse the material used for the application in a clean basin that contains pieces of ice and a small amount of water. Wring the compress thoroughly before applying it to avoid dripping. Dripping is uncomfortable for the patient and may result in wetting the patient's clothing or bed linens. Change the compress frequently, continuing the application for 20 minutes. Repeat the application every 2 to 3 hours as ordered. Ice bags or commercial devices are available for keeping the compresses cold, helping to decrease the frequency with which they must be changed.

Evaluating

The expected outcomes for applying heat and cold when included as part of a plan of care are used to evaluate the effectiveness of the planned interventions. Although the specific outcomes depend on the purpose of the application, nursing care is considered effective if the patient is able to:
- Verbalize increased comfort
- Verbalize increased ability to rest and sleep
- Demonstrate evidence of wound healing
- Demonstrate a decrease in symptoms of muscle spasms, inflammation, and edema
- Verbalize and demonstrate safe hot and cold applications

Developing Critical Thinking Skills

1. How would you individualize your teaching about needed supplies, wound care, and resources for the following patients:
   - A homeless man admitted to the hospital for gangrene of the big toe. The toe has been amputated.
   - A teenage gang member treated in the emergency department for a superficial (but long) knife wound
   - An infant who has had abdominal surgery and is now having diarrhea
   - A frail, 80-year-old man who needs daily dressing changes on a draining wound, who lives with his blind wife

2. Describe the nursing interventions you would include in a plan of care to prevent pressure ulcers in the following patients:
   - A middle-aged woman, 70 pounds over normal body weight, who has a fractured femur and is recovering at home (she lives alone)
   - A 90-year-old man with cognitive impairment who is confined to bed
   - A 17-year-old girl who is paralyzed from the waist down after a diving accident and is wheelchair dependent

Practicing for NCLEX

1. After a surgical incision, a patient often has an elevated body temperature and generalized malaise. These manifestations most often occur during which phase of wound healing?
   a. Inflammatory
   b. Primary
   c. Fibroplasia
   d. Maturation

2. Which term would the nurse use to document wound drainage that is thick, odorous, and green?
   a. Serous
   b. Sanguineous
   c. Serosanguineous
   d. Purulent

3. A patient who has a large abdominal wound suddenly calls out for help because she feels as though something is falling out of her incision. Inspection reveals a gaping open wound with tissue bulging outward. You immediately report this as:
   a. An overproduction of granulation tissue
   b. Wound dehiscence with evisceration
   c. A normal response to a large wound
   d. An unknown complication

4. Sara Liu, age 16, was in an automobile accident and received a wound across her nose and cheek. After surgery to repair the wound, Sara says, "I am so ugly now." Based on this statement, what nursing diagnosis would be most appropriate?
   a. Pain
   b. Impaired Skin Integrity
   c. Disturbed Body Image
   d. Disturbed Thought Processes

5. Which action is believed to be most useful in preventing wound infections?
   a. Using sterile dressing supplies
   b. Suggesting dietary supplements
   c. Applying antibiotic ointment
   d. Performing careful hand hygiene

6. During a dressing change, inspection of the wound reveals what appears to be reddish-pink tissue in the wound. The nurse interprets this as most likely indicating:
   a. A sign of infection
   b. Eschar
   c. Exudate
   d. Granulation tissue

7. Which intervention would the nurse expect to use for applying moist heat?
   a. Sitz bath
   b. Aquathermia pad
   c. Heat lamp
   d. Commercial hot pack

8. When assessing a patient at risk for pressure ulcer formation, which site would the nurse identify as being most common?
   a. Occipital area
   b. Sacrum
   c. Sternum
   d. Humerus

9. When explaining about factors contributing to pressure ulcers, which factor would the nurse describe as key?
   a. Moisture
   b. Incontinence
   c. Pressure
   d. Malnutrition

10. Which hospitalized patient is most at risk for a pressure ulcer?
    a. A 70-year-old patient with a fractured hip
    b. A 45-year-old woman recovering from gallbladder surgery
    c. A 16-year-old male who suffered a spinal cord injury
    d. A 50-year-old patient who suffered a mild stroke

11. After an initial assessment, the nurse documents the presence of a reddened area that has blistered. According to recognized staging systems, this ulcer is classified as:
    a. Stage I
    b. Stage II
    c. Stage III
    d. Stage IV

12. An older confused patient sits and slumps in her chair most of the day. She is most likely to develop a pressure ulcer because of:

a. Malnutrition
b. Shearing forces
c. Edema
d. A chronic disease

13. The nurse assesses a stage III pressure ulcer manifested as:
    a. Redness that persists when pressure is relieved
    b. An open lesion with subcutaneous tissue exposed
    c. A necrotic area extending through the fascia to bone
    d. A reddened area with an abrasion

14. Which action would be a priority in preventing a patient from developing a pressure ulcer?
    a. Using waterproof material on the bed
    b. Massaging any reddened area frequently
    c. Using an air-inflated ring to relieve pressure on areas
    d. Using a mild soap when cleansing the skin

15. Which treatment would the nurse expect to institute for a patient with a stage II pressure ulcer?
    a. A moisture-retentive dressing
    b. Surgical débridement
    c. Exposure to a heat lamp four times daily
    d. Whirlpool treatment twice daily

incontinence, and malnutrition predispose a patient to impaired skin integrity, making the skin more susceptible to injury.

10. The correct answer is *a*. An older patient with a fractured hip already has age-related skin changes that, coupled with some degree of immobility, make that person a likely candidate.

11. The correct answer is *b*. A stage II pressure ulcer is superficial and presents clinically as an abrasion, ulcer, or shallow crater.

12. The correct answer is *b*. Sitting slumped in a chair for an extended period can easily result in shearing force, causing a pressure ulcer. Malnutrition, edema, and the presence of chronic disease may certainly be risk factors for the development of a pressure ulcer, but the most likely cause in this situation is shearing force.

13. The correct answer is *b*. A stage III pressure ulcer is an open lesion that exposes subcutaneous tissue. Redness that persists is stage I; a reddened area that has an abrasion is stage II; and a necrotic area extending through the fascia to the bone is stage IV.

14. The correct answer is *d*. A mild soap is less irritating. The skin should be rinsed and dried thoroughly.

15. The correct answer is *a*. A moisture-retentive dressing provides a moist environment for wound healing.

Answers With Rationale

1. The correct answer is *a*. Systemic manifestations occur as a result of the inflammatory response to the altered skin and tissue integrity. Systemic manifestations do not usually continue into the fibroplasia and maturation phases of wound healing.

2. The correct answer is *d*. Purulent drainage is the result of an infection and is thick, odorous, and colored.

3. The correct answer is *b*. The wound complications of dehiscence and evisceration are manifested by a wound that opens up and has viscera protruding.

4. The correct answer is *c*. Wounds cause emotional as well as physical stress.

5. The correct answer is *d*. Although all of the answers may help in preventing wound infections, careful handwashing (medical asepsis) is the most important.

6. The correct answer is *d*. Granulation tissue is new tissue composed of many small blood vessels, is pinkish red, and fills an open wound when it starts to heal.

7. The correct answer is *a*. A sitz bath is a moist heat application. All the other responses are examples of dry heat.

8. The correct answer is *b*. All sites involve bony prominences, but the sacrum is the most common area where pressure ulcers develop.

9. The correct answer is *c*. Pressure is a key factor contributing to a pressure ulcer. It interferes with circulation to the cell, resulting in cell death. Moisture,

Bibliography

Atkinson, A. (2002). Body image considerations in patients with wounds. *Journal of Community Nursing, 16*(10), 32, 34, 36.

Bergstrom, N., Braden, B., Laguzza, A., & Holman, V. (1987). The Braden scale for predicting pressure sore risk. *Nursing Research, 36*(4), 205–210.

Braden, B., & Ayello, E. (2002). How and why to do pressure ulcer risk assessment. *Advances in Skin & Wound Care: The Journal for Prevention and Healing, 15*(3), 125–131.

Bullock, B. (1996). *Pathophysiology: Adaptations and alterations in function* (4th ed.). Philadelphia: Lippincott.

Bullock, B., & Henze, R. (1999). *Focus on pathophysiology.* Philadelphia: Lippincott.

Carpenito, L. (2002). *Nursing diagnosis: Application to clinical practice* (9th ed.). Philadelphia: Lippincott.

Davidson, M. (2002). Sharpen your wound assessment skills. *Nursing, 32*(10), 32hn1.

Franz, R., Gardner, S., Specht, J., et al. (2001). Integration of pressure ulcer treatment protocol into practice: Clinical outcomes and care environment attributes. *Outcomes Management for Nursing Practice, 5*(3), 112–120.

Krasner, D. (1995). Wound care: How to use the red-yellow-black system. *American Journal of Nursing, 5*(95), 44–47.

Mayo Clinic Geriatric Medicine. (2001). *Pressure Ulcers: Prevention and Management.* Available at http://www.mayo.edu/geriatrics-rst/PU.

McCloskey, J. C., & Bulechek, G. M. (2000). *Iowa Intervention Project: Nursing Interventions Classification (NIC)* (3rd ed.). St. Louis: C. V. Mosby.

North American Nursing Diagnosis Association. (2002). *NANDA nursing diagnoses: Definitions and classification 2002–2003*. Philadelphia: Author.

Ovington, L., & Schaum, K. (2001). Wound care products: How to choose. *Home Healthcare Nurse, 19*(4), 224–232, 240.

Pieper, B., Templin, T., Dobal, et al. (2002). Home care nurses' ratings of appropriateness of wound treatments and wound healing. *Journal of WOCN, 29*(1), 20–28.

Pieper, B., Sugrue, M., Weiland, M., Sprague, K., & Heitman, C. (1998). Risk factors, prevention methods, and wound care for patients with pressure ulcers. *Clinical Nurse Specialist, 12*(1), 7–14.

Porth, C. M. (2002). *Pathophysiology: Concepts of altered health states*. Philadelphia: Lippincott.

Stitik, T., & Nadler, S. (1999). Sports injuries: When—and how—to apply the heat. *Consultant, 39*(1), 144–157.

Stotts, N. (1990). Seeing red, yellow, and black: The three-color concept of wound care. *Nursing, 20*(2), 59–61.

Stotts, N. (1999). Evidence-based practice: What is it and how is it used in wound care? *Nursing Clinics of North America, 34*(4), 955–963.

U.S. Department of Health and Human Services, Agency for Health Care Policy and Research (1992). *Pressure ulcers in adults: Prediction and prevention*. Rockville, MD: Author. Also available at http://www.ahcpr.gov/clinic/cpgoline.htm

U.S. Department of Health and Human Services, Agency for Health Care Policy and Research. (1994). *Treatment of pressure ulcers*. Rockville, MD: Author. Also available at http://www.ahcpr.gov/clinic/cpgoline.htm

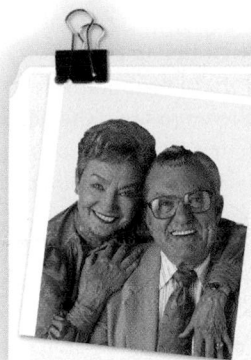

Genevieve Augustus is caring for her aging husband in their home since his stroke approximately 2 months ago. She states "My bones and joints hurt all the time. It's quite a bit of work caring for Josef. He needs a lot of help turning, moving and getting out of bed."

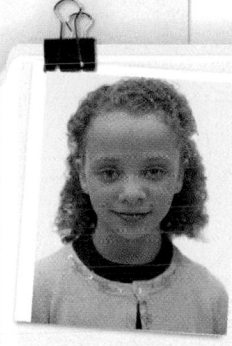

Kelsi Lester is a 10-year-old girl in the pediatric unit as a result of a skiing accident. Unconscious at present, she may or may not regain consciousness. She is on complete bed rest and requires both frequent positioning to maintain correct body alignment and attention to her range of motion.

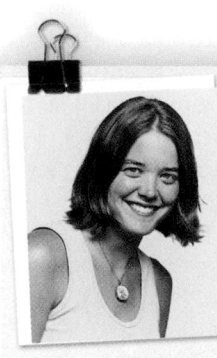

Maggie Wyatt, a woman in her 30s with a fractured right tibia, is being treated with an external fixation device that has caused an infection. Following therapy for the infection, the patient is being discharged and requires transfer from the wheelchair to her mother's car.

Focusing on Blended Skills

The types of blended skills you'll need to respond to the case scenarios include:

Cognitive Skills

- Basic knowledge of the physiology of movement, the principles of body mechanics and factors affecting body alignment and mobility, and complications related to immobility
- Knowledge of common problems associated with mobility and activity
- Knowledge of proper use of body mechanics
- Knowledge of how to design and implement a plan of care to prevent complications related to immobility and to treat mobility problems
- Ability to identify possible complications associated with immobility for a patient who is comatose and confined to bed
- Ability to integrate knowledge of the effects of activity, exercise, and immobility on a patient's functional status
- Knowledge of factors affecting mobility, including age, physical changes, and therapeutic devices
- Ability to integrate knowledge of measures used to transfer patients to ensure patient safety and comfort
- Ability to identify patients with impaired mobility, and develop and implement appropriate plans to address these impairments
- Ability to work with individuals with wide-ranging problems involving mobility, including an older woman caring for her husband, a young girl who is comatose, and a woman with an external device to treat a fracture

Technical Skills

- Strong assessment skills to identify problems related to mobility for an older woman caring for her ill husband at home, a child in a coma confined to bed, and a woman with a fractured tibia
- Ability to use correctly the protocols, products, and equipment necessary to promote body alignment and to prevent or treat complications related to immobility
- Ability to provide the technical nursing assistance necessary to meet the mobility and activity needs of patients
- Ability to demonstrate active and passive range-of-motion techniques
- Ability to demonstrate correct technique when performing passive range of motion with a patient who is comatose and confined to bed
- Demonstration of proper body mechanics when meeting the mobility needs of a patient caring for her ill husband at home, a child who is comatose and confined to bed, and a woman with a fractured tibia
- Ability to adapt techniques as necessary to meet the needs of patients, including a woman with an external device used to treat a fractured tibia

- Ability to ask for assistance when faced with new, unfamiliar, or challenging situations, such as transferring a woman with an external fixation device to the car at discharge

Interpersonal Skills

- Demonstration of strong people skills, including the ability to communicate and interact effectively with patients and their caregivers while assisting with mobility and activity
- Ability to interact effectively and work collaboratively with other members of the healthcare team to meet the needs of patients requiring assistance with mobility
- Demonstration of knowledge related to personal limitations, with a willingness to seek out help when needed
- Ability to demonstrate respect for a patient's human dignity and autonomy, regardless of whether the patient is an older woman caring for her ill husband at home, a child in a coma, or a woman who is to be discharged with an external fixation device in place
- Ability to encourage patients and their caregivers to maximize their mobility and functional status

Ethical and Legal Skills

- A strong sense of accountability for the health and well-being of patients (such as an older woman caring for an ill husband, a child in a coma, and a woman being discharged with a fractured femur)
- Ability to integrate knowledge of ethical and legal principles underlying safe mobility and activity in the home, prevention of complications in a comatose child, and discharge of a patient from the hospital
- Commitment to implementing safe, quality nursing care to patients with different mobility needs within the standards of care and scope of nursing practice
- Willingness to hold one's self accountable for safe, high-quality care for patients at different developmental stages with differing mobility impairments; a willingness to hold colleagues accountable for safe, quality practice
- Demonstration of a strong sense of responsibility and accountability
- Ability to act as a patient advocate to promote the maximum level of patient functioning
- Familiarity with nursing responsibilities to prevent and treat complications related to immobility as specified by agency policy
- Ability to document nursing care related to problems of mobility or activity intolerance according to agency policy and in a legally defensible manner

Learning Outcomes

After completing the chapter, the learner should be able to accomplish the following:

1. Describe the role of the skeletal, muscular, and nervous systems in the physiology of movement.
2. Identify seven variables that influence body alignment and mobility.
3. Differentiate isotonic, isometric, and isokinetic exercise.
4. Describe the effects of exercise and immobility on major body systems.
5. Assess body alignment, mobility, and activity tolerance, using appropriate interview questions and physical assessment skills.
6. Develop nursing diagnoses that correctly identify mobility problems amenable to nursing therapy.
7. Use proper body mechanics when positioning, moving, lifting, and ambulating patients.
8. Design exercise programs.
9. Plan, implement, and evaluate nursing care related to selected nursing diagnoses involving mobility problems.

Key Terms

active exercise
ankylosis
atrophy
body mechanics
cartilage
contractures
dangling
exercise
flaccidity
footdrop
isokinetic exercise
isometric exercise
isotonic exercise
ligaments
negative nitrogen balance
neurons
orthopedics
osteoporosis
paresis
passive exercise
range of motion
spasticity
tendons
tonus

Most healthy individuals take the ability to move for granted. People simply expect our amazingly complex musculoskeletal and nervous systems to work together smoothly and on command to enable us to stand upright, to walk, and to reach for and grasp what we want. People usually give little thought to caring for the systems that promote and coordinate healthy movement until disuse, trauma, or illness interferes with some aspect of movement. (See the accompanying Reflective Practice box for an example.) Although some people value exercise and fitness, many people live inactive lifestyles that limit their ability to experience and enjoy life to its fullest and that openly invite degenerative and chronic diseases such as hypertension, ischemic heart disease, or diabetes.

The ability to move is closely related to the fulfillment of other basic human needs. Although breathing continues during rest, movement facilitates pulmonary functioning and increases peripheral blood flow. Because regular exercise contributes to the healthy functioning of each body system and, conversely, immobility negatively affects each body system, nurses actively promote exercise to promote wellness, prevent illness, and restore health. It is generally accepted that the consequences related to a sedentary lifestyle are more serious than are the risks associated with exercise.

This chapter describes the physiology of movement, the principles of body mechanics, and factors affecting body alignment and mobility. A comprehensive section on exercise differentiates the types of exercise, explores the role of exercise in disease prevention and health promotion, notes risks related to exercise, and assists in the design of individualized

exercise programs. The effects of immobility on body systems are discussed along with related nursing interventions. A practical guide for assessing body alignment and mobility states is included, with pertinent interview questions and physical assessment techniques. Analysis of patient mobility data may lead to the nursing diagnoses of Impaired Physical Mobility or Activity Intolerance or to diagnoses identifying effects of mobility problems on other areas of human functioning. Examples of nursing diagnoses are included. Expected outcomes are identified, and specific nursing strategies are presented. The concluding nursing plan of care illustrates how the nurse uses knowledge of body mechanics and mobility along with specific nursing interventions to promote fitness and to resolve mobility problems.

PHYSIOLOGY OF MOVEMENT

Purposeful, coordinated movement of the body requires the integrated functioning of the musculoskeletal and nervous systems. The following sections review the physiology of movement.

Skeletal System

The framework of bones and cartilage that protects our organs and allows us to move is called the skeletal system. Functions of this system include the following:

- Supporting the soft tissues of the body (maintains body form and posture)

Reflective Practice
Challenge to Technical Skills

Last year during my medical–surgical clinical experience, I was taking care of Maggie Wyatt, a female patient in her 30s, with an external fixation device on her right leg. The patient had broken her tibia, and this was the third surgery to try to correct the fracture. The external device had caused an infection for which Maggie was being treated. I was assigned to care for her on the day that she was being discharged. Throughout the day, I formed a close bond with her, and the nurse asked me to bring Maggie to her car when she was ready to leave. I was a little apprehensive about being able to help her into the car with the external fixator in place because she could not bend her leg at all. I had a couple of choices—I could take her down to the car myself and hope that there wouldn't be any problem helping her get into the car or I could tell the nurse I didn't feel comfortable bringing the patient to the car because I didn't have any experience transferring patients with a device such as this one. However, I really wanted to bring this patient down and see her through the final stage of discharge.

Thinking Outside the Box: Possible Courses of Action

- Take the patient down to the car by myself and do the best I can to help transfer her to the car.
- Explain to the nurse that I don't feel that I have the skills to bring this patient down on my own and ask her to do it.
- Explain to the nurse that I would really like to bring the patient down to the car but that I do not feel that I have the experience to do it on my own; ask her to assist me.
- Ask the nurse, before bringing the patient down, what is the best way to transfer the patient to the car.

Evaluating a Good Outcome: How Do I Define Success?

- Patient receives the highest quality of care and has the least amount of pain possible during the transfer.
- I learn from the experience and gain skills and knowledge for the future.
- Patient is at least not harmed and is possibly benefited by my action.

Personal Learning: Here's to the Future!

Unfortunately, in this case I did not make the right decision. I convinced myself that it could not be that difficult to transfer this very cooperative patient to her car with her mother's assistance. However, I was very wrong. I definitely should have asked for assistance. The car was extremely small, and it was hard to get her to sit across the back seat while keeping her leg completely straight. The patient was experiencing a fair amount of pain from the device. So, every time we tried to get her into the car, she experienced more pain. Fortunately, a physical therapist came outside to help another patient and then also helped us. I realized

that not only did I not have the skills to transfer her myself, but also that this was really a two-person job. The physical therapist taught me the best way to transfer this patient, and I learned a great deal from the experience. I was very lucky that my patient was very understanding and accommodating in this situation. I learned how to transfer a patient properly, but most importantly, I realized how important it is to trust your instincts and ask for help when you think you may need it—it's always better to be overprepared than underprepared.

Reflection

How do you think you would respond in a similar situation? Why? What does this tell you about yourself and about the adequacy of your skills for professional practice? Can you think of other ways to respond? What other skills (cognitive, interpersonal, technical, ethical/legal) would you need to respond well in this situation? What factors do you think might have influenced the nursing student's actions? Suppose that the patient was using crutches or a walker instead of having the fixation device in place.

How might the nursing student's actions been different? Imagine that the physical therapist did not arrive on the scene. What would have been the nursing student's next best action? Do you agree with the criteria to evaluate a successful outcome? Did the nursing student meet the criteria? Please explain your response.

Catherine Barrell, Georgetown University

- Protecting the delicate structures of the body (brain, lung, heart, spinal cord)
- Furnishing surfaces for the attachments of muscles, tendons, and ligaments, which, in turn, pull on the individual bones and produce movement
- Providing storage areas for mineral salts and fat
- Producing blood cells (hematopoiesis)

The 206 bones in the human body are classified by their shape. Long bones, found in the upper and lower extremities (eg, humerus and femur), contribute to height and length. Short bones, located in the wrist and ankle, contribute to movement. Flat bones are relatively thin (eg, ribs and several of the skull

bones) and contribute to shape (structural contour). Irregular bones are all those bones not included in the preceding classifications (eg, bones of the spinal column and jaw).

Bones are too rigid to bend without damage. Therefore, all movements that change the positions of the bony parts of the body occur at joints. The terms articulation and joint refer to the area where a bone comes into close contact with another bone. Joints are classified according to the amount of movement they permit. Of concern are the freely movable joints, called diarthroses or synovial joints, in which there is a space between the articulating bones. Movements possible at diarthric joints include abduction, adduction, flexion, extension, and rotation. Special movements of the forearm, ankle, and clavicle include supination, pronation, inversion, and eversion. These movements are defined in Table 39-1 and illustrated in Skill 39-2 later in the chapter.

Several types of freely movable joints are found in the body. These include the following:

- *Ball-and-socket joint:* The rounded head of one bone fits into a cuplike cavity in the other; flexion–extension, abduction–adduction, and rotation can occur (eg, shoulder and hip joints).
- *Condyloid joint:* The oval head of one bone fits into a shallow cavity of another bone; flexion–extension and abduction–adduction can occur (eg, wrist joint).
- *Gliding joint:* Articular surfaces are flat; flexion–extension and abduction–adduction can occur (eg, carpal bones of wrist and tarsal bones of feet).
- *Hinge joint:* A spool-like surface of one bone fits into a concave surface of another bone; only flexion–extension can occur (eg, elbow, knee, and ankle joints).
- *Pivot joint:* A ringlike structure that turns on a pivot; movement is limited to rotation, for example, turning a doorknob (eg, joints between the atlas and axis

and between the proximal ends of the radius and the ulna).
- *Saddle joint:* Bone surfaces are convex on one side and concave on the other; movements are side to side and back and forth (eg, joint between the trapezium and metacarpal of the thumb).

The strength and flexibility of the skeletal system also depend on ligaments, tendons, and cartilage. **Ligaments** are tough fibrous bands that bind joints together and connect bones and cartilage. **Tendons** are strong, flexible, inelastic fibrous bands that attach muscle to bone. **Cartilage** is nonvascular connective tissue found in the joints as well as in the nose, ear, thorax, trachea, and larynx.

Muscular System

The muscular system is composed of three types of muscles: (1) skeletal, (2) cardiac, and (3) smooth or visceral muscles. The skeletal muscle system includes the skeletal muscle tissue and connective tissue that comprise individual muscle organs, such as the biceps. Bones and joints provide form to the body and serve as the levers and fulcrums that make body move-

TABLE 39-1 Terms Commonly Used to Describe Body Positions and Movements

Term	Definition and Example
Abduction	Lateral movement of a body part away from the midline of the body. *Example:* A person's arm is abducted when it is moved away from the body.
Adduction	Lateral movement of a body part toward the midline of the body. *Example:* A person's arm is adducted when it is moved from an outstretched position to a position alongside the body.
Circumduction	Movement of the distal part of the limb to trace a complete circle while the proximal end of the bone remains fixed. *Example:* The leg is outstretched and moved in a circle.
Flexion	The state of being bent. *Example:* A person's cervical spine is flexed when the head is bent forward chin to chest.
Extension	The state of being in a straight line. *Example:* A person's cervical spine is extended when the head is held straight on the spinal column.
Hyperextension	The state of exaggerated extension. It often results in an angle greater than 180 degrees. *Example:* A person's cervical spine is hyperextended when looking overhead, toward the ceiling.
Dorsiflexion	Backward bending of the hand or foot. *Example:* A person's foot is in dorsiflexion when the toes are brought up as though to point them at the knee.
Plantar flexion	Flexion of the foot. *Example:* A person's foot is in plantar flexion in the footdrop position.
Rotation	Turning on an axis; the turning of a body part on the axis provided by its joint. *Example:* A thumb is rotated when it is moved to make a circle.
Internal rotation	A body part turning on its axis toward the midline of the body. *Example:* A leg is rotated internally when it turns inward at the hip and the toes point toward the midline of the body.
External rotation	A body part turning on its axis away from the midline of the body. *Example:* A leg is rotated externally when it turns outward at the hip and the toes point away from the midline of the body.
Special Movements	
Pronation	The assumption of the prone position. *Example:* A person is in the prone position when lying on the abdomen; a person's palm is prone when the forearm is turned so that the palm faces downward.
Supination	The assumption of the supine position. *Example:* A person is in the supine position when lying on the back; a person's palm is supine when the forearm is turned so that the palm faces upward.
Inversion	Movement of the sole of the foot inward (occurs at the ankle)
Eversion	Movement of the sole of the foot outward (occurs at the ankle)

ment possible. Movement results from a skeletal muscle contracting and exerting force on a tendon, which, in turn, pulls on a bone. Muscles have two differing points of attachment: (1) the attachment of a muscle to the more stationary bone is called the point of origin, and (2) the attachment to the more movable bone is the point of insertion. Between these two points is the fleshy "belly" of the muscle. The excitability, contractility, extensibility, and elasticity of muscles enable them to perform three important functions for the body through contraction:

- Motion
- Maintenance of posture (skeletal muscle contractions hold the body in stationary positions)
- Heat production (skeletal muscle contractions produce heat and help maintain body temperature)

Figure 39-1 illustrates the relationship of skeletal muscles to bones and the use of bones as levers and of joints as fulcrums to produce body movement.

Nervous System

The skeletal and muscular systems cannot produce purposeful movement without a functioning nervous system. Nerve impulses stimulate muscles to contract. More specifically:

- The afferent nervous system conveys information from receptors in the periphery of the body to the central nervous system (CNS) (eg, light pressure on nose).
- Nerve cells called **neurons** conduct impulses from one part of the body to another.
- This information is processed by the CNS, leading to a response (eg, "There is a fly on my nose. I want to brush it off.").
- The efferent system conveys the response from the CNS to skeletal muscles by way of the somatic nervous system (eg, muscles in the arm, wrist, and hand contract, and the fingers brush the fly from the face).

BODY MECHANICS

Body mechanics is the efficient use of the body as a machine and as a means of locomotion. Body mechanics is directly related to the effective functioning of the body. The principles of body mechanics should be correctly used in every activity and even during rest periods, to prevent injury and to prevent sore muscles and joints.

Because correct use of body mechanics is another phase of illness prevention and health promotion, the nurse has a major responsibility to teach good body mechanics both directly and indirectly by example. The accompanying box, Promoting Health 39-1: Activity, reflects on self-care behaviors vital for maintaining a healthy level of activity. Ability to evaluate the patient's musculoskeletal needs requires a sound knowledge base and use of correct body mechanics. In addition, every activity in which the nurse engages, from as simple an activity as moving a chair to lifting a patient out of bed, requires understanding and using these principles. Nurses who con-

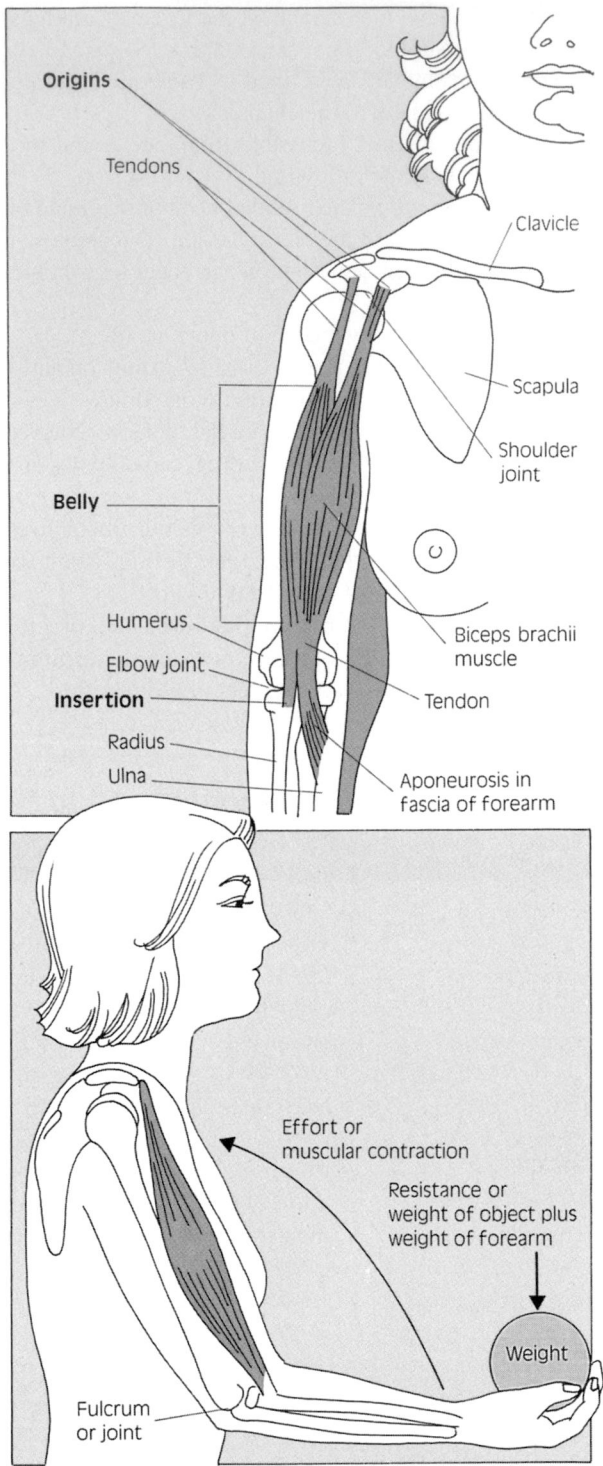

FIGURE 39-1 Relationship of skeletal muscles to bones. (*Top*) Skeletal muscles produce movements by pulling on bones. (*Bottom*) Bones serve as levers, and joints act as fulcrums for the levers. The lever and fulcrum principle is illustrated by the movement of the forearm lifting a weight.

sciously develop good habits can demonstrate to others proper ways of using the musculoskeletal system. In the home, nurses can model proper body mechanics when they assist patients to dress, help them move, or perform care. Caregivers in the home need reminders that preventing back problems is more effective than treating them after they occur.

Promoting Health 39-1 Activity

Use the following assessment checklist to determine how well you are meeting your need for exercise. Then develop a prescription for self-care by choosing appropriate behaviors from the list of suggestions.

ASSESSMENT CHECKLIST

almost always / sometimes / almost never

1. My lifestyle demonstrates that I place a high value on exercise as a component of wellness (eg, I use stairs instead of elevators).
2. I exercise for 30 to 45 minutes three or four times per week.
3. I have sufficient energy for each day's tasks.
4. I maintain my target weight/BMI.

SELF-CARE BEHAVIORS

1. Decide to make the most of everyday opportunities for exercise: use stairs instead of elevators, walk instead of ride, park the car farther from your destination than usual and walk the distance briskly, and so forth.
2. Choose exercise activities you enjoy and plan three or four 30- to 45-minute exercise sessions weekly.
3. Obtain medical clearance for exercise if you fall in a high-risk group. Learn and observe the appropriate exercise safeguards (eg, wear running shoes with the proper support).
4. Alternate types of exercise to avoid boredom.
5. Use part of your lunchtime for brisk walking or other exercise.
6. Invite a friend to exercise with you so you have the added support of a buddy or join a spa, health club, or exercise group.
7. Consistently use sound principles of body mechanics in both leisure and work activities.
8. Build up exercise sessions gradually to avoid overexertion and injury to muscles.
9. Evaluate your lifestyle to see what prevents you from exercising regularly and address these factors (low value attached to health or exercise, low motivation, lack of time, lack of rest, or faulty nutrition).

Think back to Genevieve Augustus, caring for her older husband at home after his stroke. She complains of bone and joint pain. The nurse would need to assess her mobility status including her use of body mechanics to determine if the possible cause of her discomfort is related to improper use. The nurse would also role model proper body mechanics during the home visits to teach and reinforce their proper use.

Orthopedics refers to the correction or prevention of disorders of body structures used in locomotion. Nurses have long recognized that basic orthopedic principles apply in all areas of nursing, not just to patients with bone fractures or other pathologic skeletal changes. For example, a person who has a sedentary occupation and engages in little physical activity may have poorly developed muscles. A patient who is on complete bed rest is in danger of losing muscle tonus. **Tonus** is the term used to describe the state of slight contraction—the usual state of skeletal muscles. If bed rest is prolonged, there is danger of developing **contractures** (permanent contraction of a muscle) if the patient does not have exercise and joint motion and if good posture is not maintained. The functioning of various internal body processes is also influenced by position and movement or by their absence.

Concepts of Body Mechanics

Concepts most helpful to the understanding of body mechanics include body alignment, balance, and coordinated movement.

Body Alignment or Posture

Good posture, or good body alignment, is that alignment of body parts that permits optimal musculoskeletal balance and operation and promotes healthy physiologic functioning. A person in correct alignment is experiencing no undue strain on the joints, muscles, tendons, or ligaments while balance is maintained.

Consider Maggie Wyatt, the woman being discharged with an external fixation device in place. Although the device is heavy and awkward and requires her to keep her right leg extended, body alignment is crucial for Maggie to prevent undue strain on other parts of her body.

The criteria for correct alignment in the standing, sitting, and reclining positions are described in the assessment section later in this chapter.

Balance

A body in correct alignment is balanced. An object is balanced when its center of gravity is close to its base of support, the line of gravity goes through the base of support, and the object has a wide base of support. The center of gravity of an object is the point at which its mass is centered. In humans, the center of gravity when standing is located in the center of the pelvis about midway between the umbilicus and the symphysis pubis. The line of gravity is a vertical line that passes through the center of gravity. The base of support is the foundation that provides for an object's stability. The wider the base of support and the lower the center of gravity, the greater the stability of the object. Figure 39-2 illustrates body balance.

Body balance increases when individuals spread the feet farther apart, thereby broadening the base of support, and by flexing the hips and knees, thus lowering the center of gravity. These two simple maneuvers are important principles in body mechanics that can decrease musculoskeletal strain that occurs with excessive stretching or overexertion of a muscle or muscle–tendon unit. Musculoskeletal strain most commonly affects the lower back and cervical spine region. Trauma to the musculoskeletal system is discussed later in the chapter.

Coordinated Body Movement

Providing direct patient care requires nurses to use their body frequently to assist in positioning, turning, and lifting both patients and equipment. Doing these actions correctly is necessary to avoid musculoskeletal strain and injury. Using major muscle groups rather than weaker ones and taking advantage of the body's natural levers and fulcrums facilitates these actions. For example, rather than attempt to push a patient to the opposite side of the bed, the nurse flexes the knees, positions the forearms above and below the patient's buttocks (preferably under a pull sheet), and rocks backward, sliding the patient toward self. This one coordinated movement illustrates the following principles:

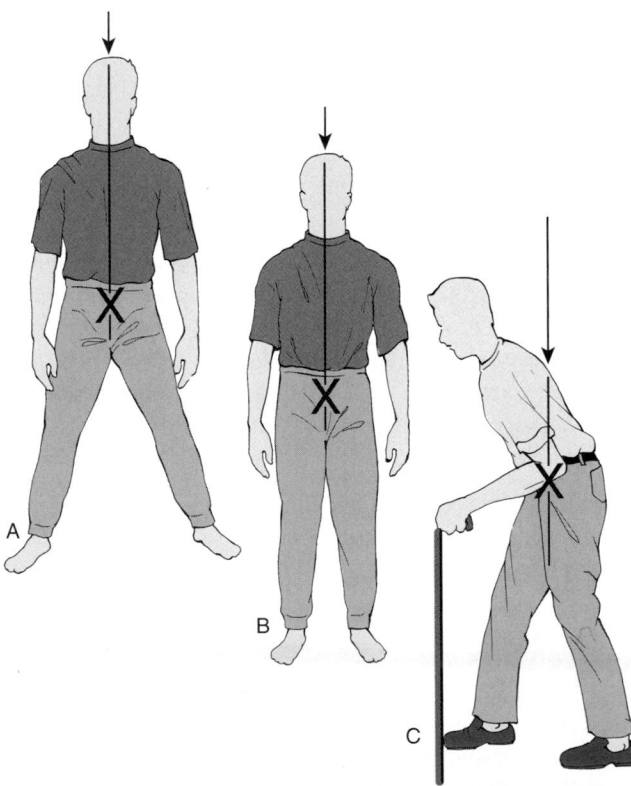

FIGURE 39-2 The effect of the base of support and gravity on balance is shown. (**A**) The line of gravity passes through the wide base of support. This person is the most stable of the three. (**B**) The line of gravity also passes through the base support, although the base is narrower. This person is less stable than the person in *A*. (**C**) The line of gravity does not pass through the base of support. This person is unstable.

- The nurse is using major muscle groups—flexors, extensors, and abductors of the thighs; flexors and extensors of the knees; flexors and extensors of the upper and lower arms—rather than weaker ones.
- Use of the arm bones as levers and the elbows as fulcrums facilitates lifting a weight against resistance (force of gravity)—the lever and fulcrum principle (see Fig. 39-1).
- Using a pull sheet and smooth, dry, firm bed foundation decreases the effects of friction, which increases the amount of effort required to move an object. Rough, wet, or soiled surfaces can contribute to friction's effect.
- By positioning the arms under the patient's center of gravity (hips) and sliding the body back toward himself or herself, the nurse is working close to the object to be moved and decreasing the effort involved.

Postural Reflexes

Integrated functioning of the musculoskeletal and nervous systems is essential for body alignment and balance. Postural tonus, the sustained contraction of select skeletal muscles that keeps the human body in an upright position against the force of gravity, depends on the functioning of several postural reflexes:

- *Labyrinthine sense:* This sense of position and movement is provided by the sensory organs in the inner ear, which are stimulated by body movement (changes in head position) and transmit these impulses to the cerebellum.
- *Proprioceptor or kinesthetic sense:* This informs the brain of the location of a limb or body part as a result of joint movements stimulating special nerve endings in muscles, tendons, and fascia.
- *Visual or optic reflexes:* Visual impressions contribute to posture by alerting the person to spatial relationships with the environment (nearness of ceilings, walls, furniture, condition of floor, etc.).
- *Extensor or stretch reflexes:* When extensor muscles are stretched beyond a certain point (eg, when knees buckle under), their stimulation causes a reflex contraction that aids a person to reestablish erect posture (eg, straighten the knee).

Application of Body Mechanics

The guidelines listed below for body mechanics are important to anyone, including nurses, who are engaged in physical activity both at home and at work. Nurses who are retiring or leaving the profession commonly cite back injuries as an influencing factor. Overexertion injuries to workers' necks, shoulders, and backs are the most costly work-related injury for healthcare facilities (Converso & Murphy, 2004; Owen, 2000).

Techniques to prevent back stress that should be included routinely in injury-prevention programs include the following:

- Develop a habit of erect posture (correct alignment) and, whenever necessary, begin activities by broadening the base of support and lowering the center of gravity.
- Use the longest and the strongest muscles of the arms and the legs to help provide the power needed in strenuous

activities. The muscles of the back are less strong and more easily injured when used improperly.

- Use the internal girdle and a long midriff to stabilize the pelvis and to protect the abdominal viscera when stooping, reaching, lifting, or pulling. The internal girdle is made by contracting the gluteal muscles in the buttocks downward and the abdominal muscles upward. It is helped further by making a long midriff by stretching the muscles in the waist. Figure 39-3 illustrates the internal girdle.
- Work as closely as possible to an object that is to be lifted or moved. This brings the body's center of gravity close to that of the object being moved, thereby permitting most of the burden to be borne by the leg and arm muscles rather than the back. Figure 39-4 illustrates a proper and an improper way to pick up an object.
- Use the weight of the body as a force for pulling or pushing, by rocking on the feet or leaning forward or backward. This reduces the amount of strain placed on the arms and the back.
- Slide, roll, push, or pull an object rather than lift it to reduce the energy needed to lift the weight against the pull of gravity.
- Use the weight of the body to push an object by falling or rocking forward and to pull an object by falling or rocking backward.
- Spread the feet apart to provide a wider base of support when increased stability of the body is necessary.
- Flex the knees, put on the internal girdle, and come down close to an object that is to be lifted.

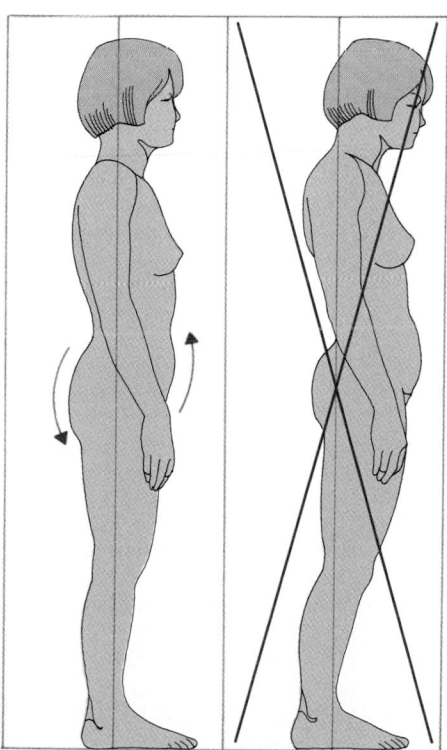

FIGURE 39-3 (*Left*) Internal girdle "on." Abdominal muscles contracted, giving a feeling of upward pull, and gluteal muscles contracted, giving a downward pull. (*Right*) Slouch position, showing abdominal muscles relaxed and body out of good alignment.

Recall Genevieve Augustus, the older woman caring for her husband at home after his stroke? The nurse would incorporate these principles of body movement and body mechanics when teaching Mrs. Augustus how to properly maneuver her husband in and out of bed. Doing so may help to alleviate some of the stress and strain on her body, thus helping to reduce her complaints of pain.

FACTORS AFFECTING BODY ALIGNMENT AND MOBILITY

Numerous factors, including growth and development, physical health, mental health, lifestyle variables, attitude and values, fatigue and stress, and external factors such as weather, influence an individual's posture, movement, and daily activity level.

Developmental Considerations

A person's age and degree of neuromuscular development markedly influence body proportions, posture, body mass, movements, and reflexes. To promote neuromuscular development in patients of all ages and to facilitate each patient's use of the body to perform self-care actions, nurses need to be familiar with developmental variations in body proportions and neuromuscular development. These variations are presented in Table 39-2 with related nursing assessment priorities and nursing interventions.

Recall Kelsi Lester, the 10-year-old girl in a coma? Typically, children of this age are highly active and mobile. However, Kelsi is confined to bed due to her accident. The nurse would obtain a history of Kelsi's activity level before the accident to determine her neuromuscular development. The nurse would then use this information to develop an age-appropriate plan of care to maximize Kelsi's level of function.

Physical Health

Problems in the musculoskeletal or nervous systems can have a negative influence on body alignment and movement. Similarly, illness or trauma involving other body systems may interfere with movement because of either the underlying pathology or the treatment regimen. Be sensitive to how both acute and chronic health problems affect a patient's general appearance (posture, body proportions, and movements) and ability to move purposefully to perform the ADLs. When assessing a patient's response to a mobility deficit, work to:

- Reinforce behaviors that promote healthy functioning (eg, congratulate a patient who manages transfers well despite left-sided weakness or paralysis)

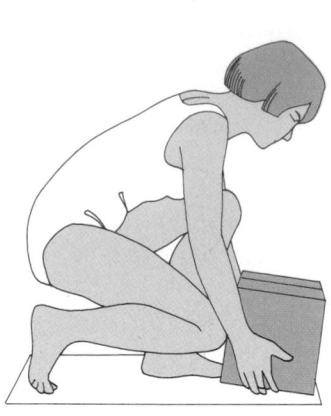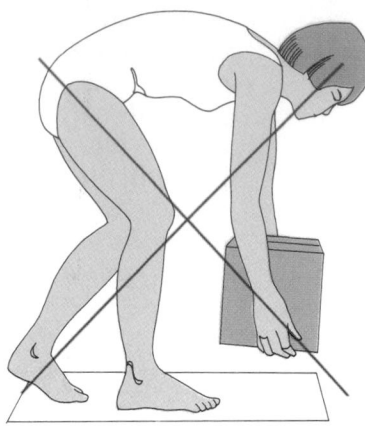

FIGURE 39-4 (*Left*) A good position for lifting is illustrated. This person is using the long and strong muscles of the arms and legs and holding the object so that the line of gravity falls within the base of support. (*Right*) This is an incorrect position for lifting because pull is exerted on the back muscles and leaning causes the line of gravity to fall outside the base.

• Correct behaviors that compound the mobility deficit over time (eg, a patient with arthritis who severely restricts movement because of joint stiffness and tenderness learns successful adaptive strategies that can be shared with other patients and families; or energy-conservation measures are used by patients with emphysema who have greatly decreased activity tolerance)

Muscular, Skeletal, or Nervous System Problems
Congenital or Acquired Postural Abnormalities

A newborn with developmental hip dysplasia or a clubfoot, a teenager with scoliosis (lateral curvature of the spine), and an older person with kyphosis (increased convexity in the curvature of the thoracic spine) are all experiencing postural ab-

TABLE 39-2 Activity Variations Based on Developmental Level: Assessment Priorities and Nursing Interventions

Developmental Level	Assessment Priorities	Nursing Interventions
Infant • Periods of activity and alertness alternate with quiet periods and sleep. • At 3 months: may raise chest and head when prone • By 5 months: head control usually achieved	Assess the following key developmental milestones at these ages: **3 to 6 mo** • Ability to sit • Head control **6 to 9 mo** • Sits steadily • Rolls over • Creeps on all fours • Pulls to a standing position • Has improved hand–eye coordination **9 to 12 mo** • Progresses toward unassisted walking • Is able to pick up small objects	• Encourage parents to examine their baby (eg, count fingers and toes). • Respond to concerns that parents have about minor variations in newborn's appearance or behavior. • Emphasize that individual variation in activity patterns and neuromuscular development should be expected. • Account for any prematurity when discussing normal developmental progression of preterm infants.
Toddler • Gross and fine motor development continue rapidly. • By 15 months: most can walk unassisted • At 18 months: most can run • At 2 years: can jump • At 3 years: most can stack blocks, string large beads, work simple puzzles, and dress themselves	• Assess progress in walking, running, and jumping. • Assess small muscle coordination (eg, ability to dress themselves, wash hands, brush teeth). • Distinguish slow developers who fall within normal range from those with developmental lags.	• Help parents to learn and accept their child's uniqueness. • Teach parents the importance of providing a safe environment. • Enthusiastically reinforce and praise toddler's mastery of new skills. • Set limits so that toddler does not overextend himself or herself in drive for mastery of skills. *(continued)*

TABLE 39-2 (Continued)

Developmental Level	Assessment Priorities	Nursing Interventions
Child • Muscles, bones, and nervous system develop, allowing greater gross and fine motor control	• Use developmental charts to assess gross and fine motor development.	• Teach parents that attitudes about the body and exercise are developed during this period. • Counsel as appropriate.
Common Activities • By age 4: negotiate stairs, walk backward, and hop on one foot • By age 5: skip, jump rope, and jump off heights of several steps • Able to manipulate writing materials • Has acquired all basic mechanisms for physical locomotion	• Determine activity level and types of play which involve physical exertion.	• Encourage physical activity and limitation of sedentary hobbies.
Adolescent • Size increases: growth spurt • Secondary sex characteristics appear • If physically fit: can be a time of boundless energy and great athletic performance • If inactive: may begin a lifelong pattern of unhealthy behavior	• Determine activity level and type of regular exercise. • Evaluate safety of recreational choices. • Screen for scoliosis (lateral curvature of the spine). • Examine muscle mass, tone, and strength and joint mobility.	• Lifestyle counseling regarding the importance of exercise and fitness is critical. • Encourage to exercise regularly if necessary. • Caution about gauging physical limits and not "pushing too hard."
Adult • Stands and sits erect and is capable of balanced and coordinated, purposeful movement • During pregnancy: center of gravity shifts because of developing fetus • Activity levels vary greatly	• Assess balance between activity and rest in person's lifestyle. • Note any lifestyle factors or illnesses that interfere with mobility or ability to carry out activities of daily living.	• Fitness counseling is important. • Clarify misconceptions about exercise. • Design and monitor safe exercise programs. • Those with mobility alterations may require special care.
Older Adult • Increased convexity in the thoracic spine (kyphosis) from disk shrinkage and decreased height • Flexed posture • Loss of muscle tone • Subcutaneous fat loss • Arthritic joint changes may be present	• Assess general ease of movement and gait. • Assess alignment. • Check joints and their function. • Assess muscle mass, tone, and strength.	Teach and counsel about: • Importance of regular exercise • Need to maintain proper weight • Need for high protein, calcium, and vitamin D–enriched diet • Pacing activities • Using assistive devices safely when needed • Safety-proof homes to reduce falls

normalities that affect their appearance and mobility. Nursing responsibilities may include the following:

- Early detection of and referral for these problems
- Exploration and selection of patient education, counseling, and support as treatment options
- Careful attention to positioning, transfers, and exercise
- Education of the patient and family regarding safe self-care activities

Problems With Bone Formation or Muscle Development

Problems with bone formation may include any of the following:

- Congenital problems, such as achondroplasia, in which premature bone ossification leads to dwarfism, or osteogenesis imperfecta, which is characterized by excessively brittle bones and multiple fractures both at birth and later in life

- Diet-related problems, for example, vitamin D deficiency, which results in deformities of the growing skeleton (rickets)
- Disease-related problems, such as Paget's disease, in which excessive bone destruction and abnormal regeneration result in skeletal pain, deformities, and pathologic fractures
- Age-related problems, such as osteoporosis, in which bone destruction exceeds bone formation and in which the resultant thin, porous bones fracture easily

The muscular dystrophies are a group of genetically transmitted disorders that share a common progressive degeneration and weakness of skeletal muscles. They vary in terms of the muscle groups involved and their clinical course. Myasthenia gravis is a weakness of the skeletal muscles caused by an abnormality at the neuromuscular junction that prevents muscle fibers from contracting.

Nursing responsibilities for patients with problems of bone formation and muscle development and functioning include the following:

- Careful collaboration with the physician and healthcare team to determine the motor capacities of the individual
- Patient and family education aimed at developing optional mobility

The nurse must be knowledgeable about the underlying disease process and be able to position, lift, transfer, and exercise the patient safely, with attention to patient comfort.

Problems Affecting Joint Mobility

Inflammation, degeneration, and trauma can all interfere with joint mobility. The term arthritis describes more than 20 diseases, all characterized by inflammation in one or more joints and possibly pain and stiffness in adjacent body parts. Degenerative joint disease, also termed osteoarthritis, is a noninflammatory, progressive disorder of movable joints, particularly weight-bearing joints, characterized by the deterioration of articular cartilage and pain with motion. Once the articular cartilage is damaged, bony deposits (bone spurs) may form in the joints causing more pain with movement of the joint.

Remember Genevieve Augustus, the older woman caring for her husband at home? The nurse would need to consider the impact of possible age-related problems as contributing to Genevieve's current complaints of bone and joint pain. Due to her older adult status, the likelihood of osteoporosis and degenerative joint disease is high. Therefore, teaching to minimize stress on the joints when assisting with her husband's care would be important in preventing possible bone and joint injuries and reducing pain.

Trauma to a joint may result in either a sprain, in which the wrenching or twisting of a joint results in a partial tear or rupture to its attachments, or a dislocation, the displacement of a bone from a joint with tearing of ligaments, tendons, and capsules. Any condition restricting joint mobility has potentially crippling effects.

Nurses caring for patients with joint problems work collaboratively with physicians and physical therapists to maintain joint mobility. Patient education is directed to the patient's mastery of an exercise and care program, which fosters tissue repair and maximal independence in activities of daily living (ADLs).

Think back to Maggie Wyatt, the woman being discharged after treatment for a fractured tibia. The nurse would need to work closely with other members of Maggie's healthcare team to ensure that joint mobility is maintained, even with the device in place. The discharge teaching plan would include measures to maintain function of the right leg while the external fixation device immobilizes the fractured area.

Problems Affecting the Central Nervous System

A problem in any of the principal parts of the brain or spinal cord involved with skeletal muscle control can affect mobility: The cerebral motor cortex assumes the major role of controlling precise, discrete movements. A cerebrovascular accident (stroke) or head trauma may damage the motor cortex and produce temporary or permanent voluntary motor impairment. Basal ganglia integrate semivoluntary movements such as walking, swimming, and laughing. In Parkinson's disease, there is progressive degeneration of the basal ganglia of the cerebrum. Unnecessary skeletal movements result in tremors and muscle rigidity, which interfere with voluntary movement. The cerebellum assists the motor cortex and basal ganglia by making body movements smooth and coordinated. In multiple sclerosis, the myelin sheaths of neurons in the CNS deteriorate to hardened scars or plaques. Plaque formation in the cerebellum may produce lack of coordination of one hand.

The pyramidal pathways convey voluntary motor impulses from the brain through the spinal cord by way of two major pathways: (1) the pyramidal pathway and (2) the extrapyramidal pathway. With trauma to the spinal cord, transection of these motor pathways results in complete bilateral loss of voluntary movement below the level of the trauma.

The overwhelming complaint of patients with injury to the CNS is that no one talks with them (or with their families) about how the disease may progress and affect their functioning. Nurses caring for these patients need to be knowledgeable about the pathology and clinical course of these diseases to provide appropriate patient education and counseling.

Recall Kelsi Lester, the 10-year-old in a coma after a skiing accident? Although she is unconscious, the nurse must communicate with Kelsi, making sure to explain all that is happening to her and all that is being done. In addition, the nurse would need to communicate with Kelsi's family to ensure that they understand what is happening. For example, the nurse needs to explain the reasons for frequent turning, position changes, and exercises while Kelsi is unconscious.

Trauma to the Musculoskeletal System

Injury to the musculoskeletal system can result in fractures and soft tissue injuries. A fracture, a break in the continuity of a bone or cartilage, may result from a traumatic injury or some underlying disease process. Healing requires realignment of the bone fragment, immobilization, and restoration of the bone's function. Soft tissue injuries include sprains, strains, and dislocations (dislocations and sprains are discussed above under Problems Affecting Joint Mobility). A strain, the least serious of these injuries, is a stretching of a muscle. Nurses need to be knowledgeable in first-aid measures for musculoskeletal trauma as well as in acute and rehabilitative care.

Problems Involving Other Body Systems

The pathology of numerous other acute and chronic illnesses may also affect mobility. Chronic obstructive lung disease and conditions such as ascites may alter posture. Any illnesses that interfere with oxygenation at the cellular level decrease the amount of oxygen available to the muscles for work and thus decrease activity tolerance. These illnesses include anemia, angina, cardiac arrhythmias, heart failure, and chronic obstructive pulmonary disease. Diseases characterized by a larger breakdown of protein than that which is manufactured leads to a **negative nitrogen balance** (eg, anorexia nervosa and certain cancers) that results in muscle wasting and decreased physical energy for movement and work. Symptoms accompanying many illnesses, such as fatigue, muscle aches, and pain, may also lead to immobility. Bed rest is an important component of treatment for many diseases or trauma states, such as myocardial infarction, surgery, and fractures. Although rest is essential for the healing process, immobility associated with bed rest may cause its own problems (Table 39-3). Nurses

TABLE 39-3 Comparison of Effects of Exercise and Immobility on Body Systems

Effects of Exercise	Effects of Immobility
Cardiovascular System ↑Efficiency of heart ↓Resting heart rate and blood pressure ↑Blood flow and oxygenation of all body parts	**Cardiovascular System** ↑Cardiac workload ↑Risk for orthostatic hypotension ↑Risk for venous thrombosis
Respiratory System ↑Depth of respiration ↑Respiratory rate ↑Gas exchange at alveolar level ↑Rate of carbon dioxide excretion	**Respiratory System** ↓Depth of respiration ↓Rate of respiration Pooling of secretions Impaired gas exchange
Gastrointestinal System ↑Appetite ↑Intestinal tone	**Gastrointestinal System** Disturbance in appetite Altered protein metabolism Altered digestion and utilization of nutrients
Urinary System ↑Blood flow to kidneys ↑Efficiency in maintaining fluid and acid–base balance ↑Efficiency in excreting body wastes	**Urinary System** ↑Urinary stasis ↑Risk for renal calculi ↓Bladder muscle tone
Musculoskeletal System ↑Muscle efficiency ↑Coordination ↑Efficiency of nerve impulse transmission	**Musculoskeletal System** ↓Muscle size, tone, and strength ↓Joint mobility, flexibility Bone demineralization ↓Endurance, stability ↑Risk for contracture formation
Metabolic System ↑Efficiency of metabolic system ↑Efficiency of body temperature regulation	**Metabolic System** ↑Risk for electrolyte imbalance Altered exchange of nutrients and gases
Integument Improved tone, color, turgor, resulting from improved circulation	**Integument** ↑Risk for skin breakdown and formation of decubitus ulcers
Psychological Well-Being Energy, vitality, general well-being Improved sleep Improved appearance Improved self-concept Positive health behaviors	**Psychological Well-Being** ↑Sense of powerlessness ↓Self-concept ↓Social interaction ↓Sensory stimulation Altered sleep–wake pattern ↑Risk for depression

need to be vigilant in determining the effects of any injury or illness on mobility and in providing care to facilitate optimal mobility.

Mental Health

Just as an individual's physical health influences body appearance and movement, so also does the person's mental health. Body processes tend to slow down in depression, and there is a lack of visible energy and enthusiasm. Body posture also may be affected. For example, the person with depression often sits with head bowed and shoulders slumped and may lack the energy to eat or even to use the toilet. Even facial movement may be decreased to the point at which the individual's face registers no emotion (termed a flat affect). On the other hand, individuals who are not depressed are more likely to have erect posture and animated facial features.

Lifestyle

An individual's lifestyle, whether active or sedentary, is influenced by many variables. Among the most important are the individual's occupation, leisure activity preferences, and cultural influences. Commonly, activities in many occupations along the socioeconomic ladder are sedentary. Therefore, individuals wishing to exercise regularly need to plan for these leisure activities. In addition, culture may play a role, encouraging or discouraging exercise. For example, it is popular for both male and female professionals to engage in aerobic exercise. In the not-so-distant past, women being involved in most sports activities were looked upon with disdain. A person's diet and smoking history are other lifestyle variables that influence mobility.

Nurses, particularly those involved in community health activities, need to consider appropriate forms of exercise and geographic location before making recommendations to patients from diverse cultures. Commonly prescribed exercises, such as jogging, tennis, or even walking, may be viewed as acceptable choices. However, these activities may pose a threat to the individual in unsafe environments, such as high-crime areas. For example, an exercise prescription for a Native American might include suggestions for exploring nearby mountain areas, hunting, or even participating in Native American dances as more acceptable methods to increase activity level.

Attitude and Values

In some families, such as those who hike, swim, or play ball together, children learn early to value regular exercise. As these children mature, they often continue to value exercise and find new ways to incorporate regular exercise into their daily routine. Similarly, children may be raised in families who are sedentary and where watching sports is the closest anyone comes to exercise. This attitude may also be internalized for a lifetime. Many individual values also influence the exercise options people make. Older people who integrate a planned exercise regimen into their daily routine benefit physiologically and report improved self-esteem.

Individuals who place a high value on physical attractiveness may be highly committed to regular exercise because it helps produce the body they want. Another individual may exercise because of the desire for physical strength, relating strength with power. Someone more disposed to intellectual pursuits may perceive body development as simply wasting time that could be better used to develop the mind.

Fatigue and Stress

Chronic stress may deplete body energy to the point that fatigue makes even the thought of exercise overwhelming. Ironically, regular exercise is energizing and can better equip a person to deal with daily stresses. At the same time, excessive exercise may stress the body and lead to injury as well as to fatigue.

External Factors

Many external factors can influence activity and mobility. Among these, weather probably exerts the greatest influence. A brisk, clear day is invigorating and invites increased activity. High humidity and high temperatures, on the other hand, discourage extra movement. Sufficient financial resources for exercise memberships and equipment, safe outdoor parks and sports areas, the availability of malls for early-morning walkers, support people, and occupational or insurance rewards for exercise can all encourage regular exercise. Discouraging factors include insufficient funds, air pollution, unsafe neighborhoods, lack of free time, and lack of support and reinforcement.

EXERCISE

Active exertion of muscles involving the contraction and relaxation of muscle groups is termed **exercise.** Each of the many different types of exercise can produce different physiologic and psychological benefits.

Types of Exercise

Exercise can be divided into two major groups. One group is based on the type of muscle contraction occurring during the exercise. The second group is based on the type of body movement occurring and the health benefits achieved.

Muscle Contraction

Exercise may be categorized according to the type of muscle contraction involved as being isotonic, isometric, or isokinetic (Fig. 39-5).

Isotonic exercise involves muscle shortening and active movement. Examples include carrying out ADLs, independently performing range-of-motion exercises, and swimming, walking, jogging, and bicycling. Potential benefits include

Isometric exercise involves muscle contraction without shortening (ie, there is no movement or only a minimum shortening of muscle fibers). Examples include contractions of the quadriceps and gluteal muscles. Potential benefits are increased muscle mass, tone, and strength, increased circulation to the exercised body part, and increased osteoblastic activity. Nurses encourage both isotonic and isometric exercises for hospitalized patients with limited mobility.

Isokinetic exercise involves muscle contractions with resistance, varying at a constant rate produced by a device with a capacity for variable resistance. Examples include rehabilitative exercises for knee and elbow injuries and lifting weights. Using the isokinetic device, the person takes the muscles and joint through a complete range of motion without stopping, meeting resistance at every point.

> *Consider Maggie Wyatt, the woman being discharged with an external fixation device in place. A specific exercise routine that includes isometric and isotonic exercises would most likely be prescribed for Maggie. Later in the course of Maggie's treatment after her fracture has healed, isokinetic exercises may be included to strengthen her right leg.*

Body Movement

Exercise activities may also be categorized according to the type of body movement involved and the health benefits they produce. Types of exercise involving body movement include aerobic exercises, stretching exercises, strength and endurance exercises, and movement and ADLs.

Aerobic exercise refers to sustained (often rhythmic) muscle movements that increase blood flow, heart rate, and metabolic demand for oxygen over time, promoting cardiovascular conditioning. Examples of aerobic activities include swimming, walking, jogging, cross-country skiing, aerobic dance, bicycling, jumping rope, and racquetball. Aerobic exercise may be further distinguished as having high or low impact. The number of injuries, such as shin splints, related to high-impact aerobic workouts led to the development of low-impact workouts that place less stress on the musculoskeletal system.

Stretching exercises involve movements that allow muscles and joints to be stretched gently through their full range of motion, increasing flexibility. Specific warm-up and cool-down exercises, hatha yoga, and some forms of dance are examples. Benefits include increased range-of-joint movements, improved circulation and posture, and relaxation.

Strength and endurance exercises are components of a variety of muscle-building programs. Weight training, calisthenics, and specific isometric exercises can build both strength and endurance, increasing the power of the musculoskeletal system and generally improving the whole body. They may or may not have aerobic benefit.

Movement and ADLs include housecleaning, running after playful toddlers, climbing stairs instead of riding in elevators, and so on. Household activities can also contribute to an active lifestyle.

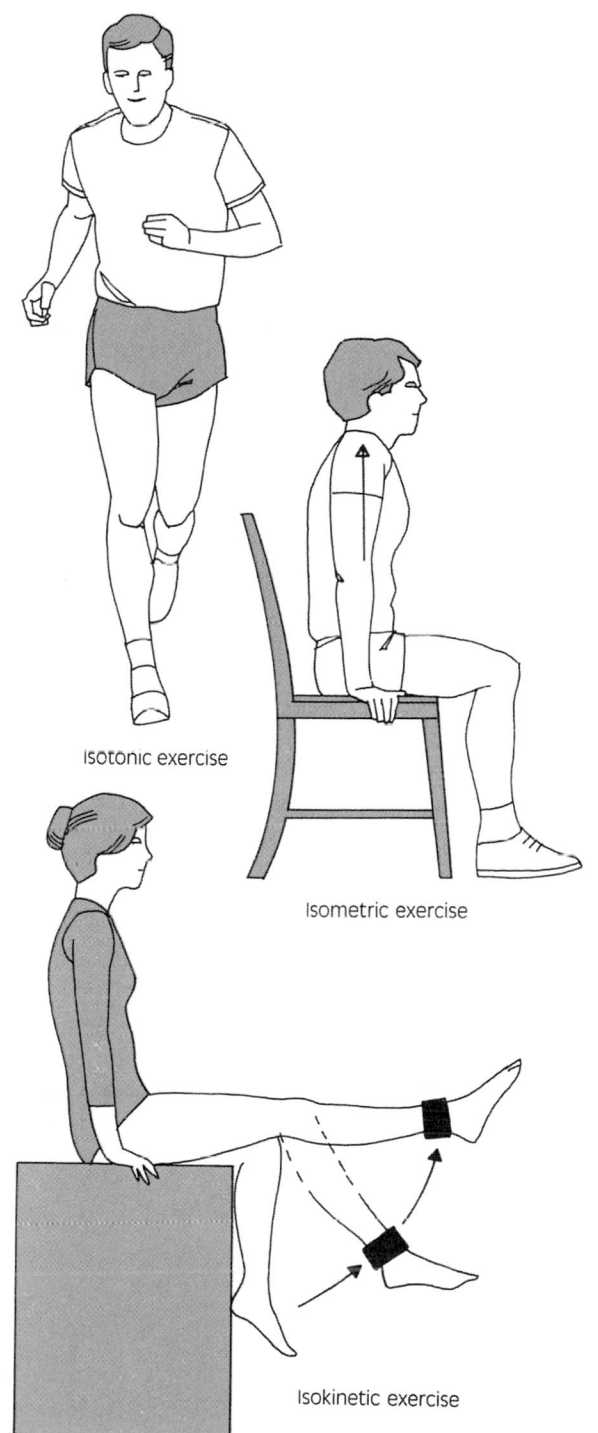

Isotonic exercise

Isometric exercise

Isokinetic exercise

FIGURE 39-5 Three types of exercise. *Isotonic exercise* involves muscle shortening and active movement. *Isometric exercise* involves muscle contraction without shortening. *Isokinetic exercise* involves muscle contraction with resistance.

increased muscle mass, tone, and strength; improved joint mobility; increased cardiac and respiratory function; increased circulation; and increased osteoblastic or bone-building activity. When the nurse or family member performs passive range-of-motion exercises for a patient, the patient's muscles do not exert effort. Therefore, although still beneficial, the overall potential benefits are reduced.

Effects of Exercise on Major Body Systems

The human body was designed for motion, and regular exercise is necessary for its healthy functioning. Individuals who choose inactive lifestyles or who are forced into inactivity by illness or injury place themselves at high risk for serious health problems. The effects of regular exercise on major body systems are explored in the following sections and outlined in Table 39-3. Individuals differ in the benefits they receive from exercise based on the patient's age and overall health status.

Cardiovascular System

To meet the demand for oxygen created by the rhythmic contraction and relaxation of skeletal muscle groups, the supply of oxygenated blood to skeletal muscle needs to be increased. The cardiovascular system meets this challenge by increasing the heart rate, increasing the contractile strength of the myocardium, and increasing stroke volume (volume of blood ejected), thus increasing cardiac output. Arterial (systolic) blood pressure is increased, and blood is shunted from the nonexercising tissues to the heart and muscles. Exercise also improves venous return because the contracting muscles compress superficial veins and push blood back to the heart against gravity. Over time, with cardiovascular conditioning, regular exercise produces the following benefits:

- Increased efficiency of the heart
- Decreased heart rate and blood pressure
- Increased blood flow to all body parts
- Increased circulating fibrinolysin (substance that breaks up small clots)

The amount of exercise has been found to be a greater factor in exerting a positive effect on the cardiovascular system than the type of exercise performed. See Research in Nursing: Making a Difference.

Respiratory System

The respiratory and cardiovascular systems work together to make increased oxygen available to the muscles. During exercise, the depth of respiration, respiratory rate, gas exchange at the alveolar level, and rate of carbon dioxide excretion are increased. Over time, regular exercise leads to improved pulmonary functioning.

Musculoskeletal System

The rhythmic contraction and relaxation of muscle groups during exercise result in increased muscle mass, tone, strength, and increased joint mobility. The more a person exercises, the more strength he or she has to exercise or work in the future. Regular exercise produces the following benefits:

- Increased muscle efficiency (strength) and flexibility
- Increased coordination
- Increased efficiency of nerve impulse transmission

Regular exercise is also believed to slow the effects of aging (ie, it helps prevent osteoporosis associated with aging).

Metabolic Processes

The metabolic rate increases during exercise so that sufficient glucose and fatty acids can be converted to provide the energy needed for increased muscle function. During strenuous exercise, the metabolic rate can increase to up to 20 times normal. Increased body heat and waste products are also produced. With regular exercise the body develops the following:

- Increased efficiency of metabolic system
- Increased efficiency of body temperature regulation

Gastrointestinal System

During exercise, blood is shunted away from the stomach and intestines to the exercising muscles. With regular exercise:

- Appetite is increased.
- Intestinal tone is increased, which improves digestion and elimination.
- Weight may be controlled.

Research in Nursing Making a Difference

Exercise to Lower Coronary Heart Disease Risk Factors

The positive effects of exercise have often been documented. An active lifestyle is particularly important for older adults as they strive to stay healthy and independent.

Many times nurses help patients begin an exercise routine that is individualized.

Related Research

Lee, I., Rexrode, K. M., Cook, N. R., Manson, J. E., & Buring, J. E. (2001). Physical activity and coronary heart disease in women: Is "No pain, no gain" passé? *JAMA, 285*(11), 1447–1454.

In this cohort study, 39,372 healthy female health professionals aged 45 years or older, participated in this study. Before beginning the study, participants reported their recreational activi-

ties. During the study, the women were surveyed to find out the amount and type of physical activity in which they participated monthly. The women also took a placebo pill. The participants of the study thought that the main focus was the pill and its effects. The participants were followed for 5 years. During this 5-year period, 244 confirmed cases of coronary heart disease were reported.

Implications for Nurses

This study confirms that physical activity in women decreases coronary heart disease rates in women. A beneficial finding of the study is that time spent walking is a more reliable indicator for predicting lower risk than the pace of walking. Encouraging women to become active at any level can have a positive impact on their health.

Urinary System

Regular exercise increases blood circulation, including improved blood flow to the kidneys. This allows the kidneys to maintain the body's fluid balance and acid–base balance more efficiently and to excrete body wastes.

Skin

Increased circulation resulting from regular exercise nourishes the skin. Thus, regular exercise aids in promoting the overall general health of the skin.

Psychosocial Outlook

Some of the most important benefits of regular exercise are psychological. These benefits include:

- Increased energy, vitality, and general well-being
- Improved sleep
- Improved appearance (body image)
- Improved self-concept
- Increased positive health behaviors

Role of Exercise in Preventing Illness and Promoting Wellness

According to Healthy People 2010, regular physical activity helps prevent certain chronic diseases such as hypertension, type 2 diabetes, cardiovascular disease, obesity, and osteoporosis (U.S. Department of Health and Human Services, 2000). Vigorous physical activity is not always needed to achieve positive results. A recent study has shown that the amount of time spent walking has a bigger effect on the outcome than the pace of the walking (Lee et al., 2001; see Research in Nursing box earlier in this chapter).

Promoting exercise and emphasizing wellness behaviors are challenging opportunities for nurses. Nurses are committed to assisting and supporting patients to make lifestyle changes that improve the patients' health and well-being. As researchers focus on the potential of regular exercise activities to slow the aging process, nurses intervene to prevent the deleterious effects associated with decreased physical activity. See the accompanying box, Focus on the Older Adult, for a summary of the benefits of exercise and specific precautions related to exercise for this age group.

Risks Related to Exercise

Most commonly, exercise is viewed as too much of a chore. As a result, individuals avoid exercise. Offer suggestions for how to incorporate exercise into the person's daily routine, thus making exercise less of a chore. Another common reason many people offer for not exercising is fear of experiencing personal harm. Personal harm can include muscle injuries, falling, or cardiovascular events. Be responsive to these fears with realistic knowledge of the risks associated with exercise and specific prevention strategies.

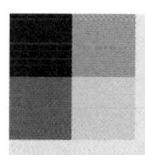

Focus on the Older Adult
Nursing Strategies to Promote Exercise and Activity for Age-Related Changes in the Older Adult

Age-Related Changes	Nursing Strategies
Activity Intolerance	
• Decreased respiratory vital capacity	• Encourage patient to gradually increase physical activity and to listen to cues from his or her own body.
• Decreased transport of oxygenated blood to tissue (as in chronic obstructive pulmonary disease or decreased cardiac output)	• Instruct patient to avoid sudden position changes that may cause dizziness. • Instruct patient to avoid extreme temperatures if exercising. • Provide for sufficient hydration. • Encourage patient to avoid exercise if weak or ill. • Instruct patient to stop exercising if chest pain occurs, and consult with physician before resuming activity. • Instruct patient to respect fatigue. Do not push to the point of exhaustion.
Impaired Physical Mobility	
• Decreased range of motion • Decreased stability of gait	• Encourage patient to warm up before beginning exercises and to cool down after exercising. • Encourage patient to modify exercises versus forcing joints beyond the natural range of motion. • Discuss safety precautions that patient may take when exercising, such as walk in a gym or mall versus on an uneven sidewalk. • Recommend that patient wear proper footwear when exercising.

Precipitation of a Cardiac Event

Although the risk of exercise precipitating a major cardiac event in a healthy individual is minimal, the risk is much higher for individuals with known or suspected cardiovascular disease. Thus, a preexercise medical examination, medical supervision during exercise, and an individually designed exercise plan are recommended for sedentary people older than 35 years of age and for any person with a past or current cardiovascular condition.

Orthopedic Discomfort and Disability

Orthopedic problems caused by irritation of bones, tendons, ligaments, and sometimes muscles are the most common injuries associated with exercise. This irritation may result from added weight-bearing stress or from collision with the ground, an object, or another person. Teach patients to follow the guideline of rest, ice, compression, and elevation (RICE) if injury occurs. While the injured area is rested, recommend the application of ice to minimize pain and edema, an elastic bandage for compression, and elevation of the injured area to help reduce edema. Advise the patient to contact a physician immediately to diagnose the extent of the injury. Instruct the patient to discontinue exercise until the injury is healed.

Other Health Problems

Other types of health problems may be associated with different types of exercise, depending to a large extent on external factors (temperature on a given day, humidity, pollution index, safety of the neighborhood) as well as internal factors (age, history of previous injury, overuse, obesity, health history). Examples of other health problems related to exercise include heat exhaustion or heat stroke, exercise-induced asthma, and chest pain related to overexertion.

Effects of Immobility on the Body

Lack of exercise, inactivity, or immobility related to illness or injury place a person at high risk for serious health problems. Immobility can affect the major body systems. Like the benefits a person receives from exercise, complications resulting from immobility differ in their occurrence and severity based on the patient's age and overall health status.

Cardiovascular System

The primary and serious effects of immobility on the cardiovascular system include increased cardiac workload, orthostatic hypotension, and venous thrombosis. Immobility results in an increased workload for the heart. It has been demonstrated that the heart works more when the person is immobile because the skeletal muscles that normally compress valves in the leg veins and help to pump the blood back to the right side of the heart do not adequately contract. There is less resistance offered by the blood vessels and blood pools in the veins, thus increasing the venous blood pressure and changing the distri-

bution of blood in the immobile person. As a result, the heart rate, cardiac output, and stroke volume increase.

Immobility predisposes the patient to thrombi formation because of venous stasis, especially in the legs, where normal muscular activity helps move blood toward the central circulatory system. Thrombus formation is also caused by an increased rate in the coagulation of blood, one reason being that during periods of immobility, calcium leaves bones and enters the blood, where it influences blood coagulation.

A person who is immobile is more susceptible to developing orthostatic hypotension. The person tends to feel weak and faint when this condition occurs. See Chapter 24 for additional discussion of orthostatic hypotension.

Respiratory System

The effects of immobility on the respiratory system are related to decreased ventilatory effort and increased respiratory secretions. Immobility causes a decrease in the depth and rate of respirations, in part because of a reduced need for oxygen by body cells. When areas of lung tissues are not used over time, atelectasis (incomplete expansion or collapse of lung tissue) may occur. Immobility results in a poor exchange of carbon dioxide and oxygen, upsets their balance in the body, and eventually causes an acid–base imbalance.

When a person is immobile, the movement of secretions in the respiratory tract is decreased, causing secretions to pool and leading to respiratory congestion. These conditions predispose the person to respiratory tract infections. Hypostatic pneumonia is a type of pneumonia that results from inactivity and immobility. The situation worsens when the person is dehydrated or using pharmacologic agents that increase the tenacity of secretions, depress the coughing mechanism, and depress respirations.

Decreased movement in the thoracic cage during respirations also occurs with immobility. This decrease may be due to loss of tonus in muscles involved with respirations, pressure on the chest wall because of the patient's position in bed, or depression of the respiratory apparatus by various pharmaceutical agents.

Musculoskeletal System

Effects of immobility on the musculoskeletal system are rapidly seen in patients confined to bed. People attempting to walk after several days of bed rest are often surprised to find how weak their legs have become. Immobility (musculoskeletal disuse) leads to decreased muscle size (**atrophy**), tone, and strength; decreased joint mobility and flexibility; bone demineralization; and limited endurance, resulting in problems with ADLs.

Immobility is often the cause of contractures and **ankylosis** (a consolidation and immobilization of a joint). Contractures result from atrophy of muscles with resulting incompetence and from a decrease in the muscle's strength, coordination, and endurance. A joint can be permanently fixed when ankylosed.

The process of bone demineralization (**osteoporosis**) is also increased in immobile patients. Normally, the stress and strain of weight-bearing activity stimulate bone formation and balance it with the natural destruction of bone. With immobility, however, bone formation slows while breakdown increases, resulting in a net loss of bone calcium, phosphorus, and matrix. This condition, disuse osteoporosis, is characterized by bones that may be either spongy or brittle. Bone demineralization may result in pathologic fractures related to the bone's brittleness; bone deformities related to the bone's sponginess; arthropathy (joint disease) related to calcium depletion in the joints; or renal calculi (stones) related to the excessive excretion of calcium through the kidneys and urinary tract.

Metabolic Processes

Because the resting body requires less energy, the cellular demand for oxygen is decreased, leading to a decreased metabolic rate. In many immobilized patients, however, factors such as fever, trauma, chronic illness, or poor nutrition can actually increase the body's metabolic demands and increase catabolism (the breakdown of the body's protein stores to provide energy to meet the body's energy requirements). If unchecked, this process results in muscle wasting and a negative nitrogen balance. Anorexia, or decreased appetite, often accompanies and compounds this problem. Negative nitrogen balance and poor nutrition thus worsen the muscle atrophy and weakness already resulting from immobility. Numerous fluid and electrolyte imbalances, alterations in the exchange of nutrients and gases at the cellular level, and gastrointestinal (GI) problems can all result from metabolic disturbances.

Gastrointestinal System

Immobility leads to disturbances in appetite, decreased food intake, altered protein metabolism, and poor digestion and utilization of food. If individuals increase food intake while decreasing energy expenditure, weight gain will result. Obesity and physical inactivity have been linked to colorectal cancer (Price, 2003).

Normal muscular activity in the GI tract also slows down in an immobile person, which often results in constipation, poor defecation reflexes, and an inability to expel feces and gas adequately.

Urinary System

In a nonerect patient, the kidneys and ureters are level, and urine remains in the renal pelvis for a longer period of time before being gravity causes it to move into the ureters and bladder. Urinary stasis favors the growth of bacteria that, when present in sufficient quantities, may cause urinary tract infections. Poor perineal hygiene, incontinence, decreased fluid intake, or an indwelling urinary catheter can increase the risk for urinary tract infection in an immobile patient.

Immobility also predisposes the patient to renal calculi, or kidney stones, which are a consequence of high levels of urinary calcium; urinary retention and incontinence resulting from decreased bladder muscle tone; the formation of alkaline urine, which facilitates growth of urinary bacteria; and decreased urine volume.

Skin

In patients who are immobile, especially those who are older or debilitated, the impaired circulation that accompanies immobility may result in serious skin breakdown. Prolonged pressure over bony prominences produces areas of breakdown, leading to pressure ulcers. Pressure ulcers can progress from stage 1, redness, to stage 4, destruction of subcutaneous tissue and muscle. Pressure ulcers are described in detail in Chapter 38.

Psychosocial Outlook

When a person can no longer move the body purposefully and needs to depend on someone else for assistance with simple self-care activities, the person's sense of self is often threatened. Skeletal deformities can influence body image; an inability to meet role expectations can decrease self-concept; and a prolonged period of lying dependent in bed can lead to feelings of worthlessness and diminished self-esteem.

Immobility can produce exaggerated emotional responses to the stresses of everyday living. Patients can become apathetic, possibly because of decreased sensory stimulation, and develop altered thought processes. Lack of mobility can also diminish an individual's opportunities to interact socially and deprive that person of normal support systems. Coping difficulties are common for both immobilized patients and their families. Furthermore, the amount of time immobilized patients spend resting often disrupts their usual sleep–wake patterns and may interfere with both the quantity and quality of their sleep.

Remember Kelsi Lester, the 10-year-old girl who is unconscious? Due to her current state, Kelsi is at high risk for developing any or all of the possible complications associated with immobility, including thrombi, pneumonia, constipation, urinary tract infection, and skin breakdown. Although she is unconscious, the effects of immobility ultimately can affect her psychosocial outlook. The nurse would integrate knowledge of the effects of immobility when developing Kelsi's plan of care that would include close frequent assessment, early detection, and prompt intervention to prevent any possible complications. Vigilant nursing care is essential.

THE NURSING PROCESS

Assessing

The comprehensive nursing assessment uses both interview and physical assessment skills to elicit data about the patient's mobility status. When alterations in a patient's physical or mental health state result in impaired mobility, additional specific assessment skills are needed to determine the patient's physical limitations.

Nursing History

During the nursing history, interview patients regarding their daily activity level, endurance, exercise and fitness goals, mobility problems, physical or mental health alterations that affect mobility, and external factors affecting mobility. Questioning patients about their fitness goals is important to provide an indication of the patient's view of health. This interviewing strategy communicates to patients that you expect them to be exercising and is itself a powerful teaching tool.

The accompanying Focused Assessment Guide illustrates elements common to obtaining a mobility status history. When a problem exists, assess the nature of the problem, its onset and frequency, known causes, severity and symptoms, effects on everyday functioning, the interventions attempted by the patient, and the results.

Physical Assessment

Physical assessment of mobility status includes an assessment of general ease of movement and gait; alignment, joint structure, and function; muscle mass, tone, and strength; and endurance. Table 39-4 provides normal findings and significant alterations. During this assessment, direct attention to both structure and function. The patient's ability to stand, walk, sit

Focused Assessment Guide 39-1

Mobility and Exercise

Factors to Assess	Questions and Approaches
Daily activity level	Describe the activities you normally carry out during a routine day. What type of physical exercise is a part of your daily lifestyle? • Activities of daily living • Type, frequency, duration of physical exercise • Past history of activity and exercise; recent changes
Endurance	Describe how much and what type of activity makes you tired. • History of dizziness, dyspnea, frequent pauses in activity to rest, or marked increase in respiratory rate after moderate activity
Exercise/fitness goals	What exercise or fitness goals are you currently working on? • Attitudes about exercise and physical fitness • Knowledge of the benefits of exercise • Motivation to exercise • Current exercise and fitness goals
Mobility problems	Do you experience any problems with movement or with more vigorous activity or exercise? If yes, please describe these problems. • Nature of the problem • Onset of disturbance and frequency • Known causes • Severity • Symptoms • Effect of problem on everyday functioning • Interventions attempted and results
Physical or mental health alterations	Are there any physical or mental health problems that may be affecting your mobility? Tell me about them. • Decrease of strength or endurance (eg, myocardial infarction, congestive heart failure, cardiomyopathy, chronic obstructive pulmonary disease, cancer, gastrointestinal disorders) • Neuromuscular impairment (multiple sclerosis, Parkinson's disease, spinal injuries) • Musculoskeletal impairment (arthritis, fractures, muscular dystrophy) • Perceptual or cognitive impairment (cerebrovascular accident, brain tumor or trauma, vision disorders) • Pain or discomfort (burns, rheumatoid arthritis, chronic pain syndrome, postoperative pain) • Depression or severe anxiety (neurosis, schizophrenia)
External factors affecting mobility	Is there anything else you can think of that limits your ability to get around? • Environmental factors (stairs, lack of railings or other assistive devices, unsafe neighborhood) • Financial resources

TABLE 39-4 Overview of the Physical Assessment of Mobility Status

Component	Normal Finding	Significant Alterations
General ease of movement	Body movements are: • Voluntarily controlled (purposeful) • Fluid • Coordinated	Involuntary movements: • Tremors • Tics • Chorea • Athetosis • Dystonia • Fasciculations • Myoclonus • Oral–facial dyskinesias
Gait and posture	Head erect, vertebrae are straight Knees and feet point forward Arms at side with elbows flexed Arms swing freely in alternation with leg swings While one leg is in the stance phase, the other is in the swing phase	Abnormalities of gait and posture: • Spastic hemiparesis • Scissors gait • Steppage gait • Sensory ataxia • Cerebellar ataxia • Parkinsonian gait • Gait of old age • Use of assistive devices for ambulation
Alignment	Independent maintenance of correct alignment: • In the standing and sitting position, a straight line can be drawn from the ear through the shoulder and hip • In bed, the head, shoulders, and hips are aligned	Abnormal spinal curvatures Inability to maintain correct alignment independently
Joint structure and function	Absence of joint deformities Full range of motion	Limitation in the normal range of motion Increased joint mobility Swelling or tenderness in or around the joint Heat or redness Crepitation Deformities Muscle atrophy, nodules, skin changes Asymmetry of involvement
Muscle mass, tone, and strength	Adequate muscle mass, tone, and strength to accomplish movement and work	Atrophy, hypertrophy Hypotonicity (flaccidity), spasticity Paresis or paralysis
Endurance	Ability to turn in bed, maintain correct alignment when sitting and standing, ambulate, and perform self-care activities	Physiologic or psychological inability to tolerate an increase in activity: • Significantly increased pulse, respiration, blood pressure after rest • Shortness of breath, dyspnea • Weakness • Pallor • Confusion • Vertigo • Pain

up, and grasp are important because these enable the patient to wash, dress, and feed himself or herself and perform other basic ADLs.

General Ease of Movement and Gait

Begin the physical assessment of an ambulatory patient the moment the patient walks into the room. Voluntarily controlled, fluid, and coordinated body movements are keys to the integrated functioning of the skeletal, muscle, and nervous systems. Common involuntary movements that may be observed include tremors (continuous quivering of whole muscles or major portions of a muscle) and tics (irregularly occurring spasmodic movements such as winking, grimacing, or shoulder shrugging).

Also note whether the patient's body movements are quick and sure or slow and deliberate. These observations communicate both a sense of the person's emotional status and self-care abilities.

Note the gait of patient who is ambulatory. The patient's movements while walking should be coordinated and the posture well balanced. The arms should swing freely in a rhythm alternating with the legs. Figure 39-6 illustrates stance and swing, the two phases of the normal gait. The heel of the right foot strikes the ground (stance), while the toe of the left foot pushes off and leaves the ground, moving the leg from behind to in front of the body (swing). While one leg is in the stance phase, the other is in the swing phase. Gait abnormalities are important because they may place the individual at risk for injury and also because they may indicate intoxication or a neuromuscular disorder.

If a patient uses any assistive devices such as wheelchair, brace, cane, walker, or crutches to aid in ambulation, note this. Also determine whether this aid is meeting the patient's needs, if this aid is required for mobility, and is this aid being used safely.

Alignment

Correct body alignment permits optimal musculoskeletal balance and operation and promotes good physiologic functioning. Deviations in body alignment may result from chronic poor posture, trauma, muscle damage, or nerve dysfunction. Fatigue and a person's mental and emotional status may also influence alignment. Alignment may be observed when a patient is standing, sitting, or lying (Fig. 39-7). Note whether the patient is able to maintain correct alignment independently.

A patient's body is in correct body alignment when standing when:

- The head is held erect.
- The face is in the forward position, in the same direction as the feet.
- The chest is held upward and forward.
- The spinal column is upright, and the curves of the spine are within normal limits.
- The abdominal muscles are held upward and the buttocks downward.
- The knees are extended—not bent or hyperextended in the knee-locked position.
- The feet are at right angles to the lower legs.
- The line of gravity goes through the center of the knees and in front of the ankle joints.
- The base of support is on the soles of the feet, and weight is distributed through the soles and heels.

Correct body alignment when sitting is similar to correct alignment when standing except that the hips are flexed, the knees are flexed and not crossed, and the base of support is on the buttocks and upper thighs. The popliteal area should be free of the edge of the chair to prevent circulatory stasis and possible nerve injury.

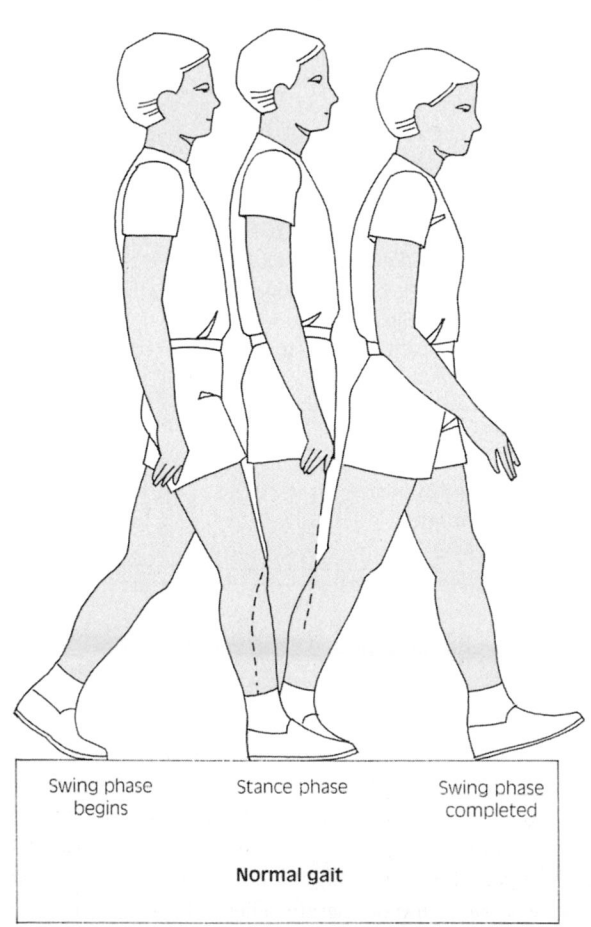

Swing phase begins   Stance phase   Swing phase completed

Normal gait

FIGURE 39-6 The stance and swing phases of normal gait.

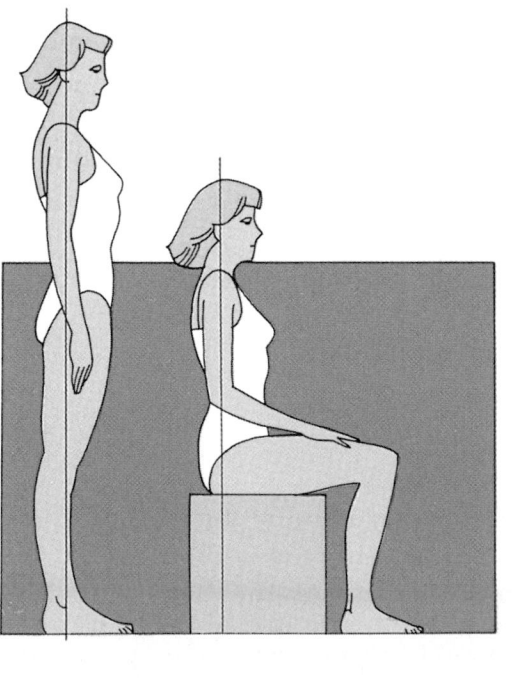

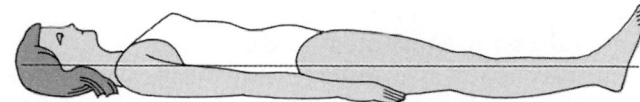

FIGURE 39-7 Adequate posture. In the sitting and standing positions, a straight line can be drawn from the ear through the shoulder and hip. In bed, the head, shoulders, and hips are aligned.

Joint Structure and Function

Use inspection and palpation to examine joints, their range of motion, and the surrounding tissue. **Range of motion** is the complete extent of movement of which a joint is normally capable. Skill 39-2 later in this chapter illustrates the range of motion of selected joints. When assessing joint mobility, note the following:

- Size, shape, color, and symmetry of joints. Note any masses, deformities, or muscle atrophy.
- Range of motion of each joint
- Any limitation in the normal range of motion or any unusual increase in the mobility of a joint (instability). Range of motion varies among individuals and decreases with aging.
- Muscle strength when performing range-of-motion exercises against resistance
- Any swelling, heat, tenderness, pain, nodules, or crepitation (palpable or audible crunching or grating sensation produced by motion of the joint)
- Compare findings in one joint with those of the opposite joint.

Muscle Mass, Tone, and Strength

Adequate skeletal muscle mass, tone, and strength are prerequisites to body movement and work performance. Mass refers to muscle size. Atrophy describes muscle mass that is decreased through disuse or neurologic impairment. Hypertrophy refers to increased muscle mass resulting from exercise or training. The examiner assesses muscle mass throughout the body and may also compare one muscle group to another using tape measurements. Patients experiencing muscle wasting as a result of a chronic disease process such as cancer may report visible changes in muscle mass.

The slight residual tension that remains in a resting normal muscle with an intact nerve supply is termed muscle tone. Muscle tone may be assessed by flexing and extending the elbow or knee and noting the degree of resistance to these movements. Decreased tone, hypotonicity, or **flaccidity** results from disuse or neurologic impairments. **Spasticity,** increased tone that interferes with movement, is also caused by neurologic impairments.

> *The nurse would need to assess closely the muscle tone of Kelsi Lester, the 10-year-old girl who is unconscious. Due to her current neurologic status of being unconscious, this assessment information would provide a means to evaluate her nervous system function. In addition, the nurse would be alert for evidence of flaccidity, which could result from lack of use or possibly impairment of her nervous system due to the accident.*

Muscle strength varies greatly from one individual to another and within the same individual and is affected by muscle use. Muscle strength is tested by asking the patient to move actively against resistance. For example, the patient may be instructed to push the examiner's palms apart or to push the foot against the examiner's palm. When comparing muscle groups, remember that a person's dominant side tends to be stronger.

Impaired muscle strength or weakness is termed **paresis.** The absence of strength secondary to nervous impairment is called paralysis. Hemiparesis refers to weakness of one half of the body, and hemiplegia is paralysis of one half of the body. Paraplegia is paralysis of the legs, and quadriplegia is paralysis of the arms and legs.

The patient's muscle strength should be adequate for the performance of tasks the patient deems necessary. For example, a patient whose primary means of ambulation is a wheelchair requires upper body strength.

Endurance

When assessing endurance, evaluate the patient's ability to turn in bed, maintain correct alignment when sitting or standing, ambulate, and perform self-care activities. When a physical or psychological factor is believed to be affecting endurance, accomplish the following:

- Obtain vital signs while the patient is at rest.
- Instruct the patient to perform the activity (eg, ambulation).
- Observe the patient's response during and after the activity.
- Take the vital signs immediately after the activity.
- Reassess the vital signs after the patient has rested for 3 minutes.

Significant findings indicating that a person's exercise tolerance has been reached include noticeably increased pulse, respirations, and blood pressure; shortness of breath; dyspnea; weakness; pallor; confusion; and vertigo.

Diagnosing

Recognizing cues that indicate both potential and actual problems is essential when analyzing data about a patient's mobility status. Because the problems associated with immobility can seriously undermine the patient's well-being and often require complex and costly treatment, prepare to direct interventions aimed at preventing these problems whenever possible. The plan of care for the patient with an alteration in mobility should include nursing diagnoses that identify the complications of immobility for which the patient is at greatest risk.

Nursing diagnoses specifically addressing problems of mobility include Activity Intolerance and Impaired Physical Mobility. Examples of related factors and defining characteristics are listed in the accompanying Examples of NANDA Nursing Diagnoses box. Examples of nursing diagnoses that describe the effect of immobility on body systems along with assessment priorities, expected outcomes, and nursing interventions are included in Table 39-5.

A patient's mobility status also may affect other areas of human functioning. Examples of possible nursing diagnoses may include:

Pain related to inability to change body position independently, limited range of motion and muscle atrophy

Examples of NANDA Nursing Diagnoses | Mobility

Nursing Diagnoses	Related Factors	Sample Defining Characteristics
Activity Intolerance	Any condition that interferes with the transport of oxygenated blood to tissue (eg, cardiac problems such as congestive heart failure and arrhythmias; respiratory problems, especially chronic obstructive pulmonary disease; circulatory problems; diabetes mellitus) Any condition that causes fatigue (depression, pain, sleep disturbances, prolonged bed rest, sedentary lifestyle)	Decreased ability to perform basic self-care activities: turning in bed, changing position, ambulating, washing, dressing, eating, and so on Altered response to activity: • Dyspnea, shortness of breath, excessive increase in respiratory rate • Weak pulse, excessive increase in pulse rate, change in rhythm • Blood pressure that fails to increase with activity or that decreases • Weakness, pallor, confusion, vertigo
Impaired Physical Mobility	• Neuromuscular impairment (arthritis, stroke, Parkinson's disease) • Musculoskeletal impairment • Decreased strength and endurance • Pain or discomfort • Depression	• Physical inability to move purposefully or a reluctance to move • Limited range of motion • Decreased muscle mass, tone, or strength • Therapy-related restrictions on movement (eg, an order for bed rest, traction, cast, or splints)

Impaired Walking related to development of footdrop

Impaired Transfer Ability related to generalized weakness

Ineffective Health Maintenance related to lack of mobility to procure needed services—no support people

Impaired Home Maintenance Management related to immobility

Noncompliance With Exercise Prescription related to decreased endurance, decreased motivation

Bathing/Hygiene, Feeding, Dressing/Grooming, Toileting Self-Care Deficit related to physical weakness (decreased muscle mass and strength), altered mobility (upper or lower extremities)

Sexual Dysfunction related to neuromuscular impairment

Outcome Identification and Planning

If the patient is not experiencing any mobility problems, expected patient outcomes are directed toward the promotion of physical fitness. For example, the patient will:

• Follow a program of regular physical exercise that improves cardiovascular function, endurance, flexibility, and strength

To achieve this long-term expected outcome, numerous short-term expected outcomes may be needed. An example follows.

By the next visit, 8/20/06, the patient will:

• Identify four personal benefits of regular exercise
• Describe an exercise program (activities, frequency, duration) the patient is willing to follow
• Identify his or her own target heart range

• Obtain medical clearance for the exercise program if at high risk for complications
• List support systems that will reinforce exercise efforts

Patients at high risk for specific mobility problems require different expected outcomes. For example, the patient will:

• Demonstrate correct body alignment whenever observed (alignment)
• Adhere to an every-2-hour positioning schedule (alignment)
• Demonstrate full range of joint motion (joint mobility)
• Demonstrate adequate muscle mass, tone, and strength to perform functional ADLs (muscle mass, tone, and strength)

Specific expected outcomes for patients at risk for complications related to immobility may be found in Table 39-5. Outcomes need to be individualized for more specific problems (eg, for the patient learning to walk with crutches or needing to master transfer techniques with only upper body mobility).

Consider Maggie Wyatt, the woman being discharged after treatment for a fracture. An appropriate outcome for Ms. Wyatt would be that she demonstrates ability to transfer herself from the bed to the chair and then to the car, with the assistance of a support person.

Implementing

Nursing strategies designed to promote correct body alignment, mobility, and fitness are described in the following sections. Techniques for positioning patients, performing range-of-motion exercises, moving, lifting, and ambulating patients, and designing exercise programs are included.

TABLE 39-5 Selected Nursing Diagnoses, Assessment Priorities, Expected Outcomes, and Nursing Interventions

Nursing Diagnoses Related to Immobility	Etiologies	Assessment Priorities	Expected Outcomes	Nursing Interventions
Cardiovascular				
Activity Intolerance: Increased Cardiac Workload	Supine position contributes to greater volume of circulating blood, which must be pumped by the heart; decreased vascular resistance	Assess apical and peripheral pulses. Note increased heart rate, weakened peripheral pulses. Note presence of edema.	Patient will maintain baseline vital signs. Patient will show signs of adequate venous return (absence of dependent edema, thrombi, emboli).	Encourage patient to sit in Fowler's position. Avoid activities that increase intrathoracic pressure (eg, Valsalva maneuver).
Ineffective Tissue Perfusion: Thrombus Formation	Venous stasis due to lack of muscle contraction in the legs. Increased blood coagulation because calcium moves from bones into circulation. External pressure on the veins (eg, from knee gatch on bed)	Assess for complaints of pain, especially calf pain, and signs of inflammation. Compare one extremity to the other. Measure calf or thigh circumference daily (mark place to measure).		Encourage active exercise of legs three to four times daily. Elevate legs periodically. Avoid prolonged knee and hip flexion. Apply TEDS if ordered. Never rub or massage the legs—especially if patient complains of pain.
Risk for Injury: Orthostatic Hypotension	Skeletal muscle weakness and decreased vessel tone. Hypovolemia	Assess for complaints of dizziness or fainting. Compare BP before position change with BP after position change.	Patient will change from a lying to a sitting or standing position safely, without injury.	Have patient sleep sitting up or in an elevated position (if not contraindicated). Change position gradually. Encourage leg exercises. Avoid Valsalva maneuver.
Respiratory				
Ineffective Breathing Pattern	Limited chest expansion. Prolonged sitting or lying. Muscle disuse or atrophy. Loss of muscle coordination. Medications that decrease respiratory effort	Assess rate, rhythm, quality of respirations. Assess symmetry of chest wall movements.	Patient will maintain baseline respiratory rate and depth. Patient coughs and deep breathes every 1 to 2 hours.	Change position every 2 hours. Encourage deep breathing and coughing every 1–2 hours. Remove abdominal binders every 2 hours to allow for deep breathing.
Ineffective Airway Clearance	Altered function of mucous membranes and cilia. Decreased position changes. Ineffective coughing due to weakness, pain. Dehydration	Assess breath sounds over the entire lung region. Note any adventitious breath sounds. Assess sputum (C&S may be ordered). Percuss chest.	Patient's lungs will be clear to auscultation. Patient will remain free of signs of respiratory infection.	See nursing interventions for Ineffective Breathing Pattern. Keep patient well hydrated. Initiate chest physiotherapy. Suction as needed.
Impaired Gas Exchange (O_2/CO_2 ratio)	Decreased respiratory movement. Pooling of secretions	Note any changes in behavior or mental status. Compare clinical picture with changes in ABGs, pulse oximetry, PFTs.	Patient will maintain an adequate O_2/CO_2 exchange.	See nursing interventions for Ineffective Breathing Pattern and Ineffective Airway Clearance.

(continued)

TABLE 39-5 (Continued)

Nursing Diagnoses Related to Immobility	Etiologies	Assessment Priorities	Expected Outcomes	Nursing Interventions
Musculoskeletal Risk for Activity Intolerance (Self-Care Deficits) Impaired Physical Mobility	Decreased muscle mass, tone, and strength (atrophy) Contractures Stiffness and pain in the joints Limited range of motion Decreased endurance	Assess for weakness, fatigue, muscle, or joint pain or tenderness. Assess for decreased muscle mass, decreased muscle tone and strength. Note contractures of ankyloses.	Patient will maintain adequate muscle strength and joint mobility to perform basic self-care activities.	Incorporate ROM exercises and isometric setting exercises into daily routine (at least three to four times daily).
Risk for Injury: Pathologic Fractures	Excessive bone demineralization (disuse osteoporosis)	Bone demineralization is not detectable through physical assessment. Relate clinical picture to blood chemistries (note elevated serum calcium and phosphorus levels).	Patient will remain free of contractures, ankyloses, pathologic fractures.	Increase patient's activity tolerance gradually. Progress to independence in all self-care activities.
Metabolic Imbalanced Nutrition: Less Than Body Requirements Imbalanced Nutrition: More Than Body Requirements Fluid Volume Excess: Dependent Edema	Negative nitrogen balance Anorexia Imbalance between calories ingested and burned off Fluid shifts because of negative nitrogen balance	Assess diet history. Monitor intake and output. Compare clinical picture to laboratory studies that evaluate fluid and electrolyte status. Evaluate muscle atrophy. Assess skin turgor and wound healing.	Patient will maintain appropriate weight for height. Patient's fluid input will approximately equal output. Patient's electrolyte values and serum protein will fall within normal range. Patient's skin will demonstrate adequate turgor.	Provide patient with high-protein, high-calorie diet. Explore parenteral and enteral alternatives if patient is unable to eat. Serve small, frequent feedings in pleasant environment. Monitor intake and output.
Gastrointestinal Constipation	Decreased gastric motility and muscle tone Decreased fluid intake	Assess frequency and consistency of bowel movements. Examine for bowel sounds, abdominal tone, and anal sphincter tone.	Patient will have a formed, semisolid stool every 1 to 3 days. Patient will be free of signs of fecal impaction.	Respect usual elimination schedule. Offer assistance with bedpan or commode and provide privacy. Increase fluid intake and roughage.
Urinary Altered Urinary Elimination Urinary Retention Risk for Infection: Urinary Tract	Renal calculi Urinary stasis	Assess voiding patterns—time and amount. Question about urgency, dysuria, pain. Monitor fluid output. Examine for bladder distention. Examine urine for cloudiness or odor (C&S if indicated).	Patient will maintain usual voiding pattern. Patient will be free of renal calculi. Patient will be free of signs of urinary tract infection.	Keep patient well hydrated. Maintain usual voiding pattern. If needed, provide assistance with bedpan or urinal—respect patient's privacy.

(continued)

TABLE 39-5 (Continued)

Nursing Diagnoses Related to Immobility	Etiologies	Assessment Priorities	Expected Outcomes	Nursing Interventions
Skin				
Impaired Skin Integrity (pressure ulcer)	Decreased local blood circulation to the tissues Prolonged pressure on the skin	Examine skin, especially pressure points, for beginning stages of breakdown with each position change (at least every 2 hours). Assess for factors that place patient at high risk for breakdown (eg, malnutrition and incontinence).	Patient's skin will show no signs of breakdown.	Reposition patient in correct alignment at least every 1–2 hours. Protect pressure points (eg, heel and elbow protectors). Decrease effects of shearing force. Keep skin clean and dry. Keep bed linens dry and free of wrinkles.
Psychological and Social				
Low Self-Esteem Powerlessness Impaired Social Interaction Disturbed Thought Processes Deficient Knowledge Ineffective Coping Ineffective Family Coping Disturbed Sleep Pattern	Inability to move voluntarily Dependency on others Inability to fulfill role expectations Pain experience Skeletal deformities Exaggerated emotional and behavioral responses Decreased ability to learn and retain information Increased need for sleep and napping	Assess patient for changes in behavior, emotional status, and mental abilities. Assess adequacy of the patient's and family's coping. Assess sleep–wake patterns. Explore with patient and family possible reasons for these changes.	Patient will identify personal strengths. Patient will verbalize positive body image. Patient will describe successful coping strategies. Patient will demonstrate ability to problem solve.	Explore immobility effects on mental status and behavior. Explore means to meet needs for socialization. Increase stimuli to maintain orientation. Encourage patient to be as independent as possible. Challenge patient intellectually. Explore impact of patient's illness on family and counsel appropriately.

BP, blood pressure; TEDS, thromboembolis disease stockings; C&S, culture and sputum; ABGs, arterial blood gas levels; PFTs, pulmonary function tests; ROM, range of motion.

Positioning Patients

Positioning that maintains correct body alignment and facilitates physiologic functioning contributes to the patient's psychological and physical well-being. The force of gravity pulls parts of the body out of alignment unless adequate support is provided. Various positions are therefore protective in nature only when the patient is positioned properly.

Common Devices to Promote Correct Alignment

Many devices can help maintain good body alignment and muscle tonus while the patient is in bed and can alleviate discomfort or pressure on various parts of the body.

Pillows

Pillows are used primarily to provide support or to elevate a body part. Pillows of different sizes are useful for different parts. Those intended for the head are usually full-sized or large-sized pillows. Small pillows are ideal for support or ele-

vation of the extremities, shoulders, or incisional wounds. Specially designed heavy pillows are useful to elevate the upper part of the body when an adjustable bed is unavailable, such as at home.

Mattresses

For a mattress to be comfortable and supportive, it must be firm but have sufficient "give" to permit good body alignment. A patient who must remain in a bed with a nonsupportive mattress may complain of backache and other discomforts.

A well-made and well-supported foam-rubber mattress retains a uniform firmness. This mattress is made of natural or synthetic rubber or a combination of both. A large volume of air is incorporated. The foam-rubber mattress conforms to the contours of the body and provides support at all points. Its greatest advantage is that it does not form slopes and valleys as innerspring mattresses are likely to do. Moreover, foam-rubber mattresses do not create as much pressure against bony prominences, such as the ankles, the elbows, the scapulae, and the coccyx. Special mattresses, pads, and types of beds used to help prevent pressure ulcers are discussed in Chapter 38.

Adjustable Beds

The head of an adjustable bed can be elevated to the desired degree. This positioning is discussed later in the chapter. The foot of an adjustable bed can also be elevated as desired. Some adjustable beds allow the bed to be "broken," or gatched, so that the mattress is flexed at the level of the knees. This position is rarely recommended. However, it may be used only for brief periods because it can cause pressure on the popliteal space behind the knee, resulting in impaired circulation to the lower extremity and an increased risk for clot formation.

The adjustable bed can also be changed so that the distance of the bed to the floor can be altered. The patient can get in and out of bed more easily when the bed is in the lowest position. The higher positions are used by healthcare workers so that they do not strain their backs while giving bed care. General guidelines for safe use of beds are discussed in Chapter 37.

> *Consider Genevieve Augustus, the older woman caring for her husband after his stroke. If necessary and not already in the home, an adjustable bed could be recommended to help Genevieve provide care to her husband. This would be beneficial to both Genevieve and her husband.*

Bed Side Rails

A major nursing concern is patient safety and preventing patients from falling out of bed. The use of side rails helps to ensure safety when a patient is in bed. Side rails remind patients that they are not in their usual environment or that medical equipment is in place, should they awaken during the night and wish to get out of bed. Side rails also make it possible for a patient to roll from one side to the other or to sit up without calling for assistance. In addition to providing safety, using side rails helps the patient retain or regain muscle efficiency. When using side rails, be sure to explain their use to patients and their families and follow the protocol of the healthcare agency. If a patient requests that side rails be raised for additional security, the patient must have the ability to raise and lower the side rails independently.

Unfortunately, bed side rails may not deter some patients from getting out of bed. Many a patient has crawled over the foot of the bed. Side rails also place a patient at risk for serious injury should he or she become lodged or trapped between the bed and the side rail or in the side rail itself. Safe use of side rails is discussed in Chapter 26.

Trapeze Bar

A trapeze bar (Fig. 39-8) is a hand grip suspended from a frame near the head of the bed. The patient can grasp the bar with one or both hands and then raise the trunk from the bed. The trapeze makes moving and turning considerably easier for many patients and facilitates transfers into and out of bed.

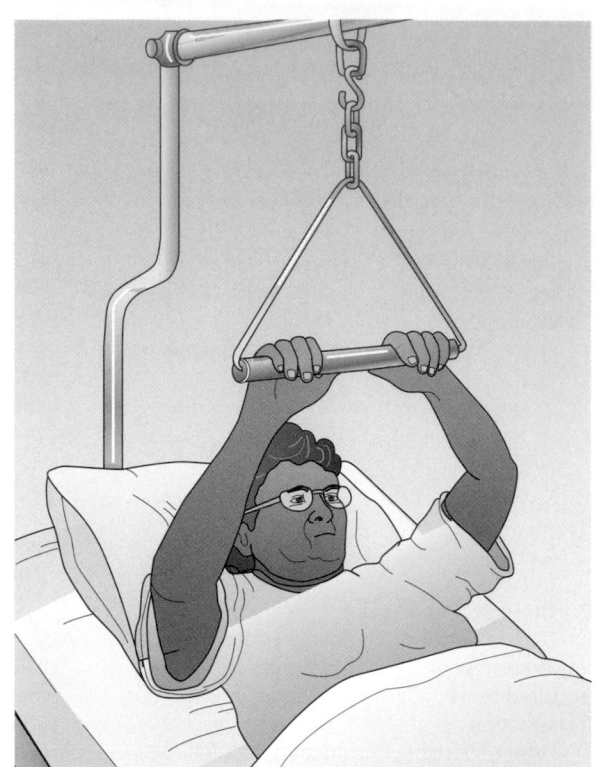

FIGURE 39-8 A trapeze device makes it possible for the patient to lift part of the body from the bed, thus facilitating turning and moving up in bed.

It can also be used when a patient needs to perform exercises that strengthen some muscles of the upper extremities (eg, biceps).

Additional Equipment

The greatest danger to the feet occurs when they are unsupported in the dorsiflexion position. The toes drop downward, and the feet are in plantar flexion. Because of the pull of gravity, this position of the feet occurs naturally when the body is at rest. If maintained for extended periods, plantar flexion can cause an alteration in the length of muscles, and the patient may develop a complication called **footdrop.** In this position, the foot is unable to maintain itself in the perpendicular position, heel–toe gait is impossible, and the patient experiences extreme difficulty in walking. The use of a foot support, such as a foot boot, helps avoid this complication. Figure 39-9 demonstrates a foot in plantar flexion versus the dorsiflexion position maintained by wearing a high-top canvas sneaker.

If top bedding must be kept off the patient's lower extremities, a device called a cradle is used. A cradle is usually a metal frame that supports the bed linens away from the patient while providing privacy and warmth. There are a number of sizes and shapes of cradles. If used, the cradle should be fastened securely to the bed so that it does not slide or fall on the patient.

Sandbags, highly valuable when available in various sizes, can be used to immobilize an extremity and support body alignment. When properly filled, they should be pliable enough to

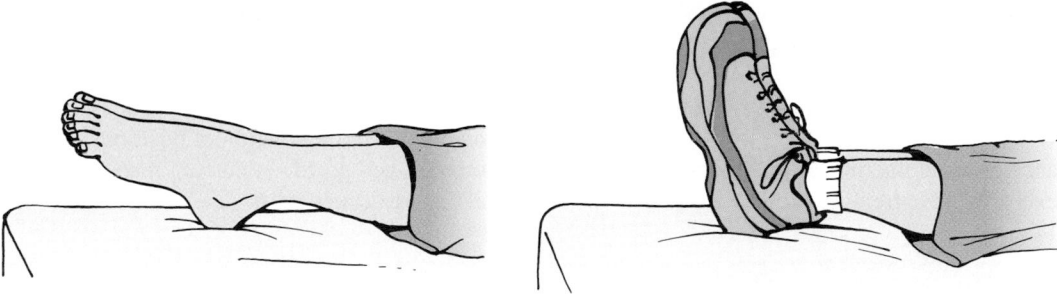

FIGURE 39-9 (*Left*) Plantar flexion occurs when the foot is not supported. (*Right*) When high-top sneakers support the feet, the dorsiflexion position is maintained.

be shaped to body contours to provide support. Avoid hard or firmly packed sandbags. Position a sandbag to avoid creating pressure on a bony prominence.

Trochanter rolls are used to support the hips and legs so that the femurs do not rotate outward. Figure 39-10 illustrates and describes how to use trochanter rolls. Properly placed pillows can also be used to help prevent the thighs from turning outward, but they tend to slip out of place and require frequent adjustment to be effective.

If a patient is paralyzed or unconscious, hand–wrist splints or hand rolls may be necessary to provide a means for keeping the thumb in the correct position, that is, slightly adducted and in apposition to the fingers. A hand roll can be created by folding a washcloth, rolling it, and securing it in place with tape. Once placed against the palm of the hand, it can effectively keep the hand in a functional position (Fig. 39-11). A

commercial plastic or aluminum splint also may be used to hold the thumb in place regardless of the hand position. Encourage patients who are not moving their fingers to do finger exercises, with special attention to having the thumb touch the tip of each finger.

> *Remember Kelsi Lester, the 10-year-old girl who is unconscious after a skiing accident? The nurse would assess Kelsi closely and then determine which devices would be most appropriate to use with her. Pillows for positioning, an adjustable bed, possibly a specialized mattress to prevent skin breakdown, and side rails may be appropriate. In addition, if Kelsi's neurologic status improves, a trapeze bar may help in moving her and allowing Kelsi to participate in her own care. If Kelsi remains unconscious, the nurse would anticipate the need for other devices such as trochanter rolls, foot support, and wrist splints or hand rolls to prevent complications.*

Protective Positioning

Patients accustomed to an active lifestyle who generally use a bed only for sleep are often unaware of the importance of correct body alignment and regular position changes when on

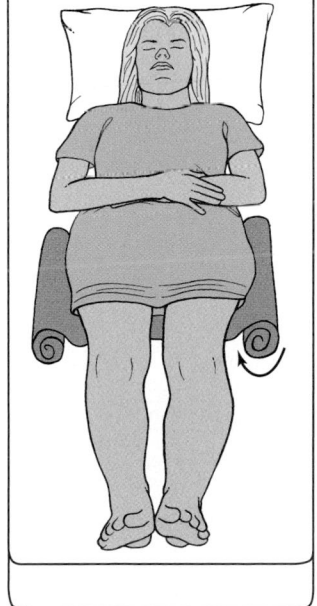

FIGURE 39-10 Trochanter rolls prevent the external rotation of the hips of a bedridden patient. The patient is placed on a folded sheet so that the top edge is at the hips and the lower edge is about one third of the way down the thighs. Towels or a bath blanket is rolled under each side until the roll is snugly against the patient's hips and thighs. The support cannot unroll, and the weight of the patient keeps it secure.

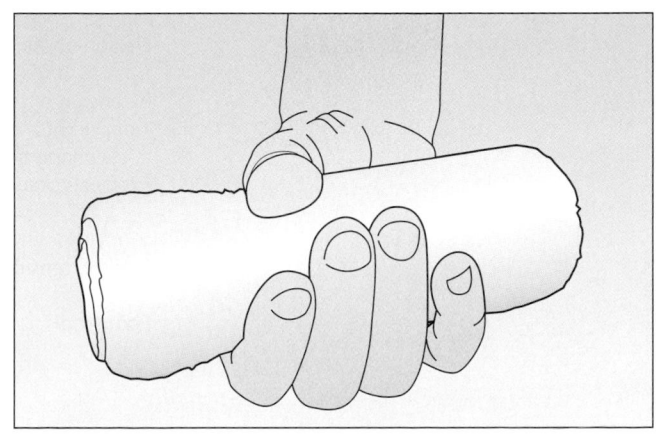

FIGURE 39-11 A hand roll holds the hand in functional position.

prescribed bed rest. Whenever possible, nurses should teach both the patient and family the following:

• Correct positioning techniques
• The need to change positions frequently, at least every 2 hours
• The importance of using the time allotted to position changes to exercise the extremities and to assess and

massage pressure areas (reddened areas should not be massaged)

When the patient is unable to change position independently, use a turn schedule, posted at the bedside to assist with and document the rotation of positions. Table 39-6 describes common bed positions nursing measures to prevent complications associated with these positions.

TABLE 39-6 Common Bed Positions and Protective Nursing Actions

Position	Complication to Be Prevented	Suggested Preventive Actions
Fowler's Position 	Flexion contracture of the neck	Allow the head to rest against the mattress or be supported by a small pillow only.
	Exaggerated curvature of the spine	Use a firm support for the back; position the patient so that the angle of elevation starts at the hips.
	Dislocation of the shoulder	Support the forearms on pillows to elevate them sufficiently so that no pull is exerted on the shoulders.
	Flexion contracture of the wrist	Support the hand on pillows so that it is in natural alignment with the forearm.
	Edema of the hand	Support the hand so that it is slightly elevated in relation to the elbow.
	Flexion contractures of the fingers and abduction of the thumbs	Provide hand–wrist splints if necessary.
	Impaired lower extremity circulation and knee contracture, pressure on heels	Elevate the knees for only brief periods; place one or two pillows under the lower legs from below the knees to the ankles; avoid pressure on the popliteal vessels; avoid using the knee gatch.
	External rotation of the hips	Use trochanter roll.
	Footdrop	Support the feet in dorsal flexion. Use footboard; high-top sneakers can also be used.
Protective Supine Position 	Exaggerated curvature of the spine and flexion of the hips	Provide a firm supportive mattress; use a bed board if necessary.
	Flexion contracture of the neck	Place pillows under the upper shoulders, the neck, and the head so that the head and the neck are held in the correct position.
	Internal rotation of the shoulders and extension of the elbows (hunch shoulders)	Place pillows or arm supports under the forearms so that the upper arms are alongside the body and the forearms are pronated slightly.
	Flexion of the lumbar curvature	Place rolled towel or small pillow under lumbar curvature if needed.
	Extension of the fingers and abduction of the thumbs (clawhand deformities)	Use hand–wrist splints if appropriate.
	External rotation of the femurs	Place sandbags or a trochanter roll alongside the hips and the upper half of the thighs.
	Hyperextension of the knees	Place a pillow under the lower legs from below the knees to the ankles.
	Footdrop	Use a footboard or make an improvised firm foot support to hold the feet in dorsal flexion; high-top sneakers may also be recommended.

(continued)

TABLE 39-6 (Continued)

Position	Complication to Be Prevented	Suggested Preventive Actions
Protective Side-Lying or Lateral Position	Lateral flexion of the neck	Place a pillow under the head and the neck.
	Inward rotation of the arm and interference with respiration	Place a pillow under the upper arm; lower arm should be flexed and positioned comfortably.
	Extension of the finger and abduction of the thumbs	Provide hand–wrist splint if necessary.
	Internal rotation and adduction of the femur	Use one or two pillows as needed to support the leg from the groin to the foot.
	Twisting of the spine	Ensure that the two shoulders are aligned with the two hips.
Protective Sims' Position	Lateral flexion of the neck	Place a small pillow under the head unless the drainage of oral secretions is desired.
	Damage to nerves and blood vessels in the axillae of the lower arm	Carefully position lower arm behind and away from the patient's back.
	Internal shoulder rotation and adduction	Abduct the upper shoulder slightly so that shoulder and elbow are flexed; place a pillow between the chest and upper arm.
	Internal rotation and adduction of the hip; lumbar lordosis	Place a pillow under the upper flexed leg from the groin to the foot.
	Twisting of the spine	Ensure that the two shoulders are aligned with the two hips.
	Footdrop	Support the lower foot in dorsal flexion with a sandbag.
Protective Prone Position	Flexion on the cervical spine	Place a small pillow under the head.
	Hyperextension of the spine; impaired respirations	Place some suitable support under the patient between the end of the rib cage and the upper abdomen if this facilitates breathing and if there is space there.
	Footdrop	Move the patient down in bed so that the feet are over the mattress, or support the lower legs on a pillow just high enough to keep the toes from touching the bed.

Fowler's Position

The semisitting position, or Fowler's position calls for the head of the bed to be elevated 45 to 60 degrees. This position is often used to promote cardiac and respiratory functioning because abdominal organs drop in this position, thereby providing maximal space in the thoracic cavity. This is also the position of choice for eating, conversation, vision, and urinary and intestinal elimination.

Variations of Fowler's position include high Fowler's and low Fowler's or semi-Fowler's position. In the high Fowler's position, the head of the bed is elevated 90 degrees. When a bedside table with a pillow on top of it is placed in front of the patient in high Fowler's position, the patient can lean forward and rest the arms on the pillow, assuming a posture that allows for maximal lung expansion. In low Fowler's or semi-Fowler's position, the head of the bed is elevated only 30 degrees.

In Fowler's position, the buttocks bear the main weight of the body. In this position, the heels, sacrum, and scapulae are at risk for skin breakdown and require frequent assessment. See Table 39-6 for information about correct positioning and nursing actions to prevent complications associated with this position.

Supine or Dorsal Recumbent Position

In the supine position, the patient lies flat on the back with the head and shoulders slightly elevated with a pillow unless contraindicated, such as spinal anesthesia or surgery on the spinal vertebrae. Correct alignment in the supine position is illustrated in Table 39-6.

Side-lying or Lateral Position

In the side-lying position, the patient lies on the side and the main weight of the body is borne by the lateral aspect of the lower scapula and the lateral aspect of the lower ilium. Because many people routinely fall asleep in the side-lying position, this is a comfortable alternate to the supine position for the patient on bed rest. Although it relieves pressure on the scapulae, sacrum, and heels and allows the legs and feet to be comfortably flexed, support pillows are needed for correct positioning (see Table 39-6).

The oblique position is recommended as an alternative to the side-lying position because it places significantly less pressure on the trochanter region. The patient turns toward the side with the hip of the top leg flexed at a 30-degree angle and the knee flexed at 35 degrees. The calf of the upper leg is positioned slightly behind the body's midline. Pillows support the patient's back and calf of the top leg (Fig. 39-12).

A variation of the lateral position is Sims' position. In this position, the patient again lies on the side, but the lower arm is behind the patient and the upper arm is flexed at both the shoulder and the elbow. In this position, the main body weight is borne by the anterior aspects of the humerus, clavicle, and ilium. Thus, the major pressure points differ from those in the lateral and other bed-lying positions (see Table 39-6).

Prone Position

In the prone position, the person lies on the abdomen with the head turned to the side. The body is straightened out in the prone position because the shoulders, head, and neck are in an erect position, the arms are easily placed in correct alignment with the shoulder girdle, the hips are extended, and the knees can be prevented from flexing or hyperextending. When patients on bed rest use this position periodically, it helps to prevent flexion contractures of the hips and knees. However, the pull of gravity on the trunk when the patient lies prone produces a marked lordosis or forward curvature of the lumbar spine. The position is thus contraindicated for people with spinal problems. The pull of gravity on the feet may result in plantar flexion unless the legs and feet are positioned carefully (see Table 39-6). Placing a patient in the prone position requires that the nurse and an assistant to move the person as far as is safely possible onto his or her side, facing the direction that the person will be turned, and near the edge of the level bed. While maintaining the patient securely in that position, pillows can be situated alongside the trunk and upper and lower extremities. Once the patient is gently turned face down, the pillows can be readjusted for comfort and support.

Turning the Patient in Bed

Frequently, a patient cannot turn in bed without assistance. Nurses need to use their knowledge of correct body mechan-ics and correct alignment to turn the patient from the back onto the side, from the back onto the abdomen, and from the abdomen onto the back. The technique for turning a patient in bed is described and illustrated in Skill 39-1. Mastering this turning technique helps nurses adhere to an every-2-hour turn schedule for an immobile patient.

> *Consider Genevieve Augustus, the older woman caring for her husband at home and Kelsi Lester, the 10-year-old girl who is unconscious. Teaching Mrs. Augustus how to properly turn her husband in bed and assist him in doing so would be crucial to minimize stress and strain on Mrs. Augustus' back and legs. Turning Kelsi every 2 hours would be essential to prevent skin breakdown.*

Assisting With Range-of-Motion Exercises

Range of motion is the complete extent of movement of which a joint is normally capable. Engaging in routine tasks, such as bathing, eating, dressing, and writing, helps use muscle groups that keep many joints in effective range of motion. When all or some of normal ADLs are impossible, attention should be given to the joints not being used at all or to those that are limited in their use.

Unless contraindicated, active, active-assistive, or passive range-of-motion exercises should be encouraged regularly and included in the patient's plan of care. In **active exercise,** the patient independently moves joints through their full range of motion (isotonic exercise). In active-assistive exercise, the nurse may provide minimal support, whereas in **passive exercise,** the patient is unable to move independently, and the nurse moves each joint through its range of motion. Both active and passive exercises improve joint mobility and increase circulation to the affected part, but only active exercise increases muscle mass, tone, and strength and improves cardiac and respiratory functioning. Thus, exercises should be as active as the patient's physical condition permits. It is also helpful to teach isometric exercises to patients to increase muscle mass, tone, and strength.

Include directives in the nursing plan of care for range-of-motion exercises, specifying what, how, and when, so that all who care for the patient observe the same routine. In some institutions, nurses work closely with physiotherapists in designing and implementing exercise programs. The following

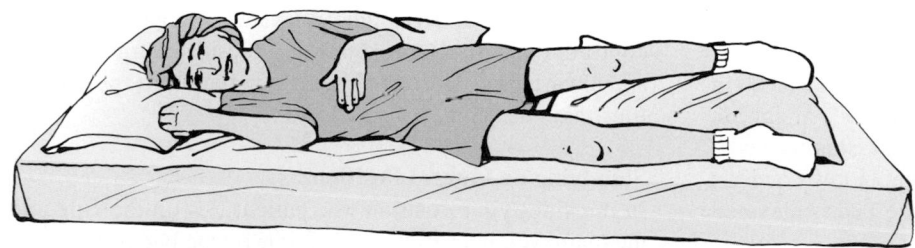

FIGURE 39-12 Modified lateral position (oblique position) is an alternative to the side-lying position and results in significantly less pressure on the trochanter area.

SKILL 39-1 Turning a Patient in Bed

ACTION	RATIONALE
1. Explain the procedure to the patient.	This facilitates the cooperation of the patient.
2. Perform hand hygiene.	Hand hygiene deters the spread of microorganisms.
3. Raise the bed to your waist level. Adjust to flat position or as low as the patient can tolerate. Lower side rail nearest you and raise the opposite side.	This position facilitates the turning maneuver and minimizes strain on the nurse yet keeps the patient safe.
4. Position the patient closer to the far side of the bed in the supine position.	The patient will be in the center of the bed after turning is accomplished.
5. Place the patient's arms across the chest and cross the patient's far leg over the near one.	This facilitates the turning motion and protects the patient's arms during the turn.
6. Stand opposite the patient's center with your feet spread and one foot ahead of the other. Tighten your gluteal and abdominal muscles and flex your knees.	This positions the turner opposite the center of the body mass. It places the nurse in a stable position with good body alignment and prepared to use large muscle masses to turn the patient.

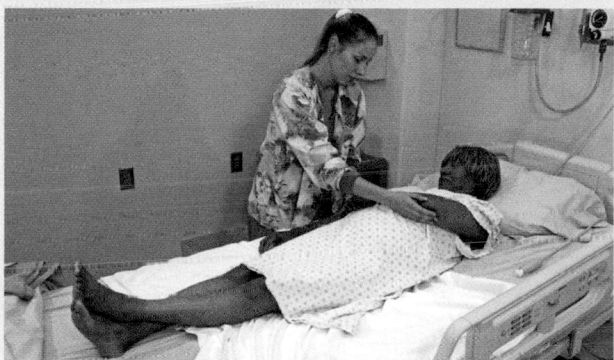

Action 5: Positioning patient's arms and legs.   (Photo by Rick Brady.)

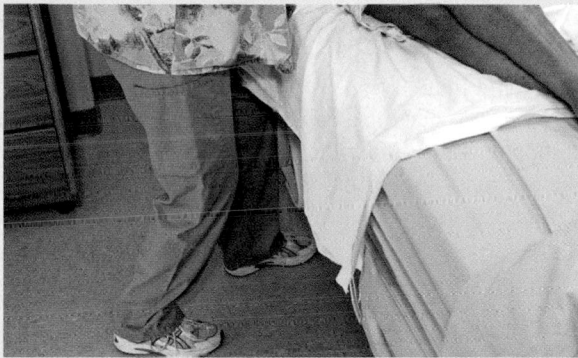

Action 6: Preparing to turn patient.   (Photo by Rick Brady.)

ACTION	RATIONALE
7. Position your hands on the patient's far shoulder and hip and roll the patient toward you.	This maneuver supports the patient's body and makes use of the nurse's weight to assist with turning.
8. Make the patient comfortable and position in proper alignment.	This ensures that the patient will be able to maintain desired position.

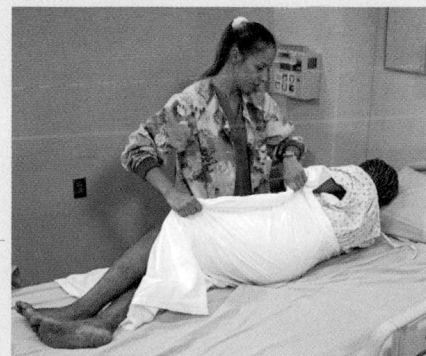

Action 7: Turning patient.   (Photo by Rick Brady.)

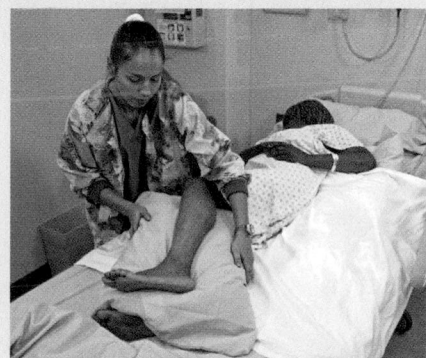

Action 8: Making patient comfortable.   (Photo by Rick Brady.)

ACTION	RATIONALE
9. Readjust the bed height and position and raise side rail if appropriate. Ensure that call light is within patient's reach.	This ensures the patient's safety.
10. Perform hand hygiene.	Hand hygiene deters the spread of microorganisms.

are basic guidelines when helping to put the patient's joints through range of motion:

- Teach the patient what exercise is being undertaken, why, and how it will be done. A show-and-tell technique is often helpful.
- Avoid overexertion and using exercises to the point that the patient develops fatigue. The exercises are not to exhaust or tax the patient. Certain exercises may need to be delayed until the patient's condition allows.
- Avoid neck hyperextension and attempts to achieve full range of motion in all joints with older patients. These movements may prove painful. Encourage adequate range of motion in those joints necessary to perform ADLs.
- Start gradually and work slowly. All movements should be smooth and rhythmic. Irregular and jerky movements are uncomfortable for patients.
- Move each joint until there is resistance but not pain. Uncomfortable reactions should be reported and exercises halted until further instructions are obtained.
- While exercising joints, use a variety of support measures to prevent muscle strain or injury to the patient as demonstrated in Figure 39-13:
  - *Cupping*—placing a cupped hand under the joint to support it (eg, under the elbow)
  - *Cradling*—supporting the joint with one hand while cradling the distal portion of the extremity with the remaining arm (eg, the calf or forearm might be cradled while the knee or elbow is supported)
  - *Supporting* the joint by holding the adjacent distal and proximal muscular areas (indicated when a joint is painful); grasping muscle groups or major tendons is likely to cause injury to the tissues
- Return the joint to a neutral position, that is, its normal position of alignment, when finishing each exercise.
- Keep friction at a minimum when moving extremities to avoid injuring the skin.
- Use range-of-motion exercises twice a day, and do the exercises regularly to build up muscle and joint capabilities. Each exercise is carried out two to five times. Many of the exercises can be carried out when the patient is being bathed and become part of that procedure. Encourage routine tasks such as eating, dressing, self-bathing, and writing to help to put certain joints through range of motion.
- Expect the patient's respiratory and heart rate to increase during exercising, which is good. These rates should return to usual resting levels within 3 minutes. If they do not, the exercises are probably too strenuous for the patient.
- Use passive exercises as necessary, but encourage active exercises of the same kind when the patient is able to do so independently. Exercises should

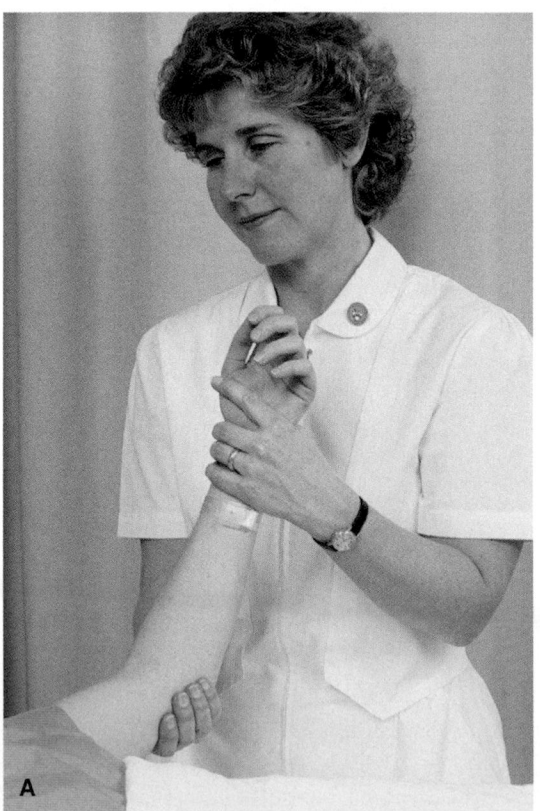
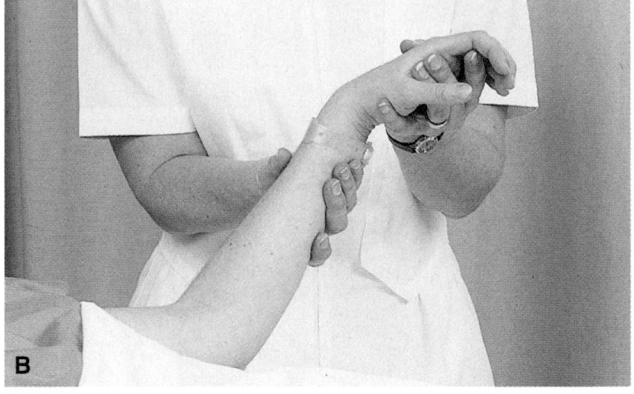
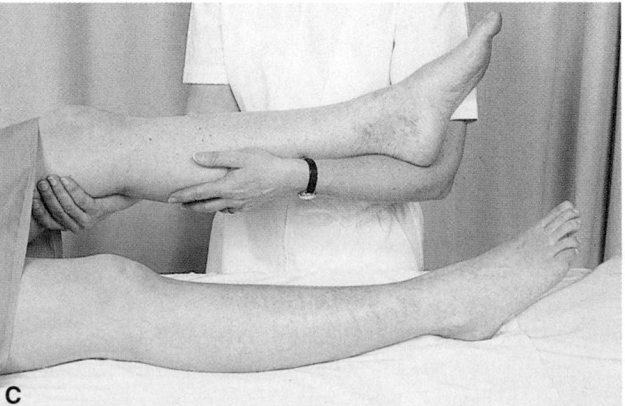

FIGURE 39-13 Support measures used to prevent muscle strain or injury to the patient during range-of-motion exercises. (**A**) Using a cupped hand to support a joint. (**B**) Supporting the joint by holding the distal and proximal areas adjacent to the joint. (**C**) Cradling the distal portion of a lower extremity.

continue at home after a period of hospitalization, as necessary.

> *Think back to Maggie Wyatt, the woman being discharged after treatment for a fracture. Range-of-motion exercises are essential for Maggie to maintain function. Although physical therapy would probably develop the exercise regimen, the nurse would need to reinforce these instructions with Maggie before discharge. In addition, the nurse would observe Maggie performing the active range-of-motion exercises and would assist with the passive exercises until she goes home.*

The goal of range-of-motion exercises is to keep the patient in the best possible physical state when bed rest is necessary. When range-of-motion exercises are not considered as routine measures, the patient's physician should be consulted. Skill 39-2 illustrates the normal movements incorporated in passive range-of-motion exercises.

Moving and Lifting the Patient

Frequently, it is necessary to move a patient who is weak or unable to move himself or herself. Keep the patient in good alignment and protect from injury while being moved. Follow these recommended guidelines when moving and lifting patients:

- Know the patient's medical diagnosis, capabilities, and any movement not allowed. Put in place braces or any device the patient wears before helping from bed.
- Plan carefully what you will do before moving or lifting a patient. Assess the mobility of attached equipment. You may injure the patient or yourself if you have not planned well. If necessary, enlist the support of another nurse. This reduces the strain on everyone involved.
- Explain to the patient what you plan to do. Then use what abilities the patient has to assist you. This technique often decreases the effort required and the possibility of injury to you.

SKILL 39-2 　Assisting With Passive Range-of-Motion (ROM) Exercises

ACTION	RATIONALE
1. Explain the procedure to the patient.	This facilitates the patient's cooperation.
2. Perform hand hygiene.	Hand hygiene deters the spread of microorganisms.
3. Raise the bed to your waist level. Adjust to flat position or as low as patient can tolerate.	This position minimizes strain on the nurse.
4. Begin ROM exercises at the patient's head and move down one side of the body at a time.	Systematic progression ensures that all body parts are exercised.
5. Perform each exercise two to five times, moving each joint in a smooth and rhythmic manner.	Repeated movement of muscles and joints improves flexibility and increases circulation to the body part.
6. Protect joint during ROM exercises (see Fig. 39-13).	This prevents muscle strain or injury to the joint.
7. Progress through ROM exercises for each joint.	

HEAD

- *Flexion*—move chin down to rest on chest.
- *Extension*—return head to normal upright position.
- *Lateral flexion*—tilt head as far as possible toward each shoulder.

NECK

- *Rotation*—move the head from side to side bringing chin toward shoulder.

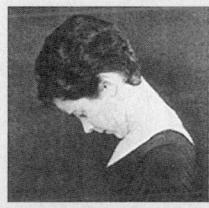
Flexion

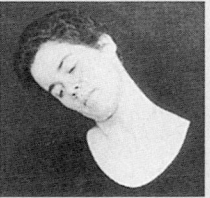
Lateral flexion

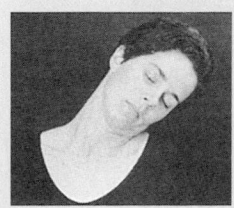
Lateral flexion

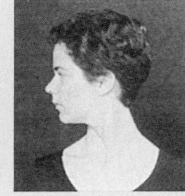
Rotation

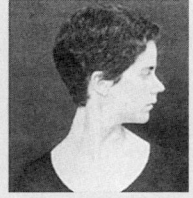
Rotation

(continued)

SHOULDER

- *Flexion*—start with arm at side and lift arm forward to above head.
- *Extension*—return arm to starting position at side of body.

- *Abduction*—start with arm at side and move laterally to upright position above head.
- *Adduction*—lower arm to original position and move across body as far as possible.
- *Internal and external rotation*—raise arm at side until upper arm is on line with shoulder. Bend elbow at a 90-degree angle and move forearm upward and downward.

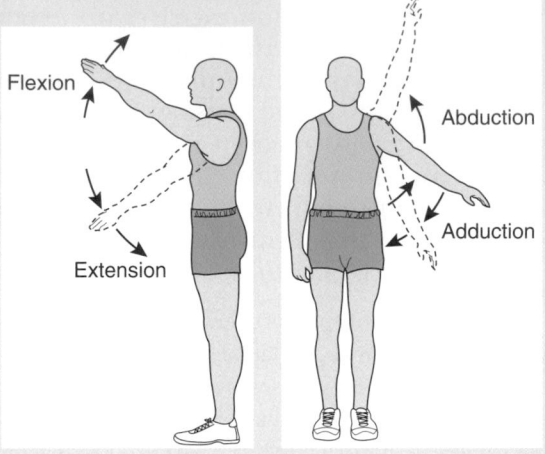

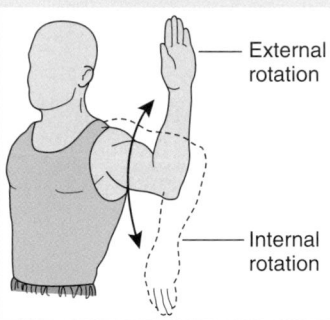

ELBOW

- *Flexion*—bend elbow and move lower arm and hand upward toward shoulder.
- *Extension*—return lower arm and hand to original position while straightening elbow.

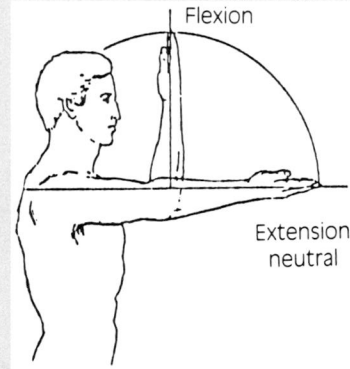

FOREARM

- *Supination*—rotate lower arm and hand so palm is up.
- *Pronation*—rotate lower arm and hand so palm is down.

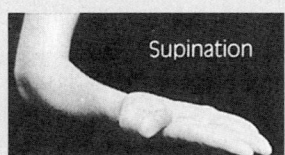
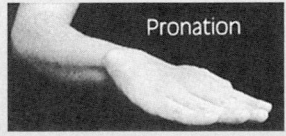

WRIST

- *Flexion*—move hand downward toward inner aspect of forearm.
- *Extension*—return hand to neutral position even with forearm.
- *Hyperextension*—move dorsal (upper) portion of hand backward as far as possible.

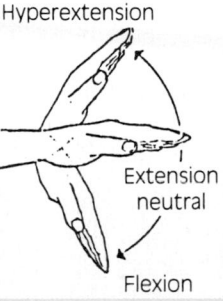

(continued)

Assisting With Passive Range-of-Motion (ROM) Exercises (continued)

FINGERS

- *Flexion*—bend fingers in to make a fist.
- *Extension*—straighten fingers out.
- *Abduction*—spread fingers apart.
- *Adduction*—return fingers until they are together.
- *Opposition of thumb to fingers*—touch thumb to each finger on hand.

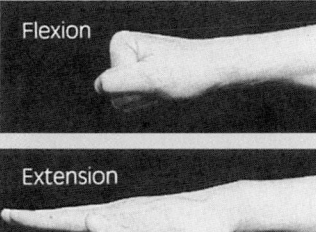

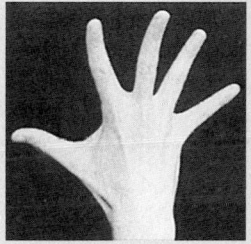

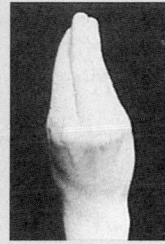
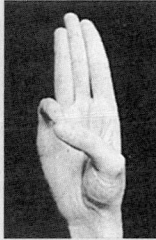

Abduction   Adduction   Opposition of thumb to finger

HIP

- *Flexion*—with leg extended, lift upward.
- *Extension*—return leg to original position next to other leg.
- *Abduction*—lift leg laterally away from body.
- *Adduction*—return leg toward other leg and lift beyond it if possible.
- *Internal rotation*—turn foot and leg toward other leg.
- *External rotation*—move foot and leg outward away from other leg.

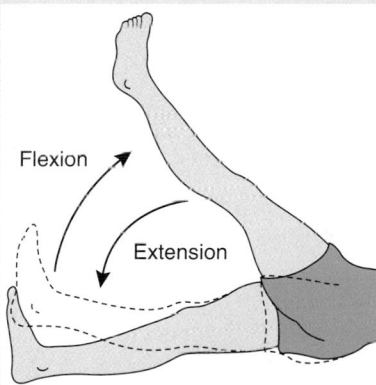

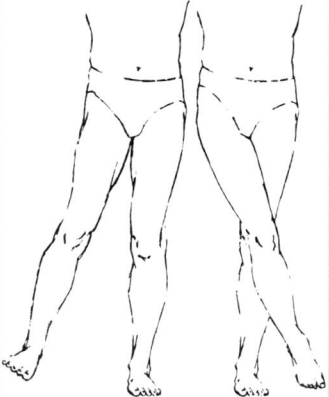
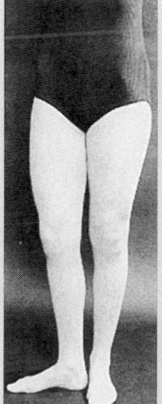
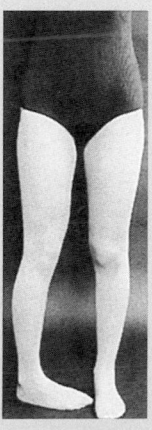

Abduction   Abduction   External rotation   Internal rotation

(continued)

KNEE

- *Flexion*—bend leg, bringing heel toward back of leg.
- *Extension*—return leg to straight position.

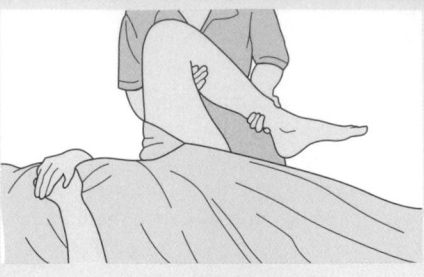

Flexion

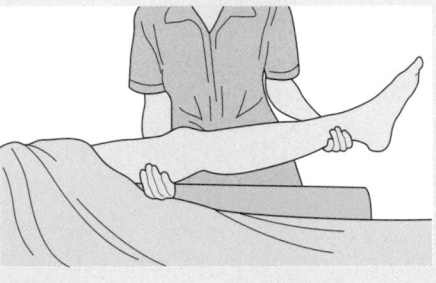

Extension

ANKLE

- *Dorsiflexion*—move foot up and back until toes are upright.
- *Plantar flexion*—move foot with toes pointing downward.
- *Inversion*—turn sole of foot toward the middle.
- *Eversion*—turn sole of foot outward.

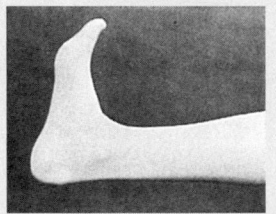

Dorsiflexion

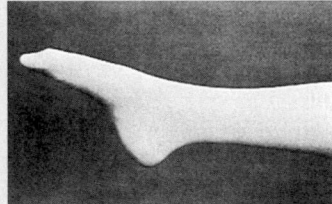

Plantar flexion

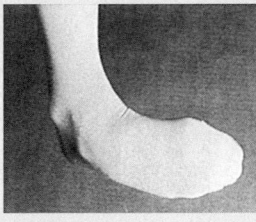

Inversion

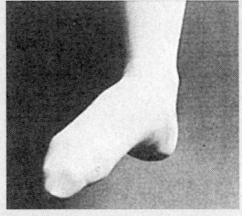

Eversion

TOES

- *Flexion*—curl toes downward.
- *Extension*—straighten toes out.
- *Abduction*—spread toes apart
- *Adduction*—bring toes together.

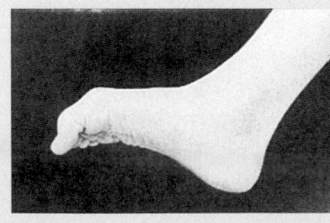

Flexion

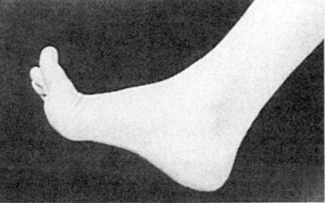

Extension

(continued)

Assisting With Passive Range-of-Motion (ROM) Exercises (continued)

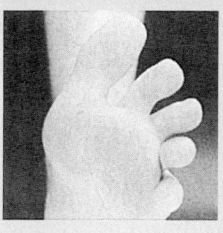
Abduction

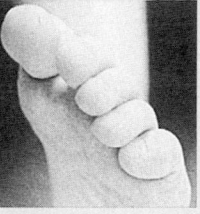
Adduction

ACTION	RATIONALE
8. Return patient to comfortable position.	This promotes rest and sleep.
9. Readjust the bed height and position and raise side rail if it is appropriate. Ensure that call bell is within patient's reach.	This ensures the patient's safety.
10. Perform hand hygiene.	Hand hygiene deters the spread of microorganisms.

- If the patient is in pain, administer the prescribed analgesic sufficiently in advance of the transfer to allow the patient to participate in the move comfortably.
- Remove any obstacles that may make moving and lifting inconvenient.
- Elevate the bed as necessary so that you are working at a height that is comfortable and safe for you.
- Lock the wheels of the bed, wheelchair, or stretcher so that they do not slide while you are moving the patient.
- Observe the principles of body mechanics to prevent injuring yourself while you work.
- Be sure the patient is in good body alignment while being moved and lifted to protect the patient from strain and muscle injury.
- Support the patient's body well. Avoid grabbing and holding an extremity by its muscles.
- Avoid friction on the patient's skin during moving. Friction can be reduced by sprinkling powder or cornstarch on bed linens and on the patient's skin.
- Move your body and the patient in a smooth, rhythmic motion. Jerky movements tend to put extra strain on muscles and joints and are uncomfortable for the patient.
- Use mechanical devices such as lifts, slides, transfer chairs, or gait belts when available for moving patients. Be sure that you understand how the device operates and that the patient is properly secured and informed of what will occur. Patients who do not understand or are afraid may be unable to cooperate and may suffer injury as a result.
- Be realistic about how much you can safely do without injury. Two small people cannot lift or move an obese patient without risking muscle strain and injury.

Consider Genevieve Augustus, the woman caring for her husband at home. The nurse would incorporate these guidelines when role modeling the proper techniques for moving and lifting Mr. Augustus. In addition, the nurse would use these guidelines to develop a teaching plan for Mrs. Augustus to ensure safety for all involved when moving and lifting Mr. Augustus.

Preventing Back Injury

Nurses who retire from or leave nursing often cite back injuries as an influencing factor. Forty-seven percent (47%) of nurses in the United States have reported injuries to their back (Nelson, Fragala, et al., 2003). Nurses may incur back injuries as a result of poor body mechanics or become injured when a patient falls. Many nurses say they have had episodes of occupation-related back problems and accept back pain as a routine consequence of the job—which it need not be. Variables that can lead to back injuries or back pain for healthcare workers include:

- Uncoordinated lifts
- Height–weight differential among the lifters
- Lifting when fatigued
- Lifting after recent recovery from a back injury
- Lack of training in proper body mechanics
- Standing for long periods of time
- Transferring patients from beds to stretchers, wheelchairs, or operating tables

Recent research conducted at a Veterans Administration medical center has suggested that consistent use of standardized protocols and mechanical lifting devices is a more effective approach than just using proper body mechanics to decrease the risk of back injury for healthcare workers (Nelson, Fragala, et al., 2003, and Nelson, Owen, et al., 2003). Even routine repetitive care activities such as changing bed linens and bathing patients have the potential to cause back injury. Preventive measures should also focus on careful assessment of the patient care environment so that patients can be moved safely and effectively. Based on experiences in some hospitals in the United Kingdom, several U.S. hospitals attempted to implement a "no lift" policy. Without adequate purchase of necessary lifting equipment, cooperation of the staff, and re-engineering of the environment, "no lift" policies have proved unenforceable and ineffective. There is also no evidence that the use of a back belt safeguards a nurse from back injury. In some institutions, specially trained staff members who function as "back injury resource nurses" are responsible for assisting nurses to assess patients and use step-by-step protocols or algorithms to prevent injury (Fig. 39-14).

Techniques to prevent back stress should be included routinely in injury-prevention programs.

Moving a Patient Up in Bed

Children and adults who are lighter in weight or who can assist with movement are relatively easy to slide toward the head of the bed without the assistance of a second person. The patient assists movement either by pushing with the feet flat against the bed or by using an overbed trapeze. A technique used to move a patient up in bed when the patient is able to assist and two nurses are available is described and illustrated in Skill 39-3.

Moving the Patient From Bed to Stretcher

Considerable care must be taken when moving a patient from a bed to a stretcher, or vice versa, to prevent injury to the patient and injury to the nurse's back. If the patient is unconscious or weakened, additional nurses are needed to support the extremities and the head. These actions are described in Skill 39-4. For patients who are obese, use of a transfer board or roller board facilitates the move from stretcher to bed and helps ensure that the patient's body is properly aligned during the transfer (see Special Considerations in Skill 39-4). When returning the patient to the bed from the stretcher, the same techniques are used. The carriers first move the patient from the stretcher onto the edge of the bed. Then one member of the team supports the patient on the edge of the bed to ensure the patient does not fall off while the other two team members go around to the opposite side of the bed and place their arms underneath the patient. After the two people on the opposite side of the bed have a good grip on the patient, the third person joins them and assists in sliding the patient to the center of the bed.

In an emergency, sometimes, patients must be lifted and carried. This can be done by means of a three-carrier lift. If done properly, the patient will feel secure, and those lifting will

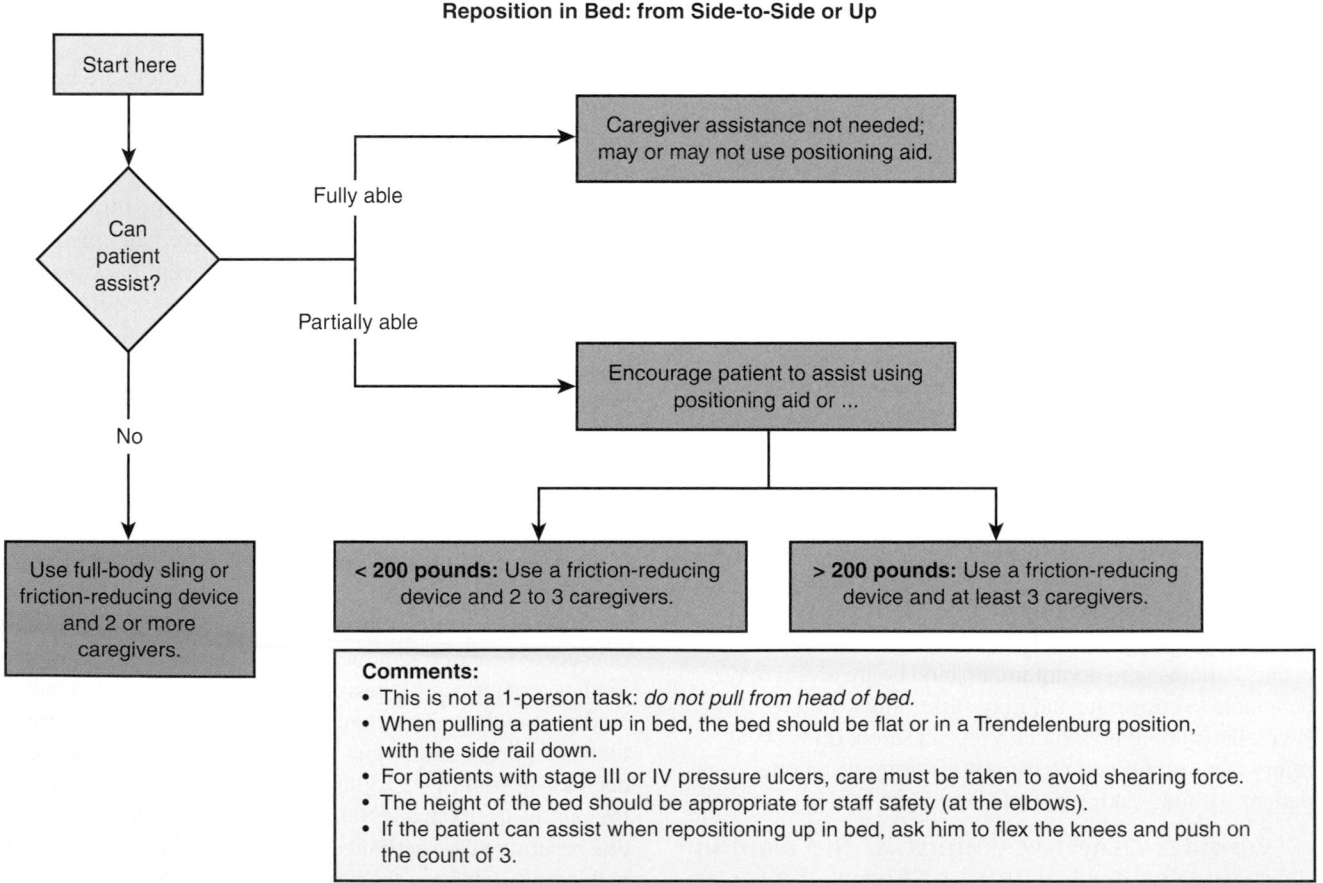

FIGURE 39-14 Step-by-step procedure or algorithm used to outline safe technique for repositioning a patient in bed. (From Nelson, A., Owen, B., Lloyd, J., Fragala, G., Matz, M., et al. [2003]. Safe patient handling & movement. *American Journal of Nursing, 103* [3], 32–43.)

SKILL
39-3

Assisting a Patient Up in Bed (Two Nurses)

ACTION	RATIONALE
1. Explain the procedure to the patient.	This facilitates cooperation of the patient.
2. Perform hand hygiene.	Hand hygiene deters the spread of microorganisms.
3. Raise the bed to a comfortable position for you. Adjust the bed to flat position if the patient can tolerate it. With two nurses on opposite sides of the bed, lower the side rails.	This position facilitates moving the patient and minimizes strain on the nurse.
4. Remove the pillow and place it at the head of the bed.	This reduces friction and protects the patient's head from striking the top of the bed.
5. Place drawsheet on bed under the patient's midsection.	Drawsheet supports the patient's weight and reduces friction during the lift.
6. If able to assist, have the patient flex the knees and place feet flat on the bed.	The patient is prepared to push upward by using a major muscle group.
7. Fold the patient's arms across the chest and instruct patient to flex the neck with chin on the chest.	This provides assistance, reduces friction, and prevents hyper-extension of the neck.
8. Stand opposite the patient's center with your feet spread and turned toward the head of the bed. Position one foot slightly forward.	This positions the mover opposite the center of the body mass. It places both nurses in a stable position with good alignment.
9. Fold or bunch drawsheet close to the patient before grasping it securely and preparing to move patient.	This brings the patient's center of gravity closer to each nurse and provides for a secure hold.

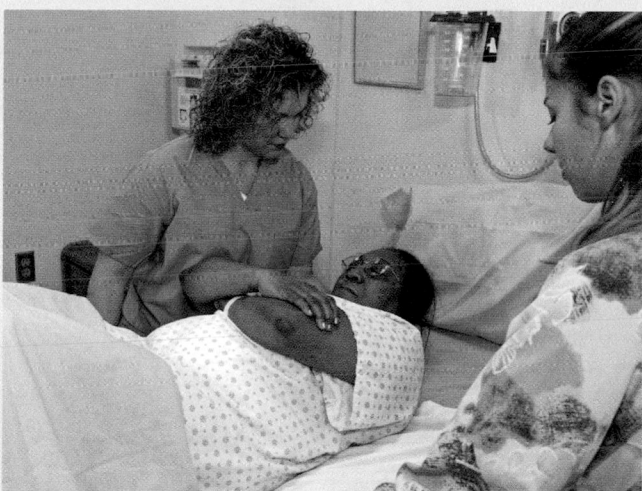

Action 7: Patient with arms folded across chest and neck flexed with chin on chest.   (Photo by Rick Brady.)

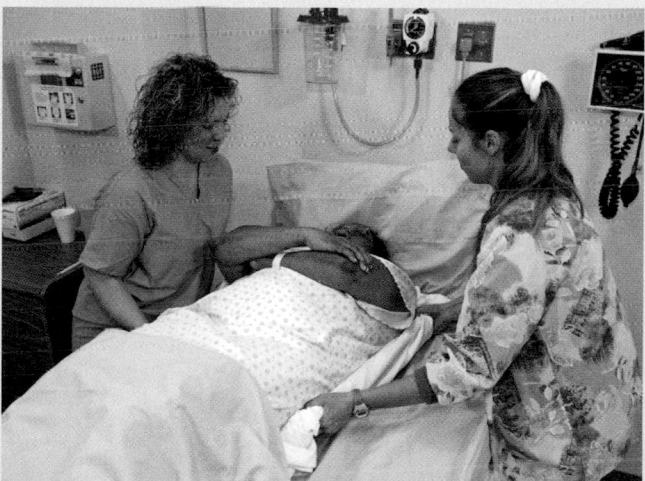

Action 9: Folding drawsheet in preparation for moving patient. (Photo by Rick Brady.)

10. Shift your weight back and forth from back leg to front leg, and on count of three, move the patient upward in bed. If possible, the patient can assist the move upward by pushing with the legs. Repeat if necessary.	The rocking motion uses the nurses' weight to counteract the patient's weight as the nurses move the patient up in bed. If the patient assists, less effort is required by the nurses.
11. Assist the patient to a comfortable position. Reposition the pillow. Raise the side rail and adjust the bed position if necessary. Place call light within patient's reach.	This ensures the patient's safety.
12. Perform hand hygiene.	Hand hygiene deters the spread of microorganisms.

Special Considerations   If two nurses are available, consider moving a patient up in bed by interlocking arms under the patient's shoulders and thighs and lifting as described above. The most serious back injuries can occur when the nurse attempts to move a patient without help, and twists and lifts at the same time (Converso & Murphy, 2004).

If patient is small, determine how much strength to use when lifting. Although the pillow will protect the head, if the patient is lifted with too much force, a neck injury may occur.

SKILL 39-4   Transferring a Patient From Bed to Stretcher

ACTION	RATIONALE
1. Explain the procedure to the patient.	This facilitates the cooperation of the patient.
2. Perform hand hygiene.	Hand hygiene deters the spread of microorganisms.
3. Move the bed and equipment in the room to make room for the stretcher. Make sure that assistants are available. Close the door or curtain.	This facilitates transfer movement and provides for privacy.
4. Raise the bed to the same height as the stretcher and adjust the head of the bed to the flat position if the patient can tolerate it. Lower side rails.	Pushing and pulling require less effort than lifting, This position facilitates moving the patient.
5. Place a drawsheet under the patient if one is not already there. Use the drawsheet to move the patient to the side of the bed where the stretcher will be placed.	This facilitates movement of the patient to the stretcher.
6. Position stretcher next to the bed and parallel to it. Lock wheels on the stretcher and bed. Remove the pillow from the bed and place it on the stretcher.	Positioning of the stretcher and locking the wheels facilitate safe transfer of patient.
7. To move the patient:	
a. The first nurse should kneel on far side of the bed away from the stretcher. Position the knee at the upper torso closer to the patient than the other knee. Grasp the drawsheet securely.	The nurse uses a major muscle group to assist in movement. The nurse's flexed hips help avoid back injury.
b. The second nurse should reach across the stretcher and grasp the drawsheet at the head and chest areas of the patient.	This promotes safe transfer by supporting the patient's head and upper body.
c. The third nurse should reach across the stretcher and grasp the drawsheet at the patient's waist and thigh area. Ask the patient to fold arms across the chest.	This supports the lower part of the patient's body for safe transfer.
d. At a signal given by the first nurse, the second and third nurses pull while the first nurse lifts the patient from the bed to the stretcher.	Working in unison distributes the work of moving the patient and facilitates the transfer.

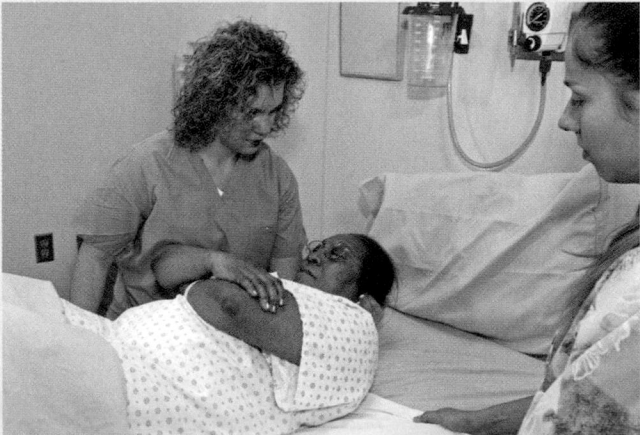

Action 5: Using drawsheet to move patient to side of bed.   (Photo by Rick Brady.)

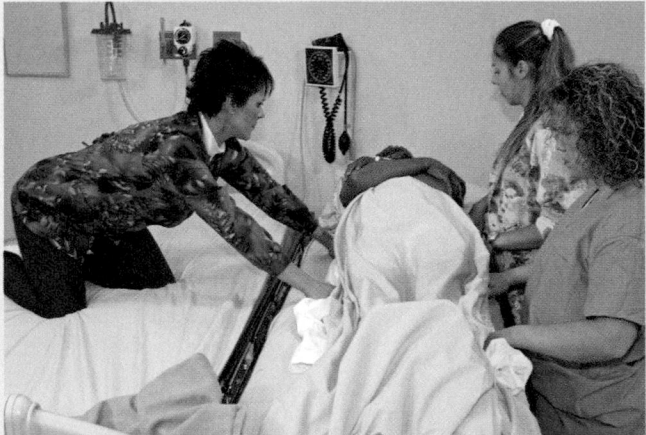

Action 7: Moving patient to stretcher.   (Photo by Rick Brady.)

8. Secure the patient on the stretcher until side rails are raised. Assist the patient to a comfortable position with the covering in place. Leave the drawsheet in place for transfer back to bed.	This ensures patient safety and comfort.
9. Perform hand hygiene.	Hand hygiene deters the spread of microorganisms.

(continued)

SKILL 39-4 Transferring a Patient From Bed to Stretcher (continued)

Special Considerations

- A long polyethylene board with handgrips on the edges may be used to assist with the transfer:
  - Turn the patient on his or her side with the back toward the stretcher.
  - Position the transfer board lengthwise and midway between the bed and stretcher.
  - Return the patient to his or her back with a bottom sheet or drawsheet between the patient and the board.
  - Using the sheet, slide the patient across the transfer board and onto the stretcher.
  - Reposition the patient on the stretcher, remove the board, and secure with safety belts and side rails.

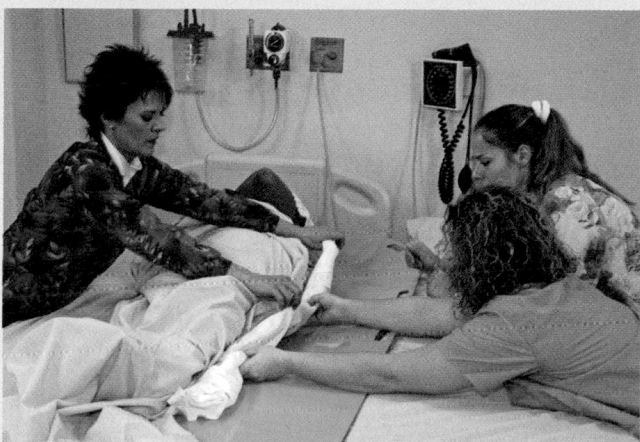

Special Considerations: Using a transfer board to facilitate moving the patient from bed to stretcher. (Photo by Rick Brady.)

- In an emergency, a three-carrier lift may also be done to move a patient from bed to stretcher:
  - Each person must support one section of the patient's body—head, shoulders, and chest; hips; and thighs and legs.
  - Slide your arms under the patient as far as possible and on signal, simultaneously roll the patient toward your chests.
  - On signal, stand up and steady the patient against your chests.
  - Step back together, pivot around to the stretcher, and, on signal, lower the patient onto the stretcher.

not suffer strain. The three-carrier lift is described in Skill 39-4 under Special Considerations.

For patients who present special problems because of their excessive weight or a cast, it may be necessary to have an additional person to support the heaviest or most cumbersome part of the patient. The people distribute their arms while carrying so that the heaviest part is well supported.

Moving the Patient From Bed to Chair

Safety and comfort are key concerns when the nurse assists the patient out of bed. Preliminary assessment of vital signs provides baseline data, and subsequent recordings determine the effect of this activity on the patient. The position of the nurse as he or she prepares to move the patient and placement of the chair are critical elements in the transfer. The patient's apparel should be sufficient to prevent embarrassment and provide warmth yet not impede movement. The technique for assisting a patient to transfer from bed to chair is described in Skill 39-5.

It is possible for only one person to help a weakened patient transfer from a bed to a chair. However, it is safer and simpler with two people present. The one-person technique

is valuable for nurses to know when providing care for the patient in the home and an emergency exists. More than one person should be available if the bed and chair seat are not the same height. In addition, if the patient is dependent and requires total assistance, two nurses are necessary. The technique for two nurses transferring a dependent patient is described in Skill 39-6.

Recall Maggie Wyatt, the woman being discharged with an external fixation device in place? In assessing the situation, the nurse would need to determine how much Maggie can help with the transfer. From there, the nurse would then determine if another person is needed to help transfer Maggie. Realizing that the device is heavy and cumbersome, the nurse would determine that most likely two persons are needed.

Logrolling a Patient

When a patient has a spinal injury or is recovering from neck, back, or spinal surgery, it is necessary to keep the body in

SKILL 39-5   Assisting a Patient to Transfer From Bed to Chair

ACTION	RATIONALE
1. Explain the procedure to the patient. Offer bedpan.	This facilitates cooperation of the patient. Empty bladder will increase patient comfort.
2. Perform hand hygiene.	Hand hygiene deters the spread of microorganisms.
3. Assess the patient's ability to assist with transfer. Move equipment as necessary to make room for the chair. Close the door or curtain.	This ensures patient safety and facilitates the transfer. Closing the door or curtain provides for privacy.
4. Place the bed in the low position.	This facilitates transfer to chair.
5. Assist the patient to put on a robe and slippers with nonskid soles.	These provide warmth. Slippers provide protection and stability.
6. Position the chair at the bedside: a. *For a patient with unimpaired mobility:* Bring chair close to the bedside facing the foot of the bed and, if possible, brace the back of the chair against a bedside table.	This increases stability and ensures patient safety during the transfer.
b. *For a patient with impaired mobility:* Position the chair facing the head or foot of the bed. When sitting on the side of the bed, the patient should be able to steady self by using the hand on the unaffected side to grasp the arm of the chair.	This uses the strong side to provide balance and improve stability during the transfer.

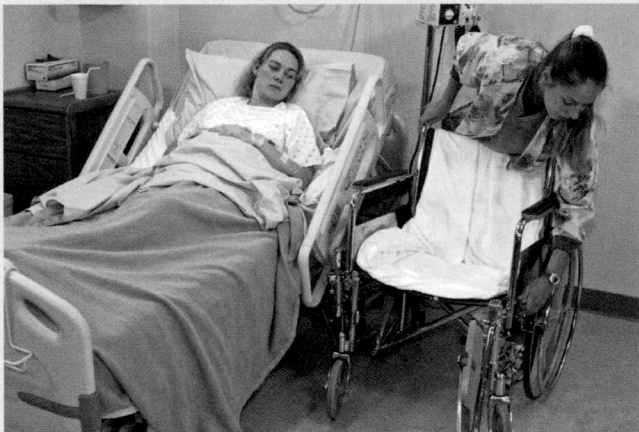

Action 6: Placing chair at bedside.   (Photo by Rick Brady.)

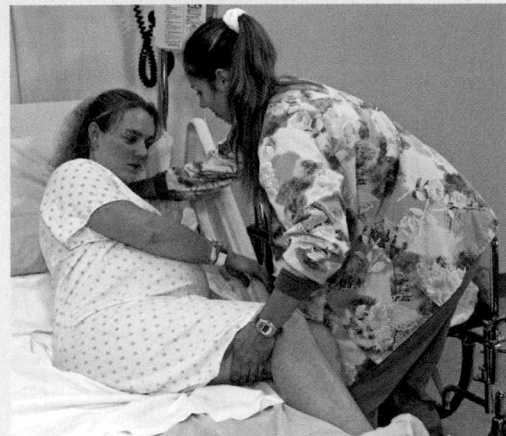

Action 9: Supporting patient while moving legs off bed. (Photo by Rick Brady.)

ACTION	RATIONALE
7. Lock the wheels on the chair and bed if appropriate. Raise the foot pedals on the wheelchair to the up position.	This ensures patient safety.
8. Raise the head of the bed to the highest position.	Moving from the sitting to the standing position requires less energy.
9. Assist the patient to sit on the side of the bed by supporting the patient's head and neck while moving the patient's legs off the bed to dangle. Steady the patient in that position for a few minutes.	The sitting position facilitates transfer to the chair and allows the circulatory system to adjust to a change in position.
10. Assist the patient to the standing position: a. *For a patient with unimpaired mobility:* Face the patient and brace your feet and knees against the patient. Place your hands around the patient's waist while the patient holds onto you between the shoulders and the waist. Use your legs to help you raise the patient to the standing position.	This provides for stability and for use of major muscle groups to facilitate movement. Allowing the patient to grasp the nurse around the neck could injure the nurse if the patient should fall.
b. *For a patient with impaired mobility:* Face the patient and brace your feet and knees against the patient, especially against the affected extremity. Place your hands around the patient's waist. The patient may place the unaffected arm around your shoulder or use the unaffected arm to reach for the arm of the chair and to push up while raising to the standing position.	This provides for stability and makes use of the unaffected extremities to facilitate movement.

(continued)

SKILL
39-5 Assisting a Patient to Transfer From Bed to Chair (continued)

ACTION	RATIONALE
11. Pivot the patient (on the unaffected limb if applicable) into position in front of the chair with legs positioned against the chair.	This provides security and proper position before sitting.
12. The patient may use one arm (the unaffected limb if applicable) to place on the arm of the chair and steady self while slowly lowering to the sitting position. Continue to brace the patient's knees with your knees and flex your own hips and knees when seating the patient.	The patient uses own arm for support and stability. The nurse flexes the knees and hips to use a major muscle group to aid in movement and reduce strain on the back.

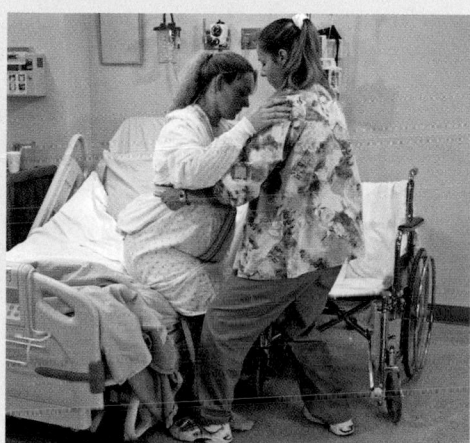

Action 10b: Assisting patient to stand.   (Photo by Rick Brady.)

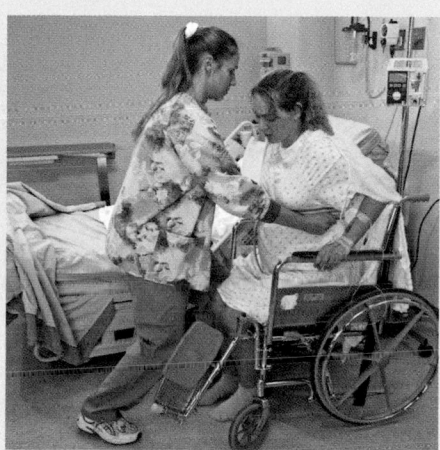

Action 12: Bracing patient's knees while lowering patient to chair.   (Photo by Rick Brady.)

13. Adjust the patient's position using pillows where necessary. Cover the patient and use restraint if necessary. Position the call bell so it is available for use.	This maintains proper body alignment and provides for comfort and safety.
14. Perform hand hygiene.	Hand hygiene deters the spread of microorganisms.
15. Document the patient's tolerance of the procedure and length of time in the chair.	This provides accurate documentation and ensures continuity of care.

Special Considerations
- A walking or transfer belt may be used to assist the transfer. With the belt secure around the patient's waist, the nurse can grasp the belt on both sides (or use handles if they are available) and assist the patient to stand and move to the chair.
- A sliding board may also be used to ease the patient who cannot stand into a chair.

straight alignment when turning the patient. Two or three nurses can accomplish this safely by logrolling a patient (Fig. 39-15). Following are guidelines for using this technique:
- Use a drawsheet if possible to facilitate smooth movement.
- Have the patient cross his or her arms on the chest.
- Place a pillow between the knees.
- Have two nurses stand on one side of the bed opposite the direction the patient will be turned. The third helper stands on the other side.
- Fanfold or roll the drawsheet tightly against the patient and carefully slide him or her to the side of the bed toward the two nurses.

- Have one helper then move to the other side of the bed.
- Holding the rolled drawsheet taut to support the body, turn the patient as a unit toward the two nurses. Everyone moves on a predetermined signal.
- Use pillows to support the patient on his or her side in straight alignment.
- Raise the side rails, lower the bed, and place the call signal within the patient's reach.

Using a Hydraulic Lift
A hydraulic device, such as the Hoyer lift, can help to transfer an immobile or obese patient safely from bed to chair. One

SKILL 39-6   Transferring a Dependent Patient From Bed to Chair (Two Nurses)

ACTION	RATIONALE
1. Explain the procedure to the patient.	This facilitates cooperation of the patient.
2. Perform hand hygiene.	Hand hygiene deters the spread of microorganisms.
3. Move equipment as necessary to make room for the chair. Close the door or curtain. Assist the patient to put on a robe and slippers.	This ensures patient safety and facilitates transfer. It provides for privacy and warmth.
4. Move the patient to the near side of the bed and cross the patient's arms across the chest if possible. Lock the wheels of the bed.	This requires less effort to move the patient. Locked wheels will prevent the bed from moving if the patient leans against it.
5. Position the chair next to the bed near the upper end and with the back of the chair parallel to the head of the bed. (If wheelchair, remove the armrest closer to the bed if possible.) Lock the wheels if appropriate.	Positioning the chair next to the bed facilitates easier movement into the chair.
6. Adjust the bed to a comfortable level for nurses or at the level of the armrest if one is present on the chair.	This facilitates transfer with minimal muscle strain on the nurses.
7. Prepare to lift the patient from the bed to the chair: a. The first nurse should stand behind the chair. Slip the arms under the patient's axillae and grasp the patient's wrists securely. b. The second nurse should face the wheelchair and support the patient's knees by placing the arms under them. c. On a predetermined signal, both nurses flex their hips and knees and simultaneously lift the patient gently to the chair.	Two people lifting the patient distributes weight and decreases the effort needed for transfer.

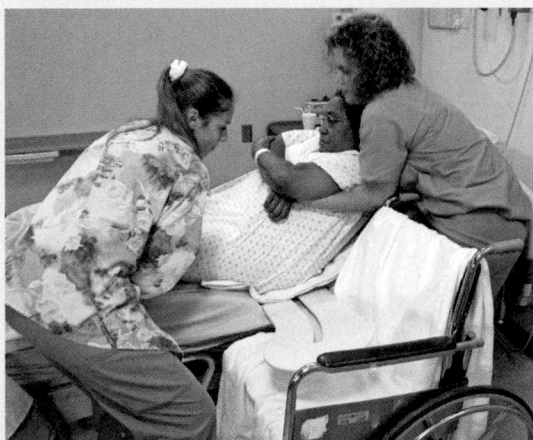

Action 7a & b: First nurse slips arms under patient's axillae and grasps wrists; second nurse support patient's knees. Use of a chair transfer board may be helpful.   (Photo by Rick Brady.)

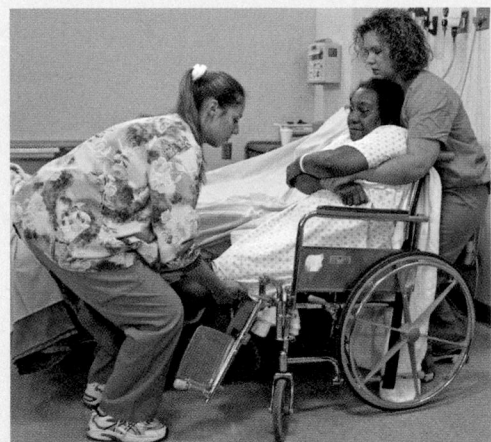

Action 7c: Lowering patient into chair. Use of a chair transfer board may be helpful.   (Photo by Rick Brady.)

ACTION	RATIONALE
8. Adjust the patient's position using pillows where necessary. Cover the patient and use restraint if necessary. Position the call bell so it is available for use.	This maintains proper body alignment and provides for comfort and safety.
9. Perform hand hygiene.	Hand hygiene deters the spread of microorganisms.
10. Document the patient's tolerance of the procedure and length of time in the chair.	This provides accurate documentation and ensures continuity of care.

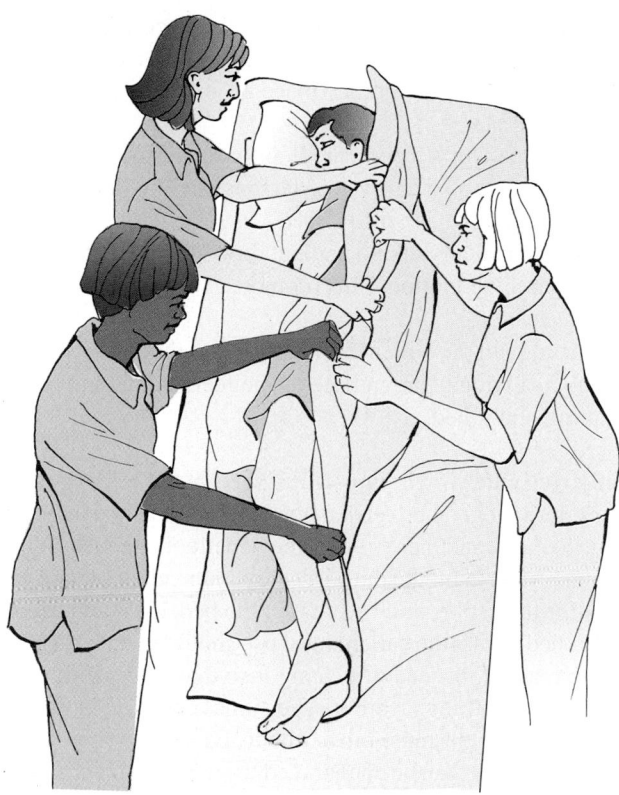

FIGURE 39-15 Logrolling by two or three nurses aids in turning a patient with a spinal injury. One nurse stands on the side, holding the drawsheet taut. The patient is moved toward the other two nurses on a predetermined signal.

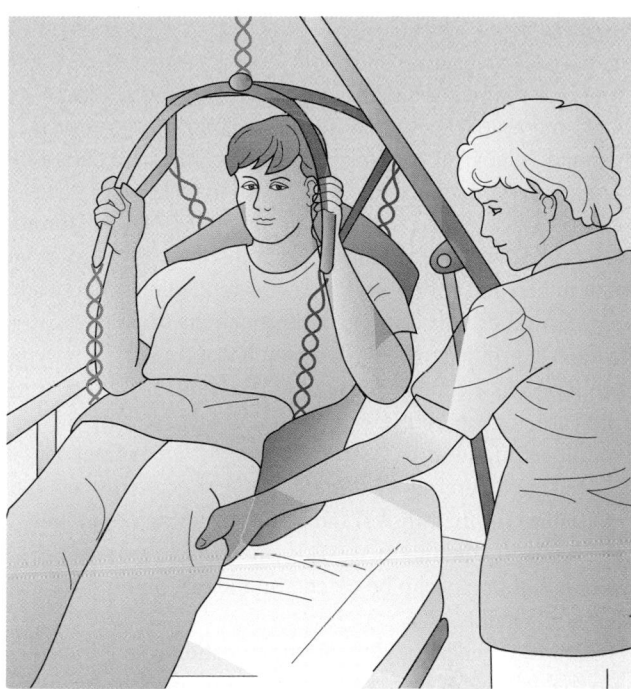

FIGURE 39-16 A hydraulic lift is used to transfer an immobile or obese patient. The patient is raised to a sitting position suspended just above the bed. Then the patient is transferred, and the sling with the patient is lowered onto the seat.

person may operate the device, but two are preferable. Carefully review the manufacturer's instructions before using the device. Generally, position the patient supine in the center of the sling. Attach chains or straps from the hydraulic mechanism to the sling; then raise the patient to a sitting position, lift clear of the bed, and slowly lower the patient into the chair (Fig. 39-16). Many caregivers do not readily use a hydraulic lift because the lift was not readily available or they view the procedure as too time-consuming.

Helping Patients Ambulate

Fortunately for most patients, prolonged periods of bed rest are no longer considered necessary during most illnesses. Activity, even as mild as a short walk around the room, down the hall, from the bedroom to the living room, or out into the yard, is a protective measure for the body.

Physical Conditioning

Patients who are not confined to bed for long periods, who sleep well, and who experience possibly short periods of rest during the day may not require special considerations for increased physical activity in preparation for ambulation. However, others have to be prepared for the day when ambulation is resumed. Certain exercises that strengthen the overall efficiency of the musculoskeletal system can be done in bed.

Quadriceps and Gluteal Setting Drills (Sets)

Quadriceps drills are an isometric exercise—an exercise in which muscle tension occurs without a significant change in the length of the muscle. One of the most important muscle groups used in walking is the quadriceps femoris. This muscle group helps extend the leg and flex the thigh. To help reduce weakness and make first attempts at walking easier, encourage bedridden patients to contract this muscle group frequently. Following are techniques for quadriceps drills:

- Have the patient contract or tighten the muscles on the front of the thighs. The patient has the feeling of pushing the knees downward into the mattress and pulling the feet upward.
- Have the patient hold the position just described while counting slowly to 4, and then relax the muscles for an equal count. Emphasize that relaxation is important to prevent muscle fatigue.
- Caution the patient not to hold his or her breath during these exercises to avoid straining the heart.
- Teach the patient to do quadriceps drills two or three times each hour, four to six times a day.
- Instruct the patient to stop the exercise short of muscle fatigue.

The muscles in the buttocks can be exercised in the same way by pinching the buttocks together and then relaxing them. This is called gluteal setting. Tightening and holding the abdominal muscles for 6 seconds and then relaxing them also strengths this muscle group to facilitate walking.

Pushups

The muscles of the arms and shoulders may also need strengthening before the patient is ready to be out of bed. Exercises should improve the strength needed to hold onto or get into a chair and to move about with greater ease. They are part of the preparation for patients who must learn to walk on crutches.

A trapeze attached to the bed of a patient who has limited use of the lower part of the body helps the patient to move about in bed and strengthens muscles in the upper part of the body. However, this does not strengthen the triceps, which is the muscle group necessary for crutch walking or for moving from a bed to a chair. More suitable exercises are pushups, which are done as follows:

- While sitting up in bed without support, the patient can do pushup exercises to strengthen the triceps. Instruct the patient to lift the hips off the bed by pushing down with the hands on the mattress. If the mattress is too soft, a block of books can be placed on the bed under the patient's hands.
- Pushups may also be done with the patient lying in bed on the abdomen. Instruct the patient to place the hands near the outstretched body at about shoulder level, with palms down on the mattress and elbows bent sharply. Then have the patient straighten the elbows to lift the head and shoulders off the bed.
- Pushups may also be done when the patient sits in an armchair or wheelchair. The patient places the hands on the arms of the chair and then raises the body out of the seat.
- Pushups should be done three or four times a day at first, with the number increased as upper body strength is increased.

Remember Maggie Wyatt, the woman with a fracture being discharged? Due to bedrest, her physical conditioning may be less than what it was before the fracture. Therefore, exercises, such as quadriceps and gluteal setting exercises, and pushups in bed could help to improve Maggie's conditioning, allowing her to participate more fully in her care, including when she transfers from the bed to the chair or from the chair to the car.

Dangling

Dangling refers to the position in which the person sits on the edge of the bed with legs and feet over the side of the bed. This exercise helps prepare patients for being out of bed. It is carried out as follows:

- Place the patient in the sitting position in bed for a few minutes. This will accustom the patient to this position and help prevent feelings of faintness.
- Place the bed in the low position or have a footstool handy on which the patient can rest the feet while dangling.
- Move the patient toward the side of the bed near you so that you do not stretch and strain while turning the patient.

- Pivot the patient a quarter of a turn by supporting the shoulders and legs. Swing the patient's legs over the side of the bed. The patient may place his or her hands on your shoulders.
- Rest the patient's feet on the floor or on a footstool. This gives a sense of security, and lessens the likelihood that the patient will slide off the bed.
- Have the patient pick up and put down the feet alternately in a marching motion. This promotes circulation in the legs.
- Remain with the patient and be ready to place the patient back to a lying position if he or she feels faint, to prevent falling out of bed.

Daily Activities for Purposeful Exercise

Many activities can be carried out in ways that encourage patients to move and thereby gain the benefit of exercise. When patients understand the purpose, they often adopt other exercises for themselves. For example, the bedside stand can be positioned so that the patient must use shoulder and arm muscles to reach it, instead of placing it so that little effort is required to take things from it. The signal cord can be placed so that the patient must move either the arm or shoulder to reach it. Patients can be encouraged to sit up and reach for the overbed table, to pull it close, and then to push it back in place. Patients can be encouraged to try to wash their back independently. Patients can put on socks while still in bed.

In a hospital setting, ADLs may be one of the few independent activities that a patient can perform. Allowing the patient to do as much as he or she can accomplish independently is vital. Be sure to offer encouragement and praise. "Learned dependency," which often occurs with the older adult population, can lead to a decrease in self-esteem and depression. Collaborate with the occupational therapist when necessary to determine types of adaptive equipment that would help the patient achieve maximal functional independence. Box 39-1 provides examples of available adaptive equipment. Providing the necessary adaptive tools, coupled with encouraging independence, will create the optimal outcome.

BOX 39-1 Adaptive Equipment to Assist With Activities of Daily Living

- Long-handled bath sponges
- Reachers
- Long-handled shoe horns and sock aids
- Elastic shoe laces
- Utensils that are enlarged, specially angulated, or have special grips
- Velcro® devices
- Feeding devices such as plates or bowls with suction-cup bottoms
- Splints and positioning equipment
- Environmental adaptations

Assistance With Walking

Many patients who have been confined to bed for an extended period find that they must almost learn to walk all over again. Often, nurses play a major role in the patient's recovery, mental outlook, hope, and faith, especially when the patient must adhere to a rigid and often difficult schedule of reeducating muscle groups. A patient who is able to raise the leg only 2.5 cm (1 inch) from the bed possesses sufficient power to begin walking.

Because muscle reeducation is a major task, the patient needs the assistance of experts in physical medicine. However, nurses can assist patients out of bed and help them walk when a physical therapist is not present. Nurses should also plan to walk with a patient who is walking for the first few times after a period of bed rest.

Before getting the patient out of bed, do the following:

- Assess the patient's ability to walk and the need for assistance (one nurse, two nurses, walker, cane, walking belt, or crutches).
- Explain to the patient exactly what is to be done: transfer technique from bed to erect position, projected distance to be ambulated, assistance available and the correct manner of using it. Instruct the patient to alert the nurse immediately if feeling dizzy or weak.
- Ensure that the patient has a clear path for ambulation.

Assist the patient to an erect position for ambulation, pausing after the patient is seated at the edge of the bed and again after the patient first stands, to ensure that the patient feels steady. Reinforce the need to stand erect and to hold the head high to achieve the full benefits of walking. Patients who are fearful of walking often tend to look at their feet. Remind the patient to take deep breaths to aerate the lungs while walking. Because patients who are walking for the first time after prolonged bed rest often feel faint or weak, plan ambulation for a short distance, gradually increasing the distance as tolerated. As this distance is increased, have chairs readily available

should the patient need to rest. Should a patient faint or begin to fall while walking, stand with feet apart to create a wide base of support and rock the pelvis out on the side facing the patient. With arms under the patient's axillae and encircling the patient, slide the patient down one's body to the floor, carefully protecting the patient's head (Fig. 39-17A). If the patient is wearing a walking belt, use the belt to ease the patient backward against one's own body and gently ease the patient to the floor while protecting the patient's head. When two nurses are assisting a patient who starts to fall or faint, they both should use one hand to support the patient under the axillae and grasp the patient's hand or wrist with their other hand. After they have steadied the patient, they can slowly lower him or her to a chair or the floor (Fig. 39-17B). Practice these maneuvers before they are needed in an emergency situation.

One-Nurse Assist

Patients who require minimal nursing assistance may walk well with the nurse walking alongside. Provide support by standing at the patient's side and placing both hands at the patient's waist. Supporting the patient at the waist helps the patient to maintain an erect posture and prevents unintentionally pulling the patient to one side. Use of a walking belt snugly secured around the patient's waist also provides this type of support. Grasp the belt securely in the back and walk behind and slightly to the side of the patient (Fig. 39-18).

Frequently, it is necessary to assist the patient with intravenous (IV) therapy equipment to walk. Secure a portable IV pole that moves easily. The patient walks with the assistance of the nurse and the portable IV pole. Ensure that all the equipment is secure before walking and be alert for any tension or sudden action that might dislodge or interfere with the infusion (Fig. 39-19A). Also consider reviewing this technique with family members who are assisting with ambulation and are unfamiliar with how to steady the patient, maneuver equipment, and navigate through crowded or narrow areas.

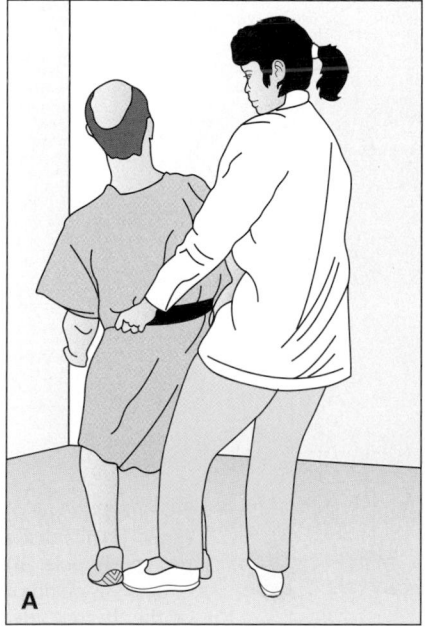
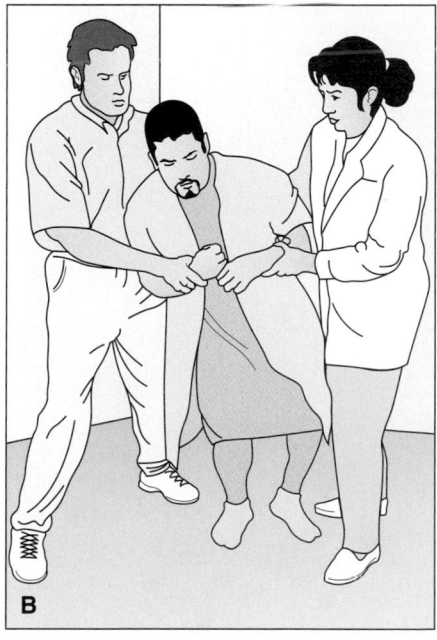

FIGURE 39-17 (**A**) One nurse guiding a patient to the floor. (**B**) Two nurses lowering a patient to the floor.

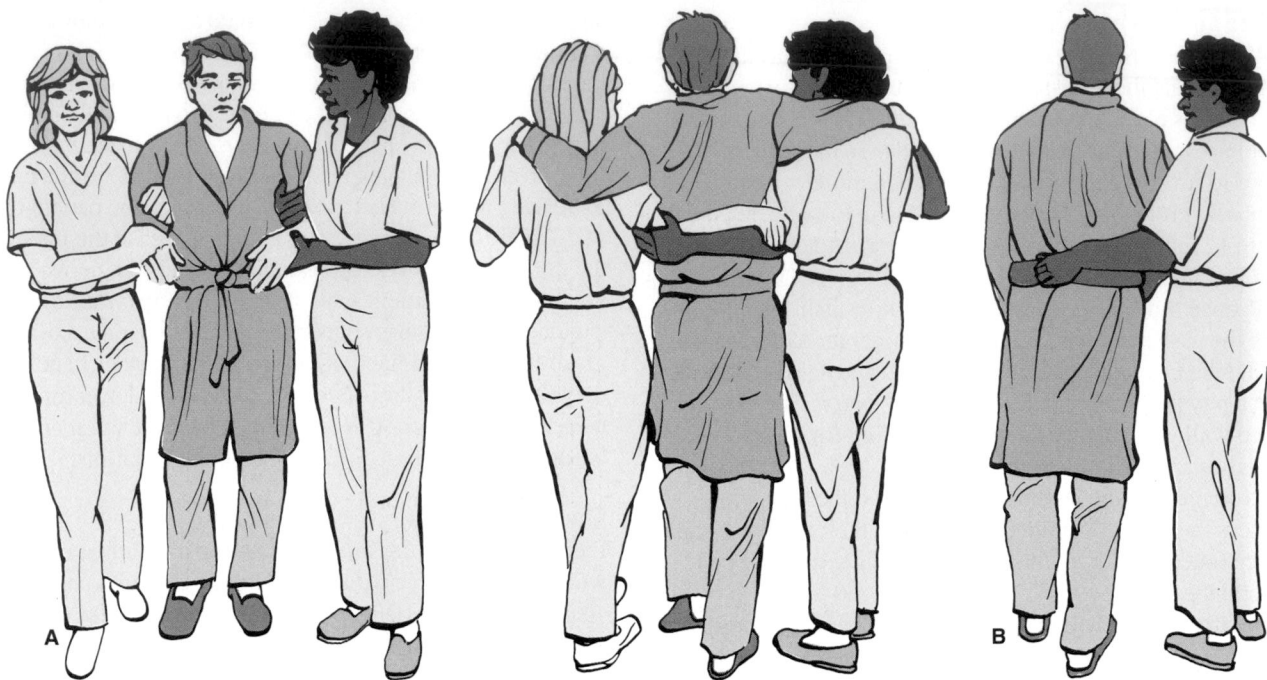

FIGURE 39-18 Assisting a patient to ambulate. (**A**) Two techniques for two nurses to safely assist a patient to ambulate. (**B**) The nurse using a walking belt to support a patient while walking.

When a patient has weakness or paralysis on one side, stand on the weaker or affected side and stabilize the patient by putting one arm around the patient's waist. Support the patient's weak arm by placing one's other arm around the inner aspect of the patient's upper arm in the axilla area or use one's hand to support the patient's forearm and hand (see Fig. 39-19B). Supporting the patient's weak arm in the axillary area allows the nurse to support the patient's weight more easily and ease him or her to the floor should the patient feel faint. Always use a transfer belt with patients who are unstable.

Two-Nurse Assist

A two-nurse assist is the safer method to use when there is uncertainty about the patient's ability to walk. Two methods

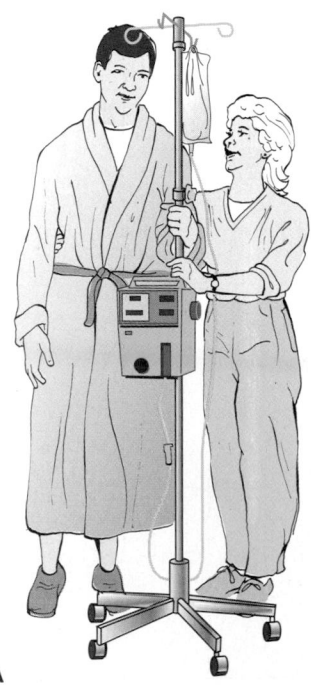

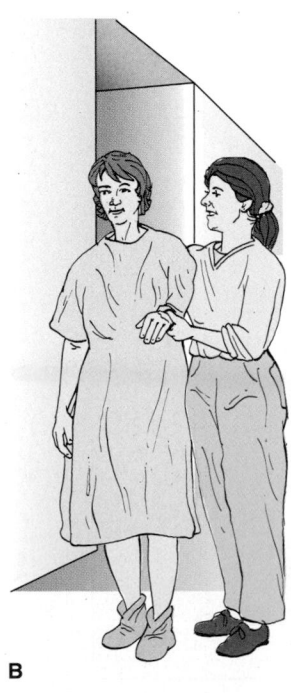

FIGURE 39-19 (**A**) Ambulating a patient who needs additional support. The nurse assists the patient to ambulate with a portable IV pole. (**B**) The nurse assists the patient with weakness or paralysis on one side to ambulate by supporting the patient on the affected side.

of ambulation can be used by two nurses to support a patient safely. In the first, the nurses stand at the patient's sides with their near hands grasping the inferior aspect of the patient's near upper arm and their far hands holding the patient's lower arm or hand. The second position provides more support to the patient but requires the three people involved to be of similar height. The nurses again position themselves at the patient's sides, slipping their near arms under the patient's arms and around the patient's back, grasping one another's wrists. The patient stretches the arms around the nurses' shoulders and the nurses grasp the patient's hands with their far hands. In both positions, the nurses and the patient step in unison (see Fig. 39-18).

Mechanical Aids for Walking

Various devices can assist a patient with walking. The most common are walkers, canes, braces, and crutches. Typically, a patient is fitted for a device and instructed in its use in the department of physical medicine or physical therapy. In this instance, nursing's concern is chiefly to reinforce the teaching the patient has received and to ensure that the patient continues to use the device properly to assist in safe ambulation. In some healthcare settings, however, nurses may be responsible for fitting patients with the device. Whenever you assess a patient who has been using a walker, cane, brace, or crutches for a period of time, determine whether the device is still needed, whether it continues to meet the patient's needs, and whether the patient continues to use it properly.

Some older patients consider the use of a mobility aid a visible symbol of weakness or an indication of decline in capabilities and loss of independence. Many patients refuse to use them and keep them out of sight. If the mobility aid is intended for short-term use (eg, after hip replacement surgery), the response is usually more positive. Be sensitive to a patient's perspective regarding these devices and focus on the meaning the aid has for the patient rather than simply emphasizing how to use it. Allow patients some control over their mobility decisions while still ensuring a safe environment. General guidelines for helping patients who need the assistance of a walker, cane, brace, or crutches include the following:

- Whenever possible, instruct the patient and family members in the correct use of the device before it is needed (eg, before surgery). If family members are knowledgeable, they can reinforce the teaching as needed.
- When ready to begin walking with the new device, make sure the patient is wearing rubber-soled, well-fitting shoes and that there is a clear path for ambulation (clean, flat, dry, and well lit). If the patient is at high risk for falls, use a walking belt for added support.
- Before moving, make sure the patient is steady on the feet when standing; instruct the patient to stand erect, looking straight ahead. The nurse should walk behind and slightly to one side of the patient (in cases of hemiparesis or hemiparalysis, walk on the patient's affected side). Should the patient lose balance, be prepared to grasp the patient's shoulder and the transfer belt to steady the patient.

Walker

A walker is a lightweight metal frame (usually aluminum) with four legs (Fig. 39-20A). The walker provides a sense of

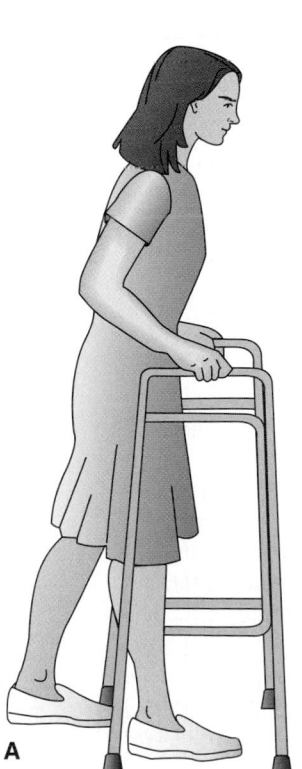
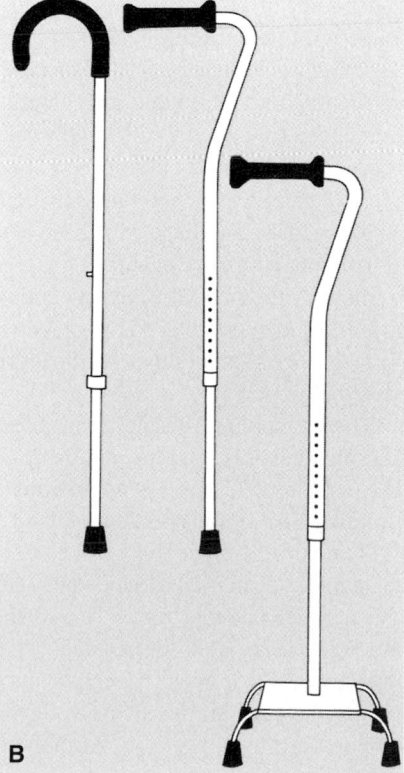

FIGURE 39-20 Mechanical aids to walking. (**A**) A walker is a lightweight metal frame with a broad, four-point base of support. The walker should be adjusted to the height of the patient's hip joint so that the patient's elbows are flexed about 30 degrees. (**B**) Three types of canes. Single-ended canes with half-circle handles are recommended for patients requiring minimal support. Single-ended canes with straight handles are recommended for patients with hand weakness. Three- or four-prong canes are recommended for patients with poor balance.

A   B

security and support. There are several types of walkers, specified according to the arm strength and balance of the patient.

When the patient stands between the back legs of the walker, the walker should extend from the floor to the patient's hip joint; the patient's elbows should be flexed about 30 degrees. The walker's rubber tips should be intact to prevent slipping. Generally, the patient lifts the walker ahead of himself or herself and steps into it. Instruct a patient using a walker to do the following:

- Wear nonskid shoes or slippers.
- When rising from a seated position, use the chair arms for support. Once standing, place one hand at a time on the walker and move forward into it.
- If one leg is impaired, move that leg and the walker forward together for 6 to 8 inches. Move the unaffected leg forward once body weight is securely supported by the walker and the impaired leg. Older patients frequently develop dangerous walking patterns with a walker and may require close observation.
- Never attempt to use a walker on stairs.

> *Recall Genevieve Augustus, the older woman caring for her husband at home? The nurse would need to assess the functional status of Mr. Augustus carefully to determine his limitations and need for any assistive devices, such as a walker or quad cane. These devices would be helpful in promoting safety and providing support for Mr. Augustus while also providing support for Genevieve.*

Canes

Canes come in three variations (see Fig. 39-20B): single-ended canes with half-circle handles (recommended for patients requiring minimal support and those who will be using stairs frequently); single-ended canes with straight handles (recommended for patients with hand weakness because the handgrip is easier to hold but not recommended for patients with poor balance); canes with three (tripod) or four prongs (quad cane) or legs to provide a wide base of support (recommended for patients with poor balance).

Instruct the patient to use a cane with as small a base as possible and eventually to progress to a single-ended cane if possible. The smaller the base, the less the patient relies on the cane for support.

Many canes are adjustable and should be fitted so that when the patient stands with the cane's tip 4 inches (10 cm) to the side of the foot, the cane extends from the floor to the patient's hip joint. The elbow should be flexed 30 degrees when holding the cane. Rubber tips on the cane prevent slipping and accidents and should be inspected regularly to ensure they are intact. Teach patients to stand erect when walking with a cane and not to lean out over the cane.

When walking with a cane, patients are generally instructed to hold the cane on the unaffected side to provide additional support for the weaker leg. Ambulation proceeds in the following fashion:

1. The patient stands with weight evenly distributed between the feet and the cane.
2. The cane is held on the patient's stronger side and is advanced 4 to 12 inches (10–30 cm).
3. Supporting weight on the stronger leg and the cane, the patient advances the weaker foot forward, parallel with the cane.
4. Supporting weight on the weaker leg and the cane, the patient next advances the stronger leg forward ahead of the cane (heel slightly beyond the tip of the cane).
5. The weaker leg is moved forward until even with the stronger leg, and the cane is once again advanced as in step 2.

When less support is required from the cane, the patient can advance the cane and weaker leg forward while the stronger leg supports the patient's weight. Patients should be taught to position their canes within easy reach when they sit down so that they can rise easily.

Braces

Braces that support weakened leg muscles are available in many variations. Nursing responsibilities include learning with the patient when the brace is to be worn and the correct technique for applying the brace; monitoring the patient's correct use of the brace; and observing for any untoward problems the brace might cause (eg, skin irritation). Muscle changes such as those occurring with growth and development or brought about by illness (atrophy) may require the brace to be refitted to maintain its effectiveness.

Crutches

Sometimes it is necessary for patients to use crutches for a time to avoid using one leg or to help strengthen one or both legs. The two types of crutches most commonly used are the underarm or axillary crutches and the forearm support crutches (Fig. 39-21).

Forearm support crutches have no axillary support. A supportive frame extends beyond the handgrip for the lower arm to help guide the crutch. These crutches are more likely to be used by patients who have permanent limitations and will always need crutch assistance for ambulation.

The procedure for crutch walking is taught best by a physical therapist. However, nurses are often called on to measure patients for axillary crutches and to teach them to use them. Even if a patient is receiving instructions for crutch walking by a physical therapist, be knowledgeable about the patient's progress and the gait being taught. Be prepared to guide the patient at home or in the hospital after the initial teaching is completed.

Measuring for Axillary Crutches. The following techniques can be used to measure the patient for axillary crutches:

- Have the patient lie flat in bed on the back wearing the shoes to be used when walking.
- Measure the distance from the anterior fold of the axilla straight down to the heel, and then add 2.5 cm (1 inch).
- With the patient standing, position the crutch pad three finger-widths below the axilla, with the bottom tip of the

Promoting Exercises to Prepare for Crutch Walking. Before trying to use the crutches, several exercises will help the patient become more confident and skillful. The patient begins by strengthening the arm and the shoulder muscles. The pushup exercise described earlier is most helpful. The muscles of the hand must also be strengthened. Squeezing a rubber ball 50 times a day by flexing and extending the fingers helps to do this.

Assist the patient into a chair that is close to the wall and then help the patient to stand against the wall, with the crutches placed in the patient's hands. Next, standing slightly away from the wall, have the patient sway on the crutches from side to side. This accustoms the hands and the arms to weight bearing.

Next, ask the patient to lean against the wall and pick one crutch up about 15 cm (6 inches) from the floor and then place it down. Have the patient repeat this motion with the other crutch, and then perform the entire exercise six to eight times. Then, still leaning against the wall, instruct the patient to pick up both crutches from the floor and place them down. Have the patient repeat this motion several times.

These exercises make it possible to judge the patient's ability to hold and manage the crutches without the risk of moving. If judged capable, the patient then begins to practice a gait. If possible, it is recommended that the patient begin with the four-point gait. Patients using axillary crutches need to be carefully screened for cardiovascular problems and advised to ambulate slowly to reduce cardiovascular stress.

Crutch Gaits. Before moving into one of the gaits, the patient assumes the tripod position, or basic crutch stance (Fig. 39-22). Placing the crutches 15 cm (6 inches) in front of the feet and 15 cm to the side of each foot creates a triangle that provides a wide base of support. Instruct the patient to maintain erect posture with the head held straight and eyes facing forward.

Five crutch gaits can be used: four-point, three-point, two-point, swing-to, and swing-through. These gaits are described here and their patterns outlined in Figure 39-23.

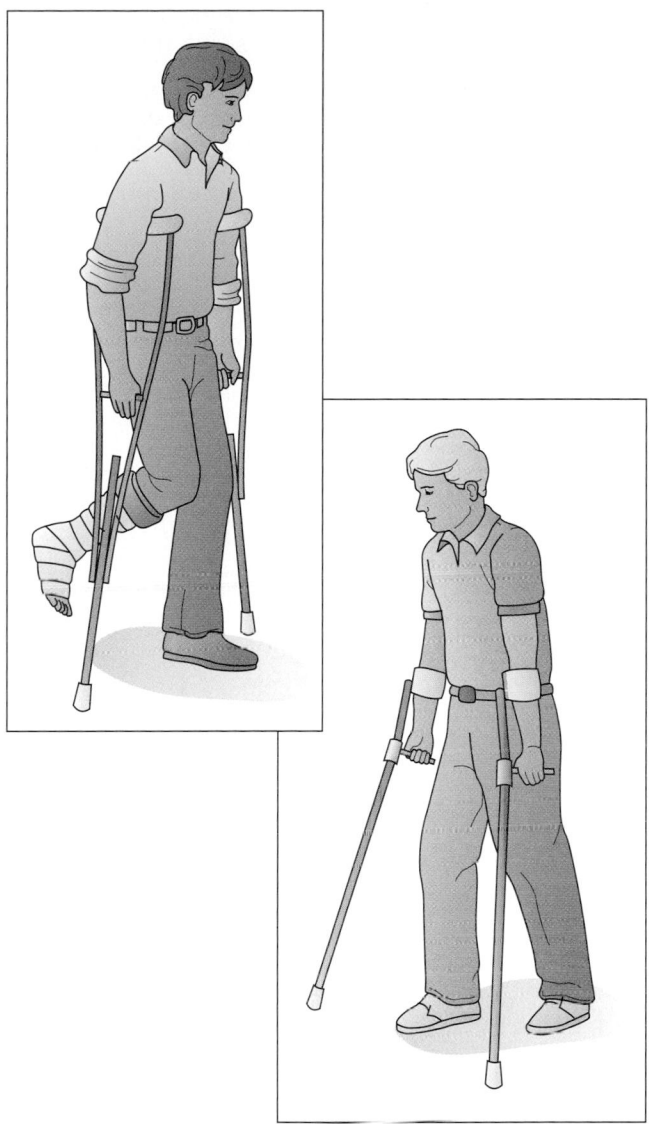

FIGURE 39-21 Axillary and forearm support crutches.

crutch placed diagonally out to a point 10 to 15 cm (4–6 inches) to the side of the heel.

- To obtain an approximate crutch length, use the patient's height and subtract 16 inches (40 cm).
- After the crutches have been adjusted to the proper length, have the patient stand to adjust the handgrips. Secure the handgrips while the patient grasps them in the hands, with elbows slightly bent and wrists bent backward.
- Teach the patient that the support of body weight should come primarily on the hands and arms while using the crutches, not in the axillary areas, where pressure may damage nerves and cut off circulation. Also, the crutches should not be forced into the axillae each time the body moves forward.

Ensuring that axillary crutches are properly fitted and used correctly is crucial to prevent damage to nerves and to prevent cutting off circulation. In addition, properly fitted crutches provide well-balanced support.

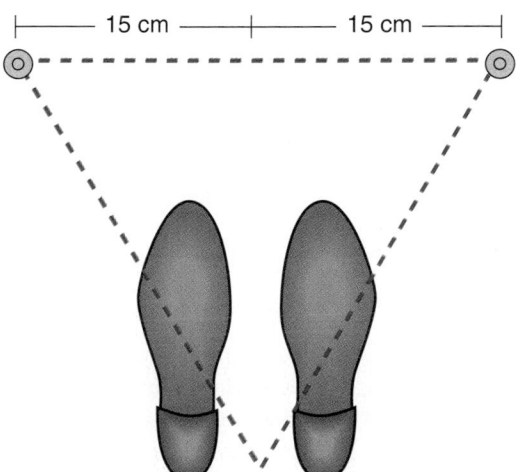

FIGURE 39-22 The tripod position is the initial crutch stance from which the person advances.

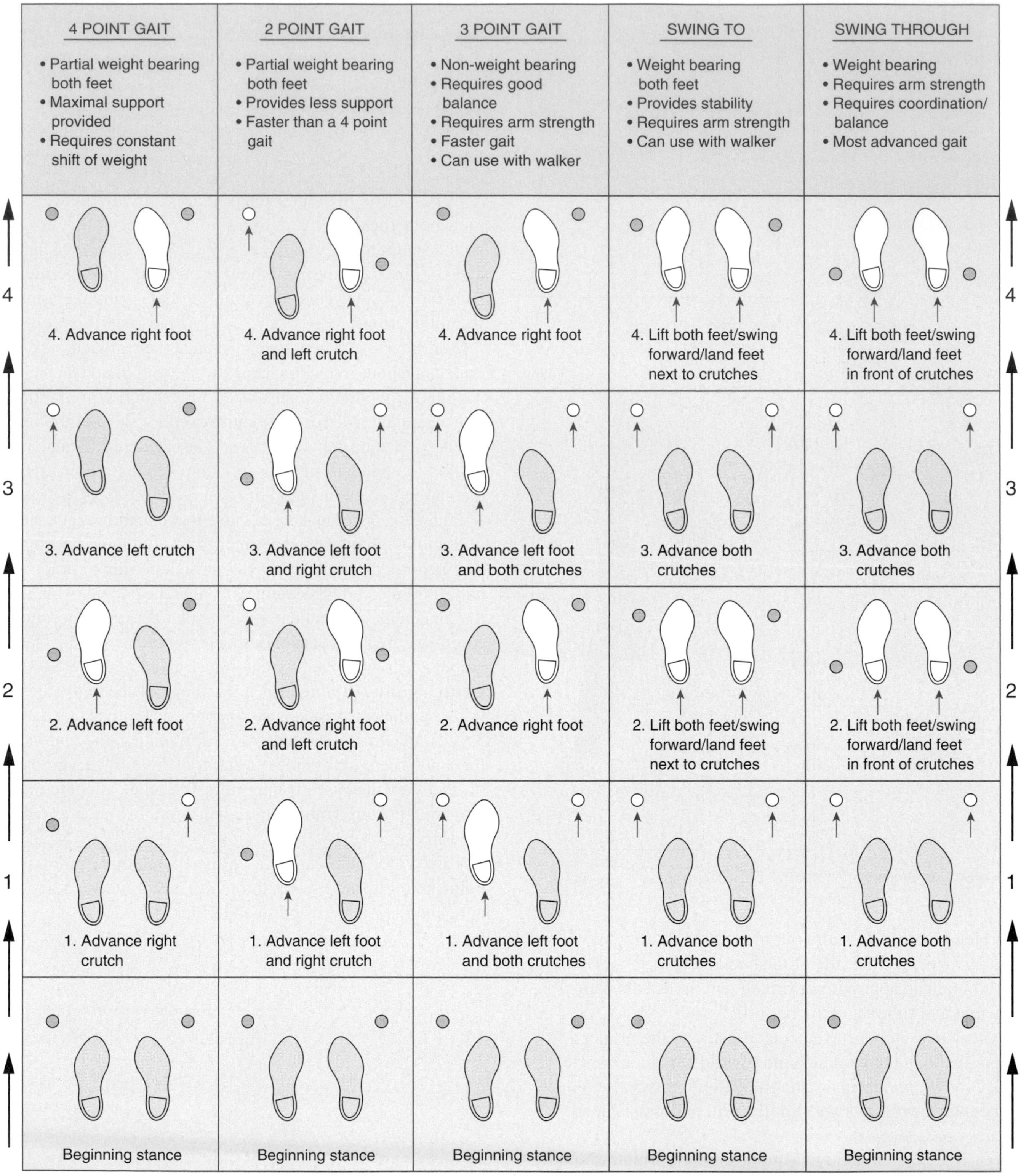

4 POINT GAIT	2 POINT GAIT	3 POINT GAIT	SWING TO	SWING THROUGH
• Partial weight bearing both feet • Maximal support provided • Requires constant shift of weight	• Partial weight bearing both feet • Provides less support • Faster than a 4 point gait	• Non-weight bearing • Requires good balance • Requires arm strength • Faster gait • Can use with walker	• Weight bearing both feet • Provides stability • Requires arm strength • Can use with walker	• Weight bearing • Requires arm strength • Requires coordination/ balance • Most advanced gait
4. Advance right foot	4. Advance right foot and left crutch	4. Advance right foot	4. Lift both feet/swing forward/land feet next to crutches	4. Lift both feet/swing forward/land feet in front of crutches
3. Advance left crutch	3. Advance left foot and right crutch	3. Advance left foot and both crutches	3. Advance both crutches	3. Advance both crutches
2. Advance left foot	2. Advance right foot and left crutch	2. Advance right foot	2. Lift both feet/swing forward/land feet next to crutches	2. Lift both feet/swing forward/land feet in front of crutches
1. Advance right crutch	1. Advance left foot and right crutch	1. Advance left foot and both crutches	1. Advance both crutches	1. Advance both crutches
Beginning stance	Beginning stance	Beginning stance	Beginning stance	Beginning stance

FIGURE 39-23 Crutch gaits. *Shaded areas* are weight-bearing. *Arrow* indicates advance foot or crutch.

In four-point gait, weight bearing is permitted on both legs. In two-point gait, weight bearing is also permitted on both feet, but the pattern is a speed-up version of the four-point gait. In three-point gait, weight bearing is permitted on only one foot; the other foot cannot support, but acts as a balance. The swing-to gait requires that both crutches move ahead to-gether and the body weight is lifted by the arms and swung to the crutches. In swing-through gait, the body weight is swung through and beyond the crutches. The swing gaits require strength and coordination and are frequently used by patients with hip and leg paralysis. A disadvantage of these two gaits is that they do not simulate normal walking. Extended use leads to atrophy of the muscles in the lower extremity that are not being used.

Instructions for crutch walking should also include practice and demonstration of the safe technique for moving up and down stairs. One technique involves advancing the unaffected leg first up the stairs and past the crutches. The patient's body weight is then transferred to the unaffected leg and the crutches are then positioned on either side of the unaffected leg. When coming down the stairs, move the affected leg and crutches first, followed by the unaffected one (Fig. 39-24). An easy way to teach the patient to remember this technique is the statement "The good leg goes up, the bad leg goes down."

When a railing is available, the patient can use another technique to climb and descend stairs. This technique involves using one hand to grasp the railing firmly while the other hand grasps both crutches held together at the handgrips and under the axilla and uses them for support. While holding securely onto the rail, move the uninjured leg up one step, straighten it, and move the injured leg and the crutches onto the same step. When moving down the stairs, one hand should always be on the railing, while the other hand again steadies both crutches under the arm using the handgrips. The crutches and the injured leg move together down one step, followed by the uninjured leg. Teaching to Promote Health at Home 39-1 summarizes the important content to be included when teaching crutch walking.

Designing Exercise Programs

The benefits of exercise for each of the major body systems are so significant that designing individualized exercise programs for patients is an important nursing responsibility. Such a program should incorporate ADLs and planned exercise sessions. Depending on the patient's physical condition, exercise is designed to promote optimal fitness.

The individual's commitment to a program of regular exercise depends on the following:
- Knowledge of the benefits of exercise and the problems related to immobility
- Appreciation of the fact that in society, sedentary lifestyles are common and most people must consciously choose to exercise
- Belief that each person is responsible for his or her own health and that exercise is essential to one's well-being

Foster a commitment to regular exercise by teaching and counseling patients about exercise. To do this, be knowledgeable about the types and benefits of exercise as well as the risks associated with exercise.

When working with a patient to develop an individualized exercise prescription, use the following guidelines:
- Explore the patient's fitness goals, interests, skills, exercise opportunities, and exercise capacity.
- Assist the patient in obtaining medical clearance for exercise.
- Explore feasible exercise activities with the patient, considering the health benefits sought, the time involved, cost, any need for special equipment, precautions, and risks.
- Develop an exercise program that specifies warm-up and cool-down activities (walking, stretching) and three or four major exercise activities from which the patient can choose. Specify the frequency, duration, and intensity of the exercise activity. The recommended frequency for most types of exercise is at least three times a week (but may work up to five or six times a week). For recommended duration and

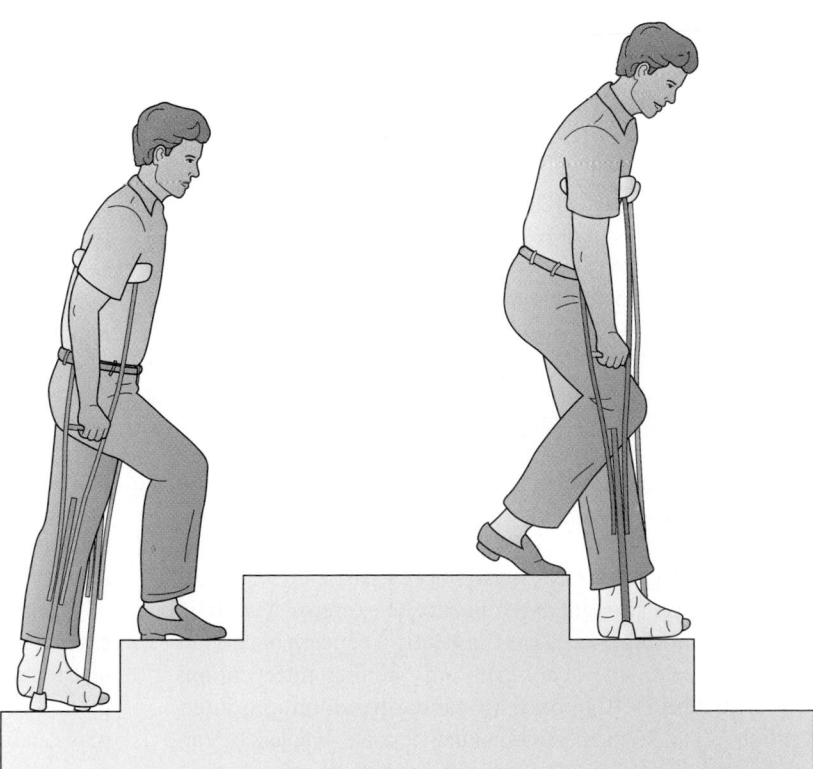

FIGURE 39-24 Stairs can be dangerous for the person navigating them with crutches; therefore, the proper method must be learned. Illustrated here is one of the methods, using both crutches: the good leg goes up, the bad leg comes down.

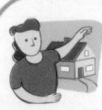

Teaching to Promote Health at Home 39-1
Crutch Walking

Health Topic	Teaching Tip	Why is This Important?
Correct positioning for use of crutches	Prevent pressure on the axillae.	Pressure placed on the axillae can cause damage to nerves and circulation.
	Keep elbows close to sides.	This helps stabilize the crutches to prevent the patient from falling.
	Prevent crutches from getting closer than 3 inches to feet.	This prevents the patient from tripping over the crutches.
The correct gait for the patient	Use the four-point, three-point, two-point, *or* swing-to gait.	Each gait is used for specific reasons. The four-point gait is used for patients who may weight bear on both feet. The three-point gait is used for patients who may not weight bear on either foot. The two-point gait is for patients who may weight bear on one foot. The swing-to or swing-through gaits are used for patients who may weight bear on both feet. The nature of the injury determines whether the patient may weight bear.
Functioning at home	To rise from a chair: Slide forward to the edge of the chair. Extend the injured leg to prevent any weight bearing. Place crutches on unaffected side, lean forward, and push off using the crutches. To climb stairs: Advance unaffected leg past crutches, then place weight on unaffected leg. Advance affected leg and then crutches to the step. Continue with this order until top of stairs is reached. To descend stairs: Move crutches and affected leg first, followed by the unaffected leg.	Patient needs to learn that everyday occurrences may be challenging and, if not done correctly, may end up with injury to affected leg.

intensity, a person should be able to speak normally without getting out of breath or should maintain a target heart rate (60%–90% of maximal heart rate [220 minus age]).

- Encourage the patient to complement the exercise program with everyday activities that require exercise.
- Try to identify with the patient any potential threats to the exercise program's successful implementation. Plan support strategies.
- Use ongoing evaluation to determine whether the exercise prescription is meeting the patient's needs and whether the patient is adhering to the prescription.

Box 39-2 identifies characteristics of a successful exercise program and prevention strategies to avoid the risks associated with exercise.

Advanced age has traditionally been associated with a decline in muscle strength and reticence to exercise. Maintaining balance during exercise is frequently a concern of patients and caregivers. The accompanying Nursing Interventions Classification (NIC) box lists standardized nursing interventions that help the patient maintain a sense of balance. Various studies have shown several positive outcomes to physical

activity: increased bone density, decreased incidence of colorectal cancer, and decreased risk of coronary heart disease, to name a few. An ongoing program of exercise for older patients also promotes confidence, offers opportunities for socialization, and fosters continued independence, while lessening the potential for falls and other factors that often lead to nursing home admission.

Teaching Exercise Benefits to Populations at Risk

Nurses can significantly contribute to the well-being of all populations by promoting health and wellness. Assessment and intervention priorities that promote positive health behaviors for each developmental stage were outlined in Table 39-2 earlier in this chapter. As life expectancy continues to extend, nursing activities will increasingly focus on teaching that regular exercise is a positive factor contributing to longevity. In addition to improving the quality of life, exercise plays an important role in the prevention or slowing of osteoporosis. According to the National Osteoporosis Foundation

BOX 39-2 Characteristics of a Successful Exercise Program

- The program is individually designed (considers the individual's fitness goals, interests, skills, exercise opportunities, and exercise capacity).
- The program specifies warm-up and cool-down activities and a variety of major exercise activities— variety is preferable to a single-exercise activity.
- The program specifies frequency, intensity, and duration of exercise.
- The program is convenient to perform, compatible with the individual's lifestyle, and fun!
- The individual in such a program should understand the program and feel confident that exercise will result in definite health benefits.

Prevention Strategies to Avoid Risks Associated With Exercise

People beginning exercise programs should be familiar with the following guidelines:

- Obtain a preexercise medical examination and medical supervision during exercise if older than age 35 years and sedentary or if there is any past or current cardiovascular condition.
- Begin a new exercise program slowly and allow your body's support structure time to accommodate to the new stress.
- Know your body and respect its limitations. Never force a joint beyond its natural range of motion.
- Respect fatigue. Whenever you feel tingling, pain, or burning in a muscle, stop and rest the muscle for 15 minutes before continuing to exercise.
- Follow the safety guidelines for specific exercises; for example, joggers are advised to run on soft surfaces as opposed to cement or asphalt, to wear well-constructed shoes with thick soles and arch supports, and to run in a safe environment with a low pollution index.

Examples of Nursing Interventions Classification (NIC)
Exercise Therapy: Balance

- Determine patient's ability to participate in activities requiring balance.
- Evaluate sensory functions (eg, vision, hearing, and proprioception).
- Dress patient in nonrestrictive clothing.
- Provide safe environment for practice of exercises.
- Encourage patient to maintain wide base of support, if needed.
- Assist to stand (or sit) and rock body from side to side to stimulate balance mechanisms.
- Assist patient to practice standing with eyes closed for short periods at regular intervals to stimulate proprioception.
- Monitor patient's response to balance exercises.

(From McCloskey, J., & Bulechek, G. [2000]. *Nursing interventions classification [NIC]* [3rd ed]. [p. 321]. St. Louis: C. V. Mosby. A full listing of nursing activities for each nursing intervention can be found in this book.)

(2004, February), 10 million Americans suffer from osteoporosis and another 34 million have low bone mass, which increases the risk for osteoporosis. Nurses can help older patients use physical exercise to avert or to alleviate the effects of this debilitating aging process.

Evaluating

When evaluating the effectiveness of a plan of care designed to help patients enhance, maintain, or regain mobility and fitness goals, the nurse uses each nurse–patient interaction to evaluate the patient in the following respects:

- General ease of movement and gait
- Body alignment
- Joint structure and function
- Muscle mass, tone, and strength
- Endurance

An excellent time to assess these essential ingredients of well-being is when the patient is performing simple everyday tasks such as walking, undertaking hygiene measures, dressing, and eating. Because illness and enforced inactivity can affect these tasks negatively, ongoing evaluation is necessary if serious problems are to be avoided. See Nursing Plan of Care 39-1 for Quan Hong Nguyen.

NURSING PLAN OF CARE 39-1   *for Quan Hong Nguyen*

Quan Hong Nguyen is an alert, 57-year-old married man who was admitted to the hospital with a diagnosis of right cerebrovascular accident or brain attack secondary to thrombosis. He has a history of hypertension. This is his 2nd hospital day, and the attending physicians have termed the stroke a *completed stroke*; that is, Mr. Nguyen's neurologic deficits have been unchanged for 2 days, and he is believed to be ready for more aggressive rehabilitative treatment. On hospital day 2, an assessment of Mr. Nguyen's mobility status and ability to participate in activities of daily living revealed the following data:

- *Mental status*—basically alert and able to follow simple commands; expresses his needs verbally when encouraged, but speech is slow; seems forgetful of usual routine for basic self-care activities
- *Neuromuscular status*—hemiplegia; severe motor and sensory deficits of the left side of the face and the left arm and leg

- *Muscle mass, tone, and strength*—well-developed muscles in all extremities; history of a lifetime of sports, most recently played tennis two to four times weekly; decreased muscle tone (hypotonicity, flaccidity) in left arm and leg motor function is absent in left arm and very weak in left leg; strong motor function on right extremities; incapable of weight-bearing on left side; incapable of independent turning, sitting, standing, transferring, or ambulation
- *Joint mobility*—decreased on left side; otherwise full range of motion; no contractures
- *Endurance*—fatigues quickly (eg, during complete bath)
- Some deficit in spatial–perceptual orientation (eg, ignores objects on his left side), but it is difficult to assess this completely yet

NURSING DIAGNOSIS

Impaired Physical Mobility (turning in bed, sitting, standing, transferring, and ambulating) related to left hemiplegia and weakness as manifested by: motor function absent in left arm and weak in left leg, decreased joint mobility in left extremities, fatigue

EXPECTED OUTCOME

1/25/06   Whenever observed, the patient will:
- Be in correct body alignment with (1) each joint on the left side higher than the joint proximal to it and (2) supportive devices in place (bed board, footboard, trochanter roll, hand–wrist splint, shoulder sling, pillows)

Nursing Interventions

At each position change (as dictated by every-2-hour turn schedule posted at the bedside), make sure that the patient is in correct alignment. Follow agency positioning guidelines for the supine, side-lying (lies on unaffected side), and prone positions.

Use the following supportive devices: firm mattress, footboard, trochanter roll, shoulder sling when patient is in upright position, volar resting splint, and pillows.

Rationale

Correct positioning prevents contractures, relieves pressures, and maintains alignment.
- Positioning each joint higher than the preceding one prevents edema and its resulting fibrosis.
- Placing the patient in the prone position for 30 minutes two or three times daily helps prevent knee and hip flexion contractures.

Support devices aid in maintaining the patient in correct positioning.
- Firm mattress provides skeletal support.
- Footboard during flaccid period prevents footdrop, heel cord shortening, and plantar flexion.
- Trochanter roll prevents external rotation of hip when patient is in dorsal position.
- Shoulder sling during flaccid period prevents shoulder subluxation and shoulder–hand syndrome.
- Volar resting splint supports the wrist and hand in a functional position.
- A pillow in the axilla of the left side prevents adduction of the affected side.

Evaluative Statement

1/27/06   Outcome being met. Every-2-hour positioning schedule being followed with patient in correct body alignment to prevent contractures.

S. Beecher, RN

(continued)

NURSING PLAN OF CARE 39-1   *for Quan Hong Nguyen* (continued)

Nursing Interventions	Rationale	Evaluative Statement
Teach both the patient and family the importance of correct positioning. Allow the family to participate in helping the patient to get comfortable in the different positions.	Teaching promotes self-care and lays the foundation for successful rehabilitation. Involving the family in the patient's care facilitates the coping process.	

EXPECTED OUTCOME

By hospital day 7, 1/30/06, the patient will:
• Replace the passive range-of-motion exercises the nurse is now performing four times daily to all joints with (1) the patient's active exercise of the left arm and left leg and (2) the patient's active range-of-motion exercises for all other joints

Nursing Interventions	Rationale	Evaluative Statement
Assess the patient's knowledge of the importance of exercise and ability and motivation to exercise. Teach the patient how to exercise his left arm and leg by using his unaffected (right) extremities. Demonstrate a complete set of range-of-motion exercises to the patient and family and have the patient return the demonstrations.	Unless the patient understands the reason for exercise and is physically, mentally, and attitudinally capable of exercise, he will not follow through. Active exercise maintains joint mobility, prevents contracture development in the paralyzed extremity, prevents further deterioration of the neuromuscular system, helps to regain motor control, and increases circulation. Involving the family helps ensure the success of the exercise program because it requires a big time and effort commitment.	1/30/06 Outcome partially met. Patient has successfully demonstrated complete set of range-of-motion exercises (to both left and right sides); however, he tires during the exercises and stops unless verbally encouraged. *Revision:* Monitor patient's exercise four times daily; continue to enlist family's support. *S. Beecher, RN*

EXPECTED OUTCOME

By hospital day 7, 1/30/06, the patient will:
• Perform quadriceps, gluteal, and abdominal settings five times daily

Nursing Interventions	Rationale	Evaluative Statement
Teach the patient and family how to tighten the quadriceps, gluteal, and abdominal muscles and hold them for 6 seconds (slow count to 4) before relaxing. A 2-minute rest should be allowed between contractions and the patient cautioned not to hold his breath during these exercises because this places strain on the heart. The exercises should be stopped short of muscle fatigue.	These exercises will maintain muscle mass, tone, and strength (while the patient is on bed rest); and prevent atrophy. They also increase circulation to the exercised body parts.	1/30/06 Outcome partially met. Patient has demonstrated exercises correctly; however, he needs to be reminded to perform them. Family is effective in this regard. *Revision:* Compliment family on excellent job they are doing and reinforce importance of exercise to maximize rehabilitative potential. *S. Beecher, RN*

EXPECTED OUTCOME

By hospital day 7, 1/30/06, the patient will:
• Participate in the every-2-hour positioning schedule by assisting with turning to the degree he is able

(continued)

NURSING PLAN OF CARE 39-1   *for Quan Hong Nguyen* (continued)

Nursing Interventions	Rationale	Evaluative Statement
Teach the patient how he can help to reposition himself by grabbing onto the side rail with his right hand and also by placing his unaffected leg under the left one to move himself.	The more the patient can do independently, the more in control he will feel. These activities will pave the way to increasing independence in self-care activities.	1/27/06 Outcome met. Patient consistently assists in repositioning. Seems pleased to be able to help the nurses in this way. *S. Beecher, RN*

EXPECTED OUTCOME   By hospital day 7, 1/30/06, the patient will:
• Demonstrate a safe pivot transfer from bed to chair and chair to bed

Nursing Interventions	Rationale	Evaluative Statement
Assess the stage of recovery of muscle function.	Most patients will begin to show signs of spasticity with exaggerated reflexes within 48 hours—this denotes progress. If muscles are still flaccid after several weeks, prognosis for regaining function if poor.	1/30/06 Outcome met. Patient can safely transfer from bed to chair and chair to bed but requires nursing assistance. *S. Beecher, RN*

EXPECTED OUTCOME   By hospital day 7, 1/30/06, the patient will:
• Demonstrate standing balance

Nursing Interventions	Rationale	Evaluative Statement
Assess activity tolerance by taking vital signs before attempting balance training and transfers.	Vital signs and the patient's physical condition should be assessed before a new activity, during the activity, and shortly afterward to assess activity tolerance.	1/30/06 Outcome not met. Patient has not demonstrated standing balance; falls to left side without nursing support. *Revision:* Allow more time for goal achievement. *S. Beecher, RN*
Precede transfers with balance training. Assist the patient to a sitting position at the edge of the bed and observe for steadiness and the ability to maintain an erect posture.	The patient needs sitting and standing balance before progressing to harder tasks. Dizziness or syncope may signal vasomotor instability.	
Place the chair by the bed on the patient's unaffected side and assist the patient to dress. Initially, the nurse helps the patient to stand by placing his or her right knee against the patient's strong knee, grasping the patient around the waist with both arms, and pulling the patient forward while rocking back on the left leg (nurse's knees are slightly flexed).	This prevents the patient's knees from buckling and the pressure of the nurse's knee forces the patient to straighten the strong knee and bear weight on it. In this position, the patient's feet cannot slip forward. In this position, the nurse is using good principles of body mechanics.	

(continued)

NURSING PLAN OF CARE 39-1

for Quan Hong Nguyen (continued)

Nursing Interventions	Rationale	Evaluative Statement
Once the patient is standing, assess standing balance and observe for signs of activity intolerance (pallor, shortness of breath, excessive increase in pulse rate, perspiration). Direct the patient to (1) grab the far arm of the chair with his strong arm, (2) turn on his strong foot, and (3) sit down. The nurse's right leg and the patient's strong leg are used as a pivot.	Using the unaffected extremity facilitates movement and provides stability.	
Pivot patient out of bed to chair three times a day (may pivot out of bed to bedside commode). Gradually increase time in chair based on patient's tolerance. Correctly align patient in chair using supportive devices as necessary.	Increasing exercise to the patient's tolerance level promotes improved muscle strength and maintenance of range of motion.	

EXPECTED OUTCOME

On discharge to rehabilitation center, the patient will:
• Be free of contractures

Nursing Interventions	Rationale	Evaluative Statement
Implement previously stated nursing actions.	These actions promote independence and return to activities of daily living.	1/30/06 Outcome met. Patient has no contractures. *S. Beecher, RN*

NURSING DIAGNOSIS

Self-Care Deficit (all basic self-care activities) related to decreased alertness and left-sided motor and sensory deficits as manifested by: inability to use left arm (is right-handed), inability to ambulate, forgetfulness, fatigue.

EXPECTED OUTCOME

By hospital day 7, 1/30/06, the patient will:
• Demonstrate beginning ability to resume self-care activities despite motor and sensory deficits of left side; use right arm to (1) assist in morning hygiene; (2) feed himself (finger foods, beverages); and (3) exercise

Nursing Interventions	Rationale	Evaluative Statement
Continue to assess extent of patient's motor and sensory deficits and ability to perform self-care activities.	This facilitates recognition of any recovery of function and allows setting of appropriate goals.	1/29/06 Outcome met. For the past 2 days, patient has washed his left arm, abdomen, and legs; combed his hair; fed himself; and performed range-of-motion exercises. *S. Beecher, RN*
Set realistic short-term goals for each sessions with patient and reward progress: "This morning we'll see how much of your bath you are able to manage yourself!" "It must feel good to be able to do this for yourself again."	Adding *realistic* new tasks for each day gives the patient a goal to work toward; a pattern of *noticed* success encourages continued efforts.	

(continued)

NURSING PLAN OF CARE 39-1 for Quan Hong Nguyen (continued)

Nursing Interventions	Rationale	Evaluative Statement
Approach patient from his unaffected side, and place call light, bedside table, phone, and so on, on this side.	This helps the patient to compensate for alterations in sensory perception.	
Teach patient how to transfer all self-care activities to the unaffected side and how to use one-handed techniques and adaptive equipment.	There is never only one way to do anything.	
Encourage patient to brush his teeth, comb his hair, bathe and feed himself, and to assist in toileting. Explain to the family why it is critical to allow him to do these things himself, even if movements are tiring, clumsy, and initially frustrating.	This improves the patient's sense of control of his own activities of daily living and improves morale.	
Continually reevaluate the patient's need for gentle care versus firm, directive encouragement. Involve the family in this process.	Emotional lability is common after stroke. Patients fluctuate between heroic efforts toward independent self-care and whining demands to be totally cared for. The appropriate nursing response varies from moment to moment and runs the range of tender care to unrelenting firm direction. All nursing responses need to communicate the nurse's sincere care for the patient and commitment to developing his best potential.	

EXPECTED OUTCOME

On discharge to rehabilitation center, the patient will:
• Show signs of physical and mental readiness to acquire increasing independence in self-care

Nursing Interventions	Rationale	Evaluative Statement
Implement previously stated nursing actions.	These actions help the patient toward regaining control of his daily living and improve morale.	1/31/06 Outcome met. Patient's muscle strength and joint mobility maintained during hospitalization. Patient is now participating in self-care activities and is eager to learn skills to become more independent. *S. Beecher, RN*

SAMPLE DOCUMENTATION

1/25/06   3 PM, Nursing

Dr. Steel examined the patient at 1 PM and noted he is now in "completed stroke stage and ready for more aggressive rehabilitative treatment." This was explained to patient, his wife, and son. The patient smiled and seemed to understand that he is out of immediate danger. Initial instructions given to the patient on how he can assist with position changes and actively exercise his left arm and leg. Correctly demonstrated these maneuvers with verbal cuing. Motor function still absent in left arm and weak in left leg. Plan of care revised to incorporate new exercise goals.

S. Beecher, RN

Developing Critical Thinking Skills

1. Pretend that you have a mobility impairment (ie, you have to use crutches or a walker, cane, or wheelchair), and attempt to perform your usual daily activities, ideally including visiting a public place such as a school or mall. How did you feel about the restriction of your movement? How can nurses best assist patients who are coping with these restrictions? How did the public respond to your impairment, and what effects might such responses have on individuals with mobility impairments? Are public spaces adequately adapted to meet the needs of those with mobility impairments? What measures are needed to address any deficiencies? Did you identify any safety needs?

2. Suppose a friend is confined to bed for several months after a motorcycle accident that resulted in severe orthopedic and internal injuries. What nursing measures would you recommend to avoid the hazards of immobility?

Practicing for NCLEX

1. When describing the strong, flexible, inelastic fibrous bands that attach muscle to bone, the nurse would refer to these as:
   a. Tendons
   b. Ligaments
   c. Cartilage
   d. Joints

2. The underlying rationale for nurses to spread their feet apart when they prepare to help raise a patient from a chair would be to:
   a. Use the body's weight to assist movement
   b. Make a long midriff
   c. Provide a wide base of support
   d. Facilitate use of the stronger back muscles

3. A patient performs rehabilitative exercises with resistance after a knee injury. The nurse interprets this type of exercise as which of the following?
   a. Isotonic
   b. Isokinetic
   c. Isometric
   d. Aerobic

4. Which of the following would the nurse expect to assess when a patient experiences a greater breakdown of protein than that which is manufactured?
   a. Fluid volume excess
   b. A contracture
   c. Osteoporosis
   d. Negative nitrogen balance

5. An immobile patient experiences multiple urinary tract infections. Urinary bacteria are more likely to grow when urine is
   a. Alkaline
   b. Dilute
   c. Aromatic
   d. Acidic

6. Mr. Brown is experiencing some difficulty breathing. The nurse most appropriately assists him into the
   a. Dorsal recumbent position
   b. Lateral position
   c. Fowler's position
   d. Sims' position

7. While doing range-of-motion exercises with a patient who is bedridden, the nurse is aware that
   a. Neck hyperextension should be encouraged, particularly in older people.
   b. Exercises should be continued until the patient is fatigued.
   c. Exercises should be done frequently to lessen pain for the patient.
   d. Each joint is exercised to the point of resistance but not pain.

8. The nurse is assisting a patient with conditioning exercises to prepare for ambulation. The nurse correctly instructs the patient to
   a. Do full-body pushups in bed six to eight times daily
   b. Breathe in and out smoothly during quadriceps drills
   c. Dangle on the side of the bed for 30 to 60 minutes
   d. Allow the nurse to bathe the patient completely to prevent fatigue

9. In many situations, a patient has sufficient strength to walk if he or she can
   a. Lie prone for 1 hour
   b. Bathe himself or herself
   c. Raise the foot off the bed 1 inch
   d. Sit up in bed for 1 hour

10. Mrs. Eden tells the nurse she feels faint while walking in the corridor with the nurse. The nurse
    a. Instructs the patient to quicken her pace so they can return to her room
    b. Leaves her momentarily to find another nurse to help
    c. Advises her to look down at her feet to help maintain her balance
    d. Guides her to a nearby chair, easing her onto it to rest

11. When using a cane for maximal support, the nurse is aware that the patient should
    a. Hold the cane on the weaker side
    b. Distribute weight evenly between the feet and the cane
    c. Keep the elbow that is holding the cane straight and stiff
    d. Advance the weaker foot ahead of the cane

12. One technique the nurse can use when measuring a patient for axillary crutches is
    a. Measure from axilla to heel while the patient is lying on his back in bed with his shoes on and add 1 inch
    b. Have the patient stand with feet separated 12 inches and arms extended at shoulder height

c. Measure the distance from the shoulder to the heel and add 4 inches

d. Measure the distance from the anterior fold of the axilla diagonally to a point 12 inches from the heel

13. When using the swing-through crutch gait, the patient should
   a. Bear weight on the unaffected foot
   b. Bear weight on both feet
   c. Simulate normal walking as closely as possible
   d. Move the right crutch and left foot forward at the same time

14. When working with an older patient to develop an exercise program, the nurse would recommend
   a. A frequency of six times a week
   b. Exercising to the point of breathlessness when trying to speak
   c. Maintaining a target heart rate of 220 plus age
   d. Medical clearance before beginning the program

15. A bedridden patient who is blind is admitted to a healthcare facility from his or her home with pressure ulcers on the sacral area. Which nursing diagnosis would be a priority?
   a. Risk for Imbalanced Body Temperature related to stage 2 pressure ulcer
   b. Impaired Skin Integrity related to immobility
   c. Feeding Self-Care Deficit related to blindness
   d. Activity Intolerance related to prolonged bed rest

Answers With Rationale

1. The correct response is *a*. Tendons are the strong fibrous bands that attach muscle to bone. Ligaments (*b*) bind joints together and connect bones and cartilage, whereas cartilage (*c*) is nonvascular connective tissue found in the joints as well as in the nose, ear, thorax, trachea, and larynx. Joints (*d*) are areas in which one bone comes into close contact with another bone.

2. The correct response is *c*. Spreading the feet apart broadens the base of support and lowers the center of gravity. The muscles of the back (*d*) are not as strong as the long muscles of the arms and legs, and making a long midriff (*b*) is accomplished by stretching the muscles in the waist. Rocking on the feet or leaning forward or backward uses the weight of the body as a moving force (*a*).

3. The correct response is *b*. Isokinetic exercise involves muscle contraction with resistance, whereas isotonic exercise (*a*) involves muscle shortening and active movement. Isometric exercise (*c*) involves muscle contraction without shortening, and aerobic exercise (*d*) is sustained muscle movements that increase blood flow, heart rate, and metabolic demand for oxygen over time, promoting cardiovascular conditioning.

4. The correct response is *d*. Negative nitrogen balance results when the body excretes more nitrogen than it takes in. Contractures (*b*) are permanent contraction states of muscles, and osteoporosis (*c*) involves bone demineralization. Fluid volume excess (*a*) is indirectly related to protein manufacture or breakdown.

5. The correct response is *a*. Bacteria grow more easily in alkaline urine than acidic urine (*d*). Normally urine is acidic. Whether urine is dilute (*b*) or aromatic (*c*) is not a factor in bacteria growth.

6. The correct response is *c*. Fowler's position promotes maximal breathing space in the thoracic cavity and is the position of choice when someone is having difficulty breathing. Lying flat on the back or side (*a, b*) or Sims' position (*d*) would not facilitate respiration and would be difficult for the patient to maintain.

7. The correct response is *d*. Joints should be exercised slowly, smoothly, and rhythmically to the point of resistance but not pain. Joints should never be exercised to the point of pain or fatigue (*b*). Neck hyperextension (*a*) should be avoided in older patients and may prove painful.

8. The correct response is *b*. Breathing in and out smoothly during quadriceps drills maximizes lung inflation. The patient should never hold his or her breath during exercise drills because this places a strain on the heart. Pushups are usually done three or four times a day and involve only the upper body (*a*). Dangling for 30 to 60 minutes is unsafe (*c*). The nurse encourages the patient to be as independent as possible to prepare for return to normal ambulation and ADLs.

9. The correct response is *c*. Being able to raise the foot 1 inch off the bed frequently indicates sufficient strength for walking. Lying prone (*a*), bathing himself or herself (*b*), or sitting up in bed (*d*) do not necessarily indicate the muscle coordination and strength necessary in the lower limbs for walking.

10. The correct response is *d*. Guiding the patient to a chair in the hall and easing her into it is the safest action. Asking her to walk faster (*a*) and leaving her alone (*b*) are definitely unsafe actions. If the patient looks down at her feet, she may become dizzy and unbalanced (*c*).

11. The correct response is *b*. The patient's weight should be evenly distributed between his or her feet and the cane. Holding the cane on the weaker side (*a*) is difficult and unsafe. The elbow should be flexed at a 30-degree angle when holding the cane. The cane is advanced first, then the weaker foot.

12. The correct response is *a*. Axillary crutches should be measured when the patient is lying flat in bed with his or her walking shoes on. The distance is measured from the anterior fold of the axilla straight down to the heel, and then adding 2.5 cm (1 inch). Or, measure the distance from the anterior fold of the axilla diagonally out to a point 10 to 15 cm (4–6 inches) away from the heel, allowing 3 finger-

widths distance from the crutch top to the axilla. Any other measurements would be incorrect.

13. The correct response is *a*. With the swing-through gait, weight-bearing is permitted only on one foot. A disadvantage of this gait is that is does not simulate normal walking (*c*). Both crutches are brought forward at the same time, and then both legs swing through and between the crutches, with weight-bearing returning to the unaffected leg.

14. The correct response is *d*. Patients older than 35 years should always get medical clearance before initiating an exercise program. Frequency is initially three times a week, and exercise should be maintained so that the patient is able to talk without becoming breathless. The target heart rate is calculated as 60% to 90% of the maximal heart rate (220 minus age).

15. The correct response is *b*. The priority nursing diagnosis for this patient at this moment is Impaired Skin Integrity related to immobility. An end result of the immobility is the development of a pressure ulcer. The other nursing diagnoses may be appropriate but are not the priority on admission to the healthcare facility.

Bibliography

Bennett, J., Stewart, A., Kayser-Jones, J., & Glaser, D. (2002). The mediating effect of pain and fatigue on level of functioning in older adults. *Nursing Research, 51*(4), 254–265.

Boyd, L. (2001). Clinical highlights. *RN, 64*(6), 16, 18.

Burns, K., Camaione, D., & Chatterton, C. (2000). Prescription of physical activity by adult nurse practitioners: A national survey. *Nursing Outlook, 48*(1), 28–33.

Converso, A., & Murphy, C. (2004). Winning the battle against back injuries. *RN, 67*(2), 52–57.

Janz, K., Burns, T., Torner, J., Levy, S., Paulos, R., et al. (2001). Physical activity and bone measures in young children: The Iowa bone development study. *Pediatrics, 107*(6), 1387–1393.

Laufer, Y. (2001). Effects of one-point and four-point canes on balance and weight distribution in patients with hemiparesis. *Clinical Rehabilitation, 16*(10), 141–148.

Lee, I., Rexrode, K., et al. (2001). Physical activity and coronary heart disease in women. *JAMA, 285*(11), 1447.

McCloskey, J., & Bulechek, G. (2000). *Nursing interventions classification* (3rd ed.). St. Louis: C. V. Mosby.

McConnell, E. (2001). Clinical do's & don'ts: Teaching your patient to use a stationary walker. *Nursing, 31*(10), 17.

National Osteoporosis Foundation. (2004, February). *Disease statistics.* Retrieved March 11, 2004, from http://www.nof.org.

Nelson, A., Fragala, G., & Menzel, N. (2003). Myths and facts about back injuries in nursing. *American Journal of Nursing, 103*(2), 32–40.

Nelson, A., Owen, B., Lloyd, J., Fragala, G., Matz, M., et al. (2003). Safe patient handling & movement. *American Journal of Nursing, 103*(3), 32–43.

Nies, M., & Kershaw, T. (2002). Psychosocial and environmental influences on physical activity and health outcomes in sedentary women. *Journal of Nursing Scholarship, 34*(3), 243–249.

North American Nursing Diagnosis Association. (2003). *NANDA nursing diagnoses: Definitions & classification 2003–2004.* Philadelphia: Author.

Owen, B. (2000). Preventing injuries using an ergonomic approach. *AORN, 72*(6), 1031–1033, 1035–1036.

Price, A. (2003). Primary and secondary prevention of colorectal cancer. *Gastroenterology Nursing, 26*(2), 73–81.

Robbins, L., Pender, N., Conn, V., Frenn, M., Neuberger, G., et al. (2001). Physical activity research in nursing. *Journal of Nursing Scholarship, 33*(4), 315–321.

U.S. Department of Health and Human Services. (2000). *Healthy People 2010,* conference edition. Washington DC: U.S. Department of Health and Human Services. Available at http://www.health.gov/healthypeople/Document/HTML/Volume2/22Physical.htm. Accessed September 19, 2003.

U.S. Preventive Services Task Force. (2003). Behavioral counseling in primary care to promote physical activity: Recommendation and rationale. *American Journal of Nursing, 103*(4), 101–107.

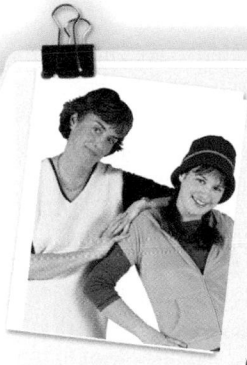

Jeanette Clark accompanies her 15-year-old daughter to the clinic. While the daughter is having some routine laboratory testing done in another department, Mrs. Clark says, "She always seems to be tired. When she was small, I could never get her to sleep. Now all she wants to do is sleep. It's all I can do to get her up for school each morning."

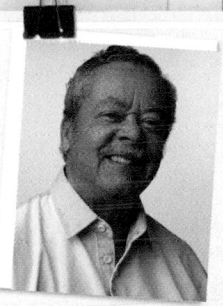

Charlie Singer, an older man who lives in a long-term care facility, says, "I don't know why they give me these pills. They don't do anything. I'm up half the night trying to fall asleep, and then I'm no sooner asleep when I wake up and spend the rest of the early morning trying to fall back asleep. I wish you could find something to knock me out for at least a couple of hours."

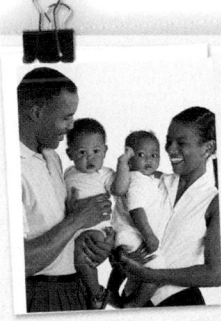

Lydia Omeara asks whether she should let her infant twins sleep in bed with her and her husband. "They have their own beds, of course, but at night, when they get up, they like to be in bed with us. Plus, I still breastfeed my babies, so having them nearby would really make it easier for me."

Focusing on Blended Skills

The types of blended skills you'll need to respond to the case scenarios include:

Cognitive Skills

- Knowledge of the physiology of sleep
- Ability to identify circadian rhythms, stages of sleep, and the sleep cycle for patients across the lifespan
- Knowledge of the factors that influence rest and sleep, including developmental variables
- Ability to apply knowledge of the nursing process to identify patients at risk for sleep disorders and to implement a plan of care to prevent or resolve sleep problems
- Knowledge of pharmacologic and nonpharmacologic measures to promote rest and sleep
- Knowledge of the research process to ensure the use of scientifically sound rationales

Technical Skills

- Strong assessment skills to identify possible and actual problems with sleep
- Competence in the skills required to assess sleep and implement measures to promote sleep
- Ability to provide technical nursing assistance to assess and meet the needs of patients across the lifespan with differing needs for sleep and experiencing sleep problems
- Ability to adapt techniques to address changes in sleep and rest needs for patients across the lifespan
- Ability to seek assistance as necessary when caring for an adolescent patient who is reported to be sleeping a lot, an older adult voicing problems with sleep medication, and a mother of two young children who wake during the night

Interpersonal Skills

- Strong interpersonal skills to establish trusting relationships and build rapport with patients of various developmental stages who are experiencing disturbed sleep patterns

- Demonstration of a nonjudgmental, caring attitude to help facilitate assessment and identification of problems associated with sleep
- Ability to assist patients of various developmental stages to develop methods to promote adequate sleep and cope with disturbed sleep patterns
- Ability to communicate and interact effectively with patients experiencing disturbed sleep patterns
- Ability to provide clear information about research related to children sleeping with their parents
- Demonstration of respect for each patient's human dignity and autonomy regardless of whether the patient is the mother of an adolescent, an older man living in a long-term care facility, or the mother of two young children

Ethical and Legal Skills

- Demonstration of a strong sense of accountability for the health and well-being of patients experiencing disturbed sleep patterns, regardless of the underlying cause
- Commitment to patient advocacy, including getting patients the help they need to achieve their rest and sleep goals—within the scope of your nursing responsibilities and available resources
- Willingness to hold colleagues accountable for safe and quality practice, especially related to promotion of sleep
- Ability to integrate knowledge of ethical and legal principles concerning sleep in the plan of care for the mother of an adolescent, an older man reporting ineffectiveness of sleep medications, and a mother with questions about her two children sleeping in their parents' bed
- Ability to practice in an ethically and legally defensible manner when providing care to patients experiencing various degrees of disturbed sleep patterns

Learning Outcomes

After completing the chapter, the learner should be able to accomplish the following:

1. Describe the functions and physiology of sleep.
2. Identify variables that influence rest and sleep.
3. Describe nursing implications that address age-related differences in the sleep cycle.
4. Perform a comprehensive sleep assessment using appropriate interview questions, a sleep diary when indicated, and physical assessment skills.
5. Describe common sleep disorders, noting key assessment criteria.
6. Develop nursing diagnoses that correctly identify sleep problems that may be treated through independent nursing interventions.
7. Describe nursing strategies to promote rest and sleep based on scientific rationale.
8. Plan, implement, and evaluate nursing care related to select nursing diagnoses involving sleep problems.

Key Terms

circadian rhythm
delta sleep
dyssomnias
enuresis
hypersomnia
insomnia
narcolepsy
nocturnal myoclonus
non–rapid eye movement (NREM) sleep
parasomnias
rapid eye movement (REM) sleep
rest
restless leg syndrome
sleep
sleep apnea
sleep cycle
sleep deprivation
somnambulism

In this chapter, rest connotes a condition in which the body is in a decreased state of activity, with the consequent feeling of being refreshed. Many factors affect a person's ability to rest. Adults juggling the demands of their job and family responsibilities often find little opportunity for rest and relaxation during the course of a day. Children involved in numerous extracurricular activities, as well as trying to excel academically, also do not have the opportunity to rest and relax during the day. Even when rest is possible, the environment is not always conducive to physical and mental relaxation. Suggestions for preparing a restful environment and promoting relaxation are discussed later in the chapter.

Sleep is a state of rest accompanied by altered consciousness and relative inactivity. Sleep is a complex rhythmic state involving a progression of repeated cycles, each representing different phases of body and brain activity. Although sensitivity to external stimuli is diminished during sleep, this sensitivity can be readily reversed.

Most people can fall asleep easily and remain asleep until the desired waking time. Conversely, others rarely fall asleep without a struggle, and then when they do, sleep is fragmented. Many people have sleep disturbances that go undetected for years, progressively undermining their energy and destroying their sense of self. Sleep loss that results in fatigue and decreased competence may be a contributing factor in accidents. The National Highway Traffic Safety Administration, in collaboration with the National Center on Sleep Disorder Research (NHTSA & NCSDR, 1999), estimated that 71,000 nonfatal injuries and 1,550 fatalities annually can be attributed to drowsy drivers. Also, the discomfort produced by illness and the need for hospitalization and treatment may interfere dramatically with a patient's ability to sleep. Consequently, nurses need to be vigilant in detecting and treating sleep disturbances (see the accompanying Reflective Practice box for an example).

This chapter provides the nurse with knowledge of the functions and physiology of sleep and factors affecting sleep. Practical suggestions for performing a comprehensive sleep assessment are included. Sample interview questions for a general sleep history are presented, along with information on sleep diaries and pertinent physical assessment data. The importance of analyzing these data is explained and numerous examples of nursing diagnoses are given. Expected patient outcomes and specific nursing strategies for promoting rest and sleep are described. The concluding nursing plan of care illustrates how the nurse's knowledge of rest and sleep, combined with skilled nursing interventions and caring, can resolve sleep problems.

PHYSIOLOGY OF SLEEP

Two systems in the brain stem, the reticular activating system (RAS) and the bulbar synchronizing region, are believed to work together to control the cyclic nature of sleep. The RAS extends upward through the medulla, the pons, the midbrain, and into the hypothalamus. It comprises many nerve cells and

fibers. The fibers have connections that relay impulses into the cerebral cortex and spinal cord. The RAS facilitates reflex and voluntary movements as well as cortical activities related to a state of alertness. During sleep, the RAS experiences few stimuli from the cerebral cortex and the periphery of the body. Wakefulness occurs when this system is activated with stimuli from the cerebral cortex and from periphery sensory organs and cells (Fig. 40-1). For example, an alarm clock awakens us from sleep to a state of consciousness where we realize that we must prepare for the day. Sensations such as pain, pressure, and noise produce wakefulness by means of peripheral organs and cells.

The hypothalamus has control centers for several involuntary activities of the body, one of which concerns sleeping and waking. Injury to the hypothalamus may cause a person to sleep for abnormally long periods.

Various neurotransmitters are involved with the sleeping process. Norepinephrine and acetylcholine, followed by dopamine, serotonin, and histamine, are involved with excitation. Gamma-aminobutyric acid (GABA) appears to be necessary for inhibition. However, research has yet to prove exactly how biochemical changes and hormones function in sleep.

Circadian Rhythms

Rhythmic biologic clocks are known to exist in plants, animals, and humans. Influenced by both internal and external factors, they regulate certain biologic and behavioral functions in humans. Some cycles are monthly, such as a woman's menstrual cycle. Circadian rhythms complete a full cycle every 24 hours. "Circa" in Latin means "approximately" and "diem" is the Latin word for "day"; circadian represents approximately one day (Wolf, 2002). Fluctuations in a person's heart rate, blood pressure, body temperature, hormone secretions, metabolism, and performance and mood depend in part on circadian rhythms.

Sleep is one of the body's most complex biologic rhythms. Circadian synchronization exists when an individual's sleep–wake patterns follow the inner biologic clock. When physiologic and psychological rhythms are high or most active, the person is awake; when these rhythms are low, the person is asleep. Although light and dark appear to be powerful regulators of the sleep–wake circadian rhythm, they do not exert primary control. The regulating mechanism is the person's individual biologic clock, which is subject to numerous influences, such as occupational demands and social pressures.

Think back to Charlie Singer, the older man living in a long-term care facility. The nurse would need to assess Mr. Singer, gathering data about his circadian rhythm. This knowledge would be important in developing an individualized plan of care for the patient to promote adequate sleep.

For example, nurses who work the night shift may routinely sleep from 2 to 8 p.m., and peak physiologic activity

Reflective Practice
Challenge to Intellectual Skills

I was working in our well-baby clinic today when a mother, Lydia Omeara, asked my advice about letting her infant twins sleep in bed with her and her husband: "They have their own beds, of course, but at night, when they get up, they seem to like to be in bed with us. Plus, I still breastfeed my babies, so having them nearby would really make it easier for me." She mentioned reading an article recently about this, noting that while this custom is usual in other countries, it had been discouraged until recently in the United States. According to the article, she said that it seems that more and more U.S. parents are doing this now. She asked for my advice, and I had no idea how to respond. Clearly, anything that resulted in better rest for the parents—who are up many times each night if the babies aren't sleeping well—would seem to be a good idea. However, I vaguely remembered learning that small children are at increased risk for sudden infant death syndrome in an adult bed. I needed to find the best way to respond to Mrs. Omeara.

Thinking Outside the Box: Possible Courses of Action

- Make up an answer: "Yes, it's OK" or "No way! What are you, crazy?"
- Refer her to a nurse with more experience.
- Tell her that I honestly don't know the answer but I will find out more about this and then get back to her.

Evaluating a Good Outcome: How Do I Define Success?

- A decision is made about where the children sleep that protects them and promotes rest, health, and well-being for each member of the family.
- I learn more about what science dictates is the best recommendation.
- I am faithful to my professional obligations to be knowledgeable about matters like this.

Personal Learning: Here's to the Future!

Since I don't have children myself and couldn't ever remember spending the night in my parents' bed or having a conversation with them about this, I certainly couldn't draw on personal experience in responding to this mother. In addition, we had never studied anything about this topic. I did remember a recent article in "Newsweek" magazine raising the issue, but I didn't remember this article proposing a scientifically grounded recommendation. As a result, I did some research on this issue and learned that there is a wide range of opinion on this matter. I did my best to summarize the arguments, pro and con, and then I shared these with Mrs. Omeara so that she and her husband could make an informed decision.

This little experience has taught me a lot about the power of my profession to influence—literally—how people are born, live, and die. I want to have enough knowledge to help people make the best possible life choices, never leading them astray by virtue of my ignorance!

Reflection

How do you think you would respond in a similar situation? Why? What does this tell you about yourself and about the adequacy of your skills for professional practice? Can you think of other ways to respond? Research the Internet for the "Newsweek" article referred to by the nursing student. What information does this article provide? Would this article be a reliable research article? Please explain why or why not. What other skills (cognitive, interpersonal, technical, ethical/legal) would you need to respond well in this situation? What information would be necessary for the nursing student to obtain from the patient to provide an overall picture of the family situation? Create a sleep history tool that the nursing student could use to assess the patient's sleep. Do you agree with the criteria to evaluate a successful outcome? Did the nursing student meet the criteria? Please explain your answer.

Amy Norris, Georgetown University

---

may occur between 10 p.m. and 6 a.m. during work. Problems of desynchronization occur when sleep–wake patterns are frequently altered and the person attempts to sleep during high-activity rhythms or to work when the body is physiologically prepared to rest.

Stages of Sleep

Research reveals that there are two major stages of sleep: **non–rapid eye movement (NREM) sleep** and **rapid eye movement (REM) sleep.** These stages have been studied and analyzed with the help of the electroencephalograph (EEG), which receives and records electrical currents from the brain; the electrooculogram (EOG), which records eye movements;

and the electromyograph (EMG), which records muscle tone (Fig. 40-2).

NREM Sleep

NREM sleep consists of four stages. Stages I and II, consuming about 5% and 50% of a person's sleep time, respectively, are light sleep. During these stages, the person can be aroused with relative ease. Stages III and IV, each representing about 10% of total sleep time, are deep-sleep states, termed **delta sleep** or slow-wave sleep. The arousal threshold (intensity of stimulus required to awaken) is usually greatest in stage IV NREM. Throughout the stages of NREM sleep, the parasympathetic nervous system dominates, and decreases in pulse, respiratory rate, blood pressure, metabolic rate, and body tem-

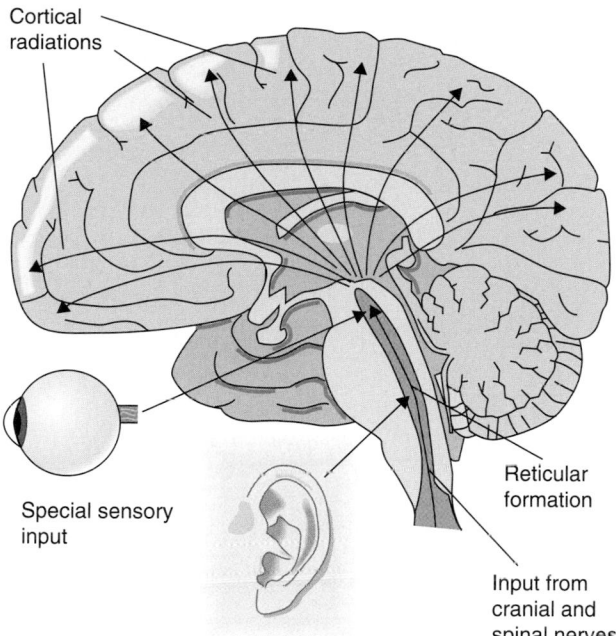

Cortical
radiations

Special sensory
input

Reticular
formation

Input from
cranial and
spinal nerves

FIGURE 40-1 Nerve impulses from all the sensory tracts reach the reticular activating system (RAS), which then selectively allows certain impulses to reach the cerebral cortex and to be perceived.

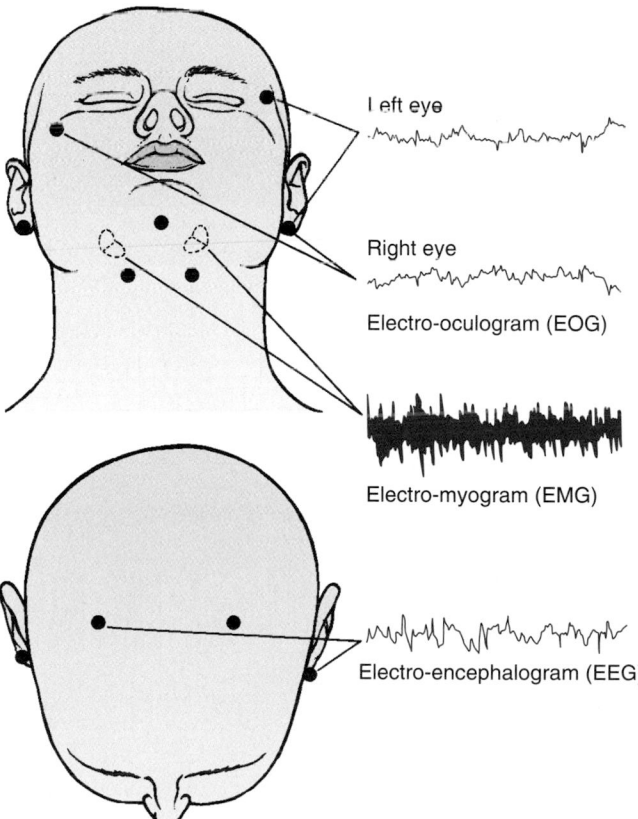

Left eye

Right eye

Electro-oculogram (EOG)

Electro-myogram (EMG)

Electro-encephalogram (EEG)

FIGURE 40-2 Sleep is determined in the laboratory by measuring the electrical activity of the brain and muscles and the movement of the eyes, using techniques of electro-oculography, electromyography, and electroencephalography.

perature are observed. Characteristics of the four stages of NREM sleep are summarized in Table 40-1.

REM Sleep

It is more difficult to arouse a person during REM sleep than during NREM sleep. In normal adults, the REM state consumes 20% to 25% of a person's nightly sleep time. People

TABLE 40-1 Characteristics of NREM and REM Sleep

NREM Sleep

Stage I	The person is in a transitional stage between wakefulness and sleep
	The person is in a relaxed state but still somewhat aware of the surroundings.
	Involuntary muscle jerking may occur and waken the person.
	The stage normally lasts only minutes.
	The person can be aroused easily.
	This stage constitutes only about 5% of total sleep.
Stage II	The person falls into a stage of sleep.
	The person can be aroused with relative ease.
	This stage constitutes 50% to 55% of sleep.
Stage III	The depth of sleep increases, and arousal becomes increasingly difficult.
	This stage composes about 10% of sleep.
Stage IV	The person reaches the greatest depth of sleep, which is called *delta sleep*.
	Arousal from sleep is difficult.
	Physiologic changes in the body include the following:
	Slow brain waves are recorded on an EEG.
	Pulse and respiratory rates decrease.
	Blood pressure decreases.
	Muscles are relaxed.
	Metabolism slows and the body temperature is low.
	This constitutes about 10% of sleep.

REM Sleep

	Eyes dart back and forth quickly.
	Small muscle twitching, such as on the face
	Large muscle immobility, resembling paralysis
	Respirations irregular; sometimes interspersed with apnea
	Rapid or irregular pulse
	Blood pressure increases or fluctuates
	Increase in gastric secretions
	Metabolism increases; body temperature increases
	Encephalogram tracings active
	REM sleep enters from stage II of NREM sleep and reenters NREM sleep at stage II: arousal from sleep difficult
	Constitutes about 20% to 25% of sleep

who are awakened during the REM state almost always report that they have been dreaming. Everyone dreams. Some people repress their dreams because the content is too painful; others forget their dreams because the content did not seem pertinent (Gilbert, 2002).

During REM sleep, the pulse, respiratory rate, blood pressure, metabolic rate, and body temperature increase, whereas general skeletal muscle tone and deep tendon reflexes are depressed. REM sleep is believed to be essential to mental and emotional equilibrium and to play a role in learning, memory, and adaptation.

A person who is deprived of REM sleep for several nights generally then spends more time in REM sleep on successive nights. This phenomenon, termed REM rebound, allows the total amount of REM sleep to remain fairly constant over time. Characteristics of REM sleep are included in Table 40-1.

Sleep Cycle

Normally during a **sleep cycle,** a person passes consecutively through the four stages of NREM sleep. This pattern is then reversed, and the person returns from stage IV to stage III to stage II. Instead of reentering stage I and awakening, the person enters into the REM stage of sleep, after which he or she reenters NREM sleep at stage II and returns to stages III and IV. If a person is awakened from sleep at any time, he or she returns to sleep again by starting at stage I of NREM sleep.

> *Consider Charlie Singer, the long-term care resident described at the beginning of the chapter. When evaluating Mr. Singer's sleep cycle, the nurse would need to keep in mind that each time Mr. Singer awakes, his sleep cycle is starting all over again. Subsequently, he is experiencing light sleep, characteristic of sleep stages I and II.*

Most people go through four or five cycles of sleep each night. On average, each cycle lasts about 90 to 100 minutes. The cycles tend to become longer as morning approaches. Ordinarily, more sleep occurs in the delta stage in the first half of the night, especially if one is tired or has lost sleep.

Figure 40-3 illustrates the normal sleep pattern of young adults. Variations in the sleep cycle occur according to age, as Figure 40-4 illustrates.

Sleep Requirements and Patterns

For no known reason, 8 hours of sleep a night has been the accepted standard for adults, despite obvious variations seen in the general population. No rigid formula exists for normal periodicity and duration of sleep. It is important, however, that each person follow a pattern of rest that maintains well-being.

Despite individual variations, some generalities can be stated. On the average, infants sleep 14 to 20 hours each day. Growing children require from 10 to 14 hours of sleep.

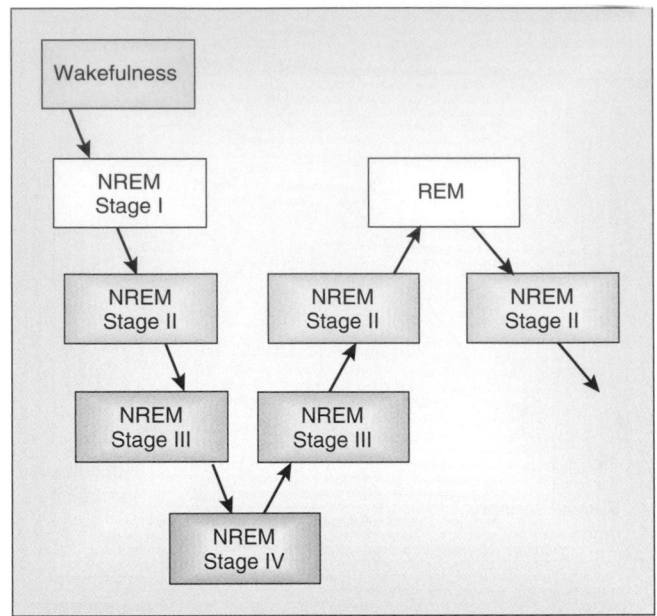

FIGURE 40-3 A single normal sleep cycle. In the normal nocturnal pattern, the shaded cycle is repeated four or five times. Periods of REM sleep generally increase in duration, and periods of deep sleep (stage IV) progressively decrease as morning approaches.

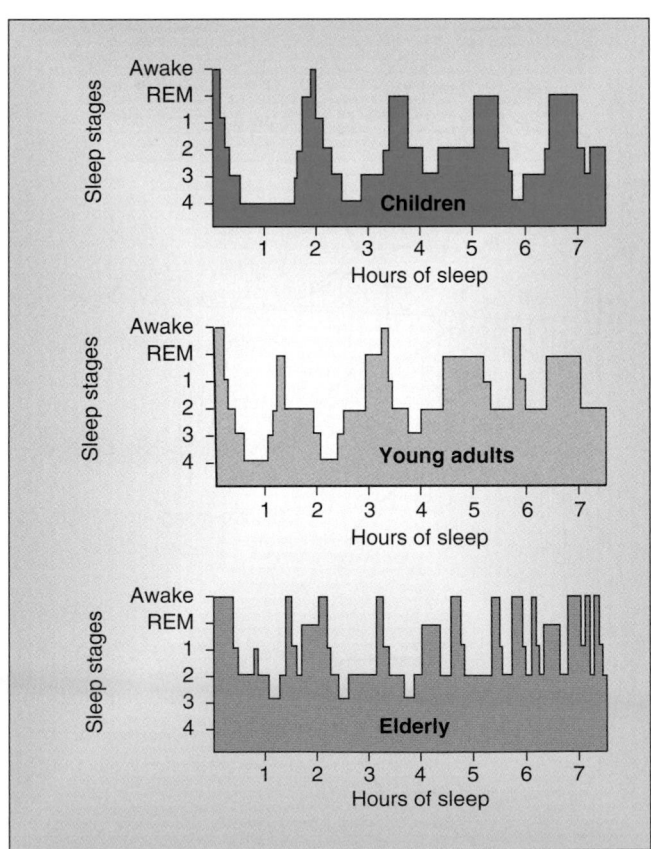

FIGURE 40-4 A comparison of developmental differences in NREM and REM cycles during nocturnal sleep for children, young adults, and older people.

Recall Jeanette Clark, the mother of an adolescent girl who seems to want to sleep all the time. When discussing this issue with Mrs. Clark, the nurse would need to keep integrate information about the adolescent's developmental stage—that is, that adolescence is a period of tremendous growth.

Adults average 7 to 9 hours. Those who are able to relax and rest easily, even while awake, often find that less sleep is needed, whereas others may find that more sleep is required to overcome fatigue. Fatigue can be considered a normal, protective body mechanism and nature's warning that sleep is necessary. Chronic fatigue, however, is abnormal and is often a symptom of illness.

Sleep patterns of older adults vary. However, older people often need more time to fall asleep, wake earlier and more frequently during the night, and are less able to cope with changes in their usual sleep patterns than younger people are. Many older individuals nap during the day, which often results in sleeping fewer hours at night. Illnesses in older adults may also affect their sleep patterns. For instance, many older men suffer from enlargement of the prostate gland, which may cause them to awaken throughout the night to use the bathroom.

Patterns of sleep periodicity appear to be learned. For example, most people learn to sleep at night and to be awake and work during the day. However, many night workers learn to sleep equally well during the day.

FACTORS AFFECTING SLEEP

A variety of factors influence both the quality and quantity of sleep.

Developmental Considerations

Variations in sleep patterns are related to age. Table 40-2 highlights these variations and associated nursing implications.

TABLE 40-2 Developmental Patterns of Sleep

Sleep Pattern	Nursing Implications
Infants • *Newborn:* sleeps an average of 16 hours/24 hours; averages about 4 hours at a time • Each infant's sleep pattern is unique. On the average, infants sleep 10–12 hours at night with possibly several naps during the day. • Usually by 8–16 weeks of age, an infant sleeps through the night. • REM sleep constitutes much of the sleep cycle of a young infant.	• Teach parents to position infant on the back. Sleeping in the prone position increases the risk for sudden infant death syndrome (SIDS). • Advise parents that eye movements, groaning, grimacing, and moving are normal activities at this age. • Encourage parents to have infant sleep in a separate area rather than their bed. • Caution parents about placing pillows, quilts, stuffed animals, etc. in the crib because this may pose a suffocation risk.
Toddlers • Need for sleep declines as this stage progresses. May initially sleep 12 hours at night with two naps during the day and end this stage sleeping 8-10 hours a night and napping once during the day. • Toddlers may begin to resist naps and going to bed at night. • They may move from crib to youth bed or regular bed around 2 years.	• Establish a regular bedtime routine (eg, reading a story, singing a lullaby, saying prayers). • Advise parents of the value of a routine sleeping pattern with minimal variation. • Encourage attention to safety once child moves from crib to bed. If child attempts to wander out of room, a folding gate may be necessary across the door of their room.
Preschoolers • Children in this stage generally sleep 9–16 hours at night, with 12 hours being the average. • The REM sleep pattern is similar to that of an adult. • Daytime napping decreases during this period and most children by the age of 5 years no longer nap. • This age-group may continue to resist going to bed at night.	• Encourage parents to continue bedtime routines. • Advise parents that waking from nightmares or night terrors (awakening screaming about 20 minutes after falling asleep) are common during this stage. Waking the child and comforting him or her generally helps. Sometimes use of a night-light is soothing.
School-Aged Children • Younger school-aged children may require 10–12 hours nightly, whereas older children in this stage may average 8 to 10 hours • Sleep needs usually increase when physical growth peaks.	• Discuss the fact that the stress of beginning school may interrupt normal sleep patterns. • Advise that a relaxed, bedtime routine is most helpful at this stage.

(continued)

TABLE 40-2 (Continued)

Sleep Pattern	Nursing Implications
	• Inform parents about child's awareness of the concept of death possibly occurring at this stage. Encourage parental presence and support to help alleviate some of the child's concerns.
Adolescents • Sleep needs of teenagers vary widely. The growth spurt that normally occurs at this stage may necessitate the need for more sleep; however, the stresses of school, activities, and part-time employment may cause adolescents to have a restless sleep. • Many adolescents do not get enough sleep.	• Advise parents that complaints of fatigue or inability to do well in school may be related to not enough sleep. *Excessive daytime sleepiness (EDS)* may also make the teenager more vulnerable to accidents and behavioral problems.
Young Adults • The average amount of sleep required is 8 hours, but in fact, many young adults require less sleep. • Sleep is affected by many factors: physical health, type of occupation, exercise. Lifestyle demands may interfere with sleep patterns. • REM sleep averages about 20% of sleep.	• Reinforce that developing good sleep habits has a positive effect on health, particularly as an individual ages. • If loss of sleep is a problem, explore lifestyle demands and stress as possible causes. • Suggest use of relaxation techniques and stress-reduction exercises rather than resorting to medication to induce sleep. Sleep medications decrease REM sleep, may be habit forming, and frequently lose their effectiveness over time.
Middle-Aged Adults • Total sleep time decreases during these years with a decrease in stage IV sleep. • The percentage of time spent awake in bed begins to increase.	• Individuals become more aware of sleep disturbances during this period. • Encourage adults to investigate consistent sleep difficulties to exclude pathology or anxiety and depression as causes. • Encourage adults to avoid use of sleep-inducing medication on a regular basis.
Older Adults • An average of 5–7 hours of sleep is usually adequate for this age group. • Sleep is less sound, and stage IV sleep is absent or considerably decreased. Periods of REM sleep shorten. • Elderly people frequently have great difficulty falling asleep and have more complaints of problems sleeping. • Decline in physical health, psychological factors, effects of drug therapy (eg, nocturia), or environmental factors may be implicated as causes of inability to sleep.	• A comprehensive nursing assessment and individualized interventions may be effective in the long-term care of this age group. • Emphasize concern for a safe environment because it is not uncommon for older people to be temporarily confused and disoriented when they first awake. • Use sedatives with extreme caution because of declining physiologic function and concerns about polypharmacy. • Encourage people to discuss sleep concerns with their physicians.

Psychological Stress

Illness and various life situations that cause psychological stress tend to disturb sleep. Generally, psychological stress affects sleep in two ways: (1) the person experiencing stress may find it difficult to obtain the amount of sleep he or she needs, and (2) REM sleep decreases in amount, which tends to add to anxiety and stress.

> *Consider Mrs. Omeara, the mother described in the Reflective Practice example. The nurse would need to gather additional information about Mrs. Omeara's current situation, including any stressors that may be affecting her ability to obtain adequate rest and sleep. Areas to address may include her typical daily activities, amount of time spent caring for each child, employment, and amount of assistance and support from others. In addition, the nurse would need to investigate the reasons underlying Mrs. Omeara's question.*

Motivation

A desire to be wakeful and alert helps overcome sleepiness and sleep. For example, a tired person may be wakeful and alert when at a party or when attending an interesting play or concert. The opposite is also true: when there is minimal motivation to be awake, sleep generally follows. For example, a student who is bored and disinterested in a lecture or class may doze during the lecture.

Culture

An individual's cultural beliefs and practices can influence rest and sleep. Although developmental stages are similar, children's bedtime rituals, sleeping place, and pattern of sleep may vary based on culture. Methods to enhance or foster sleep may also be culturally influenced. For example, an older Asian patient may choose herbal tea rather than a sleeping medication to promote relaxation and sleep. A cultural orientation toward privacy and quiet makes sleep difficult in a busy special care unit where male and female patients sleep in close proximity. Sensitivity to a patient's culture must be included in the plan of care for preparing the patient for an evening's sleep.

> *Think back to Mrs. Omeara, the mother of infant twins, who is wondering whether she should let her twins sleep in their parents' bed. The nurse would need to investigate the family's cultural background to determine any influences it may have on the patient's question. The nurse would then use this information to develop an individualized, culturally appropriate plan of care for dealing with this question.*

Lifestyle and Habits

Various lifestyle factors can affect a person's ability to sleep well. People working a shift other than the day shift must reorganize their priorities, or sleep difficulties may occur. Sleep disorders are the major problem associated with shift work, but shift work can also result in anxiety, personal conflicts, loneliness, depression, gastrointestinal symptoms, and substance abuse. Developing a sleep pattern is especially difficult if the shift changes periodically. Sleep can be affected by watching some types of television shows, participating in stimulating outside activities, and taking part in activity or exercise. One's abilities to relax from work-related pressures and to put aside home stresses are also important factors in the ability to fall asleep (see Promoting Health 40-1: Rest and Sleep).

Physical Activity and Exercise

Activity and exercise increase fatigue and, in many instances, promote relaxation that is followed by sleep. It appears that physical activity increases both REM and NREM sleep.

Moderate exercise is a healthy way to promote sleep, but exercise that occurs within a 2-hour interval before normal bedtime can hinder sleep. The fatigue that results from normal work activities or exercise is believed to contribute to a restful sleep, whereas excessive exercise or exhaustion can decrease the quality of sleep.

> *Remember Jeanette Clark, the mother of the adolescent girl who seems to be sleeping all the time. As part of the health promotion teaching plan, the nurse would need to explain to Mrs. Clark about the changes occurring during adolescence. In addition to this stage being a period of rapid growth, it is also a time of increased activity, physically, emotionally, and socially. All of these may be affecting her daughter's sleep patterns.*

Dietary Habits

It has long been believed that the dietary amino acid L-tryptophan acts to promote sleep. A small protein-containing snack before bedtime used to be recommended for patients with insomnia. However, as nutritionists have studied the effects of various foods on mood, new information has emerged. Protein may actually increase alertness and concentration, whereas carbohydrates appear to affect brain serotonin levels and promote calmness and relaxation. A small protein- and carbohydrate-containing snack may be effective.

Promoting Health 40-1 Rest and Sleep

Use the assessment checklist to determine how well you are meeting needs for rest and sleep. Then develop a prescription for self-care by choosing appropriate behaviors from the list of suggestions.

ASSESSMENT CHECKLIST

almost always / sometimes / almost never

1. I feel rested and refreshed when I get up in the morning.
2. I have energy to carry out normal activities of daily living.
3. I understand the normal changes in sleep and rest requirements and patterns that occur with aging.
4. I set aside time for quiet recreation and restful activities each day.

SELF-CARE BEHAVIORS

1. Follow a regular routine for bedtime and morning awakening.
2. Accept individual differences in need for sleep.
3. Use relaxation exercises to relax before bedtime, especially if feeling stressed.
4. Avoid caffeine, smoking, and alcohol before bedtime.
5. Adjust bedcoverings, room temperature, and lighting to your preferences.
6. Eat a small carbohydrate snack before going to bed.
7. Be aware of the potential dangers of sleeping pills.
8. Use some part of each day for quiet, enjoyable activities, such as crafts, hobbies, reading, watching television, listening to music, visiting with friends.
9. Incorporate three or four periods of regular exercise into each week.

Alcohol Intake

Alcoholic beverages, when used in moderation, appear to induce sleep in some people. However, large quantities have been found to limit REM and delta sleep. This effect may partially explain the phenomenon of a hangover after excessive alcohol consumption.

Caffeine-Containing Beverages

Caffeine is a central nervous system stimulant. For many people, beverages containing caffeine interfere with the ability to fall asleep. Examples of beverages containing caffeine include coffee, tea, and most cola drinks. Chocolate also contains caffeine.

Smoking

Nicotine has a stimulating effect, and smokers usually have a more difficult time falling asleep. They are more easily aroused once asleep and may describe themselves as light sleepers. Eliminating cigarette smoking after the evening meal appears to improve the smoker's ability to fall asleep. People usually report improved sleep patterns after discontinuing nicotine use. Total withdrawal from smoking may be associated with temporary sleep disturbances. Patients who stop smoking often have more daytime sleepiness and report significantly more restlessness at night. Whether this is a short-term effect or is related to nicotine's effect on the central nervous system is uncertain.

Environmental Factors

Most people sleep best in their usual home environments. Sleeping in a strange or new environment tends to influence both REM and NREM sleep. People accustomed to sleeping in a noisy environment such as the middle of a large city may actually have a hard time falling asleep in an area that is extremely quiet. By turning on a radio or other noise, the person may actually be able to rest in the new environment. Likewise, if a patient is accustomed to sleeping in a quiet environment, choosing a room next to a high-traffic area such as the nurse's desk may not be the best place for this patient to rest.

Illness

Illness, a physiologic and psychological stressor, influences sleep. Certain illnesses are more closely related to sleep disturbances than others. For example:

- Gastric secretions increase during REM sleep. Many people with peptic ulcers wake at night with pain. They find that eating a snack or using antacids to neutralize stomach acidity often relieves discomfort and promotes sleep.
- The pain associated with coronary artery disease and myocardial infarction is more likely with REM sleep.
- Epilepsy seizures are most likely to occur during NREM sleep and appear to be depressed by REM sleep.
- Liver failure and encephalitis tend to cause a reversal in day–night sleeping habits.

- Hypothyroidism tends to decrease the amount of NREM sleep, especially stages II and IV.

Chronotherapeutics is a growing field of study that involves the strategic use of time in the administration of medicine. Researchers have determined that certain treatments for disease are more effective when body rhythms are taken into account. A larger midafternoon dose of asthma medication may be more effective in preventing attacks that commonly occur at night during sleep. The timing of antihypertensive medication administration may need to be adjusted to provide peak protection during early-morning hours, when heart attacks are more common. Cancer chemotherapy appears to be less toxic when administered at certain times of the day. Paying attention to biologic rhythms may influence drug tolerance and medication effectiveness.

Medications

Sleep quality is also influenced by certain drugs. Drugs that decrease REM sleep include barbiturates, amphetamines, and antidepressants. Diuretics, antiparkinsonian drugs, some antidepressants and antihypertensives, steroids, decongestants, caffeine, and asthma medications are seen as additional common causes of sleep problems. Chloral hydrate and zolpidem tartrate (Ambien) appear to influence the quality of sleep least and promote normal sleep.

> *Consider Charlie Singer, the older man receiving a sleeping medication that is not working. The nurse needs to investigate what type of medication the patient is receiving and how it may be affecting his sleep. In addition, the nurse would need to determine whether other factors, such as the patient's diet, activity level, or environment, may be contributing to his sleeping difficulty.*

COMMON SLEEP DISORDERS

A nurse who interviews a patient to obtain a sleep history needs to understand common sleep disturbances to recognize significant data. The most recent classification of sleep disorders devised by the American Sleep Disorders Association includes four major categories of disturbances:

- Dyssomnias
- Parasomnias
- Sleep disorders associated with medical or psychiatric disorders
- Other proposed disorders

This classification system has been developed based on current and ongoing research, and not all disorders have been clearly defined. The more common sleep disorders are the dyssomnias and parasomnias. **Dyssomnias** are sleep disorders characterized by insomnia or excessive sleepiness. **Parasomnias** are patterns of waking behavior that appear during sleep. A brief description of these disturbances follows.

Dyssomnias

Insomnia

Insomnia is characterized by difficulty falling asleep, intermittent sleep, or early awakening from sleep. It is the most common of all sleep disorders. People older than 60 years of age, women (especially after menopause), and persons with a history of depression are more likely to experience insomnia. This sleep disorder can also occur during periods of stress, in situations involving some change in the normal environment, after traveling across time zones (jet lag), and as a result of the side effects of medications.

Usually, people complaining of insomnia have been observed to fall asleep more quickly and sleep more than they report they do. However, the condition can lead to such distress that further wakefulness results. A person with insomnia often reports feeling tired, lethargic, and irritable during the day. Difficulty concentrating is also a common manifestation.

Hypersomnia is a condition characterized by excessive sleep, particularly during the day. Although this may result from a medical condition, it frequently occurs as a coping mechanism in someone who has no desire or energy to face a new day.

Treatment of insomnia is usually unnecessary because most episodes last for only a short period. Chronic insomnia lasts for longer than 3 to 4 weeks and may even continue throughout life. Depression is a common cause of chronic insomnia. Behavioral factors such as the misuse of alcohol or caffeine are also frequently implicated. Identifying and stopping these behaviors may reduce or eliminate the insomnia.

Pharmacologic therapy may include the use of sedatives and hypnotics; however, only short-term use is recommended, at the lowest dose. Nonpharmacologic therapies may include stimulus control, sleep restriction, sleep hygiene, cognitive therapy, multicomponent therapy, and relaxation therapy (Petit et al., 2003).

Stimulus control involves using the bedroom for sex and sleep only. People with insomnia who have problems initiating sleep should stay in the bedroom for only 15 to 20 minutes. If after this time they cannot fall asleep, they should leave the room and return only when they feel sleepy. Getting up at the same time every day, no matter what time the patient fell asleep, and refraining from napping during the day are recommended.

Sleep restriction is based on the theory of limiting the time in bed to actual sleep time. It is thought that excessive time in bed may result in fragmented sleep, which may exacerbate the insomnia (Petit et al., 2003). The time in bed should not be decreased to less than 5 hours per night. Brief midday naps are permitted with this type of therapy.

Sleep hygiene involves reviewing and changing the person's lifestyles and environment. This includes restricting the intake of caffeine, nicotine, and alcohol, especially later in the day; not engaging in activities that may stimulate the person after 5 p.m., and avoiding any other factors that may affect the sleep pattern. Sleep hygiene has not been as effective as other measures when used by itself but is very successful when used in conjunction with another complementary therapy.

Cognitive therapy involves meeting with a therapist and working through maladaptive sleep beliefs. This includes discussing what is normal and abnormal. Cognitive therapy also does not work well by itself but when used in conjunction with another complementary therapy is very successful.

Multicomponent therapy is a combination of two or more therapies. The choice of which therapies to combine depends on what is best for the patient. The benefits of this type of therapy do not outweigh those of other therapies.

Relaxation therapy involves any type of relaxation, such as progressive muscle relaxation, imagery training, or meditation. Not all relaxation methods are beneficial for all patients.

Narcolepsy

Narcolepsy is a condition characterized by an uncontrollable desire to sleep. A person with narcolepsy can literally fall asleep standing up, while driving a car, in the middle of a conversation, or while swimming. Individuals with narcolepsy tend to fall asleep quickly, find it difficult to wake up, sleep fewer hours than others, and sleep restlessly. Narcolepsy is considered a neurologic disorder. The condition usually begins in susceptible people during adolescence or early adulthood and continues through life.

Sleepiness during the day is often the first symptom of narcolepsy and usually precedes by several years any difficulty with nighttime sleep. Common features of narcolepsy include the following:

- Sleep attacks: irresistible urge to sleep regardless of the type of activity in which the patient is engaged
- Cataplexy: sudden loss of motor tone that may cause the person to fall asleep
- Hypnagogic hallucinations: nightmares or vivid hallucinations
- Sleep-onset REM periods: during a sleep attack, the person moves directly into REM sleep
- Sleep paralysis: skeletal paralysis that occurs during the transition from wakefulness to sleep

The presence of any two symptoms helps to confirm the diagnosis. Undiagnosed, a person with narcolepsy is potentially dangerous to himself or herself and others. In some countries a person diagnosed with narcolepsy is not permitted to drive a motor vehicle. A central nervous system stimulant (eg, methylphenidate [Ritalin]) that causes wakefulness is used to control narcolepsy. People using such drugs should take them faithfully because if they are discontinued, the uncontrollable desire to sleep returns.

Sleep Apnea

Sleep apnea is a condition in which the patient experiences the absence of breathing between snoring intervals. Breathing may cease for 10 to 20 seconds, possibly as long as 2 minutes. During long periods of apnea, the oxygen level in the blood drops, the pulse usually becomes irregular, and the blood pressure often increases. Many people experience sleep apnea without symptoms. Although it occurs most commonly in middle-aged men who are obese and have short thick necks, women and people of other ages may also experience it.

Obstructive sleep apnea can result when the airway is occluded due to the collapse of the hypopharynx (Fig. 40-5) or from other structural abnormalities, such as enlarged tonsils and adenoids, a deviated nasal septum, and thyroid enlargement. Another factor that contributes to sleep apnea is the narrowing of nasal passageways, as caused by allergic rhinitis (Virkkula et al., 2003). Some investigators have theorized that sleep apnea may explain certain cases of death that occur during sleep.

Polysomnography is the only method that can confirm the diagnosis of sleep apnea. This overnight sleep study consists of an EEG recording of the stages of sleep and any episodes of apnea; an electrooculogram that detects eye movements; and an electromyographic recording of muscle movement (Tate & Tasota, 2002). Cardiopulmonary monitoring of the arterial oxygen saturation and an electrocardiogram (ECG) to detect any cardiac arrhythmias can also assist in the diagnosis of obstructive sleep apnea.

People with obstructive sleep apnea may become irritable during the day, fall asleep during monotonous activities, have difficulty concentrating, and exhibit slower reaction times. They are also more likely to be involved in motor vehicle accidents. Alcohol, tobacco, and sleeping pills increase the breathing disruption that occurs in sleep apnea and should be avoided.

Treatment of moderate obstructive sleep apnea may consist of removing the tonsils or using an oral appliance when sleeping. If this is ineffective, continuous positive airway pressure (CPAP) may be recommended. CPAP is noninvasive and consists of a mask connected to an air pump that is worn during sleep. This device delivers positive air pressure that holds the airway open. Many patients discontinue use of CPAP because of a sensation of claustrophobia, discomfort exhaling against air inflow, or dryness and skin irritation. If conservative treatment methods fail, surgery to remove soft tissue at the back of the mouth may be an option. This surgery is not without risks, and people with obstructive sleep apnea need continued support.

Restless Leg Syndrome

People with **restless leg syndrome** cannot lie still and report unpleasant creeping, crawling, or tingling sensations in the legs. Usually, these sensations are in the calf, but they may occur anywhere from the ankle to the thigh. Patients describe an irresistible urge to move the legs when these sensations occur. Massaging the legs, walking, doing knee bends, and moving the legs sometimes bring relief. Although restless leg syndrome is a common sleep disorder that affects millions, many healthcare workers are unaware of its existence. Research continues into additional treatment options, but the following may prove effective:

- Eliminate use of caffeine, tobacco, and alcohol.
- Take a mild analgesic at bedtime (provided it is compatible with the current medical regimen).
- Use antiembolism stockings at the onset of symptoms (Boucher, 1997).

The Restless Legs Syndrome Foundation (http://www.rls.org) is a support group available for the millions of people with this disorder who suffer from chronic sleep loss.

Sleep Deprivation

Sleep deprivation refers to a decrease in the amount, consistency, or quality of sleep. It may result from decreased REM sleep or NREM sleep. Total sleep deprivation is rarely seen other than in experimental settings. There are many causes, and the manifestations progress from irritability and impaired mental abilities to a total disintegration of personality. In general, the effects of sleep deprivation become increasingly apparent after 30 hours of continual wakefulness. Partial sleep deprivation may result in loss of concentration, inattention, and impaired information processing and pose serious safety risks. Excessive daytime sleepiness, a form of partial sleep deprivation, impairs performance at times when individuals need to be alert. The strange environment of the hospital, physical discomfort and pain, the effects of medications, and the need for 24-hour nursing care may also contribute to sleep deprivation in hospitalized patients.

It is unclear whether irreversible damage to body tissue results from prolonged or chronic sleep deprivation. However, sleep deprivation clearly produces changes in physical and mental functioning, supporting the belief that sleep is essential for well-being. Sleep deprivation may be caused by shorter periods of sleep, which over time can cause impairment. Researchers reported that for 14 nights in a row, subjects slept between 4 and 6 hours per night. These same subjects showed cognitive performance equal to going without sleep for 3 days in a row, and yet the subjects did not realize the extent of their impairment (Dinges et al., 2003).

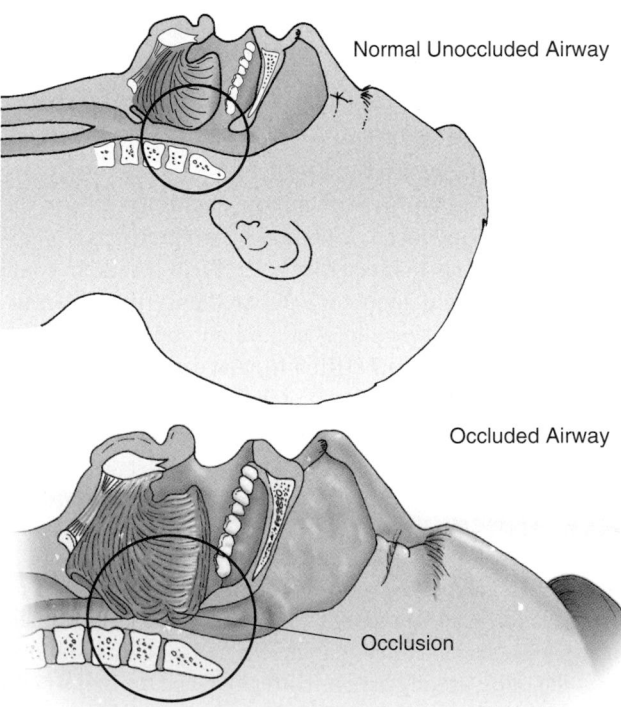

Normal Unoccluded Airway

Occluded Airway

Occlusion

FIGURE 40-5 Obstructive sleep apnea occurs when the airway is occluded due to collapse of the hypopharynx. Normally the airway remains open during sleep (*see inset*).

Recall Charlie Singer, the long-term care facility resident complaining of sleep problems. From the patient's statements, the nurse would identify that Mr. Singer is at risk for developing sleep deprivation. Therefore, the nurse would work with Mr. Singer to establish measures that would promote effective sleep patterns.

Parasomnias

Parasomnias are patterns of waking behavior that appear during sleep. Common examples are **somnambulism** (sleepwalking); sleeptalking; nocturnal erections; bruxism (grinding of teeth during sleep); and **enuresis** (urinating during sleep). They are more commonly seen in children. Although parasomnias are commonly outgrown before adulthood, safety and prevention of injury are paramount concerns.

A type of parasomnia that is gaining more attention is sleep-related eating disorder, which is when the patient eats but does not remember eating in the morning. People with sleep-related eating disorder can gain weight and experience injury either from cooking in their sleep or eating potentially dangerous raw food. They also may experience sleep disruption.

THE NURSING PROCESS FOR REST AND SLEEP

Assessing

Sleep History

Interview questions help identify the patient's sleep–wakefulness patterns, the effect of these patterns on everyday functioning, the patient's use of sleep aids, and the presence of sleep disturbances and contributing factors. The sleep history may be brief (four questions) if the patient's sleep is adequate and poses no problems, or it may be more detailed. When the patient's response to any of the interview questions indicates a potential problem, open-ended questions may be used to gather more data (see the Focused Assessment Guide).

If the patient is being admitted to a care facility, assess his or her usual times for retiring and waking, bedtime rituals, and preferences regarding sleep environment so that these can be incorporated into the plan of care, if possible. Research has shown that patients in hospitals receive fragmented sleep. However, over time patients become accustomed to the hospital routine and report an improvement in the quality of sleep (Tranmer et al., 2003). Paying attention to small matters can make the difference between a patient's good night's sleep and no sleep.

When a sleep disturbance is noted, ask about the following when obtaining the history:
- The nature of the problem
- Its cause
- The related signs and symptoms
- When it began and how often it occurs
- How it affects everyday living

- The severity of the problem and whether it can be treated independently by nurses or needs to be referred to another professional
- How the patient is coping with the problem and the success of any treatments attempted

Think back to Lydia Omeara, the mother of two infants who was asking about allowing the infants to sleep in their parents' bed. The nurse would need to obtain a sleep history from Mrs. Omeara to ascertain her sleep pattern. This information would be helpful in determining the reasons for allowing the children to sleep in their parents' bed.

Assistance from the patient's bed partner may be needed to aid in data collection and provide more accurate information regarding his or her sleep patterns. The patient's record may also contain pertinent information (eg, a history of illnesses that influence sleep).

Sample records of a sleep history in a comprehensive nursing assessment are as follows:

Reports needs 8 to 9 hours of sleep to feel his best and usually gets this without problem.

Generally retires at 11:30 p.m. and rises at 7:30 a.m. No special sleep rituals.

Mother reports toddler has erratic sleep patterns. May nap at any time in the afternoon or evening and sleep from 1 to 3 hours. Depending on nap, goes to bed anywhere from 7 to 11 p.m. and sleeps about 11 to 13 hours. Resists falling asleep and wants "water, story, snack, kisses, etc." Parents' lifestyle is constantly changing—little consistency for the child regarding sleep expectations.

Sleep Diary

A sleep diary or log provides more specific data on the patient's sleep–wakefulness patterns over a long period. It summarizes information about these patterns, possibly indicating activities and behaviors that affect the quality and quantity of sleep. The diary generally is kept for 14 days and typically includes a graph of the total number of hours of sleep per day. Depending on the nature of the problem, graphs may be made of the number of undisturbed hours of sleep, number of awakenings, and so forth. In addition, a daily record is completed addressing the following:
- Time patient retires
- Time patient tries to fall asleep
- Approximate time patient falls asleep
- Time of any awakenings during the night and when sleep was resumed
- Time of awakening in the morning
- Presence of any stressors patient believes are affecting his or her sleep
- A record of any food, drink, or medication patient believes has positively or negatively influenced his or her sleep (include time of ingestion)
- Record of physical activities—type, duration, and time
- Record of mental activities—type, duration, and time

Focused Assessment Guide 40-1

Rest and Sleep

Factors to Assess	Questions and Approaches
Usual sleep–wakefulness pattern:	Do you set an alarm and hit "snooze" before getting up?
Recent changes	
Usual sleeping and waking times	How many hours of sleep do you usually get in a day?
	Do you wake up earlier in the morning than you would like and find it difficult to fall back asleep?
	Have there been any recent changes in your usual sleep–wake patterns? If yes, describe them and tell me if they are causing any problems for you.
	Do you usually go to bed and wake up about the same time each day?
Number of hours of undisturbed sleep	How have you been sleeping?
	Do you have any difficulty falling asleep?
	Do you wake up frequently during the night?
	Do you dream at night?
	Are your dreams frightening?
Quality of sleep	How much sleep do you think you need to feel rested?
Number and duration of naps	Do you take naps throughout the day?
Effect of sleep pattern on everyday functioning	In what way does the sleep you get each day affect your everyday living?
	Has this sleep disturbance caused any change in your sex life?
Energy level (ability to perform activities of daily living)	Do you feel rested and ready to start the day when you wake up?
	Are there times during the day or certain activities when you feel especially tired?
	What happens when you don't get enough sleep?
	Are you having difficulty concentrating?
Sleep aids	
Means of relaxing before bedtime	What do you do to relax before you get ready for bed?
Bedtime rituals	Describe what you usually do to help yourself fall asleep.
Sleep environment	Tell me how you like your room (lights, noises, ventilation, position of door, temperature) and bed (mattress, pillows, blankets) when you are sleeping.
Pharmacologic aids	Do you take any medications to help you sleep?
	Are you taking any medicine at all?
Sleep disturbances and contributing factors	
Nature of the sleep disturbance	Tell me about your sleep problem.
Onset of disturbance	How often does it occur?
Causes (physical, psychosocial, medicine related)	Are you doing anything differently now that might be causing the problem?
Severity	Do you wake up gasping for air?
Symptoms	Do you snore?
	Do you recall changing your position frequently during the night?
Interventions attempted and results	What have you been doing to deal with the problem?

- Record of activities performed 2 to 3 hours before bedtime, bedtime rituals, changes in sleep environment
- Presence of any worries or anxieties patient believes are affecting his or her sleep

Remember Jeanette Clark, the mother of the adolescent girl who seems to be sleeping all the time. Having Mrs. Clark's daughter complete a sleep diary might be helpful in obtaining a better picture of what is happening and helping rule out other causes for the daughter's increased fatigue and sleeping. These underlying causes could be wide ranging, including such conditions as depression, physical illness, or increased activity or schoolwork.

It is helpful if the patient has a bed partner who can assist with the diary. The patient needs to understand that the diary is simply a diagnostic tool. If keeping the diary causes too much stress for the patient and further interferes with his or her ability to sleep restfully, it should be discontinued.

Physical Assessment

The findings in the physical assessment may either confirm that the patient is getting sufficient rest to provide energy for the day's activities or validate the existence of a sleep disturbance that is decreasing the quantity or quality of sleep. Key findings include energy level (presence of physical weakness, fatigue, lethargy, or decreased energy), facial characteristics (narrowing or glazing of eyes, swelling of eyelids, decreased animation), or behavioral characteristics (yawning, rubbing eyes, slow speech, slumped posture). Physical data suggestive of potential sleep problems (eg, obesity, enlarged neck, deviated nasal septum) may also be noted.

If the nurse or a bed partner can observe the patient sleeping, other sleep characteristics to assess include restlessness, sleep postures, and sleep activities such as snoring or leg jerking (nocturnal myoclonus).

Snoring

Snoring is caused by an obstruction to airflow through the nose and mouth. Other than disturbing others in the same bedroom, snoring is not ordinarily a sleeping disorder, but snoring accompanied by apnea can present a problem. When snoring changes from the characteristic sawing-wood sound to a more irregular silence followed by a snort, this indicates obstructive apnea.

Nocturnal Myoclonus

Observed in 10% to 20% of chronic insomniacs, **nocturnal myoclonus** involves marked muscle contractions that result in the jerking of one or both legs during sleep. The jerking lasts about 28 seconds on the average, may arouse the sleeper, and contributes to insomnia.

Diagnosing

Disturbed Sleep Pattern as the Problem

When assessment data point to a sleep problem that is amenable to nursing therapy, it receives the label Disturbed Sleep Pattern if the problem is time limited or Sleep Deprivation if the problem is prolonged. Common etiologies for these nursing diagnosis may include the following:
- Physical discomfort or pain
- Emotional discomfort or pain caused by anxiety and stress
- Changes in bedtime rituals or sleep environment
- Disruption of circadian rhythm
- Exercise just before sleep
- Caffeine, nicotine, or alcohol intake after dinner
- Drug dependency and withdrawal
- Symptoms of physical illness

Examples of nursing diagnoses in which the disturbed sleep pattern is the primary problem are presented in the accompanying NANDA box.

Disturbed Sleep Pattern as the Etiology

The disturbed sleep pattern may affect many other areas of human functioning. In the nursing diagnoses that follow, the disturbed sleep pattern is the cause of another problem:

Anxiety related to inability to fall asleep, inability to control behavior while asleep, and sleep apnea (threat of death)

Activity Intolerance related to sleep deprivation

Fatigue related to prolonged excessive role demands

Ineffective Coping related to insomnia: insufficient quantity and quality of sleep

Fear related to narcoleptic patient's potential to harm self or others

Impaired Gas Exchange related to sleep apnea (oxygen saturation of the blood)

Risk for Injury related to somnambulism, narcolepsy, sleep apnea

Deficient Knowledge (eg, nonpharmacologic remedies for insomnia) related to misinformation, lack of interest in learning, cognitive limitation

Low Self-Esteem related to effects of sleep deprivation (eg, sleep apnea syndrome)

Anxiety related to nocturnal enuresis

Impaired Social Interaction related to excessive daytime sleeping, sleep deprivation

Disturbed Thought Processes related to chronic insomnia, sleep deprivation

Important Distinctions

Because the problem statement of the nursing diagnosis identifies what is wrong with the patient and suggests the expected outcomes and the etiology of the problem directs nursing interventions, analysis of the assessment data is essential when deciding whether the sleep data indicate the problem, contribute to a different problem, or are signs or symptoms of the problem. Sleep data potentially fit in all three categories. For example, when a disturbed sleep pattern involving altered sleep–wake patterns is assessed in a graduate nurse who is getting adjusted to a new full-time job, shift work, and increased independence, three different diagnoses might be written:

Disturbed Sleep Pattern associated with altered sleep–wake patterns related to shift work and stress of new job as manifested by complaints of always feeling tired and not getting enough sleep: The disturbed sleep pattern involving the altered sleep–wake pattern is the problem statement; priority nursing energies are directed toward changing this pattern and helping the patient achieve both the necessary quantity and quality of sleep.

Ineffective Coping related to multiple stresses of new job and altered sleep–wake pattern (sleep deprivation) as manifested by statements such as, "I don't know how much longer I can do this," "I'm always tired, and all I want to do is sleep," "I'm so grouchy—people must hate me!" Here, the altered sleep–wake pattern is just one of the factors contributing to the patient's problem of ineffective coping; priority nursing energies are directed toward improving the patient's coping skills by teaching the patient how to increase the quantity and quality of sleep.

Ineffective Coping related to multiple stressors and lack of stress-relieving rituals as manifested by inability to fall asleep, excessive fatigue, and feelings that personality is changing: In this instance, the altered sleep–wake pattern is merely a symptom of the patient's actual problem—

Examples of NANDA Nursing Diagnoses | Sleep

Nursing Diagnoses	Related Factors	Sample Defining Characteristics
Disturbed Sleep Pattern: Difficulty Falling Asleep	Worries about family and lack of destressing rituals	• "At least four or five nights a week I lay in bed awake for 3 or 4 hours before I finally fall asleep. Sometimes it is 2 or 3 in the morning and I'm still awake worrying about the kids. I've tried getting up and reading or paying my bills, but even that doesn't make me sleepy." • Reports problem falling asleep for past 6 months; is widowed and very concerned about two teenage sons. Never sleeps until both sons are home. States she does nothing special to relax. Feels her worries are "her business"—no support person with whom she shares these.
Disturbed Sleep Pattern: Difficulty Remaining Asleep	Noise of hospital environment and need for periodic treatments	• Admitted to hospital 3/6/04; cholecystectomy 3/7/04 • "I don't think I've had one decent night's sleep since my surgery. I've been falling asleep about 9 pm and then someone wakes me up for my medicine. I just about get back to sleep and someone's putting the light on to poke at my dressing or to check this tube. I know I'm getting grouchy." • Orders include every-4-hour vital signs; nursing assessment of the incision, nasogastric tube, intravenous therapy; and medication for pain and for sleep.
Disturbed Sleep Pattern: Premature Awakening	Barbiturate dependency and lack of knowledge of non-pharmacologic aids for insomnia	• Patient has history of mild to moderate depression, related to loss of job and perceived role inadequacy, for the past 3 years; has been taking secobarbital (Seconal), a barbiturate hypnotic, 100 mg by mouth nightly for the past year and a half. • "I seem to be waking up earlier and earlier, can't fall back asleep, and I start each day feeling like I have a hangover." • "I'd like to get off these drugs, but I'm terrified that without them I won't sleep at all."
Disturbed Sleep Pattern: Excessive Daytime Sleeping	Effects of biologic aging (moderate increase in stage I and II sleep; slow-wave sleep, stages III and IV, decreases by 50% or more)	• Male patient aged 74, complains during his annual physical that he seems to be napping more during the day, yet when he tries to fall asleep at night he often cannot. • "I'm spending more time in bed, but I'm less rested. Worst of all is not knowing whether or not I'll be awake enough to drive my car or enjoy a good card game."
Disturbed Sleep Pattern: Altered Sleep–Wake Patterns	Frequent rotations of shift and overtime	• Graduate nurse, 24 years old, who has been working on a busy medical floor for 6 months; rotates 11–7 and 7–3 shifts; recently a problem with staffing has necessitated frequent rotations. Patient often volunteers (two or three times a week) for overtime. • "I don't know what is wrong with me. I'm so tired anymore and don't feel at all like myself. All I want to do when I'm off is to sleep—but often I can't fall asleep when I lay down. Please help!"

ineffective coping. The expectation is that when the coping problem is resolved, the symptom will disappear.

None of the preceding diagnoses is more correct than the others. With each patient, the nurse must review each cluster of significant data and identify the key problem, contributing factors, and related signs and symptoms. The exact nature of the nursing diagnosis directs the nursing interventions.

Outcome Identification and Planning

Rest and sleep are essential components of well-being. Planning for patient care, especially in a healthcare facility, involves planning with the patient suitable measures to promote rest and sleep. Whenever nurses care for a patient, nursing measures support the following expected patient outcomes: The patient will:

- Maintain a sleep–wake pattern that provides sufficient energy for the day's tasks
- Demonstrate self-care behaviors that provide a healthy balance between rest and activity
- Identify stress-relieving rituals that enable the patient to fall asleep more easily
- Demonstrate decreased signs of sleep deprivation
- Verbalize feeling less fatigued and more in control of life activities

Implementing

In most cases, sleep problems are not the primary reason for a patient's interaction with the healthcare system. Communicating with the patient while displaying a nonjudgmental, caring attitude often is the key to detecting a patient's sleep problem. Patients who believe the nurse is generally concerned about their well-being are not reluctant to discuss their insomnia or their concern about a child who is a bedwetter. In order to correct a sleep problem, the patient needs to believe that the nurse cares and will provide extra help to promote rest and sleep. The accompanying box lists a selection of standardized nursing interventions from the Nursing Interventions Classification (NIC) that aid in sleep promotion.

Examples of Nursing Interventions Classification (NIC)
Sleep Enhancement

- Approximate patient's regular sleep–wake cycle in planning care.
- Determine the effects of the patient's medications on sleep pattern.
- Adjust environment (eg, light, noise, temperature, mattress, and bed) to promote sleep.
- Encourage patient to establish a bedtime routine to facilitate transition from wakefulness to sleep.
- Facilitate maintenance of patient's usual bedtime routines, presleep cues/props, and familiar objects (eg, for children, a favorite blanket/toy, rocking, pacifier, or story; for adults, a book to read, etc.) as appropriate.
- Instruct patient to avoid bedtime foods and beverages that interfere with sleep.
- Instruct patient how to perform autogenic muscle relaxation or other nonpharmacologic forms of sleep inducement.
- Initiate/implement comfort measures of massage, positioning, and affective touch.
- Discuss with patient and family comfort measures, sleep-promoting techniques, and lifestyle changes that can contribute to optimal sleep.

McClosky, J., & Bulechek, G. (2000). *Nursing interventions classification (NIC)* (3rd ed.). St. Louis: C. V. Mosby Inc. A full listing of nursing activities for each nursing intervention can be found in this book.

Preparing a Restful Environment

A comfortable bed helps promote rest and sleep. The bottom linen should be tight and clean. The upper linen, while secure, should allow freedom of movement and should not exert pressure, especially over the legs and feet. Good body alignment is conducive to relaxation. For patients who must assume unusual positions because of their illness, ingenuity and skill are necessary to minimize muscle strain and discomfort. For example, patients who must remain in the orthopneic position to aid breathing should be well supported in a manner that relieves muscle strain.

A quiet and darkened room with privacy is relaxing for nearly everyone. In a strange environment, unfamiliar noises, such as people walking by or entering and leaving the room and the sounds of elevator doors, bring complaints from most hospitalized patients. Although some of these sounds are difficult to control, make every effort to reduce disturbances and to promote relaxation and sleep. In an effort to modify noise and promote sleep, Cmiel et al. (2004) recommend that nurses identify sources of noise, adjust care to limit interruptions to sleep, and modify equipment to create a quieter environment.

The temperature of the room, the amount of ventilation, and the amount of bed covering are matters of individual choice. Meet the patient's wishes when at all possible. Many older patients cannot sleep if they feel cold. Thermal blankets or comforters, insulated bed socks, cotton flannel sheets, leg warmers, long underwear, and a stockinette cap help patients stay warm and promote comfort and sleep. See Focus on the Older Adult for additional suggestions.

> *Recall Charlie Singer, the older man living in a long-term care facility. The nurse would work with Mr. Singer to ensure that his sleeping area is as comfortable and restful as possible. Making sure that he is warm enough, dimming the lights, closing the door (as much as allowed), and minimizing disturbances outside his room would be key.*

Promoting Bedtime Rituals

Most people have bedtime rituals to help them relax and promote sleep. Reading, listening to the radio, watching television, talking to a family member, and praying are common before-sleep activities. Children may take a favorite doll, stuffed toy, or blanket to bed; listen to a bedtime story; kiss everyone good night; and say prayers before bed. Readiness for sleep follows a personal hygiene routine for many people, such as brushing teeth, washing hands and face, voiding, or taking a bath or shower. Snacks are important elements in the bedtime rituals of many children and adults. Although eating the wrong foods may produce a bad night's sleep, going to bed hungry may also interfere with sleep.

> *Teaching Mrs. Omeara about the importance of bedtime rituals for her two small children may promote the children's sleep. In addition, the nurse would need to reinforce the need for her own bedtime rituals to ensure that the sleep she obtains is restful.*

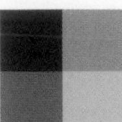

Focus on the Older Adult
Age-Related Changes and Nursing Strategies for Rest and Sleep

Age-Related Changes	Nursing Strategies
Disturbed Sleep Pattern: Initiation of Sleep	
• Decreased physical activities	• Encourage patient to engage in some type of physical activity, such as walking or water aerobics.
• Tired and fatigued throughout day	• Discourage napping throughout day.
• Depression	• Arrange for assessment for depression and treatment.
• Polypharmacy	• Review medications that patient is taking and assess for any side effects of sleep pattern disturbances.
Disturbed Sleep Pattern: Maintaining Sleep	
• Nocturia	• Decrease fluids during the evening.
	• Take diuretics in the morning or early evening.
• Sleep-related movement disturbances (eg, restless leg syndrome)	• Discuss problems with healthcare provider.

To promote relaxation and sleep, be alert to the patient's bedtime rituals and observe them as much as possible. Include these rituals in the patient's plan of care so that all health personnel can observe them.

Offering Appropriate Bedtime Snacks and Beverages

Because carbohydrates seem to promote sleep, there appears to be justification for offering a snack or beverage high in carbohydrates before bedtime, such as toast, a small bagel, crackers, or a glass of fruit juice, if this is allowed in the patient's regimen. An alcoholic beverage helps to promote sleep for some people, but generally alcohol after dinner should be avoided because it may interrupt the normal sleep cycle and interfere with deep sleep. For most patients, beverages containing caffeine should be avoided for at least 4 to 5 hours before bedtime. Recommend that the patient take fluids during the day but avoid excessive fluid intake before bedtime so that he or she will not have to use the bathroom during the night.

Promoting Relaxation

One can relax without sleeping, but sleep rarely occurs until one is relaxed. Stress and anxiety interfere with a person's ability to relax, rest, and sleep. Means for dealing with worries include dealing with problems as they arise; conditioning yourself to consider stressful issues only at certain times; teaching yourself that worrying never solves problems and is counterproductive; and giving the worries over to another (eg, a trusted family member, friend, caregiver, or God). The distraction and relaxation techniques described in Chapter 32, Stress and Adaptation, and Chapter 41, Comfort, may be beneficial for a patient whose worries are contributing to a sleep disturbance. A backrub, a warm bath, and washing the face if the patient is bedridden are typical nursing measures to help patients relax. The technique for back massage is described in Skill 41-1 in Chapter 41.

Promoting Comfort

One of the greatest deterrents to rest and sleep is pain, and pain commonly occurs in illness. Depending on the cause and severity of the discomfort or pain, appropriate nursing measures include remaining with a lonely and frightened child or adult, using the simple strategy of caring presence and touch, offering a back massage, obtaining an extra blanket, or administering an analgesic. These and other nursing techniques to promote comfort are described in Chapter 41. Be sensitive to the patient's discomfort to recognize and relieve it.

Respecting Normal Sleep–Wake Patterns

Make every effort to allow the patient to experience his or her normal period of sleep. In many instances, insisting that all patients retire and awaken at specific times is not necessary. For example, is there a good reason to wake a patient at 7 a.m. if the patient ordinarily sleeps until 9 a.m.? The patient's normal napping habits should also be followed when possible. REM sleep is more common during morning naps, whereas NREM sleep is more common during naps later in the day. With this knowledge, help the patient plan napping periods that best fit his or her needs and least interfere with nighttime sleeping.

Scheduling Nursing Care to Avoid Unnecessary Disturbances

Many patients complain that they are awakened to take sleeping pills and are aroused in the early morning to prepare for breakfast long before it is served. Consider these common complaints when developing the patient's plan of care to promote rest and sleep.

Whenever possible, provide care during periods when the patient is normally awake. When this is not feasible, avoid awakening the patient during REM sleep, when the rapid eye movements can be observed. Because a patient's need for sleep is important, examine priorities for nursing care. For example, consider whether checking a vital sign or carrying out a particular nursing measure is more important than the patient's sleep (see Focused Critical Thinking Guide 40-1).

Using Medications to Produce Sleep

Medications for sleep are often ordered for patients. Sedative-hypnotics induce sleep; antianxiety drugs reduce anxiety and tension. The sleep produced by sedative-hypnotics is an unnatural sleep, however. All these drugs disturb either REM or NREM sleep to some degree. Although most sedative-hypnotics provide several nights of excellent sleep, the med-

ication often loses its effect after 1 or 2 weeks. At this point, many people increase the dosage of the medication or complement the drug with alcohol. Vigorous nursing intervention is needed to prevent a patient from developing a pattern of drug dependency and alcohol abuse. The combination of a sedative-hypnotic and an over-the-counter antihistamine (eg, diphenhydramine [Benadryl]) may intensify central nervous system depression, leading to additional safety concerns. Because of its sedative effect, the antidepressant trazodone (Desyrel) is often prescribed for older adults. This drug has a low incidence of cardiovascular and anticholinergic effects, making it a safe alternative for insomnia in this age group.

 # Focused Critical Thinking Guide 40-1

Sleep

You have just arrived on the unit and checked your clinical assignment. You have two patients today and about 30 minutes before preconference. Your routine is to review their charts for pertinent information, go and introduce yourself to them, and take their morning vital signs before preconference. With 10 minutes to spare, you visit your second patient and find that he is sound asleep. Remembering that he had a fractured hip repaired 2 days ago and that the night nurse had stated in his note that the patient was restless and awake until 4:00 a.m., you are reluctant to awaken him. On the other hand, at your midterm conference your instructor commented that you need to improve your organizational skills. If you don't have your vital signs recorded until after preconference, then breakfast arrives, doctors make rounds, and you're that much further behind in your morning care and documentation. When you look at the flow sheet at the foot of the bed, you note that the last set of vitals were taken at midnight and were within normal limits. You're attempting to reconcile several things—the importance of these morning vital signs, the patient's need for sleep, and your need to accomplish your tasks on time and receive a good evaluation. What should you do?

1. **Identify Goal of Thinking**
   Determine whether it is more important to awaken your patient for morning vital signs or let him sleep at least until after your preconference.

2. **Assess Adequacy of Knowledge**
   Pertinent circumstances: Your patient had major surgery 2 days ago, did not have a restful night, but is sleeping peacefully now. You realize that his vital signs can be an important indicator of a complication. You also need to accomplish your tasks in a timely and organized manner.
   Prerequisite knowledge: To make your decision, you need knowledge about his postoperative condition, and assessment data that indicate he is recovering or developing a complication. You are aware that sleep is vital to promote tissue repair, physical recovery, and mental well-being. You also need to review the tasks that you need to accomplish this morning and decide how and if priorities could be shifted.

Room for error/time constraints: Will a delay in taking vital signs cause injury to this patient? You are not planning to omit this task but just questioning whether to postpone it and allow the patient to have some additional sleep.

3. **Address Potential Problems**
   Waking your patient for vital signs may be disturbing for him and interfere with his need for rest. A decision to postpone morning vital signs might also cause several problems. If the patient has developed a complication such as an infection, his elevated temperature may go undetected for at least another hour. By the time you come out of preconference, the patient may be eating his breakfast, which further delays recording of vital signs. You perceive that you are already falling behind on your schedule and are really intent on completing your responsibilities on time today.

4. **Consult Helpful Resources**
   Before you make your decision, you should check the patient's flow sheet and note whether the previous set of vital signs were within normal limits. The primary nurse and your instructor may also help you sort through your priorities in this situation.

5. **Critique Judgment/Decision**
   You have two choices here. If you wake your patient up and take his vital signs, you are disturbing him when he is sleeping soundly, risking the fact that he may be angry with you but are on schedule for the day's activities. By postponing his vital signs at least until after postconference, you provide additional rest for the patient but know that you are already behind schedule and worry that your instructor will view you as disorganized. After reviewing your options and checking his chart again, you decide to allow him to sleep and plan to take them as soon as possible after your preconference. During preconference, when your instructor reviews your priorities for the day, she comments positively that you have individualized care based on your particular patient's needs at the moment. In your mind, you determine that the vital signs are your next priority and will take minimal time, and you should still be able to complete care and documentation in a competent manner and on time.

Also be alert to the dangers of withdrawal symptoms that can accompany the abrupt cessation of barbiturate sedative-hypnotics. Progressive withdrawal symptoms include weakness, tremulousness, restlessness, insomnia, increased pulse and heart rates, anxiety, convulsions, psychosis, continued seizures, and death.

Medications used to induce sleep may produce daytime drowsiness and a morning hangover effect. Some people counteract this side effect by taking illicit drugs such as amphetamines ("uppers"). The antianxiety medications, once hoped to be the answer to the sleeping pill dilemma, are increasingly found to cause physical and psychological dependence.

Sleep medications are often ordered on a p.r.n. (as needed) basis. Administer these medications only when indicated and always with full knowledge of their limitations. Provide thorough patient education about these medications. In addition, help patients develop other self-care strategies, including developing healthy sleep and lifestyle behaviors. Use alternative nonpharmacologic measures to promote sleep when appropriate.

Remember Charlie Singer, the older man living in the long-term care facility. Nonpharmacologic measures would be helpful to promote sleep. Having Mr. Singer consume a warm beverage before bedtime, listen to soft music, or receive a backrub may promote relaxation, thereby enhancing the effectiveness of the prescribed sleep medication (see Research in Nursing: Making a Difference).

Teaching About Rest and Sleep

A well-informed person is better able to cope with distressing situations. Teach patients and their families about the nature of rest and sleep and their importance to well-being. Also include information about normal variations in sleep patterns and common measures to promote relaxation and sleep (see Teaching to Promote Health at Home 40-1). Discuss the plan of care with the patient and make sure it is acceptable to him or her. If a sleep disorder becomes a problem and common nursing measures are inadequate, the nurse may need to refer the patient to a health practitioner prepared to deal with it.

Evaluating

The nurse evaluates the effectiveness of the plan of care to promote rest and sleep by checking whether the patient has met the individualized expected outcomes specified in the plan. Nursing care is considered effective if the following are achieved: The patient is able to:

- Verbalize feeling rested or having had a restful night's sleep
- Identify factors that interfere with or disrupt the normal sleep pattern
- Use techniques that promote sleep and provide a restful environment
- Concentrate and function effectively during waking hours
- Eliminate behaviors related to sleep deprivation
  See the Nursing Plan of Care for an example.

Research in Nursing Making a Difference
Using Music to Promote Sleep in Older Women

Although sleep disturbances occur at any age, it has been documented that older adults, especially women, often experience difficulty obtaining a restful sleep. The most common complaint is initiating and maintaining restful sleep. Many times, healthcare providers prescribe a sedative-hypnotic drug (SHD). This medication helps for a short period, but then the dose usually needs to be increased to sustain the same restful sleep. Over time, the patient may notice a need for the medication to obtain sleep as well as impaired psychomotor and cognitive functioning.

Related Research
Johnson, J. E. (2003). The use of music to promote sleep in older women. *Journal of Community Health Nursing, 20*(1), 27–35.

Fifty-two women over the age of 70 years were recruited into this study. Participants had recently complained to their healthcare provider about sleep disturbances occurring at least 3 times per week for over 6 months. All the participants lived in their own home and had not used SHDs within 3 months of the study.

Each participant chose her own music, ranging from classical to gospel to new age. Data were collected for 10 nights prior to music therapy and for 10 nights after the initiation of music therapy. Effectiveness was evaluated through a sleep log kept by the participant and the Stanford Sleepiness Scale. The Stanford Sleepiness Scale asks the participant to rate the level of sleepiness–alertness on a scale ranging from 1 (feeling active and alert) to 7 (lost the struggle to stay awake).

Results showed that with music therapy, there was a significant increase in level of sleepiness at bedtime, a significant decrease in time to falling asleep, and a decrease in the number of nighttime awakenings.

Relevance to Nursing Practice
By incorporating simple measures such as providing soothing music at bedtime, nurses can provide nonpharmacologic alternatives for older patients who are at increased risk for side effects from SHDs. By individualizing the type of music, the nurse may help promote sleep initiation as well as enabling a person to maintain sleep.

Health Topic	Suggested Content	Why Is This Important?
Activity	• Find an activity that can be done daily and involves physical exertion, such as walking. • Do not participate in any physical activities right before bedtime.	• Sleep is easier to obtain if some physical activity has been completed. • Many people find it hard to rest and sleep right after a physical activity.
Diet	• Avoid food, beverages, or OTC medications that contain caffeine in the evening. • Eat a light dinner. • Eat a light carbohydrate-containing snack at bedtime if hungry.	• Caffeine is a stimulant and may prolong the time it takes to fall asleep. • Eating a large meal before bedtime may produce heartburn, delaying sleep. • Carbohydrates may affect the serotonin levels in the brain and thus promote sleep.
Sleep Patterns	• Keep to usual waking time every day, even if previous night's bedtime was later than usual or sleep was restless. • Get out of bed if unable to fall asleep within 30 minutes, and go into another room.	• Keeping the same pattern helps the body's circadian rhythms. • By using the bedroom for only sleep and sexual activity, the mind begins to associate this room with sleep.

NURSING PLAN OF CARE 40-1 *for Mr. Bitner*

Mr. Bitner is an alert, widowed, 86-year-old African American man who was admitted to a nursing home 2 months ago. He is ambulatory and performs most of his self-care. His admitting medical diagnoses include diabetes mellitus and hypertension. He adds to this list "a touch of arthritis." His daughter complains to the charge nurse that her father seems to be spending more and more time during the day napping and that he says he does not sleep well at night. A comprehensive sleep assessment of Mr. Bitner after his daughter's expression of concern reveals the following data.

SLEEP–WAKEFULNESS PATTERN
• Patient goes to bed between 8 and 9 p.m. and gets out of bed between 7 and 8 a.m. because the staff are getting his roommate out of bed at this time. He states he never falls asleep before midnight because he always watched the late news at home. He usually wakes twice during the night to void and often cannot go back to sleep.
• During the day, patient is frequently observed dozing in his chair. If not discouraged, he returns to his room midmorning and afternoon for a 1-hour nap.

EFFECT OF SLEEP PATTERN ON EVERYDAY LIVING
• Patient states: "I'm always tired. I don't seem to have much energy anymore."

• Patient has not socialized yet with other residents and, without strong encouragement, does not participate in group activities.
• From his point of view, life holds little reason for him to be awake. "I worked for the railroad for almost 50 years and I never overslept once."

SLEEP AIDS
• Patient denies ever using medication to fall asleep. States he often relaxed at home in the evening with a couple of beers.
• Patient likes a dim light on during the night so that he can find the bathroom easily and likes his bedroom door ajar.
• Patient sleeps with two blankets and is often still cold.

SLEEP DISTURBANCES AND CONTRIBUTING FACTORS
• Patient states: "Ever since my wife died, I'm just not getting enough sleep, and since I came here it's worse. I don't know why I don't fall asleep when I go to bed or why I wake up so much. It sure makes the nights long."
• Patient has no regular periods of exercise and drinks black coffee with every meal and one or two diet colas in the evening.

NURSING DIAGNOSIS	Disturbed Sleep Pattern: involving difficulty falling asleep and remaining asleep related to new sleep environment and schedule, evening caffeine intake, and insufficient meaningful daytime activity
EXPECTED OUTCOME	By the next monthly assessment, 1/20/06, the patient will: • Retire after viewing the 11 pm news in the TV room with Mr. Sparter

(continued)

NURSING PLAN OF CARE 40-1

for Mr. Bitner (continued)

Nursing Interventions

Assess advisability of reestablishing Mr. Bitner's usual retiring pattern of going to bed after the 11 p.m. news. Assess how patient spends the time from the evening meal to 11 p.m.—explore relaxing alternatives with him. Investigate possibility that he and Mr. Sparter might become social partners.

Rationale

Strengthens the natural rhythm of his sleep–wake cycle. Elimination of evening naps will facilitate his falling asleep more easily.

Evaluative Statement

1/18/06   Outcome met. Patient does not go to bed until after the news and has been observed talking with Mr. Sparter.

Recommendation: Continue to develop evening activities with him—he finds that the time after supper "drags."

M. LeBon, RN

EXPECTED OUTCOME

By the next monthly assessment, 1/20/06, the patient will:
• Report that he falls asleep within 1 hour of getting into bed

---

Nursing Interventions

Continue to assess how long it takes patient to fall asleep after getting into bed.

Explore with patient means to relax before falling asleep—deep breathing, imagery, prayer.

Teach the importance of using the bed only as a place to sleep. Advise patient when he cannot sleep to get out of bed and to go to another room where he can perform some monotonous activity (watching television, listening to radio).

Rationale

In elderly patients, stage I time is increased.

Activities that calm and relax the person prepare the body for sleep.

This maintains the bed as a powerful stimulus for sleep and helps to prevent "conditioned" insomnia ("Well, here I am in bed now and I know sleep won't come").

Evaluative Statement

1/18/06   Outcome partially met. Three or four nights a week, he falls asleep within 30 minutes of going to bed. States he really misses comfort of his wife.

Revision: Investigate patient's sense of loss and need for touch. May be a good candidate for pet therapy program.

M. LeBon, RN

EXPECTED OUTCOME

By the next monthly assessment, 1/20/06, the patient will:
• Decrease nighttime awakenings to one, after which he returns to a sound sleep

---

Nursing Interventions

Assess and manipulate factors that contribute to nighttime awakenings:
• Need to void (time of day diuretic is taken, amounts of fluid intake in the evening)
• Roommate's wakefulness, snoring, or need for care
• Uncomfortableness in strange environment
• Comfort (eg, temperature)

Teach patient how, on awakening, to concentrate on breathing until he falls back to sleep.

Rationale

Individualizing the patient's bedtime environment and meeting comfort needs (warmth, soft light, and so forth) promote sleep onset and maintenance.

This uses the power of positive thinking to facilitate return to sleep.

Evaluative Statement

1/18/06   Outcome partially met. Nighttime awakenings vary from none to three nightly. See previous revision.

M. LeBon, RN

EXPECTED OUTCOME

By the next monthly assessment, 1/20/06, the patient will:
• Attend the center's exercise sessions Monday through Friday at 10 a.m.

(continued)

NURSING PLAN OF CARE 40-1   *for Mr. Bitner* (continued)

Nursing Interventions	Rationale	Evaluative Statement
Assess whether patient understands the relation between daily exercise and his ability to sleep.	Regular exercise throughout the day is known to increase physical fatigue and to promote sleep. Exercise or stimulating activities immediately before retiring interfere with sleep's onset.	1/20/06 Outcome met. Patient has become an enthusiastic participant in exercise sessions—attends daily. *M. LeBon, RN*
Determine how his exercise needs can best be met (ie, through a group program or an individualized program of walking, or other program)	Exercise program must be individualized based on physical state and interests of patient.	
Use positive verbal reinforcement to communicate to patient that someone cares that he is using positive means to remedy his sleep disturbance and increase his well-being.	Activity provides the opportunity for socialization and improvement of a self-image.	
Encourage patient's daughter to go for walks with him when she visits and to question him about his exercise program.	Communications and interaction with family members helps the elderly patient to maintain self-esteem and to feel valuable and loved.	

EXPECTED OUTCOME

By the next monthly assessment, 1/20/06, the patient will:
- Substitute caffeine-free beverages for coffee and cola at supper and evening snack

Nursing Interventions	Rationale	Evaluative Statement
Assess patient's willingness to substitute caffeine-free beverages for coffee and cola.	Caffeine is a stimulant that can cause difficulty sleeping.	1/20/06 Outcome met. Patient now drinks decaffeinated coffee with meals and milk in the evening. Dislikes caffeine-free sodas. *M. LeBon, RN*
Consult with dietary department and his daughter about options. Experiment with options until his preferences are determined.	Caffeine-free versions of beverages are often available and can be used based on patient acceptance.	
Gradually reduce his caffeine intake, especially from evening meal onward. Offer a carbohydrate evening snack.	Carbohydrate snack appears to promote sleep.	

SAMPLE DOCUMENTATION

12/20/06   Nursing

Family conference to discuss Mr. Bitner's sleep disturbance—initiated by daughter's concern. Present were Mr. Bitner and his daughter (A. Jelner), K. Behner (social worker), W. Quing (activity director), and M. LeBon (primary nurse). Primary nurse presented findings from comprehensive sleep assessment: Nursing diagnosis: Disturbed Sleep Pattern: difficulty falling asleep and remaining asleep related to new sleep environment and schedule, evening caffeine intake, and insufficient meaningful daytime activity. Discussion centered on strategies to help Mr. Bitner develop interests in the center, including possibilities for increased physical exercise; decrease his evening caffeine intake (daughter to bring noncaffeine colas); and reestablish usual retiring and waking times. See plan of care. Patient's progress will be evaluated at next monthly assessment, 1/20/06.

M. LeBon, RN

Developing Critical Thinking Skills

1. Interview three adults of varying ages (young, middle, and elderly) about their sleep and rest patterns, using the Focused Assessment Guide in this chapter. Explore the special problems experienced by each of the adults, the efficacy of the self-help measures they use to cope, and helpful nursing interventions.

2. Interview three practicing nurses who are recent graduates, using the Focused Assessment Guide in the text. Ask them if they are getting adequate rest, what factors are compromising their rest (eg, working double or rotating shifts), how any lack of rest is affecting their practice, and what self-help measures are indicated. Discuss with your classmates the situation of practicing nurses with sleep alterations, the factors that place nurses at risk for sleep alterations, and what students can learn to lower their risk.

Preparing for NCLEX

1. A patient's body temperature is 37.2°C (99°F) in the late afternoon. This is most likely:
   a. A sign of an infection
   b. Result of a normal circadian rhythm
   c. Hyperpyrexia
   d. Due to a warm environment
2. Muscle tone is recorded by the:
   a. Electroencephalograph (EEG)
   b. Electrocardiogram (ECG)
   c. Electrooculogram (EOG)
   d. Electromyograph (EMG)
3. The nurse observes some involuntary muscle jerking in a sleeping patient. The patient is most likely in:
   a. Stage I NREM sleep
   b. Stage II NREM sleep
   c. Stage IV NREM sleep
   d. REM sleep
4. The nurse observes a slight increase in a patient's vital signs while he is sleeping during the night. According to his stage of sleep, the nurse expects that:
   a. He is aware of his surroundings at this point
   b. He is in delta sleep at this time
   c. It would be most difficult to awaken him at this time
   d. This is most likely an NREM stage
5. How many cycles of sleep does a person typically go through each night?
   a. 2
   b. 4 or 5
   c. 10
   d. 20 to 25
6. While discussing with an older woman the factors that induce sleep, the nurse teaches her that:
   a. A cup of regular tea may induce sleep.
   b. Large quantities of alcohol promote a deep sleep.

   c. The amount of REM sleep decreases with age.
   d. Physical activity decreases REM and NREM sleep.
7. A patient falls asleep in the middle of a conversation. This disorder is called:
   a. Hypersomnia
   b. Narcolepsy
   c. Somnambulism
   d. Sleep apnea
8. A sleep diary is a diagnostic tool that:
   a. Is generally kept for 1 week
   b. Includes a record of daily physical activity
   c. Includes a record of body temperature taken each evening
   d. Reports only subjective information about sleep activities
9. To help a patient get to sleep, the nurse suggests that he:
   a. Follow his usual bedtime routine if possible
   b. Drink two or three glasses of water at bedtime
   c. Have a large snack at bedtime
   d. Take a sedative-hypnotic every night at bedtime
10. The most common complaint of patients visiting sleep disorder clinics is:
    a. Hypersomnia
    b. Narcolepsy
    c. Chronic insomnia
    d. Enuresis
11. A prolonged pattern of REM deprivation may result in:
    a. Symptoms of psychosis
    b. Increased episodes of dreaming
    c. Decreased sensitivity to pain
    d. Increased mental alertness
12. Active dreaming occurs during:
    a. Stage II NREM sleep
    b. Stage III NREM sleep
    c. Stage IV NREM sleep
    d. REM sleep
13. Illness is a stressor and can influence sleep during various stages. An example is that:
    a. Asthma attacks appear to occur less frequently during stage IV NREM sleep.
    b. A person with heart disease is more likely to have chest pain during NREM sleep.
    c. An epileptic patient is more likely to have seizures during REM sleep.
    d. An increase in gastric secretions in a person with an ulcer will most likely occur during NREM sleep.
14. Caffeine is a known stimulant, and its intake should be:
    a. Avoided at least 30 minutes before bedtime
    b. Combined with milk to counteract its effect
    c. Avoided at least 4 to 5 hours before bedtime
    d. Encouraged during waking hours to counteract the effects of sleeplessness

15. Medications that induce sleep (sedative-hypnotics) may disturb REM or NREM sleep. The nurse should be aware that:
    a. They should be taken with alcohol for increased effect.
    b. They usually become ineffective after several weeks.
    c. They can usually be given at intervals during the night.
    d. They should be combined with daytime use of amphetamines to counteract any hangover effect.

■ Answers With Rationale

1. The correct answer is *b*. A slight increase in body temperature in the late afternoon is a normal circadian rhythm. This slight variation from normal does not necessarily mean an infection is present, nor is it hyperpyrexia (high fever). A warm environment might cause an elevation in body temperature, but the most likely cause is normal circadian rhythm.
2. The correct answer is *d*. An EMG measures muscle tone, an EEG records electrical currents from the brain, an EOG records eye movements, and an ECG records cardiac activity.
3. The correct answer is *a*. Involuntary muscle jerking occurs in stage I NREM sleep. In the other stages, the muscles proceed from a relaxed state to large muscle immobility.
4. The correct answer is *c*. During REM sleep, it is difficult to arouse a person, and the vital signs increase. Delta sleep is NREM stages III and IV sleep.
5. The correct answer is *b*. A person goes through probably four or five cycles of sleep each night, with each cycle lasting 90 to 100 minutes.
6. The correct answer is *c*. Regular tea contains caffeine and increases alertness. Large quantities of alcohol limit REM and delta sleep. Physical activity increases both REM and NREM sleep.
7. The correct answer is *b*. Narcolepsy is an uncontrollable desire to sleep. Hypersomnia refers to excessive sleep, somnambulism is sleepwalking, and sleep apnea is a condition in which breathing ceases for a period of time between snoring.
8. The correct answer is *b*. A sleep diary includes activities during the day because they have an effect on sleep, is usually kept for at least 14 days, and is more helpful if objective comments from a bed partner are included. A record of body temperature is insignificant.
9. The correct answer is *a*. Drinking two or three glasses of water at bedtime will probably cause the patient to awaken during the night to void. A large snack may be uncomfortable right before bedtime. Taking a sedative-hypnotic every night disturbs REM and NREM sleep, and sedatives also loses their effectiveness quickly.
10. The correct answer is *c*. Chronic insomnia is the most common reason people visit a sleep disorder clinic.
11. The correct answer is *a*. Prolonged episodes of REM deprivation may cause symptoms of psychosis. With REM deprivation, dreaming is absent, sensitivity to pain increases, and mental alertness decreases.
12. The correct answer is *d*. Active dreaming occurs during REM sleep.
13. The correct answer is *a*. Chest pain occurs more frequently during REM sleep. Epileptic seizures occur more frequently during NREM sleep. Gastric secretions increase during REM sleep.
14. The correct answer is *c*. Caffeine should be avoided at least 4 to 5 hours before bedtime. Milk does not counteract its effect, and caffeine use is never recommended, even during waking hours.
15. The correct answer is *b*. Sedative-hypnotics should never be taken with alcohol because alcohol potentiates their effect. They are usually ordered only at bedtime and may have one repeat order if the patient cannot fall asleep, but they are not given at intervals during the night. Amphetamine use is never recommended.

Bibliography

Boucher, M. (1997). Restless legs syndrome. *Home Healthcare Nurse, 15*(8), 551–556.

Brooks, L. J., & Topol, H. I. (2003). Enuresis in children with sleep apnea. *Journal of Pediatrics, 142*(5), 515–518.

Cmiel, C., Karr, D., Gasser, D., Oliphant, L., & Neveau, A. (2004). Noise control: A nursing team's approach to sleep promotion. *American Journal of Nursing, 104*(2), 40–48.

Colson, E. R., & Joslin, S. C. (2002). Changing nursery practice gets inner-city infants in the supine position for sleep. *Archives of Pediatrics & Adolescent Medicine, 156*(7), 717–720.

Dinges, P., et al. (2003). Sustained reduced sleep can have serious consequences. *Connecticut Nursing News, 76*(2), 22.

Finkelstein, Y., Stein, G., Ophir, D., Berger, R., & Berger, G. (2002). Laser-assisted uvulopalatoplasty for the management of obstructive sleep apnea. *Archives of Otolaryngology-Head & Neck Surgery, 128*(4), 429–434.

Gilbert, T. (2002). The spiritual art of working with dreams. *Journal of Holistic Nursing, 20*(3), 305–310.

Johnson, J. E. (2003). The use of music to promote sleep in older women. *Journal of Community Health Nursing, 20*(1), 27–35.

Malow, B. A. (2002). Paroxysmal events in sleep. *Journal of Clinical Neurophysiology, 19*(6), 522–534.

McCloskey, J., & Bulechek, G. (2000). *Nursing interventions classification (NIC)* (3rd ed.). St. Louis: Mosby, Inc.

McMillan, D. E. (2002). Interpreting heart rate variability sleep/wake patterns in cardiac patients. *Journal of Cardiovascular Nursing, 17*(1), 69–81.

Neal, S. C. (2001). Sleep it off? That's just the problem. *Nursing Spectrum: Florida, 11*(13), 26.

NHTSA & NCSDR Program to Combat Drowsy Driving (1997). Report to the House and Senate Appropriations Committees describing collaboration between National Highway Traffic Safety Administration and National Center on Sleep Disorders research. National Heart, Lung, and Blood Institute. http://www-rd.nhtsa.dot.gov/departments/nrd-01/summaries/ITS_11.html

North American Nursing Diagnosis Association. (2003). *NANDA nursing diagnoses: Definition & classifications, 2003–2004.* Philadelphia: Author.

Overeem, S., Mignot, E., GertvanDijik, J., & Lammers, G. J. (2001). Narcolepsy: Clinical new features, new pathophysiologic insights, and future perspectives. *Journal of Clinical Neurophysiology, 18*(2), 78–105.

Parthasarathy, S., & Tobin, M. J. (2002). Effect of ventilator mode on sleep quality in critically ill patients. *American Journal of Respiratory and Critical Care Medicine, 166*(11), 1423–1429.

Petit, L., Azad, N., Byszewski, A., Sarazan, F., & Power, B. (2003). Non-pharmacological management of primary and secondary insomnia among older people: Review of assessment tools and treatments. *Age and Ageing, 32*(1), 19–25.

Phipps, W., Monahan, F., Sands, J., Marek, J., & Neighbors, H. (2002). *Medical-surgical nursing: Health & illness perspectives* (7th ed.). St. Louis: C. V. Mosby.

Smyth, C. (2003). The Pittsburgh Sleep Quality Index. *Dermatology Nursing, 15*(2), 195–196.

Stansberry, T. T. (2001). Narcolepsy: Unveiling a mystery: New discoveries may explain this puzzling disorder. *American Journal of Nursing, 101*(8), 50–53.

Tate, J., & Tasota, F. (2002). More than a snore: Recognizing the danger of sleep apnea. *Nursing, 32*(8), 46–49.

Tranmer, J. E., Minard, J., Fox, L. A., & Rebelo, L. (2003). The sleep experience of medical surgical patients. *Clinical Nursing Research, 12*(2), 159–173.

Tsay, S. L., Rong, J. R., & Lin, P. F. (2003). Acupoints massage in improving the quality of sleep and quality of life in patients with end-stage renal disease. *Journal of Advanced Nursing, 42*(2), 134–142.

Virkkula, P., Maasilta, P., Hytonen, M., Salmi, T., & Malmberg, H. (2003). Nasal obstruction and sleep-disordered breathing: The effect of supine body position on nasal measurements in snorers. *Acta Oto-Laryngologica, 123*(5), 648–654.

Weinger, M. B., & Ancoli-Israel, S. (2002). Sleep deprivation and clinical performance. *Journal of the American Medical Association, 287*(8), 955–957.

Wolf, G. (2002). Three vitamins are involved in regulation of the circadian rhythm. *Nutrition Reviews, 60*(8), 257–260.

Comfort

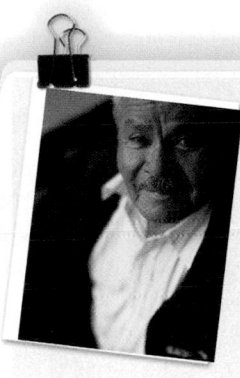

Ernesto Plachutta, an older man experiencing severe pain related to a diagnosis of cancer, believes that his pain is punishment for sins in his past life. When different measures are suggested to alleviate his pain, he rejects these suggestions, stating "I can bear the pain."

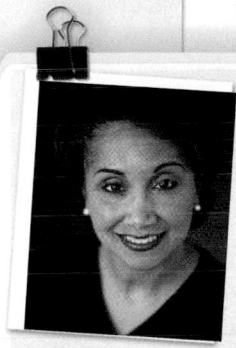

Sheree Lincoln, who has just undergone abdominal surgery, returns to the medical-surgical unit. Patient-controlled analgesia (PCA) is prescribed. Approximately 2 hours after returning from surgery, the patient is complaining of pain. Assessment reveals that she has not been using the PCA device.

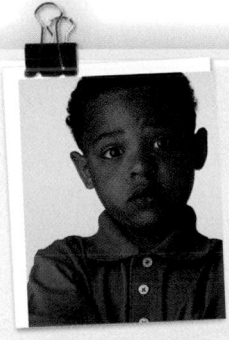

Xavier Malton, a 5-year-old boy diagnosed with ulcerative colitis, is in the bathroom with his mother. He suddenly grabs his belly while on the toilet and starts to scream "Something hurts really bad!" His mother pulls the emergency call light. He is doubled over in pain and can't get off the toilet. After being assisted back to his bed and receiving the smallest dose of pain medication possible as per the physician's order, Xavier continues to scream for half an hour more as he curls up in a fetal position on his bed. "The pain is so bad, it will never go away!"

Focusing on Blended Skills

The types of blended skills you'll need to respond to the case scenarios include:

Cognitive Skills

- Knowledge about the pain experience, pain process, and factors influencing the pain experience, including culture, age, gender for patients across the lifespan, such as an older adult with severe cancer pain, a woman who has had surgery, and a child experiencing acute pain
- Knowledge of the different types of pain
- Ability to identify misconceptions about pain and knowledge of strategies to correct these misconceptions
- Knowledge of the effects on pain on various body systems
- Knowledge of the different types of responses to pain
- Knowledge of effective pharmacologic and nonpharmacologic pain relief measures
- Knowledge of how to use the nursing process to identify patients at risk for pain and to implement a plan of care to prevent or resolve pain problems

Technical Skills

- Strong assessment skills related to pain assessment, including the ability to identify responses to pain, and how to use appropriate pain assessment tools for an older adult with severe cancer pain, a woman who has had surgery, and a 5-year-old child
- Ability to provide technical nursing assistance to assess and meet the needs of patients across the lifespan with different needs for comfort and experiencing different types of pain
- Ability to adapt techniques to address changes in patients' needs related to comfort and pain relief
- Knowledge of PCA and ability to demonstrate use of the PCA device for a postoperative patient
- Knowledge of how to use and to document use of the equipment and protocols related to effective pain management protocols
- Ability to seek out assistance as necessary when caring for patients at various developmental stages and experiencing different types of pain

Interpersonal Skills

- Strong people skills, to establish trusting relationships with an older adult patient experiencing severe cancer pain, a woman experiencing postoperative pain, and a child experiencing acute abdominal pain
- Special interpersonal competence to relate to 5-year-old Xavier, who most likely has limited understanding of why he hurts, and to Mr. Plachutta, who may believe that he does not deserve compassionate care
- Demonstration of a nonjudgmental, caring attitude to help facilitate assessment and care of an older adult patient with severe cancer pain and a 5-year-old child with acute pain
- Ability to assist patients of various developmental stages to use pharmacologic and nonpharmacologic methods of pain relief to promote optimal comfort
- Ability to communicate and interact effectively with patients experiencing pain
- Demonstration of respect for a patient's human dignity and autonomy regardless of whether the patient is an older adult rejecting suggestions for pain relief, a woman who has had surgery and is not using the prescribed PCA device, or a young child experiencing acute pain
- Ability to confront members of the healthcare team who are demonstrating judgmental attitudes about a child's pain

Ethical and Legal Skills

- Demonstration of a strong sense of accountability for the health and well-being of patients experiencing pain, regardless of the underlying cause
- A commitment to patient advocacy, including getting patients the help they need to achieve comfort—within the scope of your nursing responsibilities and available resources
- A willingness to hold colleagues accountable for safe and good quality practice—especially for a young child in acute pain
- Ability to integrate knowledge of the ethical and legal principles that guide decision making about pain management and appropriate treatment modalities
- Ability to practice in an ethically and legally defensible manner when providing care to patients experiencing different types of pain

Learning Outcomes

After completing the chapter, the learner should be able to accomplish the following:

1. Describe specific elements in the pain experience.
2. Compare and contrast acute and chronic pain.
3. Identify factors that may affect an individual's pain experience.
4. Obtain a complete pain assessment using appropriate interviewing and physical assessment skills.
5. Develop nursing diagnoses that correctly identify pain problems and demonstrate the relation between pain and other areas of human functioning.
6. Demonstrate the correct use of nonpharmacologic pain relief measures.
7. Administer analgesic agents safely to produce the desired level of analgesia without causing undesirable side effects.
8. Collaborate with the members of other health disciplines, using different treatment modalities to promote pain relief.
9. Use teaching and counseling skills to empower patients to direct their own pain management programs.

Key Terms

acute pain
addiction
allodynia
analgesic
breakthrough pain
chronic pain
cutaneous pain
dynorphin
endorphins
enkephalins
exacerbation
gate control theory
intractable
neuromodulators

neuropathic pain
neurotransmitters
nociceptive
opioid
pain threshold
pain tolerance
phantom pain
physical dependence
placebo
psychogenic pain
referred pain
remission
somatic pain
visceral pain

A person in pain often experiences it as an all-consuming reality and wants only one intervention—pain relief. If pain relief were as simple as rubbing a back or administering a prescribed analgesic, nursing's task would be easy. However, no two people experience pain exactly the same way. Differences in individual pain perception and response to pain, as well as the multiple and diverse causes of pain, require the use of highly specialized abilities to promote comfort and to relieve pain. The most essential of these are the nurse's belief that the patient's pain is real, the willingness to become involved in the patient's pain experience, and a competence in developing effective pain management regimens. (See the accompanying Reflective Practice box for an example.)

Although pain is often an all-consuming priority for patients, it can be easily missed because it is intangible. As a result, it becomes easier to overlook a patient's poorly communicated pain than it is to ignore a dressing that needs to be changed, or the need for assistance with walking, or the administration of a prescribed medication. Nurses who somehow manage to practice nursing while remaining insensitive to the comfort needs of their patients do a grave disservice to these patients and to the nursing profession itself.

Nurses are not alone in undervaluing the need for pain management. Although pain is a common reason for seeing a physician and for taking medication, medical science still is ill equipped to deal with its widespread occurrence. Pain also affects the body in many ways, including hyperglycemia, immune system dysfunction, altered coagulation, gastrointestinal (GI) ileus, urinary retention, decreased lung volume, sympathetic nervous system stimulation, and psychological

distress (Stoelting & Miller, 2000). Scientists and clinicians have united in their efforts to ensure that pain management is a high priority in our healthcare system. New advances in understanding and treating pain have focused on the real possibility of controlling most human pain. The Joint Commission on Accreditation of Healthcare Organizations (JCAHO) supports the patient's right to pain management and published revised standards for assessment and management of pain in hospitals, ambulatory care settings, and home care settings (Acello, 2000). The JCAHO recommendations include teaching all patients to use a pain-rating scale and determining a pain-rating goal with each patient. Also, according to the JCAHO guidelines, if a facility does not have the resources to treat a patient's pain adequately, the patient must be referred to a facility that does (Acello, 2000).

This chapter discusses the pain experience and factors that influence it. A detailed guide to assessing pain is presented, along with numerous examples of nursing diagnoses and specific nursing strategies for promoting comfort and assisting patients to achieve pain management goals. The concluding nursing plan of care illustrates how to use specific nursing interventions based on knowledge of and sensitivity to the patient's pain experience to resolve pain problems successfully.

THE PAIN EXPERIENCE

Pain is an elusive and complex phenomenon, and despite its universality, its exact nature remains a mystery. It is one of the human body's defense mechanisms that indicates the person is experiencing a problem. Margo McCaffery (1979, p. 11)

Reflective Practice
Challenge to Interpersonal and Ethical Skills

While working as a childcare technician one summer, I took my job quite seriously. As a nurse-in-training, I saw this job as an extension of my nursing education. I believed that the standards of care to which I held myself in my clinical rotations, and to which my professors held me, applied just as diligently in this job. I quickly found that I was the only childcare technician on the floor who held myself, let alone everyone else, to such high standards. In addition, I was quite dismayed to find that my standards for quality were actually higher than those of most of the registered nurses (RNs) employed on that unit. Nonetheless, I did not let that dissuade me. I sought out the few RNs whose standards were on par with mine, and I tried to work with them as often as possible.

One particular evening, about 15 minutes before our 12½-hour shift was finally over, I was very grateful to be working with one such nurse. The quality of care that one of my patients was receiving from the physicians during an episode of acute pain was what I could only kindly call substandard.

I was caring for Xavier Malton, a 5-year-old boy diagnosed with ulcerative colitis, a form of inflammatory bowel disease (IBD). Suddenly, at the end of this relatively quiet shift, the emergency call bell alarm sounded. Frantically searching the switchboard for the source of the alarm, I realized that it was coming from Xavier's bathroom. As I ran the 10 feet to his room, thoughts of him bleeding internally or perforating his bowel ran through my head. I got there at the same time his nurse did, only to discover that his mother had pulled the alarm because her son had suddenly grabbed his belly while on the toilet and had started screaming that something was hurting very much. He was so doubled over in pain that he could not even get off the toilet. Having Crohn's disease myself, another form of IBD, I knew that the pain this boy was experiencing was excruciating and not imagined.

Over the course of the next half hour, his physicians reluctantly allowed us to drag them into his room, but they would only examine him after we insisted it was necessary because they could be dealing with an obstruction or a perforated bowel that might need surgery. Their attitude was that since he had IBD, abdominal pain was part of that, and that we should just "Let it pass" uneventfully, giving him the smallest dose of pain medication possible—which we did.

However, Xavier continued to scream, literally, for half an hour more, as he lay curled up in a fetal position on his bed. From across the hallway, I could hear him screaming that the pain was "so bad" and that it would never go away.

Thinking Outside the Box: Possible Courses of Action

- I can "give up" and try not to care since this system clearly is not committed to meeting comfort needs. But this means abandoning my patients.
- I could be persistent about advocating for this patient until his pain is relieved—trying to get as many healthcare professionals on my side as possible.
- I can consult with a colleague whom I respect about the best way to accomplish the above, since I don't want to alienate caregivers with whom I will need to continue to work.

Evaluating a Good Outcome: How Do I Define Success?

- Patient's pain is relieved and patient reports feeling comfortable.
- Colleagues are newly committed to the responsibility of EVERYONE to adequately manage pain.
- My working relationships with other professional caregivers are not compromised by my fierce advocacy for this patient.
- My personal and professional integrity remains intact.

Personal Learning: Here's to the Future!

Forty-five minutes after our shift had ended, Xavier's nurse and I were still following the physicians around, demanding that they reassess the patient and prescribe additional pain medication for him. Finally, we simply refused to leave the hospital until Xavier's pain was properly treated. We threatened to report them to JCAHO for substandard care, for allowing a 5-year-old child to scream and writhe in pain when all they needed to do was write a p.r.n. order for additional pain medication.

Finally, they wrote the order. Unfortunately, the narcotic they ordered was in short supply in the hospital, and we had none on the floor. The pharmacy had none to give. We spent the next 15 minutes tracking some down. Finally, we did give Xavier additional pain medication—and ultimately, it did relieve his pain and he was able to fall asleep. However, we left the hospital almost an hour and a half after our shift had ended, time which was lost to Xavier and time for which we would receive compensation.

Transforming the culture of healthcare is a daunting task. Challenging the traditionally all-powerful physician takes courage and commitment. Demanding an unacceptable situation be remedied requires an absolute belief in the rights of the patient. The situation was indeed unacceptable—even when everyone else thinks it is acceptable. Any RN facing a situation that has the potential to transform the culture of healthcare for the better has the responsibility to take advantage of that situation, no matter what the professional risk. I would recommend that any RN in a similar situation take the same steps that Xavier's nurse and I did. Fight for what you believe is right. Do not be afraid to challenge others whom you think are wrong, even physicians. Be confident in your opinions. Refuse to back down. Remember that if you do not ensure that your patient's needs are met, maybe no one else will either. Advocate at all times for high-quality care, never settling for less.

(continued)

Reflective Practice
Challenge to Interpersonal and Ethical Skills (Continued)

Reflection

How do you think you would respond in a similar situation? Why? What does this tell you about yourself and about the adequacy of your skills for professional practice? What responses to pain did Xavier exhibit that would indicate to the nurse and nursing student that Xavier was in pain? What factors and misconceptions may have played a role in this situation? Propose possible strategies that might be appropriate to remedy these factors or correct these misconceptions. Can you think of other ways to respond? What other skills (cognitive, interpersonal, technical,

ethical/legal) would you need to respond well in this situation? Explain how the nurse and nursing student advocated for Xavier. Would you use the same methods to advocate for Xavier? If so, why? If not, please explain why not. Do you agree with the criteria to evaluate a successful outcome? Did the nursing student meet the criteria? Please explain.

Tracey Sara Miller, Georgetown University

offers the definition of pain that is probably of greatest benefit to nurses and their patients: "Pain is whatever the experiencing person says it is, existing whenever he (or she) says it does." This definition rests on the belief that the only one who can be a real authority on whether, and how, an individual is experiencing pain is that individual.

Pain is present whenever a person says it is, even when no specific cause of the pain can be found. Health practitioners must rely on the patient's description of the pain because it is a subjective symptom that only the patient can identify and describe.

> *Consider Xavier Malton, the 5-year-old boy with ulcerative colitis who suddenly develops acute pain. The nurse demonstrates understanding that Xavier is indeed experiencing pain because of his screaming that something hurts. Furthermore, his screaming is validated by his body posture and inability to get off the toilet.*

Categories of Pain

Pain may be classified according to source (nociceptive, neuropathic, and psychogenic), area to which it is referred, or duration (acute and chronic).

Source of Pain

Pain that is usually acute and transmitted after normal processing of noxious stimuli is termed **nociceptive.** It may be categorized as cutaneous, deep somatic, or visceral in nature. **Cutaneous** (or superficial) **pain** usually involves the skin or subcutaneous tissue. A paper cut that produces sharp pain with a burning sensation is an example of cutaneous pain. Deep **somatic pain** is diffuse or scattered and originates in tendons, ligaments, bones, blood vessels, and nerves. Strong pressure on a bone or damage to tissue that occurs with a sprain causes deep somatic pain. **Visceral pain** is poorly localized and originates in body organs in the thorax, cranium, and abdomen. This pain occurs as organs stretch abnormally and become distended, ischemic, or inflamed.

> *Think back to Sheree Lincoln, the woman who has had abdominal surgery. Based on the nurse's understanding of the sources of pain, the nurse would identify that Sheree is most likely experiencing visceral pain, secondary to the effects of surgery on the abdominal organs.*

A reflex contraction or spasm of the abdominal wall, called guarding, may occur as a protective mechanism to prevent additional trauma to underlying structures.

Neuropathic pain results from an injury to or abnormal functioning of peripheral nerves or the central nervous system (CNS). The exact cause of neuropathic pain is unknown, and it can occur in many forms. Neuropathic pain can be of short duration or lingering and is often described as burning or stabbing. **Allodynia,** a characteristic feature of neuropathic pain, is pain that occurs after a normally weak or nonpainful stimuli, such as a light touch or a cold drink. Numerous pain syndromes have been identified that produce neuropathic pain. Several common examples are included in Table 41-1. All of these pain syndromes are capable of causing severe pain. Because appropriate treatment of these syndromes is often delayed as a result of misdiagnosis, nursing can play an important role in their early detection.

Pain may originate from physical causes; that is, a physical cause for the pain can be identified. Pain may also have a psychogenic origin (**psychogenic pain**); that is, a physical cause for the pain cannot be identified. However, it has been observed that a pure origin is probably rare, and pain usually has both physical and psychogenic components. Furthermore, pain that results from a mental event can be just as intense as pain that results from a physical event.

Referred Pain

Referred pain is pain that is perceived in an area distant from its point of origin. Pain associated with a myocardial infarction, or heart attack, is frequently referred to the neck, shoulder, or arms (often the left arm). Referred pain is transmitted to a cutaneous (skin) site different from where it originated. This is possible because the pain can travel to other areas of the body innervated by the affected nerve root. Figure 41-1

TABLE 41-1 Common Pain Syndromes

Pain Syndrome	Description
Complex regional pain syndrome (causalgia)	Pain occurs in the area of a partially injured peripheral nerve (the most common lesions are of the brachial plexus or median or sciatic nerve). The pain is described as burning, severe, diffuse, and persistent and is elicited by minimal movement or touch of the affected area. It increases with repeated stimulation and continues even after stimulation ceases.
Postherpetic neuralgia	Pain syndrome follows an acute central nervous system infection, such as herpes zoster (shingles). The herpes syndrome is characterized by a vesicular eruption and neuralgic pain, which is usually unilateral and encircles the body in bandlike clusters. The severity of the pain may be mild to severe. Intractable pain may persist for months to years.
Phantom limb pain	May occur in any person who has had a body part amputated either surgically or traumatically. Pain varies and may be a severe, burning, fiery sensation; crushing; cramping; a sense that the limb is edematous; or a sensation that the limb is being twisted and distorted. It may be triggered by the sensation of touching the stump, the occurrence of another illness, fatigue, atmospheric changes, and emotional stress.
Trigeminal neuralgia	Paroxysms of lightening-like stabs of intense pain in the distribution of one or more divisions of the trigeminal nerve, the fifth cranial nerve. Pain is usually experienced in the mouth, gums, lips, nose, cheek, chin, and surface of the head and may be triggered by everyday activities like talking, eating, shaving, or brushing one's teeth.
Diabetic neuropathy	A common complication of long-term diabetes mellitus. Metabolic and vascular changes result in damage to peripheral and autonomic nerves. Sensory loss can result when peripheral nerves are involved and eventually leads to injury progressing to infection and gangrene. Symptoms include sensations of numbness, prickling, or tingling (paresthesias).

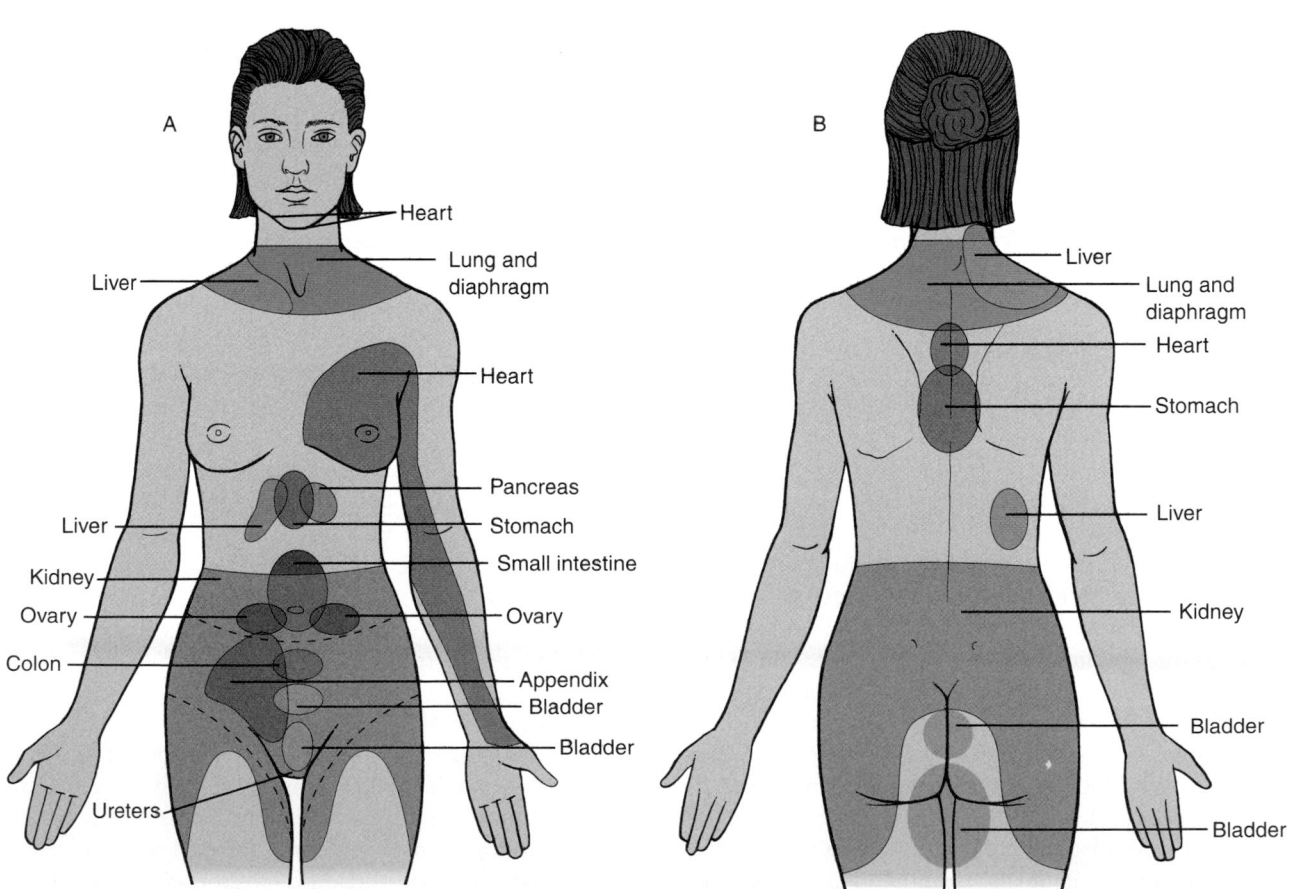

FIGURE 41-1 These drawings representing the anterior (**A**) and posterior (**B**) views of the body illustrate areas to which various organs refer pain.

illustrates cutaneous areas to which pain from various organs is usually referred.

Duration of Pain

Perhaps the most common distinction is between acute and chronic pain. **Acute pain** is generally rapid in onset, varies in intensity from mild to severe, and may last from a brief period to any period less than 6 months. Acute pain is protective in nature; that is, it warns the individual of tissue damage or organic disease. After its underlying cause is resolved, acute pain disappears. Causes of acute pain include a pricked finger, sore throat, or surgery.

Chronic pain is pain that may be limited, intermittent, or persistent but that lasts for 6 months or longer and interferes with normal functioning. Commonly, people with chronic pain experience periods of **remission** (when the disease is present but the person does not experience symptoms) or **exacerbation** (the symptoms reappear). Pain associated with cancer or other progressive disorders is termed chronic malignant pain. Pain in people whose tissue injury is nonprogressive or healed is termed chronic nonmalignant pain. When pain is resistant to therapy and persists despite a variety of interventions, it is referred to as **intractable.** Patients have difficulty describing chronic pain because it may be poorly localized. Moreover, healthcare personnel have difficulty assessing it accurately because of the unique responses of individual patients to persistent pain. Loeb (1999) states that about 45% to 80% of older adult patients residing in long-term care facilities have significant pain that negatively affects the quality of life. Approximately 40% of all patients with cancer have inadequate pain control, and 25% of older adult patients with cancer who live in nursing homes do not receive any form of pain relief treatment for the pain that accompanies the cancer (Clinical Update, 2001). Unlike acute pain, chronic pain is often perceived as meaningless and may lead to withdrawal, depression, anger, frustration, and dependency. In addition, the misconceptions and personal biases of caregivers can adversely affect the management of patients with chronic pain. Individuals with chronic pain may be viewed in general by healthcare personnel as hysterical personalities, malingerers, or hypochondriacs. On the other hand, nurses who have experienced chronic pain or struggled through the experience with a loved one have a special awareness of its debilitating, destructive nature. Nurses need an awareness of their own personal feelings toward pain and the factors that affect pain if they are to assess and manage their patient's pain creatively and effectively. See Promoting Health 41-1 for a checklist of behaviors to foster one's self-awareness of comfort needs and pain.

The Pain Process

The mechanism or process of pain is believed to involve four stages: transduction, transmission, modulation, and perception of pain (Phipps et al., 2002).

Transduction

The activation of pain receptors is referred to as transduction. It involves conversion of painful stimuli into electrical impulses that travel to the spinal cord at the dorsal horn. Additionally, when the threshold of perception for pain has been reached and when there is injured tissue, it is believed that the injured tissue releases chemicals that excite or activate nerve endings. For example, a damaged cell releases histamine, which excites nerve endings. Lactic acid accumulates in tissues injured by lack of blood supply and is believed to excite nerve endings and cause pain or to lower the threshold of nerve endings to other stimuli (eg, heat or pressure). Other substances are also released that stimulate nociceptors or pain receptors. These include bradykinin, prostaglandins, and substance P:

Promoting Health 41-1 Comfort

Use the assessment checklist to determine how well you are meeting comfort needs. Then develop a prescription for self-care by choosing appropriate behaviors from the list of suggestions.

ASSESSMENT CHECKLIST

almost always / sometimes / almost never

1. I seek medical attention when pain persists.
2. I am aware of my usual behavioral responses to pain.
3. I use stress reduction techniques regularly.
4. I am able to have a restful sleep at night.
5. I have a positive outlook about my present situation.
6. I am aware of how to use distraction strategies to deal with pain.

SELF-CARE BEHAVIORS

1. Obtain a medical evaluation when acute or chronic pain is present.
2. Respect pain as the body's means of signaling that all is not well.
3. Control stress in the environment.
4. Avoid excessive fatigue.
5. Practice stress reduction or diversionary behaviors when pain is present.
6. Become aware of personal preconceived notions that affect your perception of pain in others.

- Bradykinin, a powerful vasodilator that increases capillary permeability and constricts smooth muscle, plays an important role in the chemistry of pain at the site of an injury even before the pain message gets to the brain. It also triggers the release of histamine and, in combination with histamine, produces the redness, swelling, and pain typically observed when an inflammation is present.
- Prostaglandins are hormone-like substances that send additional pain stimuli to the CNS.
- Substance P sensitizes receptors on nerves to feel pain and also increases the rate of firing of nerves (McHugh & McHugh, 2000).

Prostaglandins, substance P, and serotonin (a hormone that can act to stimulate smooth muscles, inhibit gastric secretion, and produce vasoconstriction) are **neurotransmitters,** substances that either excite or inhibit target nerve cells.

Receptors in the skin and superficial organs, although incapable of responding selectively, may also be stimulated by mechanical, thermal, chemical, and electrical agents. Friction from bed linens and pressure from a cast are mechanical stimulants. Sunburn and cold water on a tooth with caries are thermal stimulants. An acid burn is the result of a chemical stimulant. The jolt of a static charge is an electrical stimulant.

Stretching of the hollow viscera, pulling on the omentum, and muscle spasms result in perceived pain. Some investigators believe that at least some of the deep-lying organs have their own individual pain receptors, the uterus being an example. Some organs, such as the lungs, are insensitive to pain because of the absence of nociceptors or pain receptors.

It has been observed that pain may be present without injury and may not be present with injury. Therefore, tissue injury does not accompany pain in all instances. For example, tissue injury is present when the patient experiences pain because of a first- or second-degree burn. On the other hand, although physiologic changes do occur, tissue injury or destruction is not necessarily present when the patient has a headache caused by psychological tension. In addition, the intensity of pain may not be correlated to the seriousness of a particular condition giving rise to the pain. For example, a patient may not experience pain until the ravages of a malignancy are beyond control, whereas the severe pain that usually accompanies a bunion does not indicate a very serious pathology.

Transmission of Pain Stimuli

Pain sensations are conducted along pathways that have been rather clearly defined in certain areas but are still somewhat unclear in other areas. No specific pain organs or cells exist in the body. Rather, an interlacing network of undifferentiated free nerve endings receives painful stimuli. Free nerve ending pain receptors include the afferent (those fibers carrying impulses from the pain receptors toward the brain) fast-conducting A-delta-fibers and the slow-conducting C-fibers. The larger A-delta-fibers transmit acute, well-localized pain, whereas the smaller C-fibers convey diffuse, visceral pain that is often described as burning and aching. It is estimated that there are several million of these nerve endings in the body, numerous in the layers of the skin and in some internal tissues, such as

the joint surfaces. In the deeper tissues of the body, the pain receptors are diffusely but unevenly spread.

A protective pain reflex is responsible for withdrawal of an endangered tissue from a damaging stimulus. Sensory impulses travel over A-fibers through the dorsal root ganglion to the dorsal horn of the spinal cord. At this point, the sensory nerve impulse synapses with a motor neuron, and the impulse is carried along efferent nerve pathways back to the site of the painful stimulus in a reflex arc. This results in an immediate muscle contraction that removes the injured part from the source of the pain.

Somatic sensation is carried to the dorsal gray horn cells of the spinal cord, then to the spinothalamic tract, and eventually to the cerebral cortex. Although the autonomic nervous system is an efferent system—that is, it carries impulses from the CNS—pain sensations from the viscera apparently course along the autonomic system. Through that system, these sensations from deep-lying structures reach the spinal cord by way of the dorsal roots and then continue along the same pathways as sensations from the skin and superficial body structures. Pain impulses are also carried by the cranial nerve to the CNS. There is integration of the sensory impulses of pain along its entire CNS route, but the highest level of integration occurs in the cortex. Figure 41-2 illustrates the transmission of the pain sensation, the initiation of the protective reflex response, and conscious awareness of the location, intensity, and quality of the pain after the impulse reaches the cortex.

Stimulation of sensory receptors and intactness of their nerve supply are neither necessary nor sufficient conditions for pain. It would appear that a receptor for pain and a nerve route that eventually carries the impulse to the brain are necessary when pain is present. However, it is well known that this is not always necessary. The pain that is often referred to an amputated leg where receptors and nerves are clearly absent is a real experience for the patient. This type of pain is called **phantom pain** or phantom limb pain and is without demonstrated physiologic or pathologic substance. One theory suggests that sensory misrepresentations from the missing limb may still remain in the brain thereby causing phantom pain.

Gate Control Theory of Pain

The **gate control theory** of pain describes the transmission of painful stimuli and recognizes a relation between pain and emotions. The theory states that certain nerve fibers, those of small diameter, conduct excitatory pain stimuli toward the brain, but nerve fibers of a large diameter appear to inhibit the transmission of pain impulses from the spinal cord to the brain. There is a gating mechanism that is believed by some to be located in substantia gelatinosa cells in the dorsal horn of the spinal cord. The exciting and inhibiting signals at the gate in the spinal cord determine the impulses that eventually reach the brain. Thus, only a limited amount of sensory information can be processed by the nervous system at any given moment. When too much information is sent through, certain cells in the spinal column interrupt the signal as if closing a gate.

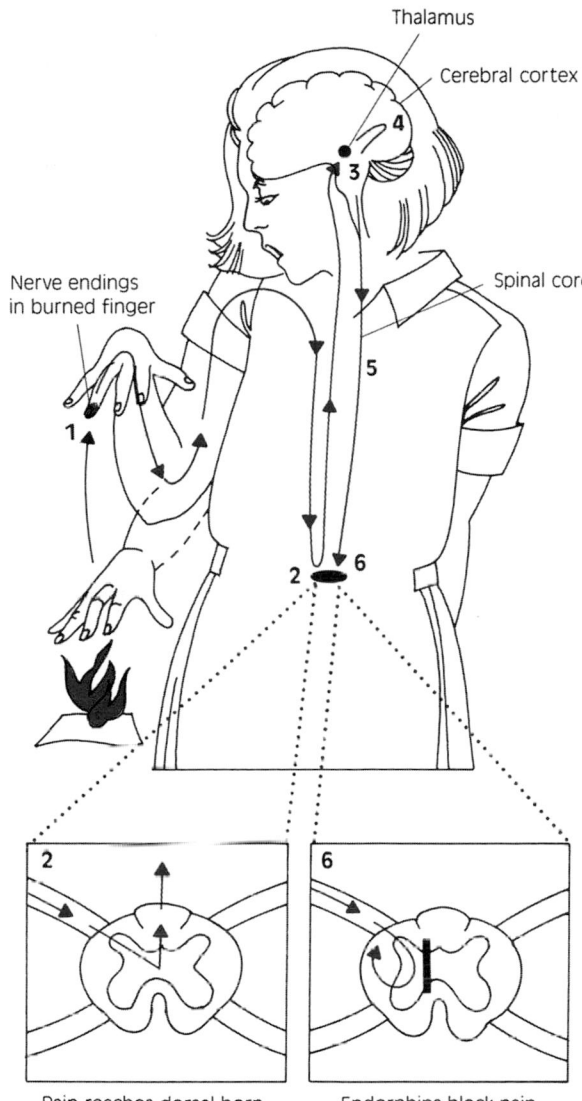

FIGURE 41-2 Pain sensation and relief. (1) Pain's path begins as a message and is received by nerve endings in a burned finger. Potent chemicals (substance P, bradykinin, prostaglandins) are released, sensitizing the nerve endings, helping to transmit the pain message from the injured finger toward the brain, and setting the stage for healing (inflammatory response). (2) The pain signal from the burned finger travels as an electrochemical impulse along the length of the nerve to the dorsal horn on the spinal cord, a region that runs the length of the spine and receives signals from all over the body. (3) The message is relayed to the thalamus, a sensory center in the brain where sensations like heat, cold, pain, and touch first become conscious. (4) It then travels on to the cortex, where the intensity and location of pain are perceived. Little is known about factors that influence the individual's perception of pain at this point, the meaning attributed to the pain, and the voluntary responses elicited. (5) Pain relief begins as a signal from the brain descends by way of the spinal cord. (6) In the dorsal horn, chemicals like endorphin S are released to diminish the pain message from the injured finger. (Adapted from Unlocking pain's secrets. [1984, June 11]. Time, pp. 58–66.)

The brain can also influence the gating mechanism. Past experiences and learned behaviors, which are interpreted by the brain, regulate or adjust the eventual behavioral responses to pain. Thus, the gating mechanism appears to be influenced by the amount of activity in large and small afferent fibers in

addition to nerve impulses that descend from the brain. This helps explain why similar painful stimuli are interpreted differently by different people. Although not everyone accepts the gate control theory, it appears to explain why mechanical and electrical interventions or heat and pressure may provide effective pain relief. Nursing measures, such as massage or a warm compress to a painful lower back area, stimulate large nerve fibers to close the gate, thus blocking pain impulses from that area. Figure 41-3 illustrates the gate control theory of pain.

Perception of Pain

The perception of pain involves the sensory process that occurs when a stimulus for pain is present. It includes the person's interpretation of the pain. The threshold of perception, the **pain threshold,** is the lowest intensity of a stimulus that causes the subject to recognize pain. This threshold is remarkably similar for everyone, but according to Criste (2002), many studies have reached the conclusion that women have lower thresholds than men. Still, it is theorized by at least some authorities that the phenomenon of adaptation does occur, that is, the pain threshold can be changed within a certain range. This phenomenon has been studied, for example, when prisoners of war reported that the pain of repeated torture was not as acute as it would have been under different circumstances. Many factors might well have played a role, but at least some adaptation appears likely.

Adaptation may also be demonstrated when a person's hand is immersed in warm water. A sensation of pain eventually occurs as the water is heated. However, the person can tolerate a higher temperature as water is gradually heated to the pain level than if the hand had been plunged into hot water without any preparation.

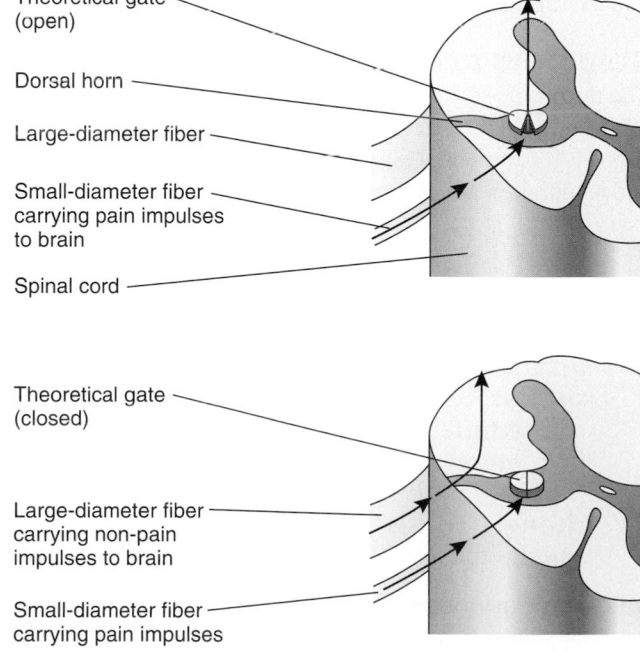

FIGURE 41-3 An illustration of the gate control theory of pain.

Modulation of Pain

The sensation of pain appears to be regulated or modified by substances called neuromodulators. **Neuromodulators** are endogenous opioid compounds, meaning they are naturally present, morphine-like chemical regulators in the spinal cord and brain. They appear to have analgesic activity and alter the perception of pain. These endogenous opioid compounds are believed to produce their analgesic effects by binding to specific opioid receptor sites throughout the CNS, blocking the release or production of pain-transmitting substances. Both pain and stress appear capable of activating the endogenous opiate system.

Endorphins and enkephalins are opioid neuromodulators. **Endorphins** are produced at neural synapses at various points in the CNS pathway. They are powerful pain-blocking chemicals that have prolonged analgesic effects and produce euphoria. It is suggested that endorphins may be released when certain measures are used to relieve pain, such as skin stimulation and relaxation techniques, and when certain pain-relieving drugs are used. The endorphin, **dynorphin,** has the most potent analgesic effect. However, many questions remain about endorphins.

Enkephalins, which are widespread throughout the brain and dorsal horn of the spinal cord, are considered less potent than endorphins. Enkephalins are thought to reduce pain sensation by inhibiting the release of substance P from the terminals of afferent neurons.

Pain is a highly personal experience. A person learns to know what causes unpleasantness and what to interpret as pain. Each person's interpretation is influenced by background, such as how he or she has experienced and dealt with pain in the past, and what culture has taught about pain. Through past experiences, each person also learns to differentiate among the various types of pain and to associate pain with certain descriptive words. Table 41-2 lists common definitions for additional terms used by patients to describe pain.

Responses to Pain

The three types of responses to pain are physiologic, behavioral, and affective. Examples of these responses are listed in Box 41-1, Common Responses to Pain. The severity of pain and its duration affect responses to pain.

> Recall Xavier Malton, the child with ulcerative colitis experiencing an acute episode of pain? The nurse assesses that Xavier is in pain first by his screams. Additionally, the nurse interprets his behavioral and affective responses, such as his body posture, inability to get off of the toilet, and later his fetal position in bed. Moreover, the nurse would validate these findings with physiologic responses, noting changes in his vital signs, skin color, and muscle tension.

Mild pain experienced briefly may produce little or no behavioral response, whereas intense pain experienced briefly usually results in reflex action to escape the cause. Pain that

TABLE 41-2 Additional Terms Used to Describe Pain

Quality

Sharp	Pain that is sticking in nature and that is intense
Dull	Pain that is not as intense or acute as sharp pain, possibly more annoying than painful. It is usually more diffuse than sharp pain.
Diffuse	Pain that covers a large area. Usually, the patient is unable to point to a specific area without moving the hand over a large surface, such as the entire abdomen.
Shifting	Pain that moves from one area to another, such as from the lower abdomen to the area over the stomach.

Other terms used to describe the quality of pain include sore, stinging, pinching, cramping, gnawing, cutting, throbbing, shooting, viselike pressure.

Severity

Severe or excruciating / Moderate / Slight or mild	These terms depend on the patient's interpretation of pain. Behavioral and physiologic signs help assess the severity of pain. On a scale of 1 to 10, slight pain could be described as being between about 1 and 3; moderate pain, between about 4 and 7; and severe pain, between about 8 and 10.

Periodicity

Continuous	Pain that does not stop
Intermittent	Pain that stops and starts again
Brief or transient	Pain that passes quickly

continues for a relatively short time, such as for a few days or a week, is often accepted by the patient without its being all consuming. The patient expects relief and believes the cause is self-limiting. However, anxiety is ordinarily present. On the other hand, chronic pain tends to consume the entire person. It demands total attention so that the patient has limited resources to take care of other matters of daily living. It is physically and emotionally exhausting and tends to result in depression and irritability. Chronic fatigue usually accompanies chronic pain.

Lack of an obvious response to pain does not mean the patient is without pain. Careful assessment is especially important to understand what the patient is experiencing.

FACTORS AFFECTING THE PAIN EXPERIENCE

Many factors influence the comfort status of a person at any given moment. When an individual experiences pain, almost anything can influence how the painful stimulus is transmit-

---

BOX 41-1 Common Responses to Pain

Behavioral (Voluntary) Responses
Moving away from painful stimuli
Grimacing, moaning, and crying
Restlessness
Protecting the painful area and refusing to move

Physiologic (Involuntary) Responses
Typical Sympathetic Responses When Pain Is Moderate and Superficial
Increased blood pressure
Increased pulse and respiratory rates
Pupil dilation
Muscle tension and rigidity
Pallor (peripheral vasoconstriction)
Increased adrenalin output
Increased blood glucose

Typical Parasympathetic Responses When Pain Is Severe and Deep
Nausea and vomiting
Fainting or unconsciousness
Decreased blood pressure
Decreased pulse rate
Prostration
Rapid and irregular breathing

Affective (Psychological) Responses
Exaggerated weeping and restlessness
Withdrawal
Stoicism
Anxiety
Depression
Fear
Anger
Anorexia
Fatigue
Hopelessness
Powerlessness

---

ted to the brain, how it is perceived, and the response that is made to it.

Culture

Because cultural norms dictate much of our daily behavior, attitudes, and values, it is natural that culture influences the individual's response to pain. Nurses need to understand that there are ways other than their own of responding to pain. Nurses, as a subculture, value self-control and the ability to function under stress. As a result, nurses may expect patients in pain to display a similarly calm, objective, uncomplaining approach to pain. It is particularly important to avoid stereotyping responses to pain because the nurse frequently encounters patients who are in pain or anticipating that it will develop. A form of pain expression that is frowned on in one culture may be desirable in another cultural group. Be knowledgeable about cultural variations and develop an understanding of cultural influences on pain tolerance, expressions of pain, and alternative practices used to manage pain.

Ethnic Variables

Much research has been done on ethnic and cultural influences on pain. The classic study on behavioral responses to pain in people of similar ethnic origin was done by Zborowski (1969). He studied men in the 1950s and 1960s in four cultural groups—"Old American" (American-born, white, Protestant, and without identification with any foreign group), Jewish, Italian, and Irish. According to Zborowski, Old American and Irish men typically minimized and controlled their expression of pain, whereas Jewish and Italian men tended to be more vocal and outwardly emotional with their expressions of pain. Today the ethnic heritage of many people is mixed, thereby making it more difficult to anticipate individual responses to pain. Healthcare providers increase their respect and sensitivity for diversity if they understand the effects of culture and ethnicity on the pain experience. Table 41-3 describes typical pain responses in selected ethnocultural groups. The nurse working with other ethnic groups can find pertinent studies in the literature. Additional information on cultural influences on pain is presented in Chapter 3.

Family, Gender, and Age Variables

Other culturally related variables are family, gender, and age. An individual's response to pain or symptoms may be affected or influenced by the response of family members. Spouses also may reinforce pain behavior in their partners. Children growing up in different families may learn to "be brave" and ignore pain or to use the pain experience to secure attention and service from family members. Family size and birth order do not appear to be significant in distinguishing chronic pain sufferers.

Similarly, children may learn that there are gender differences in pain expression—it may be acceptable for a little girl to run home crying with a scraped knee, but a little boy may be told that he should be brave and not cry. Adult men and women may hold on to gender expectations regarding pain communication and incorrectly interpret the presence or absence of pain expressions in others. Women are more comfortable communicating the discomfort associated with pain, but this ability to verbalize may cause some to view the pain as emotionally or psychologically based (Criste, 2002). Several studies report that pain in women needs to be addressed more aggressively because their pain management is consistently reported as inadequate.

In addition, different age groups have different beliefs and norms regarding pain sensation and response. At one time, the infant's inability to communicate pain led healthcare practitioners to the erroneous assumption that pain sensation was diminished or absent. More recently, it has been demonstrated that infants and small children are sensitive to and experience pain. Among older people, pain has often been viewed as a natural component of the aging process, being ignored or undertreated by healthcare providers. On the other hand, conditions

TABLE 41-3 Pain Expression in Selected Ethnocultural Groups

Ethnic Group	Response to Pain
African Americans	Often viewed as a sign of illness or disease Some believe that suffering and pain are inevitable. Spiritual and religious beliefs may contribute to high tolerance for pain. Some believe that praying and laying on of hands may aid in deliverance from pain and suffering.
Arab Americans	Often view pain as unpleasant and something that should be controlled Tend to express pain openly with family members but may act in a more restrained manner in the presence of health professionals Usually expect positive response from Western medical interventions to control pain
Chinese Americans	Expressions of pain are usually similar to those of Americans Often believe pain is related to the influence of imbalances in the yin and yang Usually cope with pain by using externally applied oils and massage as well as warmth, sleeping on the area of pain, relaxation, and aspirin
Greek Americans	Ponos (pain) is viewed by most as an evil that needs to be eradicated. Physical and emotional pain are usually shared with the family. Family is considered a resource for pain relief because they act as advocates and provide emotional support.
Mexican Americans	Most delay seeking medical help for pain and hope, instead, that it will go away; consider it a necessary part of life Seem to experience more pain than other ethnic groups but report it less frequently Often see a direct relationship between pain and suffering and immoral behavior
Navajo Indians	Do not usually openly express their pain or request pain medication Adequate pain control is often difficult because they may mask the actual intensity of their pain. May prefer herbal medicines and use them without the knowledge of the healthcare provider

Adapted from Purnell, L., & Paulanka, B. (1998). *Transcultural health care.* Philadelphia: F. A. Davis.

normally painful in young adults (eg, myocardial infarction) may result in minimal pain complaints in older people. That an older person does not complain of pain may indicate that he or she fears the treatment for the pain or just refuses to give in to the pain. For many older adults, pain has become accepted as a daily occurrence and is regarded as part of the normal aging process. These variables, which influence pain sensation, perception, and response, make pain assessment a complex task for the nurse.

Religious Beliefs

Religious beliefs can be a powerful influence on the individual's experience of pain. In some religions, individuals view pain and suffering as a "lack of goodness" in themselves. Thus pain and suffering are viewed as a means of purification or of making up for individual and community sin. This meaning helps the individual to cope with pain and becomes a source of strength. Patients with this belief may refuse analgesics and other pain relief measures, feeling that this lessens their suffering. On the other hand, illness and pain may also be viewed as punishment from a vengeful God. Individuals may find their faith shaken and question the existence of a loving God. How can belief in a loving God be compatible with their present experience of pain? Anger, resentment, and depression may compound the pain experience. Patients may find it helpful to confer with a spiritual adviser about their pain experience.

Think back to Ernesto Plachutta, the older man with severe cancer pain. Mr. Plachutta believes that his pain is a punishment from God for his past sins and therefore rejects measures to relieve the pain to atone for these sins. The nurse would need to gather additional data surrounding this belief to develop an individualized plan of care for Mr. Plachutta. Such a plan of care would respect his beliefs while at the same time provide him with some comfort. Contacting Mr. Plachutta's religious or spiritual person or referring him to pastoral care may be helpful in providing him with support.

Environment and Support People

An individual's environment and the presence or absence of caring support people may also influence the experience of pain. Many people find that the strangeness of the healthcare environment, especially the lights, noise, lack of sleep, and constant activity of a critical care unit, compounds the experience of pain. The sense of powerlessness that accompanies admission to an institution may decrease the individual's ability to cope with pain.

Remember Sheree Lincoln the postoperative patient in pain described at the beginning of the chapter? In addition to the pain related to surgery, the nurse would need to assess the effect of the environment on Sheree's pain. For example, she may be frightened by equipment being used postoperatively. Additionally, she may feel alone and powerless due to her current condition. Assessment also would need to include information about past experiences with pain, support persons available, and teaching she received preoperatively.

Depersonalization or separation from a favorite pillow, pet, or source of music may further decrease the person's sense of comfort. For some, the presence of a loved family member or friend is essential to their sense of well-being. Others prefer to be alone when in pain and may become agitated in the presence of a family member.

Some patients may use their pain to acquire secondary gains, such as special attention and services from their families. If unchecked, this tendency usually leads to resentment and anger in family members and their eventual avoidance of the patient. Intervening and attempting an honest discussion of this problem is important.

Anxiety and Other Stressors

Anxiety, which is almost always present when pain is anticipated or being experienced, tends to increase the perceived intensity of pain. The threat of the unknown is ordinarily more devastating and anxiety producing than a threat for which one has been prepared. Studies have indicated that patients who were taught preoperatively about what to expect postoperatively did not require as much medication for pain as those who had similar operative procedures but did not receive this teaching.

Ordinarily, pain is aggravated with anxiety, muscular tension, and fatigue. A vicious circle can easily develop when pain interferes with rest and relaxation, and tension and fatigue almost always aggravate the discomfort. The rested and relaxed person can often cope with more discomfort than someone who is suffering from a lack of sleep.

An individual who is greatly fatigued and who has no competing demands requiring attention may experience pain acutely. For example, many people have discovered that the pain of a foot ache or an ingrown toenail that was only mildly annoying during the day's work becomes unbearable at night when there is nothing else to distract the mind from the pain.

Past Pain Experience

An individual's experience of pain in the past and the qualities of that experience profoundly affect new pain experiences:

- Some patients have never known severe pain and have no fear of pain, not realizing how intense the sensation can be.
- Some patients have experienced severe acute or chronic pain in the past but received immediate and adequate pain relief. These patients are generally unafraid of pain and initiate appropriate requests for assistance.
- Some patients have known severe pain in the past and were unable to secure relief. Even the suggestion of new pain can lead to acute feelings of fear, despair, and hopelessness.
- An individual whose past pain experience led to correction of unhealthy behavior and produced a greater sense of health and well-being may respect and value pain and consider the meaning and significance of a new pain carefully.
- In general, people who have experienced more pain than usual in their lifetimes tend to anticipate more pain and to exhibit increased sensitivity to pain.
- Some pain memories are virtually unerasable; new contact with conditions similar to those that caused the earlier pain can provoke a violent response.

THE NURSING PROCESS FOR COMFORT

Assessing

Because the pain experience is unique to each individual, the nurse who wants to help the patient achieve comfort and pain control needs sophisticated pain assessment skills. Assessing all factors that affect the pain experience—psychological, emotional, and sociocultural, as well as physiologic—is essential. Pain is complex and difficult to interpret and requires a reliable assessment tool.

Pain as the Fifth Vital Sign

In an effort to improve patients' quality of life and make pain management a priority, the American Pain Society is encouraging caregivers to include assessment for pain as the fifth vital sign. Routine measurement of vital signs accompanied by a pain assessment raises awareness of the existence of pain, places additional emphasis on optimizing pain relief, and moves patients more quickly toward comfort and recovery.

The JCAHO is also attempting to improve pain management and has developed accreditation standards that include the following (JCAHO, 2000):

- Patients have the right to appropriate assessment and management of their pain.
- Ongoing assessment of the existence of pain should also include the nature and intensity of the pain.
- Assessment results should be recorded in a manner that promotes regular reassessment and follow-up.
- Staff must be oriented and competent in assessment and management of pain.
- Policies and procedures that support prescription or ordering of pain medications must be in place.
- Patients and families require education about effective pain management.
- Discharge planning should address the patient's needs for management of pain symptoms.

Common Misconceptions

Many patient misconceptions interfere with the patient's ability to communicate pain:

- The doctor has ordered pain-relieving medication for me, which I will be given routinely.
- If I ask for something for my pain, I may become addicted to the medication.
- Sometimes it's better to put up with the pain than to deal with the side effects of the pain medication.
- I should somehow be able to control my pain. It is immature to talk about pain.
- It is better to wait until the pain gets really bad before asking for help. If I take the medication now for moderate pain, it won't relieve severe pain later on.
- I don't want to bother anyone—I know how busy they are.

- It's natural for me to have pain after surgery. After a few days, I should notice it lessening.

> *Recall Sheree Lincoln, the woman who has undergone abdominal surgery? It would be important for the nurse to investigate Sheree's understanding of her postoperative pain and what her expectations are. Doing so would provide clues for the nurse indicating possible patient misconceptions about pain and pain relief, thereby providing a basis for teaching and correcting these misconceptions.*

Additional misconceptions and prejudices about pain and pain relief that hamper the nurse's assessment and treatment of the patient with pain have been summarized by McCaffery and Pasero (1999) and are presented in Table 41-4.

TABLE 41-4 Barriers to the Assessment and Treatment of Pain

Misconception	Correction
1. The best judge of the existence and severity of a patient's pain is the physician or nurse caring for the patient.	The patient is the authority about his or her pain. The patient's self-report is the most reliable indicator of the existence and intensity of pain.
2. Clinicians should use their personal opinions and beliefs about the truthfulness of the patient to determine the patient's true pain status.	Allowing each clinician to act on personal beliefs presents the potential for different pain assessments by different clinicians, leading to different interventions from each clinician. This results in inconsistent and often inadequate pain management. It is essential to establish the patient's self-report of pain as the standard for pain assessment.
3. The clinician must believe what the patient says about pain.	The clinician must accept and respect the patient's report of pain and proceed with appropriate assessment and treatment. The clinician is always entitled to his or her personal opinion, but this cannot be allowed to guide professional practice.
4. Comparable noxious stimuli produce comparable pain in different people. The pain threshold is uniform.	Findings from numerous studies have failed to support the notion of a uniform pain threshold. Comparable stimuli do not result in the same pain in different people. After similar injuries, one person may suffer moderate pain and the other severe pain.
5. Patients with a low pain tolerance should make a greater effort to cope with pain and should not receive as much analgesia as they desire.	A stoic response to pain is valued in this society and many others. Research shows that clinicians often do not like patients with a low pain tolerance. However, imposing these values on the patient and withholding analgesics is inappropriate.
6. There is no reason for patients to hurt when no physical cause for pain can be found.	Pain is a new science, and it would be foolish of us to think that we will be able to determine the cause of all the pains that patients report.
7. Patients should not receive analgesics until the cause of pain is diagnosed.	Pain is no longer the clinician's primary diagnostic tool. Symptomatic relief of pain should be provided while the investigation of cause proceeds. Early use of analgesics is now advocated for patients with acute abdominal pain.
8. Visible signs, either physiologic or behavioral, accompany pain and can be used to verify its existence and severity.	Even with severe pain, periods of physiologic and behavioral adaptation occur, leading to periods of minimal or no signs of pain. Lack of pain expression does not necessarily mean lack of pain.
9. Anxiety makes pain worse.	Anxiety is often associated with pain, but the cause-and-effect relationship has not been established. Pain often causes anxiety, but it is not clear that anxiety necessarily makes pain more intense.
10. Patients who are knowledgeable about opioid analgesics and who make regular efforts to obtain them are "drug seeking" (addicted).	Patients with pain should be knowledgeable about their medications, and regular use of opioids for pain relief is not addiction. When a patient is accused of "drug seeking," it may be helpful to ask, "What else could this behavior mean? Might this patient be in pain?"

(continued)

TABLE 41-4 (Continued)

Misconception	Correction
11. When the patient reports pain relief after a placebo, this means that the patient is a malingerer or that the pain is psychogenic.	About one third of patients who have obvious physical stimuli for pain (eg, surgery) report pain relief after a placebo injection. Therefore, placebos cannot be used to diagnose malingering, psychogenic pain, or any psychological problem. Sometimes, placebos relieve pain, but why this happens remains unknown.
12. The pain rating scale preferred for use in daily clinical practice is the VAS.	For patients who are verbal and can count from 0 to 10, the NRS pain rating scale is preferred. It is easy to explain, measure, and record, and it provides numbers for setting pain-management goals.
13. Cognitively impaired elderly patients are unable to use pain rating scales.	When an appropriate pain rating scale (eg, 0–5) is used and the patient is given sufficient time to process information and respond, many cognitively impaired elderly patients can use a pain rating scale.

May be duplicated for use in clinical practice. From McCaffery, M., & Pasero, C. (1999). *Pain: Clinical manual* (p. 37). St. Louis: Mosby, Inc.

Components of a Pain Assessment

Various forms used to help guide the assessment of pain have been described in the nursing literature. The primary purposes of using a guide to assess pain are to eliminate guesswork and biases when dealing with the patient's pain, to understand what the person is experiencing, to analyze findings that will help prepare an appropriate nursing response to the patient's pain, and to facilitate improved outcomes, such as fewer complications, shorter hospital stays, and improved quality of life.

Characteristics of pain generally assessed include the following:
- Patient's verbalization and description of the pain
- Duration of the pain
- Location of the pain
- Quantity and intensity of the pain
- Quality of the pain
- Chronology of the pain
- Aggravating factors
- Alleviating factors
- Physiologic indicators of pain
- Behavioral responses
- Effect of the pain experience on activities and lifestyle

A comprehensive pain assessment must also include discussion of the patient's expectations for pain relief. The patient and healthcare team need to select a realistic goal or a number on the pain scale that is acceptable and satisfactory and that facilitates recovery. This helps the patient recognize and report pain that is unacceptable and also allows caregivers to evaluate more readily the effectiveness of their pain management techniques. The accompanying Focused Assessment Guide suggests questions or approaches helpful in assessing the various pain factors.

Pain centers commonly ask patients to complete a self-questionnaire. The McGill–Melzack Pain Questionnaire is one commonly used example. The individual checks words that fit the description of the pain experience and then places marks on a body figure to designate the location of the pain. Comparison of changes on subsequent questionnaires aid in determining an individual's improvement or regression. This comprehensive pain assessment is time-consuming and should be performed when the patient is more comfortable and better able to respond to questions.

An example of a pain assessment tool that is brief and easily administered is shown in Figure 41-4. For continued assessment of pain and evaluation of pain control measures, a pain scale allows the patient to rate effectively the pain he or she is experiencing on a continual basis. Figure 41-5 shows examples of several pain-intensity rating scales.

When assessing an individual's pain, McCaffery and Pasero (1999) lists these basic methods:
- Patient's self-report
- Report of family member, other person close to the patient, or caregiver who is familiar with the patient
- Behaviors (restlessness, grimacing, crying, protecting the painful area)
- Physiologic measures (increased blood pressure and pulse)

Another easy assessment tool to use is the WILDA pain measurement scale. The WILDA scale, developed by Fink as cited in Salmore (2002), consists of an acronym that prompts the nurse to ask all needed questions regarding pain:
- **W**ords that describe the pain
- **I**ntensity of pain (using a 0–10 scale with 0 being no pain and 10 worst pain)
- **L**ocation of pain
- **D**uration of pain
- **A**ggravating or alleviating factors

Assessment in the Cognitively Impaired Patient

Assessment of pain in people who are cognitively impaired presents special challenges to nurses. It is generally recognized that cognitively impaired individuals are frequently under treated because they may be unable to report pain verbally or describe the dimensions of their pain. Special efforts are needed to identify accurate methods for assessing their pain. Parke (1998) concluded that gerontologic nurses used intuition, experience, and their long-term relationships with patients as a guide to validating pain cues and recognizing the

Focused Assessment Guide 41-1

The Pain Experience

Factors to Assess	Questions and Approaches
Characteristics of the pain Location	*"Where is your pain? Is it external or internal?"* (Asking the patient with acute pain to point to the painful area with one finger may help to localize the pain. Patients with chronic pain may have difficulty trying to localize their pain, however.)
Duration	*"How long have you been experiencing pain? How long does a pain episode last? How often does a pain episode occur?"*
Quantity	Ask the patient to indicate the degree (amount) of pain currently experienced on the scale below:

0	1	2	3	4	5	6	7	8	9	10
No pain		Mild		Moderate			Severe			Pain as bad as it can be

	It is also helpful to ask how much pain the patient has (on the same scale) when the pain is at its least and at its worst: Least _____ Worst _____
Quality	*"What words would you use to describe your pain?"*
Chronology	*"How does the pain develop and progress?"* (If pattern can be identified, interventions early in a pain sequence will often be far more effective than those used after the pain is well established.) *"Has the pain changed since it first began? If so, how?"*
Aggravating factors	*"What makes the pain occur or increase in intensity?"*
Alleviating factors	*"What makes the pain go away or lessen? What methods of relief have you tried in the past? How long were they used? How effective were they?"* (Methods of relief currently in effect for hospitalized patients should be apparent from the chart. It is important to verify the use of current orders and their effectiveness with the patient. Outpatients may need to be asked to record a medication profile, a thorough and accurate account of all medications they are taking.)
Associated phenomena	*"Are there any other factors that seem to relate consistently to your pain? Any other symptoms that occur just before, during, or after your pain?"*

Physiologic responses
  Vital signs (blood pressure, pulse, respirations)
  Skin color
  Perspiration
  Pupil size
  Nausea
	Signs of sympathetic stimulation commonly occur with acute pain. Signs of parasympathetic stimulation (decreased blood pressure and pulse, rapid and irregular respirations, pupil constriction, nausea and vomiting, and warm, dry skin) may be present, especially in prolonged, severe pain, visceral, or deep pain.

Muscle tension	Observe. Ask the patient whether he or she is aware of any tight, tense muscles.
Anxiety	Are signs of anxiety evident? (May include decreased attention span or ability to follow directions, frequent asking of questions, shifting of topics of conversation, avoidance of discussion of feelings, acting out, somatizing.)
Behavioral responses Posture, gross motor activities	Does patient rub or support a particular area? Make frequent position changes? Walk, pace, kneel, or assume a rolled-up position? Does patient rest a particular body part? Protect an area from stimulation? Lie quietly? (In acute pain, postural and gross motor activities are often altered; in chronic pain, the only signs of change may be postures characteristic of withdrawal.)
Facial features	Does the patient have a pinched look? Are there facial grimaces? Knotted brow? Overall taut, anxious appearance? (A look of fatigue is more characteristic of chronic pain.)
Verbal expressions	Does the patient sigh, moan, scream, cry, repetitively use the same words?
Affective responses Anxiety	*"Do you feel anxious? Are you afraid? If so, how bad are these feelings?"*

(continued)

Focused Assessment Guide 41-1

The Pain Experience (Continued)

Factors to Assess	Questions and Approaches
Depression	*"Do you feel depressed, down, or low? If so, how bad are these feelings? Are your feelings about yourself mostly good or bad? Do you have feelings of failure? Do you see yourself or your illness as a burden to those you care about?"*
Interactions with others	How does the patient act when he or she is in pain in the presence of others? How does the patient respond to others when he or she is not in pain? How do significant others and caregivers respond to the patient when the patient is in pain? When the patient is not in pain?
Degree to which pain interferes with patient's life (use past performance as baseline)	*"Does the pain interfere with sleep? If so, to what extent? Is fatigue a major factor in the pain experience? Is the conduct of intimate or peer relationships affected by the pain? Is work function affected? Participation in recreational–diversional activities?"* (An activity diary is often helpful—sometimes crucial. One to several weeks of hourly activity recorded by the patient may be necessary. Levels of pain, intake of food, and sleep–rest periods are noted along with activities performed. Separate diaries for inpatient and outpatient episodes may be necessary because hospitalization markedly affects the nature and type of activities performed.)
Perception of pain and meaning to patient	*"Are you worried about your illness? Do you see any connection between your pain and the nature or course of illness? If so, how do you see them as related? Do you find any meaning in your pain? If so, is this beneficial or detrimental to you? Are you struggling to find some meaning for your pain?"*
Adaptive mechanisms used to cope with pain	*"What do you usually do to relieve stress? How well do these things work? What techniques do you use at home to help cope with the pain? How well have they worked? Do you use these in the hospital? If not, why not?"*
Outcomes	*"What would you like to be doing right now, this week, this month, if the pain were better controlled? How much would the pain have to decrease (on the 0–10 scale) for you to begin to accomplish these goals?"*

presence of pain in a group of cognitively impaired older adults. Pain has been demonstrated as a possible cause of aggressive behavior in cognitively impaired older adults. The combination of a history of pain, observations of a patient's pain by families and caregivers, and the presence of medical diagnoses associated with pain facilitated the development of a model for pain assessment in this population. To manage pain effectively, nurses must rely on their own careful assessments, their empathic qualities, and the expectation that a cognitively impaired patient will experience pain if a verbal patient usually reports this event as painful. The accompanying Research in Nursing box presents information on a pain scale developed to monitor sedated patients who are temporarily cognitively impaired.

Assessment in a Child

In recent years, healthcare personnel have become much more concerned about addressing pain relief in infants and children. Previously, it was believed that young children lacked the neurologic development to sense pain the way adults do. Thus, pain relief was not a priority when children were hospitalized. Young children frequently received no treatment for pain during their entire hospital stay. Current thinking is that inadequately controlled pain during infancy and childhood may

alter a person's response to pain in adulthood. Pain is frustrating for children because they are unable to understand the concept and cause of pain and may have difficulty describing it. Depending on age, the child may see the pain as a form of punishment for something that he or she has done. Current methods of assessing and measuring children's pain frequently involve use of more than one technique for assessment. A pain history provides information about the language the child uses to indicate pain, how and to whom this pain is usually reported, and indications of previous pain experiences and coping strategies. Self-report is usually the most reliable account of pain. Communication with parents, guardians, or other important family members is vital for accurate pediatric pain assessment and management. In addition, the following observations may provide an indication of the presence and severity of pain in a child:

- Irritability and restlessness
- Crying, screaming, or other verbal expression of pain
- Grimacing, grinding of teeth, or clenching fists
- Touching or grabbing of painful body part
- Kicking, thrashing, or attempting to move away from a painful stimulus

One commonly used pain assessment scale asks children to compare their pain to a series of faces ranging from a broad

Date _____

Patient's name _____ Age _____ Room _____

Diagnosis _____ Physician _____

Nurse _____

1. LOCATION: Patient or nurse marks drawing.

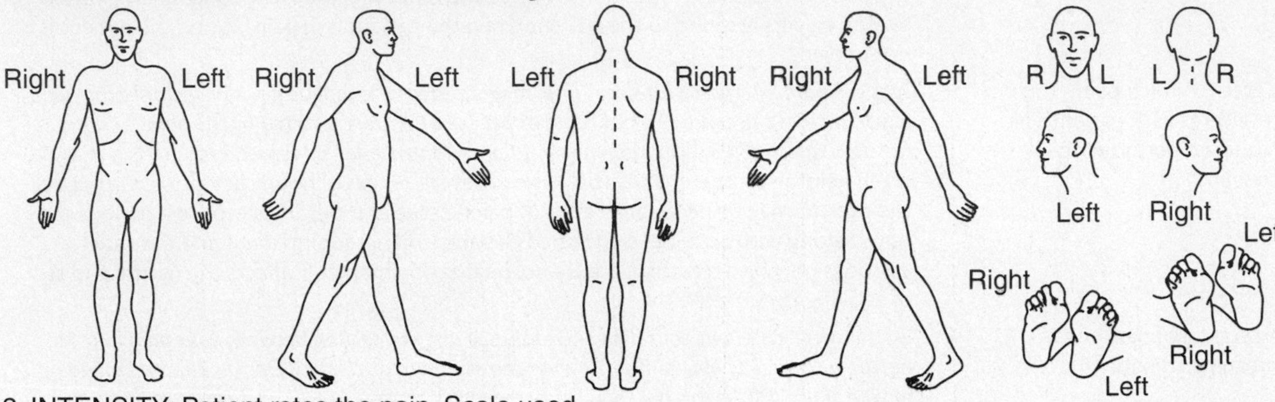

Right   Left   Right   Left   Left   Right   Right   Left   R) L   L) R

Left   Right

Right   Left

Right

Left

2. INTENSITY: Patient rates the pain. Scale used _____
   Present: _____
   Worst pain gets: _____
   Best pain gets: _____
   Acceptable level of pain: _____
3. QUALITY: (Use patient's own words, e.g., prick, ache, burn, throb, pull, sharp)

   _____
4. ONSET, DURATION, VARIATION, RHYTHMS: _____

   _____
5. MANNER OF EXPRESSING PAIN: _____
6. WHAT RELIEVES THE PAIN? _____
7. WHAT CAUSES OR INCREASES THE PAIN? _____
8. EFFECTS OF PAIN: (Note decreased function, decreased quality of life.)
   Accompanying symptoms (e.g., nausea) _____
   Sleep _____
   Appetite _____
   Physical activity _____
   Relationship with others (e.g., irritability) _____
   Emotions (e.g., anger, suicidal, crying) _____
   Concentration _____
   Other _____

9. OTHER COMMENTS: _____

   _____
10. PLAN: _____

   _____

FIGURE 41-4 Initial pain assessment tool. May be duplicated for use in clinical practice.
(Adapted from McCaffery, M., and Pasero, C. [1999]. *Pain: Clinical manual* [p. 37]. St. Louis: Mosby.)

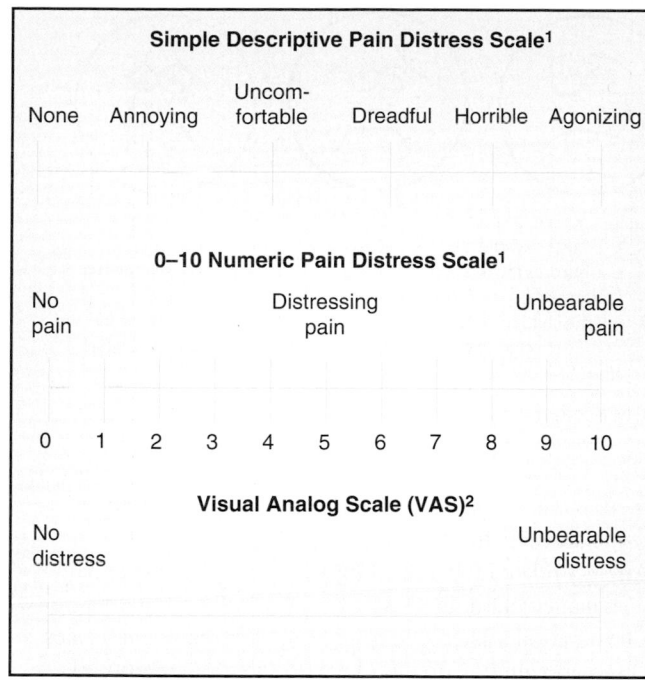

Simple Descriptive Pain Distress Scale¹

None   Annoying   Uncom-   Dreadful   Horrible   Agonizing
                   fortable

0–10 Numeric Pain Distress Scale¹

No   Distressing   Unbearable
pain   pain   pain

0   1   2   3   4   5   6   7   8   9   10

Visual Analog Scale (VAS)²

No   Unbearable
distress   distress

¹ If used as a graphic rating scale, a 10-cm baseline is recommended.
² A 10-cm baseline is recommended for VAS scales.

FIGURE 41-5 Pain distress scales. (From AHCPR, Acute Pain Management Guide Panel, 1992.)

smile to a tearful grimace (Fig. 41-6 is an example of a pediatric pain assessment scale). The Oucher pain scale, developed by Beyer and others (1992) for use in young patients, combines a 0-to-100 scale with six photographic images of children in pain that older children can use. Children may also be asked to record their pain experiences in a daily diary. Detecting and accurately assessing pediatric pain have resulted in new and innovative approaches toward pain control in children.

Think back to Xavier Malton, the 5-year-old with acute pain. Incorporating the use of an age-appropriate pain assessment tool would be crucial in assessing Xavier's pain. Since Xavier is 5 years old, he may have difficulty describing his pain and its severity. For example, according to Xavier, "Something was hurting very much." Using the faces scale or the Oucher scale would help the nurse to quantify the severity of Xavier's pain, providing objective evidence from which to intervene appropriately. The tool also would be extremely useful in determining the effectiveness of pain relief interventions, providing objective evidence denoting any changes in the pain's severity. This evaluation would serve as a basis for continuing pain management.

Assessment in the Older Patient

Assessing pain in the elderly can be challenging. As previously mentioned, many see pain in the elderly as being part of the normal aging process. Because many older people have chronic disease, pain is a prevalent occurrence. Visual or hearing impairments may influence the assessment format. Multiple-drug regimens that are common in older people can also affect reliable reporting of pain. One myth held by many is that older patients have a decreased sensitivity to pain and therefore a heightened pain tolerance. Pain is seen by many elderly patients as a forecast of serious illness or death. Boredom, loneliness, and depression may affect an older person's perception and report of pain.

Experts agree that pain can be adequately assessed in most older adults using common rating scales. The Wong/Baker Faces Rating Scale (see Fig. 41-6), recommended for pain assessment in children, may also be effective for this age group because a 0-to-5 scale is easier to use. Special attention and consideration of an older patient's and the younger patient's pain can positively affect the nurse's ability to assess pain accurately.

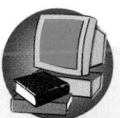

Research in Nursing Making a Difference
Assessing Sedated Patients for Pain

Many times the words *sedated* and *pain control* are used synonymously. This is not always accurate. Just because a person is sedated does not mean that he or she is not experiencing pain. The challenge for the nurse is to assess patients who cannot verbalize their pain due to sedating medication.

Related Research

Salmore, R. (2002). Development of a new pain scale: Colorado behavioral numerical pain scale for sedated adult patients undergoing gastrointestinal procedures. *Gastroenterology Nursing*, 25(6), 257–262.

Thirty patients who were undergoing a gastrointestinal procedure were used in the study. Nurses who were experienced with GI procedures monitored the sedated patients during the procedure using the Colorado Behavioral Numerical Pain Scale (CBNPS). (The pain scale uses a scale of 0 to 5, with a 0 reflecting a patient quietly at rest with no facial expression, and a 5 indicating a combative patient.) A second and third nurse also assessed the patient's pain level. In 82% of the cases, the nurses agreed completely on the assessment of the patient's pain. In 17% of the cases, two of the three nurses agreed on the pain level, and in the remaining 1% there was no agreement.

The CBNPS is an effective pain-measurement tool. It is easy to use and results can be documented quickly. If the rated score indicates that the patient is experiencing pain, additional medication can be administered to relieve the pain, thus demonstrating caring by healthcare providers to ensure that pain management is taken seriously.

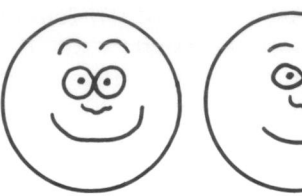 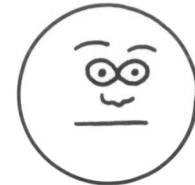   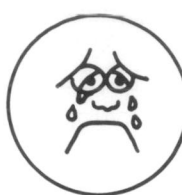

1. Explain to the child that each face is for a person who feels happy because he or she has no pain (hurt, or whatever word the child uses) or feels sad because he or she has some or a lot of pain.
2. Point to the appropriate face and state, "This face . . .":
   0—"is very happy because he [or she] doesn't hurt at all."
   1—"hurts just a little bit."
   2—"hurts a little more."
3—"hurts even more."
4—"hurts a whole lot."
5—"hurts as much as you can imagine, although you don't have to be crying to feel this bad."
3. Ask the child to choose the face that best describes how he or she feels. Be specific about which pain (eg, "shot" or incision) and what time (eg, Now? Earlier before lunch?)

FIGURE 41-6 Wong/Baker Faces Rating Scale for use with children. (From Wong, D. L., et al. [2001]. *Wong's essentials of pediatric nursing* [6th ed.]. St. Louis: Mosby.)

Diagnosing

Pain is such a complex phenomenon that its analysis often requires multidisciplinary collaboration. Although nursing has much to offer individuals experiencing both acute and chronic pain, the data collected by the nurse during the comprehensive pain assessment benefit the patient most when shared with physicians and other members of the healthcare team.

Attempting to intervene before an accurate assessment has been completed may mask the real cause of the patient's pain and lead to false assumptions and even further progression of symptoms and the disease process. The nurse who notes a pattern of headaches in a patient and relates this to the patient's description of recent stress (divorce, relocation, new job) may erroneously assume that the headaches are merely stress related and devise and implement a plan of relaxation exercises. A more careful analysis of patient data, however, may reveal that the headaches are of vascular origin, are migraine in nature, and that medical intervention is indicated. The headaches may also be symptomatic of intracranial disease such as a brain tumor, in which case delay in diagnosis could decrease the possibility of treatment and cure.

When a nursing diagnosis of acute or chronic pain is developed, the diagnostic statement and plan of care should identify the following:

- Type of pain
- Etiologic factors, to the extent that they are known and understood
- Patient's behavioral, physiologic, and affective responses
- Other factors affecting pain stimulus, transmission, perception, and response

Pain or Chronic Pain as the Problem

Many diagnoses can be developed for pain problems. The importance of identifying these problems and including them as priorities in the plan of care cannot be overstated. See the accompanying box for examples of NANDA nursing diagnoses.

Pain or Chronic Pain as the Etiology

Because the experience of pain affects so many other aspects of human functioning, pain may be the etiology of numerous other nursing diagnosis statements such as:

Ineffective Airway Clearance related to postoperative incisional pain

Anxiety related to pain anticipation and inadequate pain management in the past

Constipation related to chronic use of narcotic analgesics

Disabled Family Coping related to father's inability to allow family to share his pain experience

Ineffective Coping related to failure of chronic pain management strategies to date

Ineffective Health Maintenance related to loss of will to live secondary to prolonged chronic pain

Hopelessness related to belief that present pain means imminent death

Risk for Injury related to decreased pain sensation

Deficient Knowledge: Angina Pain Management related to belief that nothing will help the pain

Fatigue related to lack of relief from chronic pain

Fear related to possible significance of pain

Impaired Physical Mobility related to arthritic pain

Imbalanced Nutrition: Less Than Body Requirements related to gastrointestinal distress

Dressing/Grooming Self-Care Deficit related to painful movement of joints

Ineffective Sexuality Patterns related to painful intercourse

Disturbed Sleep Pattern from inability to fall asleep related to pain's worsening at night

Risk for Spiritual Distress related to belief that God is unfairly causing this pain as some sort of undeserved punishment

Disturbed Thought Processes related to effects of chronic pain and overmedication

Risk for Self-Directed Violence related to loss of will to live with unrelieved chronic pain

Outcome Identification and Planning

After the diagnosis of a pain problem is made, developing a plan of care that, when implemented, demonstrates nursing's commitment to assist the patient to develop effective pain-management strategies is crucial.

> ## Examples of NANDA Nursing Diagnoses | Pain
>
> | Nursing Diagnoses | Related Factors | Sample Defining Characteristics |
> |---|---|---|
> | Pain: Acute Postoperative | Fear of taking prescribed analgesics | • Recent cholecystectomy
• Face is pale and drawn; vital signs elevated from baseline
• States, "I don't like to ask for anything for pain because I know people often get addicted." |
> | Pain: Left Leg | Fractured femur and multiple lacerations; unsuccessful attempts to determine effective analgesic | • Recent motor vehicle accident
• Grimaces whenever left leg is moved
• Directs abusive language to anyone who touches left leg
• Refused to have dressing changed on left leg
• Reports analgesic "only takes the edge off" the pain |
> | Pain | Prolonged labor (dystocia) and commitment to natural childbirth | • Admitted to labor unit 18 hours ago with moderate contractions 2 minutes apart
• Strength of contractions weakening; progress of dilation and effacement slow; failure to progress
• "I'll feel like a failure if I take anything for pain. I want to 'go natural.' I know I can do it. Besides, the drugs would only hurt my baby." |
> | Pain: Heightened Anticipation | Child's history of undergoing frequent painful procedures | • Child diagnosed at age 3 years with acute nonlymphoid leukemia
• History of bone marrow aspirations, spinal taps, platelet transfusions, chemotherapy, and other such procedures
• Child "freezes" when unfamiliar healthcare worker enters room |
> | Pain: Chest | Decreased blood supply to myocardium (angina) and fear | • "I never know when it will grab me next. I get this crushing pain in my chest and can't do anything. Usually one or two of those nitro tablets bring me relief. I'm always scared, though, that the pain won't go away." |
> | Chronic Pain: Headaches | Inadequate pain management secondary to belief that somehow patient "deserves this pain" | • Reports history of migraine headaches for past 5 years
• Never sought treatment
• "My mother told me that we all get the pain in life that we deserve—goodness, I've been no saint." |
> | Chronic Pain | Inadequate pain management of metastatic cancer involving bone | • "I can't help feeling, though, that no one is meant to live like this."
• Diagnosed with cancer of bladder 2 years ago; presently metastatic spread to spine
• Rates pain 10 on a scale of 1 (minimal) to 10 (greatest)
• "I haven't been taking as much of this pain medicine as the doctor said I could because if I get used to it now nothing will work when the pain gets even worse later."
• "When I told the nurse in the hospital about my pain she said I'd have to get used to it."
• "I don't want to burden my wife and kids with my pain." |
> | Chronic Pain | Rheumatoid arthritis and inappropriate activity during exacerbations | • Stiffness of joints, limitation of motion, heat, swelling, and tenderness
• States pain is often intense after activity
• "I can't accept not being able to do all I want to do for my husband and children." |

Nursing measures are directed toward the achievement of the following patient outcomes for individuals whose pain is acute in nature (ie, it is expected that with healing the pain will subside and eventually disappear). The patient will:
• Describe a gradual reduction of pain, using a scale ranging from 0 (no pain) to 10 (pain as bad as it can be)

• Demonstrate competent execution of successful pain management program (specify)

For patients whose pain is chronic in nature, an expected outcome may be contacting a hospice or a pain clinic. Hospice care (also mentioned in Chaps. 8 and 10) addresses the physical, spiritual, social, and economic needs of terminally ill patients and their families either in the home or a hospice center. Pain relief is a priority in this setting. Numerous outpatient centers are also available to support patients with chronic pain and to improve their pain management through a variety of approaches. The physician, nurse, and other members of the healthcare team collaborate to develop the optimal pain treatment plan for each patient with chronic pain.

Implementing

After the plan of care is developed, the nurse implements the nursing strategies that are most likely to assist the patient to achieve pain relief outcomes, whether at home or in a healthcare facility. Nursing interventions described in this chapter include establishing a trusting nurse–patient relationship, manipulating factors that affect the pain experience, initiating nonpharmacologic pain relief measures, managing pharmacologic interventions, reviewing additional pain control measures, considering ethical and legal responsibility to relieve pain, and teaching the patient about pain.

Establishing a Trusting Nurse–Patient Relationship

Most patients with pain feel better, suffer less, and experience less anxiety when they believe that a competent nurse cares about their experience of pain and is available for help and support. Without the confidence developed in a good nurse–patient relationship, nothing seems to work. With it, often amazing results have been obtained by using measures that ordinarily are only modestly effective. Measures that help strengthen the nurse–patient relationship and promote pain relief include discussing pain with the patient, allowing the patient to help choose a method of pain relief, and visiting and remaining with the patient in pain. These measures promote a collaborative relationship in which the patient's pain is treated with respect (see the accompanying box, Through the Eyes of the Patient).

> Consider Ernesto Plachutta, the older man with severe cancer pain. Establishing a therapeutic relationship would be crucial to promote Mr. Plachutta's comfort. Listening to the patient and understanding his beliefs would provide the nurse with a solid foundation on which to develop an appropriate plan of care collaboratively with the patient to achieve mutually acceptable outcomes.

Manipulating Factors Affecting the Pain Experience
Removing or Altering the Cause of Pain

Removing or altering the cause of the pain is ideal and sometimes possible. Possible measures that promote comfort and help in pain relief include removing or loosening a tight binder, if permissible; seeing to it that a distended bladder is emptied; taking steps to relieve constipation and flatus; chang-

Through the Eyes of a Patient

I've always thought of myself as a "take charge" kind of person. It's important for me in my business to be calm and always in control of my emotions. The "big C" changed everything for me. A recent hospitalization made me take time to think about what's happening to me.

Even in the hospital, I had a steady stream of visitors—some friends and some business associates. Even the mayor stopped by to see me! For all of them, I was my usual self—smiling, joking, and acting as if everything was normal. I made sure I took my pain medicine before they came. I kept all my fears about cancer and dying hidden behind my smiling face. I never broke down—not even in front of my wife! Men aren't supposed to cry, you know!

One nurse's simple gesture changed all that. One evening after all my visitors, my wife, and my son had left, she must have sensed something. She came over, stood next to me, put her arm around my shoulders and quietly said, "You know, Bob, it's alright to cry." It was like the dam opened up. I looked at her, my face cracked, and all of a sudden I couldn't stop sobbing. She must have known that I needed to talk about what was happening to me. I needed to say those words out loud to someone—"I'm afraid the pain will get too bad! I'm afraid of dying. I can't let my family see me this way!" She just let me cry, kept holding my hands, and just by being there and listening, helped me at that particular moment in ways that you will never know.

ing body positions and ensuring correct body alignment; and changing soiled linens and dressings that may be irritating the skin. A hungry or thirsty patient may need a snack or a drink to feel more comfortable.

Certain drugs are useful for removing or altering the intensity of painful stimuli. For example, drugs that decrease smooth muscle spasms in the GI tract and those that decrease contractions of skeletal muscles reduce discomfort.

Altering Factors Affecting Pain Tolerance

As a result of the pain assessment and the trusting relationship he or she has established, the nurse is better able to identify those factors that are increasing the patient's pain experience and decreasing his or her pain tolerance. **Pain tolerance** is the point beyond which a person is no longer willing to endure pain. These factors should be alleviated whenever possible. For example, patients whose families have never acknowledged their pain and who have repeatedly been told that their pain is all in their head may experience a greater ability to deal with their pain when someone finally takes the pain seriously. Nursing measures include communication to the patient that responses to pain are acceptable and education of the patient's family.

Fatigue tends to increase pain, therefore, promoting rest is helpful. The patient in pain usually feels more comfortable when the environment is quiet and restful. Although sensory restrictions, such as eliminating unnecessary noise and bright lights, are usually indicated, it is rarely helpful to leave the patient alone in an environment with little sensory input. The patient is then more likely to focus on self and the discomfort.

Lack of knowledge, finding no meaning in the pain, being pessimistic about its relief, and fear may also interfere with the patient's ability to deal with pain. Common fears include a loss of control and embarrassment by being unable to deal with the pain maturely. Another fear may be a fear of taking pain relief medication. The patient may view the need for medication as a sign of weakness or may fear addiction or loss of the effectiveness at a later date. Older patients, in particular, are frequently frustrated by similar concerns about pain management.

Initiating Nonpharmacologic (Complimentary and Alternative) Relief Measures

Although analgesics are usually the primary treatment measure for pain, a growing trend is seen involving integration of complementary, nonpharmacologic measures with conventional medical treatment. These interventions are varied and can be practiced in all healthcare settings by most members of the healthcare team.

Distraction

Conscious attention often appears to be necessary to experience pain, whereas preoccupation with other things has been observed to distract the patient from pain. Distraction requires the patient to focus attention on something other than the pain. It is not entirely clear whether distraction raises the threshold of pain or increases pain tolerance. Many patients whose pain is relieved by distraction report being able to place pain in the periphery of awareness. This is compatible with the theory that if the reticular formation in the brainstem receives sufficient sensory input, it can ignore or block out select sensations such as pain. The Lamaze method of childbirth is one common example involving the use of distraction.

Distraction alone may relieve mild pain. However, it is most effective when used before pain begins or soon thereafter. It has also been proven effective when used with analgesics for treatment of a brief episode of severe pain (eg, pain that accompanies a diagnostic procedure). Distraction may also be used successfully with children.

> *Recall Xavier Malton, the child with ulcerative colitis in severe pain? The nurse could incorporate the use of nonpharmacologic measures for pain relief, such as distraction, to enhance the effectiveness of analgesics.*

Techniques that distract attention include the following:
- Visual distractions: counting objects, reading, or watching TV
- Auditory distractions: listening to music
- Tactile kinesthetic distractions: holding or stroking a loved person, pet, or toy; rocking; slow rhythmic breathing
- Project distractions: playing a challenging game, performing meaningful play or work

Humor

Humor can be an effective distraction, can help an individual cope with pain, and may even have a positive effect on the immune system. It has been proven particularly effective before painful procedures, and many pain, cancer, and ambulatory care centers encourage patients to view humorous videos before a painful, tedious procedure (Pasero, 1998b). Rothrock (1999) discussed guidelines for using humor with patients (Box 41-2). Remember to use humor only with patients who are responsive to its use and wish to use it. Humor should not be used in

---

BOX 41-2 Using Humor to Help Patients Cope With Pain

Laughter is good medicine for our patients. Twenty years ago, Norman Cousins wrote his book, *Anatomy of an Illness as Perceived by the Patient: Reflections on Healing and Regeneration.* In this book, he recounted the value of humor and how 10 minutes of laughter gave him hours of pain-free sleep. Since then, there have been a number of studies on laughter in patient care situations. In one study, patients with chronic cancer pain rated laughter as the most effective self-initiated, nonpharmacologic measure they used to cope with pain. In another study, patients who listened to laughter-inducing tapes had higher pain thresholds, and this persisted for 10 minutes after the chuckling subsided. Some healthcare institutions have humor carts, humor baskets, and even humor rooms for patients. These may contain CDs, audiotapes, and videotapes of situation comedies; movies; stand-up comedy acts; and reading materials such as comic books and humorous magazines. Some carts even contain playful items, such as soap bubbles, wind-up toys, games, magic tricks, puppets, fingerpaints, and playdough—and this is not reserved for the pediatric ward. However, sources of humor should not be offensive (it is suggested that they have a "G" rating—for general audiences—and be age appropriate).

General guidelines for using humor with patients include using it only with those who are responsive to its use and wish to use it. Humor should not be used in patients with moderate to severe pain, nor should it be a replacement for pharmacologic analgesia. It is important, as it is in most nursing interventions, that the humor be patient specific. Thus, the nurse will need to determine what (or who, like Jack Benny or Lucille Ball or a Disney character) makes a patient laugh, how the patient has used humor or play in the past, and how it helped. Let the patient select the humorous materials, and when possible, incorporate strategies that include the patient's family and friends.

Nurses are often involved in procedures that are painful to their patients. Using humor is one nursing intervention that can be initiated after assessing the patient's interest and willingness and then evaluating its effectiveness.

Adapted from Rothrock, J. C. (1999). Laughter: The attitude worth catching. *First Hand, 14*(1), 5–6.

patients with moderate to severe pain, nor should it be a replacement for pharmacologic analgesia. In addition, humor must be patient specific. Thus, the nurse will need to determine what makes a patient laugh, how the patient has used humor or play in the past, and how it helped. Let the patient select the humorous materials, and when possible, incorporate strategies that include the patient's family and friends.

Music

Listening to music can relax, soothe, decrease pain, and provide distraction. By stimulating the release of endorphins, music enhances one's sense of well-being and decreases the need for pain medication. Patients can select the music they prefer to be used for relaxation before, during, and after surgical experiences, or to help focus on breathing techniques during labor. It has also been proven effective for soothing agitated newborns and comatose patients.

Imagery

Patients who use imagery (an example of mind–body interaction) to decrease pain sensation imagine something that involves one or all of the senses, concentrate on that image, and gradually become less aware of the pain. Imagery may be as simple as a child thinking of "happy things" (a beloved pet, lollipops, Christmas morning, Grandmom's lap), or as involved as an adult recreating a favorite place and then experiencing the healing presence or touch of a loved person or the healing energies of nature in that setting. The imagery technique has also been used to create an image in which the cause of the pain is visualized and then overcome or counteracted by some more powerful image.

Imagery has been found to be more effective for patients with chronic pain than for patients with acute, severe pain. General techniques for successfully guiding a patient to use imagery include the following:

- Help the patient to identify the problem or goal.
- Suggest that the patient begin the imagery with several minutes of focused breathing, relaxation, or meditation.
- Help the patient to develop images of the problem, as well as personal internal resources (eg, coping strategies) and external healing therapies (eg, medications, treatments).
- Encourage images of the desired state of well-being at the end of the session.

If the patient becomes restless or upset, the imagery experience is terminated and attempted later when the patient seems better disposed. Guided imagery is also discussed in Chapter 32.

Relaxation

Relaxation techniques reduce skeletal muscle tension and lessen anxiety. By assisting the patient with relaxation techniques, the nurse acknowledges the patient's pain and expresses a willingness to help the patient relieve the distress caused by his or her pain. The positive effects of relaxation for the person with pain include the following (LeMone & Burke, 2004):

- Improved quality of sleep
- Distraction from the pain
- Decreased fatigue
- Increased confidence and sense of self-control in coping with pain
- Lessening of the detrimental physiologic effects of continued or repeated stress from pain
- Increased effectiveness of other pain relief measures
- Improved ability to tolerate pain
- Decreased distress or fear during anticipation of pain
- Reassurance that the nurse is aware of his or her problem and wants to help

Relaxation is most effective as a pain alleviator when combined with slow, deep, easy breathing from the abdomen or diaphragm, with the patient's eyelids closed or with the individual focusing on a real or imagined fixed spot. Relaxation techniques are also discussed in Chapter 32.

Cutaneous Stimulation

The success of cutaneous stimulation (techniques that stimulate the skin's surface) in relieving pain is often explained using the gate control theory. The gate control theory of pain postulates that cutaneous nerve fibers are large-diameter fibers carrying impulses to the CNS. When the skin is stimulated, pain is believed to be controlled by closing the gating mechanism in the spinal cord. This decreases the number of pain impulses that reach the brain for perception. These techniques can be used in all healthcare settings to supplement a pain-control regimen. Some forms of cutaneous stimulation include the following:

- Massage (with or without analgesic ointments or liniments containing menthol); see Skill 41-1
- Application of heat or cold, or both intermittently (explained in detail in Chap. 38)
- Acupressure
- Transcutaneous electrical nerve stimulation (TENS)

Acupressure, a modern-day Western descendant of acupuncture, involves the use of the fingertips to create gentle but firm pressure to usual acupuncture sites. This technique of holding and releasing various pressure points has a calming effect, most likely related to the body's release of endorphins and enkephalins. Acupressure is easily taught to patients and families. Since the patients can perform acupressure on themselves, it gives them a feeling of control in their care.

TENS is a noninvasive alternative technique that involves electrical stimulation of large-diameter fibers to inhibit transmission of painful impulses carried over small-diameter fibers. The TENS unit consists of a battery-powered portable unit, lead wires, and cutaneous electrode pads that are applied to the painful area (Fig. 41-7). It requires a physician's order. TENS therapy has reportedly been effective in reducing postoperative pain and improving mobility after surgery. Positive results have also been noted when it is used as an adjunct with physical therapy and for patients with low back pain. The TENS unit may be applied intermittently throughout the day or worn for extended periods of time, depending on the physician's order.

SKILL 41-1   Giving a Back Massage

EQUIPMENT

Massage lubricant or lotion
Powder

Bath blanket
Towel

ACTION	RATIONALE
1. Explain the procedure and offer back massage to the patient.	Back massage can facilitate circulation and promote relaxation.
2. Perform hand hygiene.	Hand hygiene deters the spread of microorganisms.
3. Close the curtain or door.	Privacy increases relaxation.
4. Assist the patient to the prone position or side-lying position with the back exposed from the shoulders to the sacral area. Use the bath blanket to drape the patient. Raise the bed to the high position and lower the side rail closest to you.	This position exposes an adequate area for massage with privacy and warmth maintained. Having the bed in the high position reduces back strain for the nurse.
5. Warm the lubricant or lotion in the palm of your hand or place the container in warm water.	Cold lotion causes chilling and uncomfortable sensation.
6. Using light gliding strokes (*effleurage*), apply lotion to patient's shoulders, back, and sacral area.	Effleurage relaxes the patient and lessens tension.
7. Place your hands beside each other at the base of the patient's spine and stroke upward to the shoulders and back downward to the buttocks in slow, continuous strokes. Continue for several minutes.	Continuous contact is soothing and stimulates circulation and muscle relaxation.
8. Massage the patient's shoulders, entire back, areas over iliac crests, and sacrum with circular stroking motion. Keep your hands in contact with the patient's skin. Continue for several minutes, applying additional lotion as necessary.	A firmer stroke with continuous contact promotes relaxation.
9. Knead the patient's skin by gently alternating grasping and compression motions (*pétrissage*).	Kneading increases blood circulation to areas.
10. Complete the massage with additional long stroking movements.	Long stroking motion is soothing and promotes relaxation.
11. During massage, observe the patient's skin for reddened or open areas. Pay particular attention to the skin over bony prominences.	Pressure may interfere with circulation and lead to development of decubitus ulcers. Backrub stimulates circulation to these areas.
12. Use the towel to pat the patient dry and to remove excess lotion. Apply powder if the patient requests it.	This provides additional comfort for the patient.
13. Perform hand hygiene.	Hand hygiene deters the spread of microorganisms.
14. Assess the patient's response and record your observations on the patient's chart.	This provides accurate documentation of the procedure and condition of the patient's skin.

Use of cutaneous stimulation is limited because the pain must be localized. Otherwise it is most likely too diffuse to be effective. In addition, most individuals cannot tolerate stimulation of the painful area; they may, however, be helped by stimulation of the surrounding or contralateral area.

Acupuncture

Acupuncture is a technique that uses needles of various lengths inserted into specific parts of the body to produce insensitivity to pain. The technique was developed in China and has been used for centuries in many Asian countries. It has gained acceptance in the Western world as an alternative intervention to help control discomfort from disorders such as headaches, menstrual cramps, postoperative dental pain, low back pain,

and carpal tunnel syndrome. The relief of pain by acupuncture is generally explained on the basis of the gate control theory. Self-hypnosis may also account for some of acupuncture's success. Repeated treatments are often needed.

Percutaneous electrical nerve stimulation (PENS) is a complementary therapy used particularly for the management of acute and chronic pain syndromes. This form of acupuncture combines the advantages of both electroacupuncture and TENS and consists of needle probes being placed into soft tissue to stimulate peripheral sensory nerves that relate to the area of injury or pain. The electrical stimulus that is delivered bypasses the skin barrier and goes directly to the involved nerve. PENS has been shown to be effective when dealing with chronic low back pain as well as diabetic neuropathy pain.

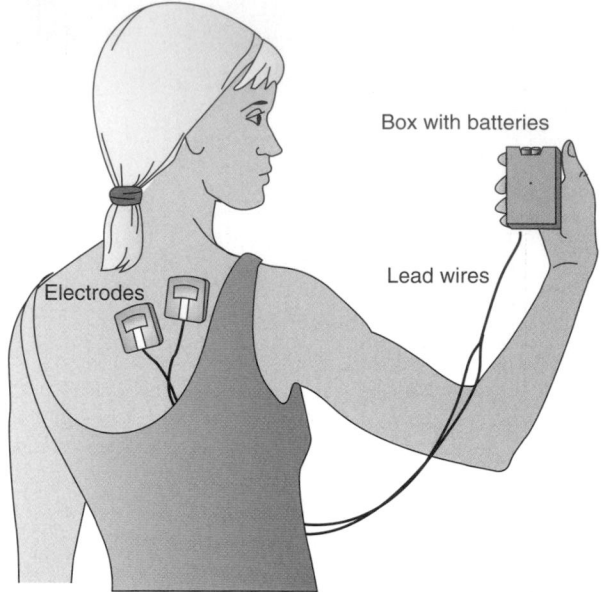

FIGURE 41-7 Three major components of a TENS unit with two electrodes placed on the upper back of the patient to relieve shoulder pain. This shows the size of the TENS unit in relation to an adult body, illustrating that it is small and portable. (From McCaffery, M., & Beebe, A. [1989]. *Pain: Clinical manual for nursing practice* (p. 158). St. Louis: C. V. Mosby.)

Hypnosis

Hypnosis, a technique that produces a subconscious state accomplished by suggestions made by a hypnotist, has been used successfully in many instances to control pain. The person's state of consciousness is altered by suggestions so that pain is not perceived as it normally would be. According to many hypnotists, it also alters the physical signs of pain. Many people can be taught autohypnosis, that is, self-induced hypnosis, for the control of pain. It is generally believed that a successful response to hypnosis is related to the individual's openness to suggestion, belief that hypnosis will work, and emotional readiness.

Biofeedback

Biofeedback is a technique that uses a machine to monitor physiologic responses through electrode sensors on the patient's skin. The feedback signal or unit transforms the physiologic data into a visual display. Upon seeing pain-related responses, such as increased muscle tension or elevated blood pressure, the patient is taught to regulate this physiologic response and control pain by practicing techniques such as deep-breathing exercises, progressive relaxation exercises, or visual imagery. Biofeedback decreases the individual's pain by reducing the anxiety associated with lack of control over bodily functions, distracts the person's attention from the pain to concentration on the person's inner state and the feedback signal, and reduces the cause of the pain. Eventually, the desired effect is for an individual to produce the expected effect without the use of the biofeedback machinery. Limitations of this method include the high degree of motivation needed and difficulty of maintaining control after the training program.

Therapeutic Touch

Therapeutic touch is an alternative therapy that involves using one's hands to direct an energy exchange consciously from the practitioner to the patient to facilitate healing or pain relief. It is viewed by many as a powerful adjunct to pain relief therapy. Patients who have received therapeutic touch state that it helps with feelings of comfort, calmness, and well-being (Newshan & Schuller-Civitella, 2003). It is derived from the ancient practice of laying on of hands, but nurses skilled in therapeutic touch never actually touch their patients when using this technique. Therapeutic touch was developed by nurses, does not require a physician's order, and can be used in any setting. Nurses caring for patients with terminal diseases relate that therapeutic touch complements their efforts to alleviate suffering and can be used to promote comfort during the final stages of life.

Managing Pharmacologic Relief Measures

Whether pain is acute or chronic, measures exist to control most pain experiences. However, many misconceptions still exist about pain relief and, because of this, many people still receive inadequate pain treatment and suffer needlessly. To make informed decisions and individualize care, nurses need updated information and ongoing education about drug therapy, the cornerstone of many pain-treatment regimens.

Analgesic Administration

An **analgesic** is a pharmaceutical agent that relieves pain. Analgesics function to reduce the person's perception of pain and to alter the person's responses to discomfort. There are three general classes of drugs used for pain relief:
- Nonopioid analgesics (acetaminophen and nonsteroidal anti-inflammatory drugs [NSAIDs])
- Opioids or narcotic analgesics (all controlled substances; eg, morphine, codeine, meperidine, methadone)
- Adjuvant drugs (anticonvulsants, antidepressants, and multipurpose drugs)

The nurse administering analgesics needs to combine a healthy respect for the drug being administered with a thorough knowledge of its mechanism of action, side effects, and administration guidelines. This combination of knowledge of and respect for the drug should result in analgesics being used wisely to produce their desired effect.

Knowledge of common analgesics enables the nurse to tailor the patient's regimen and communicate professionally with physicians about a patient who is being undermedicated or who needs a different drug or route of administration. Nurses should not refrain from using analgesics or reduce their doses because of an unrealistic fear of their potency and side effects.

Repeated studies have demonstrated that pain is frequently undertreated. Physician, nurse, and patient variables all contribute to this situation. Physicians often prescribe insufficient analgesic doses because of a tendency to overestimate the efficacy and duration of analgesics, underestimate the pain experience, and worry excessively about the possibility of respiratory problems and addiction. Nurses, who ideally spend the most time with the patient and who are supposed experts in human responses (eg, the response to pain), often compound this problem by further reducing the insufficient analgesic dose or by not administering the medication at all. Nurse variables include the low priority given to pain management; arbitrary pain assessments and erroneous judgments about a patient's pain and need for analgesia; and fear of being the person who administers the drug that causes respiratory depression or another serious side effect. The inability of many patients to discuss their pain and to request pain assistance perpetuates this problem.

Opioid Analgesics

Opioids are generally considered the major class of analgesics used in the management of moderate to severe pain because of their effectiveness. In sufficient dosage, they are considered capable of relieving pain of virtually every nature. **Opioids** produce analgesia by attaching to opioid receptors in the brain. Morphine, the prototype opioid, is available in multiple dosage forms, has a fairly predictable action, and is relatively inexpensive. The most common side effects associated with opioid use are sedation, nausea, and constipation. Most side effects disappear with prolonged use, but if constipation persists, it usually responds to treatment with increased fluids and fiber and use of a mild laxative.

Respiratory depression is a commonly feared side effect of opioid use. In reality, it is an uncommon occurrence in long-term therapy because patients have usually developed a tolerance to the drug and its respiratory depressant effects. If respiratory depression is suspected, it is usually preceded by sedation. Nursing assessment using the numeric sedation scale that follows can determine those patients at risk for respiratory depression (McCaffery and Pasero, 1999).

1 = awake and alert; no action necessary
2 = occasionally drowsy but easy to arouse; requires no action
3 = frequently drowsy and drifts off to sleep during conversation; decrease the opioid dose
4 = somnolent with minimal or no response to stimuli; discontinue the opioid and consider use of naloxone

If respiratory depression is suspected and the opioid dose is withheld, the patient may be physically stimulated by shaking or using a loud sound, along with reminders every few minutes to breathe deeply. If this is ineffective, naloxone (Narcan), an opioid antagonist that reverses the respiratory-depressant effect of an opioid, can be used. Naloxone is administered intravenously very slowly. Within 1 to 2 minutes, the patient usually opens his or her eyes and is able to respond to the nurse. When the patient is alert again and the respiratory rate is greater than 9 breaths/min, the opioids may be resumed.

Many myths and irrational fears persist concerning the use of opioid analgesics. Patients and caregivers cite fear of addiction as a reason for ineffective treatment of pain. Because of this, nurses are concerned about administering prescribed doses of opioids, physicians underprescribe pain medication, and patients refuse or take less than prescribed doses of the drugs. **Physical dependence** and tolerance are frequently confused with **addiction.** Physical dependence is a phenomenon in which the body physiologically becomes accustomed to the opioid and suffers withdrawal symptoms if the opioid is suddenly removed. Tolerance occurs when the body becomes accustomed to the opioid and needs a larger dose each time for pain relief. Addiction is a pattern of compulsive opioid use for means other than pain control. McCaffery and Ferrell (1999) report that fewer than 1% of patients with pain become addicted to opioids, yet many nurses surveyed seriously overestimated the likelihood of addiction when opioids are used for pain relief. Opioid tolerance and physical addiction are common with chronic opioid use, but this is not the same as the psychological dependence of addiction. The tolerance and physical dependence that can occur after 4 weeks of regular opioid use and result in a decrease in analgesic effect can be treated by increasing the dose until pain control is again apparent. The American Pain Society recommends that opioid doses that are safe but ineffective can be increased by 25% to 50% to control pain that is unrelieved (McCaffery & Ferrell, 1999).

Nonopioid Analgesics

Nonopioid analgesics are usually the drugs of choice for mild to moderate pain. The simplest dosage schedules and least invasive pain management modalities should be used first. Many times, these drugs alone can provide adequate pain relief. Nonsteroidal anti-inflammatory drugs (NSAIDs) also have an anti-inflammatory effect. Many of these medications are over-the-counter (OTC) products, whereas some are available by prescription only. Some can cause gastric side effects, but these symptoms may be preventable if the drug is taken with food or antacids. Individual responses to the NSAIDs vary, but these agents are contraindicated in patients with bleeding disorders (their action may interfere with platelet function) or probable infections (NSAIDs can mask the signs of an infection). The combination of nonopioid analgesics and opioids provides more analgesia than either drug taken alone.

Adjuvant Drugs

Adjuvant drugs or analgesics are used to enhance the effect of opioids by providing additional pain relief. They may also reduce side effects from prescribed opioids or lessen anxiety about the pain experience. Commonly used adjuvant drugs include corticosteroids, anticonvulsants, and antidepressants.

General Principles for Analgesic Administration

When using medications for pain relief, the nurse must first assess the patient's pain and understand the patient's goals for pain relief. In the home as well as in acute care settings, nurses provide quality nursing care when they empower patients to take charge of their own pain relief measures. The following guidelines are recommended for effective, individualized pain management in any setting (Salmore, 2002):

• Review the pain scale of choice thoroughly.
• Discuss the benefits of using a pain scale.
• Try various pain control measures.
• Use pain control measures before pain increases in severity.
• Ask the patient what has proved effective for pain relief in the past.

- Select and modify pain control measures based on the patient's response.
- Encourage the patient to try the pain treatment several times before labeling it ineffective.
- Be open-minded about alternative pain relief strategies.
- Be persistent.
- Be a safe practitioner.

Various organizations and groups have made recommendations for pain control in a variety of settings. These include the American Pain Society, the National Institutes of Health National Center for Nursing Research, and the American Nurses Association. The revised JCAHO standards ensure that pain management is a quality-assurance issue in healthcare agencies (Pasero, Gordon, & McCaffery, 1999).

In the home, oral morphine is still the drug of choice to control chronic pain and to moderate severe acute pain. This method is less expensive and easy to administer but requires that the patient is able to swallow and retain food and fluids. Accurate documentation is imperative to determine effectiveness of the current regimen or the need to change pain control measures if relief is not obtained. Effective patient and family teaching is the cornerstone of pain relief therapy in the home.

Ongoing Assessment

Just as the pain experience of each patient is unique, so too is the response of each patient to a prescribed analgesic. The nurse continually needs to evaluate whether the medication is producing the desired analgesic effect; identify changes in the patient's condition (correction or worsening of pathology, increased drug tolerance) that necessitate changes in the analgesic agent, dose, or route of administration; and identify the development of side effects of the analgesic that may warrant its discontinuance. As long as the patient's pain exists, ongoing assessment and documentation of pain control is imperative. Figure 41-8 depicts an example of a pain control record used in a home setting. Fundamental to this assessment is the knowledge of the basic action, doses, routes of administration, side effects, and administration guidelines of the analgesic being administered.

Timing is an important consideration when administering analgesics. To time analgesics appropriately, know the average duration of action for the drug and time administration so that the peak analgesic effect occurs when the pain is expected to be most intense. For example, an analgesic would be offered before ambulating a patient postoperatively.

A p.r.n. (as needed) drug regimen has not been proven effective for people experiencing acute pain. In the early postoperative period, when pain is expected, this protocol may result in an intense pain experience for the patient. Later, however, in the postoperative course, a p.r.n. schedule may be acceptable to relieve occasional pain episodes. Continuous intravenous infusion of opioids has proved effective for the relief of acute postoperative pain. Patient-controlled analgesia and epidural analgesia are discussed later in the chapter.

The p.r.n. protocol is totally inadequate for patients experiencing chronic pain. Regular administration of analgesics, or around-the-clock (ATC) administration (at regularly scheduled intervals), has been shown to offer superior pain management

for chronic cancer pain. Long-acting controlled-release oral morphine or use of a fentanyl patch have been proven effective for this type of pain.

Breakthrough pain (a temporary flare-up of moderate to severe pain that occurs even when the patient is taking ATC medication for persistent pain) is treated more effectively with supplemental doses of an opioid taken on a p.r.n. basis rather than an increase in the dose of the ATC medication. However, the frequent need for rescue pain medication when taking a long-acting opioid may necessitate an increase in the ATC medication dose. It is best if the rescue or breakthrough drug is the same as that used for ATC pain control. Breakthrough pain can be classified as either incident pain (eg, pain caused by movement) or end-of-dose pain, where the pain occurs before the next dose of analgesic is due. Although it usually occurs in patients with chronic pain, it can occur in acute situations, such as a patient with postoperative pain. The dose of the breakthrough drug is usually calculated as 10% to 15% of the total daily ATC dose. If there is an increase in the ATC dose, it is important to recalculate the breakthrough dose to provide adequate pain control (McCaffery & Pasero, 2003).

Acute Pain Management Treatment Regimens

As a patient's advocate, ensure that a strong emphasis is placed on the need for aggressive, individualized strategies that can minimize or eliminate acute pain and promote positive patient outcomes. Preventing pain is easier than treating it once it has occurred. Discuss pain control options with patients before surgery, and address the patient's responsibility regarding reporting pain. Additional nursing interventions that can eliminate acute postoperative pain include maintaining a steady serum level of the analgesic (PCA or epidural analgesia can help here), treating side effects quickly and aggressively, encouraging use of nondrug complementary therapies as adjuncts to the medical regimen, and expecting incident pain and dealing with it.

Undertreatment of pain that accompanies procedures, whether performed in a hospital, home, or outpatient clinic, is a common occurrence. If there is any doubt about the likelihood of pain resulting from a procedure, analgesia should be provided. In some instances, for example, if the patient is unable to communicate verbally, it may be necessary to provide a method for the patient to indicate that pain is occurring during a procedure. A simple raising of a finger or hand or squeeze of a squeak toy can alert the caregiver that analgesia is needed.

Cancer or Chronic Pain Management Treatment Regimens

Individuals with cancer sometimes suffer needlessly from pain. This pain, surprisingly, remains undertreated in both children and adults, and nurses need to act as advocates for pain relief for these patients. The major principles that guide treatment for chronic pain include:

- Give medications orally, if possible.
- Administer medication ATC rather than on a p.r.n. basis.
- Adjust the dose to achieve maximum benefits with minimal side effects.

Pain Control Record

This is a record of how your pain medicines are working. Please keep this record until you and your nurse/doctor find the dose and frequency of medicine that provides satisfactory pain relief for you most of the time. After that, you only need to keep this record when you have problems related to your pain medicines.

Name: _Martin_   Date: _Friday_

GOALS Satisfactory pain rating: _5_   Activities: _Sleep through the night; walk around the house_

My pain rating scale:

```
|---|---|---|---|---|---|---|---|---|---|
0   1   2   3   4   5   6   7   8   9   10
No              Moderate            Worst
pain              pain             possible
                                     pain
```

Directions: Rate your pain before you take pain medicine and 1 to 2 hours later.

Time:	Pain rating:	Medicine I took:	Side effects (drowsy, upset stomach?)	Other:
12:15 a.m.	6	30 MS IR	No	
3	6	30		can't sleep
5:15	5	30		
8:30	6	30 + ibuprofen + MS Contin		staying in bed
10:30	4			MS IR 45 8 p.m. MS Contin 150 mg
11	6	45		
12	3			

If Pain is greater than _5_ , or if you have other problems with your pain medicine, call:

Nurse: Name/phone _C. Adams   555-1234_

Doctor: Name/phone _Jones   555-4321_

This patient has been receiving the following analgesics ATC every day: ibuprofen, 400 mg qid; amitriptyline, 100 mg HS; MS Contin, 100 mg q12h (8 AM and 8 PM). His supplemental (breakthrough, rescue) dose is morphine immediate release (MS IR), 30 mg PO q2h. He usually takes two supplemental doses a day. This has relieved his pain to a 3 or less, and he has been able to sleep through the night uninterrupted by pain and walk around his home. The record reveals that his pain ratings are now greater than 3 and that he is taking supplemental doses every 3 to 4 hours. Pain keeps him awake and he stays in bed. The patient talks with the nurse at 10:30 AM. The nurse contacts the physician and the decision is to increase his morphine doses by 50% to 45 mg MS IR q2h and to MS Contin 150 mg q12h. (This dose of MS Contin requires five 30-mg tablets. However, depending on the tablet strength the patient has on hand, the MS Contin dose may be slightly more or less than 150 mg.) When an opioid dose is safe but ineffective, a 50% increase will usually produce a moderate increase in pain relief. When the patient takes more than two supplemental doses during a 12-hour period, the controlled-release should be increased.

FIGURE 41-8 Patient pain control record: patient example. (From McCaffery, M., & Pasero, C. [1999]. *Pain: Clinical manual* [p. 37]. St. Louis: Mosby, Inc.). May be duplicated for use in clinical practice.

- Allow patients as much control as possible over their medication regimen.

In an effort to alleviate unnecessary pain and suffering, the World Health Organization (WHO) has devised a three-step analgesic ladder (Fig. 41-9) that recommends the appropriate progression of drugs and dosages that should be used to manage chronic pain effectively. Emphasis is on individualizing treatment and using the analgesic ladder to provide attentive, aggressive pain relief.

Pain Treatment in Special Populations

Children

Effective pain management in children requires careful assessment; good communication between patient, family, and caregivers; and understanding of the actions and side effects of drugs used to relieve pain. The child is still the best source of information about the pain, and various assessment tools mentioned previously help to measure the intensity of the pain.

Remember Xavier Malton, the child with ulcerative colitis in acute pain? The nurse needs to assess Xavier continually for effectiveness of the prescribed analgesic and request changes in any orders if the analgesic is not effective. Considering Xavier's current state, suggesting that the physician change the analgesic administration from p.r.n. dosing to around the clock dosing may be appropriate for a short period of time.

In postoperative situations, children need analgesics ATC or by continuous infusion, and opioids are the drug of choice for mod-

erate to severe pain. Pain management for cancer pain or chronic pain in children follows the prescription outlined in the WHO analgesic ladder. Withholding opioid drugs from children with cancer because of fear of addiction is unjustified because current knowledge does not indicate they are vulnerable to this problem. Children also require pain management to minimize or alleviate the pain and distress associated with some procedures. Adequate education before the procedure and using drug and nondrug therapies to complement each other can take the pain and fear out of the experience. This is especially important for children with a chronic disease who must undergo multiple procedures as part of the treatment regimen.

Older Adults

Little research exists about pain management in older adults. Many healthcare providers, and older individuals as well, expect that pain is a natural outcome of the aging process. Opioid drugs can be used safely for these patients as long as appropriate precautions are taken, pain is conscientiously assessed, and potential side effects are monitored. The recommendation is to start opioid doses at 50% to 75% of the normal dose for a younger adult, with adjustments upward based on the older patient's response (Pasero, 1998a). The accompanying box, Focus on the Older Adult, describes additional strategies pertinent to this age group.

Additional Methods for Administering Analgesics

Patient-Controlled Analgesia

Patient-controlled analgesia (PCA) provides effective individualized analgesia and comfort. This drug delivery system may be used to manage acute and chronic pain in a healthcare facility or the home. PCA effectively relieves pain associated with operative procedures, labor and delivery, trauma situations, and cancer. This device is most commonly used to deliver analgesics intravenously, but the subcutaneous route is also an option. The most frequently prescribed drug for PCA administration is morphine.

The PCA system consists of a portable infusion pump containing a reservoir or chamber for a syringe that is prefilled with the prescribed opioid. When the sensation of pain occurs, the patient pushes a button that activates the PCA device to deliver a small preset bolus dose of the analgesic. A lockout interval that is programmed into the PCA unit (usually, 5–10 minutes) prevents reactivation of the pump and administration of another dose during that period of time. The pump mechanism can also be programmed to deliver only a specified amount of analgesic within a given time interval (most commonly every hour or, occasionally, every 4 hours). These safeguards limit the possibility of possible overmedication. In addition, time is provided for the patient to evaluate the effect of the previous dose. PCA pumps also have a locked safety system that prohibits any tampering with the device.

PCA has many advantages including the following:

- Consistent analgesic blood level is maintained rather than the inconsistent analgesia obtained with periodic intramuscular injections, which results in sharp rises and falls of serum opioid levels.

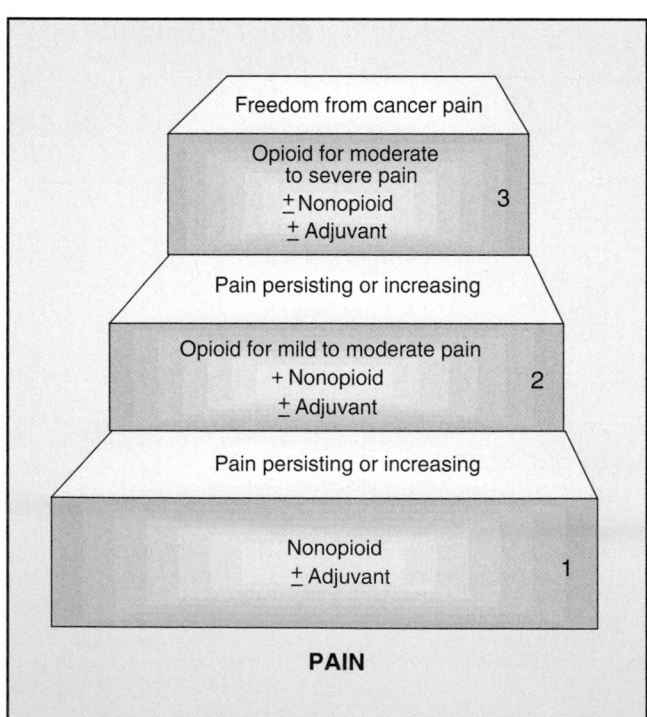

FIGURE 41-9 The WHO three-step analgesic ladder. (From World Health Organization. [1990]. *Cancer pain relief and palliative care: Report of a WHO expert committee.* WHO Tech Rep Series, No. 804. Geneva: WHO.)

Focus on the Older Adult
Nursing Strategies to Address Physiologic Changes Affecting Comfort

Age-Related Changes	Nursing Strategies
Communication Difficulties	• Observe carefully for any behavioral manifestations or indications of pain (eg, change in activity level or grimacing with movement). • Use open-ended questions to solicit information about pain. • Rely on family or caregiver to assist with information-gathering process. • Monitor for any behavior changes or confusion after medication has been taken.
Denial of Pain	• Clarify terms used to describe pain or discomfort. • Emphasize importance of reporting pain to caregivers. • Express concern about pain and a willingness to help. Explain that pain is not a normal consequence of aging.
Altered Physiologic Response to Analgesics	• Be aware of dosage and frequency to avoid oversedation and toxicity. • Monitor carefully for oversedation and respiratory depression. • Explain side effects of analgesics to patient. • Use memory aid if necessary to avoid overdosing. • Discourage self-medication. • Caution about use of alcohol with analgesics. • Caution about driving or operating machinery when taking analgesics.

• The analgesic is delivered intravenously so that absorption is faster and more predictable than with the intramuscular route.

• The patient is in charge of the pain management program.

• The patient tends to use less medication because it is self-administered before the pain becomes too severe.

• The patient is more satisfied and has improved pain relief.

An individual or child who is cognitively or physically unable to operate the PCA device may rely on a family member to act as pain manager. The nurse may also function in this role if a patient is incapable of managing PCA yet requires the consistent pain relief that this delivery system offers. A chemically dependent patient may qualify as a candidate for this pain relief strategy provided that expectations for its use are clearly stated. Careful documentation is required, indicating specifically who is responsible and how the individual's pain is being managed.

Standardized nursing responsibilities are summarized in the accompanying Examples of Nursing Interventions Classification (NIC) box. Patients need instruction preoperatively if they are expected to use the PCA device postoperatively. Suitable candidates for this type of delivery system include individuals who are alert and capable of controlling the unit. Setting up the PCA system and ensuring that it is functioning properly are additional nursing activities. Figure 41-10 demonstrates a PCA device.

Recall Sheree Lincoln, the postoperative woman who is to use PCA system for pain control? Two hours after surgery, the patient is complaining of pain but has not used the PCA system. The nurse would need to determine the underlying reasons for not using the device. This assess-ment would include investigation of Sheree's knowledge base and what, if any, teaching she received preoperatively. For example, Sheree may have received teaching on how to use PCA, but not have understood when or why to use it.

Examples of Nursing Interventions Classification (NIC) Patient-Controlled Analgesia (PCA) Assistance

• Collaborate with physicians, patient, and family members in selecting the type of narcotic to be used.

• Avoid use of meperidine (Demerol).

• Ensure that patient is not allergic to analgesic to be administered.

• Teach patient and family to monitor pain intensity, quality, and duration.

• Teach patient and family to monitor respiratory rate and blood pressure.

• Teach patient and family members how to use the PCA device.

• Assist patient or family member to administer an appropriate bolus loading dose of analgesic.

• Consult with patient, family members, and physician to adjust lockout interval, basal rate, and demand dosage, according to patient responsiveness.

• Document patient's pain, amount and frequency of drug dosing, and response to pain treatment in a pain flow sheet.

McClosky, J., & Bulechek, G. (2000). *Nursing interventions classification (NIC)* (3rd ed.) (p. 496). St. Louis: C. V. Mosby. A full listing of nursing activities for each nursing intervention can be found in this book.

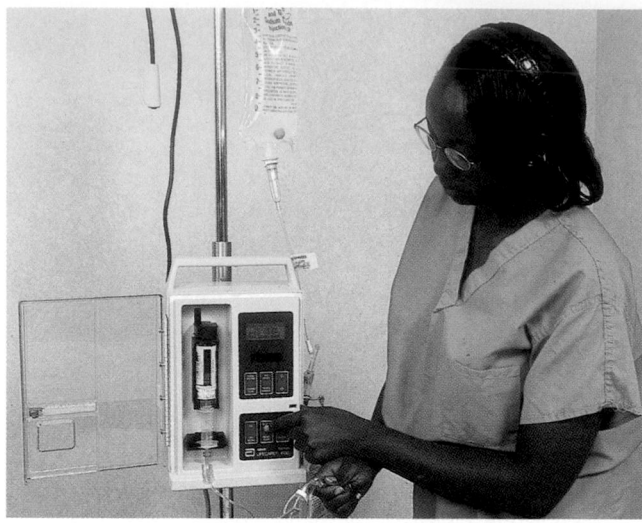

FIGURE 41-10 A patient-controlled analgesia unit allows the patient to regulate the intravenous infusion of small amounts of analgesic as needed.   (Photo by Rick Brady.)

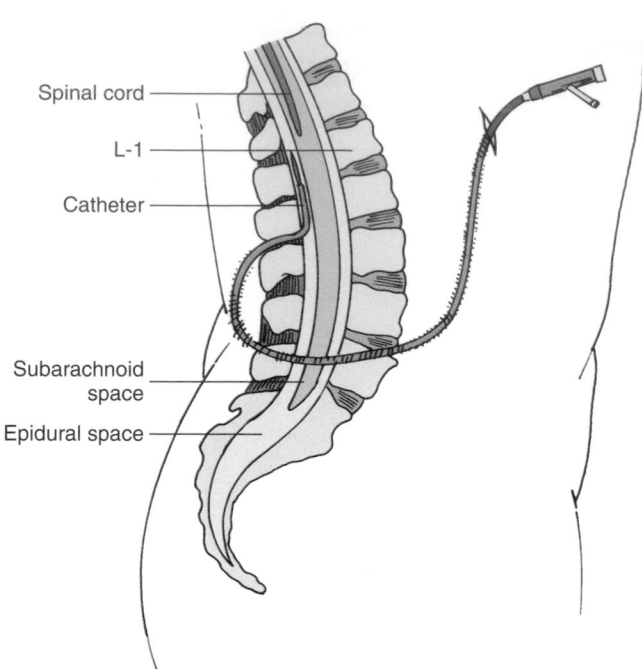

FIGURE 41-11 Placement of an epidural catheter for long-term use.

Possibly she may be wanting to avoid use of any medication. The nurse would use this opportunity to reinforce instructions for using PCA and also for other nonpharmacologic measures for pain relief, such as distraction, relaxation, massage, or imagery.

Epidural Analgesia

Epidural analgesia is being used more commonly to provide pain relief during the immediate postoperative phase (particularly after thoracic, abdominal, orthopedic, and vascular surgery) and for chronic pain situations. Epidural pain management is also being used for children with terminal cancer and for children undergoing hip, spinal, or lower extremity surgery. The anesthesiologist usually inserts the catheter in the midlumbar region into the epidural space between the walls of the vertebral canal and the dura mater or outermost connective tissue membrane surrounding the spinal cord. For temporary therapy, the catheter exits directly over the spine, and the tubing is positioned over the patient's shoulder, with the end of the catheter taped to the person's chest. For long-term therapy, the catheter is usually tunneled subcutaneously and exits on the side of the body or on the abdomen (Fig. 41-11). The narcotic or opioid acts directly on the opiate receptors in the spinal cord, and pain relief is achieved with smaller doses and less severe side effects. The epidural analgesia can be administered as a bolus dose (either one time or intermittent) via a continuous infusion pump, or by means of a patient-controlled epidural analgesia (PCEA) pump (Pasero, 2003b). The drug of choice is usually preservative-free morphine or fentanyl (Sublimaze). Since the epidural space contains blood vessels, nerves, and fat, lipid-soluble fentanyl is readily dissolved, has a rapid onset of action (5 minutes), but a short duration of action (approximately 2 hours). Morphine is a hydrophilic opioid, meaning that this drug has a high affinity for water. It has a slower onset of action but may exert its analgesic effect for as long as 24 hours because it remains longer in the cerebrospinal fluid (CSF) and spinal tissue (Pasero, 2003). Epidural catheters used for the management of acute pain are typically removed between 36 and 72 hours after surgery, when oral medication can be substituted for relief of pain.

Nursing responsibilities vary among institutions but must include careful monitoring of the patient's response to therapy, with particular attention to the respiratory rate and pattern (see Guidelines for Nursing Care 41-1). Too much narcotic or a displaced catheter may allow the medication to have a depressant effect on the brainstem center, causing life-threatening respiratory depression. Other potential side effects include hypotension, pruritus, urinary retention, nausea and vomiting, and infection or contamination.

Local Anesthesia

Anesthetic agents may be applied topically to the skin or mucous membranes or injected into the body to produce a temporary loss of sensation and motor and autonomic function in a localized area. The agents work by chemically blocking the nerve pathways involved in pain sensation and response and are sometimes called nerve blocks. Many people have experienced nerve blocks during dental work, when having a wound sutured, during delivery of a newborn, or for some minor surgical procedures. Nursing measures include noting any allergic responses the patient has had in the past to anesthetic agents, alerting the patient to the pain associated with the initial injection of the anesthetic if the physician does not numb the area first, offering emotional support to the patient during the procedure, observing for any untoward effects, and protecting the patient from injury until sensory and motor functions return. Two topical anesthetic creams (EMLA, which contains 2.5% lidocaine and 2.5% prilocaine, and ELA-Max, a 4%-lidocaine cream) provide safe, effective analgesia for

Guidelines for Nursing Care 41-1
Caring for Patients Receiving Epidural Opioids

Nursing Action	Rationale
Verify the physician's order for analgesia, drug preparation, and rate of infusion with another RN.	Verification provides for safe administration of the correct dose at the correct rate.
Keep an ampule of 0.4 mg of naloxone (Narcan) and a syringe at the bedside.	Naloxone reverses the respiratory depressant effect of opioids.
Label tubing and pump apparatus "For Epidural Infusion Only."	Labeling prevents inadvertent administration of other intravenous medications through this setup.
Assess and record sedation level (using a sedation scale) and respiratory status q 1 h for the first 24 hours followed by q 4 h intervals (or according to agency policy). Notify MD for the following: sedation rating of 3, ↓ in depth and respiratory rate below 8 breaths/min.	Opioids can depress respiratory center in the medulla. Change in level of consciousness is usually the first sign of altered respiratory function.
Keep head of bed elevated 30 degrees unless this is contraindicated.	Elevation of the patient's head minimizes upward migration of opioid in the spinal cord, thus decreasing risk for respiratory depression.
Record level of pain and effectiveness of pain relief.	Referencing helps in determining need for subsequent "breakthrough" pain medication.
Monitor urinary output and assess for bladder distention.	Opioids can cause urinary retention.
Assess motor strength q 4 h.	Catheter may migrate into the intrathecal space and allow opioids to block transmission of nerve impulses completely through the spinal cord to the brain.
Monitor for side effects (pruritus, nausea, and vomiting).	Opioids may spread into the trigeminal nerve causing itching or result in nausea and vomiting due to slowed gastrointestinal function or stimulation of a chemoreceptor trigger zone in the brain. Medications are available to treat these side effects.
Assess for signs of infection at the insertion site.	Inflammation or local infection may develop at the catheter insertion site. Strict aseptic technique and sterile dressing and tubing changes according to agency policy can prevent this complication.
Do not administer any other narcotics or adjuvant drugs without approval of clinician responsible for epidural injection.	Additional medication may potentiate the action of the opioid, thus increasing the risk for respiratory depression.

children before painful procedures such as phlebotomy, spinal tap, or bone marrow aspiration. EMLA cream is prescribed by the physician and must be covered by an occlusive dressing for at least 1 hour before the procedure to provide local pain relief. After the time period, the cream is removed. ELA-Max is an OTC preparation that does not require an occlusive dressing to cause analgesia (Wong, 2003).

Teaching the Patient and Family About Pain

Often, a well-informed person can cope better with the distress of pain and tends to experience less anxiety about pain. Teaching about pain should include family members so that they understand the concept of pain and are able to help the person in pain. The patient and family need information about the nature and causes of pain, explanation about a pain scale that can be used easily, practice with this assessment tool, and assistance to set goals for comfort and either optimal function

or recovery. Teaching to Promote Health at Home 41-1 includes specific suggestions related to safety concerns about pain control in the home setting.

Play may be used effectively to discover a child's experience of pain and to teach the child how to cope with pain. Children are usually receptive to using dolls to act out pain experiences.

Ensuring the Ethical and Legal Responsibility to Relieve Pain

Quality pain management results when patients have access to safe, effective pain relief measures. Healthcare providers, in addition to monitoring, delivering, and documenting administration of analgesics, also have responsibility to inform patients that effective pain relief is vital to their treatment. Patients also have the right to expect that their statements of pain will be heeded quickly. Institutions must assign and educate clinicians to address these issues in a timely, knowl-

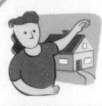

Teaching to Promote Health at Home 41-1
Comfort

Health Topic	Teaching Tip	Why Is This Important?
Safety	Do not drive vehicle or operate heavy machinery after taking pain medication.	Reflexes may be slowed and cognitive thinking decreased due to pain medications.
	Avoid alcohol and other CNS depressants while taking pain medication.	Alcohol may interact with the pain medication and further depress the CNS, leading to respiratory failure.
	Do not smoke without someone else present while taking pain medication.	The patient may become tired due to the medication, fall asleep while smoking, and start a house fire.
	Do not walk without assistance while taking pain medication.	Some pain medications can cause drowsiness, dizziness, and blurred vision.
Diet	Do not take pain medication on an empty stomach.	Many patients become nauseated if pain medication is taken on an empty stomach.
Miscellaneous	Do not breastfeed without checking with your physician while taking pain medication.	Many pain medications can be found in breast milk and may harm the baby.

edgeable manner. The Rights of Patients with Pain highlighted in Box 41-3 recognizes the multidimensional aspects of the pain experience and an individual's right to have pain controlled as soon as possible. Also, as mentioned previously in this chapter, a patient's right to effective pain control is a focus of the JCAHO.

Consider Xavier Malton, the child with acute pain. The nurses in the scenario advocated for Xavier, reinforcing his rights to have pain controlled as soon as possible.

The Placebo Controversy

The term **placebo** comes from the Latin word meaning "I shall please." It consists of an inactive substance often given to satisfy a person's demand for a drug. The person, unaware of the placebo's properties, may find it to be effective for the relief of pain because of the perception that it will provide comfort and because of belief in the person administering it. It is an injustice to judge a person experiencing relief from pain after the use of a placebo as a malingerer or as mentally ill. Various researchers have reported that a positive placebo effect may be related to a physiologic response (release of endorphins) or the patient's cultural expectations, attitudes, health beliefs, or anticipation of a positive response.

The use of placebos, however, raises serious ethical questions. Is lying to a patient justifiable? A nurse who administers a placebo must be willing to risk the possible consequence of the patient becoming aware of the duplicity and then refusing to trust the nurse or any other healthcare professional again. Patients who feel themselves to be in pain are vulnerable. If such a patient discovers a seeming plot to trick him or her into feeling better, it is unlikely that the patient will respect or appreciate the intentions of the physicians and nurses involved. The long-term effects of this practice far outweigh any of its benefits. Two nursing organizations, the Oncology Nursing Society and the American Nurses Association, oppose placebo use, and this practice may even violate state board of nursing policies. The nurse has firm legal and ethical grounds for refusing to administer a placebo.

BOX 41-3 **The Rights of Patients With Pain**

A Bill of Rights for People With Pain

1. I have the right to have my reports of pain accepted and acted on by healthcare professionals.
2. I have the right to have my pain controlled, no matter what its cause or how severe it may be.
3. I have the right to be treated with respect at all times. When I need medication for pain, I should not be treated like a drug abuser.

May be duplicated for use in clinical practice. From McCaffery, M., & Pasero, C. (1999). *Pain: Clinical manual* (p. 13). Copyright © 1999, Mosby, Inc. St. Louis.

Evaluating

As soon as a pain problem is identified and a treatment plan developed and implemented, evaluation becomes ongoing. Evaluation is directed toward the changing nature of the pain experience, the treatment modalities (pain management program), and the patient's and family's response to the plan of care, all of which overlap.

The Pain Experience

The pain the patient is experiencing may change in many ways, and the nurse must be careful not to make a judgment about this too quickly. For example, if the pain lessens in intensity or disappears, it may mean that the underlying cause of the pain is diminished or absent and that treatment should be stopped, or it may mean that the pain management program is effective and should be continued. When pain intensity increases, it may simply indicate the need for more aggressive therapy, or it may be a warning that the underlying pathology has changed or worsened and that new medical intervention is required. Often, a new problem amenable to treatment is masked by "old pain," and its detection may be delayed to the point that treatment is useless.

Treatment Modalities

The use of both noninvasive and invasive therapies must be continually evaluated to determine whether they are the best possible means the patient could use to obtain pain relief and whether they are effective with only minimal risk to the patient. Too often, a patient stays with the first analgesic prescribed without questioning whether it is the most effective drug for the particular pain, whether the dosage and timing guidelines are correct for the patient, and whether the analgesic is per-haps producing annoying or even harmful side effects that another drug would not produce. Similarly, one patient may take to progressive relaxation exercises and find them helpful, whereas another patient may obtain similar benefits from a daily walking program. Nursing time spent evaluating the effectiveness of each pain relief therapy is well spent and results in a pain management program that is truly individualized to the patient.

Patient and Family Response

Ultimately, the plan of care is unsuccessful unless the patient and family are satisfied with the results. A successful plan of care results in the achievement of specified patient outcomes valued by the patient. Whenever possible, nursing care should terminate when the patient and family can independently direct the pain management program with the assistance of appropriate resources. See the accompanying Nursing Plan of Care for Carla Potter.

NURSING PLAN OF CARE 41-1 — for Carla Potter

Carla Potter is a 26-year-old white woman. She is unmarried and has no children. She is employed at a large company as a computer programmer. During the past 7 months, she has been experiencing periodic fatigue, anxiety, irritability, depression, and mood swings. Her general health is excellent. The nurse practitioner at the gynecologist's office believes Ms. Potter may be suffering from premenstrual syndrome. The nurse practitioner who interviewed Ms. Potter noted the following data:

• Patient has generalized discomfort—fatigue, anxiety, irritability, depression, and mood swings—about 1 week before her menses; discomfort subsides after onset of menses.

• Discomforts are believed to be heightened by stress at work but do not depend on this. Patient denies any new or unusual stress in life but believes symptoms are affecting her job performance and relationships.

• Patient relates history of "bad cramps" ever since periods started. Patient lacks knowledge of appropriate dietary and stress management techniques.

• Patient relates she has occasionally taken some of her friend's "tranquilizers" to ease her through a bad day—but she prefers not to take medication.

NURSING DIAGNOSIS	Ineffective Coping related to discomforts of premenstrual symptoms as manifested by reports of fatigue, anxiety, irritability, depression, and mood swings
EXPECTED OUTCOME	By the next monthly assessment, 10/30/06, patient will: • Use relaxation techniques during periods of anxiety

Nursing Interventions	Rationale	Evaluative Statement
Assess patient's knowledge of relaxation techniques and motivation to use them.	Effective use of relaxation techniques requires a motivated patient.	10/30/06 Outcome partially met, patient used relaxation techniques during two periods of anxiety. Was driving on expressway during another period of anxiety, which made relaxation difficult.
Instruct patient regarding the use of progressive relaxation exercises and controlled breathing during periods of anxiety. For example, "Find a quiet, comfortable place and sit down. Consciously contract and relax the muscles of the whole body starting at the head and neck and working down to the feet until completely relaxed. At the same time, take slow, rhythmic breaths. Continue until anxiety passes."	Relaxation and controlled breathing are used to decrease anxiety and increase coping mechanisms.	*R. Gordon, RNC*

(continued)

NURSING PLAN OF CARE 41-1 for Carla Potter (continued)

EXPECTED OUTCOME

By the next monthly assessment, 10/30/06, the patient will:
- Use a meal plan that includes three balanced meals per day and excludes caffeine, sugar, and sodium

Nursing Interventions	Rationale	Evaluative Statement
Assess patient's nutritional intake. Have patient identify current food preferences high in caffeine, sugar, and sodium and discuss substitutes. Teach patient rationale for decreasing intake of caffeine, sugar, and sodium.	Refined sugar and caffeine contribute to feelings of tension and irritability. Sodium contributes to water retention in the body.	10/30/06 Outcome met. Patient used meal plan for three balanced meals per day and eliminated all sugar, caffeine, and sodium from diet. *R. Gordon, RNC*
Instruct patient in developing a meal plan that includes three balanced meals per day.	Balanced meals provide optimal nutrition.	

EXPECTED OUTCOME

By the next monthly assessment, 10/30/06, the patient will:
- Incorporate exercise into routine

Nursing Interventions	Rationale	Evaluative Statement
Assess value patient attaches to physical fitness and regular periods of aerobic exercise; explore preferences.	Exercise can alleviate symptoms of depression, tension, anxiety, fatigue, and irritability. Exercise also serves as a distraction from discomforts.	10/30/06 Outcome met. Patient includes daily brisk walk around her neighborhood in her routine. *R. Gordon, RNC*
Instruct patient in use of regular daily exercise; design exercise prescription.	The fitness produced by regular exercise contributes to self-esteem.	

EXPECTED OUTCOME

By the next monthly assessment, 10/30/06, the patient will:
- Supplement her diet with 50 mg of vitamin B_6 daily

Nursing Interventions	Rationale	Evaluative Statement
Instruct patient on daily use of vitamin B_6.	Vitamin B_6 may be effective in relieving symptoms of irritability, fatigue, and depression.	10/30/06 Outcome met. Patient supplements her diet daily with 50 mg of vitamin B_6. *R. Gordon, RNC*

EXPECTED OUTCOME

By the next monthly assessment, 10/30/06, the patient will:
- Continue use of daily record of premenstrual syndrome (PMS) symptoms

Nursing Interventions	Rationale	Evaluative Statement
Instruct patient to continue use of daily record of PMS symptoms throughout the menstrual cycle.	Record keeping allows evaluation of the effectiveness of care plan.	10/30/06 Outcome met. Patient continued daily record, which illustrated drastic reduction in occurrence of PMS symptoms. Patient expressed delight in greater feeling of control she now has over how she feels. "I never realized that so many things affect my comfort level and health." *R. Gordon, RNC*

(continued)

NURSING PLAN OF CARE 41-1   *for Carla Potter* (continued)

SAMPLE DOCUMENTATION

8/13/06   Nursing

Consultation with patient regarding apparent symptoms of PMS. She stated she experiences fatigue, anxiety, irritability, depression, and mood swings about 1 week before her menses. She states these symptoms interfere with her job performance and relationships. She also states that these symptoms seem to subside after onset of her menses. Patient admits to use of tranquilizers but prefers not to use medication. Advised patient to keep daily record of symptoms for one complete menstrual cycle. Patient indicated understanding of all instructions. She will return to office after completion of daily record for its analysis and to begin treatment, if indicated.

R. Gordon, RNC

Courtesy of Ruth E. Gordon, RNC, CRNP, DEd, Assistant Professor, Department of Nursing, Millersville University, Millersville, PA.

Developing Critical Thinking Skills

1. Interview a nurse who specializes in pain management. Ask the nurse to describe the various physiologic and emotional responses to pain that she has observed in patients with acute and chronic pain. Question her about the different nursing interventions most likely to be effective for patients in general experiencing either acute or chronic pain. Inquire about specific pain management information and guidelines that she usually includes in discharge planning and teaching.

2. Consider what you personally believe about pain: what it is, what causes it, what is most likely to relieve it. Determine how pain is currently being managed within the tradition of Western medicine and what role nursing plays in keeping patients pain free. Visit nontraditional health centers where practitioners use a variety of noninvasive pain relief modalities, such as acupressure, relaxation techniques, imagery, and massage. In what ways, if any, has this new learning experience modified your beliefs about pain? Will it change your ability to design effective pain management regimens for your patients?

Preparing for NCLEX

1. A patient complains of abdominal pain that is difficult to localize. The nurse categorically interprets this as
   a. Causalgia
   b. Visceral
   c. Superficial
   d. Psychogenic

2. A patient complains of pain in a cutaneous site that is different from where it originates. The nurse documents this as
   a. Transient pain
   b. Superficial pain
   c. Phantom pain
   d. Referred pain

3. A patient who has fallen and injured his wrist carefully cradles it with the other hand. The patient is demonstrating which of the following responses to pain?
   a. Behavioral
   b. Affective
   c. Physiologic
   d. Involuntary

4. To help relieve her pain, Ann concentrates on a favorite vacation setting. The nurse interprets this technique as
   a. Distraction
   b. Relaxation
   c. Recall
   d. Imagery

5. The nurse best describes intractable pain as being
   a. Intermittent in nature
   b. Resistant to treatment
   c. Excruciating
   d. Widespread

6. Applying the gate control theory of pain, an effective nursing intervention for a patient with lower back pain would be
   a. Encouraging regular use of analgesics
   b. Applying a moist heating pad to the area at prescribed intervals
   c. Reviewing the pain experience with the patient
   d. Ambulating the patient after medicating him or her

7. Which of the following would the nurse expect to assess as a physiologic response to moderate pain?
   a. Increased blood pressure
   b. Restlessness
   c. Decreased pulse rate
   d. Protection of the painful area

8. Mrs. Young is receiving ATC medication for treatment of terminal cancer. She has recently reported several episodes of breakthrough pain. What treatment is most effective to manage these sudden flare-ups of pain?

a. Increasing the dose of her ATC medication
b. Restricting her physical activity
c. Doing nothing more since her cancer is terminal
d. Supplementing with doses of a short-acting opioid

9. When assessing pain in a child, the nurse needs to be aware that
   a. Immature neurologic development results in reduced sensation of pain.
   b. Inadequate or inconsistent relief of pain is widespread.
   c. Reliable assessment tools are currently unavailable.
   d. Narcotic analgesic use should be avoided.

10. Mr. Wright is recovering from abdominal surgery. When the nurse assists him to walk, she observes that he grimaces, moves stiffly, and becomes pale. She is aware that he has consistently refused his pain medication. A priority nursing diagnosis would be
    a. Acute Pain related to fear of taking prescribed medications in the postoperative period
    b. Impaired Physical Mobility related to surgical procedure
    c. Anxiety related to outcome of surgery
    d. Risk for Infection related to surgical incision

11. When planning strategies for pain control in older patients, the nurse should be aware that
    a. Pain is a natural outcome of the aging process.
    b. Sensitivity to pain increases with age.
    c. Narcotic use should be avoided.
    d. Denial of pain may occur.

12. Chronic pain is most effectively relieved when analgesics are administered
    a. On a p.r.n. (as needed) basis
    b. Conservatively
    c. Around the clock (ATC)
    d. Intramuscularly

13. Using a placebo for pain control is
    a. A widespread practice
    b. Consistently effective
    c. Deceptive and unethical
    d. Justified to determine whether the pain is real

14. The patient receiving epidural analgesia requires careful monitoring to prevent the occurrence of
    a. Pruritus
    b. Urinary retention
    c. Nausea and vomiting
    d. Respiratory depression

15. When assessing a patient receiving a continuous opioid infusion, the nurse immediately notifies the physician when the patient has
    a. A respiratory rate of 10 with respirations of normal depth
    b. A sedation level of 4
    c. Mild confusion
    d. Reported constipation

Answers With Rationale

1. The correct response is *b*. Visceral pain is poorly localized and can originate in body organs in the abdomen. Complex regional pain syndrome (causalgia) (*a*) is pain that occurs in the area of injured peripheral nerves, whereas cutaneous pain is superficial (*c*) and usually involves the skin or sub-cutaneous tissue. When a physical cause for the pain cannot be identified, it is known as psychogenic pain (*d*).

2. The correct response is *d*. Referred pain is perceived in an area distant from its point of origin, whereas transient pain (*a*) is brief and passes quickly. Superficial pain (*b*) originates in the skin or subcutaneous tissue. Phantom pain (*c*) may occur in a person who has had a body part amputated, either surgically or traumatically.

3. The correct response is *a*. Protecting or guarding a painful area is a behavioral response. Affective responses (*b*) are psychological ones, and examples of a physiologic (*c*) or involuntary (*d*) response would be increased blood pressure and dilation of the pupils.

4. The correct response is *d*. Imagery is a mind–body interaction that decreases pain sensation by focusing on pleasurable images. Distraction (*a*) involves pre-occupation with other things to relieve pain, and relaxation (*b*) is a technique that reduces skeletal muscle tension and lessens anxiety. Recall (*c*) is not a noninvasive relief measure.

5. The correct response is *b*. Intractable pain is severe pain that is resistant to relief measures. The other terms do not describe this resistance to treatment.

6. The correct response is *b*. Nursing measures such as applying warmth to the lower back stimulate the large nerve fibers to close the gate and block the pain. The other choices do not involve attempts to stimulate large nerve fibers that interfere with pain transmission as explained by the gate control theory.

7. The correct response is *a*. Increased blood pressure is a physiologic or involuntary response to moderate pain, whereas decreased pulse rate (*c*) occurs when pain is severe and deep. Restlessness (*b*) and protection of the painful area (*d*) are behavioral responses.

8. The correct response is *d*. Breakthrough pain is best addressed by administering a short-acting opioid similar to her ATC medication. Increasing the dose of her ATC medication (*a*) also increases her risk for developing side effects. All pain can be treated effectively, and limiting physical activity (*b*) will not affect her breakthrough pain but may negatively affect her current lifestyle and self-esteem.

9. The correct response is *b*. Healthcare personnel are only now becoming aware of pain relief as a priority for children in pain. The evidence supports the fact that children do indeed feel pain (*a*), and reliable assessment tools (*c*) are available specifically for use with children. Opioid analgesics may be safely

used with children as long as they are carefully observed (*d*).

10. The correct response is *a*. Mr. Wright's immediate problem is his pain that is unrelieved because he refuses to take his pain medication for an unknown reason. The other nursing diagnoses are plausible but not a priority in this situation.

11. The correct response is *d*. Older people frequently deny pain because they view it as an ominous sign that may interfere with their independence. Pain sensitivity (*b*) may decrease with age, but even this assumption is unsafe. Pain is not a natural outcome of the aging process (*a*). Opioid medications (*c*) can be used if the older patient's response is carefully monitored and evaluated.

12. The correct response is *c*. The p.r.n. protocol (*a*) is totally inadequate for patients experiencing chronic pain. ATC doses of analgesics are more effective, whereas conservative pain management (*b*) for whatever reason may also prove ineffective. Intramuscular administration (*d*) is not practical on a long-range basis for a patient with chronic pain.

13. The correct response is *c*. Using a placebo to control pain creates distrust in the nurse–patient relationship and is considered unethical behavior. It is not a widespread practice, is ineffective, and is never used to determine whether pain is real. Pain exists when the patient says it does.

14. The correct response is *d*. Too much of an opioid drug given by way of an epidural catheter or a displaced catheter may result in the occurrence of respiratory depression. Pruritus (*a*), urinary retention (*b*), and nausea and vomiting (*c*) may occur but are not life-threatening.

15. The correct response is *b*. Sedation level is more indicative of respiratory depression because it usually precedes it. A sedation level of 4 calls for immediate action because the patient has minimal or no response to stimuli. A respiratory level of 10 with normal depth of breathing (*a*) is usually not a cause for alarm. Mild confusion (*c*) may be evident with the initial dose and then disappear; additional observation is necessary. Constipation (*d*) should be reported to the physician, but is not the priority in this situation.

Bibliography

Acello, B. (2000). Meeting JCAHO standards for pain control. *Nursing, 30*(3), 52–54.

Arnstein, P. (2002). Optimizing perioperative pain management. *AORN, 76*(5), 812–818.

Beyer, J., et al. (1992). The creation, validation, and continuing development of the Oucher: A measure of pain intensity in children. *Journal of Pediatric Nursing, 7*(5), 335.

Clinical Update: New standards for assessment and treatment of pain instituted by JCAHO. (2001), *The American Journal for Nurse Practitioners, 5*(1), 43–44.

Criste, A. (2002). AANA Journal course update for nurse anesthetists. *AANA Journal Course, 70*(6), 475–480.

Donovan, H., & Ward, S. (2001). A representational approach to patient education. *Journal of Nursing Scholarship, 33*(3), 211–216.

Dooks, P. (2001). Diffusion of pain management research into nursing practice. *Cancer Nursing, 24*(2), 99–103.

Ellis, J. (2003). Keeping pediatric patients comfortable. *Nursing, 33*(7), 22.

Griffie, J. (2003). Addressing inadequate pain relief: Effective communication among the health care team is essential. *American Journal of Nursing, 103*(8), 61–63.

Hseish, R., & Lee, W. (2002). One shot percutaneous electrical nerve stimulation vs transcutaneous electrical nerve stimulation for low back pain: Comparison of therapeutic effects. *American Journal of Physical Medicine and Rehabilitation, 81*(11), 838–843.

Joint Commission on Accreditation of Healthcare Organizations. (2000). *Joint Commission on Accreditation of Healthcare Organizations pain standards for 2001.* Available at http://jcaho.org.

Kettelman, K. (1999). Why give more morphine to a dying patient? *Nursing, 29*(11), 54–55.

Krieger, D. (1999). Therapeutic touch in hospice care. *American Journal of Nursing, 99*(4), 46.

LeMone, P., & Burke, K. (2004). *Medical-surgical nursing: Critical thinking in client care* (3rd ed.). Upper Saddle River, NJ: Pearson/Prentice Hall.

Loeb, J. (1999). Pain management in long-term care. *American Journal of Nursing, 99*(2), 48–52.

Love, G. (2000). Electrifying news about iontophoresis. *Nursing, 30*(1), 48–49.

McCaffery, M. (1979). *Nursing management of the patient with pain* (2nd ed.). Philadelphia: J. B. Lippincott.

McCaffery, M. (2003). Switching from IV to PO: Maintaining pain relief in the transition. *American Journal of Nursing, 103*(5), 62–63.

McCaffery M., & Beebe, A. (1989). *Pain: Clinical manual for nursing practice.* St. Louis: C. V. Mosby.

McCaffery, M., Ferrell, B., & Pasero, C. (1998). When the physician prescribes a placebo. *American Journal of Nursing, 98*(1), 52–53.

McCaffery, M., & Ferrell, B. (1999). Opioids and pain management: What do nurses know? *Nursing, 29*(3), 48–52.

McCaffery, M., & Pasero, C. (1999). *Pain: clinical manual* (2nd ed.). St. Louis: C. V. Mosby.

McCaffery, M. & Pasero, C. (2003). Breakthrough pain. *American Journal of Nursing, 103*(4), 83–86.

McClosky, J., & Bulechek, J. (2000). *Nursing interventions classification (NIC)* (3rd ed.). St. Louis: C. V. Mosby.

McHugh, J. M. & McHugh, W. (2000). Pain: Neuroanatomy, chemical mediators, and clinical implications. *AACN Clinical Issues, 11*(2), 168–178.

Melzak, R., & Wall, P. (1968). Gate control theory of pain. In A. Soulairac, J. Cahn, & J. Carpentier (Eds.). *Pain: Pro-*

ceedings of the international association on pain. Baltimore: Williams & Wilkins.

Newshan, G., & Schuller-Civitella, D. (2003). Large clinical study shows value of therapeutic touch program. *Holistic Nursing Practice, 17*(4), 189–192.

Nichols, R. (2003). Pain management in patients with addictive disease: A new position paper provides guidance. *American Journal of Nursing, 103*(3), 87, 89–90.

Nisbet, A. (2003). Alternative approach. Some like it hot! Closing the gate on pain with superficial heat application. *Virginia Nurses Today, 11*(2), 10.

North American Nursing Diagnosis Association. (2003). *NANDA nursing diagnosis: Definitions & classification: 2003–2004.* Philadelphia: Author.

Parke, B. (1998). Realizing the presence of pain in cognitively impaired older adults. *Journal of Gerontological Nursing, 24*(6), 21–28

Pasero, C. (1998a). How aging affects pain management. *American Journal of Nursing, 98*(6), 12–13.

Pasero, C. (1998b). Is laughter the best medicine? *American Journal of Nursing, 98*(12), 12–14.

Pasero, C. (2003a). Pain in the emergency department: Withholding pain medication is not justified. *American Journal of Nursing, 103*(7), 73–74.

Pasero, C. (2003b). Epidural analgesia for postoperative pain: Excellent analgesia and improved patient outcomes after major surgery. *American Journal of Nursing, 103*(10), 62–64.

Pasero, C., Gordon, D., & McCaffery, M. (1999). JCAHO on assessing and managing pain. *American Journal of Nursing, 99*(7), 22.

Pasero, C., & McCaffery, M. (1999). Providing epidural analgesia. *Nursing, 29*(8), 34–39.

Peloso, P. (2000). NSAIDs: A Faustian bargain. *American Journal of Nursing, 100*(6), 34–39.

Phipps, W., Monahan, F., Sands, J., Marek, J., & Neighbors, H. (2002). *Medical-surgical nursing: Health & illness perspectives* (7th ed.). St. Louis: C. V. Mosby.

Pullen, R. (2003). Managing IV patient-controlled analgesia. *Nursing, 33*(7), 24.

Rothrock, J. C. (1999). Laughter: The attitude worth catching. *First Hand, 14*(1), 5–6.

Rush, S. L., & Harr, J. (2001). Evidence-based pediatric nursing: Does it have to hurt? *AACN Clinical Issues, 12*(4), 597–605.

Salmore, R. (2002). Development of a new pain scale: Colorado behavioral numerical pain scale for sedated adult patients undergoing gastrointestinal procedures. *Gastroenterology Nursing 25*(6), 257–262.

Shea, R., Brooks, J., Dayhoff, N., & Keck, J. (2002). Pain intensity and postoperative pulmonary complications among the elderly after abdominal surgery. *Heart & Lung, 31*(6), 440–449.

Sherwood, G., McNeill, J., Starck, P., & Disnard, G. (2003). Changing acute pain management outcomes in surgical patients. *AORN, 77*(2), 374, 377–380, 384, 386–388, 390, 393–395.

Steefel, L. (2001). Treat pain in any culture. *Nursing Spectrum (Philadelphia), 10*(25), 20–21.

Stoelting, R., & Miller, R. (2000). *Basics of anesthesia* (4th ed.). Philadelphia: Churchill Livingstone.

Tanabe, P., & Buschmann, M. (2000). Emergency nurses' knowledge of pain management principles. *Journal of Emergency Nursing, 26*(4), 299–305.

Wong, D. (2003). Topical local anesthetics. *American Journal of Nursing, 103*(6), 42–44.

World Health Organization. (1990). *Cancer pain relief and palliative care: Report of a WHO expert committee.* WHO Tech Rep Series, No, 804. Geneva: WHO.

Zborowski, M. (1969). *People in pain.* San Francisco: Jossey-Bass.

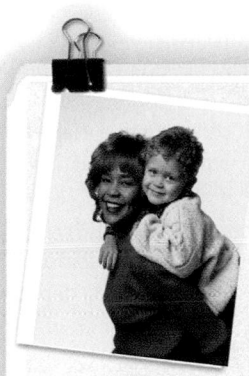 **Sophia Vincent,** the mother of a 3-year-old boy, states "I'm at my wits' end trying to get him to eat a balanced diet. My daughter ate whatever I placed in front of her. My son will go a whole day eating only bananas or something else he likes, even when I threaten him!"

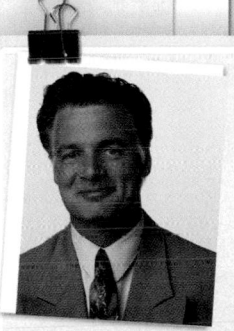 **William Johnston,** a 42-year-old executive, is newly diagnosed with high blood pressure and high cholesterol. He confides that his health has been the last thing on his mind and that his health habits are less than admirable. "I usually eat on the run, often fast food, or big dinners with lots of alcohol. I can't remember the last time I worked out or did any exercise, unless running from my car to the train counts! I guess it's no wonder I've gained a few pounds over the years!"

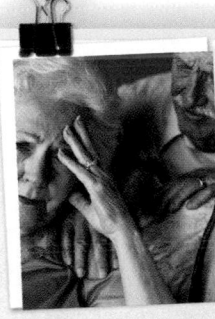 **Charles Gallagher** is the husband of a 67-year-old woman in the end stages of advanced dementia. She had a percutaneous endoscopic gastrostomy (PEG) inserted during her last hospitalization 6 weeks ago due to recurrent episodes of aspiration pneumonia from an inability to swallow. He states "I was talking to the chaplain at the nursing home, and he questioned the wisdom of this tube. I respect him but we really don't have an option here, do we? I mean, if they take the tube out she'll starve to death, no?"

Focusing on Blended Skills

The types of blended skills you'll need to respond to the case scenarios include:

Cognitive Skills

- Ability to incorporate knowledge of the nursing process to identify and care for patients with nutritional problems
- Knowledge of nutrients and nutritional requirements for patients across the lifespan
- Knowledge of hypertension, high cholesterol, and advanced dementia
- Knowledge of normal and abnormal assessment findings, such as bowel sounds and eating patterns
- Basic knowledge about nutritional theory and the factors and variables affecting nutrition
- Knowledge about age-related considerations influencing nutrition and eating habits
- Knowledge of ethical and legal principles underlying withdrawal of nutritional support
- Ability to incorporate knowledge of teaching and learning principles for the mother of a young child at her "wits' end" and a middle-aged executive with poor health habits
- Ability to think critically about how to best respond to the husband of a woman receiving enteral nutrition, and when and how to confer

Technical Skills

- Strong nutritional assessment skills to identify problems involving nutrition
- Demonstration of competence in technical assistance to meet the needs of patients across the lifespan with problems involving nutrition
- Ability to adapt technical assistance to meet the needs of patients at various ages with different nutritional needs
- Ability to use appropriate teaching strategies, adapting them as necessary for patients at different developmental stages
- Ability to seek out assistance in new, unfamiliar, or complex situations to meet the needs of patients, such as the husband of a patient with advanced dementia receiving enteral nutrition

Interpersonal Skills

- Strong people skills to establish trusting nurse–patient relationships with the mother of a young child, a middle-aged man with hypertension and high cholesterol, and the family of a woman with advanced dementia receiving enteral nutrition
- Special interpersonal competence to help the executive see the value in making lifestyle changes necessary to improve his nutritional status
- A good working relationship with colleagues to make sure that the needs of the family of a woman with advanced dementia are met
- Ability to communicate with other members of the healthcare team to promote effective and informed decision making for the family of a woman with advanced dementia
- Demonstration of respect for the patient's human dignity and autonomy throughout the patient's care

Ethical and Legal Skills

- A strong sense of accountability for the health and well-being of individuals, with a commitment to getting them the help needed to achieve their health goals—within the scope of nursing responsibilities and available resources
- A willingness to hold colleagues accountable for safe, ethical, and legal quality practice
- Ability to integrate knowledge of the ethical and legal principles that guide decision making about initiating or withholding nutritional support
- Ability to act as a trusted and effective patient advocate
- Ability to practice in an ethically and legally defensible manner consistent with the nursing code of ethics and the scope of legal practice

Learning Outcomes

After completing the chapter, the learner should be able to accomplish the following:

1. List the six classes of nutrients, explaining the significance of each.
2. Evaluate a diet using the Food Guide Pyramid.
3. Identify risk factors for poor nutritional status.
4. Describe how nutrition influences growth and development throughout the life cycle.
5. Discuss the components of a nutritional assessment.
6. Develop nursing diagnoses that correctly identify nutritional problems that may be treated by independent nursing interventions.
7. Describe nursing interventions to help patients achieve their nutritional goals.
8. Plan, implement, and evaluate nursing care related to selected nursing diagnoses that involve nutritional problems.
9. Differentiate between enteral and parenteral nutrition.

Key Terms

anorexia
anorexia nervosa
anthropometric
basal metabolism
body mass index (BMI)
bulimia
calorie
carbohydrate
cholesterol
clear liquid diet
enteral
full liquid diet
ketosis
lipid
minerals
nasogastric (NG) tube
nasointestinal (NI) tube
NPO
nutrient

nutrition
obesity
parenteral
partial peripheral nutrition (PPN)
percutaneous endoscopic gastrostomy tube (PEG)
peripheral parenteral nutrition (PPN)
protein
recommended dietary allowance (RDA)
residual
soft diet
total parenteral nutrition (TPN)
trans fat
triglycerides
vitamins

Nutrition is a basic human need that changes throughout the life cycle and along the wellness–illness continuum. Food provides nutrition for both the body and the mind. Eating has evolved from being simply a necessity—it may be a source of pleasure, a pastime, a social event, a political statement, a religious symbol, a cultural emblem, or an integral component of medical treatment. As such, food, eating, and nutrition take on different meanings to different people, and changing a person's eating behaviors may be a difficult and slow process. Because nutrition is vital for life and health, and because poor nutrition can seriously decrease one's level of wellness, it is a vital component of nursing. (See the accompanying Reflective Practice box for an example.)

This chapter provides information about basic nutrition theory, focusing on the six classes of nutrients, energy balance, choices for an adequate diet, food patterns and habits, and factors affecting nutrition. Components of simple screening and in-depth nutritional assessments are outlined. Two sets of nursing diagnoses are provided, and patient outcomes for healthy nutrition are discussed. The accompanying plan of care illustrates the significance of nutrition in nursing care.

PRINCIPLES OF NUTRITION

The science of **nutrition** encompasses the study of nutrients and how they are handled by the body as well as the impact of human behavior and environment on the process of nourishment. As such, this discipline involves physiology, psychology, and socioeconomics.

Nutrients are specific biochemical substances used by the body for growth, development, activity, reproduction, lactation, health maintenance, and recovery from illness or injury. The metabolic processes involved in these functions are complex. Subsequently, most nutrients work better together than they do alone. Also, nutrient needs change throughout the life cycle in response to changes in body size, activity, growth, development, and state of health.

Some nutrients are considered *essential* because they either are not synthesized in the body or are made in insufficient amounts. Essential nutrients must be provided in the diet or through supplements. Essential nutrients that supply energy and build tissue (such as carbohydrates, fats, and protein) are referred to as *macronutrients. Micronutrients,* such as vitamins and minerals, are required in much smaller amounts to regulate and control body processes.

Nonessential nutrients do not have to be supplied through exogenous sources because they either are not required for body functioning or are synthesized in the body in adequate amounts. Some nutrients can be converted to others in the body. For instance, the body converts excess carbohydrates and protein into fat and stores them as triglycerides.

Of the six classes of nutrients, three supply energy (carbohydrates, protein, and lipids) and three are needed to regulate body processes (vitamins, minerals, and water).

Reflective Practice
Challenge to Legal and Ethical Skills

Mrs. Constance Gallagher is only 67 years old but she is in the end stages of advanced dementia. She can no longer swallow and has had several hospitalizations in the past year for aspiration pneumonia. She lives in a nursing home (where I am doing a clinical rotation for my gerontologic nursing experience) and has a devoted family, husband, son, and daughter, who all visit regularly. For the last 6 weeks she has received enteral feedings from a percutaneous endoscopic gastrostomy (PEG) tube that was placed during her last hospitalization. Mrs. Gallagher's husband confided to me that the chaplain at the nursing home, whom he respects and likes, questioned the wisdom of the feeding tube. He then asked me "But we really don't have an option here, do we? I mean, if they take the tube out, she'll starve to death, no?" I had no idea how to respond.

Thinking Outside the Box: Possible Courses of Action

- Simply refer Mr. Gallagher to someone more experienced about these things (since I am clearly over my head).
- Find out more about this myself and then get back to him.
- Request an ethics consult to explore how we can best respond to the husband's questions about what is in his wife's best interests, especially given the role the home's chaplain is playing.

Evaluating a Good Outcome: How Do I Define Success?

- The patient's medical goals are met, including, if the family wishes, a dignified death.
- The Gallagher family feels at peace with their decisions and the results of these decisions.
- An ethically justified decision is made about continuing or withdrawing artificial nutrition and hydration that is respect-
ful of Mrs. Gallagher's wishes (to the extent that these are known) and compatible with her beliefs and interests.
- I develop skill in assisting with tough end-of-life decisions and learn more about how an ethics consult functions.

Personal Learning: Here's to the Future!

When I reported my exchange with Mr. Gallagher to the charge nurse, she said we might want to call an ethics consult because there were actually a few similar situations pending and not everyone on the unit seemed comfortable with the lead role the chaplain was taking in recommending the withdrawal of nutritional support. The consult was a great experience. All of the patient's family members attended, plus the medical director of the home, the nurses on the patient's unit, as well as the chaplain, the social worker, the home's ethicist, and myself. After the medical director described the natural progression of advanced dementia, the ethicist noted that there is a difference between dying of starvation (which only happens if food is withdrawn but fluids continue to hydrate) and dying of dehydration (which will happen if we pull the PEG tube and discontinue all enteral feedings, and which is not

believed to be painful). The ethicist then asked the family if they knew what the patient would want done if she could be asked if the benefits of continuing nutritional support outweighed the accompanying burdens of having her wrists restrained so she wouldn't pull out the tube, skin problems, etc. After some discussion, they were in agreement that she would not want to live this way. Since the Gallaghers were Catholic, the Catholic chaplain was invited to describe what the Roman Catholic Church teaches about this. After a rather lengthy discussion, a decision was made to withdraw enteral feedings. The family seemed at peace with their decision.

Through this experience, I learned how an ethics consult works and can see the advantages of tapping this resource in the future.

Reflection

How do you think you would respond in a similar situation? Why? What does this tell you about yourself and about the adequacy of your skills for professional practice? How did the ethics consult facilitate decision making? What ethical and legal principles were maintained? Investigate your agency for this service. What other services or resources might be available to aid in this type of decision-making process? Can you think of other ways to respond?

What other skills (cognitive, interpersonal, technical, ethical/legal) would you need to respond well in this situation? How did the nursing student act as a patient advocate? Was the human dignity of the patient and the patient's family maintained? Why or why not? Do you agree with the criteria to evaluate a successful outcome? Did the nursing student meet these criteria?

Energy Balance

The body needs energy to function. Energy is derived or obtained from foods consumed. Energy in the diet is measured in the form of kilocalories, commonly abbreviated as **calories,** or cal. Only carbohydrates, protein, and fat provide energy. Vitamins and minerals, needed for the metabolism of energy, do not provide calories.

Total energy intake for a meal, a day, or longer can be calculated by using food composition tables: the values given for total calories for each food eaten can simply be added, or the grams of carbohydrate, protein, and fat for each food eaten can be added and multiplied by the appropriate calorie level (4, 4, and 9 cal, respectively).

Energy in the body is used to carry on any kind of activity, whether voluntary or involuntary. A person's total daily energy expenditure is the sum of all the calories used to perform physical activity, maintain basal metabolism, and digest, absorb, and metabolize food.

If a person's daily energy intake is equal to their total daily energy expenditure, the person's weight will remain stable. However, if the energy intake is less than the energy expended, the person's weight will decrease. If the energy intake exceeds energy expenditure, weight will increase.

Metabolic Requirements

Basal metabolism is the amount of energy required to carry on the involuntary activities of the body at rest, such as maintaining body temperature and muscle tone, producing and releasing secretions, propelling food through the gastrointestinal (GI) tract, inflating the lungs, and contracting the heart muscle. As the amount of energy used on physical activity declines, the proportion of calories used for basal metabolism increases; it accounts for more than half of most people's total energy requirements. Because of their larger muscle mass, men have a higher basal metabolic rate (BMR) than women. BMR is about 1 cal/kg of body weight per hour for men and 0.9 cal/kg per hour for women.

> Think back to William Johnston, the middle-aged man with hypertension and high cholesterol. Based on the patient's sex, the nurse would expect his BMI to be greater than that for a woman. The nurse would need to consider this fact when planning the patient's care.

Other factors that increase BMR include growth, infections, fever, emotional tension, extreme environmental temperatures, and elevated levels of certain hormones, especially epinephrine and thyroid hormones. Aging, prolonged fasting, and sleep all decrease BMR. Most nutritionists agree that fasting or following a very-low-calorie diet (VLCD) defeats a weight-loss plan because the body interprets this eating pattern as starvation and compensates by slowing down the resting metabolic rate, making it even more difficult to lose weight.

Body Weight Standards

As previously discussed, if a person's energy intake does not equal energy expenditure, weight will fluctuate. Ideal body weight (IBW) or healthy body weight is an estimate of optimal weight for optimal health. A general guideline, often called the rule-of-thumb (ROT) method, determines ideal weight based on height. This formula is as follows:

For adult females:

100 lb (for height of 5 ft) + 5 lb for each additional inch over 5 ft

For adult males:

106 lb (for height of 5 ft) + 6 lb for each additional inch over 5 ft

(Add or deduct 10% from this figure based on body frame size.)

Using this method can result in unrealistically low figures for adults who are very short or very tall. (Height and weight tables commonly are used for infants and children.)

In the past, the 1983 Metropolitan Life Insurance Company height and weight table had consistently been the standard reference that nurses used to determine healthy body weight. The weight standards on the chart represent survey results of Americans who purchased life insurance. The values are adjusted according to height and frame size for the 25- to 59-year age bracket. However, this measurement chart is problematic. Minority populations are not represented. Additionally, the most recent edition, 1983, lists heavier mortality weights (weights at the 25- to 59-year age bracket that are associated with the lowest death rate), not ideal weights (Dudek, 2001).

Although numerous tables and approaches have been devised for determining healthy body weight, many health experts now consider the **body mass index (BMI)** to be the most precise parameter. The BMI is a ratio of height to weight, providing a more accurate reflection of total body fat stores in the general population. The BMI does not differentiate according to sex and is calculated in the following manner:

Using kilograms and meters:

$$\frac{\text{Weight in kilograms}}{\text{Height}^2 \text{ in meters}} \quad \begin{array}{l}(2.2 \text{ lb} = 1 \text{ kg}) \\ (39.37 \text{ inches} = 1 \text{ m})\end{array}$$

Using pounds and inches:

$$\frac{\text{Weight in pounds}}{\text{Height in inches}} \times 704.5$$

A quick method of determining BMI is displayed in Figure 42-1. Many health practitioners use this more accurate weight calculation as an initial assessment of nutritional status. BMI also provides an estimation of relative risk factors for diseases such as heart disease, diabetes, and hypertension. However, the BMI may not be accurate for people such as athletes, with a large muscle mass, or people with edema (Dudek, 2001).

According to these most recent BMI guidelines published by the National Heart, Lung, and Blood Institute, a person with a BMI of 25 is considered overweight, whereas a BMI of 30 or greater indicates obesity. For individuals with a BMI of 25 to 29, cessation of weight gain is the initial step. If risk factors are present (eg, high blood pressure or high cholesterol), a weight loss of 10% is desirable.

Caloric Requirements

Just as healthy body weight or IBW can be determined in a variety of ways, so can a person's calorie requirements. Box 42-1 illustrates one method. After calorie requirements have been determined, adjustments can be made for weight gain or loss as needed. For instance, 1 lb (0.45 kg) of body fat equals

Body Mass Index (BMI)														
	19	20	21	22	23	24	25	26	27	28	29	30	35	40
Height Weight (pounds)														
4'10"	91	96	100	105	110	115	119	124	129	134	138	143	167	191
4'11"	94	99	104	109	114	119	124	128	133	138	143	148	173	198
5'0"	97	102	107	112	118	123	128	133	138	143	148	153	179	204
5'1"	100	106	111	116	122	127	132	137	143	148	153	158	185	211
5'2"	104	109	115	120	126	131	136	142	147	153	158	164	191	218
5'3"	107	113	118	124	130	135	141	146	152	158	163	169	197	225
5'4"	110	116	122	128	134	140	145	151	157	163	169	174	204	232
5'5"	114	120	126	132	138	144	150	156	162	168	174	180	210	240
5'6"	118	124	130	136	142	148	155	161	167	173	179	186	216	247
5'7"	121	127	134	140	146	153	159	166	172	178	185	191	223	255
5'8"	125	131	138	144	151	158	164	171	177	184	190	197	230	262
5'9"	128	135	142	149	155	162	169	176	182	189	196	203	236	270
5'10"	132	139	146	153	160	167	174	181	188	195	202	207	243	278
5'11"	136	143	150	157	165	172	179	186	193	200	208	215	250	286
6'0"	140	147	154	162	169	177	184	191	199	206	213	221	258	294
6'1"	144	151	159	166	174	182	189	197	204	212	219	227	265	302
6'2"	148	155	163	171	179	186	194	202	210	218	225	233	272	311
6'3"	152	160	168	176	184	192	200	208	216	224	232	240	279	319
6'4"	156	164	172	180	189	197	205	213	221	230	238	246	287	328
	Normal						Overweight					Obese		

FIGURE 42-1 Select your correct height, and move across the chart to your approximate weight. The appropriate body mass index is listed directly above this line. (From the National Heart, Lung, and Blood Institute, 2001.)

BOX 42-1 Method of Calculating Caloric Requirements

- Calculate the *resting energy equivalent* (REE), or the amount of calories necessary to maintain the body at rest. Because men usually have a greater muscle mass than women, their caloric requirements are slightly higher (1 cal/kg versus 0.9 cal/kg). A weight of 143 lb or 65 kg, is used for purposes of this calculation.

Male
65 kg × 1 cal/kg × 24 hr = 1560 cal/day

Female
65 kg × 0.9 cal/kg × 24 hr = 1404 cal/day

- Determine the calories needed for a specific activity level. The REE is multiplied by one of the following: light activity (REE × 0.55 to 0.65), moderate activity (REE × 0.65 to 0.7), heavy activity (REE × 0.75 to 1.0). Charts are available in most nutrition textbooks that define and give examples of each of the specific activity levels. For purposes of this calculation, 0.55 calories for light activity is used.

Male
1560 × 0.55 = 858 calories

Female
1404 × 0.55 = 772 calories

- Total the REE and calories needed based on activity level.

Male
1560 + 858 = 2418 calories

Female
1404 + 772 = 2176 calories

This is one method for calculating the energy requirements for a lightly active 143 pound man or woman.

(Adapted from Dudek, S. G. [2001]. *Nutrition handbook for nursing practice* [4th ed.]. Philadelphia: Lippincott Williams & Wilkins.)

about 3500 cal. Therefore, to gain or lose 1 lb (0.45 kg) in a week, daily calorie intake should be increased or decreased, respectively, by 500 cal (3500 cal divided by 7 days = 500 cal/d). Similarly, a weight gain or loss of 2 lb (0.9 kg) per week would require an adjustment of 1000 cal/d. Because it becomes increasingly difficult to plan an adequate diet as the calorie level drops, diets that result in more than a 2-lb (0.9-kg) weight loss per week are not recommended.

Consider William Johnston, the man with poor health habits. The nurse would work with Mr. Johnston to develop an appropriate weight-loss plan that would contain adequate calories yet still foster a weight loss of 1 to 2 lb/week. Doing so would promote weight loss while still allowing for adequate nutritional intake.

Energy Nutrients

Carbohydrates

Carbohydrates, commonly known as sugars and starches, are organic compounds composed of carbon, hydrogen, and oxygen. They serve as the structural framework of plants. The only animal source of carbohydrate in the diet is lactose, or "milk sugar."

The significance of carbohydrates cannot be overstated. They are relatively easy to produce and store, making them the most abundant and least expensive source of calories in the diet worldwide. In countries where grains are the dietary staple, carbohydrates may contribute as much as 90% of total calories. Table 42-1 summarizes the sources, functions, and significance of dietary carbohydrates.

In addition, carbohydrate intake is correlated to income. As income increases, carbohydrate intake decreases and protein intake, a more expensive form of energy, increases.

TABLE 42-1 Sources, Functions, and Significance of Carbohydrates, Protein, and Fat

Nutrient	Sources	Functions	Significance
Carbohydrates Simple sugars and starch	Fruits Vegetables Grains: rice, pasta, breads, cereals Dried peas and beans Milk (lactose) Sugars: white and brown sugar, honey, molasses, syrup	Provide energy Spare protein so it can be used for other functions Prevent ketosis from inefficient fat metabolism	Provide about 46% of the calories in the typical American diet; many believe carbohydrate intake should be increased to 50%–60% of total calories. Low carbohydrate intake can cause ketosis; high simple sugar intake increases the risk for dental caries.
Cellulose and other water-insoluble fibers	Whole wheat flour and wheat bran Vegetables: cabbage, peas, green beans, wax beans, broccoli, brussels sprouts, cucumber skins, peppers, carrots Apples	Absorb water to increase fecal bulk Decrease intestinal transit time	Are nondigestible; therefore, are excreted Help relieve constipation North Americans are urged to eat more of all types of fiber Excess intake can cause gas, distention, and diarrhea.
Water-soluble fibers	Oat bran and oatmeal Dried peas and beans Vegetables Prunes, pears, apples, bananas, oranges	Slow gastric emptying Lower serum cholesterol level Delay glucose absorption	Help improve glucose tolerance in diabetics
Protein	Milk and milk products Meat, poultry, fish Eggs Dried peas and beans Nuts	Tissue growth and repair Component of body framework: bones, muscles, tendons, blood vessels, skin, hair, nails Component of body fluids: hormones, enzymes, plasma proteins, neurotransmitters, mucus Helps regulate fluid balance through oncotic pressure Helps regulate acid–base balance Detoxifies harmful substances Forms antibodies Transports fat and other substances through the blood Provides energy when carbohydrate intake is inadequate	Most North Americans consume twice the RDA (RNI) for protein. Experts recommend that we eat less animal protein and more vegetable protein. Protein deficiency is characterized by edema, retarded growth and maturation, muscle wasting, changes in the hair and skin, permanent damage to physical and mental development (in children), diarrhea, malabsorption, numerous secondary nutrient deficiencies, fatty infiltration of the liver, increased risk for infections, and high mortality. Except for elderly people, fad dieters, hospitalized patients, and people of low income, protein deficiency is rare in the United States and Canada.
Fat	Butter, oils, margarine, lard, salt pork, salad dressings, mayonnaise, bacon Whole milk and whole milk products High-fat meats Nuts	Provides energy Provides structure Insulates the body Cushions internal organs Necessary for the absorption of fat-soluble vitamins	Fat supplies about 37% of total calories in the typical North American diet; experts suggest a reduction to 30% or less of total calories. High-fat diets increase the risk for heart disease and obesity and are correlated with an increased risk for colon and breast cancers.

(Dudek, S. G. [2001]. *Nutrition handbook for nursing practice* [4th ed.]. Philadelphia: Lippincott Williams & Wilkins.)

Classification and Metabolism

The number of molecules within the structure determines the classification of carbohydrates. They are classified as simple (monosaccharides and disaccharides) or complex (polysaccharides) sugars.

Carbohydrates are more easily and quickly digested than protein and fat. Ninety percent of carbohydrate intake is digested. This percentage decreases as fiber intake increases. All carbohydrates are converted to glucose for transport through the blood or for use as energy. Glucose is an efficient fuel that certain tissues, particularly the central nervous system, rely on almost exclusively for energy. Glucose is transported from the GI tract, through the portal vein, to the liver. The liver stores glucose and regulates its entry into the blood. Hormones, especially insulin and glucagon, are responsible for keeping serum glucose levels fairly constant during both feasting and fasting.

Through a series of steps, cells oxidize (burn) glucose to provide energy, carbon dioxide, and water. Depending on a person's state of energy balance, the period between when carbohydrate is consumed and when it is used for energy may vary from minutes to months or longer. Unlike protein and fat, glucose is burned efficiently and completely and does not leave a toxic product for the kidneys to excrete.

When the supply of glucose exceeds what is needed for energy and for maintaining serum levels, it is stored. If muscle or liver glycogen stores are deficient, glucose is converted to glycogen and stored (glycogenesis). Conversely, glycogen is broken down in time of need to supply a ready source of glucose (glycogenolysis). When glycogen stores are adequate, the body converts excess glucose to fat and stores it as triglycerides in adipose tissue.

Functions and Recommended Dietary Allowance

The primary function of carbohydrates is to supply energy. Except for undigestible fiber, all carbohydrates provide 4 cal/g, regardless of the source.

The **recommended dietary allowance (RDA)** of essential nutrients refers to recommendations for average daily amounts that healthy population groups should consume over time. Although an exact requirement for carbohydrates has not been established, at least 50 to 100 g is needed daily to prevent **ketosis** (an abnormal accumulation of ketone bodies that is frequently associated with acidosis). In terms of an optimal diet, most health experts recommend that carbohydrates provide 50% to 60% of the diet's total calories, mostly in the form of complex carbohydrates. (See Table 42-1 for more information regarding the sources, functions, and significance of carbohydrates.)

Protein

Protein is a vital component of every living cell. Within the human body, more than 1000 different proteins are made by combining various amounts and proportions of the 22 basic building blocks known as amino acids. Although amino acids, like carbohydrates, contain carbon, hydrogen, and oxygen, they differ in that amino acids also contain nitrogen. Nine amino acids are classified as essential because they cannot be synthesized in the body; the remaining amino acids are no less important, but because the body can make them if a supply of nitrogen is available, they are termed nonessential. Proteins are required for the formation of all body structures, including genes, enzymes, muscle, bone matrix, and hemoglobin.

Classification and Metabolism

Dietary proteins may be labeled complete (high quality) or incomplete (low quality), based on their amino acid composition. Complete proteins contain sufficient amounts and proportions of all the essential amino acids to support growth, whereas incomplete proteins are deficient in one or more essential amino acids. Generally, animal proteins (eggs, dairy products, and meats) are complete, and plant proteins (grains, legumes, and vegetables) are incomplete. The only exception is soy, a plant protein which is considered a complete protein. Because different sources of plant proteins lack different amino acids, a plant protein can be complemented by combining it with a different plant protein or by adding a small amount of an animal protein to supply a complete protein. Examples of complementary vegetable proteins include corn tortilla and refried beans and lentil rice soup. Complementary proteins that use a small amount of animal protein include cereal with milk, rice pudding, and a cheese sandwich.

Dietary protein is broken down into amino acid particles by pancreatic enzymes in the small intestine. These are absorbed through the intestinal mucosa to be transported to the liver. In the liver, amino acids are recombined into new proteins or are released into the bloodstream for use in protein synthesis by tissues and cells. Excess amino acids are converted to fatty acids, ketone bodies, or glucose and are stored or used as metabolic fuel.

The body's protein tissues are in a constant state of flux. Tissues are continuously being broken down (catabolism) and replaced (anabolism). Nitrogen balance, a comparison between catabolism and anabolism, can be measured by comparing nitrogen intake (protein intake) and nitrogen excretion (nitrogen lost in urine, urea, feces, hair, nails, and skin). When catabolism and anabolism are occurring at the same rate, as in healthy adults, the body is in a state of neutral nitrogen balance (ie, nitrogen intake equals nitrogen excretion). A positive nitrogen balance occurs when nitrogen intake is greater than excretion—for example, during periods of growth, pregnancy, lactation, and recovery from illness. A negative nitrogen balance, an undesirable state that occurs in situations such as starvation and the catabolism that immediately follows surgery, illness, trauma, and stress, indicates that more nitrogen is being excreted than consumed.

Functions and Recommended Dietary Allowance

The major function of protein is to maintain body tissues that break down from normal wear and tear and to support the growth of new tissue. Protein can be oxidized to provide 4 cal/g. Using protein for energy is more expensive both financially and physiologically than using carbohydrates. The nitrogen remaining after protein is metabolized burdens the kidneys. In addition, energy must be used to excrete the nitrogen. Like carbohydrates, protein consumed in excess of need can be converted to and stored as fat.

The RDA for protein for adults is 0.8 g/kg of desirable body weight, or about 56 g for the average woman and 63 g for the average man. Most health experts recommend that protein intake should contribute 10% to 20% of total caloric intake (Dudek, 2001; see Table 42-1 for more information about the sources, functions, and significance of protein).

The stress of illness, surgery, or prolonged periods of time on simple intravenous (IV) solutions without oral intake places hospitalized patients at risk for developing protein-calorie malnutrition (PCM), resulting in weakness, poor wound healing, mental apathy, and edema (Dudek, 2001). In addition, an increase in infant deaths may occur when PCM is combined with low calorie intake over a period of time (marasmus). Kwashiorkor, the most severe form of protein deficiency, is more common in developing countries.

Fats

Fats in the diet, or **lipids,** are insoluble in water and, therefore, insoluble in blood. Like carbohydrates, they are composed of carbon, hydrogen, and oxygen. Ninety-five percent of the lipids in the diet are in the form of **triglycerides,** the predominant form of fat in food and the major storage form of fat in the body. Compound lipids (such as phospholipids, in which a lipid is combined with another substance) and derived lipids (such as cholesterol) constitute the remainder of the lipids ingested.

Classification and Metabolism

Food fats contain mixtures of saturated and unsaturated fatty acids. The difference in degree of saturation depends on the amount of hydrogen in fat molecules. Saturated fats contain more hydrogen than unsaturated fats. Most animal fats are considered saturated and have a solid consistency at room temperature. Conversely, most vegetable fats are considered unsaturated, remain liquid at room temperature, and are referred to as oils. Saturated fats tend to raise serum cholesterol levels, whereas unsaturated fats lower serum cholesterol levels. When manufacturers partially hydrogenate liquid oils, they become more solid and more stable. This substance is referred to as **trans fat.** Trans fat raises serum cholesterol. Therefore, it is to be counted in with the total number of saturated fats in a day. The U.S. Food and Drug Administration (FDA) has announced that effective January 1, 2006, food nutrition labels must list trans fat so that consumers may make healthy choices in their diet.

Cholesterol is a fatlike substance found only in animal products. It need not be provided in the diet because the body synthesizes about twice as much cholesterol as most people in North America eat. Cholesterol is an important component of cell membranes and is especially abundant in brain and nerve cells. It also is used to synthesize bile acids and is a precursor of the steroid hormones and vitamin D. Although cholesterol serves many important functions in the body, high serum levels are clearly associated with an increased risk

for atherosclerosis. To help lower serum cholesterol levels, researchers recommend limiting cholesterol intake, eating less total fat—especially saturated and trans fat—eating more unsaturated fat, and increasing fiber intake, which increases fecal excretion of cholesterol.

> *Remember William Johnston, the middle-aged executive with hypertension and high cholesterol? Due to Mr. Johnston's "on-the-run" lifestyle, developing an individualized nutritional plan might be somewhat challenging. Based on an assessment of Mr. Johnston's eating habits, likes, and dislikes, the nurse would work with him to develop a plan that promotes weight loss and includes limiting cholesterol and total fat intake and consuming more foods containing unsaturated fats and fiber. Adapting the plan will help to promote adherence to it, thereby increasing the chances for success.*

Fat digestion occurs largely in the small intestine. Bile, secreted by the gallbladder, emulsifies fat to increase the surface area so that pancreatic lipase can break down fat more effectively. Through a complex series of events, most fats are absorbed into the lymphatic circulation with the help of a protein carrier and are transported to the liver. Of 100 g eaten, only about 3 g are excreted in the feces.

Functions and Recommended Dietary Allowance

Fats are the most concentrated source of energy in the diet, providing 9 cal for every gram. Fat increases the palatability of the diet (eg, to most people, filet mignon tastes better than flank steak) and has a high satiety value because it delays gastric emptying time. In the body, fat aids in the absorption of the fat-soluble vitamins and provides insulation, structure, and temperature control. (See Table 42-1 for more information about the sources, functions, and significance of fat.)

Because the body can synthesize fat from carbohydrates and protein, an RDA for fat has not been established. Americans consume about 34% of their total caloric intake in the form of fat. Most experts agree that fat should not contribute more than 30% of the day's caloric intake, and saturated or trans fat intake should be limited to less than 10% of total fat calories (Dudek, 2001).

Regulatory Nutrients

Vitamins, minerals, and water are regulatory nutrients because they are needed by the body for the metabolism of energy nutrients.

Vitamins

Vitamins are organic compounds needed by the body in small amounts. Most vitamins are active in the form of coenzymes, which, together with enzymes, facilitate thousands of chemical reactions in the body. Although vitamins do not provide energy (calories), they are needed for the metabolism of carbohydrates, protein, and fat. Vitamins are essential in the diet because most are not synthesized in the body or are made in insufficient quantities.

Vitamins are present in foods in only small amounts. Fresh foods are higher in vitamins than processed foods because vitamins may be destroyed by light, heat, air, and during preparation. The exception is when vitamins not naturally occurring in a food are added, such as vitamin D-fortified milk. This process is called fortification.

In the United States, severe vitamin deficiencies are uncommon. Mild or subclinical deficiencies of vitamin A, vitamin C, folate, and vitamin B_6, however, may affect a significant proportion of the population, especially those who (1) are members of certain age groups or patient groups (infants, adolescents, pregnant and lactating women, and older people); (2) smoke, abuse alcohol, or use medications on a long-term basis; (3) are chronically ill, either physically or psychologically; or (4) are poor or finicky eaters, such as chronic dieters, strict vegetarians, and food faddists.

Vitamins are classified as either water soluble or fat soluble. Water-soluble vitamins include vitamin C and the B-complex vitamins. They are absorbed through the intestinal wall directly into the bloodstream. Although some tissues are able to hold limited amounts of water-soluble vitamins, they usually are not stored in the body. Deficiency symptoms are apt to develop quickly when intake is inadequate; therefore, a daily intake is recommended. However, because water-soluble vitamins are not stored, amounts consumed in excess of need are excreted in the urine. Toxicities are not likely, although megadoses of certain water-soluble vitamins can be harmful.

Vitamins A, D, E, and K, the fat-soluble vitamins, are absorbed with fat into the lymphatic circulation. Like fat, they must be attached to a protein to be transported through the blood. Secondary deficiencies of the fat-soluble vitamins can occur anytime fat digestion or absorption is altered, such as during malabsorption syndromes and pancreatic and biliary diseases. The body stores excesses of the fat-soluble vitamins mostly in the liver and adipose tissue. Because they are stored, a daily intake is not imperative and deficiency symptoms may take weeks, months, or years to develop. Excessive intake, particularly of vitamins A and D, are toxic.

Many studies have attempted to evaluate the relationship of vitamin intake to diseases ranging from cardiovascular disease, osteoporosis, and neural tube defects to some types of cancers (Fairfield & Fletcher, 2002). At least 30% of Americans have stated that they use vitamin supplementation on a regular basis (Balluz et al., 2000). Many nutrition experts still believe that adequate amounts of most vitamins can be obtained from a healthy diet, but a growing body of scientific research indicates that benefits are achieved with use of certain vitamin supplements. Although scrutiny and research continue about vitamin supplements and their long-term effects, most nutritionists agree that vitamins will never be a substitute for good nutrition and healthy lifestyle practices. Table 42-2 summarizes water- and fat-soluble vitamins.

Think back to Sophia Vincent, the mother of the 3-year-old concerned about her son's eat-

ing habits. After a thorough assessment, the nurse may consult with the physician about the possibility of using a vitamin supplement if the assessment reveals a definite nutritional deficiency.

Minerals

Minerals are inorganic elements found in all body fluids and tissues in the form of salts (eg, sodium chloride) or combined with organic compounds (eg, iron in hemoglobin). Some minerals function to provide structure within the body, whereas others help to regulate body processes. Minerals, which are elements, are not broken down or rearranged in the body but, rather, are contained in the ash that remains after digestion. Excessive soaking and cooking in water can cause loss of minerals from food. However, minerals are commonly not destroyed by food processing.

Macrominerals, minerals needed by the body in amounts greater than 100 mg/day, include calcium, phosphorus, and magnesium. RDAs have been established for calcium and magnesium. A safe dose has been suggested for phosphorus. Microminerals, or trace elements, are minerals needed by the body in amounts less than 100 mg/day. Microminerals include iron, zinc, manganese, and iodine. RDAs have been established for some trace elements, including iron, iodine, selenium, and zinc. Ranges of estimated safe and adequate daily intakes have been suggested for manganese, fluoride, chromium, and molybdenum. However, no recommendations have been made for cobalt, nickel, vanadium, arsenic, and silicon. Macrominerals and microminerals are summarized in Table 42-3.

Water

As the major body constituent present in every body cell, water accounts for between 50% and 60% of the adult's total weight. Infants have proportionately more water accounting for body weight. About two thirds of the body's water is contained within the cells (intracellular fluid [ICF]); the remainder is called extracellular fluid (ECF), which includes all other body fluids, such as plasma and interstitial fluid. Total body water and ECF decrease with age; ICF increases with an increase in body mass. (See Chapter 46 for more information on body water.)

Water is more vital to life than food because it provides the fluid medium necessary for all chemical reactions, it participates in many reactions, and it is not stored in the body. Water acts as a solvent that dissolves many solutes, thereby aiding digestion, absorption, circulation, and excretion. Through evaporation from the skin, water helps to regulate body temperature. As a lubricant, water is needed both for mucous secretions and for movement between joints.

Think back to Charles Gallagher, husband of the woman with advanced dementia receiving enteral nutrition. During the group meeting about continuing or withdrawing the enteral nutrition, Mr. Gallagher learns that with-

TABLE 42-2 Summary of Vitamins

Nutrient and Adult RDA	Sources	Functions	Signs and Symptoms of Deficiency	Signs and Symptoms of Excess
Water-Soluble Vitamins				
Vitamin C (ascorbic acid) 60 mg (60–100 mg for smokers)	Citrus fruits, broccoli, green pepper, strawberries, greens	Collagen formation, antioxidant, enhances iron absorption	Scurvy, hemorrhaging, delayed wound healing	Kidney stones, scurvy on withdrawal, nausea, diarrhea
Vitamin B Complex				
Thiamin 1–1.4 mg	Pork, liver, whole and enriched grains, legumes	Coenzyme in key reactions that produce energy from glucose	Beriberi, mental confusion, fatigue	None known
Riboflavin 1.2–1.7 mg	Milk, organ meats, enriched grains, greens	Carbohydrate, protein, and fat metabolism	Ariboflavinosis—symptoms related to inflammation and poor wound healing	None known
Niacin 13–19 mg	Kidney, grains, lean meat, nuts	Carbohydrate, protein, and fat metabolism	Pellagra, dermatitis	Flushing and itching, nausea, vomiting
B_6 (pyridoxine) 1.6–2 mg	Yeast, banana, cantaloupe, broccoli, spinach	Coenzyme in protein, fat, carbohydrate metabolism	Anemia, CNS problems	Difficulty walking, numbness of feet and hands
Folate 180–200 µg	Green leafy vegetables, liver	RNA and DNA synthesis, formation and maturation of RBC	Macrocytic anemia: fatigue, weakness, pallor	None known
B_{12} (cobalamin) 2 µg	Only animal foods: organ meats, seafood	Coenzyme in protein metabolism and formation of heme portion of hemoglobin	Pernicious anemia (B_{12} deficiency related to impaired absorption due to lack of intrinsic factor)	None known
Pantothenic acid 4–7 mg	Liver, egg yolk, yeast	Carbohydrate, protein, and fat metabolism	None known	None known
Biotin 30–100 µg	Liver, egg yolk	Carbohydrate, protein, and fat metabolism	Deficiency produced by adding large amounts of raw egg white to a biotin-deficient diet	None known
Fat-Soluble Vitamins				
Vitamin A (retinol, retinal, retinoic acid) 800–1000 RE	Liver, carrots, egg yolk, fortified milk	Visual acuity in dim light, formation and maintenance of skin and mucous membranes	Night blindness, rough skin	Anorexia, loss of hair, dry skin, bone pain
Vitamin D (cholecalciferol, ergosterol) 5–10 µg	Sunlight, fortified milk, fish liver oils	Calcium and phosphorus metabolism, stimulates calcium absorption	Retarded bone growth, bone malformation	Excessive calcification of bones, renal calculi, nausea, headache
Vitamin E (tocopherol) 8–10 µg	Vegetable oils, wheat germ, whole grain products	Antioxidant, protects vitamin A, heme synthesis	Increased RBC hemolysis and macrocytic anemia in premature infants	Relatively nontoxic, although large doses can cause fatigue, diarrhea
Vitamin K 65–80 µg	Dark, green leafy vegetables; synthesized in intestines from gut bacteria	Synthesis of certain proteins necessary for blood clotting	Hemorrhagic disease of newborn, delayed blood clotting	Hemolytic anemia and liver damage with synthetic vitamin K

(Dudek, S. G. [2001]. *Nutrition handbook for nursing practice* [4th ed.]. Philadelphia: Lippincott Williams & Wilkins; Williams, S. and Schlenker, E. [2002]. *Essentials of nutrition and diet therapy* [8th ed.]. St. Louis: C. V. Mosby.)

TABLE 42-3 Summary of Macrominerals and Microminerals

Nutrient and Adult RDA	Sources	Functions	Signs and Symptoms of Deficiency	Signs and Symptoms of Excess
Macrominerals				
Calcium 800 mg (18–24 yr: 1200 mg)	Milk and dairy products, canned fish with bones, greens	Bone and tooth formation, blood clotting, nerve transmission, muscle contraction	Tetany, osteoporosis	Renal calculi in susceptible people
Phosphorus 800 mg (11–24 yr: 1200 mg)	Milk and milk products, soft drinks, processed foods	Bone and tooth formation, acid–base balance, energy metabolism	Hypophosphatemia: anorexia, muscle weakness	Hyperphosphatemia: symptoms of hypocalcemic tetany
Magnesium 280–350 mg	Green leafy vegetables, nuts, beans, grains	Bone and tooth formation, protein synthesis, carbohydrate metabolism	Hypomagnesemia: weakness, muscle pain, poor heart function	Hypermagnesemia: CNS depression, coma, hypotension
Sulfur (provided by adequate amounts of protein)	Meat, eggs, milk, dried peas and beans, nuts	Promotes certain enzyme reactions and detoxification reactions	None known	None known
Sodium 500 mg	Salt, processed foods	Major ion of extracellular fluid, fluid balance, acid–base balance	Hyponatremia: muscle cramps, cold and clammy skin	Edema, weight gain, high blood pressure if susceptible
Potassium 1600–2000 mg	Whole grains, fruits, leafy vegetables	Major ion of intracellular fluid, fluid balance, acid–base balance	Hypokalemia: muscle cramps and weakness, irregular heart beat	Hyperkalemia: irritability, anxiety, cardiac arrhythmia, heart block
Chlorine 750 mg (minimum requirement)	Salt	Component of HCl in stomach, fluid balance, acid–base balance	Hypochloremia: muscle spasms, alkalosis, depressed respirations	Hyperchloremia: acidosis
Microminerals				
Iron 10–15 mg	Liver, lean meats, enriched and whole-grain breads and cereals	Oxygen transport by way of hemoglobin, constituent of enzyme systems	Microcytic anemia, pallor, decreased work capacity, fatigue, weakness	Hemosiderosis; acute iron poisoning from accidental overdose leads to GI symptoms and possible shock
Iodine 150 mg	Iodized salt, seafood, food additives	Component of thyroid hormones	Goiter	Acne-like lesions
Zinc 12–15 mg	Oysters, liver, meats, dried peas and beans, nuts	Tissue growth, sexual maturation, immune response	Impaired growth, sexual maturation, immune system functioning	Anorexia, nausea, vomiting, diarrhea, muscle pain, lethargy
Copper 1.5–3 mg	Liver, shellfish, grains, dried peas and beans	Aids in iron metabolism and activity of some enzymes	Anemia, altered bone formation, hypercholesterolemia	Nervous system disturbances, vomiting
Manganese 2–5 mg	Whole grains, nuts, dried peas and beans, fruit	Part of enzymes needed for protein and energy metabolism	Poor reproductive performance, growth retardation	None known
Fluoride 1.5–4 mg (estimated safe, adequate intake)	Fluoridated water, fish, tea	Tooth formation and integrity, bone formation and integrity	Tooth decay; may increase risk for osteoporosis	Mottling and discoloration of tooth enamel

(continued)

TABLE 42-3 (Continued)

Nutrient and Adult RDA	Sources	Functions	Signs and Symptoms of Deficiency	Signs and Symptoms of Excess
Chromium 50–200 µg	Whole grains, meats	Cofactor for insulin, proper glucose metabolism	Impaired glucose tolerance, insulin resistance	None known
Selenium 55–70 µg	Wheat (if grown in high-selenium soil), organ meats	Antioxidant	None known	Loss of hair, brittle fingernails, fatigue
Molybdenum 75–250 mg (estimated safe, adequate intake)	Liver, whole grains, dried peas and beans, organ meats	Oxidizes sulfur and products of sulfur metabolism	None known	Interferes with copper metabolism
Cobalt Unknown— apparently minute	Organ meats	Essential component of vitamin B_{12}	None known	None known

(Dudek, S. G. [2001]. *Nutrition handbook for nursing practice* [4th ed.]. Philadelphia: Lippincott Williams & Wilkins; Williams, S. and Schlenker, E. [2002]. *Essentials of nutrition and diet therapy* [8th ed.]. St. Louis: C. V. Mosby.)

drawal of the feedings would also involve limited water intake. This information is important in helping Mr. Gallagher and his family arrive at an informed decision about whether or not to continue the enteral feedings.

Sources of water in the diet include not only beverages but also solid foods, which contain from 10% to 98% water. Water is also produced through the metabolism of carbohydrates, protein, and fat. It leaves the body through urine, feces, expired air, and perspiration. Water intake (an average of 2000–2500 mL/day for adults) usually equals water output. Water balance may be seriously affected when intake (such as in individuals who are elderly or in comatose states) or output (such as in patients with altered renal function, profuse perspiration, diarrhea, vomiting, fistulas, drainage tubes, hemorrhage, and severe burns) is altered.

ADEQUATE DIET SELECTION

An adequate diet provides a balanced intake of all essential nutrients in appropriate amounts. However, what constitutes an adequate diet is less obvious. Although a major problem in developing countries, malnutrition related to poor dietary intake is uncommon in the United States. Rather, nutritional concerns focus more on problems of overnutrition. Tools for planning or evaluating a diet for adequacy include the Food Guide Pyramid, the RDA, and dietary recommendations and guidelines issued from health and U.S. governmental agencies. The task of promoting health through proper nutrition has been made easier by labeling regulations that provide specific information about food contents and their comparison to recommended daily intakes.

Food Guide Pyramid

In response to the concerns of nutritionists and health officials, coupled with public interest in fitness and health, the U.S. Department of Agriculture developed the Food Guide Pyramid (Fig. 42-2). This graphic device illustrates the importance of specific food groups in the diet. The Food Guide Pyramid was designed to represent a total diet and to provide a firm foundation for health. At the time it was developed, it represented a focus on wellness and recognition of the role that food plays in prevention of such chronic disease threats as heart disease, high blood pressure, some types of cancer, diabetes, and obesity. The Food Guide Pyramid was instituted to give people guidelines in making healthier, more nutritious food selections.

Grain and cereal group are at the base of the pyramid, followed by the fruit and vegetable group, the meat and dairy groups, and a fat, oil, and sweets group at the peak. The intent of the pyramid is to emphasize the grain and cereal group as the basic food in the diet, with the less desirable groups playing a much smaller nutritional role. Each of these groups provides some nutrients, but all are required, in proper proportions, for a healthy diet. Typical serving sizes are displayed in Box 42-2.

Ongoing research conducted since the current Food Guide Pyramid was developed indicate that its food recommendations are misleading. Based on these findings, a revised pyramid is expected to be released in 2004. Rather than emphasize the elimination of fats from the diet, expected changes include a greater emphasis on the consumption of monounsaturated and polysaturated fats. Rather than recommending a high intake of carbohydrates, nutritionists now emphasize including high-quality whole grain foods with each meal. It is expected that these dietary changes can have a significant impact

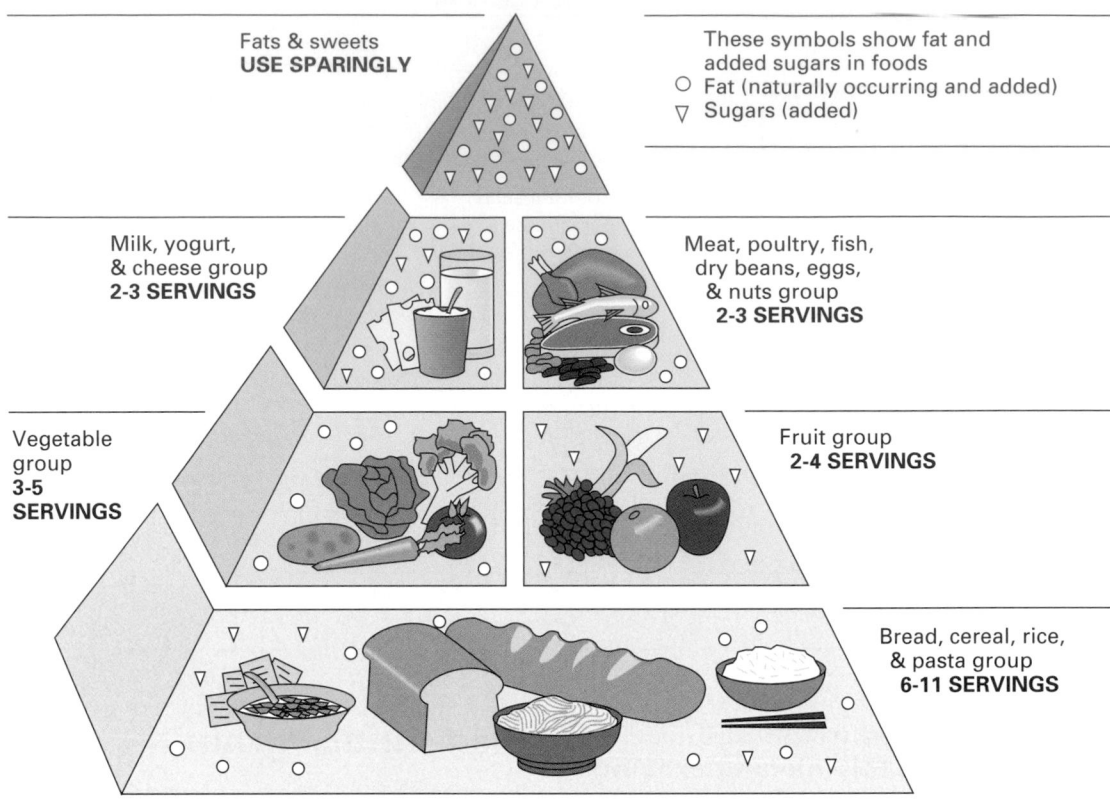

FIGURE 42-2 The Food Guide Pyramid.   (Source: U.S. Department of Agriculture, October, 1996.)

on the reduction of cardiovascular disease and obesity in men and women.

Recommended Dietary Allowance

The RDA, prepared by the Committee on Dietary Allowances of the Food and Nutrition Board, represents average daily amounts of nutrients considered to be adequate to meet the known nutritional needs of practically all healthy people. Un-

like a requirement, which is the amount of a nutrient needed to prevent a deficiency, an allowance has a safety factor built in to account for individual variations. Because the RDA is intended for populations and not individuals, some people may not be able to meet their individual requirements, despite consuming the RDA. Likewise, it is possible for some people to eat less than the RDA and still avoid deficiencies. Although the RDA is defined for age and sex and is revised about every 5 years as new information becomes available, it has not been

---

BOX 42-2 **Food Guide Pyramid: Typical Serving Size**

Bread, Cereal, Rice, & Pasta Group
1 slice of bread
$^1/_2$ cup of cooked rice, pasta, or cereal
1 ounce of ready-to-eat cereal
$^1/_2$ English muffin

Vegetable Group
$^1/_2$ cup of chopped raw or cooked vegetables
1 cup of leafy raw vegetables

Fruit Group
1 medium piece of fruit or melon wedge
$^3/_4$ cup of juice
$^1/_2$ cup of canned fruit
$^1/_4$ cup of dried fruit

Milk, Yogurt, & Cheese Group
1 cup of milk or yogurt
$1^1/_2$ ounces of natural cheese
2 ounces of processed cheese

Meat, Poultry, Fish, Dry Beans, Eggs, & Nut Group
$2^1/_2$ to 3 ounces of cooked lean meat, poultry, or fish
Count $^1/_2$ cup of cooked beans, or 1 egg, or 2 tablespoons of peanut butter as 1 ounce of lean meat.

Fats & Sweets
Limit calories from these, especially if you need to lose weight.

(U.S. Department of Agriculture and the U.S. Department of Health and Human Services, 1996.)

established for all nutrients. Like the food pyramid approach, variety is recommended.

Dietary Recommendations

The dietary recommendations and guidelines proposed by numerous governmental and health agencies complement the Food Guide Pyramid approach to diet planning and the RDA through their focus on avoiding nutritional excesses. Although these diet recommendations are not guaranteed to prevent diseases, many experts believe that most Americans can reduce their risk for chronic diet-related diseases, such as diabetes, certain types of cancer, and heart disease, by modifying the typical diet. The Public Health Service of the Department of Health and Human Services and the U.S. Department of Agriculture together update the "Dietary Guidelines for Americans" every 5 years. This document, entitled *Healthy People 2010,* includes broad nutritional challenges as part of overall strategies for health promotion. These guidelines, updated in 2000, are listed in Box 42-3.

Food Labeling

Food labels provide a significant amount of nutritional information for the consumer. Regulations that control food labels have always been controversial. In 1975, the FDA, a federal agency charged with protecting the U.S. food and drug supply, enacted legislation for a standardized label format that was considered a positive step toward educating the consumer about nutrition. Confusion and misinformation resulted as food manufacturers oversimplified or exaggerated health claims for

their products. In 1990, Congress passed the Nutritional Labeling and Education Act, which required all foods, including fruits and vegetables, to be clearly labeled. Four broad categories are addressed in this legislation. They include nutrition labeling, serving sizes, descriptors, and health claims (Dudek, 2001). Consumers should be easily able to identify the amount of saturated fat and dietary fiber included in a product, the number of calories from fat, in addition to viewing a listing of other nutritional information. Figure 42-3 illustrates a sample label with explanation of terms. All professional organizations agree that the food label is primarily a tool to educate the public about nutrition. A move is underway to ensure that nutritional labeling is responsible and accurate.

FACTORS AFFECTING NUTRITION

Although nutritional adequacy is an important consideration in planning a diet, a person's food patterns and habits may have a greater impact on overall food intake. Food habits are a product of many evolving variables, such as physical factors (eg, geographic location, food technology, and income), physiologic factors (eg, health, hunger, and stage of development), and psychosocial factors (eg, culture, religion, tradition, education, politics, social status, food ideology [the meaning of food for an individual] and learned aversions). These variables alone or in combination also can affect nutrition. Although not static, conservative traditional influences, like culture, geographic region, and religion, have a stabilizing effect on food habits.

Physiologic and Physical Factors That Influence Nutrient Requirements

There are various reasons why a person's nutrient requirements may differ. Some are permanent, such as gender, while others are temporary, such as with pregnancy.

Developmental Considerations

Throughout the life cycle, nutrient needs change in relation to growth, development, activity, and age-related changes in metabolism and body composition. Periods of intense growth and development, such as during infancy, adolescence, pregnancy, and lactation, cause an increase in nutrient needs. Nutrient needs stabilize during adulthood, although older people may need more or less of some nutrients. Age influences not only nutrient requirements but also food intake. The consistency of food, eating patterns, and the significance of food change with physical and psychosocial development.

Remember Sophia Vincent, the mother of the 3-year-old and William Johnston, the executive with hypertension and high cholesterol described at the beginning of the chapter? The

---

BOX 42-3 Dietary Guidelines for Americans: The ABCs for Your Health

Aim for Fitness
- Aim for a healthy weight.
- Be physically active each day.

Build a Health Base
- Let the Pyramid guide your food choices.
- Choose a variety of grains daily, especially whole grains.
- Choose a variety of fruits and vegetables daily.
- Keep food safe to eat.

Choose Sensibly
- Choose a diet that is low in saturated fat and cholesterol and moderate in total fat.
- Choose beverages and food that limit your intake of sugars.
- Choose and prepare foods with less salt.
- If you drink alcoholic beverages, do so in moderation.

(U.S. Department of Health and Human Services. [2002]. *Report of the Dietary Guidelines Advisory Committee on The Dietary Guidelines for Americans.* Washington, DC: Author.)

Total Fat

Aim low: Most people need to cut back on fat! Too much fat may contribute to heart disease and cancer. Try to limit your calories from fat. For a healthy heart, choose foods with a big difference between the total number of calories and the number of calories from fat.

Saturated Fat

A new kind of fat? No — saturated fat is part of the total fat in food. It is listed separately because it's the key player in raising blood cholesterol and your risk of heart disease. Eat less!

Cholesterol

Too much cholesterol — a second cousin to fat — can lead to heart disease. Challenge yourself to eat less than 300 mg each day.

Sodium

You call it "salt," the label calls it "sodium." Either way, it may add up to high blood pressure in some people. So, keep your sodium intake low — 2,400 to 3,000 mg or less each day.*

* The AHA recommends no more than 3,000 mg sodium per day for healthy adults.

Daily Value

Feel like you're drowning in numbers? Let the Daily Value be your guide. Daily Values are listed for people who eat 2,000 or 2,500 calories each day. If you eat more, your personal daily value may be higher than what's listed on the label. If you eat less, your personal daily value may be lower.

For fat, saturated fat, cholesterol and sodium, choose foods with a low **% Daily Value**. For total carbohydrate, dietary fiber, vitamins and minerals, your daily value goal is to reach 100% of each.

g = grams (About 28 g = 1 ounce)
mg = milligrams (1,000 mg = 1 g)

Nutrition Facts

Serving Size 1/2 cup (114g)
Servings Per Container 4

Amount Per Serving

Calories 90   Calories from Fat 30

	% Daily Value*
Total Fat 3g	5%
Saturated Fat 0g	0%
Cholesterol 0mg	0%
Sodium 300mg	13%
Total Carbohydrate 13g	4%
Dietary Fiber 3g	12%
Sugars 3g	
Protein 3g	

Vitamin A 80%	•	Vitamin C 60%
Calcium 4%	•	Iron 4%

* Percent Daily Values are based on a 2,000 calorie diet. Your daily values may be higher or lower depending on your caloric needs:

	Calories	2,000	2,500
Total Fat	Less than	65g	80g
Sat Fat	Less than	20g	25g
Cholesterol	Less than	300mg	300mg
Sodium	Less than	2,400mg	2,400mg
Total Carbohydrate		300g	375g
Fiber		25g	30g

Calories per gram:
Fat 9   •   Carbohydrate 4   •   Protein 4

* More nutrients may be listed on some labels.

Serving Size

Is your serving the same size as the one on the label? If you eat double the serving size listed, you need to double the nutrient and caloric values. If you eat one-half the serving size shown here, cut the nutrient and caloric values in half.

Calories

Are you overweight? Cut back a little on calories! Look here to see how a serving of the food adds to your daily total. A 5'4", 138-lb. active woman needs about 2,200 calories each day. A 5'10", 174-lb. active man needs about 2,900. How about you?

Total Carbohydrate

When you cut down on fat, you can eat more carbohydrates. Carbohydrates are in foods like bread, potatoes, fruits and vegetables. Choose these often! They give you nutrients and energy.

Dietary Fiber

Grandmother called it "roughage," but her advice to eat more is still up-to-date! That goes for both soluble and insoluble kinds of dietary fiber. Fruits, vegetables, whole-grain foods, beans and peas are all good sources and can help reduce the risk of heart disease and cancer.

Protein

Most Americans get more protein than they need. Where there is animal protein, there is also fat and cholesterol. Eat small servings of lean meat, fish and poultry. Use skim or low-fat milk, yogurt, and cheese. Try vegetable proteins like beans, grains and cereals.

Vitamins & Minerals

Your goal here is 100% of each for the day. Don't count on one food to do it all. Let a combination of foods add up to a winning score.

FIGURE 42-3 Sample nutritional label with explanation of terms.   (Source: American Heart Association.)

nurse would need to incorporate knowledge of each patient's developmental level when planning care.

Infants

The period from birth to 1 year of age is the most rapid period of growth. Birth weight doubles in 4 to 6 months and triples by 1 year of age. Length increases 50% in the first year. Muscle control and the development of hand–eye coordination allow the infant to progress to sitting upright and self-feeding. The iron stores present at birth start to become depleted between 3 and 4 months of age. The immune system matures between 4 and 6 months of age.

Nutritional needs per unit of body weight are greater than at any other time in the life cycle. Breastfeeding is recommended as the major source of nutrition for the first 6 to 12 months of life. If the infant is not breastfed, the infant should receive one of the commercially prepared infant formulas that contain iron. Cow's milk is not recommended for infants under the age of 1 year. Supplemental vitamins may be prescribed. Generally, solid foods are not introduced until 6 months of age because solid foods given too early may trigger allergic reactions. By 1 year of age, the infant typically is eating table food. Iron-fortified foods are recommended.

Toddlers and Preschoolers

During this stage, the decrease in growth is dramatic. Mobility, autonomy, and coordination increase, as do muscle mass and bone density. Language skills improve, and the 3- to 5-year-old child also develops attitudes toward food.

Nutritionally, toddlers and preschoolers can feed themselves, verbalize food likes and dislikes, and occasionally use food to manipulate their parents. Appetite dramatically decreases and becomes erratic. Inappropriate use of food (ie, to punish, reward, bribe, or convey love) may lead to inappropriate food attitudes.

> *Remember Sophia Vincent, the mother of the 3-year-old concerned about her son's eating? The nurse would develop a teaching plan that addresses developmental changes associated with this age group, such as the distinct food attitudes, likes and dislikes, and the strive for autonomy. In addition, the nurse needs to alert the mother about how this age group can use food to manipulate parents.*

School-Aged Children

The 6- to 12-year-old child has an uneven, individualized, sometimes erratic growth pattern. Permanent teeth erupt as the digestive system matures. Socialization and independence increase. At this stage, the body accumulates reserves in preparation for the upcoming adolescent growth spurt.

Nutritional implications for the school-aged child focus on health promotion. Increasing energy requirements need to be balanced with foods of high nutritional value. The appetite improves but still may be irregular. The parents' role as the primary regulator of food intake diminishes, and advertising has more of an impact on the child's food choices.

Adolescents

Adolescence is a period of rapid physical, emotional, social, and sexual maturation. The growth spurt begins at different ages among individuals. Girls begin menstruation and experience fat deposition, whereas males experience an increase in muscle mass, lean body tissue, and bones. Adolescence is also marked by intense psychosocial growth, family conflict, and social and peer pressure.

Nutrient needs, especially for calories, protein, calcium, and iron, increase to support growth. Weight consciousness becomes compulsive in 1 of 100 teenaged girls and results in **anorexia nervosa,** an eating disorder characterized by extreme weight loss, muscle wasting, arrested sexual development, refusal to eat, and bizarre eating habits. **Bulimia,** another eating disorder characterized by gorging followed by purging with self-induced vomiting, diuretics, and laxatives, also becomes more common in this age group. Although contrasts exist, there is also some overlap between these diseases. Both conditions are serious health and nutritional problems, and individuals with these disorders require professional medical help and counseling.

If a teenage pregnancy occurs, both mother and child are at increased nutritional risk due to competition for the nutrients between the adolescent mother's body and that of the infant. Nutritional needs may be harder to meet because fewer meals are eaten at home, and peer influence and busy schedules have an impact.

Adults

With adulthood, growth ceases. This age is also marked by a decline in the BMR with each decade. Adults may become more aware of the preventive role of exercise, or pressures of work and family may lead to a decline in physical activity and exercise.

Nutritional needs level off in adulthood, and fewer calories are required because of the decrease in BMR. If adjustments in caloric intake are not made, weight gain results.

Pregnant and Lactating Women

During pregnancy, the fetus, maternal tissues, and placenta grow dramatically. Weight gain occurs, and GI changes as a result of the pregnancy may result in nausea, vomiting, heartburn, or constipation. The quantity of breast milk produced depends on an adequate supply of nutrients.

Nutrient needs during pregnancy increase to support growth and maintain maternal homeostasis, particularly during the second and third trimesters. Key nutrient needs include protein, calories, iron, folic acid, calcium, and iodine. Caloric needs are higher for lactation than pregnancy, and the nutritional quality of breast milk is maintained at the expense of maternal nutrition if dietary intake is inadequate.

Older Adults

Because of the decreases in BMR and physical activity and loss of lean body mass, energy expenditure decreases. Loss of teeth and periodontal disease may make chewing more difficult. A decrease in peristalsis can result in constipation. Loss of taste between sweet and salty begins between 55 and 59 years of age, but discrimination between bitter and sour remains intact. The sensation of thirst also decreases. Degenerative diseases and the use of medications are more common with aging. It is not uncommon for social isolation, poor self-esteem, or loss of independence to affect nutritional intake negatively.

Because of the changes related to aging, the caloric needs of the body decrease. Foods that are difficult to chew may need to be eliminated, whereas an increase in fiber and fluid intake can relieve constipation. Elderly people are also prone to dehydration, and lack of interest in eating is common. Nutrient intake, digestion, absorption, metabolism, or excretion may be altered because of the physiologic changes common to this age.

The U.S. Department of Agriculture Human Nutrition Center on Aging at Tufts University developed a modified Food Pyramid for adults 70 years of age and older who are relatively healthy and active. The base of the food pyramid is narrower to reflect the lower energy needs of this age group. Emphasis is on consuming nutrient-dense and high-fiber foods and water (Fig. 42-4). The flag atop the food pyramid serves as a reminder that calcium, vitamin D, and vitamin B_{12} supplements are frequently recommended for optimal nutrition in this population.

Sex

Men differ from women in their nutrient requirements due to differences in body composition and reproductive function. Their larger muscle mass translates into higher caloric and pro-

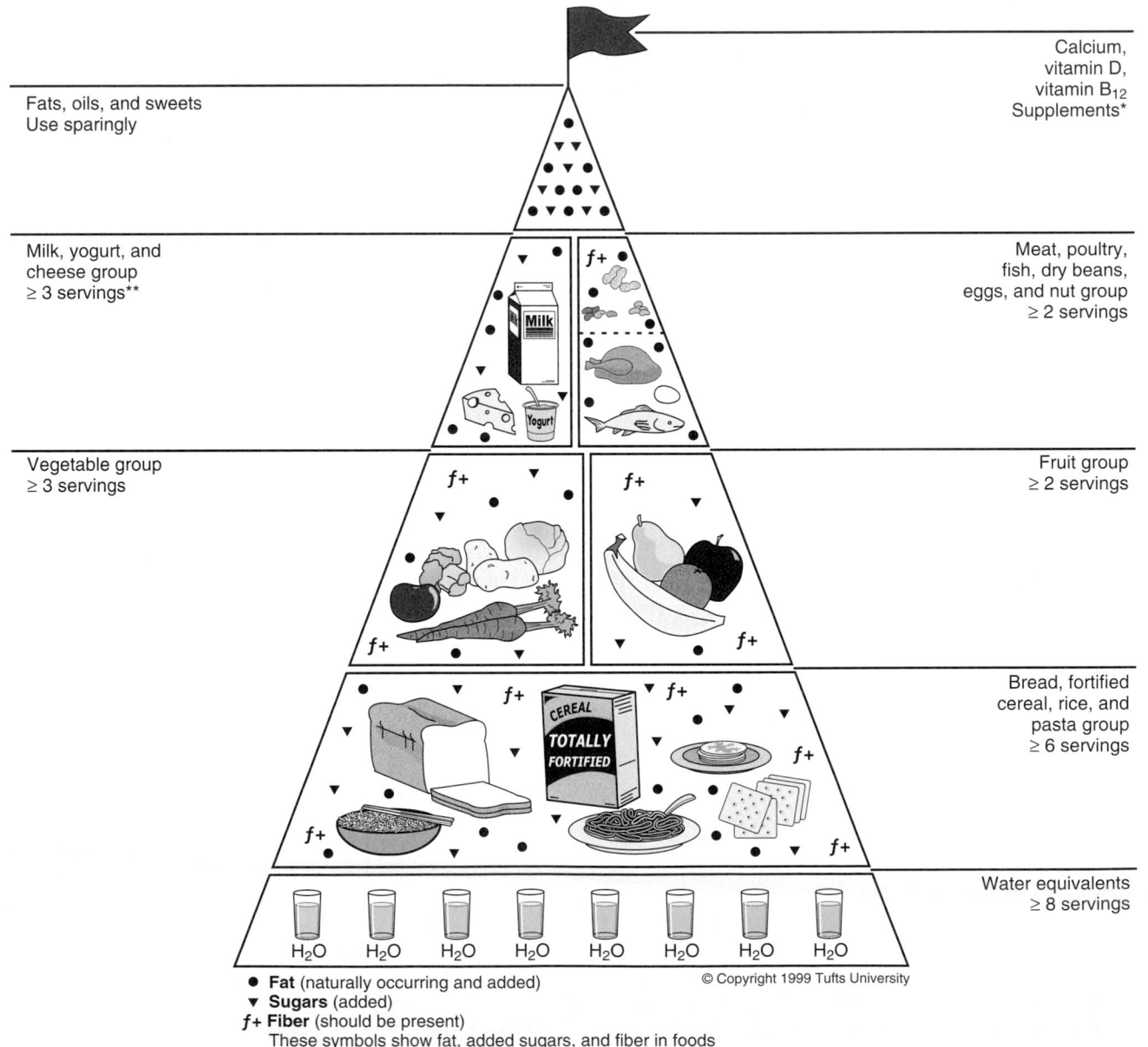

FIGURE 42-4 Modified food pyramid for adults age 70 and above.

tein requirements (and therefore slightly higher needs for B vitamins that metabolize calories and protein) because muscle is more metabolically active than adipose tissue (women have proportionately more adipose tissue). Women of childbearing age have higher iron requirements related to menstruation.

State of Health

The alteration in nutrient requirements that results from illness and trauma varies with the intensity and duration of the stress. For instance, fevers increase the need for calories and water. Unlike fevers related to septicemia, however, fevers caused by a mild case of the flu require few dietary adjustments.

Trauma, like major surgery, burns, and crush injuries, is followed by hormonal changes that profoundly affect the body's use of nutrients. To preserve or replenish body nutrient stores and to promote healing and recovery, nutrient requirements increase dramatically in the adaptive phase after stress. In some cases of severe trauma, such as major burns, the rehabilitative phase of recovery, characterized by the gradual normalization of nutrient needs, may last for years.

Chronic disorders, like diabetes mellitus, renal disease, hypertension, heart disease, GI disorders, and cancer, can alter nutrient requirements by influencing nutrient intake, digestion, absorption, metabolism, utilization, or excretion.

Alcohol Abuse

Alcohol can alter the body's use of nutrients, and thereby its nutrient requirements, by numerous mechanisms. The toxic effect of alcohol on the intestinal mucosa interferes with normal nutrient absorption; thus, requirements increase as the efficiency of absorption decreases. Need for B vitamins increases because they are used to metabolize alcohol. Alcohol can also influence nutrient metabolism by impairing nutrient storage, increasing nutrient catabolism, and increasing nutrient excretion. Alcohol abuse that results in liver damage has profound effects on the body's nutrient metabolism and requirements.

Medication

Many drugs have the potential to influence nutrient requirements. Nutrient absorption may be altered by drugs that (1) change the pH of the GI tract, (2) increase GI motility, (3) damage the intestinal mucosa, or (4) bind with nutrients, rendering them unavailable to the body. Nutrient metabolism can be altered by drugs that (1) act as nutrient antagonists, (2) alter the enzyme systems that metabolize nutrients, or (3) alter nutrient degradation. Some drugs alter the renal reabsorption of nutrients and therefore may increase or decrease nutrient excretion.

Megadoses of Nutrient Supplements

Because some nutrients compete against each other for absorption, an excess of one nutrient can lead to a deficiency (or increase the requirement) of another, especially if one is absorbed preferentially. For instance, a delicate balance exists between zinc and copper. People who take therapeutic levels of zinc run the risk of developing a copper deficiency—which is otherwise rare—unless they also increase their intake of copper.

Sociocultural and Psychosocial Factors

Dietary choices or restrictions also are influenced by culture, religion, and personal feelings and meanings associated with food. Diverse lifestyles and eating habits directly impact a person's nutritional health and well-being.

Religion

Dietary restrictions associated with religions might affect a patient's nutritional requirements. For example, during the Lenten season, Roman Catholics fast on Ash Wednesday and Good Friday in addition to abstaining from meat on every Friday. Alternative food choices or meal patterns may be necessary. Kosher dietary laws require special food preparation techniques and prohibit intake of pork and shellfish. Thus, a patient's religious affiliation may impact his or her nutritional regimen. Patients should be asked regarding any preferences or restrictions. Kosher diets and other special diets are available in hospitals, nursing homes, retirement homes, and programs such as Meals on Wheels.

Economics

The adequacy of a person's food budget affects dietary choices and patterns. The increasing cost of food, coupled with limited purchasing power, may result in a decrease in the nutritional quality of the diet. Many variables influence the types of foods purchased. Creative use of the food dollar means using unit pricing to determine cost per serving (eg, comparing the unit price of 39¢ per serving with a similar product's 45¢ per serving), selecting foods that contain adequate nutrients, and buying seasonal foods that are more economical and can be prepared easily at home. Avoiding convenience foods and meals purchased away from home saves food dollars.

Meaning of Food

Food means different things to different people, with food playing multiple roles in the lives of most individuals. In addition to satisfying hunger and providing nutrition, food may signify a celebration, a social gathering, or a reward. Some people use various foods to indicate caring or to give comfort and reassurance during times of stress or unhappiness. Mealtime may evoke memories of family discussions, laughter, and enjoyable times. Some may remember conflicts associated with eating or avoid eating because it reminds them of their loneliness and isolation. Others, because of society's emphasis on being thin, may resort to fad or crash-reducing diets to resolve eating conflicts and lose weight rapidly. This initial weight reduction seldom is sustained for an extended period, and a cycle of yo-yo dieting frequently results. Drastic weight loss is followed by an eating binge that causes the dieter to regain all the lost weight and, possibly, some additional weight each time the sequence occurs. Nutritional deficiencies may occur and place the person at risk for other diseases. Losing weight and keeping it off require a change in eating habits as part of the overall commitment to health.

Culture

Nutritional diversity is common among cultural or ethnic groups. The variety and selections are unique to each group and represent their personal beliefs and customs. Culture influences what is eaten or considered edible, how it is prepared, and what combinations of food are permitted. The varia-tions in food choices within a culture also depend on income levels and availability of foods. If a patient of a different culture is to be placed on a specific diet, discussing food choice options is necessary to customize the diet to meet the person's cultural demands. Many institutions have developed culturally sensitive food pyramids. Figure 42-5 shows a food guide pyramid developed for a Native American patient. Table 42-4 summarizes the food patterns of common ethnic groups.

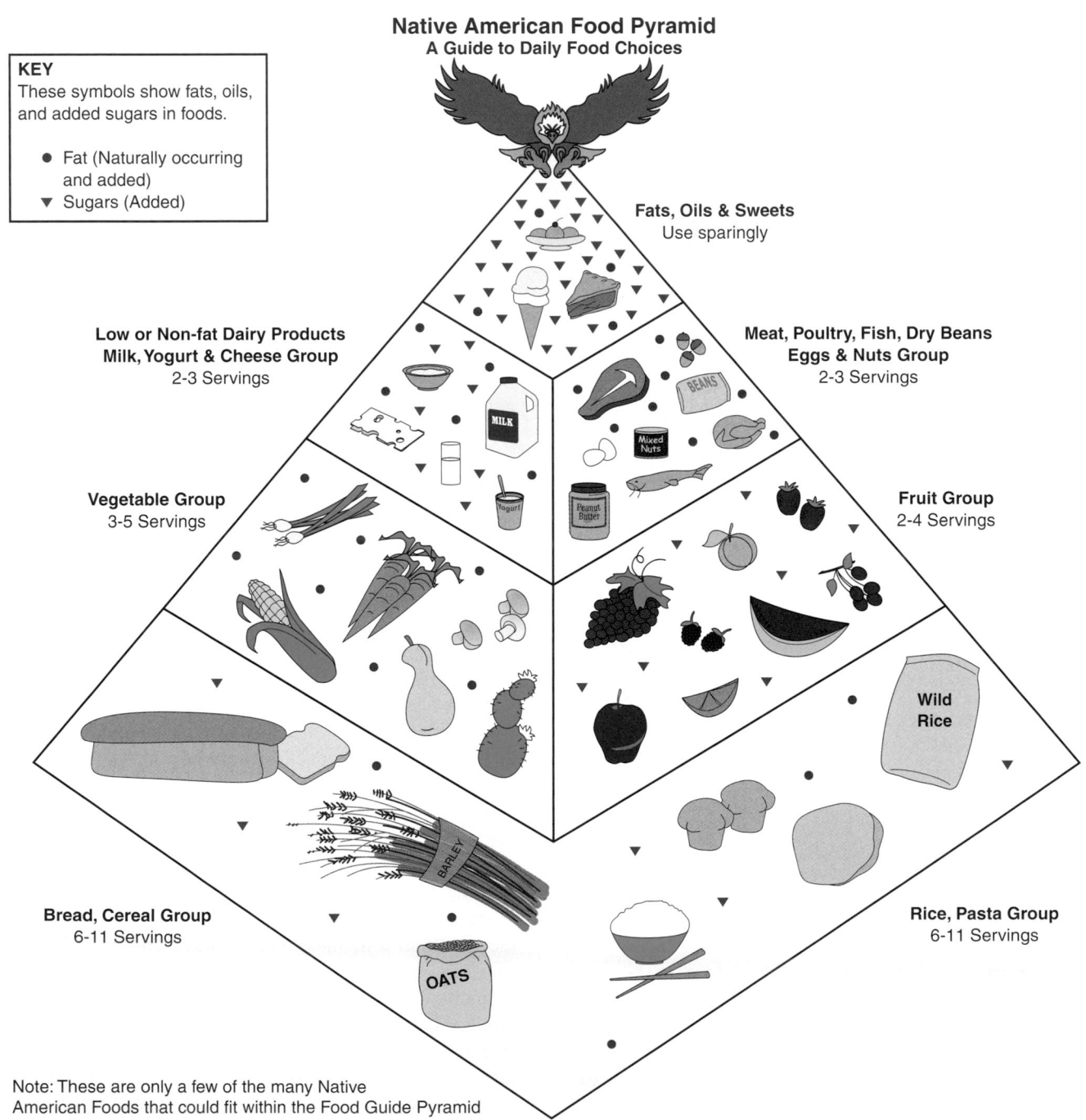

Native American Food Pyramid
A Guide to Daily Food Choices

KEY
These symbols show fats, oils, and added sugars in foods.

● Fat (Naturally occurring and added)
▼ Sugars (Added)

Fats, Oils & Sweets
Use sparingly

Low or Non-fat Dairy Products
Milk, Yogurt & Cheese Group
2-3 Servings

Meat, Poultry, Fish, Dry Beans
Eggs & Nuts Group
2-3 Servings

Vegetable Group
3-5 Servings

Fruit Group
2-4 Servings

Wild Rice

Bread, Cereal Group
6-11 Servings

Rice, Pasta Group
6-11 Servings

Note: These are only a few of the many Native American Foods that could fit within the Food Guide Pyramid

FIGURE 42-5 Native American Food Pyramid. (Adapted from California Adolescent Nutrition and Fitness Program. Available at http://www.nal.usda.gov/fnic/Fpyr/NAmFGP.html. Designed by CANFit Youth Leadership Committee & Project Staff, Escondido Community Health Center.)

TABLE 42-4 Cultural Variations on Nutrition

Culture	Food Patterns	Additional Comments
African/American	• Favorite meats are pork and chicken. • Intake of milk and dairy foods is low. • Intake of dark green, leafy vegetables.	• Diet tends to be high in fat and sodium. • Frying is a common method of preparation. • Obesity is common.
Chinese	• Little milk or cheese is used. • Rice is consumed with most meals. • Fresh foods are used and stir-fried before serving. • Unsweetened green tea is a common drink.	• Diet is high in fiber, low in fat, and may be deficient in protein. • Moderation is valued, and obesity is rare.
Greek	• Cheese is a favorite food. • Yogurt is a popular source of calcium. • Lamb is the favorite meat.	• Relatively large quantities of sweets and snacks are consumed. • Consumption of meat is on the increase. • A meal is a family ritual.
Italian	• Bread and pasta are basic foods. • Olive oil is used to prepare meats. • Cheese is main source of calcium.	• Milk is rarely consumed as a beverage. Red or white wine is consumed with dinner.
Japanese	• Rice may be eaten with every meal. • Seafood, especially raw fish, is the main protein source. • Main seasoning is soy sauce. • Tea is main beverage.	• Diet is low in fat but high in sodium. • Common methods of food preparation include broiling, steaming, boiling, and stir-frying.
Latino	• Many varieties of beans are consumed; little meat is used. • Milk intake is small but large quantities of coffee are consumed. • Corn is the basic grain.	• Selection of hot and cold foods plays a role in body equilibrium. • Lactose intolerance is possible. • Diet is high in fiber and starch. • Lard is a basic cooking fat, and obesity is common.
Puerto Rican	• Steamed white rice is a staple. • Starchy vegetables (eg, breadfruit and viandas) and fruits such as plantains are popular. • Legumes are a good source of protein.	• Milk is rarely consumed as a beverage. • Food is frequently fried and cooked for a long period of time.

(Adapted from Dudek, S. G. [2001]. *Nutrition handbook for nursing practice* [4th ed.]. Philadelphia: Lippincott Williams & Wilkins; Purnell, L., & Paulanka, B. [1998]. *Transcultural health care*. Philadelphia: F. A. Davis.)

Factors Affecting Nutritional Intake

At times, a combination of factors can affect an individual's nutritional intake. Subsequently, these factors can result in a decrease or increase in food intake.

Decreased Food Intake

Food intake may decrease for various reasons. **Anorexia,** or the lack of appetite, may be related to systemic and local diseases; numerous psychosocial causes, such as fear, anxiety, depression, pain; and impaired ability to smell and taste—or it may occur secondary to drug therapy or medical treatments. Others who may have limited food intake include those who have difficulty chewing and swallowing, those who experience chronic GI problems or undergo certain surgical procedures, and those on inadequate food budgets.

> *Consider Charles Gallagher, whose wife is receiving enteral feedings. The underlying reason for insertion of the PEG tube was her inability to swallow and subsequent development of aspiration pneumonia that required numerous hospitalizations. The nurse would need to communicate this information to Mr. Gallagher to ensure that he understands the rationale for the feeding. This understanding is important for decision making.*

Increased Food Intake

Increased food intake may lead to obesity. Obesity presents a serious health problem physically, socially, and emotionally. **Obesity** is defined as body weight 20% or more above ideal weight or having a BMI of 30 or more. A positive caloric balance, resulting from an excess caloric intake or a decrease in energy expenditure, leads to the gradual accumulation of weight. This excess weight increases the risk for numerous medical problems; increases the risks associated with surgery; increases the risk for complications during pregnancy, labor, and delivery; and increases morbidity and mortality. People who are obese are often discriminated against in social, educational, and employment settings. In a society that values thinness, obesity can cause one to feel desperate, frustrated, depressed, and rejected, and to perceive oneself as a failure.

Numerous theories about the cause of obesity have been proposed. According to genetic theories, a low resting metabolic rate or an inherited family tendency contribute to obesity. Physiologic factors that have been implicated include an increased number of fat cells, a lowered basal metabolic rate set-point, a decreased amount of brown fat that burns kilocalories, insulin resistance, and hormone imbalance. A food and family environment that encourages overeating, a lifestyle where exercise is minimal, and the availability of foods in a multitude of settings at all times are environmental factors that contribute to obesity (Liebman, 2001). Additionally, many identify psychological reasons for obesity, including compulsiveness, using food to satisfy emotional needs, relying on food for compensation for lack of affection and companionship, and overeating as a release mechanism for boredom, anxiety, and feelings of inadequacy.

About 30.5% of Americans are considered obese (have a BMI ≥ 30)—a decade ago this number was only 22.9% (Flegal, Carroll, Ogden, & Johnson, 2002). In addition, approximately 15% of school-aged children are overweight today, in comparison to 11% identified in the early 1990s. Obesity is resistant to treatment, and weight loss is temporary at best unless behavior modification and exercise are incorporated into the dietary plan.

THE NURSING PROCESS

Assessing

Nutritional status has a significant impact on both health and disease. For well patients, good nutritional status can help to maintain health, promote normal growth and development, and protect against disease. During illness, good nutritional status can reduce the risk for complications and speed recovery time. Conversely, poor nutritional status can increase the risk for illness or death.

The nature of the nurse–patient relationship affords nurses the opportunity to incorporate nutritional assessment into the nursing process. Like other aspects of nursing care, nutritional assessment is a systematic approach used to identify the patient's actual or potential needs, formulate a plan to meet those needs, initiate the plan or assign others to implement it, and evaluate the effectiveness of the plan. The level of assessment may range from simple screening to a comprehensive, in-depth assessment, depending on individual circumstances. Regardless of the level of assessment, nutritional assessment is appropriate for all patients. Nurses can collect assessment data through history taking (dietary, medical, and socioeconomic data), physical assessments (anthropometric and clinical data), and laboratory data. When performing a nutritional assessment, nurses need to be aware of the specific changes in older people that may reflect on the accuracy of the assessment process (Box 42-4).

BOX 42-4 Nutritional Assessment Considerations for Older Adults*

Biochemical Data
- Low serum albumin level (below 3.5 mg/dL) may be a reflection of the aging process rather than a nutritional risk factor. Albumin synthesis declines with age.
- Hemoglobin levels that are lower than normal may only reflect anemia observed in elderly people as part of the aging process.

Anthropometric Data
- Because of age-related changes in body composition, skin-fold measurements should be taken from several body sites.

Dietary Data
- Dietary recall may be inaccurate because of vision and memory problems.
- Question use of vitamin and mineral supplements.
- Gather information concerning medication regimen (prescribed and over-the-counter) to assess for food–drug interactions and adverse effects of medications.

* Specific clinical data for older adults may be found in the Focus on the Older Adult display.

Nurses, by nature of their caring role and personal encounters, serve as nutritional role models and are ideally situated to identify nutritional needs and assess and monitor for nutritional risks. See Promoting Health 42-1: Nutrition.

Dietary Data

Dietary data may be collected from the patient or family and can be evaluated according to the Food Guide Pyramid, dietary guidelines, or the RDA, depending on the purpose of the assessment. Statistics indicate that as many as 50% of elderly people living independently may have nutritional deficiencies, and 20% of this group may, in fact, skip at least one meal a day (Dudek, 2001).

Discussion continues among health experts about the most effective method to assess for the risk for nutritionally related complications. Some nutritionists state that a thorough physical assessment and nutritional history can more accurately determine the presence of malnutrition than a series of laboratory test results. Guigoz, Lauque, & Vellas (2002) developed the Mini Nutritional Assessment tool (MNA). The MNA is used to detect elderly persons at risk for malnutrition prior to changes in albumin level and the BMI. The MNA is a combination of screening questions followed by anthropometric measurements, including BMI, mid-arm and calf circumference, and weight loss. The MNA is fast and easy, and the authors recommend performing the MNA on all elderly patients, whether community dwelling, hospitalized, or in nursing homes.

After a screening tool identifies a patient at risk, such as in a group of older adults, it is imperative that a nutritional

Promoting Health 42-1 *Nutrition*

Use the assessment checklist to determine how well you are meeting your nutritional needs. Then develop a prescription for self-care by choosing appropriate behaviors from the list of suggestions.

ASSESSMENT CHECKLIST

almost always / sometimes / almost never

1. I know and use the recommended dietary guidelines and servings.
2. My weight is within 10% of the ideal for my height and body frame.
3. I maintain an appropriate balance between exercise and food intake.
4. I limit my fat, sugar, salt, and red meat intake.
5. I limit my caffeine intake.
6. I use alcoholic beverages in moderation.
7. I make an effort to eat high-fiber foods.

SELF-CARE BEHAVIORS

1. Maintain desirable weight, eating a variety of foods in adequate amounts from each of the four food groups.
2. Eat slowly, take smaller portions, and avoid second helpings if trying to control overeating.
3. Eat a variety of foods low in calories and high in nutrients to lose weight.
4. Obtain medical clearance before starting a weight-loss program.
5. Avoid too many foods high in cholesterol (milk, egg yolk, organ meats, fats, oils); instead choose lean meat, fish, poultry, and beans.
6. Eat foods high in fiber: whole-grain breads and cereals, fruits, vegetables, dry beans.
7. Avoid excess use of salt and sugar.
8. Begin an exercise program, and maintain it.
9. Learn healthy eating habits; read labels, become familiar with healthy fast-food and restaurant menus, drink alcohol moderately (if at all).
10. Substitute healthy rewards for yourself that do not include high-calorie, low-nutrition snacks and beverages.

---

assessment be completed as a follow-up. When this is combined with other methods of assessing nutritional status, the nurse is better prepared to coordinate a focused strategy to combat malnutrition.

24-Hour Recall Method

The easiest way to collect dietary data is to obtain a 24-hour recall of all food and beverages the patient normally consumes during an average day. It includes the patient's usual portion sizes, meal and snack patterns, meal timing, and location where food is eaten. Because this method relies on memory and accurate interpretation of portion sizes, the information may not be reliable.

Food Diaries

Food-frequency questionnaires or food diaries may provide a better overall picture of nutrient intake because the patient records all food and beverages consumed in a specified period, usually 3 to 7 days.

Diet History

A more comprehensive approach to diet assessment is a full diet history. In addition to a 24-hour food recall and food-frequency record, interview questions are geared to provide information on past and present food intake and habits. Sample questions are included in the accompanying Focused Assessment Guide 42-1.

Consider Sophia Vincent, the mother of a 3-year-old boy who is concerned about his eating. The nurse could use a diet history to obtain specific information about the child's actual intake. Analysis of this information would reveal the extent of the child's problem and the possibility that an actual nutritional problem exists.

The following findings are considered dietary risk factors for malnutrition and are spelled out in the acronym DETERMINE (Nutrition Initiative Screening, retrieved from http://www.aafp.org/x16087.xml). This is part of a larger nutrition screening tool.

- **D**isease
- **E**ating Poorly
- **T**ooth Loss/Mouth Pain
- **E**conomic Hardship
- **R**educed Social Contact
- **M**ultiple Medicines
- **I**nvoluntary Weight Loss/Gain
- **N**eeds Assistance in Self-Care
- **E**lder Years Above Age 80

Medical and Socioeconomic Data

Medical, social, and economic factors, as well as cultural and psychological influences, require evaluation for their impact on nutritional requirements and food choices. A nutritional assessment should include information about the following (Dudek, 2001):

MEDICAL DATA

- Current illness as well as medical and surgical history
- Past and current drug history
- History of drug dependence or abuse
- Ability to chew and swallow, including condition of mouth, missing teeth, or dentures
- Appetite, food intolerance and allergies, and bowel habits

Focused Assessment Guide 42-1

Nutrition

Factors to Assess	Questions and Approaches
Usual dietary intake	Does your current intake differ from your usual intake? If so, is the reason a loss of appetite, changes in smell or taste, difficulty chewing and swallowing, hospitalization, a modified diet? With whom do you usually eat meals?
Food allergies or intolerances	Do you have any food allergies or intolerances?
Food preparation and storage	Who does the food shopping? Who prepares the meals? How is the food normally prepared? For instance, is food usually fried, baked, or broiled? Do you have adequate food storage space and preparation equipment?
Type of diet	Do you now or have you in the past followed a modified diet prescribed by a physician?
Dietary practices	Do you now or have you in the past used a fad diet, health foods, or self-prescribed supplements?
Eating disorder patterns	Do you view yourself as overweight? Do you weigh yourself frequently during one day? How is your appetite? Do you binge on large amounts of food in a short period? Have you ever caused yourself to vomit after eating a meal? Have you used laxatives, diuretics, herbal supplements or over-the-counter weight loss pills to lose weight?

SOCIAL DATA

- Age, gender, family history, lifestyle (eg, those at extremes in age are most at risk)
- Educational background
- Information about occupation, exercise, and sleep patterns
- Religious affiliation, cultural, and ethnic background
- Use of alcohol and tobacco

ECONOMIC DATA

- Source of income
- Food budget

Anthropometric Data

Anthropometric measurements are used to determine body dimensions. In children, anthropometric measurements are used to assess growth rate; in adults, they can give indirect measurements of body protein and fat stores. For the data to be accurate and reliable, standardized equipment and procedures must be used, and the data must be compared with the appropriate reference standards for the patient's age and sex.

Height and weight, the most common anthropometric measurements, are obtained when the patient is admitted to the healthcare facility and periodically thereafter or assessed in a home care environment. Weigh a patient on the same scale each time and at the same time of day, preferably before breakfast. Usual body weight is compared with the BMI standard. Because actual weight may be increased if the patient has edema, hydration status must be considered. Although self-reported weight may be recorded when actual weight is

unobtainable, it is highly inaccurate and must be noted. An actual weight is recorded as soon as feasibly possible.

Additional anthropometric measurements include triceps skin-fold measurements, a measure of subcutaneous fat stores; midarm circumference, a measure of skeletal muscle mass; and midarm muscle circumference, a measure of both skeletal muscle mass and fat stores. (Fig. 42-6). Reference standards have been determined for men and women for all three measures, as have figures representing 90%, 80%, 70%, and 60% of standard.

Clinical Data

Although signs and symptoms of altered nutrition may be observed during a physical assessment (Table 42-5), they usually do not appear until the condition is advanced. In addition, further investigation is necessary to determine whether abnormal findings are actually caused by a nutritional deficiency, are possibly related to a nutritional deficiency, or are unrelated to nutritional status.

Biochemical Data

Laboratory tests, which measure blood and urine levels of nutrients or biochemical functions that depend on an adequate supply of nutrients, can objectively detect nutritional problems in their early stages. Most routine biochemical tests measure protein status; measures of body vitamin, mineral, and trace element status are also available.

Hemoglobin, the oxygen-carrying protein of the red blood cells, and hematocrit, the volume of red blood cells packed by

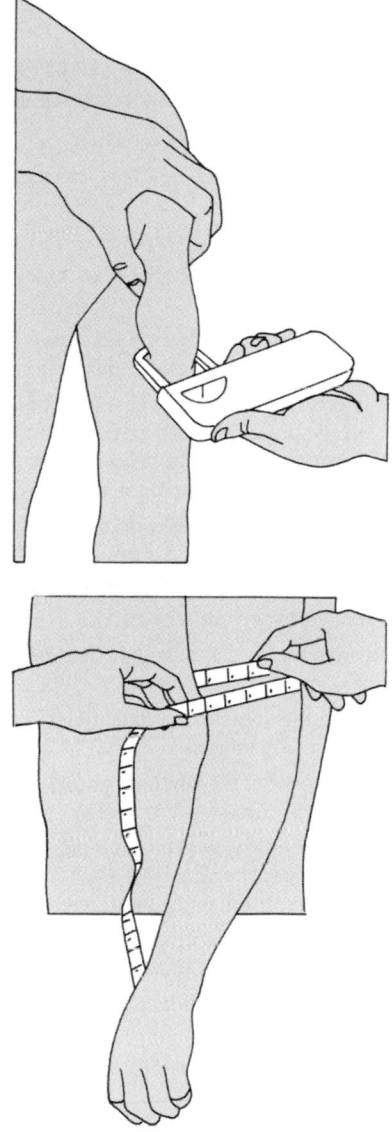

FIGURE 42-6 Two anthropometric measurements to assess nutritional status: triceps skin-fold measurement (*top*) and midarm muscle circumference (*bottom*).

centrifugation in a given volume of blood, are measures of plasma protein that also reflect a person's iron status. Protein status can also be determined by measuring serum albumin and transferrin levels and by a total lymphocyte count. The total lymphocyte count reflects immune status and is directly affected by impaired nutritional states. Albumin is an important laboratory value to assess over a period of time. The albumin level does not change with increasing age, but malnutrition and various disease states cause its level to decrease.

Twenty-four-hour urine tests used to measure protein metabolism include urine creatinine excretion and urine urea nitrogen. Urea, a breakdown product of amino acids, can be measured in the urine and blood. It reflects protein intake and the body's ability to detoxify and excrete this metabolic by-product. Creatinine levels are directly proportional to the body's muscle mass, and a reduction in this value reflects severe mal-

nutrition. These biochemical indicators with nutritional implications are summarized in Box 42-5.

Recall Sophia Vincent, the mother voicing frustration and concern about her child's nutrition? If a diet history reveals the possibility of a nutritional problem, the nurse would anticipate obtaining biochemical tests to provide additional information to support or refute the existence of a problem.

Diagnosing

Assessment data may reveal actual or potential nutritional problems.

Imbalanced Nutrition as the Problem
The following nursing diagnoses may be made when imbalanced nutrition is the cause of the patient's disorder:
Imbalanced Nutrition: Less Than Body Requirements related to nothing by mouth (NPO), inadequate tube feeding, prolonged use of a clear liquid diet, numerous food intolerance or allergies, excessive dieting, anorexia, chewing or swallowing difficulties, nausea, vomiting, chronic diarrhea, malabsorption, psychological eating disorders (anorexia nervosa, bulimia), alcoholism, metabolic and endocrine disorders, inappropriate use of supplements
Imbalanced Nutrition: More Than Body Requirements related to overeating, inactivity, metabolic and endocrine disorders, inappropriate use of supplements
Risk for Imbalanced Nutrition: More Than Body Requirements related to inappropriate eating, closely spaced pregnancies, metabolic and endocrine disorders, inappropriate use of supplements
See specific examples in the accompanying NANDA Nursing Diagnoses box.

Imbalanced Nutrition as the Etiology
Nutritional problems may affect other areas of human functioning. In the following nursing diagnoses, the nutritional problem is the cause of another problem.
Activity Intolerance related to inadequate caloric intake, obesity, iron-deficiency anemia
Impaired Dentition related to nutritional deficits
Ineffective Health Maintenance related to lack of knowledge about adequate nutrition
Anxiety related to obesity
Constipation related to inadequate fluid or fiber intake
Diarrhea related to overeating, excessive fiber intake, excessive sorbitol intake (sugar alcohol)
Deficient Fluid Volume related to inadequate fluid intake
Risk for Infection related to inadequate calorie intake, inadequate protein intake
Impaired Home Maintenance Management related to inability to purchase, store, or prepare food for family
Impaired Skin Integrity related to protein malnutrition, vitamin A deficiency

TABLE 42-5 Clinical Observations for Nutritional Assessment

Body Area	Signs of Good Nutritional Status	Signs of Poor Nutritional Status
General appearance	Alert, responsive	Listless, apathetic, and cachexic
General vitality	Endurance, energetic, sleeps well, vigorous	Easily fatigued, no energy, falls asleep easily, looks tired, apathetic
Weight	Normal for height, age, body build	Overweight or underweight
Hair	Shiny, lustrous, firm, not easily plucked, healthy scalp	Dull and dry, brittle, loss of color, easily plucked, thin and sparse
Face	Uniform skin color; healthy appearance, not swollen	Dark skin over cheeks and under eyes, flaky skin, facial edema (moon face), pale skin color
Eyes	Bright, clear, moist, no sores at corners of eyelids, membranes moist and healthy pink color, no prominent blood vessels	Pale eye membranes, dry eyes (xerophthalmia); Bitot's spots, increased vascularity, cornea soft (keratomalacia), small yellowish lumps around eyes (xanthelasma), dull or scarred cornea
Lips	Good pink color, smooth, moist, not chapped or swollen	Swollen and puffy (cheilosis), angular lesion at corners of mouth or fissures or scars (stomatitis)
Tongue	Deep red, surface papillae present	Smooth appearance, beefy red or magenta colored, swollen, hypertrophy or atrophy
Teeth	Straight, no crowding, no cavities, no pain, bright, no discoloration, well-shaped jaw	Cavities, mottled appearance (Fluorosis), mal-positioned, missing teeth
Gums	Firm, good pink color, no swelling or bleeding	Spongy, bleed easily, marginal redness, recessed, swollen and inflamed
Glands	No enlargement of the thyroid, face not swollen	Enlargement of the thyroid (goiter), enlargement of the parotid (swollen cheeks)
Skin	Smooth, good color, slightly moist, no signs of rashes, swelling, or color irregularities	Rough, dry, flaky, swollen, pale, pigmented, lack of fat under the skin, fat deposits around the joints (xanthomas), bruises, petechiae
Nails	Firm, pink	Spoon shaped (koilonychia), brittle, pale, ridged
Skeleton	Good posture, no malformations	Poor posture, beading of the ribs, bowed legs or knock-knees, prominent scapulas, chest deformity at diaphragm
Muscles	Well developed, firm, good tone, some fat under the skin	Flaccid, poor tone, wasted, underdeveloped, difficulty walking
Extremities	No tenderness	Weak and tender, presence of edema
Abdomen	Flat	Swollen
Nervous system	Normal reflexes, psychological stability	Decrease in or loss of ankle and knee reflexes, psychomotor changes, mental confusion, depression, sensory loss, motor weakness, loss of sense of position, loss of vibration, burning and tingling of the hands and feet (paresthesia)
Cardiovascular system	Normal heart rate and rhythm, no murmurs, normal blood pressure for age	Cardiac enlargement, tachycardia, elevated blood pressure
GI system	No palpable organs or masses (liver edge may be palpable in children)	Hepatosplenomegaly

(Adapted from Dudek, S. G. [2001]. *Nutrition handbook for nursing practice* [4th ed.]. Philadelphia: Lippincott Williams & Wilkins.)

Deficient Knowledge related to new medical diet, nutrition misinformation, lack of interest in nutrition, intellectual deficit

Noncompliance to a particular diet order related to lack of motivation, misinformation

Chronic Low Self-Esteem related to obesity

Disturbed Sleep Pattern related to excessive caffeine intake

Social Isolation related to obesity

Wellness Diagnosis

For patients who are incorporating sound nutritional practices in their daily routine, the following wellness diagnosis may

BOX 42-5 Biochemical Data With Nutritional Implications

- Hemoglobin (normal = 12–18 g/dL)
  decreased → anemia
- Hematocrit (normal = 40%–50%)
  decreased → anemia
  increased → dehydration
- Serum albumin (normal = 3.3–5 g/dL)
  decreased → malnutrition (prolonged protein depletion), malabsorption
- Transferrin (normal = 240–480 mg/dL)
  decreased → anemia, protein deficiency
- Total lymphocyte count (normal = greater than 1800)
  decreased → impaired nutritional intake, severe debilitating disease
- Blood urea nitrogen (normal = 17–18 mg/dL)
  increased → starvation, high protein intake, severe dehydration
  decreased → malnutrition, overhydration
- Creatinine (normal = 0.4–1.5 mg/dL)
  increased → dehydration
  decreased → reduction in total muscle mass, severe malnutrition

(Fischbach, F. [2003]. *A manual of laboratory and diagnostic tests* [7th ed.]. Philadelphia: Lippincott Williams & Wilkins.)

be appropriate: Readiness for Enhanced Nutrition associated with Low-Fat Diet Regimen.

Outcome Identification and Planning

Expected outcomes are derived from the actual or potential nutritional problems diagnosed. General patient outcomes follow. The patient will:

- Attain and maintain ideal body weight.
- Eat a diet adequate but not excessive in all nutrients.
- Eat a variety of food in each of three or more meals.
- Follow the appropriate modified diet, when necessary, to restore health, avoid disease recurrences, and prevent or delay potential complications.

Remember Charles Gallagher, the husband of the woman receiving enteral nutrition? Initially, outcomes would focus on maintaining his wife's nutritional status. However, the informed decision made to withdraw the nutritional support would lead the nurse to revise the outcomes. Therefore, the outcomes then would focus on emotional comfort for the Gallagher family and a peaceful, dignified death for Mrs. Gallagher.

Examples of NANDA Nursing Diagnoses | Nutrition

Nursing Diagnoses	Related Factors	Sample Defining Characteristics
Imbalanced Nutrition: Less Than Body Requirements	Malabsorption	• "I seem to eat all day long and yet I keep losing weight." • Reports losing 15 lb within the past 3 weeks. Has 8 to 10 bowel movements daily of frothy, odorous stools that float. Fecal fat excretion test indicates steatorrhea. Patient appears fatigued and undernourished; muscle wasting is evident. Laboratory data reveal low serum albumin level (protein deficiency) and iron-deficiency anemia.
Imbalanced Nutrition: More Than Body Requirements	Decreased thyroid function leading to a decrease in metabolism	• "I don't eat enough to keep a bird alive, but I just keep getting fatter and fatter. I don't know what else to do unless I stop eating altogether." • Patient reports a 10-lb weight gain within the past month despite following a 1200-calorie diet. Other symptoms noted include fatigue, amenorrhea, and dry skin. Laboratory data indicate low serum thyroxine (T_4) level, protein-bound iodine, and elevated serum thyroid-stimulating hormone and cholesterol levels. Radioactive iodine uptake was low.
Risk for Imbalanced Nutrition: More Than Body Requirements	Inappropriate use of supplements	• "I sent a sample of my hair away for a nutritional analysis, and the report came back saying that I should take supplements of zinc, iron, potassium, and magnesium." • For the past week, patient has been taking supplements of 500% of the RDA for zinc and magnesium. She takes twice as much iron as recommended, and large doses of potassium ad lib.

Implementing

Providing proper and adequate nourishment to the patient is a team effort implemented in a variety of settings. Diet orders are written by the physician, confirmed by the dietitian, and frequently explained to the patient by the nurse. The nurse may also be responsible for screening patients at home who are at nutritional risk, observing intake and appetite, evaluating the patient's tolerance, assisting the patient with eating, administering enteral and parenteral feedings, consulting with the dietitian and physician when dietary problems arise, addressing the potential for drug–nutrient reactions, obtaining more food or snacks for the patient when appropriate, monitoring food brought by visitors, and participating in nutrition education efforts.

Teaching Nutritional Information

For the greatest chance of success, tailor diet instructions individually to the patient's lifestyle, culture, intellectual ability, and level of motivation.

> *Recall William Johnston, the patient with hypertension and high cholesterol? The nurse would need to consider Mr. Johnston's lifestyle when developing a teaching plan for him. As a result of his "on-the-run" lifestyle, the nurse would need to adapt the teaching plan, making sure that it is realistic for his needs. For example, the nurse might teach Mr. Johnston about reading food labels to ensure that his selections, when he is 'on the run' are low in fat and cholesterol. In addition, the nurse would also provide Mr. Johnston with appropriate suggestions for choices when dining out. Doing so will help communicate to him that the plan is workable, enhancing the chances of Mr. Johnston complying with the plan, thereby achieving success.*

Although strict guidelines and printed handouts may seem ideal, in practice, simplicity and compromise are often the keys to patient compliance. The accompanying box suggests standardized nursing interventions for nutritional counseling using the Nursing Interventions Classification (NIC) terminology.

Monitoring Nutritional Status

Nurses are aware that malnourished patients are more likely to have slower wound healing and to develop complications. Prevention of malnutrition can have a positive effect on patient outcomes. In the hospital, shortened stays limit the time available for nutritional screening and intervention. Patients are often acutely ill and uninterested or unable to absorb and retain any nutritional instruction. It may also be difficult to include a family member or caregiver responsible for food preparation in scheduled teaching sessions. In many situations, the home healthcare nurse has the opportunity to have a significant impact on nutritional health. Instruction can be provided in a relaxed setting that allows insight into a patient's

---

Examples of Nursing Interventions Classification (NIC) Nutritional Counseling

- Determine patient's food intake and eating habits.
- Establish realistic short-term and long-term goals for change in the nutritional status.
- Provide information, as necessary, about the health need for diet modification: weight loss, weight gain, sodium restriction, cholesterol reduction, fluid restriction, and so on.
- Help patient to consider factors of age, stage of growth and development, past eating experiences, injury, disease, culture, and finances in planning ways to meet nutritional requirements.
- Discuss patient's food likes and dislikes.
- Discuss food-buying habits and budget constraints.
- Discuss the meaning of food to the patient.
- Praise efforts to achieve goals.
- Provide referral or consultation with other members of the healthcare team, as appropriate.

(From McCloskey, J., & Bulechek, G. [2000]. *Nursing interventions classification [NIC]* [3rd ed.]. [p. 476]. St. Louis: C. V. Mosby. A full listing of nursing activities for each nursing intervention can be found in this book.)

---

cultural orientation and family patterns and traditions. This environment also encourages modification and adjustments in the nurse's approach to nutritional instruction. The variety of community services and programs that are available to provide nutritional support to patients at home should be investigated. The accompanying box, Focus on the Older Adult, includes teaching content and strategies for the specific nutritional challenges facing the older adult.

Stimulating Appetite

Pain, illness, anxiety, and medications can contribute to anorexia and poor intake when in a healthcare facility or in the home. To the hospitalized patient, food and eating may take on much greater meaning. Loss of control over food choices, the way food is prepared, when and how food is served, and eating alone may do little to encourage normal eating. Every effort must be made to ensure that the proper food is not only served but also eaten. The additional time and attention spent when encouraging a person to eat may have a positive effect on dietary intake. The following measures may help to stimulate appetite in any setting:

- Serve small, frequent meals to avoid overwhelming the individual with large amounts of food.
- Solicit food preferences and encourage favorite foods from home or prepared when at home, if possible.
- Provide encouragement and a pleasant eating environment.
- Be sure that any prepared food looks attractive.
- Schedule procedures and medications at times when they are least likely to interfere with appetite.
- Control pain, nausea, or depression with medications.

Focus on the Older Adult
Nursing Strategies to Address Age-Related Changes Affecting Nutrition

Age-Related Changes	Nursing Strategies
Altered ability to chew related to loss of teeth, ill-fitting dentures, and gingivitis	• Encourage and instruct patient to care for and retain own teeth and dentures. • Encourage proper tooth-brushing and use of special toothpaste if gums and teeth are sensitive. • Chop, shred, or puree foods that are difficult to chew. • Select ground meat, fish, or poultry as protein sources more easily chewed.
Loss of senses of smell and taste	• Serve food that is attractive and at proper temperature. • Eat one food at a time rather than mixing foods. • Serve foods with different textures and aromas.
Decreased peristalsis in the esophagus	• Avoid cold liquids. • Avoid emotional upsets and stress-producing situations. • Take anticholinergic drugs as ordered by physician.
Gastroesophageal reflux	• Avoid overeating. • Avoid juices, chocolate, and fat. • Avoid alcohol and smoking. • Elevate the head of the bed 30 to 40 degrees when sleeping. • Lose weight if necessary. • Avoid bending over. • Take antacids or other medications as ordered by physician. • Avoid eating right before bedtime.
Decreased gastric secretions	• Chew food thoroughly. • Eat meals on a regular schedule. • Use antacids or other medications as prescribed by physician. • Be alert for symptoms of deficiency of nutrients, particularly iron, calcium, fat, protein, and vitamin B_{12}.
Slowed intestinal peristalsis	• Eat a high-fiber diet. • Remain as active as possible. • Increase fluid intake. • Avoid laxative use. • Eat meals at a regular time. • Drink prune juice or eat prunes every morning.
Lowered glucose tolerance	• Eat more complex carbohydrates. • Avoid sugar-rich foods.
Reduction in appetite and thirst sensation	• Offer fluids at regular intervals and at preferred temperature. • Be alert for symptoms of dehydration and electrolyte imbalance. • Offer small meals at frequent intervals.
Nutritional deficiencies related to alcohol intake	• Encourage diet high in protein and carbohydrates. • Offer small, frequent meals to maintain caloric intake. • Restrict sodium and fluids if edema is present. • Take multivitamin supplements as ordered by physician.
Loss of appetite associated with depression and loneliness	• Promote mealtime as a social event. • Set an attractive table in a pleasant setting. • Eat outdoors whenever possible. • Invite guests as often as possible. • Participate in special programs for senior citizens.
Physical handicaps	• Open cartons and assist with setup of meal. • Arrange for home-delivered meals. • Conserve energy when preparing meals (sit on a stool, etc.). • Provide transportation and assistance to obtain food.
Low income	• Buy specials when available at food store. • Use generic brands. • Use coupons.

(continued)

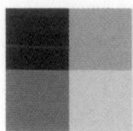

Focus on the Older Adult (Continued)
Nursing Strategies to Address Age-Related Changes Affecting Nutrition

Age-Related Changes	Nursing Strategies
Low income *(cont'd.)*	• Cook larger quantities than necessary and freeze the leftovers for future use. • Substitute eggs, skim milk powder, and beans for meat. • Check for any community resources available to elderly.
Malnutrition	• Eat essential foods first. • Select nutrient-dense foods. • Monitor for signs of nutritional deficiencies. • Encourage eating by planning special events.
Increased risk for drug–nutrient interactions	• Avoid unnecessary drugs; monitor for polypharmacy. • Be aware of drug actions and interactions. • Check with pharmacist to determine if medication may or may not be taken with food. • Assess for confusion and inability to manage medication regimen.

- Offer alternatives for items that a person cannot or will not eat.
- Encourage or provide good oral hygiene.
- Remove clutter from the eating area.
- Keep eating area free from irritating odors.
- Arrange food tray so that an individual can easily reach food.
- Provide a comfortable position.
- Ask about any rituals during mealtimes at home and include them if possible.

Assisting With Eating

The loss of independence that comes with the inability to self-feed can be a severe blow to a person's self-esteem. The following measures may help a person maintain dignity while being fed:

- Involve the person as much as possible. Solicit his or her preferences regarding the order of items eaten and the eating pace.
- Engage the individual in pleasant conversation to ease tension.
- Place a napkin, not a bib, over the person's clothes for protection.
- Use straws or special eating utensils whenever possible.
- Ensure that if a person wears dentures, hearing aids, or glasses, they are in place before mealtime.
- Open containers, cut meat, or apply condiments to the prepared food only if the person wishes.

Providing Nutrition in Special Situations

A variety of normal and modified diets are available in healthcare settings and may be prescribed for use at home. Normal, regular, or house diets are designed to maintain optimal nutritional status by providing adequate amounts of all nutrients. The diet's actual composition varies with the quantity and types of food selected; the average calorie content ranges from 1400 to 2500 cal.

Liquid diets are used most often as transitional diets when eating resumes after acute illness, surgery, or parenteral nutrition. **Clear liquid diets** contain only foods that are clear liquids at room or body temperature—gelatin, fat-free broth, bouillon, ice pops, clear juices, carbonated beverages, regular and decaffeinated coffee, and tea. Because clear liquid diets are inadequate in calories, protein, and most nutrients, progression to more nutritious alternatives is recommended as soon as possible. **Full liquid diets** contain milk, plain frozen desserts, pasteurized eggs, cereal gruels, and milk and egg substitutes in addition to clear liquids. A full liquid diet contains liquids that can be poured at room temperature. High-calorie, high-protein supplements are recommended if a full liquid diet is used for more than 3 days.

Soft diets are usually regular diets that have been modified to eliminate foods that are hard to digest and to chew, including those that are high in fiber, high in fat, and highly seasoned. Soft diets are adequate in calories and nutrients and may be used on a long-term basis. Many nutritionists substitute low-fiber vegetables in place of purees.

Vegetarian Diets

Some patients may prefer a vegetarian diet for a variety of reasons, such as religious preference, ethical belief that killing animals for food is unjust, fear of contamination with pesticides, or health concerns about the cholesterol and saturated fats found in meats. Due to the different degrees of vegetarian diets, the population of people claiming to be vegetarian in the United States varies from 4.8 million (Vegetarian Resource Group, 2000) to 12 million (Peckenpaugh & Poleman, 1999). Meats are usually replaced with legumes, grains, and vegetables, and, if well planned, this type of diet can satisfy all nutritional requirements. Vegetarian diets have a variety of formats and are more commonly followed by younger people. An individual who eats any animal product except red meat is at one end of the spectrum, with a Zen macrobiotic who consumes only brown rice and herb tea at the other end. Vitamin B_{12}, vitamin A, and iron are nutrients that may require supplementation in some vegetarian diets, but most vegetarian diets are not deficient in any nutrients. Support patients who follow a vegetarian diet by assisting them or their caregiver to select nutritious food items from the large variety of foods available within their dietary framework.

Nothing By Mouth

In some cases, such as before surgery to prevent aspiration related to anesthesia, and after surgery until bowel sounds return, patients may be ordered nothing by mouth (**NPO**). NPO may also be necessary for patients undergoing certain medical tests, for patients experiencing severe nausea and vomiting, an inability to chew or swallow, or various acute or chronic GI abnormalities, for those who are comatose, and for women during labor and delivery.

The following measures may provide comfort to patients who are ordered NPO:

- Encourage or provide good oral hygiene.
- Provide the patient with ice chips or sips of water as allowed.
- Urge the patient to avoid watching others eat. Suggest alternate activities at mealtimes.

Well-nourished patients can easily withstand the stress of NPO for a short period, but being NPO for an extended period of time poses a nutritional challenge for many individuals. Patients with increased nutritional requirements and those who will be NPO for more than 2 days may require nutritional support from **enteral,** administering nutrients directly into the stomach, or **parenteral,** providing nutrition via IV therapy, nutrition.

Providing Enteral Nutrition

Oral feeding is the preferred and most effective method of feeding patients. The next best method is the enteral route. Enteral nutrition involves passing a tube into the GI tract to administer a formula containing adequate nutrients. This alternate feeding method may deliver total or supplemental nutrition over a short-term period or for longer intervals.

Short-Term Nutritional Support

For short-term use (less than 6 weeks), a nasogastric or nasointestinal route is usually selected. A **nasogastric (NG) tube** is inserted through the nose and into the stomach, whereas **nasointestinal (NI) tube** is passed through the nose and into the upper portion of the small intestine. Nasogastric feedings have the advantage of allowing the stomach to be used as a natural reservoir, regulating the amount of foods and liquids released into the small intestine. It is also thought that the presence of gastric acid in the stomach may decrease the risk for infection. However, the patient is at risk for aspirating the tube feeding solution into the lungs, a disadvantage for using this route. Patients with a dysfunctional gag reflex and those who are unable to have the head of the bed elevated during feedings are not candidates for nasogastric feeding. Occasionally, a smaller, softer, more pliable tube (eg, Dobhoff tube) may be inserted via the nose into the stomach or small intestine. This type of tube is advantageous, providing greater patient comfort and less trauma to the nares. However, checking tube placement is more difficult. The method of inserting a nasogastric feeding tube is described in Skill 42-1. Insertion,

---

SKILL 42-1 — Inserting a Nasogastric Tube

EQUIPMENT

Nasogastric tube of appropriate size (8–18 French)
Small basin filled with ice or warm water (optional)
Water-soluble lubricant
Tongue blade
Flashlight
Topical analgesic (optional)

Stethoscope
Normal saline solution (for irrigation only)
Asepto bulb syringe or Toomey syringe (20–50 mL)
Nonallergenic tape (1 inch wide)
Tissues
Glass of water with straw

Suction apparatus (if ordered)
Bath towel or disposable pad
Safety pin and rubber band
Clamp
Emesis basin
Disposable gloves
Tincture of benzoin

ACTION	RATIONALE
1. Check physician's order for insertion of nasogastric tube.	This clarifies procedure and type of equipment required.
2. Explain procedure to patient.	Explanation facilitates patient cooperation.
3. Gather equipment.	This provides for organized approach to task.
4. If nasogastric tube is rubber, place it in a basin with ice for 5 to 10 minutes or place a plastic tube in a basin of warm water if needed.	Cold stiffens the rubber tube, making it easier to insert. Plastic tube may be placed in warm water to make it more flexible.
5. Assess patient's abdomen.	Assessment determines presence of bowel sounds and amount of abdominal distention.

(continued)

ACTION	RATIONALE
6. Perform hand hygiene. Don disposable gloves.	Hand hygiene deters the spread of microorganisms. Gloves protect from exposure to blood or body fluids.
7. Assist the patient to high Fowler's position, or 45 degrees, if unable to maintain upright position, and drape chest with bath towel or disposable pad. Have emesis basin and tissues handy.	Upright position is more natural for swallowing and protects against aspiration, if the patient should vomit. Passage of tube may stimulate gagging and tearing of eyes.
8. Check the nares for patency by asking the patient to occlude one nostril and breathe normally through the other. Select the nostril through which air passes more easily.	Tube passes more easily through the nostril with the largest opening.
9. Measure the distance to insert the tube by placing tip of tube at patient's nostril and extending to tip of earlobe and then to tip of xiphoid process. Mark tube with a piece of tape.	Measurement ensures that the tube will be long enough to enter the patient's stomach.

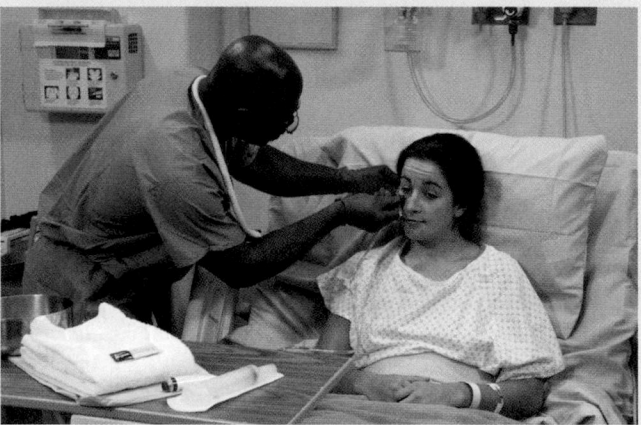

Action 9a: Measuring distance from nostril to tip of earlobe.
(Photo by Rick Brady.)

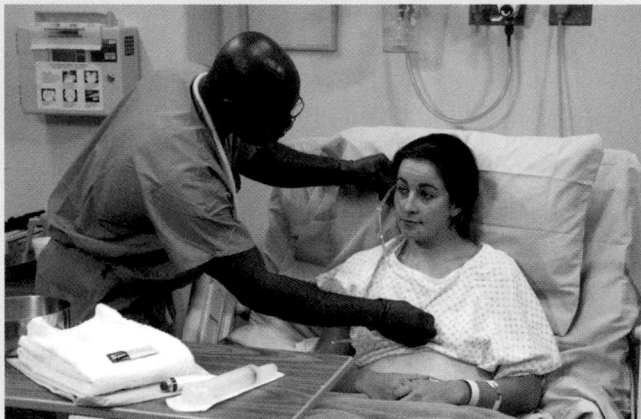

Action 9b: Measuring distance from earlobe to tip of xiphoid process.
(Photo by Rick Brady.)

ACTION	RATIONALE
10. Lubricate the tip of the tube (at least 1–2 in) with a water-soluble lubricant. Apply topical analgesic to nostril and oropharynx or ask patient to hold ice chips in mouth for several minutes (according to physician's preference).	Lubrication reduces friction and facilitates passage of the tube into the stomach. Water-soluble lubricant will not cause pneumonia if tube accidentally enters the lungs. Topical analgesic or ice acts as a local anesthetic, reducing discomfort.
11. Ask the patient to lift the head, and insert the tube into the nostril while directing the tube downward and backward. The patient may gag when the tube reaches the pharynx.	Following the normal contour of the nasal passage while inserting the tube reduces irritation and the likelihood of mucosal injury. The gag reflex is readily stimulated by the tube.
12. Instruct the patient to touch his chin to his chest. Encourage him or her to swallow even if no fluids are permitted. Advance the tube in a downward and backward direction when the patient swallows. Stop when the patient breathes. Provide tissues for tearing or watering of eyes. If gagging and coughing persist, check placement of tube with a tongue blade and flashlight. Keep advancing the tube until the tape marking is reached. Do not use force. Rotate the tube if it meets resistance.	Bringing the head forward helps close the trachea and open the esophagus. Swallowing helps advance the tube, causes the epiglottis to cover the opening of the trachea, and helps to eliminate gagging and coughing. Tears are a natural response as the tube passes into the nasopharynx. Excessive coughing and gagging may occur if the tube has curled in the back of throat. Forcing the tube may injure mucous membranes.
13. Discontinue the procedure and remove the tube if there are signs of distress, such as gasping, coughing, cyanosis, and the inability to speak or hum.	The tube is not in the esophagus if the patient shows signs of distress and is unable to speak or hum.
14. While keeping one hand on the tube, determine that the tube is in the patient's stomach.	Keeping one hand on the tube stabilizes it while the position is being determined.
a. Attach the syringe to the end of the tube and aspirate small amount of stomach contents.	The tube is in the stomach if its contents can be aspirated; pH of aspirate can then be tested to determine gastric placement.

(continued)

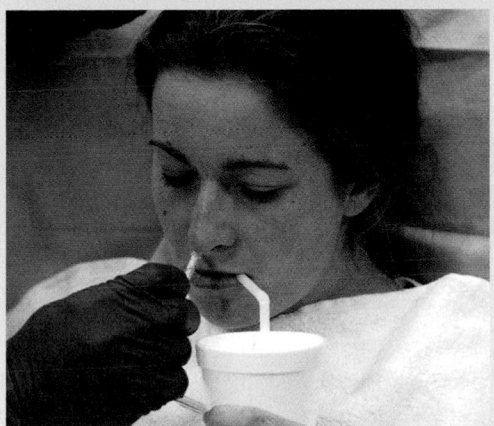

Action 12: Advancing tubing while patient has chin to chest and is swallowing.
(Photo by Rick Brady.)

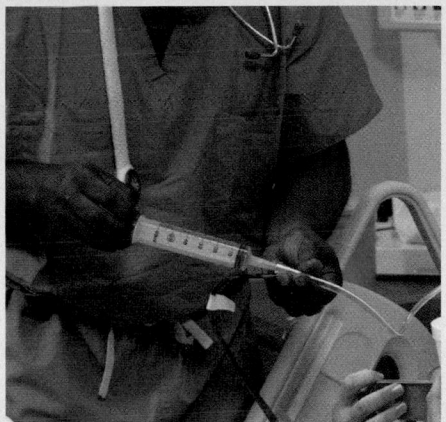

Action 14a: Aspirating to obtain gastric fluid.   (Photo by Rick Brady.)

ACTION	RATIONALE
b. Measure the pH of aspirated fluid using pH paper or a meter.	The pH of gastric contents is acidic (4 or less), compared with an average pH of 7.0 or greater for respiratory fluid. Because pH of intestinal fluid also is slightly basic, this method will not effectively differentiate between intestinal fluid and pleural fluid.
c. Visualize aspirated contents, checking for color and consistency.	Gastric fluid can be green with particles; brown if old blood is present, clear, or straw colored. Tracheobronchial fluid is usually off-white to tan. Pleural fluid can be straw colored and is usually watery. Intestinal fluid is usually light to dark-golden yellow or brownish-green (Metheny & Titler, 2001).
d. Obtain radiograph of placement of tube (as ordered by physician).	Radiographic visualization is the most definitive measure to determine tube placement.
15. Apply tincture of benzoin to tip of nose and allow to dry. Secure the tube with tape to the patient's nose. Be careful not to pull the tube too tightly against the nose: a. Cut a 4-inch piece of tape and split bottom 2 inches or use packaged nose tape for nasogastric tubes. b. Place unsplit end over bridge of patient's nose. c. Wrap split ends under the tubing and up and over onto the nose.	Tincture of benzoin facilitates attachment of tape. Constant pressure of the tube against the skin and mucous membranes causes tissue injury.
16. Attach tube to suction or clamp the tube and cap it according to the physician's orders.	Suction provides for decompression of stomach and drainage of gastric contents.
17. Secure tube to the patient's gown by using a rubber band or tape and a safety pin. If double-lumen tube is used, secure vent above stomach level. Attach at shoulder level.	This prevents tension and tugging on the tube. Securing the double-lumen tube above stomach level prevents seepage of gastric contents and keeps the lumen clear for venting air.
18. Assist with or provide patient with oral hygiene at regular intervals.	Oral hygiene keeps mouth clean and moist and promotes comfort.
19. Perform hand hygiene. Remove all equipment and make patient comfortable.	Hand hygiene deters the spread of microorganisms.
20. Record the insertion procedure, type and size of tube, and measure the tube from the tip of the nose to the end of the tube. Also document a description of gastric contents, which nare is used, and patient's response.	This facilitates documentation and provides for comprehensive care. Measurement of tube provides a baseline for future comparison.

(continued)

Special Considerations   *For insertion of a nasointestinal tube:*

- Measure tube from tip of nose to ear lobe and from ear lobe to xiphoid process. Add 8 to 10 inches for intestinal placement. Mark tubing at desired point.
- Place patient on his or her right side. Nasointestinal tube is usually placed in the stomach and allowed to advance through peristalsis via the pyloric sphincter (may take up to 24 hours).
- Administer GI motility medications (metoclopramide) if ordered.
- Test pH of aspirate when tube has advanced to marked point to confirm placement in the intestine. Check position by radiograph. Tape in place when confirmed.

which requires skill and accuracy, is frequently done by the nurse.

A patient with a nasointestinal tube is at minimal risk for aspiration. When formula is delivered directly into the intestine, a type of dumping syndrome may develop because the pyloric valve in the stomach, which normally slows transit of food into the intestine, is bypassed. The volume of feeding distends the intestine and, combined with a hypoglycemic reaction as the body adjusts to the rapid entry of a high-carbohydrate formula, may result in symptoms of gas, bloating, crampy pain, weakness, and dizziness. Some medical conditions (delayed gastric emptying, gastric tumor) also necessitate the use of a nasointestinal tube.

Long-Term Nutritional Support

When enteral feeding is required for a long-term period, an enterostomal tube may be placed through an opening created into the stomach (gastrostomy) or into the jejunum (jejunostomy) (Noble, 2003). The methods of accomplishing long-term feeding into the stomach include **percutaneous endoscopic gastrostomy (PEG)** or a surgically or laparoscopically placed gastrostomy tube. PEG tube insertion is popular because, unlike a gastrostomy tube, it usually does not require general anesthesia, can be safely inserted and removed at the bedside or in an outpatient setting, and, therefore, is more economical (Bowers, 2000). Simply stated, positioning a PEG tube involves local anesthesia, passage of an endoscope into the stomach, a small incision or stab wound through the skin of the abdomen, pushing a cannula through the small incision, insertion of a guide wire or suture material through the cannula, and introduction and placement of the PEG tube through one of several methods (Fig. 42-7 illustrates a PEG tube in place in the stomach). Use of a PEG tube or other type of gastrostomy tube requires an intact, functional GI tract.

In long-term feeding situations in which gastric problems exist, the jejunostomy is an alternate method through which nutrition can be delivered. These tubes may be inserted surgically or with endoscopic or laparoscopic guidance (Fig. 42-8 illustrates a PEG/J tube in the jejunum). Gastrostomy or jejunostomy tubes are not easily dislodged.

For patients who are active yet require long-term continuous or intermittent feedings, a low-profile gastrostomy device (LPGD) may be an option. Children are also excellent candidates for LPGDs. The external apparatus is minimal and consists of a button or skin disk that is stable, less irritating to the skin, and has no external tubing so it is easier to conceal with clothing. Additional advantages include the fact that it can be immersed in water, is less noticeable, and is less likely to migrate or become dislodged.

Confirmation of Tube Placement

After the initial insertion of a feeding tube, before beginning a feeding or instilling liquids, and at regular intervals during continuous feedings, the placement of a nasogastric or nasointestinal tube must be verified. The most common malposition location is the lungs, but tubes have also been inadvertently placed in the esophagus and the brain (Metheny & Titler, 2001). A misplaced feeding tube in the lungs or pulmonary tissue places the patient at risk for aspiration. In addition, enteral feedings also are associated with nosocomial infections.

Radiographic examination is the standard procedure to verify initial placement of a feeding tube (Fellows, Miller, Frederickson, Bly, & Felt, 2000; Metheny & Stewart, 2002; Metheny & Titler, 2001). This is especially a priority when a small-bore tube has been used or when patients are at high risk for aspiration.

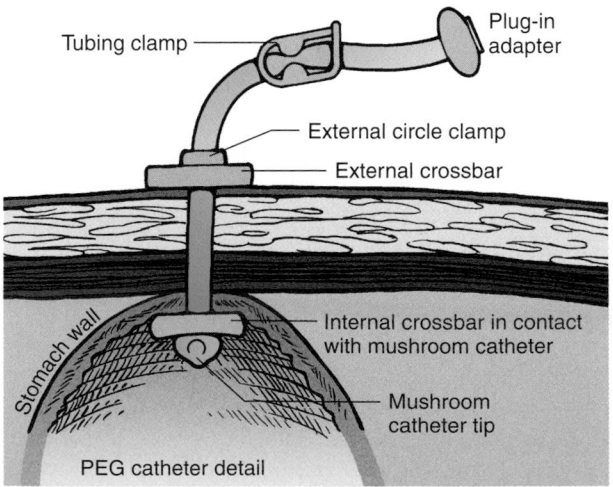

FIGURE 42-7 Percutaneous endoscopic gastrostomy tube in place in the stomach. (Smeltzer, S. C., & Bare, B. G. [2004]. *Brunner and Suddarth's textbook of medical surgical nursing* [10th ed., p. 998.]. Philadelphia: Lippincott Williams & Wilkins.)

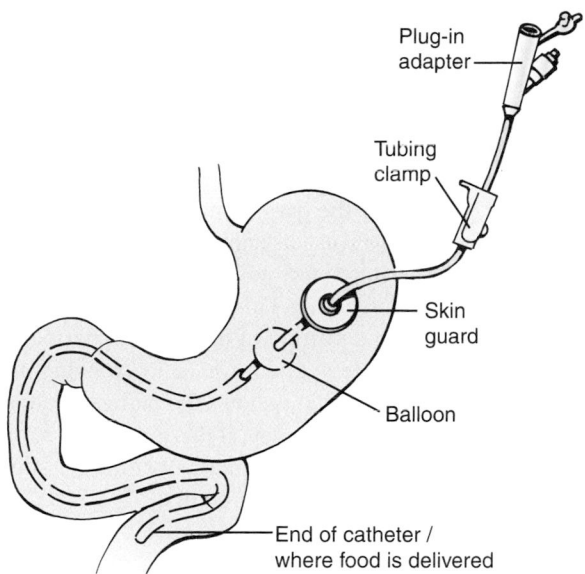

FIGURE 42-8 PEG/J tube inserted in the jejunum.

Other methods may be used to check for tube placement because radiographs expose the patient to radiation, must be interpreted by a physician, are costly if done on a routine basis and may be inaccessible. These include aspirating gastric contents and measuring the pH of the aspirate (Guidelines for Nursing Care 42-1). After radiographic examination, measurement of pH is the recommended method for determining correct placement of a feeding tube. Some clinicians remain reluctant to abandon the auscultatory method of checking tube placement (injecting 10–30 cc of air into the tube while listening with stethoscope placed over the epigastrium for a "whooshing" sound). This procedure has proved unreliable and may result in tragic consequences if used as the sole indicator of tube placement.

Small-bore tubes are associated with a lower risk of aspiration than larger feeding tubes because the smaller tubes place less pressure on the esophageal sphincter, thus decreasing the risk of reflux (Bowers, 2000). Because they are less rigid, they may be more likely to collapse when negative pressure is applied during aspiration. More than likely, the difficulty is a result of a blocked tube. Additionally, the ports on the tip of the tube may not be positioned in fluid. Research by clinicians has demonstrated that aspiration is easier in small-bore tubes if there are multiple ports rather than a single port. Several attempts may be necessary to aspirate gastric contents. If repeated instillations of 30 mL of air and repositioning prove ineffective, tube placement should be checked by radiograph after obtaining a physician's order.

If the patient is at high risk for aspiration, for example, due to a diminished gag reflux or slow gastric motility, the physician may specifically want the tube placed into the small intestine. After an initial x-ray for placement, the nurse can validate that the tube is still in the small intestine by checking the pH and also by checking for bilirubin, the major bile component. The gastric level of bilirubin should be none to a small amount due to reflux from the small intestine (Metheny & Titler, 2001).

Guidelines for Nursing Care 42-1
Measuring pH of Gastric Fluids

- Allow 1-hour interval after patient has received medication or completed an intermittent feeding before testing pH of gastric fluid. If feeding is continuous, plan pH testing at a time when feeding can be withheld.
- Irrigate tube with 30 mL of warm water after medications or feeding.
- Insert 30 mL of air into tube before aspirating GI contents to flush out contents of tube.
- Withdraw small amount (5–10 mL) of gastric secretions.
- If unable to obtain specimen, reposition the patient and flush tube again with 30 mL of air. It may be necessary to retry several times, especially if a small-bore feeding tube is in place.
- Place drop of gastric secretions onto pH test paper or place small amount in plastic cup and dip the pH paper into it. Within 30 seconds, compare the color on the paper with the chart supplied by the manufacturer. (A pH meter and color chart are also an option.)
- Document results in the patient's chart. The following are indications of placement:

pH
- Stomach: pH 0–4.0 (If patient is taking an acid-inhibiting agent [eg, Zantac], the range may be 4.0–6.0)
- Intestines: pH 7.0 or higher
- Respiratory tract: pH 6.0 or higher

Color of Aspirate
- Stomach: grassy green, tan, off-white, bloody, or brown
- Intestines: medium to deep golden yellow (may be greenish-brown if stained with bile)
- Respiratory tract: off-white and tinged with mucus

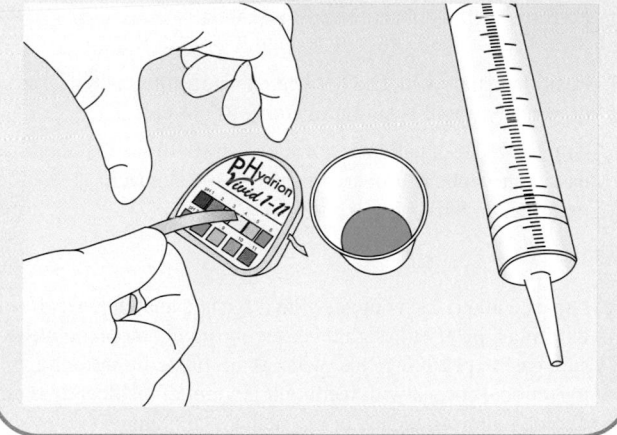

Checking placement of a gastrostomy or jejunostomy tube requires regular comparisons (according to agency policy) of the tube length to the measurement (inches or centimeters) that was documented after insertion. An indelible marker can be used to identify the exit point of the tube from the nares.

Feeding tubes with built-in pH sensors are available. These tubes have been shown to be helpful when distinguishing between gastric and small intestine placement. The cost of these tubes have inhibited their use by many hospitals.

Tube Feeding Administration

Feeding Schedule

Based on the patient's physical, medical, and nutritional condition, the nutritionist usually makes recommendations concerning the feeding pattern or schedule. Continuous feedings allow gradual introduction of the formula into the GI tract, promoting maximal absorption. They require use of an enteral feeding pump, which limits the patient's mobility and increases cost. Feedings into the intestine are always continuous to avoid triggering the dumping syndrome (thought to be triggered by overdistention of the small intestine), by introducing a large amount of formula quickly, leading to diarrhea, cramping, and light headedness (Bowers, 2000). Continuous

feeding into the stomach is controversial because of the risk for reflux and aspiration.

Intermittent feedings are delivered at regular intervals, introducing the formula gradually over a set period of time via gravity or a feeding pump. Bolus intermittent feedings, whereby a syringe is used to deliver the formula quickly into the stomach, may place the patient at risk for aspiration or cause distention. They are usually not recommended but may be used in long-term situations if tolerated by the patient. Another option is cyclic feeding. This involves administering continuous feeding for a portion of the 24-hour period. The usual routine is to feed the patient for 12 to 16 hours, most often overnight. Cyclic feeding allows the patient to attempt eating regular meals during the day, if this is possible making ambulation and activity easier. The basic method for administering a tube feeding is outlined in Skill 42-2.

SKILL 42-2   Administering a Tube Feeding

EQUIPMENT

Tube feeding at room temperature	Clamp (Hoffman or butterfly)	Rubber band
Stethoscope	Disposable pad or towel	Enteral feeding pump (if ordered)
Feeding bag or prefilled tube feeding set	Sterile water for irrigation	IV pole
Alcohol preps	Asepto or Toomey syringe	Disposable gloves

ACTION	RATIONALE
1. Explain procedure to patient. Use stethoscope to assess bowel sounds.	This facilitates cooperation and provides reassurance for patient. Presence of bowel sounds may indicate functional GI tract.
2. Assemble equipment. Check amount, concentration, type, and frequency of tube feeding on patient's chart. Check expiration date of formula.	This provides for organized approach to task. Ensures that correct feeding will be administered. Outdated formula may be contaminated.
3. Perform hand hygiene. Don disposable gloves.	Hand hygiene deters the spread of microorganisms. Gloves protect from exposure to blood or body fluids.
4. Position patient with head of bed elevated at least 30 degrees or as near normal position for eating as possible.	This position minimizes possibility of aspiration into trachea.
5. Unpin tube from patient's gown and check to see that the nasogastric tube is properly located in the stomach, as described in Skill 42-1, Action 14.	Even when initially positioned correctly, a nasogastric tube left in place can become dislodged between feedings. The instillation of water or nourishment could lead to serious respiratory problems if a gastric tube is in the trachea or a bronchus, rather than in the stomach.
6. Aspirate all gastric contents with a syringe and measure. Return immediately through tube, saving small amount to measure gastric pH. Flush tube with 30 mL of sterile water for irrigation. Proceed with feeding if amount of residual does not exceed policy of agency or physician's guideline. Disconnect syringe from tubing.	This indicates gastric emptying time. A residual of more than 100 mL from a gastrostomy tube or 200 mL from a nasogastric tube, or more than 10% to 20% above the hourly feeding rate must be reported to physician. Fluid should be returned to stomach so as not to cause any fluid or electrolyte losses.

For Intermittent Feedings

ACTION	RATIONALE
7. When using a feeding bag (open system):	
a. Hang bag on IV pole and adjust to about 12 inches above the stomach. Clamp tubing.	Formula displaces air in the tubing.
b. Cleanse top of feeding container with alcohol before opening it. Pour formula into feeding bag and allow solution to run through tubing. Close clamp.	Cleansing container top with alcohol minimizes risk for contaminants entering feeding bag. Formula displaces air in tubing.

(continued)

SKILL 42-2　Administering a Tube Feeding (continued)

ACTION	RATIONALE
c. Attach feeding setup to feeding tube, open clamp, and regulate drip rate according to physician's order or allow feeding to run in over 30 minutes.	Introducing the formula at a slow, regular rate allows the stomach to accommodate to the feeding and decreases GI distress.
d. Add 30 to 60 mL (1–2 oz) of sterile water for irrigation to feeding bag when feeding is almost completed and allow it to run through tube.	Water rinses the feeding from the tube and helps to keep it patent.

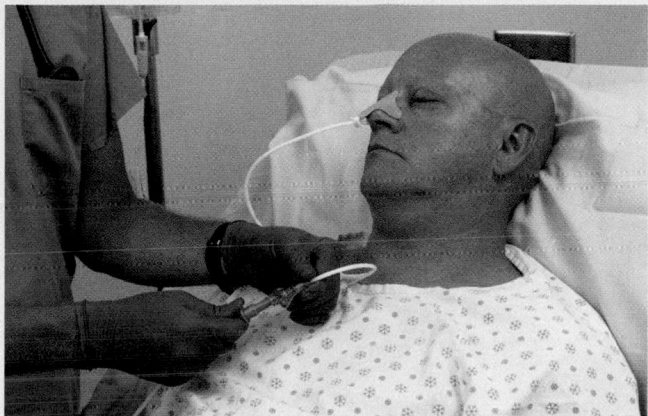

Action 7c: Attaching feeding-bag tubing to tube.　(Photo by Rick Brady.)

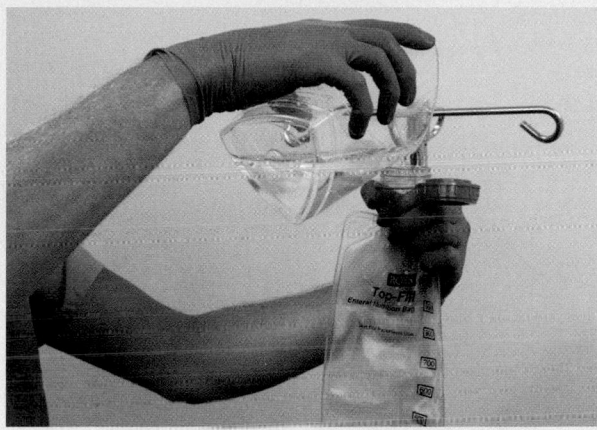

Action 7d: Adding water to rinse feeding tube.　(Photo by Rick Brady.)

ACTION	RATIONALE
e. Clamp the tubing immediately after water has been instilled. Disconnect from tube. Clamp tube and cover end with sterile gauze secured with a rubber band or apply cap.	Clamping the tube prevents air from entering the stomach. Cover on end of tube deters entry of microorganisms and protects patient and linens from fluid leakage from tube.
8. When using a large syringe (open system):	
a. Remove plunger from 30-mL or 60-mL syringe.	Removing the plunger allows feeding to be added directly to the syringe and flow in by gravity.
b. Attach syringe to feeding tube, pour pre-measured amount of tube feeding into syringe, open clamp, and allow feeding to enter tube. Regulate the rate by raising or lowering the height of the syringe. Do not push feeding with syringe plunger.	Introducing the formula at a slow regular rate allows the stomach to accommodate to the feeding and decreases GI distress. The higher the syringe is held, the faster the formula flows.
c. Add 30 mL to 60 mL (1–2 oz) of water for irrigation to syringe when feeding is almost completed and allow it to run through the tube.	Water rinses the feeding tube and helps to maintain tube patency.
d. When syringe has emptied, hold the syringe high and disconnect from the tube. Clamp the tube and cover end with a sterile gauze secured with a rubber band or apply a cap.	The syringe does not have a clamp. Holding the tube high prevents backflow of feeding until the tube is clamped. Clamping the tube prevents air from entering the stomach. Covering the end of the tube deters the entry of microorganisms and protects the patient and linens from fluid leakage.
9. When using prefilled tube feeding set-up (closed system):	
a. Remove screw-on cap and attach administration set-up with drip chamber and tubing. Hang set on IV pole and adjust to about 12 inches above the stomach. Clamp tubing and squeeze drip chamber to fill one third to one half of capacity. Release clamp and run formula through tubing. Close clamp.	Formula displaces air in tubing.
b. Follow Actions 7c, 7d, and 7e. Feeding pump may be used with tube feeding set-up to regulate drip.	

(continued)

SKILL 42-2 Administering a Tube Feeding (continued)

ACTION	RATIONALE
10. When using a feeding pump (continuous feeding): a. Close flow-regulator clamp on tubing and fill feeding bag with prescribed formula. The amount used depends on agency policy. Place label on container.	Feeding intolerance is less likely to occur with smaller volumes. Hanging smaller amounts of feeding also reduces risk for bacteria growth and contamination of feeding at room temperature.
b. Hang feeding container on IV pole and allow solution to flow through tubing.	This prevents air from being forced into the stomach or intestines.
c. Connect to feeding pump following manufacturer's directions. Set rate.	Smaller volume of feeding is infused continuously and is more easily tolerated by patient.
d. Check residual every 4 to 8 hours.	Checking verifies placement of the tube and proper absorption of the feeding.

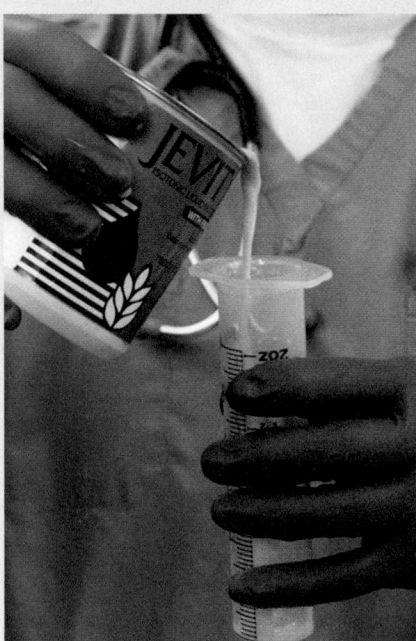

Action 8b: Pouring feeding from container into syringe.   (Photo by Rick Brady.)

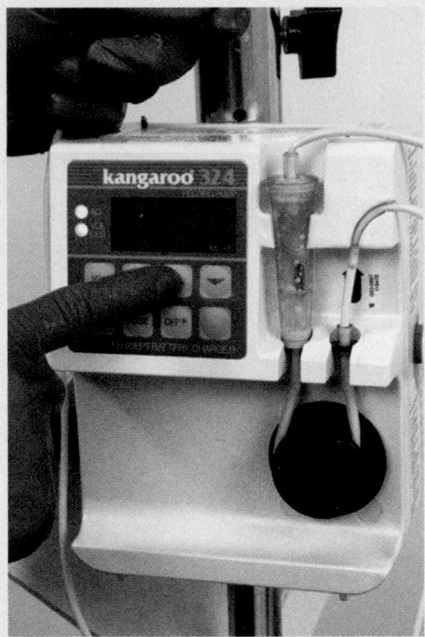

Action 10c: Setting up feeding pump with feeding bag and primed tubing.   (Photo by Rick Brady.)

ACTION	RATIONALE
11. Observe patient's response during and after tube feeding.	Pain may indicate stomach distention, which may lead to vomiting.
12. Have patient remain in upright position for at least 30 minutes to 1 hour after feeding.	This position minimizes risk for backflow and discourages aspiration, if any vomiting should occur.
13. Wash and clean equipment or replace according to agency policy. Remove gloves and perform hand hygiene.	This prevents contamination and deters spread of microorganisms.
14. Record type and amount of feeding and patient's response. Monitor blood glucose, if ordered by physician.	This provides accurate documentation of procedure. Many feedings contain high amounts of carbohydrates.

Feeding Formulas

Many enteral feeding formulas are available. The nutritional composition of tube feedings depends on the feeding route, the patient's ability to digest and absorb nutrients, and his or her nutrient and fluid requirements. Other considerations include the availability and cost of the formula, medical conditions that require diet modifications, food intolerance, and allergies. The typical feeding formula has the following caloric breakdown: 16% protein, 54% carbohydrate, and 30% fat (Dudek, 2001). Protein is the most critical component; the patient's needs will determine the complexity of the protein that is required. In addition to being nutritionally balanced, formulas may be high in calories, contain fiber, contain additional protein, or be especially formulated for patients with respiratory, renal, or other health problems. Detailed information on their composition and caloric value (most formulas contain 1 cal/mL, although 2 cal/mL concentrations are available) can be obtained from the product label.

Enteral Feeding Pumps

An enteral feeding pump regulates the amount of feeding solution that is delivered to the patient. The newer pumps are user friendly, have built-in safeguards that protect the patient from complications, and can be used in both institutions and the home. Safety features include automatic tube flush, cassettes that prevent free-flow of formula, safety tips that prevent accidental attachment to an IV setup, and various audible and visible alarms. Most pumps can operate for up to 8 hours on battery. However, manufacturers recommend using the pump plugged into an electrical outlet for recharging whenever the patient is seated or resting for a period of time (Bauer, 2003).

Nursing Considerations With Tube Feeding

Agency protocols may differ and should be followed, but nursing actions that contribute to successful tube feedings focus on patient safety, monitoring for complications, comfort, and education.

Promote Patient Safety

To promote patient safety when administering a tube feeding, be sure to do the following:

- Check tube placement before administering any fluids, medications, or feeding (for technique for testing gastric pH, see Guidelines for Nursing Care 42-1). The practice of adding food dye or coloring to the tube feeding as a means of detecting aspirated fluid is not recommended (Dudek, 2001; Fellows et al., 2000; Maloney et al., 2002). Reports over a period of time continue to implicate FD & C Blue No. 1 dye in deaths related to absorption of the dye. Case reports also indicate that addition of this dye to enteral feedings can lead to serious injury, and its use for the purpose of detecting aspiration of tube feeding has not been validated (Fellows et al., 2000; Maloney et al., 2002). The coloring may also be contaminated with bacteria because it usually sits by the bedside. Additionally, it has been shown to cause allergic reactions, can cause diarrhea because it contains sorbitol, and can interfere with guaiac and pH testing of stool. It is safer and more reliable to test pulmonary secretions with a glucose reagent strip. Unless blood is present in pulmonary secretions, they usually do not contain any glucose.
- Check **residual** (feeding remaining in the stomach) before each feeding or every 4 to 6 hours during a continuous feeding (according to institution policy). Record residuals on flow sheet or progress notes. Check agency procedure, but a residual of more than 200 mL for nasogastric tubes and 100 mL for a gastrostomy tube or more than 10% to 20% above the hourly rate for the feeding may indicate that the feeding should be interrupted or delayed for 30 minutes to 1 hour. The difference between the residuals for nasogastric and gastrostomy tubes is due to the gastrostomy tubes port being high on the anterior gastric wall (Edwards & Metheny, 2000). Some experts now recommend that the patient's pattern of residual is more important than the amount. Refer to the accompanying box, Through the Eyes of a Student, for a student nurse's experience with residual and a tube feeding.
- Assess for bowel sounds at least once per shift to check for the presence of peristalsis and a functional intestinal tract. Experts, however, have recently concluded that it is common for acutely ill patients to have delayed or absent

Through the Eyes of a Student

She looked lost in that big hospital bed, so thin and frail. Her hair was as white as her pillowcase and blankets, and her skin looked almost transparent. And then I saw it. Snaking under her blankets into her belly was the feeding tube surrounded by thick, green, smelly discharge.

During preconference my instructor had told me that I needed to check residual every 2 hours to monitor her absorption rate. The first time, with my instructor standing beside me like my guardian angel (or my patient's guardian angel, I'm not sure which), the procedure naturally went off without a hitch. I could do this, I thought, feeling more confident.

Because my patient had chronic diarrhea as well as skin breakdown at her sacrum, the next 2 hours flew by in a whirlwind of bathing. But now the time had come. This is it, I thought. I'm on my own for the second residual check. And, again, I breathed a sigh of relief when the procedure was completed with no problems.

As the day progressed, I got myself a little behind schedule because I was determined to remove the hardened crusts from underneath her nails. Before I knew it, I got the message from another student that it was postconference time. Oh no! I didn't do my last residual check yet. Quickly, I emptied the basin I was using on her fingernails and grabbed the plunger. I reached into my pocket for my hemostat to clamp off the line and the next thing I saw was Jevity squirting all over the bed, my patient, the clean Chux and me! I had cut the line instead of clamping it!

I quickly pinched both ends to stop the Jevity from squirting and frantically called for help. While waiting for rescue, I checked on my patient's response, not knowing how she was going to react. Thankfully, she was sound asleep, soothed by her recent nail massage. It seemed like forever before my instructor rushed in. With my eyes filling up, I attempted to explain that I had grabbed the scissors from my pocket instead of the hemostat. Guardian angel that she was (I think she was both of ours), my instructor calmly and efficiently proceeded to attach both ends of the tube together with the use of an adapter.

Many lessons were learned that day, such as don't attempt a procedure in haste, and have all your supplies readily at hand. But the one thing I'll never, ever forget is that the scissors are the crooked ones!

—Eileen Cooper
Delaware County Community College, Media, PA

gastric emptying; therefore, delaying enteral feedings based on the absence of bowel sounds may place a patient at risk for malnutrition. Gastric distention or pain may be a better indicator of how well a patient is tolerating a tube feeding (Grant & Martin, 2000).

- Prevent contamination during enteral feedings by maintaining the integrity of the feeding system and using proper technique. Closed systems, consisting of a sterile, prefilled, ready-to-hang container, reduce the opportunity for bacterial contamination of the feeding formula. An open system exists when formula from a can or bottle is added to a feeding setup. Always check the expiration date of formula and perform hand hygiene (also a deterrent to microbial contamination of enteral feeding apparatuses) before touching the equipment. Label all equipment with the patient's name, date, and time the feeding was hung, and cap or cover any disconnected tubing. Clean a reusable feeding system with soap and hot water every 24 hours; replace a disposable feeding apparatus every 24 hours. (See the accompanying Research in Nursing box.)

Monitor for Complications

Patients receiving tube feedings are at risk for several complications. Guidelines for Nursing Care 42-2 summarize nursing measures to prevent selected complications. In addition, prevent the tube from becoming clogged or obstructed. Common causes of clogged enteral tubes include aspirated stomach contents, residue from medications, feeding flow rate of less than 50 mL/h, infrequent or inadequate addition of water to the system, and using a tube with a small lumen (Dudek, 2001). Flush tube with 30 to 50 mL of water before and after each feeding or introduction of medications, at least every 4 hours during a continuous feeding, and after aspirating a tube for gastric contents. After flushing the tube, be sure to document the amount on the intake and output record. For neonates or small children, a flush using air in a syringe may be used instead of water to avoid adding fluid to the fluid intake, thereby allowing for more formula to be delivered (Grant & Martin, 2000). Use of a feeding pump helps to prevent clogging. If an occlusion occurs, fill a large piston syringe with warm water and use a gentle push-and-pull motion. Carbonated beverages have not proved effective in unclogging a feeding tube (Kohn-Keeth, 2000).

Provide Comfort Measures

To ensure the patient's comfort, perform these interventions:

- Administer oral hygiene frequently (every 2–4 hours) to prevent drying of tissues and to relieve thirst. Offer the patient the opportunity to rinse the mouth with warm water and mouthwash solution frequently. Lubricate the lips generously.
- Keep the nares clean, especially around the tube, where secretions tend to accumulate. Using a lubricant after cleaning the nares is recommended.
- Help control local irritation from the tube in the throat. Analgesic throat lozenges or anesthetic sprays may be effective.
- Encourage the patient, if able, to verbalize concerns about tube feeding and presence of tube. A visit from another person who has learned to cope with this alternate feeding method may prove helpful.
- Ensure that the tube is taped securely to the nose to prevent trauma to the nares.
- Be aware that some studies indicate that patients report being able to taste the feedings even though they are being fed through a gastric tube. If available and not contraindicated, offer the patient a choice of flavors.

Recall Charles Gallagher, the husband of the woman with advanced dementia receiving enteral nutrition? The nurse could teach

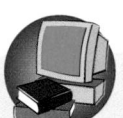

Research in Nursing Making a Difference
Contamination of Enteral Feeding

Many experts agree that enteral feeding is the better choice over parenteral nutrition in upholding gut structure and function. Enteral nutrition is cheaper, has less adverse effects, and the patient can fully use the nutrients. However, enteral feedings have been related to nosocomial infections. Contamination of enteral feedings can lead to abdominal distention, aspiration pneumonia, and colonization of the patient by the contaminant. Previous research has shown that the contamination can occur in the tube feeding itself, as well as nasogastric tubes.

Related Research

Matlow, A., Wray, R., Goldman, C., et al. (2003). Microbial contamination of enteral feed administration sets in a pediatric institution. *American Journal of Infection Control, 31*(1), 49–53.

The authors hypothesized that the enteral feeding administration sets could become contaminated by external microbes present in the enteral tube hub, and the administration sets would then serve as a reservoir for the organism. The study entailed culturing the external enteral feeding administration set and the hub of nasogastric, gastric, or gastrojejunal tubes in patients receiving enteral feeds. The samples were obtained from 37 pediatric patients in a tertiary-care pediatric hospital. Thirty-six of 37 hubs cultured showed bacterial growth. Twenty-nine of 36 administration sets (78%) cultured had at least one microbe isolated that was also cultured from the hub.

Relevance to Nursing Practice

Results of this nursing research study indicate that standard precautions, including good hand hygiene, are indicated while administering enteral feedings and checking for residual volumes. By taking these measures, cross contamination from one patient to another can be prevented, thus protecting our patients as well as reducing healthcare costs.

Guidelines for Nursing Care 42-2
Preventing Complications of Enteral Feeding

Potential Complications for Aspiration
- Use appropriate measures to check tube placement.
- Elevate head of bed at least 30 degrees during feeding and for 1 hour afterward.
- Give small, frequent feedings.
- Avoid oversedation of patient.
- Check residual volume per policy.

Potential Complications for Clogged Tube
- Flush tube before and after feeding, every 4 hours during continuous feeding, and after withdrawing aspirate.
- Instill 30 mL of water with 50-mL or 60-mL syringe.

Potential Complications for Nasal Erosion With Nasogastric or Nasointestinal Tubes
- Check nostrils every shift for signs of pressure.
- Clean and moisten nares every 4 to 8 hours.

Potential Complication for Diarrhea
- Start feeding at slow rate.
- Prevent contamination in both open and closed systems:
  - Change delivery set every 12 to 24 hours according to agency policy.
  - Refrigerate opened cans of formula and discard after 24 hours.
  - Limit hang time to 8 hours when using open system.
- Use aseptic technique for patients who are immunosuppressed or acutely ill.
- Assess for fecal impaction.

Potential for Other GI Symptoms (Nausea, Vomiting, Distention)
- Check residual prior to intermittent feedings and every 4 hours during continuous feedings.

- Avoid oversedating client (delays gastric emptying).
- Administer GI motility medications (Metoclopramide) as ordered.

Potential Complication for Unplanned Extubation
- Anchor tube adequately with tape.
- Check on patient frequently.
- Measure external length of tubing at regular intervals.
- Restrain patient only if necessary, with physician's order.

Potential Complication for Gastrostomy or Jejunostomy: "Buried Bumper" Syndrome (bumper or retaining disc presses too tightly against abdominal wall)
- Notify physician for complaints of bloating, abdominal discomfort, or signs of tube malfunction or bleeding.

Potential Complication for Stoma Infection
- Clean skin every shift with soap and warm water. Dry thoroughly.
- Use topical antibiotics as ordered.
- Assess for signs of infection.
- Request consult with wound care specialist.

Potential Complication for Refeeding Syndrome (electrolyte and metabolic disorder that can occur when a nutritionally depleted patient is fed enterally or parenterally)
- Monitor for muscle weakness that can progress to respiratory failure (due to decreased phosphorus in the cells).
- Assess for potassium depletion.
- Administer phosphorus and potassium supplements as ordered by physician.

Mr. Gallagher how to provide oral hygiene for his wife, including lubricating her lips. Doing so would allow Mr. Gallagher to feel some control over the situation. In addition, he would be helping to meet his wife's comfort needs and his own needs.

Provide Instruction

Often patients will continue to receive enteral feedings at home. (See Teaching to Promote Health at Home 42-1.) Provide the patient and family with individualized instructions in written form as a reference for the patient and caregivers. Be sure to include the following in the teaching plan (Dudek, 2001):
- Information about the administration of feedings, operation of the pump, formula, instructions regarding rate and how to check for tube placement, as well as what to do if the tube becomes dislodged
- Care of the tube insertion site and possible complications that need to be reported
- Proper preparation, cleaning, and disposal of equipment

- Emergency telephone numbers, including the number for the home healthcare agency and the physician
- Arrangements for follow-up from the home health nurse as soon as possible after discharge

Removal of Tube

Removing the tube as carefully as it is inserted is important to avoid causing the patient undue discomfort. After the tube is removed, provide for oral hygiene, which is especially important to remove disagreeable tastes and odors. Thorough oral hygiene is crucial when the tube has been in the intestinal tract and in contact with intestinal contents. Directions for removing the nasogastric tube are given in Skill 42-3.

Nasoenteric Tubes for Decompression

In addition to providing enteral feedings, nasogastric tubes can be used for other purposes. They may be inserted to decompress or drain the stomach of fluid, unwanted stomach contents such as poison or medication and air, allowing it to rest, or before or after surgery, to promote healing. Nasogastric tubes may also be used to monitor GI bleeding and prevent intestinal obstruction.

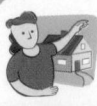

Teaching to Promote Health at Home 42-1
Tube Feedings

Health Topic	Teaching Tip	Why is This Important?
Cleaning around a gastric tube insertion site	Use of soap and water, making sure that area is adequately rinsed Rotation of the guard after cleaning around it	If soap is left under the gastric tube guard, it can lead to skin irritation. The guard can put pressure on the skin, leading to skin breakdown.
Checking residuals	Method and reason for checking residual contents, as well as what to do with residual contents	Residual contents should not be routinely discarded to prevent an acid–base imbalance; however, the patient should know when discarding is appropriate to prevent aspiration of stomach contents.
Delivering tube feedings	Head elevation while delivering a gastric feeding and for approximately an hour after the feeding Method of administration such as delivering the feedings via continuous or bolus method, and steps for carrying out the feeding	Keeping the head elevated helps to prevent aspiration of gastric tube feedings. Some patients do not tolerate the bolus method without vomiting. The patient should know how to operate the machinery if it is to be delivered via continuous method or how to set up for a bolus feeding.
Leaking of gastric contents	Method of checking for problems (is guard too loose or balloon not filled adequately) if gastric tube is leaking stomach contents around insertion site	If gastric tube is leaking acidic stomach contents, the area around the insertion site can quickly break down.

SKILL 42-3   Removing a Nasogastric Tube

EQUIPMENT
Tissues
Bath towel or disposable pad
Disposable plastic bag

50-mL syringe (optional)
Normal saline solution for irrigation
  (optional)

Disposable gloves

ACTION	RATIONALE
1. Check physician's order for removal of nasogastric tube.	This ensures correct implementation of physician's order.
2. Explain procedure to patient and assist to semi-Fowler's position.	Explanation facilitates patient cooperation. Sitting position decreases risk of aspiration, if vomiting should occur.
3. Gather equipment.	This provides for organized approach to task.
4. Perform hand hygiene. Don clean disposable gloves.	Hand hygiene deters the spread of microorganisms. Gloves protect hands from contact with abdominal secretions.
5. Place towel or disposable pad across patient's chest. Give tissues to patient.	Precautions protect patient from contact with gastric secretions. Tissues are necessary if patient wants to blow his or her nose when tube is removed.
6. Discontinue suction and separate tube from suction. Unpin tube from patient's gown and carefully remove adhesive tape from patient's nose.	Disconnecting tube allows for its unrestricted removal.
7. Attach syringe and flush with 10 mL normal saline solution or clear with 30 to 50 cc of air (optional).	Air or saline solution clears the tube of feeding or debris.
8. Instruct patient to take a deep breath and hold it.	This prevents accidental aspiration of gastric secretions in tube.
9. Clamp tube with fingers by doubling tube on itself. Quickly and carefully remove tube while patient holds breath.	Careful removal minimizes trauma and discomfort for patient. Clamping prevents drainage of gastric contents in tube.
10. Place tube in disposable plastic bag. Remove gloves and place in bag.	This prevents contamination with microorganisms.

(continued)

Removing a Nasogastric Tube (continued)

ACTION	RATIONALE
11. Offer mouth care to patient and facial tissue to blow nose.	Provides for comfort.
12. Measure nasogastric drainage. Remove all equipment and dispose according to agency policy. Perform hand hygiene.	Measuring nasogastric drainage provides for accurate recording of output. Hand hygiene and proper disposal deter spread of microorganisms.
13. Record removal of tube, patient's response, and measurement of drainage. Continue to monitor patient for 2–4 hours after tube removal for gastric distention, nausea, or vomiting.	Facilitates documentation and provides for comprehensive care.

Single- and double-lumen tubes (the lumen is the inner open space) are available. A single-lumen Levin tube lacks a venting system, and mucosal damage can occur when suction is applied continuously. Double-lumen sump tubes are a tube within a tube (eg, the Salem sump tube). One lumen empties the stomach, and the second lumen provides for a continuous flow of air. The airflow lumen controls suction by preventing the drainage lumen from pulling stomach mucosa into the tube's eyes and irritating the stomach lining. Tubes for decompression typically are attached to suction. Suction can be continuous rather than intermittent, as is required when a single-lumen tube is used. Nasogastric tubes used for decompression require irrigation with 30 to 60 mL of normal saline solution (0.9% sodium

chloride) to maintain patency and compensate for electrolytes that are lost in the gastric fluids removed by suction. This is different from tubes used for feeding purposes, which are cleared before and after use with sterile water or tap water according to the physician's order. Skill 42-4 outlines techniques for irrigating a nasogastric tube that is being used for decompression.

Providing Parenteral Nutrition

Patients who have nonfunctional GI tracts, who are comatose, or who cannot consume a nutritionally adequate diet enterally (eg, patients undergoing aggressive cancer therapy and those recovering from extensive burns, surgery, sepsis, or multiple fractures) may require parenteral nutrition. **Total parenteral**

Irrigating a Nasogastric Tube Connected to Suction

EQUIPMENT

Nasogastric tube connected to continuous or intermittent suction
Irrigation set (Asepto or Toomey syringe and container for irrigating solution) or 60 mL catheter tip syringe and cup

Normal saline solution (0.9% sodium chloride solution) for irrigation
Stethoscope

Disposable pad or bath towel
Clamp
Disposable gloves

ACTION	RATIONALE
1. Check physician's order for irrigation. Explain procedure to patient.	This clarifies schedule and irrigating solution. An explanation encourages patient cooperation and reduces apprehension.
2. Gather necessary equipment. Check expiration dates on irrigating saline solution and irrigation set.	This provides for organized approach to task. Agency policy dictates safe interval for reuse of equipment.
3. Perform hand hygiene.	Hand hygiene deters the spread of microorganisms.
4. Assist patient to semi-Fowler's position, unless this is contraindicated.	This position minimizes risk for aspiration.
5. Check placement of nasogastric tube (refer to Skill 42-1, Action 14).	
6. Pour irrigating solution into container. Draw up 30 mL of saline solution (or amount ordered by physician) into syringe. Don non-sterile gloves.	This delivers measured amount of irrigant through tube. Saline solution compensates for electrolytes lost through nasogastric drainage. Gloves ensure adherence to standard precautions.

(continued)

ACTION	RATIONALE
7. Clamp suction tubing near connection site. Disconnect tube from suction apparatus and lay on disposable pad or towel or hold both tubes upright in nondominant hand.	This protects patient from leakage of nasogastric drainage.
8. Place tip of syringe in tube. If Salem sump or double-lumen tube is used, make sure that syringe tip is placed in drainage port and not in air vent. Hold syringe upright and gently insert the irrigant (or allow solution to flow in by gravity if agency or physician indicates). Do not force solution into tube.	Position of syringe prevents entry of air into stomach. Gentle insertion of saline solution (or gravity insertion) is less traumatic to gastric mucosa.

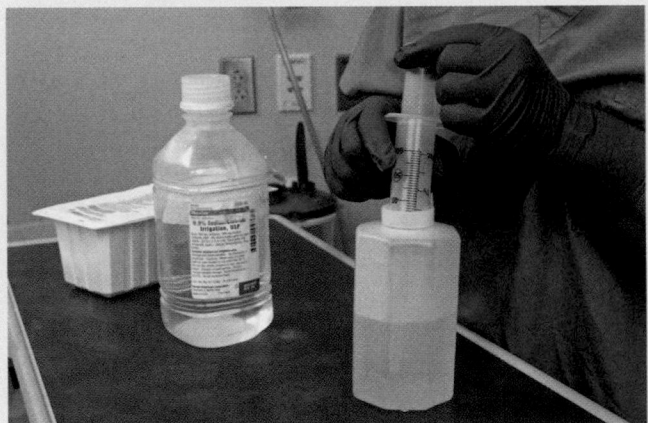

Action 6: Preparing syringe with 30 mL saline for irrigation.   (Photo by Rick Brady.)

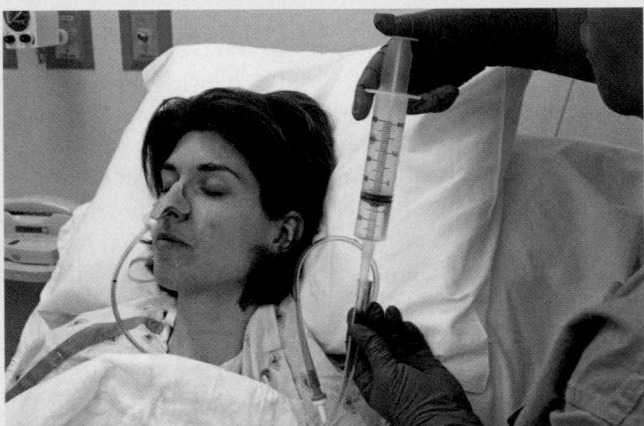

Action 8: Gently instilling irrigation.   (Photo by Rick Brady.)

ACTION	RATIONALE
9. If unable to irrigate tube, reposition patient and attempt irrigation again. Check with physician if repeated attempts to irrigate tube fail.	Tube may be positioned against gastric mucosa, making it difficult to irrigate.
10. Withdraw or aspirate fluid into syringe. If no return, inject 20 cc of air and aspirate again.	Injection of air may reposition the end of tube.
11. Reconnect tube to suction. Observe movement of solution or drainage. Remove gloves.	Observation determines patency of tube and correct operation of suction apparatus.
12. Measure and record amount and description of irrigant and returned solution.	Irrigant placed in tube is considered intake; solution returned is recorded as output.
13. Rinse equipment if it will be reused.	This promotes cleanliness and prepares equipment for next irrigation.
14. Perform hand hygiene.	Hand hygiene deters the spread of microorganisms.
15. Record irrigation procedure, description of drainage, and patient's response.	This facilitates documentation of procedure and provides for comprehensive care.

nutrition (TPN) provides complete nutrition via bypassing the GI tract for patients who are unable to take fluid orally. TPN meets the patient's nutritional needs by way of nutrient-filled solutions administered intravenously through a central line, usually the subclavian or internal jugular veins. Hyperalimentation is another term used synonymously with parenteral nutrition.

Enteral nutrition, instead of parenteral nutrition, was the treatment of choice for the wife of Charles Gallagher, the older man described *in the Reflective Practice display. His wife had a functioning GI tract, but was unable to swallow. Thus, she was unable to consume anything orally.*

Assessment of serum albumin level is the best indicator of a patient in need of TPN. Patients whose levels are 2.5 g/dL or less are at severe risk for malnutrition. Therefore, they are candidates for TPN.

TPN therapy is costly, requires constant monitoring, and has the potential for causing infectious, metabolic, and mechanical complications. It should be used only when enteral intake is inadequate or contraindicated and should be gradually discontinued as soon as possible. **Partial parenteral nutrition** or **peripheral parenteral nutrition (PPN)** is prescribed for patients who require nutrient supplementation through a peripheral vein because they have an inadequate intake of oral feedings.

Parenteral Nutrition Solutions and Administration

Solutions used for PPN typically are isotonic, whereas solutions used for TPN are hypertonic solutions. Thus, TPN must be administered through a central vein.

TPN contains the three primary components necessary to maintain nutrition: proteins, carbohydrates, and fats. Additional components of parenteral nutrition include electrolytes, vitamins, and trace elements. Medications such as insulin (because TPN contains large concentrations of glucose) and heparin (to prevent formation of a blood clot on the tip of the catheter) may also be added to the solution. Due to the high glucose concentration, usually about 25% (thus a hypertonic solution), TPN solutions must not be stopped suddenly. Otherwise, the patient may experience a sudden decline in glucose levels, causing a hypoglycemic reaction. In addition, blood glucose levels must be monitored (Skill 42-5). Fat or lipid

---

SKILL 42-5 Monitoring the Blood Glucose Level

EQUIPMENT

Blood glucose meter	Sterile lancet	Alcohol swab or soap and water
Testing strips	Cotton balls	Disposable gloves

ACTION	RATIONALE
1. Check physician's order for monitoring schedule.	This confirms times for checking blood glucose.
2. Gather equipment.	This provides an organized approach to the task.
3. Explain procedure to patient.	Explanation encourages patient cooperation.
4. Perform hand hygiene. Don disposable gloves.	Hand hygiene deters the spread of microorganisms. Gloves protect from exposure to blood or body fluids.
5. Prepare lancet.	Aseptic technique maintains sterility.
6. Remove test strip from the vial and recap container immediately. Turn monitor on and check that code number on strip matches the code number on the monitor screen.	Immediate recapping protects strips from exposure to humidity, light, and discoloration. Matching code numbers on the strip and glucose monitor ensure that machine is calibrated correctly.
7. Massage side of finger for adult (or heel for child) toward puncture site.	Massage encourages blood flow to the area.

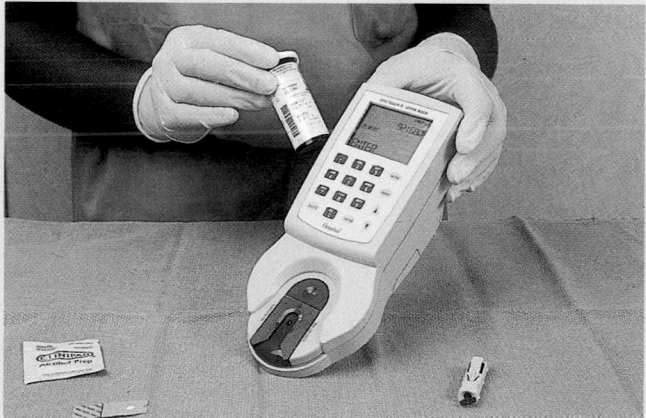

Action 6: Comparing the code number on the strip to the code number on the monitor screen.

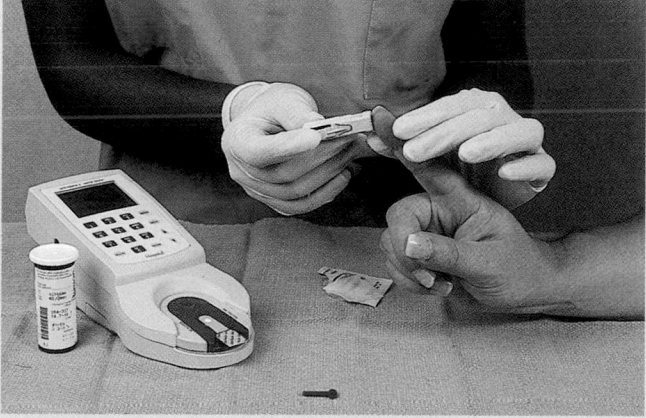

Action 9: Using the lancet to prick the skin.

8. Have patient wash hands with soap and warm water or cleanse area with alcohol. Dry thoroughly.	Washing with soap and water or alcohol cleanses the puncture site. Warm water also helps to cause vasodilation.
9. Hold lancet perpendicular to skin and prick site with the lancet.	Holding lancet in proper position facilitates proper skin penetration.

(continued)

SKILL 42-5 Monitoring the Blood Glucose Level (continued)

ACTION	RATIONALE
10. Wipe away first drop of blood with cotton ball if recommended by manufacturer of monitor.	Some feel first drop of blood may be contaminated by serum or cleansing product and produce an inaccurate reading.
11. Lightly squeeze or milk the puncture site until a hanging drop of blood has formed (check instructions for monitor).	Large droplet facilitates accurate test results.
12. Gently touch drop of blood to pad on test strip without smearing it.	Smearing blood on strip may result in inaccurate test results.
13. Insert strip into the meter according to directions for that specific device. Some devices require that the drop of blood is applied to a test strip that has already been inserted in the monitor.	Correctly inserted strip allows meter to read blood glucose level accurately.
14. Press timer if directed by manufacturer.	Timing produces accurate results.

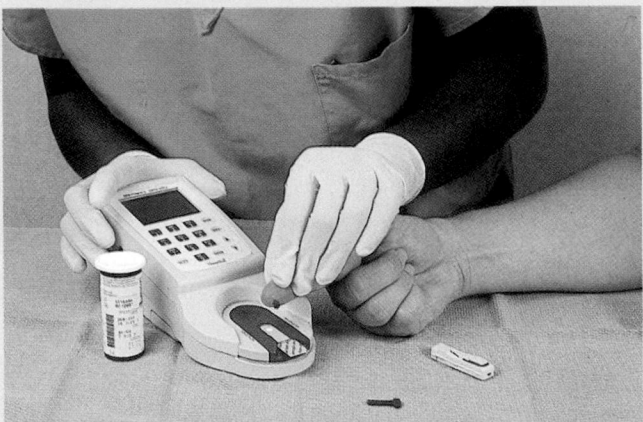

Action 12: Preparing to place a drop of blood on the strip.

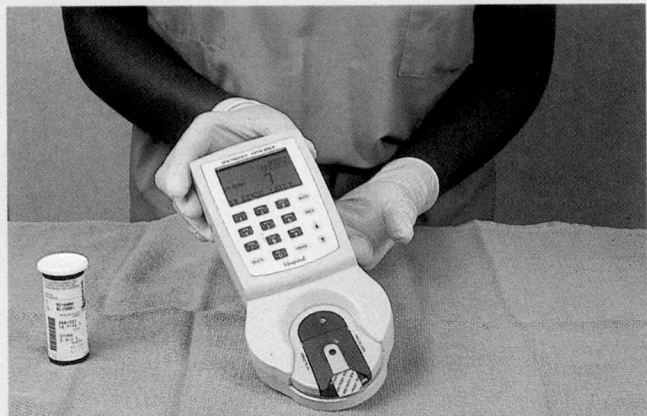

Action 14: Awaiting test results while the timer counts down.

ACTION	RATIONALE
15. Apply pressure to puncture site. Do not use alcohol wipe.	Pressure causes hemostasis. Alcohol stings and may prolong bleeding.
16. Read blood glucose results and document appropriately at bedside. Inform patient of test result.	Timing when awaiting results depends on type of meter.
17. Turn meter off, dispose of supplies appropriately, and place lancet in sharps container.	Proper disposal prevents exposure to blood and accidental needle sticks.
18. Remove gloves and perform hand hygiene.	Hand hygiene prevents the spread of microorganisms.
19. Record blood glucose on chart or medication record.	This facilitates documentation of procedure and provides for comprehensive care.

emulsions and the dextrose add caloric value that the body needs to meet energy requirements. TPN can be given for extended periods of time (up to 3 months) through a peripherally inserted central catheter (PICC; refer to Chap. 46 for additional discussion of PICCs).

PPN solutions provide fewer calories and supplement a patient's inadequate oral intake. This solution usually contains 10% glucose, which is suitable for administration into a peripheral vessel. The accompanying Guidelines for Nursing

Care box lists nursing guidelines for monitoring administration of parenteral nutrition.

Although the benefits of parenteral nutrition are extensive, return to oral or enteral nutrition is recommended as soon as possible. Doing so reduces the risk for sepsis, decreases cost, and prevents wasting and deterioration of the GI tract. Prevention of potential complications associated with total parenteral nutrition requires vigilance and careful monitoring by the nurse. They include the following (Smeltzer & Bare, 2004):

Guidelines for Nursing Care 42-3
Monitoring Administration of Parenteral Nutrition

- Use the same catheter lumen for administration of parenteral nutrition each time the tubing is changed.
- Use a pump to administer infusion of parenteral nutrition.
- If administration of parenteral nutrition is interrupted, administer a 5% to 10% dextrose solution to prevent hypoglycemia.
- Discard unused parenteral nutrition solution within 24 hours of starting its administration.
- Check vital signs every 4 hours to monitor for development of infection or sepsis.
- Monitor blood glucose levels every 6 hours. (Skill 42-5 explains the technique for monitoring serum glucose levels.)
- Use aseptic technique when changing solution, tubing, filter, or dressings according to agency policy. Most infec-

tion control practitioners recommend changing infusion administration sets every 24 hours. Dressings should be changed at least every 72 hours or according to agency protocol.
- Check that all connections are securely taped, catheter is clamped before opening the system, and insertion site is covered with sterile dressing.
- Compare the patient's daily weight to fluid intake and output. Total weight gain should not be greater than 3 lb per week.
- Assess serum protein and electrolyte levels for signs of imbalance.
- Due to the high glucose concentration, use tubing with an in-line filter.

- Insertion problems, such as pneumothorax, air embolism, and thromboembolism
- Infection
- Metabolic alterations, such as hyperglycemia or hypoglycemia when infusion is discontinued or interrupted
- Fluid, electrolyte, and acid–base imbalances
- Phlebitis

Many patients, however, require long-term parenteral nutrition and continue this therapy in the home. Individuals with acquired immunodeficiency syndrome (AIDS), advanced cancer, difficulty swallowing, or chronic bowel problems are candidates for this type of nutritional support. Nurses are involved in educating the patient and caregiver about the techniques and responsibilities associated with parenteral nutrition, providing technical and psychological support, and documenting the assessments that allow parenteral nutrition to be continued in the home.

Evaluating

The effectiveness of the plan of care is evaluated as the last step in the nursing process. On an ongoing basis, the nurse accomplishes the following:

- Evaluates the patient's progress toward meeting nutritional outcomes
- Evaluates the patient's tolerance and adherence to the diet, when appropriate
- Assesses the patient's level of understanding of the diet and the need for further diet instruction or reinforcement
- Communicates findings to other members of the healthcare team
- Revises the plan of care, as needed, or terminates nursing care

See the accompanying Nursing Plan of Care 42-1 for Susan Oakland.

NURSING PLAN OF CARE 42-1 for Susan Oakland

Susan Oakland, a 21-year-old student, was seen at the prenatal clinic for her first pregnancy at 5 weeks' gestation. On her next visit, 4 weeks later, she complained of nausea and vomiting and had lost 3 lb (1.4 kg).

ASSESSMENT FINDINGS
A comprehensive nutritional assessment revealed the following data:

Anthropometric Data
Usual body weight: 112 lb (50.8 kg)
Weight at 9 weeks' gestation 109 lb (49.4 kg)
Height: 5 feet 5 inches (165.1 cm)

Ideal body weight: 125 lb (56.7 kg; range is 113 to 137 lb [51.3 to 62.1 kg])
Expected weight gain for 9 weeks' gestation: 1 to 2 lb (0.45 to 0.9 kg)

Biochemical Data
Laboratory data revealed low hemoglobin level and hematocrit.

Medical and Socioeconomic Data
- Patient complains of nausea and vomiting, which begin in the morning and continue until midafternoon. Her appetite is poor. She also states, "I'm always tired."

(continued)

NURSING PLAN OF CARE 42-1 · for Susan Oakland (continued)

- Patient and her husband are first-semester graduate students; their source of income is graduate assistantships, and their food budget is limited.
- Patient states that she did not intend to become pregnant, but both she and her husband are excited about becoming parents. She plans to take a leave of absence from school for one semester when the baby is born; she wants to breastfeed.

Clinical Data

Patient appears pale. No other abnormal physical findings were noted.

Dietary Data

- Patient's 24-hour recall revealed an inadequate intake from the milk group and a marginal intake from the grain and meat groups. She skips breakfast because of a hurried schedule, which is now complicated by nausea; lunch comprises soup, salad, and fruit; dinner usually comprises chicken; cooked vegetables; pasta, rice, or potatoes; and fruit. Patient dislikes red meat and eats it only once or twice a month. She also dislikes milk and substitutes sugar-free soft drinks and water. Before becoming pregnant, she drank five or six cups of black coffee a day, but now she avoids it. Her snacks usually consist of fresh fruit and vegetables.
- Patient is very weight conscious; she periodically crash diets to maintain her weight at 112 lb (50.8 kg).
- Patient does not take vitamins, medications, or drugs; she drinks socially, one or two times per month.
- Nutritional problems and contributing factors include the following:
  - Inadequate intake of milk and calories contributed to by nausea and vomiting, dislike for milk, limited food budget, weight consciousness
  - Poor iron intake contributed to by lack of good sources of iron in her diet, no supplemental iron intake
  - Meal-skipping contributed to by nausea and vomiting, hurried schedule
  - Underweight or weight loss contributed to by weight consciousness, nausea, and vomiting

NURSING DIAGNOSIS

Imbalanced Nutrition: Less than Body Requirements related to increased requirements imposed by pregnancy, nausea and vomiting, weight consciousness, hurried schedule, food dislikes as manifested by: reports of anorexia, fatigue, 3-lb weight loss in 4 weeks' time, pale color, and low hemoglobin and hematocrit values.

OUTCOME IDENTIFICATION

By the next monthly assessment, 6/26/06, the patient will:
- Eat three or more small meals a day

Nursing Interventions	Rationale	Evaluative Statement
Determine how the patient's schedule may be altered to allow time for meals. Encourage the patient to have easy-to-eat foods available for quick snacks, like cartons of yogurt, cheese and crackers, muffins, and fresh fruit.	Patient complained that her current schedule prevents regular meals. Easy-to-eat foods may be more acceptable and can be nutritionally comparable to traditional meals.	6/26/06 Outcome met. Patient eats three meals daily. Tries snacking on easy-to-eat foods when possible. *Recommendation:* Encourage more snacking to increase overall food intake. *L. Swift, RN*
Advise the patient that nausea may be lessened by avoiding periods of hunger, and that later in the pregnancy, avoiding hunger will help ensure a steady supply of nutrients to the fetus.	Low blood glucose may contribute to nausea early in pregnancy; later in pregnancy, low blood glucose and resultant ketosis may be harmful to the fetus.	

EXPECTED OUTCOME

By the next monthly assessment, 6/26/06, the patient will:
- Eat dry crackers, bread sticks, or dry cereal 30 minutes before rising.

Nursing Interventions	Rationale	Evaluative Statement
Advise the patient to eat a source of dry carbohydrates before getting up in the morning.	Eating dry carbohydrates 30 minutes before rising helps avoid nausea.	6/26/06 Outcome met. Patient eats dry crackers every morning 30 minutes before getting out of bed. Reports that it prevents morning nausea. *L. Swift, RN*

(continued)

NURSING PLAN OF CARE 42-1

for Susan Oakland (continued)

EXPECTED OUTCOME

By the next monthly assessment, 6/26/06, the patient will:
• Eat 6 small meals per day.

Nursing Interventions	Rationale	Evaluative Statement
Advise the patient to eat 6 small meals per day.	Small meals are easier to digest. Low glucose may contribute to nausea.	6/26/06 Outcome met. Patient eats at least 6 small meals per day. Nausea is occurring less frequently throughout the day.

EXPECTED OUTCOME

By the next monthly assessment, 6/26/06, the patient will:
• Avoid diet soft drinks

Nursing Interventions	Rationale	Evaluative Statement
Advise the patient to avoid diet soft drinks. Recommend acceptable nutritional alternatives to the patient.	Saccharin and aspartame have not been proved safe for the fetus. The diet sodas are filling but offer no calories for fetus.	6/26/06 Outcome partially met. Patient reports that she drinks two or three cans of diet soft drinks a week at school to relieve thirst because nothing else is available. *Recommendation:* Encourage the patient to bring something to drink during the day from home, such as frozen drink boxes of 100% fruit juice, which will thaw at room temperature, or an insulated container of ice water or milk flavored with vanilla (dislikes plain milk). *L. Swift, RN*

EXPECTED OUTCOME

By the next monthly assessment, 6/26/06, the patient will:
• Eat the recommended number of servings from each food group as suggested by the daily food guide for pregnancy.

Nursing Interventions	Rationale	Evaluative Statement
Provide the patient with a daily food guide for pregnancy, and explain the rationale for the increased recommendations. Investigate acceptable alternatives for red meat and milk, which the patient normally does not consume.	Because this is the patient's first pregnancy, she is not aware of the recommendations for eating during pregnancy. Although no one particular food is essential during pregnancy, red meat is essential during pregnancy and an excellent source of iron, and milk is an excellent source of calcium, two minerals important for the developing fetus. If the patient is not provided with nutritionally equivalent alternatives, her diet may not be optimal, even if she consumes the recommended number of servings from the meat and milk groups (ie, patient may not be getting as much iron as she can from	6/26/06 Outcome partially met. Patient's intake is improved: intake from the grain and meat groups is adequate instead of marginal. However, the patient still has difficulty consuming enough items from the milk group. *Recommendation:* Continue encouraging the patient to consume more items from the milk group, such as cheese, yogurt, and pudding. Will advise the patient to add skim milk powder whenever possible to fortify home-cooked and home-baked products. Will recommend that the patient increase her intake of nondairy sources of calcium, such as broccoli, spinach, and

(continued)

NURSING PLAN OF CARE 42-1

for Susan Oakland (continued)

Nursing Interventions	Rationale	Evaluative Statement
	her diet if she relies on fish, cheese, and white-meat poultry to satisfy the meat group recommendations).	greens or breakfast cereal, fruit juice, and soy beverages with added calcium. Iron may also be consumed through turkey dark meat, shellfish or spinach. *L. Swift, RN*

EXPECTED OUTCOME

By the next monthly assessment, 6/26/06, the patient will:
• Gain 1 to 2 lb

Nursing Interventions	Rationale	Evaluative Statement
Advise the patient on the recommended rate and amount of weight gain. Stress the importance of quality weight gain.	Patient needs to understand that a 25- to 35-lb gradual weight gain is considered optimal for fetal development, and results in little gain in maternal fat tissue. However, because the fetus and maternal tissues require nutrients along with calories, it is essential that the weight gain comes from eating nutrient-dense calories instead of empty calories.	6/26/06 Outcome met. Noting a relief from nausea and an increase in the number of daily meals, the patient gained 2 lb. *L. Swift, RN*

EXPECTED OUTCOME

By the next monthly assessment, the patient will:
• Take prenatal vitamins as prescribed by the physician.

Nursing Interventions	Rationale	Evaluative Statement
Advise the patient to take the supplement as prescribed and that the supplements are not a substitute for an adequate diet.	Supplements are intended to be used in conjunction with an optimal diet, not in place of one, because they do not provide optimal amounts of all required nutrients. Because the requirements for folic acid and iron during pregnancy are usually not met through diet alone, supplements of these two nutrients in particular are necessary.	6/26/06 Outcome met. Patient reports taking supplement as prescribed. No adverse effects noted. *Recommendation:* Will continue to monitor patient's tolerance of supplement. Will continue to implement plan and reassess at next monthly appointment, 7/28/06. *L. Swift, RN*
Advise the patient that the iron content in the supplements may cause constipation and the stools to become black.	Common adverse effects of large iron doses are constipation and black stools.	

SAMPLE DOCUMENTATION

5/22/06   Nursing

Mrs. Oakland was seen for routine prenatal checkup at 9 weeks' gestation. Assessment findings reveal that the patient is underweight, has lost 3 lb (1.4 kg) in the past 4 weeks, is experiencing nausea and vomiting, has a deficient hemoglobin and hematocrit, and is fatigued. Other contributing factors include weight consciousness, hurried schedule, and food dislikes. Discussion centered on maintaining good dietary habits, improving overall intake and meal patterns to meet the demands of pregnancy and subsequent lactation, initiating dietary changes aimed at avoiding nausea and vomiting, and increasing iron intake. See plan of care. Patient's progress will be evaluated at the next monthly visit, 6/26/06. *L. Swift, RN*

■ Developing Critical Thinking Skills

1. Prepare a diet for an economically disadvantaged family consisting of a single working mother and three children, ages 3 to 14 years, taking into consideration the family's culture (specify a minority culture in your locale) and yearly income (below poverty level).

2. Prepare a 1-day menu that meets the recommended daily allowance of essential nutrients for the following patients:
   - An obese teenager
   - A child vegetarian
   - An executive with high blood pressure who dines out frequently with clients
   - A woman running a minimum of 12 miles daily as she trains for a marathon

■ Practicing for NCLEX

1. When reviewing a patient's dietary intake, the nurse would identify which nutrient as providing the most concentrated source of energy in the body?
   a. Protein
   b. Carbohydrates
   c. Fat
   d. Macrominerals

2. Which of the following would the nurse need to keep in mind when teaching a patient about the current Food Guide Pyramid?
   a. Meat and dairy products are located at the peak.
   b. All food groups are equally emphasized.
   c. Consumption of all complex carbohydrates is promoted.
   d. The Pyramid focuses on deficiencies in our diet.

3. Which laboratory test result would the nurse interpret as indicating that a patient is at risk for poor nutritional status?
   a. Decreased serum albumin level
   b. Increased lymphocyte count
   c. Decreased blood urea nitrogen level
   d. Increased platelet count

4. Mr. Yow is refusing to eat. Which intervention would be most helpful in stimulating his appetite?
   a. Administering pain medication after meals
   b. Encouraging food from home when possible
   c. Scheduling his respiratory therapy before each meal
   d. Reinforcing the importance of his eating exactly what is delivered to him

5. Mrs. James has progressed to a full liquid diet. Which items would the nurse expect to see on the patient's meal tray?
   a. Apple juice and bouillon
   b. Water ice and ginger ale
   c. Puréed beef and cream of broccoli soup
   d. Custard and a glass of milk

6. When explaining parenteral nutrition, the nurse would describe this method as providing nutrients to the patient by way of which of the following?
   a. Gastrostomy tube
   b. Intravenous route
   c. Nasointestinal route
   d. Jejunostomy tube

7. The nurse completing anthropometric measurements for a patient collects which of the following information?
   a. Height and weight
   b. Serum hemoglobin and hematocrit levels
   c. Diet history
   d. Intake and output

8. When discussing a weight-reduction plan with Mrs. Young, the nurse would explain that 1 lb of body fat is equal to about
   a. 1500 cal
   b. 2400 cal
   c. 3500 cal
   d. 5000 cal

9. Mr. White has been admitted to the alcoholic referral unit in the local hospital. Based on an understanding of the effects of alcohol on the GI tract, which of the following would the nurse be most alert for nutritionally?
   a. Vitamin B malnutrition
   b. Obesity
   c. Dehydration
   d. Vitamin C deficiency

10. A patient has a nasogastric tube inserted for feeding purposes. Using the stomach as a reservoir for food is advantageous in preventing what complication?
    a. Dumping syndrome
    b. Duodenal ulcers
    c. Hyperglycemia
    d. Gastric ulcers

11. The nurse connects a patient's single-lumen nasogastric tube to intermittent suction for which purpose?
    a. Drain the stomach more effectively
    b. Prevent electrolyte losses
    c. Help to prevent dumping syndrome
    d. Help to prevent the tube from suctioning the mucosa

12. Mr. Lang is receiving continuous tube feedings through a small-bore nasogastric tube. Which method would the nurse expect as the most accurate in verifying correct tube placement?
    a. Auscultatory method
    b. Measurement of the gastric aspirate pH
    c. Measurement of the amount of residual
    d. Radiographic examination

13. Saline solution is used to irrigate a nasogastric tube used for decompression based on which rationale?
    a. Irrigating with water is a contaminated procedure.
    b. Saline solution is a hypertonic solution.

c. Saline solution replaces electrolytes lost through nasogastric suction.

d. Saline solution is less irritating to the gastric mucosa.

14. A patient's history reveals gorging followed by purging with self-induced vomiting. The nurse interprets this as suggesting which disorder?
    a. Anorexia
    b. Morbid obesity
    c. Bulimia
    d. Cachexia

15. Which plant protein contains all the essential amino acids necessary to support growth?
    a. Grains
    b. Soy
    c. Vegetables
    d. Legumes

■ Answers With Rationale

1. The correct response is *c*. Fat provides 9 cal for every gram compared with 4 cal/g each for protein (*a*) and carbohydrates (*b*). Macrominerals (*d*) are regulatory nutrients, not energy nutrients.

2. The correct response is *c*. The focus of the Food Guide Pyramid (*d*) is on wellness and prevention of nutritionally related diseases. Fats are at the peak of the pyramid (*a*), whereas the greatest focus is on grains and cereals as the basic food group. Future pyramids will address selection of high-quality whole grain foods with each meal.

3. The correct response is *a*. A decreased serum protein level places a patient at nutritional risk. The other test results do not represent a nutritional risk.

4. The correct response is *b*. Food from home that the patient enjoys may stimulate him to eat. Pain medication (*a*) should be given before meals, respiratory therapy (*c*) should be scheduled after meals, and telling the patient what he must eat (*d*) is no guarantee that he will comply.

5. The correct response is *d*. Custard and milk are items found in a full liquid diet. Apple juice, bouillon, (*a*) water ice, and ginger ale (*b*) are clear liquids, and puréed beef and cream of broccoli soup (*c*) are more likely to be found in a soft diet.

6. The correct response is *b*. Parenteral nutrition is given intravenously. Gastrostomy tube (*a*), nasointestinal route (*c*), and jejunostomy tube (*d*) are routes for enteral feedings.

7. The correct response is *a*. Height and weight are the most common anthropometric measurements obtained. Intake and output measurements (*d*) indicate fluid balance, hemoglobin and hematocrit (*b*) are biochemical data, and a diet history (*c*) is used to complete dietary data.

8. The correct response is *c*. One pound of body fat is equal to about 3500 cal.

9. The correct response is *a*. The need for B vitamins is increased in alcoholics because these nutrients are used to metabolize alcohol, thus depleting their supply. Alcohol abuse specifically affects the B vitamins. Obesity (*b*), dehydration (*c*), and vitamin C (*d*) deficiency may be present but these are not directly related to the effect of alcohol on the GI tract.

10. The correct response is *a*. When the stomach is used as a reservoir, the formula is released at a controlled rate, preventing the occurrence of the dumping syndrome. Duodenal (*b*) or gastric (*d*) ulcers are not commonly associated with enteral nutrition. Feeding solutions would not precipitate hyperglycemia (*c*) because they contain balanced amounts of nutrients.

11. The correct response is *d*. Intermittent suction prevents damage to the mucosa of the stomach, and that is the primary purpose for using it with a single-lumen tube. Intermittent suction does help remove stomach contents (*a*); however, intermittent suction is not considered to be more effective in doing so. Suction promotes electrolyte loss and has no effect on the dumping syndrome (*c*).

12. The correct response is *d*. Although a radiographic examination exposes the patient to radiation and is costly, it is still the most accurate method to check correct tube placement. Other methods that can be used are aspiration of gastric contents (*b*) and measurement of the pH of the aspirate (*c*). The auscultatory method (*a*) is considered inaccurate and unreliable.

13. The correct response is *c*. Saline solution reduces loss of electrolytes through nasogastric suction and is, therefore, the irrigant of choice. Water (*a*) does not cause contamination but it does upset the electrolyte balance. Saline solution (*b*) is isotonic, not hypertonic. However, it is not considered to be less irritating to the mucosa.

14. The correct response is *c*. Bulimia is the only eating disorder mentioned that involves the cycle of gorging and purging. Anorexia (*a*) refers to a lack of appetite, while cachexia (*c*) reflects a state of malnutrition and wasting. Morbid obesity (*b*) indicates extreme obesity that interferes with normal activities.

15. The correct response is *b*. Soy is considered a complete plant protein that contains all of the essential amino acids. Grains (*a*), vegetables (*c*), and legumes (*d*) are incomplete proteins.

Bibliography

Balluz, L., Kiezak, S., Philen, R., & Mulinare, J. (2000). Vitamin and mineral supplement use in the United States. Results from Third National Health and Nutrition Examination Survey. *Archives of Family Medicine, 9*(3), 258–262.

Barr, S., & Chapman, G. (2002). Perceptions and practices of self-defined current vegetarian, former vegetarian, non-vegetarian women. *Journal of the American Dietetic Association, 102*(3), 354–360.

Bauer, J. (2003). Enteral feeding pumps. *RN, 66*(8), 69–70.

Bowers, S. (2000). All about tubes: Your guide to enteral feeding devices. *Nursing, 30*(12), 41–47.

Dudek, S. (2001). *Nutrition handbook for nursing practice* (4th ed.). Philadelphia: Lippincott Williams & Wilkins.

Edwards, S., & Metheny, N. (2000). Measurement of gastric residual volume: State of the science. *MEDSURG Nursing, 9*(3), 125–128.

Eisenberg, P. (2002). An overview of diarrhea in the patient receiving enteral nutrition. *Gastroenterology Nursing, 25*(3), 95–104.

Fairfield, K., & Fletcher, R. (2002). Vitamins for chronic disease prevention in adults: Scientific review. *JAMA, 287*(23), 3116–3126.

Fellows, L., Miller, E., Frederickson, M., Bly, B., & Felt, P. (2000). Evidence-based practice for enteral feedings: Aspiration prevention strategies, bedside detection, and practice change. *MEDSURG Nursing, 9*(1), 27–31.

Fischbach, F. (2004). *A manual of laboratory and diagnostic tests* (6th ed.). Philadelphia: Lippincott Williams & Wilkins.

Flegal, K., Carroll, M., Ogden, C., & Johnson, C. (2002). Prevalence and trends in obesity among U.S. adults, 1999–2000. *JAMA, 288*(14), 1723–1727.

Grant, M., & Martin, S. (2000). Delivery of enteral nutrition. *AACN Clinical Issues, 11*(4), 507–516.

Guigoz, Y., Lauque, S., & Vellas, B. (2002). Identifying the elderly at risk for malnutrition: The mini nutritional assessment. *Clinics in Geriatric Medicine, 18*(4), 735–757.

Kohn-Keeth, C. (2000). How to keep feeding tubes flowing freely. *Nursing, 30*(1), 58–59.

Liebman, B. (2001). Defensive eating: Staying lean in a fattening world. *Nutrition Action Health Letter, 28*(10), 1–8.

Lord, L. (2001). How to insert a large-bore nasogastric tube. *Nursing, 31*(9), 46–48.

Mackie, S. (2001). PEGS and ethics. *Gastroenterology Nurse, 24*(3), 138–142.

Maloney, J., Ryan, T., Brasel, K., Binion, D., Johnson, D., et al. (2002). Food dye use in enteral feedings: A review and a call for a moratorium. *Nutrition in Clinical Practice, 17*(3), 168–181.

Matlow, A., Wray, R., Goldman, C., Streitenberger, L., Freeman, R., & Kovach, D. (2003). Microbial contamination of enteral feed administration sets in a pediatric institution. *American Journal of Infection Control, 31*(1), 49–53.

McCloskey, J., & Bulechek, J. (2000). *Nursing interventions classification (NIC)* (3rd ed.). St. Louis: C. V. Mosby.

Metheny, N. (2002). Inadvertent intracranial nasogastric tube placement. *American Journal of Nursing, 102*(8), 25–27.

Metheny, N., & Stewart, B. (2002). Testing feeding tube placement during continuous tube feedings. *Applied Nursing Research, 15*(4), 254–258.

Metheny, N., & Titler, M. (2001). Assessing placement of feeding tubes. *American Journal of Nursing, 101*(5), 36–45.

Moore, B. (2003). Supersized America: Help your patients regain control of their weight. *Cleveland Clinic Journal of Medicine, 70*(3), 237–240.

Noble, K. (2003). Name that tube. *Nursing, 33*(3), 56–62.

North American Nursing Diagnosis Association. (2003). *NANDA nursing diagnoses: Definitions & classification, 2003–2004.* Philadelphia: Author.

Peckenpaugh, N., & Poleman, C. (1999). *Nutrition essentials and diet therapy* (8th ed.). Philadelphia: W. B. Saunders.

Purnell, L., & Paulanka, B. (1998). *Transcultural health care.* Philadelphia: F. A. Davis.

Russell, R., Rasmussen, H., & Lichtenstein, A. (1999). Modified food guide pyramid for people over seventy years of age. *Journal of Nutrition, 129*(3), 751–753.

Schiff, L. (2000). Enhanced enteral feeding formulas. *RN, 63*(9), 77–79.

Smeltzer, S. C., & Bare, B. G. (2004). *Brunner and Suddarth's textbook of medical surgical nursing* (10th ed.) Philadelphia: Lippincott Williams & Wilkins.

Stahl, P. (2000). Informing consumers about trans fat labeling. *Journal of the American Dietetic Association, 100*(10), 1132, 1134.

United States Department of Agriculture. (October, 1996). The food guide pyramid. Accessed July 6, 2003 at http://www.usda.gov/cnpp/pyrabklt.pdf.

Vegetarian Resource Group. How many vegetarians are there? Accessed July 6, 2003 at http://www.vrg.org/journal/vj2000may/2000maypoll.htm

Jewel Carson delivered healthy twin girls several hours ago and has not voided yet. Her bladder is palpably full and distended, but she has been unable to void on her own.

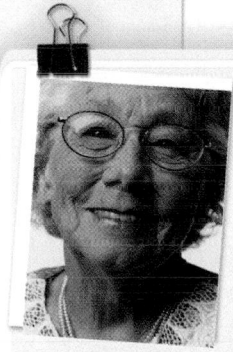

Anna Galinski, age 85, is frail and has numerous medical problems. She lives in a nursing home and like many of the residents was on a toileting regimen. Not long after a new charge nurse arrived, Anna and the other residents who used to be on toileting regimens had indwelling catheters inserted.

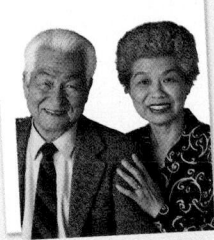

Midori Morita, age 69, is taking care of her 70-year-old husband at home. She asks, "Should I talk with my husband's doctor about getting him a urinary catheter? Ever since he came back from the hospital this last time, he seems unable to use the urinal. He dribbles constantly and I can't keep up with the sheets. He had a catheter in the hospital."

Focusing on Blended Skills

The types of blended skills you'll need to respond to the case scenarios include:

Cognitive Skills

- Knowledge of the anatomy and physiology of the urinary system and variables that influence urination
- Knowledge of medical and surgical asepsis
- Knowledge of measures to promote urinary elimination, including maintaining normal habits, promoting fluid intake, strengthening muscle tone, stimulating urination, and assisting with toileting
- Ability to integrate knowledge of factors affecting urinary elimination as a basis for developing the plan of care for a postpartum woman, the wife of a patient with incontinence, and an elderly woman on a toileting program who now has an indwelling catheter
- Ability to incorporate knowledge of specific conditions that may affect the urinary tract into the plan of care for a patient experiencing an alteration in urinary elimination
- Ability to apply knowledge of the nursing process to identify and care for patients with diagnoses associated with urinary problems

Technical Skills

- Strong assessment skills to determine problems related to urinary elimination and possible contributory factors
- Ability to use the equipment and protocols necessary to diagnose and treat urinary problems
- Demonstration of proper techniques for infection control and asepsis
- Demonstration of appropriate measures to assist with diagnostic studies involving the urinary tract
  - Ability to help patients use the toilet, bedpan, urinal, and commode; perform catheterizations; and assist with urinary diversions
  - Demonstration of competence in technical nursing assistance, including measuring urine output, collecting urine specimens, assisting with toileting, and catheterizing, to meet the needs of patients experiencing alterations in urinary elimination
  - Ability to adapt technical nursing assistance to meet the needs of patients experiencing problems with urinary elimination

Interpersonal Skills

- Strong people skills to establish trusting relationships with patients experiencing problems with urinary elimination
  - Ability to use therapeutic communication skills to obtain assessment data about a personal and private subject matter
  - Ability to use therapeutic communication skills to meet the needs of patients experiencing a disturbed body image related to urinary elimination problems
  - Ability to mobilize supportive resources to provide needed services, such as for a wife caring for her husband with incontinence at home
  - Ability to work collaboratively with other members of the healthcare team to develop the most appropriate plan of care
  - Demonstration of respect for the patient's human dignity as a key component in the plan of care

Ethical and Legal Skills

- Strong sense of accountability for the health and well-being of patients experiencing urinary problems
- Ability to incorporate knowledge of ethical and legal responsibilities involved with measures to promote urinary elimination
- Adherence to safety when performing nursing interventions to promote and maintain urinary elimination
- Ability to communicate respect to promote the patient's and family's sense of worth
- Ability to serve as a trusted and effective patient advocate
- Ability to consult with other members of the healthcare team to ensure the patient's safety and promote safe, quality care
- Ability to practice in an ethically and legally defensible manner, maintaining the patient's rights
- Commitment to secure the patient's well-being within the bounds of professional responsibilities and scope of practice

Learning Outcomes

After completing the chapter, the learner should be able to accomplish the following:

1. Describe the physiology of the urinary system.
2. Identify variables that influence urination.
3. Assess urinary elimination, using appropriate interview questions and physical assessment skills.
4. Perform the following assessment techniques: measure urine output, collect urine specimens, determine the presence of select abnormal urine constituents, determine urine specific gravity, and assist with diagnostic tests and procedures.
5. Develop nursing diagnoses that correctly identify urinary problems amenable to nursing therapy.
6. Demonstrate how to promote normal urination; facilitate use of the toilet, bedpan, urinal, and commode; perform catheterizations; and assist with urinary diversions.
7. Describe nursing interventions that can be used to manage urinary incontinence effectively.
8. Describe nursing interventions that can prevent the development of urinary tract infections.
9. Plan, implement, and evaluate nursing care related to selected nursing diagnoses associated with urinary problems.

Key Terms

bacteriuria
condom catheter
enuresis
functional incontinence
hematuria
hesitancy
ileal conduit
indwelling urethral catheter
intermittent catheter
Kegel exercises
micturition
mixed incontinence
nephrotoxic
overflow incontinence
postvoid residual (PVR)
specific gravity
stress incontinence
suprapubic catheter
urge incontinence
urinary diversion
urinary incontinence
urinary retention

A properly functioning urinary system is essential to the body's physical well-being, to life itself, and to a person's general sense of well-being. Elimination from the urinary tract helps to rid the body of waste products and materials that exceed bodily needs. Problems involving urinary elimination can be so embarrassing to patients that they may no longer participate in activities outside the home. Nurses assisting a patient with urinary elimination problems or intervening to resolve health problems related to urination need many specialized skills (see the accompanying Reflective Practice box for an example).

This chapter describes the anatomy and physiology of the urinary system and the many factors that affect urination. A practical guide for assessing urinary elimination is included, along with detailed information on specific assessment measures, such as monitoring fluid intake, collecting urine specimens, testing urine, and assisting with other diagnostic procedures. Analysis of urinary assessment data may lead to the identification of one or more nursing diagnoses or, when reported to the physician, to the early detection of a medical problem. When planning care, expected patient outcomes are established for which specific nursing strategies are presented. The concluding patient care study illustrates how the nurse's knowledge of the urinary system and urinary pathology forms the foundation for specific nursing interventions to resolve urinary problems.

ANATOMY AND PHYSIOLOGY

Kidneys and Ureters

The kidneys are located on either side of the vertebral column behind the peritoneum, in the posterior portion of the abdominal cavity. One of the more significant functions of the kidneys is to help maintain the composition and volume of body fluids. About once every 30 minutes, the body's total blood volume passes through the kidneys for waste removal. The kidneys filter and excrete blood constituents that are not needed and retain those that are. Despite varying kinds and amounts of food and fluids ingested, body fluids remain relatively stable if the kidneys are functioning properly. Urine, the waste product excreted by the kidneys, contains organic, inorganic, and liquid wastes.

The nephron is the basic structural and functional unit of the kidneys. There are about 1 million nephrons in each kidney. Nephrons remove the end products of metabolism, such as urea, creatinine, and uric acid, from the blood plasma and form urine. Each nephron consists of a complicated system of arterioles, capillaries, and tubules. The nephrons maintain and regulate fluid balance through the mechanisms of selective reabsorption and secretion.

Once formed, urine from the nephrons empties into the pelvis of each kidney. From each kidney, urine is transported

Reflective Practice
Challenge to Ethical Skills

We had a strange experience during our rotation in a community nursing home. I was assigned to care for Anna Galinski, an 85-year-old frail woman with numerous medical problems. She, like many of the residents, was on a toileting regimen. In the middle of our 7-week experience, a new charge nurse started working on our unit. All of a sudden Anna and the other residents who used to be on toileting regimens were given indwelling catheters. Knowing the greatly increased risk of infections with indwelling catheters, we suspected that the decision to rely on indwelling catheters was more a matter of convenience for the staff than what was in the best interests of the residents. The problem, how do you challenge a charge nurse?

Thinking Outside the Box: Possible Courses of Action

- Don't rock the boat! In 3 weeks we'd be out of there. Keep our mouths shut and don't challenge authority.
- Ask for a meeting with the new charge nurse to explain our concerns, bringing our instructor for support. Be willing to go higher if the charge nurse cannot justify her decision and refuses to respond to our concerns.
- Work around the problem and try to get the residents' families to raise the issue.

Evaluating a Good Outcome: How Do I Define Success?

- Decisions are made about indwelling catheters that benefit and do not harm residents.
- I am faithful to my advocacy responsibilities within the current scope of my practice as a third-year student.
- I learn how to make the healthcare system work for patients/residents.
- I learn how to constructively challenge a physician or colleague.

Personal Learning: Here's to the Future!

This turned into a painful experience that made me realize just how difficult it can be to be an effective advocate for patients and residents. I am also newly aware of just how vulnerable nursing home residents are. A group of four students and myself asked to meet with the charge nurse. When we told her our concerns, she tried to justify her decision, but we still couldn't see any proof that the decision was made to benefit residents. Regrettably, she didn't respond to our concerns about infections at all. Because she was adamant about keeping the catheters, we told her that we would take the matter higher. Ultimately, we had to go all the way to the medical director, after thoroughly researching our concerns and getting lots of support for the argument we were making. In the process, the charge nurse made horrible accusations about us, threatening to ensure that students from our school would never work in this home again. Eventually, all was well that ended well. The charge nurse was "relieved of her administrative responsibilities" and our good names were restored. However, the process that we went through was difficult.

Reflection

How do you think you would respond in a similar situation? Why? What does this tell you about yourself and about the adequacy of your skills for professional practice? Can you think of other ways to respond? Did the nursing students act appropriately? Legally? Ethically? Why or why not? What issues or factors might have played a role in the charge nurse's response? The students' responses? Do you think that the charge nurse would have responded differently if the students had included their instructor in the meeting? What other skills (cognitive, interpersonal, technical, ethical/legal) would you need to respond well in this situation? Do you agree with the criteria to evaluate a successful outcome? Did the nursing student meet the criteria? Please explain your answer.

---

by rhythmic peristalsis through the ureters to the urinary bladder. The ureters enter the bladder obliquely. A fold of membrane in the bladder closes the entrance to the ureters so that urine is not forced up the ureters to the kidneys when pressure exists in the bladder. Figure 43-1 shows the male and female urinary systems and the position of the kidneys and ureters in the abdomen.

Bladder

The urinary bladder is a smooth muscle sac that serves as a reservoir for urine. It is composed of three layers of muscle tissue: the inner longitudinal layer, the middle circular layer, and the outer longitudinal layer. These three layers are called the detrusor muscle. At the base of the bladder, the middle circular layer of muscle tissue forms the internal, or involuntary, sphincter, which guards the opening between the urinary bladder and the urethra. The urethra conveys urine from the bladder to the exterior of the body.

The urinary bladder muscle is innervated by the autonomic nervous system. The sympathetic system carries inhibitory impulses to the bladder and motor impulses to the internal sphincter. These impulses cause the detrusor muscle to relax and the internal sphincter to constrict, retaining urine in the bladder. The parasympathetic system carries motor impulses to the bladder and inhibitory impulses to the internal sphincter. These impulses cause the detrusor muscle to contract and the sphincter to relax. The female and male urinary bladders are shown in Figure 43-1.

The bladder normally contains urine under very little pressure. As the volume of urine increases, the pressure increases only slightly. The bladder wall adapts to pressure, apparently because of the muscle tissue in the bladder. This makes it possible for urine to continue to enter the bladder from the ureters

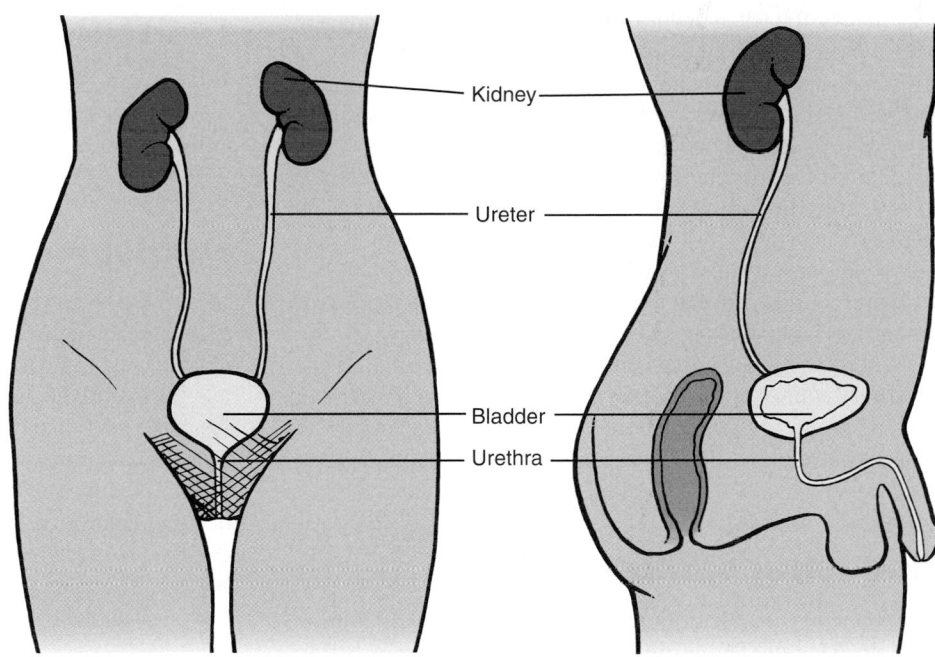

FIGURE 43-1 Frontal view of the female urinary tract *(left)* and lateral view of the male urinary tract *(right)*.

against low pressure. When the pressure becomes sufficient to stimulate nerves, called stretch receptors, in the bladder wall, the person feels a desire to empty the bladder.

Urethra

The urethra's function is to convey urine from the bladder to the exterior of the body. The anatomy of the urethra differs in males and females. The male urethra functions in the excretory system and the reproductive system. It is about 5-½" to 6-¼" (13.7 to 16.2 cm) long and consists of three parts: the prostatic, the membranous, and the cavernous portions (Fig. 43-2). The external urethral sphincter consists of striated muscle and is located just beyond the prostatic portion of the urethra. The external sphincter is under voluntary control.

In contrast, the female urethra is about 1-½" to 2-½" (3.7 to 6.2 cm) long. The external, or voluntary, sphincter is located about in the middle of the urethra. No portion of the female urethra is external to the body, as in the male, although the muscle at the meatus is usually called the external sphincter.

Act of Micturition

The process of emptying the bladder is known as **micturition,** voiding, or urination. The nerve centers for micturition are situated in the brain and the spinal cord. Voiding is largely an involuntary reflex act, but its control can be learned.

When stretch receptors in the bladder are stimulated as the urine collects, the person feels a desire to void. This usually occurs when the bladder fills to about 100 to 200 mL in a child or about 200 to 300 mL in an adult. With micturition, the pressure within the bladder is many times greater than it is during the time the bladder is filling. When micturition is initiated, the detrusor muscle contracts, the internal sphincter relaxes, and

urine enters the posterior urethra. The muscles of the perineum and the external sphincter relax, the muscle of the abdominal wall contracts slightly, the diaphragm lowers, and micturition occurs.

The act of micturition is normally painless. The voluntary control of voiding is limited to initiating, restraining, and interrupting the act.

Restraint of voiding is thought to occur subconsciously when the volume of urine in the bladder is small. If voiding is delayed, however, the bladder continues to fill. Discomfort

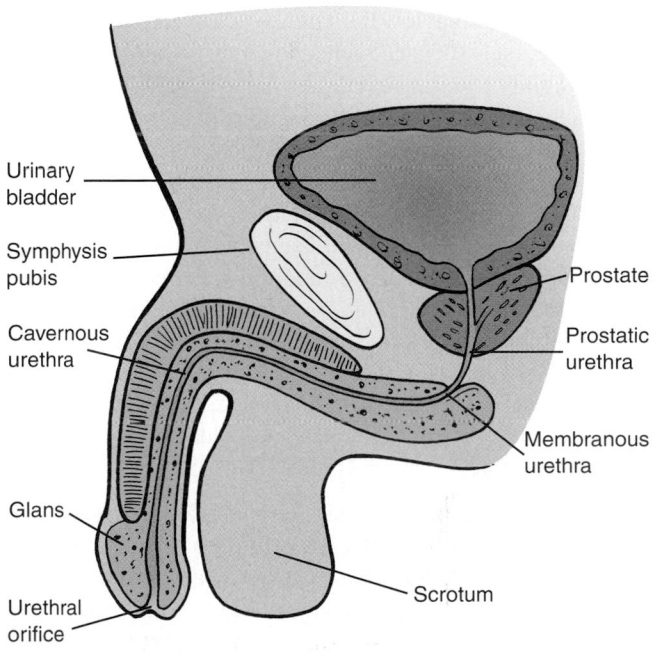

FIGURE 43-2 Parts of the male urethra.

may then be felt when undue distention occurs, and the urgency to void becomes paramount.

Sometimes increased abdominal pressure, such as occurs during coughing and sneezing, forces an involuntary escape of urine, especially in females, because the urethra is shorter. Any involuntary loss of urine that causes such a problem is referred to as **urinary incontinence.** Strong psychological factors, such as marked fear, also may result in involuntary urination. In certain conditions, it may be difficult for a person to relax the restraining muscles sufficiently to void, such as when a shy or embarrassed person needs to give a urine specimen.

When the higher nerve centers develop after infancy, the voluntary control of micturition develops also. Until that time, voiding is purely a reflex action. People whose bladders are no longer controlled by the brain because of injury or disease also void by reflex only. This is called autonomic bladder.

Frequency of Micturition

The frequency of micturition depends on the amount of urine being produced. The more urine produced, the more often voiding is necessary. Except when fluid intake is very large, most healthy people do not void during normal sleeping hours. The first voided urine of the day is usually more concentrated than other urine excreted during the day. Because the first urine of the day is not fresh, but rather an accumulation of a number of hours of kidney output, this urine may or may not be used as a specimen for certain tests.

Some people normally void small amounts at frequent intervals because they habitually respond to the first early urge to void. This habit usually is meaningless and is not necessarily an indication of disease. On the other hand, if this pattern occurs as a change in urination routine, it may indicate illness.

Other people have habits of infrequent voiding. For example, some people go 8 to 12 waking hours or longer without urinating. A habitual low fluid intake or a decrease in the sensation of thirst associated with aging may be one reason. The inaccessibility of toilet facilities owing to travel, work circumstances, or illness, as well as limitations in mobility, can also lead to infrequent urination. People who habitually urinate infrequently develop more urinary tract infections and kidney disorders than those who urinate at least every 3 to 4 hours. The reason for this is believed to be stagnation of urine in the bladder, which serves as a good medium for bacterial growth. Newly occurring infrequent voiding can also indicate a decreased production of urine caused by a kidney or circulatory disorder. **Urinary retention** occurs when urine is produced normally but is not excreted completely from the bladder. Factors associated with urinary retention include medications, an enlarged prostate, or vaginal prolapse.

Think back to Jewel Carson, the postpartum woman who cannot void. The nurse's assessment of a full distended bladder indicates that the patient is producing urine. As a result, the nurse would suspect that Ms. Carson is experiencing urinary retention because she has been unable to void.

FACTORS AFFECTING MICTURITION

Numerous factors affect the amount and quality of urine produced by the body and the manner in which it is excreted.

Developmental Considerations

Infants are born without voluntary control of micturition and with little ability to concentrate urine. An infant's urine is usually very light in color and without odor. At about 6 weeks of age, the infant's nephrons are able to control reabsorption of fluids in the tubules and effectively concentrate urine. Most children develop urinary control between the ages of 2 and 5 years. Daytime control precedes nighttime control, and girls generally develop control earlier than boys. Older children and adults control urination voluntarily. They seldom wake to void at night because their kidneys are able to concentrate urine and produce less urine at night as a result of decreased renal blood flow.

Toilet Training

Most children begin to control urination voluntarily at 18 to 24 months of age. Involuntary urination that occurs after an age when continence should be present is termed **enuresis.** Enuresis is estimated to occur in 40% of 3-year-old children and is not seen as a medical problem until the child reaches 6 years of age (Burns et al., 2000).

Toilet training should not begin until the child is able to:

- Hold urine for 1 to 2 hours
- Recognize the feeling of bladder fullness
- Communicate the need to void and control urination until seated on the toilet

The child's desire to gain control is also important. Wanting to be like a parent or older sibling often provides adequate motivation. Lifelong attitudes toward urination, the body, and cleanliness may develop during the time of toilet training. Even after toilet training has been completed, the child may continue to have nocturnal enuresis (bedwetting). Although humiliating for the older child, nocturnal enuresis is not generally treated medically until after age 6 years.

Cultures approach toilet training differently. In some cultures, toilet training begins before the child is 1 year old; in other cultures, it may not be considered until the child is near 5 years of age. Nurses must recognize cultural influences on this parenting responsibility while promoting flexibility. Parents also need reassurance that any regression of toileting skills that occurs during a child's hospitalization is to be expected and is usually short-lived.

Effects of Aging

Physiologic changes that accompany normal aging may affect urination in older adults. These changes include the following:

- The diminished ability of the kidneys to concentrate urine may result in nocturia.
- Decreased bladder muscle tone may reduce the capacity of the bladder to hold urine, resulting in increased frequency of urination.

- Decreased bladder contractility may lead to urine retention and stasis, which increase the likelihood of urinary tract infection.
- Neuromuscular problems, degenerative joint problems, alterations in thought processes, and weakness may interfere with voluntary control and the ability to reach a toilet in time.

Individuals who view themselves as old, powerless, and neglected may cease to value voluntary control over urination and simply find toileting too much bother no matter what the setting. Incontinence is often the result.

Consider Midori Morita, the wife of a 70-year-old man who has been experiencing urinary problems since his last hospitalization. The nurse would need to keep in mind these age-related changes during assessment to determine if Mrs. Morita's husband was experiencing urinary problems related to these changes or something else.

Food and Fluid Intake

When the body is functioning well, the kidneys help the body maintain a careful balance of fluid intake and output, which should be about equal. When the body is dehydrated, the kidneys reabsorb fluid. The urine produced is more concentrated and is decreased in amount. Conversely, with fluid overload, the kidneys excrete a large quantity of dilute urine.

Caffeine-containing beverages (cola, coffee, and tea) have a diuretic effect and increase urine production. Alcohol produces the same effect by inhibiting the release of antidiuretic hormone. Foods high in water may increase urine production. Foods and beverages with high sodium content cause sodium and water reabsorption and retention, thereby decreasing urine formation. Certain foods may affect the odor of the urine (asparagus, onions) or its color (beets). Promoting Health 43-1 suggests behaviors to maintain healthy urinary elimination patterns.

Psychological Variables

Many individual, family, and sociocultural variables influence a person's normal voiding habits. For some people, voiding is a personal and private act—something one does not talk about. Needing assistance with a bedpan or urinal provokes great embarrassment and anxiety, especially when the bedpan is offered by a nurse of the opposite sex. For others, voiding is a natural act that does not cause embarrassment, and these people readily excuse themselves to void whenever the urge presents.

Many people who experience stress void smaller amounts of urine at more frequent intervals. Stress can also interfere with the ability to relax the perineal muscles and the external urethral sphincter. When this happens, the person may feel an urge to void, but emptying the bladder completely becomes difficult or impossible.

Activity and Muscle Tone

Among the many benefits of regular exercise are increased metabolism and optimal urine production and elimination. During prolonged periods of immobility, decreased bladder and sphincter tone can result in poor urinary control and urinary stasis. People with indwelling urinary catheters lose bladder tone because the bladder muscle is not being stretched by the bladder filling with urine. Other causes of decreased muscle tone include childbearing, muscle atrophy due to decreased estrogen levels as seen with menopause, and damage to muscles from trauma.

Pathologic Conditions

Certain renal or urologic problems can affect both the quantity and the quality of urine produced. Diseases associated with renal problems include congenital urinary tract abnormalities, polycystic kidney disease, urinary tract infection, urinary calculi (kidney stones), hypertension, diabetes mellitus, gout, and certain connective tissue disorders.

Promoting Health 43-1 Urine Elimination

Use the assessment checklist to determine how well you are meeting your need for urine elimination. Then develop a prescription for self-care by choosing appropriate behaviors from the list of suggestions.

ASSESSMENT CHECKLIST

	almost always	sometimes	almost never	
	☐	☐	☐	1. I urinate at regular intervals throughout the day.
	☐	☐	☐	2. I have an adequate fluid intake.
	☐	☐	☐	3. I limit my sodium intake.
	☐	☐	☐	4. My urine volume remains relatively constant.

SELF-CARE BEHAVIORS

1. Maintain a normal voiding pattern and volume.
2. Respond as soon as possible to the urge to void.
3. Drink 8 to 10 glasses of water daily.
4. Avoid foods that contain excess sodium.
5. Monitor use of caffeine, alcohol, or medication schedules that promote voiding and may interfere with sleep.
6. Seek medical assistance for any change in the characteristics of urine or presence of pain on urination.

Diseases that reduce physical activity or lead to generalized weakness, such as arthritis, Parkinson's disease, and degenerative joint disease, may interfere with toileting. Cognitive deficits and certain psychiatric problems can interfere with a person's ability or desire to control urination voluntarily. Fever and diaphoresis (profuse perspiration) result in body fluid conservation by the kidneys. Urine production is decreased, and the urine is highly concentrated. Other pathologic conditions, such as congestive heart failure, may lead to fluid retention and decreased urine output. High blood glucose levels, such as with diabetes mellitus, may lead to an increase in urine output secondary to an osmotic diuretic effect.

Medications

Medications have numerous effects on urine production and elimination. Of gravest concern are the many prescription and nonprescription drugs known to be **nephrotoxic** (capable of causing kidney damage). Abuse of analgesics, such as aspirin or ibuprofen (Advil), can cause nephrotoxicity; some antibiotics, such as gentamicin, can be nephrotoxic.

Diuretics (water pills), which commonly are used in the treatment of hypertension and other disorders, prevent the reabsorption of water and certain electrolytes in the tubules. Depending on their strength, they cause moderate to severe increases in production and excretion of dilute urine. Cholinergic medications stimulate contraction of the detrusor muscle and produce urination. Some analgesics and tranquilizers suppress the central nervous system, interfering with urination by diminishing the effectiveness of the neural reflex.

Certain drugs cause urine to change color, including the following:

- Anticoagulants may cause **hematuria** (blood in the urine) or a red color.
- Diuretics can lighten the color of urine to pale yellow.
- Phenazopyridine (Pyridium), a urinary tract analgesic, can cause orange or orange-red urine.
- The antidepressant amitriptyline (Elavil) or B-complex vitamins can turn urine green or blue-green.
- Levodopa (L-dopa), an antiparkinson drug, and injectable iron compounds can lead to brown or black urine.

THE NURSING PROCESS FOR URINARY ELIMINATION

Assessing

A comprehensive nursing assessment of the functioning of a patient's urinary system includes the following:

- Collection of data about the patient's voiding patterns, habits, and difficulties and a history of current or past urinary problems
- Physical examination of the kidneys, bladder, and urethral meatus; assessment of skin integrity and hydration; and examination of the urine
- Correlation of these findings with the results of diagnostic tests and procedures for examining the urine and the urinary tract

Recall Anna Galinski, the 85-year-old frail woman living in a nursing home. Initially she was placed on a toileting regimen, but now she and other patients on the unit have indwelling catheters. In determining how to respond to the situation, it would be helpful for the nurse to perform a comprehensive assessment of the patient. Doing so would provide information to substantiate whether or not catheter insertion was indicated.

Nursing History

In the initial nursing history, the patient (or caregiver) is questioned about usual voiding habits and any current or past voiding difficulties. Box 43-1 lists some additional terms to use to describe several urinary problems. Use terminology that the patient (or caregiver) understands. Focused Assessment Guide 43-1: Urinary Elimination lists elements of a urinary elimination history to be incorporated into the initial nursing assessment.

With infants and young children, assess whether the child has achieved bladder control during both day and nighttime. Be sure to indicate on the nursing history and plan the words that the child uses to indicate the need to void.

With older adults, decreased bladder tone may be a problem. Note on the nursing history any problems, how the per-

---

BOX 43-1 Additional Terms Used to Describe Urinary Problems

Anuria: Technically, no urine voided; 24-hour urine output is less than 100 mL; synonyms are complete *kidney shutdown or renal failure*

Dysuria: Difficulty in voiding; may or may not be associated with pain; a feeling of warm local irritation occurring during voiding is called *burning*

Frequency: Increased incidence of voiding

Glycosuria: Presence of sugar in the urine; if due to an unusually large intake of sugar or to marked emotional disturbances and is temporary, there is little cause for alarm

Nocturia: Frequency of urination during the night

Oliguria: Scanty or greatly diminished amount of urine voided in a given time; 24-hour urine output is 100 to 400 mL

Orthostatic albuminuria: Presence of albumin in urine that is voided after periods of standing, walking, or running; phenomenon of the circulatory system and not necessarily a symptom of kidney disorders

Pneumaturia: Passage of urine containing gas

Polyuria: Excessive output of urine (diuresis)

Proteinuria: Albumin in the urine; indication of kidney disease

Pyuria: Pus in the urine; urine appears cloudy

Suppression: Stoppage of urine production; normally the adult kidneys produce urine continuously at the rate of 60 to 120 mL/h

Urgency: Strong desire to void

Focused Assessment Guide 43-1

Urinary Elimination

Factors to Assess	Questions and Approaches
Usual patterns of urinary elimination	How often do you urinate (pass your water) during the day? Do you awaken at night to empty your bladder? How would you describe your urine?
Recent changes in urinary elimination	Have you noticed any changes in your usual voiding patterns (frequency, amount, force of stream, difficulty, comfort)? Do you ever leak urine (eg, on your way to the bathroom or when you sneeze or cough)? Do you ever notice that your undergarments are wet or damp?
Aids to elimination	Is there anything you do that helps you to urinate?
Present or past occurrence of voiding difficulties (nature of problem, onset, frequency, causes, severity, symptoms, intervention attempted, and results)	Tell me about any problems you are having now when you urinate (urgency, pain or burning, difficulty starting or stopping stream, dribbling, incontinence). If there is a problem, describe what you feel like before you urinate and while you are urinating. Have you had any urinary problems in the past (any history or urinary tract infections, kidney or bladder disease or problems)? Do you use any type of absorbent pad or product to protect your clothes?
Presence of artificial orifices (normal routine, history of problems)	Tell me about your usual routine with your ureterostomy.

son normally handles these problems, and your judgment of the adequacy of the solution.

People with limited or no bladder control and those with urinary diversions usually have well-established routines for emptying the bladder. **Urinary diversions** involve the surgical creation of an alternate route for excretion of urine and are discussed later in the chapter. Assess the procedures and equipment used by patients to make sure they follow accepted guidelines and do not predispose themselves to infection or other risk. Record in both the history and the nursing plan of care any special routine, equipment, or supplies the patient uses for urinary elimination.

When a patient (or caregiver) reports a problem with voiding, explore its duration, severity, and precipitating factors. Also note the patient's perception of the problem and the adequacy of the patient's self-care behaviors.

Remember Midori Morita, the wife of the 70-year-old man experiencing problems with dribbling. The nurse would need to question Mrs. Morita about the problem, obtaining specific information such as when it started, how often it occurs, how much the patient is voiding, events of the previous hospitalization, and any factors associated with it, such as use of medications, increased fluid intake, or changes in mobility.

Physical Assessment

The physical assessment of urinary functioning includes an examination of the kidneys, urinary bladder, urethral meatus, skin, and urine.

Kidneys

The kidneys are normally well protected by considerable fat and connective tissue and are difficult to palpate. The right kidney is at the level of the 12th rib, lower than the left kidney. The right kidney can sometimes be palpated if it is pushed down by the diaphragm when the patient inhales. Standing to the right of the supine patient, place the left hand under the patient's flank while the right hand palpates the abdominal wall. This technique requires deep palpation and should be practiced only under supervision. The left kidney is palpated similarly. The contour and size of the kidneys are noted along with any lumps or complaints of tenderness.

The examination of the kidneys includes checking for costovertebral tenderness. The costovertebral angle is formed by the 12th rib and the spine. Place one palm flat over the costovertebral angle and strike the back of this hand with the other fist. When the kidneys are inflamed, the patient feels pain when this angle is percussed. If the patient complained of pain on palpation, avoid striking too strongly when assessing the costovertebral angle.

Bladder

The bladder is normally positioned below the symphysis pubis and cannot be palpated or percussed when empty. When the bladder is distended, it rises above the symphysis pubis and may reach to just below the umbilicus (Fig. 43-3). Before palpating the bladder, always ask the patient when he or she voided last. Then observe the lower abdominal wall, noting any swelling, and palpate this area for tenderness, also noting the smoothness and roundness of the bladder. The height of the edge of the bladder above the symphysis pubis may be measured, and the bladder may also be percussed. A full bladder produces a dull sound.

A bedside scanner is another way to assess the bladder. The scanner is a small, handheld ultrasound scanner that estimates the amount of urine in the bladder, thus giving a more exact measurement than traditional percussion methods. This method is noninvasive and not painful.

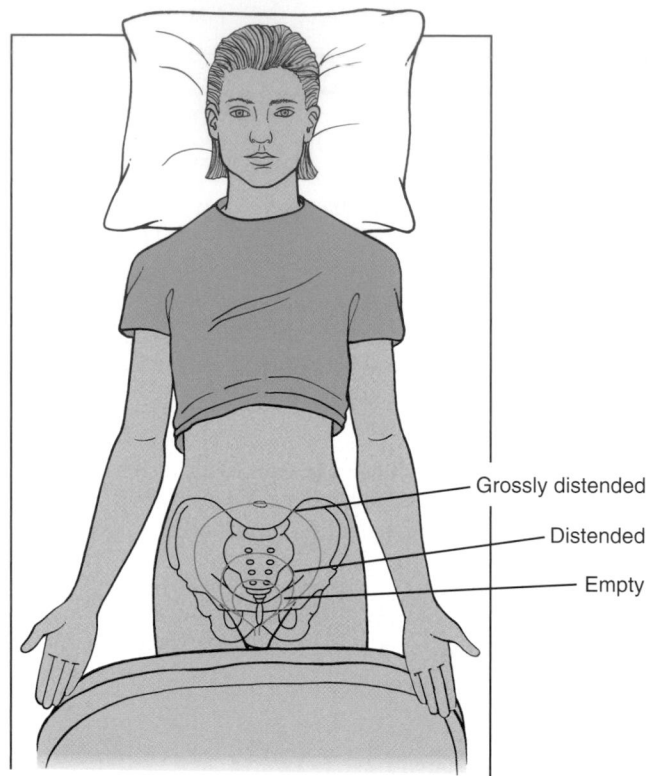

— Grossly distended

— Distended

— Empty

FIGURE 43-3 Position of bladder when empty and distended.

Urethral Orifice

Inspect the urethral orifice for any signs of inflammation, discharge, or foul odor. In females, the urethral meatus is a pink, slitlike opening below the clitoris and above the vaginal orifice. Place female patients in the dorsal recumbent position with the inner labia retracted for good visualization of the meatus. In males, the meatus is at the tip of the penis. If the male patient is uncircumcised, retract the foreskin to visualize the meatus.

Skin Integrity and Hydration

Because problems with urinary functioning may result in disturbances in hydration and excretion of body wastes, assess the skin carefully for color, texture, turgor, and the excretion of any wastes. Also assess the integrity of the skin in the perineal area. Problems with incontinence may result in severe excoriation.

> *Inspecting the perineal area would be extremely important when assessing the husband of Ida Fleming, the woman described at the beginning of the chapter. Mrs. Fleming has reported that her husband constantly dribbles and soils the bed linens, and this places the patient at risk for skin breakdown.*

Urine

Assess the patient's urine for color, odor, clarity, and the presence of any sediment. Note any abnormalities. In select patients, the pH and specific gravity of the urine are monitored and the urine is checked for abnormal constituents such as pro-

tein, blood, glucose, ketone bodies, and bacteria. The normal characteristics of urine are detailed in Table 43-1.

Assessment Techniques

In addition to the nursing history and physical examination, the nurse gathers data about urinary elimination through the following assessment measures: measuring urine output, collecting urine specimens, determining the presence of abnormal constituents in the urine, and assisting with diagnostic procedures. These are discussed in the following sections.

Measuring Urine Output

Measuring the patient's intake and output is an important nursing responsibility. Accuracy of the total fluid intake and output from all sources is essential for planning the patient's nursing and medical care. The measurement of intake and output is described further in Chapter 46. Gloves are required when handling urine to prevent exposure to pathogenic microorganisms or blood that may be present in the urine. Goggles also are worn whenever there is a concern of urine splashing.

The Patient Who is Voiding

The procedure for measuring the urine output of a patient who is voiding is as follows:

1. Ask the patient to void into a bedpan, urinal, or specimen hat, either in bed or in the bathroom. Urinary devices used to collect or measure urine are shown in Figure 43-4.
2. Pour the urine from the collection device into the appropriate measuring device provided by the agency. The devices are calibrated in milliliters.
3. Place the calibrated container on a flat surface, such as a shelf, for an accurate reading. Reading at eye level, note the amount of urine voided and record it on the appropriate form. Figure 43-5 shows a form commonly used for recording urine output. The form is usually kept at the patient's bedside. The total amount voided during each shift and 24-hour period is recorded on the patient's permanent record.
4. Discard the urine in the toilet unless a specimen is required. If a specimen is required, pour the urine into an appropriate specimen container.

To ensure that all urine voided is measured, be sure to tell ambulatory patients when their urine output is to be measured and recorded. A specimen hat is a valuable device that can be placed under the toilet seat to collect and measure voided urine for ambulatory patients (see Fig. 43-4). Patients who are willing and able can be taught to measure and record their own output.

The Patient With an Indwelling Catheter

For patients with an indwelling catheter, the procedure for measuring urine output is as follows:

1. Put on clean gloves.
2. Place a calibrated measuring device beneath the collection bag at the bedside.

TABLE 43-1 **Characteristics of Urine**

Characteristic	Normal Findings	Special Considerations
Color	A freshly voided specimen is pale yellow, straw-colored, or amber, depending on its concentration.	Urine is darker than normal when it is scanty and concentrated. Urine is lighter than normal when it is excessive and diluted. Certain drugs, such as cascara, L-dopa, and sulfonamides, alter the color of urine.
Odor	Normal urine smell is aromatic. As urine stands, it often develops an ammonia odor because of bacterial action.	Some foods cause urine to have a characteristic odor; for example, asparagus causes urine to have a strong, musty odor. Urine high in glucose content has a sweet odor. Urine that is heavily infected has a fetid odor.
Turbidity	Fresh urine should be clear or translucent; as urine stands and cools, it becomes cloudy.	Cloudiness observed in freshly voided urine is abnormal and may be due to the presence of red blood cells, white blood cells, bacteria, vaginal discharge, sperm, or prostatic fluid.
pH	The normal pH is about 6.0, with a range of 4.6 to 8. (Urine alkalinity or acidity may be promoted through diet to inhibit bacterial growth or urinary stone development or to facilitate the therapeutic activity of certain medications.) Urine becomes alkaline on standing when carbon dioxide diffuses into the air.	A high-protein diet causes urine to become excessively acid. Certain foods tend to produce alkaline urine, such as citrus fruits, dairy products, and vegetables, especially legumes. Certain foods tend to produce acidic urine, for example, meat and cranberry juice. Certain drugs influence the acidity or alkalinity of urine; for example, ammonium chloride produces acidic urine, and potassium citrate and sodium bicarbonate produce alkaline urine.
Specific gravity	This is a measure of the concentration of dissolved solids in the urine. The normal range is 1.010 to 1.025.	Concentrated urine will have a higher than normal specific gravity, and diluted urine will have a lower than normal specific gravity. In the absence of kidney disease, a high specific gravity usually indicates dehydration and a low specific gravity indicates overhydration.
Constituents	*Organic* constituents of urine include urea, uric acid, creatinine, hippuric acid, indican, urene pigments, and undetermined nitrogen. *Inorganic* constituents are ammonia, sodium, chloride, traces of iron, phosphorus, sulfur, potassium, and calcium.	*Abnormal constituents* of urine include blood, pus, albumin, glucose, ketone bodies, casts, gross bacteria, and bile.

3. Place the drainage spout from the collection bag above, but not touching, the calibrated measuring device, and open the clamp.
4. Allow the urine to flow from the collection bag into the measuring device.
5. Reclamp the drainage tube, wipe the spout of the tube with an alcohol pad, and replace the tube into the slot on the drainage bag. Then proceed with measurement as described above.

To prevent the spread of infection, each patient should have his or her own calibrated measuring device.

Catheterized patients who are acutely ill may require hourly measurements of urine. This is facilitated by using a special collection bag that has a built-in calibrated measuring chamber called a urimeter. After assessing and recording the amount of urine produced hourly, tilt the measuring chamber so that this urine flows into the general collection bag. This empties the measuring chamber, making it ready to collect the next hour's urine.

Collecting Urine Specimens

Nurses have specific responsibilities for diagnostic tests pertaining to urinary elimination. They routinely collect clean and sterile urine specimens, measure the specific gravity of urine, and assess urine for abnormal constituents.

Routine Urinalysis

The collection of urine specimens for urinalysis is a nursing responsibility. A sterile urine specimen is not required for a routine urinalysis. Urine is collected by having the patient void into a clean bedpan, urinal, or receptacle such as a specimen hat in the toilet bowl. Care is taken to avoid contamination with feces. If a woman is menstruating when a urine sample is obtained, note this on the laboratory slip, because red blood cells may appear in the urine. When patients are voiding into a

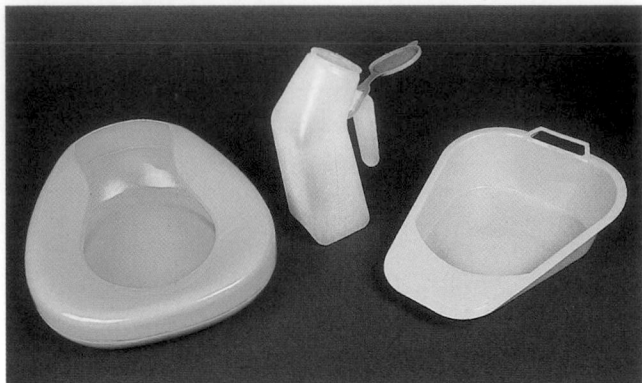

Bedpan and fracture pan: containers used to collect urine from nonambulatory patients.
Urinal: container used to collect urine from nonambulatory male patients.

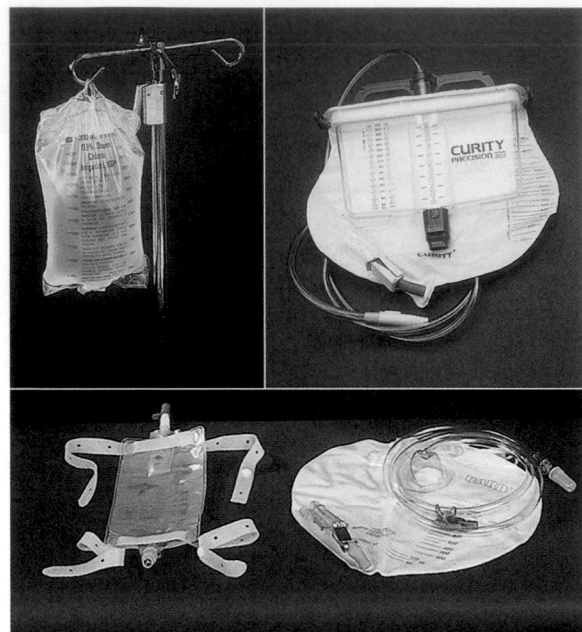

Bladder irrigation fluid for continuous bladder irrigation.
Large urine collection bag with urometer for use with patients who have indwelling urinary catheters and require frequent urine output measurements, such as hourly.
Small urine collection bag, commonly called a leg bag, for use by ambulatory patients who have an indwelling urinary catheter.
Large urine collection bag.

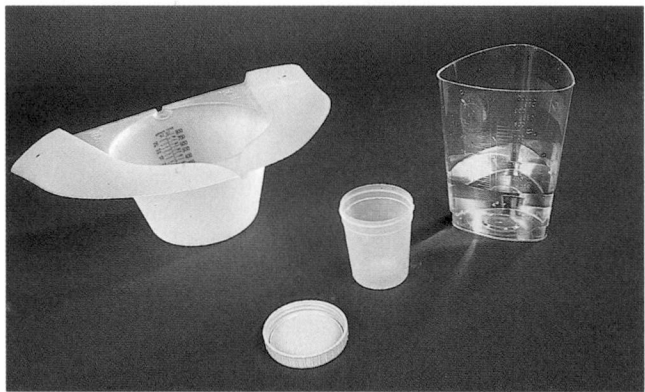

Specimen hat: container that is placed anteriorly on the toilet, underneath the seat. Used to collect urine.
Specimen cup: container that holds urine.
Calibrated measuring device: makes possible the recording of an accurate urine output.

FIGURE 43-4 Devices for collecting and measuring urine.

bedpan or collection device on the toilet, instruct them not to place toilet tissue into the urine because this makes analysis more difficult. Using aseptic technique, pour the urine into an appropriate container; label it with the patient's name, date, and time of collection; package it appropriately; and send it to the laboratory for examination. Do not leave urine standing at room temperature for a long period before sending it to the laboratory because this may alter both the appearance and chemistry of the urine.

Specimens From Infants and Children. Plastic disposable collection bags are available for infants and young children who have not achieved voluntary bladder control (Fig. 43-6). Follow the manufacturer's instructions and take care when applying and removing the bag to avoid irritating the sensitive perineal skin.

Clean-Catch or Midstream Specimen. A clean-catch specimen of urine is required in some situations. Most health agencies specify that a clean-catch specimen be collected during midstream. This means that the patient voids a small amount of urine, which is discarded; then the specimen is collected during midstream in a sterile specimen container, with the last amount of urine in the bladder also being discarded.

The first small amount of urine voided helps to flush away any organisms near the meatus because the urinalysis findings may be inaccurate if these organisms enter the specimen. Additionally, it is generally thought that urine voided at midstream is most characteristic of the urine the body is producing. A clean-catch midstream specimen from a male is considered sterile. If a sterile specimen is needed from a female patient, the patient may be catheterized. (Catheterization is discussed later in this chapter.)

A patient who can carry out the technique properly may collect his or her own clean-catch midstream urine specimen and often prefers to do so. The nurse provides the appropriate equipment and instructions for the procedure. Refer to Guidelines for Nursing Care 43-1: Obtaining a Clean-Catch or Midstream Urine Specimen for the steps.

Sterile Specimen From an Indwelling Catheter. Sterile urine specimens may be obtained by catheterizing the patient's bladder (see Skills 43-2 and 43-3 later in this chapter) or by taking the specimen from an indwelling catheter already in place.

When it is necessary to collect a urine specimen from a patient with an indwelling catheter, always obtain it from the catheter itself using the special port for specimens. A specimen

Intake and Output Chart

7:00 AM _11-18-06_ to 7:00 AM _11-19-06_

		I.V.		Blood	Other	Comments	Urine	Stool	Gastric tube	Drainage tubes		Vomitus	Other	Comments
	Oral													
7-8	250					Force fluids to 1100cc/shift	300							
8-9														
9-10	120													
10-11	60													
11-12	100						250							
12-1	300													
1-2	240													
2-3	100						200							
8 hr Tot	1170						750							voiding s discomfort
3-4														
4-5														
5-6														
6-7														
7-8														
8-9														
9-10														
10-11														
8 hr Tot														
11-12														
12-1														
1-2														
2-3														
3-4														
4-5														
5-6														
6-7														
8 hr Tot														
24 hr Tot														
Total intake							**Total output**							

FIGURE 43-5 An example of a form commonly used for recording intake and output.

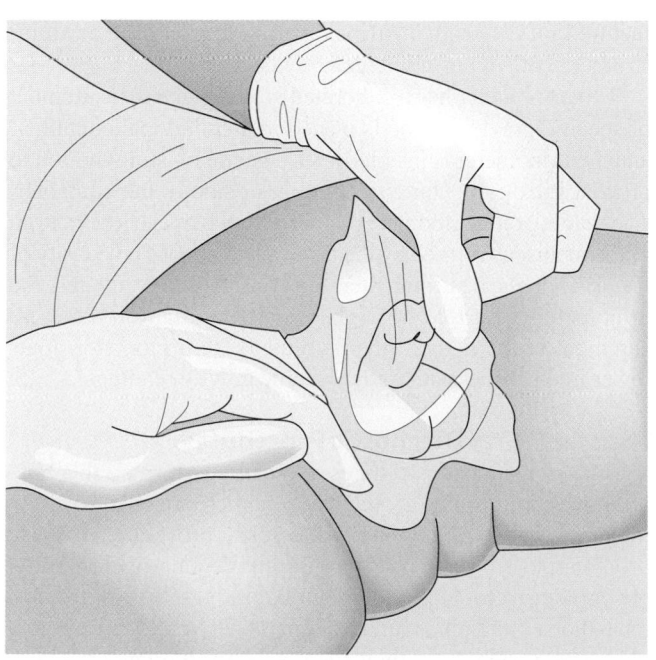

FIGURE 43-6 Disposable plastic urine collection device for infants.

from the collecting receptacle (drainage bag) may not be fresh urine and could result in an inaccurate analysis. Sterile technique also must be observed.

The size of the syringe for the specimen depends on the specific laboratory test. A urine culture requires about 3 mL, whereas routine urinalysis requires at least 10 mL of urine. A sterile 21- to 25-gauge needle, an antiseptic swab, a specimen container, and possibly a clamp are required. Wearing gloves protects the nurse from any contact with the specimen.

If urine is not present in the tube, clamp the tube below the collection port briefly (not to exceed 30 minutes) to allow urine to accumulate. Most catheters have a self-sealing area designed for a needle puncture. Clean the entry port with an antiseptic swab, and carefully insert the sterile needle into the catheter (Fig. 43-7). Aspirate urine into the syringe, remove the syringe, release the clamp if one was used, and transfer the specimen into the appropriate container. Place the uncapped needle and syringe in the sharps container. Then package and transport the specimen according to agency policy. It is unsafe to puncture a Silastic or plastic catheter because leakage will probably occur.

Guidelines for Nursing Care 43-1
Obtaining a Clean-Catch or Midstream Urine Specimen

Female
- Wear clean gloves.
- Clean the area at the meatus with soap and water.
- Have patient void about 30 mL, and discard this urine.
- Position the sterile specimen container near, but not touching, the meatus, and ask the patient to void forcibly if she is lying down to prevent urine from dribbling across the perineum.
- Stop collecting urine before the patient empties the bladder. Allow patient to continue voiding into a bedpan or the commode and discard this urine.
- Use a sterilized bedpan to collect the midstream specimen if the patient has difficulty voiding into the container, and then transfer the urine into the sterile specimen container.
- Label the specimen container, package it appropriately, and send the specimen to the laboratory.

Male
- Wear clean gloves.
- Retract the foreskin to expose the glans penis in the uncircumcised male patient.
- Clean the area of the external meatus with soap and water.
- Have the patient void about 30 mL, and discard this urine.
- Have the patient void directly into the sterile container.
- Stop collecting urine before the patient empties his bladder. Allow the patient to void the remaining urine in his bladder and discard it.
- Return the foreskin to its normal position in an uncircumcised patient to prevent swelling and irritation of the glans penis.
- Use a sterile urinal to collect the midstream specimen if the patient has difficulty voiding into the container, and then transfer the urine into the sterile specimen container.
- Label the specimen container appropriately, and send the specimen to the laboratory.

24-Hour Urine Specimens. For some laboratory studies, 24-hour specimens are required. The patient and the entire nursing team must understand the importance of collecting all the urine voided in a 24-hour period. A sign posted on the patient's bathroom door is a helpful reminder not to discard urine. The collection is initiated at a specific time (which is recorded) by asking the patient to empty his or her bladder. This urine is discarded. All urine voided for the next 24 hours is collected. At the end of the 24 hours, the patient is asked to void. This urine is added to the previously collected urine, and then the entire specimen is sent to the laboratory.

Depending on the type of examination, the urine from each voiding may be kept in a separately marked container and the time of each voiding recorded, or all urine voided may be collected in a common receptacle. The laboratory usually specifies whether a preservative is used to retard decomposition and whether the specimen is to be refrigerated or kept on ice. In some situations, the patient may be required to collect the specimen at home. Many laboratories have a transport service that picks up specimens from a patient's home and returns them to the laboratory within the appropriate time frame.

Determining Abnormal Constituents in the Urine

In some situations the nurse may perform tests on urine specimens, especially when specimens are being tested repeatedly for known abnormalities, when screening tests are being used, or when laboratory facilities are not readily available. For example, a nurse may test urine for the presence of glucose, protein, bilirubin, bacteria, and blood. The results of the test are recorded on the patient's record. Many commercially prepared diagnostic kits are available for such tests and can be used in the home or the healthcare facility. Although these tests are economical and fast, laboratory analysis is recommended when precise results are needed.

Most commercially prepared diagnostic kits contain all needed equipment and the appropriate reagent, a substance used in a chemical reaction to detect another substance. Reagents are available as tablets, fluids, impregnated paper, and plastic strips with a special coating. When the reagent contacts the urine, a chemical reaction occurs, causing a color change. This color is then compared with an accompanying chart that describes the significance of the color.

The precise directions for the amount of the specimen, the time allowed for the chemical reaction, and the interpretation of the color vary with the manufacturer. Therefore, it is important to follow the directions accompanying the diagnostic kit exactly.

Determining Specific Gravity

The **specific gravity** of urine can be determined with manufactured plastic reagent strips (as described above) or an instrument called a urinometer or hydrometer.

The urinometer has a calibrated scale for the measurement of specific gravity. Urine is placed in a cylindrical container, and the urinometer is inserted with a gentle twisting motion to prevent it from touching the bottom or side of the container. The reading on a urinometer is made at eye level at the bottom of the meniscus formed by the urine (Fig. 43-8). The density of the urine floats the urinometer. If the urine is concentrated, the urinometer is buoyed up high, registering high on the measurement scale. If the urine is diluted, the urinometer floats lower in the urine, with a low specific gravity reading.

Assisting With Diagnostic Procedures

Various diagnostic procedures, typically performed in a hospital operating room or outpatient facility, are used to study the urinary system. Common diagnostic procedures include urodynamic studies, cystoscopy, intravenous pyelography, retrograde pyelography, computed tomography (CT) scans, renal biopsy, and ultrasound examination. Nurses are responsible for preparing the patient and giving appropriate aftercare.

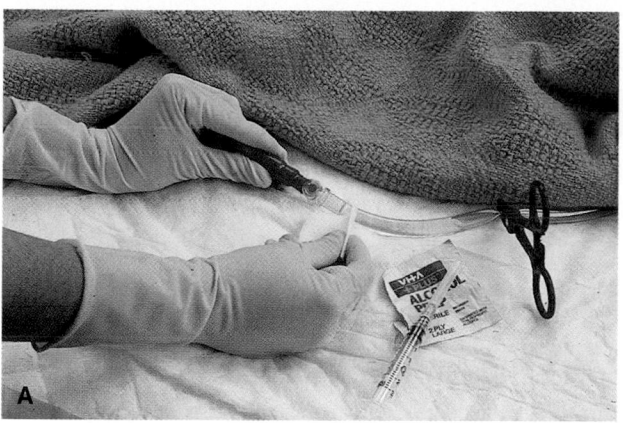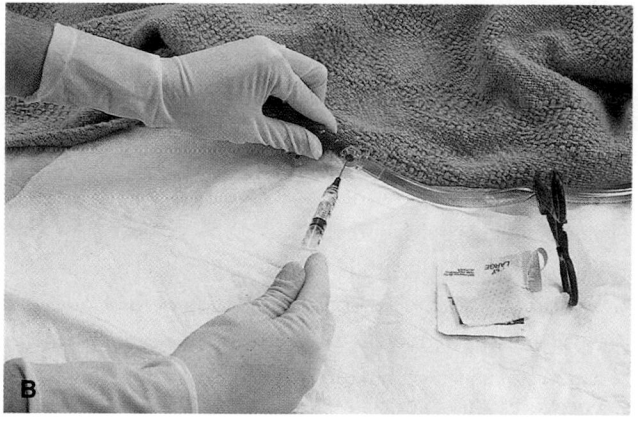

FIGURE 43-7 Obtaining a urine specimen from a patient with an indwelling catheter. (**A**) First, use a swab moistened with an antiseptic to clean the area where the sterile needle will be introduced. (**B**) Then insert the needle and withdraw a specimen of urine. Standard precautions require that gloves be used when contact with urine is probable.   (Photos © B. Proud.)

Explaining the procedure helps reduce the patient's anxieties. The preparation and aftercare of the patient for each of these procedures are described in Table 43-2.

Diagnosing

The data collected about the patient's urinary functioning may lead to one or more nursing diagnoses. Some data are appropriately reported to the physician and may contribute to the physician's identification of a medical diagnosis. Nurses must identify significant urinary findings, record these appropriately, and report them to the proper people.

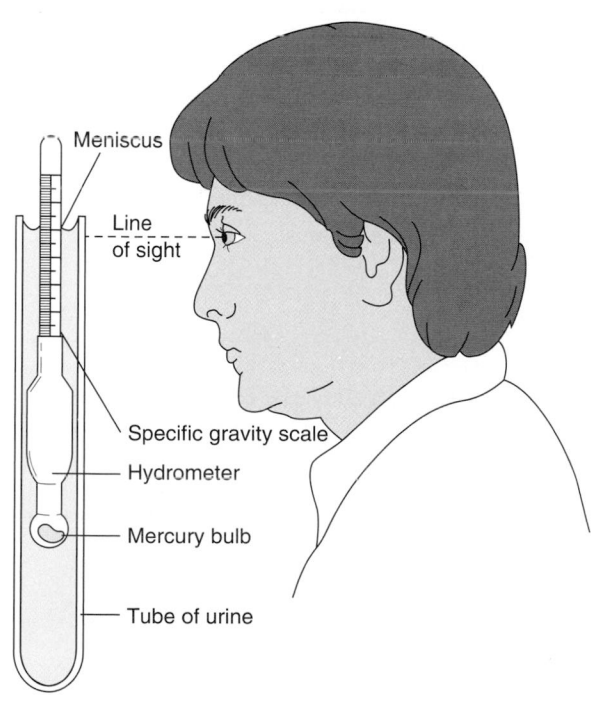

FIGURE 43-8 To determine specific gravity, read the urinometer at eye level at the base of the meniscus formed by the urine.

Urinary Functioning as the Problem

Nursing diagnoses that specifically address problems in urinary functioning include problems of incontinence, pattern alteration, and urinary retention. Sample defining characteristics for these diagnoses appear in the box Examples of NANDA Nursing Diagnoses: Urinary Elimination.

Urinary Functioning as the Etiology

Difficulty with urination or changes in normal voiding patterns may affect other areas of human functioning. Examples of nursing diagnoses related to urinary problems include the following:

- Anxiety related to incontinence, diagnostic procedures
- Caregiver Role Strain related to incontinence of family member
- Risk for Infection related to indwelling urinary catheter
- Impaired Skin Integrity (Actual, Risk for) related to incontinence
- Deficient Knowledge related to any existing or new urinary disease or disorder, lack of information about personal hygiene
- Noncompliance With Medication Regimen related to misunderstanding the need to finish all doses of medication for urinary tract infection
- Acute Pain related to bladder spasms, dysuria, urinary retention, cancer of the bladder, diagnostic procedures
- Low Self-Esteem related to urinary incontinence, urinary diversion
- Sexual Dysfunction related to urinary incontinence, urinary diversion
- Disturbed Sleep Pattern related to nocturia
- Toileting Self-Care Deficit related to parent's lack of knowledge or motivation to toilet train child, neuromuscular impairment or musculoskeletal disorders, immobility, trauma or surgical procedures, confusion, disorientation

The nurse's challenge is to identify human responses to alterations in urinary elimination that pose specific health problems for the patient and family.

(*text continues on page 1304*)

TABLE 43-2 Common Diagnostic Procedures Used to Study the Urinary Tract

Preparation	Aftercare
Urodynamic Studies: A group of tests that measure how urine flows, is stored, and is eliminated in the lower urinary tract	
Usually no fluid or food restrictions are necessary before the test.	Drink 8 to 10 glasses of water in the 24 hours after the test.
Bladder should be full before the test.	Teach patient the signs and symptoms of a urinary tract infection.
Patient is informed that a catheter will be inserted during the test.	
Cystoscopy: The direct visual examination of the bladder, ureteral orifices, and urethra with a cystoscope	
The patient is allowed liquids on the morning of the examination.	Know that tissue swelling, dysuria, and hematuria may occur owing to trauma from the procedure.
Sedation and analgesics are usually prescribed before the procedure.	Encourage a generous fluid intake, and observe and measure urine output for at least 24 hours.
A signed consent form is required for the procedure.	Observe the patient for urinary retention and for signs of infection; nosocomial infection after a cystoscopy is common.
The procedure is ordinarily painless.	
Intravenous Pyelography (excretory urography): The radiographic examination of the kidney and ureter after a contrast material is injected intravenously	
Fluids and food are withheld or limited prior to testing. Patient's allergy history is obtained focusing on sensitivity to iodine, shellfish, or seafood (contrast may contain iodine). Elderly, debilitated, or young patients may not tolerate this dehydration, and compromises may need to be made.	Fluids and food may be given immediately after the examination.
A laxative the evening before the examination and an enema the morning of the examination are given so that stool and gas do not interfere with visualization.	Observe the patient for signs of a reaction to the contrast material, such as a rash, nausea, and hives. Contrast may initiate acute renal failure. Monitor intake and output.
The patient should void before the examination.	
Retrograde Pyelography: The radiographic examination of the kidney and ureters after a contrast material is injected into the renal pelvis through the ureter	
No fluids or food are given after midnight before the examination.	Foods and fluids may be given, but if anesthesia has been used, this is delayed for several hours.
A laxative the evening before the examination and an enema the morning of the examination are given so that stool and gas do not interfere with visualization.	Check the vital signs regularly if anesthesia has been used.
The patient should void before the examination.	Observe the patient for signs of a reaction to the contrast material, such as a rash, nausea, and hives.
A signed consent form is recommended for the procedure.	Be aware that ureteral catheters may be in place and should be connected to drainage receptacles so that the amount and character of drainage from each catheter can be noted.
Ultrasonography: A noninvasive procedure that involves the use of ultrasound to produce an image or photograph of an organ or tissue	
A signed consent form is required.	Know that no special care is required after the test.
Food and fluids are restricted for 8–12 hours before an abdominal ultrasound.	Inform patient that results are usually available 1–2 days after the study.
The patient should not smoke or chew gum before the procedure to prevent swallowing air.	
The procedure is painless.	
Computed Tomography (CT Scanning): A noninvasive radiographic procedure whereby a body part can be scanned from different angles with an x-ray beam and a computer that calculates varying tissue densities and records a cross-sectional image on paper	
A consent form should be signed.	Observe for a delayed reaction to the contrast dye (skin rash, urticaria, headache, vomiting). An oral antihistamine may be given for mild reactions.
The patient is usually NPO for 8 hours before the test if a contrast dye is used.	Be supportive to patient and family. Test can be frightening.
Obtain patient's history of any allergic reaction or hypersensitivity to shellfish, iodine, or any contrast dyes (contrast may contain iodine).	Instruct patient to resume usual diet and activity unless otherwise indicated.
All metal objects need to be removed before the test.	
Medications may usually be taken until 2 hours before the test.	*(continued)*

TABLE 43-2 (Continued)

Preparation	Aftercare
Renal Biopsy: Invasive procedure that involves obtaining a small piece of renal tissue for microscopic examination. Tissue sample may be obtained by needle and syringe through a skin puncture or small incision, during an open surgical procedure during which a wedge of tissue is removed, or through a cystoscope during which a brush is used to obtain a tissue fragment.	
Coagulation studies and hematocrit must be obtained.	Instruct patient to lie quietly for 4 hours.
Baseline vital signs must be obtained.	Monitor urine for hematuria during the first 24 hours. Collect each voided specimen in a separate cup labeled with the time.
Food and fluid are withheld before the procedure.	
A signed consent form is required.	Monitor vital signs and dressing for any indication of shock or bleeding.
Sedation may be necessary, depending on the type of procedure.	Instruct patient to avoid strenuous activities or heavy lifting for several days and to report any flank pain, hematuria, or dizziness.

Examples of NANDA Nursing Diagnoses | Urinary Elimination

Nursing Diagnoses	Related Factors	Sample Defining Characteristics
Impaired Urinary Elimination	Dysuria Urinary tract infection	Small bladder capacity, less than 300 mL "It hurts when I pass my water." Urinalysis reveals hematuria and proteinuria.
Functional Urinary Incontinence	Altered environment Sensory, cognitive, or mobility deficits	"I don't know why Johnny started wetting since he's been hospitalized. He has been toilet trained for 6 months now." "When I remember to take mother to the toilet she urinates fine. But if I don't remember, I find her wet."
Reflex Urinary Incontinence	Neurologic impairment	Patient with spinal cord lesion reports no awareness of bladder filling, no urge to void or feelings of bladder fullness, involuntary loss of urine at somewhat regular intervals.
Stress Urinary Incontinence	Age-related degenerative changes High intra-abdominal pressure Incompetent bladder outlet Overdistention between voidings Weak pelvic muscles and structural supports	Obese mother of four reports involuntary dribbling of urine with coughs, sneezes, hearty laughter. Patient "too busy to void" during day reports involuntary leakage of urine with sudden movement, cough, and so on.
Total Urinary Incontinence	Neurologic impairment Trauma or disease affecting spinal cord nerves	Constant flow of urine at unpredictable times without distention or uninhibited bladder contractions Nocturia
Urge Urinary Incontinence	Decreased bladder capacity Bladder spasms Increased intake of caffeine or alcohol Increased urine concentration Overdistention of bladder	"I can never make it to the bathroom in time." Urgency, frequency, nocturia, bladder contracture or spasm
Urinary Retention	High urethral pressure caused by weak detrusor Inhibition of reflex arc Strong sphincter Blockage	Elderly man diagnosed with benign prostatic hypertrophy complains of inability to urinate despite feeling bladder is full. Woman 6 hours after delivery has had no urine output since labor; 800 mL IV fluids infused; fundus of uterus is displaced to the right by a full bladder.

Outcome Identification and Planning

When the patient is ambulatory and not experiencing difficulties with the urinary system, normal voiding is usually not a problem. Trauma or illness, however, may result in the patient's need for nursing assistance with voiding. Nursing interventions should support planned patient goals. The patient will achieve the following:

• Produce urine output about equal to fluid intake
• Maintain fluid and electrolyte balance
• Empty the bladder completely at regular intervals
• Report ease of voiding
• Maintain skin integrity

Implementing

Any alteration in urinary elimination invariably invokes anxiety and fear in people. Nursing interventions focus on maintaining and promoting normal urinary patterns regardless of the healthcare setting, improving or controlling urinary incontinence, preventing potential problems associated with bladder catheterization, and assisting with care of urinary diversions. Nurses can assist the patient and family to achieve desirable outcomes for their urination needs.

> *Think back to Anna Galinski, the frail woman in a nursing home. The toileting program focused on maintaining and promoting the patient's normal urinary patterns. However, now that the patient has an indwelling catheter, the nurse needs to focus on preventing problems associated with catheterization. Weighing the risks and benefits of catheterization for this patient would be crucial.*

Promoting Normal Urination
Maintaining Normal Voiding Habits

If the patient's voiding habits are adequate, the nurse provides care or teaches the patient to maintain these habits to ensure comfort and satisfactory urine output. Attention to the following variables is helpful:

Schedule: Some patients report voiding on demand in no apparent pattern. Others have inflexible patterns that have developed over the years and become anxious if these are interrupted. Some patients need assistance voiding and may experience urgency. Nursing actions should support the patient's usual voiding pattern as much as possible.

Privacy: Many adults and children cannot void in the presence of another person. Unless the patient is extremely weak and requires assistance, provide privacy in the healthcare facility and in the home.

Position: Helping patients assume their usual voiding position may be all that is necessary to resolve an inability to void. Some male patients cannot use a urinal while lying down or sitting; encourage them to void while standing at the bedside unless this is contraindicated. Similarly, some female patients cannot void easily on a bedpan but respond favorably with a bedside commode.

Hygiene: Patients who are confined to bed find it difficult to perform their usual genital hygiene. Careful cleansing of the perineal and genital areas is needed for patient comfort and to prevent infection. This is easily accomplished for patients on bed rest by using a bedpan and then pouring warm soapy water over the perineal area, followed by clear water. Families providing care for ill members at home may be taught this technique.

Because many people customarily wash their hands after toileting, offer patients confined to bed a moistened towelette or soap and water to wipe their hands after removing the bedpan. Specific recommendations for urinary elimination problems that affect older adults are listed in the accompanying box Focus on the Older Adult.

> *Recall Anna Galinski, the frail older woman in the nursing home. Ideally, before the charge nurse had inserted the catheter into Mrs. Galinski, these strategies should have been attempted to determine their effectiveness in promoting urinary elimination. In addition, when advocating for the patient, the nurse would strongly urge incorporating these strategies into the patient's plan of care to determine their effectiveness, ultimately substantiating that catheterization was not necessary.*

Promoting Fluid Intake

Many people routinely drink less fluid than is optimal to promote healthy urinary functioning. Adults with no disease-related fluid restrictions should drink 2,000 to 2,400 mL (8 to 10 8-oz glasses) of fluid daily. A common misperception is that drinking this much fluid causes water retention and contributes to weight gain. If a good proportion of the daily fluid intake is water, the kidneys and urinary structures are well flushed and waste products, including potentially harmful bacteria, are removed. Monitor fluid intake for excessive amounts of caffeine-containing beverages, high-sodium beverages such as diet sodas, and high-sugar beverages.

Provide fresh water, juices, and fluids of preference to patients confined to bed. Patients who are confused and children may need to be reminded to drink. Fluid restrictions may be ordered by the physician for patients with certain diseases. For others, forced fluids (above-average intake of fluids) are prescribed. This information needs to be incorporated in the plan of care and explained to the patient.

Strengthening Muscle Tone

Pelvic floor muscle training (PFMT) can improve voluntary control of urination and significantly reduce or eliminate problems with stress incontinence by strengthening perineal and abdominal muscle tone. Weakening of the pelvic floor muscles is a common cause of urinary incontinence. PFMT, more commonly called **Kegel exercises,** targets the inner muscles that lie under and support the bladder. These muscles can be toned, strengthened, and actually made larger by a regular routine of tightening and relaxing. Often patients have difficulty determining which muscles to exercise. These are the same muscles that the patient contracts to stop urinating in midstream or to

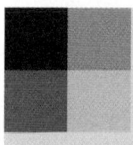

Focus on the Older Adult
Nursing Strategies for Urinary Elimination Problems Affecting Older Adult

Nocturia, Frequency, and Urgency
- Ensure easy access to the bathroom or commode.
- Discourage fluid intake at bedtime.
- Discourage alcohol use before bedtime.
- Evaluate medication regimen and schedule, particularly diuretics and drugs that produce sedation or confusion.
- Use a night light.
- Use clothing that is easily removed for voiding.
- Keep assistive ambulatory devices (walkers, canes, etc.) readily available.
- Provide call bell if assistance is necessary.
- Evaluate gait and ability to ambulate safely.
- Assess for urinary tract infection.

Incontinence
- Maintain a fluid intake of 1,500 to 2,000 mL/day.
- Discourage use of alcohol, NutraSweet, and caffeine.
- Provide easy access to the bathroom.
- Assess factors that influence voiding.
- Use assistive devices when necessary (raised toilet seat, grab bars, walker).
- Use collection devices when necessary (urinal or bedpan).
- Ensure safety when ambulating (eg, skid-proof slippers).
- Encourage use of whole, unprocessed, coarse wheat bran to prevent constipation and fecal impaction.
- Perform Kegel exercises several times daily.
- Encourage participation in a bladder retraining program.
- Consider insertion of an indwelling catheter as the last resort.

Urinary Tract Infections
- Maintain a liberal fluid intake
- Encourage shower instead of tub bath to decrease opportunity for bacteria in bath water to enter urethra.
- Void at frequent intervals.
- Void immediately after sexual intercourse.
- Assess for signs of urinary tract infection (may be non-specific in elderly patient).
- Use dipstick (Microstix) if recommended to monitor bacteria count in urine.
- Continue antimicrobial therapy as ordered.

control defecation. Instruct patients to contract the pelvic floor muscles for 10 seconds and to relax them for 10 seconds. Encourage the patient to perform Kegel exercises without involving the muscles in the abdomen, inner thigh, and buttocks. When the patient is familiar with these sensations, he or she should perform these exercises 30 to 80 times a day for at least 6 weeks and possibly longer, depending on the response (Loughrey, 1999). The exercises can be done anywhere. Assist patients to incorporate them into their daily activities.

PFMT can also be accomplished by using vaginal weights. The patient inserts a small weighted cone into her vagina. She then contracts her pelvic floor musculature to prevent the cone

from falling out. The cones can be gradually increased in weight as the muscles are strengthened.

Stimulating Urination and Resolving Urinary Retention

When urinary retention occurs, the bladder continues to fill with up to 3,000 to 4,000 mL of urine. Retention is often temporary and is common after surgery involving the lower abdomen, pelvis, bladder, or urethra, especially if ambulation is delayed, fluid intake is minimal, or epidural analgesia is used for pain control. Any mechanical obstruction, such as swelling at the meatus, which often occurs after childbirth, or an enlarged prostate in men, may cause retention.

Remember Jewel Carson, the postpartum woman who has not yet voided after delivery. The nurse needs to review her labor and delivery record for information about the use of epidural anesthesia and analgesia during labor and delivery. This, coupled with the most likely limited fluid intake during labor and the typical swelling of the urinary meatus after childbirth, places the patient at high risk for retention.

Many people experience **hesitancy** (delay or difficulty in initiating voiding). Routinely delaying urination may result in difficulty initiating a stream; therefore, always assist the patient to void when he or she first feels the urge to void. This problem may be resolved through additional measures that can be used by the nurse in the healthcare facility or caregivers at home (see Examples of Nursing Interventions Classification [NIC]: Urinary Retention Care).

Occasionally, a physician may request the patient to perform Credé's maneuver, a manual bladder compression technique used to stimulate urination by creating a sensation of bladder fullness and relaxing the urethral sphincter. The patient is taught to place both hands flat on the abdomen, between the umbilicus and the symphysis pubis, with fingers pointing downward. The patient or caregiver applies pressure over the bladder while holding the abdomen tight and holding his or her breath. This maneuver is performed only in cases of

Examples of Nursing Interventions Classification (NIC)
Urinary Retention Care

- Provide privacy for elimination.
- Use the power of suggestion by running water or flushing the toilet.
- Stimulate the reflex bladder by applying cold to the abdomen, stroking the inner thigh, or running water.
- Provide enough time for bladder emptying (10 min).
- Use spirits of wintergreen in bedpan or urinal.
- Monitor degree of bladder distention by palpation and percussion.
- Assist with toileting at regular intervals, as appropriate.

From McClosky, J., & Bulechek, G. (2000). *Nursing interventions classification (NIC)* (3rd ed.) (p. 692). St. Louis: C.V. Mosby. A full listing of nursing activities for each nursing intervention can be found in this book.

bladder flaccidity when the patient is not expected to regain voluntary control. It usually requires a physician's order.

Assisting With Toileting

Toilet

Even when the patient can use the bathroom toilet, the nurse may be responsible for noting any abnormalities of urinary elimination. In some instances, patients must be taught to report abnormalities to the nurse and instructed not to flush the toilet until the nurse checks the urine. In other instances, when the urine volume is to be calculated, the patient may need to urinate in a bedpan or a specimen hat placed in the toilet so that the urine can be measured before it is discarded. Although many patients can easily be taught to measure their urine output, the nurse is responsible for observing urine at least once during a shift and more frequently if warranted.

Assist weakened patients to the bathroom. If there is any danger of the patient falling, remain in attendance. Never lock the bathroom, and ensure that a signal bell is within easy reach so that the patient can summon help easily if he or she feels weak and needs assistance. A hand rail near the toilet also is helpful.

Commode

Commodes are chairs, straight-back chairs, or wheelchairs with open seats with a shelf or a holder underneath that holds a bedpan or bucket. They can be used for patients who can get out of bed but cannot use the bathroom toilet. The commode can be placed adjacent to the bed, and the patient can be assisted to it with minimal exertion. If the patient has a roommate, family and friends may be asked to exit the room while the patient uses the commode.

Bedpan and Urinal

Male patients confined to bed usually use the urinal for voiding and the bedpan for defecation; female patients use the bedpan for both (see Fig. 43-4). Many patients find it embarrassing and difficult to use the bedpan and the urinal. When a patient uses a bedpan or urinal, maintain the patient's privacy.

A special bedpan called a fracture bedpan is frequently used by people with fractures of the femur or lower spine. Smaller and flatter than the ordinary bedpan, it is helpful for patients who cannot easily raise themselves onto the regular bedpan. Very thin or elderly patients often find it easier and more comfortable to use the fracture bedpan. Skill 43-1 shows how to help a patient use a bedpan or urinal.

Preventing Urinary Tract Infections

Urinary tract infections (UTIs) are a leading cause of morbidity and health care expenditures in persons of all ages (Orenstein & Wong, 1999). UTIs are the leading cause of systemic infections in older adults (Mouton et al., 2001). Because the female

(*text continues on page 1308*)

SKILL 43-1   Offering and Removing a Bedpan or Urinal

EQUIPMENT

Bedpan or urinal	Handwashing supplies	Cover for bedpan or urinal (use Chux or disposable cover if others not available)
Toilet tissue	Disposable gloves	

ACTION	RATIONALE
1. Bring the bedpan or urinal and equipment to bedside. Don disposable gloves.	Having equipment on hand saves time by avoiding unnecessary trips to the storage area. Gloves protect against exposure to blood and body fluids.
2. Warm the bedpan, if it is made of metal, by rinsing it with warm water.	A cold bedpan feels uncomfortable and may make it difficult for the patient to void. Plastic bedpans do not require warming.
3. Place an adjustable bed in the high position.	Having the bed in the high position reduces strain on the nurse's back while assisting the patient onto the bedpan.
4. Place the bedpan or urinal on the chair next to the bed or on the foot of the bed. Fold the top linen back just enough to allow for placement of bedpan or urinal.	Folding back the linen in this manner prevents unnecessary exposure while still allowing the nurse to place the bedpan or urinal.
5. If the patient needs assistance to move onto the bedpan, have him or her bend the knees and rest some of his or her weight on the heels. Lift the patient by placing one hand under the lower back, and slip the bedpan into place with the other hand.	The patient uses less energy as the nurse assists by lifting him or her onto the bedpan. The nurse uses less energy when the patient can assist by placing some of his or her weight on the heels.
6. If the patient is unable to help, use two people to lift him or her onto the bedpan. Or, the patient may be placed on his or her side, the bedpan is placed against the buttocks, and the patient is rolled back onto the bedpan, as shown.	Having two people lift a patient causes less strain on the nurse's back. Rolling the patient takes less energy than lifting the patient onto a bedpan.

(continued)

ACTION

RATIONALE

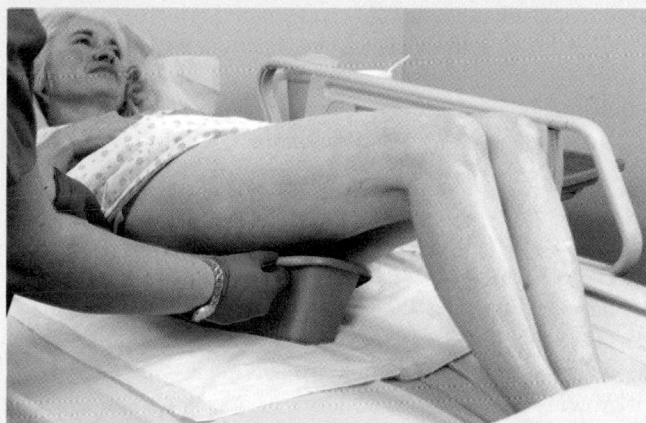

Action 5: Patient raising self in bed for bed pan.   (Photo by Rick Brady.)

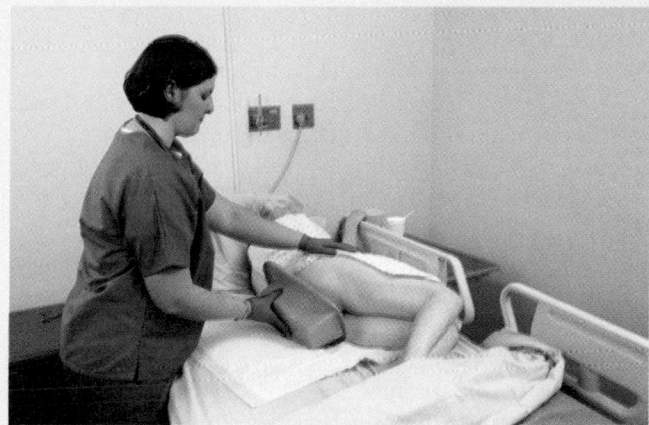

Action 6: Placing bedpan against buttocks while patient is on his side.
(Photo by Rick Brady.)

7. Ensure that the bedpan is in the proper position, the patient's buttocks rest on the rounded shelf of the bedpan. For male patients, the urinal is properly placed between slightly spread legs with the penis positioned in it and with the urinal resting on the bed.

Having the bedpan or urinal in the proper position prevents spilling contents onto the bed and prevents injury to the skin from a misplaced bedpan.

8. If permitted, raise the head of the bed as near to the sitting position as tolerated.

This position makes it easier for the patient to void or defecate, avoids strain on the patient's back, and allows gravity to aid in elimination.

9. Place call device and toilet tissue within easy reach. Leave the patient if it is safe to do so. Use side rails appropriately.

Falls can be prevented when the patient does not have to reach for items he or she needs. Side rails are an additional safety precaution. Leaving patient alone, if possible, promotes self-esteem and respects privacy.

10. Don disposable gloves. Remove the bedpan in the same manner in which it was offered, being careful to hold it steady. If necessary to assist the patient, wrap tissue around the hand several times, and wipe the patient clean, using one stroke from the pubic area toward the anal area. Discard tissue, and use more until the patient is clean. Place the patient on his or her side, and spread the buttocks to clean the anal area. Cover bedpan.

Holding the pan steady prevents spilling its contents. Cleaning an area from front to back minimizes fecal contamination of the vagina and urinary meatus. Cleaning the patient after he or she has used the bedpan prevents offensive odors and irritation to the skin.

11. Do not place toilet tissue in the bedpan if a specimen is required. Have a receptacle handy for discarding the tissue.

Toilet tissue mixed with a specimen makes laboratory examination more difficult and interferes with accurate output measurement.

12. Offer the patient supplies to wash and dry his or her hands, assisting as necessary.

Washing hands after using the bedpan or urinal helps prevent the spread of organisms.

13. Empty and clean the bedpan and urinal. Perform hand hygiene. Record according to agency procedure.

Hand hygiene helps prevent the spread of organisms. Documentation is important to maintain communication.

Nursing Considerations   If it is difficult to slide patient onto the bedpan, apply powder on the resting surfaces of the pan to eliminate friction. However, do no use powder if a specimen is required because contamination could result.

urethra is shorter and in closer proximity to the vagina and rectum, women are especially vulnerable. UTIs can affect both the upper (kidneys and ureters) and lower (bladder and urethra) urinary tract. *Escherichia coli,* bacteria commonly found in the gastrointestinal tract, are the most common causal organism (Stockert, 1999).

Risk Factors

Those at greatest risk for a UTI include the following:
- *Sexually active women:* During intercourse, perineal bacteria can migrate into the urethra and bladder.
- *Women who use diaphragms for contraception:* The spermicide used with a diaphragm decreases the amount of normally protective vaginal flora.
- *Postmenopausal women:* Urinary stasis, which is common at this age, provides an optimal environment for bacteria to multiply; in addition, decreased estrogen contributes to loss of protective vaginal flora.
- *Individuals with an indwelling urinary catheter in place:* About half of all patients with an indwelling catheter become infected within 1 week after its insertion. Although a break in sterile technique during placement can lead to an infection, most pathogens are introduced via handling of the catheter and drainage device after placement.
- *Individuals with diabetes mellitus:* Glucose in the urine acts as an excellent medium for bacteria to proliferate.
- *Elderly people:* The physiologic changes associated with aging (listed earlier in the chapter) predispose older people to development of UTIs (Mouton et al., 2001; Stockert, 1999).

> *Consider Anna Galinski, the frail older adult woman in the nursing home. Her risk for developing a UTI is increased due to her age. This risk now is further increased because of the catheter insertion.*

Diagnostic Evaluation

In addition to the nursing history and physical examination, laboratory findings can identify the presence of a UTI. Clinicians believe that the presence of bacteria in a clean-catch midstream or sterile urine specimen, accompanied by symptoms (eg, dysuria, urinary frequency or urgency, or cloudy urine with a foul odor), indicates a UTI. Red blood cells and nitrates also may be present in the urine.

Treatment

Various protocols are used to treat UTIs. A short-course antibiotic regimen (1 large dose versus 3 or 7 days of smaller doses) usually eradicates infections of the lower urinary tract, whereas longer antimicrobial therapy is required for upper tract infections. Patient education can help prevent UTI recurrence. Teaching the patient about measures such as the following that promote health and decrease the severity and incidence of UTIs is a major nursing responsibility:
- Drink 8 to 10 8-oz glasses of water daily.
- Observe the urine for color, amount, odor, and frequency. Report any sign of infection to your healthcare provider.
- Dry the perineal area after urination or defecation from the front to the back, or from the urethra toward the rectum.

- Drink two glasses of water before and after sexual intercourse and void immediately after intercourse.
- Take showers rather than baths.
- Wear underwear with a cotton crotch, and avoid clothing that is tight and restrictive on the lower half of the body.
- Drink 10 oz of cranberry juice daily. Cranberries contain chemicals that prevent *E. coli* from adhering to uroepithelial cells and urinary catheters (Maloney, 2002).
- Use an estrogen vaginal ring or cream as prescribed (for postmenopausal women who are prone to UTIs).

Nursing interventions for a patient with an indwelling catheter are discussed later in the chapter.

Caring for a Patient Who is Incontinent

Urinary incontinence, the inability to retain urine in the bladder, is widely underreported and underdiagnosed. It is a common but treatable health problem that is not an inevitable result of growing old or bearing children. Many people self-manage this life-altering condition for many years before seeking assistance from a healthcare provider. Urinary incontinence may affect as many as 200 million people, young and old, around the world (Ekerdt, 2001). The additional yearly cost of care associated with urinary incontinence is $700 to $4,000 per year per person (Langa et al., 2002). Although urinary incontinence is more prevalent in older women, 10% to 25% of women between the ages of 15 and 65 years report this condition (Johnson, 2000). Twice as many women as men are incontinent.

As the statistics indicate, urinary incontinence is a special problem for older adults who may experience decreasing control over micturition and who may find it more difficult to reach a toilet in time to void because of mobility problems or dexterity problems in undressing. The discomfort, odor, and embarrassment of urine-soaked clothing can greatly diminish a person's self-concept, causing him or her to feel like a social outcast. Age-related changes do affect urinary function, but urinary incontinence can be treated and individualized interventions can help the patient lead a normal life. Of those who seek treatment, 80% are cured or have their symptoms notably improved. Advertisements for adult disposable undergarments have increased public awareness about urinary incontinence, but they fail to mention possible treatment strategies (see Focused Critical Thinking Guide 43-1).

> *Review the scenario at the beginning of the chapter describing Midori Morita and her husband. It would be important for the nurse to assess the feelings of Ida and also of her husband related to the problems associated with urinary dribbling and incontinence. Ida may be feeling overwhelmed and possibly upset or angry. Her husband most likely would be feeling embarrassed, and possibly disgusted. Helping them resolve these feelings is essential for effective care.*

Types of Urinary Incontinence

The four major types of urinary incontinence are stress, urge, mixed, and overflow; three minor classes are functional, transient, and unconscious incontinence (Loughrey, 1999;

Focused Critical Thinking Guide 43-1

Urinary Incontinence

You have been assigned to care for an 80-year-old patient who was admitted with a recurrent leg ulcer and is due to be discharged the following day. Her nursing notes indicate that she has had two or three episodes of urinary incontinence every day while in the hospital and her plan of care states "use adult diapers." You go into the room to answer Mrs. Bartowski's call bell and help her into the bathroom. She is wearing an adult diaper, and a half-used package of diapers is on the chair. After voiding 150 mL of urine, she tearfully begs, "Please don't put that diaper back on me; I'm not a child." According to her chart, Mrs. Bartowski is mentally alert, lives at home with her daughter who visits frequently, and appears able to identify her need to urinate. You're aware that there are effective alternative therapies to resolve or minimize urinary incontinence rather than relying on absorbent products. However, the nurses have obviously made a decision to use diapers in this situation. You prefer to leave the diaper off, try some other measures, and, possibly, discuss this with her daughter; but as a student nurse you are only here for 2 days. You want to be a patient advocate and do the right thing. What should you do?

1. **Identify Goal of Thinking**
   Determine whether it is more important to replace the diaper against the patient's wishes or leave it off and discuss the possibility of using behavioral strategies with the staff.

2. **Assess Adequacy of Knowledge**
   Pertinent circumstances: Mrs. Bartowski is alert and oriented and obviously upset that diapers are being used. She has used her call light when she feels the urge to urinate, but incontinent episodes have also been documented. The nursing staff have decided that diapers are appropriate for this patient. Her daughter, with whom she lives, appears supportive and attentive. Discharge is scheduled for tomorrow.
   Prerequisite knowledge: Before you decide what to do in this situation, you need to discuss your options with your instructor. Of primary importance is whether the patient and her daughter are interested in pursuing alternatives. They can also provide invaluable information about her elimination pattern at home. The physician must be consulted to determine the etiology of the incontinence and validate that her urinary tract is intact and functioning adequately. You will also need to review the various treatment options for incontinence because these will have to be communicated to the patient and her daughter before discharge.

Room for error/time constraints: Absorbent products can provide a sense of security and are widely used for incontinence. There is, however, an 80% chance that continence can be restored once incontinence is assessed, recognized, and addressed. Early dependence on absorbent products can remove motivation to seek treatment and promote acceptance of the condition. The treatment options should be discussed with Mrs. Bartowski and her daughter before discharge tomorrow.

3. **Address Potential Problems**
   Continuing to use absorbent products offers a temporary solution to the problem. They protect the patient from embarrassment and provide a sense of security, although they do nothing to prevent incontinent episodes. Using behavioral techniques to control incontinence will require health teaching before discharge and a long-term commitment to follow-up in the home.

4. **Consult Helpful Resources**
   The patient's motivation to restore continence is your most valuable resource. The primary nurse or case manager, the physician, and your instructor can also help you sort through your priorities in this situation. The latest research and recommends use of behavioral techniques first to treat incontinence.

5. **Critique Judgment/Decision**
   If you decide to reapply a diaper against the patient's wishes, you may, in fact, be supporting the myth that incontinence is inevitable and untreatable. Long-term use of absorbent products can place the patient at risk for skin breakdown and a urinary tract infection if used improperly. You decide to leave the diaper off and establish regular intervals for voiding for the 2 days you will be caring for Mrs. Bartowski. In this short time, you hope to demonstrate to the patient, her daughter, and the staff that it is possible for Mrs. Bartowski to maintain a pattern of continence. Because she will most likely be discharged tomorrow, you also discuss the possibility of referral to home care or a continence expert who will instruct, support, and follow through with the necessary components of care. When you discuss your situation at postconference, your clinical group supports your decision.

Vapnek et al., 2001). **Stress incontinence** occurs when there is an involuntary loss of urine related to an increase in intra-abdominal pressure during coughing, sneezing, laughing, or other physical activities. Childbirth, menopause, obesity, or straining from chronic constipation can also result in urine loss. The leakage usually does not occur when the person is supine. **Urge incontinence** is the involuntary loss of urine associated with an abrupt and strong desire to void (urgency). It is usually associated with instability or involuntary contractions of the detrusor muscle that may or may not be associated

with a neurologic disorder. A diagnosis of **mixed incontinence** indicates that symptoms of urge and stress incontinence are present, although one type may predominate. With **overflow incontinence**, the involuntary loss of urine is associated with overdistention and overflow of the bladder. The signal to empty the bladder may be underactive or absent, the bladder fills, and dribbling occurs. It may be due to a secondary effect of some drugs, fecal impaction, or neurologic conditions. **Functional incontinence** is urine loss caused by factors outside the lower urinary tract, such as chronic impairments of physical or cognitive functioning. A temporary reversible loss of bladder control (transient incontinence) may result from a UTI or certain medications, such as diuretics. The mnemonic "DIAPPERS" is helpful in remembering the causes of transient incontinence:

• Delirium
• Infection (urinary)
• Atrophic urethritis and vaginitis
• Pharmaceuticals
• Psychological disorders
• Excessive urine output
• Restricted mobility
• Stool impaction (Resnick, 1984)

Unconscious incontinence, occurring when the patient is unaware, is common in patients with paraplegia and those with multisystem failure (Loughrey, 1999).

Diagnostic Evaluation

In addition to the assessment strategies mentioned earlier in the chapter, physical examination and specific diagnostic tests aid in identifying urinary incontinence. Palpate the patient's abdomen for a distended bladder, any masses, or tenderness. Pelvic and rectal examinations can determine muscle and sphincter tone and detect any irregularities. The **postvoid residual (PVR)** urine (the amount of urine remaining in the bladder immediately after voiding) can be measured by the traditional method of catheterization or use of a portable ultrasound device that scans the bladder. A bladder scan can be performed at the bedside, poses no risk for infection, and is a safer alternative. Results are most accurate when the patient is in the supine position during the scanning. A PVR less than 50 mL indicates adequate bladder emptying; a volume greater than 200 mL is considered inadequate bladder emptying. A PVR between this range indicates the need for further evaluation. If a bladder scan measures a urine volume of greater than 300 mL, catheterization should be performed to relieve distention.

A voiding record or diary provides information about the frequency, timing, and amount of voiding. By noting any patterns to voiding, either continent or incontinent, the nurse may find correlations with medications, fluid intake, or other causes of incontinence and may be able to prevent any further incontinent episodes. Voiding diaries can also be used to evaluate the effectiveness of interventions.

Treatment

Many patients incorrectly believe that surgery is the only treatment option for urinary incontinence. Surgical intervention is considered only if behavioral and pharmacologic measures prove ineffective. Nursing skills and creativity can help patients become continent again before surgery is used. Box 43-2 summarizes the recommended treatment regimen for urinary incontinence.

Patients frequently turn to absorbent products for protection when they are incontinent of urine if they have not had this condition properly diagnosed and treated. Many types of products are available, including adult diapers, liners, pads, pant

---

BOX 43-2 Treatment Options for Urinary Incontinence

Behavioral Techniques
• Pelvic floor exercises: Kegel exercises to strengthen pelvic floor muscles and sphincter muscles. Kegels can be done alone, with weighted cones, or with biofeedback.
• Biofeedback: Measuring devices are used to help patient become aware of when pelvic floor muscles are contracting.
• Electrical stimulation: Electrodes are placed in the vagina or rectum that then stimulate nearby muscles to contract.
• Timed voiding or bladder training: May be used with biofeedback. Patient keeps track of when voiding and leaking occur so that he or she may plan when to void. Bladder training involves biofeedback and muscle training.

Pharmacologic Treatment
• Treatment dependent on type of incontinence. Some medications inhibit contractions of the bladder, others may relax muscles, and some tighten muscles at the bladder neck and urethra.
• Estrogen may be used in postmenopausal women to relieve atrophy of involved muscles.
• Collagen may be injected into the tissue around the urethra to add bulk and help close the urethral opening.

Mechanical Treatment
• Pessaries: A stiff ring that is inserted into the vagina, where it helps to reposition the urethra. The pessary may be placed by the patient or by a nurse.
• External barriers: Adhere to the urethral opening to stop urine leakage but must be removed prior to voiding
• Urethral insert: Fits into the urethra; an inflated balloon keeps it in place and blocks the flow of urine.
• Surgical intervention: Used as a last resort. Type of surgery depends on cause of incontinence.

Adapted from National Institute of Diabetes & Digestive & Kidney Disease. (2002). *Urinary incontinence in women.* Retrieved Dec. 26, 2002, from http://www.niddk.nih.gov/health/urolog/pubs/uiwomen/uiwomen.htm

---

systems, and drip collectors. When used improperly, such products may cause skin breakdown and place the patient at risk for a UTI. Long-term use of these products is not recommended until the following factors have been considered and discussed with a healthcare provider:
• Functional disability of the patient
• Type and severity of incontinence
• Gender
• Availability of caregivers
• Failure of previous treatment programs
• Patient preference

Through careful assessment and planned interventions, continence can be restored, possibly helping to postpone a caregiver's decision to place a family member in a costly healthcare facility. Carefully assess environmental factors. Equipment that gives the person better access to toileting facilities (eg, walker, cane, wheelchair, Velcro closings on clothing) may be necessary. Dietary habits, such as excess caffeine intake or insufficient fluid intake, both of which can irritate the bladder and contribute to incontinence, indicate the need for teaching about nutrition.

> *Think back to Ida Fleming, the woman caring for her husband who had urinary problems at home. The nurse would need to carefully assess all aspects of the patient's current status, including the environment, and develop a patient-specific teaching plan for Ida and her husband.*

Noninvasive, low-risk behavioral interventions are the first line of therapy. The home setting is ideally suited for using these interventions. Nurses can identify patients who are incontinent and use these techniques or refer them to nurse or physician continence experts in the community. All nurses caring for older adults need to be familiar with education about urinary incontinence.

Catheterizing the Patient's Bladder

Urinary catheterization is the introduction of a catheter through the urethra into the bladder for the purpose of withdrawing urine. A catheter is a tube used for injecting or removing fluids. Catheterization is considered the most common cause of nosocomial infections (infections acquired in a hospital), so whenever possible catheterization should be avoided. When it is deemed necessary, it should be performed using careful, strict aseptic technique.

Facts About the Lower Urinary Tract

The following basic facts about the lower urinary tract system should be considered when catheterization is planned:

- The bladder is normally a sterile cavity.
- The external opening to the urethra can never be sterilized.
- The bladder has defense mechanisms. It empties itself of urine regularly and maintains an acidic environment, which has antibacterial advantages. These help to maintain a sterile bladder under normal circumstances and also help in clearing an infection if it occurs.
- Pathogens introduced into the bladder can ascend the ureters and cause bladder and kidney infections.
- A healthy bladder is not as susceptible to infection as an injured one is. A state of lowered resistance, present in many diseases and stressful situations, predisposes the patient to urinary infection.

Types of Catheters

If a catheter is to remain in place for continuous drainage, an **indwelling urethral catheter** is used. Indwelling catheters are also called retention or Foley catheters. The indwelling urethral catheter is designed so that it does not slip out of the bladder. A balloon is inflated to ensure that the catheter remains in the bladder once it is inserted.

Indwelling catheters are used for the gradual decompression of an overdistended bladder, for intermittent bladder drainage and irrigation, and for continuous bladder drainage. Several types of indwelling catheters are available, but the principles on which they operate are similar.

The indwelling catheter has more than one lumen or open tube within the catheter. In a double-lumen catheter, one lumen is connected directly to the balloon, which is inflated with sterile water; the other is the lumen through which the urine drains. The triple-lumen catheter provides an additional lumen for the instillation of irrigating solution.

Intermittent catheters, or straight catheters, are used to drain the bladder for shorter periods (5 to 10 minutes). Patients can be taught to insert and remove intermittent catheters themselves. Intermittent catheters are discussed later in this section. Figure 43-9 illustrates a triple-lumen, double-lumen, and straight catheter.

A **suprapubic catheter** is occasionally used for continuous drainage. This type of catheter is surgically inserted through a small incision above the pubic area (Fig. 43-10). Suprapubic bladder drainage diverts urine from the urethra when injury, stricture, prostatic obstruction, or gynecologic or abdominal surgery has compromised the flow of urine through the urethra. Care of the patient with a suprapubic catheter is more appropriately discussed in clinical texts.

Urologic Stents

When a patient has a urinary tract obstruction and is not a candidate for surgery, a urologic stent may be inserted. The stent may be temporary (when placed in the ureters) or permanent (when positioned in the urethra). Temporary stents are usually made of a pliable material such as radiopaque silicone, whereas permanent stents are stronger and typically are made of a flexible metal mesh. They are inserted during a cystoscopic procedure, and in most cases the patient receives only a local anesthetic and sedation. Urologic stents relieve urinary obstructions and provide a path for the flow of urine. Major nursing responsibilities include assessment, measurement, and documentation of urinary output. Never irrigate a blocked stent (Phipps et al., 2003). Instruct the patient with a urologic stent to notify the physician immediately if the urine becomes bright red, severe pain occurs, the drainage pattern changes, or any sign of infection is present. Also encourage the patient to wear a medical alert bracelet at all times.

Reasons for Catheterization

Common reasons for urinary catheterization include:

- Relieving urinary retention
- Obtaining a sterile urine specimen
- Measuring the PVR. The patient is first asked to void and is then catheterized to determine how much urine remains in the bladder after normal voiding.
- Obtaining a urine specimen when a specimen cannot be secured satisfactorily by other means. Examples include collecting an uncontaminated specimen from a woman who is menstruating or from an incontinent patient.
- Emptying the bladder before, during, or after surgery and before certain diagnostic examinations
- Monitoring of critically ill patients

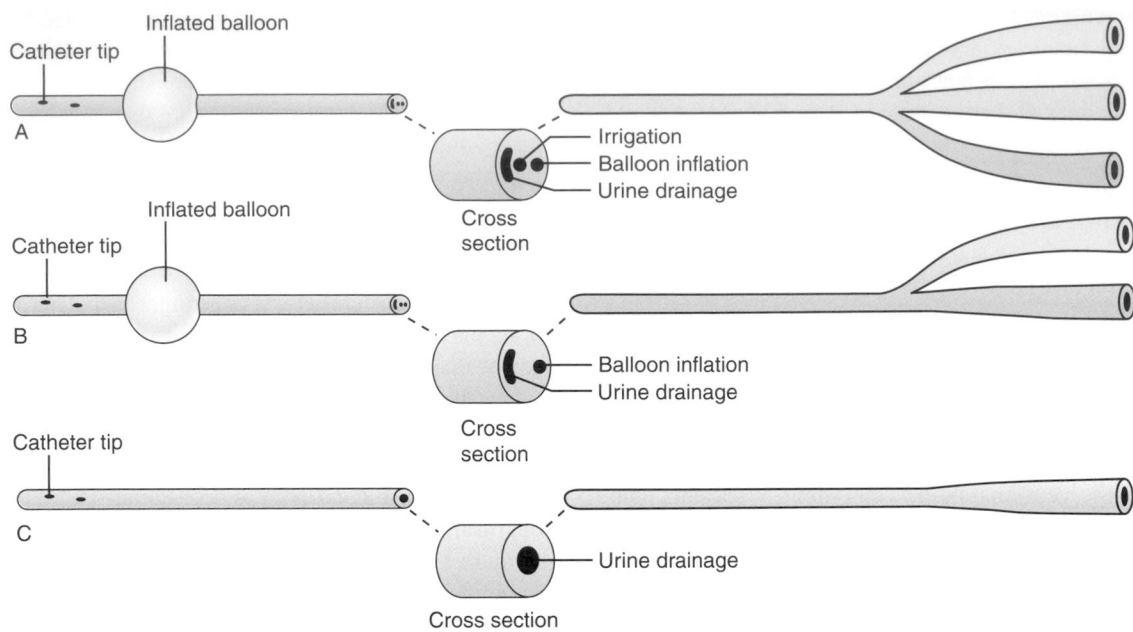

FIGURE 43-9 (**A**) Triple-lumen indwelling catheter. (**B**) Double-lumen indwelling catheter. (**C**) Straight catheter.

Hazards of Catheterization

Sepsis and trauma are the two major hazards of introducing an instrument such as a catheter into the bladder. The male urethra is especially vulnerable to injury because of its longer length. An object forced through a stricture or an irregular opening from the wrong angle can seriously damage the urethra. Although the female urethra is shorter than the male urethra, it is also susceptible to damage if a catheter is forced

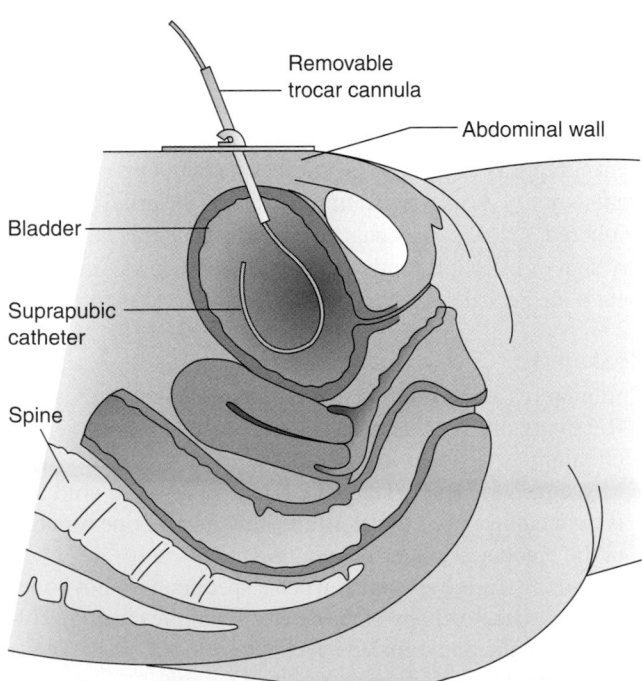

FIGURE 43-10 A suprapubic catheter positioned in the bladder. (From Smeltzer S., & Bare, B. [2004]. *Brunner & Suddarth's textbook of medical surgical nursing* [10th ed.]. Philadelphia: Lippincott Williams & Wilkins.)

through it. The mucous membrane lining the urethra is delicate and easily damaged by the friction resulting from the insertion of a catheter. Bacteria can enter the bladder when the catheter is inserted. When the catheter is left in place, the organisms may move up the catheter lumen or the space between the catheter and the urethral wall. This asymptomatic condition in which bacteria is present in the urine is known as **bacteriuria.** Most patients with an indwelling catheter in place for more than 4 weeks develop bacteriuria (Evans, 1999; Sienty & Dawson, 1999).

Intermittent catheterization, performed by the patient or a caregiver in the home, may be necessary for patients with spinal cord injuries or other neurologic conditions. Although the risk for UTI is always present, most research supports the use of clean rather than sterile technique in this environment. The procedure for self-catheterization is essentially the same as that used by the nurse to catheterize a patient. Initially a female patient may use a mirror to locate the meatus, but eventually she can learn to insert the catheter using just touch. Self-catheterization is recommended at regular intervals to prevent overdistention of the bladder and decreased blood flow through the wall of the bladder (Smeltzer & Bare, 2004).

Equipment

The equipment used for catheterization is usually prepackaged in a sterile, disposable tray. Most kits already contain a standard-sized catheter. The trays used for catheterizing male and female patients are the same. Catheters are graded on the French (F) scale according to lumen size. For long-term use for an adult, a 12F to 14F catheter with a 5- to 10-mL balloon is commonly used. Smaller catheters usually are not necessary, and a smaller-sized lumen would be so small that it would increase the time necessary for emptying the bladder. Larger catheters distend the urethra and increase the discomfort of the procedure. Size 8F or 10F catheters are commonly used for children.

Patient Preparation

Before the catheterization, explain to the patient the procedure and the reason for it. Tell the patient that catheter insertion produces a sensation of pressure and some discomfort. Explain that measures will be taken to avoid exposure and embarrassment. The more relaxed the patient is, the easier it will be to insert the catheter.

The most common patient position for catheter insertion is the dorsal recumbent position, with the patient preferably on a solid surface such as a firm mattress or a treatment table. Catheterizing a patient in a bed with a soft mattress, especially a female patient, is not as satisfactory because the patient's pelvic surfaces are not firmly supported and visualization of the meatus is difficult. Also, the patient may sink into the bed, causing the bladder to be lower than the outlet of the catheter. If the patient is in bed, supporting the buttocks on a firm cushion is helpful.

The Sims, or lateral, position is an alternate position for catheter insertion in female patients. This position may allow better visualization and be more comfortable for the patient, especially if hip and knee movements are difficult. The smaller area of exposure is also less stressful for the patient. Allow the patient to lie on either side, depending on which position is easiest for the nurse and best for the patient's comfort. Place the patient's buttocks near the edge of the bed with her shoulders at the opposite edge and her knees drawn toward her chest. Lift the upper buttock and labia to expose the urinary meatus (Fig. 43-11).

Remember Jewel Carson, the postpartum mother who has not voided. For a patient who fails to void, intermittent catheterization may be ordered to relieve bladder distention and urinary retention. If this becomes necessary, the nurse may choose to perform the procedure with Jewel in the side-lying position to enhance her comfort because the patient's perineum is probably sore and edematous.

Procedure

Catheterization of the urinary bladder in female and male patients is described in Skills 43-2 and 43-3. Adhering to surgical asepsis is of utmost importance to help prevent a UTI. See the accompanying Through the Eyes of a Student for a student's account of catheterization.

Indwelling Catheters
Inserting and Connecting to the Drainage System

Nurses are responsible for inserting indwelling catheters and caring for the patient. The procedure for inserting an indwelling catheter is similar to that for inserting a straight single-lumen catheter, with a few differences (see Skill 43-2).

An inflated balloon holds the indwelling catheter in position in the bladder. The prefilled syringe included in the catheter kit contains the amount of sterile water needed to inflate the balloon to the desired spherical shape. If only 5 mL is injected into a catheter with a 5-mL balloon, some solution would remain in the tubing leading to the balloon, not completely inflating the balloon. A balloon that is only partially inflated could cause irritation and erosion to the mucosa in the bladder. Usually 7 to 10 mL of fluid is necessary to inflate a 5-mL balloon completely. If a patient complains of pain with catheter insertion that occurs immediately after the balloon is inflated, allow the balloon to empty and replace the catheter with another one; the balloon was probably in the urethra and caused discomfort because of the distention of the urethra.

The practice of inserting an indwelling catheter in a male patient until there is urine return is also no longer recommended. See the accompanying Research in Nursing box. The technique of applying lubricant to the catheter before inserting it in a male patient is no longer recommended either.

(text continues on page 1319)

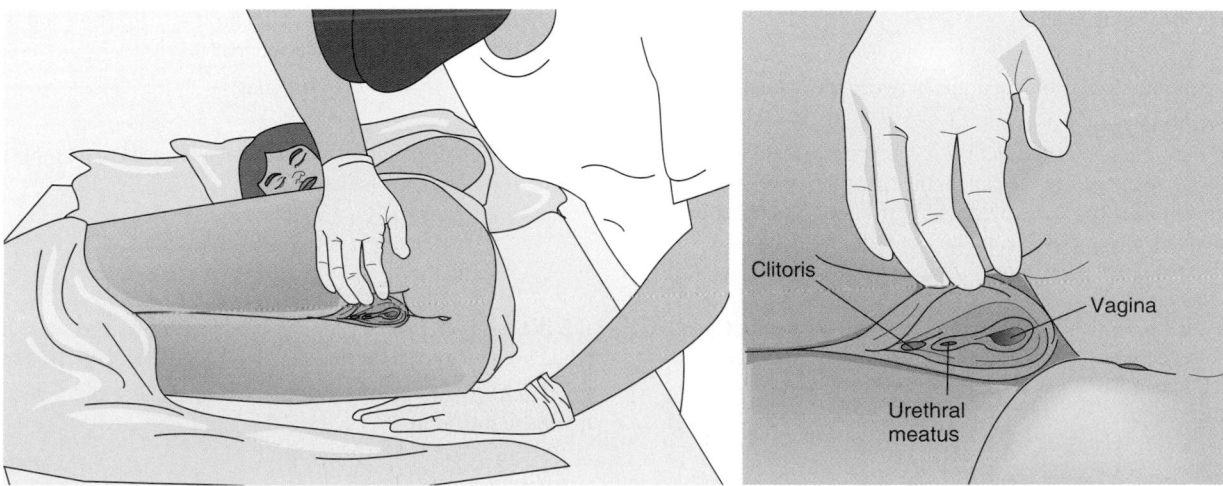

FIGURE 43-11 Demonstration of the side-lying position *(left)* and of how to expose the urinary meatus when catheterizing a female patient in the side-lying position *(right)*.

EQUIPMENT

Sterile catheterization kit that contains:
   Sterile gloves
   Sterile drapes (one of which is
    fenestrated)
   Antiseptic solution
   Lubricant
   Cotton balls or gauze squares

Forceps
Straight or indwelling catheter (size
  must be appropriate for patient)
Prefilled syringe
Basin (base of kit usually serves as this)
Specimen container
Flashlight or lamp

Urine collection bag and drainage tubing
  (may be connected to sterile indwelling
  catheter if a closed drainage system is
  used)
Velcro leg strap or tape
Disposal bag
Waterproof pad or Chux

ACTION	RATIONALE
1. Assemble equipment. Perform hand hygiene. Explain the procedure and its purpose to the patient. Discuss any allergies with patient, especially iodine or latex.	Organization facilitates performance of the task. Hand hygiene deters spread of microorganisms. An explanation encourages patient cooperation and reduces apprehension. Most catheters and gloves are latex. Some antiseptic solutions contain iodine.
2. Provide for good light. Artificial light is recommended (use of a flashlight requires an assistant to hold and position it).	Good lighting is necessary to see the meatus clearly.
3. Provide for privacy by closing the curtains or door.	The procedure may be embarrassing for the patient.
4. Assist the patient to the dorsal recumbent position with the knees flexed and the feet about 2 feet apart and drape the patient. Or, if preferable, the patient can be placed in the side-lying position as shown. Slide the waterproof drape under the patient.	Good visualization of the meatus is important. Embarrassment, chilliness, and feeling tense can interfere with introducing the catheter. The patient's comfort will promote relaxation. The drape will protect bed linens from moisture.
5. Clean the genital and perineal area with warm soap and water. Rinse and dry. Perform hand hygiene again.	Clean technique decreases the possibility of introducing organisms into the bladder.
6. Prepare urine drainage setup if indwelling catheter is to be inserted and separate urine collection system is used. Secure to bed frame according to manufacturer's directions.	This facilitates connection of the catheter to the drainage system and provides for easy access.
7. Open the sterile catheterization tray on overbed table using sterile technique.	Placement of equipment near the work site increases efficiency. Sterile technique protects the patient and prevents the spread of microorganisms.
8. Put on sterile gloves. Grasp the upper corners of the drape and unfold the drape without touching unsterile areas. Fold back a cuff over gloved hands. Ask the patient to lift her buttocks and slide the sterile drape under her with gloves protected by cuff.	The drape provides a sterile field close to the meatus. Covering the gloved hands will help keep the gloves sterile while placing the drape.
9. A fenestrated sterile drape may be placed over the perineal area, exposing the labia.	The drape expands the sterile field and protects against contamination. Use of a fenestrated drape may limit visualization and is considered optional by some practitioners.
10. Place the sterile tray on the drape between the patient's thighs.	This provides easy access to supplies.
11. Open all supplies: a. *If the catheter is to be indwelling,* test the catheter balloon. Remove the protective cap on the tip of the syringe and attach the syringe prefilled with sterile water to injection port. Inject appropriate amount of fluid. If the balloon inflates properly, withdraw fluid and leave the syringe attached to the port.	A balloon that does not inflate or that leaks needs to be replaced before insertion in the patient.
b. Pour antiseptic solution over cotton balls or gauze. Open the specimen container if specimen is to be obtained.	It is necessary to open all supplies and prepare for the procedure while both hands are sterile.
c. Lubricate 1 to 2 inches of the catheter tip.	Lubrication facilitates the insertion of the catheter and reduces trauma to the tissues.

(continued)

ACTION   RATIONALE

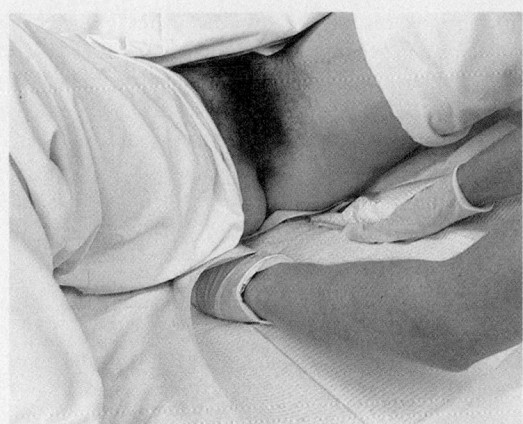

Action 8: Keeping sterile gloves protected while positioning drape under patient.

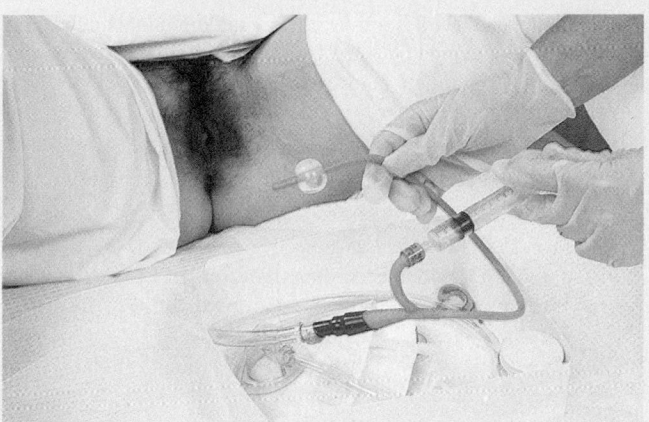

Action 11a: Testing the balloon.

12. With the thumb and one finger of your nondominant hand, spread the labia and identify the meatus, as shown in figure. Be prepared to maintain separation of the labia with one hand until urine is flowing well and continuously.

13. Using cotton balls held with forceps, clean both labial folds and then directly over the meatus. Move the cotton ball from above the meatus down toward the rectum. Discard each cotton ball after one downward stroke.

Smoothing the area immediately surrounding the meatus helps to make it visible. Allowing the labia to drop back into position may contaminate the area around the meatus, as well as the catheter. Your nondominant hand is now contaminated.

Moving from an area where there is likely to be less contamination to an area where there is more contamination helps prevent the spread of organisms. Cleaning the meatus last helps reduce the possibility of introducing organisms into the bladder.

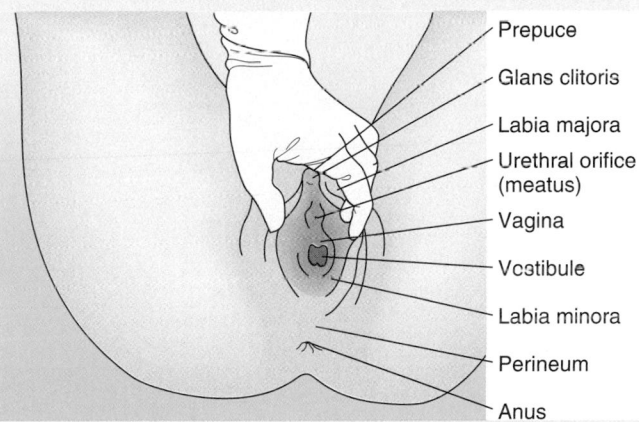

Prepuce
Glans clitoris
Labia majora
Urethral orifice (meatus)
Vagina
Vestibule
Labia minora
Perineum
Anus

Action 12: Spreading the labia with nondominant hand to identify the meatus.

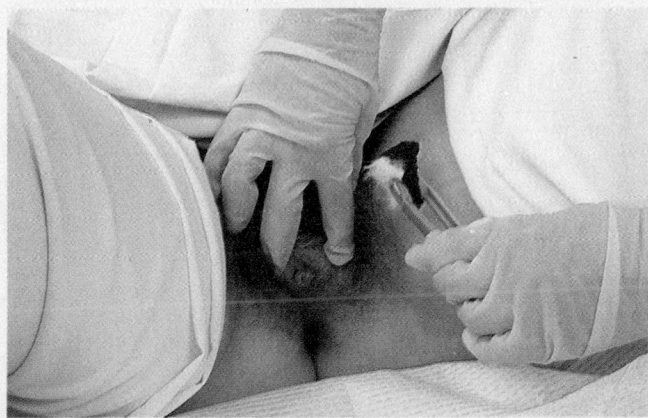

Action 13: Preparing to clean the labial folds.

14. With the uncontaminated gloved hand, place the drainage end of the catheter in the receptacle. *For insertion of an indwelling catheter that is preattached to sterile tubing and drainage container (closed drainage system), position the catheter and setup within easy reach on the sterile field.*

15. Insert the catheter tip into the meatus 5 to 7.5 cm (2–3 in) or until urine flows. Do not use force to push the catheter through the urethra into the bladder. Ask the patient to breathe deeply, and rotate the catheter gently if slight resistance is met as the catheter reaches the external sphincter. *For an indwelling catheter,* once urine drains, advance the catheter another 2.5 to 5.0 cm (1–2 in).

This facilitates drainage of urine and minimizes risk of contaminating sterile equipment.

The female urethra is about 3.7 to 6.2 cm (1½–2½ in) long. Applying force on the catheter is likely to injure mucous membranes. The sphincter relaxes, and the catheter can enter the bladder easily when the patient relaxes. Advancing an indwelling catheter an additional 1.3 to 2.5 cm (½ to 1 in) ensures placement in the bladder and facilitates inflation of the balloon without damaging the urethra.

(continued)

ACTION

RATIONALE

16. Hold the catheter securely with the nondominant hand while the bladder empties. Collect a specimen if required. Continue drainage according to agency policy.

Withdrawing and reinserting the catheter increases the chances of contaminating it. In general, no more than 750 mL of urine should be removed at one time. Pelvic floor blood vessels may become engorged from the sudden release of pressure leading to possible hypotensive episode.

17. Remove the catheter smoothly and slowly if a straight catheterization was ordered.

This causes less discomfort to the patient.

18. *If the catheter is to be indwelling:*

a. Inflate the balloon according to the manufacturer's recommendations. Inject the entire volume supplied in the pre-filled syringe.

The balloon anchors the catheter in place in the bladder. Sterile water is used to inflate the balloon as a precaution in case the balloon ruptures.

b. Tug gently on the catheter after the balloon is inflated to feel resistance.

Improper inflation can cause patient discomfort and malpositioning of catheter.

c. Attach the catheter to the drainage system if necessary.

Closed drainage system minimizes the risk for organisms being introduced into the bladder.

d. Secure to the upper thigh with a Velcro leg strap or tape. Leave some slack in the catheter to allow for leg movement.

Proper attachment prevents trauma to the urethra and meatus from tension on the tubing.

e. Check that the drainage tubing is not kinked and that movement of side rails does not interfere with catheter or drainage bag.

This facilitates drainage of urine and prevents the backflow of urine.

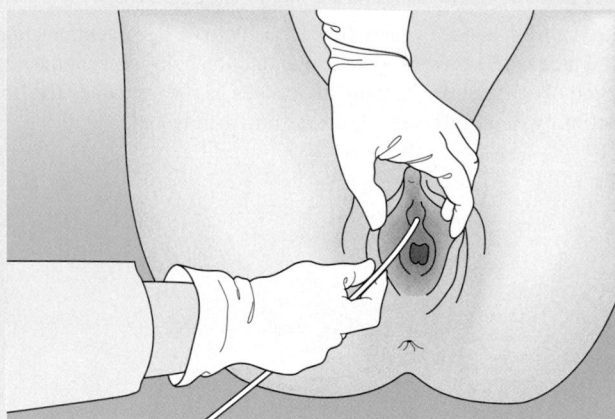

Action 15: Inserting the tip of the catheter into the meatus, using the uncontaminated gloved hand.

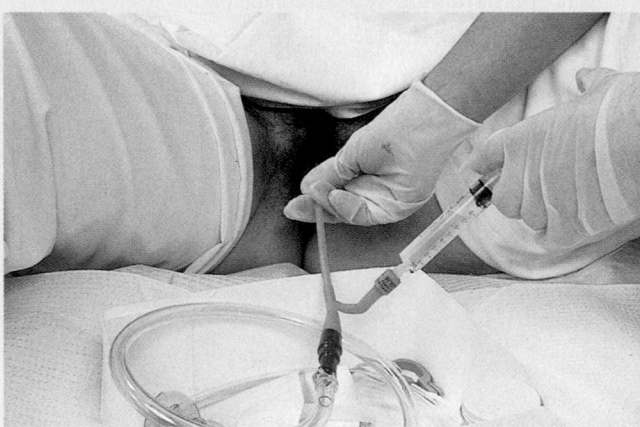

Action 18a: Injecting sterile water to inflate balloon.

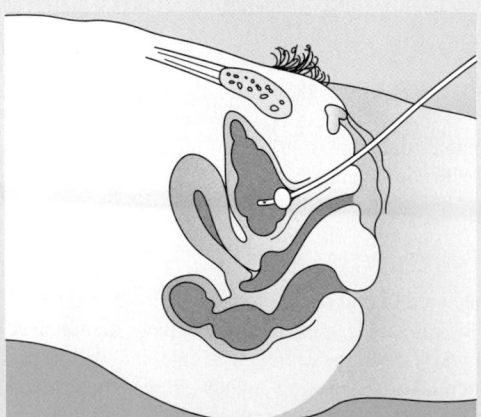

Action 18b: Tugging gently on catheter after balloon is in place to feel resistance.

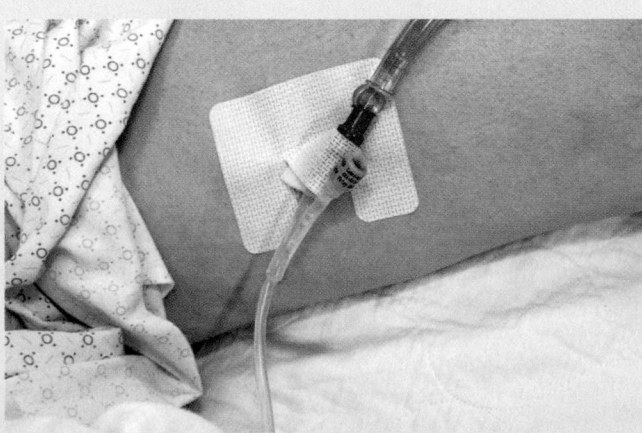

Action 18d: Attaching catheter to leg.   (Photo by Rick Brady.)

SKILL
43-2   **Catheterizing the Female Urinary Bladder (Straight and Indwelling)** (continued)

ACTION	RATIONALE
19. Remove the equipment and make the patient comfortable in bed. Clean and dry the perineal area, if necessary. Care for the equipment according to agency policy. Send the urine specimen to the laboratory promptly or refrigerate it.	Urine kept at room temperature may cause organisms, if present, to grow and distort laboratory findings.
20. Perform hand hygiene.	Hand hygiene deters the spread of microorganisms.
21. Record the time of the catheterization, the amount of urine removed, a description of the urine, the patient's reaction to the procedure, and your name.	A careful record is important for planning the patient's care.

Home Care Considerations   If self-catheterization must be performed in the home, clean technique is appropriate. The bladder's natural resistance to microorganisms normally found in the home make sterile technique unnecessary. Rubber catheters must be washed thoroughly before boiling for 20 minutes. Dry and store properly for next usage.

A shower rather than a tub bath is recommended for patients with an indwelling catheter. Sitting in the bathtub may allow for easier access of bacteria into the urinary tract.

Special Considerations   If there is not an immediate flow of urine after the catheter has been inserted, several measures may prove helpful:

- Have the patient take a deep breath, which helps to relax the perineal and abdominal muscles.
- Rotate the catheter slightly because a drainage hole may be resting against the bladder wall.
- Raise the head of the patient's bed to increase pressure in the bladder area.
- Placed a gloved finger in the vagina to feel digitally for the position of the catheter through the anterior vaginal wall.
- Temporarily leave a catheter that has inadvertently been placed in the vagina in place as a guide while the nurse regloves and inserts another sterile catheter directly above it into the urinary meatus.

SKILL
43-3   **Catheterizing the Male Urinary Bladder (Straight and Indwelling)**

EQUIPMENT
Sterile catheterization kit that contains:
  Sterile gloves
  Sterile drapes (one of which is
    fenestrated)
  Antiseptic solution
  Lubricant in 10 mL syringe
  Cotton balls or gauze squares
  Forceps

Straight or indwelling catheter
Prefilled syringe
Basin (base of kit usually serves as this)
Specimen container
Flashlight or lamp
Urine collection bag and drainage tubing
  (may be connected to sterile indwelling

catheter if a closed drainage system is
  used)
Velcro leg strap or tape
Disposal bag
Waterproof pad or Chux

ACTION	RATIONALE
1. Assemble equipment and follow actions 1 through 3 for female catheterization in Skill 43-2.	
2. Position the patient on his back with the thighs slightly apart. Drape the patient so that only the area around the penis is exposed.	This prevents unnecessary exposure.
3. Follow actions 5 to 7 for female catheterization in Skill 43-2.	

(continued)

ACTION	RATIONALE
4. Put on sterile gloves. Open the sterile drape and place on the patient's thighs. Place the fenestrated drape with the opening over the penis.	This maintains a sterile working area.
5. Place the catheter set on or next to the patient's legs on the sterile drape.	The sterile setup should be arranged so that the nurse's back is not turned to it, nor should it be out of the nurse's range of vision.
6. Open all supplies: a. *If the catheter is to be indwelling,* test the catheter balloon. Remove the protective cap on the tip of the syringe and attach the syringe prefilled with sterile water to the injection port. Inject appropriate amount of fluid. If balloon inflates properly, withdraw fluid and leave syringe attached to port. b. Pour antiseptic solution over cotton balls or gauze. Open the specimen container if specimen is to be obtained. c. Remove the cap from the syringe prefilled with lubricant.	A balloon that does not inflate or that leaks must be replaced before insertion in the patient. It is necessary to open all supplies and prepare for the procedure while both hands are sterile.
7. Lift the penis with your nondominant hand, which is then considered contaminated. Retract the foreskin in the uncircumcised male patient. Clean the area at the meatus with a cotton ball held with a forceps. Use a circular motion, moving from the meatus toward the base of the penis for three cleansings.	The hand touching the penis becomes contaminated. Cleansing the area around the meatus and under the foreskin in the uncircumcised male patient helps prevent infection. Moving from the meatus toward the base of the penis prevents bringing organisms to the meatus.
8. Hold the penis with slight upward tension and perpendicular to the patient's body. Gently insert the tip of the syringe with lubricant into the urethra and instill the 10 mL of lubricant.	The lubricant causes the urethra to distend slightly and facilitates passage of the catheter without traumatizing the lining of the urethra.

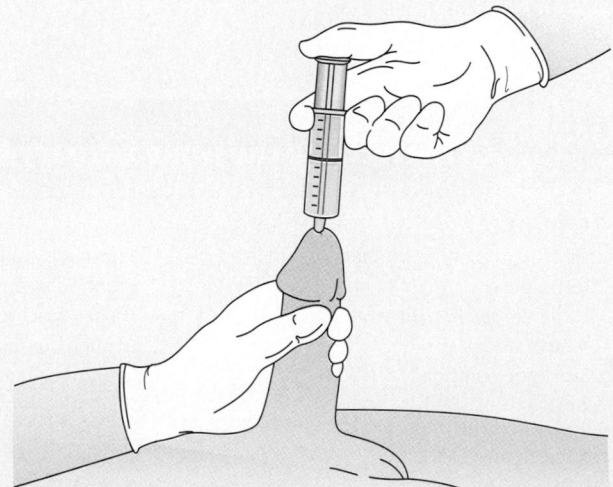

Action 7: Cleaning area of the meatus.   Action 8: Instilling lubrication before male catheterization.

9. Ask the patient to bear down as if voiding. With your dominant hand, place the drainage end of the catheter in the receptacle. *For insertion of an indwelling catheter* that is preattached to sterile tubing and a drainage container (closed drainage system), position the catheter and setup within easy reach on the sterile field.	Bearing down eases the passage of the catheter through the urethra.

(continued)

SKILL
43-3 **Catheterizing the Male Urinary Bladder (Straight and Indwelling)** (continued)

ACTION	RATIONALE
10. Insert the tip into the meatus. Advance the intermittent catheter 15 to 20 cm (6–8 in) or until urine flows. Do not use force to introduce the catheter. If the catheter resists entry, ask the patient to breathe deeply and rotate the catheter slightly. *For an indwelling catheter,* advance the catheter to the bifurcation of the catheter. Once the balloon is inflated, the catheter may be gently pulled back into place. Replace the foreskin in uncircumsized patient. Lower the penis.	The male urethra is about 20 cm long. Deep breaths or slight twisting of the catheter may ease the catheter past resistance at the sphincters. Advancing an indwelling catheter to the bifurcation ensures its placement in the bladder and facilitates inflation of the balloon without damaging the urethra.
11. Follow Actions 16 through 21 for female catheterization in Skill 43-2 except that the catheter may be secured to the upper thigh or lower abdomen with the penis directed toward the patient's chest. Slack should be left in the catheter to prevent tension.	This is done to prevent irritation at the angle of the penis and scrotum. Slack left in the catheter allows for penile erection, which can occur naturally during sleep.

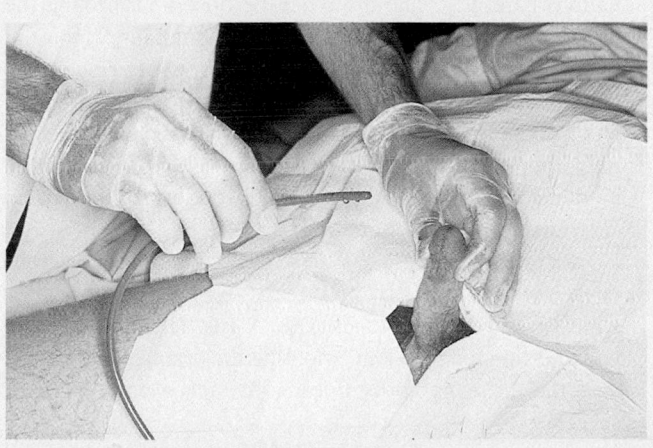

Action 9: Preparing to insert the catheter.

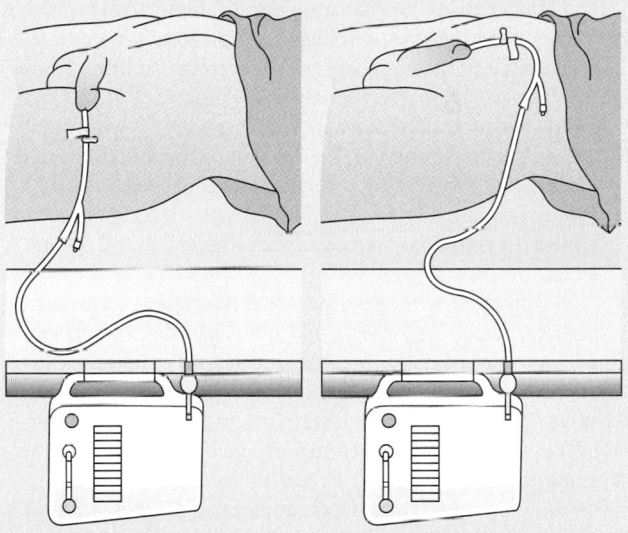

Action 11: Secure the catheter to the upper thigh or lower abdomen, allowing slack to prevent tension.

Special consideration If resistance is met while inserting the catheter and rotating the catheter does not help, do not use force. Enlargement of the prostate gland is commonly seen in men over the 50 years. A special crook-tipped catheter called a coudé catheter may be required to maneuver past the prostate gland.

Lubricant applied externally to the catheter remains at the meatus, essentially allowing an unlubricated catheter to cause trauma to the lining of the urethra. Currently, the recommendation is to gently insert the tip of a syringe prefilled with lubricant into the male urethra before inserting the catheter (see Skill 43-3). If the prepackaged kit does not contain a syringe with lubricant, the nurse may need assistance in filling a syringe while keeping the lubricant sterile. Some institutions use lidocaine jelly for lubrication prior to insertion of the catheter. The jelly comes prepackaged in a sterile syringe and serves a dual purpose of lubricating and numbing the urethra. A physician's order is necessary for the use of lidocaine jelly.

Once inserted, the indwelling catheter is connected to a drainage and collection system that must be properly posi-

tioned and secured to minimize the risk for infection. The following technique is used to complete the closed urinary drainage system:

- Check to see that the patient is not lying on the drainage tubing and compressing it.
- Keep the catheter drainage bag below the level of the bladder at all times.
- Keep the drainage bag off the floor at all times to reduce the risk of infection. The floor is grossly contaminated!
- Check that all connections are secure and that no leakage is occurring.

An indwelling catheter must be properly secured to prevent injury or friction (see Skills 43-2 and 43-3 for appropriate methods).

Through the Eyes of a Student

Remembering my first hospital experiences, I would have to say that doing my first catheterization was the scariest. I was working with a nurse on the maternity floor. Our patient had not voided in more than 8 hours and seemed to be in great discomfort. We palpated her abdomen to see if her bladder was distended, and it was. Because she didn't have an urge to void, we decided to straight cath her to lessen her discomfort. The nurse I was working with turned and handed me the kit. She said, "You know what to do, right?" Automatically I replied, "Sure."

My heart began to race. Of course I knew the procedure, but I never actually did it on a real person. Not only was I nervous about doing the procedure, but I also didn't want to make her labor more painful. The nurse, out of courtesy, asked the patient if she minded if I did the procedure. Thank God the patient had a soft side for a beginner. Smiling, she looked at me and said, "You know what you're doing, right?" Again I said, "Sure." I began setting up to begin my mission. To my amazement, I really did remember how to prepare for a catheterization. I even was amazed that my sterile procedure wasn't bad for the first time. When it was time to insert the catheter, I took a deep breath. Thankfully, it went in nice and smooth, and I reached the bladder in seconds. The urine began flowing through rapidly. It seemed like it would never stop. Amazingly, it filled the container. I removed the catheter, cleaned up, and let out my breath.

In summary, I was glad that I had the experience to do a catheterization. The nurse told me that I did a good job, which made me feel good. Also, my patient thanked me for relieving some of her discomfort and gave me a reassuring smile. As I look back now, it wasn't as bad as I had myself believed it would be. Even though it's invasive to the patient, sometimes it's necessary. I want to do everything I can to help my patients. Now, I look at all my new adventures as helping my patients feel better.

—Alysia Paxson,
Holy Family College, Philadelphia

Irrigating the Indwelling Catheter or Bladder

The flushing of a tube, canal, or area with solution is called irrigation. The purpose of catheter irrigation is to restore or maintain its patency. A bladder irrigation rinses out the bladder and can also instill medication that acts directly on the bladder wall. Skill 43-4 describes how to irrigate an indwelling catheter using the closed system.

Continuous or frequent irrigations may be ordered when blood clots or other debris threaten to block the catheter. In the past, an open procedure was done routinely for almost all indwelling catheters, but because this is another means of introducing pathogens, the closed system is now recommended. Natural irrigation of the catheter through increased fluid intake by the patient is preferred.

Preferably, the patient who needs frequent irrigation so that the catheter and tubing remain patent will have a triple-lumen catheter using continuous irrigation (Fig. 43-12). Skill 43-5 describes continuous bladder irrigation.

Caring for Patients With an Indwelling Catheter

The following are nursing measures used to care for patients with an indwelling catheter:

- Wash hands before and after caring for a patient with an indwelling catheter, and wear gloves and goggles to protect against exposure to blood and body fluids.
- Clean the perineal area thoroughly, especially around the meatus, daily and after each bowel movement.
- Cleanse the catheter by cleaning gently from the meatus outward.
- Use mild soap and water or a perineal cleanser to clean the perineal area; rinse the area well. Do not use powders and lotions after cleaning.
- Make sure that the patient maintains a generous fluid intake. This helps prevent infection and irrigates the catheter naturally by increasing urine output.
- Encourage the patient to be up and about, as ordered.
- Note the volume and character of urine, and record observations carefully. The urine can be observed through the drainage tubing and in the collecting container. The usual procedure is to note and record the amount of urine on the patient's intake-and-output record every 8 hours. The collecting container is calibrated, but the volume markings are only approximations. The urine should be emptied into a graduated container that is accurately calibrated for correct determination of output.
- Do not open the drainage system to obtain urine specimens or to measure urine. If the tubing becomes disconnected, wipe the ends of both tubes with antiseptic solution before reconnecting them. When emptying the drainage bag, make sure the drainage spout does not touch a contaminated surface.
- Teach the patient the importance of personal hygiene, especially the importance of careful cleaning after having a bowel movement and thorough, frequent hand hygiene.
- Promptly report any signs or symptoms of infection. These include a burning sensation and irritation at the meatus, cloudy urine, a strong odor to the urine, an elevated temperature, and chills.
- Help keep the urine acidic, because acidity retards bacterial growth. As mentioned earlier, plain water in increased amounts and cranberry juice are helpful for acidifying urine.
- Help the patient take a tub or shower bath when permitted. Clamp the catheter temporarily if the collecting container is higher than the bladder at any time. In a tub, with the catheter clamped, the container can be hung over the side of the tub. Take care that the catheter does not remain clamped after the bath. In a shower, the catheter can be attached to a smaller urinary drainage bag that can be secured to the patient's leg, in which case clamping the tube is usually unnecessary.
- Change indwelling catheters only as necessary. If rolling the drainage tubing between the hands frees the tubing of sandy

Research in Nursing Making a Difference

Ensuring a Safe Catheter Placement in the Male

Many aspects of nursing care rely on tradition and internship-type clinical learning. Unfortunately, this can be a disadvantage at times. When asked how far they insert a urinary catheter for males, many nurses reply, "I advance until I get urine, then another 1 to 2 inches." Studies have now shown that this is not an appropriate technique to use. Many times the catheter balloon is still in the urethra when it is inflated. Because of the male anatomy, urine can return even when the tip of the catheter is well below the external sphincter.

using fluoroscopy. Placement of the catheter was checked at 6″ and 8″ from the meatus with penis on full stretch and relaxed and completely on insertion to the bifurcation. Ten subjects were used, ranging in age from 33 to 80 years old. None of the catheters were noted to be fully in the bladder at 6″ or 8″ relaxed or stretched. All of the catheters were noted to be fully into the bladder when inserted to the bifurcation. There was no significant difference in penis length between the subjects of the study.

Related Research

Daneshgari, F., Krugman, M., Bahn, A., & Lee, R. (2002). Evidence-based multidisciplinary practice: Improving the safety and standards of male bladder catheterization. *MedSurg Nursing*, *11*(5), 236–242.

All patients had urinary catheters placed with fluoroscopy. As the catheters were inserted, catheter tip placement was checked

Relevance to Nursing Practice

To prevent urethral tears in the male population requiring indwelling urinary catheter insertion, all indwelling urinary catheters should be inserted to the bifurcation. This is an example of where evidence-based practice can save our patients from unnecessary pain.

SKILL 43-4 Irrigating the Catheter Using the Closed System

EQUIPMENT

Sterile basin or container
Gauze squares or cotton balls with disinfectant or alcohol swabs
Waterproof drape

30- to 50-mL syringe with 18- or 19-gauge needle
Sterile irrigating solution (at room temperature or warmed to body temperature)

Bath blanket
Disposable gloves

ACTION	RATIONALE
1. Assemble equipment. Perform hand hygiene. Explain the procedure and its purpose to the patient.	Organization facilitates performance of task. Hand hygiene deters spread of microorganisms. An explanation encourages patient cooperation and reduces apprehension.
2. Provide for privacy by closing the curtains or door and draping the patient with the bath blanket.	The procedure may be embarrassing for the patient.
3. Assist the patient to a comfortable position and expose the aspiration port on the catheter setup. Place the waterproof drape under the catheter and aspiration port.	This provides for adequate visualization. The drape protects the patient and the bed from leakage.
4. Open the sterile supplies. Pour sterile solution into the sterile basin. Aspirate irrigant (30 to 50 mL) into the sterile syringe and attach the capped sterile needle. Don gloves.	This prevents the spread of microorganisms and contact with blood or body fluids.
5. Wipe the aspiration port with alcohol swabs or gauze square with antiseptic solution.	This prevents the spread of microorganisms.
6. Clamp or fold the catheter tubing distal to the aspiration port.	This directs the irrigating solution into the bladder.
7. Remove the cap and insert the needle into the port. Gently instill solution into the catheter.	Gentle irrigation prevents damage to the lining of the bladder.
8. Remove the needle from the port. Unclamp or unfold the tubing and allow irrigant and urine to drain. Repeat the procedure as necessary.	Gravity aids drainage of urine and irrigant from the bladder.
9. Assess the patient's response to the procedure and the quality and amount of drainage. Document on the patient's chart.	This provides accurate documentation of the procedure.
10. Remove equipment and discard uncapped needle and syringe in appropriate receptacle. Remove gloves and perform hand hygiene. Make patient comfortable.	Hand hygiene deters the spread of microorganisms. Proper disposal of needle prevents the nurse accidentally puncturing self.
11. Record the amount of irrigant used on the intake and output record. Subtract this from the urine output when totaled.	Subtracting irrigant total from drainage in urine collection bag provides accurate recording of urine output.

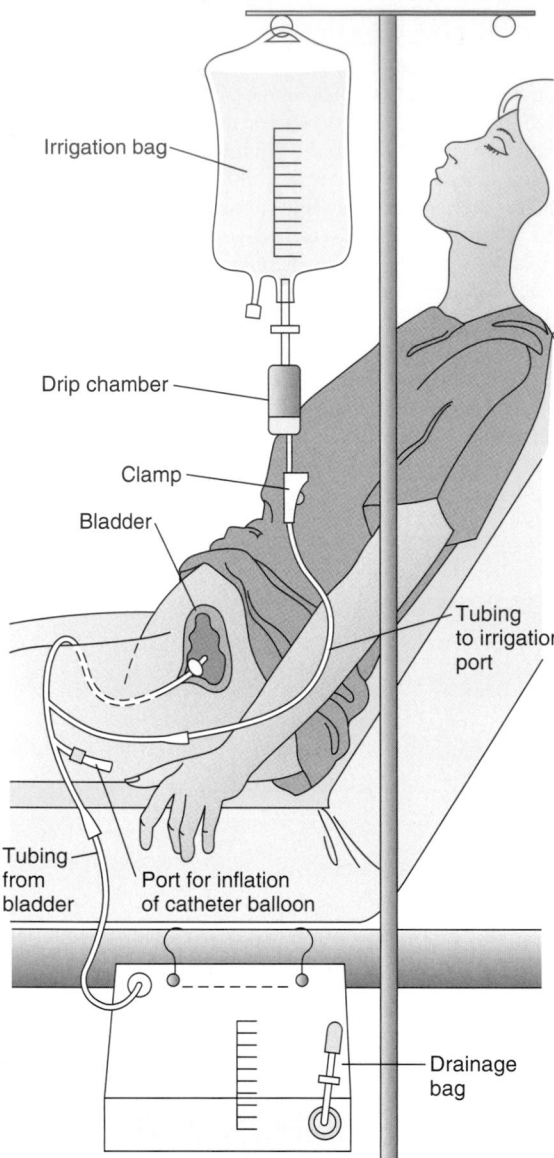

FIGURE 43-12 A continuous bladder irrigation (CBI) setup.

Labels in figure: Irrigation bag; Drip chamber; Clamp; Bladder; Tubing to irrigation port; Tubing from bladder; Port for inflation of catheter balloon; Drainage bag

particles, it is time to change the catheter. The interval between catheter changes varies and should be individualized for the patient. The less often a catheter is changed, the lower the likelihood of an infection developing.

Removing the Indwelling Catheter
The removal of an indwelling catheter and the aftercare of the patient should include the following nursing measures:
- Wash hands before and after the procedure, and wear gloves.
- Be sure the balloon is deflated before attempting to remove the catheter. This is done by inserting a syringe into the balloon valve and aspirating the fluid used to inflate the balloon. Always verify the size of the balloon, which is printed either on the catheter or documented in the chart, so that you know how much fluid to remove before proceeding. Do not cut the tubing with scissors.

- Ask the patient to take several deep breaths to relax while you gently remove the catheter. Wrap the catheter in a towel or disposable waterproof drape.
- Clean the perineal area after the catheter is removed.
- Ensure that the patient's fluid intake is generous, and record the patient's intake as well as time and amount of output for at least 24 hours or according to agency policy. Instruct the patient to void into the bedpan or urinal. If patient does not void within 8 hours of removal of the indwelling catheter, notify the physician promptly.
- Inform the patient that it may take a little while for the bladder to reestablish voluntary control and that an accident now is not unusual.
- Tell the patient that there may be a slight burning sensation when voiding the first one or two times after catheter removal.
- Observe the urine carefully for any abnormalities.
- Record and report any unusual signs or symptoms, such as discomfort, a burning sensation when voiding, bleeding, or changes in vital signs, especially the patient's temperature. Be alert to any signs or symptoms of infection, and report them promptly.

The current standard technique for catheter removal is under investigation by clinicians. Some believe that a totally deflated, wrinkled balloon may cause urethral trauma. A recommendation to wait 30 to 60 seconds after deflating the balloon and then to instill 0.5 to 1 mL of water into the balloon before removing it is a subject of research. The hypothesis is that the addition of this small amount of fluid creates a smoother surface (Evans, 1999).

Patient Education
Teach patients who have an indwelling catheter how the system functions and how they can assist with their care. Teaching points include keeping the tubing free of kinks, maintaining a constant downward flow of urine, maintaining an adequate fluid intake, and promptly reporting any unusual symptoms.

If the patient is ambulatory, the indwelling catheter can be connected to a smaller drainage bag that can be secured to the lower leg. Instructions for patients who use this apparatus include the following:
- Empty the leg bag at regular intervals. A full drainage bag may cause reflux of urine into the bladder or may pull away from its attachment on the leg.
- Wash hands before and after emptying the leg bag. Use an antiseptic solution to cleanse the connections.
- Disinfect the leg bag at regular intervals with a chlorine solution consisting of 2 oz bleach mixed with 5 oz water (Evans, 1999).

Condom Catheters
When voluntary control of urination is not possible for male patients, an alternative to an indwelling catheter is the **condom catheter.** This soft, pliable device made of plastic or rubberized material is applied externally to the penis. It is connected to tubing and a leg bag during the day and a drainage bag

SKILL 43-5 Administering a Continuous Bladder Irrigation

EQUIPMENT

Sterile irrigating solution (at room temperature or warmed to body temperature), usually 200-mL bags

Sterile tubing with drip chamber and clamp for connection to irrigating solution

IV pole

Three-way Foley catheter in place in patient's bladder

Foley drainage setup (tubing and collection bag)

Bath blanket

Disposable gloves

ACTION	RATIONALE
1. Explain the procedure and its purpose to the patient.	An explanation encourages patient cooperation and reduces apprehension.
2. Assemble the equipment.	Organization facilitates performance of tasks.
3. Perform hand hygiene.	Hand hygiene deters the spread of microorganisms.
4. Provide for privacy by closing the curtains or door and draping the patient with the bath blanket.	The procedure may be embarrassing for the patient.
5. Prepare the sterile irrigation bag for use as directed by the manufacturer. Secure the clamp and attach the sterile tubing with drip chamber to the container. Hang the bag on IV pole 2½ to 3 feet above the level of the patient's bladder. Release the clamp and remove the protective cover on the end of the tubing without contaminating it. Allow the solution to flush the tubing and remove air. Reclamp.	Irrigation solution continuously bathes the lining of the bladder and keeps the catheter patent. Flushing the tubing before irrigation clears air from the tubing that might cause bladder distention.
6. Using sterile technique, attach the irrigation tubing to the irrigation port of the three-way Foley catheter. If a closed system is used, tubing may already be connected to the irrigation port on the catheter.	Sterile technique prevents the spread of microorganisms into the bladder.

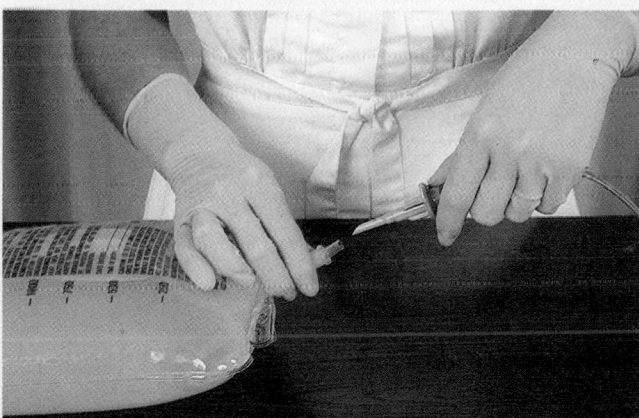

Action 5: Inserting spike into container of irrigating solution.

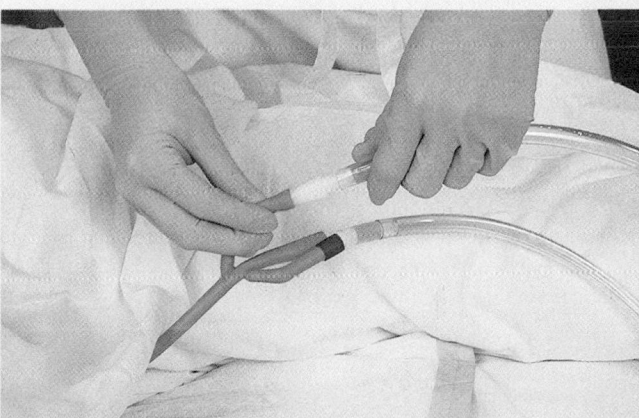

Action 6: Attaching irrigation tubing to irrigation port of three-way Foley catheter using sterile technique.

7. Release the clamp on the irrigation tubing and regulate the flow according to the physician's order.	This allows for continual gentle irrigation without causing discomfort to the patient.
8. As irrigation is completed, clamp the tubing. Do not allow the drip chamber to empty. Disconnect the empty bag and attach a full irrigation bag. Continue as ordered by the physician.	This eliminates the need to separate tubing from the catheter and clear air from the tubing. Opening the drainage system provides access for introduction of microorganisms.
9. Assess the patient's response to the procedure and the quality and amount of drainage. Document on the patient's chart.	This provides accurate documentation of the procedure.
10. Record the amount of irrigant used on the intake and output record. Don gloves and empty the drainage collection bag as each new container is hung and record.	This ensures accurate recording of urine output. Gloves protect against exposure to blood, body fluids, and microorganisms.
11. Perform hand hygiene.	Hand hygiene deters the spread of microorganisms.

at night, thus allowing the patient to be dressed and to participate in activities without problems.

> *Think back to Ida Fleming, the woman described at the beginning of the chapter who is caring for her husband at home. The nurse might anticipate using a condom catheter for Mrs. Fleming's husband as a possible alternative rather an indwelling catheter, which would increase his risk for infection.*

Steps for applying a condom catheter are described in Skill 43-6.

Nursing care of a patient with a condom catheter includes vigilant skin care to prevent excoriation. Remove the condom daily and wash the penis with soap and water, dry it carefully, and inspect the skin for irritation. Always follow the manufacturer's instructions for applying the condom because there are several variations. In all cases, care must be taken to fasten the condom securely enough to prevent leakage, yet not so tightly as to constrict the blood vessels in the area. Self-

SKILL 43-6 Applying a Condom Catheter

EQUIPMENT
Condom sheath in appropriate size
Basin of warm water and soap
Washcloth and towel

Bath blanket
Disposable gloves (optional)
Elastic strip or Velcro strap (optional)

Reusable leg bag with drainage
tubing or urinary drainage setup

ACTION	RATIONALE
1. Explain the procedure to the patient. Ask if the patient is aware of any allergy to latex.	This provides reassurance and promotes patient cooperation. If the patient is allergic to latex, a latex-free condom catheter must be used.
2. Assemble the equipment. Prepare urinary drainage setup or reusable leg bag for attachment to the condom sheath.	This provides for an organized approach to the task.
3. Perform hand hygiene.	Hand hygiene deters the spread of microorganisms.
4. Assist the patient to the supine position. Close the curtain or door. Use the bath blanket and sheet to expose only the patient's genital area.	This provides privacy for the patient.
5. Don disposable gloves. Trim any long pubic hairs that are in contact with the penis	Trimming pubic hairs prevents any unnecessary pulling of hair by adhesive without risk of infection associated with shaving.
6. Wash the genital area with soap and water, rinse, and dry thoroughly. If uncircumsized, retract foreskin and clean. Replace foreskin.	Washing removes urine, secretions, and microorganisms. The penis must be clean and dry to minimize skin irritation.
7. Roll the condom sheath outward onto itself. Grasp the penis firmly with your nondominant hand. Apply the condom sheath by rolling it onto the penis with your dominant hand. Leave 2.5- to 5-cm (1- to 2-inch) space between the tip of the penis and the end of the condom sheath.	Rolling the condom sheath outward allows for easier application. The space prevents irritation to the tip of the penis and allows for free drainage of urine.

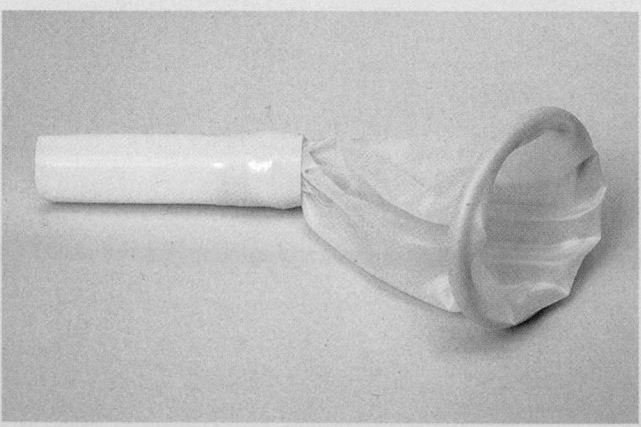

Condom sheath.

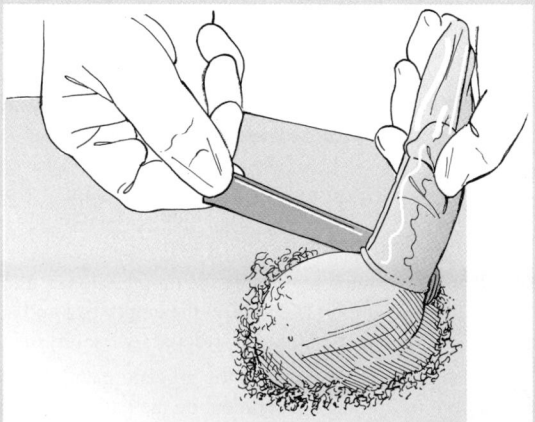

Action 7: Application of a Velcro strap at the base of the condom sheath.

(continued)

SKILL 43-6   Applying a Condom Catheter (continued)

ACTION	RATIONALE
8. Apply the elastic or Velcro strap snugly but not too tightly. Do not allow the elastic or Velcro to come in contact with the skin.	The elastic or Velcro strap should secure the condom sheath but not interfere with blood circulation to the penis.
9. Connect the condom sheath to the drainage setup. Avoid kinking or twisting of the drainage tubing.	The collection device keeps the patient dry. Kinked tubing encourages backflow of urine.
10. Remove the equipment. Place the patient in a comfortable, safe position. Perform hand hygiene.	This provides a safe, comfortable setting for the patient. Hand hygiene deters the spread of microorganisms.
11. Assess the patient's response and record observations on the patient's chart.	This provides accurate documentation and observation of urine output.

adhesive condom catheters are also available. The tip of the tubing should be kept 1″ to 2″ (2.5 to 5 cm) beyond the tip of the penis to prevent irritation to the sensitive glans area. Maintaining free urinary drainage is another nursing priority. Institute measures to prevent the tubing from becoming kinked and urine from backing up in the tubing. Urine can lead to excoriation of the glans, so position the tubing that collects the urine from the condom to draw urine away from the penis.

For some men, the condom catheter may not be an option because of penis retraction. For these patients, the retracted penis pouch may be appropriate. This is a baglike appliance in which the penis is placed. The pouch can then be connected to a leg bag.

Assisting With Urinary Diversions

Obstructions or tumors in the urinary tract may require some patients to have urinary flow diverted surgically. An **ileal conduit** is a surgical diversion of the ureters to the ileum rather than the bladder. This separated section of the small intestine is then brought to the abdominal wall, where urine is excreted through a stoma, a surgically created opening on the body surface. Figure 43-13 shows how the ureters are diverted in an ileal conduit. Such diversions are usually permanent, and the patient wears an external appliance to collect the urine because elimination of the urine from the stoma cannot be voluntarily controlled.

Patients with an ileal conduit must adapt to an altered body image and usually need assistance in coping. The time required for adaptation varies. The adjustment can often be assisted with the support of family, friends, nurses, physicians, and people with a similar health problem. Most of all, the patient needs to understand that an active, useful life is compatible with a urinary diversion.

Another option is a continent urostomy (eg, the Kock continent ileal reservoir). This is a surgical alternative that creates, from a section of the intestines, an internal reservoir that holds urine. The external stoma or outlet must be catheterized at regular intervals to drain the urine that has collected in this reservoir.

Another type of surgical intervention is the Mitrofanoff procedure, in which a tract is formed surgically from the umbilicus to the bladder by using the appendix. The patient must intermittently catheterize the bladder via the umbilicus. This allows patients who normally could not intermittently catheterize themselves through the urethra to provide self-care or decrease the embarrassment of having a second person perform the catheterization.

Appliances to Collect Urine

With a urinary diversion, the external appliance to collect the urine is typically a soft rubber or plastic pouch that is either reusable or disposable. The upper part of the pouch has a firm

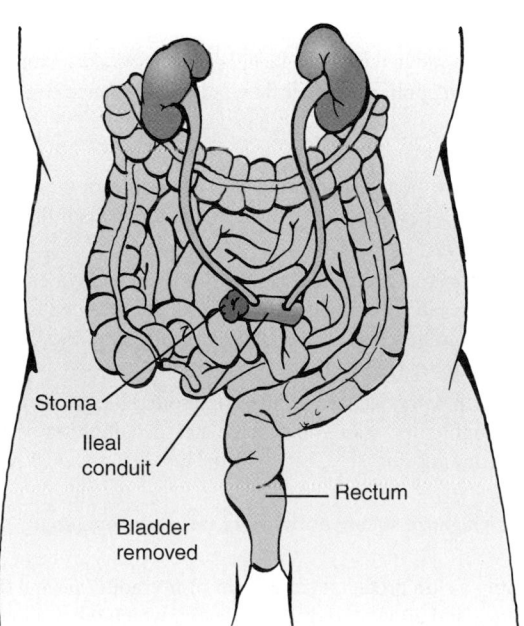

FIGURE 43-13 Location of an ileal conduit. The ureters are brought to the ileum of the small intestine and a stoma is made where the urine is excreted. (Redrawn after *Types of Ostomies.* Copyright 2000. Hollister Inc. All rights reserved.)

faceplate several inches in diameter, with an opening the size of the stoma. Some faceplates are detachable from the pouch. The plate surface is firmly secured around the stoma opening with a moisture-proof adherent so that no urine leakage occurs. Many patients also wear an elasticized belt around the waist for added support. The lower end of the pouch may have a drainage valve, which is used for emptying.

The patient needs to empty the pouch before it becomes heavy with the weight of urine, which might cause the seal to loosen. For most people, this means emptying the appliance several times a day. Urine-collection receptacles designed to be placed under the bed can be used at night.

Urinary Appliance Application and Removal

The frequency of changing the appliance depends on the type being used. The appliance usually is changed after a time of low fluid intake, such as in the early morning. Urine production is less at this time, making changing the appliance easier. Skill 43-7 describes how to change an appliance worn over an ileal conduit.

SKILL
43-7

Changing a Stoma Appliance on an Ileal Conduit

EQUIPMENT

Basin with warm water, soap, towel, washcloth or cotton balls
Graduated container
Skin protectant or barrier

Sterile 2″ × 2″ gauze squares
Ostomy bag cut to the correct stomal size (with adhesive-backed faceplate, if available)

Ostomy belt (optional)
Adhesive cement (optional for reusable pouches)
Disposable gloves

ACTION	RATIONALE
1. Explain the procedure and encourage the patient to observe or participate if possible. Provide for privacy.	Observing or assisting with procedure encourages self-acceptance.
2. Assemble the equipment.	Organization facilitates performance of task.
3. Perform hand hygiene and don disposable gloves.	Hand hygiene deters the spread of microorganisms. Gloves protect the nurse from blood, body fluids, and microorganisms.
4. Have the patient sit or stand if able to assist with procedure or assume supine position in bed.	These positions result in less abdominal folds and facilitate removal and application of the device.
5. Empty the pouch being worn into the graduated container (before removing if it is reusable and not attached to straight drainage).	Having the pouch empty before handling it reduces the likelihood of spilling the excretions. The physician may have ordered recording of intake and output.
6. Gently remove the pouch faceplate from the skin by pushing skin from appliance rather than pulling appliance from skin.	The seal between the surface of the faceplate and the skin must be broken before the faceplate can be removed. Harsh handling of the appliance can damage the skin and impair the development of a secure seal in the future.
7. Discard the pouch appropriately if disposable, or wash reusable pouch in lukewarm soap and water and allow to air dry.	Thorough cleaning and airing of the appliance reduce odor and deterioration. For aesthetic and infection-control purposes, used appliances should be discarded appropriately.
8. Clean the skin around the stoma with soap and water or a commercial cleaner using a washcloth or cotton balls. Make sure you remove all of old adhesive from the skin. An adhesive remover may be used.	Cleaning the skin removes excretions and old adhesive and skin protectant. Excretions or a buildup of other substances can irritate and damage the skin.
9. Gently pat dry. Make sure the skin around the stoma is thoroughly dry. Assess the stoma and the condition of the surrounding skin.	Careful drying prevents trauma to the skin and stoma. An intact, properly applied urinary collection device protects skin integrity. Any change in the color and size of the stoma may indicate circulatory problems.
10. Place a gauze square or two over the stoma opening.	Continuous drainage must be absorbed to keep the skin dry during the appliance change.
11. Apply a skin protectant to a 5-cm (2-in) radius around the stoma, and allow it to dry completely, which takes about 30 seconds.	The skin needs protection from the excoriating effect of the excretion and appliance adhesive. Allowing the protectant to dry completely enhances its effectiveness.

(continued)

Changing a Stoma Appliance on an Ileal Conduit (continued)

ACTION	RATIONALE
12. If necessary, enlarge the size of the faceplate opening to fit the stoma.	The appliance should fit snugly around the stoma, with only ¹⁄₁₆ to ⅛ inch of skin visible around the opening. A faceplate opening that is too small can cause trauma to the stoma. Exposed skin will be irritated by urine if the opening is too large.
13. Apply adhesive to the faceplate or remove the protective covering from the disposable faceplate, carefully position the appliance, and press it in place, moving from the center outward. Remove the gauze squares from the stoma before applying the pouch.	The appliance is effective only if it is properly positioned and securely adhered. Commercial deodorants may be used if odor is a problem.
14. Secure the optional belt to the appliance and around the patient.	An elasticized belt helps support the appliance for some people.
15. Remove or discard the equipment and assess the patient's response to the procedure. Perform hand hygiene and remove gloves.	The patient's response may indicate acceptance of the ostomy as well as the need for health teaching. Hand hygiene deters the spread of microorganisms.
16. Record the appearance of the stoma and the surrounding skin as well as the patient's reaction to the procedure.	A careful record is important for planning the patient's care.

Patient Education

Nursing care includes patient education for the achievement of optimal self-care. As the patient assumes responsibility for self-care, he or she should be taught to make the necessary observations, to be aware of indications of problems, and to recognize when to seek assistance. For these goals to be met, the patient needs to be able to do the following:

- Explain the reason for the urinary diversion and the rationale for treatment.
- Demonstrate self-care behaviors that effectively manage the diversion.
- Describe follow-up care and existing support resources.
- Report where supplies may be obtained in the community.
- Verbalize related fears and concerns.
- Demonstrate a positive body image.

The assistance of a Wound, Ostomy, and Continence nurse can help the patient achieve these outcomes. The patient may also be referred to the United Ostomy Association for further information and helpful periodicals. Detailed discussion of other aspects of caring for a patient with a urinary diversion can be found in clinical texts.

Evaluating

The nurse evaluates the effectiveness of a plan of care to promote healthy urinary functioning by checking whether the patient has met the individualized patient goals specified in the plan. Nursing care is considered effective if the patient expresses satisfaction with the regular voiding pattern and is able to achieve the following:

- Produce a sufficient quantity of urine to maintain fluid, electrolyte, and acid–base balance
- Empty the bladder completely at regular intervals without discomfort
- Provide care for urinary diversion and know when to notify the physician
- Develop a plan to modify any factors that contribute to current urinary problems or that might impair urinary functioning in the future
- Correct unhealthy urinary habits, such as delaying voiding, drinking insufficient fluids, or abusing diuretics

See the Nursing Plan of Care 43-1 for Mrs. Jaspers.

NURSING PLAN OF CARE 43-1   *for Elana Jaspers*

Mrs. Elana Jaspers is an alert, 83-year-old woman whose husband of 59 years died 6 months ago. Although Mrs. Jaspers was adamant about wanting to live independently in her own home, arthritis severely restricted her movement and ability to manage. After a hospitalization for pneumonia, she was transferred to a nursing home 1 month ago. The admitting medical diagnoses included hypertension, osteoarthritis, and depression. A comprehensive nursing assessment of Mrs. Jaspers performed 1 month after her admission to the nursing home included the following notations:

- Continent of urine on admission
- At present, incontinent of urine one or two times a day; often found wet in the morning; states it is "too much bother to get into the bathroom"
- Sits in chair in room unless encouraged and assisted to walk, although capable of independent ambulation with care; progressive muscle atrophy and joint stiffness
- No identifiable pathology underlying incontinence
- Medications include a diuretic for hypertension and a tricyclic antidepressant
- Reddened skin in the perineal area

NURSING DIAGNOSIS   Functional Urinary Incontinence related to difficult transition to nursing home and mobility deficit as manifested by incontinence of urine one or two times a day; feeling toileting is too much bother; mobility deficits secondary to osteoarthritis; taking a diuretic and antidepressant.

EXPECTED OUTCOME   By the next monthly assessment, 5/1/06, the patient will:
- Verbalize the importance of getting to bathroom or toilet when she first feels the need to void.

Nursing Interventions	Rationale	Evaluative Statement
Assess the value the patient attaches to voluntary control of urination and urinary continence; counsel appropriately.	Unless the patient is committed to the plan of care, goal achievement is impossible.	5/1/06 Outcome partially met. Patient has commented on the importance of regular toileting but still finds this "too much trouble" some days.
Teach the importance of complete bladder emptying at regular intervals and the harmful effects of ignoring the urge to void.	Patient understanding of the causes and harmful effects of urinary incontinence may motivate desire for reestablishment of voluntary control.	*Revision:* Reinforce value. *D. Mora, RN*
Assess patient's normal voiding habits at home and assist her to reestablish these. Initial reminders to toilet herself may be necessary.	Respect for the patient's normal voiding schedule and patterns communicates nursing's sincere concern for the individual and encourages patient achievement of goals.	

EXPECTED OUTCOME   By the next monthly assessment, 5/1/06, the patient will:
- Demonstrate the ability to walk to the bathroom using cane to toilet herself.

Nursing Interventions	Rationale	Evaluative Statement
Assess the patient's ability to toilet herself independently. Work consistently with her to increase activity tolerance: encourage short walks throughout the day to increase mobility.	One response to experiencing the multiple losses associated with aging is to surrender all control and become increasingly dependent. Non–pathology-based incontinence is less likely to occur if the daily living of the person keeps her more mobile, flexible, oriented, and motivated. An older person who seeks to take control and has a positive self-image is more continent.	5/1/06 Outcome met. Patient can safely walk to bathroom using cane and toilet herself when she wants to. *D. Mora, RN*
Refer patient to occupational therapy for assistance with diagnosis and treatment if necessary.		

(continued)

NURSING PLAN OF CARE 43-1

for Elana Jaspers (continued)

Nursing Interventions	Rationale	Evaluative Statement
Communicate clearly that the patient is expected to use the toilet to urinate. Refrain from using incontinent briefs or pads. Talk with family about patient's having sufficient undergarments to allow changes as needed until control is reestablished. Assess patient's motivation and ability to be clean, dry, and comfortable. Teach perineal hygiene.	The specialized skills of the occupational therapist may facilitate relearning toileting skills. Understanding that the staff expects continence and is committed to working with the patient to achieve it is a powerful patient motivator. Patient may not understand how easily skin irritation can occur and danger of pressure ulcers. Keeping the perineal area clean and dry promotes intact skin around the urinary meatus and the perineal area. Proper hygiene measures also decrease the possibility of bacteria or organisms migrating into the bladder.	5/1/06 Outcome not met. Patient repeatedly neglects a.m. perineal care. *Revision:* Reteach both the importance and procedure of perineal care. Assess each a.m. *D. Mora, RN*

EXPECTED OUTCOME

By the next monthly assessment, 5/1/06, the patient will:
• Decrease urinary incontinent episodes to less than three or four per week

Nursing Interventions	Rationale	Evaluative Statement
Communicate to patient that the nurses *care* about her reestablishing urinary continence and believe she can do this. Use verbal reinforcement to reward "dry" days. Chart incontinent episodes and monitor progress; discuss this with patient.	A common feeling of recently institutionalized elderly people is *abandonment* and the sense that no one cares; response: "Why should I?" Communicating that the patient's progress toward goal achievement is valued by the nurses is an excellent encouragement to continue progress. This records progress with incontinent episodes and provides positive reinforcement.	5/1/06 Outcome met. Patient in last week was completely dry for 4 of 7 days. Recorded four incontinent episodes. *D. Mora, RN*

NURSING DIAGNOSIS

Impaired Skin Integrity related to functional urinary incontinence as manifested by reddened perineal area (skin still intact)

EXPECTED OUTCOME

By the next monthly assessment, 5/1/06, the patient will:
• Demonstrate healing of reddened perineal area

Nursing Interventions	Rationale	Evaluative Statement
Assess skin for breakdown each a.m. and p.m. and after each incontinent episode.	Perineal care is often neglected or assigned to the least trained personnel in care settings. Skin irritation not detected and treated early may progress to serious pressure ulcers.	5/1/06 Outcome partially met. Perineal area is less inflamed. *Revision:* Continue to monitor perineal hygiene. No need for protective ointment. *D. Mora, RN*

(continued)

NURSING PLAN OF CARE 43-1

for Elana Jaspers (continued)

Nursing Interventions	Rationale	Evaluative Statement
Teach the patient the importance of washing this area carefully with soap and water each a.m. and after incontinent episodes. Teach the importance of always cleaning and wiping the perineum from front to back to prevent autoinfection. Until incontinent episodes are eliminated, a protective waterproof ointment may be indicated.	The woman who is doing self-care may neglect it entirely or use incorrect technique.	
Encourage use of cotton underwear and avoidance of nylon pantyhose, girdles, tight-fitting pants.	Nylon products tend to hold moisture and may minimize airflow to the perineal area.	

SAMPLE DOCUMENTATION

4/3/06   Nursing

This a.m., after an incontinent episode, Mrs. Jaspers began to talk about how hard it is to get adjusted to living here, and commented, "I feel like just giving up." We talked about the importance of being as independent as possible and the dangers of becoming passively dependent. Nursing teaching and counseling included values of independently adhering to usual toileting schedule and importance of perineal hygiene. Two hours later, after lunch, Mrs. Jaspers walked to bathroom and toileted herself. Progress with urinary incontinence will continue to be monitored. Ability definitely present but encouragement needed.

D. Mora, RN

■ Developing Critical Thinking Skills

1. The daughter of an older patient who is about to be discharged to the daughter's home requests that a catheter be inserted in her mother to make home care easier. The mother knows when she needs to void but needs assistance to get to the bathroom. How do you respond to the daughter's request?
2. If you noted the following when assessing a patient, what would you do?
   - A 6-year-old refuses to give a urine sample.
   - Frank blood appears in urine of a patient who has no history of urinary problems.
   - When you ask for a urine sample, a teenager asks, "This won't reveal drugs, will it?"
   - A young woman complains of painful urination with burning.
   - An older man reports frequency and pain when voiding.

■ Practicing for NCLEX

1. When collecting a urine specimen for routine urinalysis from a patient, the nurse keeps in mind which of the following?

a. A sterile specimen is required for collection.
b. Leaving the sample standing at room temperature for a prolonged period may alter the urine chemistry.
c. The external meatus requires cleaning with antiseptic soap and water before voiding.
d. A clean-catch midstream specimen is necessary.

2. Which of the following would the nurse incorporate into the teaching plan for a patient to promote healthy urinary functioning?

a. Drinking more than 2,000 mL of fluid per day will cause fluid retention.
b. The healthy adult should drink four to six 8-ounce glasses of water per day.
c. Because of greater thirst sensitivity, children drink required amounts of fluid without being reminded.
d. Caffeine-containing beverages should be monitored to prevent excess intake.

3. When a person has a fever or diaphoresis, the urine output will be which of the following?

a. Decreased and highly concentrated
b. Decreased and highly dilute
c. Increased and concentrated
d. Increased and dilute

4. The physician has ordered an indwelling catheter inserted in a hospitalized male patient. The nurse is aware that:
   a. The male urethra is more vulnerable to injury during insertion.
   b. Normally a clean technique is required for catheter insertion.
   c. The catheter is inserted 2″ to 3″ into the meatus.
   d. Smaller catheters are usually necessary because of the size of the urethra.

5. Nursing care for a patient with an indwelling catheter includes which of the following?
   a. Irrigation of the catheter with 30 mL of normal saline solution every 4 hours
   b. Disconnecting and reconnecting the drainage system quickly to obtain a urine specimen
   c. Encouraging a generous fluid intake if permitted
   d. Informing the patient that burning and irritation at the meatus are normal, subsiding within a few days

6. After surgery, Ms. Young is having difficulty voiding. Which nursing action would most likely lead to an increased difficulty with voiding rather than stimulation of voiding?
   a. Pouring warm water over Ms. Young's fingers
   b. Having Ms. Young ignore the urge to void until her bladder is full
   c. Using a warm bedpan when Ms. Young feels the urge to void
   d. Stroking Ms. Young's leg or thigh

7. Mr. Cheng, a hospitalized patient with diabetes mellitus, has developed a UTI. He is 80 years old and has an indwelling catheter in place. Which factor is most likely the cause of his UTI?
   a. The close proximity of the male genitalia to the rectum
   b. Decreased immunity
   c. A high urine glucose level
   d. The indwelling urinary catheter

8. Which of the following terms denotes a patient's inability to void even though the kidneys are producing urine that enters the bladder?
   a. Urgency
   b. Retention
   c. Oliguria
   d. Dysuria

9. Mrs. D'Ambrosia, an alert, ambulatory, older nursing home resident, voids frequently and has difficulty making it to the bathroom in time. The nurse planning her care is aware that:
   a. Incontinence is to be expected in a woman Mrs. D'Ambrosia's age.
   b. One of every 10 nursing home residents is incontinent.
   c. Kegel exercises performed at regular intervals throughout the day may be helpful.

   d. An indwelling catheter should be inserted as soon as possible.

10. The priority treatment option for Mrs. D'Ambrosia would most likely involve:
    a. Behavioral techniques
    b. Pharmacologic measures
    c. Surgical intervention
    d. Use of absorbent products

11. A patient taking phenazopyridine (Pyridium, a urinary tract analgesic) should be cautioned that her urine color may change to:
    a. Pale yellow
    b. Green
    c. Orange-red
    d. Brown

12. Mr. Bales is 60 years old and alert. He is timid and reluctant to talk about his urinary retention problem. Which part of this plan could create stress for Mr. Bales and possibly increase his inability to urinate?
    a. Assisting him in assuming his normal voiding position
    b. Pulling curtains around him to provide privacy during voiding
    c. Staying with him while voiding
    d. Offering the urinal on a regular schedule

13. Which of the following is a nursing priority when caring for a male patient with a condom catheter?
    a. Preventing the tubing from kinking to maintain free urinary drainage
    b. Not removing the catheter for any reason
    c. Fastening the condom tightly to prevent the possibility of leakage
    d. Maintaining bed rest at all times to prevent the catheter from slipping off

14. If you read the nursing diagnosis Impaired Urinary Elimination related to maturational enuresis, you would recognize that your patient is which of the following?
    a. An adult older than 65 years of age who is incontinent
    b. A child older than 4 years of age who has involuntary urination
    c. A 12-month-old child who has involuntary urination
    d. A patient with neurologic damage resulting in bladder dysfunction

15. Data must be collected to evaluate the effectiveness of a plan to reduce urinary incontinence in an older adult patient. Of the information below, which is least important for the evaluation process?
    a. The incontinence pattern
    b. State of physical mobility
    c. Medications being taken
    d. Age of the patient

■ Answers With Rationale

1. The correct answer is *b*. Urine chemistry is altered after urine stands at room temperature for a long period of time. For a routine urinalysis, a clean specimen is adequate. The external meatus does not need to be cleaned with an antiseptic, as is required for a clean-catch midstream specimen.

2. The correct answer is *d*. Caffeine intake should be limited because it is irritating to the bladder mucosa. It is recommended that a healthy adult drink 8 to 10 8-oz glasses of fluid daily. Unless a disease process is present, this will not cause fluid retention. Children frequently need to be reminded to drink fluids.

3. The correct answer is *a*. Fever and diaphoresis cause the kidneys to conserve body fluids. Thus, the urine is concentrated and decreased in amount.

4. The correct answer is *a*. Because of its length, the male urethra is more prone to injury and requires that the catheter be inserted 6″ to 8″. This procedure requires surgical asepsis to prevent introducing bacteria into the urinary tract. Larger catheters are used for male catheterization.

5. The correct answer is *c*. A generous fluid intake promotes healthy urinary tract functioning. Irrigation may introduce bacteria into the urinary tract and is not routinely ordered. The drainage system should never be disconnected to obtain a specimen because this may allow bacteria to enter the urinary tract. Burning and irritation may indicate that an infection is present and should never be disregarded.

6. The correct answer is *b*. Ignoring the urge to void makes urination even more difficult and should be avoided. The other activities are all recommended nursing activities to promote voiding.

7. The correct answer is *d*. Most UTIs in hospitalized patients are caused by the presence of an indwelling catheter. Additional, although less significant, causes of UTI include a decrease in immunity common in elderly people and the presence of glucose in the urine, as seen in diabetes.

8. The correct answer is *b*. Urgency is a strong desire to void. Oliguria is scanty or a greatly diminished amount of urine voided in a given time. Dysuria is difficulty urinating.

9. The correct answer is *c*. Kegel exercises may help a patient regain control of the micturition process. Incontinence is not a normal consequence of aging, and at least half of nursing home residents may be incontinent. An indwelling catheter is the last choice of treatment.

10. The correct answer is *a*. The least invasive interventions should be attempted first. Pharmacologic and surgical interventions are not recommended until behavioral techniques have been attempted. Using absorbent products may remove motivation from the patient and caregiver to seek evaluation and treatment of the incontinence. They should be used only after careful evaluation by a healthcare provider.

11. The correct answer is *c*. Pyridium is noted for turning the urine orange-red, and the patient needs to be aware of this.

12. The correct answer is *c*. Mr. Bales will probably be embarrassed if the nurse remains with him as he attempts to void and is more likely to have difficulty voiding.

13. The correct answer is *a*. The catheter should be allowed to drain freely through tubing that is not kinked. It also should be removed daily to prevent skin excoriation and should not be fastened too tightly, or restriction of blood vessels in the area is likely. Confining a patient to bed rest increases the risk for other hazards related to immobility.

14. The correct answer is *b*. Maturational enuresis is involuntary urination after an age when continence should be present. A 12-month-old child is not expected to be continent, and incontinence and neurologic damage are not maturational problems.

15. The correct answer is *d*. Incontinence is not a natural consequence of the aging process. All the other factors are necessary information for the plan of care.

Bibliography

Blazys, D. (1999). Clinical nurses forum: Urinary catheterization. *Journal of Emergency Nursing, 25*(4), 300–301.

Burns, C., Brady, M., Dunn, A., et al. (2000). *Pediatric primary care: A handbook for nurse practitioners* (2nd ed.). Philadelphia: W. B. Saunders.

Daneshgari, F., Krugman, M., Bahn, A., & Lee, R. (2002). Evidence-based multidisciplinary practice: Improving the safety and standards of male bladder catheterization. *Med-Surg Nursing, 11*(5), 236–242.

Ekerdt, D. (Ed.). (2002). *Encyclopedia of aging* (Vol. 4, 1st ed., pp. 1441–1443). New York: Macmillan.

Evans, E. (1999). Indwelling catheter care: Dispelling the misconceptions. *Geriatric Nursing, 20*(2), 85–88.

Gray, M. (2000). Urinary retention: Management in the acute care setting. *American Journal of Nursing, 100*(7), 40–47.

Hanchett, M. (2002). Techniques for stabilizing urinary catheters: Tape may be the oldest method, but it's not the only one. *American Journal of Nursing, 102*(3), 44–48.

Johnson, S. (2000). From incontinence to confidence. *American Journal of Nursing, 100*(2), 69–75.

Kniest, K., & McGovern, P. (2002). Using the umbilicus for catheterization. *RN, 65*(8), 26–30.

Kolcaba, K., Dowd, T., Winslow, E., et al. (2000). Kegel exercises. *American Journal of Nursing, 100*(11), 59.

Langa, K., Fultz, N., Saint, S., et al. (2002). Informal caregiving time and costs for urinary incontinence in older individuals in the United States. *Journal of the American Geriatrics Society, 50*(4), 733–737.

Loughrey, L. (1999). Taking a sensitive approach to urinary incontinence. *Nursing, 29*(5), 60–61.

Lyons, S., & Specht, J. (2000). Prompted voiding protocol for individuals with urinary incontinence. *Journal of Gerontological Nursing, 26*(6), 5–13.

Maloney, C. (2002). Estrogen & recurrent UTI in postmenopausal women. *American Journal of Nursing, 102*(8), 44–53.

McCloskey, J., & Bulechek, J. (2000). *Nursing interventions classification* (NIC) (4th ed.). St. Louis: C. V. Mosby.

McConnell, E. (2001). Applying a condom catheter. *Nursing, 31*(1), 70.

Mouton, C., Bazaldua, O., Pierce, B., et al. (2001). Common infections in older adults. *American Family Physician, 63*(2), 257–268.

National Institute of Diabetes & Digestive & Kidney Disease. (2002). *Urinary incontinence in women.* Retrieved Dec. 26, 2002, from http://www.niddk.nih.gov/health/urolog/pubs/uiwomen/uiwomen.htm

Newman, D. (2003). Stress urinary incontinence in women. *American Journal of Nursing, 103*(8), 46–55.

North American Nursing Diagnosis Association. (2003). *NANDA nursing diagnoses: Definitions & classification, 2003–2004.* Philadelphia: Author.

Orenstein, R., & Wong, E. (1999). Urinary tract infections in adults. *American Academy of Family Physicians, 59*(5), 1225–1237.

Phipps, W., Sands, J., & Marek, J. (2003). *Medical-surgical nursing: Concepts & clinical practice* (7th ed.). St. Louis: C. V. Mosby.

Resnick, N. M. (1984). Urinary incontinence in the elderly. *Medical Grand Rounds 3:*281–290.

Shultz, J. (2002). Urinary incontinence: Solving a secret problem. *Nursing, 32*(11), 53–55.

Sienty, M., & Dawson, N. (1999). Preventing urosepsis from indwelling urinary catheters. *American Journal of Nursing, 99*(1), 24C—24H.

Slugg, A. (2000). A scanner can help restore continence in LTC patients. *RN, 63*(2), 16.

Smeltzer, S., & Bare, B. (2004). *Brunner & Suddarth's textbook of medical-surgical nursing* (10th ed.). Philadelphia: Lippincott Williams & Wilkins.

Smith, D. (1999). Gauging bladder volume. *Nursing, 29*(12), 52–53.

Stockert, P. (1999). Getting UTI patients back on track. *RN, 62*(3), 49–52.

Vapnek, J., Leipzig, R., & Edelberg, H. (2001). Urinary incontinence: Screening and treatment of urinary dysfunction. *Geriatrics, 56*(10), 25–30.

Wooldridge, L. (2000). Ultrasound technology and bladder dysfunction. *American Journal of Nursing,* June (suppl.), 3–14.

Wyman, J. (2000). Management of urinary incontinence in adult ambulatory care populations. *Annual Review of Nursing Research,* 171–194.

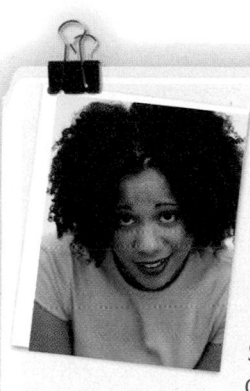

Sally Germaine, a college junior with Crohn's disease, has frequent episodes of diarrhea. "It's so embarrassing," she says. "Sometimes I don't make it fast enough to the bathroom. If I have one more accident in a public place, I think I'll die. Sometimes I think I should never go out in public again."

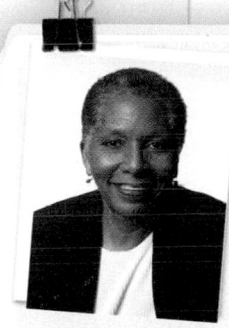

Alberta Franklin, age 55, has recently undergone abdominal surgery and creation of a sigmoid colostomy. Her stoma is bright red and moist and draining semi-soft brown stool. Her ostomy appliance needs to be changed.

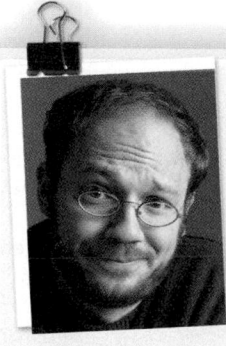

Leroy Cobbs, newly diagnosed with cancer, is taking acetaminophen (Tylenol) with codeine for pain. He is hospitalized for fecal impaction. "Nobody told me I would get so constipated," he says. "It's been almost a week and I'm still not moving my bowels normally. I didn't know anything could hurt so bad. I'll take my chances with the cancer pain in the future rather than take more pain meds and have this happen again."

The types of blended skills you'll need to respond to the case scenarios include:

Cognitive Skills

- Knowledge of the anatomy and physiology of bowel elimination and variables that influence bowel elimination
- Knowledge of how to promote regular bowel habits; how to use cathartics, laxatives, and antidiarrheals; how to empty the colon of feces; how to design and implement bowel training programs; and how to use comfort measures to ease defecation
- Knowledge of the actions of medications, specifically narcotic analgesics, and the effects on GI system functioning
- Ability to incorporate knowledge of specific disease conditions affecting the gastrointestinal tract into the plan of care for a patient experiencing an alteration in bowel elimination
- Knowledge of the various types of bowel diversions and effect on gastrointestinal functioning and the patient's self-esteem
- Ability to incorporate knowledge of the nursing process to identify and care for patients with bowel problems

Technical Skills

- Demonstration of strong history and physical assessment techniques to determine problems related to bowel elimination and possible contributory factors
- Ability to use the equipment and protocols necessary to diagnose and treat bowel problems
- Ability to demonstrate appropriate measures to assist with diagnostic studies involving the gastrointestinal tract
- Ability to demonstrate competence in technical nursing assistance to meet the needs of patients experiencing alterations in bowel elimination

- Ability to adapt technical nursing assistance to meet the needs of patients experiencing problems with bowel elimination

Interpersonal Skills

- Demonstration of strong people skills to establish trusting relationships with patients experiencing alterations in bowel elimination patterns
- Ability to interact nonjudgmentally and professionally when interacting in situations involving bowel elimination, a typically private matter
- Ability to use therapeutic communication skills effectively to meet the needs of patients experiencing a disturbed body image related to bowel elimination problems
- Ability to mobilize supportive resources to provide needed services, especially for patients with bowel diversion such as ostomies

Ethical and Legal Skills

- Demonstration of a strong sense of accountability for the health and well-being of individuals experiencing problems with bowel elimination
- Ability to demonstrate a commitment to getting patients the help they need to achieve their health goals—within the scope of nursing responsibilities and available resources
- Adherence to safety and quality when performing nursing interventions to promote bowel elimination
- Knowledge of ethical and legal responsibilities involved with measures for promoting bowel elimination that are within the scope of nursing responsibilities

Learning Outcomes

After completing the chapter, the learner should be able to accomplish the following:

1. Describe the physiology of bowel elimination.
2. Identify variables that influence bowel elimination.
3. Assess bowel elimination using appropriate interview questions and physical assessment skills.
4. Assist with stool collection for laboratory analysis and direct and indirect visualization studies of the gastrointestinal tract.
5. Develop nursing diagnoses that identify bowel elimination problems amenable to nursing therapy.
6. Describe how to: (1) promote regular bowel habits (timing, positioning, privacy, nutrition, exercise); (2) use cathartics, laxatives, and antidiarrheals; (3) empty the colon of feces (enemas, rectal suppositories, rectal catheters, digital removal of stool); (4) design and implement bowel training programs; and (5) use comfort measures to ease defecation.
7. Describe nursing care for a patient with an ostomy.
8. Plan, implement, and evaluate nursing care related to select nursing diagnoses that involve bowel problems.

Key Terms

bowel incontinence
bowel training program
cathartic
defecation
colostomy
constipation
diarrhea
endoscopy
enema
fecal impaction
feces
flatulence
flatus
hemorrhoids
ileostomy
laxative
occult blood
ostomy
paralytic ileus
peristalsis
stoma
stool
suppository
Valsalva maneuver

Elimination of the waste products of digestion is
a natural process critical for human functioning. Patients differ widely in their expectations about bowel elimination, their usual pattern of defecation, and the ease with which they speak of bowel problems. Although most people have experienced minor acute bouts of diarrhea or constipation, some patients experience severe or chronic alterations in bowel elimination that affect their fluid and electrolyte balance, hydration, nutritional status, skin integrity, comfort, and self-concept. Moreover, many illnesses, diagnostic tests, medications, and surgical treatments can affect bowel elimination. Nurses need to be knowledgeable about measures for preventing and managing bowel elimination problems.

This chapter discusses the physiology of bowel elimination and the multiple factors that influence this process. A practical guide for assessing bowel elimination, including diagnostic studies of the gastrointestinal tract and their associated nursing responsibilities, is presented. Numerous examples of nursing diagnoses are included.

The chapter describes goals for both the nurse and the patient and nursing strategies to meet those goals (for an example addressing bowel diversions, see the accompanying Reflective Practice: Challenge to Technical Skills). The concluding patient care study illustrates the use of specific nursing interventions to resolve bowel elimination problems.

ANATOMY AND PHYSIOLOGY

The gastrointestinal tract, also known as the alimentary tract or canal, extends from the mouth to the anus. The anatomy of the gastrointestinal tract is shown in Figure 44-1. The major organ involved with bowel elimination is the large intestine.

Large Intestine

The large intestine, the primary organ of bowel elimination, is the lower, or distal, part of the gastrointestinal (alimentary) tract. It extends from the ileocecal valve to the anus. Functions of the large intestine include the completion of absorption, the manufacture of certain vitamins, the formation of feces, and the expulsion of feces from the body.

The large intestine in adults is about 1.5 m long (about 59 inches), but variations in length are normal. The width of the colon also varies. At its narrowest point, the colon is about 2.5 cm (1 inch) wide; at its widest point, it is about 7.5 cm (3 inches). The diameter of the colon decreases from the cecum to the anus.

The connection between the ileum of the small intestine and the large intestine is the ileocecal, or ileocolic, valve. This valve normally prevents contents from entering the large intestine prematurely and prevents waste products from returning to the small intestine.

Waste products of digestion, called chyme, move from the small intestine, passing through the ileocecal valve, and enter the cecum, the first part of the large intestine. The cecum is situated on the right side of the body, and to it is attached the vermiform process, or appendix.

Approximately 1,500 mL of chyme enters the large intestine daily. Its contents are liquid or watery. While passing through the large intestine, most water is absorbed. About 800 to 1,000 mL of liquid is absorbed daily by the intestinal tract, allowing for the formed, semisolid consistency of the normal stool. When absorption does not occur properly, such as when the waste products pass through the large intestine rapidly, the stool is soft and watery.

Recall Sally Germaine, the college student with Crohn's disease described at the beginning of the chapter. Knowledge of normal gastrointestinal function would help the nurse in developing a teaching plan for this patient about her disease.

Conversely, if the stool remains in the colon too long, or if too much water is absorbed, the stool becomes dry and hard.

From the cecum, the digestive contents enter the colon, which consists of several segments. The ascending colon extends from the cecum upward toward the liver, where it turns to cross the abdomen. This turn is called the hepatic flexure. Upon turning, this portion of the colon becomes the transverse colon, crossing the abdomen from right to left. The colon then turns at the splenic flexure to become the descending colon. The descending colon passes down the left side of the body to the sigmoid, or pelvic, colon.

The sigmoid colon contains **feces,** waste products that have reached the distal end of the colon and are ready for excretion. Once excreted, feces are called **stool.** The sigmoid colon empties into the rectum, the last part of the large intestine. The rectum is about 12 cm (5 inches) long, 2.5 cm (1 inch) of which is the anal canal. In the rectum, three transverse folds of tissue are present that may help to hold the fecal material in the rectum temporarily. Vertical folds also are present, each of which contains an artery and a vein. If the veins become abnormally distended, **hemorrhoids** occur.

The rectum is empty except immediately before and during **defecation** (the process of bowel elimination; a bowel movement). Feces are excreted from the rectum through the anal canal and the anus, which is approximately 1 to 1.5 inches (2.5 to 3.8 cm) long.

Nervous System Control

The autonomic nervous system innervates the muscles of the colon. The parasympathetic nervous system stimulates movement, while the sympathetic system inhibits movement. Contractions of the circular and longitudinal muscles of the intestine (**peristalsis**) occur every 3 to 12 minutes, moving waste products along the length of the intestine continuously (Fig. 44-2). Mass peristaltic sweeps occur one to four times each 24-hour period in most people, propelling the fecal mass forward. This movement is different from the frequent peristaltic rushes that occur in the small intestine. Mass peristalsis often occurs after food has been ingested, accounting for the urge to defecate that often occurs after meals. Timing nursing interventions to

Reflective Practice
Challenge to Technical Skills

Nursing school is filled with learning technical skills. The type and difficulty of these skills vary greatly throughout the 4 years, from learning how to monitor blood pressure in freshman year to learning how to perform suctioning in junior year. Although nursing students learn the technologies in the simulation practice laboratory, it is often quite a different situation when they are asked to perform the technology for the first time independently. I found this to be true the first time that I had to perform colostomy care independently.

I met Alberta Franklin while working as a nursing extern this summer. She was a 55-year-old woman who had recently undergone abdominal surgery and creation of a sigmoid colostomy. She required a new colostomy bag, and I was asked to change the bag. Although colostomies do not require the computerized technology found in an ICU, they do require technical skills. I had practiced changing colostomy bags in lab and had observed nurses changing the colostomy bag in the hospital. I had even previously changed a colostomy bag while being supervised by a nurse. Although I was not completely comfortable with the situation, I agreed to change the bag. I quickly reviewed the steps in the protocol book and went into the patient's room. I measured the colostomy and then cut the bag to the appropriate size. Unfortunately, I had measured the colostomy incorrectly, and the bag was too large, so I had to leave the room and get more supplies. After a few more obstacles, I was able to adhere a properly fitting bag to the patient—but not before the patient correctly guessed that this was the first time I had performed this skill! Her ability to guess that I had never performed this skill before illustrates my technical incompetence.

Thinking Outside the Box: Possible Courses of Action

- Refuse to provide the care and ask another nurse to change the colostomy bag.
- Observe a nurse performing the care one more time.
- Check protocol and perform the care, knowing that I could call a nurse if needed.
- "Wing it" and hope that I remember what I had learned in lab.

Evaluating a Good Outcome: How Do I Define Success?

- Patient receives safe care.
- Patient's needs are met.
- Nurse demonstrates technical competency with the skill.

Personal Learning: Here's to the Future!

I think that my actions were appropriate. Although I was unsure about my technical skills regarding colostomy care, I performed the skill adequately. In addition, I reviewed the appropriate steps and I knew that I could summon the assistance of a nurse in case I needed to do so. I also made sure that I knew where the nurse was so that if I did need help, I wouldn't waste any time looking for help. Therefore, I ensured that the patient's safety would not be compromised. Although at that time I would have preferred to have another nurse perform the colostomy change, I am glad that I completed this technical skill independently. Observing another person performing a skill can be beneficial, but there comes a point when you must "spread your wings" and complete the skill on your own. Of course, this philosophy regarding spreading your wings applies only to certain technologies: it would be inappropriate to use this philosophy if it compromised patient safety. However, in incidences like this one, where patient safety is not compromised and the appropriate teaching and training have been completed, I think it is appropriate to take action. If you don't, the various technologies in the hospital can become extremely intimidating and overwhelming. As a result, fear increases, which can possibly threaten a patient's safety and lead to injury.

Reflection

How do you think you would respond in a similar situation? Why? What does this tell you about yourself and about the adequacy of your skills for professional practice? Did the nursing student's actions adhere to ethical and legal principles? If not, describe what principles were violated. Could the nursing student have done anything more to deal with this situation? Explain your answer. What actions or behaviors by the nursing student might have provided clues to the patient that this was the nursing student's first independent attempt at the skill? Can you think of other ways to respond? What other skills (cognitive, interpersonal, technical, ethical/legal) would you need to respond well in this situation? Do you agree with the criteria to evaluate a successful outcome? Are there any other criteria that would need to be included? If so, specify these criteria. Did the nursing student meet the criteria listed?

Elizabeth Nalli, Georgetown University

evacuate bowel contents with this natural urge to defecate is helpful. One third to one half of ingested food waste is normally excreted in the stool within 24 hours, and the remainder within the next 24 to 48 hours.

After passing through the sigmoid colon, the waste products enter the rectum, where they are stopped from exiting by the anal sphincters. The internal sphincter in the anal canal and the external sphincter at the anus control the discharge of feces and intestinal gas (**flatus**). The internal sphincter consists of involuntary smooth muscle tissue that is innervated by the autonomic nervous system. Motor impulses are carried by the sympathetic system (thoracolumbar) and inhibitory impulses by the parasympathetic system (craniosacral). These two divisions of the autonomic nervous system function antagonistically in a dynamic equilibrium. The external sphincter at the anus has striated muscle tissue and is under voluntary control. The levator ani muscle reinforces the action of the external sphincter and is controlled voluntarily (Fig. 44-3).

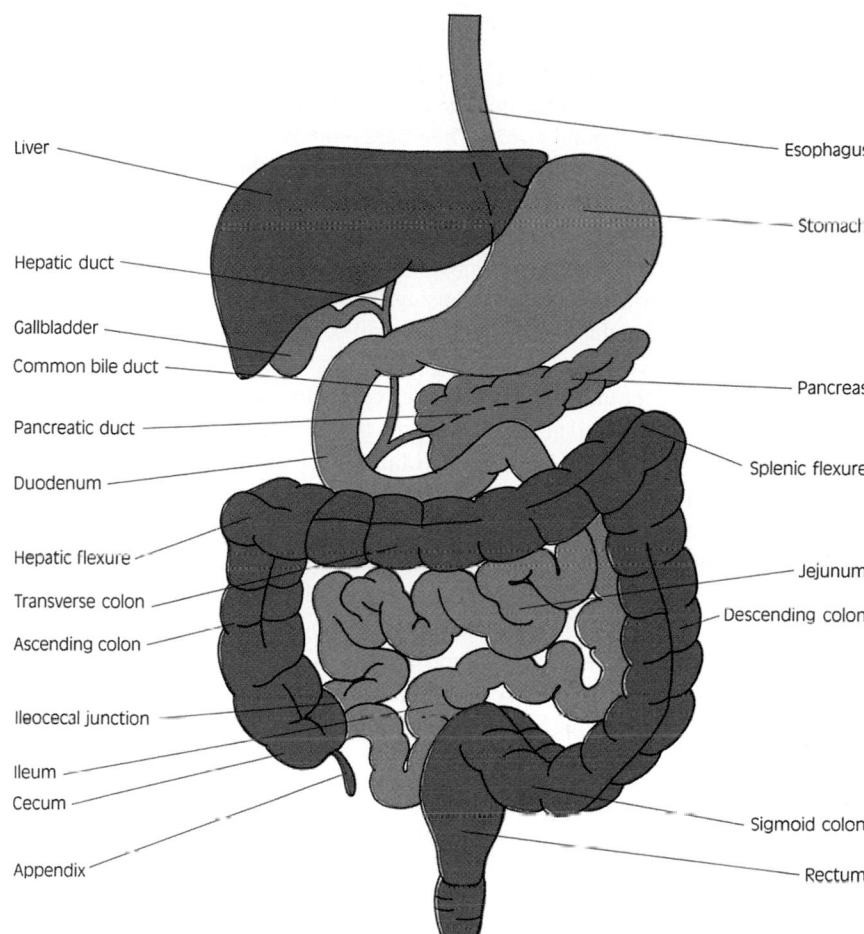

FIGURE 44-1 Organs of the gastrointestinal system

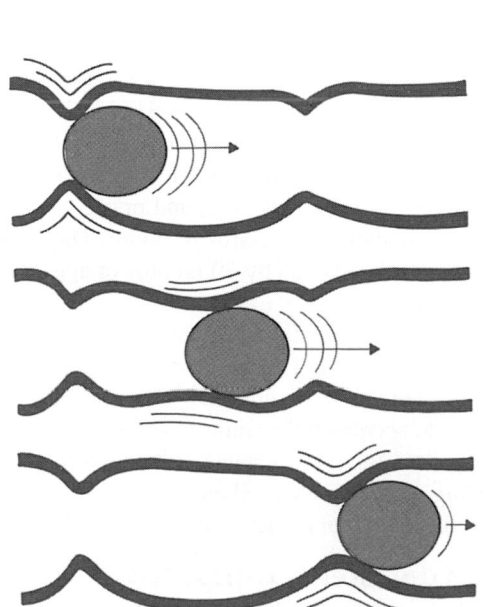

FIGURE 44-2 Peristaltic movements in the intestine.

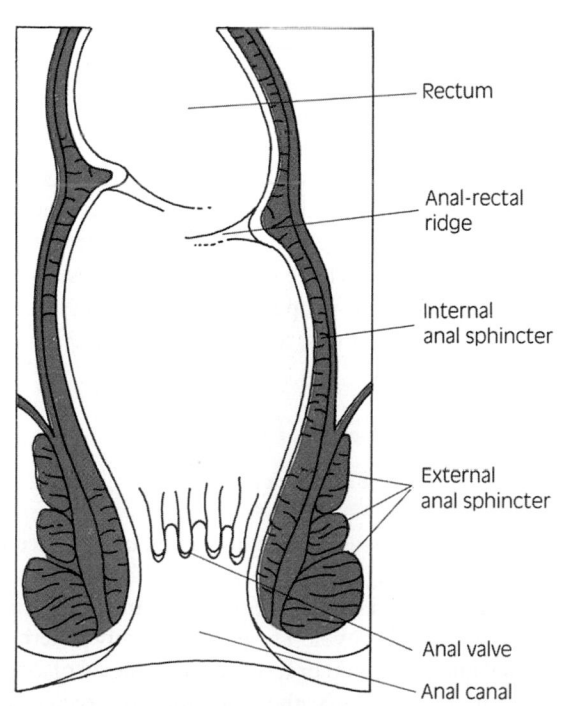

FIGURE 44-3 Interior view of the rectum and anal canal.

Act of Defecation

Defecation refers to the emptying of the large intestine. Two centers govern the reflex to defecate, one in the medulla and a subsidiary one in the spinal cord. When parasympathetic stimulation occurs, the internal anal sphincter relaxes and the colon contracts, allowing the fecal mass to enter the rectum.

The rectum becomes distended by the fecal mass, the primary stimulus for the defecation reflex. Rectal distention leads to an increase in intrarectal pressure, causing the muscles to stretch and thereby stimulating the defecation reflex and subsequently the urge to eliminate.

The external anal sphincter, which is under voluntary control, is constricted or relaxed at will. If the urge to defecate is ignored, defecation often can be delayed voluntarily.

During the act of defecation, several additional muscles aid in the process. Voluntary contraction of the muscles of the abdominal wall by holding one's breath, contracting the diaphragm, and closing the glottis increases intra-abdominal pressure up to four or five times the normal pressure, which helps expel feces. Simultaneously, the muscles on the pelvic floor contract and aid in expulsion of the fecal mass. Defecation is eased by flexing the thigh muscles, which increases abdominal pressure, and by the sitting position, which increases downward pressure on the rectum.

When an individual bears down to defecate, the increased pressures in the abdominal and thoracic cavities result in a decreased blood flow to the atria and ventricles, thus temporarily lowering cardiac output. Once bearing down ceases, the pressure is lessened, and a larger than normal amount of blood returns to the heart; this may dangerously elevate the blood pressure in an already hypertensive individual (Smeltzer & Bare, 2000). Therefore, this technique of bearing down, termed the **Valsalva maneuver,** may be contraindicated in people with cardiovascular problems and other illnesses.

The act of defecation is usually painless. If the bowels move at regular intervals and the stools are formed and soft, functional problems involving frequency of elimination seldom occur. Many people become concerned if they do not have a daily bowel movement, but there is no "normal" frequency of bowel movements. Although many adults pass one stool each day, other healthy people have more frequent or less frequent bowel movements. Some people have a bowel movement two or three times a week; others, two or three times a day.

FACTORS AFFECTING BOWEL ELIMINATION

Various factors can affect bowel elimination. Interference with the normal functioning of elimination from the intestines can occur in health as well as during illness. Elimination can be affected by a person's developmental stage, daily patterns, the amount and quality of fluid or food intake, the level of activity, lifestyle, emotional states, pathologic processes, medications, and procedures, such as diagnostic tests and surgery.

Developmental Considerations

Age affects what a person eats and the body's ability to digest nutrients and eliminate wastes. The stools of an infant are markedly different from those of an older person. Because patients are often reluctant to discuss their bowel habits and stool characteristics, nurses need to be familiar with bowel concerns pertinent to each developmental group.

Infant

The stool characteristics depend on whether the infant is being fed breast milk or formula. Breast milk is easier for the intestines to break down and absorb. Breastfed babies have more frequent stools, and the stools are yellow to golden and loose and usually have little odor. With formula or cow's milk feedings, the infant's stools vary from yellow to brown, are pastelike in consistency, and have a stronger odor because of the decomposition of protein. Both stools may have curds and mucus. Infants have no voluntary control over bowel elimination.

The number of stools infants pass varies greatly. For example, breastfed infants can pass from two to ten stools daily, whereas bottle-fed infants typically pass one or two stools daily. At the age of 1 year, all infants commonly pass one stool a day. Parents may mistakenly interpret the infant's liquid stool as **diarrhea** (excessively liquid stool). Loose stools may be related to overfeeding or too much corn syrup in formula. True diarrhea, however, requires evaluation. Some children have bowel movements only once every 2 to 3 days. Teach parents that as long as the stools are soft, the child is not constipated. If **constipation** (dry, hard stool) occurs, dietary manipulation is the initial treatment. The consistent use of suppositories and laxatives is discouraged. Infants with persistent constipation require evaluation for structural defects.

Toddler

Between the ages of 18 and 24 months, the nerve fibers innervating the internal and external anal sphincters become fully developed, and voluntary control of defecation becomes possible. Voluntary defecation requires intact muscular, sensory, and nervous structures. Successful bowel training also includes an awareness by the toddler of the need to defecate, the ability to communicate this need, the wish to please the significant person involved in bowel training, and praise and reinforcement for the toddler's successful behavior. Daytime bowel control is normally attained by 30 months of age, but the age varies with each child.

Help parents to understand that physiologic maturity is the first priority for successful bowel training. Discourage the use of punishment or shame for elimination accidents or for a lack of readiness to become toilet-trained. Toddlers who are toilet-trained often regress and experience soiling when hospitalized, and scolding or acting disgusted only reinforces this behavior. The only constructive approach is to seek the underlying cause.

Child, Adolescent, and Adult

From childhood into adulthood, defecation patterns vary in quantity, frequency, and rhythmicity. Many people may not understand the significance of changes in bowel habits or may worry needlessly about normal stool characteristics or bowel habits. Emphasize that the use of over-the-counter laxatives and enemas can have serious consequences, and that any problems prompting such use need to be evaluated.

Older Adult

Constipation is often a chronic problem for older adults. Diarrhea, fecal impaction, or fecal incontinence can also result from physiologic or lifestyle changes (see the accompanying box Focus on the Older Adult).

Daily Patterns

Most people have individual patterns of bowel elimination involving frequency, timing considerations, position, and place. Changes in any of these may upset a person's routine and lead to constipation. For example, many people defecate after breakfast, when the gastrocolic and duodenocolic reflexes cause mass propulsive movements in the large intestine. If this urge to defecate is ignored because the person finds the time inconvenient, the feces remain in the rectum until the defecation reflex is again initiated. Meanwhile, water continues to be absorbed from the unexpelled feces, which makes stool dry, hard, and painful to pass.

Most people assume the squatting or slightly forward-sitting position with the thighs flexed. In either position,

increased pressure is placed on the abdomen, as well as downward pressure on the rectum; both facilitate defecation. Obtaining the same results when seated on a bedpan is difficult. Embarrassment may further inhibit defecation.

For most people, defecation is a private affair experienced easily only in the comfort of one's own bathroom. Defecation may be difficult in a shared hospital room with only a curtain for privacy.

Food and Fluid

Both the type and the amount of foods eaten and the amount of fluids ingested affect elimination. A high-fiber diet and a daily fluid intake of 2,000 to 3,000 mL facilitate bowel elimination. High-fiber foods increase the bulk in fecal material. Bulkier feces increase pressure on the intestinal wall, which serves as a stimulus for peristalsis. As a result, feces move more quickly through the colon, allowing less time for water to be reabsorbed. Subsequently, the stool is soft and easy to pass. There is also less time for toxins to be absorbed from feces by the colon. Many believe that such toxins play an important role in promoting the development of colon cancer.

People digest and tolerate foods differently. This variation is determined in part by one's culture. For example, travelers to a foreign country who eat native foods or drink the water may suffer severe indigestion and elimination problems, such as diarrhea. Food intolerance may alter bowel elimination,

---

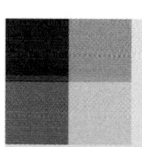

Focus on the Older Adult
Bowel Elimination Problems

Older adults frequently experience problems with bowel elimination. These can be due to a variety of causes and can have serious implications for the elderly patient.

Bowel Elimination Problem	Related Factors and Implications

Chronic constipation	Can be caused by:
	    Decreased gastrointestinal motility
	    Effect of medications (eg, antacids, opioids, antihypertensives)
	    Decreased fluid intake
	    Less active lifestyle
	    Inadequate fiber intake
	    Incomplete emptying of the bowel
	Can lead to laxative abuse

Diarrhea	Can be caused by:
	    Laxative abuse
	    Effect of medications/tube feedings
	Can lead to life-threatening dehydration and electrolyte imbalance

Fecal impaction	Can result from chronic constipation May be preceded by oozing of liquid feces—often mistaken for diarrhea Can lead to distended abdomen, abdominal pain, and complete bowel obstruction

Fecal incontinence	Can be caused by:
	    Decreased muscle tone
	    Alteration in nervous system innervation to rectum
	    Altered cognition
	Can lead to skin breakdown and depression

possibly resulting in diarrhea, gaseous distention, and cramping. For example, people who lack the enzyme lactase, which helps to break down the simple sugar lactose found in milk and milk products, cannot digest milk; this is called lactose intolerance. These people often experience excessive intestinal gas and diarrhea when they ingest milk.

Certain foods have been associated with specific effects on bowel elimination. These include:

- Constipating foods: processed cheese, lean meat, eggs, pasta
- Foods with laxative effect: certain fruits and vegetables (eg, prunes), bran, chocolate, spicy foods, alcohol, coffee
- Gas-producing foods: onions, cabbage, beans, cauliflower

Activity and Muscle Tone

Regular exercise improves gastrointestinal motility and muscle tone, whereas inactivity decreases both. Adequate tone in the abdominal muscles, the diaphragm, and the perineal muscles is essential for ease of defecation. Patients on prolonged bed rest are prime candidates for constipation.

Lifestyle

Many individual, family, and sociocultural variables influence a person's usual elimination habits. The long-term effects of bowel training may result in a person's (1) acceptance of bowel elimination as a normal life process, (2) preoccupation with bowel elimination, or (3) feeling that bowel elimination is a "dirty" process. Rituals associated with bowel elimination, cleanliness considerations, the language used to talk about bowel elimination or reluctance to discuss it, individual responses to involuntary passage of flatus (gas), and so on vary widely among people. A person's daily schedule, occupation, and leisure activities may contribute to a habit of defecating at regular times or to an irregular pattern (see the accompanying box Promoting Health 44-1).

Psychological Variables

Psychological stress affects the body in many ways. In some people, anxiety seems to have a direct effect on gastrointestinal motility, and diarrhea accompanies periods of high anxiety. In the fight-or-flight response, when the body mobilizes itself for intense action, blood is shunted away from the stomach and intestines, resulting in a slowing of gastrointestinal motility. Persons who chronically worry and those with certain personality types who tend to hold onto problems and negative feelings may experience frequent constipation.

Pathologic Conditions

Numerous pathologic processes may change a person's usual bowel elimination habits. Changes in stool characteristics or frequency may be one of the first clinical manifestations of a disease, and their evaluation may lead to the diagnosis of the disease. For example, when a patient reports that his or her stool has become narrower or ribbon-like, a tumor may be obstructing normal stool passage through the colon. The nurse should report this finding to the physician. Similarly, a parent's report that a child's stools are frequent, bulky, greasy, and foul-smelling suggests cystic fibrosis and would require further evaluation, especially if other clinical manifestations are present.

Diarrhea may result from pathologic conditions such as diverticulitis, infection, malabsorption syndromes, neoplastic diseases, diabetic neuropathy, hyperthyroidism, and uremia.

Think back to Sally Germaine, the college student with Crohn's disease. Adequate understanding of this disorder is crucial in developing an appropriate plan of care for the patient. Additionally, this information is important in assisting the patient to adjust to her condition, thereby helping to minimize the effects of the disorder on her body image.

Promoting Health 44-1 Bowel Elimination

Use the assessment checklist to determine how well you are meeting your need for bowel elimination. Then develop a prescription for self-care by choosing appropriate behaviors from the list of suggestions.

ASSESSMENT CHECKLIST

almost always / sometimes / almost never

1. I have a regular bowel elimination pattern, satisfactory to support comfort and activities of daily living.
2. I eat a diet high in fiber.
3. I exercise regularly.
4. I have an adequate intake of fluids.

SELF-CARE BEHAVIORS

1. Accept individual patterns of defecation as normal.
2. Eat a balanced diet, including high-fiber foods, such as fruits, vegetables, and nuts.
3. Follow a regular exercise program with 30 to 45 minutes of activity three to four times a week.
4. Do not ignore the urge to defecate.
5. Establish a routine, if needed (1 hour after meals is usually best).
6. Avoid prolonged use of over-the-counter medications or enemas to treat constipation.
7. Drink 8–10 glasses of water per day.
8. Seek medical assistance for any change in the characteristics of stool or presence of blood in stool.

Constipation may be the result of conditions such as diseases within the colon or rectum, injury to or degeneration of the spinal cord, and megacolon. Changes in color, contents, odor, and appearance of stool may be related to conditions that traumatize the stomach or intestines or that interfere with normal digestion. Thus, stool assessment is an important diagnostic task for the nurse.

Recall Leroy Cobbs, the patient with fecal impaction secondary to the use of narcotic analgesics to control his cancer pain. Frequent follow-up assessments of the patient's stool would provide valuable information for the nurse in the determining the effectiveness of interventions to relieve his impaction.

Outbreaks of food poisoning can result in severe gastrointestinal symptoms, including diarrhea. Infections caused by certain types of *Escherichia coli,* particularly dangerous for young children (under 10 years of age) and older adults, can progress quickly to life-threatening hematologic and renal complications ("Wisconsin center cracks. . . .," *Nursing Spectrum,* 2001). Severe abdominal cramping followed by watery or bloody diarrhea may signal a microbial infection, which can be confirmed by a stool sample. Supportive treatment, careful monitoring, and attentive nursing care are essential.

Medications

Medications are available that can promote peristalsis (cathartics and laxatives) or inhibit peristalsis (antidiarrheal medications). These are discussed later in the chapter.

Other types of medications may affect bowel elimination and stool characteristics. Opioids, antacids containing aluminum, iron sulfate, and anticholinergic medications decrease gastrointestinal motility, resulting in constipation.

Remember Leroy Cobbs, the patient described at the beginning of the chapter who developed fecal impaction resulting from the narcotic analgesics he was using to control his cancer pain. Had the possible adverse effects of narcotics for pain control been addressed in the patient's medication teaching plan when the drug was first prescribed, the risk for fecal impaction could have been reduced. Additionally, the teaching plan could have addressed measures to counteract the effects of the medication.

Many medications can cause diarrhea as a side effect. For example, diarrhea is seen in 10% to 25% of patients treated with amoxicillin clavulanate (Augmentin), an antibiotic (Bartlett, 2002). In this situation, using antidiarrheal drugs is not recommended because their use would prolong the exposure of the intestinal mucosa to the irritating effect of the antibiotic or toxin. If diarrhea is severe enough, the drug may need to be discontinued.

Medications may also influence the appearance of the stool, for a variety of reasons. Any drug with the potential to cause gastrointestinal bleeding (eg, anticoagulants, aspirin products) may cause the stool to appear pink to red to black. Iron salts result in a black stool from the oxidation of iron. Antacids may cause a white discoloration or speckling in the stool. Antibiotics may cause a green-gray color because of impaired digestion.

Diagnostic Studies

A patient's usual bowel elimination pattern may be affected by diagnostic studies. For example, patients may need to fast for diagnostic studies. Additionally, the stress of hospitalization and waiting for the results of the study, combined with changes in food intake, can severely alter a patient's usual elimination patterns. The cathartics or enemas used for bowel cleansing before certain diagnostic studies of the gastrointestinal tract can interfere with the normal timing of a patient's bowel movements (see Table 44-2 later in this chapter).

Surgery and Anesthesia

Direct manipulation of the bowel during abdominal surgery inhibits peristalsis, causing a condition termed **paralytic ileus.** This temporary stoppage of peristalsis normally lasts 24 to 48 hours; during this time, food and fluids are withheld. Many times, the patient is receiving narcotics for pain relief, which can exacerbate the situation. If this condition persists, distention and symptoms of acute obstruction may occur, possibly resulting in the need for surgical intervention. Inhaled general anesthetic agents also inhibit peristalsis by blocking the parasympathetic impulses to the intestinal musculature. However, local and regional anesthetics have little effect on peristalsis.

THE NURSING PROCESS FOR PATIENTS WITH BOWEL ELIMINATION DISTURBANCES

Assessing

Nursing History

Because many patients are reluctant to initiate a conversation about their bowel status, include pertinent bowel elimination questions in each comprehensive nursing history. See the Focused Assessment Guide 44-1.

If the patient is experiencing any disturbance in bowel elimination, conduct a more detailed assessment, directing attention to the factors described earlier that may influence bowel elimination.

Patients who are critically ill or who have impaired cognition may be incapable of reporting their bowel status accurately. A person who is color-blind may not be able to visualize frank (bright red) blood in stool (Reiss, Labowitz, Forman & Wormser, 2001). Record the patient's daily bowel status to look for clues to impending problems. While making

Focused Assessment Guide 44-1

Bowel Elimination

Factors to Assess	Questions and Approaches
Usual patterns of bowel elimination	How often do you move your bowels? Any special time of the day? What does your stool look like: • Frequency • Time of day • Description of usual stool characteristics (amount, consistency, shape, color, odor)
Aids to elimination	Do you use anything to help move your bowels? • Natural aids (liquids, food) • Pharmacologic aids (laxatives) • Enemas
Recent changes in bowel elimination	Have you noticed any changes in your stool recently? Have you noticed any blood in your stool? (May need to ask patient about color blindness) Have you noted a difference in the appearance of your stool (narrowing, presence of mucus)?
Problems with bowel elimination	Are your bowels causing you any problem now? • Nature of disturbance • Onset and frequency • Causes (*physical:* food and fluid intake, exercise status, history of surgery or illnesses influencing gastrointestinal tract; psychosocial; medicine related) • Severity • Symptoms • Interventions attempted and results
Presence of artificial orifices	What is your usual routine with your colostomy or ileostomy? Do you have any problems with it?

daily rounds, ask patients who can give reliable answers, "Did you move your bowels yesterday or today?" and chart the response. If the patient cannot provide this information, the nurse who is assisting with bowel elimination records the daily stools.

Physical Assessment

Assessment of bowel elimination includes physical assessment of the abdomen, anus, and rectum (discussed in Chap. 25). Described below are examination techniques that may be helpful when assessing the functioning of the gastrointestinal tract.

Abdomen

The sequence for abdominal assessment proceeds from inspection, auscultation, and percussion to palpation. Inspection and auscultation are performed before palpation because palpation may disturb normal peristalsis and bowel motility. Place the patient comfortably in the supine position with the abdomen exposed, the chest and pubic area draped, and the knees slightly flexed. Encourage the patient to urinate so that the bladder is empty.

Inspection

First, observe the contour of the abdomen, noting any masses, scars, or areas of distention. Peristalsis is usually not visible except in very thin patients. When an intestinal obstruction is pre-

sent, the visible waves of peristalsis to the point of the obstruction may be observed on the abdomen.

Auscultation

Using the diaphragm of a warmed stethoscope, listen for bowel sounds in all abdominal quadrants, using a systematic, clockwise approach. If the patient has a nasogastric tube in place, disconnect it from suction during this assessment to allow for accurate interpretation of sounds. Keep in mind that the timing of the patient's most recent meal or a full bladder may also affect the examination.

Note the frequency and character of bowel sounds, audible clicks and gurgles produced by the movement of air and flatus in the gastrointestinal tract. They are usually high-pitched, gurgling, and soft. Their frequency may range from 5 to 34 bowel sounds per minute, depending on the rate of peristalsis ("Interpreting abnormal abdominal sounds," 2000). Significant findings include absent or infrequent bowel sounds, indicating hypoperistalsis or paralytic ileus (evidenced only after listening for 5 minutes) or abnormally intense and frequent bowel sounds (borborygmus), indicating hyperperistalsis. Describe bowel sounds as audible, hyperactive, hypoactive, or inaudible.

Percussion

Percuss all quadrants of the abdomen in a systematic, clockwise manner to identify any masses, fluid, or air in the abdomen. Expect a resonant sound or tympany over the abdomen and stomach because these are hollow organs. With practice, learn to distinguish normal resonance from the hyperresonance that occurs when excess flatus is trapped in the intestines. An intestinal obstruction sounds dull on percussion. Areas of increased dullness may be caused by fluid, a mass, or a tumor.

Palpation

Both light palpation and deep palpation in each quadrant are performed next by a skilled nurse. Note any muscular resistance, tenderness, enlargement of organs, and masses. The beginning nurse quickly learns the feel of a distended abdomen. If the patient is in pain, administer medication before proceeding with the palpation.

Anus and Rectum

The nurse's skill level determines the extent of the rectal examination. Perform a superficial examination each time you wash a patient's anal area or assist with bowel evacuation. Position the patient in the left Sims' position.

Inspection and Palpation

First, examine the anal area for cracks, nodules, distended veins (hemorrhoids), masses, or polyps. Observe for a fecal mass, which may distend the anus. Insert a gloved, lubricated finger through the anus into the rectum to assess sphincter tone and smoothness of the mucosal lining; note any masses, polyps, hardened stool, bleeding, or abnormal discharge. Also inspect the perineal area for areas of skin irritation or breakdown secondary to diarrhea or fecal incontinence.

Stool Characteristics

Nurses are responsible for observing and recording information about the patient's stool. Table 44-1 describes the characteristics of a normal stool, along with special considerations used when observing a stool. Report and record anything unusual, including the passage of little or no gas or unusual amounts.

Note and record (usually on the patient's bedside flow sheet) the frequency, amount, and characteristics of the patient's bowel movements. Frequency is recorded as I, II, III, or i, ii, iii, to indicate the number of bowel movements in a given period of time. Describe any additional unusual observations, such as lightheadedness or straining, on the patient's medical record. When auxiliary personnel or the patient assumes this responsibility, check with the patient at regular intervals to see that it is being done correctly.

Ideally, populations at high risk for bowel elimination problems are identified before problems occur, and such problems are prevented or minimized through vigilant nursing care. Also, be aware of the clinical manifestations of colon cancer, because early detection significantly improves survival (Box 44-1).

Diagnostic Studies

The nurse is often responsible for caring for patients with elimination problems who are undergoing diagnostic testing.

Following are specific guidelines for the nurse's role in stool collection and direct and indirect visualization studies.

Stool Collection

The nurse is responsible for obtaining the specimen according to agency procedure, labeling the specimen, and ensuring that the specimen is transported to the laboratory in a timely manner. The institution's policy and procedure manual or laboratory manual identifies specific information about the amount of stool needed, the time frame during which stool is to be collected, and the type of specimen container to use.

Use of medical aseptic techniques is imperative. Always wear disposable gloves when any contact or handling of a stool specimen is likely. Hand hygiene, before and after glove use, is essential. Also, take care not to contaminate the outside of the specimen container with stool. Package, label, and transport specimens according to agency policy to ensure that no leakage of the specimen occurs.

Patients may need specific instructions about collecting a stool specimen. These instructions may include the following:
- Void first, because the laboratory study may be inaccurate if the stool contains urine.
- Defecate into the required container, such as clean or sterile bedpan or the bedside commode (depending on the specimen required), rather than the toilet, because the analysis results may be affected by the water in the toilet bowl.
- Do not place toilet tissue in the bedpan or specimen container, because contents in the paper may influence laboratory results.
- Notify the nurse when the specimen is available, so that it may be collected and transported to the laboratory as required.

When placing a specimen in a laboratory container, put on gloves and use two clean tongue blades. Usually, 1 inch (2.5 cm) of formed stool or 15 to 30 mL of liquid stool is sufficient. If portions of the stool include visible blood, mucus, or pus, include these with the specimen. Also be sure that the specimen is free of any barium or enema solution. Because a fresh specimen produces the most accurate results, send the specimen to the laboratory immediately. If this is not possible, refrigerate it unless contraindicated.

To test the stool for pH or blood, use a commercial tape, dipstick, or solution according to the manufacturer's directions. **Occult blood** in the stool (blood that is hidden in the specimen or cannot be seen on gross examination) can be detected with simple screening tests. Certain conditions, such as ulcer disease, inflammatory bowel disorders, and colon cancer, place the patient at high risk for intestinal bleeding. The color of the stool may reflect the source of the bleeding. Generally, black stools indicate upper gastrointestinal bleeding, such as from a peptic ulcer, due to a reaction between hemoglobin and gastric acid. Lower gastrointestinal bleeding (eg, hemorrhoids) may produce bright-red blood in the stool. Certain foods and medications can also cause a black or reddish stool.

TABLE 44-1 The Stool: Normal Characteristics and Special Considerations for Observation

Characteristic	Normal Finding	Special Considerations for Observation
Volume	Variable	The volume of the stool depends on the amount the person eats and the nature of the diet. For example, a diet high in roughage produces more feces than a soft, bland diet. Consistently large diarrheal stools suggest a disorder in the small bowel or proximal colon; small, frequent stools with urgency to pass them suggest a disorder of the left colon or rectum.
Color	Infant: Yellow to brown Adult: Brown	The brown color of the stool is due to stercobilin, a bile pigment derivative. The rapid rate of peristalsis in the breastfed infant causes the stool to be yellow. The color of the stool is influenced by diet. For example, the stool will be almost black if the person eats red meat and dark green vegetables, such as spinach. The stool will be light brown if the diet is high in milk and milk products and low in meat. The absence of bile may cause the stool to appear white or clay-colored. Certain drugs influence the color of the stool. For example, iron salts cause the stool to be black. Antacids cause it to be whitish. Bleeding high in the intestinal tract causes a stool to be black owing to the digestion of the blood. Bleeding low in the intestinal tract results in fresh blood in the stool. The stool darkens with standing.
Odor	Pungent; may be affected by foods ingested	The characteristic odor of the stool is due to indole and skatole, caused by putrefaction and fermentation in the lower intestinal tract. The odor of the stool is influenced by its pH value, which normally is neutral or slightly alkaline. Excessive putrefaction causes a strong odor. The presence of blood in the stool causes a unique odor.
Consistency	Soft, semisolid, and formed	The consistency of the stool is influenced by fluid and food intake and gastric motility. The less time stool spends in the intestine (or the shorter the intestine), the more liquid the stool. Many pathologic conditions influence consistency.
Shape	Formed stool is usually about 1 inch (2.5 cm) in diameter and has the tubular shape of the colon, but may be larger or smaller, depending on the condition of the colon.	A gastrointestinal obstruction may result in a narrow, pencil-shaped stool. Rapid peristalsis thins the stool. Increased time spent in the large intestine may result in a hard, marblelike fecal mass.
Constituents	Waste residues of digestion: bile, intestinal secretions, shedded epithelial cells, bacteria, and inorganic material (chiefly calcium and phosphates); seeds, meat fibers, and fat may be present in small amounts	Internal bleeding, infection, inflammation, and other pathologic conditions may result in abnormal constituents. These include blood, pus, excessive fat, parasites, ova, and mucus. Foreign bodies also may be found in the stool.

BOX 44-1 Warning Signs of Colon Cancer

- Change in the bowel elimination pattern
- Blood in the stools
- Rectal or abdominal pain
- Change in the character of the stool
- Sensation of incomplete emptying after bowel movement

Tests for occult blood in the stool may be performed quickly by nurses within an institution or by patients at home. These simple tests use reagent substances to detect the enzyme peroxidase in the hemoglobin molecule. The Hematest and guaiac test are chemical tests commonly used to determine occult blood in the stool. Guidelines for Nursing Care 44-1 gives additional nursing considerations for fecal occult blood testing, and Figure 44-4 demonstrates the procedure for a Hemoccult test.

Guidelines for Nursing Care 44-1
Testing for Fecal Occult Blood

- Instruct the patient about food and drug restrictions for at least 2 to 3 days before the test, if they apply.
- Review manufacturer's directions for collecting the specimen. Equipment may include a specimen card, collection tissues, or test paper.
- Avoid mixing the specimen with urine or water.
- Inform the patient that multiple or serial specimens are usually collected from different bowel movements to verify results.
- Collect the amount recommended for the particular test (usually only a small amount is required).
- Wear gloves and perform thorough hand hygiene if collecting a specimen from a bedpan, commode, or plastic receptacle.
- Use tongue blades to transfer the stool to the test tape or folder.
- Follow instructions based on type of test. Hemoccult slide test requires placing 2 drops of developer solution on the back side of the specimen paper. The tablet test directions include placing 2 to 3 drops of tap water on the tablet, which is centered on the stool specimen.
- Document the test results according to agency policy. *A blue color is a positive result and needs to be reported.*
- Inform the patient of the test results.

The ingestion of rare or raw meat, processed meats, or liver, horseradish, certain fruits and vegetables, and certain medications (eg, salicylate intake of more than 325 mg daily, steroids, iron preparations, and anticoagulants) may result in a false-positive reading (Ahmed, Karch & Karch, 2000). The ingestion of vitamin C for 3 days prior to testing can produce false-negative results even if bleeding is present. For home testing, recommendations usually include the following:

- Before stool testing, avoid the foods (for 3 days) and drugs (for 7 days) that may alter test results.
- In a woman who is menstruating, postpone the test until 3 days after her period has ended.
- Delay the test if hematuria or bleeding hemorrhoids are present.
- Caution a person who is color-blind to the color blue not to attempt to interpret the test results.

In clinical settings, these restrictions are usually not practical.

Timed Specimens
Consider the first stool passed by the patient as the start of the collection period. Collect a specimen of every stool passed within the designated period (the test may require saving the entire stool passed or only a sample). Follow instructions for sending stools to the laboratory.

Specimens for Pinworms
Use clear cellophane tape to collect a specimen for pinworms (frosted tape makes examination difficult). Apply gloves and press the tape against the anal opening, remove it immediately, and then place it on a slide. Collect this specimen in the morning, immediately after the patient awakens and before the patient has a bowel movement or bath. Pinworms tend to come to the anal area during the night to deposit eggs and retreat into the anal canal during the day. They can be seen with the naked eye by spreading the buttocks and visualizing the anus while the child is asleep. Pinworm eggs can usually be detected on the tape under a microscope. For accurate results, this test may need to be repeated on consecutive days.

Direct Visualization Studies
Endoscopy is the direct visualization of the lining of a hollow body organ. Most commonly this is done using a fiber optic endoscope, a long, flexible tube containing glass fibers that transmit light into the organ and return an image that can be viewed. Pincers may be inserted through the tube to obtain a tissue sample for biopsy. An endoscope enables the physician to view the integrity of the mucosa, blood vessels,

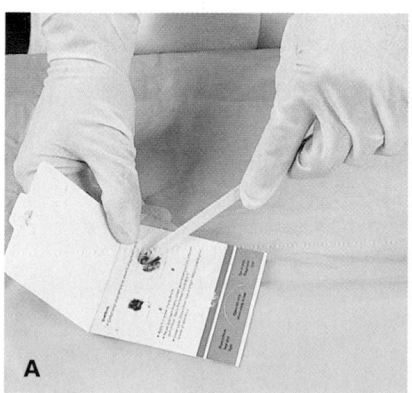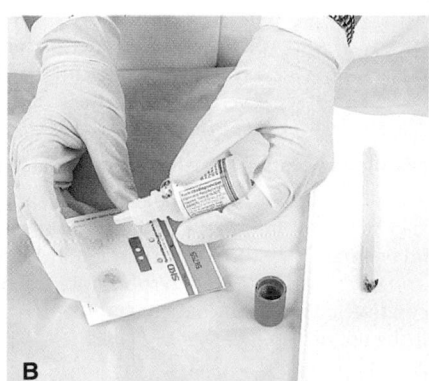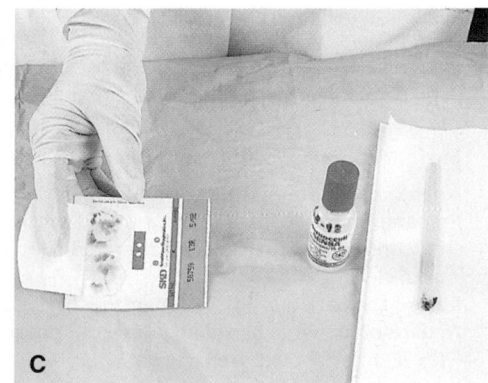

FIGURE 44-4 Testing a stool specimen for occult blood. (**A**) Applying a stool specimen to the test paper. (**B**) Adding developing solution to the back side of the paper according to directions. (**C**) *Blue coloration* indicating positive results. (Photos © B. Proud.)

and specific organ parts and is helpful for diagnosing in-flammatory, ulcerative, and infectious diseases; benign and malignant neoplasms; and other lesions of the esophageal, gastric, and intestinal mucosa. Endoscopic studies include the following:

Esophagogastroduodenoscopy: visual examination of the lin-ing of the esophagus, the stomach, and the upper duode-num with a flexible fiber optic endoscope

Colonoscopy: visual examination of the lining of the large in-testine with a flexible fiber optic endoscope

Sigmoidoscopy: visual examination of the lining of the dis-tal sigmoid colon, the rectum, and the anal canal using either a flexible or rigid instrument. The tube has an at-tached light source and is equipped to allow biopsy. The rigid sigmoidoscope may be more uncomfortable for the patient, especially one who is not relaxed.

Nursing responsibilities before and after these studies are de-scribed in Table 44-2.

A newer procedure is wireless capsule endoscopy. In this procedure the patient swallows a capsule, about the size of a

TABLE 44-2 Common Diagnostic Studies for the Gastrointestinal Tract

Preparation	Aftercare
Esophagogastroduodenoscopy: Allows visual examination of the esophagus, stomach, and upper duodenum by means of a long, flexible, fiberoptic-lighted scope	
A signed consent form is required for this procedure. Fasting is required 6 to 12 hours before the test (check agency policy). Dentures need to be removed before the test. Remind the patient that he will be awake but sedated and that a local anesthetic will be sprayed into the mouth and throat to depress the gag reflex.	Withhold food and fluids until the gag reflex returns. Check vital signs according to the protocol. Observe for signs of perforation: pain, persistent difficulty swallowing, vomiting blood, or black, tarry stools. Explain to the patient that it is normal to sense throat soreness and hoarseness for several days; saline gargles and lozenges may be helpful.
Colonoscopy: Allows visual examination of the rectum, colon, and distal small bowel using a long, flexible, fiberoptic-lighted scope	
Ensure that an informed consent is signed. Preparation prior to test may involve: • Clear liquid diet (24–48 h before test) • 2 day bowel preparation—strong cathartic and Dulcolax on day 1 and enema the day of the test, *or* • 1 day bowel preparation—ingestion of a gallon of bowel cleanser such as GoLytely in a short period of time Sedation will be given before the test.	May experience flatulence or gas pains because air was used to distend the intestines for better visibility. Usual diet may be resumed once patient recovers from the sedation. Check vital signs according to agency protocol. Observe for signs of bowel perforation: rectal bleeding, abdominal pain and distention, fever, malaise.
Sigmoidoscopy: Allows visual examination of the distal sigmoid colon, the rectum, and the anal canal through a flexible or rigid sigmoidoscope	
Obtain an informed consent for this procedure. Preparation usually consists of light meal before the test and two Fleet enemas. Sedation is not usually required.	May experience flatulence or gas pains because air was used to distend the intestines for better visibility. Observe for signs of bowel perforation. If biopsy was performed, patient should be informed that slight rectal bleeding may occur.
Upper Gastrointestinal (UGI) and Small Bowel Series: Fluoroscopic examination of the esophagus, stomach, and small intestine after ingestion of barium sulfate	
Ensure that an informed consent is signed. Keep patient NPO after midnight the day of the test. Inform patient that a chalky-tasting barium contrast mixture will be given to drink before the test.	A posttest cathartic (eg, Milk of Magnesia) is usually prescribed to prevent fecal impaction from barium sulfate that has hardened. Explain that the barium may lighten the color of stools for the next several days. After the barium is expelled, the stool color will return to normal.
Barium Enema: A series of radiographs that examine the large intestine after rectal instillation of barium sulfate	
An informed consent must be signed. Preparation may consist of dietary modifications, increased fluid intake, a cathartic, NPO after midnight, and enemas until clear before the test. Review the patient's history for any history of ulcerative colitis or active GI bleeding that would prohibit the use of the standard bowel preparation.	Encourage fluids to prevent dehydration. Inform the patient that the barium may lighten the color of the stools. A cathartic may be prescribed. Encourage rest because the bowel preparation and the test exhaust many patients.

Adapted from Fischbach, F. (2003). *A manual of laboratory diagnostic tests* (7th ed.). Philadelphia: Lippincott Williams & Wilkins; and Pagana, K., & Pagana, T. (2002). *Manual of diagnostic and laboratory tests* (2nd ed.). St. Louis: C. V. Mosby.

vitamin, that contains a small camera that emits a radio signal. The capsule is propelled through the small intestine via peristalsis. Several wires on the patient's abdomen pick up the radio signal from the capsule, and the data are recorded on a data recorder, which the patient can wear on a belt. The information is downloaded from the recorder to a computer and can be transferred to a videotape for easy viewing by the physician.

The patient is normally NPO for 6 hours before the wireless capsule endoscopy. During the first 2 hours of the study, the patient is not allowed to eat or drink anything. After the first 2 hours, the patient may consume small amounts of liquids. After 4 hours, the patient may have a small meal. The patient may resume normal activities while the camera is passing through the small intestine. The patient returns to the physician after 8 hours to have the belt and wires removed, and the capsule is excreted naturally in 24 to 48 hours (Buchman, 2002). Since there is no sedation or discomfort and a normal day can be planned, many patients prefer this method of endoscopy. Additionally, no air is needed to expand the small intestine, as it is in traditional endoscopy; therefore, the patient does not feel uncomfortable and bloated.

Indirect Visualization Studies

Indirect visualization of the gastrointestinal tract is commonly performed through radiography. The passage of x-rays through the patient creates a radiograph or film depicting body structures. This technique is useful for detecting obstructions, strictures, inflammatory disease, tumors, ulcers, and other lesions and for diagnosing hiatal hernia and other structural changes in the gastrointestinal tract. Use of a radiopaque contrast medium, such as barium sulfate, accentuates the body structures being visualized. In the upper gastrointestinal examination and small bowel series, the patient drinks the barium sulfate like a milkshake. The barium coats the esophagus, stomach, and small intestine to enhance visualization. In the barium enema or lower gastrointestinal examination, barium sulfate is instilled into the large intestine through a rectal tube inserted through the anus. Fluoroscopy projects consecutive x-ray images onto a screen for continuous observation of the flow of the barium. The specific nursing responsibilities are included in Table 44-2.

Scheduling for Diagnostic Studies

Nurses are commonly involved in scheduling diagnostic studies when a patient is to undergo multiple studies. Use the following guidelines for scheduling studies of the gastrointestinal tract:

1. Follow a logical sequence when more than one test is required for accurate diagnosis:

    Fecal occult blood tests: to detect gastrointestinal bleeding

    Barium studies: to visualize gastrointestinal structures and reveal any inflammation, ulcers, tumors, strictures, or other lesions

    Endoscopic examinations: to visualize an abnormality, locate a source of bleeding, and if necessary provide biopsy tissue samples

2. A barium enema and routine radiography should precede an upper gastrointestinal series, because retained barium from an upper gastrointestinal series could take several days to pass through the gastrointestinal tract and cloud anatomic detail on the barium enema studies.

3. Noninvasive procedures usually take precedence over invasive procedures, such as endoscopic studies, when sufficient diagnostic data can be obtained from them. (In some instances, endoscopic studies may be done before barium studies to ensure visualization.)

Diagnosing

Bowel Elimination as the Problem

When the analysis of assessment data points to a bowel elimination problem that can be prevented or resolved by independent nursing intervention, a nursing diagnosis is developed. If alterations in bowel elimination require new self-care behaviors, for example colostomy management, Deficient Knowledge may be an appropriate nursing diagnosis. (See the accompanying box, Examples of NANDA Nursing Diagnoses.)

Bowel Elimination as the Etiology

Problems of bowel elimination may also affect other areas of human functioning. In the nursing diagnoses that follow, problems of bowel elimination are the etiology for other problems:

Delayed Growth and Development related to child's inability to attain bowel control secondary to inconsistency and lack of adequate parental knowledge

Imbalanced Nutrition: Less Than Body Requirements related to loss of appetite from flatulence or impaction, prolonged diarrhea

Anxiety related to lack of voluntary control of fecal elimination and significant others' response to ostomy

Disturbed Body Image related to ostomy, need to wear disposable adult briefs, continuous episodes of diarrhea

Deficient Fluid Volume related to prolonged diarrhea

Impaired Skin Integrity related to prolonged diarrhea, fecal incontinence

Ineffective Coping related to inability to accept permanent ostomy

Deficient Knowledge: Bowel Training related to no previous experience

Pain related to intestinal distention, prolonged constipation or impaction, fecal incontinence, hemorrhoids

Self-Care Deficit: Toileting related to mobility deficit, weakness, confusion

Low Self-Esteem related to need for assistance with toileting, fecal incontinence

Sexual Dysfunction related to perceived change in body image, lack of interest, loss of self-esteem

Examples of NANDA Nursing Diagnoses | Bowel Elimination

Nursing Diagnoses	Related Factors	Sample Defining Characteristics
Constipation	Decreased fiber in diet Decreased fluid intake Inactivity Delaying defecation when urge is present Abuse of laxatives Use of constipating medications (antacids, narcotic analgesics [opioids], anticholinergics) Change in routine Pain associated with defecation	*"I feel bloated and know I have to move my bowels but I can't."* *"Whenever I'm constipated I feel lethargic and lose my appetite."* • Reports straining during defecation with little result • Passes small "marbles" of dry, hard stool • Decreased frequency • Decreased frequency of bowel sounds or changes in abdominal growling • Straining often results in small amount of bleeding from swollen external hemorrhoids • Reports feeling rectal fullness or pressure in rectum • Headache
Risk for Constipation	Habitually ignores urge to defecate Inactivity Decreased fiber in diet Inadequate fluid intake Use of pharmacologic agents that can result in constipation (iron, opioids, anticholinergics) Stress, confusion	• *"I'm in such a rush in the morning that I never take time to go to the bathroom."* • Reports straining during defecation • Passes small, hard, dry stool • Reports feeling bloated
Perceived Constipation	Culture Family health beliefs Faulty appraisal Impaired thought processes	• Expectation of daily bowel movement with resulting abuse of laxatives, enemas, suppositories • Expected passage of stool at the same time every day
Diarrhea	Food intolerance (coarse, greasy, or spicy foods) Food or drug allergies Abuse of laxatives Alteration in normal bacterial flora of the intestine (antibiotic therapy) Emotional stress Intestinal infection Colon disease and other diseases Surgical alterations	• Loose liquid stools, increased frequency • Urgency with soiling • Reports of abdominal pain and cramping • Increased frequency of bowel sounds
Bowel Incontinence	Gross constipation with impaction and subsequent overflow Organic changes in neural innervation of the rectum Local causes (inflammation, cancer of rectum, prolapsed anus, semifluid stool) Extreme debilitation Cognitive impairment	• Involuntary passage of stool (stool characteristics vary) • *"I'm sorry, I couldn't get into the bathroom (or onto the bedpan) quickly enough."* • *"It came so fast I couldn't hold it back."* • History of constipation with sudden development of oozing diarrheal stool

Outcome Identification and Planning

Planning interventions for patients without specific bowel elimination problems are directed toward the patient's achievement of the following outcomes. The patient will:

• Have a soft, formed bowel movement every 1 to 3 days without discomfort
• Explain the relationship between bowel elimination and dietary fiber, fluid intake, and exercise
• Relate the importance of seeking medical evaluation if changes in stool color or consistency persist

Implementing

Promoting Regular Bowel Habits

Regular bowel habits can be promoted in well and ill patients by attention to timing, positioning, privacy, nutrition, and exercise.

Timing

Once the time that a patient usually experiences the urge to defecate (often about an hour after meals, when mass colonic peristalsis occurs) is known, offer whatever assistance is needed to help the patient to the bathroom, commode, or bedpan at this time. Do not schedule nursing care or treatments during this time. Because many patients feel uncomfortable about requesting time for elimination, inform all patients about the importance of heeding this natural urge, explaining that postponing it only results in constipation and other problems.

Positioning

The squatting position best facilitates defecation, but most patients routinely use a sitting position while leaning a bit forward. Most patients who are able to use the bedside commode or bathroom toilet have little difficulty assuming this position, although they may need support. An elevated toilet seat may be ordered for patients with orthopedic problems who cannot lower themselves to a toilet seat.

Patients who need to use a bedpan in bed often benefit from having the head of the bed elevated 30 degrees, unless this is contraindicated. This eliminates the hyperextension of the back that occurs when a patient who is lying flat attempts to lift his or her hips onto the pan. After the head of the bed is elevated, the patient raises the hips by bending the knees, digging in the heels, and lifting the hips upward. An overhead trapeze may be helpful for patients with weak lower extremities. Do not raise the head of the bed more than 45 degrees because this makes it harder for the patient to lift the hips straight up (see Skill 43-1 for more information about positioning a patient on a bedpan). Many patients on bed rest appreciate having moistened hand wipes at the bedside to substitute for handwashing after toileting. Always empty, clean, and return bedpans to the patient's bedside stand promptly.

Privacy

Because most people consider elimination a private act, always respect the patient's need to be alone while defecating, unless the patient's condition makes this impossible. Pull the bedside drapes around a patient using a bedside commode or bedpan. If any visitors are present, ask them to step outside for a few minutes. For well patients who cannot defecate in a public restroom (with multiple toilets) or strange environment, suggest that they use a private restroom with only one toilet.

Nutrition

Patients with bowel elimination problems may need a dietary analysis to determine which foods and fluids are contributing to their problem and which may help in its treatment. General dietary recommendations to promote regular defecation include a fluid intake of 2,000 to 3,000 mL and high fiber intake. Water is recommended as the fluid of choice because fluids containing large amounts of caffeine and sugar may have a diuretic effect. Increasing fiber intake without sufficient fluid intake can result in severe gastrointestinal problems, including fecal impaction. Specific recommendations are discussed in the sections that follow.

Exercise

Regular exercise improves gastrointestinal motility and aids in defecation. Encourage well patients to exercise regularly three to five times a week. Ambulate patients who are ill as soon as possible, instructing them about how inactivity can lead to constipation, distention, and impaction. Bedside exercises may be helpful for patients who are immobile.

The following exercises may help patients with weak abdominal and perineal muscles who are using a bedpan:

Abdominal setting: The patient, lying in a supine position, tightens and holds the abdominal muscles for 6 seconds and then relaxes them. Repeat several times each waking hour.

Thigh strengthening: The thigh muscles are flexed and contracted by slowly bringing the knees up to the chest one at a time and then lowering them to the bed. Perform this exercise several times for each knee each waking hour.

Preventing and Treating Constipation

Constipation is the passage of dry, hard stools. Decreased gastric motility slows the passage of feces through the large intestine, resulting in increased fluid absorption from the fecal mass and causing dry, hard stool. Straining often accompanies defecation. Some people may be constipated and yet have a daily bowel movement, whereas others who regularly defecate no more than three times a week are not constipated. Individuals at high risk for constipation include (1) patients on bed rest who take constipating medications (opioids, anticholinergics), (2) patients with reduced fluids or bulk in their diet, (3) people who are depressed, and (4) patients with central nervous system disease or local lesions that cause pain.

Teaching About Nutrition

Promoting healthy behaviors can assist the patient and family to achieve mutually desirable outcomes for preventing constipation. A combination of high-fiber foods, 8 to 10 glasses of water daily, and exercise has been shown to be as effective as medications in controlling constipation (Selig & Boyle, 2001). Caution the patient to avoid increasing fiber intake without drinking enough fluids; this can lead to a bowel obstruction. Foods that contain high amounts of fiber include bran, fruits, vegetables, and whole grains.

Think back to Leroy Cobbs, the patient who developed fecal impaction from using narcotic analgesics. The nurse should list in the teaching plan foods that stimulate peristalsis to prevent future episodes of constipation. If the patient knows to include these foods in his diet, he will be less worried about future problems and may be more amenable to using the medication to control his pain.

Teaching About Cathartics and Laxatives

Cathartics and **laxatives** are drugs that induce emptying of the intestinal tract. Although these terms are sometimes used interchangeably, cathartics exert a stronger effect on the intestines than laxatives do. Some of these drugs, such as castor oil, cascara, senna, phenolphthalein, and bisacodyl (Dulcolax), act chemically by stimulating peristalsis. Others, such as magnesium sulfate and psyllium hydrophilic mucilloid (Metamucil), act by increasing the intestinal bulk, which promotes additional mechanical stimulation on the intestine. Still others, such as mineral oil and docusate sodium (Colace), soften the fecal material. Another frequently used laxative is Milk of Magnesia. It has antacid properties in small dosages and laxative properties in larger doses. Table 44-3 summarizes the types of laxatives.

Laxatives are sometimes necessary for people with limited activity or poor food intake. They are also used to empty the intestinal tract in preparation for surgery or diagnostic tests. Laxatives such as docusate sodium (Colace) may be used in conjunction with some prescribed medications to counteract the medications' constipating properties. Occasional use of laxatives is not harmful for most people, but people should not become dependent on them. Because many laxatives are available as nonprescription drugs, and advertising promotes their use, many people take them frequently on their own initiative, whether they need them or not.

Because of their chemical action, laxatives should not be taken when there is abdominal pain because an intestinal pathologic condition could be harmed by the increased peristalsis. Although many people take laxatives because they believe they are constipated, most are unaware that habitual use of laxatives is the most common cause of chronic constipation.

Nurses play a key role in helping patients who abuse laxatives. Breaking the physical and psychological habit of using laxatives is not easy for a person who has come to depend on them: it often requires much patience, support, and

TABLE 44-3 Classification of Laxatives

Type	Action	Advantages	Caution
Bulk-forming (eg, Metamucil)	Psyllium, grain, or synthetic product that causes stool to absorb water and swell, thus stimulating peristalsis	Usually acts within 24 hours	May interfere with absorption of calcium and iron and certain drugs Should not be given to bedridden patients or those with intestinal strictures May be expensive
Emollient/stool softener (eg, Colace)	Agents with detergent activity that allow water and fat to penetrate and lubricate the stool	Recommended for those who must avoid straining	Has lubricant component of drug that may interfere with absorption of fat-soluble vitamins
Lubricant (eg, mineral oil)	Lubricant is absorbed from intestinal tract and softens stool, making it easier to pass.	Usually effective within 8 hours	May interfere with absorption of fat-soluble vitamins Can be aspirated, possibly resulting in a lipid pneumonia
Stimulant (eg, Dulcolax)	Drug promotes peristalsis by irritating the intestinal mucosa or stimulating nerve endings in intestinal wall.	Works more quickly than bulking agents	Are the most abused laxatives on the market Causes lazy bowel syndrome May affect absorption of vitamin D and calcium Not recommended for elderly patients because of prolonged action Alters electrolyte transport
Saline-osmotic (eg, Fleet)	Drug draws water into intestine and stimulates peristalsis.	Is used when rapid cleansing desired	Should not be used by elderly people Can produce dehydration Not recommended in patients with kidney disease or heart failure

teaching. The person also frequently needs assistance with his or her diet, fluid intake, activity, and regularity of habits (see the accompanying Research in Nursing box).

Preventing and Treating Diarrhea

Diarrhea is the passage of excessively liquid, unformed stools. Frequent bowel movements are not always indicative of diarrhea, but patients with diarrhea usually pass stools more frequently. Diarrhea is often associated with intestinal cramps. Nausea and vomiting may occur; blood also may be noted. Diarrhea is a protective response when the cause is irritants in the intestinal tract. Regardless of the cause, however, large amounts of fluids and electrolytes may be lost relatively quickly through diarrhea, especially in infants and young children. If diarrhea is untreated, this loss of fluids and electrolytes places the child at high risk for life-threatening complications. If oral intake is possible, cold fluids and rich foods, especially sweets, should be avoided.

Additional nursing measures for the patient with diarrhea include the following:

- Answer the patient's call bell immediately, or ensure that a bedpan or commode is within easy reach. Diarrhea can be embarrassing, and the patient needs to know that the nurse is there to help.
- Whenever possible, remove the cause of the diarrhea. Discontinuing medications that cause diarrhea usually results in a return to normal defecation within 1 to 3 days.
- If there is any indication of an impaction, obtain a physician's order for a rectal examination before using antidiarrheal medications.

- Give special care to the region around the anus, where skin irritation is common. Keep the area clean and dry. Use skin creams, ointments, or powders as necessary.

> *Skin care measures would be important to include in the plan of care for Sally Germaine, the college junior experiencing episodes of diarrhea. Doing so reduces her risk for perianal excoriation and breakdown, which could further impair her body image.*

- After the diarrhea stops, suggest the intake of fermented dairy products such as buttermilk or yogurt to promote the return of normal bowel flora.

Teaching About Nutrition

The first precaution is to ensure that food is safe for consumption and prepared and stored properly. Food poisoning and the diarrhea that frequently accompanies it can be prevented by these common measures (Goldrick, 2003):

- Never purchase food with damaged packaging. Items that require refrigeration should be taken home immediately.
- Never use raw eggs in any form because of the danger of infection with the *Salmonella* bacillus. When cooking eggs, use only fresh ones that have been purchased within 3 to 5 weeks and kept in the refrigerator.
- Cook ground meat thoroughly. It should not have a pink center and should not drain pink juices. Avoid placing cooked meat on platters or cutting boards that held uncooked meat. Do not use knives previously used to cut uncooked meat.

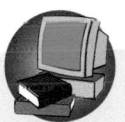

Research in Nursing Making a Difference

Managing Chronic Constipation in Long-Term Care Residents

Changes in bowel elimination patterns are distressing to patients and caregivers. Laxatives, enemas, and manual removal of fecal impactions are commonly prescribed to alleviate constipation in long-term care residents. In addition to being unpleasant for the resident, they are also costly and require additional nursing assistance. Nursing interventions that can help to alleviate the hopelessness and stress associated with constipation promote the emotional as well as the physical well-being of an individual. The results of previous studies supported the use of bran to treat constipation, but controlled research is necessary to define an effective bran protocol and decrease reliance on pharmacologic and invasive measures.

Related Research

Howard, L., West, D., & Ossip-Klein, D. (2000). Chronic constipation management for institutionalized older adults. *Geriatric Nursing, 21*(2), 78–82.

The subjects in this study were 12 male residents of a Veterans Administration Medical Center who had chronic constipation (two or fewer stools per week) and regularly used laxatives or enemas. They were paired into groups of two: one resident in the control group continued with the usual treatments and medications, and the other participated in the bran-treatment regimen.

During a 4-month period, as the amount of bran was gradually increased to a maximal dose of 6 tablespoons per day, laxative use was significantly reduced in the bran-treatment group. At the conclusion of this study, oral laxatives were totally discontinued for this test group, and the use of other bowel medication was reduced by 80%. Nurses also reported a decrease in patient discomfort with bowel elimination in the bran-treatment group. The control group did not experience any change in bowel habits or their medication and treatment regimen.

Relevance to Nursing Practice

This study verified that a simple dietary measure, over time, can have a dramatic effect on bowel elimination. Bran that is added slowly to the diet usually has minimal adverse effects and results in positive outcomes. Additional investigations will be necessary to compare the bran protocol with other treatment measures for constipation. The amount of bran and the length of time it is used merit additional study. Problems in bowel elimination are commonly identified and treated by nurses, and the nurse can play an essential role in helping a vulnerable population to regain control of this body function and maintain their dignity.

- Never cut meat on a wooden surface.
- Do not eat seafood raw. Do not eat seafood if it has a strong, unpleasant odor.
- Thoroughly clean all vegetables and fruit before eating.
- Refrigerate leftovers within 2 hours of preparation.
- Give only pasteurized fruit juices to small children.

Additional measures for preventing or treating diarrhea include avoiding highly spiced foods and foods with laxative effects such as raw fruits and vegetables. Encourage the patient to eat foods with a low fiber content. Replace lost fluids and electrolytes with weak tea, water, bouillon, clear soup, and gelatin. If diarrhea is severe, intravenous therapy may be needed.

Teaching About Treatment for Diarrhea

Treatment for diarrhea typically depends on whether the problem is acute or chronic. Acute diarrhea may result from a viral or bacterial infection, a reaction to medication, or alterations in diet. It is characterized by its sudden onset and lasts several hours to several days. Rehydration is key with acute diarrhea. Oral liquids may be used if the patient can tolerate them; otherwise, intravenous fluid replacement may be necessary. Stress the importance of hand hygiene with the patient and family. Antidiarrheal agents are avoided in acute diarrhea until a bacterial causative agent has been ruled out.

Chronic diarrhea typically lasts for more than 3 to 4 weeks. It has many possible causes, such as secondary disease states, surgery, laxative and alcohol abuse, and radiation and chemotherapeutic agents, and usually necessitates pharmacologic intervention along with fluid and electrolyte replacement. Antidiarrheal medications are usually reserved for treatment of chronic diarrhea. Whatever the type of diarrhea, every effort must be made to identify and eliminate the underlying cause.

Several types of antidiarrheal medications are available. Medications such as camphorated opium tincture (Paregoric), loperamide (Imodium), and diphenoxylate hydrochloride (Lomotil) act directly on the smooth muscle of the gastrointestinal tract. Kaolin and pectin (Kaopectate) is thought to act as an absorbent and demulcent. Bismuth subsalicylate (Pepto-Bismol) has a antimicrobial action and an antisecretory effect. Table 44-4 highlights the major antidiarrheal agents.

The focus of nursing care is on eliminating the cause of the diarrhea and replacing lost fluids as well as treating the symptoms. Some commercial fluid and electrolyte replacement

TABLE 44-4 Classification of Antidiarrheal Medications

Category	Name	Action	Advantages	Cautions
Action on gastrointestinal smooth muscle	Opium (Paregoric)	Increases smooth muscle tone Decreases GI motility Diminishes GI secretions	Effective	May be addictive due to morphine content May cause drowsiness and lightheadedness Should be discontinued as soon as diarrhea has diminished
	Diphenoxylate and atropine (Lomotil)	Slows gastric motility through local effect on gastrointestinal wall	Effective	Is chemically related to morphine; atropine added to prevent addiction but in high doses can become addictive May cause drowsiness
	Loperamide (Imodium)	Inhibits peristalsis via direct effect on gastrointestinal wall muscles	Not addictive Longer duration than Lomotil	May cause drowsiness Must be discontinued if no improvement in 48 hours with acute cases
Absorbent	Kaolin-pectin (Kaopectate)	Absorbs and soothes	No drowsiness	May interfere with absorption of other oral medications May interfere with absorption of nutrients with prolonged use
Antisecretory/ antimicrobial	Bismuth subsalicylate (Pepto-Bismol)	Decreases gastrointestinal tract secretion Has antimicrobial action against bacterial and viral pathogens	No drowsiness	Contains salicylates, so check with physician before giving to children or administering with aspirin May decrease absorption of some medications

products, such as Gatorade, may be helpful. Oral rehydration therapy using fluid and electrolyte replacement and water for adults is cost-effective and replaces fluid loss without the challenges associated with intravenous fluid therapy. It is particularly important that fluid balance be maintained in older patients because of their increased risk for dehydration, fluid overload, and electrolyte imbalances.

Infants and children require more water than adults. Based on size, children have a larger volume of output and intake than adults do, and infants and young children also have a larger extracellular fluid volume. When infants and children become ill, they lose a majority of the fluids from their extracellular compartment, which quickly leads to dehydration (Wong, Perry & Hockenberry, 2002). Encourage fluids, especially soy formula and Pedialyte (an oral electrolyte solution for children that is low in sugar), and make them accessible for the child. Special diets for dehydration such as the BRAT diet (bananas, rice cereal, applesauce, and toast) are no longer recommended because they lack sufficient calories.

Decreasing Flatulence

Excessive formation of gases in the stomach or intestines is known as **flatulence.** When the gas is not expelled but accumulates in the intestinal tract, the condition is referred to as intestinal distention or tympanites. Gas-producing foods, such as beans, cabbage, onions, cauliflower, and beer, often predispose a person to flatulence and distention.

> *Recall Alberta Franklin, the patient described in Reflective Practice. The nurse should include information about gas-producing foods in this patient's teaching plan to avoid excess gas formation and accumulation, which could cause her colostomy bag to overfill and possibly lead to detachment and leakage.*

In addition to avoiding irritating foods, other nursing interventions are helpful in decreasing flatus. To promote peristalsis and the escape of flatus, the patient should avoid reclining after meals and should move around in bed and ambulate.

When ambulation to relieve flatulence is unsuccessful, the physician may order a rectal tube to be inserted. The tube helps to stimulate peristalsis and provides a passageway for the escape of flatus. When inserting a rectal tube, follow these steps:

1. Use a 22 to 34 French tube for adults (use a smaller size for children).
2. Position the patient on his or her side, and drape the patient properly.
3. Lubricate the rectal tube to reduce irritation to mucous membranes.
4. Separate the buttocks so that the anus is in plain view. Insert the tube, introducing it beyond the anal canal into the rectum for about 10 cm (4 inches). It may be inserted a bit further if no flatus is being removed.
5. Secure a dressing or waterproof pad to the end of the rectal tube, or place the end of the tube in a specimen con-

tainer or urinal placed between the patient's legs. These techniques allow any discharge that empties through the rectal tube to be caught.
6. Leave the rectal tube in place for no longer than about 20 minutes; the tube no longer acts as a stimulant for peristalsis if left in place longer. If distention is not relieved, use the rectal tube intermittently every 2 to 3 hours, as necessary.
7. Have the patient assume various positions to help move flatus along the intestinal tract toward the anus. Because gas is lighter than fluids and solids, it will rise. Helpful positions include lying on the abdomen, assuming the knee-chest position, and positioning the upper part of the body over the edge of the bed while the lower part rests across the bed. Do not use these positions if they are contraindicated or unsafe for the patient.
8. Confer with the physician if these measures bring no relief. An enema, a suppository, or a medication may be prescribed to help bring relief.

Emptying the Colon of Feces

Several methods are used to help promote elimination of feces: enemas, suppositories, oral intestinal lavage, and digital removal of stool.

Enemas

An **enema** is the introduction of a solution into the large intestine, usually to remove feces. The instilled solution distends the intestine and may irritate the intestinal mucosa, thus increasing peristalsis. Enemas are classified as cleansing, retention, or return-flow enemas.

Cleansing Enemas

Cleansing enemas are given to remove feces from the colon, commonly to:
- Relieve constipation or fecal impaction
- Prevent involuntary escape of fecal material during surgical procedures
- Promote visualization of the intestinal tract by radiographic or instrument examination
- Help establish regular bowel function during a bowel training program

The most common types of solutions used for cleansing enemas are tap water, normal saline solution, soap solution, and hypertonic solution. Commonly used enema solutions are described in Table 44-5.

Hypotonic (tap water) and isotonic (normal saline solution) enemas are large-volume enemas that result in rapid colonic emptying. However, using such large volumes of solution (adults, 500 to 1,000 mL; infants, 150 to 250 mL) may be dangerous for patients with weakened intestinal walls. These solutions often require special preparation and equipment.

Hypertonic solution preparations are available commercially and are administered in smaller volumes (adult, 70 to 130 mL). These solutions draw water into the colon, which stimulates the defecation reflex. They may be contraindicated in patients for whom sodium retention is a problem.

TABLE 44-5 Commonly Used Enema Solutions

Solution	Amount	Action	Time to Take Effect	Adverse Effects
Tap water (hypotonic)	500–1,000 mL	Distends intestine, increases peristalsis, softens stool	15 min	Fluid and electrolyte imbalance, water intoxication
Normal saline (isotonic)	500–1,000 mL	Distends intestine, increases peristalsis, softens stool	15 min	Fluid and electrolyte imbalance, sodium retention
Soap	500–1,000 mL (concentrate at 3–5 mL/1,000 mL)	Distends intestine, irritates intestinal mucosa, softens stool	10–15 min	Rectal mucosa irritation or damage
Hypertonic	70–130 mL	Distends intestine, irritates intestinal mucosa	5–10 min	Sodium retention
Oil (mineral, olive, or cottonseed oil)	150–200 mL	Lubricates stool and intestinal mucosa	30 min	

Retention Enemas

Retention enemas are retained in the bowel for a prolonged period for different reasons.

Oil-retention enemas: lubricate the stool and intestinal mucosa, making defecation easier. About 150 to 200 mL of solution is administered to adults.

Carminative enemas: help to expel flatus from the rectum and provide relief from gaseous distention. Common solutions include the milk-and-molasses enema (equal parts) and the magnesium sulfate–glycerin–water (MGW) enema (30 mL of magnesium sulfate, 60 mL of glycerin, and 90 mL of warm water).

Medicated enemas: provide medications that are absorbed through the rectal mucosa

Anthelmintic enemas: destroy intestinal parasites

Nutritive enemas: administer fluids and nutrition rectally

Return-Flow Enemas

Return-flow, or Harris flush, enemas are occasionally prescribed to expel flatus. For an adult, 100 to 200 mL of a solution is instilled into the rectum and sigmoid colon, and then the solution container is lowered so that the solution flows back into the container. This process is repeated five or six times, and the alternating flow of solution stimulates peristalsis and aids in the expelling of flatus. The procedure is terminated when abdominal distention is relieved. If the return solution becomes thick with feces, it is replaced by fresh solution.

Equipment

Commercially prepared enema kits include a flexible bottle containing hypertonic solution with an attached prelubricated firm tip about 5 to 7.5 cm (2 to 3 inches) long. Its ease of use makes it particularly convenient in the home. Patients can readily administer their own enema in many instances.

For tap water, saline solution, or soap solution enema, a container, rubber or plastic tubing with side openings near its distal end, a tubing clamp, lubricant, and the solution are nec-

essary. Regardless of the type of enema to be given, clean or medically aseptic technique is used. Always wear or have the caregiver wear disposable gloves to protect from exposure to blood, body fluids, and microorganisms.

Patient Preparation

Because enemas are a common procedure, some patients already know why they are used and how they are administered. Reinforce this information and correct any misconceptions that they may have. For patients who have not previously had an enema, explain the purpose, what they can expect, and how they can participate. In all cases, provide for patient privacy. The procedure offers an excellent opportunity for health teaching because many people are unfamiliar with or uncomfortable talking about the functioning of the intestinal tract. Failure to provide explanations and protect privacy may result in an uncomfortable and disagreeable situation for the patient.

A reclining position for enema administration is recommended, but if the patient has a respiratory disorder or is having difficulty breathing, elevate the head of the bed slightly. Avoid the Fowler's position because the solution will remain in the rectum and expulsion will occur rapidly, resulting in minimal cleansing.

Some patients think the solution should be expelled as soon as possible. Reinforce the need to retain the solution to achieve the desired results.

Administration Using a Large Volume of Solution

The procedure for administering a cleansing enema using a large volume of solution is described in Skill 44-1.

Administration Using a Hypertonic Solution

Administering a cleansing enema using a hypertonic solution differs from the procedure described in Skill 44-1 in the following ways:

- The equipment is included in the commercially prepared set. The only additional equipment needed is a bedpan for

SKILL 44-1   Administering a Cleansing Enema

EQUIPMENT

Disposable enema set
Water-soluble lubricant
Solution as ordered by physician:
  Temperature:
  For adults: 105°–110°F (40°–43°C)
  For children: 100°F (37.7°C)

Amount: Will vary, depending on type
  of solution, age of the person, and the
  patient's ability to retain the solution.
  Average cleansing enema for an adult
  may range from 750 to 1000 mL.
Necessary additives (soap, salt, and so forth)
Bath thermometer

Waterproof pad
Bath blanket
Bedpan and toilet tissue
IV pole
Disposable gloves
Paper towel
Washcloth, soap, and towel or Handi-wipes

ACTION	RATIONALE
1. Assemble the necessary equipment. Warm solution in amount ordered, and check temperature with a bath thermometer if available. If tap water is used, adjust temperature as it flows from faucet.	Organization facilitates performance of task. If bath thermometer is not available, warm to room temperature or slightly higher, and test on inner wrist.
2. Explain the procedure to the patient and plan where he or she will defecate. Have a bedpan, commode, or nearby bathroom ready for his use.	The patient is better able to relax and cooperate if he or she is familiar with the procedure and knows everything is in readiness when the urge to defecate is felt. Defecation usually occurs within 5 to 15 minutes.
3. Perform hand hygiene.	Hand hygiene deters the spread of microorganisms.
4. Add enema solution to container. Release the clamp and allow fluid to progress through tube before reclamping.	This causes any air to be expelled from the tubing. Although allowing air to enter the intestine is not harmful, it may further distend the intestine.
5. Position waterproof pad under the patient.	This protects bed linen.
6. Provide for patient's privacy. Position and drape the patient on the left side (Sims' position) with anus exposed or on the back, as dictated by patient comfort and condition.	The patient's comfort and warmth help him or her relax. The exact position of the reclining person has not been found to alter results of an enema significantly.
7. Put on disposable gloves.	This protects the nurse from microorganisms in the feces.
8. Elevate the solution so that it is 45 cm (18 inches) above the level of the patient's anus. Plan to give the solution slowly over a period of 5 to 10 minutes. The container may be hung on an IV pole or held in the nurse's hands at the proper height.	Gravity forces the solution to enter the intestine. The amount of pressure determines the rate of flow and pressure exerted on the intestinal wall. Giving the solution too quickly causes rapid distention and pressure in the intestine, resulting in too rapid expulsion of the solution, poor defecation, or damage to the mucous membrane.
9. Generously lubricate the end of the rectal tube for 5 to 7 cm (2–3 inches). A disposable enema set may have a prelubricated rectal tube.	This facilitates passage of the rectal tube through the anal sphincter and prevents injury to the mucosa.
10. Lift the buttock to expose the anus. Slowly and gently insert the rectal tube 7 to 10 cm (3–4 inches). Direct it at an angle pointing toward the umbilicus.	Good visualization of the anus helps prevent injury to tissues. The anal canal is about 2.5 to 5 cm (1–2 inches) in length. The tube should be inserted past the internal sphincter. Further insertion may damage intestinal mucous membrane. The suggested angle follows the normal intestinal contour. Slow insertion of the tube minimizes spasms of the intestinal wall and sphincters.

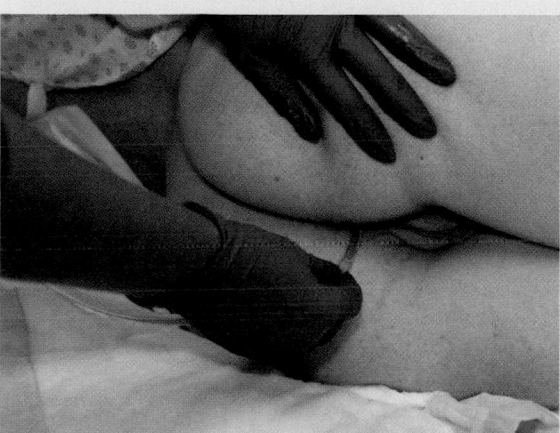

Action 10: Inserting enema tip into anus, directing tip toward umbilicus.   (Photo by Rick Brady.)

(continued)

ACTION	RATIONALE
11. If the tube meets resistance while inserting it, permit a small amount of solution to enter, withdraw the tube slightly and then continue to insert it. Do not force entry of the tube. Ask the patient to take several deep breaths.	Resistance may be due to spasms of the intestine or failure of the internal sphincter to open. The solution may help to reduce spasms and relax the sphincter, thus making continued insertion of the tube safe. Forcing a tube may injure the intestinal wall. Taking deep breaths helps relax the anal sphincter.
12. Introduce the solution slowly over a period of 5 to 10 minutes. Hold tubing all the time that solution is being instilled.	Introducing the solution slowly helps prevent rapid distention of the intestine and a desire to defecate.
13. Clamp the tubing or lower the container if the patient has the desire to defecate or cramping occurs. Patient also may be instructed to take small, fast breaths or to pant.	These techniques help relax muscles and prevent the expulsion of the solution prematurely.
14. After solution has been given, clamp the tubing and remove the tube. Have paper towel ready to receive tube as it is withdrawn. Have the patient retain the solution until the urge to defecate becomes strong, usually in about 5 to 15 minutes.	This amount of time usually allows muscle contractions to become sufficient to produce good results.
15. Remove disposable gloves from inside out and discard.	This protects the nurse from contact with any microorganisms.
16. When the patient has a strong urge to defecate, place him or her in a sitting position on a bedpan or assist to a commode or to the bathroom.	The sitting position is most natural and facilitates the act of defecation.
17. Record the character of the stool and the patient's reaction to the enema. Remind the patient not to flush commode before nurse inspects results of enema.	The nurse needs to observe and record the results. Additional enemas may be necessary if physician has ordered enemas "until clear."
18. Assist patient if necessary with cleaning of anal area. Offer washcloth, soap, and water to wash patient's hands.	Deters spread of microorganisms.
19. Leave the patient clean and comfortable. Care for the equipment properly.	There is abundant growth of bacteria in the intestine, which can be spread to others when equipment is not properly cared for.
20. Perform hand hygiene.	Hand hygiene deters the spread of microorganisms.

Older Adult Considerations

Elderly or infirm patients who are unable to retain the enema solution should receive the enema while on the bedpan in the supine position. For comfort, the head of the bed can be elevated 30 degrees if necessary and pillows used appropriately. Disposable gloves protect the hands as the enema is being expelled.

Home Care Considerations

Give enema in area that is as close to bathroom as possible. If using bedpan or commode, have it readily accessible.

Inform patient about availability of commercially prepared solutions and equipment.

Special Considerations

The limit for "enemas until clear" is usually three for an adult patient. Check with the physician before continuing with additional enemas because fluid and electrolyte imbalance can occur. Do not repeat an enema on a child or an infant without first consulting the physician.

Modify amount of solution according to patient's ability to tolerate procedure and size of patient.

Check with the physician before administering a cleansing enema to a patient who has a history of cardiac problems or one who has recently had rectal or prostate surgery. Cleansing enemas are also contraindicated for patients with glaucoma and increased intracranial pressure. Large-volume cleansing enemas have the potential to interfere with the action of the normal intestinal flora. The persistent diarrhea that may continue after the enema will usually cease once the normal flora are restored following the intake of buttermilk or yogurt with active cultures.

a bedridden patient and a disposable waterproof pad to protect bed linens.

- Do not warm the hypertonic solution. Administer it at room temperature, and warm it only if it is very cold.
- Place the patient in the side-lying position or the knee-chest position, which helps to distribute the solution throughout the lower intestinal tract and is recommended if the patient can assume it. Additional lubrication of the rectal tip is recommended, even though it is prelubricated.
- Instill the solution into the rectum by applying gentle pressure on the collapsible solution container. It should take 1 to 2 minutes to administer the enema (Fig. 44-5).
- Administer the hypertonic enema solution (Fleet enema) cautiously to a patient with hemorrhoids. The rigid tip may tear fragile rectal mucosa that is enlarged and inflamed, causing pain, torn rectal tissue, and necrosis. A rectal examination and generous lubrication are recommended before inserting the enema tip.

Administration of an Oil-Retention Enema

The procedure for giving an oil-retention enema differs from that for giving a cleansing enema in the following respects:

- A small rectal tube is used. The small size helps to reduce intestinal contractions so that the patient can retain the oil more easily. Oil enemas are available in commercial kits similar to those for hypertonic solution enemas. The kits contain a small rectal tube.
- Administer the oil-retention enema at body temperature to minimize muscle contractions caused by a warmer or cooler solution.
- Instruct the patient to retain the oil for at least 30 minutes for best cleansing results.

Rectal Suppositories

A **suppository** is a conical or oval solid substance shaped for easy insertion into a body cavity and designed to melt at body temperature. Various rectal suppositories are available. Some are fecal softeners, others have a direct action on the nerve endings in the rectal mucosa, and some liberate carbon dioxide when moistened. Fecal softeners are useful when the stool is very hard. Substances that stimulate the rectal nerves are helpful for people with weak muscle tone or poor innervation. The carbon dioxide suppositories liberate about 200 mL of gas, which causes distention, causing stimulation and elimination impulses (see Guidelines for Nursing Care 44-2).

Oral Intestinal Lavage

An oral solution, such as GoLYTELY or Colyte, can be used to cleanse the intestine of feces. This solution is prescribed by the physician and can be administered before diagnostic tests that require a clear bowel for visualization purposes or as a "bowel prep" before intestinal surgery. Evacuation of feces usually begins within 1 hour after the first glass and is completed within 4 to 6 hours. As with an enema, a clear return indicates that the bowel preparation is complete. A clear diet for 24 hours before taking this solution lessens the time needed for completion of the bowel prep, but potassium replacement may be required before surgery because of the limited potassium in a clear diet. The solution has a slightly salty taste and is easier to tolerate if it is cold and consumed quickly. Older patients require careful assessment because they are more prone to electrolyte imbalances.

Digital Removal of Stool

Fecal impaction is prolonged retention or an accumulation of fecal material that forms a hardened mass in the rectum. Fecal impaction often prevents the passage of normal stools. Small amounts of fluid may pass around the impacted mass; liquid fecal seepage with no passage of normal feces is a sign of an impaction.

If a patient with a fecal impaction cannot expel the fecal mass voluntarily and oil and cleansing enemas fail to break up the mass, the impaction must be broken up manually. A physician's order is required. This procedure may cause great discomfort to the patient as well as irritation of the rectal mucosa and bleeding. Digital removal of a fecal mass can stimulate the vagus nerve, resulting in a slowed heart rate. If this occurs, stop the procedure immediately, monitor the patient's heart rate and blood pressure, and notify the physician.

To manually remove a fecal impaction, the following technique is recommended:

1. Have a second person assist with the procedure. The second person can reassure and comfort the patient while the first person works to break up the mass.
2. Place the patient in a side-lying position.
3. Place a bedpan on the bed for depositing removed feces.
4. Drape the patient to preserve privacy yet provide easy access.
5. Use clean gloves for the procedure, because the intestinal tract is not sterile.
6. Lubricate the forefinger generously to reduce irritating the rectum, and insert the finger gently into the anal canal. The presence of the finger added to the mass tends to cause discomfort for the patient if the work is not done slowly and gently.
7. Work the finger around and into the hardened mass to break it up and then remove pieces of it. Instruct the patient to

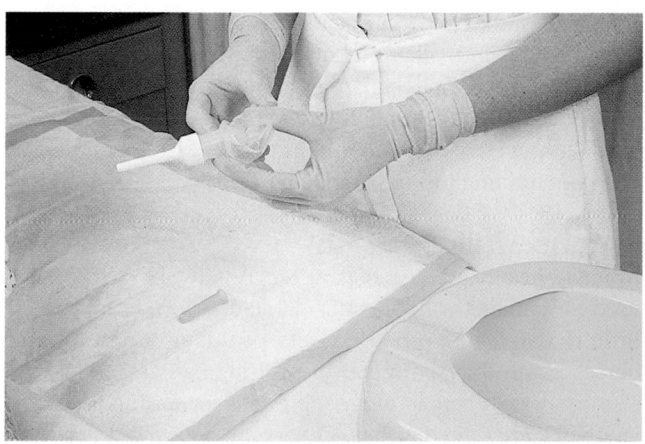

FIGURE 44-5 Technique for compressing Fleet enema container.

Guidelines for Nursing Care 44-2
Inserting a Rectal Suppository

- Use a glove for protection while inserting the suppository.
- Have the patient lie on either side, and pie-fold top linens over him or her.
- Lubricate the suppository and fingertips to reduce irritation on intestinal mucosa while inserting the suppository.
- Separate the buttocks and then have the patient relax by breathing through the mouth while the suppository is inserted.
- Using one finger, introduce the suppository well beyond the internal sphincter (4 inches for adults and 2 inches for children and infants) so that the suppository is in the rectum, where its effect is desired.
- Avoid embedding the suppository in the fecal mass. Correct placement when there is stool in the rectum is between the stool and the rectal mucosa.
- Be sure the patient understands that he or she is to retain the suppository, usually for 30 to 45 minutes after insertion.

- Encourage the patient to walk about if ambulatory; this often helps promote peristalsis.

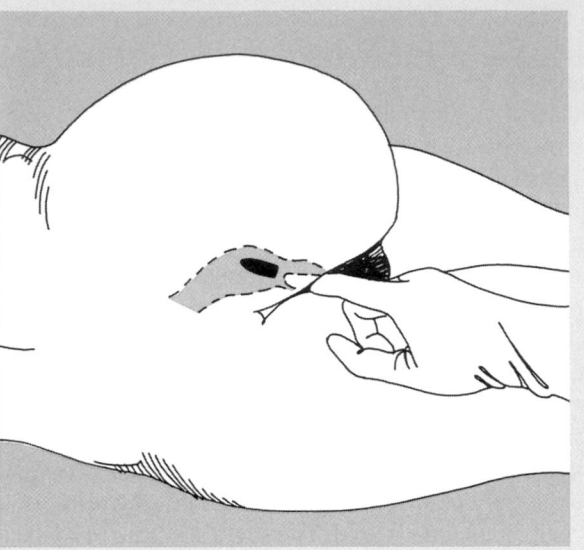

bear down, if possible, while extracting feces to ease in removal.

8. Remove the impaction at intervals if it is severe. This helps to avoid discomfort as well as irritation, which can injure intestinal mucosa.

9. Use an oil-retention enema if necessary. The enema may be given before attempts are made to break up and remove the impaction digitally, or it may be ordered after digital attempts fail. A cleansing enema is often ordered after an oil-retention enema.

It is important for the nurse caring for Leroy Cobbs, the patient with fecal impaction described at the beginning of the chapter, to demonstrate competency and care when performing manual disimpaction to decrease the patient's discomfort and embarrassment. Additionally, the nurse may need to adapt the procedure to ensure that the patient experiences relief as quickly as possible without any undue harm or injury.

Figure 44-6 demonstrates the procedure for removal of fecal impaction. Many patients find that a sitz bath or tub bath after this procedure soothes the irritated perineal area.

Managing Bowel Incontinence

Bowel incontinence is the inability of the anal sphincter to control the discharge of fecal and gaseous material. The cause of incontinence is usually an organic disease, resulting either in a mechanical condition that hinders the proper functioning of the anal sphincter or an impairment in the nerve supply to

the anal sphincter. Mental illness may also cause a patient to be indifferent to the passage of stool. Although bowel incontinence is seldom life-threatening, patients with bowel incontinence suffer embarrassment, may become depressed, and pose a challenge for nurses because of the risk for skin breakdown.

The following nursing interventions are helpful for a patient who suffers from bowel incontinence:

- Note when incontinence is most likely to occur, and place the patient on a bedpan at those times. If there is no pattern, offer a bedpan at regular intervals, such as every few hours.
- Keep the skin clean and dry by using proper hygienic measures. Pressure ulcers may develop when such measures are overlooked.
- Change bed linens and clothing as necessary to avoid odor, skin irritation, and embarrassment. Disposable bed pads and moisture-proof undergarments can be considered but should not be used until other measures have been tried.
- Confer with the physician about using a suppository or a daily cleansing enema. These measures empty the lower colon regularly and often help to decrease incontinence. Bowel training programs may be helpful.

Rectal Indwelling Catheter

In many healthcare agencies, a rectal indwelling catheter is used for patients with uncontrollable diarrhea, but relatively little research supports the safety of this procedure. Some nurses claim that the rectal indwelling catheter stimulates sensory nerve fibers in the rectum, thus increasing peristalsis and worsening the diarrhea. Others are concerned about the danger of rectal perforation and the development of mucosal

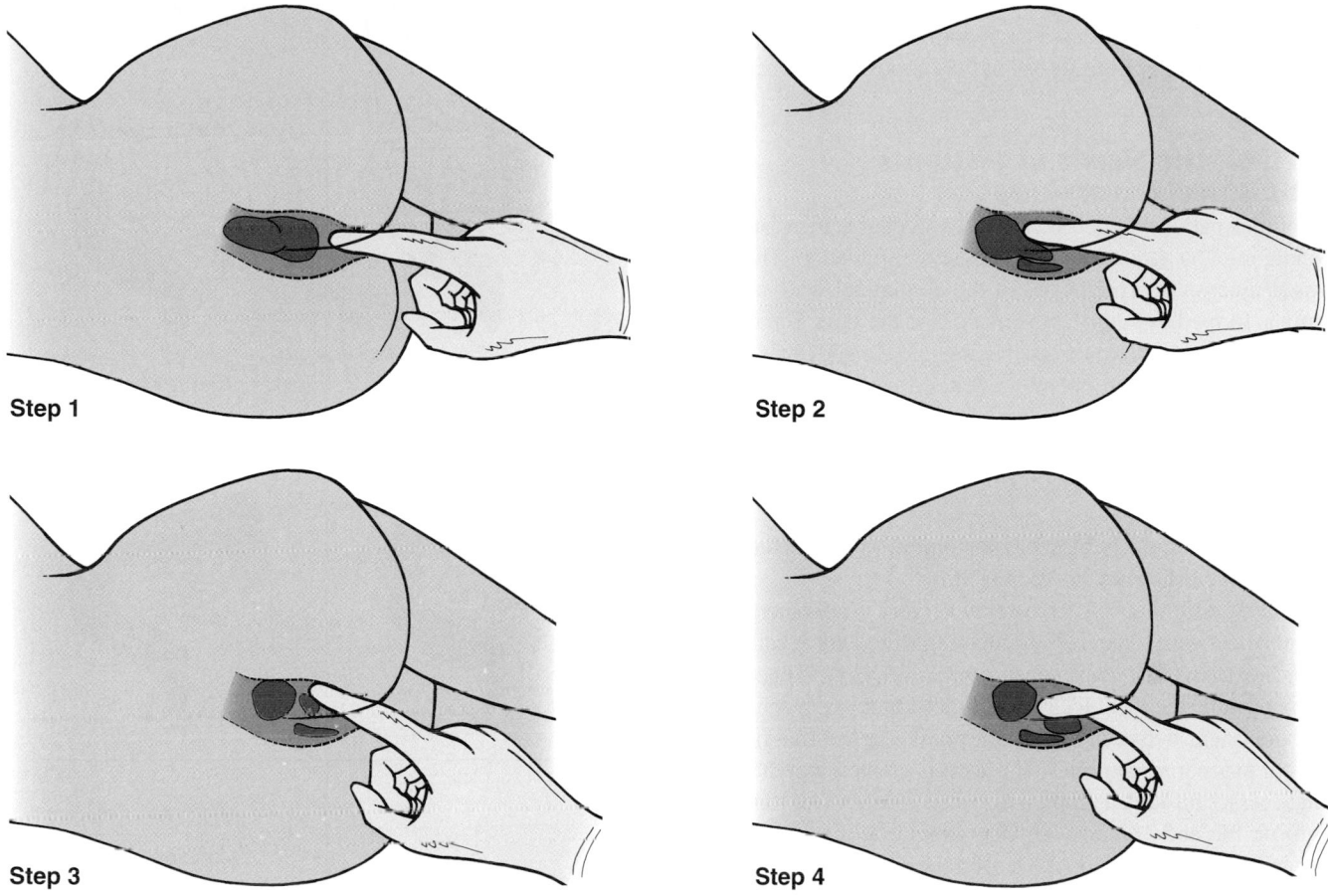

Step 1

Step 2

Step 3

Step 4

FIGURE 44-6 Digital removal of fecal impaction. *Step 1:* Inserting the gloved, lubricated finger into the fecal mass. *Step 2:* Using the finger to break up some of the hardened mass. *Step 3.* Breaking off a section of the impaction. *Step 4:* Removing a section of the impaction.

necrosis. Most experts agree that indwelling rectal catheters should not be used to manage large volumes of diarrhea.

Fecal Incontinence Pouch

An alternative measure to protect perianal skin from repeated episodes of fecal incontinence is the fecal incontinence pouch. This device can be secured via adhesive around the anal opening and attached to gravity drainage, allowing liquid stool to accumulate in a collection bag. It is best applied before the perianal area becomes excoriated. If excoriation is already present, application of a skin barrier can be effective.

Nursing responsibilities include careful regular assessment and documentation of the perianal skin condition and attentive management of the drainage system. Change the pouch at least every 72 hours, or sooner if it is not intact or leakage has occurred. Provide explanations and support to the patient and family members so that they understand the benefits of this system.

Designing and Implementing Bowel Training Programs

Patients with a history of chronic constipation and impaction and those who are incontinent of stool may benefit from a **bowel training program.** The purpose of this program is to manipulate factors within the person's control (food and fluid intake, exercise, time for defecation) to produce the elimination of a soft, formed stool at regular intervals without a laxative. This effort to regain bowel control may be initiated in the healthcare setting or the patient's home. Examples of steps in a bowel training program are described in the accompanying Examples of Nursing Interventions Classification box.

Examples of Nursing Interventions Classification (NIC)
Bowel Training

- Plan bowel program with patient and appropriate others.
- Instruct patient about which foods are high in bulk.
- Ensure adequate fluid intake.
- Initiate an uninterrupted, consistent time for defecation.
- Ensure privacy.
- Administer suppository, as appropriate.
- Evaluate bowel status regularly.
- Modify bowel program, as needed.

From McClosky, J., & Bulechek, G. [2002]. *Nursing interventions classification [NIC]* [4th ed.]. St. Louis: C. V. Mosby. A full listing of nursing activities for each nursing intervention can be found in this book.

When the patient has established a regular pattern of defecation, continue to offer assistance with toileting at the successful time, but discontinue use of the suppository if one was used.

Meeting the Needs of Patients With Bowel Diversions

Sometimes patients undergo surgical procedures to create an opening into the abdominal wall for fecal elimination. The intestinal mucosa is brought out to the abdominal wall, and a **stoma** is formed by suturing the mucosa to the skin. The word **ostomy** is a general term for an opening into the body; it is usually used to refer to an opening created for the excretion of body wastes. An **ileostomy** allows liquid fecal content from the ileum of the small intestine to be eliminated through the stoma. A **colostomy** permits formed feces from the colon to exit through the stoma. Figure 44-7 shows the location of an ileostomy and variously placed colostomies, as well as the expected stool consistency for each ostomy.

In many institutions, if the ostomy surgery is not emergent, patients meet with a specially trained registered nurse called a wound, ostomy, and continence nurse (WOCN). Together, they determine the ideal location for the stoma.

A continent ileostomy is an alternative to the traditional surgical procedure. An internal pouch is created that the patient accesses through a nipple-like valve constructed from the ileum on the abdominal wall. The patient does not need to wear an external collection device, but because the valve malfunctions frequently, this procedure has limited use at this time. Another surgical alternative that does not involve an external stoma is the creation of an ileoanal reservoir. The terminal ileum is sutured directly to the anus, a pouch is created, and the patient is able to control expulsion of feces through the intact anal sphincter (Fig. 44-8). This procedure also has complications, and candidates are carefully selected for this surgery.

An ileostomy or colostomy may be either temporary or permanent. Temporary ostomies are performed to allow the intestine to repair itself after inflammatory disease, some types of intestinal surgery, or injury. Permanent ostomies are performed for debilitating intestinal diseases or cancer of the colon or rectum.

Colostomy and Ileostomy Care

The patient with an ostomy needs physical and psychological support both preoperatively and postoperatively. This support can come from the patient's significant others as well as from members of the healthcare team and from people who have had similar experiences. The ostomy requires specific physical care for which the nurse is initially responsible. The following guidelines help to promote the ostomy patient's physical and psychological comfort:

- Keep the patient as free of odors as possible. The application of a temporary appliance after surgery or during the time of the first dressing change postoperatively can eliminate much of the fecal odor from a bulky dressing. The ostomy appliance should be emptied frequently.

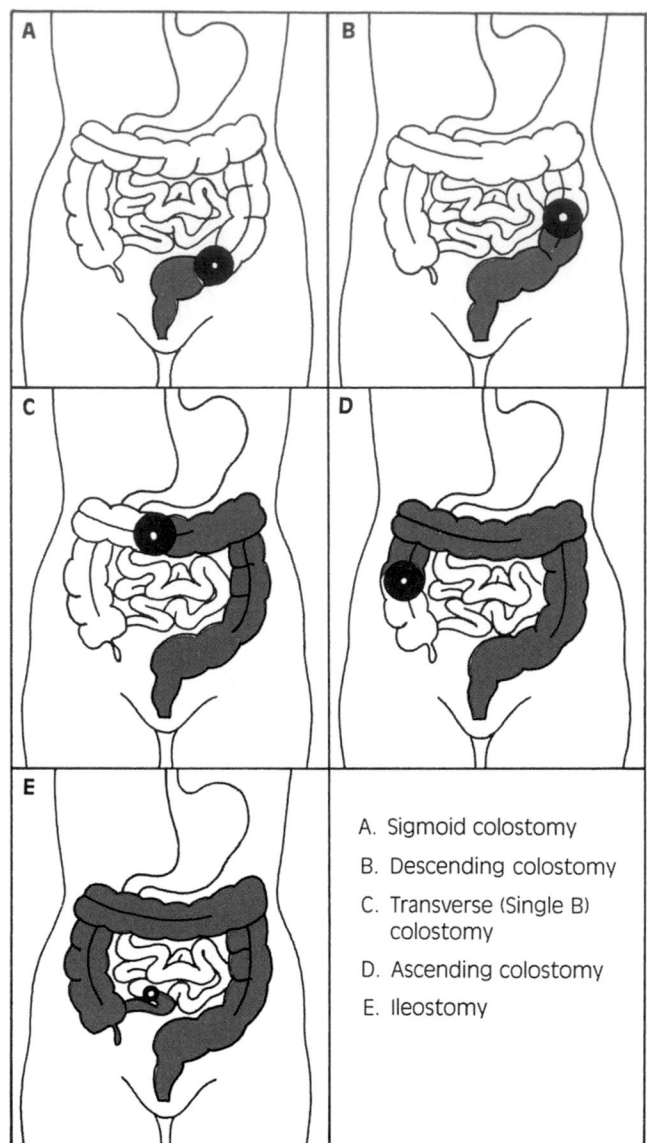

A. Sigmoid colostomy
B. Descending colostomy
C. Transverse (Single B) colostomy
D. Ascending colostomy
E. Ileostomy

FIGURE 44-7 (A–D) Location of various colostomies, and (**E**) location of an ileostomy. The *shaded portions* represent the sections of the bowel that have been removed or are currently inactive.

- Inspect the patient's stoma regularly. It should be dark pink to red and moist. A pale stoma may indicate anemia, and a dark or purple-blue stoma may reflect compromised circulation or ischemia (Fig. 44-9). Bleeding around the stoma and its stem should be minimal. Notify the physician promptly if bleeding persists or is excessive or if color changes occur in the stoma.
- Note the size of the stoma, which usually stabilizes within 6 to 8 weeks. Most stomas protrude ½ to 1 inch from the abdominal surface and may initially appear swollen and edematous. After 6 weeks, the edema has usually subsided. If an abdominal dressing is in place, check it frequently for drainage and bleeding.
- Keep the skin around the stoma site (peristomal area) clean and dry. If care is not taken to protect the skin around the stoma, irritation or infection may occur. A leaking appli-

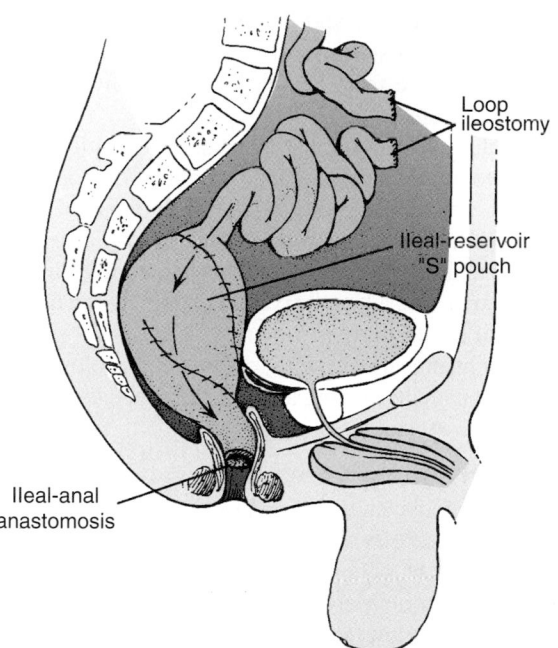

Loop ileostomy

Ileal-reservoir "S" pouch

Ileal-anal anastomosis

FIGURE 44-8 Ileoanal reservoir. (From Smeltzer, S. C., & Bare, B. G. [2004]. *Brunner & Suddarth's textbook of medical-surgical nursing* [10th ed.]. Philadelphia: Lippincott Williams & Wilkins.)

ance frequently causes skin erosion. Candida or yeast infections can also occur around the stoma if the area is not kept dry.

- Measure the patient's fluid intake and output. Check the ostomy appliance for the quality and quantity of discharge. Record intake and output every 4 hours for the first 3 days after surgery. If the patient's output decreases while intake remains stable, report the condition promptly.

- Explain each aspect of care to the patient and explain what his or her role will be when he or she begins self-care. Patient teaching is one of the most important aspects of colostomy care and should include family members when appropriate. Teaching can begin prior to surgery so that the patient has adequate time to absorb information.

- Encourage the patient to participate in care and to look at the ostomy. Patients normally experience emotional depression during the early postoperative period. The nurse can help the patient to cope by listening, explaining, and being available and supportive. A visit from a representative of the local ostomy support group may be helpful. Patients usually begin to accept their altered body image when they are willing to look at the stoma, make neutral or positive statements concerning the ostomy, and express interest in learning self-care.

Changing the Ostomy Appliance

The ostomy appliance should protect the skin, collect the fecal discharge, and control odor. Typically, a colostomy does not produce drainage until normal peristalsis returns, usually within 2 to 5 days. An ileostomy drains within 24 to 48 hours because of the liquid contents in the small intestine.

For the first few days after surgery, most patients wear an open-ended appliance or pouch that allows for drainage of fecal material without removing the appliance. The skin barrier has an adhesive barrier that protects the surrounding skin from the stoma output. Appliances are either one-piece (barrier already attached to the pouch) or two-piece (separate pouch that fastens to the barrier).

Appliances can be either drainable or closed. A pouch that can be drained is emptied when it is one-third full and replaced every 3 to 7 days, or whenever the seal comes away from the skin. The drainable pouch is cleansed by rinsing the inside

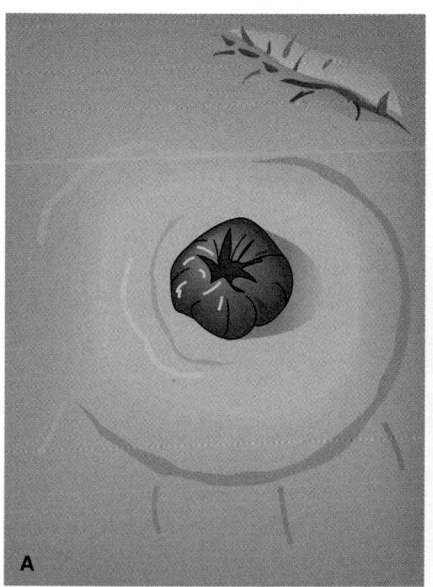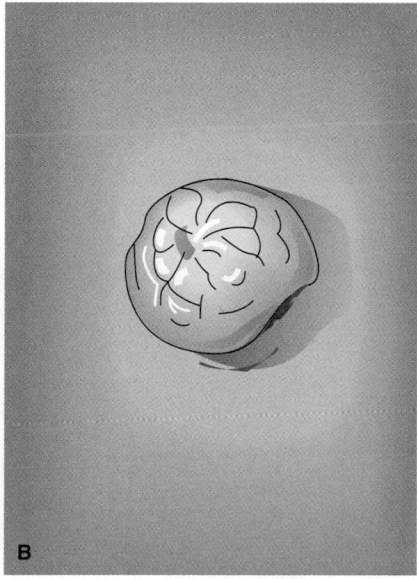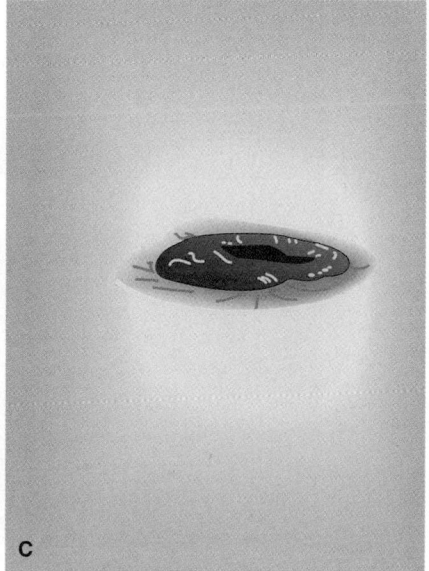

A   B   C

FIGURE 44-9 Comparison of stomal appearance. (**A**) Normal-appearing stoma is bright red, moist, and perfectly round. (**B**) A pale stoma indicates severe anemia. (**C**) Eroded skin around the area may lead to a flush stoma.

with tepid water and wiping the lower 2 inches of the pouch with tissue to remove any fecal material. Nondrainable pouches require removal and changing when they are half full. Types of ostomy equipment are illustrated in Figure 44-10 and include the following components:

- Various types of one-piece and two-piece pouches (drainable and nondrainable)
- Skin-barrier rings that surround the stoma and protect the peristomal skin
- Clamps that securely close drainable pouches

> *Recall Alberta Franklin, the patient with the new colostomy requiring a bag change. The nurse needs to demonstrate competence and dexterity when changing this patient's bag by being adequately prepared and organized. Additionally, the nurse can use the time during bag changes to teach the patient about self-care measures and to assess the patient's acceptance of the colostomy.*

If an appliance is leaking from underneath the skin barrier, ring, or wafer, the bag will have to be removed, the skin cleaned, and a new bag applied. Changing or emptying an ostomy appliance is shown in Skill 44-2.

Irrigating a Colostomy

Irrigations may be used to promote regular evacuation of some colostomies, typically those in the lower right portion of the colon. Various factors, such as the site of the colostomy in the colon and the patient's and physician's preferences, determine whether a colostomy is irrigated. Ileostomies are not irrigated because the fecal content of the ileum is liquid and cannot be controlled.

Before an irrigation is done, familiarize the patient with the technique to be used. Explain the procedure, demonstrate the equipment, and explain how the return fluid can be directed into a bedpan, commode, or toilet bowl. It may also be helpful to have a family member learn the irrigation techniques in case there are times when the patient cannot do the irrigation. Irrigation of a colostomy is shown in Skill 44-3.

In many healthcare agencies, ostomy care, colostomy irrigations, and patient teaching are done by specially trained ostomy or enterostomal therapists.

Long-Term Ostomy Care

The patient can live an active and useful life with an ostomy. He or she should be aware of community resources available for assistance, such as home healthcare nurses, special clinics, and ostomy support groups. The patient should be encouraged to seek medical follow-up care on a regular basis.

During the first 6 to 8 weeks after surgery, encourage the patient with an ostomy to avoid foods high in fiber (eg, foods with skins, seeds, and shells) as well as any other foods that cause diarrhea or excessive flatus (Box 44-2). By gradually adding new foods, the ostomy patient can progress to a normal diet. Also urge the patient to drink at least 2 quarts of fluids, preferably water, daily.

Health teaching about medication use is frequently overlooked for patients with ostomies. Some medications may dis-

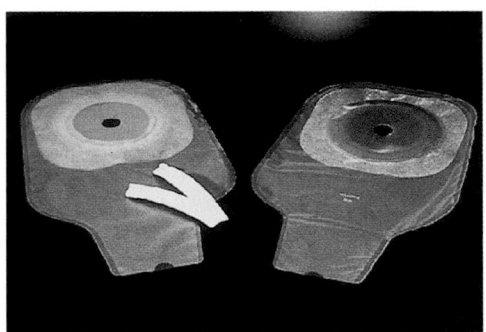

One-piece pouch

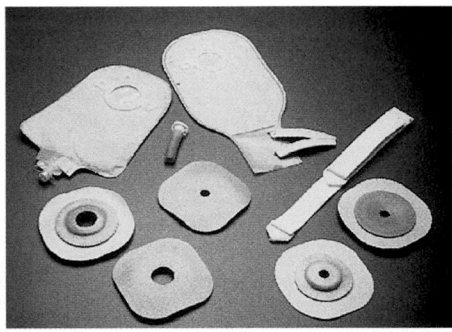

Two-piece pouch

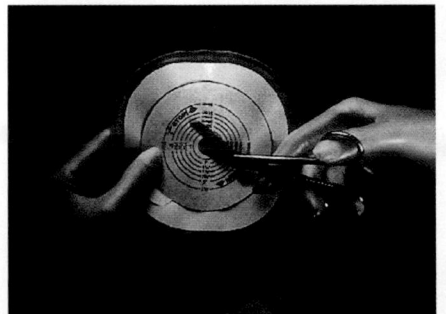

Cut-to-fit pouch

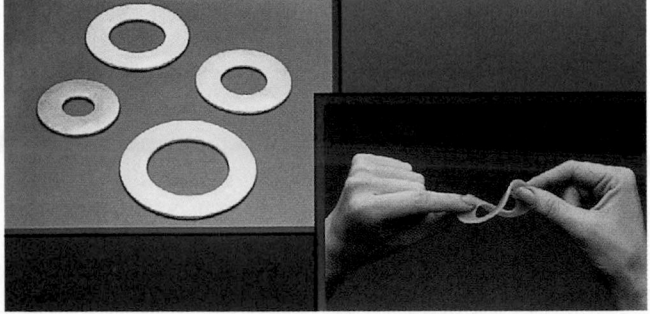

Skin-barrier rings

FIGURE 44-10 Examples of ostomy pouches, closures, and skin barriers. This equipment comes in various models and sizes. Convex pouches, belts, and other devices to prevent leaks and irritation are also available.
(Copyright Hollister Inc. Used with permission.)

SKILL 44-2

Changing or Emptying an Ostomy Appliance

EQUIPMENT

Clean ostomy appliance
Closure clamp
Stoma measuring guide
Scissors
Toilet tissue
Cleansing products (warm water, mild soap
  [optional], washcloth, and towel)

Adhesive solvent (optional)
Plastic bag
Toilet or bedpan
Water or special solution to clean pouch
Gauze pad

Disposable gloves
Disposable pad (optional)
Skin barrier (optional)
Deodorant for pouch (optional)

ACTION	RATIONALE
1. Assemble the necessary equipment	Organization facilitates performance of the task.
2. Explain the procedure to the patient.	The patient is better able to cooperate and learn the technique when he or she is aware of the procedure.
3. Perform hand hygiene and don disposable gloves.	Hand hygiene deters the spread of microorganisms. Gloves protect the nurse from exposure to blood or microorganisms in the feces.
4. Provide for patient's privacy. Assist to a comfortable sitting or lying position in bed or a standing or sitting position in the bathroom.	Either position should allow the patient to view the procedure in preparation for learning to apply it independently. Lying flat or sitting upright facilitates smooth application of the appliance.

TO CHANGE THE POUCH

ACTION	RATIONALE
5. Empty the partially filled appliance into a bedpan if it is a drainable pouch.	Emptying the contents before removal of the pouch prevents accidental spillage of fecal material. Pouches that are too full can detach or leak.
6. Slowly remove the appliance beginning at the top while keeping the abdominal skin taut. If any resistance is felt, use warm water or the adhesive solvent to facilitate removal. Discard the disposable pouch in the plastic bag.	Careful removal protects the underlying skin from damage and minimizes discomfort for the patient. Solvent is rarely necessary to ease removal of the pouch.
7. Use toilet tissue to remove any excess stool from the stoma. Cover stoma with a gauze pad. Gently wash and pat dry the peristomal skin. Mild soap or a cleansing agent may be used according to agency policy.	Soap may not be recommended because it may be irritating to the peristomal skin. Toilet tissue, used gently, will not damage the stoma. The gauze absorbs any drainage from the stoma while the skin is being prepared.
8. Assess the appearance of the peristomal skin and stoma. A moist, reddish-pink stoma is considered normal.	Any change in normal appearance may indicate either anemia (pale stoma) or altered circulation (bluish purple color), and the physician should be notified.
9. Apply the skin barrier and appliance together (wafer or disc style): • Select size for stoma opening by using the measurement guide. • Trace same size circle on the back and center of the skin barrier. • Use scissors to cut an opening ¼- to ⅛-inch larger than stoma. • Remove the backing to expose sticky side. • Remove gauze pad covering stoma. • Ease barrier and pouch over the stoma and gently press onto skin while smoothing out creases or wrinkles. Hold the pouch in place for 5 minutes.	Placing both the skin barrier disc and the appliance together over the stoma makes application easier for the patient. The opening is cut slightly larger to prevent irritation to the stoma as peristalsis occurs but not large enough to allow for skin irritation from stool. Smooth application of the pouch prevents escape of odor and feces. The warmth from the nurse's hands facilitates a tight seal.
10. Close the pouch if it is drainable by folding the end upward and using a clamp or clip (see manufacturer's directions).	A tightly sealed appliance will not leak and cause embarrassment and discomfort for the patient.

(continued)

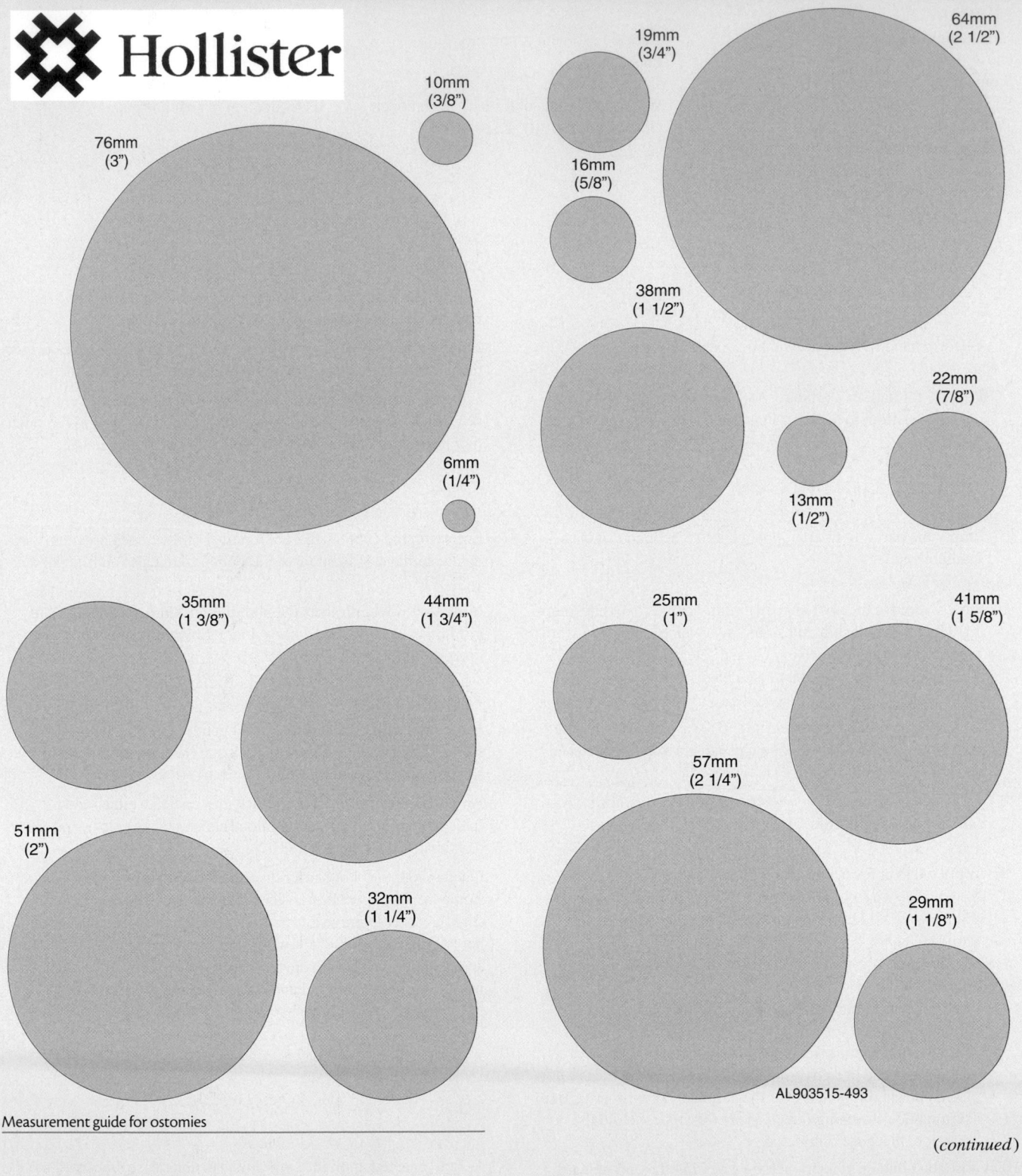

Measurement guide for ostomies

AL903515-493

(continued)

SKILL 44-2 Changing or Emptying an Ostomy Appliance (continued)

TO EMPTY THE POUCH

11. Plan to drain the pouch when it is ⅓ to ½ full. Remove clamp and fold the end of the pouch upward like a cuff.	Allowing the pouch to fill more than half-way increases its weight and makes it more likely to separate or loosen from the skin. Creating a cuff before emptying prevents additional soilage and odor.
12. Empty contents into bedpan or toilet. Rinse pouch with tepid water or water mixed with a drop of mouthwash administered with a squeeze bottle.	Rinsing the inside of the pouch provides a cleaner appearance and minimizes odor.
13. Wipe the lower 2 inches of the pouch with toilet tissue.	Drying the lower section of the pouch removes any additional fecal material.
14. Uncuff the edge of the pouch and apply the clip or clamp.	The edge of the pouch should remain clean. The clamp secures closure of the appliance.
15. Dispose of used equipment according to agency policy. Remove gloves and perform hand hygiene.	Proper disposal of equipment and hand hygiene prevent contamination from microorganisms.
16. Document appearance of stoma, condition of peristomal skin, characteristics of drainage (amount, color, consistency, unusual odor), and patient's reaction to the procedure.	Careful documentation facilitates continuity of care.

Special Considerations	Many different types of appliances are available; the nurse should always read manufacturer's instructions or check with the enterostomal therapist before handling unfamiliar equipment.
	Flatus may cause a pouch to balloon out. This requires immediate attention because if flatus is not released, the pouch may separate from the skin barrier, causing seepage of fecal contents or release of fecal odor. Open the clamp and release the flatus. Never puncture a hole in the appliance.
Older Adult Considerations	A one-piece appliance makes application easier for an older patient, particularly if impaired vision or compromised mobility from arthritis is present.
Home Care Considerations	Always send written directions home with the patient.
	Encourage patient to participate in a support group.

color the stool and cause unusual odors, some may cause constipation, and some may not dissolve or be absorbed completely because the small bowel is where most absorption occurs. The use of liquid, chewable, or injectable forms rather than long-acting, enteric-coated, or sustained-release medications is recommended. Laxatives and enemas are dangerous because they may cause severe fluid and electrolyte imbalance.

Many times, patients are embarrassed when they have to use public restrooms to empty their bag. Teach patients with ostomies about the various methods of odor control. Remind them that if the bag is clean and sealed well, odor usually is not a problem during normal activity. Encourage the intake of dark green vegetables. These vegetables contain chlorophyll, which helps to deodorize the feces. Buttermilk, cranberry juice, parsley, and yogurt can also prevent odor. Crackers, toast, and yogurt can help to reduce gas, which in turn aids in odor control. Commercial odor-control products also are available for purchase. The enterostomal therapist can help with the selection of odor-control strategies.

Some patients can achieve control over fecal elimination from a colostomy by using regular irrigations and by habitually emptying the colon at a certain time each day. Few patients with an ileostomy gain any degree of control over excretion and seldom may dispense with the use of an appliance, except for short periods.

The patient with an ostomy can resume normal activity, including work and sexual relations. However, direct physical contact sports and heavy lifting should be avoided. The patient can go swimming and may need to wear only gauze or a large adhesive bandage over the stoma. When traveling, the patient should carry a 1- to 2-day supply of equipment in a carry-on bag in case checked luggage is lost.

Providing Comfort Measures

Comfort measures related to defecation include working with the patient to develop a bowel elimination routine that results in the easy passage of a soft, formed stool; being attentive to perineal hygiene and the maintenance of skin integrity; and using warm moist heat (sitz bath or tub bath) to soothe the perineal area. Additional nonsurgical treatment options include the following (Smeltzer & Bare, 2004):

- Encouraging recommended diet (if pertinent) and exercise
- Using medications, such as laxatives and antidiarrheals, only as needed
- Applying ointments or astringents (witch hazel)
- Using suppositories that contain anesthetics

SKILL 44-3   Irrigating a Colostomy

EQUIPMENT

Disposable irrigation system
Irrigation sleeve
Water soluble lubricant
Lukewarm solution (as ordered by physi-
cian; normally tap water; amount may
vary normally 750 to 1,000 mL)

Waterproof pad
Bedpan or toilet
IV pole
Disposable gloves

Paper towel
Washcloth, soap, and towels
New appliance if needed

ACTION	RATIONALE
1. Assemble the necessary equipment. Warm solution in amount ordered. If tap water is used, adjust temperature as it flows from faucet.	If solution is too cool, patient may experience cramps or nausea.
2. Explain procedure to the patient and plan where he or she will receive irrigation. Assist patient onto bedside commode or into nearby bathroom.	Unlike a cleansing enema, the patient cannot hold the irrigation solution. A large immediate return of irrigation solution and stool usually occurs.
3. Perform hand hygiene.	Hand hygiene deters the spread of microorganisms in the feces.
4. Add irrigation solution to container. Release the clamp and allow fluid to progress through the tube before reclamping.	This causes any air to be expelled from the tubing. Although allowing air to enter the intestine is not harmful, it may distend the intestine, causing gas pains.
5. Hang container so that the bottom of bag will be at patient's shoulder level when seated.	Gravity forces the solution to enter the intestine. The amount of pressure determines the rate of flow and pressure exerted on the intestinal wall. Giving the solution too quickly causes rapid distention and pressure in the intestine, which may result in nausea or cramps.
6. Put on disposable gloves.	This protects the nurse from microorganisms in the feces.
7. Remove appliance and attach irrigation sleeve, placing the drainage end into the toilet bowl.	The irrigation sleeve helps all irrigation fluid and stool to drain into the toilet for easy disposal.
8. Lubricate the end of the cone with water-soluble lubricant.	This facilitates passage of the cone into the stoma opening.
9. Introduce the solution slowly over a period of 5 minutes. Hold or have patient hold the tubing all the time that solution is being instilled. You may control the rate of flow by closing or opening the clamp.	If the irrigation solution is administered too quickly, the patient may experience nausea and cramps.

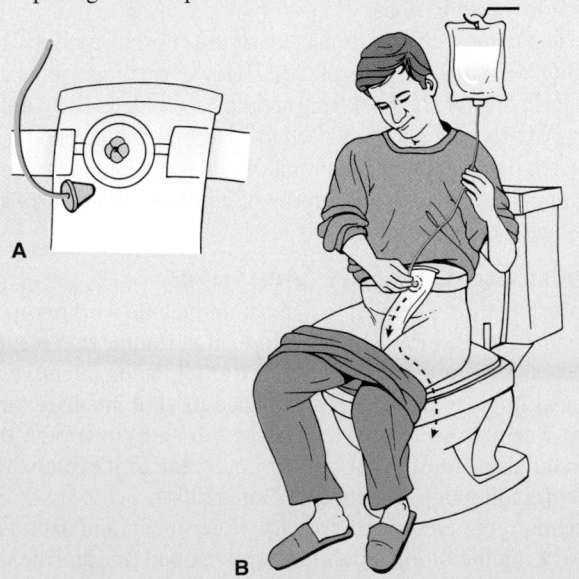

A

B

Action 9: Patient receiving colostomy irrigation. (**A**) Inserting irrigation cone. (**B**) Instilling irrigating fluid with sleeve in place.

(continued)

SKILL 44-3 Irrigating a Colostomy (continued)

ACTION	RATIONALE
10. Hold the cone in place for an additional 10 seconds after the fluid is infused.	This will allow for a small amount of dwell time of the irrigation solution.
11. Remove the cone. Assist patient to remain seated on toilet or bedside commode.	An immediate return of solution and stool will usually occur, followed by a return in spurts for up to 45 more minutes.
12. After majority of solution has returned, patient may clip the bottom of the irrigating sleeve and continue with daily activities.	An immediate return of solution and stool will usually occur, followed by a return in spurts for up to 45 more minutes.
13. After solution has stopped flowing from stoma, remove irrigation sleeve and cleanse skin around stoma opening with mild soap and water. Gently pat peristomal skin dry.	Peristomal skin must be clean and free of any liquid or stool prior to application of new appliance.
14. Attach new appliance to stoma (see Skill 44-2) if needed.	Patient has now finished colostomy irrigation and is ready to continue daily activities.

Evaluating

The nurse evaluates the effectiveness of the plan of care to promote regular bowel elimination by checking to see if the patient has met the individualized patient outcomes specified in the plan. Nursing care is considered effective if the patient expresses satisfaction with his or her regular pattern of defecation and the ability to pass a soft, formed stool comfortably without the use of medications or laxatives. The plan of care is most successful when the patient is able to accomplish the following:

- Verbalize the relationships among bowel elimination and nutrition, fluid intake, exercise, and stress management.
- Develop a plan to modify any factors that contribute to current bowel problems or that might adversely affect bowel functioning in the future.

See the accompanying Nursing Plan of Care 44-1.

BOX 44-2 Nutritional Impact on Ostomies

Foods that should be eaten in moderation for a person who has a *colostomy* or *ileostomy*:

Foods that may increase odor

Asparagus	Eggs
Broccoli	Fish
Brussels sprouts	Garlic
Cabbage	Onions
Cauliflower	Some spices

Foods and beverages that may increase gas

Beans	Cauliflower
Beer	Corn
Broccoli	Cucumbers
Brussels sprouts	Mushrooms
Cabbage	Peas
Carbonated beverages	Spinach

Foods and beverages that may thicken stools

Applesauce	Peanut butter (creamy, not chunky)
Bananas	
Buttermilk	Pretzels
Cheese	Rice
Marshmallows	Tapioca pudding
Milk (boiled)	Toast
Noodles (any type)	Yogurt

Foods and beverages that may cause loose stools

Beer or other alcohol	Green beans
Broccoli	Prunes or prune juice
Fresh fruits (except bananas)	Spicy foods
	Spinach
Grape juice	

Foods that are high in fiber and can cause blockages that may not easily pass through the stoma in the person with an *ileostomy*:

Foods that are high in fiber

Celery	Meats with casings (sausage, wieners, bologna)
Chinese vegetables	
Coconut	
Cole slaw (raw cabbage)	Mushrooms
Corn	Nuts
Dried fruits	Popcorn
Foods with nondigestible peels (apples, potatoes, grapes)	

From *Managing your colostomy* and *Managing your ileostomy* (1997). Illinois: Hollister Incorporated.

NURSING PLAN OF CARE 44-1   *for Jeremy Green*

Jeremy Green, 4 years of age, was placed in day care when his mother returned to work 6 months ago. He presents at the hospital with a diagnosis of viral gastroenteritis. A comprehensive nursing assessment included the following notations:

- Admitted with complaints of diarrhea beginning 3 days ago
- Seen today by pediatrician who recommended admission and work-up to exclude causes other than viral
- Mother reports liquid stools (no observable blood, pus, or mucus) six to seven times daily beginning 3 days ago with amounts of "one to two cups."
- Urgency results in soiling of pants.

- Child has sipped boiled skim milk and cola and eaten a small amount of broth and a few pretzels but has no appetite.
- Complained of nausea and vomited twice 3 days ago
- Child is pale and eyes are sunken.
- Skin is warm and dry with decreased turgor, dry mucous membranes.
- Hyperactive bowel sounds (52/minute)
- Height, 45 inches; weight, 36 lb; temperature, 99.8°F (rectally); pulse, 88 beats/min; respiratory rate, 18 breaths/min
- Mother reported several other children in same day care center are out sick with diarrhea.

NURSING DIAGNOSIS   Diarrhea related to unknown cause (possibly viral, rule out malabsorption of lactose and other causes) as manifested by passage of liquid stools (1–2 cups) for 3 days; urgency with fecal soiling.

EXPECTED OUTCOME   At the time of discharge, the patient will:
- Voluntarily pass a formed stool of usual consistency (experience less or no diarrhea)

Nursing Interventions	Rationale	Evaluative Statement
Assess and chart frequency and amount of diarrhea, stool characteristics, precipitating factors, and accompanying manifestations (gastrointestinal symptoms, hyperactive bowel sounds).	This assists in identifying the cause of the diarrhea.	5/8/06 Outcome partially met. No recurrence of liquid stools for 24 hours. *Revision:* Continue to monitor. *D. Lentsky, RN*

EXPECTED OUTCOME   At the time of discharge, the patient will:
- Exhibit decreased bowel sounds (5 to 34/min)

Nursing Interventions	Rationale	Evaluative Statement
Work collaboratively with the physician to identify the cause of the diarrhea. Obtain stool specimens and send to laboratory.	Correct treatment depends on identification of the cause of the diarrhea. Viral diarrhea is usually self-limiting and lasts 24 to 72 hours. Prolonged diarrhea after acute viral illness may be from temporary malabsorption of lactose or other simple sugars.	5/8/06 Outcome met. Bowel sounds are normal. *D. Lentsky, RN*
Instruct Jeremy and his parents (if they want to participate in care) on correct infection control precautions for handling stool.	Proper precautions prevent transmissions of infectious diarrhea to others.	
Increase frequency and length of rest periods and discourage strenuous activity.	Exercise and activity stimulate peristalsis.	
Administer prescribed antidiarrheal medication and observe for adverse effects.	Antidiarrheal medications may cause drowsiness and dizziness. These agents may be used in diarrhea due to viruses to slow peristalsis and passage of stool.	

SAMPLE DOCUMENTATION   5/7/06   Nursing

Liquid stools have decreased to two in the past 24 hours. Negative report on stool culture. Normal bowel sounds auscultated in all four quadrants.

Developing Critical Thinking Skills

1. If you noticed the following when assessing a patient, what would you do?
   - Patient has frank blood in stool.
   - Parent reports that child's stool is unusually foul-smelling and greasy.
   - Patient's stool is ribbon-like.
   - Patient receiving cancer pain medication reports chronic constipation.
   - Teenager reports frequent episodes of diarrhea that leave her weak and dehydrated.

2. A 52-year-old man presents with acute stomach pain and altered bowel elimination: diarrhea. Role-play with another student the interview you would use to assess his bowel elimination status. Identify variables that make you, as either the nurse or patient, uncomfortable talking about elimination. Discuss how you can best address your discomfort.

Practicing for NCLEX

1. The nurse would instruct Mr. Brown to avoid which of the following foods to prevent a laxative effect?
   a. Cheese
   b. Alcohol
   c. Eggs
   d. Pasta

2. Which of the following is a true statement about the effects of medication on bowel elimination?
   a. Diarrhea occurs with amoxicillin clavulanate use about 20% of the time.
   b. Anticoagulants cause a white discoloration of the stool.
   c. Narcotic analgesics increase gastrointestinal motility.
   d. Iron salts impair digestion and cause a green stool.

3. Mr. Jones has a fecal impaction. The nurse correctly administers an oil-retention enema by doing which of the following?
   a. Administering a large volume of solution (500 to 1,000 mL)
   b. Mixing milk and molasses in equal parts for an enema
   c. Instructing the patient to retain the enema for at least 30 minutes
   d. Following the return-flow or Harris flush procedure

4. As the nurse prepares to assist Mrs. Perez with her newly created ileostomy, she is aware that:
   a. An appliance will not be required on a continual basis
   b. The size of the stoma stabilizes within 2 weeks
   c. Irrigation is necessary for regulation
   d. Fecal drainage will be liquid

5. Which class of laxative acts by causing the stool to absorb water and swell?
   a. Bulk-forming
   b. Emollient
   c. Lubricant
   d. Stimulant

6. Mr. Toney is nervous about a colonoscopy scheduled for tomorrow. The nurse describes the test by explaining that it allows which of the following?
   a. Visual examination of the esophagus and stomach
   b. Visual examination of the large intestine
   c. Radiographic examination of the large intestine
   d. Fluoroscopic examination of the small intestine

7. A bowel training program includes which of the following?
   a. Using a diet that is low in bulk
   b. Decreasing fluid intake to 1,000 mL
   c. Administering an enema once a day to stimulate peristalsis
   d. Allowing ample time for evacuation

8. Your patient complains of excessive flatulence. When reviewing the patient's dietary intake, which food, if eaten regularly, would you identify as possibly responsible?
   a. Meat
   b. Cauliflower
   c. Potatoes
   d. Ice cream

9. A barium enema should be done before an upper gastrointestinal series because of which of the following?
   a. Retained barium may cloud the colon.
   b. Barium can cause lower gastrointestinal bleeding.
   c. The physician's orders are in that sequence.
   d. Barium is absorbed readily in the lower intestine.

10. Nurses should recommend avoiding the habitual use of laxatives. Which of the following is the rationale for this?
    a. They will cause a fecal impaction.
    b. They will cause chronic constipation.
    c. They change the pH of the gastrointestinal tract.
    d. They inhibit the intestinal enzymes.

11. When explaining the action of a hypertonic solution enema, the nurse incorporates which of the following as the basis for action?
    a. Bowel mucosa irritation
    b. Diffusion of water out of colon
    c. Osmosis of water into colon
    d. Softening of fecal contents

12. Which of the following is the rationale for discouraging use of rectal indwelling catheters?
    a. Peristalsis decreases.
    b. A physician's order is required.
    c. Rectal necrosis can occur.
    d. Draining of liquid stool is prevented.

13. During removal of a fecal impaction, which of the following could occur because of vagal stimulation?
    a. Bradycardia
    b. Atelectasis

c. Tachycardia
d. Cardiac tamponade

14. Which of the following would be a common nursing diagnosis for the patient with an ileostomy?
    a. Disturbed Body Image
    b. Constipation
    c. Delayed Growth and Development
    d. Excess Fluid Volume

15. Your patient, who is experiencing flatulence, would be helped if he were placed in which of the following positions?
    a. Trendelenburg position
    b. Knee–chest position
    c. Semi-Fowler's position
    d. Fowler's position

■ Answers With Rationale

1. The correct answer is *b*. All the foods listed except alcohol have a constipating effect.

2. The correct answer is *a*. Anticoagulants may result in the stool having a pink to red to black appearance, whereas iron salts also cause a black stool. Narcotic analgesics decrease gastric motility.

3. The correct answer is *c*. The usual amount of solution administered with a retention enema is 150 to 200 mL for an adult. The milk-and-molasses mixture is a carminative enema that helps to expel flatus, as does the Harris flush procedure.

4. The correct answer is *d*. An appliance is usually required on a continual basis because the fecal drainage is liquid. Stoma size usually stabilizes within 4 to 6 weeks, and ileostomy irrigation is not necessary because fecal matter is liquid.

5. The correct answer is *a*. Emollients lubricate the stool; lubricants soften the stool, making it easier to pass; and stimulants promote peristalsis by irritating the intestinal mucosa or stimulating nerve endings in the intestinal wall.

6. The correct answer is *b*. An esophagogastroduodenoscopy allows visual examination of the esophagus and stomach. The radiographic examination of the large intestine refers to a barium enema, and a fluoroscopic examination of the small intestine refers to an upper gastrointestinal series.

7. The correct response is *d*. For a bowel training program to be effective, the patient must have ample time for evacuation (usually 20 to 30 minutes). Fluid intake is increased to 2,500 to 3,000 mL; food high in bulk is recommended as part of the program; and a daily enema is not administered in a bowel training program. A cathartic suppository may be used 30 minutes before the patient's usual defecation time to stimulate peristalsis.

8. The correct answer is *b*. Cauliflower is a gas-producing food that results in flatulence.

9. The correct answer is *a*. The barium enema should always precede the upper gastrointestinal series because retained barium from the latter may take several days to pass through the gastrointestinal tract and may cloud anatomic detail on the barium enema studies.

10. The correct answer is *b*. Habitual use of laxatives is the most common cause of chronic constipation.

11. The correct answer is *c*. Hypertonic solutions draw water into the colon by osmosis, thus stimulating the defecation reflex. Oil solutions soften fecal contents, and soap solutions distend the intestine and irritate the bowel mucosa.

12. The correct answer is *c*. Concern for mucosal necrosis is one of the main reasons that the use of rectal indwelling catheters is discouraged. Nurses also feel that the catheter stimulates sensory nerve fibers in the rectum, thus worsening diarrhea. The catheter allows liquid feces to drain, and the need to obtain a physician's order is not a factor in determining the safety of the rectal catheter.

13. The correct answer is *a*. Removing a fecal impaction manually may result in stimulation of the vagal nerve and resulting bradycardia.

14. The correct answer is *a*. Constipation does not occur with an ileostomy because the drainage is liquid. Growth and development are not affected by the formation of an ileostomy. Excess fluid volume is unlikely to occur because the drainage is liquid and probably continual.

15. The correct answer is *b*. Because gas rises, the knee-chest position facilitates the passage of flatus.

Bibliography

Ahmed, D., Karch, A., & Karch, F. (2000). Hidden factors in occult blood testing. *American Journal of Nursing, 100*(12), 25.

Banks, N., & Razor, B. (2003). Preoperative stoma site assessment and marking: Trained RNs can improve ostomy outcomes. *American Journal of Nursing, 103*(3), 64A–64B, 64E.

Bartlett, J. (2002). Antibiotic-associated diarrhea. *New England Journal of Medicine, 346*(5), 334–339.

Black, P. (2000). Practical stoma care. *Nursing Standard, 14*(41), 47–55.

Buchman, A. (2002). Wireless endoscopy: The camera capsule. Retrieved December 26, 2002, from http://www.ccfa.org/news/wireless_endoscopy.html

Bryant, D., & Fleischer, I. (2000). Changing an ostomy appliance. *Nursing, 30*(11), 51–55.

Erwin-Toth, P. (2001). Caring for a stoma is more than skin deep. *Nursing, 31*(5), 36–40.

Fischbach, F. (2003). *A manual of laboratory diagnostic tests* (7th ed.). Philadelphia: Lippincott Williams & Wilkins.

Fries, C. (1999). Managing an ostomy. *Nursing, 29*(8), 26.

Goldrick, B. (2003). Foodborne diseases: More efforts needed to meet Healthy People 2010 objectives. *American Journal of Nursing, 103*(3), 105–106.

Hinrichs, M., & Huseboe, J. (2001). Research-based protocol: Management of constipation. *Journal of Gerontological Nursing, 27*(2), 17–27.

Hyland, J. (2002). The basics of ostomies. *Gastroenterology Nursing, 25*(6), 241–245.

Ignatavicius, D., & Workman, M. (2002). *Medical-surgical nursing* (4th ed.). Philadelphia: W. B. Saunders Company.

Interpreting abnormal abdominal sounds (2000). *Nursing, 30*(6), 28.

Kenney, S., Hubbartt, E., & Michaels, T. (2000). Keys to bowel success. *Rehabilitation Nursing, 25*(2), 66–69.

McClosky, J., & Bulechek, J. (2002). *Nursing interventions classification* (NIC) (4th ed.). St. Louis: C. V. Mosby.

McConnell, E. (2000). Myths & facts about rectal catheters. *Nursing, 30*(1), 73.

North American Nursing Diagnosis Association. (2001). *NANDA nursing diagnosis: Definitions & classification, 2001–2002* (4th ed.). Philadelphia: Author.

Pagana, K., & Pagana, T. (2002). *Manual of diagnostic and laboratory tests* (2nd ed.). St. Louis: C. V. Mosby.

Phipps, W., Monahan, F., Sands, J., Marek, J., & Neighbors, M. (2003). *Medical-surgical nursing: Health and illness perspectives* (7th ed.). St. Louis: C. V. Mosby.

Pullen, M. (2002). Management of difficult stomas. *Nursing and Residential Care, 4*(2), 76–78, 80.

Reiss, M., Labowitz, D., Forman, S., & Wormser, G. (2001). Impact of color blindness on recognition of blood in body fluids. *Archives of Internal Medicine, 161*(3), 462–465.

Secord, C., Jackman, M., Wright, L., & Winton, S. (2001). Adjusting to life with an ostomy. *Canadian Nurse, 97*(1), 29–32.

Selig, H., & Boyle, J. (2001). Bowel care and maintenance in long term care. *Canadian Nurse, 97*(8), 28–33.

Sheff, B. (2000). Minimizing the threat of *C. difficile. Nursing Management, 32*(6), 32–38.

Smeltzer, S., & Bare, B. (2004). *Brunner and Suddarth's textbook of medical-surgical nursing* (10th ed.). Philadelphia: Lippincott Williams & Wilkins.

Thompson, J. (2000). Part one: A practical ostomy guide. *RN, 63*(11), 61–68.

Wisconsin center cracks dangerous *E. coli* genome sequence. (2001). *Nursing Spectrum* (Greater Chicago/NE Illinois and NW Indiana Edition), *14*(3), 3.

Wong, D., Perry, S., & Hockenberry, M. (2002). *Maternal child nursing care.* St. Louis: C. V. Mosby.

Oxygenation

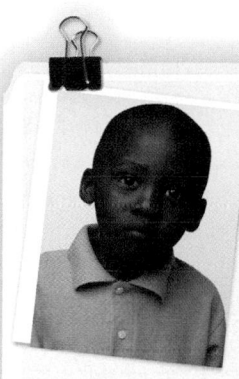

Tyrone Jacobs, age 2, is brought to the emergency room gasping for breath. His parents are frantic. "It just seemed like he had a really bad cold," his mother says. An acute asthma attack is suspected, and measures are instituted immediately to protect the child's airway.

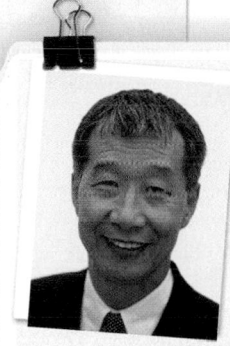

Yan Kim, age 57, developed respiratory failure from complications associated with pulmonary surgery. He is receiving oxygen therapy and mechanical ventilation via an endotracheal tube and undergoing continuous cardiac monitoring.

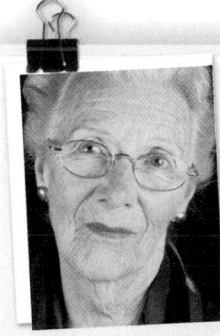

Joan McIntyre, age 72, has a tracheostomy and is receiving mechanical ventilation in the medical intensive care unit. Efforts are being made to wean her from the ventilator, but she has been unable to breathe on her own for any length of time. She has written notes asking the staff to "let me go" the next time she fails to be weaned.

Focusing on Blended Skills

The types of blended skills you'll need to respond to the case scenarios include:

Cognitive Skills

- Knowledge of the anatomy and physiology of the respiratory system and the factors that affect respiratory function
- Ability to incorporate knowledge of the nursing process to identify and care for patients with respiratory problems
- Knowledge of developmental variables affecting respiratory function
- Knowledge of normal and abnormal assessment findings such as breath sounds and respiratory parameters
- Knowledge of medications used to treat respiratory problems such as asthma
- Knowledge of measures used to treat problems involving oxygenation

Technical Skills

- Ability to use the equipment and protocols necessary to diagnose and treat respiratory problems
- Strong history and physical assessment techniques to identify problems associated with alterations in respiration and oxygenation
- Competence in particular skills, such as administration of inhaled medications, ventilatory assistance, oxygen therapy, and tracheostomy care
- Ability to ask for assistance when necessary when obtaining the nursing history or completing the physical examination or performing procedures to promote adequate oxygenation
- Ability to use measures to promote proper breathing and comfort
- Ability to adapt technical assistance related to oxygenation to meet the needs of patients at different developmental stages

Interpersonal Skills

- Strong people skills to establish trusting relationships with patients experiencing problems with respiratory functioning
- A good working relationship with colleagues to ensure competent multidisciplinary care
- Ability to communicate concern about patient, patient's complaints, and situation
- Demonstration of respect for patient's human dignity to promote patient's self-esteem
- Ability to use therapeutic communication effectively to meet the needs of patients at different developmental stages and with different abilities to communicate verbally
- Ability to interact with patients at different developmental stages, ensuring that care meets the developmental needs of each

Ethical and Legal Skills

- Strong sense of accountability for the health and well-being of patients experiencing respiratory problems and their families
- Ability to act as patient advocate to ensure competent care
- Knowledge of patients' and families' rights related to refusal of care
- Ability to consult with other members of the healthcare team to ensure the patient's safety
- Ability to practice in an ethically and legally defensible manner, maintaining the patient's rights, including the right to refuse care and the right to self-determination
- Ability to integrate ethical and legal principles into patient assessments, documentation, and communication

Learning Outcomes

After completing the chapter, the learner should be able to accomplish the following:

1. Describe the principles of respiratory physiology.
2. Describe age-related differences that influence the care of patients with respiratory problems.
3. Identify factors that influence respiratory function.
4. Perform a comprehensive respiratory assessment using appropriate interview questions and physical assessment skills.
5. Develop nursing diagnoses that correctly identify problems that may be treated by independent nursing interventions.
6. Describe nursing strategies to promote adequate respiratory functioning, giving their rationale.
7. Plan, implement, and evaluate nursing care related to select nursing diagnoses involving respiratory problems.

Key Terms

adventitious	inspiration
alveoli	metered-dose inhaler (MDI)
atelectasis	
bronchial	nasal cannula
bronchodilator	nebulizer
bronchovesicular	pleurae
cilia	pleural effusion
crackles	pneumothorax
dyspnea	pulse oximetry
endotracheal tube	spirometer
expiration	surfactant
hemothorax	thoracentesis
hyperventilation	tracheostomy
hypoventilation	ventilation
hypoxemia	vesicular
hypoxia	wheezes

Most people take respiratory functioning for granted, but adequate respiratory functioning is necessary for life. Living cells require oxygen. The air passages must remain patent (open) for oxygen to enter the system. Any condition that interferes with normal functioning must be minimized or eliminated to prevent pulmonary distress, which could lead to death. (See the accompanying Reflective Practice box for an example.)

Normal functioning depends on essentially three factors:

- The integrity of the airway system to transport air to and from the lungs
- A properly functioning alveolar system in the lungs to oxygenate venous blood and to remove carbon dioxide from the blood
- A properly functioning cardiovascular and hematologic system to carry nutrients and wastes to and from body cells

This chapter describes the respiratory system's anatomy and physiology and general factors affecting respiratory functioning. Practical suggestions for performing a comprehensive respiratory assessment are presented, including sample interview questions for both a general and focused respiratory history and a description of the nursing examination. Laboratory and radiologic studies are addressed in the assessment. After analyzing the data, nurses decide whether the respiratory data lead to a problem statement, indicate another problem, or are the possible cause of a problem. Numerous examples of nursing diagnoses are provided. Expected patient outcomes and specific nursing strategies for implementation are described. The concluding patient care study illustrates how, with knowledge of respiratory functioning and skilled nursing interventions, the nurse resolves respiratory problems.

ANATOMY AND PHYSIOLOGY OF RESPIRATION

Knowledge of the basic anatomy and physiology of the respiratory system provides a firm foundation for assessing this system and planning and implementing interventions to promote optimal respiratory function. This knowledge also helps nurses understand, interpret, and analyze assessment findings and provides the rationale for sound nursing interventions.

The Respiratory System Structures

The airway, which begins at the nose and ends at the terminal bronchioles, is a pathway for the transport and exchange of oxygen and carbon dioxide. The airway is divided into the upper and the lower airways.

The upper airway is composed of the nose, pharynx, larynx, and epiglottis. Its main function is to warm, filter, and humidify inspired air. The lower airway, known as the tracheobronchial tree, includes the trachea, right and left mainstem bronchi, segmental bronchi, and terminal bronchioles. Its major functions are conduction of air, mucociliary clearance, and production of pulmonary surfactant.

The airways are lined with mucus, which traps cells, particles, and infectious debris. This covering of mucus also helps to protect the underlying tissues from irritation and infection. To prevent an accumulation of mucus, the mucus is moved toward the oropharynx by cilia. **Cilia,** which are microscopic hairlike projections, propel mucus toward the upper airway so that the mucus can be removed (by coughing). For removal, mucus must be watery in consistency. An adequate fluid intake is necessary for the production of watery mucus normally present in the respiratory tract and for ciliary action.

The lungs, the main organs of respiration, are located within the thoracic cavity on the right and left sides (Fig. 45-1). The lungs extend from the base at the level of the diaphragm to the apex (top), which is above the first rib. The heart lies between the right and left lung.

Each lung is divided into lobes. The right lung has three lobes; the left has two. Each lobe is subdivided into segments or lobules. The right lung has 10 bronchopulmonary segments; the left has 8. The lungs are composed of elastic tissue that can stretch or recoil. Normally, the elastic fibers are partially stretched at all times, thus partially filling the thoracic cavity.

The actual lung is composed of **alveoli,** small air sacs that are lined with fluid at the end of the terminal bronchioles (Fig. 45-2). The average adult has more than 300 million alveoli. These structures are the site of gas exchange. **Surfactant,** a detergent-like phospholipid, reduces the surface tension of the fluid lining the alveoli. When surfactant production is reduced, the lung becomes stiff and the alveoli collapse.

The **pleurae** are two-layered membranes: the visceral pleura covers the lungs, and the parietal pleura lines the thoracic cavity. These two membranes are continuous with each other and form a closed sac. There is normally a potential space between them, not an actual space. Pleural fluid between the membranes acts as a lubricant and as an adhesive agent to hold the lungs in an expanded position. A few milliliters of fluid between the pleural surfaces allows the lungs to move easily along the chest wall as they expand and contract. Without this fluid, filling and emptying of the lungs are difficult.

Pressure within the pleural space (intrapleural pressure) is always subatmospheric (a negative pressure). This constant intrapleural negative pressure is essential for normal ventilation.

Pulmonary Ventilation

Ventilation is the movement of air into and out of the lungs. The process of ventilation has two phases: inspiration (inhalation) and expiration (exhalation). **Inspiration,** the active phase, involves movement of muscles and the thorax to bring air into the lungs. **Expiration,** the passive phase, is the movement of air out of the lungs. The diaphragm and the intercostal muscles are responsible for normal inspiration and expiration.

Immediately before inspiration, the air pressure in the lungs is equal to that of the surrounding atmospheric pressure. According to Boyle's law, the volume of a gas at a constant temperature varies inversely with the pressure. This means that less pressure in the lungs facilitates the movement of more air

Reflective Practice
Challenge to Technical Skills

Ventilators and telemetry have always intimidated me, so having a patient like Yan Kim was overwhelming. A 57-year-old man who had developed respiratory failure from complications secondary to pulmonary surgery, he was receiving oxygen therapy and mechanical ventilation via an endotracheal tube. Mr. Kim was also undergoing continuous cardiac monitoring. Providing care for him with all his equipment and so many alarms that could sound seemed insurmountable. The monitor had several different values on it and the continuous electrocardiogram (ECG) monitor always made me feel like the patient was on the verge of dying. We had not covered these skills yet in class, and I felt incompetent for the first 2 weeks of my critical care clinical experience. I could have voiced my concerns with these two machines, and I should have asked the first day what I should and shouldn't be worried about with critical care patients. But I didn't.

Thinking Outside the Box: Possible Course of Action

- Ask my instructor if there was any danger in having a patient who was receiving mechanical ventilation and being monitored by telemetry.
- Ask for someone to explain the ECG waveforms on the monitor and what to be concerned with when looking at them.

- Avoid caring for patients on ventilators and undergoing telemetry.

Evaluating a Good Outcome: How Do I Define Success?

- Patient is safe and receives care by a competent care provider promoting his health.
- I am confident in my technical skills and able to use technology to deliver the most helpful care.

- I continue to ask questions, challenge my practice, and learn to contribute to improved care, which will lead to enhanced nursing.

Personal Learning: Here's To the Future!

Fortunately our clinical rotations are planned so that we do not take care of critical care patients until we learn the necessary skills (telemetry and ventilation). This semester in my critical care clinical experiences, my fears have dissipated. I have learned that having patients that are being monitoring continuously via telemetry is quite reassuring: it serves as a constant monitor for me. Although I still assess the patient on my own, having continuous values to check is reassuring. As for the ventilator, I realized I knew a lot more than I thought. My instructor gave me a lesson on the ventilator during my clinical experience and connected the class lectures and book work with what I was seeing with my patient. I asked many questions and checked to see if I knew which settings would change with different scenarios. There are several settings and several values constantly being measured with the machine. Once I was able to see what all of these numbers meant and realized that I understood what each was for, I felt much more comfortable with patients on a ventilator. I realized my concerns and made sure that I provided unbiased care so that my concerns did not force me to neglect a patient.

Before, I would have been scared to get too close to the machine for fear of hitting the wrong button, fearing I would harm the patient. Now I am learning how the settings are specific to each patient. I feel comfortable reading the values and setting the controls. Still, I ask questions about the ventilator and telemetry readings because I want to know that I am interpreting them correctly. I feel it is my responsibility to obtain as much understanding and knowledge as I can so that I can provide the best care to these patients. This is very relieving and rewarding: now critical care patients don't seem so critical! My care for these patients is enhanced since I am more confident in my skills, and this enhances the care I deliver. Next time there is something new to me, I will voice my concern early on even if I am not "supposed to know" yet.

Overall, although I do not yet have much experience, I feel technically competent as a senior nursing student. I am confident because I challenge myself and I am self-motivated when it comes to searching for more information when needed.

Reflection

How would you respond in a similar situation? Why? What does this tell you about yourself and about the adequacy of your skills for professional practice? How did the nursing student apply the knowledge obtained through the lessons given by the instructor? How do you think the nursing student would have responded if the clinical experience was strictly observational? What information did the nursing student receive from the monitors? How did the nursing student use this information? What interventions did the nursing student implement to care for the patient's psychosocial status? Can you think of other ways to respond? What other skills (cognitive, interpersonal, technical, ethical/legal) would you need to respond well in this situation? Do you agree with the criteria to evaluate a successful outcome? Are there any other criteria that would be appropriate to use? Did the nursing student meet the criteria? Why or why not?

Carrie Staines, Georgetown University

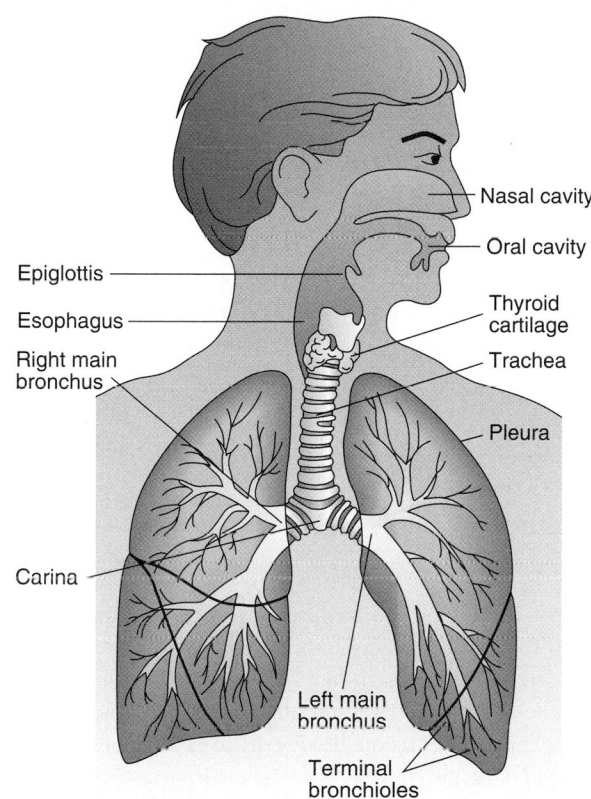

FIGURE 45-1 The organs of the respiratory tract.

Nasal cavity
Oral cavity
Epiglottis
Esophagus
Thyroid cartilage
Right main bronchus
Trachea
Pleura
Carina
Left main bronchus
Terminal bronchioles

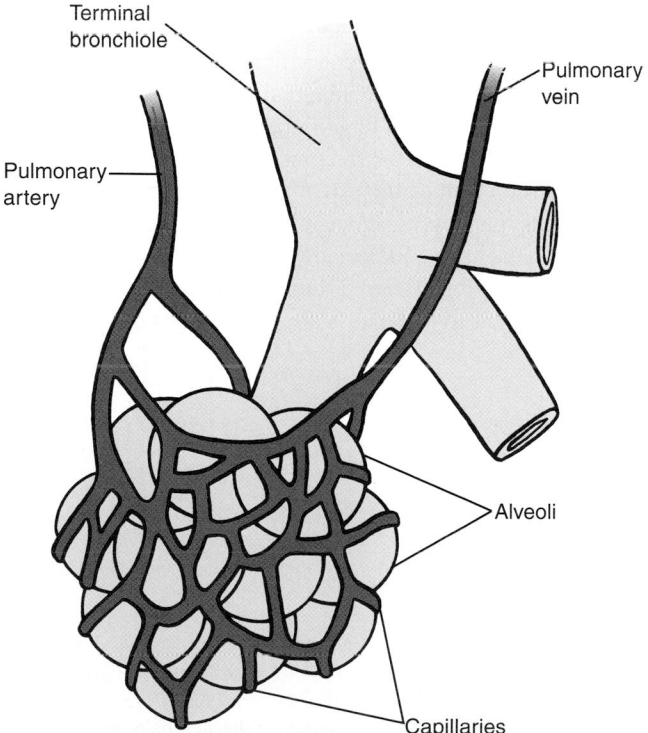

Terminal bronchiole
Pulmonary vein
Pulmonary artery
Alveoli
Capillaries

FIGURE 45-2 Alveoli and the intrapulmonary system where gas exchange occurs. The terminal bronchioles lead into the alveoli. Air in the alveoli and blood in the capillaries are separated by only a very thin partition, which is readily crossed by diffusing gases. The pulmonary artery carries unoxygenated blood to the capillaries, and the pulmonary veins return oxygenated blood to the left side of the heart.

into the lungs. The pressure within the lungs (intrapulmonic pressure) decreases as the volume of the lungs increases.

During inspiration, the following events occur: the diaphragm contracts and descends, lengthening the thoracic cavity; the external intercostal muscles contract, lifting the ribs upward and outward; and the sternum is pushed forward, enlarging the chest from front to back. This combination of an increased lung volume and decreased intrapulmonic pressure allows atmospheric air to move from an area of greater pressure (outside air) into an area of lesser pressure (within the lungs). The relaxation, or recoil, of these structures then results in expiration. The diaphragm relaxes and moves up, the ribs move down, and the sternum drops back into position. This causes a decreased volume in the lungs and an increase in intrapulmonic pressure. As a result, air in the lungs moves from an area of greater pressure to one of lesser pressure and is expired (Fig. 45-3).

The accessory muscles of the abdomen, neck, and back are used to maintain respiratory movements at times when breathing is difficult. Thus, the condition of the body's musculature can affect the process of respiration. For example, when the respiratory center is depressed and pulmonary congestion is present, normal respiratory effort is compromised. The accessory muscles help to maintain movement of air into and out of the lungs. When these muscles are used to facilitate breathing, the movement is called retractions. The most common retractions involve the intercostal, scalene, sternocleidomastoid, trapezius, and pectoralis muscles.

The compliance of lung tissue affects lung volume. Lung compliance refers to the stretchability of the lungs, the ease with which the lungs can be inflated. The varying changes in lung pressure and resulting lung compliance can be compared to differences in blowing up a new, noncompliant balloon versus one that was previously inflated. A stiff, noncompliant lung (like a new balloon) requires a greater inspiratory effort to inflate it. Emphysema, a chronic lung condition, and the normal changes associated with aging are examples of conditions that result in decreased elasticity of lung tissue, which, in turn, decreases compliance. Surfactant increases the ease of inflation or lung compliance. Without surfactant, lung inflation would be very difficult.

Any impediment or obstruction that air meets as it moves through the airway is known as airway resistance. Airway resistance during inspiration is less than during expiration because the size of the airway opening is increased. Obstruction in any part of the normal passageways impedes respiration. Obstruction can be caused by a foreign substance, such as a piece of food, a coin, or a toy, or by liquids, as in the case of a drowning victim. Obstruction can also result from secretions (eg, excessive or thickened secretions) or tissues (eg, tumors or edema of the respiratory tract). A decrease in the size of air passages resulting from constriction or poor neck positioning can also impede respiration.

Consider Tyrone Jacobs, the 2-year-old boy with suspected asthma. An understanding of the underlying pathophysiologic processes

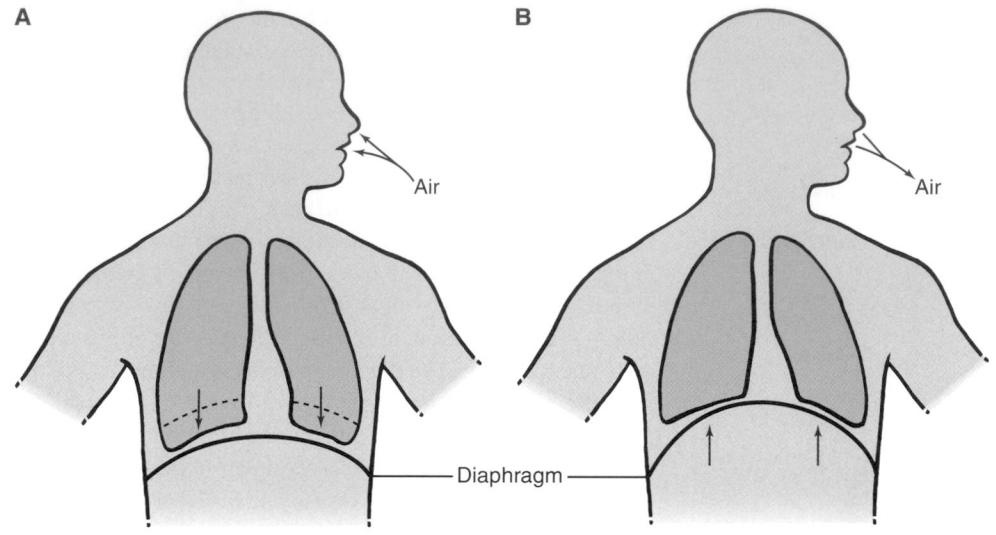

A

B

Air

Air

Diaphragm

FIGURE 45-3 Movement of the diaphragm in ventilation. With inspiration (**A**), the diaphragm contracts and descends, the thoracic cavity lengthens, intrapulmonic pressure decreases, and air rushes in. With expiration (**B**), the diaphragm relaxes and moves upward, intrapulmonic pressure increases, and air moves out of the lungs and is expired.

involved with this disorder would provide the basis for the nurse's actions to protect the child's airway.

Gas Exchange

Gas exchange in the respiratory system refers to the intake of oxygen and the release of carbon dioxide. This exchange is made possible by respiration and perfusion.

Respiration

Respiration, which refers to gas exchange, occurs at the terminal alveolar capillary system. Gases are exchanged between the air and blood via the dense network of capillaries in the respiratory portion of the lungs and the thin alveolar walls (Fig. 45-4). Gas exchange occurs via diffusion. Diffusion refers to the movement of oxygen and carbon dioxide between the air (in the alveoli) and the blood (in the capillaries). The appropriate gas moves passively from an area of higher concentration to an area of lesser concentration. The greater pressure of

oxygen in the alveoli causes the oxygen to move from the alveoli into the capillaries containing the unoxygenated venous blood. Likewise, the carbon dioxide in the returning venous blood exerts a greater pressure than the carbon dioxide in the alveoli. Therefore, carbon dioxide diffuses across the capillary into the alveoli and ultimately is exhaled.

Diffusion of gases in the lung is influenced by four factors:
- Change in surface area available
- Thickening of alveolar–capillary membrane
- Partial pressure
- Solubility and molecular weight of the gas

Any change in the surface area available for diffusion hinders diffusion. For example, removal of a lung or the presence of a disease that destroys lung tissue can decrease the surface area available, ultimately affecting gas exchange. Incomplete lung expansion or the collapse of alveoli, known as **atelectasis,** prevents the pressure changes and the exchange of gas by diffusion in the lungs. Atelectatic areas of the lung cannot fulfill a function of respiration. Examples of conditions that predispose a patient to atelectasis are obstructions of the airway

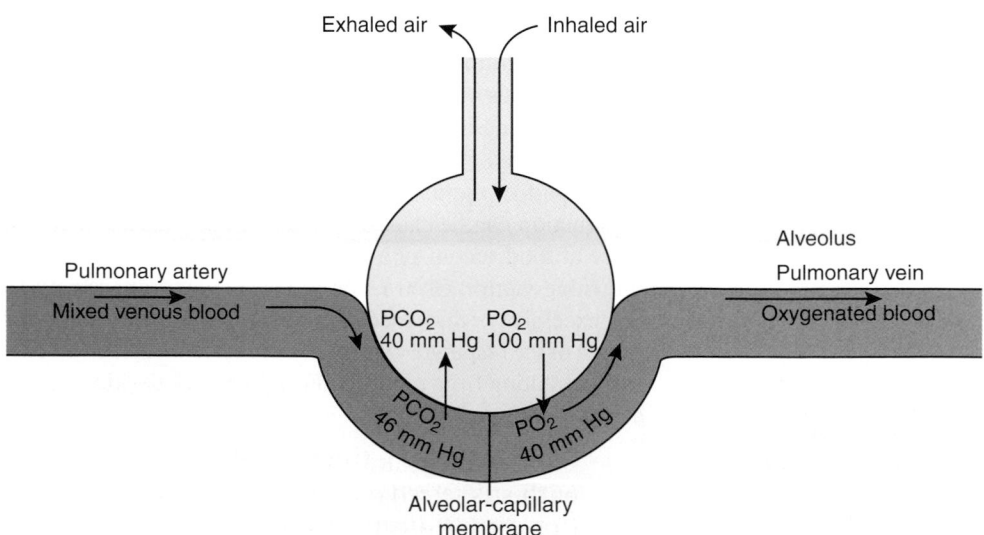

Exhaled air   Inhaled air

Pulmonary artery

Mixed venous blood

PCO_2 40 mm Hg PO_2 100 mm Hg

PCO_2 46 mm Hg PO_2 40 mm Hg

Alveolar-capillary membrane

Alveolus

Pulmonary vein

Oxygenated blood

FIGURE 45-4 Gas exchange in the alveolus. The greater pressure of the oxygen in the air inhaled into the alveoli causes the oxygen to move into the capillaries, which contain unoxygenated blood. The carbon dioxide in the returning venous blood moves from the capillaries (area of greater concentration) into the alveoli (area of lesser concentration).

by foreign bodies, mucus, airway constriction, external compression by tumors or enlarged blood vessels, and immobility. Any disease or condition that results in thickening of the alveolar–capillary membrane such as pneumonia or pulmonary edema makes diffusion more difficult.

The partial pressure, or pressure resulting from any gas in a mixture depending on its concentration, can also affect diffusion. If environmental oxygen is reduced, such as when a person is at higher altitudes or in the presence of toxic fumes, less oxygen is available for diffusion. When oxygen is administered therapeutically, the increased amount available results in greater diffusion across capillary membranes. Finally, the solubility and molecular weight of the gas are factors in diffusion; carbon dioxide has greater solubility in the respiratory membranes and diffuses more rapidly than oxygen. This allows for carbon dioxide to be released from the lungs with each exhalation.

Perfusion

This oxygenated capillary blood passes through tissue in the process called perfusion. The amount of blood flowing through the lungs is a factor in the amount of oxygen and other gases that are exchanged. The amount of blood present in any given area of lung tissue depends partially on whether the person is sitting, standing, or lying down. Perfusion is greater in dependent areas. The perfusion of lung tissue also depends on the person's activity level. Greater activity results in an increased need for cellular oxygen by the body's tissues and a subsequent increase in cardiac output and consequently in increased blood return to the lungs. In addition, perfusion to the body's tissues depends on an adequate blood supply and proper cardiovascular functioning to carry oxygen and carbon dioxide to and from the lungs. Cardiovascular function is discussed in relation to vital signs in Chapter 24.

Transport of Respiratory Gases

Oxygen and carbon dioxide must move through the alveoli and be carried to and from body cells by the blood. Oxygen is carried two ways in the body: via plasma and red blood cells. It is dissolved in plasma, but because oxygen is insoluble in liquids, little oxygen is carried in this way. The majority of oxygen is carried by the red blood cells. The hemoglobin in red blood cells has a strong affinity for oxygen. Therefore, most oxygen (97%) is carried in the body by red blood cells as part of hemoglobin in the form of oxyhemoglobin. Hemoglobin also carries carbon dioxide easily in the form of carboxyhemoglobin.

Once the red blood cells reach the tissue, internal respiration, or the exchange of oxygen and carbon dioxide between the circulating blood and the tissue cells, must occur. Any abnormality in the alveoli or in the blood's constituents affects internal respiration. A decrease in cardiac output (eg, caused by hemorrhage or loss of blood) means a reduction in the amount of circulating blood that is available to deliver oxygen to the tissues. Any decrease in the amount of red blood cells or erythrocytes is referred to as anemia. Anemia results in insufficient hemoglobin available to transport oxygen. This may lead to an inadequate supply of oxygen to the tissues of the body.

Unlike a decrease in cardiac output or anemia, exercise can improve the transport of oxygen because the heart pumps more effectively and cells are better able to use oxygen.

If a problem exists in ventilation, respiration, or perfusion, **hypoxia** (condition in which an inadequate amount of oxygen is available to cells) may occur. The most common symptoms of hypoxia are **dyspnea** (difficulty breathing), an elevated blood pressure with a small pulse pressure, increased respiratory and pulse rates, pallor, and cyanosis. Anxiety and restlessness are also common signs of hypoxia. Hypoxia is often caused by **hypoventilation** (decreased rate or depth of air movement into the lungs). Hypoxia also can occur chronically. The effects of chronic hypoxia can be detected in all body systems and are manifested as altered thought processes, headaches, chest pain, enlarged heart, clubbing of the fingers and toes, anorexia, constipation, decreased urinary output, decreased libido, weakness of extremity muscles, and muscle pain.

Control of Respirations

The medulla in the brain stem immediately above the spinal cord is the respiratory center. It is stimulated by an increased concentration of carbon dioxide and hydrogen ions and, to a lesser degree, by the decreased amount of oxygen in the arterial blood. In addition, chemoreceptors in the aortic arch and carotid bodies are sensitive to the same arterial blood gas levels and can activate the medulla.

Stimulation of the medulla increases the rate and depth of ventilation (both inspiration and expiration) to blow off carbon dioxide and hydrogen and increase oxygen levels (the patient is breathing faster and more deeply). The medulla sends an impulse down the spinal cord to the respiratory muscles to stimulate a contraction leading to inhalation. If a condition causes a chronic change in the oxygen and carbon dioxide levels, these chemoreceptors may become desensitized and not regulate ventilation adequately.

FACTORS AFFECTING RESPIRATORY FUNCTIONING

A variety of factors affect adequate respiratory functioning. Seven important factors are described in the following sections.

Levels of Health

Acute and chronic illnesses can dramatically affect a person's respiratory function. People with renal or cardiac disorders often have compromised respiratory functioning because of fluid overload. People with chronic illnesses often have muscle wasting and poor muscle tone. These problems affect all the muscles, including those of the respiratory system. Since hemoglobin also carries carbon dioxide to the lungs, anemia results in diminished carbon dioxide exchange.

Recall Yan Kim, the 57-year-old patient who developed respiratory failure from complications associated with pulmonary surgery. The acuity of the situation played a major role in the patient's current condition. The pulmonary surgery most likely reduced his respiratory function. The effects of anesthesia on his lungs and subsequently the development of complications compounded his situation.

Developmental Considerations

In addition to age-related developmental considerations (described below), physical changes such as scoliosis (curvature of the spine) influence breathing patterns and may cause air trapping. Research reveals a statistically significant correlation between obesity and chronic bronchitis. Moreover, people who are obese are often short of breath during activity, ultimately leading to less participation in exercise. As a result, the alveoli at the base of the lungs are rarely stimulated to expand fully.

Infant

Birth necessitates many adaptations by a newborn. The most obvious changes occur in the lungs, which are transformed from fluid-filled structures to air-filled organs. The normal infant's chest is small, the airways are short, and aspiration is a potential problem. The respiratory rate is more rapid in infants than at any other age (Table 45-1). As the alveoli increase in number and size, adequate oxygenation is accomplished at lower respiratory rates. Respiratory rates stabilize in young adulthood. Surfactant is formed in utero around 34 to 36 weeks. An infant born prior to 34 weeks may not have sufficient surfactant produced, leading to collapse of the alveoli and poor alveolar exchange. Synthetic surfactant can be give to the infant to help reopen the alveoli.

Respiratory activity is primarily abdominal in infants. The infant's chest wall is so thin and has so little musculature that the ribs, sternum, and xiphoid process are easily seen. Infants have a rounded chest wall in which the anteroposterior diameter (the measurement from the front to the back of the thorax) equals the transverse diameter. Occasional fine **crackles** (a sound that occurs when air moves through airways that contain fluid) at the end of deep inspiration heard on auscultation of the infant's thorax are normal.

Child

In preschool-aged and school-aged children, some subcutaneous fat is deposited on the chest wall, making landmarks less prominent than they were in infants. Muscular development is also more noticeable. The ratio of the transverse diameter to the anteroposterior diameter reaches the adult configuration of 1:2 by age 6 years.

The preschool child's eustachian tubes, bronchi, and bronchioles are elongated and less angular. Thus, the average number of routine colds and infections decreases until the child enters day-care or school and is exposed more frequently to pathogens. Young children who are not placed in day-care usually have not had the opportunity to develop antibodies for the variety of viruses and bacteria they encounter. Good hand hygiene and tissue etiquette should be encouraged. Most children at this age have colds or upper respiratory infections, but some have more serious problems of otitis media, bronchitis, and pneumonia. By the end of late childhood and during adulthood, the immune system is prepared to protect the person from most infections.

Older Adult

Specific physical changes occur in older adults that are unrelated to any pathology (see Focus on the Older Adult box). Bony landmarks are more prominent because of the loss of subcutaneous fat. Kyphosis (curvature of the spine) contributes to the older person's appearance of leaning forward. Barrel chest deformity (see Fig. 25-31 in Chap. 25) may result in an increased anteroposterior diameter. The tissues and airways of the respiratory tract (including the alveoli) become more rigid with age. The power of the respiratory and abdominal muscles is reduced, and therefore the diaphragm moves less efficiently. These alterations increase the risk for disease, especially pneumonia.

TABLE 45-1 Respiratory Variations in the Life Cycle

	Infant (Birth–1 year)	Early Childhood (1–5 years)	Late Childhood (6–12 years)	Aged Adult (65+ years)
Respiratory rate	30–60 breaths/min	20–40 breaths/min	15–25 breaths/min	16–20 breaths/min
Respiratory pattern	Abdominal breathing, irregular in rate and depth	Abdominal breathing, irregular	Thoracic breathing, regular	Thoracic, regular
Chest wall	Thin, little muscle, ribs and sternum easily seen	Same as infant's but with more subcutaneous fat	Further subcutaneous fat deposited, structures less prominent	Thin, structures prominent
Breath sounds	Loud, harsh crackles at end of deep inspiration	Loud, harsh expiration longer than inspiration	Clear inspiration is longer than expiration	Clear
Shape of thorax	Round	Elliptical	Elliptical	Barrel shaped or elliptical

Focus on the Older Adult
Nursing Strategies for Oxygen Problems Affecting Older Adults

Age-Related Changes	Nursing Strategies
Decreased Gas Exchange and Increased Work of Breathing	
• Decreased elastic recoil of the lungs	• Encourage rest periods as necessary.
• Expiration requiring use of accessory muscles	• Encourage cessation or moderation of smoking and second-hand smoke exposure.
• Fewer functional capillaries and more fibrous tissue in alveoli	• Teach breathing exercises.
	• Remind about avoiding air pollutants.
• Decreased skeletal muscle strength in thorax	• Caution about effect of extreme weather conditions.
	• Instruct to avoid narcotics and sleeping pills.
• Reduction in vital capacity and increase in residual volume	• Discuss home management with patient and family.
	• Teach avoidance of infection and preventive measures (ie, flu vaccination).
	• Use pillows as necessary to sleep.
Decreased Ventilation and Ineffective Cough	
• Less air exchange; more secretions remain in lungs	• Encourage increased fluid intake, especially water, as allowed.
• Drier mucous membranes	• Use cool-mist humidifier (teach proper cleaning technique).
• Altered pain sensation	• Encourage attendance at pulmonary exercise rehabilitation program.
• Different norms for body temperature; fever may be atypical	• Discourage use of over-the-counter medications.
	• Teach how to splint thorax and cough effectively.
• Greater risk for aspiration due to slower gastric motility	• Instruct in use of supplemental oxygen.
	• Teach avoidance of milk products if they are troublesome.
• Impaired mobility and inactivity, effects of medication	

Think back to Joan McIntyre, the 72-year-old woman who is having difficulty being weaned from the ventilator. The nurse needs to incorporate information about age-related changes when planning the patient's care. The nurse also needs to consider that some of these age-related changes may be making weaning more difficult for this patient.

Medications

Opioids are chemical agents that depress the medullary respiratory center; as a result, the rate and depth of respirations decrease. This occurs especially with the use of morphine and meperidine (Demerol). The nurse must be alert for the possibility of respiratory arrest when administering any narcotic or sedative.

Lifestyle

Activity levels and habits can dramatically affect a person's respiratory status. For example, sedentary activity patterns do not encourage the expansion of alveoli and the development of pulmonary exercise patterns (deep breathing). People who exercise (eg, aerobics, walking, swimming) three to six times per week can better respond to stressors to respiratory health. Cigarette smoking (active or passive) is a major contributor to lung disease and respiratory distress. Nurses working with patients to initiate changes in health habits that affect respiration must also examine themselves as a factor in the success of the plan. See Promoting Health 45-1: Oxygenation.

Environment

Although it is impossible to pinpoint all the effects of air pollution, researchers have demonstrated a high correlation between air pollution and cancer and lung diseases. For example, a person with adequate respiratory functioning who is exposed to air pollution experiences stinging of eyes and nasal passages, coughing, choking, headache, and dizziness. Occupational exposure to asbestos, silica, or coal dust can lead to chronic pulmonary disease. People who have experienced an alteration in respiratory functioning in the past often have difficulty continuing to perform self-care activities in a polluted environment.

Psychological Health

Individuals responding to stress may sigh excessively or exhibit **hyperventilation** (increased rate and depth of ventilation, above the body's normal metabolic requirements). Generalized anxiety has been shown to cause enough bronchospasm to produce an episode of bronchial asthma. In addition, patients with respiratory problems often develop some anxiety as a result of the hypoxia caused by the respiratory problem.

Think back to Tyrone Jacobs, the young boy described at the beginning of the chapter. The patient is gasping for breath, which is extremely frightening and anxiety producing. In addition, his parents are frantic; this would increase Tyrone's anxiety level, further limiting his ability to breathe. The nurse needs to incorporate

Promoting Health 45-1 *Oxygenation*

Patients view nurses as role models for achieving healthy lifestyles. Nurses dealing with stresses from professional and personal aspects of their own lives sometimes channel their energies into destructive behaviors. If the nurse wishes to encourage optimal respiratory functioning, he or she must demonstrate behaviors that support a healthy lifestyle.

Use the assessment checklist to determine how well you are meeting oxygenation needs. Then develop a prescription for self-care by choosing appropriate behaviors from the list of suggestions.

ASSESSMENT CHECKLIST

almost always | sometimes | almost never

1. I breathe easily, without discomfort and without feeling short of breath.
2. I exercise regularly.
3. I maintain normal weight for my height and body frame.
4. I live in an environment free of pollution.
5. I avoid substances (tobacco, chemicals) that cause respiratory problems.
6. I arrange to receive recommended immunizations.

SELF-CARE BEHAVIORS

1. Follow a regular exercise program with 30 to 45 minutes of moderate activity three or four times a week.
2. Maintain normal body weight.
3. Obtain medical evaluation for chest pain, problems with breathing, chronic cough with sputum or blood.
4. Evaluate personal use of nicotine.
5. Incorporate a plan to reduce smoking and then stop smoking on a specific target date.
6. Avoid exposure to second-hand smoke when possible.
7. Arrange to have a tuberculin test (PPD) done annually.
8. Receive yearly influenza immunization.
9. Avoid chemical substances that cause respiratory depression.
10. Maintain a pollution-free environment (as much as possible).
11. Support federal and community efforts to keep the air free of pollution.

---

an understanding of this situation and plan interventions that promote oxygenation while reducing anxiety.

THE NURSING PROCESS FOR OXYGENATION

Assessing

The patient's health history is an essential component for assessing respiratory functioning. Either the patient or a family member can provide this information. The nursing examination combined with laboratory findings can provide information to identify a patient's strengths, the nature of the problem, its course, related signs and symptoms, and its onset, frequency, and effects on activities of daily living. The nurse decides, based on these findings, what problems can be treated independently by nursing. Other problems are referred to a physician for decisions on treatment.

Nursing History

The nursing history, an important clinical tool in the early steps of the nursing process, always includes a respiratory component. The information gained provides data about why the patient needs nursing care and what kind of care is required to maintain a sufficient intake of air. Interview questions help identify current or potential health deviations, actions performed by the patient for meeting respiratory

needs and the effects of such actions, contributing factors, the use of any aids to improve the intake of air, and effects on the patient's lifestyle and relationships with others.

Before starting the interview, ascertain that the patient is not in acute distress and that family members are comfortable. If the patient is experiencing any respiratory distress, initiate appropriate actions immediately to help relieve symptoms. Enlist the aid of family members or others to help answer questions. When the patient is able, interview the patient to expand this initial database. If no emergency interventions are necessary for the patient's clinical condition, obtain a comprehensive history at this time.

When a health deviation is noted during the data collection, collect as much descriptive information as possible, including whether the problem evolved suddenly or slowly. The accompanying Focused Assessment Guide 45-1 provides some appropriate questions for assessment.

Physical Assessment

The basic examination of the lungs and respiratory status is discussed in Chapter 25. Always proceed in a well-organized manner through a sequence of inspection, palpation, percussion, and auscultation.

Recall Mr. Kim, the 57-year-old man who is receiving oxygen therapy and mechanical ventilation via an endotracheal tube. A complete assessment is necessary to identify specific prob-

Focused Assessment Guide 45-1

Respiration and Oxygenation

Factors to Assess	Questions and Approaches
Usual patterns of respiration	How would you describe your breathing patterns? Do you have allergies? Do you smoke? Do you live with a smoker or are there smokers or other pollutants in your workplace?
Recent changes	Have you noticed any changes in your breathing pattern (out of breath, cough, pain)? Do you have chest pain?
Cough	How much and how often do you cough? Is the cough related to the time of day or any activity? What is it like (dry, bubbly, hoarse)? Do you have a history of allergies? Do you ever wheeze? Are you exposed to dust? Fumes? Where do you work? What kind of work? How are you treating the cough?
Sputum	Do you ever cough up and spit out mucus? How much do you spit out and do you associate it with anything (time of day, environment)? What color is it? Is it ever blood tinged? What is its odor?
Chest pain	On a scale of 0 to 5 (5 being very painful), how severe is the pain? Where is the pain? Is the pain worse with inspiration? Expiration? Cough? Does the pain radiate? What measures are you using to relieve the pain?
Dyspnea	Is it constant or remittent or related to any activity? How do different positions affect it? How does it affect your daily activities? Is any part of your body bluish during the breathing problem? What do you do during and after the breathing attack? Have you ever been told that you have asthma? Emphysema? Tuberculosis? Heart disease? Do you think the problem is getting worse or staying the same?
Fever	Have you had pneumonia recently? Do you have any contact with people who have tuberculosis? Do you have night sweats? Are others in your household well or ill? Have you traveled anywhere recently? What medications are you using? Have you been exposed to any pollutants?
Fatigue	Have you noticed you feel more tired lately? Are you getting your normal amount of sleep at night? Has your sleep at night been affected by any difficulty breathing? Do you become easily fatigued when you climb stairs? Has your pattern of daily activity changed lately? Can you sleep lying flat? How many pillows do you use?

lems related to oxygenation as well as to determine the effectiveness of current treatments.

Inspection

Inspect the chest contour and shape. Normally, the chest contour is slightly convex, with no sternal depression. The anteroposterior diameter should be less than the transverse diameter. Describe or sketch any abnormalities in thoracic structure (see Fig. 25-30 in Chap. 25 for structures). Also note the contour of the intercostal spaces, which should be flat or depressed, and the movement of the chest, which should be symmetrical. Inspect the skin over the thorax for temperature and color. It should be warm and dry and even in color, with no cyanosis or pallor. Note any scars, recording the origin of such in the history under previous surgery or accidents.

Observe the respiratory rate and rhythm for 1 full minute. Normally, respirations are quiet and nonlabored. Note any flaring of the nostrils, muscular retractions, tachypnea, or bradypnea, suggestive of a health deviation requiring further evaluation. Refer to Figure 25-35 in Chapter 25 for illustrations of abnormal breathing patterns.

Always be alert for common clinical manifestations that may indicate an airway emergency. Specific disease processes and conditions leading to acute respiratory failure, and their associated clinical manifestations, are discussed in medical–surgical nursing textbooks.

Palpation

Palpate the trachea, which should lie equidistant from each clavicle. Skin temperature in this area typically is the same as the rest of the body.

Measure respiratory excursion by placing your hands on the patient's posterior thorax at the 10th rib, with both thumbs almost touching the vertebrae. Ask the patient to take a few deep breaths, and watch the movement of the hands. Usually the thumbs move 5 to 8 cm symmetrically at maximal inspiration (see Fig. 25-33 in Chap. 25).

Assess tactile fremitus (the capacity to feel sound on the chest wall) by placing your palm to the patient's chest wall, avoiding bony areas (eg, scapulae). Ask the patient to repeat some multisyllable word (eg, "ninety-nine") and feel for the vibration. Normally the vibrations are equal bilaterally in different areas on the chest wall. The greatest intensity is noted at the anterior and posterior base of the neck and along the trachea and large bronchi. Increased fremitus occurs in patients with pneumonia because solid tissue conducts sound well. Conversely, patients with chronic obstructive pulmonary disease (COPD) have decreased fremitus because air does not conduct sound as well. Note the presence or absence of crepitation, masses, edema, or tenderness on palpation.

Percussion

Perform percussion posteriorly as the patient pulls the shoulders forward. Then continue with the examination proceeding down the patient's back, comparing one side to the other. Examine the anterior and lateral thorax with the patient in a supine position. Listen carefully to the intensity and quality of each sound as the chest wall and underlying structures are percussed:

- Resonance: a loud, hollow, low-pitched sound, heard over normal lungs
- Hyperresonance: a loud, low, booming sound typically heard over emphysematous lungs
- Flat sound detected over bone or heavy muscle
- Dull sound with medium pitch and intensity usually heard over the liver (fifth intercostal space at the right midclavicular line)
- Tympany: a high-pitched, loud, drumlike sound produced over the stomach

Dullness over the lung field occurs when fluid or solid tissue replaces normal lung tissue in the pleural space. This finding requires further investigation.

Auscultation

Using the diaphragm of a stethoscope, move from apex to base, comparing one side with the other side while listening to a complete respiratory cycle, inspiration and expiration. Normal breath sounds include **vesicular** (low-pitched, soft sound during expiration and heard over most of the lung); **bronchial** (high-pitched and longer sound, heard primarily over the trachea); and **bronchovesicular** (medium-pitched and medium sound during expiration, heard over the upper anterior chest and intercostal area; see Fig. 25-34 in Chap. 25). While auscultating, ask the patient to breathe through an open mouth slowly because breathing through the nose can produce falsely abnormal breath sounds. Breathing too quickly, such as with hyperventilation, may cause syncope and patient distress. If any abnormal breath sound is detected, instruct the patient to cough and auscultate again for at least two complete respiratory cycles. Record location, change in breath sounds after coughing, and phase of respiration (eg, expiration) when any abnormal sound is noted.

Adventitious, or abnormal, lung sounds are categorized as either crackles (formerly called rales) or wheezes. Crackles are discontinuous (intermittent) sounds that occur when air moves through airways that contain fluid. They are produced by a delayed reopening of deflated airways. Crackles can be further classified as fine, medium, or coarse. Fine crackles, which are high-pitched sounds similar to static that are heard toward the end of inspiration or early expiration, indicate congestion in small air passages and alveoli. Rubbing strands of hair between the fingers creates a sound similar to fine crackles. Medium crackles are louder and may sound moist, whereas coarse crackles are somewhat louder, bubbly noises heard during inspiration and possibly expiration that are not cleared by coughing. Coarse crackles result when air passes through fluid in the larger airways, increasing pulmonary congestion. Usually, coarse crackles are first detected in the lung bases; they typically cannot be cleared with coughing and may be auscultated in a patient with pneumonia.

Wheezes are continuous sounds heard on expiration and sometimes on inspiration. They originate as air passes through airways constricted by swelling, secretions, or tumors. They can be further classified as sibilant wheezes (formerly called wheezes) or sonorous wheezes (formerly known as rhonchi). Sibilant wheezes originate in smaller airways and are high pitched and whistling, whereas sonorous wheezes can be heard over larger airways and sound like a snore (Smeltzer & Bare, 2004). They are often heard in patients with asthma or emphysema.

When assessing Tyrone Jacobs, the young boy with asthma, auscultation of breath sounds is crucial. Auscultation of a child with asthma typically reveals wheezes.

A pleural friction rub is a continuous, dry grating sound caused by inflammation of pleural surfaces. It is more often heard on inspiration than expiration, is unaltered by coughing, and resembles the sound made by rubbing two leather surfaces together. This can be heard in a patient with infective pericarditis.

Common Diagnostic Methods to Assess Respiratory Functioning

In addition to the nursing history and physical examination, the laboratory and radiologic tests described in Table 45-2 provide further assessment data that can aid in the formation of nursing diagnoses.

> The nurse might anticipate diagnostic procedures such as radiography for Joan McIntyre, the older woman who is being weaned from the ventilator. This diagnostic test might provide clues to another problem that might be affecting the patient's ability to be weaned. In addition, arterial blood gases may be used to evaluate her response to weaning.

The tests described in the next sections are not distinctive for a particular disease but reflect how well the respiratory system is functioning.

Pulmonary Function Studies

Pulmonary function studies are routinely done to evaluate pulmonary status and detect abnormalities. Spirometry studies measure lung capacity, volumes, and flow rates while the patient inhales deeply and exhales forcefully into a **spirometer,** an instrument that measures these volumes and airflow. Individuals with chronic lung disease are usually exhausted after these tests. Drugs affecting the respiratory tract, such as bronchodilators, are withheld before the examination so that test results reflect the patient's present status.

Pulmonary function tests measure the following lung volumes and capacities:

- Tidal volume (TV): the amount of air inspired and expired in a normal respiration. Normal is 500 mL.
- Inspiratory reserve volume (IRV): the amount of air that can be inspired beyond tidal volume. Normal is 3,100 mL.
- Expiratory reserve volume (ERV): the amount of air that can be exhaled beyond tidal volume. Normal is 1,200 mL.
- Residual volume (RV): the amount of air remaining in the lungs after a maximal expiration. Normal is 1,200 mL.
- Vital capacity (VC): the maximal amount of air that can be exhaled after a maximal inhalation. Normal is 4,800 mL.
- Inspiratory capacity (IC): the largest amount of air that can be inhaled after a normal quiet exhalation. Normal is 3,600 mL.
- Functional residual volume (FRV): equal to the expiratory reserve volume plus the residual volume. Normal is 2,400 mL.
- Total lung capacity (TLC): the sum of the TV, IRV, ERV, and RV. Normal is 6,000 mL.

Peak Expiratory Flow Rate

Peak expiratory flow rate (PEFR) refers to the volume of air that can be forcibly exhaled. A decrease in PEFR can signal airway obstruction. PEFR is measured via a peak flow meter; this test is noninvasive, inexpensive, quick, and easy. With the patient standing or sitting with the back positioned as straight as possible, the patient takes a deep breath and places the peak flow meter in his or her mouth, closing the lips tightly around the mouthpiece. The patient forcibly exhales into the peak flow meter, and an indicator on the meter rises to a number. The patient is asked to repeat this three times, and the highest number is recorded. This produces a measurement in liters indicating the maximum flow rate during a forced expiration. Normal values are established in regard to height, age, and gender. Patients commonly measure PEFR at home to monitor airflow in conditions such as asthma. The results are brought to the clinician's office to check for severity of asthma and to track responses to any change in the medication regimen.

Pulse Oximetry

Pulse oximetry is a noninvasive technique that measures the oxygen saturation (SpO_2) of arterial blood. Pulse oximetry is useful for monitoring patients receiving oxygen therapy, those at risk for hypoxia, and postoperative patients. It indicates trends in oxygen saturation but is not a replacement for arterial blood gas analysis. However, the test can be used as an adjunct diagnostic test.

The nurse should know the patient's hemoglobin level before evaluating oxygen saturation because the test measures only the percentage of oxygen carried by the available hemoglobin. Thus, even a patient with a low hemoglobin could appear to have a normal SpO_2 because most of that hemoglobin is saturated. However, the patient may not have enough oxygen to meet body needs. A range of 95% to 100% is considered normal SpO_2; values less than 85% indicate that oxygenation to the tissues is inadequate.

> Consider Tyrone Jacobs, the young boy with asthma described at the beginning of the chapter. The nurse would use pulse oximetry initially to obtain baseline information about the patient's oxygen saturation level and then as a means to evaluate the effectiveness of therapy.

Figure 45-5 shows a nurse using a pulse oximetry unit, and Skill 45-1 outlines nursing responsibilities when using a pulse oximetry unit.

Thoracentesis

Thoracentesis is the procedure of entering the pleural cavity and aspirating fluid. The pleural cavity is a potential cavity because it is normally not distended with fluid or air. The physician usually performs thoracentesis at the bedside with the nurse assisting. The patient is required to sign a permit for this procedure. A thoracentesis may be performed to obtain a specimen for diagnostic purposes or to remove fluid that has accumulated in the pleural cavity and is causing respiratory difficulty and discomfort. Because the cavity being entered is

TABLE 45-2 Common Diagnostic Procedures Used to Assess Respiratory Functioning

Preparation	Aftercare

Arterial blood gas and pH analysis examine arterial blood to determine the pressure exerted by oxygen and carbon dioxide in the blood and the blood pH. This test measures the adequacy of oxygenation, ventilation, and perfusion. Normal results are: pH (7.35–7.45), PCO_2 (35–45 mm Hg), PO_2 (80–100 mm Hg), and HCO_3 (22–26 mEq/L).

• Explain to the patient that this test requires an arterial puncture and collection of a blood specimen.	• The arterial specimen is immediately placed on ice and taken to the laboratory.
• The radial, brachial, or femoral arteries are usually the sites of choice.	• Apply pressure for 3–5 minutes and watch for evidence of bleeding. If patient is taking anticoagulants, pressure must be applied for a longer interval.
• Perform Allen's test to ensure adequate ulnar blood flow when using radial Artex.	

A cytologic study involves a microscopic examination of sputum and the cells it contains. It is done primarily to detect cells that may be malignant, to determine organisms causing infection, and to identify blood or pus in the sputum.

• Collect the specimen, if possible, in the morning before breakfast. The test usually involves 3 successive days of sputum collection. About 1 teaspoon of sputum is needed for a specimen.	• Advise the patient to inform the nurse when the specimen has been obtained.
• Instruct the patient that saliva is not a satisfactory specimen.	• Label and package the specimen and send it to the laboratory as soon as possible.
• Patient should take a deep breath and then expel the air with a deep cough.	
• Expectorate the specimen into a sterile specimen container that contains 50% alcohol.	
• Close the container with a tight-fitting lid.	

Endoscopic studies involve direct visualization of a body cavity. A bronchoscope is used to examine the larynx, bronchi, and trachea. Bronchoscopy is used to view lesions, obtain a biopsy, improve drainage, remove foreign substances, and drain abscesses.

• Obtain an informed consent.	• Withhold food and fluids until the gag reflex returns.
• The patient should be NPO for 4–8 hours before the test.	• Check vital signs according to the protocol.
• An analgesic, sedative, and/or anticholinergic may be administered before the test.	• Observe carefully for signs of respiratory impairment. Emergency resuscitation equipment should be available.
• Local anesthetic is sprayed into the throat.	• Warm saline gargles may relieve throat irritation once the gag reflex has returned.

Skin tests determine antigen–antibody reactions. In intradermal tests, antigens (to which the patient may have previously been exposed) are injected into the superficial layer of the skin with a needle and syringe to evaluate immune response.

• Check patient's history for hypersensitivity to any of the test antigens. If positive, notify the physician before performing test.	• Instruct the patient to have the test results read at the appropriate time.
• Cleanse the test area with alcohol and allow it to dry.	• After reading the results, document the reaction, noting the amount of erythema or induration. Record the test, time, date, method, and site of administration on the patient record.

Radiography is an x-ray examination of the lungs and the thoracic cavity. Radiographic examinations of the lungs are done to help diagnose pulmonary diseases and to determine the progress or development of disease.

• Instruct patient to remove clothing to the waist and put on gown. All metal jewelry should be removed.	• No special care is required after chest radiograph.
• The patient will be required to take a deep breath and hold it during the radiograph.	

Lung scan is the recording on a photographic plate of the emissions of radioactive waves from a substance injected into a vein as it circulates through the lung. A *perfusion scan* (Q scan) is done to measure integrity of pulmonary blood vessels and evaluate blood flow abnormalities (eg, pulmonary emboli). A *ventilation scan* (V scan) is done to detect ventilation abnormalities (especially in patients with emphysema). Both scans used together provide greater and more accurate diagnostic information than either test used solely.

• Obtain an informed consent if required by agency.	• No special care is required after the lung scan.
• Explain that no fasting is required.	• Reassure patient that no radiation precautions are necessary.
• Patient should be told to remove jewelry from the chest area.	

(Adapted from Fischbach, F. [2000]. *A manual of laboratory diagnostic tests* [6th ed.]. Philadelphia: Lippincott Williams & Wilkins; and Pagana, K., & Pagana, T. [2002]. *Manual of diagnostic and laboratory tests* [2nd ed.]. St. Louis: C. V. Mosby.)

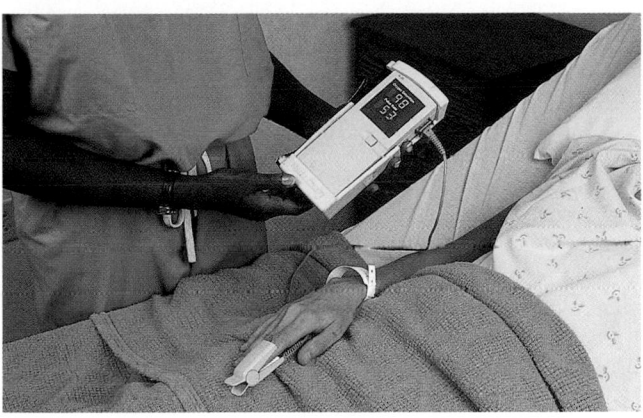

FIGURE 45-5 Portable pulse oximetry unit, used to measure oxygen saturation (SpO₂) of arterial blood.   (Photo © B. Proud)

sterile, surgical asepsis is required. Standard precautions also are used.

Procedure

A thoracentesis is usually carried out with the patient sitting on a chair or the edge of the bed with the legs supported and the arms folded and resting on a pillow on the bedside table (Fig. 45-6). If unable to sit up, the patient may lie on the unaffected side with the hand of the affected side raised above the shoulder.

The location where the needle is inserted depends on where the fluid is present and where the physician can best aspirate it. Once this spot is identified by the physician, the skin is prepared over the area. A local anesthetic is administered and then the needle is inserted between the ribs through

SKILL
45-1   Using a Pulse Oximeter

EQUIPMENT
Pulse oximeter
Nail polish remover (if necessary)

ACTION	RATIONALE
1. Explain procedure to patient.	An explanation relieves anxiety and facilitates patient cooperation.
2. Perform hand hygiene.	Hand hygiene deters the spread of microorganisms.
3. Select an adequate site for application of the sensor:	Inadequate circulation can interfere with the SpO₂ reading.
a. Use the patient's index, middle, or ring finger.	
b. Check the proximal pulse and capillary refill at the pulse closest to the site.	Brisk capillary refill and a strong pulse indicate that circulation to the site is adequate.
c. If circulation at site is inadequate, the ear lobe or bridge of nose may be considered.	These alternate sites are highly vascular alternatives.
d. Use a toe only if lower extremity circulation is not compromised.	Peripheral vascular disease is common in lower extremities.
4. Use the proper equipment:	
a. If one finger is too large for the probe, use a smaller one. A pediatric probe may be used for a small adult.	Inaccurate readings can result if probe or sensor is not attached correctly.
b. Use probes appropriate for patient's age and size.	Probes come in adult, pediatric, and infant sizes.
c. Check if patient is allergic to adhesive. A non-adhesive finger clip or reflectance sensor is available.	A reaction may occur if patient is allergic to adhesive substance.
5. Prepare the monitoring site:	Skin oils, dirt, or grime on site; polish; and artificial nails can interfere with the passage of light waves.
a. Cleanse the selected area and allow it to dry.	
b. Remove nail polish and artificial nails after checking manufacturer's instructions.	
6. Apply the probe securely to the skin. Make sure that the light-emitting sensor and the light-receiving sensor are aligned opposite each other (not necessary to check if placed on the forehead or bridge of the nose).	Secure attachments and proper alignment of the markings for the light-emitting and light-receiving sensor promote satisfactory operation of the equipment and accurate recording of the SpO₂.
7. Connect the sensor probe to the pulse oximeter and check operation of the equipment (presence of audible beep and fluctuation of bar of light or waveform on the face of the oximeter).	Audible beep represents the arterial pulse, and fluctuating waveform indicates strength of the pulse. A weak signal will produce an inaccurate recording of the SpO₂. Tone of beep reflect SpO₂ reading. If SpO₂ drops, tone becomes lower pitched.

(continued)

ACTION	RATIONALE
8. Set the alarms on the pulse oximeter. Check manufacturer's alarm limits for high and low pulse rate settings.	Alarm provides additional safeguard for patient and signals when high or low limits have been surpassed.
9. Check oxygen saturation at regular intervals as ordered by physician and necessitated by alarms. Monitor patient's hemoglobin level.	Monitoring SpO_2 provides ongoing assessment of patient's condition. A low hemoglobin level may be satisfactorily saturated yet not be adequate to meet a patient's oxygen needs.
10. Remove sensor on a regular basis and check for skin irritation or signs of pressure (every 2 hr for spring-tension sensor or every 4 hr for adhesive finger or toe sensor).	Prolonged pressure may lead to tissue necrosis and adhesive sensor may cause skin irritation.
11. Evaluate any malfunctions or problems with equipment.	
a. For absent or weak signal, check the patient's vital signs and condition. If satisfactory, check connections and circulation to site.	Hypotension makes an accurate recording difficult. Equipment (restraint, BP cuff) may compromise circulation to site and cause venous blood to pulsate, giving an inaccurate reading. If extremity is cold, cover with warm blanket.
b. For inaccurate reading, check prescribed medications and history of circulatory disorders. Try device on a healthy person to see if problem is equipment related or patient related.	Drugs that cause vasoconstriction interfere with accurate recording of oxygen saturation.
c. If bright light (sunlight or fluorescent light) is suspected of causing equipment malfunction, cover probe with a dry washcloth.	Bright light can interfere with operation of light sensors and cause unreliable report.
12. Document and report SpO_2 appropriately.	Documentation ensures continuity of care and ongoing assessment record.

Home Care Consideration   Portable units are available for use in the home or an outpatient setting.

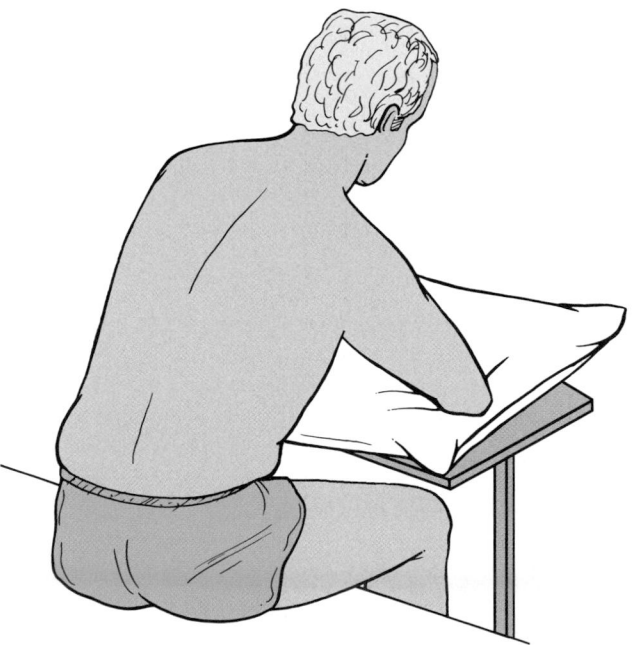

FIGURE 45-6 Position of the patient for thoracentesis.

the intercostal muscles and fascia and into the pleura. After the procedure, the needle or plastic catheter is removed and a small sterile dressing is placed over the entry site.

During thoracentesis, fluid or air can be removed from the pleural cavity with a syringe. Another method for removing fluid is to drain the fluid into a bottle in which a partial vacuum has been created. With this technique, a small plastic catheter may be threaded through the needle, allowing the needle to be withdrawn. This catheter reduces the possibility of puncturing the lung. When this method is used, the tubing connecting the needle and the bottle must be sterile. Commonly, a calibrated bottle is used to collect the drainage, allowing the amount of fluid removed to be determined. The upper limit is generally 1,000 mL.

Assisting With the Procedure

The nurse is responsible for collecting baseline data before the procedure and preparing the patient physically and emotionally for the procedure. Instruct the patient not to cough or breathe deeply during the procedure. Urge the patient to remain as still as possible to diminish the risk for accidental injury to the lung. Administer analgesics before the test as ordered.

During the procedure, observe the patient's reactions. Monitor the patient's color, pulse, and respiratory rates, reporting any deviation from the norm to the physician immediately. Fainting, nausea, and vomiting may occur. Ensure that specimens, if obtained, are taken to the laboratory immediately. Note any medications the patient is taking, particularly antibiotics, on the laboratory slip that accompanies the specimen.

After the procedure, assess the patient for changes in respirations. If a large amount of fluid was removed, respirations usually become easier. If the lung was punctured, respiratory distress becomes acute. If blood appears in the sputum or the patient has severe coughing, notify the physician promptly. A chest radiograph is usually done after the procedure to verify the absence of complications.

Diagnosing

Each nursing diagnosis statement identifies a patient problem and suggests expected patient outcomes. The etiology of the problem directs nursing interventions. In analyzing the assessment data, the nurse must determine whether the alteration in respiratory functioning:

- Is the problem
- Is contributing to a different problem
- Is a sign or symptom of a problem

Alterations in Respiratory Function as the Problem

After the assessment is completed and the data are examined, the nurse concludes either that there is no problem at this time or that there is an actual or potential respiratory problem that is amenable to independent or interdependent nursing actions. Nursing diagnoses indicating alterations in respiratory function are:

- Ineffective Airway Clearance
- Ineffective Breathing Pattern
- Impaired Gas Exchange

Common etiologies for these diagnoses include an inability to maintain proper position, pain or fear of pain, viscous secretions, fatigue, decreased level of consciousness, lack of knowledge, smoking, allergy, mechanical obstruction, medications, and decreased elasticity of the lungs. Examples of these diagnoses, etiologic factors, and defining characteris-

tics appear in Examples of NANDA Nursing Diagnoses: Oxygenation.

Alterations in Respiratory Function as the Etiology

An alteration in respiratory functioning may affect other areas of human functioning. Other nursing diagnoses resulting from alterations in respiratory functioning include:

- Activity Intolerance related to shortness of breath
- Anxiety related to feeling of suffocation
- Acute Pain related to pleural inflammation
- Impaired Verbal Communication related to endotracheal intubation
- Ineffective Coping related to frequent hospitalization resulting from acute symptoms of COPD
- Deficient Diversional Activity related to loss of ability to perform specific activities because of shortness of breath
- Fatigue related to impaired oxygen transport system
- Fear related to disabling respiratory illness
- Dysfunctional Grieving related to loss of normal respiratory functioning
- Ineffective Health Maintenance related to smoking
- Noncompliance (eg, with performance of daily respiratory exercises) related to side effects of therapy
- Imbalanced Nutrition: Less Than Body Requirements, related to difficulty breathing
- Impaired Oral Mucous Membrane related to presence of endotracheal tube
- Powerlessness related to inability for self-care because of COPD
- Chronic/Situational Low Self-Esteem related to loss of normal respiratory function

Examples of NANDA Nursing Diagnoses | Oxygenation

Nursing Diagnoses	Related Factors	Sample Defining Characteristics
Ineffective Airway Clearance	Thick yellow secretions, fever, fatigue, dehydration, poor nutrition	"I never feel as though I am getting enough air." Seventy-year-old man with a 20-year history of COPD, recent development of pneumonia. He is pale with circumoral cyanosis. His respiratory rate is 40 breaths/min and shallow. Coarse crackles are auscultated bilaterally. He does not sit quietly in chair or on bed. He cannot walk length of room without coughing episode, which produces little sputum.
Impaired Gas Exchange	Smokes one pack per day; works with asbestos in auto factory; has had a cold for 7 days	Cyanotic 50-year-old man. Using pursed-lip breathing while sitting on emergency room stretcher. Sitting hunched forward with overbed table supporting arms. Altered blood gases show respiratory acidosis. Admits to shortness of breath, nausea, and ankle edema for 1 week.
Ineffective Breathing Pattern	Anxious about results of cardiac catheterization and possible cardiac surgery	Hyperventilating, tachypneic (40 minutes). "I have a tingling feeling in my fingers."

- Disturbed Sleep Pattern related to orthopnea and bronchodilators
- Social Isolation related to inability to walk to usual "people places"
- Risk for Suffocation related to child playing with a plastic bag
- Risk for Aspiration related to reduced level of consciousness

Outcome Identification and Planning

When caring for patients with an alteration in respiratory functioning, nursing measures support the following general expected outcomes. The patient will:

- Demonstrate improved gas exchange in the lungs by an absence of cyanosis or chest pain and a pulse oximetry reading more than 95%
- Relate the causative factors, if known, and demonstrate a method of coping with these factors
- Preserve pulmonary function by maintaining an optimal level of activity
- Demonstrate self-care behaviors that provide relief from symptoms and prevent further pulmonary problems

When the patient's physical, psychosocial, and spiritual dimensions contribute to alterations in respiratory function, individualized expected outcomes are developed with the patient's input (eg, "By March 15, the patient will be able to walk up one flight of steps at home without dyspnea").

Implementing

Teaching About Pollution-Free Environments

A pollution-free environment is particularly important for individuals with respiratory problems. Teach the patient to assess the environment and make adjustments, whenever possible, to factors that impair respiratory functioning or "triggers." The patient must actively plan to prevent exposure to pollutants and triggers. This might involve a job change, use of protective equipment, requesting enforcement of laws by government agencies, or subcontracting jobs. Dusting and vacuuming the office and home must be done at least twice per week. In some situations, the patient may wear a mask to prevent some symptoms of respiratory distress. Exposure to industrial or occupational hazards (eg, paint, varnish, gaseous fumes, and asbestos) must be restricted.

In the United States, fine pollutants including carbon monoxide, sulfur dioxide, total suspended particulates, ozone, and nitrogen dioxide that pose a hazard to health are monitored closely. On days when pollutant levels are significantly elevated, morbidity and mortality rates among people with preexisting pulmonary disease are greatly increased. Thus, on days when pollution alerts are announced, persons with altered respiratory function should reduce their activities, stay indoors, and use an air conditioner, electronic air cleaner, or air filter. If pollen alters the patient's respiratory function, the same principles apply.

Cigarette smoking is the most important risk factor in pulmonary disease. The inhalation of cigarette smoke increases airway resistance, reduces ciliary action, increases mucus production, causes thickening of the alveolar–capillary membrane, and causes bronchial walls to thicken and lose their elasticity. These effects occur in both smokers and nonsmokers (children and adults) who live with smokers. Habitual smokers usually have great difficulty quitting or reducing their smoking and need much encouragement. The American Lung Association and the American Heart Association offer many free educational materials to aid and support patients who are trying to stop smoking. Their addresses and phone numbers are listed in local telephone directories. Nurses play a key role in presenting accurate information about the negative effects of smoking and to encourage the decision to stop smoking or never to start smoking.

Promoting Optimal Function

Most people with altered respiratory functioning experience anxiety as a result of their symptoms and the actual or potential loss of independence. Oxygen deficits, particularly in older people, impair all aspects of daily living. Going to get the mail or cleaning the house becomes a monumental task for people with oxygen deficits.

The nurse can create an environment that is likely to reduce anxiety. Help institute measures to alleviate discomfort immediately. Use effective listening skills and accurate observation to display a caring attitude. Attempt to understand the patient's life experiences and habits without judging them. Patients with harmful health habits often fear they will be judged, and this impedes the use of nursing interventions. Patients who believe nurses are genuinely concerned about them and their family are more willing to work toward achieving mutually desirable outcomes.

> *Think back to Joan McIntyre, the woman requesting to be "let go" the next time she fails to be weaned. The nurse needs to provide support to the patient, showing genuine concern for her welfare. In addition, the nurse needs to act ethically and legally to ensure the patient's rights.*

Promoting Proper Breathing

Breathing exercises are designed to help patients achieve more efficient and controlled ventilations, to decrease the work of breathing, and to correct respiratory deficits. The Examples of Nursing Interventions Classification (NIC) box focuses on nursing interventions that maximize oxygen and carbon dioxide exchange in the lungs.

Deep Breathing

Many people, both well and ill, have breathing habits that are not conducive to maximal respiratory functioning. Some people develop a pattern of shallow breathing or walk with a posture that makes the chest wall appear caved in. Ill people, for any number of reasons, may limit their respiratory efforts. When hypoventilation occurs, a decreased amount of air enters and leaves the lungs. However, deep-breathing exercises can be used to overcome hypoventilation.

Instruct the patient to make each breath deep enough to move the bottom ribs. Unless the patient has a nasal condition that prohibits or prevents normal breathing, have the patient start slowly taking deep ventilations nasally and then expiring slowly through the mouth. Breathing through the nose warms, filters, and humidifies the air. The patient's respiratory status, motivation, and general clinical condition dictate the timing of this exercise, which should be done hourly while awake or four times daily.

Using Incentive Spirometry

In incentive spirometry, the patient takes a deep breath and can see the results of his or her efforts on the spirometry equipment while sustaining that maximal inspiration, providing immediate positive reinforcement. Incentive spirometry forces the patient to inflate the lungs, which keeps the alveoli from collapsing so that gas exchange can occur and secretions can be cleared and expectorated. Before using incentive spirometry equipment, the patient needs instructions on using the equipment properly. Validate the patient's correct use of this equipment in both healthcare and home environments. See Chapter 30, Guidelines for Nursing Care 30-1, for additional suggestions when teaching patients to use this device.

Pursed-Lip Breathing

Patients who experience dyspnea and feelings of panic can often gain control of their respiration by using pursed-lip breathing. This exercise trains the muscles to prolong exhalation, increasing airway pressure during expiration and

reducing the amount of airway trapping and resistance. The patient inhales through the nose while counting to three and then exhales slowly and evenly against pursed lips while tightening the abdominal muscles. During exhalation, the patient counts to seven. To purse the lips, the patient should position the lips as though he or she was sucking through a straw or whistling. When walking, the patient should inhale while taking two steps and then exhale through pursed lips while taking the next four steps, and then repeat the cycle. Before teaching these techniques, practice them alone and then with a partner.

Abdominal or Diaphragmatic Breathing

Many people with COPD breathe in a shallow, rapid, and exhausting pattern. This type of upper chest breathing can be altered to another form of breathing, diaphragmatic breathing, which reduces the respiratory rate, increases tidal volume, and reduces the functional residual capacity. The patient places one hand on the stomach and the other on the middle of the chest. The patient breathes in slowly through the nose, letting the abdomen protrude as far as it will go. Then the patient breathes out through pursed lips while contracting the abdominal muscles, with one hand pressing inward and upward on the abdomen. The patient repeats these steps for 1 minute, followed by a rest for 2 minutes. Encourage the patient to practice this breathing pattern several times during the day; eventually it will become automatic.

Managing Chest Tubes

Patients with fluid (**pleural effusion**), blood (**hemothorax**), or air (**pneumothorax**) in the pleural space require a chest tube to drain these substances and allow the compressed lung to re-expand. A chest tube is a firm plastic tube with drainage holes in the proximal end that is inserted in the pleural space. Once inserted, the tube is secured with a suture and tape, covered with an airtight dressing, and attached to a drainage system that may or may not be attached to suction. Other components of the system may include a closed water-seal drainage system that prevents air from reentering the chest once it has escaped and a suction control chamber that prevents excess suction pressure from being applied to the pleural cavity. The suction chamber may be a water-filled or a dry chamber. A water-filled suction chamber is regulated by the amount of water in the chamber, while dry suction is automatically regulated to changes in the patient's pleural pressure (Lazzara, 2002). At one time, the drainage system was composed of one, two, or three bottles, but now most healthcare agencies use a molded plastic, three-compartment disposable chest drainage unit (Fig. 45-7).

The placement of the chest tube is determined by the type of drainage. When air is to be drained, the tube is placed higher in the chest; if fluid needs to be drained, the tube is inserted lower in the lung because fluids settle at the base of the lung.

Nursing responsibilities include assisting with insertion and removal of a chest tube and, once the tube is in place, monitoring the patient's respiratory status and vital signs,

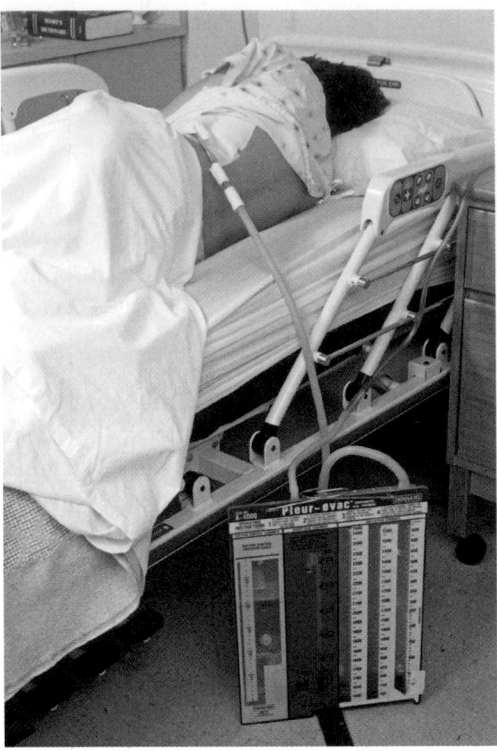

FIGURE 45-7 A chest drainage system attached to a patient. (Photo by Rick Brady.)

checking the dressing, and maintaining the patency and integrity of the drainage system. Guidelines for monitoring a patient with a chest tube are shown in Guidelines for Nursing Care 45-1.

Promoting and Controlling Coughing

A cough is a cleansing mechanism of the body. It is a means of helping to keep the airway clear of secretions and other debris. A cough that is dry is termed a nonproductive cough; one that produces respiratory secretions is termed a productive cough.

When the patient has excessive fluids or secretions in an organ or body tissue, the patient is said to be congested. Thus, a person with secretions or fluid in the lungs is said to have congested lungs. If the cough is dry, the patient is said to be congested with a nonproductive cough. If the cough produces respiratory secretions, the patient is said to be congested with a productive cough. Thick respiratory secretions are sometimes called phlegm. A patient who is coughing and does not have any congestion or secretions produced is said to be noncongested with a nonproductive cough.

A series of events produce a cough. The cough mechanism (Fig. 45-8) consists of an initial irritation; a deep inspiration; a quick, tight closure of the glottis together with a forceful contraction of the expiratory intercostal muscles; and an upward push of the diaphragm. This causes an explosive move-

---

Guidelines for Nursing Care 45-1
Monitoring a Patient With a Chest Tube

- Assess the patient's respiratory status, vital signs, and breath sounds. Monitor for any indication of change in respiratory status.
- Observe the dressing around the chest tube insertion site and ensure that it is occlusive. All connections should also be securely taped.
- Check that the drainage tube has no dependent loops or kinks. The drainage collection device must be positioned below the tube insertion site to facilitate drainage.
- Keep drainage collection device secure so that it does not tip over.
- Check that two padded Kelly clamps are available and secured at the bedside. If the drainage unit requires changing, one clamp is positioned 1½ to 2½ inches from the insertion site, and the second clamp is placed 1 inch down from the first one until the unit has been switched. The physician may order a chest tube clamped before its removal to observe the patient's tolerance when it is discontinued or the chest tube may be clamped to assess for an air leak.
- Keep bottle of sterile saline or water at bedside. If chest tube disconnects from drainage unit, submerge end in water. This is done instead of clamping to prevent another pneumothorax. Air is still allowed to escape.

- *Never* clamp the tube if the patient leaves the unit for a test or moves away from the bed. Disconnect the suction tubing from the drainage system, allowing the unit to continue to collect drainage by gravity. Take bottle of sterile normal saline or water with patient.
- Avoid milking or stripping the tube to promote drainage. This creates excessive negative pressure that can damage delicate lung tissue.
- Assess the suction control chamber if suction is in use. If water suction is used, ensure that water is at the appropriate level (fluid can evaporate); water must be added to ensure that suction is adequate. Gentle bubbling in the suction chamber indicates that suction is being applied to assist drainage.
- Assist the patient to remain in high Fowler's position (if hemothorax is present) or semi-Fowler's position (for pneumothorax) for improved drainage or evacuation.
- Measure drainage output at the end of each shift by marking the level on the container or placing a small piece of tape at the drainage level to indicate date and time. Drainage is never emptied from the collection chamber. Document color and consistency of drainage. Drainage exceeding 100 mL/hr or a change in drainage to a bright red color that indicates fresh bleeding requires immediate notification of the physician.

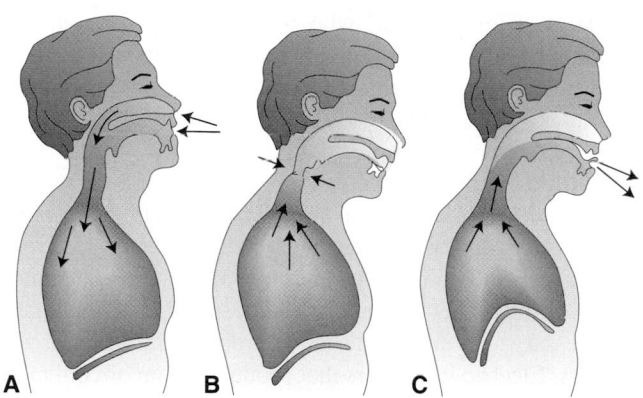

FIGURE 45-8 (**A**) A cough begins with a deep inspiration, distending the trachea and hyperinflating the lungs. (**B**) After inspiration, the glottis closes while intercostal and abdominal muscles contract forcibly. (**C**) When intrathoracic pressure reaches a high level, the glottis opens slightly, and the diaphragm is pushed up, producing an explosive movement of air.

ment of air from the lower to the upper respiratory tract. To be effective, a cough should have enough muscle contraction to force air to be expelled and to propel a liquid or a solid on its way out of the respiratory tract. Coughing is most effective when the patient is sitting upright with feet flat on the floor. Coughing can be voluntary or involuntary.

Promoting Voluntary Coughing

When a cough does not occur as a result of reflex stimulation of the cough-sensitive areas, it can be induced voluntarily. Teaching the patient to cough voluntarily is an important aspect of preoperative and postoperative care. Although teaching a patient to cough and deep breathe is relatively easy, experience has shown that it is difficult to motivate patients to follow through and perform coughing on their own. Frequently remind patients throughout the day. Develop a specific schedule for coughing on the patient's plan of care. Coughing early in the morning after rising removes secretions that have accumulated during the night. Coughing before meals improves the taste of food and oxygenation. At bedtime, coughing removes any buildup of secretions and improves sleep patterns. For a patient who is unable to cough voluntarily, manual stimulation over the trachea and prolonged exhalation can be helpful. If neither of these methods is successful, mechanical endotracheal suctioning with a catheter may be necessary.

If the patient has a neuromuscular disorder and is unable to cough physically, an assisted cough may be used. For an assisted cough, firm pressure is placed on the abdomen below the diaphragm in rhythm with exhalation. This pressure is similar to the Heimlich maneuver but with less force. This pressure is used to substitute for the weakened or paralyzed abdominal muscles.

Promoting Involuntary Coughing

Involuntary coughing often accompanies respiratory tract infections and irritations. Many times respiratory infections lead to the production of respiratory secretions. These secretions can trigger the cough mechanism. When the cough is productive, it helps clear the airway. However, when the cough is nonproductive, it can be fatiguing and irritating. Medications may control involuntary coughing. Observation of the patient's breathing and coughing characteristics is necessary to determine the appropriate type of medication.

Using Cough Medications

Various medications can be used to promote coughing, thereby aiding in the movement of mucus through the respiratory tract, and to control coughing to allow the patient to rest.

Cough Suppressants

Suppressants are drugs that depress a body function—in this case, the cough reflex. Codeine, which is present in many cough preparations, is generally considered the preferred cough suppressant ingredient. However, codeine can be addictive, and because of possible abuse, many states require a prescription for its use. Drowsiness (also common with antihistamines) is a side effect, so it may not be safe to use codeine when the person must remain alert, such as when driving a car.

A suppressant that is not addictive is dextromethorphan, which can be found in many over-the-counter cold and cough remedies.

An irritating nonproductive cough in people without congestion may be appropriately treated with suppressants. Suppression of the productive cough is usually not recommended unless the patient is trying to sleep. If a productive cough is suppressed, secretions can be retained, leading to a pulmonary infection.

Expectorants

Expectorants are drugs that facilitate the removal of respiratory tract secretions by reducing the viscosity of the secretions. Patients with extremely tenacious (thick) secretions may need the secretions liquefied for their cough to be effective. In that way, the nonproductive cough of a person with lung congestion can become productive. Use of an expectorant by a person without congestion is inappropriate. Guaifenesin is widely used as an expectorant in cold and cough preparations (eg, Robitussin). Adequate fluid intake and air humidification are considered effective expectorants by some authorities.

Lozenges

Mild, nonproductive coughs in people without congestion can often be relieved by cough lozenges. A lozenge is a small, solid medication intended to be held in the mouth until it dissolves. Lozenges generally control coughs by the local anesthetic effect of benzocaine. The local anesthetic acts on sensory and motor nerves, controlling the primary irritation and inhibiting afferent and efferent impulses.

Teaching About Cough Medications

Cough medications are readily available, and people who purchase them are usually eager for relief. Often, consumers take excessive amounts of more than one type. Teach about the appropriate choice of expectorants and suppressants and about misuse of cough mixtures. For example, cough syrups with a high sugar or alcohol content can disturb the metabolic balance of patients with diabetes mellitus or can trigger a relapse for recovering alcoholics. Preparations containing antihistamines have an anticholinergic action, which can cause serious problems for people with glaucoma or can cause urinary retention in men with prostate enlargement. Other cough preparations can be detrimental to people with hypertension or thyroid or cardiac diseases. In addition, prolonged use of self-prescribed cough preparations can conceal more serious health problems. If a cough lasts more than 7 days, urge the person to contact a physician. In addition, encourage the person to increase fluid intake if the secretions become too thick to expectorate.

Promoting Comfort

Positioning

Proper positioning—a position that allows free movement of the diaphragm and expansion of the chest wall—is important to ease respirations. For example, sitting in a slumped position permits the abdominal contents to push upward on the diaphragm, decreasing lung expansion during inspiration. People with dyspnea and orthopnea are most comfortable in a high Fowler's position because accessory muscles can then be used easily to promote respiration. Recent research has demonstrated that in patients with pulmonary disease who are acutely ill, turning to the prone position on a regular basis promotes oxygenation (Gattinoni, 2001). In this position, the posterior dependent sections of the lungs are better ventilated and perfused. A partially prone position appears to be sufficient to achieve better ventilation while at the same time allowing access to invasive lines and the airway.

Maintaining Adequate Fluid Intake

Patients can help keep their secretions thin by drinking 2 to 3 quarts (1.9 to 2.9 L) of clear fluids daily. Fluid intake should be increased to the maximum that the patient's health state can tolerate. Increased fluids are needed by patients who have an elevated temperature, who are breathing through the mouth, who are coughing, or who are losing excessive body fluids in other ways. In patients with right-sided heart failure, fluid intake should not exceed 1.5 quarts (1.4 L) daily.

Providing Humidified Air

Inspiring dry air removes the normal moisture in the respiratory passages that protects against irritation and infection. This is especially troublesome for patients who cannot breathe through their nose. When air humidity is low, it may be necessary to humidify the air with room humidifiers or vaporizers. Electric vaporizers that produce steam or cool mist are also useful, but neither device has been demonstrated to have greater therapeutic value than the other. Although a cool-mist vaporizer reduces the danger of burns because it does not generate heat or hot water, it can be a medium for pathogen growth if it is not adequately cleaned. A steam vaporizer does not present this risk for infection because the heat kills most pathogens.

Performing Chest Physiotherapy

Chest physiotherapy helps loosen and mobilize secretions. This is especially helpful for patients with large amounts of secretions or an ineffective cough. Chest physiotherapy includes percussion, vibrating, and providing postural drainage.

Percussing

Percussing lung areas involves the use of a cupped palm to loosen pulmonary secretions so that they can be expectorated with greater ease. With the hand held in a rigid, dome-shaped position (Fig. 45-9), the area over the lung lobes to be drained is struck in a rhythmic pattern. Usually the patient is positioned supine or prone and should not experience any pain. Cupping is never done on bare skin or performed over surgical incisions, below the ribs, or over the spine or breasts because of the danger of tissue damage. Typically, each area is percussed for 30 to 60 seconds several times a day. If the patient has tenacious secretions, the area may be percussed for up to 3 to 5 minutes several times per day. Patients may learn

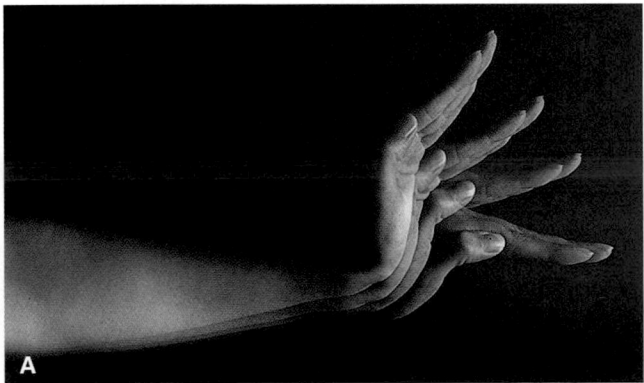
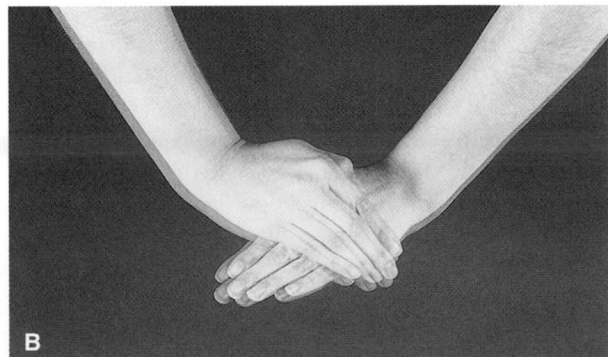

FIGURE 45-9 (A) The cupping position and action of the hand on manual percussion of the lung area. **(B)** The position and action of the hands necessary to use vibration to loosen respiratory secretions in the lungs. (Photos © B. Proud.)

how to percuss the anterior surfaces of their own chest wall. In addition, family members can be taught how to percuss posterior surfaces. Mechanical devices as well as manual handheld cupping devices also are available for percussion on the chest wall.

Vibrating

In vibration, the nurse uses rhythmic contraction and relaxation of his or her arm and shoulder muscles while holding the hands flat on the patient's chest wall as the patient exhales. The purpose is to help loosen respiratory secretions so that they can be expectorated with ease. Vibration (at a rate of about 200 per minute) can be done for several minutes several times a day. To avoid causing patient discomfort, vibration is never done over the patient's breasts, spine, sternum, and lower rib cage. Vibration (see Fig. 45-9) can also be taught to family members or accomplished using a mechanical device.

Providing Postural Drainage

In postural drainage, gravity is used to drain secretions from the lungs. The patient is positioned in a way that promotes the drainage of secretions from smaller pulmonary branches into larger ones, where they can be removed by coughing (Fig. 45-10).

Postural drainage is often preceded by vibration, percussion, or both. Postural drainage is carried out as follows:
- Have tissues and an emesis basin close at hand for the patient to use when coughing and expectorating secretions.
- Place the patient in an appropriate position to promote drainage from the lobes of the lungs, as follows:

Use high Fowler's position to drain the apical sections of the upper lobes of the lungs.

Place the patient in a lying position, half on the abdomen and half on the side, right and left, to drain the posterior sections of the upper lobes of the lungs.

Place the patient lying on the left side with a pillow under the chest wall to drain the right lobe of the lung.

Place the patient in Trendelenburg's position to drain the lower lobes of the lungs.
- Carry out postural drainage two to four times a day for 20 to 30 minutes. Discontinue the drainage if the patient begins to feel weak or faint.

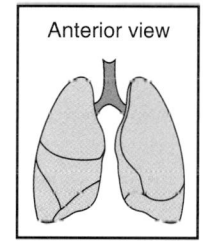
Anterior view

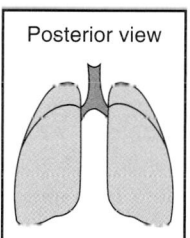
Posterior view

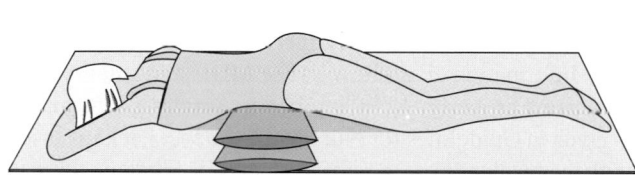
Posterior lower lobes

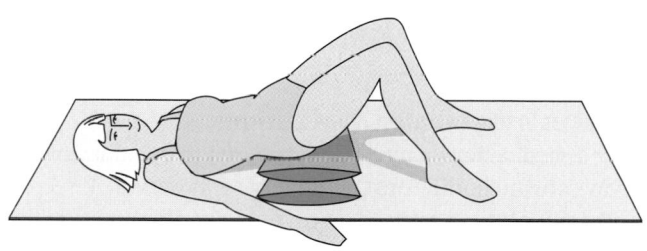
Anterior lower lobes

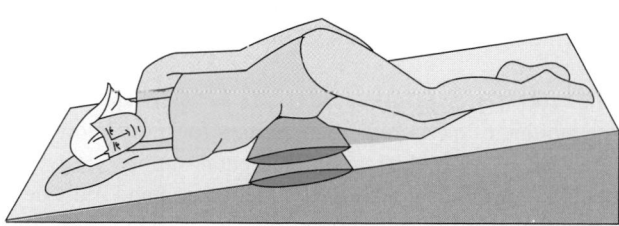
Left lower lobe

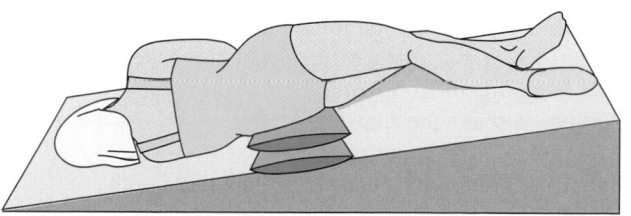
Right lower lobe

FIGURE 45-10 Postural drainage. Shown are four positions that use the force of gravity to assist the drainage of secretions from the smaller bronchial airways into the main bronchi and trachea so the patient is able to cough them up.

- Delay postural drainage for 1 to 2 hours after meals to avoid provoking vomiting.

Maintaining Good Nutrition

People who are working hard at breathing often do not have energy for eating. Therefore, maintaining an adequate nutritional intake is crucial. Assess nutritional status by measuring the patient's height, weight, upper arm circumference, serum protein levels, and nitrogen balance. Direct interventions to ensure an adequate intake of proteins, vitamins, and minerals. Consider the use of six small meals distributed over the course of the day instead of the usual three larger meals. Provide frequent oral hygiene and rest periods before eating to help improve the patient's intake. Meals should be eaten 1 to 2 hours after breathing treatments and exercises.

In patients who have COPD or are ventilator dependent, providing nutrients in the proper balance to reduce the production of carbon dioxide (from metabolism) is essential. Fat metabolism produces the least amount of carbon dioxide, carbohydrate metabolism the most. Thus, nonprotein calories in the diet should be equally divided between fat and carbohydrates for these patients. Some healthcare facilities call this type of diet a COPD or respiratory diet (Grodner et al., 2000).

Meeting Respiratory Needs With Medications

Although treating patients with medications is a dependent nursing intervention, monitoring the patient's response and development of side effects to medications is an independent nursing action. Table 45-3 shows some common medications for respiratory functioning, their side effects, and nursing implications. Many of the drugs used to dilate bronchial airways interact with caffeine, so remind patients and caregivers about the need to avoid caffeine, which may potentiate the side effects of bronchodilators.

Administering Inhaled Medications

Inhaled medications may be administered to open narrowed airways (**bronchodilators**), to liquefy or loosen thick secretions (mucolytic agents), or to reduce inflammation in airways (corticosteroids). These medications typically are administered via nebulizer or metered-dose inhaler. **Nebulizers** disperse fine particles of medication into the deeper passages of the respiratory tract, where absorption occurs. The treatment continues until all the medication in the nebulizer cup has been inhaled. A **metered-dose inhaler (MDI)** delivers a controlled dose of medication with each compression of the canister. Common mistakes that patients make when using MDIs including the following:

- Failing to shake the canister
- Holding the inhaler upside down
- Inhaling through the nose rather than the mouth
- Inhaling too rapidly
- Stopping the inhalation when the cold propellant is felt in the throat
- Failing to hold their breath after inhalation
- Inhaling two sprays with one breath

To use an MDI, the patient must activate the device while continuing to inhale. For some patients, especially young children and older adults, a spacer or extender device may be necessary to aid delivery of medication by the inhalation route. The spacer acts as a reservoir. When the MDI is compressed, the medication is deposited in the reservoir, and the patient then inhales the medication from the spacer device. This makes administration less complicated and the dose more predictable.

> *Remember Tyrone, the 2-year-old boy with suspected asthma. During this acute attack, the nurse would anticipate administering bronchodilators via a nebulizer. Depending on the child's abilities, the physician may order bronchodilators to be administered at home using a nebulizer or possibly an MDI with a spacer.*

Dry powder inhalers (DPI) are another type of delivery method for inhaled medications. DPIs require less manual dexterity than a MDI. DPIs are actuated by the patient's inspiration, so there is no need to coordinate the delivery of puffs with inhalation (Togger & Brenner, 2001). One disadvantage of DPIs is that the medication in DPIs will clump if exposed to humidity.

A microchip-based inhaler has been developed that determines when the patient is breathing at an ideal rate to deliver a metered dose of asthma medication. This device (eg, SmartMist) delivers a standard dose with a high degree of precision. Several companies are working on similar pulmonary drug-delivery systems.

Teaching Patients About Inhaled Medications

Patients need repeated instruction on how to use inhalers and nebulizers effectively and safely. Overuse may result in serious side effects and eventual ineffectiveness of the medication. Information about how to use MDIs and small-volume nebulizers properly, including patient teaching information, is given in Guidelines for Nursing Care 45-2. Package inserts with the medication also reinforce correct technique for using inhalers.

To ensure correct administration when a spacer is used, slow, deep inspirations are necessary. To prevent inhaling too quickly, some spacers are equipped with a whistle device that sounds if inhalation is too rapid. A spacer is also recommended for patients using corticosteroid inhaled agents because it reduces the risk for an oral fungal infection.

Providing Supplemental Oxygen

The amount of oxygen the patient uses for inspiration can be increased by providing a supplemental supply via oxygen therapy. Oxygen is considered a medication and must be ordered by a healthcare provider. Oxygen therapy can frighten patients, so provide clear explanations about the procedures and purpose to help reduce this fear. Encourage patients to discuss their anxieties. If oxygen is given in an emergency, explanations concurrent with administration are appropriate.

TABLE 45-3 Selected Medications Used to Improve Respiratory Functioning

Medications	Activity	Route	Side Effects	Nursing Implications
Zafirlukast (Accolate) Montelukast (Singulair)	Bronchodilator Also inhibits leukotriene release as well as inflammatory reaction	PO	Headache, dizziness, nausea, vomiting	Not used to treat acute attacks. Do not give Accolate with meals. Singulair should be given before bedtime.
Albuterol	Bronchodilator	PO, inhalation	Tremors, anxiety, insomnia, headache, palpitations, hypertension, vomiting	Caution patient not to increase dosage without consulting physician. Be aware that children 2–6 years of age more frequently exhibit CNS stimulation.
Theophylline (Aminophylline)	Bronchodilator	PO, IV, rectally	Nausea, vomiting, tachycardia, diuresis, irritability, vertigo, convulsions, nervousness	Monitor vital signs closely. Force fluids as clinical status allows. Monitor serum theophylline levels, especially if patient does not respond to drug or if severe side effects develop.
Corticosteroids (prednisone, dexamethasone, budesonide, triamcinolone acetonide)	Reduces inflammation	PO, IV, inhalation, intranasal	Fluid retention, hypertension, mood swings, weight gain, gastritis hyperglycemia, insomnia	Reduce sodium intake. Make patient and family aware of potential for labile emotions. Weigh daily in morning. Monitor blood pressure and blood sugar.
Diphenhydramine (Benadryl)	Antihistamine H₁-receptor antagonist	PO	Drowsiness, anorexia, dry mouth, constipation, blurred vision, urinary retention	Warn patient to use only with physician's advice in presence of bronchial asthma.
Cetirizine (Zyrtec)		PO	Headache with limited sedative effect, not associated anticholinergic effects	Monitor effectiveness of drug. Contraindicated while breastfeeding.
Fexofenadine (Allegra)			Headache, not associated with anticholinergic or sedative effects	
Cromolyn sodium (Intal)	Mast cell stabilizer Asthma prophylactic agent—no bronchodilator, antihistamine, or vasoconstrictor properties	Inhalation—MDI or nasal solution	Cough, nausea, nasal stinging and burning, throat irritation	Remind patient this is used to prevent asthma attacks, not to treat acute episodes. Inform patient that drug is effective only if taken routinely (2–4 times per week). Safety not established during pregnancy and breastfeeding.

CNS, central nervous system; PO, orally; IV, intravenously.

Guidelines for Nursing Care 45-2
Using an Inhaled Medication Device

- Assess the patient's ability to manage a metered-dose inhaler or small-volume nebulizer.
- Explain, demonstrate, and encourage the patient to manipulate the inhaler or nebulizer apparatus.
- Encourage the patient to wash hands thoroughly before using device.

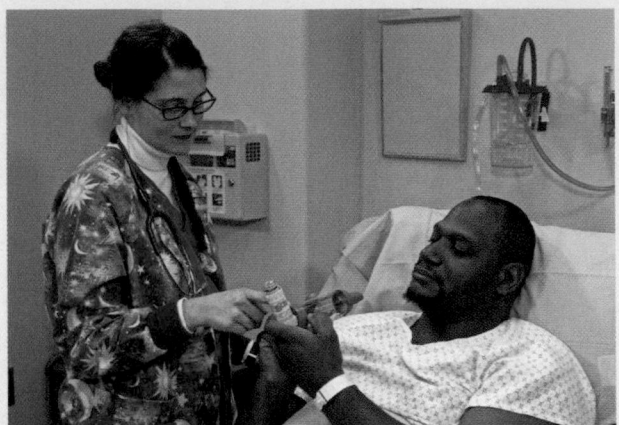

Teaching a patient about the inhaler.   (Photo by Rick Brady.)

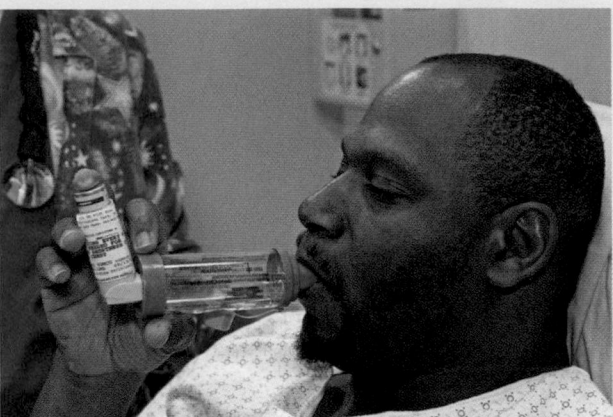

Patient using a metered-dose inhaler with an extender.   (Photo by Rick Brady.)

The Metered-Dose Inhaler

- Remove the mouthpiece cover and shake inhaler well.
- Follow caregiver's or manufacturer's recommendations for placement of the mouthpiece. Two methods are possible:
  - Hold the inhaler 1–2 inches in front of open mouth; or
  - Place mouthpiece into mouth grasping securely with teeth and lips (an MDI coupled with a spacer or extender is always placed in the mouth).
- Take a deep breath and exhale.
- Inhale slowly and deeply through the mouth. Press down on the medication canister while continuing to inhale a full breath (when using a spacer or extender, depress the canister about one fourth or one third through the inspiration).
- Hold your breath for 5 to 10 seconds or as long as possible.
- Exhale slowly through pursed lips.
- If another puff is prescribed, wait 1 to 5 minutes before the next inhalation.
- If desired, gargle with tap water and blow nose into a tissue to remove any remaining trace of medication. If MDI is a steroid this must be done to prevent oral fungal infection.
- Use mild soap and water to clean the mouthpiece, rinse it, and let it dry before replacing it.
- Follow physician's order regarding frequency of inhaler use.

The Small-Volume Nebulizer

- Remove the nebulizer cup from the device, open it, and place it on a flat working surface.
- Place premeasured unit dose medication in the bottom section of the cup or use a dropper to place concentrated dose of medication in cup and add prescribed fluid to dilute it.
- Screw the top portion of nebulizer cup back in place and attach the cup to the nebulizer.
- Attach one end of tubing to the stem on the bottom of the nebulizer cuff and the other end to the air compressor or oxygen source (if valve to control airflow is not available, a Y tube can be added to the tubing so that one branch of the Y tube connects to the nebulizer cup and the other branch is left open).
- Turn on the air compressor or oxygen.

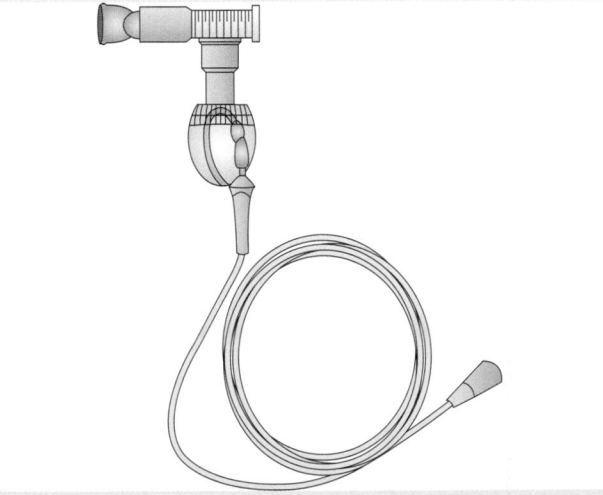

Small-volume nebulizer.

(continued)

Guidelines for Nursing Care 45-2 (Continued)

- Check that a fine medication mist is produced by opening valve or placing thumb over open branch of Y tube.
- Place mouthpiece into mouth and grasp securely with teeth and lips.
- Inhale slowly through the mouth (a nose clip may be necessary if patient is also breathing through the nose).
- Hold each breath for 5 to 10 seconds or as long as possible before exhaling.

- Continue this inhalation technique until all medication in the nebulizer cup has been aerosolized (usually about 15 minutes).
- If desired, gargle with tap water after using nebulizer.
- Rinse the equipment in warm water and allow to air dry on a clean towel.

Special Considerations

- Teach patients how to tell when their inhaler is empty. They can either count the number of times they have used the inhaler (usually about 200 sprays per container) or separate the canister from the plastic holder and place it in a bowl of water. When full, it sinks; when empty, it floats.

Home Considerations

- Once a week, MDI mouthpiece, spacer or extender, or nebulizer parts should be soaked in a vinegar solution (1 pint of water to 2 oz of vinegar) for 20 minutes. Rinse with clean water and allow to air dry.

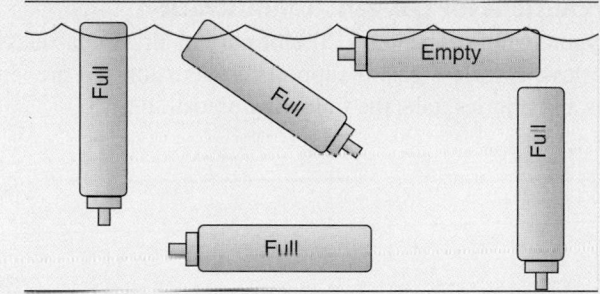

Sources of Oxygen

Therapeutic oxygen is supplied from a wall outlet or a portable cylinder. With a wall outlet source, oxygen is supplied from a central source in the agency through a pipeline, usually at 50 to 60 pounds per square inch (psi) of pressure. A specially designed flowmeter is attached to the outlet (see Skill 45-2 later in the chapter for an illustration of a flowmeter). A valve regulates the oxygen flow. The wall outlet source can be prepared for use quickly.

Oxygen also can be dispersed under pressure from portable steel cylinders or tanks. The tank is delivered with a protective cap to prevent accidental damage of the cylinder outlet. When a standard, large-sized cylinder is full, its contents are under more than 2,000 psi of pressure. The force through an outlet that has been partially opened by accident could cause the tank to take off like an uncontrolled missile. Smaller cylinders are available for emergency and ambulatory settings. The principles and precautions are the same for all size cylinders.

To release oxygen safely and at the desired rate from a cylinder or tank, a regulator is used. The regulator has two gauges. The one nearest the tank shows the pressure or amount of oxygen in the tank. The other gauge indicates the number of liters per minute of oxygen being released.

The oxygen cylinder and the regulator must be handled cautiously. The oxygen cylinder must be transported carefully, preferably strapped onto a wheeled carrier to prevent the cylinder from falling and the outlet from breaking. The cylinder also must be stabilized securely in a properly fitting stand.

Before attaching oxygen tubing to the tank, prime the tank. Turn the cylinder key counterclockwise to allow any dust or other particles that may be present to be cleaned out of the cylinder pressure gauge. Turn the cylinder key clockwise to turn the oxygen off before attaching oxygen tubing. Once oxygen tubing has been connected, turn the cylinder key counterclockwise until you meet resistance. Then turn the key back one-half turn. You may now control the flow of oxygen by turning the flow dial on the cylinder pressure gauge clockwise.

The force with which the oxygen is released from this opening causes a loud, hissing sound that can be startling. Therefore, prime the tank away from the bedside if possible, or prepare patients and visitors for the noise with an appropriate explanation.

Oxygen Flow Rate

The flow rate of oxygen, measured in liters per minute, determines the amount of oxygen delivered to the patient. The rate varies depending on the condition of the patient and the route of administration of the oxygen. The flow rate does not necessarily reflect the oxygen concentration actually inspired by the patient because there is leaking and mixing with atmospheric air. If more precise doses are necessary, they are usually prescribed in terms of percentage of inspired oxygen. To regulate the oxygen percentage concentration accurately, samples of the air mixture the patient is actually inhaling should be analyzed every 4 hours. Several types of commercial oxygen analyzers are available.

The physician's written order prescribes the rate of oxygen administration. Closely monitor the flow rate for patients with chronic lung conditions, such as emphysema. Normally, excessive levels of carbon dioxide in the blood stimulate the patient to breathe. However, the chemoreceptors of patients with chronic lung disease become insensitive to carbon dioxide and respond to hypoxia to stimulate breathing. If excessive oxygen is given, the stimulus to breathe is removed; as a result, the patient may stop breathing completely. Most patients with chronic lung disease can tolerate oxygen administered at 2 L/min (usually by nasal cannula; see discussion below). However, arterial blood gas results should be monitored closely for changes. Many times, continuous pulse oximetry also is used to monitor the patient receiving oxygen.

Humidification

Most institutions do not require humidification with very-low-flow oxygen (2 L/min or less) delivered by nasal cannula when administered to adults. However, because oxygen dries and dehydrates the respiratory mucous membranes, humidifying devices (supplying 20% to 40% humidity) are commonly used when oxygen is delivered at higher flow rates. Distilled or sterile water is commonly used to humidify oxygen. When moving patients receiving humidified oxygen, make sure that water from the humidifier does not enter the tubing through which the oxygen is flowing. Additional suggestions for transporting a patient with a portable oxygen tank are given in Guidelines for Nursing Care 45-3.

Precautions for Oxygen Administration

Oxygen, which constitutes 20% of normal air, is a tasteless, odorless, colorless gas. It supports combustion. To prevent fires and injuries, take the following precautions:

Guidelines for Nursing Care 45-3
Transporting a Patient With a Portable Oxygen Cylinder

Before the Transfer:
- Check that additional oxygen source is available where patient is being transferred.
- Check amount of oxygen in cylinder (place cylinder key or wrench on valve stem and turn fully counterclockwise until needle on gauge indicates amount of available oxygen; turn the key back a half turn; use cylinder only if gauge indicates more than 500 psi).
- Connect oxygen tubing or humidifier bottle with tubing to the flowmeter adapter and adjust the flow-control dial to the prescribed setting.
- Attach patient's oxygen cannula to transport oxygen.
- Ensure that the cylinder is secured in holder before transporting patient (it is a dangerous practice to place the cylinder between the patient's legs or next to the patient during transfer because injury to the patient may result). If humidifier is used, ensure that cylinder remains upright.
- Place coiled tubing under pillow or attach to linen or patient's gown.

After the Transfer:
- Attach patient's oxygen cannula to wall oxygen.
- Turn off the oxygen flow from the cylinder by turning the cylinder key clockwise until it is tight.
- Remove any excess oxygen in the pressure gauge by "bleeding" it. Turn the flow-control dial back on until hissing sound stops and needle on gauge has fallen to zero. Turn flow-control dial off.

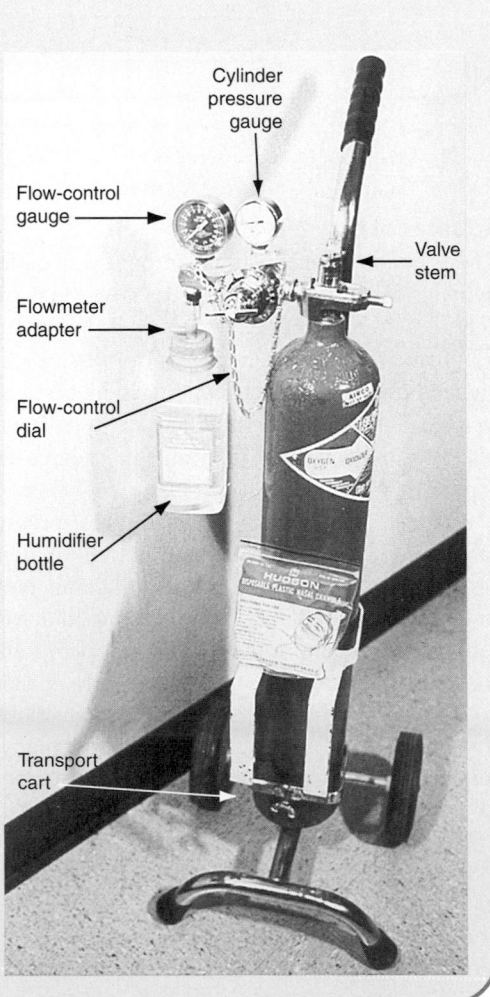

Labels: Cylinder pressure gauge, Flow-control gauge, Valve stem, Flowmeter adapter, Flow-control dial, Humidifier bottle, Transport cart

- Avoid open flames in the patient's room.
- Place "No Smoking" signs in conspicuous places in the patient's room or home. Instruct the patient and visitors about the hazard of smoking when oxygen is in use.
- Check to see that electrical equipment used in the room, such as electric bell cords, razors, radios, and suctioning equipment, is in good working order and emits no sparks.
- Avoid wearing and using synthetic fabrics that build up static electricity.
- Avoid using oils in the area. Oil can ignite spontaneously in the presence of oxygen.

Oxygen Administration

Oxygen can be administered by nasal cannula, nasal catheter, transtracheal catheter, simple mask, partial rebreather mask, nonrebreather mask, Venturi mask, and tent. Table 45-4 compares the oxygen delivery systems.

Nasal Cannula

A **nasal cannula,** also called nasal prongs, is probably the most commonly used oxygen delivery device. The cannula is a disposable plastic device with two protruding prongs that are inserted into the nostrils; the cannula is connected to an oxygen source with a humidifier and flowmeter. The cannula does not impede eating or speaking and is easily used in the home. Disadvantages of this system are that it can easily be dislodged and can cause dryness of the nasal mucosa. Skill 45-2 describes oxygen administration by nasal cannula.

Nasal Catheter

A nasal, or oropharyngeal, catheter is another efficient means for administering oxygen, but it is infrequently used because it is uncomfortable for the patient and may cause trauma to respiratory mucous membranes. It is inserted into the nose through one nostril, with the end of the catheter resting in the oropharynx. The catheter must be changed to the other nostril every 8 hours. Gastric distention often occurs because the gas flow can be misdirected into the stomach.

Face Masks

Disposable and reusable face masks are available. The mask is fitted carefully to the patient's face to avoid leakage of oxygen and should be comfortably snug but not tight against the face. The most commonly used types of masks are the simple face mask, the partial rebreather mask, the nonrebreather mask, and the Venturi mask. Skill 45-3 describes the actions and rationales involved in using face masks.

The simple face mask is connected to oxygen tubing, a humidifier, and a flowmeter, just like the nasal cannula. This mask has vents on its sides that allow room air to leak in at many places, thereby diluting the source oxygen. The vents also allow exhaled carbon dioxide to escape (see Table 45-4). Often a simple mask is used when an increased delivery of oxygen is needed for short periods (eg, less than 12 hours). The mask should fit closely to the face to deliver this higher concentration of oxygen effectively. Patients may have difficulty keeping the mask in position over the nose and mouth, and because of this pressure and the presence of moisture, skin breakdown is a possibility. Eating or talking with the mask in place

TABLE 45-4 Oxygen Delivery Systems

Method	Amount Delivered FiO$_2$ (Fraction Inspired Oxygen)	Priority Nursing Interventions
Nasal cannula	Low Flow 1 L/min = 24% 2 L/min = 28% 3 L/min = 32% 4 L/min = 36% 5 L/min = 40% 6 L/min = 44%	Check frequently that both prongs are in patient's nares. Never deliver more than 2–3 L/min to patient with chronic lung disease.
Simple mask	Low Flow 6–10 L/min = 35%–60% (5 L/min is minimum setting)	Monitor patient frequently to check placement of the mask. Support patient if claustrophobia is a concern. Secure physician's order to replace mask with nasal cannula during meal time.
Partial rebreather mask	Low Flow 6–15 L/min = 70%–90%	Set flow rate so that mask remains two-thirds full during inspiration. Keep reservoir bag free of twists or kinks.
Nonrebreather mask	Low Flow 6–15 L/min = 60%–100%	Maintain flow rate so reservoir bag collapses only slightly during inspiration. Check that valves and rubber flaps are functioning properly (open during expiration and closed during inhalation). Monitor SaO$_2$ with pulse oximeter.
Venturi mask	High Flow 4–10 L/min = 24%–55%	Requires careful monitoring to verify FiO$_2$ at flow rate ordered. Check that air intake valves are not blocked.

SKILL 45-2   Administering Oxygen by Nasal Cannula

EQUIPMENT

Flowmeter connected to oxygen supply

Humidifier with sterile distilled water (optional with low-flow system)

Nasal cannula and tubing
Gauze to pad tubing over ears (optional)

ACTION	RATIONALE
1. Explain procedure to patient and review safety precautions necessary when oxygen is in use. Place No Smoking signs in appropriate areas.	Oxygen supports combustion.
2. Perform hand hygiene.	Hand hygiene deters the spread of microorganisms.
3. Connect the nasal cannula to the oxygen setup with humidification, if one is in use. Adjust the flow rate as ordered by physician (see photo). Check that oxygen is flowing out of prongs.	Oxygen forced through a water reservoir is humidified before it is delivered to the patient, thus preventing dehydration of the mucous membranes. Low-flow oxygen does not require humidification.

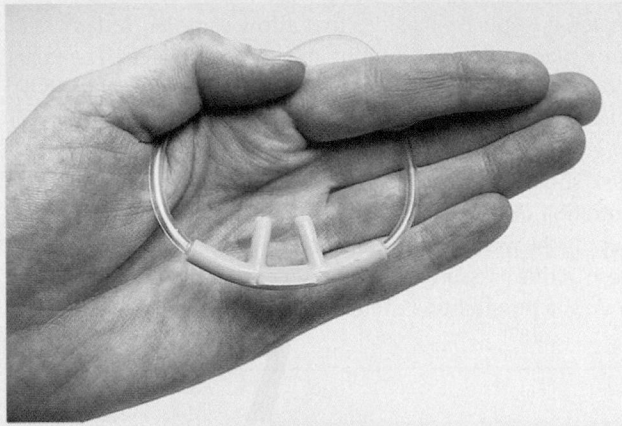

Nasal cannula.

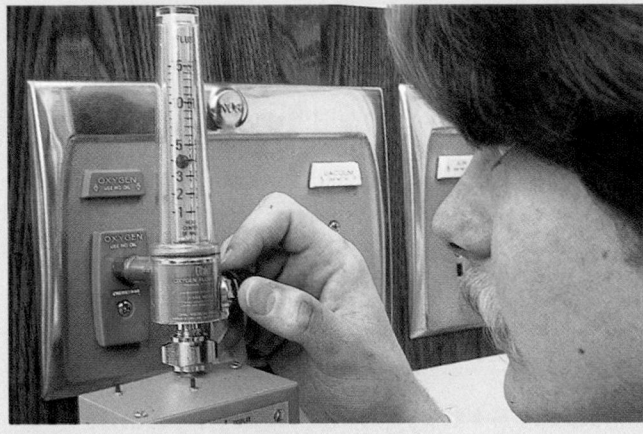

Action 3: Adjusting flow rate.

4. Place the prongs in the patient's nostrils (see photo). Adjust according to type of equipment.
   a. Over and behind each ear with adjuster comfortably under chin; or
   b. Around the patient's head
	Correct placement of the prongs and fastener facilitates oxygen administration and comfort for the patient.

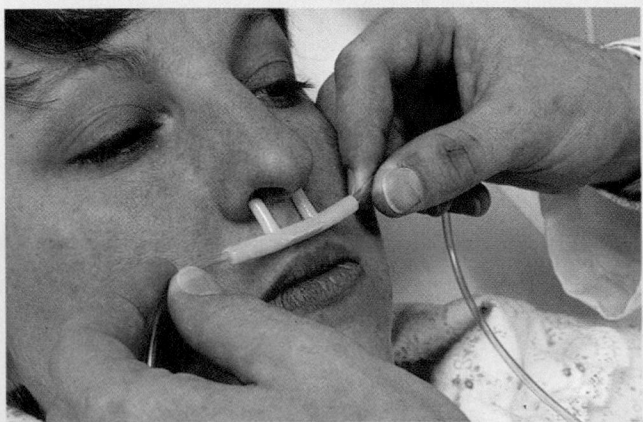

Action 4: Placing cannula prongs in nostrils.

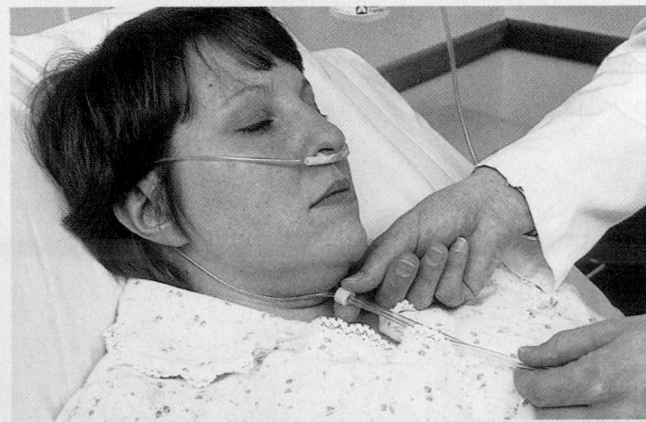

Action 4: Adjusting for comfort.

(continued)

Administering Oxygen by Nasal Cannula (continued)

ACTION	RATIONALE
5. Use gauze pads at ear beneath the tubing as necessary.	Pads reduce irritation and pressure and protect the skin.
6. Encourage patient to breathe through his or her nose with mouth closed.	Nose breathing provides for optimal delivery of oxygen to patient.
7. Perform hand hygiene.	Hand hygiene deters the spread of microorganisms.
8. Assess and chart patient's response to therapy.	Patient's respirations, color, breathing pattern, and chest movements indicate effectiveness of oxygen therapy.
9. Remove and clean the cannula and assess nares at least every 8 hours or according to agency recommendations. Check nares for evidence of irritation or bleeding.	The continued presence of the cannula causes irritation and dryness of the mucous membranes. Water-soluble lubricants can be use to counteracts the drying effects of oxygen.

Home Care Considerations   Patients may require oxygen administration to continue in the home setting. Portable oxygen concentrators are used most frequently. Caregivers require instruction concerning safety precautions with oxygen use and an understanding of the rationale for the specific liter flow of oxygen.

can be difficult. Due to the risk of retaining carbon dioxide, never apply the simple face mask with a delivery flow rate of less than 5 liters per minute.

The partial rebreather mask is similar to a simple face mask but is equipped with a reservoir bag for the collection of the first part of the patient's exhaled air. The remaining exhaled air exits through vents. The air in the reservoir is mixed with 100% oxygen for the next inhalation. Thus, the patient rebreathes about one third of the expired air from the reservoir bag. This type of mask permits the conservation of oxygen. An additional advantage is that the patient can inhale room air through openings in the mask if the oxygen supply is briefly interrupted. The disadvantages are those of any mask: eating and talking are difficult, a tight seal is required, and there is the potential for skin breakdown. Monitor the reservoir bag carefully. It should deflate slightly with inspiration; if it deflates completely, the flow rate should be increased until only a slight deflation is noted.

The nonrebreather mask delivers the highest concentration of oxygen via a mask to a spontaneously breathing patient. It is similar to the partial rebreather mask except two one-way valves prevent the patient from rebreathing exhaled air. The reservoir bag is filled with oxygen that enters the mask on inspiration. Exhaled air escapes through side vents. A malfunction of the bag could cause carbon dioxide buildup and suffocation This mask can also be used to administer other gases such as heliox.

The Venturi mask gets its name from the Venturi effect, which allows the mask to deliver the most precise concentrations of oxygen. This mask has a large tube with an oxygen inlet. As the tube narrows, the pressure drops, causing air to be sucked in through side ports. These ports are adjusted according to the prescription for oxygen concentration. Be sure that the ports are always open. If these are occluded by linens, clothing, or a patient rolling on the mask, the oxygen delivered might be at an unsafe (too high or too low) concentration.

Oxygen Tent

Oxygen also can be administered by way of a tent, a light, portable structure made of clear plastic and attached to a motor-driven unit. The motor helps to circulate and cool the air in the tent. The cooling device functions like an electric refrigeration unit. A thermostat in the unit keeps the tent at the temperature considered most comfortable for the patient. The tent fits over the top part of the bed so that the patient's head and thorax are inside. It has side openings through which nursing care can be administered. Since the tent is highly humidified and covers the majority of the patient's gown and linens, check the patient frequently to prevent the patient from lying in a wet bed. An oxygen tent is commonly used with children who need a cool and highly humidified airflow (eg, children with pneumonia). The tent does not allow the maintenance of a satisfactory or precise oxygen concentration, so it is rarely used except for children.

Oxygen Therapy in the Home

Liquid oxygen and oxygen concentrators rather than cylinders are used more commonly in the home setting. Liquid oxygen is kept inside a small thermal container that can be refilled from a larger storage tank kept in the home. An oxygen concentrator removes nitrogen from the room air and concentrates the oxygen left in the air. The oxygen concentrator needs a power source such as an electrical outlet or battery pack. Oxygen concentrators are portable, cost-effective, and easy to use but cannot deliver oxygen flow at greater than 4 L/min (fraction of inspired oxygen [FiO_2] of about 36%).

Patients using continuous supplemental oxygen therapy in the home have another alternative: transtracheal oxygen delivery (Fig. 45-11). With this type of delivery system, a small catheter is inserted into the trachea under local anesthesia, and then the catheter is attached to the oxygen source. A transtracheal catheter does not interfere with talking, eating, or drinking and delivers oxygen throughout the respiratory cycle

SKILL 45-3 Administering Oxygen by Mask

EQUIPMENT

Flowmeter connected to oxygen supply

Humidifier with sterile distilled water
Face mask specified by physician

Gauze to pad elastic band (optional)

ACTION	RATIONALE
1. Explain procedure to patient and review safety precautions necessary when oxygen is in use. Place No Smoking signs in appropriate areas.	Oxygen supports combustion. Explanation alleviates anxiety.
2. Perform hand hygiene.	Hand hygiene deters the spread of microorganisms.
3. Attach the face mask to the oxygen setup with humidification. Start the flow of oxygen at the specified rate. For a mask with a reservoir, allow O_2 to fill the bag before placing the mask over the patient's nose and mouth.	Oxygen forced through a water reservoir is humidified before it is delivered to the patient, thus preventing dehydration of the mucous membranes. A reservoir bag must be inflated with oxygen because the bag is the source of oxygen supply for the patient.
4. Position the face mask over the patient's nose and mouth. Adjust it with the elastic strap so that the mask fits snugly but comfortably on the face.	A loose or poorly fitting mask will result in oxygen loss and decreased therapeutic value. Masks may cause feeling of suffocation, and patient needs frequent attention and reassurance.
5. Use gauze pads to reduce irritation to the patient's ears and scalp.	Pads reduce irritation and pressure and protect the skin.
6. Perform hand hygiene.	Hand hygiene deters the spread of microorganisms.
7. Remove the mask and dry the skin every 2 to 3 hours if the oxygen is running continuously. Do not powder around the mask.	The tight-fitting mask and moisture from condensation can irritate the skin on the face. There is danger of inhaling powder if it is placed on the mask.
8. Assess and chart patient's response to therapy.	Patient's respiratory rate and pattern, color, and so forth indicate effectiveness of oxygen therapy.

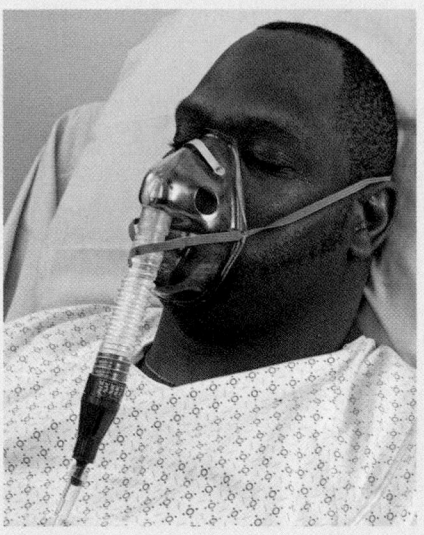

Venturi mask.

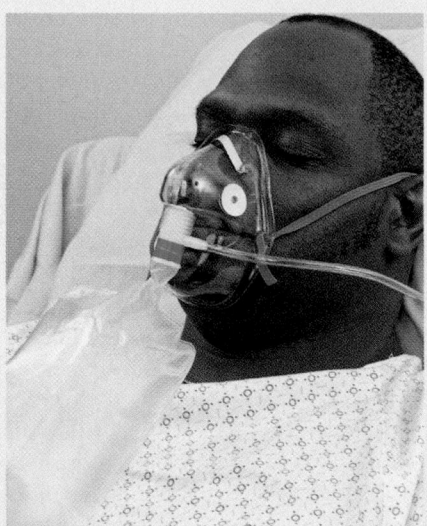

Nonrebreather mask.

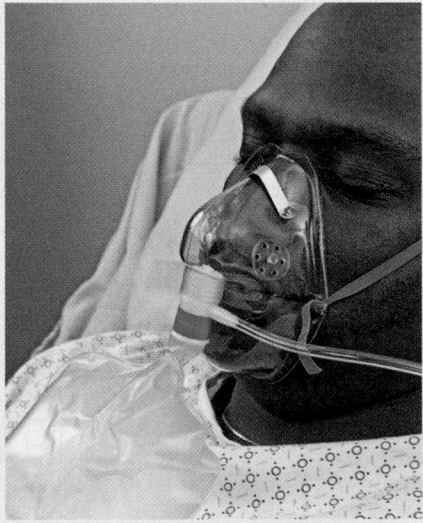

Partial rebreather mask.   (Photos by Rick Brady.)

rather than just at inspiration. The patient or family must assume responsibility for daily catheter care. Patients usually report improved mobility, comfort, and appearance and lower cost with this delivery system.

Patients using oxygen at home need instruction regarding safety precautions. See Teaching to Promote Health at Home 45-1 for information regarding the use of oxygen in the home setting.

Suctioning the Airway

If a patient is unable to remove secretions with coughing, secretions can be aspirated with a suctioning device, as

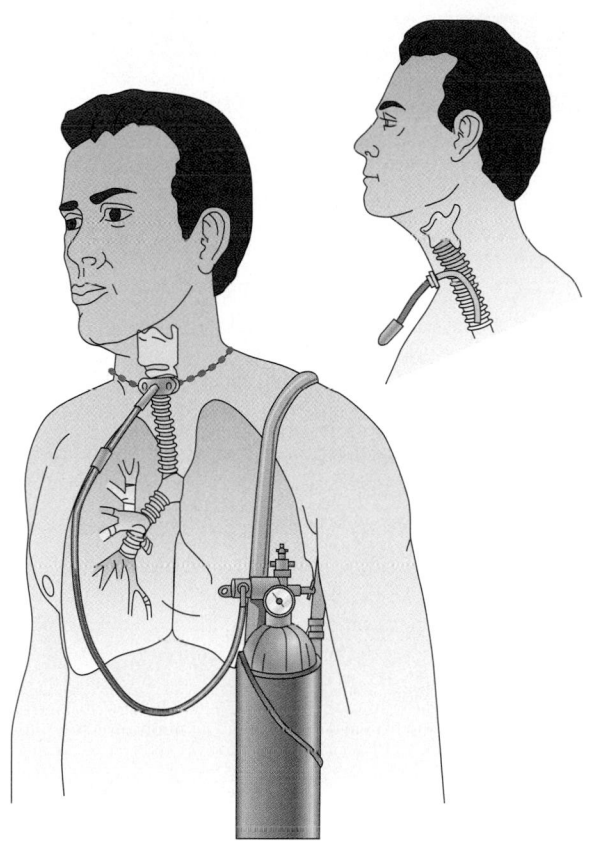

FIGURE 45-11 A transtracheal oxygen setup.

demonstrated in Skill 45-4. Suctioning to remove secretions is performed using the sterile technique as described in Chapter 27. The frequency of suctioning varies with the amount of secretions present but should be done often enough to keep ventilation effective and as effortless as possible. The suctioning catheter should be small enough not to occlude the airway being suctioned but large enough to remove secretions. Several sizes of clear plastic or red rubber catheters are available.

Suctioning irritates the mucosa and removes oxygen from the respiratory tract, possibly causing **hypoxemia** (insufficient oxygen in the blood). Thus, the patient must be hyperoxygenated before suctioning (see Skill 45-4). This is easily accomplished by having the patient take several deep breaths before inserting the catheter.

When performed correctly, suctioning provides comfort by relieving respiratory distress. When performed incorrectly, it can increase anxiety and pain and cause respiratory arrest. It is normally painless; however, anticipate administering analgesic medication to a patient who has had surgery or experienced trauma before suctioning because the cough reflex will be stimulated. Possible complications include infection, cardiac arrhythmias, hypoxia, mucosal trauma, and death.

Wear gloves on both hands, goggles, mask, and gown if necessary for protection from microorganisms. Continuously monitor the patient's color and heart rate and the color,

---

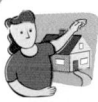

Teaching to Promote Health at Home 45-1
Using Oxygen at Home

Health Topic	Teaching Tip	Why Is This Important?
Safety	• No smoking or open flames are allowed within 10 feet of the oxygen source. Remind visitors of the restriction on smoking. • Do not use electrical equipment near oxygen administration set (eg, space heaters, blow dryers). • Use caution with gas or electric appliances when patient is receiving oxygen therapy. • Ground oxygen concentrators. • Secure the oxygen tank in a holder and away from direct sunlight or heat. • Allow adequate airflow around the oxygen concentrator (avoid placing flush against the wall). • Have patient notify local fire department of the oxygen in the home.	Oxygen is a combustible gas; a spark may ignite the oxygen.
Administration	• Follow the physician's prescription for the oxygen flow rate. • Have the physician's and nurse's phone number readily available. • Ensure enough available oxygen prior to leaving house for errands or trips. • Review with the patient the directions for reaching the oxygen equipment vendor and the reasons for contacting the vendor. • Discuss the signs and symptoms that indicate the need to call for emergency assistance or visit the local emergency room.	Too much or too little oxygen may be detrimental to the patient.

SKILL 45-4   Suctioning the Nasopharyngeal and Oropharyngeal Areas

EQUIPMENT

Portable or wall suction unit with tubing	Sterile water or saline	Sterile gloves
Sterile suction catheter with Y port	Sterile disposable container	Towel or waterproof pad

ACTION	RATIONALE
1. Determine the need for suctioning. Administer pain medication before suctioning to postoperative patient.	Suctioning should be done only when secretions have accumulated or adventitious breath sounds are audible. This minimizes trauma to airway mucosa. Suctioning stimulates coughing, which is painful for patients with surgical incisions.
2. Explain procedure to patient.	This provides reassurance and promotes cooperation.
3. Assemble equipment.	This provides for organized approach.
4. Perform hand hygiene.	Hand hygiene deters spread of microorganisms.
5. Adjust bed to comfortable working position. Lower side rail closer to you. Place the patient in a semi-Fowler's position if conscious. An unconscious patient should be placed in the lateral position facing you.	Having the patient in a sitting position helps him or her to cough and makes breathing easier. Gravity also facilitates the insertion of the catheter. Lateral position prevents the airway from becoming obstructed and promotes drainage of secretions.
6. Place towel or waterproof pad across patient's chest.	This protects bed linens.

7. Turn suction to appropriate pressure:
 a. Wall unit
   Adult: 100 to 120 mm Hg
   Child: 95 to 110 mm Hg
   Infant: 50 to 95 mm Hg
 b. Portable unit
   Adult: 10 to 15 mm Hg
   Child: 5 to 10 mm Hg
   Infant: 2 to 5 mm Hg
	Negative pressure must be at a safe level or pneumothorax may occur.

8. Open sterile suction package. Set up sterile container, touching only the outside surface, and pour sterile saline or water into it.	Sterile normal saline or water is used to lubricate the outside of the catheter, thus minimizing irritation of mucosa as it is being introduced.
9. Don sterile gloves. The dominant hand that will handle the catheter must remain sterile, while the nondominant hand is considered clean rather than sterile.	Handling the sterile catheter with a hand wearing a sterile glove helps prevent introducing organisms into the respiratory tract and the clean glove protects the nurse from microorganisms.
10. With sterile gloved hand, pick up sterile catheter and connect to suction tubing that is held with unsterile hand.	Sterilization can be maintained.
11. Moisten the catheter by dipping it into the container of sterile saline (see photo). Occlude Y tube to check suction.	Lubricating the inside of the catheter with saline helps move secretions in the catheter.

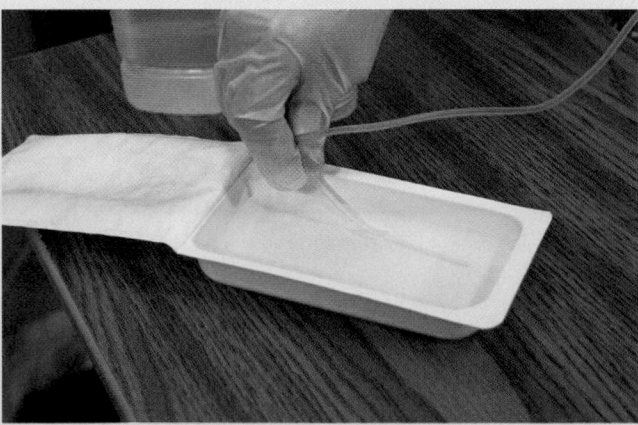

Action 11: Moistening the catheter by dipping it into the sterile saline container, and occluding Y tube to check suction.   (Photo by Rick Brady.)

(continued)

SKILL 45-4 Suctioning the Nasopharyngeal and Oropharyngeal Areas (continued)

ACTION	RATIONALE
12. Estimate the distance from the ear lobe to the nostril, and place thumb and forefinger of gloved hand at that point on the catheter.	Proper measurement ensures that catheter remains in pharynx rather than trachea.
13. Gently insert the catheter with the suction off by leaving the vent on the Y connector open (see photo). Slip the catheter gently along the floor of an unobstructed nostril toward the trachea to suction the nasopharynx. Or, insert the catheter along the side of the mouth toward the trachea to suction the oropharynx. Never apply suction as the catheter is introduced.	Using suction while inserting the catheter can cause trauma to the mucosa and removes oxygen from the respiratory tract. Coughing is induced when the trachea is touched. This helps the patient raise secretions.
14. Apply suction by occluding the suctioning port with your thumb and gently rotate the catheter as it is being withdrawn (see photo). Do not allow the suctioning to continue for more than 10 to 15 seconds at a time.	Turning the catheter as it is withdrawn helps clean all surfaces of the respiratory passageways. Suctioning the patient for longer than 10 to 15 seconds robs the respiratory tract of oxygen, which may result in hypoxia.

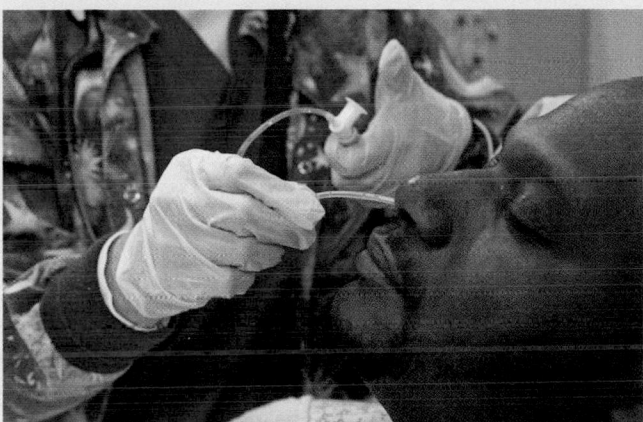

Action 13: Inserting the catheter.   (Photo by Rick Brady.)

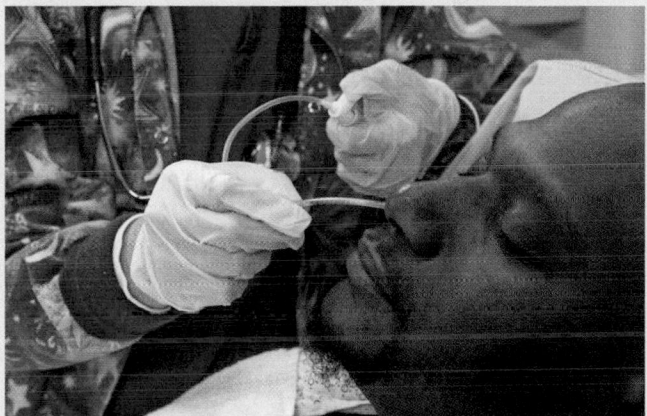

Action 14: Occluding port and rotating catheter while withdrawing.   (Photo by Rick Brady.)

15. Flush the catheter with saline and repeat suctioning as needed and according to patient's toleration of procedure.	Flushing cleans and clears catheter and lubricates it for next insertion.
16. Allow at least 20- to 30-second interval if additional suctioning is needed. The nares should be alternated when repeated suctioning is required. Do not force catheter through the nares. Encourage patient to cough and deep breathe between suctionings.	Normal breathing between suctioning helps compensate for any hypoxia induced by the previous suctioning.
17. When suctioning is completed, remove gloves inside out and dispose of gloves, catheter, and container with solution in proper receptacle. Perform hand hygiene.	Hand hygiene prevents transmission of microorganisms.
18. Use auscultation to listen to chest and breathing sounds to assess the effectiveness of suctioning (see photo).	Listening to chest and breathing sounds helps determine whether the respiratory passageways are clear of secretions.

(continued)

ACTION	RATIONALE

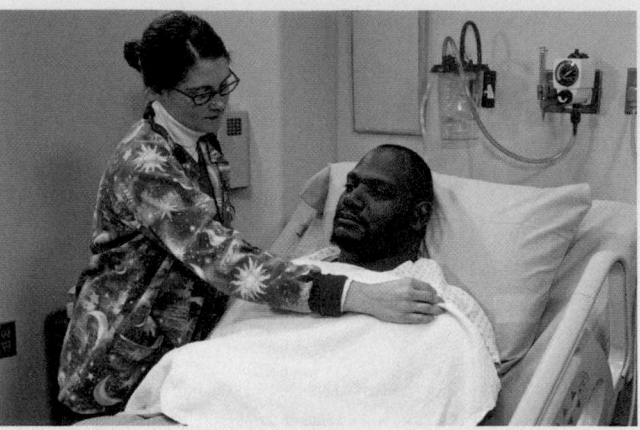

Action 18: Assessing effectiveness of suctioning.   (Photo by Rick Brady.)

19. Record the time of suctioning and the nature and amount of secretions. Also note the character of the patient's respirations before and after the suctioning.

Records of nursing measures used help assess, evaluate, and coordinate care.

20. Offer oral hygiene after suctionings.

Respiratory secretions that are allowed to accumulate in the mouth are irritating to mucous membranes and unpleasant for the patient.

---

amount, and consistency of secretions. If cyanosis, an excessively slow or rapid heart rate, or suddenly bloody secretions are noted, stop suctioning immediately, administer oxygen, and notify the physician. Cyanosis and a change in heart rate can indicate hypoxemia. Blood can indicate damage to the mucosa.

Using Artificial Airways
Oropharyngeal and Nasopharyngeal Airways

An oropharyngeal or nasopharyngeal airway is a semicircular tube of plastic or rubber inserted into the back of the pharynx through the mouth (oro) or nose (naso) in a patient who is breathing spontaneously. The oropharyngeal airway is used to keep the tongue clear of the airway. It is often used for postoperative patients until they regain consciousness. Once the patient regains consciousness, the oropharyngeal airway is removed. Tape is not used to hold the airway in place because the patient should be able to expel the airway once he or she becomes alert.

A nasopharyngeal airway, commonly called a nasal trumpet, is inserted through the nares and protrudes into the back of the pharynx. The nasal trumpet allows for frequent nasotracheal suctioning without trauma to the nasal passageway. This airway may be left in place, without much discomfort, in the patient who is alert and conscious. Techniques to use when inserting an artificial airway are given in Guidelines for Nursing Care 45-4.

Endotracheal Tube

An **endotracheal tube** is a polyvinylchloride airway that is inserted through the nose or the mouth into the trachea, using a laryngoscope as a guide. It is used to administer oxygen by mechanical ventilator, to suction secretions easily, or to bypass upper airway obstructions (eg, tongue or tracheal edema). Although uncomfortable and easy to manipulate with the tongue, orotracheal insertion is often the method of choice, especially in an emergency, because insertion is easier and a larger-sized tube can be used, making ventilation easier. Placement of the tube through the nasotracheal route, although tolerated better by patients, is more difficult and requires the use of a narrower tube. Most commonly, a cuffed endotracheal tube is used. This type of tube prevents air leakage and bronchial aspiration of foreign material while allowing more precise control of oxygen and mechanical ventilation (Fig. 45-12). However, careful monitoring of cuff pressure is necessary to decrease the risk for tracheal necrosis. The smallest amount of air that results in an airtight seal between the trachea and the tube is desirable and less likely to result in complications.

For a patient with an endotracheal tube who is receiving continuous mechanical ventilation, a closed airway suction system can be used to keep the airway patent and reduce the risk of hypoxemia or infection. The catheter (Fig. 45-13), encased in a plastic sleeve, remains connected to the patient's airway or ventilator tubing for up to 24 hours. This closed system

Guidelines for Nursing Care 45-4
Inserting an Artificial Airway

Inserting an Oropharyngeal Airway
- Use an airway that is the correct size (size 90 mm is appropriate for the average adult). Airway should reach from opening of mouth to the back angle of the jaw.
- Explain what you are doing to the patient, even though the patient appears unconscious.
- Wash your hands and don gloves (if patient is coughing, wear mask and goggles or face shield).
- Remove dentures if they are present.
- Position patient on his or her back with neck hyperextended (unless this is inappropriate).
- Open patient's mouth by using your thumb and index finger to gently pry teeth apart.
- Insert the airway with the curved tip pointing up toward the roof of the mouth.
- Slide the airway across the tongue to the back of the mouth.
- Rotate the airway 180 degrees as it passes the uvula (a flashlight can confirm the position of the airway with the curve fitting over the tongue).
- Ensure adequate ventilation by auscultating breath sounds.
- Position patient on his or her side when airway is in place.
- Remove airway for a brief period every 4 hours. Provide mouth care and rinse airway before reinserting it.

Inserting a Nasopharyngeal Airway
- Use an airway that is the correct size (size 28 French is an average adult size). Airway should reach from the tragus of the ear to the nostril plus one inch.
- Perform hand hygiene and don gloves (wear mask and goggles if patient is coughing).

- Explain the procedure to the patient.
- Lubricate the airway with the water-soluble lubricant.
- Position the patient on his or her back or in a side-lying position.
- Gently insert the airway into the naris. If resistance is met, stop and try inserting in the other naris.
- Remove the airway and place it in the other naris at least every 24 hours. Assess for any evidence of skin breakdown.
- Be aware that the airway may be used for suctioning to prevent trauma to the mucosa.

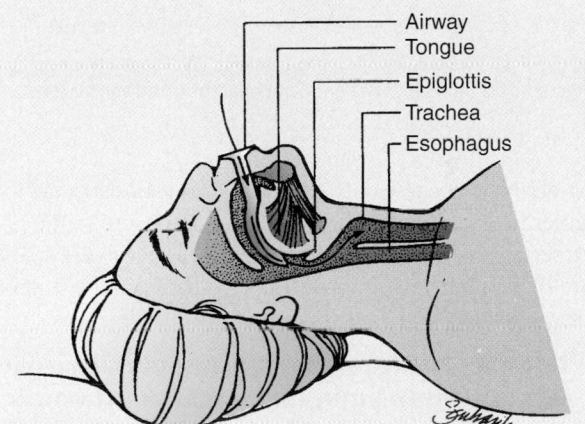

Airway in place in a patient after anesthesia. Airway allows air to pass over the tongue and into the pharynx. (Reprinted with permission from Smeltzer, S. C., & Bare, B. G. [2004]. *Brunner & Suddarth's textbook of medical-surgical nursing* [10th ed.]. Philadelphia: Lippincott Williams & Wilkins.)

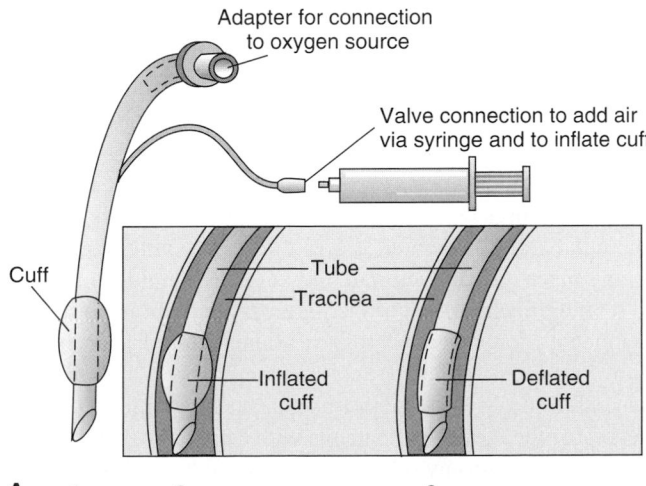
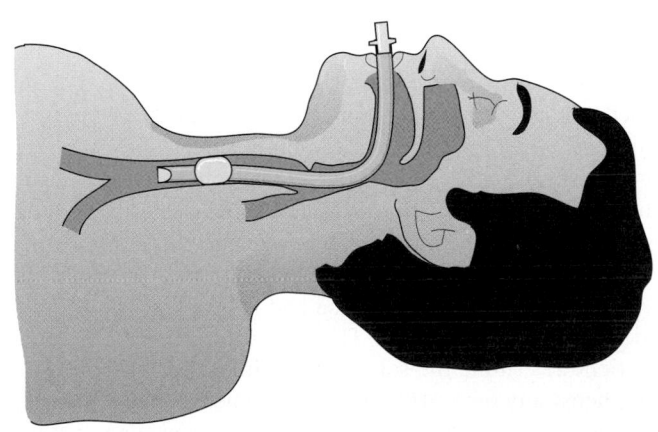

FIGURE 45-12 Endotracheal tube. (**A**) (*1*) Parts of a cuffed endotracheal tube; (*2*) tube in place with the cuff inflated; (*3*) tube in place with the cuff deflated. (**B**) Endotracheal tube in place.

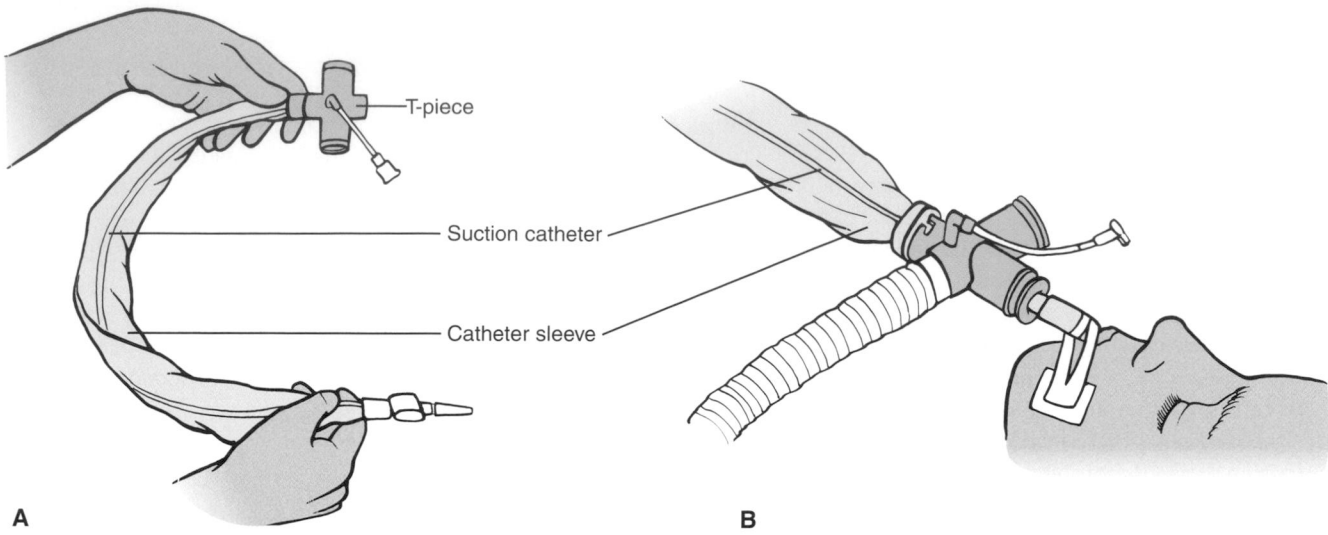

A   **B**

FIGURE 45-13 Closed airway suction system. (**A**) Closed tracheal suction system. (**B**) Closed system connected by a T-piece to the endotracheal tube and ventilator.

is cost-effective because only one catheter is used daily and the caregiver has additional protection from exposure to the patient's secretions. Some systems have an access valve, a safety feature that completely closes off access between the suction catheter and the endotracheal tube.

> *Consider Mr. Kim, the 57-year-old man receiving oxygen therapy and mechanical ventilation via an endotracheal tube. When developing the patient's plan of care, the nurse needs to assess the patient closely and frequently for signs and symptoms indicating an increase in secretions. If secretions increase, the nurse needs to suction the patient to maintain a patent airway and minimize his risk for hypoxemia and infection.*

Tracheostomy

A **tracheostomy** is an artificial opening made into the trachea through which a curved tube, called a tracheostomy tube, is inserted. A tracheostomy tube is inserted for a variety of reasons; for instance, to replace an endotracheal tube, to provide a method for mechanical ventilation of the patient, to bypass an upper airway obstruction, or to remove tracheobronchial secretions. It is inserted in the operating room or intensive care unit under sterile conditions using local anesthesia. The tracheostomy can be temporary or permanent.

The tube is made of semiflexible plastic (polyurethane or silicone), rigid plastic, or metal and is available in different sizes with varied angles. The condition and needs of the patient determine the selection of either a metal or plastic tracheostomy tube. Although metal tubes are more cost-effective for long-term use, most do not have an adapter at the neckplate that permits connection to respiratory therapy equipment (eg, an oxygen delivery system, Ambu bag, or mechanical ventilator).

A tracheostomy tube consists of an outer cannula or main shaft, an inner cannula, and an obturator. An obturator, which guides the direction of the outer cannula, is inserted into the tube during placement and removed once the outer cannula of the tube is in place (Fig. 45-14). Many tubes also have inner cannulas that may or may not be disposable. The outer cannula remains in place in the trachea, and the inner cannula is removed for cleaning or replaced with a new one. A tube with an inner cannula is necessary when patients have excessive secretions or have difficulty clearing their secretions. It also may be recommended for a patient who will be discharged with a tracheostomy tube in place.

Tracheostomy tubes may be either cuffed or cuffless (see Fig. 45-14). The inflated cuff seals the opening around the tube against air leakage, prevents aspiration, and permits mechanical ventilation. Newer tracheal cuffs are low pressure, do not require deflating for short intervals every few hours, and can be maintained at lower than tracheal capillary pressure. If a cuffed tube is used, always deflate it before oral feeding unless the patient is at high risk for aspiration. If left cuffed, the balloon can cause pressure that extends through the trachea and onto the esophagus, possibly impeding swallowing or causing erosion of the tissue.

A fenestrated tracheostomy tube has one large or several small openings or windows on its outer curve, has an inner cannula, and can be cuffed or cuffless. When the patient is being mechanically ventilated, the inner cannula is in place, blocking the small openings. After the patient is no longer connected to the ventilator, the inner cannula can be removed, the cuff deflated, and the tube plugged, allowing the patient to speak. Because the tube has these openings, it is not recommended for use in patients with a history of aspiration.

The tracheostomy tube is held in place by twill tapes or a Velcro strip fastened around the patient's neck. Usually a sterile, square gauze pad that has been precut by the manufacturer is placed between the skin and outer wings of the tube before

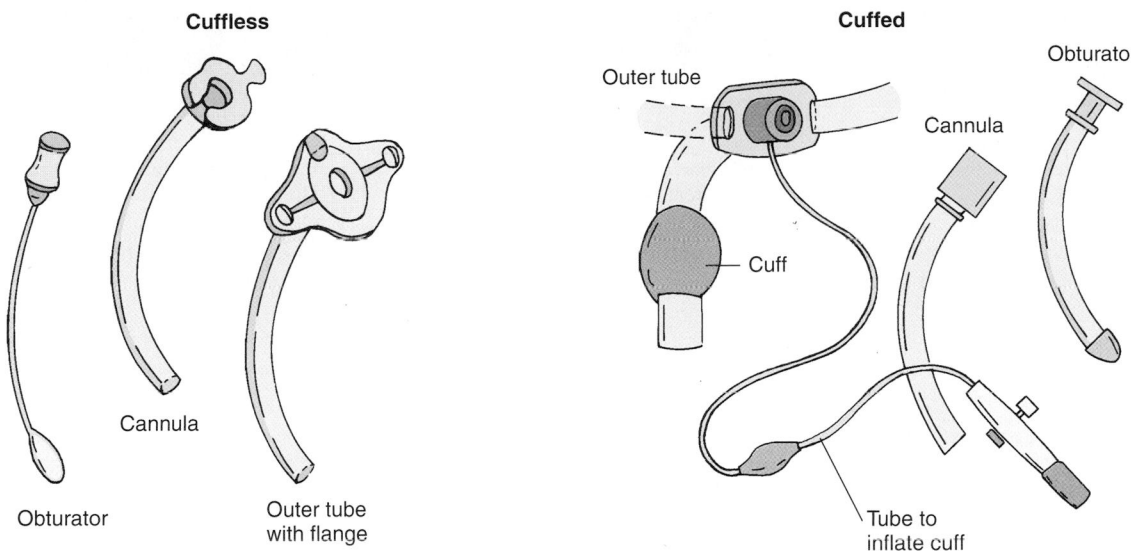

FIGURE 45-14 Two types of tracheostomy sets: cuffless and cuffed.

the tube is tied. This tracheostomy dressing must be kept dry to prevent infection and skin irritation.

Regularly check cuff pressure, although some tubes have a pressure-release valve that prevents pressure from increasing to damaging levels. Also, because the tracheostomy tube bypasses the natural humidifying and heating mechanisms in the nose and mouth, administer heated, humidified oxygen to prevent secretions from becoming dry. Also, keep the tracheostomy tube free from foreign objects and nonsterile materials, such as cotton balls, loose threads from dressings, needles, and other small objects to reduce the risk of obstruction and infection. Artificial noses, small pieces that attach over the end of the tracheostomy tube, are available for people with tracheostomies. These devices filter the air and help to warm it before it enters the trachea.

A patient who has a tracheostomy is unable to speak. Consider his or her impaired ability to communicate and keep communication tools (eg, writing board, letters, vocabulary cards) close at hand along with the call light or bell. To prevent anxiety, offer frequent reassurance and explanations and anticipate his or her needs.

> *Recall Joan McIntyre, the woman being weaned from the ventilator. Her plan of care needs to address her inability to communicate verbally. The nurse ensures that paper and pencil are readily available so that the patient can make her needs and wishes known.*

Suctioning the Tracheostomy

Skill 45-5 describes suctioning a tracheostomy. In addition to using a tracheostomy, tracheal suctioning may be performed by passing a sterile catheter through the mouth (orotracheal), through the nose (nasotracheal), or through an endotracheal tube.

Previously, it was common practice to instill a small amount of normal saline into the tracheostomy tube during the suctioning procedure to help liquefy secretions. This is no longer recommended for routine suctioning because the addition of liquid into the airway further reduces oxygenation, has no effect on thinning secretions, and may dislodge bacteria adhering to the tube and flush it into the lungs.

Providing Tracheostomy Care

In addition to suctioning the tracheostomy, the nurse is responsible for either cleaning a nondisposable inner cannula or replacing a disposable one. The inner cannula requires cleaning or replacement to prevent accumulation of secretions that can interfere with respiration and occlude the airway. Because soiled tracheostomy dressings place the patient at risk for the development of skin breakdown and infection, regularly change dressings and ties. Use gauze dressings that are not filled with cotton to prevent aspiration of foreign bodies (eg, lint or cotton fibers) into the trachea. Clean the skin around a tracheostomy to prevent buildup of dried secretions and skin breakdown. Exercise care when changing the tracheostomy ties to prevent accidental decannulation or expulsion of the tube. Have an assistant hold the tube in place during the change or keep the soiled tie in place until a clean one is securely attached. Agency policy determines specific procedures and schedules, but a newly inserted tracheostomy may require attention every 1 to 2 hours. Skill 45-6 outlines tracheostomy care.

Assisting Ventilation

Mechanical ventilators are used to assist or completely control ventilation. These machines are used with patients who have endotracheal or tracheostomy tubes in place. Mechanical ventilation can be performed in acute care facilities, in extended care settings, and in the home. Mechanical ventilation improves oxygenation and ventilation and supports the patient's breathing function during emergency or acute care episodes as well as in some long-term situations.

Many types of ventilators are available. The nurse is responsible for addressing the physical and psychological

SKILL
45-5   Suctioning the Tracheostomy

EQUIPMENT

Portable or wall suction device with
  connecting tubing
Sterile suction kit containing the following
  or gather separately:Sterile suction
  catheter of appropriate size with
  Y port

Infants: 6–8 F
Children: 8–10 F
Adults: 12–16 F
Sterile container
Sterile glove
Sterile normal saline

Clean towel or sterile drape (optional)
Goggles (or glasses) and mask
Gown (optional)
Resuscitation bag connected to 100%
  oxygen

ACTION	RATIONALE
1. Explain procedure to patient and reassure him or her that you will interrupt procedure if the patient indicates respiratory difficulty. Administer pain medication before suctioning to postoperative patient.	Explanation facilitates cooperation and provides reassurance for patient. Any procedure that compromises respiration is frightening for the patient. Suctioning stimulates coughing, which is painful for patients with surgical incisions.
2. Gather equipment and provide privacy for patient.	This provides for organized approach to task.
3. Perform hand hygiene.	Hand hygiene deters spread of microorganisms.
4. Assist the patient to a semi-Fowler's or Fowler's position if conscious. An unconscious patient should be placed in the lateral position facing you.	Sitting position helps patient to cough and breathe more easily. This position also uses gravity to aid in the insertion of catheter. Lateral position prevents the airway from becoming obstructed and promotes drainage of secretions.

5. Turn suction to appropriate pressure:
a. Wall unit
    Adult: 100 to 120 mm Hg
    Child: 95 to 110 mm Hg
    Infant: 50 mm Hg
b. Portable unit
    Adult: 10 to 15 mm Hg
    Child: 5 to 10 mm Hg
    Infant: 2 to 5 mm Hg
	Negative pressure must be at safe level or damage to tracheal mucosa may occur.

6. Place clean towel, if being used, across patient's chest. Don goggles, mask, and gown, if necessary.	Towel protects patient and bed linens. Wearing protective equipment prevents contamination of the caregiver's mucous membranes.
7. Open sterile kit or set up equipment, and prepare to suction: a. Place sterile drape, if available, across patient's chest. b. Open sterile container (see photo) and place on bedside table or overbed table without contaminating inner surface. Pour sterile saline into it.	Drape protects patient and bed linens. This maintains sterile setup.

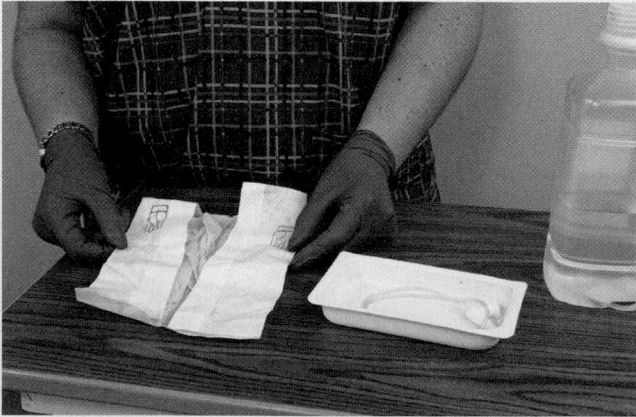

Action 7: Opening the sterile kit.   (Photo by Rick Brady.)

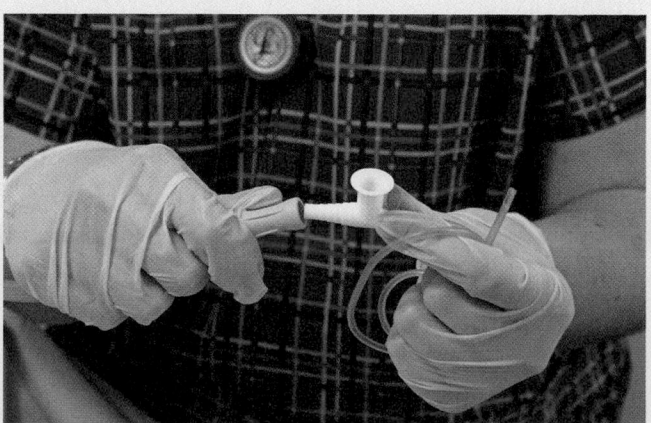

Action 7e: Connecting catheter to the suction tube.   (Photo by Rick Brady.)

(continued)

SKILL
45-5   **Suctioning the Tracheostomy** (continued)

ACTION	RATIONALE
c. Hyperoxygenate patient using manual resuscitation bag or sigh mechanism on mechanical ventilator.	This prevents hypoxemia that can occur during suctioning.
d. Don sterile gloves or one sterile glove on dominant hand and clean glove on nondominant hand.	Gloves maintain sterility of procedure and protect the nurse from microorganisms.
e. Connect sterile suction catheter to suction tubing that is held with unsterile gloved hand (see photo).	Sterile technique helps prevent introduction of organisms into the respiratory tract.
8. Moisten the catheter by dipping it into the container of sterile saline unless it is one of the newer silicone catheters that do not require lubrication.	Lubricating the inside of catheter with saline helps move secretions in the catheter. Silicone catheters do not require lubrication.
9. Remove oxygen delivery setup with unsterile gloved hand if it is still in place.	This exposes tracheostomy tube without contaminating sterile gloved hand.
10. Using sterile gloved hand, gently and quickly insert catheter into the trachea (see photo). Advance about 10 to 12.5 cm (4 to 5 inches) or until patient coughs. *Do not occlude Y port when inserting catheter.*	Using suction when inserting catheter can cause trauma to mucosa and removes oxygen from the respiratory tract.
11. Apply intermittent suction by occluding Y port with thumb of unsterile gloved hand. Gently rotate catheter with thumb and index finger of sterile gloved hand as catheter is being withdrawn. Do not allow suctioning to continue for more than 10 seconds. Hyperventilate 3 to 5 times between suctionings or encourage patient to cough and deep breathe between suctionings.	Turning the catheter while withdrawing it helps clean surfaces of respiratory tract and prevents injury to tracheal mucosa. Suctioning for longer than 10 seconds may result in hypoxia. Hyperventilation reoxygenates the lungs.
12. Flush the catheter with saline and repeat suctioning as needed and according to patient's toleration of procedure. Allow patient to rest at least 1 minute between suctionings, and replace oxygen delivery setup if necessary. Limit suctioning events to three times.	Flushing cleans and clears catheter and lubricates it for next insertion. Allowing time interval and replacing oxygen delivery setup helps compensate for hypoxia induced by the previous suctioning. Irritation from multiple suctionings results in an increased amount of secretions.
13. When procedure is completed, turn off suction and disconnect catheter from suction tubing. Remove gloves inside out and dispose of gloves, catheter, and container with solution in proper receptacle (see photo). Perform hand hygiene.	This prevents transmission of microorganisms.

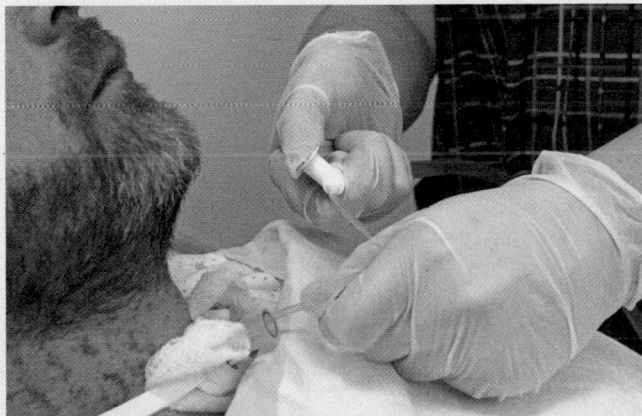

Action 10: Inserting the catheter with the Y port open.   (Photo by Rick Brady.)

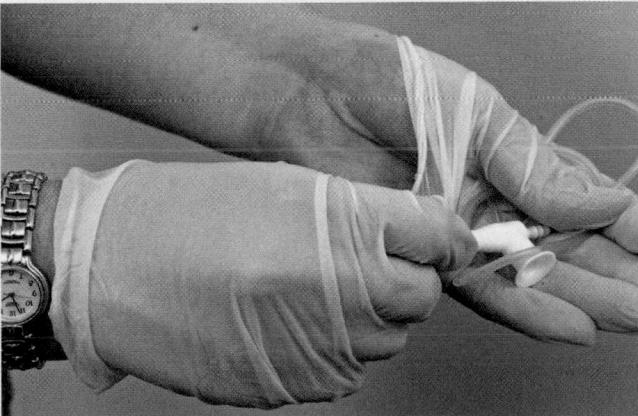

Action 13: Removing glove over the catheter.   (Photo by Rick Brady.)

14. Adjust patient's position. Auscultate chest to evaluate breath sounds.	Auscultation helps determine whether respiratory passageways are cleared of secretions.
15. Record the time of suctioning and the nature and amount of secretions. Also note the character of patient's respirations before and after suctioning.	This provides accurate documentation and provides for comprehensive care.
16. Offer oral hygiene.	Respiratory secretions that accumulate are irritating to mucous membranes and unpleasant for the patient.

Providing Tracheostomy Care

EQUIPMENT

Disposable gloves
Sterile gloves
Goggles or face shield (optional)
Sterile tracheostomy cleaning kit
  (if available) or
Sterile basins (2)
Sterile brush/pipe cleaners

Sterile cotton-tipped applicators
Sterile cleaning solutions:
  Hydrogen peroxide
  Normal saline solutions
Replacement inner cannula (if available)
Sterile suction catheter and glove set

Commercially prepared tracheostomy dress-
  ing or sterile non–cotton-filled 4" × 4"
  gauze pad, additional sterile gauze pad
Tracheostomy ties (twill tape or Velcro)
Scissors
Plastic disposal bag

ACTION	RATIONALE
1. Explain procedure to patient.	Explanation facilitates cooperation and provides reassurance for patient.
2. If tracheostomy tube has just been suctioned, remove soiled dressing from around tube and discard with gloves when they are removed.	Suctioning prevents secretions from accumulating in inner cannula and occluding airway.
3. Perform hand hygiene and open necessary supplies.	Hand hygiene deters spread of microorganisms.

Cleaning a Nondisposable Inner Cannula

ACTION	RATIONALE
4. Prepare supplies before cleaning inner cannula:	
a. Open tracheostomy care kit and separate basins touching only the edges. If kit is not available, open two sterile basins.	Basins are sterile receptacles for cleaning solutions.
b. Fill one basin ½ in (1.25 cm) deep with hydrogen peroxide.	Hydrogen peroxide facilitates removal of dry, encrusted secretions.
c. Fill other basin ½ in (1.25 cm) deep with saline.	Saline rinses and removes hydrogen peroxide and lubricates the outer surface of the inner cannula for easier reinsertion.
d. Open sterile brush or pipe cleaners if they are not already available in a cleaning kit. Open additional sterile gauze pad.	Sterile brush or pipe cleaner provides friction to clean inner surface of cannula.
5. Don disposable gloves.	Gloves protect from exposure to blood and body substances.
6. Remove the oxygen source if one is present. Rotate the lock on the inner cannula in a counterclockwise motion to release it.	Releasing the lock permits removal of the inner cannula.
7. Gently remove the inner cannula and carefully drop it in the basin with hydrogen peroxide. Remove gloves and discard.	Soaking in hydrogen peroxide loosens dry, hardened secretions.
8. Clean the inner cannula:	
a. Don sterile gloves.	Sterile gloves maintain surgical asepsis.
b. Remove inner cannula from soaking solution. Moisten brush or pipe cleaners in saline and insert into tube, using back-and-forth motion.	Movement of brush creates friction and aids in removal of accumulated secretions.
c. Agitate cannula in saline solution. Remove and tap against inner surface of basin.	Saline rinses inner cannula. Tapping tube against basin removes excess saline in inner tube.
d. Place on sterile gauze pad.	Placing on sterile gauze maintains sterility and frees both hands for suctioning.
9. Suction the outer cannula using sterile technique.	Suctioning removes any remaining secretions.
10. Replace inner cannula into outer cannula. Turn lock clockwise and check that inner cannula is secure. Reapply oxygen source if needed.	Clockwise motion secures inner cannula in place.

Replacing a Disposable Inner Cannula

ACTION	RATIONALE
11. Release lock. Gently remove inner cannula and place in disposal bag. Discard gloves and don sterile ones to insert new cannula. Replace with appropriately sized new cannula. Engage lock on inner cannula.	Disposable cannulas, although more costly, ensure that airway is clean and patent.

(continued)

SKILL 45-6 Providing Tracheostomy Care (continued)

ACTION	RATIONALE

Applying Clean Dressing and Tape

12. Dip cotton-tipped applicator in saline and clean stoma under faceplate (see photo). Use each applicator only once, moving from stoma site outward.

Saline is nonirritating to tissue. Cleansing from stoma outward and using each applicator only once promotes aseptic technique.

13. Apply hydrogen peroxide to area around stoma, faceplate, and outer cannula if secretions prove difficult to remove. Rinse area with saline.

Hydrogen peroxide may cause tissue damage and needs to be removed from skin and surrounding area.

14. Pat skin gently with dry 4" × 4" gauze.

Gauze removes excess moisture.

15. Slide commercially prepared tracheostomy dressing or pre-folded non–cotton-filled 4" × 4" dressing under faceplate (see drawing).

Lint or fiber from cotton-filled gauze pad can be aspirated into the trachea and cause irritation.

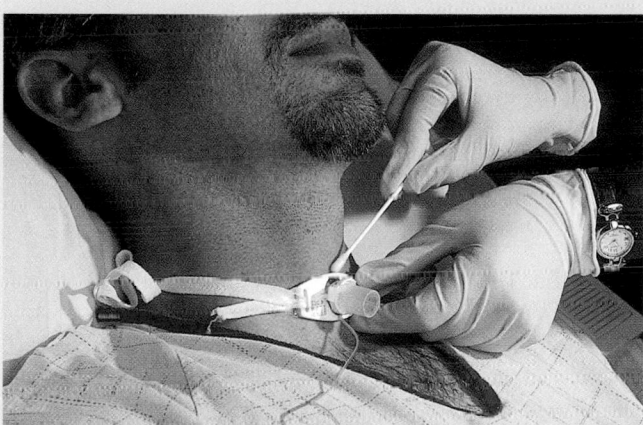

Action 12: Cleaning underneath the faceplate.   (Photo © B. Proud.)

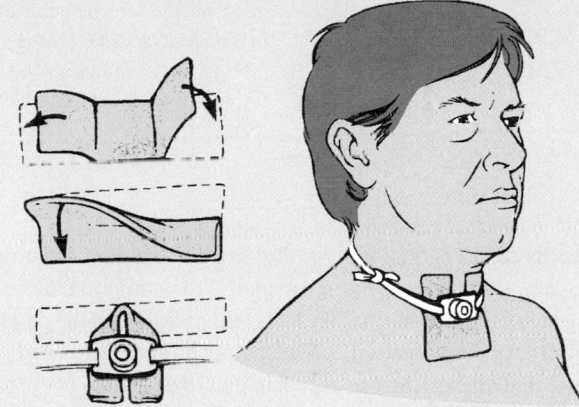

Action 15: Folding gauze square or placing commercially prepared dressing under faceplate of tracheostomy tube.

16. Change the tracheostomy tape:
    a. Leave soiled tape in place until new one is applied.

    b. Cut piece of tape that is twice the neck circumference plus 4 in (10 cm). Trim ends of tape on the diagonal.

Leaving tape in place ensures that tracheostomy will not be expelled if patient coughs or moves.
This action provides for secure attachment with knot in front at neckplate. Diagonal cut facilitates insertion of tape into openings on faceplate.

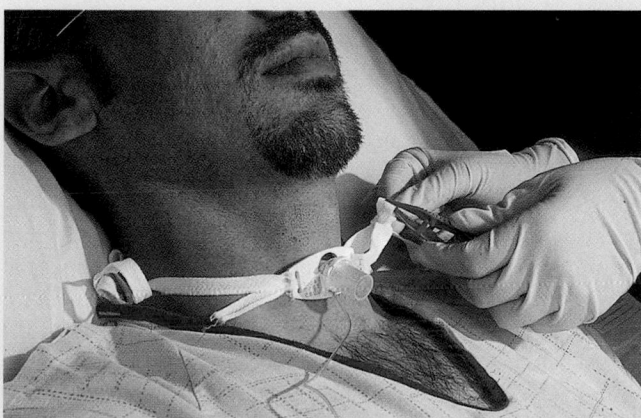

Action 16d: Inserting the tracheostomy tape through the opening and pulling through.   (Photo © B. Proud.)

(continued)

ACTION	RATIONALE
c. Insert one end of tape through faceplate opening alongside old tape. Pull through until both ends are even.	Doing so provides attachment for one side of faceplate.
d. Slide both tapes under patient's neck and insert one end through remaining opening on other side of faceplate. Pull snugly and tie ends in double square knot. Check that patient can flex neck comfortably.	A secure tape prevents accidental expulsion of the tracheostomy tube. Neck flexion that is comfortable assures that tape will not compromise circulation to the area.
e. Carefully remove old tape. Reapply oxygen source if necessary.	New tape provides for secure attachment.
17. Remove gloves and discard. Perform hand hygiene. Assess the patient's respirations. Document assessments and completion of procedure.	Assessment and accurate documentation provide for comprehensive care.

Home Care Considerations   The patient and home caregiver are given instructions on how to perform tracheostomy care. The nurse observes the return demonstration and provides feedback. Clean rather than sterile technique can be used in the home setting. Sterile saline can be made by mixing 1 teaspoon of table salt in 1 quart of water and boiling for 15 minutes. The solution is cooled and stored in a clean, dry container. Saline is discarded at the end of each day to prevent growth of bacteria. If the patient is performing self-care, the nurse recommends the use of a mirror to view the steps in the procedure.

concerns of the patient and family. In addition, key functions include evaluating the patient's response to ventilation therapy, using safe practices and techniques, and monitoring the patient carefully for complications. (See specific clinical texts and literature that discuss the use of mechanical ventilators in greater detail.)

Another mechanical device used to assist ventilation is intermittent positive-pressure breathing (IPPB). This is a method of providing a specific amount of air, oxygen, and aerosolized medication under increased pressure to the respiratory tract. The patient receiving IPPB inhales the aerosol therapy through a mouthpiece or face mask. IPPB forces deeper inspiration by positive-pressure inhalation and then permits passive exhalation. The amount of pressure varies with each patient. It is now recognized as an alternative therapy when the patient is unable or unwilling to make the effort to ventilate his or her lungs. However, conservative methods must be attempted first, such as deep-breathing and coughing exercises, percussion, vibration, and postural drainage.

In emergency situations, the manual resuscitation bag (or Ambu bag) can be used to assist ventilation in patients whose respirations have ceased.

If Joan McIntyre stops breathing during the weaning process, the nurse could intervene by reconnecting her to the ventilator. Another alternative would be to use the manual resuscitation bag to assist with ventilation temporarily.

With the patient's head tilted back, jaw pulled forward, and airway cleared, the mask is held tightly over the patient's nose and mouth. The bag also fits easily over tracheostomy and endotracheal tubes. The operator's other hand compresses the bag at a rate that approximates normal respiratory rate (eg, 16 to 20 breaths/min in adults). The one-way valve in the mask allows exhaled air to escape. Artificial ventilation can be sustained until spontaneous breathing starts, until other mechanical assistance is available, or until death is confirmed. The bag is self-inflating and may be attached to supplemental oxygen if needed.

Clearing an Obstructed Airway

Foreign-body obstruction of the airway usually occurs during eating. In adults, meat is the most common cause. In children, any variety of foods or objects can obstruct the upper airway. A patient who is semiconscious or unconscious develops airway obstruction as the tongue falls back, covering the pharynx. In fact, the tongue is the most common cause of airway obstruction.

Foreign bodies can cause either a partial or complete airway obstruction. In partial airway obstruction with good air exchange, the patient can cough forcefully. Allow the person to cough, and encourage spontaneous breathing. Do not interfere with the patient's efforts to expel the object. With a partial airway obstruction, good air exchange can progress to poor air exchange, indicated by a weak, ineffective cough; high-pitched noises while inhaling; increased breathing difficulties; and cyanosis. When this occurs, it is managed in the same way as complete airway obstruction.

With a complete airway obstruction, the victim is unable to speak or cough and may demonstrate the universal distress signal (clutching his or her throat with both hands).

Immediate action is necessary, or the patient will become unconscious as the brain becomes hypoxic. After complete airway obstruction has been determined, perform the Heimlich maneuver (abdominal thrusts). Follow the American Heart Association protocols for cardiopulmonary resuscitation and obstructed airways. These protocols are continually being developed and updated.

Administering Cardiopulmonary Resuscitation

Cardiopulmonary resuscitation (CPR) is the combination of mouth-to-mouth breathing, which supplies oxygen to the lungs, and chest compressions, which circulate blood. It is often described in terms of the ABCs of basic life support:

Airway: Tip the head and check for breathing. The respiratory tract must be opened so that air can enter.

Breathing: If the victim does not start to breathe spontaneously after the airway is opened, give two breaths lasting 1.5 to 2 seconds.

Circulation: Check the pulse. If the victim has no pulse, chest compressions are initiated to provide artificial circulation.

Start CPR in any situation in which either breathing alone or breathing and the heart beat are absent. The brain is sensitive to hypoxia and will sustain irreversible damage after 4 to 6 minutes of no oxygen. The faster CPR is initiated, the greater the chance of survival.

During CPR, standard precautions are followed even though contact with a patient's blood or body fluids does not always occur. Occupational Safety and Health Administration (OSHA) standards require healthcare facilities to provide an ample supply of ventilation masks along with other protective barriers for staff to use during resuscitation efforts.

Another device, the automated external defibrillator (AED), has also proved effective in reducing deaths attrib- uted to cardiac arrest. This easy-to-use computer-based device is designed to deliver a shock to the heart muscle quickly to interrupt ventricular fibrillation, the most common initial rhythm occurring in cardiac arrest. The AED has the ability to analyze the heart's rhythm, direct the operator to deliver a shock when appropriate or deliver one automatically, and then reanalyze the rhythm to determine whether it has returned to normal (Fig. 45-15). In healthcare facilities in which defibrillation equipment is readily available, using the AED takes priority over CPR. Despite recommendations of the American Heart Association, many hospitals have not established AED response programs, and manual defibrillator use is still most often initiated by ACLS teams. In the community, more than half of states permit healthcare workers who are not emergency medical technicians to use AEDs, and six states allow lay responders to use them. In many cases, reducing deaths from cardiac arrest appears to depend on early delivery of AED (see the Research in Nursing box).

Most professional organizations recommend and support widespread efforts to teach CPR to lay people and all health professionals. Mannequins for practice can be obtained from the American Heart Association, the American Red Cross, and health agencies. The nurse is professionally responsible for maintaining proficiency in CPR skills. This necessitates periodic practice with mannequins (adult and infant). CPR must be administered quickly and accurately, without hesitation, when cardiac arrest occurs.

Evaluating

Evaluation is an ongoing and deliberate part of the nursing process that involves the nurse, patient, family, and other healthcare team members. It compares the patient's health status with previously defined expected outcomes and exam-

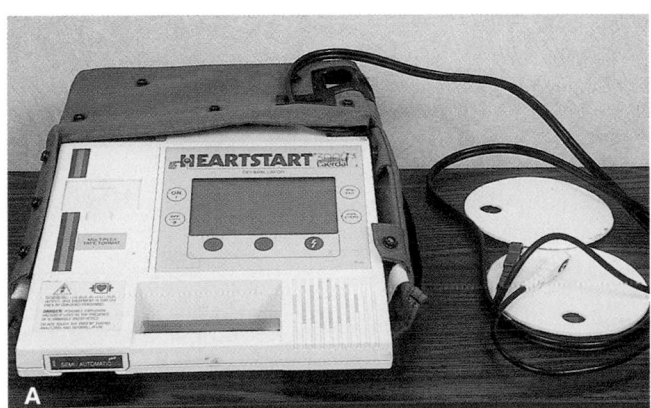
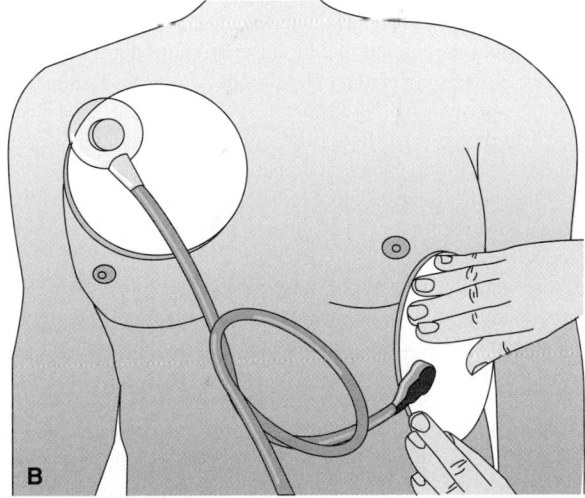

FIGURE 45-15 Placement of the automated external defibrillator (AED). (**A**) AED device. (**B**) Place the AED pad attached to the red cable connector to the left of the heart apex. To help remember where to place the pads, think "white right, red ribs." Placement of both electrode pads is the same as it is for manual defibrillation or cardioversion. (Photograph © B. Proud)

Research in Nursing Making a Difference
Use of Automated External Defibrillators by the Public

Early defibrillation in the event of a cardiac arrest has been shown to save lives. Cardiovascular disease is the most common cause of death in the United States. Many public buildings have automated external defibrillators (AEDs) available in an attempt to save lives in the future.

Related Research

Caffrey, S., Willoughby, P., Pepe, P., & Becker, L. (2002). Public use of automated external defibrillators. *New England Journal of Medicine, 347*(16), 1242–1247.

This observational study was designed to determine whether the general public would use AEDs in a public place, such as a major Midwest airport. Public service announcements were shown every half-hour including the following information: the purpose of the AED, the availability of the AED, and encour-

agement to use the AED if necessary. In a 2-year period, the AEDs were used a total of 18 times; in all but 2 of these instances the AED was initiated by a good Samaritan. Fifty-six percent of the survivors had a 1-year survival with a good neurologic outcome. This is compared to 5%, with the use of traditional cardiopulmonary resuscitation and emergency service response. The results of this study show the benefits of making AEDs available to the general public.

Relevance to Nursing Practice

Educating the general public is a major step taken to ensure the promotion of wellness. Nurses need to reassure and educate the general public regarding the use of AEDs and cardiopulmonary disease. In educating people in the use of AEDs, nurses are not only saving lives but also improving the quality of these lives.

NURSING PLAN OF CARE 45-1   *for Freddie Taft*

Freddie Taft is a 1-year-old, alert, well-developed child who has been a patient on the pediatric unit for 3 days with status asthmaticus. He has had two other hospitalizations for acute asthma, during which he responded quickly to intravenous and inhalation bronchodilators. During this hospitalization, either his mother, a teacher, or his father, a psychologist, has stayed with him. Other relatives are caring for Freddie's 9-year-old sister and 5-year-old brother.

Freddie interacts happily with staff as long as a parent is within sight. Gross and fine motor coordination are appropriate for his age. His vocabulary consists of 25 words. The history is from his mother, who is a reliable source. He has had a clear nasal discharge with slight, intermittent, nonproductive cough for 3 days with no change in appetite or activity pattern.

On the day of admission, he attended the day-care center as usual. After being there for 3 hours, his cough became more frequent, and his respirations became more labored. The caregivers were not alarmed because he continued to eat, drink, nap, and play in his usual pattern. His mother states that when she arrived in the afternoon to pick up the boys, she discovered him to be using his intercostal and neck muscles excessively with every breath. His respirations were 50 breaths/min, labored, and accompanied by a grunt. By the time she arrived home, he was pale and fitful and was crying weakly. Respirations were 60 breaths/min, and peripheral cyanosis was noted. The pediatrician advised lung evaluation in the emergency department. While there, three subcutaneous injections of epinephrine were administered 5 minutes apart. The child did not

respond satisfactorily, so he was admitted for intravenous aminophylline and steroid administration.

In addition to a history of asthma, Freddie is allergic to eggs and peanuts and has eczema on his face, arms, legs, and upper back. His current medications include albuterol every 8 hours; a topical steroid (Lidex Cream); and a multivitamin and mineral supplement (Poly-Vi-Sol drops). No one in the family smokes. The caregivers at the day-care center smoke outside the building. The day-care center is clean and had the rugs shampooed the night before this child's illness. This child had no sputum production or fever. Immunizations are current. A comprehensive assessment revealed the following findings:

Respiratory rate, 44 breaths/min

Irregular rhythm

Excessive use of accessory muscles

Nonproductive, frequent cough

Gurgles and expiratory wheezes noted

Pale, no cyanosis

Blood pressure, 100/60 mm Hg; heart rate, 120 beats/min

Restless child who naps for only 20 to 30 minutes at intervals day and night

Arterial blood gases: normal values

Chest radiograph: normal

Poor appetite, vomiting one or two times

Up early in morning

Sweat test: negative for cystic fibrosis

(*continued*)

NURSING PLAN OF CARE 45-1   *for Freddie Taft* (continued)

NURSING DIAGNOSIS

Ineffective Airway Clearance related to exposure to allergens, viral infection, broncho-spasm, overproduction of mucus as manifested by: nonproductive frequent cough, presence of sonorous wheezes (rhonchi) and sibilant wheezes on expiration, restlessness, interrupted sleep.

EXPECTED OUTCOME

By 3/20/06, the patient will:
• Have rare episodes of coughing and no vomiting

Nursing Interventions	Rationale	Evaluative Statement
Hold meals until inhalation treatments are done.	Bronchodilators stimulate coughing and often cause vomiting if given after meals.	3/19/06 Outcome met. Freddie has not vomited in 2 days and has 2-hour intervals between coughing episodes.
Offer liquids every 3 hours in a bottle or cup.	Liquids help to liquefy secretions and prevent dehydration.	*M. Jones, RN*
Perform percussion during morning and evening bath.	Percussion loosens pulmonary secretions so that they are more easily expectorated.	

EXPECTED OUTCOME

By 3/20/06, the patient's parents will:
• Remove dust collecting toys

Nursing Interventions	Rationale	Evaluative Statement
Give parents allergy pamphlets from American Lung Association.	Adequate information reinforces instruction given by healthcare providers.	3/17/06 Outcome met. Parents removed furry toys from hospital room.
Review with both parents methods to reduce exposure to possible allergens at home.	Constant exposure to allergens (dust, mold, mildew, and so forth) and irritants (perfume, smog, cleaners, and so forth) produces bronchospasm and stimulates copious mucus production. Medications are most effective when allergens are removed.	*M. Jones, RN*
Encourage parents to examine day-care environment. Explore options with them.	Environment in day-care may contain allergens. The least irritating setting is desirable.	

SAMPLE DOCUMENTATION

3/17/06 Nursing

Family and staff conference to discuss Freddie's respiratory disturbance initiated by primary nurse's concern. Present were Freddie's mother; MJ (primary nurse); TK (clinical coordinator); TR (head of respiratory department); and MM and LQ (staff nurses). Primary nurse presented findings from assessment and nursing examination. Discussion centered on strategies to control airway edema and reduce wheezes, reduce coughing episodes and control vomiting, and prevent further bronchospasms and edema resulting from exposure to allergens in environment. See plan of care. Patient progress will be evaluated in 4 days during nursing grand rounds, 3/21/06.

M. Jones, RN

ines the patient's projected progress in meeting those outcomes. Everyone involved in the evaluation process needs to identify effective interventions and reasons for any failures in achieving these expected outcomes. Adjustments in the nursing plan of care are then made accordingly. See Nursing Plan of Care 45-1 for Freddie Taft.

■ Developing Critical Thinking Skills

1. Using the Focused Assessment Guide earlier in this chapter, work with a partner to assess the respiratory functioning of the following patients. Discuss ways in which you would modify your assessment to meet the

specific needs of individual patients:

- A 6-year-old who presents with asthma and is experiencing difficulty breathing
- A 12-year-old who is brought to emergency room after illicit use of inhalants ("huffing")
- An adult dying of cancer who is receiving increasing doses of narcotics, which depress respiratory functioning
- A hospitalized young adult with a 24-pack/year history of smoking who is noted to have a persistent, hacking cough

2. A postoperative patient who is at high risk for pulmonary complications because of a long history of smoking refuses to use the incentive spirometer or to cooperate with instructions to deep breathe. How would you respond to this patient? Discuss with other students what nursing response is most likely to secure his cooperation in necessary self-care measures.

Practicing for NCLEX

1. A patient has a fractured rib and is breathing less often and with less depth because of the pain. The nurse would document this finding using which term?
   a. Fremitus
   b. Hyperventilation
   c. Pleural friction rub
   d. Hypoventilation
2. When auscultating Mr. Chang's breath sounds, the nurse detects a continuous sound heard on expiration. The nurse identifies this sound as:
   a. Crackles
   b. Wheezes
   c. Bronchial sounds
   d. Pleural friction rub
3. Air that develops in the pleural space is referred to as:
   a. Pneumothorax
   b. Pleural effusion
   c. Hemothorax
   d. Atelectasis
4. When planning care for a patient with chronic lung disease who is receiving oxygen through a nasal cannula, the nurse expects that:
   a. The oxygen must be humidified.
   b. The rate will be 2 L/min or less.
   c. Arterial blood gases will be drawn every 4 hours to assess flow rate.
   d. The rate will be 6 L/min or more.
5. Which oxygen delivery device would the nurse expect to use to provide the highest concentration of oxygen to a patient who is breathing spontaneously?
   a. Partial rebreather mask
   b. Nonrebreather mask
   c. Simple mask
   d. Venturi mask

6. When teaching a patient about pulse oximetry, which statement would the nurse most likely include in the discussion?
   a. A range of 95% to 98% is considered normal oxygen saturation.
   b. Oximetry measures the oxygen saturation of venous blood.
   c. Fasting is required for 12 hours before the test.
   d. Pulse oximetry is a replacement for arterial blood gas analysis.
7. Which action would the nurse include when performing oropharyngeal suctioning on a patient?
   a. Use clean technique.
   b. Apply suction as the catheter is introduced.
   c. Flush the catheter with saline between catheter insertions.
   d. Limit suctioning to 25- to 30-second intervals at one time.
8. Effective use of a metered-dose inhaler requires that the patient accomplish which action?
   a. Breathe in through the nose.
   b. Inhale two sprays with one breath.
   c. Hold the breath for 5 to 10 seconds after inspiration.
   d. Exhale quickly through an open mouth.
9. Mr. Parks has chronic obstructive pulmonary disease. The nurse has taught him that pursed-lip breathing helps him by:
   a. Increasing carbon dioxide, which stimulates breathing
   b. Prolonging inspiration and shortening expiration
   c. Liquefying his secretions
   d. Decreasing the amount of air trapping and resistance
10. A patient develops sudden cardiac arrest. What is the critical time that the nurse must keep in mind before irreversible brain damage occurs?
    a. 1 to 3 minutes
    b. 2 to 4 minutes
    c. 4 to 6 minutes
    d. 8 to 10 minutes
11. David White is in the hospital with a medical diagnosis of viral pneumonia. He is receiving oxygen through a simple face mask. The nurse ensures that the mask fits snugly over the patient's face for which reason?
    a. To prevent mask movement and consequent skin breakdown
    b. To help the patient feel secure
    c. To maintain carbon dioxide retention
    d. To aid in maintaining expected oxygen delivery
12. When suctioning a patient through a tracheostomy tube, the nurse was careful not to occlude the Y port when inserting the suction catheter because this would:
    a. Prevent suctioning from occurring
    b. Cause trauma to the tracheal mucosa

c. Break the sterile technique

d. Suction out all the carbon dioxide

13. The nurse follows safe technique when using a portable oxygen cylinder by:
    a. Checking the amount of oxygen in the cylinder before using it
    b. Using a cylinder for a patient transfer that indicates available oxygen is 500 psi
    c. Placing the oxygen cylinder on the stretcher next to the patient
    d. Discontinuing oxygen flow by turning cylinder key counterclockwise until tight

14. Which blood gas values would the nurse identify as within the normal range?
    a. pH, 7.25 to 7.35; $PaCO_2$, 25 to 35 mm Hg; PaO_2, 50 to 100 mm Hg
    b. pH, 7.35 to 7.45; $PaCO_2$, 45 to 50 mm Hg; PaO_2, 90 to 100 mm Hg
    c. pH, 7.35 to 7.45; $PaCO_2$, 35 to 45 mm Hg; PaO_2, 80 to 100 mm Hg
    d. pH, 7.30 to 7.40; $PaCO_2$, 30 to 45 mm Hg; PaO_2, 70 to 100 mm Hg

15. Abdominal breathing at 30 to 60 breaths/min with an irregular pattern of rate and depth would closely describe the breathing patterns of what age group?
    a. Aged adult
    b. Infant
    c. Early childhood
    d. Late childhood

■ Answers With Rationale

1. The correct answer is *d*. Hypoventilation is a decreased rate or depth of air movement into the lungs. Hyperventilation is an increased rate and depth of ventilation. Fremitus is the vibration of the chest wall that can be palpated. A pleural friction rub is a dry grating sound caused by inflammation of pleural surfaces.

2. The correct answer is *b*. Wheezes are a continuous sound heard on expiration. Crackles are not described as squeaky. The pleural friction rub is a dry, grating sound. Bronchial breath sounds are normal sounds heard over the trachea.

3. The correct answer is *a*. Air in the pleural space is termed pneumothorax. Fluid in the pleural space is referred to as a pleural effusion. Blood collection in the pleural space is referred to as a hemothorax. Atelectasis refers to an incomplete expansion or collapse of the alveoli.

4. The correct answer is *b*. A rate higher than 2 L/min may destroy the hypoxic drive that stimulates respirations in the medulla in a patient with chronic lung disease. Oxygen delivered at low rates does not necessarily have to be humidified, and arterial blood gases are not required at regular intervals to determine the flow rate.

5. The correct answer is *b*. The nonrebreather mask provides the highest concentration of oxygen to a spontaneously breathing patient. None of the other devices would provide this.

6. The correct answer is *a*. Pulse oximetry measures oxygen saturation levels of arterial blood, which normally range from 95% to 98%. Fasting is not required before the test. Pulse oximetry is an adjunct therapy, not a replacement for arterial blood gas analysis.

7. The correct answer is *c*. Flushing the catheter with saline between insertions is important to clear the catheter of secretions. The nurse should use sterile technique and should not apply suction as the catheter is being introduced; suctioning should be limited to 10- to 15-second intervals to avoid causing hypoxia.

8. The correct answer is *c*. Holding one's breath for 5 to 10 seconds after inspiration of the medication allows the drug to reach the alveoli. Correct technique for using an MDI includes breathing in through the mouth so that all the medication is properly delivered to the lungs, using one spray of medication for each breath to receive the correct dose, and exhaling slowly through pursed lips to minimize airway trapping and resistance.

9. The correct answer is *d*. Doing pursed-lip breathing correctly diminishes carbon dioxide retention. It also prolongs expiration, increases airway pressure, and lessens the amount of airway trapping and resistance.

10. The correct answer is *c*. After 4 to 6 minutes without oxygen, irreversible brain damage can occur.

11. The correct answer is *d*. A snug-fitting mask is necessary to deliver the expected rate of oxygen. A simple face mask does not trap carbon dioxide or cause retention. Patients often complain that an oxygen mask is uncomfortable. A snug fit may limit but not prevent movement of the mask.

12. The correct answer is *b*. Occluding the Y port causes suction and may traumatize the tracheal mucosa if applied when the catheter is inserted. Occluding the Y port does not prevent suction.

13. The correct answer is *a*. The cylinder must always be checked before use to ensure that enough oxygen is available for the patient. It is unsafe to use a cylinder that reads 500 psi or less because not enough oxygen remains for a patient transfer. A cylinder that is not secured properly may result in injury to the patient. Oxygen flow is discontinued by turning the valve clockwise until it is tight.

14. The correct answer is *c*. These are the normal arterial blood gas ranges for pH, carbon dioxide, and oxygen.

15. The correct answer is *b*. Respirations in the infant are more rapid and have not stabilized. As alveoli increase in number and size, the respiratory rate decreases.

Bibliography

Blazys, D. (2000). Clinical nurses forum. Teaching suctioning. *Journal of Emergency Nursing 26*(6), 584.

Bridy, M., & Burklow, T. (2002). Understanding the newer automated external defibrillator devices: Electrophysiology, biphasic waveforms, and technology. *Journal of Emergency Nursing, 28*(2), 132–137.

Carroll, P. (2001). How to intervene before asthma turns deadly. *RN, 64*(4), 52–60.

Carroll, P. (2002). A guide to mobile chest drains. *RN, 65*(5), 56–62.

Dixon, B., & Tasota, F. (2003). Inadvertent tracheal decannulation. *Nursing, 33*(1), 96.

Fischbach, F. (2000). *A manual of laboratory tests* (6th ed.). Philadelphia: Lippincott Williams & Wilkins.

Gattinoni, L., Tognoni, G., Pesenti, A., et al. (2001). Effect of prone positioning on the survival of patients with acute respiratory failure. *New England Journal of Medicine, 345*(8), 568–573.

Grodner, M., Anderson, S., & DeYoung, S. (2000). *Foundations and clinical applications of nutrition: A nursing approach* (2nd ed.). St. Louis: C. V. Mosby.

Lazzara, D. (2002). Eliminate the air of mystery from chest tubes. *Nursing, 32*(6), 36–43.

Little, C. (2000). Manual ventilation. *Nursing, 30*(3), 50–51.

McConnell, E. (2000). Suctioning a tracheostomy tube. *Nursing, 30*(1), 80.

McConnell, E. (2002a). Providing tracheostomy care. *Nursing, 32*(1), 17.

McConnell, E. (2002b). Teaching your patient to use a metered-dose inhaler. *Nursing, 32*(2), 73.

McConnell, E. (2002c). Using an automated external defibrillator. *Nursing, 32*(10), 18.

Martin, B., Llewellyn, J., Faut-Callahan, M., & Meyer, P. (2000). The use of telemetric oximetry in the clinical setting. *MedSurg Nursing, 9*(2), 71–76.

Mehta, M. (2003). Assessing respiratory status. *Nursing, 33*(2), 54.

Miracle, V. (2002). Action stat: Asthma attack. *Nursing, 32*(11), 104.

North American Nursing Diagnosis Association. (2003). *NANDA nursing diagnoses: Definitions and classification, 2003–2004.* Philadelphia: Author.

Pagana, K., & Pagana, T. (2002). *Manual of diagnostic and laboratory tests* (2nd ed.). St. Louis: C. V. Mosby.

Seay, S., Gay, S., & Strauss, M. (2002). Tracheostomy emergencies: Correcting accidental decannulation or displaced tracheostomy tube. *American Journal of Nursing, 102*(3), 59–63.

Smeltzer, S., & Bare, B. (2004). *Brunner and Suddarth's textbook of medical–surgical nursing* (10th ed.). Philadelphia: Lippincott Williams & Wilkins.

Tate, J., & Tasota, F. (2000). Using pulse oximetry. *Nursing, 30*(9), 30.

Togger, D., & Brenner, P. (2001). Metered dose inhalers. *American Journal of Nursing, 101*(10), 26–32.

Fluid, Electrolyte, and Acid–Base Balance

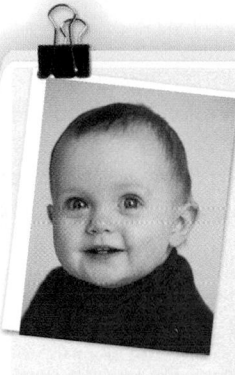

Jeremiah Kearny, a 7-month-old, is brought to the health center by his mother because he has had nausea, vomiting, and diarrhea for the past 2 days. Further assessment reveals minimal fluid intake during the past 2 days, some lethargy, and three other family members with a recent gastrointestinal virus infection. The infant is diagnosed with dehydration and electrolyte imbalance.

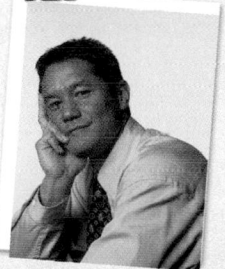

Jack Soo Park, a 58-year-old man receiving intravenous (IV) therapy with antibiotics, states "I'm having trouble breathing. It just started a little while ago." Physical examination reveals a bounding pulse, distended neck veins, and crackles and wheezes in the lungs. Excess fluid volume is suspected. Further checking reveals an IV fluid-administration error that has resulted in overhydration.

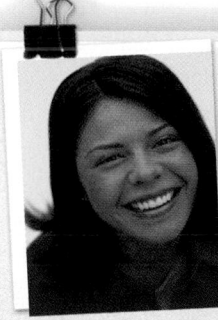

Grace Gilligan, a 28-year-old woman, arrives at the emergency department with complaints of severe bouts of nausea and vomiting. She has a past medical history of gastrointestinal (GI) problems, for which she underwent abdominal surgery several months ago. "I thought my problems were over once I had the surgery." IV therapy was ordered to restore her fluid balance.

The types of blended skills you'll need to respond to the case scenarios include:

Cognitive Skills

- Knowledge of the anatomy and physiology related to body fluids, fluid and electrolyte and acid–base balance
- Knowledge of age-related differences in body fluid content and effect on fluid balance status
- Knowledge of how to promote and maintain fluid, electrolyte, and acid–base balance
- Knowledge of specific variables that may influence fluid, electrolyte, and acid–base balance
- Ability to incorporate knowledge of specific conditions that can affect fluid, electrolyte, and acid–base balance into plan of care for a patient experiencing an imbalance
- Ability to incorporate knowledge of the nursing process to identify and to care for patients at risk for or with problems related to fluid, electrolyte, and acid–base balance

Technical Skills

- Demonstration of strong history and physical assessment techniques to determine problems related to fluid, electrolyte, and acid–base balance including possible contributory factors
- Ability to use the equipment and protocols necessary to maintain and restore fluid, electrolyte, and acid–base balance, and prevent imbalances
- Ability to demonstrate competence in technical nursing assistance, adapting it as necessary, to meet the needs of patients experiencing alterations in fluid, electrolyte, or acid–base balance
- Competence in specific skills, such as administering IV therapy, blood transfusions, and total parenteral nutrition, including adherence to proper safety and infection control precautions

Interpersonal Skills

- Strong people skills to establish trusting relationships with patients experiencing problems with fluid, electrolyte, and acid–base balance

- Ability to communicate concerns for a patient's status; for example, a woman who is visibly upset while IV insertion is being attempted or a patient who develops signs and symptoms of overhydration due to an error in IV administration
- Ability to use therapeutic communication skills effectively to meet the needs of patients experiencing a emotional upset related to repeated attempts at initiating an IV infusion
- Ability to work collaboratively with other members of the healthcare team, including a good working relationship with colleagues, essential to the unit's taking responsibility for an error in the administration of IV fluids
- Ability to identify and respond to the needs of patients of different ages requiring treatment for fluid, electrolyte, or acid–base problems
- Ability to mobilize necessary supportive resources to provide needed services, especially related to patient comfort and safety

Ethical and Legal Skills

- Strong sense of accountability for the health and well-being of patients; a commitment to getting them the help they need to achieve their health goals—within the scope of nursing responsibilities and available resources
- Ability to participate as a trusted and effective patient advocate, including a commitment to securing the best possible care for patients assigned to your care
- A willingness to hold colleagues accountable for safe quality practice
- Knowledge of how to report and to document an error in the administration of IV fluids
- Knowledge of ethical and legal responsibilities involved with measures to promote, maintain, and restore fluid, electrolyte, and acid–base balance that are within the scope of nursing responsibilities

Learning Outcomes

After completing the chapter, the learner should be able to accomplish the following:

1. Describe the location and functions of body fluids, including the factors that affect variations in fluid compartments.
2. Describe the functions, regulation, sources, and losses of the main electrolytes of the body.
3. Explain the principles of osmosis, diffusion, active transport, and filtration.
4. Describe how thirst and the organs of homeostasis (kidneys, heart and blood vessels, lungs, adrenal glands, pituitary gland, and parathyroid glands) function to maintain fluid homeostasis.
5. Describe the role of buffer systems and respiratory and renal mechanisms in achieving and maintaining acid–base balance.
6. Identify the etiologies, defining characteristics, and treatment modalities for common fluid, electrolyte, and acid–base imbalances.
7. Perform a fluid, electrolyte, and acid–base balance assessment.
8. Describe the role of dietary modification, modification of fluid intake, medication administration, IV therapy, blood replacement, and total parenteral nutrition (TPN) in resolving fluid, electrolyte, and acid–base imbalances.
9. Plan, implement, and evaluate nursing care related to select nursing diagnoses involving fluid, electrolyte, and acid–base imbalances.

Key Terms

acid	cation	hypermagnesemia	hypovolemia
acidosis	colloid osmotic pressure	hypernatremia	ion
active transport	cross-matching	hyperphosphatemia	isotonic
agglutinin	dehydration	hypertonic	osmolarity
alkalosis	diffusion	hypervolemia	osmosis
anions	edema	hypocalcemia	overhydration
antibody	electrolytes	hypokalemia	pH
antigen	filtration	hypomagnesemia	solutes
autologous transfusion	hydrostatic pressure	hyponatremia	solvents
base	hypercalcemia	hypophosphatemia	typing
buffer	hyperkalemia	hypotonic	

Fluid, comprised of water and dissolved substances in the form of electrolytes, gases, and nonelectrolytes, is the main constituent of the body. Therefore, the body's fluid balance is extremely important. The balance, or homeostasis, of water (which accounts for approximately 50%–60% of a person's body weight) and dissolved substances is maintained through the functions of almost every organ in the body. In addition, the body also contains acidic or basic substances that must be balanced. Nurses routinely care for patients with serious and even life-threatening fluid, electrolyte, and acid–base disturbances. (See the accompanying Reflective Practice box for an example.) One of nursing's most important roles is the prevention of these disturbances, especially in high-risk populations such as infants, older adults, and patients with cardiac and renal disorders.

This chapter discusses the principles of fluid, electrolyte, and acid–base balance and common disturbances. Sample interview questions for performing a fluid-balance assessment are included, with information on specific physical assessment measures and laboratory studies. Numerous examples of nursing diagnoses are provided. Expected outcomes and specific nursing interventions to promote fluid and electrolyte balance are described. These interventions include modifying dietary and fluid intake, administering medications, and assisting with IV therapy, blood replacement, and TPN. The concluding plan of care illustrates how nurses combine their knowledge of fluid, electrolyte, and acid–base balance with skilled nursing interventions and caring to resolve alterations in health status and to improve patient outcome.

Reflective Practice
Challenge to Interpersonal Skills

During my clinical rotation in the emergency department, I met Grace Gilligan. She was a 28-year-old woman who came to the emergency department with complaints of severe nausea and vomiting. She has a past medical history of gastrointestinal (GI) problems, for which she underwent abdominal surgery several months ago. "I thought my problems were over once I had the surgery." The patient was dehydrated and needed IV fluid therapy.

The ER technician attempted to insert the IV catheter in the patient's hand but was unable to thread the catheter. The technician asked my nurse to help with the situation. My nurse attempted not once, but six times. The patient was already upset by her recurrent abdominal symptoms, but now had to deal with the continuous painful stick of a needle. During the course of attempts to start the IV, the patient stated that anesthesiology always had to be called to insert her IVs. Although my nurse acknowledged the information, she continued trying to start the IV. Finally, on the sixth try, as the patient was in tears, the nurse was successful. It seemed as if the nurse was out to prove her abilities without caring for the patient. By the end, I had difficulty even watching.

Thinking Outside the Box: Possible Courses of Action

- During the regathering of supplies (outside the patient's room), mention to the nurse that maybe anesthesiology should be called, since "enough is enough!"
- Tell my clinical instructor that the patient is being abused.
- Ask the doctor if he or she could address the situation.
- Tell the patient when the nurse was out of the room to refuse any more sticks until anesthesiology was called.

(continued)

Reflective Practice
Challenge to Interpersonal Skills (Continued)

Evaluating a Good Outcome: How Do I Define Success?

• Patient is benefited by my actions. . . . or at least not harmed.
• All actions are supported by rationale.

• The patient's wishes are respected.
• Personal integrity is not compromised.

Personal Learning: Here's to the Future!

Unfortunately, I did not take any actions to protect this patient. This was my first time in the emergency room as well as my first introduction to the nurse. I was intimidated by her. Furthermore, I was scared when she continued to attempt the catheter insertion with the patient in tears. I know that it is my responsibility to advocate for the needs of my patients. In the future, I hope that I will never compromise my integrity, beliefs, and values to prove something to a student. If I fail or am not confident in my skills, I will admit this and stop before my patient is put at risk.

Reflection

How do you think you would respond in a similar situation? Why? What does this tell you about yourself and about the adequacy of your skills for professional practice? What might have prompted the emergency room nurse to act as she did? The nursing student? How could the nursing student have advocated for the patient? What other barriers (other than those listed above) might have interfered with the nursing student acting as an advocate? Can you think of other ways to respond? What other skills (cognitive, interpersonal, technical, ethical/legal) would you need to respond well in this situation? Do you agree with the criteria to evaluate a successful outcome? Were any of the criteria met?

Amy Persinger, Georgetown University

ANATOMY AND PHYSIOLOGY

Body Fluids

As the primary body fluid, water is the most important nutrient of life. Although life can be sustained for many days without food, humans can survive for only a few days without water. Water in the body functions primarily to:

• Provide a medium for transporting nutrients to cells and wastes from cells, and for transporting substances such as hormones, enzymes, blood platelets, and red and white blood cells
• Facilitate cellular metabolism and proper cellular chemical functioning
• Act as a solvent for electrolytes and nonelectrolytes
• Help maintain normal body temperature
• Facilitate digestion and promote elimination
• Act as a tissue lubricant

Body Fluid Compartments

Fluids are located in two main compartments, or spaces, in the body—the intracellular fluid (ICF) and extracellular fluid (ECF). ICF is the fluid within cells, constituting about 40% of an adult's body weight, or 70% of the total-body water. ECF is all the fluid outside the cells. It constitutes about 20% of an adult's body weight, or 30% of total-body water (Metheny, 2000). ECF includes intravascular and interstitial fluids. Intravascular fluid, or plasma, is the liquid component of the blood (ie, fluid found within the vascular system). Interstitial fluid is the fluid that surrounds tissue cells and includes lymph.

The term total-body water or fluid refers to the total amount of water in the body expressed as a percentage of body weight.

Figure 46-1A illustrates the components of total-body fluid; Figure 46-1B shows body fluid distribution on the microscopic level.

Variations in Fluid Content

In a healthy person, total-body water constitutes about 50% to 60% of the body's weight, depending on such factors as the person's age, lean body mass, and sex. Table 46-1 illustrates age-related differences in total-body water and in the various water compartments of the body. For example, an infant has considerably more total-body fluid and ECF than an adult does. Because ECF is more easily lost from the body than ICF, infants are more prone to fluid volume deficits.

Consider Jeremiah Kearny, the 7-month-old infant described at the beginning of the chapter. The nurse would need to incorporate knowledge of these age-related differences when developing Jeremiah's plan of care. In addition, the nurse would incorporate this knowledge when assessing the child, being especially alert for signs and symptoms of deficient fluid volume due to the loss of ECF.

Total-body water also differs by sex and the person's amount of fat cells. Fat cells contain little water while lean tissue is rich in water. Thus, the more obese a person is, the smaller the person's percentage of total body water is when compared with body weight. Because women tend to have proportionally more body fat than men, they also have less body fluid than men. Similarly, the decreasing percentage of body fluid in older people is related to an increase in fat cells.

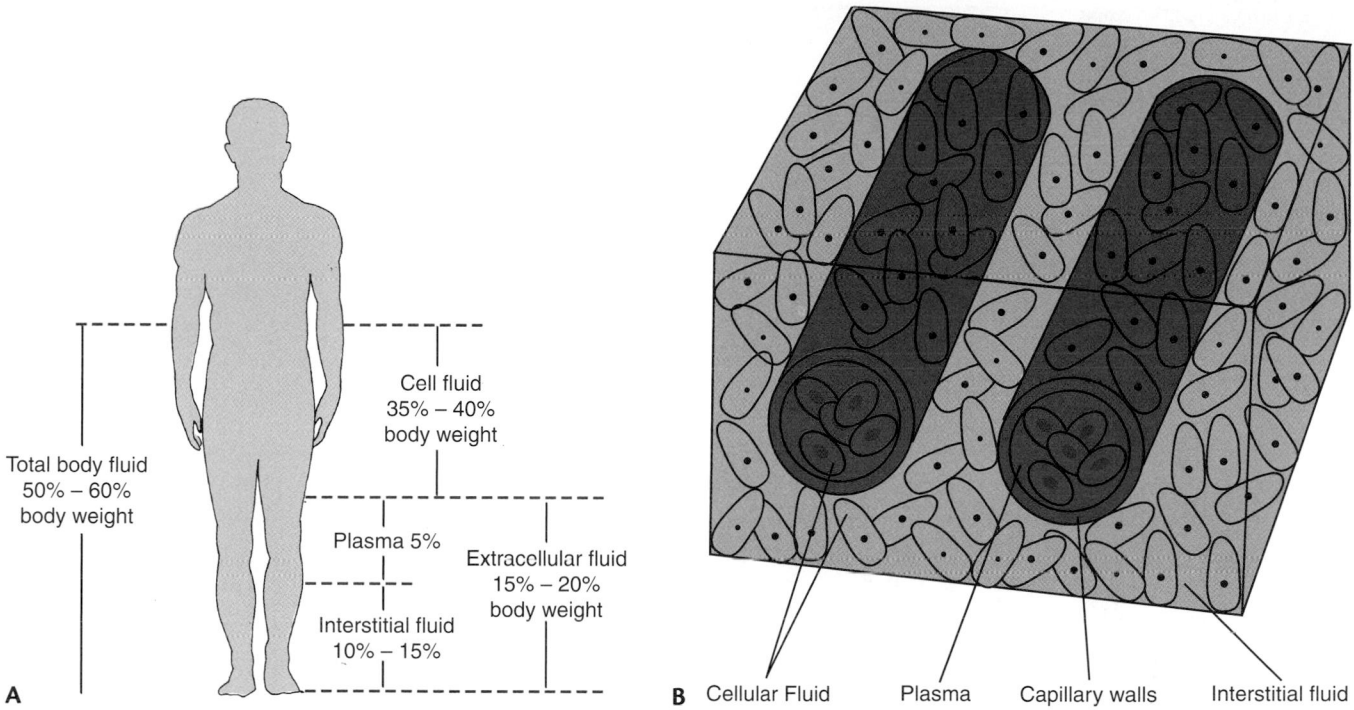

FIGURE 46-1 (A) Total body fluid represents 50% to 60% of body weight of a normal adult. **(B)** Microscopic visualization of body fluid distribution.

Electrolytes

Certain compounds dissociate in solution or separate into simpler molecules to form ions. An **ion** is an atom or molecule carrying an electrical charge. Substances capable of breaking into electrically charged ions when dissolved in a solution are called **electrolytes.** Some ions develop a positive charge and are called **cations.** Others develop a negative charge and are called **anions.** These charges are the basis of chemical interactions in the body necessary for metabolism and other functions. There are many different electrolytes in the body. The most common ones are highlighted in Table 46-2.

Other electrolytes also are present in the body. Sulfate, an anion, is found primarily within cells. The organic acid anions such as lactic acid, which is a major anion, normally have an intermediary role in cell metabolism. The anion proteinate functions in the process of diffusion to move substances to and from the capillaries. Plasma proteins include albumin, globulin, and fibrinogen. Other electrolytes are required for proper cell functioning but are found only in trace amounts in the body. One example is chromium. A well-balanced diet ordinarily ensures an adequate supply of required trace substances in the body.

Molecules in the body's chemical compounds that remain intact are called nonelectrolytes. In the human body, for example, urea and glucose are nonelectrolytes. **Solvents** are liquids that hold a substance in solution; **solutes** are substances that are dissolved in a solution. Water is the primary solvent in the body. The solutes are electrolytes and nonelectrolytes.

Fluids in various compartments of the body differ in their constituents. For example, ICF has higher concentrations of certain electrolytes than ECF. Figure 46-2 illustrates differences in the electrolyte composition of body fluids according to the compartments in which the fluids are found.

Measurement of Electrolytes

Electrolytes are measured in terms of their chemical combining power, or chemical activity. The milliequivalent (mEq) is the unit of measure that describes the chemical activity of electrolytes. One milliequivalent of either a cation or an anion is chemically equivalent to the activity of 1 mg of hydrogen. Therefore, 1 mEq of any cation is equivalent to 1 mEq of any anion.

For homeostasis, the total cations in the body are normally equal to the total anions. In healthy people, the milliequivalents per liter for electrolytes in the body vary within a relatively narrow range. When electrolytes are not in balance, the person is at risk for alterations in health because electrolytes regulate water distribution and acid–base balance, and maintain a balanced degree of neuromuscular excitability.

(text continues on page 1432)

TABLE 46-1 Water as a Percentage of Body Weight

Water Compartment	Infant (%)	Adult (%) Man	Adult (%) Woman	Elderly Person (%)
Extracellular				
Intravascular	4	4	5	5
Interstitial	25	11	10	15
Intracellular	48	45	35	25
Total-body water	77	60	50	45

TABLE 46-2 Major Electrolytes

Electrolyte	Functions	Sources and Losses	Regulation
Sodium (Na^+): chief electrolyte of ECF that moves easily between intravascular and interstitial spaces and moves across cell membranes by active transport; influential in many chemical reactions in the body, particularly in nervous tissue cells and muscle tissue cells	Controls and regulates the volume of body fluids Maintains water balance throughout the body Is the primary regulator of ECF volume Influences ICF volume Participates in the generation and transmission of nerve impulses Is an essential electrolyte in the sodium–potassium pump	The average daily requirements for sodium not known Precisely: 2,400 mg (approx. 1 tsp) as the Daily Value cited on the Nutrition Facts label; RDA for sodium for adults about 500 mg, or 0.5 g Sodium found in many foods; typically present in large amounts, particularly in bacon, ham, sausage, catsup, mustard, relish, processed cheese, canned vegetables, bread, cereal, and salted snack foods; also in table salt (sodium chloride; about 46% sodium) Sodium excesses eliminated primarily by the kidneys; small amounts lost in feces and perspiration	Sodium normally maintained in the body within a relatively narrow range; deviations quickly resulting in a serious health problem Sodium concentrations affected by salt, as well as water, intake Sodium conserved through reabsorption in the kidneys, a process stimulated by aldosterone The normal extracellular concentration of sodium: 135–145 mEq/L (mmol/L).
Potassium (K^+): major cation of ICF working in reciprocal fashion with sodium (eg, an excessive intake of sodium resulting in an excretion of potassium, and vice versa)	Is the chief regulator of cellular enzyme activity and cellular water content Plays a vital role in such processes as the transmission of electric impulses, particularly in nerve, heart, skeletal, intestinal, and lung tissue; protein and carbohydrate metabolism; and cellular building Assists in regulation of acid–base balance by cellular exchange with H^+	The average daily requirements not known precisely; an intake of 50 to 100 mEq daily enough to maintain K^+ balance Adequate quantities usually in a well-balanced diet Leading food sources: bananas, peaches, kiwi, figs, dates, apricots, oranges, prunes, melons, raisins, broccoli, and potatoes. Meat and dairy products also with adequate amounts of potassium Potassium excreted primarily by the kidneys (no effective method of conserving potassium); deficits occur if potassium excretion in excess without being replaced simultaneously. Gastrointestinal (GI) secretions containing potassium in large quantities; also some in perspiration and saliva	Conservation of cellular K^+ by the sodium pump (described later in the chapter) when Na^+ is excluded; conservation by kidneys when cellular K^+ decreased. Aldosterone secretion triggering K^+ excretion in urine Normal range for serum potassium: 3.5 to 5 mEq/L
Calcium (Ca^{2+}): most abundant electrolyte in the body, with up to 99% of the total amount of calcium in the body found in bones and teeth in ionized form; close link between concentrations of calcium and phosphorus	Is necessary for nerve impulse transmission and blood clotting Is a catalyst for muscle contraction Is needed for vitamin B_{12} absorption and for its use by body cells Acts as a catalyst for many cell chemical activities	Average daily requirement about 1 g for adults; higher amounts according to body weight required for children and pregnant and lactating women Consumption of 1,500 mg/day recommended for older adults, particularly postmenopausal women and men older than 65 years of age	Increased secretion of parathyroid hormone (PTH), to increase the release of calcium from bones into the blood and to increase reabsorption from kidneys and intestine when ECF levels are decreased

Electrolyte	Functions	Sources/Requirements	Regulation and Levels
(Calcium)	Is necessary for strong bones and teeth; Determines the thickness and strength of cell membranes	Sources including milk, cheese, and dried beans; some present in meats and vegetables; The use of calcium stimulated by vitamin D; most active form of vitamin D (calcitriol) responsible for promoting calcium absorption and limiting calcium excretion when levels are inadequate; Movement out of bones and teeth to maintain normal blood calcium levels, if necessary. Excretion via urine, feces, bile, digestive secretions, and perspiration	A high serum phosphate concentration, resulting in decreased serum calcium level; a low serum phosphate concentration leading to increased serum calcium; Calcitonin, a hormone secreted by the thyroid gland, exerting an effect on calcium opposite that of PTH. Increases in calcitonin resulting in reduced serum calcium concentration primarily by opposing osteoclast bone resorption
Magnesium (Mg^{2+}): most of cation magnesium found within body cells—heart, bone, nerve, and muscle tissues; second most important cation in the ICF	Is important for the metabolism of carbohydrates and proteins; Is important for many vital reactions involving enzymes; Is necessary for protein and DNA synthesis, DNA and RNA transcription, and translation of RNA; Maintains normal intracellular levels of potassium; Helps maintain electrical activity in nervous tissue membranes and muscle membranes	The average daily adult requirement about 18–30 mEq, with children requiring larger amounts; Magnesium found in vegetables, nuts, fish, whole grains, peas, and beans	Intestinal absorption and excretion by kidneys; Plasma concentrations of magnesium ranging from 1.3–2.1 mEq/L, with about one third of that amount bound to plasma proteins
Chloride (Cl^-): chief extracellular anion, found in blood, interstitial fluid, and lymph and in minute amounts in ICF	Acts with sodium to maintain the osmotic pressure of the blood; Plays a role in the body's acid–base balance; Has important buffering action when oxygen and carbon dioxide exchange in red blood cells; Is essential for the production of hydrochloric acid in gastric juices	The average daily requirements of chloride unknown; Found in foods high in sodium, dairy products, and meat	Normally paired with sodium; exerted and conserved with sodium by the kidneys; Chloride deficits leading to potassium deficits, and vice versa; Normal serum chloride levels: from 95–105 mEq/L (mmol/L)
Bicarbonate (HCO_3^-): an anion that is the major chemical base buffer within the body; found in both ECF and ICF	Is essential for acid–base balance; bicarbonate and carbonic acid constitute the body's primary buffer system	Losses possible via diarrhea, diuretics, and early renal insufficiency; excess possible via overingestion of acid neutralizers, such as sodium bicarbonate	Bicarbonate levels regulated primarily by the kidneys; Bicarbonate readily available as a result of carbon dioxide formation during metabolism; Normal bicarbonate levels ranging between 25–29 mEq/L (mmol/L)
Phosphate (PO_4^-): the major anion in body cells; a buffer anion in both ICF and ECF	Helps maintain the body's acid–base balance; Is involved in important chemical reactions in the body; eg, phosphorus is necessary for many B vitamins to be effective, helps promote nerve and muscle action, and plays a role in carbohydrate metabolism; Is important for cell division and for the transmission of hereditary traits	Average daily requirements for phosphorus similar to those for calcium; Found in most foods but especially in beef, pork, and dried peas and beans; Metabolism the same as calcium	Regulation by PTH and by activated vitamin D; Calcium and phosphate inversely proportional; an increase in one results in a decrease in the other; Normal range of phosphate: 2.5 to 4.5 mEq/L (mmol/L)

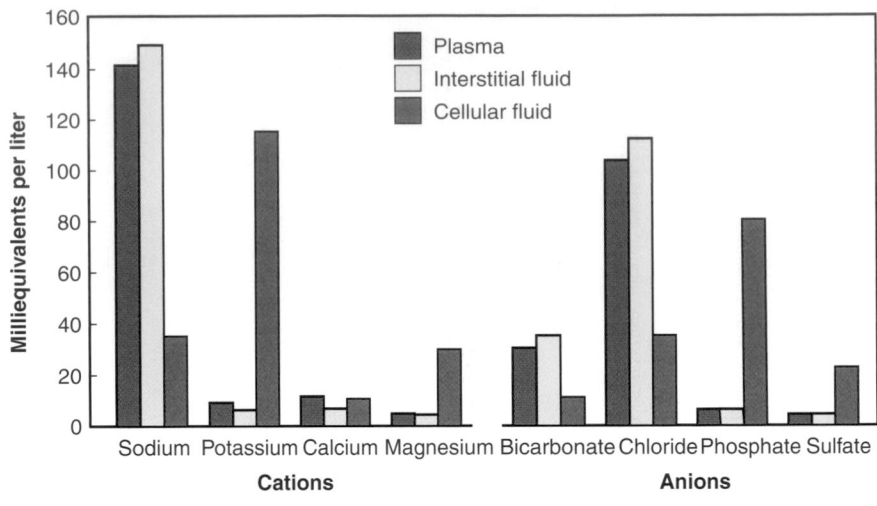

FIGURE 46-2 Electrolyte composition of body fluids according to compartment.

Consider Grace Gilligan, the young woman described in the Reflective Practice display. The nurse would need to be alert for electrolyte imbalances and possible acid–base imbalance due to the loss of gastric secretions from vomiting.

Fluid and Electrolyte Movement

The ECF provides nourishment to each body cell and receives each cell's waste products. These exchanges, which normally result in fluid balance and homeostasis, are essential to life. The most common routes for transporting materials to and from intracellular compartments are osmosis, diffusion, active transport, and filtration, described in the following sections.

Osmosis

Cell membranes are semipermeable, making it possible for water, a pure solvent, to be transported through cell walls. **Osmosis** is the major method of transporting body fluids. Water shifts and thus balance depends heavily on this route of transport.

Through the process of osmosis, the solvent, water, passes from an area of lesser solute concentration to an area of greater solute concentration until equilibrium is established. As a result, the volume of the more concentrated solution increases, and the volume of the weaker solution decreases. The greater the difference in the concentration of the two solutions on each side of a semipermeable membrane, the greater the osmotic pressure or drawing power of water.

The concentration of particles in a solution, or its pulling power, is referred to as the **osmolarity** of a solution. A solution that has about the same concentration of particles, or osmolarity, as plasma (between 275–295 mOsm/L) is considered an **isotonic** solution. An isotonic fluid remains in the intravascular compartment without any net flow across the semipermeable membrane. In contrast, a **hypertonic** solution has a greater osmolarity than plasma (>295 mOsm/L), whereas a **hypotonic** solution has less osmolarity than plasma (<275 mOsm/L). Because a hypertonic solution has a greater

osmolarity, water moves out of the cells and is drawn into the intravascular compartment, causing the cells to shrink. Due to a lower osmolarity, a hypotonic solution in the intravascular space moves out of the intravascular space and into intracellular fluid, causing cells to swell and possibly burst. Figure 46-3 illustrates the process of osmosis.

Diffusion

Diffusion is the tendency of solutes to move freely throughout a solvent. The solute moves from an area of higher concentration to an area of lower concentration (ie, "downhill")

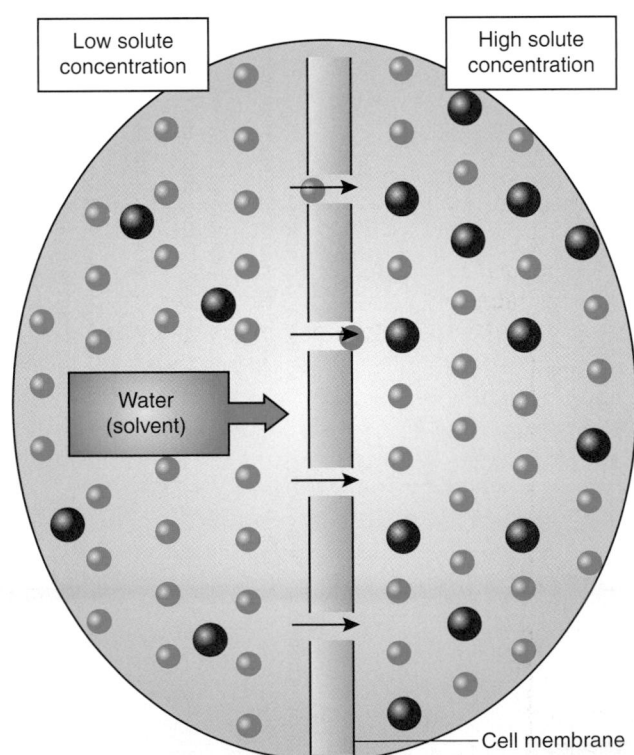

FIGURE 46-3 Body fluids are transported through cell membranes through the process of osmosis. Water, a solvent, moves from an area of lesser solute concentration to one of greater solute concentration, until equilibrium is established.

until equilibrium is established. Gases also move by diffusion. Oxygen and carbon dioxide exchange in the lung's alveoli and capillaries occurs by diffusion.

Active Transport

Active transport is a process that requires energy for the movement of substances through a cell membrane from an area of lesser solute concentration to an area of higher solute concentration. Adenosine triphosphate released from a cell makes it possible for certain substances to acquire energy needed to pass through the cell membrane. Although this process is not entirely understood, the energy requirements for active transport are affected by characteristics of the cell membrane, specific enzymes, and concentrations of ions. This process explains the so-called pump mechanism. If diffusion can be called "coasting downhill," active transport can be called "pumping uphill." Substances believed to use active transport include amino acids, glucose (in certain places only, such as in the kidneys and intestines), and ions of sodium, chloride, potassium, hydrogen, phosphate, calcium, and magnesium.

Filtration

Filtration is the passage of fluid through a permeable membrane. Passage is from an area of high pressure to one of lower pressure.

Certain substances, such as plasma proteins, which have high molecular weights, exert **colloid osmotic pressure,** or oncotic pressure, on permeable membranes in the body. **Hydrostatic pressure** is a force exerted by a fluid against the container wall. Blood hydrostatic pressure is the pressure of plasma and blood cells in the capillaries: it depends primarily on arterial blood pressure on the arteriolar side of capillaries, and on venous blood pressure on the venular side of capillaries. Filtration pressure is the difference between colloid osmotic pressure and blood hydrostatic pressure.

These pressures are important in understanding how fluid leaves arterioles, enters the interstitial compartment, and eventually returns to the venules. The filtration pressure is positive in the arterioles, helping to force or filter fluids into interstitial spaces; it is negative in the venules and thus helps fluid enter the venules. This is illustrated in Figure 46-4. Filtration is also involved in the proper functioning of the glomeruli of the kidneys.

Fluid Balance

The desirable amount of fluid intake and loss in adults ranges from 1500 to 3500 mL each 24 hours, with most people averaging 2500 mL per day. Although these figures are helpful guidelines, the individual's health state as well as balance between actual intake and loss must be considered when assessing nursing needs. A person's intake should normally be approximately balanced by output or fluid loss. A general rule is that in healthy adults, the output of urine normally approximates the ingestion of liquids, and the water from food and oxidation is balanced by the water loss through the feces, the skin, and the respiratory process. The intake–output balance may not always occur in a single 24-hour period but should normally be achieved within 2 to 3 days.

Fluid Sources

Water for the body derives from several sources, including ingested liquids, food, and metabolism.

Ingested Liquids

The ingestion of liquids makes up the largest amount of water normally taken into the body. Fluid intake is primarily regulated by the thirst mechanism. Located within the hypothalamus, the thirst control center is stimulated by intracellular dehydration and decreased blood volume.

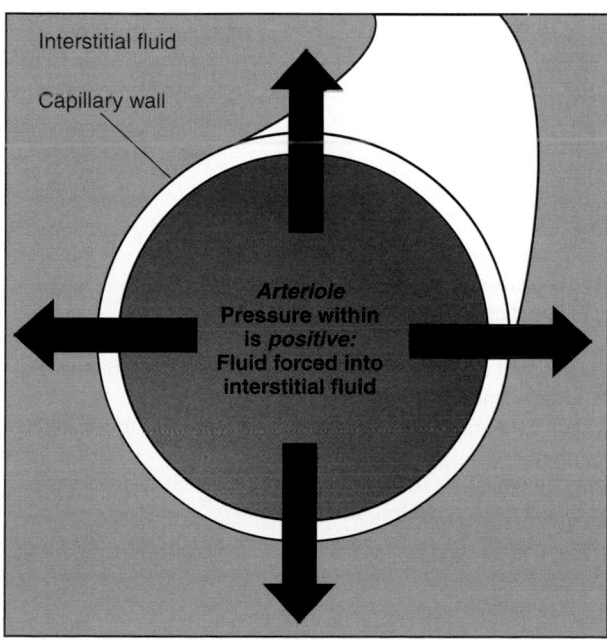

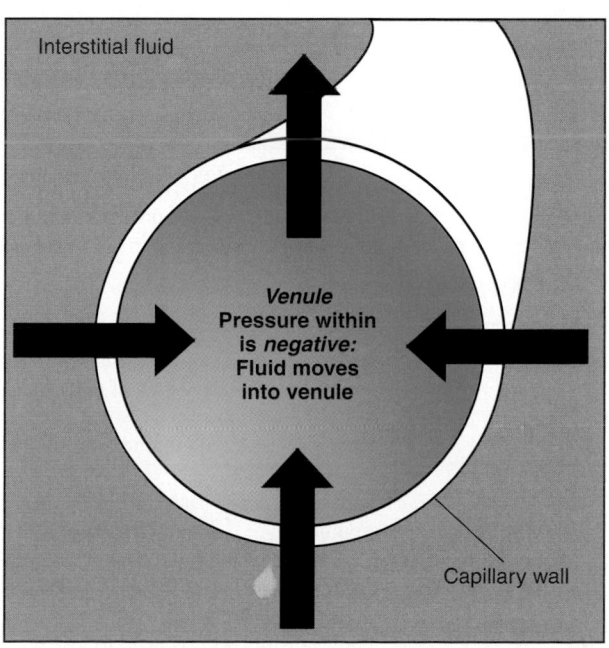

FIGURE 46-4 Filtration.

Water in Food

The water contained in food is the second largest source of water for the body. The amount ingested depends on the diet. For example, melons and citrus fruit are high in water content, whereas cereal and dried fruits have a relatively low water content.

Water From Metabolic Oxidation

Water is an end product of the oxidation that occurs during the metabolism of food substances, specifically, carbohydrates, fats, and protein. This source also varies among different types of nutrients.

Fluid Losses

Water is lost from the body through the kidneys as urine, through the intestinal tract in feces, and through the skin as perspiration. These losses are termed sensible water losses. Insensible water loss, that which is imperceptible also occurs. For example, an invisible amount of water is lost from the skin constantly through evaporation. Insensible loss from the lungs is moisture exhaled in breaths. Water losses vary according to the person and the circumstances.

Generally, fluid intake averages 2600 mL per day, with approximately 1300 mL coming from ingested water, 1000 mL coming from ingested food, and 300 mL from metabolic oxidation. Fluid output averages 2500 to 2900 mL per day, with approximately 1500 mL as urine from the kidneys, 200 to 400 mL as insensible fluid loss from the skin, and 300 to 500 mL as sensible fluid loss from the skin, 400 mL as insensible loss from the lungs, and 100 mL in feces via the GI tract (Fig. 46-5).

Any deviations from normal ranges for a balanced water intake and output should alert the nurse to potential imbalances. The accompanying Promoting Health 46-1: Fluid and Electrolyte Balance reflects on self-care behaviors vital for maintaining a healthy fluid and electrolyte balance.

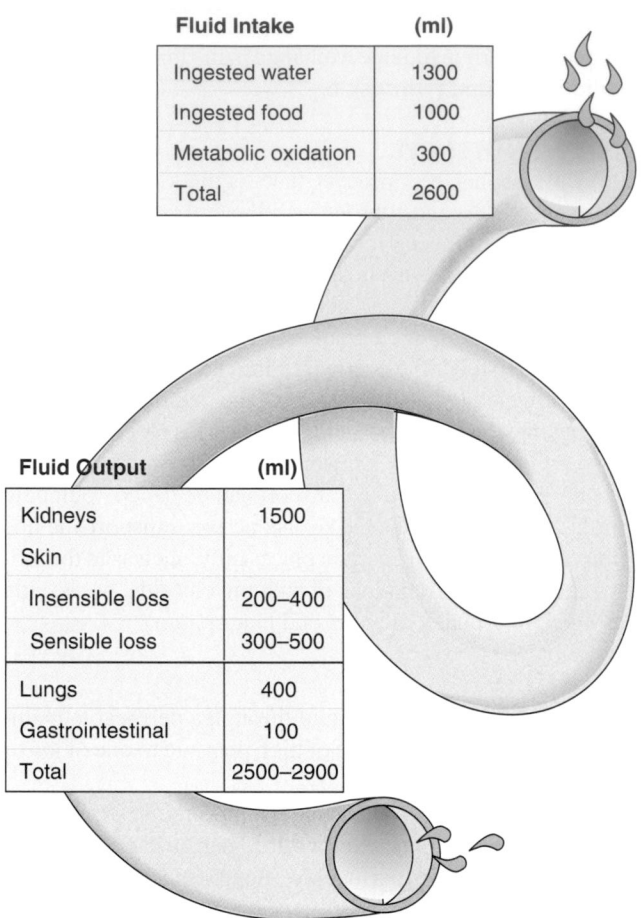

Fluid Intake	(ml)
Ingested water	1300
Ingested food	1000
Metabolic oxidation	300
Total	2600

Fluid Output	(ml)
Kidneys	1500
Skin	
Insensible loss	200–400
Sensible loss	300–500
Lungs	400
Gastrointestinal	100
Total	2500–2900

FIGURE 46-5 In health, fluid intake and fluid losses are about equal. The amounts indicated are average adult daily fluid sources and losses.

Promoting Health 46-1 Fluid and Electrolyte Balance

Use the assessment checklist to determine how well you are meeting fluid and electrolyte needs. Then develop a prescription for self-care by choosing appropriate behaviors from the list of suggestions.

ASSESSMENT CHECKLIST

almost always / sometimes / almost never

1. I drink six to eight glasses of water every day.
2. I am aware of early signs of dehydration or fluid retention.
3. I limit sugar, alcohol, and caffeine in my diet.
4. I am alert for any sudden variations in my weight.
5. I am aware of fluid and electrolyte imbalances that may be associated with intake of certain medications.
6. I diet sensibly when I need to lose weight.

SELF-CARE BEHAVIORS

1. Consume about 1½ quarts of water daily.
2. Maintain normal body weight.
3. Avoid consuming excess amounts of products high in salt, sugar, and caffeine.
4. Limit alcohol intake because of its diuretic effect.
5. Obtain medical evaluation for any ongoing indications of fluid imbalance.
6. Monitor side effects of medications, especially diuresis and diarrhea.
7. Identify situations of high risk for fluid and electrolyte imbalance and intervene appropriately.

Homeostatic Mechanisms

Fluid homeostasis normally functions automatically and effectively. Almost every organ and system in the body helps in some way to maintain fluid homeostasis. The following sections describe the primary organs of homeostasis. Their functions are highlighted in Table 46-3. Fluid balance is threatened when any organ fails to function properly.

- The kidneys, frequently referred to as the master chemists of the body, normally filter 170 L of plasma daily in the adult, while excreting only 1.5 L of urine; selectively retain electrolytes and water and excrete wastes and excesses.
- The cardiovascular system is responsible for pumping and carrying nutrients and water throughout the body.
- The lungs regulate oxygen and carbon dioxide levels of the blood; regulation of the carbon dioxide level is especially crucial in maintaining acid–base balance (see discussion later in this chapter).
- The adrenal glands secrete aldosterone, a hormone that helps the body conserve sodium, helps save chloride and water, and causes potassium to be excreted.
- Thyroxine, released by the thyroid gland, increases blood flow in the body, leading to increased renal circulation, and resulting in increased glomerular filtration and urinary output.
- The parathyroid glands secrete parathyroid hormone, which regulates the level of calcium in ECF.
- The GI tract absorbs water and nutrients that enter the body through this route.
- The nervous system, acting as a switchboard to inhibit and stimulate mechanisms that influence fluid balance, functions chiefly as the regulator of sodium and water intake and excretion.
  - Thirst center is located in the hypothalamus, and the posterior lobe of the pituitary gland stores antidiuretic hormone (ADH), a hormone manufactured in the hypothalamus.
  - Neurons, called osmoreceptors, are sensitive to changes in the concentration of ECF, sending appropriate impulses to the pituitary to release ADH or inhibit its release.

Acid–Base Balance

Body fluids must maintain an acid–base balance to sustain health and life. Acidity or alkalinity of a solution is determined by its concentration of hydrogen ions (H^+). An **acid** is a substance containing hydrogen ions that can be liberated or released. An alkali, or **base,** is a substance that can accept or trap hydrogen ions.

An acid releases hydrogen, as follows:

$$\underset{\substack{\text{Carbonic}\\\text{acid}}}{H_2CO_3} \underset{\text{releases}}{\rightarrow} \underset{\substack{\text{hydrogen}\\\text{ion}}}{H^+} \underset{\text{to form}}{+} \underset{\substack{\text{bicarbonate}\\\text{base}}}{HCO_3^-}$$

A base traps hydrogen, as follows:

$$\underset{\substack{\text{Bicarbonate}\\\text{base}}}{HCO_3^-} \underset{\text{traps}}{+} \underset{\substack{\text{hydrogen}\\\text{ion}}}{H^+} \underset{\text{to form}}{\rightarrow} \underset{\substack{\text{Carbonic}\\\text{acid}}}{H_2CO_3}$$

An acid that is strong dissociates (separates) completely in solution and releases all of its hydrogen ions, whereas a weak acid releases only a small number. A base that binds or accepts hydrogen ions easily is considered a strong base, whereas one that accepts hydrogen ions less readily is considered weak.

The unit of measure used to describe acid–base balance is **pH,** which is an expression of hydrogen ion concentration and the resulting acidity or alkalinity of a substance. The pH scale ranges from 1 to 14. A neutral solution measures 7; an example is pure water. Because pH is based on a negative logarithm, as the hydrogen ions increase and a solution becomes more acid, the pH becomes less than 7. When the concentration of hydrogen ions in a solution is reduced or accepted by another substance, the solution is alkaline, and the pH is greater than 7. Gastric secretions that are strongly acidic have an approximate pH of 1 to 1.3, whereas strongly alkaline pancreatic secretions have an approximate pH of 10.

Normal blood plasma is slightly alkaline and has a normal pH range of 7.35 to 7.45. When the blood plasma pH exceeds the normal pH range in either direction, the person develops signs and symptoms of illness, and if the condition goes on unabated, death results. **Acidosis** is the condition characterized by an excess of hydrogen ions in ECF in which the pH falls below 7.35. **Alkalosis** occurs when there is a lack of hydrogen ions and the pH exceeds 7.45. Figure 46-6 illustrates normal pH, acidosis, and alkalosis and shows the points at which death typically occurs.

The narrow range of normal pH is achieved through three major homeostatic regulators of hydrogen ions: (1) buffer systems, (2) respiratory mechanisms, and (3) renal mechanisms. A **buffer** is a substance that prevents body fluids from becoming overly acidic or alkaline. The body has three buffer systems: (1) the carbonic acid–sodium bicarbonate buffer system, (2) the phosphate buffer system, and (3) the protein buffer system, as described in the following sections.

Buffer Systems

Carbonic Acid–Sodium Bicarbonate Buffer System

The most important buffer system of the body is the carbonic acid–sodium bicarbonate system. This system buffers up to 90% of the H^+ of ECF. Buffers either act like a base and bind or soak up free hydrogen ions or act like an acid and release hydrogen ions when too few are present in a solution. Buffers attempt to bring a body fluid as close as possible to the pH of normal body fluid (7.35–7.45).

The ratio of carbonic acid (H_2CO_3), the most common acid in human body fluid, to the body's most common base, bicarbonate (HCO_3^-), is important for acid–base balance. Normal ECF has a ratio of 20 parts bicarbonate to 1 part carbonic acid. The exact quantities are unimportant for acid–base balance as long as they remain in a 20:1 ratio. Carbonic acid and bicarbonate must be carefully controlled to maintain this ratio; if either is increased or decreased, the 20:1 ratio is no longer in effect.

TABLE 46-3 Homeostatic Mechanisms That Maintain the Composition and Volume of Body Fluid Within Narrow Limits of Normal

Organs of Homeostasis	Functions
Kidneys	• Regulate extracellular fluid (ECF) volume and osmolality by selective retention and excretion of body fluids • Regulate electrolyte levels in the ECF by selective retention of needed substances and excretion of unneeded substances • Regulate pH of ECF by excretion or retention of hydrogen ions • Excrete metabolic wastes (primarily acids) and toxic substances
Heart and blood vessels	• Circulate blood through the kidneys under sufficient pressure for urine to form (pumping action of the heart) • React to hypovolemia by stimulating fluid retention (stretch receptors in the atria and blood vessels)

Lungs	• Eliminate about 13,000 mEq of hydrogen ions (H^+) daily, as opposed to only 40 to 80 mEq excreted daily by the kidneys
	• Act promptly to correct metabolic acid–base disturbances; regulate H^+ concentration (pH) by controlling the level of carbon dioxide (CO_2) in the extracellular fluid as follows:
	  1. Metabolic alkalosis causes compensatory hypoventilation, resulting in CO_2 retention (increases acidity of the extracellular fluid).
	  2. Metabolic acidosis causes compensatory hyperventilation, resulting in CO_2 excretion (decreases acidity of the extracellular fluid).
	• Remove approximately 300 mL of water daily through exhalation (insensible water loss) in the normal adult

Adrenal glands	• Regulate blood volume and sodium and potassium balance by secreting aldosterone, a mineral corticoid secreted by the adrenal cortex
	  1. The primary regulator of aldosterone appears to be angiotensin II, which is produced by the renin–angiotensin system. A decrease in blood volume triggers this system and increases aldosterone secretion, which causes sodium retention (and thus water retention) and potassium loss.
	  2. Decreased secretion of aldosterone causes sodium and water loss and potassium retention.
	• Cortisol, another adrenocortical hormone, has only a fraction of the potency of aldosterone.
	• However, secretion of cortisol in large quantities can produce sodium and water retention and potassium deficit.

Pituitary gland	• Stores and releases the antidiuretic hormone (ADH), which makes the body retain water; functions of ADH include:
	  1. Maintains osmotic pressure of the cells by controlling renal water retention or excretion
	    a. When osmotic pressure of the ECF is greater than that of the cells (as in hypernatremia—excess sodium—or hyperglycemia), ADH secretion is increased, causing renal retention of water.
	    b. When osmotic pressure of the ECF is less than that of the cells (as in hyponatremia), ADH secretion is decreased, causing renal excretion of water.
	  2. Controls blood volume (less influential than aldosterone)
	    a. When blood volume is decreased, an increased secretion of ADH results in water conservation.
	    b. When blood volume is increased, a decreased secretion of ADH results in water loss.

Nervous system	• Inhibits and stimulates mechanisms influencing fluid balance; acts chiefly to regulate sodium and water intake and excretion • Regulates oral intake by sensing intracellular dehydration, which triggers thirst (thirst center located in hypothalamus)

Parathyroid glands	• Regulate calcium (Ca^{2+}) and phosphate (HPO_4^{2-}) balance by means of parathyroid hormone (PTH); PTH influences bone reabsorption, calcium absorption from the intestines, and calcium reabsorption from the renal tubules.
	  1. Increased secretion of PTH causes:
	    a. Elevated serum calcium concentration
	    b. Lowered serum phosphate concentration
	  2. Conversely, decreased secretion of PTH causes:
	    a. Lowered serum calcium concentration
	    b. Elevated serum phosphate concentration

(Data from Metheny, N. M. [2000]. *Fluid and electrolyte balance* [4th ed.]. Philadelphia: Lippincott Williams & Wilkins.)

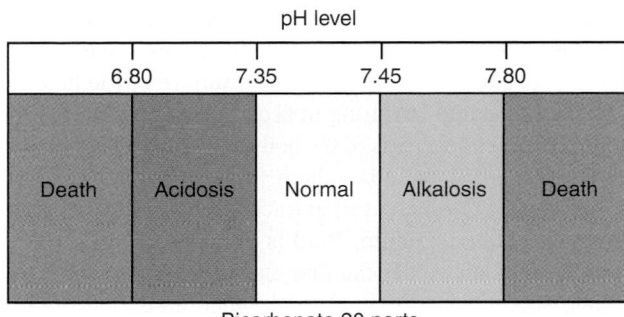

FIGURE 46-6 Acid–base balance. Note that acidosis is used to describe the condition when the pH falls below 7.35, and alkalosis describes a pH above 7.45. When the normal pH is exceeded in either direction, death can occur.

Phosphate Buffer System

The phosphate buffer system is active in intracellular fluids. It converts alkaline sodium phosphate (Na_2HPO_4), a weak base, to acid–sodium phosphate (NaH_2PO_4) in the kidneys.

Protein Buffer System

The third buffer system is a mixture of plasma proteins and the globin portion of hemoglobin in red blood cells. Because plasma proteins and hemoglobin possess chemical groups that can combine with or liberate hydrogen ions, they tend to minimize changes in pH and serve as excellent buffering agents over a wide range of pH values. For example, excess hydrogen ions in the blood cross over the plasma membrane of red blood cells and bind to the hemoglobin molecules that are plentiful in each red blood cell.

Respiratory Control of H⁺ Balance

The lungs are the primary controller of the body's carbonic acid supply. Due to the huge surface area from which CO_2 can readily diffuse, the lungs can bring about rapid changes in H⁺ when needed. Carbon dioxide, constantly produced by cellular metabolism (carbonic acid [H_2CO_3] yields CO_2 and H_2O), is excreted by exhalation. When the amount of CO_2 in the blood increases, the sensitive respiratory center in the medulla is stimulated to increase the rate and depth of respirations to eliminate more CO_2. As more CO_2 is exhaled, the H_2CO_3 level in the blood decreases, and the pH of the blood becomes more alkaline. When the blood level of CO_2 decreases, the respiratory center decreases the rate and depth of respirations to retain the CO_2 so that carbonic acid can be formed, thereby maintaining the delicate balance. This total respiratory process occurs almost as rapidly as the buffering action in the carbonic acid–sodium bicarbonate system.

Renal Control of H⁺ Balance

The concentration of bicarbonate in the plasma is regulated by the kidneys. Essentially, the kidneys excrete or retain hydrogen ions and form or excrete bicarbonate ions in response to the pH of the blood. In the presence of acidosis, the kidneys excrete hydrogen ions and form and conserve bicarbonate ions, thus raising the pH to the normal range. If alkalosis is present, the kidneys retain hydrogen ions and excrete bicarbonate ions in an effort to return to a balanced state.

Acid–base regulation by the kidneys occurs more slowly than that which occurs by the carbonic acid–sodium bicarbonate system or by respiratory regulation. It may take up to 3 days for a normal fluid pH to be restored by the kidneys. The pH of urine varies, depending on the ions that are being excreted, but generally it is between 4.5 and 8.2.

DISTURBANCES IN FLUID, ELECTROLYTE, AND ACID–BASE BALANCE

Nurses commonly encounter disturbances in fluid, electrolyte, and acid–base balance while caring for acutely or chronically ill patients. Although many of these disturbances are interrelated and may occur together, they are described here separately for learning purposes.

Fluid Imbalances

Fluid imbalances occur when the body's compensatory mechanisms are unable to maintain a homeostatic state. Fluid imbalances involve either the volume or distribution of water or electrolytes.

Fluid Volume Deficit

Fluid volume deficit can be caused by a deficiency in the amount of both water and electrolytes in the ECF when the water and electrolyte proportions remain near normal. The state is commonly known as **hypovolemia.** Both osmotic and hydrostatic pressure changes force the interstitial fluid into the intravascular space. As the interstitial space is depleted, its fluid becomes hypertonic, and cellular fluid is then drawn into the interstitial space, leaving cells without adequate fluid to function properly.

The term dehydration is sometimes used as a synonym for hypovolemia, but this is technically inaccurate. **Dehydration** refers only to a decreased volume of water, but water is not decreased without electrolyte changes also. The term hydration refers to the union of a substance with water and is often used to indicate that there is normal water volume in the body.

Fluid volume deficits result from the loss of body fluids, especially if fluid intake is simultaneously decreased. Table 46-7 later in the chapter summarizes fluid volume deficits, common assessments, and general nursing interventions.

Young children, elderly people, and people who are ill are especially at risk for hypovolemia. A weight loss of 5% in adults and 10% in infants can occur rapidly. A 5% weight loss is considered a pronounced fluid deficit; an 8% loss or more is considered severe. A 15% weight loss caused by fluid deficiency usually is life-threatening.

Recall Jeremiah Kearny, the infant with nausea and vomiting for the past 2 days? His assessment reveals that his oral intake has been minimal, further compounding his risk for deficient fluid volume. Weighing the infant would be a key nursing intervention to determine Jeremiah's extent of fluid loss.

Third-space fluid shift refers to a distributional shift of body fluids into potential body spaces such as the pleural, peritoneal, pericardial, or joint cavities; the bowel; or the interstitial space (plasma-to-interstitial shift). Once trapped in these spaces, the fluid is not easily exchanged with ECF. With third-space fluid shift, a deficit in ECF volume occurs. The fluid has not been lost but is trapped in another body space for a period of time and is essentially unavailable for use. A third-space shift may occur as a result of a severe burn, a bowel obstruction, or pancreatitis. Decreased body weight does not occur as it does with an ECF volume deficit (vomiting or diarrhea), nor can the fluid loss be measured (Metheny, 2000). Treatment is directed toward correction of the cause of the third-space shift, or third-spacing, as it is commonly called.

Fluid Volume Excess

Excessive retention of water and sodium in ECF in near-normal proportions results in a condition termed fluid volume excess. It is also called **hypervolemia.** The term overhydration is commonly used as a synonym for hypervolemia, but strictly speaking, this is inaccurate. **Overhydration** refers only to above-normal amounts of water in extracellular spaces. Common causes include malfunction of the kidneys, causing an inability to excrete the excesses, and failure of the heart to function as a pump, resulting in accumulation of fluid in the lungs and dependent parts of the body. When water is retained in excessive amounts, so is sodium.

Because of the increased extracellular osmotic pressure from the retained sodium, fluid is pulled from the cells to equalize the tonicity. By the time the intracellular and extracellular spaces are isotonic to each other, an excess of both water and sodium is in the ECF, whereas the cells are nearly depleted. The excessive ECF may accumulate in tissue spaces; this is known as **edema.** Edema can be observed around the eyes, fingers, ankles, and sacral space, and can also accumulate in or around body organs.

Remember Jack Soo Park, the patient who inadvertently received too much IV fluid? In Mr. Park's case, fluid accumulation involved his lungs and heart, exhibited by his bounding pulse, distended neck veins, and abnormal lung sounds.

It may result in a weight gain in excess of 5%. The amount or severity of edema is typically graded (Fig. 46-7). When the

1+ Pitting Edema

- Slight indentation (2 mm)
- Normal contours
- Associated with interstitial fluid volume 30% above normal

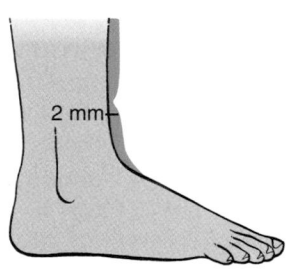

2+ Pitting Edema

- Deeper pit after pressing (4 mm)
- Lasts longer than 1+
- Fairly normal contour

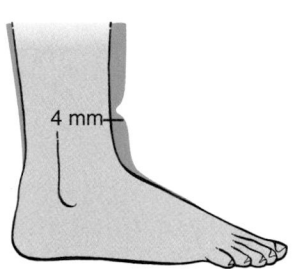

3+ Pitting Edema

- Deep pit (6 mm)
- Remains several seconds after pressing
- Skin swelling obvious by general inspection

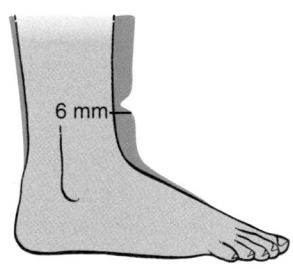

4+ Pitting Edema

- Deep pit (8 mm)
- Remains for a prolonged time after pressing, possibly minutes
- Frank swelling

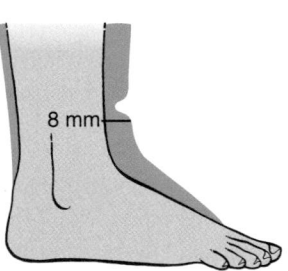

Brawny Edema

- Fluid can no longer be displaced secondary to excessive interstitial fluid accumulation
- No pitting
- Tissue palpates as firm or hard
- Skin surface shiny, warm, moist

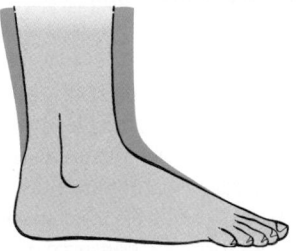

FIGURE 46-7 System for grading edema.

excess fluid remains in the intravascular space, the concentration of solids in the blood is decreased.

Interstitial-to-plasma shift is the movement of fluid from the space surrounding the cells to the blood. This shift, also called hypervolemia, is a compensatory response to volume or osmotic pressure changes of the intravascular fluid. Although the body attempts to maintain normal balance in all fluid spaces, the intravascular fluid is usually protected at the expense of interstitial fluid and ICF.

Electrolyte Imbalances

Electrolyte imbalances commonly involve a deficit or excess of the electrolyte. When patients present with deficits or excesses of sodium, potassium, calcium, magnesium, or phosphate, careful nursing assessment depends on an understanding of the effects of these imbalances.

Hyponatremia and Hypernatremia

Hyponatremia refers to a sodium deficit in ECF caused by a loss of sodium or a gain of water. Osmotic pressure changes result in ECF moving into the cells. When this occurs, prints from the examiner's fingers tend to remain on the patient's skin over the sternum when pressure is applied with the fingers. The phenomenon results from tissue plasticity as fluid moves into cells in excess amounts. **Hypernatremia** refers to a surplus of sodium in ECF that can result from excess water loss or an overall excess of sodium. Because of the increased extracellular osmotic pressure, fluids move from the cells, leaving them without sufficient fluid.

Hypokalemia and Hyperkalemia

Hypokalemia refers to a potassium deficit in ECF. When the extracellular potassium level falls, potassium moves from the cell, creating an intracellular potassium deficiency. Sodium and hydrogen ions are then retained by the cells to maintain isotonic fluids. These electrolyte shifts influence normal cellular functioning, the pH of ECF, and the functions of most body systems. Skeletal muscles are generally the first to demonstrate a potassium deficiency. Typical signs of hypokalemia include muscle weakness and leg cramps. **Hyperkalemia** refers to an excess of potassium in ECF. Although this condition occurs less frequently than hypokalemia, it can be hazardous. The transmission of stimuli through heart muscle is slowed or prevented, and cardiac arrest eventually occurs if hyperkalemia is not corrected.

Hypocalcemia and Hypercalcemia

Hypocalcemia refers to a calcium deficit in ECF. If the condition is prolonged, calcium is taken from the bones, ultimately resulting in osteomalacia, which is characterized by soft and pliable bones. Common signs of hypocalcemia include numbness and tingling of fingers, muscle cramps, and tetany. **Hypercalcemia** refers to an excess of calcium in ECF. Hypercalcemia is an emergency situation because the condition often leads to cardiac arrest.

Hypomagnesemia and Hypermagnesemia

Hypomagnesemia refers to a magnesium deficit. The body's potassium level also drops because the kidneys tend to excrete more potassium when magnesium supplies are poor. As a result, hypomagnesemia and hypokalemia often occur together. **Hypermagnesemia** refers to a magnesium excess. It can occur especially in end-stage renal failure when the kidneys fail to excrete magnesium and excessive amounts are administered therapeutically.

Hypophosphatemia and Hyperphosphatemia

Hypophosphatemia refers to a below-normal serum concentration of inorganic phosphorus. Although this may indicate phosphorus deficiency, multiple factors may lower serum phosphate levels while total-body phosphorus stores are normal. **Hyperphosphatemia** refers to above-normal serum concentrations of inorganic phosphorus.

Acid–Base Imbalances

Arterial blood gases (ABGs) are laboratory tests commonly used in the assessment and treatment of acid–base imbalances. Results from venous blood, in contrast, are only specific for the particular extremity or area where the blood was sampled and do not provide information on how well the lungs are oxygenating the blood. The pH of plasma indicates balance or impending acidosis or alkalosis. In addition, a study of the blood's oxygen and carbon dioxide gases is important. The partial pressures (indicated by "P") of these gases, or their tensions, are determined by the use of a nomogram, which reflects the chemical and physical activities of the two gases. The partial pressure of carbon dioxide is abbreviated $PaCO_2$; for oxygen, it is PaO_2. The "a" indicates an arterial specimen. When the PaO_2 is low, hemoglobin carries less than normal amounts of oxygen; when the PaO_2 is high, the hemoglobin carries more oxygen. Oxygen saturation readings (SaO_2) reveal the percentage of oxygen in the blood that combines with hemoglobin.

The $PaCO_2$ is influenced almost entirely by respiratory activity. When the $PaCO_2$ is low, carbonic acid leaves the body in excessive amounts; when the $PaCO_2$ is high, there are excessive amounts of carbonic acid in the body. Laboratory levels for ABGs are listed in Table 46-4.

Acid–base imbalances occur when the carbonic acid or bicarbonate levels become disproportionate. When there is a sin-

TABLE 46-4 Acid–Base Parameters for Arterial Blood Gas Studies

	Normal	Acid	Base
pH	7.35–7.45	<7.35	>7.45
$PaCO_2$	35–45 mm Hg	>45 mm Hg	<35 mm Hg
HCO_3^-	22–26 mEq/L	<22 mEq/L	>26 mEq/L

gle primary cause, these disturbances are known as respiratory acidosis or alkalosis and metabolic acidosis or alkalosis, which are described in the sections that follow. These disturbances are a result of an upset in acid–base balance, as follows:

- *A respiratory disturbance alters the carbonic acid portion:*
  - Respiratory acidosis and alkalosis are the results of respiratory disturbances.
  - Compensation for a respiratory disturbance occurs when the kidneys attempt to restore balance by either conserving or excreting more bicarbonate.
- *A metabolic disturbance alters the bicarbonate portion:*
  - Metabolic acidosis and alkalosis are almost entirely the result of metabolic processes.
  - The primary organs for compensation with a metabolic disorder are the lungs, which either try to conserve or excrete more carbon dioxide (available in weakly ionized carbonic acid).
  - Although compensation is the body's natural attempt to restore balance, correction may also be required. Correction involves using nursing and medical interventions to promote a return to homeostasis (eg, pharmacologic agents or mechanical ventilation).

Complicated clinical situations may occur when respiratory and metabolic imbalances coexist.

Respiratory Acidosis

Respiratory acidosis is a primary excess of carbonic acid in ECF. Any decrease in alveolar ventilation that results in retention of carbon dioxide can cause respiratory acidosis. Because the lungs are the source of the problem, they are unable to participate in compensation. As the carbonic acid content increases, the kidneys attempt to retain more bicarbonate and increase their hydrogen excretion. Thus:

$$\text{Respiratory acidosis} = \text{high PaCO}_2 \text{ because of alveolar hypoventilation}$$

Respiratory Alkalosis

Respiratory alkalosis is a primary deficit of carbonic acid in ECF. It is the result of increased alveolar ventilation and the consequent decrease in carbon dioxide. An increase in respiratory rate and depth causes the carbon dioxide loss because the carbon dioxide is excreted faster than normal.

Because of the deficit of carbon dioxide, which is a respiratory stimulant sensed in the medulla of the brain, depression or cessation of respirations eventually can occur. Because the lungs are the source of the problem, they are unable to participate in compensation. Therefore, the kidneys attempt to alleviate the imbalance by increasing the bicarbonate excretion and by retaining more hydrogen. Thus:

$$\text{Respiratory alkalosis} = \text{low PaCO}_2 \text{ because of alveolar hyperventilation}$$

Metabolic Acidosis

Metabolic acidosis is a proportionate deficit of bicarbonate in ECF. The deficit can occur as the result of an increase in acid components or an excessive loss of bicarbonate. The lungs attempt to increase the carbon dioxide excretion by increasing the rate and depth of respirations. The kidneys attempt to compensate by retaining bicarbonate and by excreting more hydrogen. If the body is unable to achieve normal balance, the person may lose consciousness as metabolic acidosis increases, and death eventually results. Thus:

$$\text{Metabolic acidosis} = \text{low bicarbonate. Nonvolatile acid is present to use up HCO}_3^- \text{ in disproportionate amounts, or HCO}_3^- \text{ is lost in similar amounts}$$

Metabolic Alkalosis

Metabolic alkalosis is a primary excess of bicarbonate in ECF. This may be the result of excessive acid losses or increased base ingestion or retention. The body attempts to compensate by retaining carbon dioxide. The respirations become slow and shallow, and periods of no breathing may occur. The kidneys attempt to excrete potassium and sodium with the excessive bicarbonate, and retain hydrogen in carbonic acid. Thus:

$$\text{Metabolic alkalosis} = \text{high bicarbonate. Nonvolatile acid is lost and is not using up HCO}_3^- \text{ or HCO}_3^- \text{ is gained in disproportionate amounts}$$

THE NURSING PROCESS FOR FLUID, ELECTROLYTE, AND ACID–BASE BALANCE

Assessing

The pathophysiology underlying acute and chronic illness, trauma, and certain therapeutic interventions may place a patient at high risk for fluid, electrolyte, and acid–base imbalances. Such imbalances can seriously compromise the patient's health status and may prove life-threatening. The nursing assessment is directed toward the following:

- Identifying patients at high risk for fluid, electrolyte, and acid–base imbalance
- Determining that a specific imbalance is present and identifying the nature of the imbalance along with its severity, etiology, and defining characteristics
- Determining the effectiveness of the plan of care

Important assessment parameters include the nursing history and physical assessment, a record of fluid intake and output, daily weights, and laboratory studies.

Nursing History

A comprehensive nursing history includes questions related to the patient's fluid, electrolyte, and acid–base balance. The accompanying Focused Assessment Guide 46-1 includes interview questions helpful in identifying the patient's usual pattern of fluid intake and elimination and the patient's evaluation of

Focused Assessment Guide 46-1

Fluid, Electrolyte, and Acid–Base Balance

Factors to Assess	Questions and Approaches
Usual patterns of fluid intake	Describe the amount and types of fluids you usually drink in a 24-hour period. Have there been any recent changes?
Usual pattern of fluid elimination	Describe your usual voiding/urination habits. Any recent changes in frequency or amount? Is your body losing fluids in any other major way? • Vomiting • Diarrhea • Excessive perspiration • Fistula
Patient's evaluation of hydration status	Do you think there is an approximate balance between your fluid intake and output? Have you noticed any signs that your body is experiencing too much or too little hydration (difficulty breathing, edema, dry skin and mucous membranes, thirst)?
History of disease process	Is there any history of disease process or injury that might disrupt fluid and electrolyte balance (eg, diabetes mellitus, cancer, burns)?
Medication/nutrition history	Do you take any medications or treatments that might disrupt fluid and electrolyte balance (eg, steroids, diuretics, total parenteral nutrition, dialysis)? Have you been trying to lose weight by dieting, using diuretics, laxatives, or diet aids? Have you been following a high-protein, low-carbohydrate diet?
Fluid, electrolyte, and acid–base imbalances and contributing factors	Are you aware of any other fluid balance problems you may be experiencing? • Nature • Onset of problem and frequency • Causes • Severity • Symptoms • Intervention attempted and results

his or her hydration status and awareness of particular problems. Interview questions are also directed toward identifying patients at high risk for imbalances. Risk factors include the following:

- The pathophysiology underlying acute and chronic illnesses (eg, diabetes mellitus, congestive heart failure, renal failure)
- Abnormal losses of body fluids (eg, prolonged or severe vomiting or diarrhea, draining wounds, fistulas). Table 46-5 lists imbalances that result from loss of specific body fluids.
- Burns
- Trauma
- Therapies that may disrupt fluid and electrolyte balance (eg, medications such as diuretics and steroids, treatments such as IV therapy and TPN)

Physical Assessment

Metheny (2000) recommends that the nurse pay attention to certain parameters when assessing a patient's fluid and electrolyte status:

- Comparison of total intake and output of fluids
- Urine volume and concentration
- Skin and tongue turgor
- Degree of moisture in oral cavity
- Body weight
- Thirst
- Tearing and salivation
- Appearance and temperature of skin
- Facial appearance
- Edema (see Fig. 46-7)
- Vital signs
- Neck and hand vein filling
- Results of hemodynamic monitoring (eg, central venous pressure [CVP] and pulmonary artery pressure [PAP])
- Neuromuscular irritability

When an imbalance of particular electrolytes is suspected, the nurse needs to understand that the associated assessment is vital. Table 46-6 presents select nursing considerations for each of these parameters, findings in a healthy adult, and significant findings.

(*text continues on page 1446*)

TABLE 46-5 Imbalances Resulting From Loss of Specific Body Fluid

Fluid Lost	Imbalances Likely to Occur	Fluid Lost	Imbalances Likely to Occur
Gastric juice	Extracellular fluid volume deficit Metabolic alkalosis Sodium deficit Potassium deficit	Pancreatic juice	Metabolic acidosis Sodium deficit Calcium deficit Extracellular fluid volume deficit
	Tetany (if metabolic alkalosis is present)	Sensible perspiration	Extracellular fluid volume deficit Sodium deficit
	Ketosis of starvation Magnesium deficit	Insensible water loss	Water deficit (dehydration) Sodium excess
Intestinal juice	Extracellular fluid volume deficit Metabolic acidosis Sodium deficit Potassium deficit	Wound exudate	Protein deficit Sodium deficit Extracellular fluid volume deficit
Bile	Sodium deficit Metabolic acidosis	Ascites	Protein deficit Sodium deficit Plasma-to-interstitial fluid shift Extracellular fluid volume deficit

TABLE 46-6 Parameters to Be Considered in Clinical Assessment for Fluid, Electrolyte, and Acid–Base Balance

Assessment Parameters	Nursing Considerations	Findings in Healthy Adult	Significant Findings
Comparison of total intake and output of fluids	• Records may be initiated by the nurse for any patient with a real or potential water or electrolyte problem. • Intake should include all fluids taken into the body. • Output should include urine, vomitus, diarrhea, drainage from fistulas, and drainage from suction apparatus. Perspiration and drainage from lesions should be noted and estimated. Prolonged hyperventilation should also be noted because it is an important route of water vapor loss.	• Fluid intake about equals fluid output—when averaged over 2 or 3 days. • Range of 1500–3500 mL fluid intake and loss; 2000 mL is average adult intake and loss per day. • Output of urine normally approximates the ingestion of liquids; water from food and oxidation is balanced by the water loss through feces, the skin, and the respiratory process.	• When the total intake is substantially less than the total output, the patient is in danger of fluid volume deficit. • When the total intake is substantially more than the total output, the patient is in danger of fluid volume excess.

Urine volume and concentration	• All fluid losses are measured according to routes.
	• A device calibrated for small volumes of urine is used when hourly urine volumes need to be measured.
	• Factors that can alter urinary output must be accounted for:
	  1. Amount of fluid intake
	  2. Losses from skin, lungs, and GI tract
	  3. Amount of waste products for excretions
		• Normal urinary output is about 1 mL/kg of body weight per hour (for the average adult: 1500 mL/24 hr, which is equivalent to about 40–80 mL/hr).
		• Stress may diminish the 24-hour urine volume in the adult to 750–1000 mL (or 30–50 mL/hr) because of increased aldosterone and ADH secretion.
			• A low urine volume with a high specific gravity indicates fluid volume deficit.
			• A low urine volume with a low specific gravity indicates renal disease.
			• A high urine volume suggests fluid volume excess.
			• Urine volume is increased in conditions with high solute loads, such as diabetes mellitus.

(continued)

TABLE 46-6 (Continued)

Assessment Parameters	Nursing Considerations	Findings in Healthy Adult	Significant Findings
	4. Renal concentrating ability 5. Blood volume 6. Hormonal influences (primarily aldosterone and ADH)	• The range of specific gravity is from 1.003–1.035. Urine osmolality ranges between 500 mOsm and 800 mOsm/kg (mmol/kg).	• Hypovolemia causes decreased renal perfusion and thus oliguria; hypervolemia causes increased urinary volume if the kidneys are functioning normally.
Body weight	• Because of the common inaccuracies in recording intake and output, body weight is believed to be a more accurate indicator of fluid gained and lost. • Guidelines for weighing patients include: 1. Using the same scale each time. 2. Measuring weight at the same time each day: in the morning before breakfast and after voiding. 3. Ensuring the patient is wearing the same or similar clothing (clothing should be dry). 4. Using a bed scale if the patient is unable to stand on a small, portable scale. • A patient may have a severe fluid volume deficit even though body weight is essentially unchanged when there is a third-space loss of body fluid.	• A patient's dry weight should remain relatively stable.	• Rapid variations in weight closely reflect changes in body fluid volume. • A rapid loss of body weight occurs when the total fluid intake is less than the total fluid output. 1. Rapid loss of 2% total body weight (TBW) indicates mild fluid volume deficit. 2. Rapid loss of 5% TBW indicates moderate fluid volume deficit. 3. Rapid loss of 8% or more of TBW indicates severe fluid volume deficit. • A rapid gain of body weight occurs when the total fluid intake is greater than the total fluid output. 1. Rapid gain of 2% TBW indicates mild fluid volume excess. 2. Rapid gain of 5% TBW indicates moderate fluid volume excess. 3. Rapid gain of 8% or more of TBW indicates severe fluid volume excess. • A rapid gain or loss of 1 kg (2.2 lb) of body weight is about equal to the gain or loss of 1 L of fluid.
Skin turgor (elasticity)	• The patient's skin over the sternum, inner aspect of the thighs, or forehead is pinched. • Some prefer to test skin turgor in children over the abdominal area and on the medial aspect of the thighs. • Skin turgor can vary with age, nutritional state, and even race and complexion.	• Pinched skin immediately falls back to its normal position when released. • Reduced skin turgor is common in older patients (those more than 55–60 years of age) because of a primary decrease in skin elasticity.	• In a person with a fluid volume deficit, the skin flattens more slowly after the pinch is released; the skin may remain elevated for many seconds. • Severe malnutrition, particularly in infants, can cause depressed skin turgor even in the absence of fluid depletion.
Tongue turgor	• Unlike skin turgor, tongue turgor is not affected appreciably by age and thus is a useful assessment for all age groups. (In an arid climate, this may not be a reliable parameter.)	• Tongue has one longitudinal furrow.	• In the person with fluid volume deficit, there are additional longitudinal furrows and the tongue is smaller. • Sodium excess causes the tongue to look red and swollen.

(continued)

TABLE 46-6 (Continued)

Assessment Parameters	Nursing Considerations	Findings in Healthy Adult	Significant Findings
Moisture and oral cavity	• A dry mouth may be the result of fluid volume deficit or of mouth breathing. (Exposure to an arid climate may result in a dry mouth.)	• Mucous membranes in oral cavity are moist.	• Dryness of the membrane where the cheek and gum meet indicates fluid volume deficit. • Dry sticky mucous membranes are noted in sodium excess. (The oral cavity feels like flypaper.)
Tearing and salivation		• Tearing and salivation decrease normally with age.	• The absence of tearing and salivation in a child is a sign of fluid volume deficit; it becomes obvious with a fluid loss of 5% of TBW.
Appearance of skin and skin temperature			• Metabolic acidosis can cause warm, flushed skin (due to peripheral vasodilation).
Facial appearance			• A person with a severe fluid volume deficit may have a pinched and drawn facial expression. • A fluid volume deficit of 10% of body weight causes decreased intraocular pressure, causing the eyes to appear sunken and to feel soft to the touch.
Edema (excessive accumulation of interstitial fluid)	• Pitting edema (see Fig. 46-7) • Measurement of an extremity or body part with a millimeter tape, in the same area each day, is a more exact method of measurement. • An excess of interstitial fluid may accumulate predominantly in the lower extremities of ambulatory patients and in the presacral region of bedridden patients. • The presence of periorbital (around the eyes) edema or pedal edema should prompt one to look for edema in other parts of the body.	• No edema	• Clinically edema is not usually apparent in the adult until the retention of 5–10 lb of excess fluid occurs. • Pitting edema is not evident until at least a 10% increase in weight has occurred. • Formation of edema may be localized (as in thrombophlebitis) or generalized (as in heart failure, cirrhosis of liver, or nephrotic syndrome). Edema of congestive heart failure, liver cirrhosis, or nephrotic syndrome is the result of sodium retention.
Body temperature	• Because fever increases the loss of body fluids, it is important that temperature elevations be detected early and appropriate interventions be taken. • Body temperature and other vital signs should be assessed as ordered and at the nurse's discretion.	• Baseline temperature: diurnal variations	• There is an elevation of body temperature in hypernatremia (dehydration) probably related to lack of available fluid for sweating. • There is a decrease in body temperature in fluid volume deficit, when uncomplicated by infection. • Fever increases the loss of body fluids.

(continued)

Chapter 46: Fluid, Electrolyte, and Acid–Base Balance

TABLE 46-6 (Continued)

Assessment Parameters	Nursing Considerations	Findings in Healthy Adult	Significant Findings
			• A temperature elevation between 101°F (38.3°C)–103°F (39.4°C) increases the 24-hour fluid requirement by at least 500 mL, and a temperature above 103°F increases it by at least 1000 mL.
Pulse		• Baseline pulse rate, rhythm, and volume	• Tachycardia is usually the earliest sign of the decreased vascular volume associated with fluid volume deficit. • Irregular pulse rates also occur with potassium imbalances and magnesium deficit. • Pulse volume is decreased in fluid volume deficit and increased in fluid volume excess.
Respirations		• Baseline respiratory rate, rhythm, and qualities	• Deep, rapid respirations may be a compensatory mechanism for metabolic acidosis or a primary disorder causing respiratory alkalosis. • Slow, shallow respirations may be a compensatory mechanism for metabolic alkalosis or a primary disorder causing respiratory acidosis. • Moist crackles, in the absence of cardiopulmonary disease, indicate fluid volume excess.
Blood pressure	• Whenever a fluid imbalance is suspected, the patient's blood pressure is checked while he or she is lying down, sitting, and standing (orthostatic).	• Baseline blood pressure	• A fall in systolic pressure greater than 15 mm Hg from the lying to the sitting or standing position (postural hypotension) usually indicates fluid volume deficit.

Neck veins and central venous pressure (CVP)	• The jugular veins provide a built-in manometer for following changes in CVP.
	• To estimate CVP, the nurse:
	  1. Positions the patient in a semi-Fowler's position (head of bed elevated to a 30- to 45-degree angle), keeping the neck straight
	  2. Removes any of the patient's clothing that could constrict the neck or upper chest
	  3. Provides adequate lighting to visualize effectively the external jugular veins on each side of the neck
	  4. Measures the levels to which the veins are distended on the neck or above the level of the manubrium
		• Normally, when the patient is supine, the external jugular veins fill to the anterior border of the sternocleidomastoid muscle. With the patient positioned sitting at a 45-degree angle, the venous distentions normally should not extend higher than 2 cm above the sternal angle.
		• Pressure in the right atrium is usually 0–4 cm H_2O; pressure in the vena cava is about 4–11 cm H_2O.
			• A low CVP may indicate:
			  1. Decreased blood volume
			  2. Drug-induced vasodilation (causing pooling of blood in peripheral veins)
			• A high CVP may indicate:
			  1. Increased blood volume
			  2. Heart failure
			  3. Vasoconstriction

TABLE 46-6 (Continued)

Assessment Parameters	Nursing Considerations	Findings in Healthy Adult	Significant Findings
	• More accurate assessments of blood volume are obtained by measuring CVP by hemodynamic monitoring.		
Neuromuscular irritability	• When imbalances in calcium, magnesium, and sodium are suspected it is important to assess patients for increased or decreased neuromuscular irritability.	• Negative response	
	• To test for *Chvostek's sign,* the facial nerve should be percussed about 2 cm anterior to the ear lobe.	• Negative response	• Patients with hypocalcemia or hypomagnesemia respond positively with a unilateral twitching of the facial muscles, including the eyelid and lips.
	• To test for *Trousseau's sign,* a blood pressure cuff is placed on the arm and inflated above systolic pressure for 3 minutes.	• The response in the prospective muscle is a sudden contraction (2+).	• A positive response is the development of carpal spasm.
	• A deep tendon reflex is elicited by briskly tapping a partially stretched tendon with a rubber percussion hammer, preferably over the tendon insertion of the muscle.		• Deep tendon reflexes may be hyperactive in the presence of hypocalcemia, hypomagnesemia, hypernatremia, and alkalosis.
	• The muscle being tested should be slightly stretched, and the patient should be relaxed.		• Deep tendon reflexes may be hypoactive in the presence of hypercalcemia, hypermagnesemia, hyponatremia, hypokalemia, and acidosis.

	• Reflexes usually are graded on a 0 to 4+ scale.
	   0 = no response
	   1+ = somewhat diminished, but present
	   2+ = normal
	   3+ = brisker than average and possibly but not necessarily indicative of disease
	   4+ = hyperactive		

Behavior
   Sensation
   Fatigue level
	• Because these changes are often vague, they are best evaluated in context with specific imbalances.		

(Data from Metheny, N. M. [2000]. *Fluid and electrolyte balance* [4th ed.]. Philadelphia: Lippincott Williams & Wilkins.)

Fluid Intake and Output

When either the physician or nurse orders that a patient's fluid intake and output be continuously measured, the patient, family, and all caregivers must be alert to the need to measure all fluids entering and leaving the body. The patient's condition dictates the strictness of these intake and output measurements. Adherence to the guidelines in the box Guidelines for Nursing Care 46-1: Measuring Fluid Intake and Output helps eliminate common errors in measuring fluid intake and output.

Daily Weights

Due to possible numerous sources of inaccuracies in fluid intake and output measurement, the record of a patient's daily weight may more accurately depict fluid balance status. As a result of the effects of medications and fluid intake on weight,

Guidelines for Nursing Care 46-1
Measuring Fluid Intake and Output

As soon as measured intake and output is ordered for the patient, the patient and family are instructed that the nurse needs a record of all fluids entering the body and all fluid output. A simple explanation of why this is being done is offered, as well as specific instructions as to how the patient can help to keep his or her record accurate. Some patients may need to be reminded each morning that this measurement will continue.

The patient's plan of care is used to communicate to nursing personnel the need to measure fluid intake and output. A sign posted in the patient's room and a bedside form for recording intake and output are helpful reminders for both the patient and nurses.

The Patient's Fluid Intake Includes the Following:

- All fluids and foods that are liquid at room temperature (ice cream, gelatin dessert [Jell-O], etc.)
  Use the agency's designation of specific volumes for common food containers (eg, juice glass = 90 mL; milk carton = 240 mL). Remind the patient that sips of water or other fluids in between meals need to be recorded; small, disposable calibrated cups at the bedside facilitate accurate measurement. Remember that liquid medications or water taken with pills may significantly increase the fluid intake of some patients.
- All parenteral fluids
- Other fluids taken into the body: subcutaneous fluids, fluids instilled into drainage tubes, enema solutions, IV flushes

The Patient's Fluid Output Includes the Following:

- Urine; vomitus; diarrhea; drainage from fistulas, wounds, and ulcers; and drainage from suctioning devices. Calibrated measuring devices should be readily available for accurate measurement. Disposable, calibrated urine collection containers that fit under the toilet seat are available for ambulatory patients. Urine or liquid feces in diapers or bed clothes, vomitus on clothing or bed linens, wound drainage saturating dressings, and so forth, need to be estimated.
- Heavy perspiration, noted on the output record, especially when the patient's clothing or bed linens are soaked
- Hyperventilation (water vapor loss) also noted on the output record. Record rate and depth of respirations.

Both intake and output should be measured whenever possible, rather than estimated. Output measurement is described in Chapter 42. Failure to record intake or output when it is measured may result in its being forgotten.

Intake and output totals are generally recorded for each 8-hour shift and totaled each 24 hours. If the nurse suspects a large difference between intake and output, the columns should be totalled earlier so that the physician can be notified. At varying intervals throughout the shift, the alert patient should be questioned about his or her intake and output.

---

weigh the patient at the same time every day. Be alert for other factors that may affect a patient's weight, such as using a different scale and weighing with the patient wearing different clothing.

Laboratory Studies

Laboratory tests are helpful in determining whether fluid, electrolyte, and acid–base balance exist. As a safety precaution and in compliance with Centers for Disease Control and Prevention guidelines, nurses must apply a "biohazard" label to all blood specimens collected from patients at home. The specimen must be transported to the laboratory as soon as possible or refrigerated if a delay of more than 1 hour is expected. Standard tests are described below (tables of normal values are given in Appendix B).

Complete Blood Count

The complete blood count, the basic screening test, determines the total number of red blood cells and values for hemoglobin and hematocrit. Significant values include the following:

- Increased hematocrit values: found in severe dehydration and shock (when hemoconcentration rises considerably)
- Decreased hematocrit values: found with acute, massive blood loss, and with hemolytic reaction after transfusion of incompatible blood or with fluid overload

- Increased levels of hemoglobin: found in hemoconcentration of the blood
- Decreased levels of hemoglobin: found with anemia states, severe hemorrhage, and after a hemolytic reaction

Serum Electrolytes

This screening test determines plasma levels of certain electrolytes such as sodium, potassium, chloride, and bicarbonate ions.

Recall Grace Gilligan, the woman described in the Reflective Practice display? Although she needs IV therapy, it would be important for the nurse to determine the patient's electrolyte levels to establish a baseline to aid in determining the best IV solution for the patient and her need for possible electrolyte replacement.

Urine pH and Specific Gravity

Both the urine pH and specific gravity may be obtained by dipstick measurement, using a fresh voided specimen or through laboratory analysis. As discussed previously, the pH of urine usually ranges between 4.5 and 8.2. Specific gravity is a measure of the urine's concentration. The range depends on the patient's state of hydration and varies with urine volume and the load of solutes to be excreted. Normal values range from 1.003 to 1.035 (concentrated urine: 1.02–1.030 or more; dilute urine: 1.001–1.010).

Arterial Blood Gases

Arterial blood gases are obtained to determine the adequacy of oxygenation and ventilation and to assess acid–base status. See Table 46-3 for the primary laboratory values used to determine acid–base balance. Additional ABG values exist but are not included in this simple interpretation of acid–base imbalances. Partial pressure of oxygen ($PaCO_2$) and oxygen saturation (SaO_2) results also directly reflect the adequacy of oxygenation and ventilation. When interpreting ABGs, follow these necessary steps:

1. Determine whether the pH is alkalotic or acidotic.
2. Check for the cause of the change in pH. Is it respiratory ($PaCO_2$) or metabolic (HCO_3^-)? In respiratory acid–base imbalances, the pH and $PaCO_2$ values are inversely abnormal (move in opposite directions):

   Respiratory acidosis:

   ↓ pH   < 7.35   ↑ $PaCO_2$ Normal HCO_3^-

   Respiratory alkalosis:

   ↑ pH   > 7.45   ↓ $PaCO_2$ Normal HCO_3^-

   In metabolic acid–base imbalances, the pH and HCO_3 values are both high or both low:

   Metabolic acidosis:

   ↓ pH   < 7.35   ↑ HCO_3^- Normal $PaCO_2$

   Respiratory alkalosis:

   ↑ pH   > 7.45   ↑ HCO_3^- Normal $PaCO_2$

3. Determine whether the body is compensating for the pH change. When the problem is respiratory, the renal system attempts to compensate either by increasing or by decreasing HCO_3^-. In contrast, the respiratory system compensates for a metabolic acid–base imbalance by regulating CO_2 levels. When compensation occurs, the $PaCO_2$ and the HCO_3^- will always point in the same direction. The focus of compensation efforts is to return the pH to the normal range:

   Respiratory acidosis:

   ↓ pH   < 7.35   ↑ $PaCO_2$ ↑ HCO_3^-
   (compensation attempt)

   Respiratory alkalosis:

   ↑ pH   > 7.45   ↓ $PaCO_2$ ↓ HCO_3^-
   (compensation attempt)

   Metabolic acidosis:

   ↓ pH   < 7.35   ↑ HCO_3^- ↓ $PaCO_2$
   (compensation attempt)

   Metabolic alkalosis:

   ↑ pH   > 7.45   ↑ HCO_3^- ↑ $PaCO_2$
   (compensation attempt)

4. Look at the total picture and determine whether compensation has occurred. Compensation is classified as follows:

   Absent if:
   pH abnormal
   One component abnormal
   Second component within normal range

   Partial if:
   pH abnormal
   One component abnormal
   Second component beginning to change

   Complete if:
   pH within normal range
   One component abnormal
   Second changed to move pH within normal range

Table 46-7 lists assessments and nursing interventions related to these acid–base disturbances.

Diagnosing

Fluid, Electrolyte, and Acid–Base Disturbances as the Problem

When assessment data point to fluid and electrolyte problems amenable to nursing therapy, they receive one of three diagnostic labels:

Excess Fluid Volume
Deficient Fluid Volume
Risk for Imbalanced Fluid Volume

Excess fluid volume may result from greatly increased fluid intake or, more frequently, from decreased excretion such as occurs in progressive renal disease and with certain cancers. Fluid volume deficits may result from decreased intake; increased excretion of fluids; fluid shifts; and the special need for fluids and electrolytes in situations involving strenuous exercise, extreme heat or dryness, and conditions (eg, fever) that increase the metabolic rate. The accompanying box presents contributing factors and defining characteristics for these diagnoses.

If nursing assessments indicate that fluid volume balance currently exists, the nursing diagnosis "Readiness for Enhanced Fluid Balance" may be appropriate. Fluid balance would be evident but certain nursing measures might contribute to maintenance or improvement of fluid volume balance (NANDA, 2003).

The nurse's analysis of assessment data may also lead to the diagnosis of specific electrolyte or acid–base disturbances that are collaborative problems because they require joint intervention by nursing and medicine. For example, potassium imbalances may be evident on the cardiac monitor.

Fluid and Electrolyte Disturbances as the Etiology

Disturbances in fluid, electrolyte, and acid–base balance may affect many other areas of human functioning. Examples of nursing diagnoses that may be appropriate include the following:

Activity Intolerance related to imbalance between oxygen supply and demand

TABLE 46-7 Acid–Base Disturbances

Risk Factors	Assessments	Nursing Interventions
Respiratory Acidosis (Carbonic Acid Excess)		

Acute respiratory disease:
  Pulmonary edema
  Aspiration of a foreign body
  Atelectasis
  Overdose of sedative or
    anesthetic
  Cardiac arrest
Chronic respiratory disease:
  Emphysema
  Bronchial asthma
  Cystic fibrosis
Inadequate mechanical
  ventilation
CNS depression
Neuromuscular disease
	Acute respiratory acidosis
	  Mental cloudiness
	  Dizziness
	  Muscular twitching
	  Unconsciousness
	  ABGs
	    pH <7.35
	    $PaCO_2$ >45 mm Hg (primary)
	    HCO_3^- normal or only slightly elevated
	Chronic respiratory acidosis
	  Weakness
	  Dull headache
	  ABGs
	    pH <7.35 or low N
	    $PaCO_2$ >45 mm Hg (primary)
	    HCO_3^- >26 mEq/L (compensatory)
		Treatment is directed at improving ventilation:
		  Pharmacologic measures
		  Pulmonary hygiene measures
		  Adequate hydration
		  Supplemental oxygen
		Mechanical ventilation may be necessary to correct disorder but must be used cautiously to decrease $PaCO_2$ slowly.

Respiratory Alkalosis (Carbonic Acid Deficit)		

Hyperventilation
Extreme anxiety (most
  common cause)
Hypoxemia
High fever
Early sepsis
Excessive ventilation by
  mechanical ventilator
CNS lesion involving the
  respiratory center
Thyrotoxicosis
	Lightheadedness
	Inability to concentrate
	Hyperventilation syndrome
	  Tinnitus
	  Palpitations
	  Sweating
	  Dry mouth
	  Tremulousness
	  Convulsions and loss of consciousness
	ABGs
	  pH >7.45
	  $PaCO_2$ <35 mm Hg (primary)
	  HCO_3^- <22 mEq/L (compensatory)
		If anxiety is the cause, the patient should be encouraged to breathe more slowly (causes accumulation of CO_2) or breathe into a closed system (paper bag). Sedative may also be necessary in extreme anxiety.
		Treatment of other causes is directed at correcting the underlying problem.

Metabolic Acidosis (Base Bicarbonate Deficit)		

Diarrhea
Intestinal fistulas
Ureterosigmoidostomy
Hyperalimentation
Excessive intake of acids, such
  as salicylates
Diabetic ketoacidosis
Renal failure
Starvational ketoacidosis
	Headache
	Confusion
	Drowsiness
	Increased respiratory rate and depth
	Nausea and vomiting
	Peripheral vasodilation
	ABGs
	  pH <7.35
	  HCO_3^- <22 mEq/L (primary)
	  $PaCO_2$ <35 mm Hg
	Hyperkalemia frequently present
		Treatment is directed toward correcting the metabolic deficit. If the cause of the problem is excessive intake of chloride, treatment obviously focuses on eliminating the source. When necessary, bicarbonate is administered.

Metabolic Alkalosis (Base Bicarbonate Excess)		

Vomiting or gastric suction
Hypokalemia
Potassium-wasting diuretics
Alkali ingestion (bicarbonate-
  containing antacids)
Renal loss of H^+ (eg, from
  steroid or diuretic use)
	Dizziness
	Tingling of fingers and toes
	Hypertonic muscles
	Depressed respirations (compensatory)
	ABGs
	  pH >7.45
	  HCO_3^- >26 mEq/L (primary)
	  $PaCO_2$ >45 mm Hg (compensatory)
	Hypokalemia may be present
		Treatment is aimed at reversal of the underlying disorder. Sufficient chloride must be supplied for the kidney to absorb sodium with chloride (allowing the excretion of excess bicarbonate). Treatment also includes administration of NaCl fluids to restore normal fluid volume.

(Adapted from Metheny, N. [2000]. *Fluid and electrolyte balance* [4th ed.]. Philadelphia: Lippincott Williams & Wilkins.)

Examples of NANDA Nursing Diagnoses

Fluid and Electrolyte Balance

Nursing Diagnoses	Related Factors	Sample Defining Characteristics
Excess Fluid Volume	Pathophysiologic factors: renal failure, decreased cardiac output, liver disease, abnormal fluid accumulations, hormonal problems	• "I've noticed that my wedding ring is tight . . . also my clothes don't fit as well as they used to. I guess I've gained some weight." • Reports dyspnea with exertion, feeling weak and fatigued • Pitting edema in feet, ankles, lower legs • Taut, shiny skin • Jugular venous distention
	Situational factors: excessive IV infusion	• Bounding pulse, increased from baseline • Shallow, rapid respirations, rales • Increased blood pressure
	Nutritional factors: excessive sodium intake, low protein intake	• 10-lb (4.5-kg) weight gain over past month • Fluid intake greater than output • "Sometimes I can't catch my breath and I feel like my heart is pounding away." • "I feel bloated."
Deficient Fluid Volume; Risk for Deficient Fluid Volume	Decreased fluid intake: imposed fluid restrictions, inability to obtain or swallow fluids (debilitation, oral pain), depression	• "After I got the flu I got so weak I couldn't get out of bed. . . . I think I was out of it for a couple of days." • Increased pulse and respirations • Dry oral mucosa, cracked lips, furrowed tongue • Scanty, dark urine output
	Abnormal fluid loss: vomiting; diarrhea; abnormal drainage; excessive use of laxative, enemas, diuretics; blood loss; diaphoresis; burns	• "I'm thirsty all the time." • "I've been vomiting and I have diarrhea—several times a day." • Weight loss: 5 lb (2–3 kg) • Urine is concentrated (specific gravity, 1.035) • Fluid output greater than fluid intake • Neck veins collapsed when lying flat • Decreased skin turgor
	Increased need for fluids: strenuous exercise, extreme heat or dryness, fever (increased metabolic rate)	• Skin is warm to touch, moist, and flushed • Increased temperature, pulse, respirations • Decreased blood pressure

Ineffective Breathing Pattern related to compensatory mechanism by lungs (hypoventilation or hyperventilation)

Decreased Cardiac Output related to decreased blood volume, shock

Risk for Injury related to neuromuscular irritability, cardiac arrhythmia

Deficient Knowledge: Harmful Effects of Abuses of Dieting, Alcohol, Diuretics, Laxatives, and Enemas related to no previous experience

Impaired Oral Mucous Membrane related to dehydration

Impaired Skin Integrity related to dehydration, edema

Disturbed Thought Processes related to cerebral edema, mental confusion or disorientation, convulsions

Ineffective Tissue Perfusion: [specify type] related to decreased cardiac output

Impaired Urinary Elimination related to decreased kidney perfusion secondary to decreased plasma volume

Outcome Identification and Planning

Nursing care supports the following expected outcomes. The healthy adult patient will:

• Maintain an approximate balance between fluid intake and fluid output (average about 2500 mL fluid intake and output over 3 days)

• Maintain a urine specific gravity within normal range (1.010–1.025)

• Practice self-care behaviors to promote fluid, electrolyte, and acid–base balance; maintain adequate intake of fluid and electrolytes; respond appropriately to the body's signals of impending fluid, electrolyte, or acid–base imbalance

When an imbalance exists, the patient will:

• Relate relief of symptoms (specify) after implementation of treatment regimen (eg, 1 month after decreasing sodium intake patient reports 4 lb [1.8 kg] weight loss)

- Exhibit signs and symptoms of restored balance or homeostasis after initiation of treatment
- Identify signs and symptoms of recurrence of imbalance with need to notify the physician

Implementing

Nursing interventions to prevent or correct fluid, electrolyte, and acid–base imbalances include dietary modification, modification of fluid intake, medication administration, IV therapy, blood and blood products replacement, and TPN.

Preventing Fluid Imbalances

An adequate fluid intake and a well-balanced, nutritious diet with appropriate adjustments throughout the life cycle are essential to promote fluid balance. Table 46-8 lists the risk factors, related assessments, and specific nursing interventions for fluid volume disturbances. Following are general measures to consider to help prevent fluid imbalances:

- Be familiar with common life events that can lead to fluid imbalances, and observe the patient carefully. Infants are particularly vulnerable to fluid imbalances because body water accounts for a greater percentage of their weight, and fluid fluctuations are more common. Loss of fluid because of an illness can cause serious and life-threatening problems in infants.

> *Think back to Jeremiah Kearny, the infant with nausea and vomiting. Although the underlying illness may be a GI virus, the nurse must assess the infant frequently to ensure that he does not develop further losses which could become life-threatening.*

- Note the patient's present fluid and food intake, and learn what his or her previous eating and drinking patterns have been. Learn whether the patient has been using a fad diet, which may lead to imbalances.
- Note whether the patient experiences excessive thirst or little or no thirst. Thirst, a subjective sensation, is an impor-

TABLE 46-8 Fluid Volume Disturbances

Risk Factors	Assessments	Nursing Interventions
Fluid Volume Deficit (Hypovolemia)		
GI: Vomiting, diarrhea, suction, fistulas	Thirst	Assess for presence or worsening of FVD.
Hemorrhage	Weight loss over short period	Administer oral fluids if indicated.
Excessive sweating	Weakness, fatigue, anorexia	If patient unable to eat and drink, anticipate TPN or tube feedings to be ordered.
Skin trauma, burns, draining wounds	Dry mucous membranes	Monitor patient's response to fluid intake, either oral or parenteral.
Third-space fluid shifts	Poor skin and tongue turgor	Be alert for signs of fluid overload.
Excessive laxative or diuretic use	Sunken eyes	Provide appropriate skin care.
Polyuria from renal disease or diuretics	Flat neck veins	
Hyperglycemia	Urine output <30 mL/hr	
Change in mental status (unable to gain access to fluids, depression, confusion)	Postural hypotension	
	Weak, rapid pulse	
	↑Urine specific gravity	
	↑Hematocrit	
	↑BUN	
	↑Serum sodium	
	Altered sensorium	
Fluid Volume Excess (Hypervolemia)		
Compromised regulatory mechanisms: renal failure, CHF, cirrhosis of liver, Cushing's syndrome	Weight gain over short period	Assess for presence or worsening of FVE.
	Peripheral edema (may be pitting)	Encourage adherence to sodium-restricted and fluid-restricted diet, if ordered.
	Increased BP	Avoid OTC drugs or check with physician or pharmacist about sodium content.
GI irrigation with hypotonic fluid	Shortness of breath	Encourage rest periods.
Excess IV fluids with sodium	Crackles and wheezes in lungs	Monitor patient's response to diuretics.
Corticosteroid therapy	Full, bounding pulse	Teach self-monitoring of weight and intake and output.
Excessive ingestion of sodium-containing substances in diet or sodium-containing medications	Neck vein distention	Attentive skin care.
	Polyuria if renal function is normal	Monitor respiratory status.
	Ascites, pleural effusion	
	Pulmonary edema	
	↓BUN (due to plasma dilution)	
	↓Hematocrit	
	↓Serum sodium	
	↓Urine specific gravity	

GI, gastrointestinal; BUN, blood urea nitrogen; FVD, fluid volume deficit; TPN, total parenteral nutrition; CHF, congestive heart failure; IV, intravenous; BP, blood pressure; FVE, fluid volume excess; OTC, over-the-counter.

tant factor determining water intake and, eventually, output through the kidneys. Although the thirst mechanism is poorly understood, both psychological and physiologic factors appear to be involved.

- Be aware of excessive losses of fluids from the body, and attempt to prevent losses when possible. Vomiting, pronounced perspiration, diarrhea, draining wounds, and excessive urinary output, for example, may cause excessive losses.
- Consider ways in which the patient's medical regimen may lead to fluid and electrolyte imbalances. For example, diuretics that stimulate urine formation may increase the elimination of potassium. If food supplements high in potassium are not included in the diet or if drug therapy is not started, hypokalemia often follows (Table 46-9 describes nursing interventions for specific electrolyte disturbances).
- Learn whether the patient has been "treating" himself or herself in some way that may threaten fluid balance. Common practices that threaten fluid balance include the indiscriminate use of enemas, laxatives, antacids, and over-the-counter drugs to promote urination.
- Consider conditions with destructive effects on the body as threats to fluid balance. Examples include immobilization, trauma, burns, surgical procedures, and exposure to toxic agents.
- Teach patients to observe for fluid imbalances and to report them promptly. Examples include rapid weight gains and losses; swollen fingers, feet, and ankles; puffy eyelids; muscle weakness; change in skin sensations; and scanty or profuse urine production.
- Help patients and their families understand the significance of maintaining fluid balance and preventing imbalances.
- Be aware that normal physiologic changes associated with aging affect elder patients' ability to maintain fluid balance. Dehydration is a common fluid and electrolyte disorder in this population. The accompanying box, Focus on the Older Adult, suggests specific nursing strategies to prevent and correct fluid and electrolyte imbalances.

Developing a Dietary Plan

Simple dietary changes may help to resolve fluid and electrolyte disturbances. After obtaining a nutritional assessment to identify actual or potential imbalances and food preferences, initiate teaching based on a nutritional plan that involves both the patient and the person who prepares the patient's meals. Include foods that help to resolve the fluid or electrolyte imbalance and that are acceptable to the patient. For example, for fluid volume deficit, increase foods with high water content (eg, citrus fruit, melons, celery); for hypokalemia, increase foods with high potassium content (eg, bananas, citrus fruits, apricots, melons, broccoli, potatoes); for hypernatremia, avoid foods high in sodium (eg, processed cheese, lunch meats, canned soups and vegetables, salted snack foods) and eliminate use of table salt.

When teaching the patient about foods to include or avoid, provide the patient with a written list for reference. Evaluate the patient's understanding of the teaching by having the patient identify those foods that can be eaten freely or moder-

ately as well as those to be avoided. Both the patient and person responsible for the patient's food preparation should be able to describe a 24-hour diet plan compatible with the recommended modifications.

Modifying Fluid Intake

Depending on the nature of the fluid or electrolyte imbalance, a patient's fluids may need to be increased, decreased, or modified in terms of types of fluids ingested. Nursing responsibilities include:

- Identifying the appropriate fluid modification (eg, with certain illnesses, the physician may order fluid directives such as "Restrict fluids to 1000 mL/d")
- Determining whether the patient understands the rationale for the fluid modification, is motivated to follow the modification, and is capable of adhering to the plan (eg, a bedridden patient who needs to increase fluid intake cannot do this independently)
- Developing and implementing a plan of care based on the preceding information

Consider these three patient scenarios. Although the three patients have the same tendency to retain fluids, each may need different nursing care. One patient has never learned that the high-sodium beverages she frequently drinks are contributing to her problem. Therefore, one teaching session may be sufficient to resolve her fluid imbalance. A second patient has a history of poor self-care behaviors. Intelligent and the recipient of much health education in the past, this patient has no need for further teaching. However, nursing time is best invested in counseling and exploring why the patient fails to value his health sufficiently to follow the treatment regimen. Until the patient values the proposed fluid modification, compliance will probably be poor. The third patient is a frail older woman with pneumonia and a history of congestive heart failure being treated with diuretic medication who depends on the nursing staff for care. Most likely, her fluid intake will be determined by the fluids offered to her by the nursing staff. In addition, diuretic medication prescribed may affect her fluid balance status further, placing her at risk for fluid deficits and potassium imbalances.

Increasing Fluids

Increasing fluids, which may be prescribed for certain patients, involves an above-average intake of fluids. The usual order reads "Force fluids" and indicates the amount of fluid the patient is to have in each 24-hour period. Typically, the plan of care specifies the amount of fluid to be ingested in 24 hours (for hospitalized patients, shift totals are helpful [eg, 7–3, 1200 mL; 3–11, 900 mL; 11–7, 300 mL]) and the patient's food preferences. Choose or assist with choosing fluids that best provide the calories and electrolytes needed by the patient.

Several techniques are recommended to help the patient take more than average amounts of fluids. Begin by explaining to the patient in understandable terms the rationale for the increased fluids and the specific goal of taking the daily amount of fluid prescribed. This explanation provides the patient with a greater understanding of why he or she needs to increase fluids. In addition, this information helps motivate the patient to

TABLE 46-9 Electrolyte Disturbances

Risk Factors	Assessments	Nursing Interventions

Hyponatremia
Loss of sodium, as in:
    Loss of GI fluids
    Use of diuretics
    Adrenal insufficiency
Gains of water, as in:
    Excessive administration of D_5W
    Water intoxication
Disease states associated with
  SIADH (a form of hyponatremia)
Pharmacologic agents that may
  impair water excretion
	Anorexia
	Nausea and vomiting
	Lethargy
	Confusion
	Muscle cramps
	Fingerprinting over sternum
	Muscular twitching
	Seizures
	Coma
	Serum Na below 135 mEq/L
	Urine specific gravity <1.010
		Monitor fluid losses and gains.
		Monitor for presence of GI and CNS symptoms.
		Monitor serum Na levels.
		Check urine specific gravity.
		If able to eat, encourage foods and fluids with high sodium content.
		Be aware of sodium content of common IV fluids.
		Avoid giving large water supplements to patients receiving isotonic tube feedings.
		Take seizure precautions when hyponatremia is severe.

Hypernatremia
Water deprivation
Increased sensible and insensible
  water loss
Ingestion of large amount of salt
Excessive parenteral administration
  of sodium-containing solutions
Profuse sweating
Diabetes insipidus
	Thirst
	Elevated body temperature
	Tongue dry and swollen, sticky mucous
	  membranes
	Severe hypernatremia
	  Disorientation
	  Hallucinations
	  Lethargy when undisturbed
	  Irritable and hyperactive
	  Focal or grand mal seizures
	  Coma
	Serum Na above 145 mEq/L
	Urine specific gravity >1.015
		Monitor fluid losses and gains.
		Observe for excessive intake of high sodium foods.
		Monitor sodium content of prescriptions and OTC drugs.
		Monitor for changes in behavior such as restlessness, lethargy, and disorientation.
		Look for excessive thirst and elevated body temperature.
		Monitor serum Na levels.
		Check urine specific gravity.
		Give sufficient water with tube feedings to keep serum Na and BUN at normal limits.

Hypokalemia
Diarrhea
Vomiting or gastric suction
Potassium-wasting diuretics
Steroid administration and certain
  antibiotics
Poor intake as in anorexia nervosa,
  alcoholism, potassium-free
  parenteral fluids
Polyuria
	Fatigue
	Anorexia, nausea, and vomiting
	Muscle weakness
	Decreased bowel motility
	Cardiac arrhythmias
	Increased sensitivity to digitalis
	Polyuria, nocturia, dilute urine
	Postural hypotension
	Serum K below 3.5 mEq/L
	ECG changes
	Paresthesias or tender muscles
		Monitor for occurrence of hypokalemia.
		Assess digitalized patients at risk for hypokalemia, which potentiates the action of digitalis
		Prevent hypokalemia by:
		  Encouraging extra K intake if possible
		  Educating about abuse of laxatives and diuretics
		Administer oral K supplements if ordered.
		Be knowledgeable about danger of IV potassium administration.

Hyperkalemia
Decreased potassium excretion:
  Oliguric renal failure
  Potassium-sparing diuretics
  Hypoaldosteronism
High potassium intake, especially
  in presence of renal insufficiency
Shift of potassium out of cells
  (acidosis, tissue trauma, malignant
  cell lysis)
	Vague muscle weakness
	Cardiac arrhythmias
	Paresthesias of face, tongue, feet, and
	  hands
	Flaccid muscle paralysis
	GI symptoms such as nausea, intermittent intestinal colic, or diarrhea may
	  occur
	Serum K above 5.0 mEq/L
		Monitor for hyperkalemia, which is lifethreatening.
		Prevent hyperkalemia by:
		  Following rules for safe administration of K
		  Avoiding giving patients with renal insufficiency K-saving diuretics, K supplements, or salt substitutes
		  Cautioning about foods high in potassium content

Hypocalcemia
Surgical hypoparathyroidism
Malabsorption
Vitamin D deficiency
Acute pancreatitis
Excessive administration of citrated
  blood
	Trousseau's and Chvostek's signs
	Numbness and tingling of fingers and
	  toes
	Mental changes
	Seizures
	Spasm of laryngeal muscles
		Take seizure precautions when hypocalcemia is severe.
		Monitor condition of airway.
		Take safety precautions if confusion is present.
		Educate people at risk for osteoporosis about need for dietary calcium intake.

(continued)

TABLE 46-9 (Continued)

Risk Factors	Assessments	Nursing Interventions
Alkalotic states	ECG changes Cramps in muscles of extremities Total serum calcium <8.5 mg/dL	Discuss calcium-losing aspects of nicotine and alcohol use.
Hypercalcemia Hyperparathyroidism Malignant neoplastic disease Prolonged immobilization Large doses of vitamin D Overuse of calcium supplements Thiazide diuretics	Muscular weakness Tiredness, lethargy Constipation Anorexia, nausea, and vomiting Decreased memory and attention span Polyuria and polydipsia Renal stones Neurotic behavior Cardiac arrest Serum calcium >10.5 mg/dL	Increase mobilization when feasible. Encourage sufficient oral intake. Discourage excessive consumption of milk products. Encourage bulk in the diet. Take safety precautions if confusion is present Be alert for signs of digitalis toxicity in hypercalcemic patients. Force fluids to prevent formation of renal stones.

Hypomagnesemia
Chronic alcoholism
Intestinal malabsorption
Diarrhea
Nasogastric suction
Drugs
  Thiazide diuretics
  Aminoglycoside antibiotics
  Excessive doses of vitamin D
  Citrate preservative in blood
	Neuromuscular irritability
	  Increased reflexes
	  Coarse tremors
	  Seizures
	Cardiac manifestations
	  Tachyarrhythmias
	  Increased susceptibility to digitalis toxicity
	Mental changes
	  Disorientation
	  Mood changes
	Serum magnesium <1.3 mEq/L
		Assess for magnesium deficit because it predisposes patient to digitalis toxicity.
		Take seizure precautions if necessary.
		Monitor condition of airway because laryngeal stridor can occur.
		Educate patient if abuse of diuretics or laxatives is a problem.
		Educate about intake of foods rich in magnesium.

Hypermagnesemia Renal failure Adrenal insufficiency Excessive magnesium administration during treatment of eclampsia Hemodialysis with hard water or dialysate high in magnesium content	Early sign is serum magnesium level of 3 to 5 mEq/L Flushing and sense of skin warmth Hypotension Depressed respirations Drowsiness, hypoactive reflexes, and muscular weakness Cardiac abnormalities	If hypermagnesemia is present, be alert for low BP and shallow respirations, lethargy, drowsiness, and coma. Do not give magnesium-containing medications to patient with renal failure or compromised renal function. Be cautious of OTC drugs. Check deep tendon reflexes frequently.
Hypophosphatemia Glucose administration Refeeding after starvation Hyperalimentation Alcohol withdrawal Diabetic ketoacidosis Respiratory alkalosis	Cardiomyopathy Acute respiratory failure Seizures Decreased tissue oxygenation Joint stiffness Serum phosphate <2.5 mg/dL	Be aware that severely hypophosphatemic patients are at greater risk for infection. Administer IV phosphate products cautiously. Introduce hyperalimentation cautiously in patients who are malnourished. Monitor for diarrhea when taking oral supplements. Sudden increase in serum phosphate level can cause hypocalcemia.

Hyperphosphatemia
Renal failure
Chemotherapy
Large intake of milk
Excessive intake of phosphate-containing laxatives (Fleet phosphosoda)
Large vitamin D intake
Hyperthyroidism
	Short-term consequences:
	  Symptoms of tetany, such as tingling of the fingertips and around the mouth, numbness, and muscle spasms
	Long-term consequences:
	  Precipitation of calcium phosphate in nonosseous sites, such as the kidneys, joints, arteries, skin, or cornea
	Serum phosphate above 4.5 mg/dL
		Monitor for signs of tetany.
		Be aware that soft tissue calcification can be a long-term complication of chronically elevated serum phosphate levels.
		Instruct patients that use of phosphate-containing laxatives can result in hyperphosphatemia.
		Avoid foods high in phosphorus content.

SIADH, syndrome of inappropriate antidiuretic hormone; ECG, electrocardiographic; CNS, central nervous system (Adapted from Metheny, N. [2000]. *Fluid and electrolyte balance* [4th ed.]. Philadelphia: Lippincott Williams & Wilkins.)

Focus on the Older Adult
Physiologic Changes and Nursing Strategies for Fluid Balance Problems

Physiologic Changes	Nursing Strategies
Altered Sense of Thirst	
• Decreased sense of thirst • Medical conditions, eg, heart failure or hypertension, requiring medications such as diuretics	• Ensure that oral intake is at least 1,500 mL for 24 hours. • Be aware of schedule for diagnostic tests (and associated dietary and fluid restrictions). • Offer fluids at regular intervals. • Replace fluids as necessary, either orally or IV. • Investigate individual fluid preferences. • Provide assistance or assistive devices for encouraging fluid intake.
Alterations in Renal Functioning	
• Loss of nephrons • Decreased renal blood flow	• Record accurate intake and output. • Note appearance and specific gravity of urine. • Check laboratory values for abnormal levels.

comply with the treatment. Together with the patient develop short-term goals for accomplishing the increased fluid intake. For example, the patient will drink a glass of water every hour, a particular beverage by the time a television program is finished, or a pitcher of water by lunch. Most patients try to reach goals that they help to set, even when they do not feel thirsty.

Ensure that a proportionately larger amount of fluid is offered during the early hours of the patient's waking day, rather than large amounts before bedtime. The patient can usually take fluids relatively easily after having few or no fluids during sleeping hours. However, large amounts of fluid at night interferes with the patient's ability to rest and sleep by being awakened during the night with the need to urinate.

Offering a variety of fluids served at the appropriate temperature is helpful, allowing the patient to choose what he or she would like, further aiding in compliance with the treatment. The likelihood for success also is increased because the patient is more likely to drink more when some liquids are iced and cold, and coffee and tea when they are hot but not hot enough to cause a burn. Variety also adds interest and makes increasing fluids more palatable. If patients dislike taking fluids (a common problem with children) or have swallowing difficulties, offering a gelatin dessert (Jell-O™), flavored frozen water (Popsicles™), water ice, and so forth, may meet with more success.

Always have fluids readily available for the patient. Take care to avoid a situation in which patients are unable to secure their own fluids (left with an unfilled water pitcher, an empty glass, a full pitcher out of reach, or a pitcher too heavy to lift). In addition, use attractive, clean, and easy-to-handle cups and glasses, a practice that helps to encourage the patient's desire to take fluids.

Patient participation in care promotes autonomy and self-esteem. Therefore, have the patient help keep a record of his or her intake when possible. This often serves as a motivating factor to increase fluid intake. Throughout, provide support, un-

derstanding, and encouragement because forcing fluid intake for the person experiencing no thirst can be uncomfortable.

Increasing the fluid intake of patients is among the most common nursing interventions. Use creativity to assist the patient and family to reach desired goals. Having a tea party may be a helpful strategy to use when encouraging a child to increase fluids. When determining the patient's increased fluid intake, be sure to include fluids replaced through nasogastric, gastrostomy, or jejunostomy tubes, and any irrigations of these tubes in the fluid balance summary (see Chap. 42).

Restricting Fluids

Restricting the patient's fluid intake is sometimes necessary. The usual order reads "Restrict fluids" and indicates the amount of fluid the patient is to have in each 24-hour period.

Several techniques are recommended to help patients restrict their intake of fluids. Similar to increasing fluids, begin by explaining to the patient in understandable terms the rationale for the fluid restriction and the specified daily amount of fluid prescribed. Then together with the patient develop short-term outcomes for accomplishing the overall task. Discuss with the patient the time intervals at which fluids will be served. Usually, offering fluids at 1- or 2-hour intervals and between meals is best because food often helps to relieve some feelings of thirst. Provide the fluid in small glasses or cups so that the container appears to contain more fluid than it actually does. Large containers partially full make the amount of fluid seem smaller than it actually is. Using ice chips also is helpful. When they melt, the water is about one half of its volume when frozen and helps to quench thirst. Remember to include the ice chips as part of the patient's fluid intake. If appropriate, encourage the patient to participate in his or her care by helping to keep a record of intake.

Consider Mr. Park, the patient who received too much IV fluid. As a result and his subsequent development of problems, the nurse would be alert to the possibility that fluid restriction may be ordered. If this occurs, the nurse needs to ensure that Mr. Park understands the reason for the restriction.

Patients restricting fluids commonly complain of thirst or dry mouth. Avoid offering patients dry, salty, or sweet foods and fluids, because they tend to increase thirst. Also attempt to divert the patients' attention from thirst by involving them in activities, and keep fluids not intended for the patient out of sight. Provide understanding, support, and encouragement, because limiting fluid intake is uncomfortable for a thirsty person.

Provide oral hygiene at regular intervals so that the patient's mouth remains clean and moist. Lubricate the lips and mucous membranes as indicated. If the patient is capable and cooperative, allow the patient to rinse his or her mouth with water without swallowing the fluid, to avoid exceeding the intake limit. At one time, offering patients hard candy or gum was thought to relieve thirst by stimulating salivation, as the sugar content increases oral tonicity and temporarily draws fluids to the mouth membranes. After about 15 to 30 minutes, however, the membranes become even drier than before. Therefore, the current recommendation is to avoid hard candy and gum. Some patients, though, may benefit from sugarless gum.

Just as with fluid increases, fluid limits should also have shift totals set. This prevents one shift from taking all of the patient's allotted fluid and prepares the patient ahead of time for the fluid limits.

Administering Medications

Patients with fluid, electrolyte, and acid–base imbalances are often prescribed medications as part of the therapeutic regimen. Be knowledgeable about the therapeutic effects of mineral–electrolyte preparations and diuretics, as well as being alert for adverse effects of other medications, such as steroids and hormone replacements.

Mineral–Electrolyte Preparations

Mineral–electrolyte preparations are frequently prescribed to correct electrolyte imbalances. Nursing responsibilities include:

- Accurately administering the medications, following manufacturer's guidelines (eg, dilute potassium supplements to disguise the unpleasant taste and decrease gastric irritation; monitor ABGs for increased pH after each 50–100 mEq of sodium bicarbonate to avoid overtreatment and metabolic alkalosis)
- Knowing and evaluating the intended therapeutic effect (eg, with magnesium sulfate, look for decreased restlessness and irritability, decreased muscle tremors, and control of convulsions)
- Assessing for adverse effects (eg, with sodium chloride injection, observe for hypernatremia and circulatory overload)
- Knowing the risks associated with administration; for example, IV potassium—never give potassium IV push, and carefully monitor the infusion rate for IV KCl solutions

(maximum rate should be 20 mEq/h). An error can result in sudden hyperkalemia leading to a fatal cardiac arrhythmia.
- Assessing for drug interactions (eg, drugs that increase the effects of minerals and electrolytes include acidifying agents, alkalinizing agents, cation exchange resin, iron salts, and potassium salts)
- Teaching patients appropriate self-care behaviors

Diuretics

Diuretics are drugs that increase renal excretion of water, sodium, and other electrolytes. Although helpful in treating patients with fluid volume excess, they increase the risk for dehydration and serious electrolyte deficiencies. Careful monitoring (eg, check urine output and serum K level) and education are essential for a patient receiving diuretic therapy.

Administering Intravenous (IV) Therapy

A relatively common form of therapy for handling fluid disturbances is the use of various solutions infused intravenously. IV therapy is delivered annually to millions of patients in homes and hospitals. The physician is responsible for prescribing the kind and amount of solution to be used. The nurse is responsible for initiating, monitoring, and discontinuing the therapy. The accompanying box lists examples of Nursing Interventions Classification (NIC) for IV therapy.

As with other therapeutic agents, the nurse must understand the patient's need for IV therapy, the type of solution being used, its desired effect, and untoward reactions that may occur. The contents of selected IV solutions are listed, along with comments about their use, in Table 46-10.

Equipment

Sterile technique must be observed when puncturing a vein. Disposable infusion tubing and needles are used to help eliminate many possible sources of contamination and to reduce the cost of equipment aftercare.

Equipment varies according to the manufacturer. Be familiar with the equipment used in the agency or patient's home

---

Examples of Nursing Interventions Classification (NIC)
Intravenous (IV) Therapy

- Maintain strict aseptic technique
- Examine the solution for type, amount, expiration date, character of the solution, and lack of damage to container
- Select and prepare an IV infusion pump, as indicated
- Administer IV fluids at room temperature
- Monitor for IV patency before administration of IV medication
- Maintain occlusive dressing
- Flush IV lines between administration of incompatible solutions

(From McClosky, J., & Bulechek, G. [2000]. *Nursing interventions classification [NIC]* [3rd ed.] [p. 409]. St. Louis: C. V. Mosby. A full listing of nursing activities for each nursing intervention can be found in this book.)

TABLE 46-10 Selected IV Solutions

Solution	Comments
Isotonic Solutions	
5% dextrose in water (D_5W)	Supplies about 170 cal/L and contains 50 g of glucose
	Should not be used in excessive volumes because it does not contain any sodium; thus the fluid dilutes the amount of sodium in the serum. Brain swelling, or *hyponatremic encephalopathy*, can develop rapidly and cause death unless it is promptly recognized and treated.
0.9% NaCl (normal saline)	Not desirable as routine maintenance solution because it provides only Na^+ and Cl^-, which are provided in excessive amounts.
	May be used to expand temporarily the extracellular compartment if circulatory insufficiency is a problem; also used to treat diabetic ketoacidosis.
Lactated Ringer's solution	A roughly isotonic solution that contains multiple electrolytes in about the same concentrations as found in plasma (note that this solution is lacking in Mg and PO_4)
	Used in the treatment of hypovolemia, burns, and fluid lost as bile or diarrhea
	Useful in treating mild metabolic acidosis
Hypotonic Solutions	
0.33% NaCl (⅓-strength saline)	A hypotonic solution that provides Na^+, Cl^-, and free water Na^+ and Cl^- allows kidneys to select and retain needed amounts
	Free water desirable as aid to kidneys in elimination of solutes
0.45% NaCl (½-strength saline)	A hypotonic solution that provides Na^+, Cl^- and free water
	Often used to treat hypernatremia (because this solution contains a small amount of Na^+, it dilutes the plasma sodium while not allowing it to drop too rapidly)
Hypertonic Solutions	
5% dextrose in 0.45% NaCl	A common hypertonic solution used to treat hypovolemia; used to maintain fluid intake
10% dextrose in water ($D_{10}W$)	Supplies 340 cal/L
	Used for peripheral parenteral nutrition (PPN)
5% dextrose in 0.9% NaCl (normal saline)	Replaces nutrients and electrolytes
	Can temporarily be used to treat hypovolemia if plasma expander is not available

(Data from Metheny, N. M. [2000]. *Fluid and electrolyte balance* [4th ed.]. Philadelphia: Lippincott Williams & Wilkins)

setting. Typically, most solutions for infusions are dispensed in 1-L or 500-mL flexible or rigid plastic containers. Because plastic bags collapse under atmospheric pressure as the solution enters the patient's vein, they do not require a vent for air to enter to replace fluid flowing from the container. Small 50-,100-, and 250-mL solution bags are available to administer intermittent IV medications (such as antibiotics given by IV piggyback).

Some medications bond with the plastic in IV bags. Therefore, glass bottles are required for certain medications. Glass bottles do not collapse under atmospheric pressure and, therefore, require a vent to allow air to enter the bottle as the fluid leaves the bottle.

Many options are available for the IV tubing that is attached to the solution container. A basic administration set is illustrated in Figure 46-8. A spike or piercing pin is inserted into the container, usually with a twisting motion. The rate of flow is manually controlled by a clamp or constricting device on the tubing. A device called a drip meter or drip chamber connects the solution bottle and tubing and permits the number of drops per minute of solution to be determined. In addition, some administration sets also have an in-line filter.

A variety of needles and catheters are commonly used for IV infusions. IV catheters are plastic tubes that have been mounted on a needle or are threaded through a needle for insertion. Once inserted, the needle is withdrawn and the flexible catheter remains in the vein. The over-the-needle catheter is easy to insert and stable, and its placement is easily detected with radiography. Single- or double-winged infusion needles (butterflies) are short-beveled, thin-walled needles with plastic flaps. They are used in pediatric settings and when short-term therapy is expected. Butterfly or scalp vein needles are not flexible and, thus, more likely to infiltrate. Other equipment necessary to start an IV infusion is listed in Skill 46-1.

The nurse is the healthcare provider most at risk for a needlestick injury. Many devices are available that minimize the potential for injury and promote safety when connecting, accessing, or disposing of IV equipment. Needleless systems

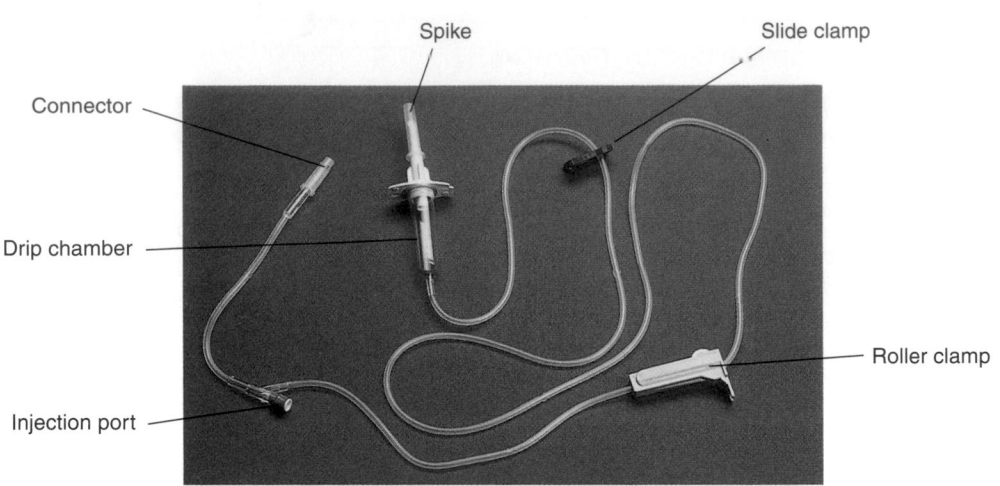

FIGURE 46-8 Basic administration set for intravenous therapy. (Courtesy of Abbott Laboratories, North Chicago, IL.)

and needle-housing systems in which the needle is recessed and protected are becoming increasingly common. Refer to Chapters 28 and 29 for additional information about these protective measures.

Vascular Access Devices

Many different options for vascular access devices are available for delivery of solutions and medications into a vein. The length of time the infusion therapy is needed, the type of medication or product that will be delivered intravenously, and the patient's health status as well as individualized needs determine which option is used. The nursing care required depends on the type of device.

Peripheral Venous Catheters

Over-the-needle catheters, which were previously discussed, are the most common type of peripheral vascular catheter used. When infusion therapy will be brief, a short (<3 inches) peripheral catheter may be ordered by the physician. The insertion site should be rotated at least every 72 to 96 hours (CDC, 2002).

SKILL 46-1   Starting an Intravenous Infusion

EQUIPMENT

IV solution
IV infusion set
IV tubing
IV catheter (over-the-needle, angiocath) or butterfly needle
Tourniquet
Cleansing swabs (alcohol, povidone-iodine)

Towel or disposable pad
Gauze or transparent dressing (according to agency policy)
Time tape or label (for IV container)
Site protector or tube-shaped elastic netting (optional)

Nonallergenic tape
Electronic infusion device (if ordered)
Armboard, if needed
Disposable gloves
IV pole

ACTION	RATIONALE
1. Gather all equipment and bring to bedside. Check IV solution and medication additives with physician's order.	Having equipment available saves time and facilitates accomplishment of task. Ensures that patient receives the correct IV solution and medication as ordered by physician.
2. Explain procedure to patient.	Explanation allays client's anxiety.
3. Perform hand hygiene.	Hand hygiene deters the spread of microorganisms.
4. Prepare IV solution and tubing:	
a. Maintain aseptic technique when opening sterile packages and IV solution	This prevents spread of microorganisms.
b. Clamp tubing, uncap spike, and insert into entry site on bag as manufacturer directs.	This punctures the seal in the IV bag.
c. Squeeze drip chamber and allow it to fill at least half way.	Suction effect causes fluid to move into drip chamber. Also prevents air from moving down the tubing.
d. Remove cap at end of tubing, release clamp, and allow fluid to move through tubing. Allow fluid to flow until all air bubbles have disappeared. Close clamp and recap end of tubing, maintaining sterility of setup.	This removes air from tubing that can, in larger amounts, act as an air embolus.

Starting an Intravenous Infusion (continued)

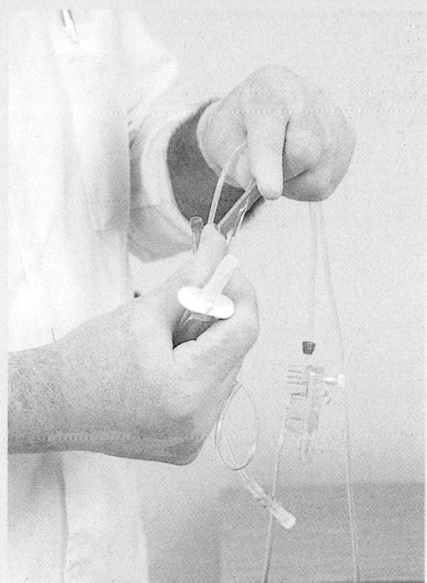

Action 4b: Clamping tubing.

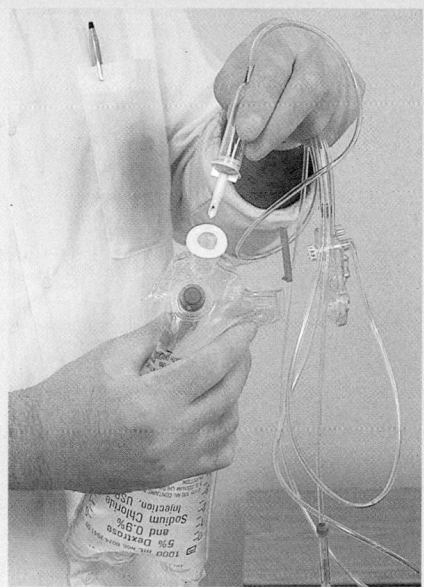

Action 4b: Inserting spike.

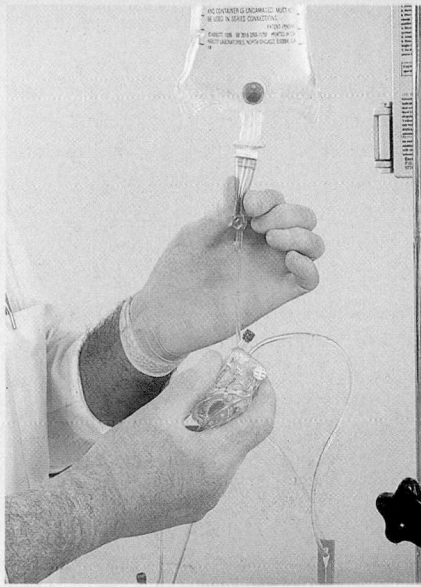

Action 4c: Squeezing drip chamber.

ACTION	RATIONALE
e. If an electronic device is to be used, follow manufacturer's instructions for inserting tubing and setting infusion rate.	This ensures correct flow rate and proper use of equipment.
f. Apply label if medication was added to container (pharmacy may have added medication and applied label).	This provides for administration of correct solution with prescribed medication or additive.
g. Place time-tape on container as necessary and hang on IV pole.	This permits immediate evaluation of IV according to schedule.
5. Have the patient in a low Fowler's position in bed. Place protective towel or pad under patient's arm.	The supine position permits either arm to be used and allows for good body alignment. The low Fowler's position is usually most comfortable for the patient.
6. Select an appropriate site and palpate accessible veins.	The selection of an appropriate site decreases discomfort for the patient and possible damage to body tissues.
7. If the site is hairy and agency policy permits, clip a 2-inch area around the intended site of entry.	It is difficult to clean the site of entry in the presence of hair because hair can harbor microorganisms.
8. Apply a tourniquet 5–6 inches above the venipuncture site to obstruct venous blood flow and distend the vein. Direct the ends of the tourniquet away from the site of entry. Check to be sure that the radial pulse is still present.	Interrupting the blood flow to the heart causes the vein to distend. Interruption of the arterial flow impedes venous filling. Distended veins are easy to see, palpate, and enter. The end of the tourniquet could contaminate the area of injection if directed toward the site of entry.
9. Ask the patient to open and close his or her fist. Observe and palpate for a suitable vein. Try the following techniques if a vein cannot be felt:	Contraction of the muscles of the forearm forces blood into the veins, thereby distending them further. Lowering the arm below the level of the heart, tapping the vein, and applying warmth help distend veins by filling them with blood.
a. Release the tourniquet and have the patient lower his or her arm below the level of the heart to fill the veins. Reapply tourniquet and gently tap over the intended vein to help distend it.	
b. Remove tourniquet and place warm moist compresses over the intended vein for 10–15 minutes.	
10. Don clean gloves.	Care must be used when handling any blood or body fluids to prevent transmission of HIV and other blood-borne infections.

(continued)

Starting an Intravenous Infusion (continued)

ACTION	RATIONALE
11. Cleanse the entry site with an antiseptic solution (alcohol swab) followed by antimicrobial solution (povidone-iodine) according to agency policy. Use a circular motion to move from the center outward for several inches.	Cleansing that begins at the site of entry and moves outward in a circular motion carries organisms away from the site of entry. Organisms on the skin can be introduced into the tissues or the bloodstream with the needle.
12. Use the nondominant hand, placed about 1 or 2 inches below entry site, to hold the skin taut against the vein. Avoid touching the prepared site.	Pressure on the vein and surrounding tissues helps prevent movement of the vein as the needle or catheter is being inserted. The needle entry site and catheter must remain free of contamination from unsterile hands.
13. Enter the skin gently with the catheter held by the hub in the dominant hand, bevel side up, at a 10- to 30-degree angle. The catheter may be inserted from directly over the vein or the side of the vein. While following the course of the vein, advance the needle or catheter into the vein. A sensation of "give" can be felt when the needle enters the vein.	This allows needle or catheter to enter the vein with minimal trauma and deters passage of the needle through the vein.

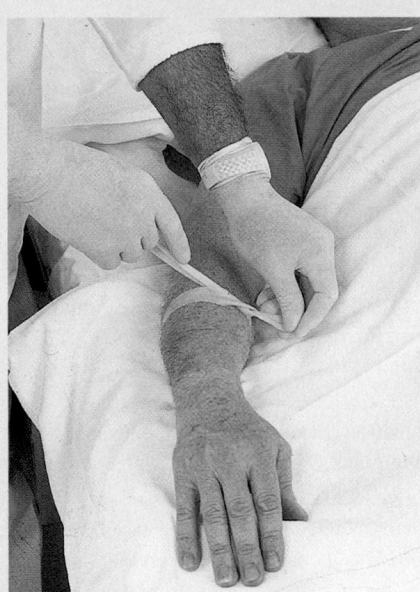

Action 8: Applying tourniquet.

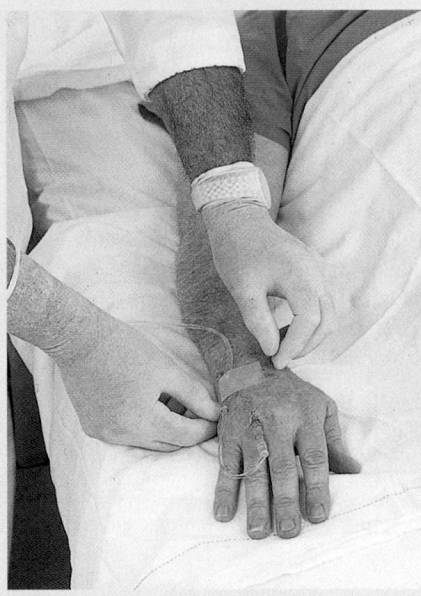

Action 18: Looping and anchoring tubing.
(Photos © B. Proud.)

14. When blood returns through the lumen of the needle or the flashback chamber of the catheter, advance either device ⅛ to ¼ inch farther into the vein. A catheter needs to be advanced until the hub is at the venipuncture site, but the exact technique depends on the type of device used.	The tourniquet causes increased venous pressure resulting in automatic backflow. Having the catheter placed well into the vein helps to prevent dislodgement.
15. Release the tourniquet. Quickly remove protective cap from the IV tubing and attach the tubing to the catheter or needle. Stabilize the catheter or needle with nondominant hand.	Bleeding is minimized and patency of the vein is maintained if the connection is made smoothly between the catheter and tubing.
16. Start the flow of solution promptly by releasing the clamp on the tubing. Examine the tissue around the entry site for signs of infiltration.	Blood clots readily if IV flow is not maintained. If catheter accidentally slips out of vein, solution will accumulate and infiltrate into surrounding tissue.
17. Secure the catheter with narrow nonallergenic tape (½ inch) placed sticky side up under the hub and crossed over the top of the hub.	The smooth structure of the vein does not offer resistance to the movement of the catheter. The weight of the tubing is sufficient to pull it out of the vein if it is not well anchored. Nonallergenic tape is less likely to tear fragile skin.

(continued)

ACTION	RATIONALE
18. Place sterile dressing over venipuncture site. Agency policy may direct nurse to use gauze dressing or transparent dressing. Apply tape to dressing if necessary. Loop the tubing near the site of entry, and anchor to dressing.	Transparent dressing allows easy visualization of site but may place patient at increased risk for infection. Gauze dressing absorbs drainage and may have a decreased infection rate. Discussion continues about effectiveness of types of dressings.
19. Mark the date, time, site and type and size of the catheter used for the infusion on the tape anchoring the tubing.	Personnel working with the infusion will know what type of device is being used, the site, and when it was inserted. Protects patient and IV site from infection.
20. Remove all equipment and dispose in proper manner. Remove gloves and perform hand hygiene.	Hand hygiene deters the spread of microorganisms.
21. Anchor arm to an armboard for support if necessary or apply a site protector or tube-shaped mesh netting over the insertion site.	An armboard or site protectors help to prevent change in the position of the catheter in the vein.
22. Adjust the rate of solution flow according to the amount prescribed or follow manufacturer's directions for adjusting flow rate on infusion pump.	The physician prescribes the rate of flow.
23. Document the procedure and patient's response. Chart time, site, device used, and solution.	This provides accurate documentation and ensures continuity of care.
24. Return to check flow rate and observe for infiltration 30 minutes after starting infusion.	This documents patient's response to infusion.

SPECIAL CONSIDERATIONS

Older adult considerations:
Avoid vigorous friction at the insertion site and using too much alcohol. Both can traumatize fragile skin and veins in the elderly.

Infant and children considerations:
Hand insertion sites should not be the first choice for children because nerve endings are very close to the surface of the skin and it is more painful.

- Scalp and feet can be used as alternate insertion sites for infants.
- Do not use the feet if the child is able to walk.
- Do not replace peripheral catheters in pediatric patients unless clinically indicated (CDC, 2002).
- Experienced nurses may elect to omit use of a tourniquet on individuals with prominent but especially fragile veins. This decreases trauma to the vessel.

The smallest-gauge device is usually selected to minimize trauma to the vein, and a dextrose solution that is 10% or less may be administered by this route (see Chap. 29, Medications, for more discussion on gauges).

Midline Peripheral Catheter

Midline catheters are inserted peripherally, normally through the antecubital fossa, but are longer (>3 inches) than peripheral venous catheters. These are not considered to be central lines and should not be used to infuse vesicants, hyperosmolar or irritating solutions (Klein, 2001). There are no set guidelines for the length of time that a midline catheter can remain in place. However, the CDC, via the *Morbidity and Mortality Weekly Report* (CDC, 2002), reports this length of time as a median of 7 days, but possibly as long as 49 days. Follow agency policy for rotation of midline catheter insertion site.

Central Venous Access Devices

Central venous access devices (CVADs) are now an integral component of patient care in acute, ambulatory, and subacute care settings, as well as in the home and long-term care facilities. They provide access for a variety of IV fluids, medications, blood products, and nutritional solutions and allow a means for hemodynamic monitoring and blood sampling. CVAD is usually introduced into the subclavian or internal jugular vein and passed to the superior vena cava just above the right atrium. All CVADs require radiographic confirmation of position. The patient's diagnosis, the type of care that is required, and other factors (eg, limited venous access, irritating drugs, patient request, or the need for long-term intermittent infusions) determine the type of CVAD used. Types of CVADs include the following:

- Peripherally inserted central catheters (PICCs)
- Nontunneled percutaneous central venous catheters
- Tunneled central venous catheters
- Implanted ports

PICCs are a type of CVAD that can be introduced into a peripheral vein (usually the basilic or cephalic veins), ideally above or below the antecubital space, and advanced as far as

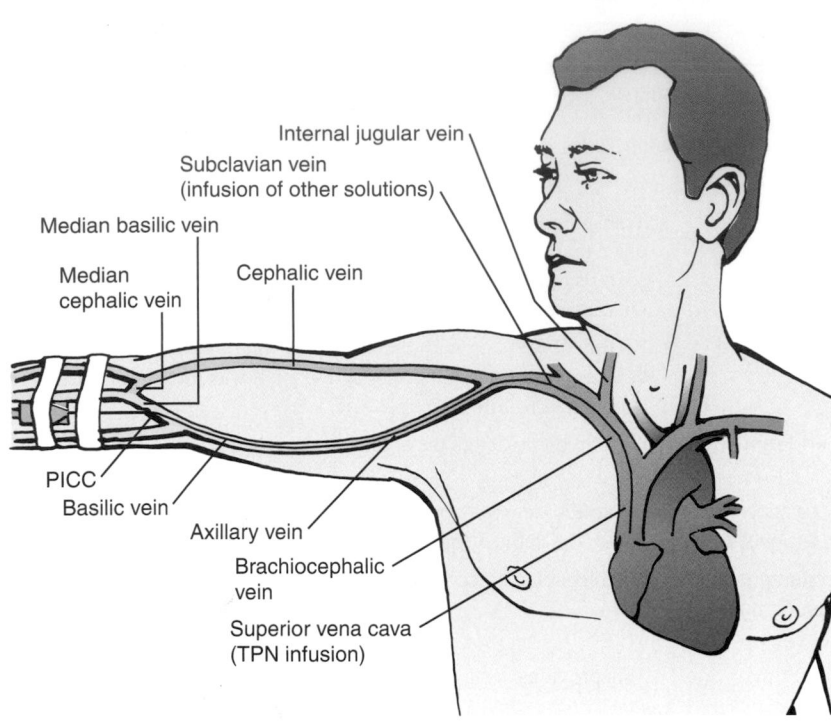

Internal jugular vein

Subclavian vein
(infusion of other solutions)

Median basilic vein

Median
cephalic vein

Cephalic vein

PICC

Basilic vein

Axillary vein

Brachiocephalic
vein

Superior vena cava
(TPN infusion)

FIGURE 46-9 Placement of peripherally inserted central catheter (PICC).

the superior vena cava (Fig. 46-9). A specially trained registered nurse or physician can insert this type of catheter. Both the Intravenous Nurses Society and the National Association of Vascular Access Networks agree that complications are less prevalent when the PICC tip rests in the superior vena cava. Radiographic verification is always required before use. PICCs may have single or dual lumens. They are used extensively in the home for IV therapy and have become an increasingly popular venous access device in acute care settings. PICCs are normally replaced as needed, that is, the catheter is no longer patent or the site looks infected. Klein (2001) reports that PICCs have been left in place for up to 1 year.

Indications for use of PICCs include administration of IV antibiotics for an extended period (2–6 weeks), infusion of parenteral nutrition, chemotherapy, continuous narcotic infusions, vesicants, hyperosmolar solutions, blood components, other specific medications (eg, vasopressors, anticoagulants), and long-term rehydration. PICC is advantageous because it can be inserted at the bedside. Additionally, the risk for pneumothorax is decreased because the catheter is inserted peripherally. PICCs are also cost-effective and provide adequate hemodilution for medications.

Nursing responsibilities include sterile dressing changes per agency schedule and protocol, routine heparin or saline flushes to maintain patency, and careful observation for any complications of PICC therapy, such as phlebitis, cellulitis, infiltration, and infection or sepsis. Guidelines for Nursing Care 46-2 provides additional information related to nursing care for a patient with a PICC.

Nontunneled percutaneous central venous catheters (Fig. 46-10) have a shorter dwell time (3–10 days) and are introduced through the skin into the jugular, subclavian, or

femoral veins and sutured into place. These catheters can have double-, triple-, or quadruple-lumens. The catheter tip rests in the superior vena cava. They may be inserted at the bedside or in outpatient settings. This type of central venous catheter has a high risk for complications, particularly infection and pneumothorax if placed in the subclavian.

A *tunneled central venous catheter,* intended for long-term use, is placed through a small incision into the jugular or subclavian vein (where the tip of the catheter lies) and tunneled in subcutaneous tissue under the skin (usually the midchest area) for 3 to 6 inches to its exit site. It is initially sutured into place, but after 7 to 14 days, the sutures are removed. Subcutaneous tissue attaches to a Dacron™ polyester cuff around the catheter, helping to stabilize the catheter and minimize the risk for infection.

Another type of long-term CVAD is an *implanted port.* The catheter tip is placed in the subclavian or jugular vein, but the proximal end or port is usually implanted in a subcutaneous pocket of the upper chest wall, and no external parts of the system are visible. Implanted ports placed in the antecubital area of the arm are referred to as peripheral access system ports. Initially used for chemotherapy, implanted ports are now used for any patient requiring long-term intermittent infusions. A special angled noncoring needle is inserted through the skin and rubber septum and into the port reservoir (Fig. 46-11).

Implanted ports require minimal care, but the discomfort of accessing the port may be a disadvantage for some patients. Some patients may request that a numbing cream be applied to the site before needle insertion. If this technique is used, ensure that all of the cream is removed and the skin adequately cleaned before accessing the port.

Guidelines for Nursing Care 46-2
Caring for a Client With a PICC

Maintenance

Always check agency policy for specific guidelines.

- Use sterile technique when changing dressings (24 hours after insertion and at least once a week thereafter). Also change dressing if soiled or loose.
- When accessing port or changing dressing, know that many agencies require nurse and patient to wear a mask.
- Keep external portion of catheter coiled under dressing.
- Change catheter caps every 3 to 7 days based on frequency of access and agency policy. Many agencies have a policy to replace caps once they have been removed (eg, when blood is drawn).
- Flush: Using a 10-mL syringe, flush *open-ended catheter* with heparin solution after intermittent use or every 12 hours if catheter is not currently in use. Using a 10-mL syringe, flush a *close-ended catheter* with saline after each intermittent use or once a week if not in use. After withdrawing a blood specimen, flush PICC with 20 mL of normal saline and follow with a final flush of heparin solution.

- Avoid blood pressure measurement in the involved arm.
- Document:
    - Appearance of site
    - Length of external part of catheter
    - Dates of dressing and cap change
    - Flushing frequency and routine
    - Any problems

Client Instruction

- Demonstrate procedures, care, and maintenance of PICC catheter as well as potential complications.
- Provide simple, written instructions for patient/caregiver at home. Instruct concerning reasons to notify nurse or doctor.
- Emphasize that there are minimal activity restrictions.
- Instruct to protect insertion site when showering or bathing.
- Advise to wear a Medic-Alert tag if use is long-term.
- Instruct to have repair kit on hand at home.
- Avoid strenuous physical activity that may cause displacement of the catheter.

Adapted from Klein, T. (2001). PICC and midlines. Fine-tuning your care. *RN, 64*(8), 26–29.

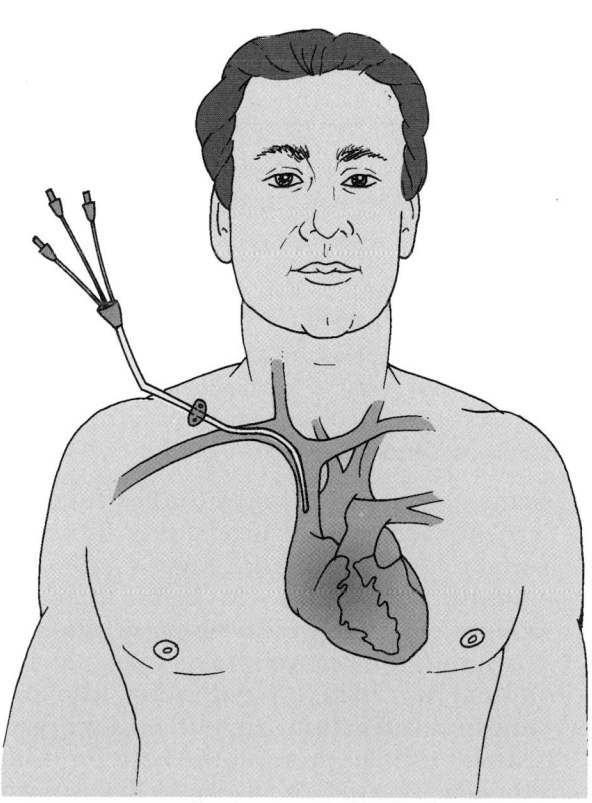

FIGURE 46-10 Placement of triple-lumen nontunneled percutaneous central venous catheter.

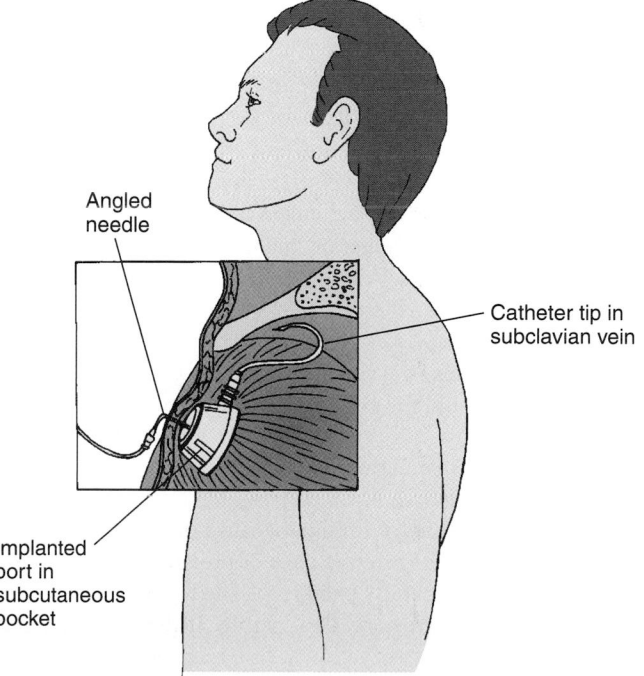

FIGURE 46-11 Placement of an implanted port with the tip in the subclavian vein. Angled needle is inserted through skin and rubber septum into port.

Nursing responsibilities with central venous catheters include using sterile technique, changing the dressing according to agency policy, carefully assessing for any sign of infection, changing injection caps on the lumens, and flushing with a prescribed solution (usually saline and heparin) to prevent clotting and blockage of the lumen. Many agencies have a policy to discard the injection cap once it is removed (eg, when blood is drawn) and replace it with a sterile cap because contaminated caps have been implicated as a cause of systemic infections. While caring for patients with CVADs, use the opportunity for health teaching about medical and surgical asepsis and meticulous skin care.

Site Selection

The suitability of particular veins for IV infusions varies with individual circumstances. Selection should be determined after considering the following factors.

Accessibility of a Vein

Keep in mind the following guidelines for accessibility:

• Determine the most desirable accessible vein. The lower cephalic vein, accessory cephalic vein, and basilic vein are good sites for infusion. The superficial veins on the dorsal aspect of the hand can also be used successfully for some people. Figure 46-12 illustrates common infusion sites on the arm and hand. Either arm may be used for IV therapy. If the patient is right-handed and both arms appear equally usable, usually the left arm is selected to free the right arm for the patient's use.

• Determine accessibility based on the patient's condition. For example, a person with severe burns on both forearms does not have vessels available in these areas, or a patient with a history of axillary node dissection should not have venipunctures in the affected arm.

• Do not use the antecubital veins if another vein is available. They are not a good choice for infusion because flexion of the patient's arm can displace the IV catheter over time. By avoiding the antecubital veins for peripheral venous catheters, a PICC line may be inserted at a later time if needed.

• Do not use veins in the leg, unless other sites are inaccessible, because of the danger of stagnation of peripheral circulation and possible serious complications. Some institutions require a physician's order to insert an IV catheter in an adult patient's lower extremity.

• Do not use veins in surgical areas. For example, infusions in the arm should not be given on the same side as recent extensive breast surgery, because of vascular disturbances in the area, or in an arm that has a device inserted for dialysis (eg, fistula or shunt).

• Select scalp veins for infants because of their accessibility and because of relative ease of preventing dislocation of the needle. Carefully palpate the site before insertion. Infant's scalp arteries are also visible. If the site is pulsating do not use.

Think back to Jeremiah Kearny, the infant with nausea and vomiting. The nurse would incorporate knowledge of appropriate site selection

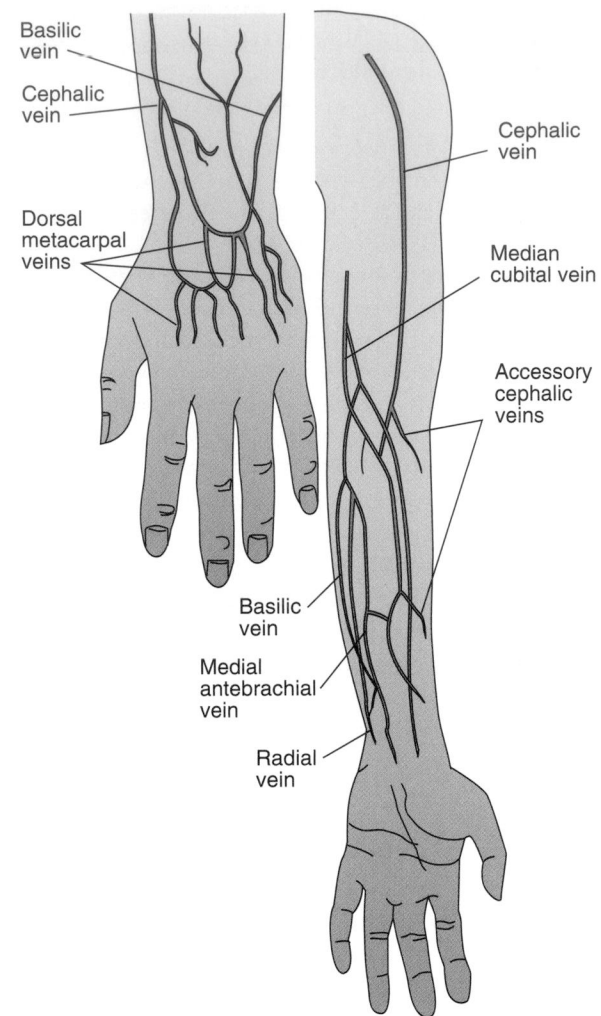

FIGURE 46-12 Infusion sites on the ventral and dorsal aspects of the lower arm and hand.

for infants when determining the location for Jeremiah's IV.

Condition of the Vein

The condition of the patient's vein is extremely important. Often, experience is necessary to acquire skill in palpating a patient's vein to determine its condition. Thin-walled and scarred veins, especially in some older patients, make continued infusion a problem.

Remember Grace Gilligan, the patient who experienced several unsuccessful IV catheter insertion attempts? The nurse's ability to palpate the patient's veins before attempting venipuncture might have been helpful in determining the best vein to be used. The information provided by palpation also could have indicated that the patient's veins were scarred, thus suggesting the need for a more experienced team member, such as someone from anesthesiology (as the patient had requested) to perform the procedure.

Type of Fluid to Be Infused

Keep in mind the following about the type of IV fluid to be infused:

- Select a vein appropriate for the solution. Hypertonic solutions, those containing irritating medications, those administered at a rapid rate, and those with a high viscosity should be given in a large vein to minimize vessel trauma and to facilitate the rate of flow.
- Advise the patient that some medications administered intravenously in a peripheral vein may cause irritation and pain (eg, potassium chloride and certain antibiotics) and urge the patient to report any complaints.

Anticipated Duration of Infusion

Consider the anticipated duration of the infusion. Always select a site where restriction in movement is kept to a minimum if this is a consideration. In addition, change peripheral venous catheter sites every 72 to 96 hours, if possible, starting with sites as distal as possible and moving in a proximal direction on the alternate arms.

Other Considerations

- Select the catheter with the smallest gauge and shortest possible length that will maintain the ordered infusion. Insert it into the largest vein available.
- Select a site that is naturally splinted by bone, such as the back of the hand or the forearm. If the site is not splinted, such as the wrist, use an immobilizer, if appropriate, to prevent movement and subsequent trauma to the vein.
- Select a site distal to the heart and move proximally, as necessary, to find an appropriate injection site.
- Select a site while moving toward the heart and away from a damaged vein.

Initiation of an IV Infusion

Before the infusion is started, perform a final check of the solution to ensure that it is clear and contains no particles or precipitates. This check is especially important when substances have been added to the solution because some additives create precipitates. Commercially available in-line filters help reduce the risk for contamination by filtering the solution immediately before it enters the patient's vein. Filters are routinely recommended for any patient receiving long-term IV therapy, TPN, or IV chemotherapy (see Skill 46-1 for techniques for starting an IV infusion, earlier in the chapter).

Some adults and young children have a fear of needles. In these situations, it may be advisable to use a product that eases the discomfort of venipuncture. One such system (eg, Numby Stuff™) uses a mild electrical current to apply local analgesia to the skin. The analgesic takes effect in 10 minutes. Lidocaine (EMLA) cream also numbs the skin, but it must be applied at least 60 minutes before the procedure to be effective. In addition, the cream must be removed before starting the venipuncture. A subcutaneous injection of local anesthetic may effectively ease insertion pain but is likely to be rejected by a patient with a fear of needles (see the accompanying Research in Nursing box).

Regulation and Monitoring

The nurse is responsible for maintaining the proper flow rate while ensuring the comfort and safety of the patient. The physician prescribes the amount of solution to be infused

Research in Nursing Making a Difference

Using Lidocaine for Peripheral IV Insertions: Patients' Preferences and Pain Experiences

The need for an IV raises the anxiety level of most patients. Whether patients have had a previous IV or not, they perceive an IV start as a painful procedure. Since the placement of an intravenous catheter is a fairly common invasive procedure, nurses should know what methods can be used to alleviate some of the pain and anxiety.

Related Research

Brown, J. (2003). Using lidocaine for peripheral IV insertions: Patients' preferences and pain experiences. *MEDSURG Nursing, 12*(2), 95–101.

This study included 188 subjects ranging in age from 19 to 82 years with an average age of 64.5 years. Eligibility for being placed into the study consisted of being 18 years of age or older, alert and oriented, able to understand English, and with a peripheral IV in place at the time of the study. Eighty-nine percent, or 160 of the 188 participants, had had previous IV catheters placed. Of the 89% with prior IV history, only 29% of the IV catheters were placed while using intradermal lidocaine.

The participants were interviewed regarding whether they had ever received intradermal lidocaine for an IV start, whether they were offered intradermal lidocaine with the placement of this IV, and if they had refused intradermal lidocaine in the past and for what reason. They were asked to rate the pain of receiving the intradermal lidocaine (if applicable) and the pain of the IV insertion.

The study showed that 79 of the participants had received intradermal lidocaine with a previous IV placement. Women rated the pain of the intradermal lidocaine as a mean of 2.28 (0–10 range) and the pain of IV insertion as a 2.4 (0–10 range), while men rated the pain of intradermal lidocaine as a mean of 1.1 (0–4 range) and the pain of IV insertion as a 1.6 (0–5 range). Out of 180 participants, 134 (74%) will request intradermal lidocaine for future IV insertions. Eight participants were excluded from the study because of insufficient data.

Relevance to Nursing Practice

This study shows that many patients would like a local anesthetic for peripheral IV insertion. Nurses should be made aware of all options so that they can inform patients. By making patients aware of all options, nurses increase the quality of care as well as improve patient satisfaction.

within a specified period. The rate is then determined on the basis of the amount of solution to be infused over 1 hour. This is called the drip rate.

The drop factor, or drops per milliliter of solution, is determined by the size of the opening in the infusion apparatus. It varies among different products from different companies. Most health agencies use the products of a single company. The most common drop factors are macrodrop systems (10, 15, 20 drops per mL), a microdrip (60 drops per mL), and a blood administration set (10 drops per mL). Microdrip or 60 drops per milliliter is used most often when small fluid volumes are administered, such as a rate less than 75 mL per hour. Macrodrop tubing is commonly used for rates greater than 75 mL per hour. A method for determining flow rate is described in the accompanying Guidelines for Nursing Care 46-3.

A buretrol, or volume-control device, as shown in Figure 46-13, can also be used to reduce the risk for fluid overload or medication overdose. These are commonly used in the pediatric area. They may also be used to deliver intermittent medications that need to be further diluted and given over a specific time.

A time tape can be placed on the container of solution to provide a quick reference for the nurse to monitor the rate at which the solution is entering the patient. The tape gives an

hourly indication of where the fluid level should be, based on the nurse's calculation of the drip rate.

Many factors can alter the rate of flow of an IV infusion, such as the height of the container in relation to the patient, the patient's blood pressure, the patient's position, the patency of the IV catheter, infiltration, and any knot or kink in the tubing. Check the infusion every hour or more frequently, if indicated, to determine if the solution is being infused at the proper hourly rate. If it is not, the nurse again regulates the flow. Because the patient's movements, disturbances of the regulation mechanism, or change in the height of the infusion bottle or bed can alter the flow rate, even after it is regulated, continually check on the infusion at regular intervals. It has been reported that standard IV administration sets lose up to one half of their initial flow rate during the first hour of infusion because of tubing flexibility; therefore, the rate may need to be adjusted.

Maintenance of the flow rate is important because it can directly affect the patient's fluid balance. Too slow a flow may result in a fluid volume deficit because the input is not balancing fluid lost or it may delay the restoration of the balance. Infusing IV fluid too rapidly can overtax the body's capacities to adjust to the increase in the water volume or the electrolytes it contains, and lead to fluid volume excess. Allowing an infusion to get behind schedule and then increasing the rate to catch

Guidelines for Nursing Care 46-3
Regulating IV Flow Rate

Follow agency's guidelines to determine if infusion should be administered by electronic pump or by gravity.
- Check physician's order for IV solution.
- Check patency of IV line and needle.
- Verify drop factor (number of drops in 1 mL) of the equipment in use.
- Calculate the flow rate:
  EXAMPLE—Administer 1000 mL D$_5$W over 10 hours (set delivers 60 gtt/1 mL).

a. **Standard formula**

$$gtt/min = \frac{volume\,(mL) \times drop\,factor\,(gtt/mL)}{time\,(in\,minutes)}$$

$$gtt/min = \frac{1000\,mL \times 60}{600\,(60\,min \times 10\,h)}$$

$$= \frac{60,000}{600}$$

$$= 100\,gtt/min$$

b. **Short formula using milliliters per hour**

$$gtt/min = \frac{milliliters\,per\,hour \times drop\,factor\,(gtt/mL)}{time\,(60\,min)}$$

Find milliliters per hour by dividing 1000 mL by 10 hours:

$$\frac{1000}{10} = 100\,mL/hr$$

$$gtt/min = \frac{100\,mL \times 60}{60\,min}$$

$$= \frac{6,000}{60}$$

$$= 100\,gtt/min$$

c. **Dimensional analysis**

$$gtt/min = \frac{gtt}{mL} \times \frac{mL}{hr} \times \frac{hr}{min}$$

$$gtt/min = \frac{60\,gtt}{1\,mL} \times \frac{1000\,mL}{10\,hr} \times \frac{1\,hr}{60\,min}$$

$$= \frac{60,000\,gtt}{600\,min}$$

$$= 100\,gtt/min$$

- Count drops per minute in drip chamber (number of gtt/15 sec interval × 4 = gtt/min). Hold watch beside drip chamber.
- Adjust IV clamp as needed and recount drops per minute.
- Mark IV container according to agency policy and manufacturer's recommendations. Use a time tape or label if indicated to measure amount to be infused at timed intervals.
- Monitor IV flow rate at frequent intervals. Document patient's response to infusion at prescribed rate.

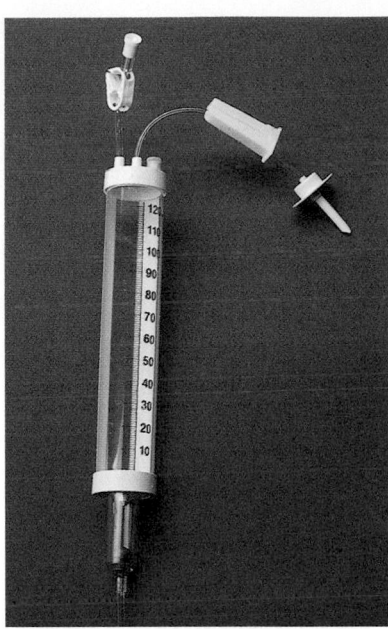

FIGURE 46-13 Volume-controlled set.

up might seriously insult the patient's compensatory mechanisms and jeopardize the patient's well-being.

Electronic infusion-control devices limit the amount of fluid to be infused at any one time and, in some healthcare facilities, are used to regulate all IV infusions. They can automatically regulate the flow rate at preset limits. An alarm sounds when air is in the tubing, the flow is obstructed, the solution level of the bottle or bag is getting low, or there is increased pressure in the system, such as occurs when an IV infiltrates and fluid flows into the tissues. Either a pump or controller may be used, but many healthcare facilities use pumps because their accuracy is greater, they deliver fluids against gravity or resistance, and there are fewer IV-related problems. Pumps totally control the delivery rate by exerting positive pressure based on preset limits when resistance develops. Controllers do not rely on pressure to control solution flow but, rather, rely on the height of the IV container in relation to the IV site to affect flow rate over time. JCAHO has listed "safe use of infusion pumps" as one of their 2004 National Patient Safety Goals. The specific concern is to prevent free-flow on all general use and PCA IV infusion pumps (JCAHO, 2003).

> *Consider Jack Soo Park, the patient who received too much IV fluid. When planning Mr. Park's care, the nurse would need to include frequent assessments of the IV infusion to ensure that it is infusing at the proper flow rate. In addition, the nurse should double-check the flow-rate calculation to ensure its accuracy, thereby minimizing the risk for error. Possibly placing the infusion on an infusion-control device, such as a pump, might have prevented this error.*

Syringe pumps are also available. They deliver small amounts of fluid, 100 mL or less, and are particularly useful with infants and children. Syringe pumps are also useful in delivering small amounts of medications over a set amount of time, as is needed with some antibiotics. Portable models are also available and are useful in ambulatory and home settings.

Candidates for infusion pump IV therapy in the home should meet certain criteria. They should be medically stable, have a full- or part-time caregiver, have access to a telephone, and have a refrigerator available for storage of prefilled medication cartridges. Patients can receive insulin infusions, pain medication, antibiotic therapy, cancer chemotherapy, or TPN through portable infusion pumps at home. Skill 46-3 later in this chapter illustrates the use of an infusion pump.

Solution and Tubing Changes

If more than one container of solution is ordered for the patient, attach additional containers using the method determined in the agency. Some IV equipment is designed to simplify the procedure by making it possible to attach additional solutions with a tandem-like arrangement. Because infusions are often continued after the responsibility for a patient's care changes from one nurse to another, it is a good practice to agree on one common method for managing infusions. Without such uniformity, serious errors can occur, or valuable time is lost in checking and rechecking. One method for changing the solution and tubing is presented in Skill 46-2.

The frequency of tubing changes varies. Most IV fluids require tubing to be changed on the average of every 72 hours. However, other fluids, such as TPN solutions, require tubing changes every 24 hours, while still other solutions with medications may require tubing changes every 6 hours. Check your agency's policy.

Infusion Site Care

Scrupulous care of the infusion site is necessary to help control contamination and to help prevent the introduction of microorganisms into the bloodstream. Catheter contamination can occur from the following sources:

- Hands of the caregiver
- Skin bacteria that contaminate the catheter during insertion
- Disconnection of the tubing or injection cap from the catheter hub, allowing bacteria to enter the closed system or multiple-lumen catheters
- Poor insertion technique
- An IV solution that becomes contaminated when solutions are changed, a medication is added, or the solution is allowed to infuse for too long a period

> *Think back to Grace Gilligan, the woman described in the Reflective Practice display. The numerous attempts at venipuncture increase the patient's risk for possible infection.*

Regular dressing changes and tubing replacements are important means of preventing infection. Gauze and transparent membrane dressings are used most commonly to protect the insertion site. Transparent dressings (eg, Tegaderm or OpSite IV) allow easy inspection of the IV site, permit evaporation of

SKILL 46-2   Changing IV Solution and Tubing

EQUIPMENT

For solution change:
   IV solution as ordered by physician

For tubing change:
   Administration set
   Sterile gauze
   Timing tape or label

Sterile dressings and antiseptic solutions
   (according to agency recommendations)
Disposable gloves

ACTION	RATIONALE
1. Gather all equipment and bring to bedside. Check IV solution and medication additives with physician's order.	Having equipment available saves time and facilitates accomplishment of task. Ensures that patient receives the correct IV solution and medication as ordered by physician.
2. Explain procedure to patient.	Explanation allays patient's anxiety.
3. Perform hand hygiene.	Hand hygiene deters the spread of microorganisms.
To Change IV Solution	
4. Carefully remove protective cover from new solution container and expose entry site.	This maintains sterility of IV solution.
5. Close clamp on tubing.	Clamping stops the flow of IV fluid during change of solution.
6. Lift container off IV pole and invert it. Quickly remove the spike from the old IV container, being careful not to contaminate it (see photo, p. 1469).	This maintains sterility of IV setup.
7. Steady new container and insert spike. Hang on IV pole.	This allows for uninterrupted flow of new solution.
8. Reopen clamp on tubing and adjust flow.	Opening clamp regulates flow rate into drip chamber.
9. Label container according to agency policy. Record on intake and output record and document on chart according to agency policy. Discard used equipment in proper manner. Perform hand hygiene.	This ensures accurate continuation and administration of correct IV solution. Hand hygiene deters the spread of microorganisms.
To Change IV Tubing and Solution	
10. Follow actions 1 through 4.	This maintains sterility of IV setup. Once clamp is closed, the bag can be spiked without loss of solution.
11. Open the administration set and close clamp on new tubing. Remove protective covering from infusion spike. Using sterile technique, insert into new container.	
12. Hang IV container on pole and squeeze drip chamber to fill at least halfway.	Gravity and suction effect cause fluid to move into drip chamber.
13. Remove cap at end of tubing, release clamp, and allow fluid to move through tubing until all air bubbles have disappeared. Close clamp and recap end of tubing maintaining sterility of setup.	This removes air from tubing that can, in larger amounts, act as an air embolus.
To Change Tubing on a Short Extension Set	
14. Close the clamp on the existing IV tubing. Also close the clamp on the short extension tubing connected to the IV catheter in the patient's arm.	A short closed tubing set (extension set) with an injection port and closure clamp between the catheter or angiocath hub and the tubing reduces the risk for blood exposure. Clamping the existing IV tubing prevents leakage of fluid. Clamping the tubing on the extension set prevents introduction of air into the line.
15. Remove the current infusion tubing from the resealable cap on the short extension IV tubing (see photo, p. 1469). Using an alcohol wipe, swab the resealable cap and insert the new IV connector into the cap. Proceed to Action 2.	Cleansing the port reduces the risk of contamination.
To Change Tubing Connected Directly into the Hub of the IV Access Catheter	
16. Loosen tape at IV insertion site. Don clean gloves. Carefully remove dressing and tape.	Removing dressing provides access to needle hub necessary for tubing change. Gloves must be worn when blood contact is possible. This prevents transmission of HIV and other blood-borne infections.

(continued)

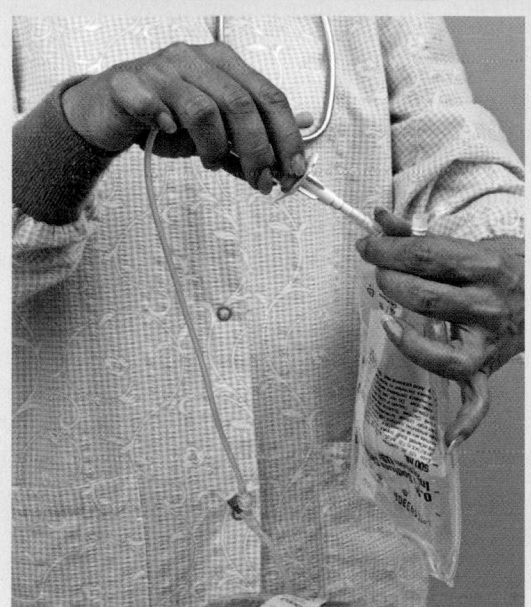

Action 6: Invert solution bag and remove spike.
(Photo by Rick Brady.)

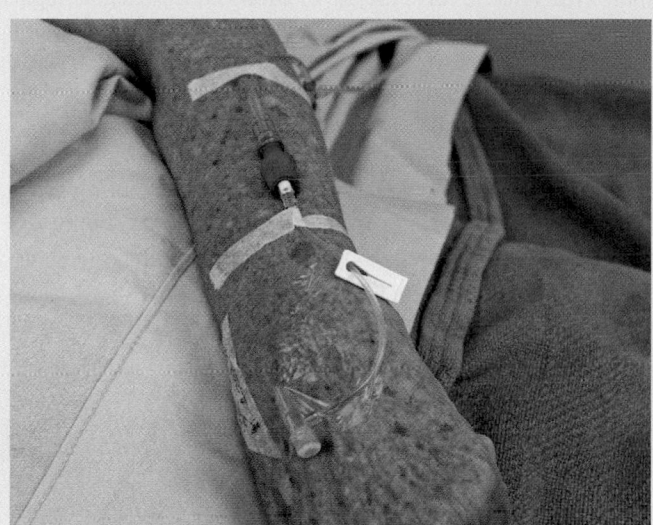

Action 15: Remove old administration set tubing.   (Photo by Rick Brady.)

ACTION	RATIONALE
17. Place sterile gauze square under needle hub.	Gauze absorbs any leakage when tubing is disconnected from needle.
18. Place new IV tubing close to patient's IV site and slightly loosen protective cap.	This facilitates removal of cap and attachment to needle hub.
19. Clamp the old IV tubing. Steady the needle hub with nondominant hand until change is completed. Remove tubing with dominant hand using a twisting motion.	This stabilizes needle and prevents inadvertently dislodging it.
20. Set old tubing aside. While maintaining sterility, carefully remove covering or cap from the new administration set and insert sterile end of tubing into the needle hub. Twist to secure it. Remove gauze square from under needle hub. Remove soiled gloves.	This maintains sterility of IV setup. Use of gentle pressure helps prevent blood from exiting the hub when tubing is removed.
21. Open the clamp on the IV tubing and check the flow.	Opening clamp allows solution to flow to patient.
22. Reapply sterile dressing to site according to agency protocol (see Skill 46-4).	This deters entry of microorganisms at site.
23. Regulate the IV flow according to physician's order.	This ensures that patient receives IV solution at the prescribed rate.
24. Attach to IV tubing tape or label that states date, time, and your initials. Label container and record procedure according to agency policy. Discard used equipment in proper manner and perform hand hygiene.	This documents IV tubing change. Hand hygiene deters the spread of microorganisms.
25. Record patient's response to IV infusion.	This ensures accurate documentation of patient's response.

moisture that accumulates under the dressing, and help to secure the catheter. Additional IV securement systems include plastic shields and adhesive anchors. Hard plastic shields that are ventilated and secured with tape are often used in pediatric settings. Adhesive anchors eliminate the need for tape but are more costly and involve the use of strong adhesives that might make it difficult to change the dressing without dislodging the catheter. Agency policy generally determines the type of dressing and the intervals for dressing change. The Intravenous Nurses Society recommends an IV dressing change every 48 hours, whereas the CDC suggest changing them every 48 to 72 hours. All guidelines state that any dressing that is damp, loosened, or soiled should be changed immediately. Skills 46-3 and 46-4 explain how to monitor an IV site and how to change an IV dressing.

A controversial aspect of the care of a central line concerns irrigation of the needle with an antithrombolytic such as t-PA (tissue plasminogen activator; Alteplase). An irrigation is sometimes used when the needle begins to clog with blood and the patient does not have other good sites for starting another infusion. The procedure requires a physician's order and should not be used unless agency policy recommends it.

Complications

The patient can be an important source of information regarding the possibility of complications associated with IV therapy. If the patient is uncomfortable, check that the infusion is entering the vein as intended, that the flow rate is not too rapid, and that the patient's position is satisfactory. Anxiety about receiving an infusion can also cause discomfort for the patient.

Local complications, such as infiltration, phlebitis, and thrombophlebitis, occur more frequently than systemic complications. Systemic complications (eg, fluid overload, embolus, sepsis), however, are more serious and may be life-

---

SKILL 46-3   Monitoring an IV Site and Infusion

EQUIPMENT
Watch with second hand (if monitoring IV
  by gravity flow)

ACTION	RATIONALE
1. Monitor IV infusion several times a shift. More frequent checks may be necessary if medication is being infused:	This promotes safe administration of IV fluids and medication. Too rapid administration of medications can result in the development of speed shock.
a. Check physician's order for IV solution.	This ensures that correct solution is being given at the correct rate and in the proper sequence with the correct medications.
b. Check drip chamber and time drops (see photo) if IV is not regulated by an infusion control device.	This ensures that flow rate is correct.
c. Check tubing for anything that might interfere with flow. Be sure that clamp is in the open position. Observe dressing for leakage of IV solution.	Any kink or pressure on tubing may interfere with flow. Leakage may occur at connection of tubing with hub of needle or catheter and allow for loss of IV solution.
d. Observe settings, alarm, and indicator lights on infusion control device if one is being used (see photo).	Observation ensures that infusion control device is functioning and that alarm is in on position.

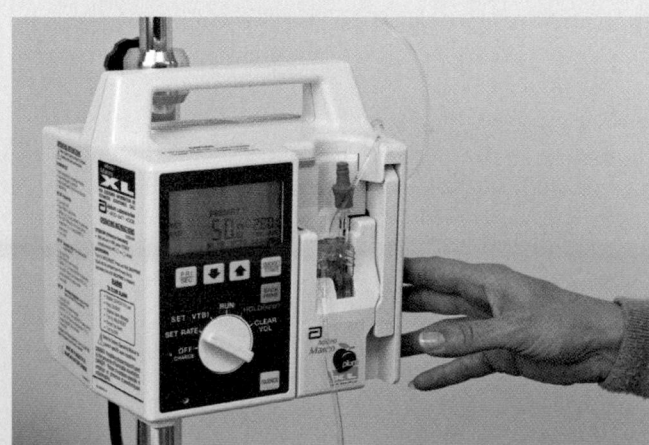

Action 1b: Timing the drops.   Action 1d: Setting up the pump.

(continued)

SKILL 46-3   Monitoring an IV Site and Infusion (continued)

ACTION	RATIONALE
2. Perform hand hygiene.	Hand hygiene deters the spread of microorganisms.
3. Inspect site for swelling, pain, coolness, or pallor at site of insertion, which may indicate infiltration of IV. This necessitates removing IV and restarting at another site.	Catheter may become dislodged from vein, and IV solution may flow into subcutaneous tissue.

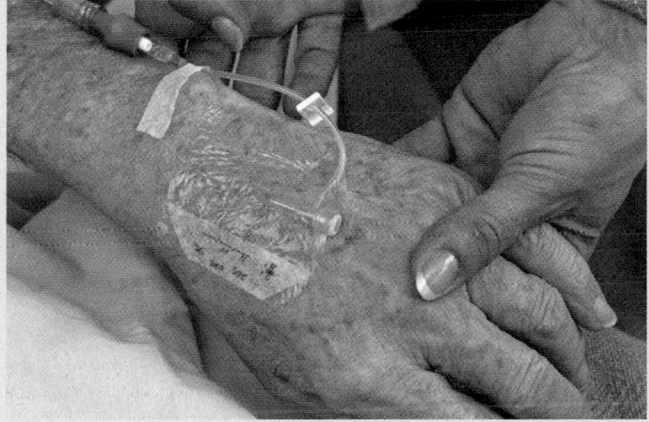

Action 3: Checking inflammation surrounding infusion site.   (Photos © B. Proud.)

ACTION	RATIONALE
4. Inspect site (see photo) for redness, swelling, heat, and pain at the IV site, which may indicate phlebitis is present. IV will need to be discontinued and restarted at another site. Notify physician if you suspect that phlebitis may have occurred.	Chemical irritation or mechanical trauma cause injury to the vein and can lead to the development of phlebitis.
5. Palpate site.	Palpation helps to detect firmness or pain suggesting a complication.
6. Check for local or systemic manifestations that indicate an infection is present at the site. IV will be discontinued and physician notified. Be careful not to disconnect IV tubing when putting on patient's hospital gown.	Poor aseptic technique may allow bacteria to enter the needle or catheter insertion site or tubing connection.
7. Be alert for additional complications of IV therapy.	
a. Circulatory overload can result in signs of cardiac failure and pulmonary edema. Monitor intake and output during IV therapy.	Infusing too much IV solution results in an increased volume of circulating fluid.
b. Bleeding at the site is most likely to occur when the IV is discontinued.	Bleeding may be caused by anticoagulant medication.
8. If possible, instruct patient to call for assistance if any discomfort is noted at site, solution container is nearly empty, or flow has changed in any way.	This facilitates cooperation of patient and safe administration of IV solution.
9. Document IV infusion, any complications of therapy, and patient's reaction to therapy.	This provides accurate documentation and ensures continuity of care.

threatening. Table 46-11 defines these complications, noting common causes, signs and symptoms, and pertinent nursing considerations.

Capping of a Primary Line for Intermittent Use

When a continuous IV is no longer necessary, the primary IV line can be capped and converted to an intermittent infusion device, commonly referred to as a heparin or saline lock, which provides venous access for intermittent or emergency medications. A heparin or saline lock consists of a plastic tube with a sealed injection port on the end that is connected to an indwelling IV catheter. Blunt cannula systems and other needleless adapters are also commonly used in healthcare facilities to cap a primary line. Periodic injection with heparin

SKILL
46-4**Changing an IV Dressing**

EQUIPMENT

Sterile gauze (2″ × 2″ or 4″ × 4″) or transparent occlusive dressing
Povidone-iodine (Betadine) swabs

Adhesive remover (optional)
Alcohol swabs
Tape

Clean gloves
Towel or disposable pad
Masks for nurse and patient (optional)

ACTION	RATIONALE
Peripheral	
1. Assess patient's need for dressing change.	Agency policy determines interval for dressing change (every 24 to 72 hours). The presence of moisture or a nonadhering dressing increases risk for bacterial contamination at the site.
2. Gather equipment and bring to bedside. Place towel or disposable pad under extremity.	Having equipment available saves time and facilitates the performance of the task.
3. Explain procedure to patient.	Explanation allays patient's anxiety.
4. Perform hand hygiene. Don clean gloves.	Hand hygiene deters the spread of microorganisms. Gloves prevent transmission of HIV and other blood-borne infections.
5. Carefully remove old dressing but leave tape that anchors IV needle or catheter in place. Discard in proper manner.	This prevents dislodging of IV needle or catheter.
6. Assess IV site for presence of inflammation or infiltration. Discontinue and relocate the IV if noted.	Inflammation or infiltration causes trauma to tissues and necessitates removal of the IV needle or catheter.
7. Loosen tape and gently remove, being careful to steady catheter with one hand. Use adhesive remover if necessary.	Tape stabilizes needle and prevents inadvertently dislodging it.
8. Cleanse the entry site with an alcohol swab using a circular motion moving from the center outward. Allow to dry. Follow with povidone-iodine swab using the same process.	Cleaning in a circular motion while moving outward carries organisms away from the entry site. Use of antiseptic solutions reduces the number of microorganisms on the skin surface.
9. Reapply tape strip to needle or catheter at entry site.	Tape anchors needle or catheter to prevent dislodgement.
10. Apply sterile gauze or transparent polyurethane dressing over entry site. Remove gloves and dispose of properly.	Dressing protects site and deters contamination with microorganisms.
11. Secure IV tubing with additional tape if necessary. Label dressing with date, time of change, and initials. Check that IV flow is accurate and system is patent.	Label documents IV dressing change.
Central Venous Access Device	
12. Follow Actions 1–5.	
13. Remove gloves and perform hand hygiene. If agency requires, nurse and patient should put on a mask. Open dressing kit using sterile technique. If patient does not wear mask, have patient turn head away from site until new dressing is applied.	Unclean hands and improper technique are potential sources for infecting a central venous access device. Most facilities have all sterile dressing supplies gathered in a single unit. Masks or turning head away helps to minimize risk of infection.
14. Put on sterile gloves.	Use of sterile gloves maintains surgical asepsis.
15. Using the alcohol swabs, move in a circular fashion from the insertion site outward (1½- to 2-inch area). Allow to dry.	The alcohol kills *Staphylococcus aureus* and *epidermis*, which are the most common causes of central line infections.
16. Follow alcohol cleansing with povidone-iodine swabs using the same technique. Allow to dry.	Povidone-iodine kills fungi that are responsible for 25% of central line infections.
17. Reapply sterile dressing or securement device according to agency policy. Secure tubing or lumens to prevent tugging on insertion site. Dressing should be occlusive.	New sterile dressing prevents contamination of the IV catheter and protects insertion site. An occlusive dressing decreases the risk for infection.
18. Note date, time of dressing change, size of catheter, and initials on tape or dressing.	This documents that dressing change occurred.
19. Discard equipment properly and perform hand hygiene.	Hand hygiene protects against spread of microorganisms.
20. Record patient's response to dressing change and observation of site.	This provides accurate documentation and ensures continuity of care.

(continued)

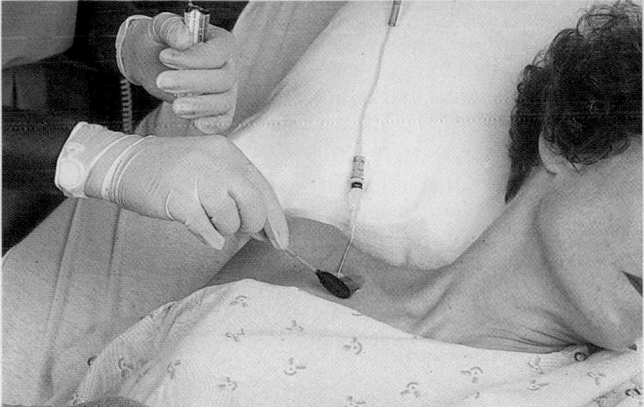

Action 16: Cleaning with povidone-iodine swabs.

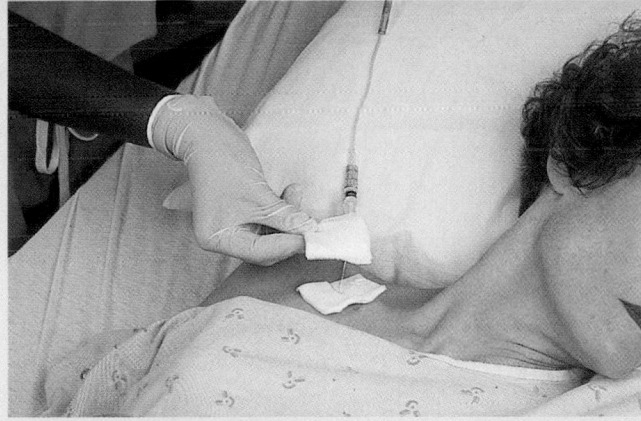

Action 17: Applying a sterile dressing.

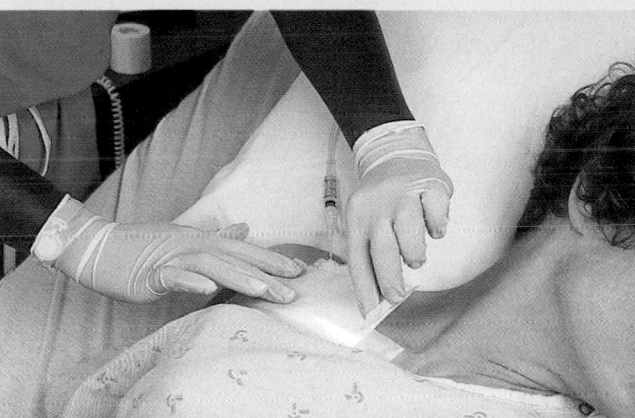

Action 17: Securing the dressing with tape.

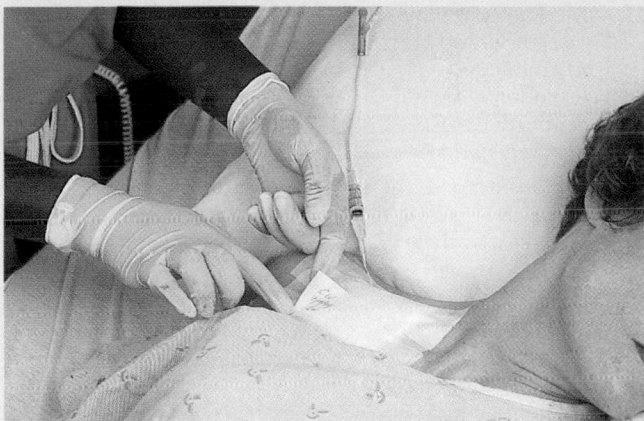

Action 18: Labeling the dressing.

or saline according to agency policy is required to keep the catheter patent. Skill 46-5 describes this technique.

Discontinuation of the Infusion

When the amount of solution the physician has ordered has been infused or when the insertion site shows signs of local complications, the nurse assumes responsibility for discontinuing the infusion. If the catheter is to be removed, the tubing is clamped, and the adhesive strips and sterile dressing are removed. The catheter is withdrawn in line with the vein, and pressure is immediately applied to the area just above the insertion site. Apply pressure using a dry sterile gauze pad rather than using an alcohol preparation; alcohol tends to burn and does not stop blood flow from the puncture wound. If the patient can do so, he or she may be asked to hold the pressure for a minute or more.

Nurses also have responsibility for removing a PICC line. Specific protocols must be followed to prevent breaking or fracture of the catheter. Guidelines for removal of a PICC are as follows:

- Wear clean gloves unless a culture of the catheter tip is ordered; then use sterile gloves. Be sure to have a pair of sterile scissors to cut the catheter tip and a sterile container readily available.
- Place the patient in supine position, with the arm straight and the catheter insertion site below heart level (to prevent the risk for an air embolus).
- Remove the dressing carefully and clip and remove any sutures if they are present.
- Remove the catheter slowly. Two methods are suggested:
  - Grasp the catheter close to the insertion site and slowly ease the catheter out, 1 inch at a time, keeping it parallel to the skin. Continue removing 1-inch segments, using a smooth and regular motion (Macklin, 2000).
  - Slowly remove the catheter with a hand-over-hand technique. Removal may take up to 2 minutes.
- Apply pressure to the site with a sterile dressing and then apply a small sterile dressing to the site.
- Measure the catheter and compare it with the length listed in the chart when it was inserted. This ensures that the entire catheter was removed.

TABLE 46-11 Complications Associated With Intravenous Infusions

Complication/Cause	Signs and Symptoms	Nursing Considerations
Infiltration: the escape of fluid into the subcutaneous tissue Dislodged needle Penetrated vessel wall	Swelling, pallor, coldness, or pain around the infusion site; significant decrease in the flow rate	Check the infusion site several times per shift for symptoms. Discontinue the infusion if symptoms occur. Restart the infusion at a different site. Limit the movement of the extremity with the IV.
Sepsis: microorganisms invade the bloodstream through the catheter insertion site Poor insertion technique Multilumen catheters Long-term catheter insertion Frequent dressing changes	Red and tender insertion site Fever, malaise, other vital sign changes	Assess catheter site daily. Notify physician immediately if any signs of infection. Follow agency protocol for culture of drainage. Use scrupulous aseptic technique when starting an infusion.
Phlebitis: an inflammation of a vein Mechanical trauma from needle or catheter Chemical trauma from solution Septic (due to contamination)	Local, acute tenderness; redness, warmth, and slight edema of the vein above the insertion site	Discontinue the infusion immediately. Apply warm, moist compresses to the affected site. Avoid further use of the vein. Restart the infusion in another vein.
Thrombus: a blood clot Tissue trauma from needle or catheter	Symptoms similar to phlebitis IV fluid flow may cease if clot obstructs needle	Stop the infusion immediately. Apply warm compresses as ordered by the physician. Restart the IV at another site. *Do not rub or massage the affected area.*
Speed shock: the body's reaction to a substance that is injected into the circulatory system too rapidly Too rapid a rate of fluid infusion into circulation	Pounding headache, fainting, rapid pulse rate, apprehension, chills, back pains, and dyspnea	If symptoms develop, discontinue the infusion immediately. Report symptoms of speed shock to the physician immediately. Monitor vital signs if symptoms develop. Use the proper IV tubing. Carefully monitor the rate of fluid flow. Check the rate frequently for accuracy. A time tape is useful for this purpose.
Fluid overload: the condition caused when too large a volume of fluid infuses into the circulatory system Too large a volume of fluid infused into circulation	Engorged neck veins, increased blood pressure, and difficulty in breathing (dyspnea)	If symptoms develop, slow the rate of infusion. Notify the physician immediately. Monitor vital signs. Carefully monitor the rate of fluid flow. Check the rate frequently for accuracy.
Air embolus: air in the circulatory system Break in the IV system above the heart level allowing air in the circulatory system as a bolus	Respiratory distress Increased heart rate Cyanosis Decreased blood pressure Change in level of consciousness	Pinch off catheter or secure system to prevent entry of air. Place patient on left side in Trendelenburg position. Call for immediate assistance. Monitor vital signs and pulse oximetry.

• Document the procedure and how the patient tolerated it in the chart.

After the infusion has been discontinued, record the date and time the infusion was completed, the kind and amount of solution infused, the name of the person discontinuing the infusion, and symptoms of any adverse reactions.

Education About Home Infusion

Many patients return to their home from a healthcare facility with IV infusions. Portable infusion pumps and the availability of home care nurses have made this an acceptable alternative. After a patient has been identified as a candidate for home infusion therapy, begin assessment and education to ensure a

**SKILL
46-5**   **Capping a Primary Line for Intermittent Use**

EQUIPMENT

Lock device
Clean gloves
4″ × 4″ gauze pad

Normal saline or heparin flush prepared in
a syringe (1–3 mL) according to agency
policy

Alcohol wipe
Tape
Extension tubing (optional)

ACTION	RATIONALE
1. Gather equipment and verify physician's order. Fill lock and extension tubing with normal saline or heparin flush. Recap syringe for use in number 10.	Having equipment available saves time and facilitates the task; ensures that the procedure has been ordered by the physician. Flush maintains patency of lock and tubing.
2. Explain the procedure to the patient.	Explanation allays the patient's anxiety.
3. Perform hand hygiene.	Hand hygiene deters the spread of microorganisms.
4. Assess the IV site.	Complications such as infiltration or phlebitis necessitate discontinuation of the IV infusion at that site.
5. Clamp off primary line.	Clamping protects patient and nurse from inadvertent blood loss when IV and tubing are disconnected.
6. Don clean gloves.	Gloves protect the nurse from contact with the patient's blood.
7. Place gauze 4″ × 4″ sponge underneath IV connection hub between IV catheter and tubing.	Gauze absorbs any blood leakage when IV and tubing are disconnected.
8. Stabilize hub of IV catheter with nondominant hand. Use dominant hand to quickly twist and disconnect IV tubing from the catheter, discard it, and attach prefilled lock device or needleless cap to hub without contaminating the tips of the catheter and lock. Extension tubing may also be attached.	This maintains sterility of IV setup.

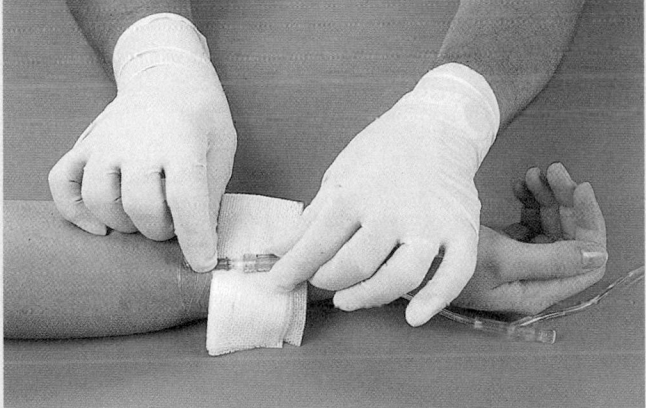

Action 8: Disconnecting tubing from an IV catheter.

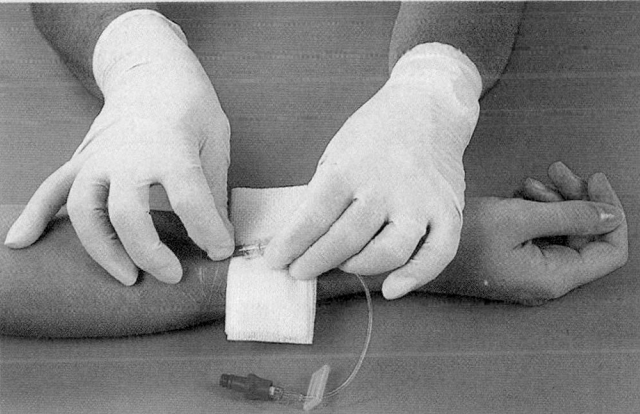

Action 8: Attaching a lock device with extension tubing to the IV catheter hub.

ACTION	RATIONALE
9. Cleanse cap with an alcohol wipe.	Cleansing removes surface bacteria at the heparin lock entry site.
10. Insert the syringe with blunt cannula or standard syringe and gently flush catheter with saline or heparin flush as per agency policy. Remove syringe carefully.	This maintains patency of the IV access line. Clinical evidence has demonstrated that a saline flush is as effective as heparin for peripheral IVs and avoids the adverse effects of heparin, is less expensive, and prevents drug incompatibilities. Most institution recommend a positive pressure flush. To do this, clamp the connecting tubing as you flush in the saline.
11. Tape lock or cap securely in place.	Tape secures the lock and IV in place.
12. Remove gloves and perform hand hygiene.	Hand hygiene deters the spread of microorganisms.
13. Chart on IV administration record or medication Kardex per institutional policy.	Accurate documentation is necessary to prevent error.

successful outcome. The patient and any caregivers must be able to perform necessary skills independently before discharge from the healthcare facility. See Teaching to Promote Health at Home 46-1.

Blood and Blood Products

A blood transfusion is the infusion of whole blood or a blood component such as plasma, red blood cells, or platelets into the patient's venous circulation. A blood transfusion is given because of red blood cell loss, such as with a major cut or when the body is not adequately producing cells such as platelets. Whole blood is infrequently used because the various components can be easily separated and used for replacement therapy. In addition, using whole blood for transfusion can lead to fluid volume overload. The person receiving the blood is the recipient. The person giving the blood is the donor. Steps in administering blood transfusions are described in Skills 46-6.

Typing and Cross-Matching

Before any blood can be given to a patient, it must be determined that the blood of the donor is compatible with the patient. If incompatible, clumping and hemolysis of the recipient's blood cells result, and death can occur. The laboratory examination to determine a person's blood type is called **typing.** The process of determining compatibility between blood specimens is **cross-matching.**

Blood Types

The four main blood types or groups in the ABO system of blood typing are A, B, AB, and O. Some groups are further broken down into subgroups.

Blood type, an inherited trait, is determined by the type of antigens and antibodies present in the blood. An **antigen** is a substance that causes the formation of antibodies. An **antibody** is a protein substance developed in the body in response to the presence of an antigen that has entered the body. An **agglutinin** is an antibody that causes a clumping of specific antigens. People who have type A blood have an A antigen on their red blood cells; those with type B blood have B antigens on their cells; those in the AB group have both A and B antigens; and people with type O blood have neither A nor B antigens on their red blood cells. People in each blood group have the agglutinins to the red blood cell antigens that they lack. Group A people have the agglutinin for B; group AB people have no agglutinins for A and B, whereas group O people have both A and B agglutinins in their blood serum. If a person with type O blood is transfused with blood from a person with either group A or group B blood, there would be destruction of the recipient's red blood cells because his or her anti-A or anti-B agglutinins would react with the A or B antigens in the donor's red blood cells. This example shows why individuals with type AB blood are often called universal recipients (because people in this blood group have no agglutinins for either A or B antigens) and group O people are often called universal donors (because they have neither A nor B antigens).

Rh Factor

The Rh factor is an inherited antigen in human blood. There are five antigens in the Rh system, but the one designated D is of first concern. A person whose blood contains a D antigen is called Rh positive; an Rh-negative person lacks this D anti-

---

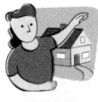

Teaching to Promote Health at Home 46-1
IV Therapy

Health Topic	Teaching Tip	Why Is This Important?
Sterile technique	• Proper handwashing technique • Dressing changes • Proper technique for infusing medications	The caregiver needs to understand the importance of sterile technique to prevent local systemic infections. If the caregiver is to administer medications, how to access the line in a sterile manner should be discussed by the nurse and then demonstrated by the caregiver.
General information	• Proper technique for using all equipment	The caregiver needs to demonstrate how to use any pumps to administer medication. The caregiver should also demonstrate how to flush the central line.
	• Assessing for any indications of an infection or other complications	The caregiver should understand signs of infection to observe for, as well as any other type of complication associated with a central line.
	• Obtaining supplies to continue home infusions	The caregiver needs to know where to obtain supplies and what supplies are needed for care at home.
	• Physician orders pertaining to the central line at home • How and why to contact the physician or nurse if questions or problems arise	Before discharge, the nurse should ensure that the caregiver understands all physician orders. The caregiver needs to know that resources are available and when it is appropriate to use these resources.

SKILL 46-6 Administering a Blood Transfusion

EQUIPMENT

Blood product
Blood administration set (tubing with in-line
  filter and Y for saline administration)

0.9% normal saline
IV pole
IV catheter (20 gauge or larger)

Disposable gloves
Tape

ACTION	RATIONALE
1. Determine whether patient knows reason for transfusion. Ask if the patient has had a transfusion or a transfusion reaction in the past.	This directs teaching before beginning transfusion.
2. Explain procedure to patient. Check for signed consent for transfusion if required by agency. Advise patient to report any chills, itching, rash, or unusual symptoms.	Explanation provides reassurance and facilitates cooperation. Prompt reporting of any reaction to transfusion necessitates stopping immediately.
3. Perform hand hygiene and put on clean gloves.	Hand hygiene deters the spread of microorganisms. Gloves protect against accidental exposure to the patient's blood.
4. Hang container of 0.9% normal saline with blood administration set to initiate IV infusion and follow administration of blood.	Dextrose may lead to clumping of red blood cells and hemolysis. Filter in blood administration set removes particulate material formed during storage of blood.

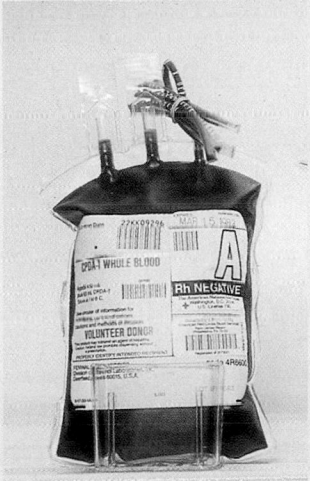

Unit of packed red blood cells.

5. Start IV with #18 or #19 catheter if not already present (see Skill 46-1). Keep IV open by starting flow of normal saline.	Large-bore needle or catheter is necessary for infusion of blood products. The lumen must be large enough not to cause damage to red blood cells. IV should be started prior to obtaining blood in case the procedure takes longer than 30 minutes.
6. Obtain blood product from blood bank according to agency policy.	Blood must be stored in refrigerated unit at carefully controlled temperature (4°C).

7. Complete identification and checks as required by agency:
a. Identification number
b. Blood group and type
c. Expiration date
 	
d. Patient's name
e. Inspect blood for clots
	Some agencies/states require two RNs to verify information:
	    Verifies that unit numbers match
	    Verifies that ABO group and Rh type are the same
	    Safe storage of blood is limited to 35 days before red blood cells begin to deteriorate.
	    Never administer blood to a patient without a name band.
	    If clots are present, blood should be returned to blood bank.

8. Take baseline set of vital signs before beginning transfusion.	Any change in vital signs during the transfusion may indicate a reaction.

(continued)

ACTION

RATIONALE

9. Start infusion of the blood product:
    a. Prime in-line filter with blood.
    b. Start administration slowly (no more than 25–50 mL for the first 15 minutes). Stay with the patient for the first 5–15 minutes of transfusion.

    c. Check vital signs at least every 15 minutes for the first half hour after the start of the transfusion. Follow the institution's recommendations for vital signs during the remainder of the transfusion.
    d. Observe patient for flushing, dyspnea, itching, hives, or rash.
    e. Use a blood warming device, if indicated, especially with rapid transfusions through a CVP catheter.

Priming is necessary if blood is to flow properly.
Transfusion reactions typically occur during this period, and a slow rate will minimize the volume of red blood cells infused. If there have been no adverse effects during this time, the infusion rate is increased.
If complications occur, they can be observed, and the blood can be stopped immediately.

These symptoms may be early indication of a transfusion reaction.
Rapid administration of cold blood can result in cardiac arrhythmias.

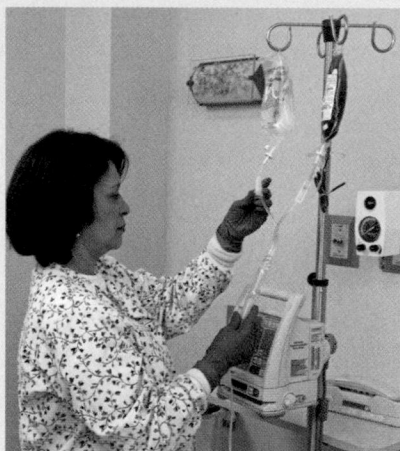

Action 9a: Priming the in-line filter.

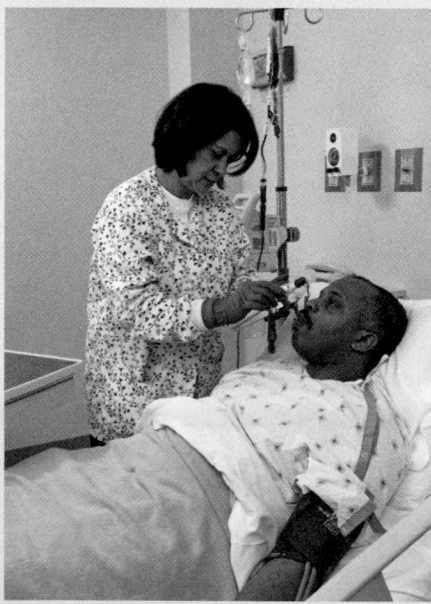

Action 9c: Checking temperature with electronic thermometer.

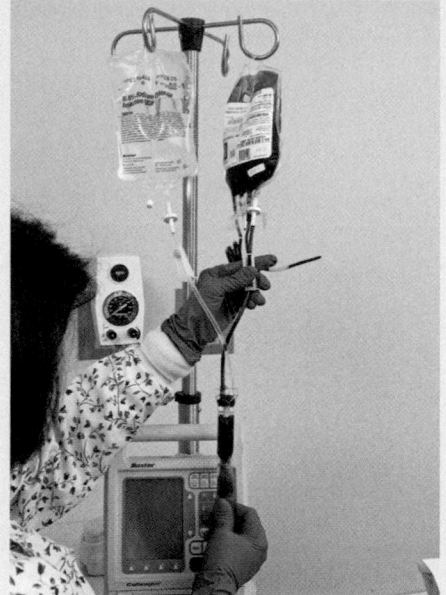

Action 9b: Starting infusion of blood slowly.

(continued)

SKILL 46-6   Administering a Blood Transfusion (continued)

ACTION	RATIONALE
10. Maintain the prescribed flow rate as ordered or as deemed appropriate by the patient's overall condition, keeping in mind the outer limits for safe administration. Assess frequently for transfusion reaction. Stop blood transfusion and allow saline to flow if you suspect a reaction. Notify physician and blood bank.	Rate must be carefully controlled, and patient's reaction must be monitored on a frequent basis.
11. When transfusion is complete, infuse 0.9% normal saline.	Saline prevents hemolysis of red blood cells and clears remainder of blood in IV line.
12. Record administration of blood and patient's reaction as ordered by agency. Return blood transfusion bag to blood bank according to agency policy.	This provides for accurate documentation of patient's response to blood transfusion.

SPECIAL CONSIDERATIONS	Electronic infusion devices may be used to maintain prescribed rate but must be specifically designed for use with blood transfusions.
HOME CARE ADMINISTRATIONS	Home care agencies evaluate patients who are candidates for a blood transfusion at home. Home transfusion is not appropriate for patients who are actively bleeding, require more than 4 hours for the transfusion, or recently had a reaction to a blood transfusion. Written consent must be obtained from the patient and the physician. The nurse transports the blood product to the patient's home in a special cooler. The nurse and patient's caregiver check serial number and other identification information together.

gen. An Rh-negative person must receive blood from another Rh-negative person. If Rh positive blood is injected into an Rh-negative person, the recipient develops anti-Rh agglutinins. Subsequent transfusion with Rh-positive blood may cause serious reactions with clumping and hemolysis of red blood cells.

Selection of Blood Donors

Blood donors must be selected with care. Not only must the donor's blood be accurately typed, but it is also important to determine that the donor is free from diseases. The blood will be tested for human immunodeficiency virus (HIV), hepatitis B virus (HBV), and other viruses that can be transmitted to the recipient. Recent information have investigators believing that West Nile virus can also be transmitted through blood transfusions (CDC, 2002). Blood donated from people who have allergies or those with a history of a chronic disease, such as tuberculosis, certain types of cancer, and hemophilia, is usually not used. As a further precaution, some blood banks do not accept blood from a donor who has been immunized recently because of a possible allergic reaction to the blood by a recipient.

The donor is examined carefully at the time of donation and receives specific information about eligibility and a confidential method to allow or disallow the distribution of the donated blood. Prospective donors are questioned about high-risk behaviors, such as unsafe sex, IV drug abuse, and the presence of any of the signs and symptoms of acquired immunodeficiency syndrome (AIDS). Individuals may give

blood only if their blood count, temperature, pulse, respiration, and blood pressure are within normal range. There is no way that donors may contract HIV or any other disease by giving blood.

Some patients who know in advance that they will need blood can donate their own blood for transfusion (**autologous transfusion**), also called autotransfusion. Autotransfusion eliminates the danger of transmitting cross-infection from donor to recipient and decreases the risk for complications from mismatched blood but requires advance planning (the blood must be donated 5 weeks before the surgery). This practice is growing in popularity. A patient's own blood can also be salvaged during surgery or collected from tubes and drains to allow for autologous transfusions.

Blood Components

Whole blood is rarely used unless blood loss has been massive. With current technology, whole blood can be easily separated into its components, and patients receive only the blood product they need. For example, a patient may need red blood cells but not the blood plasma and its constituents. Red blood cells in concentrated form, called packed red blood cells, may be used in the following situations:

- Patient with anemia suffering with a low red blood cell count
- Patient with cardiovascular failure, with a need to increase blood volume and red blood cells while avoiding cardiovascular overload

- Patient with GI bleeding, with a need to maintain adequate hemoglobin levels without increasing blood pressure, which would likely lead to more bleeding

In other situations, only plasma is required, such as when plasma protein or the blood's clotting factor is low. Fresh-frozen plasma is particularly useful in emergencies for immediate restoration of fluid because serum transfusion presents no compatibility problems and time need not be lost seeking donors and matching blood. It is also an excellent blood-volume expander when time is of essence, for example, in a patient who is severely burned and losing plasma rapidly from burn areas. Components of plasma that are used therapeutically include human albumin (used for hypovolemic shock, albuminemia, liver failure); cryoprecipitates (used for bleeding due to hemophilia or disseminated intravascular coagulation); and gamma globulins—the antibody-containing part of plasma (used for gamma globulin deficiencies).

Platelet infusion is indicated for the treatment or prevention of bleeding associated with deficiencies in the number or function of a patient's platelets. The demand for platelets has noticeably risen during the past several decades, and specialized products and preparation methods have been developed to reduce the risk for complications and improve the patient's response to platelet therapy.

Initiation of Transfusion

The procedure for starting a blood transfusion (see Skills 46-6) is basically the same as for an IV solution. If possible, select larger veins because a catheter no smaller than 20 gauge should be used. This size is necessary because of the viscosity of blood. Take and record vital signs just before starting the transfusion and during the beginning of the infusion. Institution policies vary on the frequency of vital signs. If the patient's temperature is 100°F (37.8°C) or higher, notify the physician. Blood that has not been used within 30 minutes after its arrival from the blood bank must be returned, and blood that has been infusing for more than 4 hours must be discontinued to prevent the risk for bacterial contamination.

Transfusion Reactions

When preparing and administering the transfusion, take every precaution to prevent a transfusion reaction by using meticulous technique. Table 46-12 describes potential transfusion reactions that can be serious.

TABLE 46-12 Transfusion Reactions

Reaction	Signs and Symptoms	Nursing Activity
Allergic reaction: allergy to transfused blood	Hives, itching Anaphylaxis	• Stop transfusion immediately and keep vein open with normal saline. • Notify physician stat. • Administer antihistamine parenterally as necessary.
Febrile reaction: fever develops during infusion	Fever and chills Headache Malaise	• Stop transfusion immediately and keep vein open with normal saline. • Notify physician. • Treat symptoms.
Hemolytic transfusion reaction: incompatibility of blood product	Immediate onset Facial flushing Fever, chills Headache Low back pain Shock	• Stop infusion immediately and keep vein open with normal saline. • Notify physician stat. • Obtain blood samples from site. • Obtain first voided urine. • Treat shock if present. • Send unit, tubing, and filter to lab. • Draw blood sample for serologic testing and send urine specimen to the lab.
Circulatory overload: too much blood administered	Dyspnea Dry cough Pulmonary edema	• Slow or stop infusion. • Monitor vital signs. • Notify physician. • Place in upright position with feet dependent.
Bacterial reaction: bacteria present in blood	Fever Hypertension Dry, flushed skin Abdominal pain	• Stop infusion immediately. • Obtain culture of patient's blood and return blood bag to lab. • Monitor vital signs. • Notify physician. • Administer antibiotics stat.

Administering Total Parenteral Nutrition (TPN)

Hypertonic solutions consisting of dextrose, amino acids, and select electrolytes and minerals, called total parenteral nutrition (TPN), may be infused using a central vein. TPN frequently is given for patients with malnutrition. This procedure and related nursing responsibilities are described in Chapter 42.

Evaluating

When evaluating the effectiveness of the plan of care aimed at promoting healthy fluid, electrolyte, and acid–base balance, pay attention to the following parameters:

- Are the patient's drinking and eating patterns supplying the needed fluid and electrolytes? Are food and fluid likes and dislikes interfering with the implementation of the care plan? Is the patient having any difficulties with oral fluids, tube feedings, IV therapy, or TPN?
- Is the patient's urine output about equal to the fluid intake? Does the patient void at least once each shift (except when sleeping)? Do urine characteristics (color, odor, specific gravity) indicate healthy functioning of the kidneys and excretion of fluids?
- Are abnormal sources of fluid loss (vomiting, diarrhea, draining wounds, fistula, and so forth) responding to treatment? Are these fluid losses effectively being replaced by the designated therapy? Are the signs of fluid volume deficit improving?
- Do the patient's weight and record of fluid intake and output indicate fluid balance?
- Are the signs and symptoms that initially manifested the fluid, electrolyte, or acid–base imbalances absent or improved? Has therapy led to any troublesome new signs or symptoms?
- Is the patient now able to practice self-care behaviors to maintain fluid, electrolyte, and acid–base balance? Can the patient describe appropriate responses to potential future problems?

This evaluation should be ongoing as the plan of care is implemented. As the patient achieves the expected outcomes, these should be noted and reinforced. Before nursing care is terminated, the patient and family should be able to independently promote fluid, electrolyte, and acid–base balance.

See Nursing Plan of Care 46-1.

NURSING PLAN OF CARE 46-1   for Gerry Stein

Gerry Stein is a 22-year-old Jewish man who is a senior in the premed program at a large state university. Although his grades were poor his first year in college, he currently is an honors student and plans to take the MCAT examination in 2 weeks. His overwhelming ambition is to be accepted into a prestigious medical school and to become a psychiatrist. He presents at the campus health clinic with the following assessment findings:

- History of problems with diarrhea since his junior year in high school; self-treatment with kaolin and pectin (Kaopectate) and limiting his food and fluid intake; believes diarrhea is stress related; no medical evaluation to date

- Has had two or three loose bowel movements per day for the past week with urgency and occasional incontinence; believes this is related to anxiety about performance on MCAT and his need for good grades; always thirsty but afraid to drink much; urine output is decreased, and he noted that urine is darker in color and has a stronger odor

Nursing examination: temperature, 99.8°F (37.6°C); pulse, 92 beats/min; respirations, 18 breaths/min; blood pressure, 100/60 mm Hg; skin and mucous membranes are pale and dry; weight is 4 lb less than usual (current weight, 170 lb)

NURSING DIAGNOSIS	Deficient Fluid Volume related to prolonged diarrhea and decreased fluid intake secondary to stress management as evidenced by 4-lb weight loss, dry skin and mucous membranes, and report of decreased urine output and concentrated urine
EXPECTED OUTCOME	By next week's visit, 3/24/06, the patient will: • Describe two effective means he has used to cope with stress

Nursing Interventions	Rationale	Evaluative Statement
Explore with the patient (1) what he finds most stressing at present, (2) the control he believes he has over these stressors, and (3) the adequacy of his past and present stress management strategies.	Assisting the patient to eliminate and reduce stress where possible and learn to cope better with unavoidable stress (identify and eliminate causative factors) is critical in controlling stress-related diarrhea.	3/24/06 Outcome not met. Patient reports little progress in coping with stress. With MCATs 1 week away, he feels more tense than ever before. Reports no time to explore stress management techniques.

(continued)

NURSING PLAN OF CARE 46-1   *for Gerry Stein* (continued)

Nursing Interventions	Rationale	Evaluative Statement
Assess for other factors contributing to diarrhea and fluid volume deficit.	Diarrhea may have a functional basis.	*Revision:* Goal is appropriate. Encourage visit to counseling center if not before MCATs then as soon as possible afterward.
Teach relation between stress and bouts of diarrhea.	Stress may result in increased intestinal mobility.	
Refer to counseling center on campus for assistance with stress management.	Professional assistance may facilitate identification and management of stressful situation.	*C. Ryan, RN*

EXPECTED OUTCOME   By the next week's visit, 3/31/06, the patient will:
• Report that his diarrhea is eliminated or decreased to one or two episodes per day

Nursing Interventions	Rationale	Evaluative Statement
Teach patient to link causative factors with diarrhea and to note anything that brings relief or assists in establishment of usual pattern of defecation.	Being able to make these connections helps patient to assume charge of own condition and to reinforce preventive strategies and successful relief measures.	3/31/06 Outcome met. Patient reports diarrhea decreased to one or two episodes per day.
Make sure patient understands diet: chemically and mechanically nonirritating diet high in calories, protein, and minerals; exclude foods such as cocoa, chocolate, alcohol, cold or carbonated beverages, citrus juices; try frequent, small meals.	Some patients fear eating because it stimulates the gastrocolic reflex and may result in a stool. Eating the proper diet actually reduces bowel irritation and decreases peristalsis.	*Recommendation:* Advise patient that it is important to keep appointment with gastroenterologist because relief may only be temporary.
Teach patient proper use of prescribed medications.	Loperamide hydrochloride controls diarrhea, and methylcellulose increases consistency of stool.	*C. Ryan, RN*

EXPECTED OUTCOME   By next week's visit, 3/31/06, the patient will:
• Demonstrate improved fluid and electrolyte balance as evidenced by (1) maintenance of present weight (170 lb), (2) moist mucous membranes, and (3) report of increased urinary output

Nursing Interventions	Rationale	Evaluative Statement
Explore with patient workable plan for oral replacement of fluids.	Collaboration with patient to determine acceptable sources of fluid intake may allay his fear that fluid intake causes diarrheal episodes.	3/31/04 Outcome partially met. Patient reports diarrhea decreased to once or twice a day. Two days there was no diarrhea. Weight, 169 lb. Mucous membranes are moist. Urine output is increased.
Have patient note which calorie- and electrolyte- (sodium and potassium) rich fluids he can tolerate. Increase fluid intake to maintain a normal urine specific gravity.	Increased fluid intake is necessary to compensate for excessive loss in diarrhea and to reestablish fluid balance.	*C. Ryan, RN*
Instruct patient to weigh himself every other day and to note changes in the volume or appearance of his urine.	All other things being equal, weight loss is a good indicator of continued fluid volume deficit. Other signs include decreased urinary output and high specific gravity.	
Teach patient defining characteristics of electrolyte imbalances associated with prolonged diarrhea—hyponatremia and hypokalemia.	Excreted stool pulls electrolytes with it, especially sodium and potassium.	

(continued)

> ## NURSING PLAN OF CARE 46-1
>
> ### *for Gerry Stein* (continued)
>
> **SAMPLE DOCUMENTATION**
>
> 3/31/06, nursing
>
> Mr. Stein returned to the clinic reporting that his diarrhea is decreased to one to two episodes per day and that he has an appointment with a gastroenterologist. He believes that modifying his diet, increasing rest periods, and medications (loperamide hydrochloride to control diarrhea and methylcellulose to increase the consistency of stool) were of great help. He still does not know how he can reduce his stress level. Nursing examination revealed temperature, 98.9°F (37.1°C); pulse, 88 beats/min; respirations, 18 breaths/min; blood pressure, 110/60 mm Hg; weight, 169 lb; skin and mucous membranes less dry than on previous visit. States he has not noted much change in urine output but possibly less concentrated.
>
> *C. Ryan, RN*

■ Developing Critical Thinking Skills

1. Using Table 46-6 earlier in this chapter, which describes parameters to be considered in clinical assessment for fluid, electrolyte, and acid–base balance, assess a healthy individual and then a patient whose fluid and electrolyte or acid–base balance is altered. Compare and contrast your findings.

2. Review the record of a patient who has been receiving IV fluids over a period of 3 or more days. Note the daily intake and output records, pertinent laboratory values, and clinical behaviors, and make a judgment about the patient's fluid, electrolyte, and acid–base balance. What factors complicate a hospitalized patient's usual ability to remain in balance?

■ Practicing for NCLEX

1. Plasma, the liquid constituent of blood, is correctly identified as
   a. Interstitial fluid
   b. Intravascular fluid
   c. Intracellular fluid
   d. 40% of total body fluid

2. Potassium functions as the
   a. Chief electrolyte of extracellular fluid
   b. Most abundant electrolyte in the body
   c. Major cation of intracellular fluid
   d. Chief extracellular anion

3. The movement of the solvent water from an area of lesser solute concentration to an area of greater solute concentration until equilibrium is established is known as
   a. Osmosis
   b. Diffusion
   c. Active transport
   d. Filtration

4. Which of the following would the nurse use as the most reliable indicator of a patient's fluid balance status?
   a. Intake and output
   b. Skin turgor
   c. Complete blood count
   d. Daily weight

5. Which acid–base imbalance would the nurse suspect after assessing the following arterial blood gas values (pH, 7.30; $PaCO_2$, 36 mmHg; HCO_3-, 14 mEq/L)?
   a. Respiratory acidosis
   b. Respiratory alkalosis
   c. Metabolic acidosis
   d. Metabolic alkalosis

6. Mrs. Podralski, a patient in the hospital, has been encouraged to increase her fluid intake. Which measure would be most effective for the nurse to implement?
   a. Explaining the mechanisms involved in transporting fluids to and from intracellular compartments
   b. Keeping fluids readily available for the patient
   c. Emphasizing the long-term outcome of increasing fluids when she returns home
   d. Planning to offer most daily fluids in the evening

7. Which of the following would the nurse need to keep in mind when preparing to assist the physician with insertion of a nontunneled percutaneous central venous catheter?
   a. This catheter usually remains in place for 2 to 3 months.
   b. The catheter is introduced via the basilic or cephalic veins in the antecubital space.
   c. Nursing responsibility includes accessing the catheter with an angled needle.
   d. A chest radiograph is required to confirm placement.

8. The nurse alertly assesses the acid–base balance of a patient because she is aware that the patient will be unable to effectively control his carbonic acid

supply. This is most likely a patient with badly damaged
   a. Kidneys
   b. Lungs
   c. Adrenal glands
   d. Blood vessels

9. The nurse instructs a patient to focus on breathing more slowly as the most effective intervention for which acid–base imbalance?
   a. Respiratory acidosis (carbonic acid excess)
   b. Respiratory alkalosis (carbonic acid deficit)
   c. Metabolic acidosis (base bicarbonate deficit)
   d. Metabolic alkalosis (base bicarbonate excess)

10. Which of the following is the most common etiologic factor related to the nursing diagnosis of Excess Fluid Volume?
   a. Increased need for fluids secondary to fever
   b. Abnormal fluid loss from vomiting
   c. Excessive IV infusion
   d. Decreased fluid intake secondary to depression

11. Which assessment finding would lead the nurse to suspect that a patient's IV has infiltrated?
   a. In the past hour, only 50 mL of fluid has infused.
   b. The insertion site is red, hot, and swollen.
   c. The patient's temperature has risen to 101°F (38.3°C).
   d. The site is pale, cool, swollen, and painful.

12. When developing the teaching plan for a patient at risk for hyperkalemia, which foods would the nurse instruct the patient to avoid?
   a. Carrots and squash
   b. Canned soups and potato chips
   c. Bananas and apricots
   d. Whole-grain cereals and milk

13. Which site would be most appropriate for initiating IV therapy for a patient who has sustained multiple injuries after an automobile accident and has a cast on his right arm?
   a. Left antecubital
   b. Dorsal aspect of either foot
   c. Right hand
   d. Left forearm

14. When implementing the plan of care for a patient receiving IV therapy, which intervention would be most appropriate?
   a. Changing the IV catheter and entry site daily
   b. Changing the tubing every 8 hours
   c. Increasing the rate to catch up if the correct amount has not been infused at the end of the shift
   d. Monitoring the flow rate at least every hour

15. While administering a blood transfusion, when would the nurse assess the patient for a blood transfusion reaction?
   a. 15 minutes after the infusion is started
   b. After the blood is all infused

   c. Every hour
   d. Every 15 minutes

Answers With Rationale

1. The correct response is *b*. Intravascular fluid or plasma is extracellular fluid and composes 5% of total body fluid.

2. The correct response is *c*. Potassium is the major cation of the intracellular fluid. Sodium is the chief electrolyte of extracellular fluid (*a*), calcium is the most abundant electrolyte in the body (*b*), and chloride is the chief extracellular anion (*d*).

3. The correct response is *a*. Water moves by osmosis. Gases move by diffusion (*b*). Active transport (*c*) is a process that requires energy for the movement of substances through a cell membrane from an area of lesser to higher concentration. Filtration (*d*) is the passage of fluids through a permeable membrane from an area of high pressure to one of low pressure.

4. The correct response is *d*. Daily weight is the most reliable indicator of a person's fluid balance status. Intake and output (*a*) are not always as accurate and may involve a subjective component. Measurement of skin turgor (*b*) is subjective, and the complete blood count (*c*) does not necessarily reflect fluid balance.

5. The correct response is *c*. A low pH indicates acidosis. This, coupled with a low bicarbonate, indicates metabolic acidosis. The pH and bicarbonate would be elevated with metabolic alkalosis (*d*). Decreased $PaCO_2$ in conjunction with a low pH indicates respiratory acidosis (*a*); increased $PaCO_2$ in conjunction with an elevated pH indicates respiratory alkalosis (*b*).

6. The correct response is *b*. Having fluids readily available helps promote intake. Explanation of the fluid transportation mechanisms (*a*) is inappropriate and does not focus on the immediate problem of increasing fluid intake. Meeting short-term outcomes rather than long-term ones (*c*) provides further reinforcement, and additional fluids should be taken earlier in the day.

7. The correct response is *d*. A chest radiograph is needed to ensure proper placement for any central venous access device. In addition, nontunneled percutaneous central venous catheters remain in place for 3 to 7 days, are introduced into the subclavian or internal jugular vein, and are never accessed through an angled needle (*c*) (used with an implanted port).

8. The correct response is *b*. The lungs are the primary controller of the body's carbonic acid supply and

thus, if damaged, can affect acid–base balance. The kidneys (*a*) are the primary controller of the body's bicarbonate supply. The adrenal glands (*c*) secrete catecholamines and steroid hormones. The blood vessels (*d*) act only as a transport system.

9. The correct response is *b*. Breathing more slowly causes accumulation of carbon dioxide to reverse carbonic acid deficit or respiratory alkalosis. Breathing more slowly would further increase a patient's respiratory acidosis (*a*) due to the increased carbon dioxide. Decreasing the respiratory rate would not be effective for a metabolic acid–base balance (*c*).

10. The correct response is *c*. Excessive IV infusion is the most common factor associated with excess fluid volume. The other alternatives are related to deficient fluid volume.

11. The correct response is *d*. A decrease in flow rate may indicate an infiltration but is not as significant as the other signs of a pale, cool, swollen, and painful site. Phlebitis is an inflammatory process and results in redness, warmth, and possibly a temperature elevation (*b* and *c*).

12. The correct response is *c*. Hyperkalemia is an elevated serum potassium level; bananas and apricots are foods high in potassium and should be avoided in this situation. The other foods listed would be allowed. Canned foods and potato chips (*b*) would be avoided if the patient had excess sodium levels.

13. The correct response is *d*. The left forearm is the best site selection because of the condition of the patient's right arm. The left forearm is preferable to the antecubital space of the left arm (*a*) or the lower extremities (*b*).

14. The correct response is *d*. The flow rate requires close monitoring, at least every hour. The IV catheter and entry site should be changed every 48 to 72 hours in most circumstances (*a*). The tubing is changed according to agency policy but not at the frequency of every 8 hours (*b*). Increasing the rate may lead to fluid overload (*c*).

15. The correct response is *d*. The nurse should closely observe a patient for the first 15 minutes and then check the patient thereafter every 15 minutes while he or she is receiving the blood transfusion.

Bibliography

Adrogue, H., & Madias, N. (2000). Primary care: Hyponatremia. *The New England Journal of Medicine, 342*(21), 1581–1589.

Bennett, J. (2000). Dehydration: Hazards and benefits. *Geriatric Nursing, 21*(2), 84–87.

Castialione, V. (2000). Hyperkalemia. *American Journal of Nursing, 100*(1), 55–56.

Centers for Disease Control and Prevention. (2002). Guidelines for the prevention of intravascular catheter-related infections. *Morbidity and Mortality Weekly Report, 51*(RR10), 1–32.

Centers for Disease Control and Prevention. (2003). Detection of West Nile virus in blood donations—United States, 2003. *Morbidity and Mortality Weekly Report, 52*(32), 769–772. Available at http://www.cdc.gov/mmwr/preview/mmwrhtml/mm5232a3.htm. Accessed 2/16/04.

Chang, L., Tsai, J., Huang, S., & Shih, C. (2003). Evaluation of infectious complications of the implantable venous access system in a general oncologic population. *American Journal of Infection Control, 31*(1), 34–39.

Dobson, P. (2001). A model for home infusion therapy initiation and maintenance. *Journal of Infusion Nursing, 24*(6), 385–394.

Ellenberger, A. (2002). How to change a PICC dressing. *Nursing, 32*(2), 50–52.

Fabian, B. (2000). Intravenous complication: Infiltration. *Journal of IV Nursing, 23*(4), 229–231.

Fitzpatrick, L. (2002). When to administer modified blood products. *Nursing, 32*(5), 36–42

Joint Commission on Accreditation of Healthcare Organizations. (2003). *2004 National Patient Safety Goals.* Available at http://www.jcaho.org/accredited+organizations/patient+safety/04+npsg/04_npsg.htm.

Klein, T. (2001). PICCs and midlines: Fine-tuning your care. *RN, 64*(8), 26–29.

LaRue, G., & Farnsworth, P. (2000). Silicone catheter fracture secondary to stress events and a dressing technique to reduce those events. *Journal of IV Nursing, 23*(2), 89–98.

Maag, M. (2001). An online ABG learning activity. *CIN Plus, 4*(1), 1, 4–5.

Macklin, D. (2000). Removing PICC. *American Journal of Nursing, 100*(1), 52–54.

McConnell, E. (2000). Do's & don'ts: Infusing packed RBCs. *Nursing, 30*(2), 17.

McConnell, E. (2001). Do's & don'ts: Administering total parenteral nutrition. *Nursing, 31*(11), 17.

Metheny, N. (2000). Fluid and electrolyte balance: *Nursing considerations* (4th ed.). Philadelphia: Lippincott Williams & Wilkins.

Millam, D., & Hadaway, L. (2000). On the road to successful IV starts. *Nursing, 30*(4), 34–38.

Millam, D., & Hadaway, L. (2000). From container to cannula: Trends in I.V. therapy. *Nursing, 30*(4), 39–48.

Miller, R. (2002). Blood component therapy. *Urologic Nursing, 22*(5), 331–339.

Moreau, N. (2002). IV rounds: How to remove a PICC with ease. *Nursing, 32*(5), 30.

Newell-Stokes, V., Broughton, S., Guiliano, K., et al. (2001). Developing an evidence-based procedure: Maintenance of central venous catheters. *Clinical Nurse Specialist, 15*(5), 199–204.

North American Nursing Diagnosis Association. (2003). *NANDA nursing diagnoses: Definitions and classification, 2003–2004.* Philadelphia: Author.

O'Grady, N., Alexander, M., Dellinger, E., et. al. (2002). Guidelines for the prevention of intravascular catheter related infections. *American Journal of Infection Control, 30*(8), 476–489.

Orr, M. (2002). The peripherally inserted central catheter: What are the current indications for its use? *Nutrition in Clinical Practice, 17*(2), 99–104.

Satarawala, R. (2000). Confronting the legal perils of IV therapy. *Nursing, 30*(8), 44–48.

Skokal, W. (2000). IV push at home? *RN, 63*(10), 26–30.

Smeltzer, S., & Bare, B. (2004). *Brunner and Suddarth's textbook of medical–surgical nursing* (10th ed.). Philadelphia: Lippincott Williams & Wilkins.

White, S. (2001). Peripheral intravenous therapy-related phlebitis rates in an adult population. *Journal of IV Nursing, 24*(1), 19–24.

Young, J. (2000). Transfusion reaction. *Nursing, 30*(12), 33.

Zerwekh, J. (2003). End-of-life hydration—benefit or burden? *Nursing, 33*(2), 32hn1–32hn3.

Equivalents

METRIC UNITS

The metric system, developed by the French, uses the *meter* as the basic unit. The metric system is a decimal system, with prefixes that designate the various multiples or divisibles of 10. The most commonly used prefixes in medicine are:

Milli, which means one one-thousandth (0.001)

Centi, which means one one-hundredth (0.01)

Kilo, which means one thousand (1000)

These prefixes may be affixed to any of the three basic units of measurements, which are

Meter (m), the unit of length

Gram (g), the unit of weight

Liter (L), the unit of volume

Therefore

1 millimeter (mm) = 0.001 m

1 milligram (mg) = 0.001 g

1 milliliter (mL) = 0.001 L

1 kilometer (km) = 1000 m

1 kilogram (kg) = 1000 g

1 kiloliter (kl) = 1000 L

Length

The meter (a little longer than a yard) and the kilometer (about 0.6 mile) seldom are used in medicine or nursing. The commonly used measure of length is 1 centimeter (cm) = 0.01 m = about 0.4 inch.

Volume

The most frequently used measures of volume are the *liter* and the *milliliter*. Some useful equivalents to know are

1000 milliliters (mL) = 1 liter (L)

1000 cubic centimeters (cc) = 1 liter (L)

1 milliliter (mL) = 1 cc

Weight

The gram designates the weight of 1 mL of distilled water at 4°C. The most frequently used units of weight are

1,000,000 micrograms (mcg or μg) = 1 gram (g)

1000 micrograms (mcg) = 1 milligram (mg)

1000 milligrams (mg) = 1 gram (g)

1000 grams (g) = 1 kilogram (kg) = 2.2 pounds (lb)

Metric Units and Their Household Equivalents

Household measurement is inaccurate, with wide variations in the size of teaspoons, teacups, and so forth. The generally accepted household measures are:

60 drops (gtt) = 1 teaspoon (tsp or t)

3 tsp = 1 tablespoon (Tbs or T)

12 Tbs = 1 teacup

16 Tbs = 1 glass (or a standard measuring cup)

APOTHECARY UNITS

In the apothecary system

The unit of weight is the *grain*.

The unit of volume is the *minim*.

Of the many units of measure in the apothecary system, you should know the following units, abbreviations, and equivalents.

Weight

60 grains (gr) = 1 dram (dr or ʒ)

8 drams (dr or ʒ) = 1 ounce (oz or ℥)

Volume

60 minims (min) = 1 fluid dram (fl dr or fʒ)

8 fl dr = 1 fluid ounce (fl oz or f℥)

16 fl oz = 1 pint (pt)

2 pt = 1 quart (qt)

4 qt = 1 gallon (gal)

In the apothecary system, when the symbol or abbreviation is used, the quantity is written in lowercase Roman numerals and follows the symbol. Arabic numerals are used, however, in preference to large Roman numerals. For example

5 gr = gr v

8 dr = ʒ viii

The quantity one-half may be indicated by the symbol ss.

1½ gr = gr iss

7½ gr = gr viiss

Other fractional parts are expressed as common fractions, for example, gr ½₅₀, gr ⅒.

When pint, quart, and gallon are written, the quantity is expressed in Arabic numerals, (eg, 1½ pints or 7½ quarts).

TABLE A-1 Metric and Household Equivalents

Metric Unit	Household Unit
5 mL	1 tsp
15 mL	1 Tbs
180 mL	1 full teacup
240 mL	1 full glass

Apothecary Units and Their Household Equivalents

1 drop = 1 minim (m i)

1 tsp = 1 dr (ʒ i)

1 Tbs = ½ oz (ʒ ss)

2 Tbs = 1 oz (ʒ i)

1 teacup = 6 oz (ʒ vi)

1 glass or measuring cup = 8 oz (ʒ viii)

2 measuring cups = 1 pt

TABLE A-2 Most Commonly Used Approximate Equivalents*

Metric	Apothecary	Household
0.06 g	gr i	
0.06 mL	min i	1 drop
1.0 g	gr xv	
1.0 mL	min xv	⅕ tsp
5 mL	(1 dr) ʒ i	1 tsp
15 mL	(½ oz) ʒ ss	1 Tbs
30 mL	(1 oz) ʒ i	2 Tbs
500 mL	(16 oz) ʒ 16	1 pt
1000 mL	(32 oz) ʒ 32	1 qt

* There are many discrepancies among these approximate equivalents. For example, 30 mL is the accepted equivalent for 1 oz (29.57 mL is the exact equivalent). Such discrepancies are inevitable when two systems are used whose equivalents are not exact. If the discrepancies are within a 10% margin of error, they usually are acceptable in pharmacology.

Normal Adult Laboratory Values*

COMMONLY USED ABBREVIATIONS

kg = kilogram
g = gram
mg = milligram
μg = microgram
ng = nanogram
mEq = milliequivalent
L = liter
dl = 100 milliliters
mL = milliliter
cu mm (mm^3) = cubic millimeter

nM = nanomolar
mIU = milliInternational Unit
pg = picogram
mm = millimeter
μ = micron or micrometer
mm Hg = millimeters of mercury
mU = milliunit
μU = microunit
IU = International Unit

* Laboratory values may vary according to techniques used in different laboratories.

TABLE B-1 Hematologic Values—Reference Ranges

Determination	Conventional	SI
Coagulation Factors		
Factor I (fibrinogen)	0.15–0.35 g/100 mL	4.0–10.0 μmol/L
Factor II (prothrombin)	60%–140%	0.60–1.40 μmol/L
Factor V (accelerator globulin)	60%–140%	0.60–1.40 μmol/L
Factors VII to X (proconvertin to Stuart factor)	70%–130%	0.70–1.30 μmol/L
Factor X (Stuart factor)	60%–140%	0.70–1.30 μmol/L
Factor VIII (antihemophilic globulin)	50%–200%	0.50–2.0 μmol/L
Factor IX (plasma thromboplastic cofactor)	60%–140%	0.60–1.40 μmol/L
Factor XI (plasma thromboplastic antecedent)	60%–140%	0.60–1.40 μmol/L
Factor XII (Hageman factor)	60%–140%	0.60–1.40 μmol/L
Coagulation Screening Tests		
Bleeding time (Simplate)	2–8 min	180–540 sec
Prothrombin time	9.5–12 sec	Less than 2 sec from control
Partial thromboplastin time (activated)	20–45 sec	25–37 sec
INR	1.0	none
Whole blood clot lysis	No clot lysis in 24 hr	0/day
Fibrinolytic Studies		
Euglobin lysis	No lysis in 2 hr	0 (in 2 hr)
Thrombin time		Control 15 sec
Complete Blood Count		
Hematocrit	Male: 42%–50%	Male: 0.42–0.52
	Female: 40%–48%	Female: 0.37–0.48

(continued)

TABLE B-1 (Continued)

Determination	Conventional	SI
Hemoglobin	Male: 13–18 g/dL Female: 12–16 g/dL	Male: 8.1–11.2 mmol/L Female: 7.4–9.9 mmol/L
Leukocyte count	5000–10,000/mm³	$4.3–10.8 \times 10^9$/L
Erythrocyte count	4.2 million–5.9 million/mm³	$4.2–5.9 \times 10^{12}$/L
Mean corpuscular volume (MCV)	80–94 μm³	80–94 fl
Mean corpuscular hemoglobin (MCH)	27–32 pg	1.7–2.0 fmol
Mean corpuscular hemoglobin concentration (MCHC)	33%–38%	19–22.8 mmol/L
Erythrocyte sedimentation rate (Zeta Centrifuge)	41%–54%	Male: 1–13 mm/h Female: 1–20 mm/h
Erythrocyte Enzymes		
Glucose-6-phosphate dehydrogenase	5–15 U/g Hb	5–15 U/g
Pyruvate kinase	13–17 U/g Hb	13–17 U/g
Ferritin (serum)	Females: 5–100 ng/mL Males: 10–270 ng/mL	
Folic acid, RIA	4–16 ng/mL	
Haptoglobin	50–250 mg/dL	1.0 g–3.0 g/L
Hemoglobin Studies		
Electrophoresis for A₂ hemoglobin	1.5%–3.5%	0.015–0.035
Hemoglobin, met- and sulf-	0	0
Serum hemoglobin	2–3 mg/100 mL	1.2–1.9 μmol/L

Lupus erythematosus (LE) preparation
  Heparin as anticoagulant
  Defibrinated blood
	
	0
	0
		
		0
		0

Muramidase	Serum, 3–7 μg/mL Urine, 0–2 μg/mL	3–7 mg/L 0–2 mg/L
Osmotic fragility of erythrocyte	Increased if hemolysis occurs in over 0.5% NaCl; decreased if hemolysis is incomplete in 0.3% NaCl	
Peroxide hemolysis	Less than 10%	<0.10
Platelet count	100,000–400,000/mm³	$150–350 \times 10^9$/L
Platelet Function Tests		
Clot retraction	50%–100%/2 hr	0.50–1.00/2 hr
Platelet aggregation	Full response to ADP, epinephrine and collagen	1.0
Platelet factor 3	33–57 sec	33–57 sec
Reticulocyte count	0.5%–1.5% red cells	0.005–0.15

Vitamin B₁₂	90–280 pg/mL
	  (borderline: 70–90)
		66–207 pmol/L
		  (borderline: 52–66)

TABLE B-2 Blood, Plasma or Serum Values—Reference Ranges

Determination	Conventional	SI
Acetoacetate plus acetone	0.3–2.0 mg/dL	3–20 mg/L
Aldolase	1.3–8.2 mU/mL	12–75 nmol sec⁻¹/L
Alpha amino nitrogen	3.0–5.5 mg/100 mL	2.1–3.9 mmol/L
Ammonia	80–110 μg/100 mL	47–65 μmol/L
Ascorbic acid	0.4–1.5 mg/100 mL	23–85 μmol/L
Bilirubin (van den Bergh test)	1 minute: 0.4 mg/100 mL Direct: 0.1–0.2 mg/dL Total: 1.0 mg/100 mL Indirect: 0.1–1.0 mg/dL	Up to 7 μmol/L Up to 17 μmol/L
Blood volume	8.5%–9.0% of body weight in kg Toxic level: 17 mEq/L	80–85 mL/kg
Bromsulphalein (BSP)	Less than 5% retention 45 min after 5 mg/kg IV	<0.05 L
Calcium	8.5–10.5 mg/100 mL	2.1–2.5 mmol/L
Carbon dioxide content	24 mEq–32 mEq/L	24–30 mmol/L
Carcinoembryonic antigen (CEA)	0.25 mg/mL	0–2.5 μg/L
Carotenoids	0.8–4.0 μg/mL	1.5–7.4 μmol/L
Ceruloplasmin	27–37 mg/100 mL	1.8–2.4 μmol/L
Chloride	95–105 mEq/L	100–106 mmol/L
Cholesterol	<200 mg/dL	
Cholinesterase (pseudocholinesterase)	0.5 pH U or more/hr 0.7 pH U or more/hr for packed cells	0.5 arb unit or more
Copper	Total: 100–200 μg/100 mL	16–31 μmol/L
Creatine phosphokinase (CPK)	Female: 50–250 mU/mL Male: 50–325 mU/mL	0.08–0.58 μmol sec⁻¹/L
Creatinine	0.7–1.4 mg/100 mL	60–130 μmol/L
Ethanol	0.3%–0.4%, marked intoxication; 0.4%–0.5%, alcoholic stupor; 0.5% or over, alcoholic coma	65–87 mmol/L 87–109 mmol/L >109 mmol/L
Glucose	Fasting: 60–110 mg/100 mL	3.9–5.6 mmol/L
Iron	65–170 μg/100 mL (higher in males)	9.0–26.9 μmol/L
Iron-binding capacity	250–410 μg/100 mL	44.8–73.4 μmol/L
Lactic acid	0.6–1.8 mEq/L	0.6–1.8 mmol/L
Lactic dehydrogenase isoenzymes	100–225 mU/mL	1.00–2.00 μmol sec⁻¹/L
Lead	50 μg/100 mL or less	Up to 2.4 μmol/L
Lipase	2 U/mL or less	Up to 2 arb units
Lipids, total	400–1000 mg/dL	3.10–5.69 mmol/L
Magnesium	0.33–2.4 mEq/L	0.8–1.3 mmol/L
5⁹ Nucleotidase	0.3–3.2 Bodansky U	30–290 nmol sec⁻¹/L
Osmolality	280–300 mOsm/kg water	285–295 mmol/kg
Oxygen saturation (arterial)	95%–100%	0.96–1.00 L
Pco₂	35–45 mm Hg	4.7–6.0 kPg
pH	7.35–7.45	Same
Po₂	95–100 mm Hg (dependent on age while breathing room air) Above 500 mm Hg while on 100% O₂	10.0–13.3 kPa
Phenylalanine	0–2 mg/100 mL	0–120 μmol/L

(continued)

TABLE B-2 (Continued)

Determination	Conventional	SI
Phosphorus (inorganic)	3.0–4.5 mg/100 mL	1.0–1.5 mmol/L
Potassium	3.8–5.0 mEq/L	3.5–5.0 mmol/L
Primidone (Mysoline)	Therapeutic level, 4–12 µg/mL	18–55 µmol/L
Protein, total	6.0–8.0 g/100 mL	60–84 g/L
Albumin	3.5–5.0 g/100 mL	33–50 g/L
Globulin	1.5–3.0 g/100 mL	23–35 g/L
Electrophoresis	% of total protein	% of total protein
Albumin	3.3–5.0 g/dL	0.52–0.68
Globulin		
Alpha₁	0.2–0.4 g/dL	0.042–0.072
Alpha₂	0.6–1.0 g/dL	0.068–0.12
Beta	0.6–1.2 g/dL	0.093–0.15
Gamma	0.7–1.5 g/dL	0.13–0.23
	0.3–0.7 mg/dL	0–0.11 mmol/L
Sodium	135–145 mEq/L	135–145 mmol/L
Sulfate	0.5–1.5 mg/100 mL	0.05–1.2 mmol/L
Transaminase (SGOT) (aspartate aminotransferase)	7–40 U/mL	0.08–0.32 µmol sec⁻¹/L
Urea nitrogen (BUN)	10–20 mg/100 mL	2.9–8.9 mmol/L
Uric acid	2.5–8.0 mg/100 mL	0.13–0.42 mmol/L
Vitamin A	50–220 µg/dL	0.5–2.1 µmol/L

TABLE B-3 Urine Values—Reference Ranges

Determination	Conventional	SI
Acetone plus acetoacetate (quantitative)	0	0 mg/L
Alpha amino nitrogen	64–199 mg/day; not over 1.5% of total nitrogen	4.6–14.2 mmol/day
Amylase	35–260 U/mL	24–76 arb units
Calcium	150 mg/day or less	3.8 mmol/day or less
Catecholamines	Epinephrine, 10%–40%	<55 nmol/day
	Norepinephrine, 60%–90%	<590 nmol/day
Copper	20–70 µg/day	0–1.6 µmol/day
Coproporphyrin	50–300 µg/day	80–380 nmol/day
Creatine	0–200 mg/24 hr	<0.75 mmol/day
Cystine or cysteine	0	0
Follicle-stimulating hormone		
Follicular phase	5–20 IU/day	Same
Midcycle	15–60 IU/day	
Luteal phase	5–15 IU/day	
Menopausal	50–100 IU/day	
Men	5–25 IU/day	
Hemoglobin and myoglobin	0	
5-Hydroxyindole acetic acid	2–9 mg/day (women lower than men)	10–45 µmol/day

(continued)

TABLE B-3 (Continued)

Determination	Conventional				SI		
Phenolsulfonphthalein (PSP)	At least 25% excreted by 15 min; 40% by 30 min; 60% by 120 min				0.25 L		
Phosphorus (inorganic)	Varies with intake; average 1 g/day				32 mmol/day		
Porphobilinogen	0				0		
Protein, quantitative	<150 mg/24 hr				<0.15 g/day		
Steroids							
17-Ketosteroids (per day)	Age (yr)	Male (mg)	Female (mg)		Male (μmol/day)	Female (μmol/day)	
	10	1–4	1–4		3–14	3–14	
	20	6–21	4–16		21–73	14–56	
	30	8–26	4–14		28–90	14–49	
	50	5–18	3–9		17–62	10–31	
	70	2–10	1–7		7–35	3–24	
17-Hydroxysteroids	3–8 mg/day (women lower than men)				8–22 μmol/day as hydrocortisone		
Sugar							
Quantitative glucose	0				0 mmol/L		
Identification of reducing substances							
Fructose	0				0 mmol/L		
Pentose	0				0 mmol/L		
Titratable acidity	20–40 mEq/day				20–40 mmol/day		
Urobilinogen	<0.25 mg/dL				To 1.0 arb unit		
Uroporphyrin	Up to 50 μg in 24 hr				0 nmol/day		
Vanilmandelic acid (VMA)	0.7–6.8 mg/24 hr				Up to 45 μmol/day		

TABLE B-4 Cerebrospinal Fluid Values—Reference Ranges

Determination	Conventional	SI
Bilirubin	0	0 μmol/L
Chloride	100–130 mEq/L	
Albumin	15.5–32.0 mg/dL	0.295 g/L 6 2 SD (0.11–0.48)
IgG	0–6.6 mg/dL	0.043 g/L 6 2 SD (0–0.086)
Glucose	50–75 mg/100 mL (30%–50% less than blood)	2.8–4.2 mmol/L
Pressure (initial)	70–180 mm H_2O	70–80 arb units
Protein		
Lumbar	15–45 mg/100 mL	0.15–0.45 g/L
Cisternal	15–25 mg/100 mL	0.15–0.25 g/L
Ventricular	5–15 mg/100 mL	0.05–0.15 g/L

TABLE B-5 Special Endocrine Tests—Reference Ranges

Determination	Conventional	SI
Steroid Hormones		
Aldosterone	Excretion: 5–19 µg/24 hr	14–53 nmol/day
Fasting, at rest, 210 mEq sodium diet	Supine: 48 ± 29 pg/mL	133 ± 80 pmol/L
	Upright: (2h) 65 ± 23 pg/mL	180 ± 64 pmol/L
Fasting, at rest, 110 mEq sodium diet	Supine: 107 ± 45 pg/mL	279 ± 125 pmol/L
	Upright: (2h) 239 ± 123 pg/mL	663 ± 341 pmol/L
Fasting, at rest, 10 mEq sodium diet	Supine: 175 ± 75 pg/mL	485 ± 208 pmol/L
	Upright: (2h) 532 ± 228 pg/mL	1476 ± 632 pmol/L
Cortisol		
Fasting	8 AM: 5–25 µg/100 mL	0.14–0.69 µmol/L
At rest	8 PM: below 10 µg/100 mL	0–0.28 µmol/L
20 U ACTH	4-hour ACTH test: 30–45 µg/100 mL	0.83–1.24 µmol/L
Dexamethasone at midnight	Overnight suppression test: below 5 µg/100 mL	<0.14 nmol/L
	Excretion: 20–70 µg/24 hr	55–193 nmol/day
11-Deoxycortisol	Responsive: over 7.5 µg/100 mL (after metrapone)	>0.22 µmol/L
Testosterone	Adult male: 300–1100 ng/100 mL	10.4–38.1 nmol/L
	Adolescent male: over 100 ng/100 mL	>3.5 nmol/L
	Females: 25–90 ng/100 mL	0.87–3.12 nmol/L
Unbound testosterone	Adult male: 3.06–24.0 ng/100 mL	106–832 pmol/L
	Adult female: 0.09–1.28 ng/100 mL	3.1–44.4 pmol/L
Polypeptide Hormones		
Adrenocorticotrophin (ACTH)	15–70 pg/mL	3.3–15.4 pmol/L
Calcitonin	Undetectable in normals	0
	>100 pg/mL in medullary carcinoma	>29.3 pmol/L
Growth hormone		
Fasting, at rest	Below 5 ng/mL	<233 pmol/L
After exercise	Children: over 10 ng/mL	>465 pmol/L
	Male: below 5 ng/mL	<233 pmol/L
	Female: up to 30 ng/mL	0–1395 pmol/L
After glucose	Male: below 5 ng/mL	<233 pmol/L
	Female: below 10 mg/mL	0–465 pmol/L
Insulin		
Fasting	6–26 µU/mL	43–187 pmol/L
During hypoglycemia	Below 20 µU/mL	<144 pmol/L
After glucose	Up to 150 µU/mL	0–1078 pmol/L
Luteinizing hormone	Male: 6–18 mU/mL	6–18 U/L
Preovulatory or postovulatory	Female: 5–22 mU/mL	5–22 U/L
Midcycle peak	30–250 mU/mL	30–250 U/L
Parathyroid hormone	<10 µl equiv/mL	<10 mL equiv/L
Prolactin	2–15 ng/mL	0.08–6.0 nmol/L
Renin activity		
Normal diet	Supine: 1.1 ± 0.8 ng/mL/hr	0.9 ± 0.6 nmol/L/hr
	Upright: 1.9 ± 1.7 ng/mL/hr	1.5 ± 1.3 nmol/L/hr
Low-sodium diet	Supine: 2.7 ± 1.8 ng/mL/hr	2.1 ± 1.4 nmol/L/hr
	Upright: 6.6 ± 2.5 ng/mL/hr	5.1 ± 1.9 nmol/L/hr
High-sodium diet	Diuretics: 10.0 ± 3.7 ng/mL/hr	7.7 ± 2.9 nmol/L/hr
Thyroid Hormones		
Thyroid-stimulating hormone (TSH)	0.5–3.5 µU/mL	0.5–3.5 mU/L
Thyroxine-binding globulin capacity	15–25 µg T_4/100 mL	193–322 mU/L
Total triiodothyronine by radioimmunoassay (T_3)	70–190 ng/100 mL	1.08–2.92 nmol/L
Total thyroxine (T_4) by RIA	4–12 µg/100 mL	52–154 nmol/L
T_3 resin uptake	25%–35%	0.25–0.35
Free thyroxine index (FT_4I)	1–4 ng/100 mL	12.8–51.2 pmol/L

Standard I
Nursing Practice Requires That a Conceptual Model for Nursing Be the Basis of That Practice

1. Nurses are required to have a clear idea or conception of the *distinct goal of nursing*.
2. Nurses are required to have a clear idea or conception of the *client*.
3. Nurses are required to have a clear idea or conception of their role in response to the health needs of society.
4. Nurses are required to have a clear idea or conception of the *source of client difficulty*.
5. Nurses are required to have a clear idea or conception of the *focus and modes of nursing intervention*.
6. Nurses are required to have a clear idea or conception of the expected *consequences* of nursing activities.

Standard II
Nursing Practice Requires the Effective Use of the Nursing Process

1. Nurses are required to *collect data* in accordance with their conception of the client.
2. Nurses are required to *analyze data* collected in accordance with their conception of the goal of nursing, their role, and the source of client difficulty.
3. Nurses are required to *plan* their nursing actions based upon the identified actual and potential client problems, in accordance with their conception of the focus and modes of intervention.
4. Nurses are required to perform nursing actions which *implement* the plan.
5. Nurses are required to *evaluate* all steps of the nursing process in accordance with their conceptual model for nursing.

Standard III
Nursing Practice Requires That the Helping Relationship Be the Nature of the Client–Nurse Interaction

1. Nurses are required to initiate interaction in a way that increases the likelihood that the client will perceive the health service experience as understandable, manageable, and meaningful at the onset.
2. Nurses are required to set mutually agreed upon expectations as a means of increasing the likelihood that the client will perceive the health service experience as understandable, manageable, and meaningful.
3. Nurses are required to ensure a successful termination of the helping relationship.

Standard IV
Nursing Practice Requires Nurses to Fulfill Professional Responsibilities

1. Nurses are required to respect *statutes and policies* relevant to the profession and the practice setting.
2. Nurses are required to comply with the *Code of Ethics* of their profession.
3. Nurses are required to function as members of a *health team*.

Glossary

A

Abduction: lateral movement of the body part away from the midline of the body

Absorption: process by which drugs are transferred from the site of entry into the body to the bloodstream

Accommodation: (1) ability to adjust the eye to see at various distances; (2) process by which intellectual acts are changed to handle increasingly complex information

Accreditation: process by which an educational program is evaluated and then recognized as having met certain predetermined standards of education

Acid: substance containing a hydrogen ion that can be liberated or released

Acidosis: condition characterized by a proportionate excess of hydrogen ions in the extracellular fluid, in which the pH falls below 7.35

Acquired immunodeficiency syndrome (AIDS): fatal condition in which the body's immune system is rendered ineffective as a result of infection by the retrovirus HIV

Active euthanasia: someone other than the patient commits an action with the intent to end the patient's life; for example, injecting him or her with a lethal dose

Active exercise: joint movement activated by the person

Active immunity: antibodies against harmful effects of microorganisms or toxins that are self-produced

Active transport: movement of ions or molecules across cell membranes, usually against a pressure gradient and with the expenditure of metabolic energy

Actual loss: loss that can be recognized by others as well as by the person sustaining the loss, such as loss of a limb or a spouse

Actual problems: problems that have been validated by the presence of major defining characteristics

Acupuncture: procedure consisting of placing very thin, short, sterile needles at particular acupoints, believed to be centers of nerve and vascular tissue, along a meridian to either increase or decrease the flow of chi along the meridian, restoring the balance of yin and yang, and thereby contributing to healing

Acute illness: rapidly occurring illness that runs its course, allowing the person to return to his or her previous level of functioning

Acute pain: episode of pain that lasts from seconds to less than 6 months

Adaptation: adjustment of living with other living things and environmental conditions

Addiction: a pattern of compulsive use of addictive substances for means other than those prescribed

Addictive: substance to which a person develops a psychological and physiologic dependency

Adduction: movement of a body part toward the midline of the body

Adolescence: the period of time between childhood and adulthood; a time of rapid physical change, reproductive maturity, and emotional development

Advance directive: written directive that allows people to state in advance what their choices for healthcare would be if certain circumstances should develop

Adventitious breath sounds: abnormal breath sound heard over the lungs

Advocacy: protection and support of another's rights

Aerobic bacteria: bacteria that require oxygen to live and grow

Aerobic exercise: exercise that promotes cardiovascular fitness; it increases blood flow, heart rate, and the metabolic demand for oxygen over a period of time

Afebrile: a condition in which the body temperature is not elevated

Affective learning: changes in attitudes, values, and feelings

Ageism: attitudes that stereotype the older adult on the basis of chronologic age

Agency for Health Care Policy and Research (AHCPR): a group of multidisciplinary experts who use research as well as a broad range of input from professional and consumer organizations and individuals to develop clinical practice guidelines; established by the Omnibus Budget Reconciliation Act of 1989

Agglutinin: an antibody that causes a clumping of specific antigens

Agnostic: person who believes that nothing can be known about the existence of a god

Albuminuria: albumin in the urine; an indication of kidney disease

Alkali: substance that can accept or trap a hydrogen ion; synonym for base

Alkalosis: condition, characterized by a proportionate lack of hydrogen ions in the extracellular fluid concentration, in which the pH exceeds 7.45

Allodynia: characteristic feature of neuropathic pain that occurs after a normally weak or nonpainful stimuli, such as a light touch or a cold drink

Allopathy: (biomedicine), the term generally used to describe "traditional" medical care, dominant for about 100 years, which spearheaded remarkable advances in biotechnology, surgical interventions, pharmaceutical approaches, and diagnostic tools

Alopecia: baldness

Alternative care: general term used to identify various methods of nonhospital healthcare, including residential housing, day care, respite care, hospice, and extended-care facilities

Alveoli: small air sacs at the end of the terminal bronchioles that are the site of gas exchange

Alzheimer's disease: type of dementia in which discrete patches of brain tissue degenerate; this devastating disease eventually affects all body systems

Ambulatory care: healthcare settings located in areas that are convenient for people to walk into and receive care; may be provided in hospitals, clinics, or centers

Amino acid: basic building blocks used to manufacture protein and the end products of protein digestion

Ampule: glass flask containing a single dose of medication for parenteral administration

Anaerobic bacteria: bacteria that can live without oxygen

Anaerobic exercise: exercise in which the supply of oxygen is less than the demand created by contracting muscles; oxygen debt results

Analgesic drug: pharmaceutical agent used to relieve pain

Anaphylactic reaction: severe reaction occurring immediately after exposure to a drug; characterized by respiratory distress and vascular collapse

Andragogy: the study of teaching adults

Anesthetic: agent that produces states such as loss of consciousness, analgesia, relaxation, and loss of reflexes

Anion: ion that carries a negative electric charge

Ankylosis: fixation or immobilization of a joint

Anorexia: lack or loss of appetite for food

Anorexia nervosa: eating disorder characterized by the denial of appetite and bizarre eating habits

Anoxia: absence of oxygen

Antagonistic effect: combined effect of two or more drugs that produces less than the effect of each drug alone

Anthropometric: measurements of the body and body parts

Antibacterial: agent that kills bacteria or suppresses their growth

Antibody: immunoglobin produced by the body in response to a specific antigen

Anticipatory loss: condition in which a person displays loss and grief behaviors for a loss that has yet to take place

Antigen: foreign material capable of inducing a specific immune response

Antimicrobial: antibacterial agent that kills bacteria or suppresses their growth

Antipyretic: agent that reduces fever

Antiseptic: substance that inhibits the growth of bacteria

Anuria: technically, no urine voided; 24-hour urine output is less than 100 mL; synonyms are *complete kidney shutdown* and *renal failure*

Anxiety: vague sense of impending doom or apprehension precipitated by new and unknown experiences

Apnea: absence of breathing

Applied research (practical research): research designed to directly influence or improve clinical practice

Aromatherapy: the use of essential oils of plants to treat symptoms

Arousal: condition in which the cortical area of the brain receives and responds appropriately to stimuli

Ascites: accumulation of fluid in the peritoneal cavity

Asepsis: absence of disease-producing microorganisms; being free of infection

Asphyxiation: stoppage of breathing or the lack of air reaching the lungs; synonym for suffocation

Assault: threat or an attempt to make bodily contact with another person without that person's permission

Assertiveness: ability to stand up for oneself and others using open, honest, and direct communication

Assess: systematically and continuously collect, validate, and communicate patient data

Assimilation: process by which a person interprets information to fit the current level of cognition

Assisted suicide: the act of making a means of suicide (eg, providing pills or a weapon) available to a patient with knowledge of his or her intention; in assisted suicide, someone makes the means of death available but does not act as the direct agent of death

Atelectasis: incomplete expansion or collapse of a part of the lungs

Atheist: person who denies the existence of a god

Atrophy: decrease in the size of a body structure

Attachment: active, affectionate, reciprocal relationship between two persons

Attitude: feeling or emotion, generally including a positive or negative judgment toward people, objects, or ideas

Auditory: pertaining to hearing

Aura: consists of at least seven layers of energy that surround the body and relate to the chakras

Auscultation: listening for sounds within the body

Authoritative knowledge: knowledge that comes from an expert and is accepted as truth based on a perceived level of expertise

Autocratic leadership: leadership style in which the leader assumes complete control over the decisions and activities of the group

Autologous transfusion: occurs when a patient donates his or her own blood for a transfusion

Autonomy: self-determination; being independent and self-governing

Ayurveda: a science of life that delineates the diet, medicines, and behaviors that are beneficial or harmful for life and considers that balance among people, the environment, and the larger cosmos is integral to human health

B

Bacteria: the most significant and most commonly observed infection-causing agents

Bacteriuria: an asymptomatic condition that occurs when bacteria enter the bladder during catheterization, or when organisms migrate up the catheter lumen or the urethra into the bladder

Bandage: piece of gauze or other material used to cover a wound

Basal metabolism: amount of energy required to carry out involuntary activities of the body at rest

Base: substance that can accept or trap a hydrogen ion; synonym for alkali

Base of support: foundation that provides stability for an object

Basic human needs: something essential to the health and survival of humans; common to all people

Basic research (pure research): research designed to generate and refine theory; the findings are often not directly useful in practice

Battery: assault that is carried out

Beliefs: special class of intellectual attitudes based primarily on faith as opposed to fact

Beneficence: principle of doing good

Bereavement: state of grieving or going through the grief process

Bilateral: pertaining to two sides of the body

Binder: type of bandage, usually designed to fit a large body area

Bioethics: ethics that encompass all those perspectives that seek to understand human nature and behavior, the domain of social science, and the natural world

Biologic sex: term used to denote chromosomal sexual development—male (XY) or female (XX)

Biopsy: removal of a piece of tissue for microscopic examination

Bioterrorism: the deliberate spread of pathogenic organisms into a community

Bisexuality: having sexual feelings for people of both sexes

Blended family: two single-parent families joined together to form a new family unit

Blood pressure: force of blood against arterial walls

Body image: how a person experiences his or her body

Body language: nonverbal communication

Body mass index: ratio of height to weight that provides a more accurate reflection of total body fat stores in the general population than previously existed

Body mechanics: efficient use of the body as a machine and as a means of locomotion

Body substance isolation (BSI): type of isolation that considers all body substances as potentially infective regardless of a person's diagnosis

Bolus: single injection of a concentrated solution administered intravenously

Bonding: process of initial emotional fusing of the mother and infant that occurs most often in the first few hours after birth and is necessary for later attachment

Bowel incontinence: the inability of the anal sphincter to control the discharge of fecal and gaseous material

Bowel movement: emptying of the intestinal tract; synonym for *defecation*

Bowel training program: program that manipulates factors within a person's control (timing of defecation, exercise, diet) to produce a regular pattern of comfortable defecation without medication or enemas

Bradycardia: slow heart rate

Bradypnea: abnormally slow rate of breathing

Breakthrough pain: temporary flare-up of moderate to severe pain that occurs even when the patient is taking ATC medication for persistent pain

Bronchial sounds: those heard over the trachea; high in pitch and intensity, with expiration being longer than inspiration

Bronchodilator: medication that relaxes contractions of smooth muscles of the bronchioles

Bronchoscopy: visual examination of the trachea and bronchi

Bronchovesicular: normal breath sounds heard over the upper anterior chest and intercostal area

Bruit: unusual sound, usually abnormal, heard in auscultation

Buffer: substance that prevents body fluid from becoming overly acid or alkaline

Bulimia: eating disorder characterized by episodes of gorging followed by purging; often occurs in conjunction with anorexia nervosa

Burnout: behaviors exhibited as the result of prolonged occupational stress

C

Calorie: measure of heat, or energy; *kilocalorie,* commonly referred to as a calorie, defined as the amount of heat required to raise 1 kg of water 1°C

Carbohydrate: organic compounds (commonly known as sugars and starches) that are composed of carbon, hydrogen, and oxygen; the most abundant and least expensive source of calories in the diet worldwide

Cardiac output: volume of blood pumped from the left ventricle per minute

Cardinal signs: body temperature, pulse and respiratory rates, and blood pressure; synonym for *vital signs*

Care-based approach: approach to bioethics that directs attention to the specific situations of individual patients viewed within the context of their life narrative

Caregiver burden: stress responses experienced during prolonged periods of home care by family caregivers

Caries: cavitation of the teeth

Case management: the process of coordinating an individual's healthcare for the purpose of maximizing positive outcomes and containing costs

Cathartic: medication that strongly increases gastrointestinal motility and promotes defecation

Catheter: tube for injecting or removing fluids

Cation: ion that carries a positive electric charge

Center of gravity: point at which the mass of an object is centered

Centers for Disease Control and Prevention (CDC): U.S. government agency whose responsibilities include investigation, identification, prevention, and control of disease

Central venous catheter: venous access device usually introduced into the subclavian or internal jugular veins and passed to the superior vena cava just above the right atrium

Certification: process by which a person who has met certain criteria established by a nongovernmental association is granted recognition

Cerumen: wax in the external ear canals, consisting of a heavy oil and brown pigment

Ceruminal gland: gland found in the external auditory canal that secretes a substance called *cerumen* (ear wax)

Chakra: concentrated areas of energy aligned vertically in the body, which relate to each other as well as to specific areas of the body/mind/spirit

Change: process of transforming, altering, or modifying something

Change agent: person who purposefully and systematically implements change

Change-of-shift report: communication method used by nurses who are completing care for a patient to transmit patient information to nurses who are about to assume responsibility for continuing care; may be exchanged verbally in a meeting or audiotaped

Channel: term used in communication theory to denote the medium selected to convey the message; the channel may target any of the receiver's senses

Charting by exception: shorthand method for documenting patient data that is based on well-defined standards of practice; only exceptions to these standards are documented in narrative notes

Chemical name: precise description of a drug's chemical composition

Chemical terrorism: the deliberate release of a chemical compound for the purpose of causing mass destruction

Cheyne-Stokes respirations: gradual increase and then gradual decrease in depth of respirations followed by a period of apnea

Child abuse: intentional, nonaccidental physical or mental abuse of a child by a parent or other caregiver

Chiropractic: science that investigates the relationship between structure (the spine) and function (mainly the nervous system) of the human body to restore and preserve health

Cholesterol: fat-like substance found only in animal tissues; it is important for cell membrane structure, a precursor of steroid hormones, and a constituent of bile; high serum cholesterol levels are a risk factor in the development of atherosclerosis

Chronic illness: irreversible illness that causes permanent physical impairment and requires long-term healthcare

Chronic pain: episode of pain that lasts for 6 months or longer; may be intermittent or continuous

Chyme: semifluid state that food is in when it leaves the stomach

Cilia: microscopic hairlike projections that propel mucus toward the upper airway to be removed (by coughing)

Circadian rhythm: rhythm that completes a full cycle every 24 hours; synonym for *diurnal rhythm*

Circumduction: moving the distal part of the limb to trace a complete circle while the proximal end of the bone remains fixed

Civil law: rule that regulates relationships among people; synonym for *private law*

Clear liquid diet: diet that contains only foods that are clear liquids at room or body temperature—gelatin, fat-free broth, bouillon, ice pops, clear juices, carbonated beverages, regular and decaffeinated coffee and tea

Clinical ethics: branch of bioethics concerned with ethical problem that arise within the context of caring for patients

Clinical pathway/critical path: case management tools used to communicate the standardized, interdisciplinary plan of care for a particular group of patients; care guidelines and outcomes are specified for each day of the patient's stay

Clubbing: rounding and swelling of nailbeds

Cognition: cerebral functioning; process of perceiving and understanding one's world

Cognitive development: learning that occurs as a result of the internal organization of an event, which forms a mental schema (plan) and serves as a base for further schemata as one grows and develops (Piaget's theory of cognitive development)

Cognitive learning: storing and recalling of new knowledge in the brain

Cognitively skilled: capable of thinking about the nature of things sufficiently to "make sense" of the world and to grasp conceptually what is necessary to achieve valued goals

Coitus: sexual activity in which the penis is placed in the vagina; synonym for *sexual intercourse*

Colic: acute abdominal pain caused by spasmodic contractions of the intestine during the first 3 months of life

Collaborative problem: actual or potential health problem that may occur from complications of disease, diagnostic studies, or the treatment regimen; the nurse works together with other members of the healthcare team toward its resolution

Colloid osmotic pressure: pressure exerted by plasma proteins on permeable membranes in the body; synonym for *oncotic pressure*

Colon: section of the large intestine from the cecum to the rectum

Colostomy: an opening into the colon that permits feces from the colon to exit through the stoma

Comfort measures only: an order written to indicate that the goal of treatment is a comfortable, dignified death and that further life-sustaining measures are no longer indicated

Common law: law resulting from court decisions that is then followed when other cases involving similar circumstances and facts arise; common law is as binding as civil law

Communication: process of sharing information; process of generating and transmitting meanings

Community-based healthcare: healthcare that is provided to people who live within a defined geographic region or who have common needs; designed to meet the needs of people as they move between and among healthcare settings

Complaint: legal statement of the plaintiff's claim; once filed, it initiates legal proceedings

Compliance: act of completing what is expected of one

Computer-based record: computer-generated patient data collection system that can be distributed among many caregivers in a standardized format, allowing them to compare and uniformly evaluate patient progress easily, or compare the progress of groups of patients with similar diagnoses

Computerized plans of nursing care: plans of patient care developed by computer software programs that enable the nurse to call up screens listing causes, goals, and related nursing interventions for nursing diagnoses and medical diagnoses

Concept: abstract images that are formed as impressions from the environment and organized into symbols of reality

Conceptual framework/model: set of concepts, along with the statements that arrange the concepts into an understandable pattern

Concurrent audit: evaluation of nursing care and patient outcomes conducted while the patient is receiving care; may use direct observation of nursing care, patient interview, and chart review

Concurrent evaluation: the evaluation of nursing care and patient outcomes while the patient is receiving care, conducted by using direct observation of nursing care, patient interviews, and chart review to determine whether the specified evaluative criteria are met

Condom catheter: tube for draining urine; it connects a device applied externally to the penis to a collection bag

Confidentiality: respecting privileged information

Congestion: presence of excessive fluids or secretions in an organ or body tissue

Conscious sedation/analgesia: analgesia used for short-term procedures in which the patient maintains cardiorespiratory function and can respond to verbal commands while the IV administration of sedatives and analgesics raises the pain threshold and produces an altered mood and some degree of amnesia

Constipation: passage of dry, hard, fecal material

Consultation: process in which two or more individuals with varying degrees of experience and expertise deliberate about a problem and its solution

Consumer: the person who uses healthcare services (the patient)

Continuity of care: coordination of services provided to patients before they enter a healthcare setting, during the time they are in the setting, and after they leave the setting

Continuum: graduated scale

Contraception: prevention of conception or pregnancy; also used to describe methods used for birth control

Contractual agreement: pact made between two persons or parties for the achievement of mutually set goals

Contracture: permanent contraction state of a muscle

Convalescent period: stage of an infection that represents recovery from the infection

Coping mechanism: patterns of behavior used to neutralize, deny, or counteract anxiety

Counseling: giving guidance, assisting with problem solving

Crackles: fine crackling sounds made as air moves through wet secretions in the lungs

Credentialing: general term that refers to ways in which professional competence is maintained

Crime: offense against people or property; the act is considered to be against the government, referred to in a lawsuit as "the people," and the accused is prosecuted by the state

Crisis: (1) point at which body temperature drops rapidly to normal; (2) occurs when coping and defense mechanisms are no longer effective, resulting in high levels of anxiety, disorganized behavior, and the inability to function normally

Crisis intervention: five-step problem-solving technique to promote adaptation and improve future coping

Criteria: specified behavior; for example, the measurable criteria in a patient goal specifies how the patient must perform the desired behavior

Critical/collaborative pathway: case management plan that is a detailed, standardized plan of care developed for a patient population with a designated diagnosis or procedure; it includes expected outcomes, a list of interventions to be performed, and the sequence and timing of those interventions

Critical thinking: thought that is disciplined, comprehensive, based on intellectual standards, and, as a result, well-reasoned; a systematic way to form and shape one's thinking that functions purposefully and exactly

Crossmatching: act of determining the compatibility of two blood specimens

Cue: significant data that is helpful in making decisions

Cultural assimilation: process that occurs when a minority group, living as part of a dominant group within a culture, loses the cultural characteristics that made it different

Cultural blindness: the process of ignoring differences in people and proceeding as though the differences do not exist

Cultural care deprivation: a lack of culturally assistive, supportive, or facilitative acts in the healthcare setting

Cultural diversity: diverse groups in society, with varying racial classification and national origin, religious affiliation, languages, physical size, gender, sexual orientation, age, disability, socio-economic status, occupational status, and geographic location

Cultural imposition: tendency of some to impose their beliefs, practices, and values on another culture because they believe that their ideas are superior to those of another person or group

Culturally competent care: care delivered with an awareness of the aspects of the patient's culture

Culture: sum total of human behavior or social characteristics peculiar to a specific group and passed from generation to generation or from one to another within the group

Culture shock: those feelings, usually negative, a person experiences when placed in a different culture

Cumulative effect: condition that occurs when the body cannot metabolize a drug before additional doses are administered

Cutaneous pain: superficial pain usually involving the skin or subcutaneous tissue

Cyanosis: bluish coloring of the skin and mucous membranes

Cystoscopy: direct visual examination of the bladder, ureteral orifices, and urethra with a cystoscope

Cytologic study: study of cells and fluids from the body

D

Dangling: position in which the person sits on the edge of the bed with legs and feet dangling over the side of the bed

Data: information

Data base: all the pertinent patient information that enables a comprehensive and effective plan of care to be designed and implemented for the patient

Data cluster: grouping of patient data or cues that points to the existence of a patient health problem

Day-care center: centers that provide care for infants, children, elderly people, and people with special healthcare needs

Death: termination of life and its related clinical signs

Débridement: cleaning away of devitalized tissue and foreign matter from a wound; can be accomplished by various methods

Decentralized decision-making process: autonomous, accountable professional nursing practice; a characteristic of a democratic leadership style and the heart of a self governance model of unit organization

Deductive reasoning: cognitive process in which one examines a general idea and then considers specific actions or ideas

Defamation of character: an intentional tort in which one party makes derogatory remarks about another that diminishes the other party's reputation; slander is oral defamation of character; libel is written defamation of character

Defecation: emptying of the intestinal tract; synonym for *bowel movement*

Defendant: the one being accused of a crime or tort

Defense mechanisms: forms of self-deception; unconscious process the self uses to protect itself from anxiety or threats to self-esteem

Dehiscence: separation of the layers of a surgical wound; may be partial, superficial, or a complete disruption of the surgical wound

Dehydration: decreased water volume

Delegation: the transfer of responsibility for the performance of an activity to another individual while retaining accountability for the outcome

Delta sleep: deep sleep, occurring during stage III and especially stage IV in NREM sleep

Dementia: organic impairment of intellectual functioning, gradually leading to interference with social or occupational functioning, memory, and often personality integration

Democratic leadership: leadership style characterized by a sense of equality between the leader and followers

Deontologic: ethical system in which actions are right or wrong independent of the consequences they produce

Dependent action: nursing action carried out at the instruction or order of an authorized healthcare professional other than a nurse; synonym for *physician-initiated or physician-prescribed intervention*

Dermis: underlying portion of the skin

Development: increase in the complexity of function and progression to skill advancement

Developmental crisis: predictable patterns of behavior and change occurring throughout the lifespan

Developmental delay: measure of development that lags behind the normal range for a given age

Developmental task: successful achievement of psychomotor, psychosocial, or cognitive skills at certain periods in life; failure to obtain the developmental task can lead to unhappiness and difficulty with later tasks

Development theory: theory to describe the orderly and predictable process of the growth and development of humans, individualized by social, biologic, and environmental factors

Diagnosis (nursing): analysis of patient data to identify patient strengths and health problems that independent nursing intervention can prevent or resolve

Diagnosis-related groups (DRGs): classification of patients by major medical diagnosis for the purpose of standardizing healthcare costs

Diagnostic error: failure to detect an actual unhealthy behavior

Diarrhea: passage of liquid and unformed stools

Diastolic pressure: least amount of pressure exerted on arterial walls, which occurs when the heart is at rest between ventricular contractions

Dietary Guidelines: recommendations for choosing a healthy diet made by the U.S. Department of Agriculture and the U.S. Department of Health and Human Services

Diffuse pain: pain that covers a large area

Diffusion: tendency of solutes to move freely throughout a solvent from an area of higher concentration to an area of lower concentration until equilibrium is established

Direct transfusion: infusion of blood while it is being taken from the donor

Disaster: an emergency event of greater magnitude that requires the response of people outside the involved community

Discharge planning: systematic process of preparing the patient to leave the healthcare facility and for maintaining continuity of care

Discharge summary: description of where the patient stands in relation to problems identified in the record at discharge; documents any special teaching or counseling the patient received, including referrals

Discipline: specific and unique body of knowledge that uses existing and new knowledge to creatively solve problems and meet human needs within ever-changing boundaries

Disease: pathologic change in the structure or function of the body or mind

Disinfection: process used to destroy microorganisms; destroys all pathogenic organisms except spores

Distribution: movement of drugs by the circulatory system to the site of action

Disturbed sensory perception: a state in which the individual or group experiences or is at risk for a change in the amount, pattern, or interpretation of incoming stimuli

Documentation: written, legal record of all pertinent interventions with the patient—assessments, diagnoses, plans, interventions, and evaluations

Dominant group: group within a culture that has the authority to control the value system and determine the rewards of the system; usually the largest group in a society

Donor: person who donates blood to be given to another person

Do-not-hospitalize: an order specifying that a patient, usually one who is terminally ill and anticipating death, not be admitted to the hospital in the event of a worsening of condition

Do-not-resuscitate (DNR): an order specifying that there be no attempt to resuscitate a patient in the event of cardiopulmonary arrest

Dosha: the patient's basic condition; understanding dosha is central to Ayurvedic medicine

Dressing: protective covering placed over a wound

Drug: substance that modifies body functions when taken into the living organism; synonym for *medication*

Drug allergy: hypersensitivity caused by previous exposure to a medication; may occur immediately or be delayed; manifestations range from mild to severe

Drug tolerance: tendency of the body to become accustomed to a drug over time; larger doses are required to produce the desired effects

Dynorphin: the endorphin having the most potent analgesic effect

Dysfunctional grief: abnormal or distorted grief that may be either unresolved or inhibited

Dyspnea: difficult or labored breathing

Dysrhythmia: an abnormal cardiac rhythm; synonym for *arrhythmia*

Dyssomnias: sleep disorders characterized by insomnia or excessive sleepiness

Dysuria: difficulty in voiding; may or may not be associated with pain; a feeling of warm local irritation occurring during voiding is called *burning*

E

Ecchymosis: collection of blood in subcutaneous tissues that causes a purplish discoloration

Edema: accumulation of fluid in extracellular spaces

Elective surgery: surgery that is recommended but can be omitted or delayed without catastrophe

Electrocardiogram (ECG; EKG): graphic record produced by the electrocardiograph

Electroencephalograph: instrument that measures and records electric impulses of the brain

Electrolyte: substance capable of breaking into ions and developing an electric charge when dissolved in solution

Electromyograph (EMG): instrument that records muscle tone

Electrooculogram: recording of the electric current or potential produced by eye movements

Embolism: blocking of an artery by a blood clot or by other foreign matter brought to the site by the blood flow

Embolus: foreign body or air in the circulatory system; plural form is *emboli*

Emergency assessment: assessment performed to identify life-threatening problems when a physiologic or psychological crisis presents

Emergency surgery: surgery that must be performed immediately to save the person's life or a body organ

Empathy: intellectually identifying with the way another person feels

Endogenous: infection in which the causative organism comes from microbial life the person himself or herself harbors

Endorphins: morphine-like substances released by the body that appear to alter the perception of pain

Endoscopy: direct visualization of hollow organs of the body using an endoscope or flexible, lighted tube

Endotracheal tube: polyvinyl-chloride airway that is inserted through the nose or the mouth into the trachea, using a laryngoscope as a guide

Enema: introduction of solution into the lower intestinal tract

Enkephalins: opioids that are widespread throughout the brain and dorsal horn of the spinal cord and are believed to reduce pain sensation by inhibiting the release of substance P

Enteral nutrition: alternate form of feeding that involves passing a tube into the gastrointestinal tract to allow instillation of the appropriate formula

Entry phase: phase of the home visit in which the nurse develops rapport with the patient and family members, mutually determines outcomes, makes assessments, plans and implements prescribed care, and provides teaching

Enuresis: involuntary urination; most often used to refer to a child who involuntarily urinates during the night

Epidermis: superficial portion of the skin

Epidural analgesia: means of providing pain relief with an opioid injection delivered by way of a catheter inserted in the mid-lumbar region into the epidural space

Epithelialization: stage of wound healing in which epithelial cells move across the surface of a wound; tissue color ranges from the color of "ground glass" to pink

Erection: condition that results when erectile tissue of the penis fills with blood as a result of stimulation

Erogenous zones: areas of the body that produce sexual desire and arousal when stimulated

Erythema: redness of the skin

Eschar: a thick, leathery scab or dry crust that is necrotic and must be removed for adequate pressure ulcer staging to occur

Ethical agency: the ability to behave in an ethical way; to do the ethically right thing because it is the right thing to do

Ethically and legally skilled: capable of conducting one's self in a manner consistent with a personal moral code and professional role responsibilities

Ethics: system dealing with standards of character and behavior related to what is right and wrong

Ethnicity: sense of identification that a cultural group collectively has; the sharing of common and unique cultural and social beliefs and behavior patterns, including language and dialect, religious practices, literature, folklore, music, political interests, food preferences, and employment patterns

Ethnocentrism: judgment of other people based on the standards and practices of one's own culture

Euphoria: unrealistic sense of well-being

Eupnea: normal respirations

Euthanasia: mercy killing; the deliberate termination of the life of a person

Evaluating: measurement of the extent to which the patient has achieved the goals specified in the plan of care; factors that positively or negatively influence goal achievement are identified, and the plan of care is terminated or revised

Evidence-based practice (EBP): nursing care provided that is supported by sound scientific rationale

Evisceration: protrusion of viscera through an incisional area

Exacerbation: period in an illness when the symptoms of the disease reappear

Excretion: removal of a drug from the body

Exercise: active exertion of muscles involving the contraction and relaxation of muscle groups

Exogenous: infection in which the causative organism is acquired from outside the host

Expected outcome: specific, measurable criteria used to evaluate whether the patient goal has been met

Expectorant: drug that facilitates the removal of respiratory secretions

Expert witness: nurse who explains to the judge and jury what happened based on the patient's record and who offers an opinion as to whether the nursing care met acceptable standards of practice

Expiration: act of breathing out; synonym is *exhalation*

Explicit power: power obtained by virtue of a person's position

Extended-care facility: type of care given after hospitalization of acute illness; includes residential care and intermediate or skilled nursing home care

Extended family: nuclear family and other related people

Extracellular fluid (ECF): fluid outside the cells; includes intravascular and interstitial fluids

Exudate: fluid that accumulates in a wound, may contain serum, cellular debris, bacteria, and white blood cells

F

Fact witness: nurse who has knowledge of the actual incident prompting a legal case; bases testimony on firsthand knowledge of the incident not on assumptions

Failure to thrive (FTT): physical and developmental retardation of infants or children resulting from physical or emotional neglect

Faith: (1) spiritual dimensions of a person's life regardless of religious affiliation; (2) confident belief in something for which there is no proof or material evidence

False self: a sense of self that might develop in individuals who have the emotional need to respond to the needs and ambitions significant people, such as parents, have for them

Family: any group of two or more people who live together and are emotionally involved with each other

Fasting state: abstinence from food and fluids

Fear: a feeling of dread; a cognitive response to a known threat

Febrile: condition in which the body temperature is elevated

Fecal impaction: collection in the rectum of hardened feces that cannot be passed

Feces: intestinal waste products

Feedback: verbal and nonverbal evidence that the message is received and understood

Felony: (1) crime punishable by imprisonment in a state or federal penitentiary for more than 1 year; (2) crime of greater offense than a misdemeanor

Feminist ethics: type of ethical approach that aims to critique existing patterns of oppression and domination in society, especially as these affect women and the poor

Fever: elevation above the upper limit of normal body temperature; synonym for *pyrexia*

Fiber: all dietary plant material that is not digestible by gastrointestinal tract, enzymes, and secretions

Fidelity: keeping promises and commitments made to others

Fight-or-flight response: the body prepares itself against threat, to either resist (fight) or evade (flight) the danger

Filtration: passage of a fluid through a permeable membrane whose spaces do not allow certain solutes to pass; passage is from an area of higher pressure to one of lower pressure

Fistula: an abnormal passage from an internal organ to the skin or from one internal organ to another

Flaccidity: decreased muscle tone; synonym for *hypotonicity*

Flatulence: excessive formation of gases in the gastrointestinal tract

Flatus: intestinal gas

Flexibility: ability to use a muscle through its entire range of motion

Flexion: state of being bent

Flow sheets: graphic record of abbreviated aspects of patient's condition (eg, vital signs, routine aspects of care)

Fluid balance: state in which water and its solutes in the body are in normal proportions and concentrations and are in appropriate body compartments

Fluid imbalance: state in which water and its solutes in the body are in improper proportions and concentrations or are improperly located in body compartments

Fluid volume deficit: deficiency in the amount of both water and electrolytes in extracellular fluid; water and electrolyte proportions remain near normal

Fluid volume excess: excessive retention of water and sodium in extracellular fluid in near-normal proportions

Flushing: red appearance of the skin

Focus charting: a documentation system that replaces the problem list with a focus column that incorporates many aspects of a patient and patient care; the focus may be a patient strength or a problem or need; the narrative portion of focus charting uses the data (D), action (A), response (R) format

Focused assessment: an assessment performed to gather data about a *specific problem* that has already been identified or to identify new or overlooked problems

Foley catheter: indwelling or retention catheter that remains in place to drain urine

Footdrop: complication resulting from extended plantar flexion

Formal teaching: planned teaching based on learner objectives

Frail-old: term for people over age 75; the fastest-growing segment of the population

Fraud: willful and purposeful misrepresentation that could cause, or has caused, loss or harm to people or property

Fremitus: vibration of the chest wall that can be palpated during the physical examination

Frequency: increased incidence of voiding

Friction: occurs when two surfaces rub against each other; the resulting injury resembles an abrasion and can also damage superficial blood vessels directly under the skin

Friction rub: crackling sounds heard in the chest cavity caused by inflamed pleura rubbing against the chest wall

Full liquid diet: diet that contains milk, plain frozen desserts, pasteurized eggs, cereal gruels, and milk and egg substitutes in addition to clear liquids; contains liquids that can be poured at room temperature

Functional health: level of health defined by one's ability to carry out usual and desired daily activities

Functional incontinence: state in which a person experiences an involuntary, unpredictable passage of urine

Fungi: plant-like organisms (molds and yeasts) that also can cause infection

G

Gate control theory: theory that explains that excitatory pain stimuli carried by small-diameter nerve fibers can be blocked by inhibiting signals carried by large-diameter nerve fibers

Gender identity: the inner sense a person has of being male or female, which may be the same as or different from biologic gender; synonym is *sexual identity*

Gender role behavior: the behavior a person conveys about being male or female, which may or may not be the same as biologic gender or gender identity (Pillitteri, 1995)

General adaptation syndrome (GAS): biochemical model of stress describing the body's general response to stress

General anesthesia: anesthetic drugs that produce narcosis, relaxation of skeletal muscles, and reduced or absent reflex action

Generic name: name assigned by the manufacturer who first develops a drug; it is often derived from the chemical name

Gerontologic nursing: nursing specialty concerned with the care of both the well and the ill older adult

Gerontology: study of all aspects of the aging process and their consequences

Gingivitis: inflammation of the gingivae or gums

Global self: term used to describe the composite of all the basic facts, qualities, traits, images, and feelings one holds about oneself

Glycosuria: presence of sugar in the urine; if due to an unusually large intake of sugar or to marked emotional disturbances and is temporary, there is little cause for alarm

Goal: an aim or an end

Good Samaritan law: law that holds certain health practitioners blameless when undertaking to aid a person in an emergency

Gram-negative bacteria: bacteria with chemically more complex cell walls that can be decolorized by alcohol

Gram-positive bacteria: bacteria with a thick cell wall that resists decolorization (loss of color) and are stained violet

Granulation tissue: new tissue that is pink/red in color and composed of fibroblasts and small blood vessels that fill an open wound when it starts to heal

Graphic sheet: form used to record specific patient variables

Grief: emotional response to loss. *Dysfunctional grief:* distorted or abnormal grief response, including *inhibited grief* (suppression of grief reaction) and *unresolved grief* (lengthy or denied grief reaction). *Abbreviated grief:* short but genuine grief reaction. *Anticipatory grief:* grief reaction before actual loss

Ground: conducting connection between a source of electricity and the earth

Group dynamics: study of a group's characteristics and ways of functioning

Growth: an increase in body size or changes in body cell structure, function, and complexity

Gurgles: continuous musical sounds that are audible in expiration or inspiration, or both; formerly called *rhonchi*

Gustatory: pertaining to taste

H

Half-life: the amount of time it takes for half a dose of a drug to be eliminated from the body

Halitosis: offensive breath

Healing touch: uses a collection of energy techniques to assess and treat the human energy system, thereby affecting physical, emotional, mental and spiritual health and healing

Health: state of optimal functioning or well-being

Health-belief model: what people believe to be true about themselves in relation to health

Health maintenance organization (HMO): broad term encompassing various healthcare delivery systems that use group practice and provide an incentive to use a prepaid comprehensive healthcare system

Health problem: condition related to health requiring intervention if disease or illness is to be prevented or resolved and coping and wellness are to be promoted

Helping relationship: interaction that sets the climate of movement of the participants toward common goals

Hematuria: blood in the urine; if present in large enough quantities, urine may be bright red or reddish brown

Hemolysis: process of freeing a red blood cell of its hemoglobin by destruction of the cell membrane

Hemoptysis: sputum containing blood

Hemorrhage: excessive blood loss due to the escape of blood from blood vessels

Hemorrhoids: abnormally distended rectal veins

Hemothorax: blood that develops in the pleural space

Heparin lock: intravenous needle or catheter with an injection pad attached at the end

Hesitancy: delay or difficulty in initiating voiding

Heterosexuality: having sexual feelings for a person of the opposite sex

Hierarchy of needs: as defined by Maslow, certain needs are more basic than others; a person strives to at least minimally meet certain needs before attending to others

High-level wellness: functioning to one's maximum potential while maintaining balance and purposeful direction in the environment

Holism: theory and philosophy that focuses on connections and interactions between parts of the whole

Holistic healthcare: healthcare that takes into account the whole person interacting in the environment

Holistic nursing: nursing practice built on a holistic philosophy

Home health agency: agency eligible to receive federal funds that provides home-based care; may be independent, hospital operated, or health department managed

Home healthcare: healthcare services provided in a patient's home

Homeopathy: practice of medicine based on the belief of supporting the body while the symptoms are allowed to "run their course" to stimulate and strengthen the immune system and promote healing

Homeostasis: various physiologic and psychological mechanisms respond to changes in the internal and external environment to maintain a balanced state

Homosexuality: having sexual feelings for a person of the same sex

Hospice: a type of end-of-life care for persons who are terminally ill, characterized by the following: (1) patients are kept as free of pain as possible so that they may die comfortably and with dignity; (2) patients receive continuity of care, are not abandoned, and do not lose personal identity; (3) patients retain as much control as possible over decisions regarding their care and are allowed to refuse further life-prolonging technologic interventions; and (4) patients are viewed as individuals with personal fears, thoughts, feelings, values, and hopes

Hospitals: acute-care settings that provide various healthcare services, such as emergency care, in-patient care, surgery, diagnostic tests, and patient education

Host: animal or person on or within which microorganisms live

Hydration: union of a substance with water; term often is used as the opposite of dehydration, in which case it means that there is normal intracellular and extracellular water volume

Hydrometer: instrument used to determine the specific gravity of urine

Hydrostatic pressure: force exerted by a fluid against the container wall

Hypercalcemia: excess of calcium in the extracellular fluid

Hyperkalemia: excess of potassium in the extracellular fluid

Hypermagnesemia: excess of magnesium in the extracellular fluid

Hypernatremia: excess of sodium in the extracellular fluid

Hyperphosphatemia: above-normal serum concentration of inorganic phosphorus

Hyperpyrexia: high fever, above 41°C (105.8°F)

Hypersomnia: condition characterized by excessive sleeping, especially daytime sleeping

Hypertension: blood pressure elevated above the upper limit of normal

Hyperthermia: high body temperature

Hypertonic: having a greater concentration than the solution with which it is being compared

Hyperventilation: condition in which there is more than the normal amount of air entering and leaving lungs

Hypervolemia: excess of plasma

Hypnotic: pharmaceutical agent used to induce sleep

Hypocalcemia: insufficient amount of calcium in the extracellular fluid

Hypokalemia: insufficient amount of potassium in the extracellular fluid

Hypomagnesemia: insufficient amount of magnesium in the extracellular fluid

Hyponatremia: insufficient amount of sodium in the extracellular fluid

Hypophosphatemia: below-normal serum concentration of inorganic phosphorus

Hypoproteinemia: insufficient amount of protein substances in the extracellular fluid

Hypotension: blood pressure below the lower limit of normal

Hypothermia: low body temperature

Hypotonic: having a lesser concentration than the solution with which it is being compared

Hypoventilation: decreased rate or depth of air movement into the lungs

Hypovolemia: deficiency of plasma

Hypovolemic shock: shock due to a decrease in blood volume

Hypoxemia: deficient oxygenation of blood

Hypoxia: inadequate amount of oxygen available to the cells

I

Iatrogenic infection: infection that occurs as a result of a treatment or diagnostic procedure

Ideal self: self a person would like to be or thinks he or she should be; includes aspirations, moral ideas, and values

Idiosyncratic effect: unusual, unexpected response to a drug that may manifest itself by overresponse, underresponse, or response different from the expected outcome

Ileal conduit: urinary diversion in which the ureters are connected to the ileum with a stoma created on the abdominal wall

Ileostomy: allows fecal content from the ileum to be eliminated through the stoma

Illness: abnormal process in which any aspect of the person's functioning is altered (in comparison to the previous condition of health)

Imagery: using all five senses to imagine an event or body process unfolding according to a plan

Immunization: process of rendering a person immune or resistant to particular antigenic agents or bacteria

Implement: carry out the plan of care

Implied power: power obtained by force of a person's personality that might enable him or her to have more power to influence others than designated leaders

Impotence: condition in which a man is unable to attain or maintain an erection to such an extent that he cannot have satisfactory sexual intercourse; synonym for *erectile failure*

Incentive spirometer: equipment to help maximize lung inflation

Incident report: documentation that describes any injury or potential for injury suffered by a patient in a healthcare agency

Incision: wound made with a sharp, cutting instrument

Incontinence: inability to voluntarily control the discharge of urine or feces

Independent action: (1) nursing action carried out at the instruction or order of a nurse; (2) actions within the legal scope of nursing's independent domain; synonym for *nurse-initiated* or *nurse-prescribed intervention*

Inductive reasoning: cognitive process in which one identifies a specific idea or action and then makes conclusions about general ideas

Indwelling urethral catheter: catheter that remains in place for continuous urine drainage; synonym for *Foley catheter*

Infancy: period from 1 month to 1 year of age

Infection: disease state resulting from pathogens in or on the body

Inference: the judgement reached about a cue

Infiltration: escape of fluid into subcutaneous tissue

Inflammatory response: localized response of the body to injury or infection; protective mechanism that eliminates invading pathogens and allows for tissue repair to occur

Informal teaching: unplanned teaching sessions dealing with the patient's immediate learning needs and concerns

Informed consent: knowledgeable, voluntary permission obtained from a patient to perform a specific test or procedure

Inhalation: (1) act of breathing in; synonym for inspiration; (2) administration of a drug in solution via the respiratory tract

Initial assessment: comprehensive nursing assessment resulting in baseline data that enables the nurse to make a judgment about a patient's health status, ability to manage his or her own healthcare, and need for nursing, and to plan individualized, holistic healthcare for the patient

Initial planning: planning that addresses each problem listed in the prioritized nursing diagnoses and identifies appropriate patient goals and the related nursing care

Injection: introduction of medication into the body by a syringe attached to a needle

Inpatient: person who enters a healthcare setting for a stay ranging from 24 hours to many years

Insomnia: difficulty in falling asleep, intermittent sleep, or early awakening from sleep

Inspection: purposeful and systematic observation

Inspiration: act of breathing in; synonym is *inhalation*

Integrative care: care that uses some combination of allopathic and complementary/alternative modalities

Integument: skin

Integumentary system: skin and its appendages (ie, hair, glands in the skin, and nails)

Intercessory prayer: involves praying for the benefit of another person to the Judeo-Christian God

Interdependent action: nursing action performed by the nurse in collaboration with other members of the healthcare team

Intermittent catheter: straight catheter used to drain the bladder for short periods (5–10 minutes)

Intermittent fever: body temperature that alternates between fever and normal or subnormal temperature

Intermittent pulse: normal pulse rhythm broken by periods of irregular rhythm

Interpersonal communication: communication that occurs between two or more people with a goal to exchange messages

Interpersonally skilled: capable of establishing and maintaining caring relationships that facilitate the achievement of valued goals while simultaneously affirming the worth of the participants in the relationship

Interstitial fluid: fluid between the cells

Intervention: any action performed to modify an expectation or to enhance outcomes

Interview: planned communication for a specific purpose (eg, data collection)

Interviewing techniques: communication skills specifically designed to gather and validate information

Intracellular fluid (ICF): fluid within the cell; synonym for *cellular fluid*

Intractable pain: severe pain that is extremely resistant to relief measures

Intradermal injection: injection placed just below the epidermis

Intramuscular (IM) injection: an injection into deep muscle tissue, usually of the buttock, thigh, or upper arm

Intraoperative phase: period lasting from admission to the operating room area to transfer to the postanesthesia recovery area after surgery is completed

Intrapersonal communication: communication techniques or self talk to enhance positive interaction with the patient and family

Intravascular fluid: fluid within the vascular system; synonym for *plasma*

Intravenous (IV) infusion: injection of relatively large quantities of solution into a vein

Intravenous (IV) route: injection of a solution into the vein

Intuitive problem solving: direct understanding of a situation based on a background of experience, knowledge, and skill that makes expert decision making possible

Ion: atom or molecule carrying an electric charge in solution

Irrigation: flushing of a tube, canal, or area with solution

Ischemia: deficiency of blood in a particular area

Isokinetic exercise: exercise involving muscle contractions with resistance varying at a constant rate

Isolation: protective procedure designed to prevent the transmission of specific microorganisms; also called *protective aseptic techniques* and *barrier techniques*

Isometric exercise: exercise in which muscle tension occurs without a significant change in muscle length

Isotonic: (1) having about the same concentration as the solution with which it is being compared; (2) exercise in which muscles shorten (contract) and move

J

Jaundice: yellow appearance of the skin

Justice: process that distributes benefits, risks, and costs fairly

K

Kardex nursing care plan: trade name for a care plan documentation system that encompasses (1) prescriptions for nursing care related to activities of daily living; (2) nursing diagnoses and related patient goals and nursing orders; and (3) the nursing care related to diagnostic measures and the medical regimen

Kegel exercises: repetitious contraction and relaxation of the pubococcygeal muscle to improve vaginal tone and urinary continence

Ketosis: an abnormal accumulation of ketone bodies that is frequently associated with acidosis

Kinesthesia: awareness of positioning of body parts and body movement

Korotkoff sounds: series of sounds that correspond to changes in blood flow through an artery as pressure is released

Kussmaul's respiration breathing: an extreme rate and depth of breathing

L

Laissez-faire leadership: leadership style in which the leader relinquishes all power to the group

Language: prescribed way of using words; a means to express thoughts and feelings

Law: rule of conduct established and enforced by the government of a society

Lawsuit: legal action in a court of law

Laxative: drug used to induce emptying of the intestinal tract

Leadership: ability to direct or motivate others toward the achievement of predetermined goals

Learning: increasing one's knowledge; having one's behavior changed in a measurable way as a result of an experience

Learning readiness: patient's willingness to engage in the teaching–learning process (emotional readiness) and experiential readiness to begin the challenge of learning

Liability: legal responsibility for one's acts (and failure to act); includes responsibility for financial restitution of harms resulting from negligent acts

Licensure: to be given a license to practice nursing in a state or province after successfully meeting requirements

Life review/reminiscence: universal phenomenon identified by Butler as a review of one's life through one's recollections

Ligaments: tough fibrous bands that bind joints together and connect bones and cartilage

Line of gravity: vertical line that passes through the center of gravity

Lipid: group name for fatty substances, including fats, oils, waxes, and related compounds

Literacy: ability to read and write

Litigation: process of lawsuit

Living will: advance directive specifying the medical care a person would want or refuse should he or she lack the capacity to consent to or refuse treatment himself or herself

Local adaptation syndrome (LAS): localized response of the body to stress, precipitated by trauma or pathology

Localized symptoms: symptoms that are limited or restricted to a discrete area

Long-term care: facilities for long-term care that provide healthcare and help with activities of daily living for people of any age who are physically or mentally unable to independently care for themselves

Loss: inaccessibility or change in a valued person, object, or situation. *Actual loss:* loss tangible to both the person sustaining the loss and to others. *Perceived loss:* loss tangible only to the person sustaining it. *Physical loss:* loss of life, limb, an object, person, pet, or job. *Psychological loss:* loss that affects a person's self-image. *Anticipatory loss:* loss behaviors displayed before the actual loss occurs

Love and belonging needs: understanding and acceptance of others in giving and receiving love

M

Macromineral: mineral that is needed by the body in amount greater than 100 mg/day

Macronutrient: essential nutrient that supplies energy and builds tissue, such as carbohydrate, fat, and protein

Macroshock: electric current passing through a relatively large area of a person

Malpractice: act of negligence as applied to a professional person such as a physician, nurse, or dentist

Managed care: an organized, high-quality, cost-effective system of healthcare that influences the selection and use of healthcare services of a population

Management: the act of planning, organizing, directing, and controlling available human resources and financial resources to deliver quality care to patients and families

Masturbation: self-stimulation for sexual satisfaction

Maturational loss: the loss experienced as a result of natural developmental processes

Medicaid: Title XIX (Social Security Act, 1965) to make healthcare available to those people with less than the minimum income who do not qualify for Medicare

Medical asepsis: practices designed to reduce the number and transfer of pathogens; synonym for *clean technique*

Medical diagnosis: statement about a specific disease process using terminology from a well-developed classification system accepted by the medical profession

Medicare: Title XVIII (Social Security Act, 1965) to provide a measure of health coverage to all Social Security recipients

Medication: substance that modifies body functions when taken into the living organisms; synonym for *drug*

Medication record: record documenting all medications administered to the patient, the nurse administering the drugs, and sometimes the reason the drug was administered and its effectiveness

Menarche: initiation of the menstrual cycle

Meniscus: curved surface at the top of a column of liquid in a tube

Menopause: decrease of cyclic hormonal production and cessation of menses in females, usually between ages 45 and 60 years

Menstruation: cycle of about 20 days during which the female body prepares for the presence of a fertilized ovum

Mentorship: relationship in which an experienced person (the mentor) advises and assists a less experienced person

Meridian: part of an intricate structure of 72 energy circuits that nourish and support all cells and organs of the body, through which Qi flows vertically in the body

Message: term used in communication theory to denote the actual physical product of the source or encoder (eg, a speech, interview, phone conversation, chart)

Metabolic acidosis: proportionate deficiency of bicarbonate ions in the extracellular fluid

Metabolic alkalosis: proportionate excess of bicarbonate ions in the extracellular fluid

Metabolism: (1) chemical changes in the body by which energy is provided; (2) breakdown of a drug to an inactive form; also referred to as *biotransformation*

Metered dose inhaler (MDI): instrument that delivers a controlled dose of medication to narrowed airways with each compression of the canister

Micromineral: mineral or trace element that is needed by the body in an amount less than 100 mg/day

Micronutrient: vitamin or mineral needed in much smaller amount to regulate and control body processes

Microshock: electric current passing through a relatively small area of a person, usually part of the heart

Micturition: process of emptying the bladder; urination; voiding

Middle adult: the adult between the ages of 40 and 60 years; also called *middle adulthood*

Midlife crisis: realization that the halfway point in life has been reached and youthful goals may not have been achieved

Minerals: inorganic elements found in nature

Minimum data set: a standard established by most schools of nursing and healthcare institutions that specifies the information that must be collected from every patient

Minority group: group having some physical or cultural characteristic that identifies the people within the group as different from the dominant culture

Misdemeanor: crime of lesser offense than a felony and punishable by fines, imprisonment (usually for less than 1 year), or both

Mixed incontinence: symptoms of urge and stress incontinence are present, although one type may predominate

Moral development: influence of cultural effects on one's perceptions of justice in interpersonal relationships (found in Kohlberg's theory of moral development, which occurs in levels that closely follow Piaget's theory of cognitive development)

Morals: like ethics, concerned with what constitutes right action; more informal and personal than the term ethics

Mourning: period during which a person learns to accept grief

N

Narcolepsy: condition characterized by an uncontrolled desire to sleep

Narrative: descriptive record of the patient's condition; includes patient's response to interventions by health professionals and patient's progress toward goal achievement

Nasal cannula: disposable, plastic device that delivers oxygen via two protruding prongs for insertion into the nostrils

Nasogastric tube: tube inserted through the nose and into the stomach

Nasointestinal tube: tube inserted through the nose and into the upper portion of the small intestine

National Medical Care: healthcare services in Canada, funded by taxes and provided to every Canadian citizen

Naturopathic medicine: a relatively new system of medicine that is not only a system of medicine but also a way of life, with emphasis on patient responsibility, patient education, health maintenance, and disease prevention

Nebulizer: instrument that disperses fine particles of medication into the deeper passages of the respiratory tract where absorption occurs

Necrosis: death of cells

Negative nitrogen balance: condition resulting in muscle wasting and decreased physical energy for movement and work (eg, anorexia nervosa and certain cancers)

Negative reinforcement: an ineffective teaching strategy that uses criticism or punishment

Negativism: negative verbalizations and behaviors

Negligence: performing an act that a reasonably prudent person under similar circumstances would not do, or failing to perform an act that a reasonably prudent person under similar circumstances would do

Neonate: period from birth to 1 month of age

Nephrotoxic: capable of causing kidney damage

Neuromodulator: endogenous opioid chemical regulators that appear to have analgesic activity and alter pain perception

Neuropathic pain: pain that results from an injury to or abnormal functioning of peripheral nerves or the central nervous system

Neurotransmitters: substances that either excite or inhibit target nerve cells

Nociceptive pain: pain that is categorized as cutaneous, deep somatic, or visceral in nature

Nociceptors: pain receptors

Nocturia: frequency of urination during the night

Nocturnal myoclonus: condition characterized by marked muscle contraction that results in the jerking of one or both legs during sleep

Noise: factors that distort the quality of a message and interfere with the communication process

Noncompliance: nonadherence to a therapeutic recommendation

Nonmaleficence: principle of avoiding evil

Nonproductive cough: forceful expiratory effort without production of mucus; also called a *dry cough*

Nonverbal communication: exchange of information without the use of words

Normal flora: microorganisms that normally inhabit various body sites and are part of the body's natural defense system

Nosocomial infection: hospital-acquired infection

NPO: nothing by mouth

NREM: non-rapid eye movement that characterizes four stages of sleep

Nuclear family: family unit, family of marriage, parenthood, or procreation, and their immediate children

Nuclear terrorism: intentional dispersal of radioactive materials into the environment for the purpose of causing injury and death

Nurse-initiated intervention: independent nursing actions that involve carrying out nurse-prescribed interventions written on the nursing plan of care, as well as any other actions that nurses initiate without the direction or supervision of another healthcare professional and that result from their assessment of patient needs

Nurse practice act: law established to regulate nursing practice

Nursing: profession that focuses on the holistic person receiving healthcare services and provides a unique contribution to the prevention of illness and maintenance of health

Nursing actions: any action performed by a nurse to assist patients to meet health goals: promote wellness, prevent disease or illness, restore health, or facilitate coping with altered functioning

Nursing audit: method of evaluating the outcomes of nursing care or the process by which these outcomes are achieved using a review of patient records

Nursing care conference: formal meeting of nurses to discuss some aspect of patient's care

Nursing care rounds: procedure in which a group of nurses visit patients individually at bedside to gather information that helps to plan and to evaluate nursing care

Nursing diagnosis: actual or potential health problem that independent nursing intervention can prevent or resolve. *Actual problem* is present. *Possible problem* may be present, but more data are needed to confirm or disconfirm the problem. *Potential problem* may occur; defining characteristics are present as risk factors

Nursing history: assessment of the patient by interview to identify the patient's health status, strengths, health problems, health risks, and need for nursing

Nursing intervention: any treatment, based on clinical judgment and knowledge, that a nurse performs to enhance patient outcomes; there are nurse-initiated, physician-initiated, and collaborative interventions

Nursing order: prescribes the nursing care to be given to assist patient to meet health goals

Nursing plan of care: written guide to direct the efforts of the nursing team as they work with patient to meet health goals; specifies prioritized nursing diagnoses, patient goals, and nursing orders

Nursing process: five-step systematic method for giving patient care; involves assessing, diagnosing, planning, implementing, and evaluating

Nursing research: encompasses both research to improve the care of people in the clinical setting and to study people and the nursing profession, including education, policy development, ethics, and nursing history

Nursing theory: differentiates nursing from other disciplines and activities by serving the purposes of describing, explaining, predicting, and controlling desired outcomes of nursing care practices

Nutrient: specific biochemical substance used by the body for growth, development, activity, reproduction, lactation, health maintenance, and recovery from illness or injury

Nutrition: study of the nutrients and how they are handled by the body, as well as the impact of human behavior and environment on the process of nourishment

O

Obesity: weight greater than 20% above ideal body weight

Objective data: information perceptible to the senses; may be verified by another person

Observation: conscious and deliberate use of the five senses to gather data

Occult blood: blood present in such minute quantities that it cannot be detected with the unassisted eye

Occupational Safety and Health Administration (OSHA): government agency that establishes minimum health and safety standards for workers

Official name: name by which a drug is identified in official publications

Old-old: term used to describe older adults over age 75; sometimes referred to as frail-old

Older adult: after middle age; refers to adults over age of 65

Olfactory: pertaining to smell

Oliguria: scanty or greatly diminished amount of urine voided in a given time; 24-hour urine output is 100 to 400 mL

Oncotic pressure: pressure exerted by plasma proteins on permeable membranes in the body; synonym for *colloid osmotic pressure*

Ongoing planning: planning carried out by any nurse who interacts with the patient to keep the plan up to date, to facilitate the resolution of health problems, to manage risk factors, and to promote function

Opioid: more correct term for narcotic analgesics, since these drugs act by binding to opiate receptor sites in the central nervous system

Opportunist: bacteria that may potentially be harmful

Organism: a living being

Organizational communication: process of communication that involves individuals and groups to achieve established goals

Orgasm: apex of sexual activity in which rhythmic contractions of the genital organs and many other physiologic changes occur

Orthopedics: the correction or prevention of disorders of body structures used in locomotion

Orthopnea: type of dyspnea in which breathing is easier when the patient sits or stands

Orthostatic hypotension: temporary fall in blood pressure associated with assuming an upright position; synonym for *postural hypotension*

Osmolarity: concentration of particles in a solution, or a solution's pulling power

Osmosis: passage of a solvent through a semipermeable membrane from an area of lesser concentration to an area of greater concentration until equilibrium is established

Osmotic pressure: drawing power for water or the attraction for water exerted by solute particles

Osteoporosis: condition characterized by loss of calcium from bone tissue

Ostomy: general term referring to an artificial opening; usually used to refer to an opening created for the excretion of body wastes

Outcome: end product of nursing care; patient outcomes are measurable changes in patient behavior or state of health

Outcome evaluation: evaluation that focuses on measurable changes in the health status of the patient or the end results of nursing care

Outcome identification: observation of the patient to demonstrate the resolution of the problems identified by the nursing diagnoses and general problem list, along with the time frame for accomplishing these outcomes

Outpatient: person who requires healthcare services but does not need to stay in an institution for those services

Overflow incontinence: involuntary loss of urine associated with overdistention and overflow of the bladder

Overhydration: above-normal amounts of water in extracellular spaces

Ovulation: discharge of ovum from the female ovary at about the midpoint of each menstrual cycle

Ovum: female reproductive cell, often called an *egg*

P

Pain: sensation of physical or mental suffering or hurt that usually causes distress or agony to the one experiencing it

Pain threshold: amount of stimulation required before a person experiences the sensation of pain

Pain tolerance: point beyond which a person is no longer willing to endure pain (ie, pain of greater duration or intensity)

Palliative care: (hospice care), taking care of the whole person—body, mind, spirit, heart and soul—with the goal of giving patients with life-threatening illnesses the best quality of life they can have through the aggressive management of symptoms

Pallor: paleness of the skin

Palpation: method of examining by feeling a part with the fingers or hand

Palpitation: perception of one's own heartbeat

Paracentesis: withdrawal of fluid from a body cavity, usually from the abdominal cavity

Paralytic ileus: paralysis of intestinal peristalsis

Paraplegia: paralysis of the legs

Parasomnia: patterns of waking behavior that appear during sleep (eg, sleep walking, sleep talking, nocturnal erections)

Parenteral: outside of intestines or alimentary canal; popularly used to refer to injection routes

Paresis: impaired muscle strength or weakness

Paresthesia: numbness and tingling

Partial peripheral nutrition (PPN): nutrition prescribed for patients who require nutrient supplementation through a peripheral vein because they have an inadequate intake of oral feedings

Passive exercise: manual or mechanical means of moving the joints

Paternalism: an action that is based on what a parent would do

Pathogen: disease-producing microorganism

Patient: the person receiving care

Patient-controlled analgesia (PCA): method of controlling pain that involves an infusion pump that holds a vial of an IV analgesic that the patient controls and self-administers in small doses

Patient goal: statement describing an expected patient outcome

Patient record: a compilation of a patient's health information; the patient record is the only permanent legal document that details the nurse's interactions with the patient

Peak level: highest plasma concentration of a drug

Pedagogy: science of teaching that generally refers to the teaching of children and adolescents

Pediculosis: infestation with lice

Peer review: evaluation at the closest point to the patient and an ongoing tool to use for professional growth

Perception: conscious process of organizing and interpreting data from the senses into meaningful information

Percussion: act of striking one object against another for the purpose of producing a sound; used to assess the location, shape, size, and density of body tissues

Percutaneous endoscopic gastrostomy tube (PEG): surgically or laparoscopically placed gastrostomy tube

Performance improvement: commitment to healthier patients, quality care, reduced costs, and making a difference; accomplished by discovering a problem, planning a strategy, implementing a change, and assessing the change to see if the goal is met

Perfusion: passing of fluid through body tissue

Perioperative nursing: wide variety of nursing activities carried out before, during, and after surgery

Peripherally inserted central catheter (PICC): type of venous access device that can be introduced into a peripheral vein and advanced as far as the superior vena cava

Peripheral parenteral nutrition (PPN): prescribed for patients who require nutrient supplementation through a peripheral vein because they have an inadequate intake of oral feedings

Peripheral resistance: restraint to blood flow created by arteriole walls in a partial state of contraction

Peristalsis: involuntary, progressive wavelike movement of the musculature of the gastrointestinal tract

Personal identity: an individual's conscious sense of who he or she is

Personal space: external environment surrounding a person that is regarded as being part of that person

Petechiae: small, purplish hemorrhagic spots on the skin that do not blanch with applied pressure

pH: expression of hydrogen ion concentration and resulting acidity of a substance

Phagocytosis: engulfing of microorganisms, foreign particles, or other cells by phagocytes

Phantom pain: sensation of pain without demonstrable physiologic or pathologic substance; commonly observed after the amputation of a limb

Pharmacology: study of actions of chemicals on living organisms

Philosophy: study of wisdom, fundamental knowledge, and the processes we use to develop and construct our perceptions of life

Phlebitis: inflammation of a vein

Phlegm: thick, respiratory secretions

Physical assessment: systematic examination of the patient for objective data to better define the patient's condition and to help the nurse in planning care; usually performed in a head-to-toe format

Physician-initiated intervention: dependent nursing actions, involving carrying out physician-prescribed orders

Physiologic needs: need for oxygen, food, water, temperature, elimination, sexuality, activity, and rest; these needs have the highest priority and are essential for survival

PIE charting: documentation system that is unique in that it does not develop a separate care plan; the care plan is incorporated into the progress notes in which problems are identified by number, worked up using the problem (P), intervention (I), evaluation (E) format, and evaluated each shift

Piggyback infusion: intermittent IV administration of medications through a primary IV line, with the additive container positioned higher than the primary IV solution

Placebo: Latin word meaning "I shall please"; an inactive substance that gives satisfaction to the person using it

Plaintiff: person or government bringing a lawsuit against another

Plan: establish patient goals to prevent, reduce, or resolve the problems identified in the nursing diagnoses and determination of related nursing interventions

Planned change: change agent's purposeful, systematic effort to bring about change

Plan of nursing care: written guide that directs the efforts of the nursing team as the nurses work with patients to meet health goals; it specifies nursing diagnoses, outcomes, and associated nursing interventions

Plaque: transparent, adhesive coating on teeth consisting of mucin, carbohydrate, and bacteria

Plasma: liquid constituent of blood; synonym for *intravascular fluid*

Pleurae: two-layered membranes; the visceral pleura covers the lungs, and the parietal pleura lines the thoracic cavity

Pleural effusion: fluid in the pleural space

Pneumonia: inflammation or infection of the lungs

Pneumothorax: air in the pleural space

Podiatrist: one who treats foot disorders; synonym for *chiropodist*

Poison control center: agency that handles poison exposure and provides poison prevention teaching to the general population

Polyp: tumor on a stem that bleeds easily and may become malignant

Polysomnography: sleep study consisting of an electroencephalographic recording of the stages of sleep and any episodes of apnea, continuous monitoring of arterial oxygen saturation, and an electrocardiographic recording to detect any cardiac dysrhythmias

Polyuria: excessive output of urine (diuresis)

Positive reinforcement: affirmation of the efforts of patients

Possible problems: problems the patient may experience if certain trends in the patient's condition continue unreversed

Postoperative: period lasting from admission to the postanesthesia recovery area through recovery and convalescence

Postural hypotension: temporary fall in blood pressure associated with assuming an upright position; synonym for *orthostatic hypotension*

Post-void residual (PVR): urine that remains in the bladder after the act of micturition; a synonym for *residual urine*

Power: ability to influence others to achieve a desired effect

Preceptorship: process by which an experienced person facilitates an orientee's introduction to new responsibilities through teaching and guidance

Precordium: anterior surface of the chest wall overlying the heart and its related structures

Pre-entry phase: phase of the home visit in which the nurse collects information about the patient's healthcare needs, gathers needed supplies, and evaluates safety factors

Preferred provider organization (PPO): any arrangement whereby patients are channeled to specific organizations as providers of health plans

Premenstrual (tension) syndrome (PMS): menstrual cycle–related distress; occurs a few days before the onset of menstruation

Preoperative: period lasting from the decision that surgery is necessary until the patient is transferred to the operating room area

Presbycusis: age-related hearing loss in which there is decreased ability to distinguish higher frequencies

Presbyopia: condition of aging in which decreased elasticity of the eye lens hinders accommodation to close vision

Preschooler: period from ages 3 years to 6 years

Prescription: used by physician to convey medication plans for a patient

Pressure ulcer: any lesion caused by unrelieved pressure that results in damage to underlying tissue

Primary healthcare: essential healthcare based on practical, scientifically sound, and socially acceptable methods and technology, made universally accessible through the community's full participation and at a cost the community can afford

Primary preventive care: care directed toward health promotion and specific protection against illness

Principle-based approach: an approach to bioethics that offers specific action guides

PRN (p.r.n.) order: "as needed" order for medication

Problem-oriented medical record (POR): documentation system organized according to the person's specific health problems; includes database, problem list, plan of care, and progress notes

Process: series of actions, changes, or functions to bring about a result

Process evaluation: evaluation focusing on the nature and sequence of activities carried out by nurses implementing the nursing process

Productive cough: cough that produces respiratory tract secretions

Profession: an occupation that meets specific criteria including a well-defined body of specific and unique knowledge, a code of ethics and standards, ongoing research, and autonomy

Professionalism: a way of being/commitment to secure the interests and welfare of those entrusted to one's care

Progress notes: any of a variety of methods of notes that relate how a patient is progressing toward expected outcomes

Protein: vital component of every living cell; composed of carbon, hydrogen, oxygen, and nitrogen

Proteinuria: albumin in the urine; indication of kidney disease

Protocol: written plan that details the nursing activities to be executed in specific situations

Psychogenic pain: pain for which no physical cause can be identified

Psychological loss: loss caused by an altered self-image

Psychomotor learning: acquisition of physical skills

Psychosomatic disorder: physiologic alterations and illness believed to be due to psychological influences

Puberty: period during which primary and secondary sexual characteristics develop and the capability of sexual reproduction is attained

Public health agencies: local, state, provincial, or federal agencies that provide public health services to members of communities

Pulse: wave produced in the wall of an artery with each beat of the heart

Pulse deficit: difference between the apical and radial pulse rates

Pulse oximetry: noninvasive technique that measures the oxygen saturation (SaO_2) of arterial blood

Pulse pressure: difference between systolic and diastolic pressures

Purulent: containing pus

Pyorrhea: extensive inflammation of the gums and alveolar tissues; synonym for *periodontitis*

Pyrexia: elevation above the upper limit of normal body temperature; synonym for *fever*

Pyuria: pus in the urine; urine appears cloudy

Q

Qi: represents an invisible flow of energy that circulates through plants, animals, and people, as well as the earth and sky

Qi gong: system of posture, exercise (both gentle and dynamic), breathing techniques, and visualization that regulates the Qi

Qualitative research: method of research conducted to gain insight by discovering meanings

Quality assurance program: ongoing evaluation program designed and implemented to secure the excellence of healthcare; may involve an assessment of structure, process, and outcome standards

Quality improvement: the commitment and approach used to continuously improve every process in every part of an organization, with the intent of meeting and exceeding customer expectations and outcomes (also known as continuous quality improvement [CQI] or total quality management [TQM])

Quantitative research: research involving the concepts of basic and applied research

Quantum leadership: leadership that moves beyond the traditional modes previously experienced by all levels of workers; spawned by the impact of the information age on work and the worker

R

Race: division of human beings based on distinct physical characteristics

Radiography: examination by x-ray film

Range of motion: complete extent of movement of which a joint is normally capable

Rape: sexual violation of a person by someone who uses force, threats, and abuse

Rapid eye movement sleep (REM): stage that constitutes 20% to 25% of a person's nightly sleep; person is difficult to arouse during this stage

Rapport: feeling of mutual trust experienced by people in a satisfactory relationship

Reactive hyperemia: the body's flooding of an area with blood after it has suffered from poor circulation for a period; the occurrence of a blanchable reddening of the skin when pressure is removed

Reality orientation: method of care used to promote awareness of reality in confused or disoriented patients

Receiver (decoder): term used in communication theory that specifies the person or object to which the message is directed

Reception: process of receiving data about the internal or external environment through the senses

Recommended dietary allowance (RDA): recommendations for average daily amounts of essential nutrients that healthy population groups should consume over time

Referral: process of sending or guiding someone to another source for assistance

Referred pain: pain in an area removed from that in which stimulation has its origin

Reflex pain response: automatic response of the central nervous system to the stimulus of pain

Regional anesthesia: anesthetic drug is injected or applied topically to inhibit transmission of sensory stimuli

Regression: behavior that is more characteristic of an earlier age

Rehabilitation: process of restoring a person's highest level of possible wellness and returning that person's ability to live and to work as normally as possible after a disabling illness or injury

Rehabilitation centers: centers specializing in services for patients requiring physical or emotional rehabilitation and for treatment of any type of drug dependency

Relationship: interaction of people over time

Relaxation response: an alert, hypometabolic state of decreased sympathetic nervous system arousal, which can also be viewed as the opposite of Selye's general adaptation syndrome response

Religion: organized system of beliefs about a higher power; often includes set forms of worship, spiritual practices, and codes of conduct

REM: rapid eye movement that characterizes the dream state of sleep

Remission: period in an illness when the disease is present, but the person does not experience symptoms of the disease

Reporting: oral, written, or computer-based communication of patient data with the purpose of informing others

Repression: exclusion of an anxiety-producing event from conscious awareness

Research: process that uses observable and verifiable information (data), collected in a systematic manner, to describe, explain, or predict events

Reservoir: natural habitat for the growth and multiplication of microorganisms

Residual: feeding remaining in the stomach

Residual urine: urine that remains in the bladder after the act of micturition

Respiration: act of breathing and using oxygen in body cells

Respiratory acidosis: proportionate excess of carbonic acid in the extracellular fluid

Respiratory alkalosis: proportionate deficiency of carbonic acid in the extracellular fluid

Rest: condition in which the body is in a decreased state of activity, with the consequent feeling of being refreshed

Restless leg syndrome: a condition in which patients are unable to lie still and report experiencing unpleasant creeping, crawling, or tingling sensations in the legs

Restraint: device used to limit movement or immobilize a client

Retention: inability to void although urine is produced by the kidneys and enters the bladder; excessive storage of urine in the bladder

Retention sutures: sutures used to provide extra support in wounds in obese patients or in wounds with increased risk of dehiscence

Reticular activating system: network of neurons in the core of the brain stem, with ascending and descending tracts to other areas of the brain that monitor and regulate incoming sensory stimuli and level of arousal

Retrospective audit: evaluation of nursing care and patient outcomes after the patient has been discharged (may use postdischarge questionnaires, patient interviews, or chart review)

Retrospective evaluation: evaluation of nursing care and patient outcomes after the patient has been discharged using postdischarge questionnaires, patient interviews, or chart review to collect data

Risk factor: something that increases a person's chance for illness or injury

Role performance: ability to successfully execute societal expectations regarding role-specific behaviors

S

Safety and security needs: person's need to be protected from actual or potential harm and to have freedom from fear

Sanguineous: containing or mixed with blood

Scar: connective tissue that fills a wound area

School-age: period from ages 6 to 12 years

Science: a body of knowledge gained by observing, identifying, describing, investigating, and explaining events and occurrences that are perceived in the world

Scientific knowledge: knowledge arrived at by applying scientific methods

Scientific problem-solving: systematic problem-solving process that involves (1) problem identification, (2) data collection, (3) hypothesis formulation, (4) plan of action, (5) hypothesis testing, (6) interpretation of results, and (7) evaluation resulting in conclusion or revision of the study

Scrub nurse: nurse who assists the surgeon during surgery, maintaining surgical asepsis while draping, handling instruments, and handling supplies

Scultetus binder: type of bandage with multiple tails; synonym for *many-tailed binder*

Sebaceous gland: gland found in the skin that secretes an oily substance called sebum

Secondary preventive care: care directed either to health maintenance for patients experiencing health problems or to prevention of complications or disabilities

Self-actualization: need to reach one's potential through full development of one's unique capabilities; highest level need

Self-concept: mental image or picture of self; includes body image, subjective self, ideal self, and social self

Self-esteem: person's perception of his or her total being, including self-worth and body image

Self-esteem needs: need to feel good about oneself and to believe others hold one in high regard

Self governance: employing a decentralized organizational structure for decision making; self governance at the unit level and respect for, and acknowledgement of, professional autonomy

Semantics: study of the meaning of words

Semen: seminal plasma containing sperm

Semipermeable membrane: selectively permeable membrane that allows water to pass through it but is either impermeable or selectively permeable to solutes

Sensoristasis: arousal state of the reticular activating system; general drive state

Sensory deficit: impaired or absent functioning of one or more senses

Sensory deprivation: condition resulting from decreased sensory input or input that is monotonous, unpatterned, or meaningless

Sensory overload: condition resulting from excessive sensory input to which the brain is unable to meaningfully respond

Sensory/perceptual alteration: disturbance in the body's ability to receive or process data from its internal or external environment; NANDA-approved nursing diagnosis

Sensory reception: the process of receiving data about the internal or external environment through the senses

Sentinel event: an unexpected occurrence involving death or serious physical or psychological injury, or the risk thereof

Separation anxiety: condition that occurs when a child is afraid of being sent away from caregivers who are loved and who provide security

Serous: resembling blood serum; clear and watery in appearance

Set point: level at which the hypothalamus attempts to maintain body temperature

Sexual dysfunction: condition that prevents a person or couple from engaging in or obtaining satisfaction from sexual activity

Sexual harassment: unwelcome verbal or physical advance or sexually explicit statement (eg, leers, pats, grabs, jokes, requests for dates, and even rape) that interferes with one's ability to do one's job by making one feel humiliated, intimidated, or uncomfortable

Sexual health: the integration of the somatic, emotional, intellectual, and social aspects of sexual being in ways that are positively enriching and that enhance personality, communication, and love

Sexuality: degree to which a person exhibits and experiences maleness and femaleness physically, emotionally, and mentally

Sexually transmitted disease: disease that spreads from one person to another through intimate sexual contact

Shamanism: the most widely practiced type of medicine on our planet, which believes that illness originates in the spirit world and usually involves a loss of power; treatment consists of first, restoring the individual's power, and second, treating symptoms

Shearing force: force created when layers of tissue move on one another

Shock: body's reaction to acute peripheral circulatory failure due to an abnormality of circulatory control or to a loss of circulating fluid

Situational crisis: change that results when a person faces an event or situation that causes a disruption in his or her life

Situational leadership: theory of leadership that considers the leader's style, the work group's maturity, and the situation at hand to form a comprehensive approach to management style

Situational loss: experienced as a result of an unpredictable event, including traumatic injury, disease, death, or national disaster

Sitz bath: special type of bath that applies heated water to the pelvic or rectal area

Skin sutures: used to approximate wound tissues and skin; may be silk, synthetic, wire, or metal staples

Skin tests: tests to determine antigen–antibody reaction

Sleep: state of altered consciousness throughout which varying degrees of stimuli preclude wakefulness

Sleep apnea: periods of no breathing during sleep that may last from 15 seconds to 2 minutes

Sleep cycle: passage through the four stages of NREM sleep (I, II, III, IV), then reversal (IV, III, II), and finally, instead of reentering stage I and awakening, entering REM sleep and returning to stage II

Sleep deprivation: a decrease in the amount, consistency, and quality of sleep; results from decreased REM or NREM sleep

Small-group communication: communication that occurs when two or more nurses interact with two or more individuals, allowing the members to achieve a goal through communication

SOAP format: method of charting narrative progress notes; organizes data according to subjective information (S), objective information (O), assessment (A), and plan (P)

Social isolation: sense of aloneness because of decreasing relationships with others, resulting from attitudinal, geographic, financial, or illness related factors

Social self: way a person believes that others see him or her

Soft diet: regular diet that has been modified to eliminate foods that are hard to digest and to chew, including those that are high in fiber, high in fat, and highly seasoned

Solute: substance dissolved in a solution

Solvent: liquid holding a substance in solution

Somatic pain: pain originating in structures in the body's external wall

Somnambulism: sleepwalking

Sordes: accumulation of mucus and crust formation on the teeth and around the lips

Source (encoder): term used in communication theory to specify the one who prepares and sends a message to the receiver

Source-oriented record: documentation system in which each healthcare group records data on its own separate form

Spasticity: increased muscle tone

Specific gravity: a characteristic of urine that can be determined with manufactured plastic strips or an instrument called a urinometer or hydrometer

Sperm: male reproductive cell; synonym for spermatozoan

Spermicide: chemical agent used to destroy sperm

Sphincter: circular muscle that constricts a passage or closes a natural orifice

Spiritual beliefs: practices associated with all aspects of a person's life, including health and illness that address the invisible "spirit"—a creative, mysterious, guiding power

Spiritual distress: nursing diagnosis describing an alteration in spiritual health (eg, spiritual pain, alienation, anxiety, guilt, anger, loss, despair)

Spirituality: anything that pertains to a person's relationship with a nonmaterial life force or higher power

Spiritual need: lack of anything necessary for spiritual health (eg, meaning and purpose, love and relatedness, forgiveness)

Spirometer: instrument used to measure lung capacities and volumes; one type is used to encourage deep breathing (incentive spirometry)

Standard: acceptable, expected level of performance established by authority, custom, or consent

Standardized plan of care: prepared plan of care that identifies the nursing diagnoses, patient goals, and related nursing orders common to a specific population (eg, normal neonates) or problem

Standard Precautions: new CDC precautions used in the care of all patients regardless of their diagnosis or possible infection status; this category combines universal and body substance precautions

Standards for critical thinking: clear, precise, specific, accurate, relevant, plausible, consistent, logical, deep, broad, complete, significant, adequate (for the purpose), and fair

Standing order: document that details the nursing care to be implemented in specific nursing situations, frequently when a physician is not present; may expand scope of nursing responsibilities

Statutory law: law enacted by a legislative body

Stereognosis: the sense that perceives the solidity of objects, their size, shape, and texture

Stereotyping: assigning characteristics to a group of people without considering specific individuality

Sterilization: (1) the process by which all microorganisms, including spores, are destroyed; (2) surgical procedure performed to render a person infertile

Stertorous breathing: noisy respirations

Stimulus: agent, act, or other influence capable of initiating a response by the nervous system

Stoma: artificial opening for waste excretion located on the body surface

Stool: excreted feces

Strength (muscle): ability of the muscle to move actively against resistance

Stress: condition in which the human system responds to change in its normal balanced state

Stress incontinence: state in which the person experiences a loss of urine of less than 50 mL that occurs with increased abdominal pressure

Stressor: anything causing a person to experience stress; change in the balanced state

Stridor: harsh, high-pitched sound usually heard on inspiration when upper airways become narrowed

Subculture: group of people with different interests or goals than the primary culture

Subcutaneous injection: injection into the subcutaneous tissue that lies between the epidermis and the muscle

Subjective data (symptoms, covert data): information perceived only by the affected person

Subjective self: how one sees oneself; who one thinks one is

Sublingual: area in the mouth under the tongue

Sudden infant death syndrome (SIDS): sudden death of any infant or young child without demonstrated cause

Sundowning syndrome: describes a phenomenon when a person habitually becomes confused or disoriented with darkness

Suppository: oval- or cone-shaped substance that is inserted into a body cavity and that melts at body temperature

Suprapubic catheter: catheter inserted into the bladder through a small abdominal incision above the pubic area

Surfactant: detergent-like phospholipid that reduces surface tension of the fluid lining the alveoli

Surgical asepsis: practices that render and keep objects and areas free from microorganisms; synonym for *sterile technique*

Susceptibility: degree of resistance of a host to a pathogen

Symptom: abnormality indicative of illness as experienced by the patient; synonym for *subjective data*

Syndrome (nursing diagnoses): cluster of actual or risk nursing diagnoses that are predicted to be present because of a certain event or situation

Synergistic effect: combined effect of two or more drugs is greater than the effect of each drug alone

Systemic symptoms: symptoms manifested throughout the entire body

Systolic pressure: highest point of pressure on arterial walls when the ventricles contract

T

Tachycardia: rapid heart rate

Tachypnea: abnormally rapid rate of breathing

Tactile: pertaining to touch

Tartar: hard deposit on the teeth near the gum line formed by plaque buildup and dead bacteria

Teaching: planned method or series of methods used to help someone learn

Teaching–learning process: process of patient teaching that encompasses critical steps necessary to provide teaching and to measure learning; the teaching–learning process models the nursing process

Technical competencies: skills that enable a nurse to skillfully manipulate equipment in a manner conducive to achieving a desired goal

Temperament: person's style of approaching people, situations, or events

Temperature: refers to the hotness or coldness of a substance

Tendons: strong, flexible, inelastic fibrous bands that attach muscle to bone

Teratogenic: known to have potential to cause developmental defects in the embryo or fetus

Terminal illness: illness from which there is no reasonable expectation of recovery or cure

Terminal weaning: withdrawal of life-sustaining therapy with the understanding that death may result, generally after a decision is made that the therapy in question is medically futile or disproportionately burdensome

Tertiary preventive care: care directed at helping rehabilitate patients and restore them to a maximum level of functioning after an illness

Theory: statement based on observed facts that explains or characterizes a process, an occurrence, or an event, but cannot be proved directly or absolutely as a fact

Therapeutic range: that concentration of drug in the blood serum that produces the desired effect without causing toxicity

Therapeutic touch: an alternative therapy that involves using one's hands to consciously direct an energy exchange from the practitioner to the patient to facilitate healing or pain relief

Third-space fluid shift: distributional shift and trapping of body fluids into body spaces such as the pleural, peritoneal, or pericardial, or into the interstitial space (plasma-to-interstitial shift)

Thoracentesis: aspiration of fluid or air from the pleural space

Thrill: abnormal tremor accompanying a vascular or cardiac murmur felt on palpation

Thrombophlebitis: inflammation in a vein associated with thrombus formation

Thrombus: blood clot; plural is *thrombi*

Time-lapsed assessment: an assessment that is scheduled to compare a patient's current status to baseline data obtained earlier

Toddler: period from ages 1 year to 3 years

Tonus: normal, partially steady state of muscle contraction

Topical application: application of a substance directly to a body site

Tort: wrong committed by a person against another person or his property

Total body water (TBW): total amount of water in the body, expressed as a percentage of body weight. The term total body fluid also is used; fluids usually are considered to include water and electrolytes

Total parenteral nutrition (TPN): nutritional therapy that bypasses the gastrointestinal tract for patients who are unable to take food orally; meets the patient's nutritional needs by way of nutrient-filled solutions administered intravenously through a central vein

Trace elements: minerals found in the body in quantities less than 5 g and needed in only small amounts (18 mg or less)

Tracheostomy: artificial opening made into the trachea through which a tracheostomy tube is inserted

Tracheostomy tube: curved tube inserted into an artificial opening made in the trachea that comes with varied angles and in multiple sizes

Trade name: drug name selected and trademarked by the company marketing the drug; also called *brand name* or *proprietary name*

Traditional Chinese medicine: healing system that is thousands of years old that believes the interaction of people with their environment is most significant in creating health

Traditional family: composed of a husband, wife, and their children, who live together in one house

Traditional knowledge: knowledge passed down from generation to generation

Transcultural nursing: providing nursing care that is planned and implemented in a way that is sensitive to the needs of individuals, families, and groups representing the diverse cultural populations within our society

Trans fat: fat that occurs when manufacturers partially hydrogenate liquid oils so that they become more solid and stable; trans fat raises serum cholesterol

Transformational leadership: type of leadership in which the person creates revolutionary change and commits to the personal and professional growth of self and others

Transmission-based precautions: new CDC precautions used in patients known or suspected to be infected with pathogens that can be transmitted by airborne, droplet, or contact routes; used in addition to Standard Precautions

Transsexual: person of a certain biologic gender with the feelings of the opposite sex

Transvestite: individual who desires to take on the role or wear the clothes of the opposite sex

Trauma: injury

Tremor: involuntary muscular movements

Trial: hearing of evidence in a legal case before a judge (and jury) with the intent of reaching a decision or verdict

Trial-and-error problem-solving: method of problem-solving that involves testing any number of solutions until one is found that works for that particular problem

Triglycerides: predominant form of fat in food and the major storage form of fat in the body; composed of one glyceride molecule and three fatty acids

Trough level: the point when a drug is at its lowest concentration

Turgor: tension of a cell determined by its hydration

Typing: determining a person's blood type

U

Unilateral: affecting or occurring on one side only

Universal precautions: isolation system that considers blood, body fluids containing blood, semen, and vaginal secretions of all patients as potentially infective

Unlicensed assistive personnel (UAP): individual who is trained to function in an assistive role to the licensed registered nurse in the provision of patient activities as delegated by and under the supervision of the registered professional nurse

Urge incontinence: state in which a person experiences involuntary passage of urine that occurs soon after a strong sense of urgency to void

Urgency: strong desire to void

Urinary diversion: surgical creation of an alternate route for excretion of urine

Urinary incontinence: any involuntary loss of urine that causes a problem

Urinary retention: inability to void although urine is produced by the kidneys and enters the bladder; excessive storage of urine in the bladder

Urination: process of emptying the bladder; micturition; voiding

Utilitarian: action-guiding theory of ethics that states that the rightness or wrongness of an action depends on the consequences of the action

V

Validation: act of confirming or verifying

Valsalva maneuver: forcible exhalation against a closed glottis, resulting in increased intrathoracic pressure

Values: set of beliefs that are meaningful in life and that influence relationships with others

Values clarification: process by which people come to understand their own values and value system

Value system: organization of values ranked along a continuum of importance

Variables: factors in a research study

Variance charting: documentation method in case management that records unexpected events, the cause for the event, actions taken in response to the event, and discharge planning when appropriate

Varicosity: swollen, twisted vein

Vector: nonhuman carriers, such as mosquitoes, ticks, and lice, that transmit organisms from one host to another

Ventilation: exchange of gases

Veracity: truth telling

Verbal communication: exchange of information using words

Vesicular breath sounds: normal sound of respirations heard on auscultation over peripheral lung areas

Vial: glass bottle with self-sealing stopper through which medication is removed; may be single or multiple dose

Virulence: ability to produce disease

Virus: smallest of all microorganisms; can only be seen by using an electron microscope

Visceral: pertaining to inner organs

Visceral pain: pain originating in the internal organs in the thorax, cranium, or abdomen

Visual: pertaining to sight

Vital signs: body temperature, pulse and respiratory rates, and blood pressure; synonym for *cardinal signs*

Vitamins: organic substances needed by the body in small amounts to help regulate body processes; are susceptible to oxidation and destruction

Voiding: process of emptying the bladder; also called *micturition* or *urination*

Voluntary agencies: community agencies that are often funded by private donations, grants, or fund-raising and that provide a wide variety of direct services and education

W

Wellness: an active process in which an individual progresses toward the maximum possible potential, regardless of his or her current state of health

Wellness diagnosis: clinical judgment about an individual, family, or community in transition from a specific level of wellness to a higher level of wellness

Wheeze: continuous, high-pitched squeak or musical sound made as air moves through narrowed or partially obstructed airway passages

Whistle-blowing: term generally used to refer to employees who report their employers' violation of the law to appropriate law enforcement agencies outside the employers' facilities

Wound: injury that results in a disruption in the normal continuity of a body structure

X

X-ray: high-energy electromagnetic wave capable of penetrating solid matter and acting on photographic film; synonym for *roentgen ray*

Y

Yin-yang: energy forces in Chinese teaching that must be in balance for good health; expression of strong emotions results in disharmony and imbalance between these forces

Young adult: adult between the ages of 20 and 40 years; also called *early adulthood*

Z

Z-track: zigzag technique used to administer medications intramuscularly

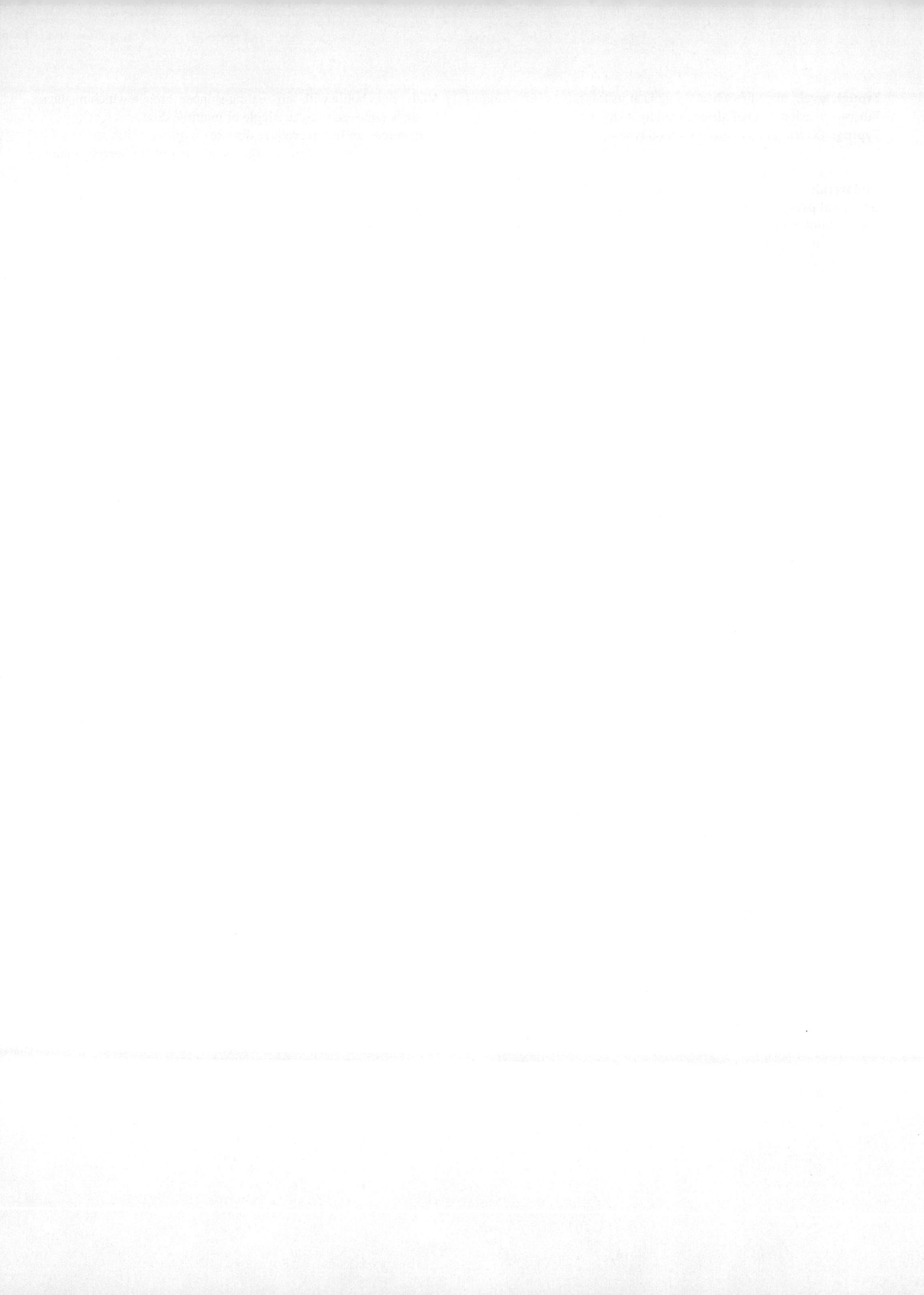

INDEX

Note: Page numbers followed by *f* indicate figures, those followed by *t* indicate tables, and those followed by *b* indicate material in boxes.

A

AACN. *See* American Association of Colleges of Nursing
Abbreviated grief, 874–875
Abbreviations
  commonly used, 340, 342*t*
  for laboratory values, 1489
Abdomen
  age-related changes in, 597
  assessment of, 595–597, 1344–1345
Abdominal breathing, 1393
Abdominal cavity, 595*f*
Abdominal exercises, for bowel elimination, 1351
Abdominal quadrants, 596*f*
Abdominal reflex, 607*t*
Abducens (VI) nerve, 605*t*
Abduction, 1105*t*, 1136, 1137, 1138, 1139
Abdullah, Faye, 80*t*
ABGs. *See* Arterial blood gas
Abortion, counseling for, 961
Abrasion, 1059*t*
Absent pulse, 538*t*
Absorption, of medications, 710–711
  intramuscular, 739
  parenteral, 727
  through skin, 760
Abstinence, 957
Abstract reasoning, assessment of, 604
Abuse
  of alcohol
    in adolescents/young adults, 410–411
    and nutrition, 1251
  of children, 376, 395, 627–628, 628*b*
  counseling for, 961–962
  domestic violence, 629
  of medications, 772–773
  physical, 395, 599–602
  sexual, 395
  substance
    in adolescents/young adults, 410–411
    and growth and development, 376
    in middle adults, 423
    by nurses, 135
    patient teaching about, 772–773
    during pregnancy, 391
Acceptance, in death and dying, 878
Access, to health care, 47
Accessory apartments, for older adults, 430*t*
Accessory muscles, and respiration, 1379
Accessory (XI) nerve, 605*t*
Accidental exposures, reporting of, 681
Accidental injuries
  in infants, 394
  in older adults, 431
Accidents
  death/death rates from, 617*t*
  equipment-related, 638–639, 639*b*
  prevention of, 621–625, 625*f* (*See also* Safety)
  procedure-related, 639, 640*b*, 640*f*
  sleepiness and, 1169
Accolate. *See* Zafirlukast
Accommodation, in cognitive development, 378
Accommodation (visual), 577, 578, 579*f*
Accountability, 213
  documentation and, 339*b*
  of home healthcare nurses, 182
  nursing diagnoses and, 256*f*
Accreditation, 117
Accuracy, of data, 238–239
ACE inhibitors, 547

Acetaminophen
  for fever reduction, 527
  in suppositories, 767
Acetoacetate plus acetone, blood values of, 1491*t*
Acetone plus acetoacetate, urine values of, 1492*t*
Acetonide, 1399*t*
Acetylcholine, and sleep, 1169
Acid, 1435
Acid-base balance, 710, 1435–1437, 1437*f*
  nursing plan of care for, 1481–1482
  nursing process for, 1440–1483
    assessing in, 1440–1448
    diagnosing in, 1448–1450
    evaluating in, 1480–1483
    implementing in, 1451–1483
    outcome identification and planning in, 1450–1451
  parameters of, in arterial blood gas studies, 1439, 1440*t*
  and respiration, 543*b*
Acid-base imbalance, 1439–1440, 1449*t*, 1456. *See also specific disorder*
Acidosis, 1435, 1437*f*
  metabolic, 1440, 1449*t*
  respiratory, 1440, 1449*t*
Acne, 1051*t*
Acoustic (VIII) nerve, 605*t*
Acquired immunodeficiency syndrome (AIDS), 412, 653, 941*t*. *See also* Human immunodeficiency virus
ACTH. *See* Adrenocorticotropin
Acting, in valuing process, 95*b*
Activated charcoal, 638
Active crying state, 392*f*
Active euthanasia, 884–885, 885*b*
Active exercise, 1132
Active transport, of body fluids, 1433
Active-assistive exercise, 1132
Activities of daily living (ADLs)
  and exercise, 1148, 1148*b*
  in preoperative care, 790
  and stress, 862–863
Activity, 1101–1162. *See also* Exercise; Movement
  and bowel elimination, 1342
  nursing plan of care for, 1158–1162
  nursing process for, 1119–1157
    diagnosing in, 1123–1124, 1125*t*–1127*t*
    evaluating in, 1157
    implementing in, 1124–1157
    outcome identification and planning in, 1124
  in older adults, 433*t*
  as physiologic need, 27
  preoperative teaching about, 796–797
  and respiratory function, 1383
  and sleep, 1175
  and urinary elimination, 1293
Activity flow sheet, with narrative notes, 347*f*
Activity theory, 427
Actovials, 729*f*, 733–734
Actual loss, 873
Actual nursing diagnoses, 264
Acuity charting forms, 357
Acupressure, 48
Acupuncture, 48, 692–693, 692*f*, 693*f*, 1217
Acute illness, 60–62
Acute pain, 1199
Acute wounds, 1057
Acute-care facility, infection control in, 659
AD. *See* Alzheimer's disease
ADA. *See* Americans with Disabilities Act
Adaptation, 849. *See also* Coping
  definition of, 850, 850*f*

factors affecting, 858 859
general adaptation syndrome, 689, 851–853, 853*f*
local adaptation syndrome, 851
in nursing profession, 859–860
and perception of pain, 1201
Adaptation theory, 78
Addams, Jane, 10*t*
Addiction, to analgesics, 1219
Adduction, 1105*t*, 1136, 1137, 1138, 1139
ADH. *See* Antidiuretic hormone
ADHD. *See* Attention deficit hyperactivity disorder
Adjustable beds, 1128
Adjuvant drugs, in pain management, 1219
ADLs. *See* Activities of daily living
Administration
  of analgesics, 1218–1220
  of general anesthesia, 784
  of medications
    assessment in, 720, 721
    buccal, 727
    diagnosing in, 720
    documentation of, 767–772, 769*f*–770*f*
    enteral, 726–727
    evaluation in, 773
    frequency of, 715–716
    implementation in, 720–773
    by inhalation, 767
    intradermal, 734, 737–738
    intramuscular, 739–747, 741*f*
    intravenous, 748–757
    nursing process for, 720–773
    nursing responsibilities for, 722*b*
    oral (*See* Oral medication administration)
    outcome identification and planning in, 720
    parenteral (*See* Parenteral medications, administration of)
    patient identification and, 720
    principles of, 714–720
    routes of, 710, 715, 716*t*
    sites of, local conditions at, 710
    subcutaneous, 734–739, 739*f*, 740–742, 742*f*
    sublingual, 727
    timing of, 714
    topical (*See* Topical medications, administration of)
Administrative law, 115
Admission
  to ambulatory care facility, 165–166
  to healthcare facility, 165–166
    and anxiety, 865
  to hospital, 166, 166*b*
  standards for, 165
Admission database information, 166, 169*f*–170*f*
ADN. *See* Associate degree nursing
Adolescence, definition of, 408
Adolescent(s)
  activity levels of, 1111*t*
  bowel elimination in, 1340–1341
  cognitive development of, 408
  communication with, 449–450
  eating disorders in, 412
  growth and development of, 408–413, 414
  health of, 410–413
  health promotion and illness prevention in, 413–414
  hygiene of, 1009
  moral development of, 410
  nutrition for, 1249
  patient learning and, 478–480
  physiologic development of, 408, 409*t*
  poisoning in, 618
  pregnancy in, 411–412, 1249

1517

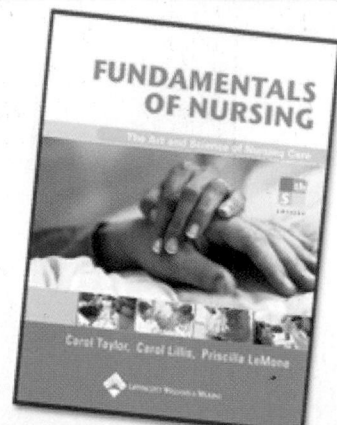
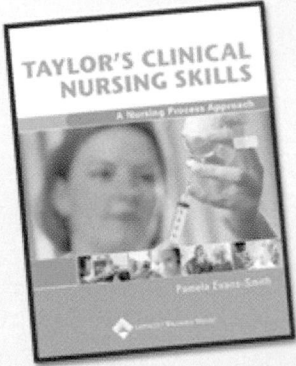
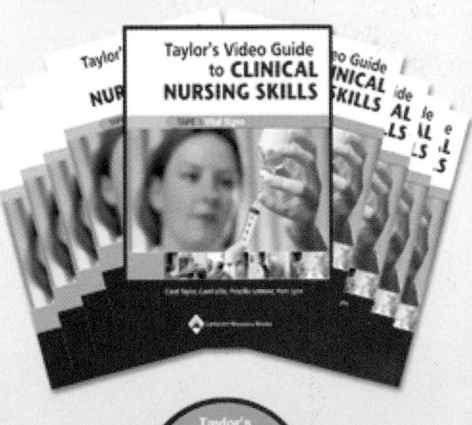
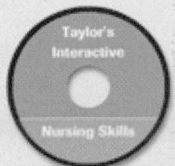
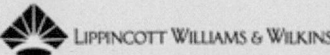